Nathan and Oski's
HEMATOLOGY
of
Infancy and Childhood

SIXTH EDITION

VOLUME

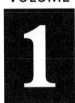

1

David G. Nathan, M.D.

President Emeritus, Dana-Farber Cancer Institute
Robert A. Stranahan Distinguished Professor of
    Pediatrics
Harvard Medical School
Boston, Massachusetts

Stuart H. Orkin, M.D.

Chairman, Department of Pediatric Oncology
Dana-Farber Cancer Institute
David G. Nathan Professor of Pediatrics
Harvard Medical School
Investigator, Howard Hughes Medical Institute
Boston, Massachusetts

David Ginsburg, M.D.

Warner-Lambert/Parke-Davis Professor of Medicine
University of Michigan
Investigator, Howard Hughes Medical Institute
Ann Arbor, Michigan

A. Thomas Look, M.D.

Professor of Pediatrics
Harvard Medical School
Dana-Farber Cancer Institute
Boston, Massachusetts

Managing Editor
Cathryn J. Lantigua

SAUNDERS
An Imprint of Elsevier Science

W.B. Saunders Company
An Imprint of Elsevier, Inc.

The Curtis Center
Independence Square West
Philadelphia, Pennsylvania 19106-3399

NOTICE

Medicine is an ever-changing field. Standard safety precautions must be followed, but as new research and clinical experience broaden our knowledge, changes in treatment and drug therapy may become necessary or appropriate. Readers are advised to check the most current product information provided by the manufacturer of each drug to be administered to verify the recommended dose, the method and duration of administration, and contraindications. It is the responsibility of the treating physician, relying on experience and knowledge of the patient, to determine dosages and the best treatment for each individual patient. Neither the publisher nor the author assumes any liability for any injury and/or damage to persons or property arising from this publication.

The Publisher

Library of Congress Cataloging-in-Publication Data

Nathan and Oski's hematology of infancy and childhood/[edited by] David G. Nathan ... [et al.].–6th ed.
    p. ; cm
  Includes bibliographical references and index.
  ISBN 0-7216-9317-2
    1. Pediatric hematology. 2. Neonatal hematology. I. Title: Hematology of infancy and childhood.
  II. Nathan, David G., 1929- III. Oski, Frank A.
  [DNLM: 1. Hematologic Diseases–Child. 2. Hematologic Diseases–Infant. WS 300 N273 2003]
  RJ411 .N37 2003
  618.92´d15–dc21

                                           2002026919

Acquisitions Editor: Delores Meloni
Developmental Editor: Jennifer Shreiner
Project Manager: Mary Stermel

Printed in the United States of America

Last digit is the print number: 9 8 7 6 5 4 3 2 1

Contributors

Estella M. Alonso, M.D.
Associate Professor of Pediatrics, Northwestern
University Medical School; Director of Hepatology and
Liver Transplantation, Children's Memorial Hospital,
Chicago, Illinois
Disorders of Bilirubin Metabolism

Blanche P. Alter, M.D., M.P.H.
Expert, Clinical Genetics Branch, Division of Cancer
Epidemiology and Genetics, National Cancer Institute;
Medical Staff, Warren Magnuson Clinical Center,
National Institutes of Health, Bethesda, Maryland
Inherited Bone Marrow Failure Syndromes

Maureen Andrew, M.D.[†]
Professor of Pediatrics, McMaster University, Hamilton
Civic Hospitals Research Centre, Hamilton; and
Hospital for Sick Children, Toronto, Ontario, Canada
*Developmental Hemostasis: Relevance to Newborns and
Infants*
Acquired Disorders of Hemostasis

Nancy C. Andrews, M.D., Ph.D.
Associate Professor of Pediatrics, Harvard Medical
School; Associate Investigator, Howard Hughes Medical
Institute, Boston, Massachusetts; Associate in Medicine,
Children's Hospital, Boston, Massachusetts
Disorders of Iron Metabolism and Sideroblastic Anemia

Kenneth A. Bauer, M.D.
Associate Professor of Medicine, Harvard Medical
School; Chief, Hematology Section, VA Boston
Healthcare System, West Roxbury, Massachusetts;
Director, Thrombosis Clinical Research, Beth
Israel Deaconess Medical Center, Boston,
Massachusetts
Rare Hereditary Coagulation Factor Abnormalities
Inherited Disorders of Thrombosis and Fibrinolysis

Richard J. Benjamin, M.B.Ch.B., Ph.D.
Assistant Professor of Pathology, Harvard University;
Chief Medical Officer, American Red Cross—
New England Region, Dedham, Massachusetts
Transfusion Medicine

Carolyn M. Bennett, M.D.
Instructor in Pediatrics, Harvard Medical School;
Assistant (Medicine), Division of Hematology/Oncology,
Children's Hospital, Boston, Massachusetts
*Myeloid Leukemia, Myelodysplasia, and Myeloproliferative
Disease in Children*

Stacey L. Berg, M.D.
Associate Professor of Pediatrics, Texas Children's
Cancer Center, Texas Children's Hospital,
Baylor College of Medicine, Houston, Texas
*Pharmacology of Antineoplastic Agents and Multidrug
Resistance*

Smita Bhatia, M.D., M.P.H.
Director, Epidemiology and Outcomes Research, City
of Hope National Medical Center, Duarte, California
Epidemiology of Leukemia in Childhood

Barbara E. Bierer, M.D.
Professor of Medicine (Pediatrics), Harvard Medical
School; Vice-President for Patient Safety, Department of
Medical Oncology, Dana-Farber Cancer Institute,
Boston, Massachusetts
*Cell-Mediated and Humoral Immunity and the Regulation of
Immune Responses*

Julie Boergers, Ph.D.
Assistant Professor of Psychiatry and Human Behavior,
Brown Medical School; Staff Psychologist, Rhode Island
Hospital, Providence, Rhode Island
Psychologic Aspects of Leukemia and Hematologic Disorders

Francisco A. Bonilla, M.D., Ph.D.
Assitant Professor of Pediatrics, Harvard Medical
School; Assistant in Medicine, Children's Hospital,
Boston, Massachusetts
Primary Immunodeficiency Diseases

Carlo Brugnara, M.D.
Professor of Pathology, Harvard Medical School;
Director, Hematology Laboratory, Department of
Laboratory Medicine, Children's Hospital, Boston,
Massachusetts
The Neonatal Erythrocyte and Its Disorders
A Diagnostic Approach to the Anemic Patient

[†]Deceased

Gustavo Charria-Ortiz, M.D.
Instructor in Neurology and Pediatrics, New York University, New York, New York
Storage Diseases of the Reticuloendothelial System

Steven C. Clark, Ph.D.
Chief Scientific Officer, GenPath Pharmaceuticals, Inc., Cambridge, Massachusetts
The Anatomy and Physiology of Hematopoiesis

Bernard A. Cooper, M.D.
Clinical Professor of Medicine (Hematology), Stanford University, Palo Alto, California; Professor of Medicine, McGill University, Montreal, Quebec, Canada
Megaloblastic Anemia

Kenneth B. DeSantes, M.D.
Associate Professor of Pediatrics, University of Wisconsin, Madison, Wisconsin
Cell, Cytokine, Monoclonal Antibody, and Gene Therapy

Mary C. Dinauer, M.D., Ph.D.
Nora Letzter Professor of Pediatrics (Hematology/Oncology), and Professor of Microbiology/Immunology and Medical and Molecular Genetics, Indiana University School of Medicine; Associate Chair for Basic Research, and Director, Herman B. Wells Center for Pediatric Research, James Whitcomb Riley Hospital for Children, Indiana University School of Medicine, Indianapolis, Indiana
The Phagocyte System and Disorders of Granulopoiesis and Granulocyte Function

Sarah S. Donaldson, M.D.
Professor of Radiation Oncology, Stanford University School of Medicine; Chief, Radiation Oncology, Lucile Salter Packard Children's Hospital, Stanford, California
The Lymphomas and Lymphadenopathy

George J. Dover, M.D.
Professor of Pediatrics, Medicine, and Oncology, Johns Hopkins University School of Medicine; Director, Department of Pediatrics and Pediatrician-in-Chief, Johns Hopkins Hospital, Baltimore, Maryland
Sickle Cell Disease

Charles T. Esmon, Ph.D.
Professor of Pathology, Biochemistry, and Molecular Biology; Lloyd Noble Chair in Cardiovascular Research; Member and Head, Cardiovascular Biology Research Program; Investigator, Howard Hughes Medical Institute, Oklahoma City, Oklahoma
Blood Coagulation

R. Alan B. Ezekowitz, M.B.Ch.B., D.Phil., F.A.A.P.
Charles Wilder Professor of Pediatrics, Harvard Medical School; Chief, Department of Pediatrics, MassGeneral Hospital for Children; Chief, Department of Pediatrics, Partners HealthCare System, Boston, Massachusetts
Hematologic Manifestations of Systemic Diseases

David Frederick Friedman, M.D.
Clinical Assistant Professor of Pediatrics, Department of Pediatrics, University of Pennsylvania; Associate Director of the Transfusion Service, Department of Pathology and Laboratory Medicine, Children's Hospital of Philadelphia, Philadelphia, Pennsylvania
Transfusion Medicine

Patrick G. Gallagher, M.D.
Associate Professor, Department of Pediatrics, Yale University School of Medicine; Attending Physician, Yale-New Haven Hospital, New Haven, Connecticut
Disorders of the Erythrocyte Membrane

Raif S. Geha, M.D.
Professor of Pediatrics, Harvard Medical School; Chief, Division of Immunology, Children's Hospital, Boston, Massachusetts
Primary Immunodeficiency Diseases

Joan Cox Gill, M.D.
Professor of Pediatrics and Medicine, Medical College of Wisconsin; Director, Comprehensive Center for Bleeding Disorders, The Blood Center, Milwaukee, Wisconsin
Hemophilia and von Willebrand Disease

Todd R. Golub, M.D.
Associate Professor of Pediatrics, Harvard Medical School, Boston, Massachusetts; Charles A. Dana Investigator, Dana-Farber Cancer Institute, Boston, Massachusetts; Director, Cancer Genomics, Whitehead Institute/Massachusetts Institute of Technology Center for Genome Research, Cambridge, Massachusetts; Associate Investigator, Howard Hughes Medical Institute
The Molecular Basis of Hematologic Malignancy

Alessandro Gozzetti, M.D., Ph.D.
Attending Hematologist and Director, Cancer Cytogenics Laboratory, Hematology Department, Ospedale Sclavo, Siena, Italy
Chromosomal Abnormalities in Childhood Hematologic Malignant Disease

John G. Gribben, M.D., D.S.C., F.R.C.P., F.R.C.Path.
Associate Professor, Harvard Medical School;
Attending Physician, Dana-Farber Cancer Institute and
Brigham and Women's Hospital, Boston,
Massachusetts
Minimal Residual Leukemia

Eva C. Guinan, M.D.
Assistant Professor of Pediatrics, Harvard Medical
School; Director, Hematopoietic Stem Cell
Transplantation, Department of Pediatric
Oncology, Dana-Farber Cancer Institute, Boston,
Massachusetts
Acquired Aplastic Anemia
Principles of Bone Marrow and Stem Cell Transplantation

Katherine Amberson Hajjar, M.D.
Professor and Chair, Department of Cell and
Developmental Biology, and Professor of Pediatrics,
Weill Medical College of Cornell University;
Professor of Pediatrics, New York Presbyterian
Hospital, New York, New York
The Molecular Basis of Fibrinolysis

W. Nicholas Haining, B.M., B.Ch.
Instructor in Pediatrics, Harvard Medical School;
Assistant in Medicine, Children's Hospital, Boston,
Massachusetts; Staff Physician, Dana-Farber Cancer
Institute, Boston, Massachusetts
Principles of Bone Marrow and Stem Cell Transplantation

Robert I. Handin, M.D.
Professor of Medicine, Harvard Medical School;
Executive Vice Chairman, Department of Medicine,
Brigham and Women's Hospital; Co-Director,
Hematology Division, Brigham and Women's Hospital,
Boston, Massachusetts
Blood Platelets and the Vessel Wall

Karl Hsu, M.D.
Instructor, Department of Medicine, Harvard
Medical School; Instructor, Department of
Pediatric Oncology, Dana-Farber Cancer Institute;
Instructor, Department of Medicine, Beth Israel
Deaconess Medical Center; Boston,
Massachusetts
Myeloid Leukemia, Myelodysplasia, and Myeloproliferative Disease in Children

Elissa Jelalian, Ph.D.
Assistant Professor of Psychiatry and Human
Behavior, Brown University Medical School;
Staff Psychologist, Rhode Island Hospital,
Providence, Rhode Island
Psychologic Aspects of Leukemia and Hematologic Disorders

Atellah Kappas, M.D.
Sherman Fairchild Professor and Physician-in-Chief
Emeritus, The Rockefeller University Hospital,
New York, New York
The Porphyrias

Andrew Y. Koh, M.D.
Clinical Fellow, Harvard Medical School; Fellow in
Infectious Disease and Hematology/Oncology, Children's
Hospital, Boston, Massachusetts; Fellow in
Hematology/Oncology, Dana-Farber Cancer Institute,
Boston, Massachusetts
Infectious Complications in Children with Hematologic Disorders

Edwin H. Kolodny, A.B., M.D.
Bernard A. and Charlotte Marden Professor and
Chairman, Department of Neurology, New York
University School of Medicine; Chairman, Department
of Neurology, Tisch Hospital and Bellevue Hospital,
New York, New York
Storage Diseases of the Reticuloendothelial System

Dominic P. Kwiatkowski, F.R.C.P., F.R.C.P.C.H., F.Med.Sci
Medical Research Council Professor, University
Department of Paediatrics, John Radcliffe Hospital,
Oxford University, Oxford, UK
Hematologic Manifestations of Systemic Diseases in Children of the Developing World

Leslie Lehmann, M.D.
Instructor of Pediatrics, Harvard Medical School;
Director, Stem Cell Transplant Unit, Children's
Hospital, Boston, Massachusetts
Principles of Bone Marrow and Stem Cell Transplantation

Helen G. Liley, M.B., Ch.B., F.R.A.C.P.
Senior Lecturer, University of Queensland School of
Medicine; Senior Staff Specialist, Neonatology, Mater
Misericordiae Mothers Hospital, South Brisbane,
Queensland, Australia
Immune Hemolytic Disease

Michael P. Link, M.D.
Professor of Pediatrics and Chief, Division of
Hematology, Oncology, and Bone Marrow
Transplantation, Stanford University School of
Medicine; Director, Center for Cancer and Blood
Diseases, Lucile Salter Packard Children's Hospital at
Stanford, Palo Alto, California
The Lymphomas and Lymphadenopathy

A. Thomas Look, M.D.
Professor of Pediatrics, Harvard Medical School; Dana-
Farber Cancer Institute, Boston, Massachusetts
Myeloid Leukemia, Myelodysplasia, and Myeloproliferative Disease in Children

Jeanne M. Lusher, M.D.
Distinguished Professor of Pediatrics and Marion I.
Barnhart Hemostasis Research Professor, Wayne State
University School of Medicine; Director, Hemophilia,
Hemostasis-Thrombosis Program and Co-director,
Hematology-Oncology Division, Children's Hospital of
Michigan, Detroit, Michigan
*Clinical and Laboratory Approach to the Patient with
Bleeding*

Samuel E. Lux, M.D.
Robert A. Stranahan Professor of Pediatrics, Harvard
Medical School; Chief, Division of Hematology-
Oncology, Children's Hospital, Boston, Massachusetts
Disorders of the Erythrocyte Membrane

Lucio Luzzatto, M.D.
Scientific Director, Istituto Scientifico Tumori, Genova,
Italy
*Glucose-6-Phosphate Dehydrogenase Deficiency and Hemolytic
Anemia*

William C. Mentzer, Jr., M.D.
Professor and Director, Division of Hematology,
Department of Pediatrics, University of California, San
Francisco; Attending Pediatrician, University of
California Hospitals and San Francisco General
Hospital, San Francisco, California
Pyruvate Kinase Deficiency and Disorders of Glycolysis

**Paul Monagle, M.B.B.S. (Hons), M.Sc.,
F.R.A.C.P., F.R.C.P.A., F.C.C.P.**
Principle Fellow, Department of Paediatrics, University
of Melbourne; Divisional Director, Laboratory Services,
Royal Children's Hospital, Melbourne, Australia
*Developmental Hemostasis: Relevance to Newborns and Infants
Acquired Disorders of Hemostasis*

Robert R. Montgomery, M.D.
Professor of Pediatric Hematology and Vice Chair for
Research, Medical College of Wisconsin; Director of
Research, The Blood Center, Milwaukee, Wisconsin
Hemophilia and von Willebrand Disease

Ronald L. Nagel, M.D.
Irving D. Karpas Professor of Medicine, Professor of
Physiology and Biophysics, and Head, Division
of Hematology, Albert Einstein College of
Medicine; Director, Bronx Comprehensive Sickle
Cell Center, Montefiore Medical Center, Bronx,
New York
Hemoglobins: Normal and Abnormal

David G. Nathan, M.D.
President Emeritus, Dana-Farber Cancer Institute;
Robert A. Stranahan Distinguished Professor of
Pediatrics, Harvard Medical School, Boston,
Massachusetts
*A Diagnostic Approach to the Anemic Patient
The Thalassemias*

**Harold J. Olney, M.D., C.M., C.S.P.Q.,
F.R.C.P.(C.)**
Assistant Professor of Medicine, University of Montreal;
Attending Hematologist and Medical Oncologist and
Director, Cancer Cytogenics Laboratory, Centre
Hospitalier de l'Université de Montréal-Notre Dame,
Montréal, Quebec, Canada
*Chromosomal Abnormalities in Childhood Hematologic
Malignant Disease*

Stuart T. Orkin, M.D.
Leland Fikes Professor of Pediatric Medicine,
Harvard Medical School; Investigator, Howard
Hughes Medical Institute; Chief, Division of
Hematology/Oncology, Children's Hospital, Boston,
Massachusetts
The Thalassemias

Frank A. Oski, M.D.†
Distinguished Service Professor, Johns Hopkins
University School of Medicine, Baltimore,
Maryland
A Diagnostic Approach to the Anemic Patient

Philip A. Pizzo, M.D.
Carl and Elizabeth Naumann Dean of the School of
Medicine; Professor of Pediatrics and Microbiology and
Immunology, Stanford University School of Medicine,
Stanford, California
*Infectious Complications in Children with Hematologic
Disorders*

Orah S. Platt, M.D.
Professor of Pediatrics, Harvard Medical School; Chief,
Department of Laboratory Medicine, Children's
Hospital, Boston, Massachusetts
*The Neonatal Erythrocyte and Its Disorders
Sickle Cell Disease*

Mortimer Poncz, M.D.
Professor of Pediatrics, University of Pennsylvania;
The Children's Hospital of Philadelphia, Philadelphia,
Pennsylvania
Inherited Platelet Disorders

---

†Deceased

David G. Poplack, M.D.
Head, Hematology-Oncology Section, Department of Pediatrics, Baylor College of Medicine; Director, Texas Children's Cancer, Texas Children's Hospital, Houston, Texas
Pharmacology of Antineoplastic Agents and Multidrug Resistance

Gregory H. Reaman, M.D.
Professor of Pediatrics, George Washington University School of Medicine and Health Sciences; Chair, Children's Oncology Group and Chief, Division of Hematology-Oncology, Children's National Medical Center, Washington, DC
Acute Leukemia in Infants

Leslie L. Robinson, Ph.D.
Professor, University of Minnesota Medical School; Associate Director, University of Minnesota Cancer Center, Minneapolis, Minnesota
Epidemiology of Leukemia in Childhood

David S. Rosenblatt, M.D.C.M., F.R.C.P.(C), F.C.C.M.G.
Professor of Human Genetics, Medicine, and Pediatrics, McGill University; Director, Division of Medical Genetics, and Director, The Hess B. and Diane Finestone Laboratory in Memory of Jacob and Jenny Finestone, Royal Victoria Hospital and Montreal General Hospital, Montreal, Quebec, Canada
Megaloblastic Anemia

Janet D. Rowley, M.D., D.Sc. (Hon.)
Blum-Riese Distinguished Service Professor of Medicine, of Molecular Genetics and Cell Biology, and of Human Genetics, University of Chicago, Chicago, Illinois
Chromosomal Abnormalities in Childhood Hematologic Malignant Disease

Stephen E. Sallan, M.D.
Professor of Pediatrics, Harvard Medical School; Chief of Staff, Dana-Farber Cancer Institute, Boston, Massachusetts
Acute Lymphoblastic Leukemia

Shigeru Sassa, M.D., Ph.D.
Medical Director, Yamanouchi Pharmaceutical Co., Ltd., Tokyo, Japan
The Porphyrias

J. Paul Scott, M.D.
Professor of Pediatrics, Medical College of Wisconsin; Attending Physician, Department of Hematology-Oncology, Children's Hospital of Wisconsin, Milwaukee, Wisconsin
Hemophilia and von Willebrand Disease

Akiko Shimamura, M.D., Ph.D.
Instructor in Pediatrics, Harvard Medical School; Assistant in Medicine, Children's Hospital and Dana-Farber Cancer Institute, Boston, Massachusetts
Acquired Aplastic Anemia

Colin A. Sieff, MB.BCh., F.R.C.Path.
Associate Professor in Pediatrics, Harvard Medical School; Associate Professor in Pediatrics, Department of Pediatric Oncology, Dana-Farber Cancer Institute; Senior Associate in Medicine, Department of Hematology, Children's Hospital, Boston, Massachusetts
The Anatomy and Physiology of Hematopoiesis

Leslie E. Silberstein, M.D.
Professor of Pathology, Harvard Medical School; Director, Joint Program in Transfusion Medicine, Children's Hospital, Boston, Massachusetts
Transfusion Medicine

Lewis B. Silverman, M.D.
Assistant Professor of Pediatrics, Harvard Medical School; Director, Pediatric Oncology Clinic, Dana-Farber Cancer Institute, Boston, Massachusetts; Assistant in Medicine, Children's Hospital, Boston, Massachusetts
Acute Lymphoblastic Leukemia

Steven R. Sloan, M.D., Ph.D.
Assistant Professor, Harvard Medical School; Blood Bank Medical Director, Children's Hospital, Boston, Massachusetts
Transfusion Medicine

Paul M. Sondel, M.D., Ph.D.
Professor and Division Head, Departments of Pediatrics, Human Oncology, and Genetics, University of Wisconsin, Madison, Wisconsin
Cell, Cytokine, Monoclonal Antibody, and Gene Therapy

Barbara M. Sourkes, Ph.D.
Associate Professor of Pediatrics and Psychiatry, Stanford University School of Medicine; Kriewall-Haehl Director of Pediatric Palliative Care, Lucile Salter Packard Children's Hospital, Stanford, California
Psychologic Aspects of Leukemia and Hematologic Disorders

Anthony Spirito, Ph.D.
Professor of Psychiatry and Human Behavior, Brown Medical School, Providence, Rhode Island
Psychologic Aspects of Leukemia and Hematologic Disorders

James A. Stockman III, M.D.
Clinical Professor of Pediatrics, University of North
Carolina, Chapel Hill, and Duke University; President,
American Board of Pediatrics
Hematologic Manifestations of Systemic Diseases

John L. Sullivan, M.D.
Professor of Pediatrics and Molecular Medicine,
University of Massachusetts Medical School; Director,
Office of Research and Rheumatologist, University of
Massachusetts Medical Center, Worcester, Massachusetts
Lymphohistiocytic Disorders

Russell E. Ware, M.D., Ph.D.
Professor of Pediatrics; Director, Duke Pediatric Sickle
Cell Program and Pediatric Hematology Research
Laboratory, Duke University Medical Center, Durham,
North Carolina
Autoimmune Hemolytic Anemia

David Weatherall, M.D., F.R.S.
Regius Professor Emeritus and former Director of the
Weatherall Institute of Molecular Medicine, University of
Oxford, Oxford, England
*Hematologic Manifestations of Systemic Diseases in Children of
the Developing World*

Iain Webb, M.D., F.R.C.P.C.
Instructor in Medicine, Harvard Medical School;
Medical Director, Cell Manipulation Core Facility,
Dana-Farber Cancer Institute Joint Program in
Transfusion Medicine, Boston, Massachusetts
Transfusion Medicine

**V. Michael Whitehead, M.A. (Cantab),
M.D.C.M., F.R.C.P.C**
Professor of Pediatrics, Medicine and Oncology, Faculty
of Medicine, McGill University; Director of Hematology,
Coordinator of Oncology, Montreal Children's Hospital,
Montreal, Quebec, Canada
Megaloblastic Anemia

Peter F. Whitington, M.D.
Sally Burnett Searle Professor of Pediatrics, The
Feinberg School of Medicine, Northwestern University;
Division Head, Gastroenterology, Hepatology, and
Nutrition, and Director of Organ Transplantation,
Siragusa Transplantation Center, Children's Memorial
Hospital, Chicago, Illinois
Disorders of Bilirubin Metabolism

David B. Wilson, M.D., Ph.D.
Associate Professor, Department of Pediatrics and
Molecular Biology and Pharmacology, Washington
University; Attending Physician, St. Louis Children's
Hospital, St. Louis, Missouri
Acquired Platelet Defects

Bruce A. Woda, M.D.
Professor and Vice-Chairman of Pathology, University of
Massachusetts Medical School; Director, Division of
Anatomic Pathology, Department of Pathology, UMass
Memorial Medical Canter, Worcester, Massachusetts
Lymphohistiocytic Disorders

Wolf W. Zuelzer, M.D.[†]
Emeritus Professor of Pediatric Research, Wayne State
University School of Medicine; Emeritus Director of
Laboratories and Hematologist-in-Chief, Children's
Hospital of Michigan, Detroit, Michigan; Emeritus
Director, Division of Blood Diseases and Resources,
National Heart, Lung, and Blood Institute, National
Institutes of Health, Bethesda, Maryland
Pediatric Hematology in Historical Perspective

[†]Deceased

Preface

This is the sixth edition of *Hematology of Infancy and Childhood*, a labor of love that has occupied us for 30 years. The task began when the late and very much lamented Frank Oski and I decided that we needed to gather our references in one place. We were steeped in the field but beginning to become victimized by the information explosion. Sharing a similar outlook, we believed in an approach to diagnosis and treatment that focuses more on basic pathophysiology and less on description and association. We believed then, and the present editors continue to hold, that the path to better care winds its way through basic biological information. So we arranged the first edition as a series of chapters on the individual diseases that began with or included a serious inquiry into what is known about their fundamental bases.

Reader acceptance proved us correct. *Hematology of Infancy and Childhood* has become the standard textbook in the field. But as the field has grown, so has the book. Its weight has become a problem to such an extent that it may be necessary to include strength tests in the selection of editors and authors.

In the preface to the fifth edition, I outlined the history of the management of the book, including the tragic loss of Frank Oski and the emergence of Stuart Orkin and David Ginsburg as co-editors. The sixth edition forced the three of us to reexamine our strategy. We realized that the book, though comprehensive and very useful, needed radical change in certain areas. The most important of these areas were in hemorrhagic disorders and thrombosis, and in cancer. Fortunately, David Ginsburg was able to take on the leadership of the hemorrhagic disease section, and we enlisted Tom Look to take on the revision of the cancer section. That left the remaining tasks to Stuart and me. In our sections, we changed or added authors quite liberally, but retained the previous successful format.

Tom Look totally reconstructed the oncology section. First he decided to eliminate the single lengthy chapter on solid tumors that our colleague Arnold Altman had written so successfully in the past three editions. Tom argued (and we finally agreed) that there are other excellent books that deal with the solid tumors of childhood and that a single chapter, no matter how excellent, could not do the subject justice. We argued that hematology and oncology are one discipline in Pediatrics, and we wanted to retain the chapter. Tom is an impressive advocate, and with reluctance we gave up the fine work that Arnold has done for us all these years. We will miss him and are grateful for his Herculean effort. Given a free hand, Tom has created a brilliant series of chapters that focuses entirely on the hematologic malignancies. He was right.

David Ginsburg retained the structure of the hemostasis section but made changes in authors and used a very strong hand in the editing process. Tragically, the world of pediatric hematology lost Maureen Andrew in the midst of the creation of this book. Her assignment was brilliantly managed by her colleague Paul Monagle, but we will deeply miss Maureen, not only in pediatric hemostasis but in pediatric research. She was a brilliant and devoted investigator, physician, and mother.

So we present this sixth edition to our colleagues around the world with the hope that they will continue to share our enthusiasm and our commitment. The book is dedicated to pediatric hematology as a discipline; to the students, house staff, fellows, and junior faculty who are trying to learn it; and to the patients who have unlocked many secrets of biology.

We could not have accomplished any of this effort without the continued assistance of Jennifer Shreiner and Dolores Meloni of WB Saunders, our managing editor Cathy Lantigua, and the man who kept me aware of deadlines, Toby Church. We thank our "old" authors who have once again shouldered the responsibility for meeting deadlines and the new ones who have joined the club. Above all we thank our own teachers, whose inspiration made us what we are.

DAVID G. NATHAN, M.D.

Contents

Nathan and Oski's

HEMATOLOGY

of

Infancy and Childhood

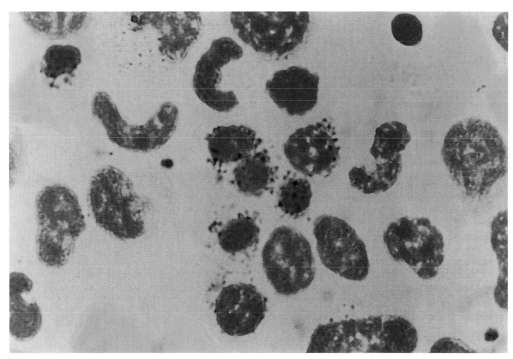

PLATE 12–7. Prussian blue stain of a bone marrow aspirate from a patient with sideroblastic anemia. The greenish blue flecks that circle the nucleus of the normoblasts are iron-laden mitochondria.

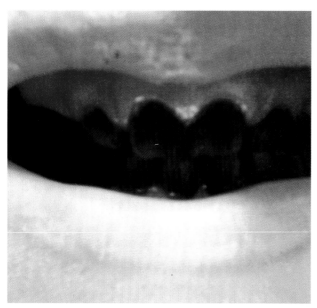

PLATE 13–6. Erythrodontia of a patient with CEP. Dark reddish-brown discoloration of the teeth is noted. When the teeth are exposed to ultraviolet light they emit the intense red fluorescence of porphyrins. Discoloration is usually more pronounced in decidual teeth than in permanent teeth. (Courtesy of H. M. Nitowsky, MD.)

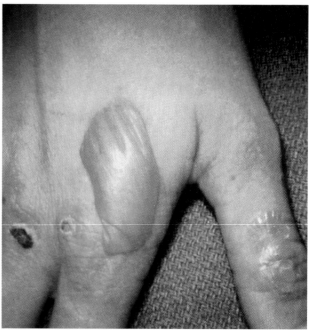

PLATE 13–8. A large fluid-like bulla, crusted erosions, and unsightly scarring are typical findings in patients with PCT. These changes may also be seen in patients with other forms of the cutaneous porphyrias, but adult onset of lesions suggests either PCT, HEP, HCP, or VP. (From Poh-Fitzpatrick MB: Porphyrin-sensitized cutaneous photosensitivity. Pathogenesis and treatment. Clin Dermatol 1985; 3:41.)

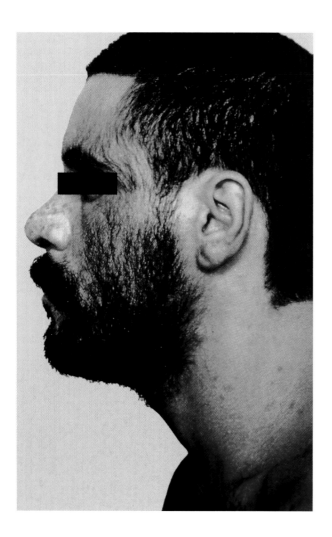

PLATE 13–9. Hypertrichosis of the face of a patient with PCT. Note the erosions and pigmentations over the nose and cheeks. (From Poh-Fitzpatrick MB: Porphyrin-sensitized cutaneous photosensitivity. Pathogenesis and treatment. Clin Dermatol 1985; 3:41.)

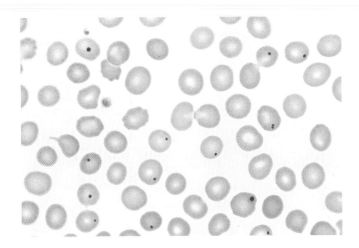

PLATE 14–4. Howell-Jolly bodies in peripheral blood erythrocytes. These nuclear remnants are identified as small inclusions within circulating erythrocytes and have several characteristic and required features by light microscopy: (1) they are spherical inclusions that are 0.5 to 2.0 μ in diameter, about the size of a small platelet; (2) they have a smooth contour and no surrounding halo, thereby distinguishing them from platelets juxtaposed to an erythrocyte; (3) they are always in the same focal plane as the erythrocyte, because they are intracellular; (4) they are never refractile, unlike talc or dust particles; and (5) they are homogeneous in appearance, unlike other intracellular inclusions such as Pappenheimer bodies or malarial parasites. Howell-Jolly bodies are normally removed when the erythrocytes pass through the cords of Billroth into the venous sinus. Their presence in the peripheral blood indicates a lack of splenic function.

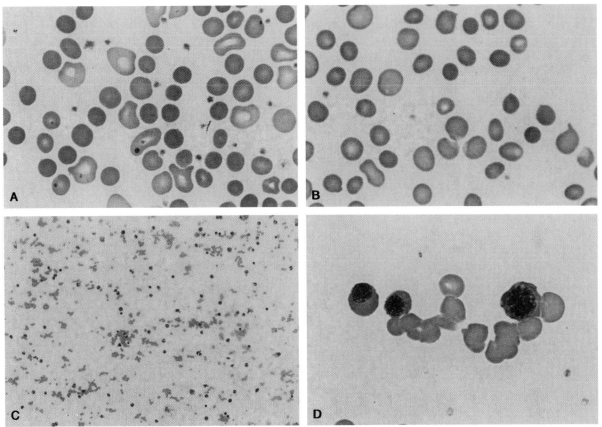

PLATE 14–5. Examination of the peripheral blood in autoimmune hemolytic anemia (AIHA). *A,* Blood from a patient with IgG (warm-reactive) AIHA illustrates many small microspherocytes and larger reticulocytes (× 1000). *B,* Blood from a patient with hereditary spherocytosis illustrates the morphologic similarities between these two conditions. *C,* Agglutinated erythrocytes from a patient with IgM (cold-reactive) AIHA are clearly visible at low power (× 400). *D,* At higher power (× 1000) the nucleated cells in the peripheral blood from this patient are identified as erythroid progenitor cells prematurely released from the bone marrow.

PLATE 14–16. Schistocytic hemolytic anemia. The peripheral blood smear (× 1000) contains several erythrocytes with characteristic triangular or crescent shapes; reflecting cells that have recently undergone fragmentation. Spherocytes are also identified, representing broken cells that have resealed their membranes and adopted a spherical shape.

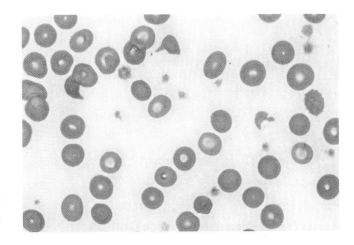

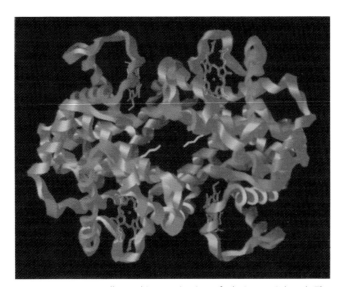

PLATE 18–14. Crystallographic examination of Hb Gower-2 ($\alpha_2\epsilon_2$). The figure was prepared by the GRASP software by Nichols and associates in 1991 on data by Sutherland-Smith et al (reference 88 in Chapter 18). The ϵ subunits are in *green* and the α subunits are in *blue*. The position of ϵ-Lys104, in *yellow*, is inside the central cavity and illustrates a difference between ϵ chains and β chains.

I | History

Pediatric Hematology in Historical Perspective

1 | Pediatric Hematology in Historical Perspective

Wolf W. Zuelzer

Wolf W. Zuelzer, who died on March 19, 1987 at the age of 77, wrote the history of pediatric hematology for the first edition of this book. We reprint it here in his memory.

As a subspecialty of pediatrics and a *sine qua non* of the modern teaching institution, pediatric hematology is a latecomer, naturally enough, for diseases of the blood were a minor problem—one is tempted to say a mere hobby of a few inquisitive and farseeing minds—compared with the great challenges of infectious and nutritional disorders that faced the pioneers of pediatrics. As a serious concern of investigators, however, pediatric hematology is as old as scientific pediatrics as a whole, though its early history is too closely interwoven with that of general hematology to be traced separately. Its tools as well as its basic concepts came largely from internal medicine and from the experimental sciences, and one needs only to mention such names as Ehrlich, Metchnikoff, Landsteiner, Chauffard, Downey, Minot, Castle, Whipple, and Wintrobe to appreciate the magnitude of this debt.

The discoveries of these and many other men were applied to the special problems of infancy and childhood by investigators who, with few exceptions, were pediatricians with diverse interests rather than hematologists with a specialized background. This is true even of those whose names are familiar through eponymic usage, such as von Jaksch, Lederer, Cooley, Blackfan, and Fanconi. Those who labored patiently in the vineyards without stumbling on a buried syndrome are mostly forgotten, though it is among them that one finds the first true pediatric hematologists. A case in point is that of Heinrich Lehndorff, who grew up in the Vienna of von Pirquet and Escherich and devoted his life to the study of both normal and abnormal hematologic conditions in childhood, publishing his first paper at the age of 29 in 1906 and his last at the age of 86 in 1963. His interest was in the blood of the newborn, in the anemias of infancy, and in leukemia. Like that of most of his contemporaries, his work was almost entirely descriptive, but he was a good morphologist and clinical observer. Lehndorff was forced to leave Vienna in 1939 at the age of 63, found temporary shelter in Birmingham with Leonard Parsons (then the leading figure in pediatric hematology in England), came to the United States during World War II, and ended his career as an octogenarian with an honorary appointment at the New York Medical College. *Sic transit gloria mundi.*

From the very beginning, the unique blood picture of the newborn received special attention. In one of the oldest hematologic texts, *Du Sang et de ses Altérations Anatomiques,* published in Paris in 1889, Hayem—known to this day as the inventor of Hayem's solution but deserving to be remembered for more important contributions—discussed the blood at birth in great detail, giving the number of red and white corpuscles and platelets on the basis of his own counts; describing macrocytosis, anisocytosis, and a tendency toward spherocytosis; and attributing the high hemoglobin level of the newborn to hyperactivity of the bone marrow. The title of a paper by E. Schiff in the *Jahrbuch für Kinderheilkunde* in 1892, "Newer contributions to the hematology of the neonate, with special reference to the time of ligation of the umbilical cord," implies the existence of earlier studies and anticipates those of Windle and his associates some 50 years later.

The hematology of the neonate remained a cardinal concern of investigators for many decades. Progress was slow, perhaps in part because of the tediousness of the methods used and in part because of variables in obstetric and pediatric practice and differences in the timing of observations. Schiff himself, working successively in Prague and Budapest, found hemoglobin levels on the first day after birth to average 104 per cent in one city and 144 per cent in the other. Much controversy arose over normal values because the early workers did not come to grips with the problems of individual variation and frequency distribution. A German author, H. Flesch,[1] wrote despairingly in 1909, "The differences in the hemoglobin values of different observers according to the ages of the children are so considerable that one is really in no position to give definite normal figures." It was difficult, moreover, to draw a line between normal and abnormal conditions. ABO hemolytic disease, for example, was unknown until 1944, when Halbrecht[2] in Hadera recognized the relationship between "icterus praecox" and incompatibility of the major blood groups of mother and child. Prior to the studies of Lippman[3] in 1924, on the other hand, the transient normoblastemia of normal full-term infants was considered pathologic, although Neumann[4] had observed it in 1871 and König[5] had written about it in 1910. Supravital staining, introduced by Ehrlich in 1880, was not used until 1925, when Friedländer and Wiedemer,[6] writing in the *American Journal of Diseases of Children*—then the only major pediatric journal in the United States—reported reticulocytosis as a regular feature of neonatal blood. Although it was known by then that reticulocytes were young cell forms, the belief still prevailed that the high hemoglobin level at birth was due solely to hemoconcentration rather than to active erythropoiesis, as postulated by Hayem.

Conversely, the postnatal drop in hemoglobin concentration was taken as evidence of accelerated hemolysis, which in turn was held by some to be the cause of physiologic jaundice. That puzzling phenomenon was long thought to signify the entry of bile into the blood as a result of temporary mechanical obstruction by a mucous plug in the common bile duct or a "desquamative catarrh" of the small radicles, or liver damage from bacterial toxins from the recently colonized intestine of the newborn. The noted Finnish neonatologist Ylppö,[7] however, had demonstrated increased bilirubin levels in the cord blood as early as 1913 and had concluded that icterus neonatorum was due to a "functional inferiority" of the liver. All theories involving the regurgitation of bile became untenable in 1922, when Erwin Schiff and E. Färber,[8] pupils of the renowned Adalbert Czerny, showed that "during the period of bilirubinemia only the indirect van den Bergh reaction is positive." The alternative that the jaundice was due to increased blood destruction, however, could not be proved. Summarizing the argument in 1928, the Viennese pediatric hematologist Eugen Stransky[9] wrote, "Although the morphologic stigmata of a hemolytic icterus (i.e., spherocytosis) are lacking and the red blood counts do not permit a firm explanation, a hematogenous origin of icterus neonatorum nevertheless seems likely. Why destruction of red corpuscles takes place is still an unsolved question."

One must sympathize with these early investigators who formulated the alternatives clearly enough but could not solve the riddle of neonatal jaundice with the means at their disposal. To them icterus meant either regurgitation of bile or increased destruction of blood. Hemolysis seemed indeed a plausible explanation for the combination of bilirubinemia of the indirect variety with a falling hemoglobin level and a regenerative blood picture, all the more because mild forms of hemolytic disease were undoubtedly included in studies of infants presumed to be normal. The life span of fetal—or, for that matter, adult—red cells remained an unknown quantity, even after Winifred Ashby in 1919 had measured it in adults, using the differential agglutination technique, as the range of 30 to 100 days reported by her was too great to be of practical value. This was also true of the blood volume of the newborn, which William Palmer Lucas and B. F. Dearing[10] of San Francisco had actually attempted to measure in the same year, using the brilliant vital red dilution method. They obtained a range of values from 107 to 195 mL per kg of body weight, almost twice that found in 1950 by Mollison and his associates[11] with a method combining isotope and dye dilution. The mere fact that they concerned themselves with such questions in 1919 puts them ahead of their pediatric contemporaries. Neither of the first two books devoted specifically to pedi-

atric hematology, that of Ferruccio Zibordi of Modena, *Ematologia Infantile Normale e Patologica*,[12] which appeared in 1925, and that of Baar and Stransky of Vienna, *Die Klinische Hämatologie des Kindesalters*,[1] published in 1928, mentioned blood volume or red cell survival. The name of Lucas deserves recognition in any survey of pediatric hematology, for, apart from looking after patients with blood diseases in the Children's Department of the University of California before such specialization had become accepted elsewhere, he was an enterprising and thoughtful investigator. His chapters on blood in Abt's *Pediatrics* of 1924, written with E. C. Fleischner,[13] are outstanding in their emphasis on physiologic processes, clarity of thought, and absence of semantic claptrap, and in these respects are superior to the two works just cited.

As for the solution to the puzzle of neonatal jaundice, the functional inferiority of the liver postulated so long ago by Ylppö could not be defined, of course, until Hijmans van den Bergh's two pigments had been identified as free and glucuronide-conjugated bilirubin by the independent studies of Billing and Lathe,[14] Schmid,[15] and Talafant[16] in 1956. The results of the preceding demonstration of the role of uridine diphosphate glucuronic acid (UDPGA) as a glucuronide donor by Dutton[17] and others could be applied to bilirubin, and the enzymatic reactions involved in the conjugation process could be investigated as a function of hepatic maturation by Brown and co-workers.[18]

Traditionally, the history of pediatric hematology begins in 1889 with von Jaksch's report[19] on the condition that bears his name, which he designated *anemia pseudoleucaemica infantum*. By an irony of fate, not only the term but the very syndrome has long since vanished from the horizon, although in its day it had an enormous vogue and was considered by some to be the anemia of infancy *par excellence*. In 1891, the condition was described independently by Hayem[20] and his compatriot Luzet,[21] so that their names were also attached to it. The clinical picture was overshadowed by severe nutritional disturbances, wasting, diarrhea, rickets, and, as a rule, chronic infections of the respiratory tract, otitis media, pyoderma, and the like. The findings suggestive of leukemia were marked splenomegaly, anemia, and that which later hematologists would call a leukemoid reaction, characterized by leukocytosis and immature granulocytes. It was Luzet who noted the normoblastemia that led to the use of the term "erythroblastic anemia," until that term was temporarily pre-empted by Cooley for the anemia that *he* described. At that time, the combination of splenomegaly and leukocytosis meant leukemia, and von Jaksch's paper was therefore a distinct step forward, though its essence was the simple observation that some of the patients survived, a remarkable fact in itself given their general condition and the paucity of therapeutic means then available.

Von Jaksch was not a hematologist, and except for a follow-up report in 1890, he made no further contributions to the understanding of the disease that made him famous. He practiced pediatrics in Prague, then the capital of the Austrian province of Bohemia, and held an appointment at the Charles University, where, as a legendary octogenarian, he was pointed out to this writer in 1934, a tall aristocratic figure with a massive white head who bore his fame with a casual elegance reminiscent of the old Hapsburg Empire. The riddle of von Jaksch's anemia was never properly solved. It was at one time common in central Europe and in France, less so in England, and still less so in the United States. Its disappearance paralleled the gradual improvement in child health and care. As Lehndorff[22] wrote many years afterward in an almost nostalgic epitaph on the extinct entity, it had been "a poor people's disease." In truth, it was not an entity at all but a convenient diagnostic wastebasket, though an interesting one. The contemporaries finally agreed that it was a nonspecific response of the infantile organism to the horrendous combinations of infectious and nutritional insults that were so common at the time and so difficult to sort out.

More lasting and far more important, of course, was the contribution made to pediatric hematology—and indeed to medical science as a whole—by Thomas B. Cooley of Detroit in 1925,[23] when he salvaged from this wastebasket the distinct entity now known as thalassemia. He soon abandoned his original designation of "erythroblastic anemia," for he realized that the conspicuous normoblastemia that had first attracted his attention was neither a specific nor a central feature of the disorder, and in his later publications he emphasized the fragmentation and shape anomalies of the red cells and the paucity and uneven distribution of the hemoglobin. He did not know, of course, that the ultimate disturbance was one of hemoglobin, let alone β chain synthesis, but he came to conceive of the disease as a fundamental disorder of hematopoiesis and was fully aware of its genetic nature from the beginning. He himself had originally proposed a recessive mode of inheritance, anticipating the classic study of Valentine and Neel of 1944.[24] Strangely enough, he failed to investigate the seemingly normal parents and siblings of the propositi. Later, unverified reports of hereditary transmission of the disorder by a single affected parent seemed to militate against a recessive mode and left him uncertain.

Cooley was, in any case, profoundly interested in the genetic aspects of the anemias and was in this respect far ahead of most contemporary hematologists. He corresponded with geneticists, used such terms as "heterozygote" for humans at a time when their use was still largely restricted to plants and *Drosophila,* and for years pondered the then wholly puzzling relationship between "sicklemia" and sickle cell anemia. He reported the first instance of sickle cell disease (which this writer later had occasion to identify as a case of sickle-thalassemia) in a Greek family.[25] He also proposed an X-linked mode of inheritance, backed by pedigree studies over five generations, for a familial hypochromic anemia in a kindred first described by him[26] and later restudied by Rundles and Falls[27] at Ann Arbor, Michigan. In accepting the term "Mediterranean anemia," which Whipple had suggested at a time when the known cases were restricted to Italian and Greek families, Cooley[28] made an interesting and prophetic reservation: "We are not inclined," he wrote in 1932, "to lay great stress on the limitation of this or any similar disease to a particular race. We have found that sickle cell anemia, formerly supposed to be peculiar to Negroes, occurs in Greeks, and it seems likely to us that any disease in which there is a hereditary element, as presumably there is in this disease, is limited more by locality and association than by race."

The style is as characteristic of the man as the thought. Cooley was articulate, well educated—he spoke or at least read four languages and maintained a global correspondence—and highly intelligent. He came from a family of distinguished jurists, the only one to eschew the law and enter the medical profession. Born in Ann Arbor, the son of a future justice of the Michigan Supreme Court, he obtained his degree in medicine at the University of Michigan, worked for 3 years in "clinical chemistry," interned at Boston City Hospital, spent a year visiting clinics in Germany, returned to Boston for prolonged training in contagious diseases, and then was appointed Assistant Professor of Hygiene at his *alma mater.* Except for a stint with the Children's Bureau of the American Red Cross during World War I, he remained in Michigan for the rest of his life, first as a practicing pediatrician and, after the death of Raymond Hoobler in 1936, as a professor of pediatrics in Detroit. Throughout these years he was closely associated with The Children's Hospital of Michigan, whose pediatrician-in-chief he ultimately became.

As mentioned, Cooley had no formal training in hematology and very little technical help. He and his faithful associate of many years, Pearl Lee, examined blood smears, roentgenograms, and, of course, the patients themselves, making sketchy notes on index cards and keeping the bulk of their observations in their heads. His equipment consisted of a monocular microscope of ancient vintage, a staining rack, a rather small card file, and—in an otherwise vacant room upstairs intended for the affairs of the Child Research Council of the American Academy of Pediatrics—a couch on which he took siestas and did much of his thinking. His daughter Emily, a gifted and artistic young woman, made the beautiful camera lucida and freehand drawings with which he illustrated his papers. She also chauffeured him about town, went to the library for him, and accompanied him to meetings. His home in Detroit's "Indian Village" and his garden, professionally landscaped by Emily, were oases of good taste. He owned a cottage on the coast of Maine where he spent his summers. He loved music, knew his wines, enjoyed good food, and was an excellent conversationalist. He knew how to live.

At times, his penchant for conversation got him into trouble. Old-time Detroiters recall the story of his house call to a well-to-do family whose child had contracted an undiagnosed illness. As a social acquaintance Dr. Cooley was led into the living room, offered refreshments, and asked his opinion on some topic of current interest. A lively discussion ensued, at the end of which the doctor, having forgotten the original purpose of his visit, grabbed his hat and coat and was out of the house before the astonished parents could remind him of the patient upstairs.

Cooley's influence extended well beyond the field of hematology. His was the conception behind a series of studies on the chemical composition of the red cell stroma carried out in the 1930s by Erickson and associates in the laboratories of Icie Macy Hoobler of the Children's Fund of Michigan, which earned high praise from Eric Ponder. He was one of the founders of the Academy of Pediatrics and, long before the time was ripe, saw the role of pediatrics in terms of preventive medicine. Politically he was a liberal, scientifically a radical, personally a patrician. Combined with a rather haughty expression, an irrepressible wit, and an utter lack of reverence for established authority, these traits were bound to earn him enmities on the part of town and gown alike, but his enemies respected and his friends admired him. He was well ahead of his time, a lucid thinker and a giant in the history of pediatric hematology.

An entirely different personality was George Guest, for many years one of the mainstays of the Children's Hospital Research Foundation in Cincinnati, whose contributions were equally important, if less spectacular. Guest was as much a physiologist as a hematologist, interested in the basic aspects of blood during growth, a stickler for precise measurements, a patient investigator who set himself longterm goals and took a systematic approach to reaching them. The meticulous studies he conducted between 1932 and 1942 on the hemoglobin levels, red blood counts, and packed cell volumes of a large group of infants and young children of widely different social and economic backgrounds are a model of intelligent and purposeful data-gathering, the purpose being both physiologic and clinical. In the face of the rather arbitrary definitions and therapeutic practices then prevailing, Guest set out to ascertain the range of normal variation and to delineate optimal values against hypoferric states. Such data were badly needed then and have remained valid to this day. In serial studies[29] involving, among other things, intrafamily and twin comparisons, he showed convincingly that a fall of the mean corpuscular volume (MCV) and mean corpuscular hemoglobin (MCH) in the presence of seemingly adequate hemoglobin levels could be reversed or altogether prevented by the administration of iron and is therefore a sensitive indicator of an incipient deficiency state rather than a physiologic phenomenon. He concluded that iron deficiency anemia was far more common among infants than had been previously thought, and advocated the general use of prophylactic measures. His earlier observations on glycolysis and the rise of inorganic phosphorus levels in stored blood[30] and his joint observations with Sam Rapoport[31] on the role of the pH in the breakdown of diphosphoglycerate were milestones in the understanding of red cell metabolism. He also made significant contributions to the knowledge of the osmometric properties of erythrocytes,[32] both normal and abnormal, devising a method that was, typically, both practical and precise and permitted simultaneous determinations of hemolysis and red cell volume at each stage of the procedure.

Apart from these accomplishments, George Guest was a delightful friend and, with the help of his wife, a perfect host, so that the house on Dana Avenue in Cincinnati became a kind of unofficial headquarters for the entertainment of the many visitors to the Children's Hospital. Here they were offered the *vin d'honneur* from a well-stocked wine cellar decorated with frescoes by an artist friend—the owners' pride and the first and last stop for the visitor—and here they would find good conversation, interesting people, and exquisite cuisine. The Guests were passionate Francophiles, and the cooking was French, unless a keg of oysters had just arrived from the East to be prepared in endless variations, or unless Jesse, the houseman, more friend than butler, just happened to have shot—illegally, of course—a fat squirrel from one of the magnificent old trees in the garden. George, a short, stocky, quiet-spoken man, understood the art of good fellowship, but the soul of the house and its social genius was his wife "M.L.," a handsome woman with red hair who had a passion for poetry and a gift for conversation. They had met in Europe after World War I as young and idealistic members of the Hoover Relief team, were drawn together by their love for all things French, and remained deeply devoted to one another. A large part of every summer was spent in France visiting friends, traveling through the countryside, and sampling wines. George Guest was the only American member of the French Pediatric Society, a fact in which he took greater pride than in all his other achievements, and though his French accent left much to be desired, he liked to attend meetings and even present papers in such delightful places as Bordeaux, Lyon, and Paris. When M.L. died about 1964, the house was sold and an era passed.

It would be instructive to trace in detail the thinking of earlier observers concerning the iron deficiency anemia of infancy, to whose definition Guest made such a solid contribution, but which remained an object of controversy, confusion, and neglect for generations of pediatricians. Although Bunge had proposed an essentially correct explanation as early as 1889, the nature of the most common anemia of infancy eluded investigators for many years. The reasons for this paradox are enlightening. One was the belief that not only mild anemia but also hypochromasia was a physiologic phenomenon. "That the hemoglobin content suffers more than the red blood count," Heinrich Baar wrote in 1928,[33] "is surely a purposeful mechanism, for the same quantity of hemoglobin can serve its function better when it is distributed over a larger number of red corpuscles." More important, no doubt, is the fact that among the clinic patients on whom most studies were conducted, pure iron deficiency anemia was rare. In the face of the multiple ailments to which such patients were prone, failure to respond to iron alone was common, and it was easy to draw erroneous conclusions from therapeutic trials. Conversely, of course, a rise of the hemoglobin level following the administration of iron was just as uncritically taken as proof of its efficacy on the principle of *post hoc propter hoc,* though it was believed that iron was a bone marrow "stimulant" rather than a specific substance effective only when correcting or preventing a deficiency.

Much of the problem was semantic in nature. Whereas French pediatricians described iron-responsive hypochromic anemia in infants as "*chlorose due jeune âge*" or "*chlorose alimentaire,*" most German and Austrian authors rejected this concept, if only because "chlorosis occurs only during puberty and only in females." The highly influential Czerny, in particular, set the clock back by stating categorically that an entire group of alimentary anemias existed that could be influenced by diet but in which iron was utterly ineffective. Baar wrote: "If it appears, *a priori*, unjustified to group together, and attribute to direct or indirect lack of iron, anemias of the most diverse origin solely because they are all hypochromic, fail to show nucleated red cells in the peripheral blood and lack splenomegaly, the notion of chlorosis of alimentary origin was definitely refuted by Czerny's findings." If this was to pour the baby out with the bathwater, Baar retreated from his a prioristic position to the extent of recognizing a "pseudochlorosis infantum," or infantile iron deficiency anemia, as an "etiologically uniform type to be separated from the rest of the alimentary anemias of infancy." This was rare, however, he asserted, in comparison with "the overwhelming majority [which] remains uninfluenced by iron administration, though nevertheless improved or cured by appropriate changes in diet." In reading such statements, one must remember that even fresh air and sunshine were still considered essential adjuncts to the treatment of anemia. Moreover, no less an authority than Haldane[34] had asserted earlier that "recovery affords no ground for assuming that iron is built up into hemoglobin," and that "in typical cases [of chlorosis] the curative factor of iron salts must be exercised otherwise than simply in building up the hemoglobin." Haldane went on to say that "The essential process in the cure of chlorosis is the reduction in the volume of the plasma [*sic*]." In addition, the notion of toxic hemolysis due to the fatty acids in cow's milk and especially in goat's milk had a prolonged vogue on the Continent, where "cow's milk anemia" and "goat's milk anemia" were accepted entities.

Related to the semantic difficulties was the problem of classification. Ever since Hayem had introduced the color index in 1877, hypochromasia had been used to characterize certain anemias. It was soon apparent that most anemias of older infants were of this type, but the difficulty of relating morphologic criteria to pathogenetic mechanisms and of recognizing in turn that different etiologic factors could operate through identical pathways proved too much. Not until the work of Minot and Castle established the characteristic response of hemoglobin and reticulocytes to specific hematinics, and Wintrobe put the morphologic classification on the firm basis of red cell measurements, did pediatric hematologists gradually abandon terms such as "alimentary-infectious" anemia. In 1936, Hugh Josephs[35] still used this term as a common denominator that, to him, included deficient hemoglobin formation, deficient erythropoiesis and deficient stimulation of erythropoiesis, deficient maturation (the "erythroblastoses"), and blood destruction. Such usage, apart from the vagueness of the etiologic concept, was bound to delay both the understanding of the pathogenesis and the development of a workable classification of the anemias. It was an internist who said that "the infant bleeds into its own increasing blood volume," and the importance of the hemoglobin mass at birth was not appreciated until later. When Blackfan and Diamond's *Atlas of the Blood in Children* finally appeared in 1944,[36] it used Wintrobe's classification and described the principal anemia of infancy under the title "iron deficiency anemia."

One cannot leave the subject of iron deficiency without reference to Hugh Josephs, a strange figure, and in his day an authority in the field of American pediatric hematology. It is remarkable that this should have been the case, for he published little and confined his work primarily to the relationship between iron metabolism and anemia in infancy. His chapters on diseases of the blood in Holt and McIntosh's textbook were excellent, but his mind had a somewhat pedantic cast and a tendency to look for profound meanings underneath simple facts. His forte was a thorough knowledge of the literature, which he analyzed in erudite but unconscionably lengthy reviews, complete with foreword, statement of scope and purpose, introduction, presentation of fundamental concepts, summary, table of contents, and a bibliography that in one instance exceeded 750 titles. He was Associate Professor of Pediatrics in Dr. Park's department at Johns Hopkins University and published mostly in the Johns Hopkins Bulletin. His manner and appearance were those of a college professor or a don—mild, pleasant, serious, single-minded, a slight, gray-haired man who smoked a pipe, wore soft collars and a velvet jacket with elbow patches, and received his visitors in a drab office in the old Harriet Lane Home cluttered with books, magazines, and reprints.

By means of a curious logic, Josephs came to the unshakable conclusion that the hypochromic iron deficiency anemia of infants was not due to depletion of iron but to its diversion to unknown sites by unknown mechanisms.[37] He based this hypothesis on theoretical calculations that proved that an anemic baby of 18 months *should* have an excess of 200 mg of unused iron—other than the necessary tissue iron—somewhere in his body; *ergo* the baby suffered from "iron deficiency without depletion." This hypothetical baby, Josephs said, "is starving in the midst of plenty. Give this baby a small amount of iron by mouth and he will utilize it avidly for hemoglobin formation, and may as a result use even more than he was given." In the absence of infection, the unavailability of iron might be due, he thought, to hormonal, histotrophic, or even emotional factors. But in 1956, 3 years after these speculations, Philip Sturgeon[38] calculated on the basis of the same data that had been available to Josephs that a seemingly normal newborn could easily have a hemoglobin mass low enough to account for severe anemia in later infancy, reflecting the expansion of the blood volume with growth. Earlier, Bruce Chown[39] of Winnipeg had documented the occurrence of massive transplacental hemorrhage. Soon afterward, Kleihauer and Betke[40] devised their ingenious method for demonstrating fetal cells in maternal blood by the acid elution technique. Subsequent studies by Cohen, Zuelzer, and associates[41] and others showed that moderate and repeated fetal bleeds were not at all rare. A mechanism for depriving the fetus of hemoglobin iron without necessarily causing overt anemia at birth but capable of explaining the later development of iron deficiency in the absence of further blood loss seemed to offer a simpler solution than the tortuous hypothesis of "iron deficiency without depletion." The modern age had arrived.

Their semantic difficulties did not keep the earlier pediatricians from devising eminently practical methods of treatment, as exemplified by the story of pediatric transfusion therapy. The technical problems of transfusing infants were overcome in various ways. In 1915, Helmholz of the Mayo Clinic advocated the use of the superior sagittal sinus, and in 1925 Hart of the Sick Children's Hospital of Toronto used this route for the first exchange transfusion ever given for "icterus gravis."[42] Though his patient recovered, exchange transfusion was not again used for this indication until Wallerstein revived it in 1946 on the grounds that "the removal of most of the Rh-positive cells and of the circulating antibody shortly after birth prevents the incidence of the more severe pathological and physiological changes." Wallerstein,[43] then Director of the Erythroblastosis Fetalis Clinic of the Jewish Memorial Hospital in New York, had used the sagittal sinus for most of his cases, but stated that "the umbilical vessels should be an excellent route for both the withdrawal and replacement procedures," with the strange proviso that they could be used "only if the decision to perform the substitution is made before birth. . . ." J.B. Sidbury,[44] a pediatrician at the Babies' Hospital in Wrightsville, North Carolina, in a little-noticed report had described a simple transfusion via the umbilical vein in the case of a bleeding newborn in 1923. It was Diamond[45] who later established the umbilical route as the safest and simplest for exchange transfusion in hemolytic disease and who, with Allen and Vaughan,[46] was the first to recognize that the prevention of kernicterus was the main rationale of the procedure. It is interesting to recall that exsanguination transfusion through the fontanelle or the femoral vein was used on a large scale at the Sick Children's Hospital in Toronto for the treatment of burns, erysipelas, and other conditions since 1921. This procedure was introduced by Bruce Robertson, who in 1916 during the campaign in France had observed two soldiers recover from severe carbon monoxide poisoning after venesections followed by transfusions. By March of 1924, when Robertson was already dead, 501 exsanguination transfusions had been performed at the Sick Children's Hospital.[47]

In the late 1950s there was a small flurry of papers reporting successful transfusions by the intraperitoneal route. This subject had been thoroughly explored in two studies, one experimental,[48] the other clinical,[49] in 1923 by a young pediatric resident in Minneapolis, David Siperstein, whose concise and accurate summary read as follows: "1. The intraperitoneal transfusion of citrated blood is a therapeutic procedure of possible merit. 2. It can apparently be utilized in cases in which transfusion is indicated, when other routes are unavailable." The author documented the effective reabsorption of the transfused cells not only with serial red counts and hemoglobin determinations but also with photomicrographs showing the dual population of hypochromic recipient and normochromic donor cells. In his review of the literature, he found that intraperitoneal transfusion was first used by Ponfick of Berlin in 1875, and that Hayem in 1884 had performed ingenious experiments involving cross transfusions of dog and rabbit blood in order to prove absorption from the peritoneal cavity. Although technical progress has since made the procedure obsolete, Siperstein's work deserves to be rescued from oblivion, if only to show that there is nothing new under the sun. He recognized a potential need, defined the problem, and solved it with an enviable economy of means (and words).

Passing mention should also be made of the use of bone marrow transfusions as a means of side-stepping technical difficulties in transfusing infants, especially for the general pediatrician with little practice in "needlework." The method had its day in England and particularly in Denmark, where Heinild[50] in 1947 described the experience of 4 years, during which 686 blood transfusions were given via the bone marrow without a single mishap. He stated that the risk of osteomyelitis was limited to patients receiving continuous infusions. One hesitates to argue with success and realizes that, in places and under conditions in which the required skills or supplies are lacking, it is better to apply unorthodox methods than to let a baby die for lack of blood.

A less desirable development that took place in the late 1920s and continued until the early 1940s was the practice of giving newborn infants intramuscular injections of adult blood as a prophylactic measure against hemorrhagic disease of the newborn. During those years, according to recollections provided by James L. Wilson, who for many years was Dr. Blackfan's right arm at The Children's Hospital in Boston, hemorrhagic disease was becoming so great a problem that this practice seemed justified. The blood was given without typing or crossmatching, and the procedure undoubtedly was responsible for a significant number of sensitizations against the Rh factor that did not come to light until these infants had grown up (and the Rh factor had meanwhile been discovered). The subsequent decline in hemorrhagic disease of the newborn coincided with both the introduction of vitamin K and a significant improvement in obstetric practices. Since the condition has now become rare and its definition was always vague and without clear distinction between traumatic hemorrhages and those primarily attributable to a coagulation difficulty, the mystery of its upsurge and the reasons for its virtual disappearance have never become quite clear.

If pediatricians proved resourceful in the matter of blood transfusions, it must be said that they showed little innovative spirit in certain other respects. It is a curious fact that the study of the bone marrow in children was neglected, especially in the United States, long after its usefulness had been amply demonstrated in adults. Thus Cooley, for example, never looked at anything but the peripheral blood, and Blackfan and Diamond's otherwise exhaustive *Atlas* of 1944 appeared without a single illustration of bone marrow. This writer remembers visiting a major pediatric center on the East Coast about 1946 and being shown half a dozen patients on the wards suspected of having leukemia and awaiting *surgical* biopsies—to be performed when and if they stopped bleeding. His own interest in the cytology of the bone marrow, which led to the recognition of megaloblastic anemia of infancy and its reversal by folic acid,[51] had been stimulated by many "curb-stone" discussions with Lawrence Berman, a student of Downey and himself an outstanding morphologist. It should be noted that Amato of Naples, Italy,[52] gave an excellent description of infantile megaloblastic anemia independently in the same year as Zuelzer and Ogden,[51] though he did not have folic acid at his disposal and concluded from the response to potent liver extract that he was dealing with true pernicious anemia or at least with a temporary deficiency of intrinsic factor. An even earlier report by Veeneklaas of Holland[53] had the misfortune of being prevented from reaching readers abroad because of World War II.

This is the place to pay tribute to the memory of Katsuji Kato, pupil and associate of Downey, a superb morphologist and illustrator, who was the first student of the infantile bone marrow in the United States. In 1937, Kato[54] published a definitive study based on bone marrow aspirations in 51 normal infants and children. He commented on the lymphocytosis in the younger subjects and gave the myeloid-erythroid ratios for the various ages. He also illustrated the diagnostic value of the procedure by citing a case of leukemia and one of Niemann-Pick disease. Kato was on the staff of Bobs Roberts Memorial Hospital in Chicago and often made the long trek to the North Side to participate in Dr. Brennemann's grand rounds at the Children's Memorial Hospital. One remembers him, a jolly, round-faced, smiling figure reminiscent of the *Hotei-Sama* statuettes of his native Japan, a rapid speaker with an atrocious accent but interesting ideas, showing off his delicate colored drawings with as much aesthetic pleasure as scientific pride and at the same time implying by his self-deprecating manner that it was all quite simple and hardly worth the honorable listener's attention. World War II put an end to his career. He returned to Japan and was lost from sight.

Perhaps it was Kato's unfortunate choice of the sternum as the site for diagnostic punctures, making the procedure unnecessarily difficult and unpleasant in pediatric practice, that kept others from emulating him. American authors virtually ignored Kato's work, except for the enterprising Peter Vogel at Mount Sinai Hospital in New York, whose study with Frank Bassen[55] in 1939 covered 113 examples of diverse conditions, including leukemia, Gaucher's disease, and metastatic neuroblastoma, illustrated with excellent photomicrographs. In Europe, and especially in Switzerland under the influence of Rohr and Moeschlin, pediatric hematologists were more curious. Zürich, where Naegeli had created a strong tradition, had already become a mecca of Continental hematology. Writing in 1937, Guido Fanconi[56] declared: "The painstaking exploration of every case [of unexplained anemia] with old and new methods, which include bone marrow puncture, handled at the Zürich [Children's] Clinic with consummate skill by my *Oberarzt, Dozent* Willi, promises to uncover new, sharply defined entities." In the short span between 1935 and 1938, H. Willi[57] published four excellent studies on the bone marrow in thrombocytopenic purpura, leukemia, and various anemias of childhood. Fanconi had the satisfaction of seeing his prophecy fulfilled, in part by his next *Oberarzt,* Conrad Gasser. In addition to megaloblastic anemia of infancy, a whole series of conditions came to light or were clarified by bone marrow studies, among them the acute erythroblastopenia described in 1949 by Gasser[58]; chronic benign neutropenia, also studied by Gasser[59] and later by Zuelzer and Bajoghli[60]; Kostmann's infantile genetic agranulocytosis[61]; "myelokathexis"[62] or "ineffective granulopoiesis"[63]; and the aplastic and hypoplastic anemias.

Hematology occupied a special place among Fanconi's far-flung interests, and in giving encouragement and support to his associates—in this respect not unlike Blackfan—he contributed as much to progress in this field as he had done earlier with the recognition of the anemia that bears his name.[64] A tall, handsome man, every inch the professor yet gracious and outgoing, capable of charming an audience in six languages, a lively and eclectic spirit, Fanconi was a superb clinician and an excellent organizer to whom pediatric hematology owes much. With Fanconi one must rank his colleague in Bern, Glanzmann,[65] whose report in 1918 on "hereditary hemorrhagic thrombasthenia" as a condition characterized by prolonged bleeding time and poor clot retraction in the presence of a normal platelet count opened the era of platelet function studies. Glanzmann postulated the existence of a platelet factor specifically involved in clot retraction. He contributed greatly to the knowledge of the various purpuras. The term "anaphylactoid purpura" stems from his studies[66] and was based partly on clinical observations and similarities with human serum sickness and partly on his interpretation of Hayem's findings in dogs injected intravenously with bovine serum.

Conrad Gasser, one of the ablest and most productive pediatric hematologists in Europe, deserves more than passing mention in this narrative. Apart from his discovery of acute erythroblastopenia—known until then only from the report of Owren[67] as a complication of congenital spherocytosis—and his study of chronic neutropenia, he added greatly to our knowledge of hemolytic anemias in childhood. His monograph *Die Hämolytischen Syndrome des Kindesalters,*[68] which appeared in 1951, ranks in quality if not in scope with Dacie's well-known book. In 1948, in a paper with Grumbach,[69] Gasser described spherocytosis as a feature of ABO hemolytic disease. In the same year he gave a detailed report of anemia with spontaneous Heinz body formation in a premature infant,[70] a condition then unknown except for a brief note by Willi. In his book, and in subsequent publications, he added a large compilation of case material, described the detailed morphologic picture of the abnormal red cells—which were identical with the "pyknocytes" later observed in full-term infants by Tuffy, Brown, and Zuelzer,[71] but which he called more graphically "ruptured eggshells"—and determined their incidence in the blood of normal premature infants. He coined the term "hemolytic-uremic syndrome," being among the first to recognize that condition.

One reports with regret that so fruitful a career was disrupted by the exigencies of an academic system that, at the time at least, provided insufficient "room at the top" and effectively eliminated key people upon the retirement of their chief (unless they happened to be chosen to succeed him). Such a system was, and to a large extent still is, in force in Switzerland and elsewhere on the Continent. Fanconi's retirement from the *Kinderspital* in Zürich almost automatically entailed that of his *Oberarzt* Gasser. The latter, a modest man with a quiet sense of humor and a *gemütlich* Alemannic temperament, maintained his interest in hematology, which came to include the treatment of childhood leukemia, but he did so as a practicing pediatrician in a private office. Similar reasons prematurely ended the academic career of Sansone in Genoa, author of a book on favism and one of the most promising pediatric hematologists in Italy.

It is manifestly impossible in the allotted space to do justice to, or even name, all those who contributed to the evolution of pediatric hematology. Among European workers one would like to dwell on the achievements of Sir Leonard Parsons of Birmingham, England, the Grand Old Man of British pediatric hematology, founder of a veritable school that attracted students from many countries, including the United States. Parsons was an original thinker who refused to accept the confused semantics of childhood anemias and created his own system along pathophysiologic lines. He was the first to recognize, in 1933, the hemolytic nature of erythroblastosis fetalis and to defend that concept[72] even against the authority of Castle and Minot. These men, along with Diamond, Blackfan and Baty, Josephs, and others, regarded erythroblastosis fetalis as a defect of hematopoiesis in a class with Cooley's anemia and other "erythroblastoses." One would like to describe the achievements of Parson's associates, Hawksley and Lightwood; of Cathie, Gairdner, Walker, Hardisty, and so many other British colleagues of Lichtenstein in Sweden—an early student of the anemia of prematurity, which he was the first to call physiologic and to separate from the later phase of iron deficiency; of his compatriots Wallgren and Vahlquist; of Plum in Copenhagen, the discoverer of vitamin K and originator of the thesis of a temporary deficiency of this substance as the cause of hemorrhagic disease of the newborn; of van Crefeld of Amsterdam, a pioneer in the study of coagulation factors in the newborn; of Betke, then in Tübingen, who with Kleihauer developed the acid elution technique for the demonstration of fetal hemoglobin in individual cells and who later, in Munich, made his department into a strong base of pediatric hematology; of Jonxis in Leyden, an imaginative investigator, who among other things organized a comparative study of the incidence of sickling in Curaçao and Dutch Guiana (now Surinam) to test Allison's hypothesis of the selective effect of malaria on two genetically similar populations exposed for centuries to different risks of the infection.

To return closer to home, credit must be given to James M. Baty as a member, with Blackfan and Diamond, of the triumvirate at Children's Hospital, Boston, that set the pattern for the development of pediatric hematology in the United States. Their collaborative effort resulted in, among other things, the recognition that hydrops fetalis, icterus gravis, and hemolytic anemia of the newborn, in spite of the differences in their clinical manifestations, were etiologically related conditions.[73] This was truly a breakthrough in the understanding of hemolytic disease. After Baty moved to the Floating Hospital and Blackfan died an untimely death, Diamond emerged as the American pediatric hematologist *par excellence*. His role cannot be described solely in terms of his publications, which are too numerous to be listed here. He became the mentor of a whole generation of pediatric hematologists who later held, and in most instances still hold, key positions in teaching institutions throughout the United States. Directly or indirectly we all owe him a debt of gratitude, even those of us who from time to time disagreed

with some of his ideas. This writer vividly remembers his first meeting with Dr. Diamond, when as a lowly intern in 1935 he consulted him in connection with a case of Cooley's anemia, then an unheard-of rarity in the small New England hospital where he served. This writer made the pilgrimage to Children's Hospital—which under Blackfan was forbidden territory to those who were not graduates of Harvard, Yale, Columbia, or Johns Hopkins—with some trepidation. His fears were not allayed when he laid eyes on Dr. Diamond, rather fierce-looking in a dark, Assyrian sort of way. But Diamond proved to be a gracious consultant, willing to discuss the case at hand without condescension or conceit with an insignificant beginner, to listen to the history and examine the blood films, and above all to confirm the beginner's diagnosis. Over the years, hundreds of colleagues and young would-be hematologists came to appreciate "L.K.'s" kindness and unfailing courtesy. Of his numerous contributions one need mention here only the "Diamond-Blackfan" syndrome of hypoplastic anemia;[74] the studies on the nature, diagnostics, and treatment of hemolytic disease; and the *Atlas,* an outstanding achievement for its day, which was his work rather than Blackfan's. But perhaps even more important was the guidance and encouragement he provided for pediatric hematologists of the next generation, of whom—at the risk of being selective—we can name here only a few: Fred ("Hal") Allen, Park Gerald, Frank Oski, N.T. Shahidi, Victor Vaughan, and William Zinkham.

Less influential, though no less respected, was the late Carl Smith of New York. His book, *Blood Diseases of Infancy and Childhood,*[75] was the first of its kind in the United States and for many years served as the major reference work in the field. Smith's most important contribution was the description of infectious lymphocytosis, an essentially asymptomatic condition associated with a blood picture reminiscent of that of whooping cough (or chronic lymphocytic leukemia), endemic and probably of viral origin. He took a great interest in thalassemia and established a model outpatient transfusion service at The New York Hospital. Carl Smith was a modest and generous man, always willing to praise and give credit, even when credit was not due. Through his untiring efforts, Cornell became one of the important centers of pediatric hematology on the East Coast.

The prime mover in the field on the West Coast was Philip Sturgeon, who created the hematology service at the Children's Hospital of Los Angeles. He emerged about 1950 as an independent investigator interested in the study of the infantile bone marrow. His research provided quantitative measurements, then badly needed,[76] and stimulated the diagnostic use of bone marrow aspiration. A great traveller and sportsman in private life, Sturgeon combined in his work the elements of common sense and scientific curiosity, establishing the outstanding hematology clinic that was later carried on by his successor, Dennis Hammond. In the midst of a productive career, Sturgeon surprised his friends and colleagues by retiring to Zermatt in Switzerland, but skiing and hiking even in the most glorious of landscapes was not enough to fill his existence, and after a few years he returned to his work, and California.

The fact that a major pediatric teaching institution in the United States (or in many European countries, for that matter) today is almost unthinkable without a pediatric hematologist reflects the influence of a few model institutions in the post–World War II era. We have noted the importance of a Diamond "school" of pediatric hematology. During this same critical era, the only other center of comparable importance was the Hematology Service at the Children's Hospital of Michigan in Detroit, which this writer was privileged to direct, and which over a quarter of a century turned out well over 100 fellows, many of them today directing services of their own in the United States and abroad, among them Audrey Brown, Flossie Cohen, Eugene Kaplan, Sanford Leikin, Jeanne Lusher, and William A. Newton. The work of this group includes contributions to the knowledge of ABO hemolytic disease, fetal-maternal hemorrhage, immune hemolytic anemia, the hemoglobinopathies, purpura and other bleeding disorders, and the therapy of childhood leukemia. The creation some time ago of a subspecialty board in pediatric hematology, whether or not it serves a practical purpose, is a sure indication that among Boston, Detroit, Los Angeles and San Francisco, New York, and more recently New Haven, Cincinnati and Syracuse, Minneapolis and Memphis, and Seattle and Houston, a sufficiency of man- (and woman-) power exists to provide service, teaching, and research at a high level of excellence today and in the future.

Throughout its history, pediatric hematology has benefited from the advances of adult hematology, and in fact some of its major achievements rest on contributions made by scientists in other fields (e.g., immunology, chemistry, genetics, and physiology). A striking example is the history of hemolytic disease of the newborn. In 1938, Ruth Darrow, a pathologist who had a deep personal interest in the subject, having experienced a series of stillbirths, reflected on the pathogenesis of what was then called erythroblastosis fetalis.[77] Assembling all of the then known facts, notably the sparing of the first child, the involvement of all or most children born after the first afflicted baby, and the range of clinical and hematologic manifestations, she discarded all the current theories and concluded that the disease could be explained only as the result of maternal sensitization to an as yet unknown fetal antigen—a splendid example of the value of intelligent speculation.

Within 3 years Darrow's hypothesis was confirmed, and the Rh factor, described in a brief communication by Landsteiner and Wiener[78] in 1940, was identified as the offending antigen. Wiener,[79] and independently Levine,[80] observed transfusion reactions after administration of ABO-compatible blood that could be attributed to Rh antibodies. It was Levine, observing such a reaction in a woman who had received no prior transfusions[81] but had received blood from her husband after delivering a stillborn fetus, who recognized the relationship between the Rh factor and hemolytic disease of the newborn.[82] He showed that mothers of affected infants possessed antibodies that reacted with most random blood samples and with blood samples of their husbands and children but not with each other's. Gentle, unassertive, and scholarly, Levine characteristically sought the opinions of those experienced in neonatal pathology before publishing his

revolutionary conclusion. This writer remembers Levine's visit to his laboratory in Detroit in this connection, which took place sometime in 1941. Bubbling with excitement yet reluctant to overturn established dogma and aware that he was venturing into uncharted seas, Levine was visibly reassured when his attention was called to Ruth Darrow's paper in the *Archives of Pathology*. But the serologic evidence was conclusive in itself, and the paper Levine and his associates published the same year bore the title "The role of isoimmunization in the pathogenesis of erythroblastosis." Levine had been an associate of Landsteiner at the Rockefeller Institute, but by this time he had withdrawn from that prestigious institution and was working at a hospital in Elizabeth, New Jersey, a modest, unpretentious man, content to pursue his research in any setting. When this writer first knew him, he was a devoted *paterfamilias,* amateur pianist, and bridge player. After the death of his wife he moved to New York City and continued his work at the Sloan-Kettering Institute, where he remains active to this day. The scope and the fruitfulness of his investigations, which extend from fetal-maternal isoimmunization to the relationship between blood group and cancer antibodies, have made him one of the most creative scientists of our time.

The names of Levine and Alexander Wiener were antithetically linked for the generation that witnessed their ascent, largely because both had been associates of Landsteiner and both contributed enormously to the knowledge of immunohematology and of human genetics, but above all because their views often clashed. This was confusing for the bystanders but in no way detracts from the achievements of each man. Wiener's role in the technical and conceptual understanding of hemolytic disease, both Rh and ABO, cannot be underestimated, but his obsession with nomenclature, his tendency to pile hypothesis upon hypothesis, usually without bothering to inform the reader that he was discarding pieces from the bottom without toppling the edifice, and most of all his imperviousness to the needs of clinicians unfamiliar with the mysteries of blood group immunology isolated him from the mainstream of clinical investigation. Of Wiener's enormous output—by 1954, when the theory of Rh isoimmunization was essentially complete, he had published more than 333 papers, and a typical Wiener bibliography might contain 60 references by A. S. Wiener (with or without et al.)—the contributions relevant to pediatric and obstetric practice were above all those dealing with the "blocking" Rh antibodies,[83] which he discovered and named "univalent," recognizing that they alone could pass the placental barrier and cause disease in the fetus.[84] He was one of the pioneers of exchange transfusion[85] and personally performed the procedure countless times at the Brooklyn Jewish Hospital, but his technique involving transection of the radial artery and the use of heparinized blood did not gain general acceptance. Less reticent to invade the domain of the clinician and the clinical pathologist than his rival Levine, he proposed ingenious but purely speculative theories of the pathophysiology of hemolytic disease that did not stand the test of time and tended to detract from his brilliant achievements in his proper field of blood group immunology. Personally a likable, friendly, unassuming man, he was always in the thick of a battle in which he was his own worst enemy.

Rh hemolytic disease has become a rarity. Within the life span of one generation the condition was defined, its etiology and pathogenesis identified, effective treatment devised, and a program of prophylaxis instituted that prevents maternal sensitization and has virtually eliminated the disease. This crowning achievement rests on the work of two teams of investigators working independently in Britain and the United States: Clarke and Finn in Liverpool,[86] and Freda, Gorman, Pollack, and their associates in New York.[87] Starting from different theoretical premises, both groups, by 1967, had demonstrated the effectiveness of passive isoimmunization of previously unsensitized mothers by means of a potent anti-Rh gamma globulin. The story of the conquest of hemolytic disease of the newborn is matched by few other chapters in the history of medicine.

The modern era of leukemia therapy begins in the 1940s with the work of Sidney Farber,[88] then pathologist at Children's Hospital of Boston and the leading pediatric pathologist in the United States and indeed the world, who in 1948 developed the concept of cancer chemotherapy. Farber had the good fortune of finding, in Subarov of Lederle Laboratories, a chemist able to give him the "antifol" compounds he needed, but the idea of disrupting the growth of malignant cells with antimetabolites was his, and he pursued and promoted it with single-minded energy. It led him to the creation of the Children's Cancer Research Foundation and to the organization of a vast program of clinical and fundamental research that in turn gave rise to the nationwide collaborative studies sponsored by the National Cancer Institute and to the efforts of countless institutions and individuals the world over. Although married to a charming woman of great artistic talent, and the father of gifted and lively children, Farber was a man of almost monastic dedication to his work, a magnificent hermit who spent day and night in his rather resplendent cell in the Jimmy Fund building planning new approaches, an indefatigable optimist who was convinced from the beginning that a cure for leukemia would come forth and who did much to bring it nearer.

It is a little known irony of fate that Farber's concept of antimetabolite therapy evolved as the result of a faulty—or at least doubtful—observation, namely the impression that the administration of folic acid accelerated the growth of leukemic cells in the bone marrow. This writer became privy to this information because it was he who, during a visit to Boston in 1946, showed his former chief slides of aspirated bone marrow from leukemic children. Farber, hitherto strictly a "tissue pathologist," became very interested in the cytologic method and switched from surgical biopsies to needle aspirations. At that time folic acid had just become available, and in view of its striking effects on the bone marrow in megaloblastic anemia, Farber decided to investigate its effects on leukemia. From sequential examinations he gained the—probably erroneous—impression that the administration of folic acid per os led to more rapid growth of the leukemic cell population. It seems unlikely that the difference, if any, between treated and untreated patients was real, given the pitfalls of quantitating the cellular elements of aspirated bone marrow, but correct or not, the observation gave rise to the idea of using folic acid antagonists, of which aminopterin was the first, and the era of cancer chemotherapy had begun.

Shortly afterward, in 1949, new ground was broken in another field. In that year, by coincidence, two papers bearing on the same subject from different angles appeared within a few months of each other; they were destined to revolutionize the study of what became known as the "hemoglobinopathies." One was the report of Linus Pauling, Harvey Itano, and their co-workers[89] identifying sickle hemoglobin as a discrete protein separable by electrophoresis from normal hemoglobin, and characterizing sickle cell anemia as a "molecular disease." The other was James V. Neel's study of the genetics of sickle cell anemia and the sickle trait, establishing the former as the homozygous and the latter as the heterozygous state for the sickling gene.[90] The findings of the two reports meshed and became the fountainhead of a veritable flood of investigations leading to the discovery of other hemoglobinopathies and enormously widening the scope of human genetics. The next major achievement was Vernon Ingram's demonstration, by means of the "fingerprinting" of hemoglobin fragments obtained by tryptic digestion, that sickle hemoglobin differs from normal adult hemoglobin (HbA) only in the replacement of a single amino acid among the more than 300 components of the half-molecule, and his subsequent identification of the abnormality as the substitution of a valine for a glutamic acid residue.[91, 92] Since then, abnormalities in the amino acid sequence of the hemoglobin molecule (for the most part involving β chain mutations) have been found in hundreds of variants, and amino acid sequencing has become a basic tool of molecular genetics.

Following the identification of point mutations affecting the amino acid skeleton of globin molecules as the basis of sickling and other hemoglobinopathies, it seemed logical to search for similar structural anomalies of hemoglobin in thalassemia and, when none were found, to postulate "silent" mutations (i.e., amino acid substitutions that did not alter the electrophoretic behavior of the hemoglobin, but inhibited the rate of its synthesis).[93] While this hypothesis proved to be incorrect, it implied the valid assumption that, in analogy to the known structural mutants, the abnormality would be specific for either the α or β chain synthesis. This assumption was made explicit in 1959 by Ingram and Stretton,[94] when they postulated two classes of thalassemia, α- and β-thalassemias, corresponding to the α and β chain variants, respectively, of the hemoglobinopathies proper. This concept proved to be extraordinarily fruitful. It soon became apparent that the thalassemias constitute a highly heterogeneous group of disorders, and that these disorders generally can be classified as either α- or β-thalassemias. Following the development of a method for separating α and β (as well as γ and δ) chains by Weatherall and co-workers,[95] it became possible—by means of incorporating radioactive amino acids into the hemoglobin of reticulocytes *in vitro*—to determine the rate of synthesis of these chains directly and to identify α- and β-thalassemias as disorders of globin chain production of one or the other type. A new explosion of knowledge began with the demonstrations by Nienhuis and Anderson,[96] and Benz and Forget[97] of reduced β chain synthesis by β messenger RNA from β-thalassemic patients, measured in a cell-free heterologous system. The emphasis now shifted to the investigation of quantitative and qualitative defects of mRNA. As additional new techniques became available—e.g., the use of DNA polymerase (reverse transcriptase) to make complementary DNA from mRNA templates, the mapping of DNA sequences by means of restriction endonucleases, and the cloning of DNA fragments—it was possible to identify coding, transcription, translation, and many other defects in the genetic machinery of both α- and β-thalassemic cells. This writer cannot trace the ramifications of this work, which is still ongoing and is discussed elsewhere in this book, nor would I presume to select the names of the investigators from among the many—in the United States, Great Britain, Greece, Thailand, and many other countries—who deserve special recognition. Suffice it to say that the elucidation of the defects in the various forms of thalassemia constitutes one of the great triumphs of biomedical and genetic research. The hoped-for conquest of these disorders surely will come from the application of this knowledge.

In yet another field, that of the enzymopathies, the red cell proved to be an almost inexhaustible source of information of equal interest to the hematologist and the geneticist. The point of departure was the 1956 report of Carson and associates[98] of a deficiency of glucose-6-phosphate dehydrogenase (G-6-PD) in primaquine-sensitive erythrocytes. Not only did this prove to be the explanation for the acute severe hemolytic anemia seen in certain adults who had received the antimalarial drug but, as shown within 2 years by Zinkham and Childs,[99] it also accounted for the then common hemolytic anemia associated with naphthalene poisoning in infants and young children (described in 1949 by this writer and Leonard Apt[100]), as well as for the previously mysterious hemolysis associated with favism, elucidated by Sansone in Genoa.[101] Through the investigations of Kirkman and co-workers[102] and those of Marks and associates,[103] it was soon apparent that G-6-PD deficiency is genetically as heterogeneous (and geographically as widespread) as are the thalassemias. Of special interest to the pediatric hematologist and to the neonatologist are the numerous reports of an association of G-6-PD deficiency and neonatal hyperbilirubinemia in certain Mediterranean and African countries, as well as in China. In addition to the many mutants of G-6-PD, all under the control of genes located on the X chromosome, other defects of the pentose pathway inherited as autosomal recessives were found, but these proved to be rare and chiefly of theoretical interest. Of greater importance for the understanding of the hereditary nonspherocytic hemolytic anemias was the discovery of a whole series of defects in the glycolytic pathway, beginning with pyruvate kinase deficiency, by Tanaka and Valentine and their co-workers.[104] Here too, an association with severe neonatal hyperbilirubinemia was observed. Here too, a high degree of genetic polymorphism soon became apparent. Today, when the well-equipped pediatric hematology laboratory must be able to perform a whole range of red cell enzyme studies as a matter of course, it seems strange that less than a generation ago the entire field of the enzymopathies was *terra incognita*.

The same can be said for several other areas of hematology that are today considered essential, but that were hardly dreamed of a few decades ago. One example is cellular immunity. During much of this writer's early career the thymus was a wholly mysterious organ, "status thymico-lymphaticus" was a widely accepted entity (and an indication for the ill-founded practice of "prophylactic" irradiation), and the different classes and functions of lymphocytes, T and B cells, and helper, suppressor, and killer cells were unknown. Similarly, immunologic tolerance, self-recognition and graft-versus-host disease, the HLA system, and the importance of these observations for bone marrow transplantation (and transplantation in general) are now such well-established concepts that it is easy to forget how recently they were elaborated. Still another example involves the origin of the various lines of blood cells. The existence of a common ancestral cell in the bone marrow, which earlier generations of hematologists so heatedly debated for so many years, was not established until the 1960s, when morphologic arguments suddenly became irrelevant in the face of Till and McCulloch's[105] demonstration of pluripotential colony-forming cells, and the subsequent studies of these and many other workers elucidating the conditions of amplification and differentiation of these precursors. A comparable quantum jump occurred in the field of blood coagulation. Only those who had to deal with the horrendous problems of hemophiliacs in the days before cryoprecipitates and factor VIII (and IX) concentrates made replacement therapy and home care possible can truly appreciate the magnitude of this progress.

It cannot be our purpose here to give a complete overview of our subject. To do so would require a book of its own and duplicate much of the information contained in the following chapters. From what has been said it is clear that pediatric hematology has come into its own. After a prolonged infancy beset by semantic and morphologic woes, it has moved out of the descriptive and empirical phase into an era of functional and physiologic concepts well beyond the fondest dreams of the pioneers. In the process, it has again become part of the mainstream of hematology, yet preserved its identity and its impetus. It seems fitting that this text, which represents the sum of current knowledge, should begin with an account of this evolution and a tribute to those who brought it about, the men and women who did the best they could with the tools available to them and on whose work the new generation is building.

ADDENDUM I

Wolf W. Zuelzer was a remarkable clinical scholar. He ends his history by reminding us that it is important to remember the investigators of an earlier period who built the foundations upon which we now do our work. Frank Oski and I were fortunate to enter pediatric hematology during a very fascinating period. When we began our work in the late 1950s and early 1960s, Cooley, Zuelzer, Blackfan, Diamond, and Smith had described nearly all the diseases with which this book is concerned. They were superb pediatricians with elephantine memories who could collect and accurately codify information about patients. We knew Dr. Diamond best and were stunned by his ability to remember almost every detail of a patient that he might have seen a decade or more before. Because he and his colleagues could reliably and reproducibly categorize their patients by clinical characteristics, we could begin to apply the rapidly developing fields of cell biology, protein chemistry, and enzymology to sort them out at a more fundamental level. We were helped immeasurably by our environment. For example, it was extraordinarily valuable to work in a hospital a block or so away from the Harvard Medical School laboratory in which Arthur K. Solomon and his students were defining the mechanisms by which water and salt are transported across the red cell membrane. At that time, unusual cases of hemolytic anemia came to our attention that could not be fitted into the categories that had been carefully established by Diamond and his aforementioned colleagues. To determine that these patients had most unusual defects in red cell water and electrolyte metabolism, we established collaborations with members of Solomon's laboratory and discovered the conditions that are today referred to as "erythrocyte hydrocytosis" and "xerocytosis." In another example of the collaboration of basic science with clinical pediatric hematology, I was introduced by my colleague Fred S. Rosen to patients with X-linked susceptibility to staphylococcal and certain gram-negative infections. These cases had already been described by Charles A. Janeway and Robert Good, but their metabolic basis was unknown. Naively wondering whether G-6-PD deficiency of the leukocyte might have something to do with the defect, Robert Baehner and I added nitroblue tetrazolium to normal and chronic granulomatous disease (CGD) leukocytes. The CGD leukocytes failed to reduce the dye. We immediately began to collaborate with Manfred L. Karnovsky, Professor of Biological Chemistry at the Harvard Medical School, who specializes in the study of the leukocyte oxidases, and discovered that CGD leukocytes are oxidase deficient. Many years later, Stuart Orkin cloned the gene for the heavy chain of the particular antimicrobial oxidase that is deficient in X-linked CGD.

Three years before I began to work at Children's Hospital, Park S. Gerald had set about to sort out the various cases of Cooley's anemia that Dr. Diamond had collected. He collaborated with Vernon Ingram at the Massachusetts Institute of Technology (MIT), who had recently discovered the molecular defect in sickle hemoglobin. Gerald's application of starch block electrophoresis to hemolysates of thalassemic blood led to the measurement of hemoglobin A_2 levels in the diagnosis of the various forms of the disorder. A burst of work in many laboratories followed. John Clegg and David Weatherall showed that one could measure the relative rates of the synthesis of hemoglobin chains in hemolysates, and this led Yuet Wai Kan, Blanche Alter, and me to the first successful application of this technique in the prenatal diagnosis of the hemoglobinopathies. However, it is the explosion in molecular biology that has been the most exciting of all. With the discoveries of restriction enzymes by Daniel Nathans and reverse transcriptase by Howard Temin and David Baltimore and the many important contributions of others, it became possible to analyze the thalassemias on a molecular level. Members of our own laboratory, including Bernard Forget, Edward Benz, and I, established most important collaborations with David Baltimore, Harvey Lodish, David Housman, and others at MIT. As a result of those collaborations and brilliant studies by Stuart Orkin, Yuet Wai Kan, Haig Kazazian, Arthur Nienhuis, and members of David Weatherall's laboratory in Oxford, huge strides were made. We now understand the various forms of thalassemia at the molecular level and have excellent molecular techniques for prenatal diagnosis. As a result of the transfer of technology, a marked decline in the incidence of new cases is already being observed in Sardinia and Greece.

Though Dr. Diamond's greatest contributions were made in erythroblastosis, he remained vitally concerned with and vexed by the problem of bone marrow failure. From the latter concern has arisen a commitment to research in experimental hematopoiesis and its clinical application in bone marrow transplantation. Today, the growth factors and receptors that govern the behavior of stem cells and committed progenitors are being identified and used to treat patients, with great effect.

So, the recent history of pediatric hematology is one of collaboration of clinical investigators with basic scientists. Our field arches into all of biology. No single individual can possibly encompass all of it. Teams are needed to solve the fundamental problems of today; but Wolf Zuelzer was right: we would have no basis to move, no logical framework with which to extend these fundamental studies, were it not for the superb clinical definitions that Zuelzer, Diamond, and the others provided. They gave us a framework without which all of our work would have been without meaning. This book is due to the great clinicians who preceded us, and its future editions will depend upon the productivity of the next generation of their students.

DAVID G. NATHAN

ADDENDUM II

The late Wolf Zeulzer's chapter on the history of pediatric hematology has been an integral part of *Hematology of Infancy and Childhood* since its first edition. In an addendum written in 1992 for the fourth edition, we attempted to bring the history up to date from a very personal perspective. Now in the 21st century, that first addendum seems barely to scratch the surface of what has happened to our field. Molecular genetics as applied to medicine began with the disorders of hemoglobin; today no aspect of hematology and the hematologic malignancies has failed to be illuminated by molecular genetics. From the arcane clotting and bleeding disorders to the immunodeficiencies and malignancies, genetics has provided both insights into pathophysiology and guides to improved prevention and therapy. All of these startling developments, most unforeseen at the time of the first edition, have had a huge impact on training programs for aspiring pediatric hematologists. The concept of a 2- or 3-year fellowship became obsolete long ago. A trainee in pediatric hematology who aspires to a significant role in this complex field must understand that one cannot amass enough clinical experience in the field without regular intermittent clinical duties fulfilled over a multiyear period. At the same time (and the proper budgeting of time is the difficulty) the trainee must be willing to devote enough effort in the wet or dry laboratory to achieve the expertise of a candidate for a doctor of philosophy degree in a chosen subsection of the field. This means intensive and prolonged focus on a subset of a fascinating and ever growing field. Just as doctoral candidates devote at least 5 years to the mastery of their craft, young pediatric hematologists must expect to devote no less time if they hope to be able to gather new knowledge independently. None of this is easy and there are practical financial problems that can cause hardship and strain on family life. Nevertheless, trainees are accepting these requirements. The quality of young people who have entered our field has never been higher. It is up to us, particularly those who knew Wolf Zeulzer and some of the great clinicians whom he describes, to provide the very best training experiences for these devoted and extraordinarily intelligent young men and women who bring so much to our patients and to the practice of pediatric hematology in the future.

The editors

REFERENCES

1. Flesch H, quoted by Baar H, and Stransky E: Die Klinische Hämatologie des Kindesalters. Leipzig, Franz Deuticke, 1928.
2. Halbrecht I: Role of hemo-agglutinins anti-A and anti-B in pathogenesis of the newborn (icterus neonatorum praecox). Am J Dis Child 1964; 45:1.
3. Lippman HS: A morphologic and quantitative study of the blood corpuscles in the new-born period. Am J Dis Child 1924; 27:473.
4. Neumann NA, quoted by Baar H, and Stransky E: Die Klinische Hämatologie des Kindesalters. Leipzig, Franz Deuticke, 1928.
5. König H: Die Blutbefunde bei Neugeborenen. Folia Haematol (Leipz) 1910; 9:278.
6. Friedländer A, and Wiedemer C, quoted by Baar H, and Stransky E: Die Klinische Hämatologie des Kindesalters. Leipzig, Franz Deuticke, 1928.
7. Ylppö A: Icterus neonatorum. Z Kinderheilk 1913; 9:208.
8. Schiff E, Färber E: Beitrag zur Lehre des Icterus Neonatorum. Jb Kinderheilk 1922; 97:245.
9. Stransky E: In Baar H, Stransky E (eds): Die Klinische Hämatologie des Kindesalters. Leipzig, Franz Deuticke, 1928.
10. Lucas WP, Dearing BF: Blood volume in infants estimated by the vital dye method. Am J Dis Child 1921; 21:96.
11. Mollison PO, Veall W, et al: Red cell volume and plasma volume in newborn infants. Arch Dis Child 1950; 24:242.
12. Zibordi F: Ematologia Infantile Normale e Patologica. Milano, Instituto Editoriale Scientifico, 1925.
13. Lucas WP, Fleischner EC: In Abt IA (ed): Pediatrics. Philadelphia, W. B. Saunders Co., 1924, p 406.
14. Billing BH, Lathe GH: The excretion of bilirubin as an ester glucuronide, giving the direct van den Bergh reaction. Biochem J 1956; 63:68.
15. Schmid R: Direct-reacting bilirubin, bilirubin glucuronide in serum, bile and urine. Science 1956; 124:76.
16. Talafant E: On the nature of direct and indirect bilirubin. V. The presence of glucuronic acid in the direct bile pigment. Chem Listy 1956; 50:1329.
17. Dutton GJ: Uridine-diphosphate-glucuronic acid and ester glucuronide synthesis. Biochem 1955; 60:XIX.
18. Brown AK, Zuelzer WW, et al: Studies on the neonatal development of the glucuronide conjugating system. J Clin Invest 1958; 37:332.
19. von Jaksch R, quoted by Baar H, and Stransky E: Die Klinische Hämatologie des Kindesalters. Leipzig, Franz Deuticke, 1928.
20. Hayem G, quoted by Baar H, and Stransky E: Die Klinische Hämatologie des Kindesalters. Leipzig, Franz Deuticke, 1928.
21. Luzet C: Etude sur L'Anémie de la Premiére Enfance et sur l'Anémie Enfantile Pseudoleucémique. Thése de Paris, 1891.
22. Lehndorff H: Jaksch-Hayem anaemia pseudoleucaemica infantum. Helv Paediatr Acta 1963; 18:1.
23. Cooley TB, Lee P: Series of cases of splenomegaly in children with anemia and peculiar bone changes. Trans Am Pediatr Soc 1925; 37:29.
24. Valentine WN, Neel JV: Hematologic and genetic study of the transmission of thalassemia (Cooley's anemia: Mediterranean anemia). Arch Intern Med 1944; 74:185.
25. Cooley TB, Lee P: Sickle cell anemia in a Greek family. Am J Dis Child 1929; 38:103.
26. Cooley TB: A severe type of hereditary anemia with elliptocytosis. Am J Med Sci 1945; 209:561.
27. Rundles LW, Falls HF: Hereditary (sex-linked) anemia. Am J Med Sci 1946; 211:641.
28. Cooley TB, Lee P: Erythroblastic anemia, additional comments. Am J Dis Child 1932; 43:705.
29. Guest GM: Hypoferric Anemia in Infancy. Symposium on Nutrition, Robert Gould Research Foundation, Inc., Cincinnati, Ohio, 1947.
30. Guest GM: Studies of blood glycolysis: sugar and phosphorus relationships during glycolysis in normal blood. J Clin Invest 1932; 11:555.
31. Guest GM, Rapoport S: Organic acid-soluble phosphorus compounds of the blood. Physiol Rev 1941; 21:410.
32. Guest GM: Osmometric behavior of normal and abnormal human erythrocytes. Blood 1948; 3:541.
33. Baar H: Die Anämien. In Baar H, Stransky E (eds): Die Klinische Hämatologie des Kindesalters. Leipzig, Franz Deuticke, 1928.
34. Haldane and Smith, quoted by Lucas WP, and Fleischner EC: In Abt IA (ed): Pediatrics. Philadelphia, W. B. Saunders Co., 1924, pp 406–623.
35. Josephs HW: Anaemia of infancy and early childhood. Medicine 1936; 15:307.
36. Blackfan KD, Diamond LK: Atlas of the Blood in Children. New York, The Commonwealth Fund, 1944.
37. Josephs HW: Iron metabolism and the hypochromic anemia of infancy. Medicine 1953; 22:125.
38. Sturgeon P: Iron metabolism: a review. Pediatrics 1956; 18:267.
39. Chown B: Anaemia in a newborn due to the fetus bleeding into the mother's circulation: proof of the bleeding. Lancet 1954; 1:1213.
40. Kleihauer E, Betke K: Praktische Anwendung des Nachweises von Hb F-haltigen Zellen in fixierten Blutausstrichen. Internist 1960; 6:292.
41. Cohen F, Zuelzer WW, et al: Mechanisms of isoimmunization. I. The transplacental passage of fetal erythrocytes in homospecific pregnancies. Blood 1964; 23:621.
42. Hart AP: Familial icterus gravis of the newborn and its treatment. Can Med Assoc 1925; 15:1008.
43. Wallerstein H: Erythroblastosis foetalis and its treatment. Lancet 1946; 2:922.
44. Sidbury JB: Transfusion through the umbilical vein in hemorrhage of the newborn. Am J Dis Child 1923; 25:290.
45. Diamond LK, Allen FH Jr, et al: Erythroblastosis fetalis. VII. Treatment with exchange transfusion. N Engl J Med 1951; 244:39.
46. Allen FH Jr, Diamond LK, et al: Erythroblastosis fetalis. VI. Prevention of kernicterus. Am J Dis Child 1950; 80:779.
47. Robertson B: Exsanguination—transfusion: a new therapeutic measure in the treatment of severe toxemias. Arch Surg 1924; 9:1.
48. Siperstein DM, Sansby TM: Intraperitoneal transfusion with citrated blood: an experimental study. Am J Dis Child 1923; 25:107.
49. Siperstein DM: Intraperitoneal transfusion with citrated blood: a clinical study. Am J Dis Child 1923; 25:203.
50. Heinild S, Søndergaard T, et al: Bone marrow infusion in childhood. J Pediatr 1947; 30:400.
51. Zuelzer WW, Ogden F: Megaloblastic anemia in infancy. Am J Dis Child 1946; 71:211.
52. Amato M: Rilievi anamnesto-clinici_._._. su 25 casi di anemie ipercromiche megaloblastiche osservate in bambini della prima infanzia. Pediatria 1946; 54:71.
53. Veeneklaas GMH: Über Megalozytäre Mangelanämien bei Kleinkindern. Folia Haematol (Leipz) 1940; 65:203.
54. Kato K: Sternal marrow puncture in infants. Am J Dis Child 1937; 54:209.
55. Vogel P, Bassen FA: Sternal marrow of children in normal and in pathologic states. Am J Dis Child 1939; 57:246.

56. Fanconi G: Die primären Anämien und Erythroblastosen im Kindesalter. Monatsschr Kinderheilkd 1937; 68:129.

57. Willi H, quoted by Rohr K: Das Menschliche Knochenmark. Stuttgart, Georg Thieme Verlag, 1949.

58. Gasser C: Akute Erythroblastopenie. Helv Paediatr Acta 1949; 4:107.

59. Gasser C: Die Pathogenese der essentiellen chronischen Granulocytopenie. Helv Paediatr Acta 1952; 7:426.

60. Zuelzer WW, Bajoghli M: Chronic granulocytopenia in childhood. Blood 1964; 23:359.

61. Kostmann R: Infantile genetic agranulocytosis (agranulocytosis infantilis hereditaria). A new recessive lethal disease in man. Acta Paediatr 1956; 45(Suppl 105):1.

62. Zuelzer WW: "Myelokathexis"—a new form of chronic granulocytopenia. Report of a case. N Engl J Med 1964; 270:699.

63. Krill CE Jr, Smith HD, et al: Chronic idiopathic granulocytopenia. N Engl J Med 1964; 270:973.

64. Fanconi F: Familiäre infantile perniciosa-artige Anämie (Perniziöses Blutbild und Konstitution). Jb Kinderheilk 1927; 117:257.

65. Glanzmann E: Hereditäre hämorrhagische Thrombasthenie. Jb Kinderheilk 1918; 88:113.

66. Glanzmann E: Die Konzeption der Anaphylaktoiden Purpura. Jb Kinderheilk 1920; 91:371.

67. Owren PA: Congenital hemolytic jaundice. The pathogenesis of the "hemolytic crisis." Blood 1948; 3:231.

68. Gasser C: Die Hämolytischen Syndrome des Kindesalters. Stuttgart, Georg Thieme Verlag, 1951.

69. Grumbach A, Gasser C: ABO-Inkompatibilitäten und Morbus Hemolyticus Neonatorum. Helv Paediatr Acta 1948; 3:447.

70. Gasser C, Karrer J: Deletäre Hämolytische Anämie mit "Spontan-Innen-Körper" Bildung bei Frühgeburten. Helv Paediatr Acta 1948; 3:387.

71. Tuffy P, Brown AK, et al: Infantile pyknocytosis, a common erythrocyte abnormality of the first trimester. Am J Dis Child 1959; 98:227.

72. Parsons LG: The haemolytic anaemias of childhood. Lancet 1938; 2:1395.

73. Diamond LK, Blackfan FD, et al: Erythroblastosis foetalis and its association with universal edema of the fetus, icterus gravis neonatorum and anemia of the newborn. J Pediatr 1932; 1:269.

74. Diamond LK, Blackfan KD: Hypoplastic anemia. Am J Dis Child 1938; 54:464.

75. Smith CH: Blood Diseases of Infancy and Childhood. 2nd ed. St. Louis, CV Mosby, 1966.

76. Sturgeon P: Volumetric and microscopic pattern of bone marrow in normal infants and children. II. Cytologic pattern. Pediatrics 1951; 7:642.

77. Darrow RR: Icterus gravis neonatorum. An examination of etiologic considerations. Arch Pathol 1938; 25:378.

78. Landsteiner K, Wiener AS: An agglutinable factor in human blood recognized by human sera for rhesus blood. Proc Soc Exp Biol Med 1940; 43:223.

79. Wiener AS, Peters HR: Hemolytic reactions following transfusions of blood of the homologous group with 3 cases in which the same agglutinogen was responsible. Ann Intern Med 1946; 13:2306.

80. Levine P, Katzin EM, et al: Atypical warm isoagglutinins. Proc Soc Exp Biol Med 1940; 45:346.

81. Levine P, Katzin EM, et al: Isoimmunization in pregnancy, its possible bearing on the etiology of erythroblastosis fetalis. JAMA 1941; 116:825.

82. Levine P, Burnham L, et al: The role of isoimmunization in the pathogenesis of erythroblastosis fetalis. Am J Obstet Gynecol 1941; 42:825.

83. Wiener AS: A new test (blocking test) for Rh sensitization. Proc Soc Exp Biol Med 1944; 56:173.

84. Wiener AS: Pathogenesis of congenital hemolytic disease (erythroblastosis fetalis) I. Theoretic considerations. Am J Dis Child 1946; 71:14.

85. Wiener AS, Wexler IB: The use of heparin in performing exchange transfusions in newborn infants. J Lab Clin Med 1946; 31:1016.

86. Clarke CA: Prevention of Rh hemolytic disease. Br Med J 1967; 4:7.

87. Freda VJ, Gorman JG, et al: Prevention of Rh isoimmunization. JAMA 1967; 199:390.

88. Farber S, Diamond LK, et al: Temporary remissions in acute leukemia in children produced by folic acid antagonist, 4-aminopteroylglutamic acid (aminopterin). N Engl J Med 1948; 238:787.

89. Pauling L, Itano AH, et al: Sickle cell anemia, a molecular disease. Science 1949; 110:543.

90. Neel JV: The inheritance of sickle cell anemia. Science 1949; 110:64.

91. Ingram VM: A specific chemical difference between the globins of normal human and sickle cell anaemia haemoglobin. Nature 1956; 178:792.

92. Ingram VM: The chemical difference between normal human and sickle cell anaemia haemoglobins. Conference on Hemoglobin. Publication No. 557, National Academy of Sciences—National Research Council, 1958, pp 233–238.

93. Itano HA: The human hemoglobins: their properties and genetic control. Adv Protein Chem 1957; 12:216.

94. Ingram VM, Stretton AOW: Genetic basis of the thalassaemia diseases. Nature 1959; 184:1903.

95. Weatherall DJ, Clegg JB, et al: Globin synthesis in thalassaemia. Nature 1965; 208:1061.

96. Nienhuis AW, Anderson WF: Isolation and translation of hemoglobin messenger RNA from thalassemia, sickle cell anemia, and normal human reticulocytes. J Clin Invest 1971; 50:2458.

97. Benz EJ, Forget BC: Defect in messenger RNA for human hemoglobin synthesis in beta thalassemia. J Clin Invest 1971; 50:2755.

98. Carson PE, Flanagan CL, et al: Enzymatic deficiency in primaquine-sensitive erythrocytes. Science 1956; 124:484.

99. Zinkham WH, Childs B: A defect of glutathione metabolism in erythrocytes from patients with a naphthalene-induced hemolytic anemia. Pediatrics 1958; 22:461.

100. Zuelzer WW, Apt L: Acute hemolytic anemia due to naphthalene poisoning, a clinical and experimental study. JAMA 1949; 141:185.

101. Sansone G, Piga AM, et al: Favismo. Torino, Minerva Medica, 1958.

102. Kirkman HW, Riley FD Jr, et al: Different enzymic expressions of mutants of human glucose-phosphate dehydrogenase. Proc Natl Acad Sci USA 1960; 46:938.

103. Marks PA, Szeinberg A, et al: Erythrocyte glucose phosphate dehydrogenase of normal and mutant subjects. Properties of the purified enzymes. J Biol Chem 1961; 236:10.

104. Tanaka KR, Valentine WN, et al: Pyruvate kinase (PK) deficiency hereditary nonspherocytic hemolytic anaemia. Blood 1962; 19:267.

105. Till JE, McCulloch EA: Direct measurement of the radiation sensitivity of normal mouse bone marrow cells. Radiation Res 1961; 14:213.

II Neonatal Hematology

2 | The Neonatal Erythrocyte and Its Disorders

Carlo Brugnara • Orah S. Platt

THE NEONATAL ERYTHROCYTE

At no other time in the life of the patient is the physician confronted with as many diagnostic considerations in the interpretation of apparent disturbances in the erythrocyte as during the neonatal period.

The erythrocytes produced by the human fetus are fundamentally different from the red cells produced by older infants and children. Fetal erythrocytes have different membrane properties, different hemoglobins, a unique metabolic profile, and a much shorter life span. In a variety of pathologic conditions, erythrocytes bearing some of the properties of fetal erythrocytes again appear in the circulation. A better understanding of the factors that regulate fetal erythropoiesis and a precise definition of the fetal erythrocyte may eventually result in the development of a unifying hypothesis that explains these acquired disorders of erythropoiesis. The interpretation of hematologic abnormalities in the neonate is confounded by the interactions of genetics, acquired disease in the neonate, and maternal factors with the gestationally related peculiarities of the fetal erythrocyte.

Development of Erythropoiesis

(See also Chapter 6)

Hematopoiesis in the embryo and fetus can be conceptually divided into three periods: mesoblastic, hepatic, and myeloid.[1, 2] All blood cells are derived from the embryonic connective tissue—the mesenchyme—and blood formation can first be detected by the 14th day of gestation. Isolated foci of erythropoiesis can be observed throughout the extraembryonic mesoblastic tissue in the area vasculosa of the yolk sac at 3 to 4 weeks after conception. Blood islands in the yolk sac differentiate in two directions. Peripheral cells in the islands form the walls of the first blood vessels, whereas the centrally located cells become the primitive blood cells, or hematocytoblasts.[3, 4]

The first blood cells produced by the embryo belong to the red cell series. Two distinct generations of erythrocytes can be observed in the developing embryo. Red cells arise as a result of either primitive megaloblastic erythropoiesis or definitive normoblastic erythropoiesis. Both megaloblasts and normoblasts apparently derive from similar-appearing hematocytoblasts and develop through roughly similar but morphologically distinct series of erythroblasts. In the very early embryo, the red cells arise from the primitive erythroblasts. These cells were called "megaloblasts" by Ehrlich because of their resemblance to the erythroid precursors found in patients with pernicious anemia.[5] Megaloblasts are large cells with abundant polychromatophilic cytoplasm, and they possess a nucleus in which fine chromatin is widely dispersed. Megaloblasts give rise to large, irregularly shaped, somewhat hypochromic erythrocytes that can be seen in circulating blood 4 to 5 weeks after conception. The primitive erythroblasts arise primarily from intravascular sites; as development continues, these cells gradually are replaced by smaller cells of the definitive or normoblastic series.

Normoblastic erythropoiesis begins at about the sixth gestational week, and enucleated macrocytes enter the circulation by the eighth week; by the 10th week of development, normoblastic erythropoiesis accounts for more than 90 percent of the circulating erythrocytic cells. Maturation of normoblastic erythroid cells resembles that seen in postnatal life, giving rise to enucleated erythrocytes and being primarily extravascular.

By about the 5th to 6th week of gestation, blood formation begins in the liver. In the period between the 5th and 10th weeks, the liver increases in size substantially, with an associated increase in the total nucleated cell count from 2.3×10^6 to 1.7×10^8 cells.[6] The fetal liver appears to be a site of pure erythropoiesis, and during the third to fifth months of gestation, erythroid precursors represent approximately 50 percent of the total nucleated cells of this organ.[7] Migration via the bloodstream of pluripotent cells and early progenitors is probably responsible for the yolk sac to liver transition.[6] However, more recently it has been proposed that circulating stem cells and progenitors do not derive from the yolk sac but from an intraembryonic site, the so-called aorta-gonad-mesonephros (AGM) region.[8, 9] This is supported by the fact that stem cells derived from the yolk sac can produce transient primitive hematopoiesis but cannot reconstitute definitive hematopoiesis.[10, 11]

The liver is the chief organ of hematopoiesis from the third to the sixth fetal month and continues to produce formed elements into the first postnatal week (Fig. 2–1). During the third fetal month, hematopoiesis also can be detected in the spleen and the thymus and shortly afterward in the lymph nodes. Blood cell formation can still be observed in the spleen during the first week of postnatal life.

Fukuda[12] used electron microscopy to examine the characteristics of hepatic hematopoiesis in 26 human embryos and fetuses from 26 days after conception to 30 weeks of gestation. The development of hepatic hematopoiesis appeared to correlate closely with the histologic development of the liver. In the earliest stages of hepatic hematopoiesis, undifferentiated mononuclear cells, presumably stem cells, were present in the intercellular spaces of the hepatocytes. With maturation of the fetus, the number of erythroid cells in the hepatic parenchyma increased, and stem cells diminished in number and eventually disappeared. These stem cells were exclusively observed in the extravascular spaces and were considered to derive from the septum transversum.

The ultrastructure of the hepatic erythroid cells was found to be quite distinct from the yolk sac-derived erythroblasts and the erythroblasts observed in the bone marrow of normal adults. The microtubules characteristic of normal bone marrow-derived erythroblasts were rarely observed in the hepatic erythroblasts.

Erythropoietic progenitors from livers of fetuses studied between 13 and 23 weeks of gestation appear more sensitive to humoral stimuli—colony-forming units-erythrocyte (CFU-E) for erythropoietin, and burst-forming units-erythrocyte (BFU-E) for burst-promoting activity—than do the progenitors from adult bone marrow.[13] Large numbers of multipotent and committed (erythroid and granulocytic-monocytic) progenitor cells have been found in blood obtained by fetoscopy at 12 to 19 weeks of gestation.[8, 14] These fetal progenitor cells are more sensitive to appropriate stimuli than are adult progenitor cells grown under the same conditions, presumably as a consequence of intrinsic differences in the progenitor cells of fetal origin.[15, 16] Functional and genetic differences between fetal and adult stem cells indicate that the hematopoietic stem cell is not an invariable cell type.[17]

The myeloid period of hematopoiesis commences during the fourth to fifth fetal month and becomes quantitatively important by the sixth fetal month. During the last 3 months of gestation, the bone marrow is the chief site of blood cell formation. Marrow cellularity becomes maximal at about the 30th gestational week, although the volume of marrow occupied by hematopoietic tissue continues to increase until term.[17] A summary of the time of the first appearance of the different blood cells in the various fetal hematopoietic organs, based on the observations of Kelemen and associates[18] from an analysis of 190 fetuses and embryos, is provided in Table 2–1.

Cord blood is rich in bone marrow progenitor cells and contains multipotential CFU granulocyte-erythroid-monocyte-macrophage (CFU-GEMM), erythroid BFU-E, and CFU granulocyte-macrophage (CFU-GM) cell lines.[19] The number of circulating CFU-GMs from the 23rd week of gestation to full term is consistently high and provides evidence that CFU-GMs are produced in the yolk sac as well as at other hematopoietic sites.[20] The number of BFU-Es is highest at midgestation, with values being threefold greater than those for cord blood and tenfold greater than those for adult bone marrow.[21] The number of CD34+ circulating progenitors also peaks at the second trimester and falls thereafter, showing an inverse relationship with gestational age between 24 and 40 weeks.[22, 23] Table 2–2 shows a comparison of the numbers of circulating hematopoietic progenitors at different gestational ages.[14]

The *in vitro* behavior of progenitor cells obtained from umbilical cord blood is substantially different from that of progenitor cells in the bone marrow of adults. In contrast to adult progenitors, which require the presence of

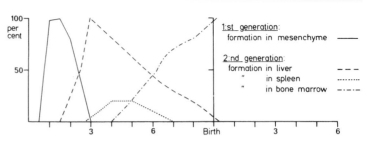

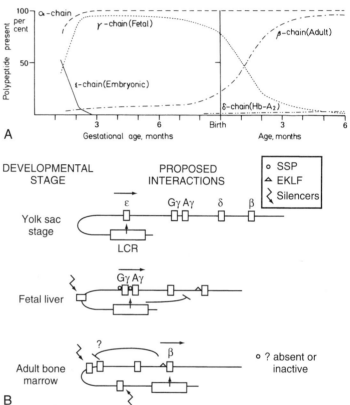

FIGURE 2–1. *A*, Hematopoietic sites and development of different globin chains during fetal life and early infancy. (*A*, After Knoll W, Pingel E: Der Gang der Erythropoese beim menschlichen Embryo. Acta Haematol 1949; 2:369, with permission of Karger, Basel; and Huehns ER, Dance N, et al: Human embryonic hemoglobins. Symp Quant Biol 1964; 29:327.) *B*, Globin gene switching in the human β-globin gene cluster. Some of the postulated interactions at each developmental stage of the human are indicated. Arcs ending in oblique lines are meant to depict competitive interactions. In the fetal liver stage, interaction of the β-globin genes with the locus control region (LCR) prevents β-globin expression, despite the presence of EKLF, a β-globin gene-specific activator. In adult bone marrow erythroid cells, interaction of the β-globin gene with the LCR may facilitate shutoff of the β-globin gene (as indicated by ?). Although it is not established, EKLF is shown to be bound to the β-globin promoter at the fetal stage to emphasize that transcription of the β-genes prevails even in its presence. The status of the stage-selector protein (SSP) complex and the postulated embryonic/fetal-specific subunit in adult cells is unknown (as shown at the bottom). It is likely that SSP is present at the yolk sac stage. If this is the case, interactions between the β-globin gene and the LCR presumably are dominant to β-globin expression. (*B*, From Orkin SH: Regulation of globin gene expression in erythroid cells. Eur J Biochem 1995; 231:271.)

multiple growth factors, fetal progenitors can mature *in vitro* with no growth factors present or with the addition of only one. Recombinant human erythropoietin (r-HuEPO),[24, 25] interleukin-6,[26] interleukin-9,[27] and interleukin-11[28] are active as single agents in fetal but not in adult progenitors. It has been shown that *in vitro* cultures of CD34+ fetal hematopoietic progenitors produce hematopoietic factors such as granulocyte-macrophage

TABLE 2–1. The First Appearance of Different Blood Cell Types in Hematopoietic Organs and in Circulating Blood, Given by Fertilization Age in Weeks

	Extraembryonic*	Liver	Thymus	Spleen	Lymph Nodes	Bone Marrow	Blood
Primitive erythroblasts	3–4	5	—	8	—	—	3–4
Definitive erythroblasts	6–7†	5	10	8	11	8–9	6–7
Granulocytes	3–4‡	5	10	8	12	8–9	7–8
Monocytes (classic)	—	?	—	11	12–13	11	7–8
Histiocytes, macrophages	3–4	5	10	8	11	8–9	3–4
Megakaryocytes, platelets	5†	5	—	11	—	8–9	6–7
Lymphocytes	6	6	8	8	9–12	10–12	7–9
Mast cells§	—	—	—	—	—	—	—

*Yolk sac, chorion, allantois, and body stalk.
†From the circulating blood?
‡Maternal origin is possible.
§The bone marrow was the only site where substantial amounts of mast cells were distinguished.
From Kelemen E, Calvo W, Filedner TM: Atlas of Human Hemopoietic Development. Berlin, Springer-Verlag, 1979.

TABLE 2–2. Hematopoietic Progenitors Circulating in Fetal Blood

Median Gestational Age (Range)	Number of Progenitors $\times$ 10^3/mL*			
	CFU-GEMM	CFU-GM	BFU-e	Total
10^{+0} weeks (7^{+6}–13^{+1})	10.5 ± 1.3	3.3 ± 0.4	5.4 ± 0.8	19.2 ± 2.1
15^{+0} weeks (14^{+5}–20^{+0})	$32.5 \pm 15.7^{\dagger}$	$31.4 \pm 12.0^{\ddagger}$	$19.7 \pm 12.6^{\dagger}$	$83.6 \pm 31.3^{\ddagger}$
39^{+0} weeks (38^{+0}–40^{+0})	5.6 ± 0.7	9.7 ± 5.7	$11.1 \pm 2.1^{\dagger}$	26.4 ± 5.6

*Mean $\pm$ SEM.
  †$P < 0.01$, comparing mean $\pm$ SEM with first trimester.
  ‡$P < 0.0001$, comparing mean $\pm$ SEM with first trimester.
  From Campagnoli C, et al: Circulating hematopoietic progenitor cells in first trimester fetal blood. Blood 2000; 95:1967–1972.

colony-stimulating factor (GM-CSF) and interleukin-3, which can sustain their growth factor-independent proliferation.[29] The exit from the G_0/G_1 phase of the cell cycle in response to stem cell factor also is accelerated in umbilical cord blood CD34$^+$ cells.[30]

The number of hematopoietic progenitors in cord blood is in the range of the requirements for successful engraftment by bone marrow cells.[19] Although the average cord blood collection contains only 14 percent of the nucleated cells present in an autologous bone marrow collection, it contains 91.6 percent of the CFU-GM colonies, 24 percent of the CFU-GEMM colonies, and 29 percent of the BFU-E colonies.[19] Studies of long-term cultures initiating cells have indicated that the number of putative stem cells in cord blood is comparable to that of allogeneic bone marrow or peripheral stem cell collections.[31]

Human umbilical cord blood has been successfully used for hematopoietic reconstitution in patients with Fanconi anemia,[32] aplastic anemia, X-linked lymphoproliferative disease, sickle cell anemia, leukemia, immune deficiency, genetic and metabolic diseases (e.g., Hunter syndrome),[33, 34] and severe hemoglobin E-β-thalassemia disease.[35] For recent reviews, see references 36 through 38.

After birth, the amount of marrow tissue continues to grow, with no apparent increase in cellular concentration. Increased cell production can occur in an infant only by more rapid turnover of cells or by an increase in the volume of hematopoietic tissue. This increase in tissue produces the marrow expansion that is most readily observed in the calvaria.

An increasing role for erythropoietin is observed during the hepatic and myeloid phases of erythropoiesis. Erythropoietin is detectable in the cord blood of nonanemic premature infants in quantities that are comparable to or greater than those in the blood of normal adults.[39] Fetal erythropoiesis is only partially influenced by maternal factors and is primarily under the control of the fetus. In the mouse, suppression of maternal erythropoiesis by hypertransfusion does not suppress fetal erythropoiesis,[40] nor does stimulation of maternal erythropoietin production result in stimulation of fetal red cell production; these findings indicate that erythropoietin is incapable of crossing the placenta.[41] The exact site of erythropoietin production in the fetus is unknown, but the liver is a likely candidate. In other animal species, nephrectomy of the fetus does not influence erythropoietin production or the erythropoietic responses to stresses such as bleeding.[42]

The development of hematopoiesis is controlled by the effect of growth factors on cell proliferation and the activation of lineage-specific genes by transcription factors (nuclear regulators).[2, 43] For each cell lineage, cell-specific transcription depends on critical deoxyribonucleic acid-binding motifs in promoters or enhancers. Differentiation in the erythroid series depends on the presence of GATA-binding and AP-1/NFE2-binding proteins and on the presence of TAL1/SCL, EKLF, and RBTN2 factors.[43, 44] The crucial role of these factors has been established with gene targeting and generation of animals with knockout mutations.[45, 46] A GATA1 mutation has been shown to be responsible for a form of familial dyserythropoietic anemia and thrombocytopenia.[47]

Stat5 is a latent cytoplasmic transcription factor, which after activation of the erythropoietin (EPO) receptor, binds to phosphorylated tyrosines on the receptor and itself becomes tyrosine-phosphorylated.[48, 49] This results in Stat5 dimerization and translocation to the nucleus, where it initiates transcription of target genes. Stat5 is critical during fetal erythropoiesis.[50] Mice mutants for both isoforms of Stat5 (Stat5a and Stat5b) show a profound alteration of fetal (definitive) erythropoiesis.[51] Fetal liver cells give rise to fewer erythroid colonies and a marked increase of apoptosis is seen *in vitro*.[51] Fetal anemia of Stat5a$^{-/-}$b$^{-/-}$ mice seems to resolve in 50 percent of adults, but adult mice are unable to generate high erythropoietic rates in response to stress.[52] Hematopoietic tissue from Stat5a$^{-/-}$5b$^{-/-}$ shows a dramatic increase in early erythroblast numbers, but these cells fail to progress in differentiation.[52] The effects seen in the Stat5a$^{-/-}$5b$^{-/-}$ mice are mostly mediated by decreased expression of bcl-x$_L$. bcl-x$_L$ is a crucial determinant of early erythroblast survival and plays a major role in fetal erythroid development and response to stress.[53] Thus, both Stat5 and bcl-x$_L$ seem to be crucial not only for fetal hematopoietic development but also for response to erythropoietic stress in adulthood.

Erythroid progenitors found in the liver, bone marrow, or peripheral blood of the fetus appear to produce identical quantities of fetal hemoglobin.[54] Fetal erythropoiesis results in the orderly evolution of a series of different hemoglobins. Developmentally, there are embryonic, fetal, and adult hemoglobins (Table 2–3). Globin genes are arranged in order of expression in the α- and β-globin clusters and are selectively activated and silenced at the various stages of erythroid development. Distal, *cis*-regulatory elements in the β-globin–like cluster are contained in the locus control region (LCR), which comprises four hypersensitivity sites[55]; additional *cis*-regulatory downstream core elements (DCE) have also been described.[56] Figure 2–1 presents some of the postulated interactions

TABLE 2–3. Globin Chain Development

Stage	Hemoglobin	Composition
Embryo	Gower 1	ε_4 or $\zeta_2\varepsilon_2$
Embryo	Gower 2	$\alpha_2\varepsilon_2$
Embryo	Portland	$\zeta_2\gamma_2$
Embryo	Fetal	$\alpha_2\gamma_2$
Fetus	Fetal	$\alpha_2\gamma_2$
Fetus	A	$\alpha_2\beta_2$
Adult	A	$\alpha_2\beta_2$
Adult	A_2	$\alpha_2\delta_2$
Adult	F	$\alpha_2\gamma_2$

involved in gene switching for the human β-globin gene cluster.

The first globin chains to be produced are the ε chains, which appear to be similar to β chains in certain aspects of their structural sequences.[57] Before the onset of other chain formation, these unpaired globin chains may form tetramers (ε_4), resulting in the presence of hemoglobin (Hb) Gower-1. Almost immediately thereafter, α and ζ chain production begins, and Hb Gower-2 ($\alpha_2\varepsilon_2$) and Hb Portland ($\zeta_2\gamma_2$) are formed. Early γ chain formation also results in the presence of fetal hemoglobin ($\alpha_2\gamma_2$). By the time the fetus has a crown-rump length of about 16 mm (about 37 days of gestation), Hbs Gower-1 and Gower-2 constitute 42 percent and 24 percent of the total hemoglobin, respectively, with fetal hemoglobin making up the remainder.[58] At a crown-rump length of about 30 mm, HbF represents 50 percent of the total hemoglobin, and at a length of 50 mm it forms more than 90 percent of the hemoglobin. Very small quantities of HbA are found beginning at 6 to 8 weeks of gestation.

Although Hb Portland may constitute as much as 20 percent of the hemoglobin at 10 weeks of gestation, only trace amounts are normally present at birth. The α chain is quite similar to the α chain in its amino acid sequences.[59] Studies of steady-state liver messenger ribonucleic acid globin levels in human embryos (gestational age, 10 to 25 weeks) indicate that levels of globin proteins are regulated by the relative amounts of each globin messenger ribonucleic acid.[60] Studies on the physiological properties of embryonal Hb will be facilitated by their recent expression in a transgenic mouse model.[61]

The absolute rate of synthesis of hemoglobin or formation of red cells during fetal life is difficult to estimate, because neither the absolute increase in circulating hemoglobin or red cells nor the absolute destruction rate is known. The absolute rate of production of red cells at birth, however, can be estimated fairly well. A value of 2.5 to 3.0 percent/day of the circulating red cell mass, or about 4.5 mL/day in a 3.5-kg infant, can be calculated on the basis of determinations of the relative number of circulating reticulocytes and determinations of the *in vitro* mean life span of reticulocytes obtained from cord blood.[62] A very similar figure was obtained on the basis of an analysis of the distribution kinetics of radioiron in the plasma and in the red cells (Fig. 2–2).[63]

Measurements of the circulating red cell volume in newborn infants at various gestational ages shown in

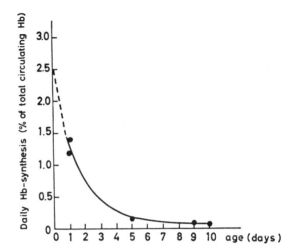

FIGURE 2–2. The relative rate of hemoglobin synthesis at birth and during the first 10 days of life. (From Garby L, Sjölin S, et al: Studies on erythrokinetics in infancy. III. Plasma disappearance and red cell uptake of intravenously injected radioiron. Acta Paediatr 1963; 52:537.)

Figure 2–3 demonstrated an increase in the red cell mass of about 1.5 percent/day.[64] Assuming a mean life span of these cells of 45 to 70 days (discussed later in this chapter), these data show a production rate of 3.6 to 4.2 percent/day of the red cell volume 2 months before term and a rate of 2.5 to 3.5 percent/day of the red cell volume at term. The combined data, therefore, indicate very strongly that the rate of red cell production during the latter part of fetal life is quite high—about three- to fivefold that of a normal adult subject. This finding is in agreement with the well-established facts that, at the same period of development, all of the bones are filled with red marrow, the concentration of red cell precursors per unit volume of marrow is markedly increased,[65–67] and the numbers of erythroid and granulocyte-monocyte progenitors in cord blood are greater than those of normal adult blood.[68]

Erythropoiesis after Birth

The rate of hemoglobin synthesis and red cell production decreases dramatically during the first few days after delivery. The production of red cells (or hemoglobin) decreases by a factor of 2 to 3 during the first few days after birth and by a factor of about 10 during the first week of life. This sudden and marked decrease in red cell production is undoubtedly initiated by the equally sudden increase in the tissue oxygen level that takes place at birth and is reflected by the virtual disappearance of erythropoietin in the plasma.[69] At the time of birth, between 55 percent and 65 percent of the total hemoglobin synthesis consists of HbF.[70] Thereafter, the synthesis of HbF decreases much more rapidly than that of HbA; the time course is shown in Figure 2–4. The switching from HbF to HbA is delayed in infants of diabetic mothers,[71] in infants with metabolic diseases characterized by the inability to metabolize propionic acid,[72] and in infants with chronic bronchopulmonary dysplasia.[73] HbF synthesis can also be "reactivated" in infants with severe anemia of prematurity.[74] The rate of production of red cells (and of hemoglobin), which reaches a minimum during

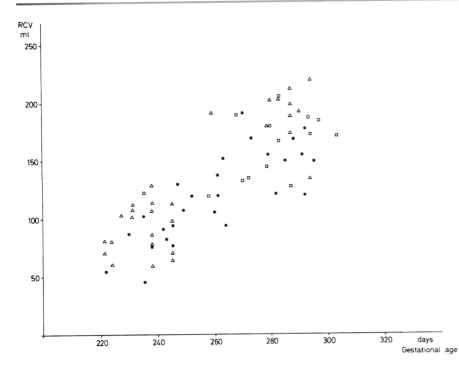

FIGURE 2–3. The circulating red blood cell mass in newborn infants in relation to the gestational age. ● = by ^{51}Cr dilution method; Δ,□ = from plasma volume measurements. (From Bratteby L-E: Studies on erythrokinetics in infancy. X. Red cell volume of newborn infants in relation to gestational age. Acta Pediatr Scand 1968; 57:132.)

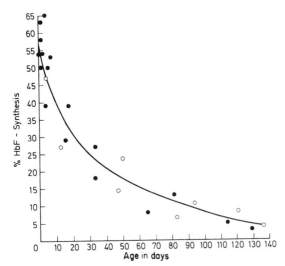

FIGURE 2–4. The time course of the relative synthesis of hemoglobin F (HbF) in normal infants during the first 140 days of life. ● = Radioiron method; ○ = reticulocyte method. (From Garby L, Sjölin S, et al: Studies on erythrokinetics in infancy. II. The relative rate of synthesis of haemoglobin F and haemoglobin A during the first months of life. Acta Paediatr 1962; 51:245.)

Because of their relative simplicity, studies using ^{51}Cr have been used most extensively. Results of numerous investigators are summarized in Table 2–4.[75] These data indicate that the mean ^{51}Cr half-life of erythrocytes from term infants is 23.3 days (range, 13 to 35 days), whereas the mean value for red cells from premature infants is 16.6 days (range, 9 to 26 days). Conversion of these fetal red cell life spans for term infants from ^{51}Cr half-life to true red cell survival indicates an actual life span of approximately 60 to 70 days. Similar calculations for the red cells of premature infants yield values of 35 to 50 days.

Wranne,[70] using the carbon monoxide technique, found that 1.5 percent of the term infant's red cell mass

TABLE 2–4. Reported ^{51}Cr Survival Data

Author(s)	No. of Cases	Range (days)	Average (days)
TERM INFANTS			
Hollingsworth	6	13–23	18.2
Giblett	10	—	20.0
Foconi and Sjölin	10	17–25	22.8
Vest	8	20–27	23.5
Gilardi and Miescher	3	21–26	23.5
Kaplan and Hsu	14	21–35	26.8
Total	51	13–35	23.3
PREMATURE INFANTS			
Foconi and Sjölin	6	10–18	15.8
Kaplan and Hsu	11	9–26	17.8
Vest	7	15–19	16.0
Gilardi and Miescher	7	15–19	16.1
Total	31	9–26	16.6

From Pearson HA: Life span of the fetal red blood cell. J Pediatr 1967; 70:166.

the second week of life, increases during the following months and reaches a maximum, at about 3 months of age, of approximately 2 mL of packed red cells per day, or about 2 percent of the circulating red cell mass per day.

Life Span of the Erythrocyte

The life span of erythrocytes obtained from term infants is somewhat shorter than that of red cells from the adult, whereas the life span of red cells obtained from premature infants is considerably shorter. The more immature the infant is, the greater the degree of reduction.

was broken down daily during the first week of life. Wranne concluded that the life span of most erythrocytes formed during the late fetal and early neonatal period is only 90 days. Equations derived from accumulated data led Bratteby and Garby[76] to the conclusion that the mean life span of cells produced during the last 60 days of fetal life was between 45 and 70 days and that the life span numbers were skewed, with a majority of the cells dying before the mean life span was achieved.[76]

No unifying hypothesis has been presented to explain why the red cells produced during fetal life have a shortened life span. Landaw and Guancial[77] demonstrated a similar shortening of the life span of erythrocytes obtained from the fetal rat. In their studies, the decrease in life span correlated with red cell rigidity, as reflected by red cell filtration studies.[78] These observations suggest that alterations in membrane function and an increased susceptibility to mechanical damage may ultimately be responsible for the decreased life span of fetal erythrocytes.[79]

Unique Characteristics of the Neonatal Erythrocyte

THE RED CELL MEMBRANE

Simple clinical laboratory studies as well as sophisticated biochemical procedures have provided evidence that the red cell membrane of fetal erythrocytes differs from that of its adult counterpart.

The red cells from normal newborns are slightly more resistant to osmotic lysis than are those of adults.[80] A minor population of cells with increased osmotic fragility also is present; however, these cells appear to be selectively destroyed within the first several days after birth.[75] The mechanical fragility of cord blood red cells also is increased.[81, 82] Neonatal reticulocytes are mostly motile R1 reticulocytes,[83] which have been shown to be capable of performing receptor-mediated endocytosis.[84] Neonatal red cells have increased total and membrane-associated myosin content compared with adult red cells[85]; possibly, this increased content is a remnant of these cells' motile machinery.

Figure 2–5 presents flow cytometric measurements of cell volume and hemoglobin concentration in neonatal red cells compared with adult red cells. Measurements of reticulocyte indices in neonatal and adult blood also are presented. Neonatal red cells have larger volumes and lower cell hemoglobin concentrations than do adult cells.[86] Neonatal reticulocytes also have larger volumes and lower hemoglobin concentrations than do adult reticulocytes. Macrocytosis is more prominent in premature newborns and appears to decrease with gestational age, probably as spleen function matures and assumes a greater role in red cell membrane remodeling. Spleen function and remodeling are major determinants of the decrease in cell volume observed when reticulocytes become mature erythrocytes. The difference in volume between reticulocytes and erythrocytes is greatly reduced in blood from premature newborns, another indication of reduced spleen function.[86]

The red cells of normal newborns also appear different by conventional light microscopy, interference phase microscopy, and electron microscopy. Zipursky and co-workers,[87] using careful analysis of wet preparations suspended in 0.2 percent glutaraldehyde, observed that 78 percent of erythrocytes from adults appeared as biconcave discs and 18 percent as "bowl" forms; in contrast, only 43 percent of cells from term infants appeared as discs and 40 percent appeared as bowl forms. In addition, only up to 3 percent of cells from normal adults appeared as assorted spherocytes and poikilocytes of various types, whereas up to 14 percent of cells from term infants showed these morphologic distortions.

In premature infants, the departure from normal adult cells was even more marked. In these infants, 40 percent of the cells were discs, 30 percent were bowls, and 27 percent displayed a variety of morphologic disturbances (Fig. 2–6). The high occurrence of dysmorphology in hematologically normal neonates creates great difficulty in diagnosing specific disorders of the red cell at birth. When the dysmorphology is severe, the condition is sometimes called *infantile pyknocytosis*. In this usually transient disorder, the red cell life span is even shorter than normal,[88] and the disorder may represent a neonatal form of hereditary ovalocytosis (see Chapter 15). Using interference phase microscopy, Holroyde and associates[89] observed that the red cells from both premature and term infants displayed the "pocked" appearance that was first observed by Nathan and Gunn[90] in splenectomized patients with thalassemia. These surface alterations are believed to reflect the presence of vacuoles and internal structures just below the red cell membrane. They were observed in greatest numbers among the most immature infants. Similar surface abnormalities are seen in patients without spleens and in patients with sickle cell hemoglobinopathies with reduced splenic function.[89, 91] The presence of these red cell "pocks" is presumed to reflect impaired splenic function in the immature infant but also may be a reflection of the tendency of fetal erythrocytes for increased vesicle formation, which overwhelms the clearance capacity of the spleen.[92, 93]

Examination of fetal red cells with electron microscopy also reveals the presence of vacuoles and internal structures just below the cell membrane.[94, 95] Freeze-etching and transmission electron microscopy of fetal erythrocyte membranes indicate that the protoplasmic fracture faces have 24 percent more intramembrane particles than do those of adult cells and that the number of particles on exoplasmic fracture faces exceeds that of the adult by 45 percent.[96]

The membrane of the fetal erythrocytes also appears to be more fluid than that of adult cells. Both ferritin-labeled anti-A antibodies[95] and concanavalin A[97] are taken up by endocytosis in the mature erythrocytes of newborn infants but not by cells from normal adults. This unique phenomenon does not appear to be the result of differences in the lipid viscosity of the membrane.[98]

Compared with adult cells, the membrane of the erythrocytes of the newborn has more binding sites for insulin,[99] more insulin-like growth factor,[100] and more prolactin[101]; however, it has fewer digoxin receptor sites[102] and a reduced amount of membrane acetylcholinesterase.[103, 104] The membrane proteins from both premature and term infants are indistinguishable from

RED CELLS

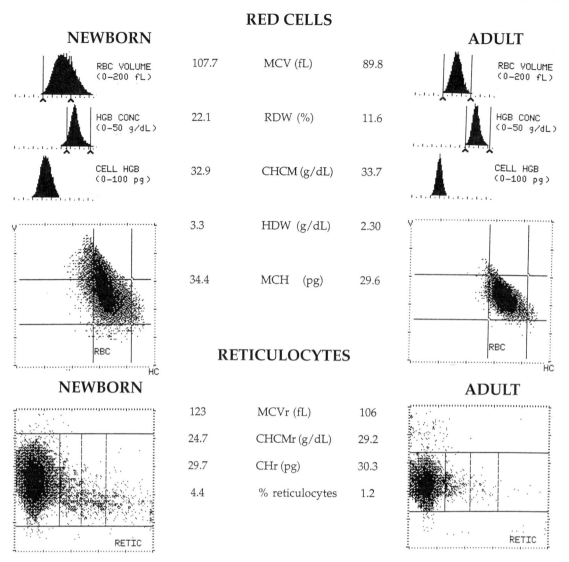

NEWBORN			ADULT
	RBC VOLUME (0–200 fL)		RBC VOLUME (0–200 fL)
107.7	MCV (fL)	89.8	
	HGB CONC (0–50 g/dL)		HGB CONC (0–50 g/dL)
22.1	RDW (%)	11.6	
	CELL HGB (0–100 pg)		CELL HGB (0–100 pg)
32.9	CHCM (g/dL)	33.7	
3.3	HDW (g/dL)	2.30	
34.4	MCH (pg)	29.6	

RETICULOCYTES

NEWBORN			ADULT
123	MCVr (fL)	106	
24.7	CHCMr (g/dL)	29.2	
29.7	CHr (pg)	30.3	
4.4	% reticulocytes	1.2	

FIGURE 2–5. Red blood cell and reticulocyte indices in neonatal and adult blood. *Top,* Histograms for red blood cell (RBC) volume, RBC hemoglobin (Hb) concentration, and RBC Hb content obtained in a newborn (*left*) and an adult (*right*). *Bottom,* Reticulocyte analysis for newborn and adult RBCs. The staining intensity of reticulocytes (*x*-axis) is plotted against the cell Hb concentration (*y*-axis).

those of the normal adult when solubilized in sodium dodecyl sulfate and analyzed with polyacrylamide gel electrophoresis.[97, 102]

The red cells of the cord blood of full-term infants contain increased quantities of total lipid, lipid phosphorus, and cholesterol per cell, although the percentages of total lipid composed of lipid phosphorus and cholesterol are similar to those found in the adult.[105] These erythrocytes have a greater percentage of their phospholipid as sphingomyelin and a lesser portion as lecithin. Phospholipid fatty acid patterns in cord blood erythrocytes show a greater percentage of palmitic, stearic, arachidonic, and combined 22- and 24-carbon fatty acids and a lesser proportion of oleic and linoleic acid. The cells are much more prone to lipid peroxidation on oxidant challenge.[106] It is likely that the relative hyposplenism of the neonate contributes to these membrane alterations.

From an immunologic perspective, the erythrocyte membrane of the newborn also is different from that of the adult. At birth, the Lewis system of absorbed serum antigens is incompletely expressed, partly because the receptor sites of the membrane are weak or absent. In the ABO system, the A antigen, particularly the A_1 antigen, and the B antigen sites are weakly expressed, and in the Ii system, the I antigen is either weak or absent. Other weakly expressed antigens are Sd[a], P1, Lu[a], Lu[b], Yt[a], Xg, and Vel.[107]

The cells are less permeable to the nonelectrolytes glycerol and thiourea,[108] they display a reduced potassium influx via the Na^+,K^+-ATPase and the Na^+, K^+,Cl^- cotransport systems[109] and altered kinetics of glucose transfer,[110] and they are prone to acid lysis.[111] The number of Na^+-K^+ pumps, estimated from ouabain binding, is increased in premature infants compared with term infants.[112] Chloride and bicarbonate transport systems of fetal and adult red cells are similar.[113]

The filtration rate of red blood cells from preterm and term infants is lower than that of adults.[114–116] This decreased filterability may be a manifestation of the larger size of the erythrocytes from the newborn rather than of their different lipid composition.

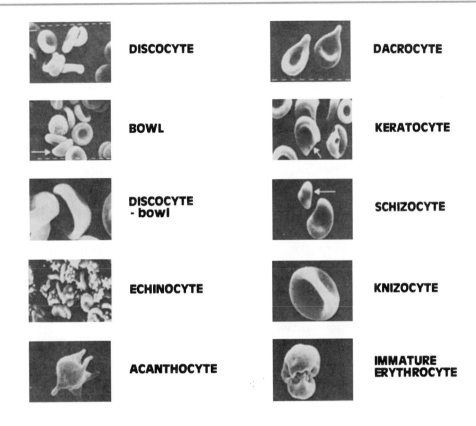

DISCOCYTE

DACROCYTE

BOWL

KERATOCYTE

DISCOCYTE - bowl

SCHIZOCYTE

ECHINOCYTE

KNIZOCYTE

ACANTHOCYTE

IMMATURE ERYTHROCYTE

THE ERYTHROCYTE DIFFERENTIAL COUNT
(Median and 5% to 95% range)

Cell Type	Premature Infant	Term Infant	Normal Adult
Discocyte	39.5 (18-57)	43 (18-62)	78 (42-94)
Bowl	29.0 (13-53)	40 (14-58)	18 (4-50)
Discocyte-Bowl	3.0 (0-10)	2 (0-5)	2 (0-4)
Spherocyte	0.0 (0-3)	0 (0-1)	0 (0-0)
Echinocyte	5.5 (1-23)	1 (0-4)	0 (0-3)
Acanthocyte	0.0 (0-2)	1 (0-2)	0 (0-1)
Dacrocyte	1.0 (0-5)	1 (0-3)	0 (0-1)
Keratocyte	3.0 (0-7)	2 (0-5)	0 (0-1)
Schizocyte	2.0 (0-5)	0 (0-2)	0 (0-1)
Knizocyte	3.0 (0-11)	3 (0-8)	1 (0-5)
Immature erythrocyte	1.0 (0-6)	0 (0-2)	0 (0-0)

FIGURE 2–6. The variety of morphologic abnormalities of the erythrocyte observed in premature infants, term infants, and normal adults. (Photomicrographs courtesy of Zipursky, Brown, and Brown.) (Adapted from Zipursky A, Brown E, et al: The erythrocyte differential count in newborn infants. Am J Pediatr Hematol Oncol 1983; 5:45.)

METABOLISM OF THE ERYTHROCYTES OF THE NEWBORN INFANT (TABLE 2–5)

Enzymes of the Embden-Meyerhof Pathway. Numerous investigators agree that the activities of the enzymes phosphoglycerate kinase and enolase in the red cells of newborn infants are much more intense than would be anticipated from the young age of their cells.[104, 117–121] The activity of the enzymes glyceraldehyde-3-phosphate dehydrogenase and glucose phosphate isomerase also is probably significantly greater than would be anticipated from the cell age.[119]

The activity of phosphofructokinase (PFK), a rate-controlling enzyme in glycolysis, has repeatedly been found to be lower than normal in the red cells of newborn infants.[118, 119, 122] The decreased PFK activity may reflect the accelerated decay of an unstable enzyme. Travis and Garvin[123] fractionated cord blood red cells into cohorts of various cell ages and compared them with adult red cells that were fractionated in a similar fashion. The rate of

TABLE 2–5. Metabolic Characteristics of the Erythrocytes of the Newborn

CARBOHYDRATE METABOLISM

Glucose consumption increased
Galactose more completely utilized as substrate both under normal circumstances and for methemoglobin reduction★
Decreased activity of sorbitol pathway★
Decreased triokinase activity★

GLYCOLYTIC ENZYMES

Increased activity of hexokinase, phosphoglucose isomerase,★ aldolase, glyceraldehyde 3-phosphate,★ phosphoglycerate kinase,★ phosphoglycerate mutase, enolase,★ pyruvate kinase, lactate dehydrogenase, glucose-6-phosphate dehydrogenase 6-phosphogluconic dehydrogenase, galactokinase, and galactose 1-phosphate uridyltransferase
Decrease activity of phosphofructokinase★
Different distribution of hexokinase isoenzymes★

NONGLYCOLYTIC ENZYMES

Increased activity of aspartate transaminase and glutathione reductase
Decreased activity of NADP-dependent methemoglobin reductase,★ catalase,★ gluthathione peroxidase, superoxide dismutase, carbonic anhydrase,★ adenylate kinase,★ and glutathione synthetase★
Presence of α-glycerol-3-phosphate dehydrogenase★

ATP AND PHOSPHATE METABOLISM

Decreased phosphate uptake,★ slower incorporation into ATP and 2,3-diphosphoglycerate★
Accelerated decline of 2,3-diphosphoglycerate upon red blood cell incubation★
Increased ATP and 2,3-diphosphoglycerate levels
Accelerated decline of APT during brief incubation

STORAGE CHARACTERISTICS

Increased potassium efflux and greater degrees of hemolysis during short periods of storage
More rapid assumption of altered morphologic forms upon storage or incubation★

MEMBRANE

Decreased ouabain-sensitive Na^+, K^+-ATPase★; decreased ouabain-resistant potassium influx★
Decreased permeability to glycerol and thiourea★
Decreased membrane deformability★
Increased sphingomyelin, decreased lecithin content of stromal phospholipids
Decreased content of linoleic acid★
Increased lipid phosphorus and cholesterol per cell
Greater affinity for glucose★
Increased number of insulin, insulin-like growth factor, and prolactin binding sites
Increased membrane-associated myosin
Reduced membrane acetylcholinestrase activity

OTHER

Increased methemoglobin content★
Increased affinity of hemoglobin for oxygen★
Glutathione instability★
Increased tendency for Heinz body formation in presence of oxidant compounds★

NADP = nicotinamide-adenine dinucleotide phosphate; ATP = adenosine triphosphate; ATPase = adenosine triphosphatase.
★Appears to be a unique characteristic of the newborn's erythrocytes and not merely a function of the presence of young red blood cells.

decline of pyruvate kinase activity was essentially the same in neonates and adults, whereas PFK activity in cord erythrocytes decreased at a significantly greater rate compared with that of adults.

The studies of Vora and Piomelli[124] have provided a clear understanding of the nature of PFK in the fetal erythrocyte. They found that human muscle and liver PFKs are homotetramers, each of which is composed of identical subunits, which they called "M_4" and "L_4." Study of adult erythrocytes revealed the presence of three heterotetramers—M_3L, M_2L_2, and ML_3. Analysis of cord blood erythrocytes revealed the presence of the three heterotetramers in adult erythrocytes; the L_4 isoenzyme was also identified. The presence of the liver homotetramer in fetal

erythrocytes may be responsible for the decreased PFK stability observed by Travis and Garvin.[123]

Differences in the distribution of other red cell isoenzymes have also been described. Hemolysates normally contain two isoenzymes of hexokinase, types I and III. Holmes and co-workers[125] found that in the cells of the newborn infant, type II hexokinase was the predominant isoenzyme. Schröter and Tillman,[126] in contrast, observed that type I predominated, although the predominance of type I was not characteristic of young cells in general but was a unique feature of the red cells of the newborn infant.[126] Chen and associates[127] also observed differences in the distribution of hexokinase isoenzymes obtained from first trimester and midtrimester fetuses.

Enolase also exists as multiple isoenzymes in erythrocytes, and the distribution of enolase isoenzymes appears to be a unique characteristic of fetal erythrocytes.[128]

Chen and associates[127] studied a total of 26 enzyme patterns in hemolysates prepared from 11 fetuses ranging in gestational age from 65 to 138 days. Six enzymes—enolase, guanylate kinase, lactate dehydrogenase, nucleoside phosphorylase, PFK, and the previously mentioned hexokinase—showed differences in the staining intensity of certain isoenzyme zones compared with adult controls. The fetal red cell zymograms contained the mitochondrial forms of isocitric dehydrogenase and aspartate transaminase as well as more definite zones of phosphoglucomutase type 3.

Glucose Consumption. Glucose consumption by the erythrocytes of both the term and the premature infant has generally been found to be greater than that observed in the cells of the normal adult.[129, 130] This would be anticipated in view of the fact that young red cells consume more glucose. However, when the cells from infants are compared with adult cell populations of similar young age, their rate of glucose consumption appears to be less than would be expected.[129]

Circumstantial evidence exists to suggest that the relative deficiency of PFK may be responsible for this relative impairment of glycolysis. All strategies designed to maximize PFK activity produce a far greater augmentation of glucose consumption in the cells of the neonate. Incubation at high phosphate concentrations causes cells of both premature and term infants to consume glucose at rates commensurate with their age.[131] Increasing the pH of the incubation medium produces a much greater increase in red cell glucose consumption in cells from the newborn infant.[129] Analysis of glycolytic intermediates reveals that as the pH increases, there is a decrease in the levels of glucose 6-phosphate and fructose 6-phosphate and an increase in the concentrations of fructose 1,6-diphosphate, glyceraldehyde 3-phosphate, dihydroxyacetone phosphate, and 2,3-diphosphoglycerate (2,3,-DPG). All of these changes are consistent with an activation of PFK. It would appear that this pH-induced augmentation of PFK obscures the relative deficiency that manifests itself as lower-than-expected glucose consumption at pH 7.4.

Further evidence that the relative deficiency of PFK may play the major role in depressing glucose consumption in the newborn comes from incubation of neonatal red cells with 10^{-6} M methylene blue. At this concentration of methylene blue, 90 percent of glucose consumption proceeds via the pentose-phosphate pathway, which bypasses the PFK step. The incubation of red cells from newborn infants in the presence of methylene blue produces a far greater acceleration of glycolysis than is observed either in the red cells of normal adults or in those of subjects with reticulocytosis.[132]

Finally, when one examines the oldest cells from the cord blood of the newborn infant, the profound PFK deficiency that was previously described is found to be associated with a marked decrease in glucose consumption and a pattern of glycolytic intermediates that suggests that a relative block in glycolysis is present at this step.

2,3-Diphosphoglycerate Metabolism. When the red cells of infants and adults are incubated under identical conditions, the concentration of 2,3-DPG declines far more rapidly in the erythrocytes of the newborn than in those of the adult.[133, 134] Three postulates have been advanced to explain this 2,3-DPG instability. Zipursky and co-workers[133] presented evidence to suggest that a relative block in glycolysis, proximal to the formation of glyceraldehyde 3-phosphate, was responsible for the failure to maintain 2,3-DPG levels. Schröter and Winter[134] proposed that in the red cells of the newborn, the synthesis of 3-phosphoglycerate was favored over the synthesis of 2,3-DPG because of the increased glycolytic rate, the increased activity of phosphoglycerate kinase, and the slight elevation in the red cell adenosine diphosphate concentration. Trueworthy and Lowman[135] proposed that the instability of 2,3-DPG resulted from an accelerated rate of hydrolysis as a consequence of increased 2,3-DPG phosphatase activity. The 2,3-DPG content of normal fetal red cells is greater than that of adult cells and is further increased in anemic fetuses, possibly as a consequence of the relative preponderance of PFK activity over pyruvate kinase activity.[136]

The Pentose-Phosphate Pathway and Response to Oxidant-Induced Injury. Oxidative stress induced by the formation of O_2, H_2O_2, or related species is handled within the red cell by the combined activities of the hexose monophosphate shunt (generating reduced nicotinamide adenine dinucleotide phosphate [NADPH]), glutathione peroxidase, catalase, and superoxide dismutase. There is general agreement that the red cells from newborn infants are more susceptible to oxidant-induced injury than are those of adults and that this susceptibility is greater for red cells from very-low-birth-weight infants.[104, 137–139]

Fetal hemoglobin is more prone than adult hemoglobin to denaturation; however, there is no relationship between the fetal hemoglobin content of the cell and the tendency to form Heinz bodies. The pentose-phosphate pathway in the cells of both the term and the premature infant is intact and responds appropriately to oxidant-induced stimulation.[132, 140] The cell content of glutathione is normal in neonatal erythrocytes.[141] The activity of glutathione peroxidase is decreased in comparison with that of adult cells[142, 143]; however, metabolic studies have failed to demonstrate a convincing direct relationship between this relative deficiency and the vulnerability to oxidants.[140, 144] Reduced levels of reduced glutathione (GSH) and increased levels of oxidized glutathione have been found in patients with retinopathy of prematurity.[145] Erythrocytes from extremely low-birth-weight infants exhibit a marked reduction in the 6-phosphogluconate dehydrogenase (6PGD)/glucose-6-phosphate dehydrogenase (G6PD) ratio, GSH peroxidase, methemoglobulin (MetHb) reductase, and catalase.[104] A slight decrease in superoxide dismutase activity has been observed in fetal red cells.[146] The relative deficiencies of glutathione peroxidase and catalase may act in concert with plasma factors to produce this metabolic handicap.[147, 148] Vitamin E plays a crucial role in limiting membrane lipid auto-oxidation. Vitamin E deficiency has been observed in the plasma of full-term and premature newborns.[149]

G6PD activity is increased in cord/neonatal blood.[118, 122, 132, 150] 6PGD activity is similar in neonatal and adult blood.[118, 151] In fetal and very low-birth-weight infant cells, 6PGD activity is markedly reduced[104, 152]; the associated reduction in 6PGD/G6PD ratio has been proposed to be a marker of developmental immaturity of erythrocytes.[104, 121]

Suggestions that other factors are implicated come from the observations that the red cells of the newborn infant, when compared with those of adults, have a decreased number of membrane SH groups,[153] that the membranes isolated from them contain more residual hemoglobin and form Heinz bodies faster,[154] and that, after the transfusion of adult cells into newborn infants, these cells also appear to be more prone to developing Heinz bodies.[155, 156]

The red cells from newborn infants, like other young red cells, consume more oxygen and produce more hydrogen peroxide than do the red cells of adults.[157, 158]

HEMATOLOGIC VALUES AT BIRTH

Several variables influence the interpretation of what might be considered normal values for hemoglobin, hematocrit, red cell indices, and reticulocyte count at the time of birth and during the early weeks of life. These variables include the gestational age of the infant, the conduct of labor and the treatment of the umbilical vessels, the site of sampling, and the time of sampling. The Appendix of this text contains a series of tables describing representative norms that have appeared in the literature. A few of these norms are highlighted in the following discussion to illustrate pertinent points.

Site of Sampling

Capillary samples obtained by skin prick, generally from the heel or toe, have a higher hemoglobin concentration than do simultaneously collected venous samples. During the first hours of life, this difference averages approximately 3.5 g/dL, as is illustrated in Figure 2–7.[159] In some instances, the capillary hemoglobin–venous hemoglobin difference may exceed 10 g/dL.[160]

The clinical importance of the site of sampling was illustrated by Moe[160] in a study of 54 infants with erythroblastosis fetalis. Simultaneously obtained cord blood and capillary samples were compared. In this study, 41 infants eventually required exchange transfusion for hyperbilirubinemia. Of these 41 infants, 25 were found to be anemic, based on determinations performed on cord blood samples, whereas only 14 could be considered anemic on the basis of the results of capillary sample analysis.

In virtually all infants, the capillary/venous hematocrit ratio is greater than 1.00. The greatest ratios, often in excess of 1.20, are observed in infants born before 30 weeks of gestation, infants with arterial blood pH values below 7.20, infants with hypotension, and infants with a red cell mass of less than 35 mL/kg.[161] In other words, the capillary hemoglobin values are falsely elevated in the sickest infants. These are the same infants in whom an accurate determination of hemoglobin concentration is most important in clinical management. The capillary/venous hematocrit ratio gradually decreases with increasing gestational age.[161] The following mean ratios have been found: infants born between 26 and 30 weeks of gestation, 1.21; infants born at 31 to 32 weeks, 1.12; infants born at 33 to 35 weeks, 1.16; and infants born between 36 and 41 weeks, 1.12. By the fifth day of life, the capillary/venous difference has decreased in healthy infants, and capillary samples may have a hematocrit that is only 2.5 percent higher when blood is obtained by deep stick from a well-warmed heel.

Several studies have shown that venipuncture is as effective and less painful than heel blood collections.[162] The use of automated incision devices for heel sticks should be encouraged, because they reduce the number of sticks needed and induce less bruising and inflammation.[163] Pain and stress are associated with the heel prick procedure,[164, 165] as well as some rare but severe permanent sequelae.[166] The use of topical anesthetics reduces the pain associated with blood drawings in infants,[167, 168] although it may transiently increase MetHb levels if prilocaine is present.[169]

Treatment of the Umbilical Vessels

At birth, the blood volume of the infant may be increased by as much as 61 percent if complete emptying of the

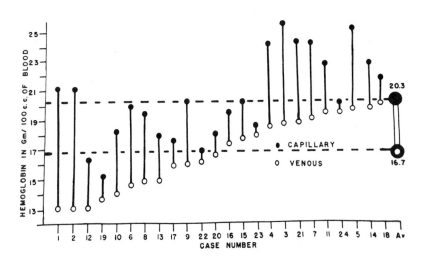

FIGURE 2–7. Simultaneous capillary and venous Hb determinations in 24 newborn infants. (From Oettinger L, Mills WB: Simultaneous capillary and venous hemoglobin determinations in newborn infants. J Pediatr 1949; 35:362.)

placental vessels is allowed before the cord is clamped.[170, 171] It has been estimated that the placental vessels contain 75 to 125 mL of blood at birth—or one quarter to one third of the fetal blood volume. Under normal circumstances, about one quarter of the placental transfusion takes place within 15 seconds of birth and one half by the end of the first minute. The ratio of blood in the neonatal and placental circulations has been found to average 67:33 at birth, 80:20 at 1 minute, and 87:13 at the end of the placental transfusion.[171]

The umbilical arteries generally constrict shortly after birth, so that no blood flows from the infant to the mother; however, the umbilical vein remains dilated, permitting blood to flow in the direction of gravity. Infants held below the level of the placenta continue to gain blood; infants held above the placenta may bleed into it.[172] Yao and co-workers[171] demonstrated that hydrostatic pressure, produced by placing the infant 40 cm below the mother's introitus, hastened placental transfusion to virtual completion in 30 seconds. In infants delivered at term by cesarean section, maximal placental transfusion is achieved within 40 seconds after birth; however, net blood flow reverses, with blood traveling from the infant back to the placenta, if the clamping is delayed for longer than 40 seconds.[173]

The effects of placental transfusion on the total blood volume of the infant are widely variable. This is partially because of the techniques used and partially because of the time at which the samples were taken. During the first hours after birth, plasma apparently leaves the circulation. It seems that the greater the placental transfusion, the greater the plasma loss. Thus, by the third day of life, there are only small differences in total blood volume, regardless of the method of cord clamping. Usher and associates[170] found that infants with delayed cord clamping had an average blood volume of 93 mL/kg at an age of 72 hours; infants with immediate cord clamping had a blood volume of 82 mL/kg.[170] Although the total blood volume may be only slightly altered by the timing of the cord clamping, more significant differences can be observed in the red cell mass or hemoglobin concentration. In the

study of Usher and associates,[170] infants with delayed cord clamping had an average red cell mass of 49 mL/kg at 72 hours of age, compared with a red cell mass of only 31 mL/kg in infants with immediate cord clamping. The results of other investigators are listed in Table 2–6.[174-176]

Infants with delayed cord clamping tend to have higher hemoglobin values during the first week of life than those for whom clamping was not delayed. A reduced volume of red blood cells is associated with an increase in mortality among premature infants affected by respiratory distress syndrome.[177] Thus, delayed cord clamping could be particularly indicated for infants born prematurely. Studies have shown that delayed cord clamping in premature infants is associated with a significant reduction in transfusion requirements and improved outcome, but not with reduced incidence of periventricular/intraventricular hemorrhages.[176, 178-180]

There have been reports of circulatory overload and congestive cardiac failure in various settings of delayed cord clamping. "Symptomatic neonatal plethora" was observed in eight premature and three full-term infants.[181] Radiologic findings of volume overload and reduced left ventricular performance have been reported in infants with delayed cord clamping.[182, 183] For infants born by cesarean sections, a delay of 3 minutes in cord clamping has been associated with signs of respiratory and metabolic acidosis (reduced oxygen tension and pH and elevated plasma lactate levels), indicating that earlier clamping may be preferable in this setting.[184]

Blood Volume

Both blood volume and red cell mass are influenced by the treatment of the cord vessels and by the clinical condition of the infant. Shortly after birth, the blood volume of term infants may range from 50 to 100 mL/kg, with the mean value being 85 mL/kg.[170, 185, 186] As previously discussed, the blood volume in infants with early cord clamping averages 78 mL/kg at 30 minutes of age, in contrast to a value of 98.6 mL/kg in infants with cords that were clamped late. By 72 hours of age, these differences are not as great;

TABLE 2–6. Effect of Cord Clamping on Hematocrit and Hemoglobin Concentration at Various Times After Delivery

Reference	Early Clamping		Delayed Clamping		Time of Study
	Hb (g/dL)	Hct (%)	Hb (g/dL)	Hct (%)	
Phillips (1941)	15.6	—	19.3	—	20–30 hr
Marsh et al. (1948)	17.4	—	20.8	—	3rd day
Colozzi (1954)	14.7	—	17.3	—	72 hr
Lanzkowsky (1960)	18.1	—	19.7	—	72–96 hr
	11.1	—	11.1	—	3 mo
Linderkamp et al. (1992)[174]		48 ± 4		50 ± 4	At birth
		47 ± 5		63 ± 5	2 hr
		43 ± 6		59 ± 5	24 hr
		44 ± 5		59 ± 6	120 hr
Kinmond et al. (1993)[176]		50.9 ± 4.5		56.4 ± 4.8	Not standardized
Nelle et al. (1993)[175]		48 ± 6		58 ± 6	2 hr
		44 ± 5		56 ± 7	24 hr
		44 ± 5		54 ± 8	5 days

Hb = hemoglobin; Hct = hematocrit.

infants with early clamping have an average blood volume of 82 mL/kg, whereas infants with late clamping have an average of 93 mL/kg.

The blood volume of the premature infant ranges from 89 to 105 mL/kg during the first few days of life.[187, 188] This increased blood volume is primarily the result of an increase in plasma volume, with the total red cell volume per kilogram of body weight being quite similar to that of the term infant. The plasma volume decreases with increasing gestational age, except in infants with intrauterine growth retardation.[189]

For infants born at term, blood volumes are approximately 73 to 77 mL/kg by 1 month of life.[190, 191]

A reduced blood volume and a reduced red cell mass are often observed in infants with hyaline membrane disease and in newborns delivered with a tight nuchal cord.[192, 193] Approximately 16 percent of infants born with a tight nuchal cord are anemic in the neonatal period.[194] Infants born after late intrauterine asphyxia tend to have a greater blood volume and red cell mass.[193]

Hemoglobin, Hematocrit, Red Cell Count, and Red Cell and Reticulocyte Indices

Representative values for these hematologic measurements are presented in Tables 2–7 to 2–10. The hemoglobin values increase gradually until approximately 32 to 33 weeks of gestation and remain relatively constant until term. The mean red cell volume (MCV) and mean reticulocyte count decline continuously during the course of

TABLE 2–7. Hematologic Values for Normal Cord Blood

Parameter	Mean	SD	n =
Hb (g/dL)	15.9	1.86	28
Hct (percent)	50.2	6.9	18
RBC count ($\times 10^6/mm^3$)	4.64	0.68	18
MCV (fL)	110	5.05	28
MCH (pg)	34.6	1.5	18
MCHC (g/dL)	31.9	1.13	18
CHCM (g/dL)	30.9	1.78	26
% Hypochromic (MCHC <28 g/dL)	12.7	12.9	18
% Hyperchromic (MCHC >41 g/dL)	0.97	0.74	28
% Microcytic (MCV <61 fL)	0.73	0.3	18
% Macrocytic (MCV >120 fL)	22.5	8.41	18
RETICULOCYTES			
%	3.69	0.95	27
MCVr (fL)	125	8.6	25
CHCMr (g/dL)	27.1	1.95	17
CHr (pg)	32.9	3.1	17

RBC = red blood cell; MCV = mean corpuscular volume; MCH = mean corpuscular hemoglobin; MCHC = mean corpuscular hemoglobin concentration; CHCM = cell hemoglobin concentration, mean; MCVr = reticulocyte MCV; CHCMr = reticulocyte CHCM; CHr = reticulocyte cell hemoglobin content.

Values obtained with an ADVIA 120 hematology analyzer (Bayer Diagnostics, Tarrytown, NY) in neonates delivered at term with weight >2500 g. These data were kindly provided by Drs. Gil Tchernia and Therese Cynober, Laboratoire d'Hematologie, Centre Hospitalier de Bicetre, Becetre, France.

TABLE 2–8. Normal Hematologic Values during First 2 Weeks of Life in Term Infant

	Cord Blood	Day 1	Day 3	Day 7	Day 14
Hb (g/dL)	16.8	18.4	17.8	17.0	16.8
Hct (%)	53.0	58.0	55.0	54.0	52.0
RBC count ($mm^3 \times 10^6$)	5.25	5.8	5.6	5.2	5.1
MCV (fL)	107.0	108.0	99.0	98.0	96.0
MCH (pg)	34.0	35.0	33.0	32.5	31.5
MCHC (g/dL)	31.7	32.5	33.0	33.0	33.0
Reticulocytes (%)	3–7	3–7	1–3	0–1	0–1
Nucleated RBC/(mm^3)	500.0	200.0	0–5	0	0
Platelets (1000/mm^3)	290.0	192.0	213.0	248.0	252.0

gestation. Hematologic values from normal fetuses with gestational ages between 18 to 30 weeks reflect this trend.[195]

In healthy term infants, no measurable decrease in hemoglobin values occurs during the first week of life (Fig. 2–8); in contrast, in infants who weigh less than 1500 g at birth but are of appropriate weight for gestational age, the hemoglobin concentration may decrease by as much as 1.0 to 1.5 g/dL during this interval (Fig. 2–9).

Considerable differences are present in the peripheral blood cell counts and indices of infants born in developing countries. A study carried out by Tchernia's group in 199 newborns in Bomako (Mali) indicated that 32 percent were anemic (hemoglobin level < 13 g/dL).[196] When compared with a control group of French newborns, the Bamako groups had lower hemoglobin levels (13.9 ± 2.0 g/dL versus 15.1 ± 1.4 g/dL), lower mean corpuscular hemoglobin levels (32.9 ± 3.0 pg versus 35 ± 1.9 pg), lower serum ferritin levels (97.5 μg/L versus 135 μg/L, geometric means), and lower erythrocyte ferritin levels (244.7 ag/cell versus 348 ag/cell, geometric means). These differences cannot be explained by hemoglobinopathies, malaria, or folate deficiency, and they are probably due to iron deficiency. However, in developed countries, there seems to be very little difference in neonatal Hb, erythrocyte zinc protoporphyrin, and cord blood serum ferritin levels between neonates born to iron-deficient and iron-replete mothers.[197]

FETAL ANEMIA

Improved diagnostic and therapeutic techniques have made possible the early identification and treatment of anemia in the fetus. The experience gained in the treatment *in utero* of hemolytic diseases of the fetus has been applied to a wide spectrum of pathologic conditions.[198] Normal fetal hematologic values also are available as a consequence of the development of percutaneous umbilical blood sampling and prenatal diagnosis (Table 2–11).[195]

A substantial portion of cases of nonimmune fetal hydrops are due to chromosomal abnormalities and thus

TABLE 2–9. Red Blood Cell Values on First Postnatal Day

	Gestational Age (weeks)							
	24–25 (7)*	26–27 (11)	28–29 (7)	30–31 (25)	32–33 (23)	34–35 (23)	36–37 (20)	Term (19)
RBC count ($\times 10^6$/mm³)	4.65† ± 0.43†	4.73 ± 0.45	4.62 ± 0.75	4.79 ± 0.74	5.0 ± 0.76	5.09 ± 0.5	5.27 ± 0.68	5.14 ± 0.7
Hb (g/dL)	19.4 ± 1.5	19.0 ± 2.5	19.3 ± 1.8	19.1 ± 2.2	18.5 ± 2.0	19.6 ± 2.1	19.2 ± 1.7	19.3 ± 2.2
Hct (%)	63 ± 4	62 ± 8	60 ± 7	60 ± 8	60 ± 8	61 ± 7	64 ± 7	61 ± 7.4
MCV (fL)	135 ± 0.2	132 ± 14.4	131 ± 13.5	127 ± 12.7	123 ± 15.7	123 ± 10.0	122 ± 10.0	119 ± 9.4
Reticulocytes (%)	6.0 ± 0.5	9.6 ± 3.2	7.5 ± 2.5	5.8 ± 2.0	5.0 ± 1.9	3.9 ± 1.6	4.2 ± 1.8	3.2 ± 1.4
Weight (g)	725 ± 185	993 ± 194	1174 ± 128	1450 ± 232	1816 ± 192	1957 ± 291	2245 ± 213	—

*Number of infants listed in parentheses.
†Mean values ± SD.
From Zaizov R, Matoth Y: Red cell values on the first postnatal day during the last 16 weeks of gestation. Am J Hematol 1976; 1:276. Copyright © 1976 Wiley-Liss. Reprinted by permission of Wiley-Liss, A Division of John Wiley and Sons, Inc.

TABLE 2–10. Normal Hematologic Values during First 12 Weeks of Life in Term Infant

Age	No. of Cases	Hb (g/dL) ± 1 SD	RBC (X10⁶/mm³) ± 1 SD	Hct (%) ± 1 SD	MCV (fL) ± 1 SD	MCHC (g/dL) ± 1 SD	Reticulocytes (%) ± 1 SD
DAYS							
1	19	19.0 ± 2.2	5.14 ± 0.7	61 ± 7.4	119 ± 9.4	31.6 ± 1.9	3.2 ± 1.4
2	19	19.0 ± 1.9	5.15 ± 0.8	60 ± 6.4	115 ± 7.0	31.6 ± 1.4	3.2 ± 1.3
3	19	18.7 ± 3.4	5.11 ± 0.7	62 ± 9.3	116 ± 5.3	31.1 ± 2.8	2.8 ± 1.7
4	10	18.6 ± 2.1	5.00 ± 0.6	57 ± 8.1	114 ± 7.5	32.6 ± 1.5	1.8 ± 1.1
5	12	17.6 ± 1.1	4.97 ± 0.4	57 ± 7.3	114 ± 8.9	30.9 ± 2.2	1.2 ± 0.2
6	15	17.4 ± 2.2	5.00 ± 0.7	54 ± 7.2	113 ± 10.0	32.2 ± 1.6	0.6 ± 0.2
7	12	17.9 ± 2.5	4.86 ± 0.6	56 ± 9.4	118 ± 11.2	32.0 ± 1.6	0.5 ± 0.4
WEEKS							
1–2	32	17.3 ± 2.3	4.80 ± 0.8	54 ± 8.3	112 ± 19.0	32.1 ± 2.9	0.5 ± 0.3
2–3	11	15.6 ± 2.6	4.20 ± 0.6	46 ± 7.3	111 ± 8.2	33.9 ± 1.9	0.8 ± 0.6
3–4	17	14.2 ± 2.1	4.00 ± 0.6	43 ± 5.7	105 ± 7.5	33.5 ± 1.6	0.6 ± 0.3
4–5	15	12.7 ± 1.6	3.60 ± 0.4	36 ± 4.8	101 ± 8.1	34.9 ± 1.6	0.9 ± 0.8
5–6	10	11.9 ± 1.5	3.55 ± 0.2	36 ± 6.2	102 ± 10.2	34.1 ± 2.9	1.0 ± 0.7
6–7	10	12.0 ± 1.5	3.40 ± 0.4	36 ± 4.8	105 ± 12.0	33.8 ± 2.3	1.2 ± 0.7
7–8	17	11.1 ± 1.1	3.40 ± 0.4	33 ± 3.7	100 ± 13.0	33.7 ± 2.6	1.5 ± 0.7
8–9	13	10.7 ± 0.9	3.40 ± 0.5	31 ± 2.5	93 ± 12.0	34.1 ± 2.2	1.8 ± 1.0
9–10	12	11.2 ± 0.9	3.60 ± 0.3	32 ± 2.7	91 ± 9.3	34.3 ± 2.9	1.2 ± 0.6
10–11	11	11.4 ± 0.9	3.70 ± 0.4	34 ± 2.1	91 ± 7.7	33.2 ± 2.4	1.2 ± 0.7
11–12	13	11.3 ± 0.9	3.70 ± 0.3	33 ± 3.3	88 ± 7.9	34.8 ± 2.2	0.7 ± 0.3

From Matoth Y, Zaizov R, et al: Postnatal changes in some red cell parameters. Acta Paediatr Scand 1971; 60:317.

FIGURE 2–8. Hb concentration and RBC count in cord blood and in venous blood in normal infants during the first week of life. NS-Blood = cord blood; Kp-Blood = capillary blood ml = million. (After Künzer W: In Kepp R, Oehlert G (eds): Blutbildung und Blutumsatz beim Feter und Neugeboreren. Stuttgart, Ferdinand Enke, 1962, p 4.)

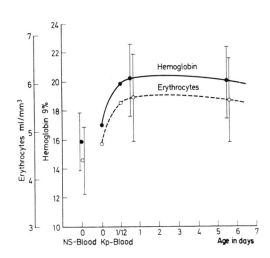

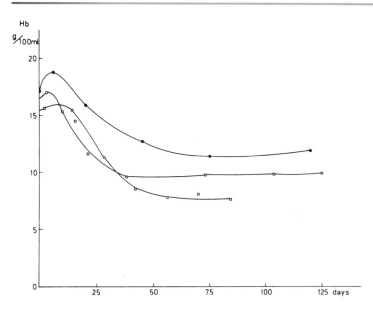

FIGURE 2–9. Hb concentration in infants of different degree of maturation at birth. ● = full-term infants; ○ = premature infants with birth weights of 1200 to 2350 g; □ = premature infants with birth weights less than 1200 g.

TABLE 2–11. Evolution of Hematologic Values of 163 Fetuses during Pregnancy*

Week of Gestation	Hb (g/dL)	Hct (%)	RBC (10⁹/L)	MCV (fL)	RDW (%)	MCH (pg)
18–20 (n = 25)	11.47 ± 0.78	35.86 ± 3.29	2.66 ± 0.29	133.92 ± 8.83	20.64 ± 2.28	43.14 ± 2.71
21–22 (n = 55)	12.28 ± 0.89	38.53 ± 3.21	2.96 ± 0.26	130.06 ± 6.17	20.15 ± 1.92	41.39 ± 3.32
23–25 (n = 61)	12.40 ± 0.77	38.59 ± 2.41	3.06 ± 0.26	126.19 ± 6.23	19.29 ± 1.62	40.48 ± 2.88
26–30 (n = 22)	13.35 ± 1.17	41.54 ± 3.31	3.52 ± 0.32	118.17 ± 5.75	18.35 ± 1.67	37.94 ± 3.67

RDW = red cell distribution width.

*Data ± SD. Studies performed with a Coulter Hematology Analyzer, model S-PLUS II.

Modified from Forestier F, Daffos F, et al: Hematological values of 163 normal fetuses between 18 and 30 weeks of gestation. Pediatr Res 1986; 20:342.

currently are not treatable.[199, 200] Fetuses with hydrops fetalis and anemia have characteristic sonographic abnormalities (thickened placenta, less pleural effusion, and less marked edema); these abnormalities aid in the distinction of infants with hydrops fetalis without anemia from those with anemia.[201] The major causes of treatable fetal anemias are listed in Table 2–12. Most of them are related to

TABLE 2–12. Fetal Anemias Treatable with Intrauterine Transfusion

IMMUNE

Hemolytic disease of the fetus

NONIMMUNE

Hemolytic: hemoglobinopathies (e.g., α-thalassemia (four-gene deletion)), G6PD deficiency
Nonhemolytic: acquired chronic pure red cell aplasia

OTHER

Severe antepartum fetomaternal hemorrhage
Twin-to-twin transfusion syndrome
Cystic hygroma with hydrops fetalis
Placenta chorioangioma
Intrauterine parvovirus B19 infection
Malaria

G6PD = glucose-6-phosphate dehydrogenase.

hemolytic disease of the fetus, hemoglobinopathies, or severe red cell enzyme defects.[202]

Cases of severe fetal anemia caused by maternal acquired chronic pure red cell aplasia[203] or congenital dyserythropoietic anemia type I[204] have been described. However, other pathologic conditions have been associated with anemia during the fetal period, such as hydrops fetalis in combination with either cystic hygroma[205] or placental chorioangioma,[206] parvovirus B19 infection,[207–212] cytomegalovirus infection,[213] and malaria.[214] Rarely, congenital mesoblastic nephromas can induce prenatal hematuria and hemorrhagic shock.[215] For a more comprehensive list of causes, management, and outcome of nonimmune hydrops fetalis see references 216 thorough 219.

Severe chronic anemia in the prenatal period may result in cutaneous manifestations, called "blueberry muffin baby,"[220] which are expressions of cutaneous hematopoiesis. They need to be distinguished from neoplastic diseases and from the angioedema in neonates caused by maternal parvovirus B19 infection.[221, 222]

ANEMIA IN THE NEONATE

Anemia present at birth or appearing during the first week of life can be broadly classified into three major categories: anemia as a result of blood loss, anemia as a result of a hemolytic process, or anemia secondary to less-than-normal red cell production. Many of the disorders producing a hemolytic process are discussed in greater detail in other sections of this text (see Chapter 3, Chapter 15, Chapter 16, Chapter 17, and Section VI).

Anemias that are unique to the newborn and that are not the result of isoimmunization are the focus of the following discussion. The reader is encouraged to consult other monographs in which the primary focus is anemia in the newborn period.[223–231]

BLOOD LOSS AS A CAUSE OF ANEMIA

Blood loss resulting in anemia may occur prenatally, at the time of delivery, or in the first few days of life. Blood loss may be the result of occult hemorrhage before birth, obstetric accidents, internal hemorrhages, or excessive blood sampling by physicians.

The many causes of blood loss in the newborn period are listed in Table 2–13. Faxelius and associates[193] estimated the red cell volume in 259 infants admitted to a high-risk unit in an attempt to determine which clinical events were most often associated with a reduction in red cell mass. They found that a low red cell volume was often associated with a maternal history of vaginal bleeding, with placenta previa or abruptio placentae, with nonelective cesarean section, and with deliveries associated with cord compression. Asphyxiated infants (Apgar score of 6 or less at 1 minute) often had low red cell volume. An early central venous hematocrit level below 45 percent correlated with a low red cell volume, but a normal or even high early hematocrit concentration did not exclude the possibility that the infant was hypovolemic. Infants with mean arterial pressures of less than 30 mm Hg and infants in whom the hematocrit value fell by more than 10 percentage points during the first 6 hours of life were also often found to have a reduced red cell mass. These findings serve to underscore the fact that much anemia in early life is the result of obstetric factors that produce blood loss in the infant.

Occult Hemorrhage before Birth

Occult hemorrhage before birth may be caused by bleeding of the fetus into the maternal circulation or by bleeding of one fetus into another when multiple fetuses are present.

FETAL-TO-MATERNAL HEMORRHAGE

In approximately 50 percent of all pregnancies, some fetal cells can be seen in the maternal circulation.[232] Nucleated fetal erythrocytes can be detected in the maternal circulation as early as the fifth gestational week,[233] and efforts to isolate these cells for prenatal diagnosis of genetic disease have progressed substantially in recent years.[234–236] Fetal DNA is also present in the maternal plasma and in amniotic fluid and represents another possible source of fetal genetic material for diagnostic testing.[237–239]

The estimated volume of fetal blood present in the maternal circulation is less than 2 mL in 98 percent of the pregnancies.[240] Fetal-to-maternal hemorrhages of 30 mL or more are observed in 3 of 1000 women, and they are

TABLE 2–13. Types of Hemorrhage in the Newborn

OCCULT HEMORRHAGE BEFORE BIRTH

Fetomaternal
Abdominal or multiple trauma
Amniocentesis in third trimester
Following external cephalic version
Placental tumors
Spontaneous

Twin-to-Twin
Velamentous cord insertion
"Stuck twin" phenomenon

OBSTETRIC ACCIDENTS, MALFORMATION OF THE PLACENTA AND CORD

Rupture of a normal umbilical cord (precipitous delivery, entanglement)
Hematoma of the cord or placenta
Rupture of an abnormal umbilical cord (varices, aneurysm)
Rupture of anomalous vessels (aberrant vessels, velamentous insertion; communicating vessels in multilobed placenta)
Intrauterine manipulation*
Manual removal of placenta*
Cesarean section*
Incision of placenta during cesarean section
Placenta previa*
Abruptio placentae*

INTERNAL HEMORRHAGE

Intracranial
Giant cephalohematoma, caput succedaneum
Retroperitoneal
Ruptured liver
Ruptured spleen

*Defined by the American College of Obstetrics and Gynecology (ACOG) as conditions associated with high risk for the development of fetomaternal hemorrhages of 30 mL or more. Additional high-risk conditions are antepartum fetal death and antepartum bleeding.

most common after traumatic diagnostic amniocentesis or external cephalic version before delivery. A study of 30,944 Rh-negative mothers showed that 1 of 1146 had fetal bleeding of at least 80 mL, whereas 1 of 2813 had bleeding of 150 mL or more.[241] The risk factors for fetal-to-maternal bleeding are summarized in Table 2–13. Traumatic injuries to the mother during pregnancy (e.g., injury secondary to motor vehicle accidents, falls, abdominal trauma),[242] third-trimester amniocentesis, placental abnormalities (abruptio placentae and placental tumors),[243] and manual removal of the placenta have also been associated with fetal-to-maternal hemorrhages.[240]

The clinical manifestations of fetal-to-maternal hemorrhages depend on the volume of the hemorrhage and the rapidity with which it has occurred. If the hemorrhage has been prolonged or repeated during the course of the pregnancy, anemia develops slowly, giving the fetus an opportunity to develop hemodynamic compensation. Such an infant may manifest only pallor at birth. After acute hemorrhage, just before delivery, the infant may be pale and sluggish, have gasping respirations, and manifest signs of circulatory shock. The typical physical findings and laboratory data that are useful in distinguishing the acute and chronic forms of fetal-to-maternal blood loss are described in Table 2–14.

TABLE 2–14. Characteristics of Acute and Chronic Blood Loss in the Newborn

Characteristics	Acute Blood Loss	Chronic Blood Loss
Clinical	Acute distress; pallor; shallow, rapid, and often irregular respiration; tachycardia; weak or absent peripheral pulses; low or absent blood pressure; no hepatosplenomegaly	Marked pallor disproportionate to evidence of distress; on occasion, signs of congestive heart failure may be present, including hepatomegaly
Venous pressure	Low	Normal or elevated
LABORATORY VALUES		
Hb concentration	May be normal initially; then drops quickly during first 24 hr of life	Low at birth
RBC morphology	Normochromic and macrocytic	Hypochromic and microcytic; anisocytosis and poikilocytosis
Serum iron level	Normal at birth	Low at birth
Course	Prompt treatment of anemia and shock necessary to prevent death	Generally uneventful
Treatment	Intravenous fluids and whole blood; iron therapy later	Iron therapy; packed RBCs may be necessary on occasion

The degree of anemia is quite variable. Usually, the hemoglobin value is less than 12 g/dL before signs and symptoms of anemia can be recognized by the physician. Hemoglobin values as low as 3 to 4 g/dL have been recorded in infants who were born alive and survived. If the hemorrhage has been acute and particularly when hypovolemic shock is present, the hemoglobin value may not reflect the magnitude of the blood loss. In such instances, several hours may elapse before hemodilution occurs and the magnitude of the hemorrhage is appreciated. In general, an acute loss of 20 percent of the blood volume is sufficient to produce signs of shock and is reflected in a decrease in hemoglobin levels within 3 hours of the event.

Examination of a peripheral blood smear provides useful diagnostic information. In acute hemorrhage, the red cells appear normochromic and normocytic, whereas in chronic hemorrhage the cells are generally hypochromic and microcytic.

In anemia that is a direct result of a fetal-to-maternal hemorrhage, the Coombs' test yields a negative result, and the infants are not jaundiced. Infants with anemia secondary to blood loss generally have much lower bilirubin values throughout the neonatal period as a consequence of their reduced red cell mass.

The diagnosis of a fetomaternal hemorrhage of sufficient magnitude to result in anemia at birth can be made with certainty only through demonstration of the presence of fetal cells in the maternal circulation. Techniques for demonstrating these cells include differential agglutination, mixed agglutination, fluorescent antibody techniques, and the acid elution method of staining cells that contain fetal hemoglobin.

The Kleihauer-Betke technique of acid elution is the simplest of these methods and the one most commonly used for the detection of fetal cells,[244, 245] although its value in monitoring patients at risk has been questioned.[246] The test is based on the resistance of fetal hemoglobin to elution from the intact cell in an acid medium. The acid elution technique can be relied on with certainty for diagnosis only when other conditions capable of producing elevations in maternal fetal hemoglobin levels are absent. These include maternal thalassemia minor, sickle cell anemia, hereditary persistence of fetal hemoglobin, and, in some normal women, a pregnancy-induced increase in fetal hemoglobin production. In the presence of these conditions, other techniques based on differential agglutination should be used.[247] In addition, flow cytometry has been shown to be an acceptable alternative to the acid elution test in the detection of fetomaternal hemorrhages.[248] However, most of the flow cytometric tests are designed to quantify D-positive fetal cells in D-negative mothers and are not applicable to D-positive mothers.[249, 250]

Diagnosis of a fetomaternal hemorrhage may be missed in situations in which the red cells of the mother and infant have incompatible ABO blood groups. In such instances, the infant's A or B cells are rapidly cleared from the maternal circulation by the maternal anti-A or anti-B antibodies and are not available for staining. A presumptive diagnosis may be made through demonstration of either marked erythrophagocytosis in smears of the maternal buffy coat or an increase in maternal immune anti-A or anti-B titers in the weeks after delivery.

TWIN-TO-TWIN TRANSFUSION SYNDROME

This form of hemorrhage is observed only in monozygotic multiple births with monochorial placentas. In approximately 70 percent of monozygotic twin pregnancies, a monochorial placenta exists.[251] The incidence of twin-to-twin transfusion syndrome (TTTS) for pregnancies in which a monochorial placenta is present has been estimated to be 13 to 33 percent in one study[252] and 6.2 percent in another.[253] Velamentous cord insertions are associated with an increased risk of TTTS, possibly as a result of compression forces, which reduce blood flow to one twin.[254] This blood exchange can produce anemia in the donor and polycythemia in the recipient. When a significant blood transfer has occurred, the difference in hemoglobin concentration between the twins exceeds 5.0 g/dL. This is in contrast to a maximal discrepancy of 3.3 g/dL in cord blood hemoglobin in dizygotic twins. The survival rate for fetuses with TTTS diagnosed before the

28th week of gestation varies between 21 and 50 percent.[252, 255, 256] Clinical characteristics, diagnostic modalities, and the possible therapeutic role of amniocentesis and cordocentesis with fetal transfusion in reducing the high perinatal mortality of this syndrome have been reviewed.[253, 256–259]

The anemic infant may develop congestive heart failure, whereas the plethoric twin may manifest symptoms and signs of the hyperviscosity syndrome, disseminated intravascular coagulation, and hyperbilirubinemia.[260] Rarely, hydrops fetalis may develop if TTTS occurs early in the pregnancy.[261]

The hemorrhage may be acute or chronic. Tan and associates[262] reviewed 482 twin pairs, among which 35 pairs were found to have TTTS. They pointed out how the difference in weight of the twins could be used to establish the timing of the hemorrhage. When the weight difference exceeded 20 percent of the weight of the larger twin, the transfusion was chronic and the smaller infant was invariably the donor. The anemic smaller twin displayed reticulocytosis. When the difference in the weight of the twins did not exceed 20 percent of the weight of the larger twin, the larger twin was the donor in almost 50 percent of all instances. In these presumably acute transfusions, significant reticulocytosis was not observed in the anemic donor. Although hemoglobin values of the recipient were increased equally with both acute and chronic transfusions, the donor twin in the chronic transfusion group was found to be more anemic than the donor in the acute transfusion group. These findings support and extend the original proposal of Klebe and Ingomar,[263] who suggested these two types of transfusions on the basis of a review of previously documented cases.

Obstetric Accidents and Malformations of the Placenta and Cord

The normal umbilical cord may rupture during precipitous deliveries. The cord also may rupture during a normal delivery when it is unusually short or is entangled around the fetus or when traction is applied to the infant with forceps.[264]

Other abnormalities of the umbilical cord that predispose to hemorrhage and the development of anemia in the infant include vascular abnormalities such as umbilical venous tortuosity and arterial aneurysm. Inflammation of the cord can weaken vessels and predispose them to rupture.

Velamentous insertion of the umbilical cord is observed in approximately 1 percent of all pregnancies. It appears to be most common in twin pregnancies and in pregnancies accompanied by low-lying placentas. It is estimated that 1 to 2 percent of pregnancies associated with velamentous insertion of the cord result in fetal blood loss.[264] The perinatal death rate in such circumstances ranges from 58 to 80 percent, with many of the infants being stillborn. Approximately 12 percent of those infants who are born alive will be anemic.

The placenta may be inadvertently incised during a cesarean section, with the incision producing a fetal hemorrhage.[265] As previously mentioned, placenta previa or abruptio placentae often results in fetal hemorrhage.[266] In women with late third-trimester bleeding, the physician may anticipate the birth of an anemic infant by examining the vaginal blood for the presence of fetal erythrocytes, using the acid elution technique of Kleihauer and Betke.[267]

Internal Hemorrhage

When internal hemorrhage takes place in the newborn, it may not be recognized until shock has occurred.

Anemia that appears in the first 24 to 72 hours after birth and that is not associated with jaundice is commonly due to internal hemorrhages. It is well recognized that traumatic deliveries may result in subdural or subarachnoid hemorrhages massive enough to result in anemia. Cephalohematomas may be of giant size and result in anemia.[268]

Blood loss into the subaponeurotic area of the scalp tends to be greater than that observed with cephalohematomas. The bleeding is not confined by periosteal attachments and thus is not limited to an area overlying a single skull bone. A subaponeurotic hemorrhage usually extends through the soft tissue of the scalp and covers the entire calvaria. Blood loss in this area can result in exsanguination.[269] Packman[270] observed a hemoglobin value of 2.2 g/dL in an infant 48 hours of age in whom a massive hemorrhage into the scalp had occurred. This form of hemorrhage most commonly occurs after difficult deliveries or vacuum extractions.[271] It also appears with vitamin K deficiency and may be seen more often in African-American infants than in those of other ethnicity. Examination of the infant reveals a boggy edema of the head extending into the frontal region and to the nape of the neck. The edema, which may have bluish coloration, obscures the fontanelles and swells the eyelids. The infant may be in shock. Robinson and Rossiter[269] have developed a formula for predicting the volume of blood loss in this condition. For each centimeter of increase in head circumference above that expected, a 38-mL loss of blood has occurred. When the products of red cell breakdown are absorbed from these entrapped hemorrhages, hyperbilirubinemia may develop.[272]

Breech deliveries may be associated with hemorrhage into the adrenal glands, kidneys, spleen, or retroperitoneal area. Blood loss of this type should be suspected in infants found to be anemic during the first few days of life after a traumatic delivery. Hemorrhage into the adrenal glands may also be observed after any difficult delivery or after birth in a large infant. In adrenal hemorrhage, the clinical picture may include sudden collapse, cyanosis, limpness, jaundice, irregular respirations, elevated or subnormal temperatures, and the presence of a flank mass accompanied by bluish discoloration of the overlying skin.

Rupture of the liver, with resultant anemia, appears to occur more often than is clinically appreciated. In stillbirths and neonatal deaths, the incidence of hepatic hemorrhages found at autopsy ranges from 1.2 to 5.6 percent.[273] In approximately half of the cases reviewed by Henderson,[274] the hemorrhage was subcapsular only; in the remainder, the capsule had ruptured, and free blood was present in the peritoneal cavity.[274]

An infant with a ruptured liver generally appears to be well for 24 to 48 hours and then suddenly goes into shock. The moment of onset of shock appears to coincide with the time when the gradually increasing hematoma finally ruptures the hepatic capsule, causing hemoperitoneum. At this time, the upper abdomen may appear distended, and often a mass contiguous with the liver is palpable. Shifting dullness can be demonstrated on abdominal percussion. Flat films of the abdomen taken with the patient in both the erect and supine positions often confirm the presence of free fluid in the abdomen. Paracentesis, performed with the infant in the lateral position, reveals free blood in the abdomen. The prognosis is poor, but infants have survived after multiple blood transfusions and prompt surgical repair of the laceration.

Splenic rupture may also occur after a difficult delivery or as a result of the extreme distention of the spleen that often accompanies severe erythroblastosis fetalis.[275, 276] The physician should always suspect a rupture of the spleen with associated hemorrhage when, at the time of exchange transfusion, the anemic and hydropic infant with erythroblastosis fetalis is found to have decreased, rather than an increased, venous pressure. Rupture of the spleen may also occur during the exchange transfusion.

Splenic rupture occurs, although uncommonly, in healthy infants born after seemingly normal deliveries.[277] Many of these infants are large. Pallor, abdominal distention, scrotal swelling, and radiographic evidence of peritoneal effusion without free air should alert the physician to the presence of splenic rupture.

Other less common causes of neonatal bleeding include maternal treatment with antiepileptic drugs during pregnancy associated with vitamin K deficiency,[278] neonatal adenovirus infection,[279] fetal cytomegalovirus infection,[280] hemangiomas of the gastrointestinal tract,[281] and hemangioendotheliomas of the skin.[282]

Bleeding into the ventricles and subarachnoid space also can produce significant anemia. Intraventricular hemorrhage may occur in half of all infants with birth weights of less than 1500 g and even more often when the mother has ingested aspirin in the week before the birth of the infant.[283] In many of these infants, no neurologic symptoms are present, and the hemorrhage is recognized on computed tomography of the head.[284]

Anemia Caused by Blood Drawing for Laboratory Analysis

Frequent drawing of blood for laboratory analysis is a major cause of anemia in critically ill neonates treated in neonatal intensive care units. In very low birth weight infants (<1500 g), a 1-mL blood volume represents 1 percent or more of the total blood volume (Fig. 2–10). In neonates weighing less than 1500 g, the total amount of blood drawn during the first 4 weeks of hospitalization may range from 5 to 45 percent of the calculated total blood volume.[285] A study in 60 very low birth weight infants (560 to 1450 g) showed an average of 4.8 punctures/day per infant, with a mean blood loss for diagnostic sampling of 50.3 mL/kg per 28-day period (range, 7 to 142 mL).[286] Increased blood loss was associated with increased number of transfusions. A more recent study showed lower blood loss (13.6 mL/kg); tests ordered most often were glucose, sodium, and potassium.[287]

Various approaches for limiting the amount of blood drawn for laboratory tests include the following:

1. Reducing the amount of blood discarded from central venous lines before blood for cultures is obtained. It has been shown that discarding only 0.3 mL in infants and 1.0 mL in children does not affect the accuracy of central venous line cultures.[288]
2. Use of micromethods that reduce blood loss from peripheral arterial catheters during sampling.[289]
3. Use of a closed method that allows return of the initial sample drawn to clear a line to the patient. This technique has been shown to reduce blood loss caused by diagnostic sampling, even in adult patients.[290, 291]

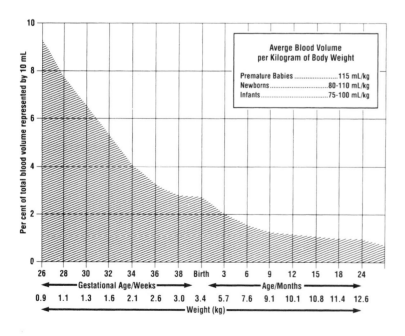

FIGURE 2–10. Average blood volume per kilogram of body weight. (From Werner M (ed): Microtechniques for the Clinical Laboratory. New York, John Wiley & Sons, 1976, p 2. Copyright © 1976. Reprinted by permission of John Wiley & Sons, Inc.)

4. Reducing the amount of blood drawn in excess of that needed for the analytic procedure (25 percent of the blood samples removed in neonatal intensive care unit settings exceed the analytic need).[285] Phlebotomy overdrawing is more common in the most critically ill infants and is greater when syringes are used.[292]

5. Reducing the need for blood drawing through the use of transcutaneous monitoring techniques (40 percent of the blood samples drawn in a neonatal intensive care unit setting are for analysis of blood gases and electrolytes).[285]

Recognition of the Infant with Blood Loss

The clinical manifestations of hemorrhage depend on the site of bleeding, on the extent of the hemorrhage, and on whether the blood loss is acute or chronic. The features that are useful in distinguishing infants with acute and chronic blood loss at the time of delivery are described in Table 2–14. Asphyxiated infants may also display pallor. Features that aid in distinguishing the infant with asphyxia from the infant with acute blood loss are presented in Table 2–15. In all circumstances associated with late third-trimester bleeding, multiple births, cesarean sections, a nuchal cord, any form of cord compression, or a difficult delivery, the infant's hemoglobin level should be obtained promptly. Even when the first value is normal, the hemoglobin should be measured again 6 to 12 hours after birth.

ANEMIA AS A RESULT OF A HEMOLYTIC PROCESS

A *hemolytic process* is generally defined as a pathologic process that results in a shortening of the normal red cell life span of 120 days. For neonates, a different definition recognizing that the normal red cell life span of term infants is only 60 to 80 days (and may be as short as 20 to 30 days in infants born at 30 to 32 weeks of gestation) must be used. A hemolytic process during the neonatal period is usually manifested by one of the following combinations of clinical and laboratory findings:

1. A persistent increase in the reticulocyte count, with or without an abnormally low hemoglobin concentration in the absence of current or previous hemorrhage.

2. A rapidly declining hemoglobin concentration without an increase in the reticulocyte count in the absence of hemorrhage.

Most infants with a hemolytic anemia have accompanying hyperbilirubinemia; however, in the majority of infants in whom the bilirubin level exceeds 12 mg/dL, an increase in red cell destruction, as reflected by an increase in blood carboxyhemoglobin levels, cannot be demonstrated.[293] Approximately 30 percent of infants with an increase in carboxyhemoglobin levels have maximum bilirubin values of less than 8 mg/dL. The major causes of a shortened red cell life span in the neonatal period are listed in Table 2–16. Only the most salient features of hereditary hemolytic anemias that manifest themselves in the neonatal period are discussed in this section. Extensive descriptions of these disorders appear in other portions of the text.

Hemoglobinopathies

Clinically significant hemoglobinopathies in the newborn may be categorized, as in the older child, as defects of structure or defects of synthesis (thalassemic syndromes). Because of the rapid evolutionary changes that occur in the fetus and newborn with respect to globin chain synthesis, a unique situation exists. Certain hereditary defects of hemoglobin may be seen at this age; some of these defects resolve spontaneously (e.g., γ chain defects), whereas other defects, clinically inapparent at birth, produce problems at a later age (e.g., β chain disorders). Other defects that might be thought to be similar in their clinical manifestations throughout life, such as α chain defects, in fact may act differently in the newborn period when paired with a γ chain rather than with a β chain.

DEFECTS OF HEMOGLOBIN STRUCTURE

Alpha Chain Structural Defects. When α chain variants of hemoglobin occur, they are present in significant concentration at birth; this is because the α chain is common to all forms of hemoglobin present at birth. In contrast, β chain variants such as HbS become quantitatively significant only as β chain synthesis replaces γ chain production during the first months after birth. When the amino acid alteration is in the α chain, the concentration of the abnormal hemoglobin will remain fairly constant during infancy and adulthood; however, during infancy, the abnormal hemoglobin will be present primarily in a fetal form ($\alpha_2^x\gamma_2$), with a lesser amount in the adult form ($\alpha_2^x\beta_2$). An example of this is HbD-St. Louis trait ($\alpha_2^{68}{}^{Asn}\rightarrow{}^{Lys}\beta_2$), in which the total concentration of abnormal hemoglobin ($\alpha_2^x\gamma_2 + \alpha_2^x\beta_2$) was found to be 27 percent in

TABLE 2–15. Differential Diagnosis of Pallor in the Newborn

Asphyxia	Acute Severe Blood Loss	Hemolytic Disease
1. Respiratory findings: retractions, response to oxygen, cyanosis 2. Moribund appearance 3. Bradycardia 4. Stable Hb	1. Decrease in venous and arterial pressure 2. Rapid shallow respirations 3. Acyanotic 4. Tachycardia 5. Drop in Hb	1. Hepatosplenomegaly, jaundice 2. Positive result on Coombs' test 3. Anemia

Adapted from Kirkman HN, Riley HD, Jr: Posthemorrhagic anemia and shock in the newborn due to hemorrhage during delivery: Report of 8 cases. Pediatrics 1959; 24:97. Copyright American Academy of Pediatrics, 1959.

TABLE 2–16. Causes of a Hemolytic Process in the Neonatal Period

A. *Immune*
    Rh incompatibility
    ABO incompatibility
    Minor blood group incompatibility
    Maternal autoimmune hemolytic anemia
    Drug-induced hemolytic anemia
B. *Infection*
    Bacterial sepsis
    Congenital infections
        Syphilis
        Malaria
        Cytomegalovirus
        Adenovirus
        Rubella
        Toxoplasmosis
        Disseminated herpes
C. *Disseminated Intravascular Coagulation*
D. *Macro- and Microangiopathic Anemias*
    Cavernous hemangioma or hemangioendothelioma
    Large vessel thrombi
    Renal artery stenosis
    Severe coarctation of the aorta
E. *Galactosemia*
F. *Prolonged or Recurrent Metabolic or Respiratory Acidosis*
G. *Hereditary Disorders of the Red Cell Membrane*
    Hereditary spherocytosis
    Hereditary elliptocytosis
    Hereditary stomatocytosis
    Hereditary xerocytosis
    Other rare membrane disorders
H. *Pyknocytosis*
I. *Red Cell Enzyme Deficiencies*
    G6PD deficiency, pyruvate kinase deficiency,
        5'-nucleotidase deficiency, glucose phosphate
        isomerase deficiency
J. *Alpha-Thalassemia Syndromes*
K. *Alpha-Chain Structural Abnormalities*
L. *Gamma-Thalassemia Syndromes*
M. *Gamma-Chain Structural Abnormalities*

neonates in comparison with adults, in whom the average concentration of HbD was 28 percent in the heterozygous state.[294]

Fortunately, most α chain mutations do not cause clinically significant disorders in adults, and the same situation appears to exist in newborns. In most infants α chain mutations are detected only as part of routine neonatal screening programs. Occasionally, the fetal form of an α chain mutation is clinically more significant than the adult form of the mutation. Hb Hasharon ($\alpha_2^{14\,Asp \to His} \beta_2$) in neonates is an example of this phenomenon. Hb Hasharon is mildly unstable: unstable mutant hemoglobins have a greater tendency to dissociate into subunits, and this increased dissociation leads to hemolysis. HbF is less stable than HbA, presumably as a result of a 10-fold greater affinity between α and β chains than that between α and γ chains. In this mildly unstable hemoglobin, the interaction between Hasharon α chains and normal β chains must be minimally decreased, but the interaction between Hasharon α chains and γ chains in the fetal form of Hb Hasharon would be expected to be considerably

less, resulting in an even more unstable form of the α chain variant. Levine and Lincoln[295] described a 965-g newborn who was heterozygous for Hb Hasharon. This infant manifested a hemolytic anemia that resolved coincidentally with the transition from the fetal to the adult form of Hb Hasharon trait at several months of age.

Beta Chain Structural Defects. The β chain mutations generally produce no clinical symptomatology in the newborn period. This does not mean that chain variants are never a problem in the neonate, nor does it mean that these variants cannot be easily detected in the laboratory.

Although HbA usually constitutes less than 30 percent of the normal hemoglobin at birth, the fraction may, under certain circumstances, be far greater. Because the γ → β chain switchover begins at about 32 weeks of gestation, any disorder that causes the fetus to destroy its existing red cell population will result in a replacement with red cells having a markedly different HbF:HbA ratio at the time of delivery. Fetomaternal blood group incompatibility and intrauterine blood loss may, for example, unmask a β chain defect earlier than it might otherwise be detected.

Sickle cell hemoglobinopathies are the most commonly encountered β chain variants in the newborn period. Homozygous sickle cell disease has presented several times clinically in the neonate. In patients with homozygous sickle cell disease, the HbS concentration at birth is usually about 20 percent.

In infants in whom sickle cell anemia has been diagnosed in the first 30 days of life because of some specific symptomatology, the most common findings are jaundice, fever, pallor, respiratory distress, and abdominal distention. Hyperbilirubinemia appears to be more common among newborns with sickle cell anemia.[296] Hegyi and Delphin[297] described a full-term newborn who developed abdominal distention during the first day of life. The cord bilirubin value was 3.1 mg/dL, the hemoglobin level was 12.7 g/dL, and the reticulocyte count was 13.3 percent. No evidence of G6PD deficiency or blood group incompatibility was found, but hemoglobin electrophoresis demonstrated 20 percent HbS and 80 percent HbF. The child rapidly improved but was later found dead in her crib on the fifth day of life. Postmortem examination revealed sickle cells in multiple organs and histopathologic findings consistent with widespread vaso-occlusion, including multifocal enterocolitis.

Of special concern is the problem of the "iatrogenic" sickle cell crisis—the exchange transfusion of neonates with respiratory distress syndrome with the blood from apparently healthy donors who happen to have sickle cell trait.[298] Such transfusions can produce death in the hypoxic infant.

Gamma Chain Structural Defects. Table 2–17 lists the most commonly observed γ chain structural hemoglobinopathies. These variants are quite interesting because they represent disorders that spontaneously resolve as γ chain production diminishes. The concentrations of these hemoglobins in cord blood average 10 to 20 percent of the total hemoglobin and appear to represent the heterozygous state of these γ chain hemoglobinopathies.[294] The structural γ defects generally present no hematologic disturbances and usually are found during newborn screening programs. HbF-Poole is an exception to this rule. HbF-Poole

TABLE 2–17. Gamma Chain Hemoglobinopathies: G_γ or A_γ

Hb Name	Residue/Substitution	% Total Hb	% Total Hb F	Notes
G_γ				
F-Malaysia	1 Gly → Cys	12.8	18.8	
F-Meinohama	5 Glu → Gly	10.0		
F-Aukland	7 Asp → Asn	19	22.5	
F-Albaicin	8 Lys → Glu or Gln	29		
F-Catalonia	15 Trp → Arg	45.5	51.5	
F-Melbourne	16 Gly → Arg	26	29	
F-Saskatoon	21 Glu → Lys	16.2	23.3	
F-Urumqi	22 Asp → Gly	21.5		
F-Granada	22 Asp → Val	22		
F-Cosenza	25 Gly → Glu	22.4		
F-Oakland	26 Glu → Lys	32		
F-Austell	40 Arg → Lys	27		
F-Lodz	44 Ser → Arg	37.1		
F-Kingston	55 Met → Arg	21		
F-Sacromonte	59 Lys → Gln	25		
F-Emirates	59 Lys → Glu	37		
F-M-Osaka	63 His → Tyr			Decreased O_2 affinity, methemoglobinemia
F-Brooklyn	66 Lys → Gln	23		
F-Kennestone	77 His → Arg	25.3	30.7	
F-Marietta	80 Asp → Asn	12.4	16.2	
F-Columbus-GA	94 Asp → Asn	30.5		
F-La Grange	101 Glu → Lys	14.0		Increased O_2 affinity, mildly unstable
F-Malta-I	117 His → Arg			
F-Carlton	121 Glu → Lys	26		
F-Port Royal	125 Glu → Ala	14–16		
F-Onoda	146 His → Tyr	26.4	35	Increased O_2 affinity,
A_γ				
F-Macedonia-I	2 His → Gln	15		
F-Texas-I	5 Glu → Lys	12		Increased acetylation (3-fold)
F-Pordenone	6 Glu → Gln	5.7	8.6	
F-Calluna	12 Thr → Arg	8.7	10.8	
F-Kuala Lumpur	22 Asp → Gly	11		
F-Pendergrass	36 Pro → Arg	6.7	8.5	
F-Bonaire-GA	39 Gln → Arg	8.3	9.8	
F-Beech Island	53 Ala → Asp	15–16		
F-Jamaica	61 Lys → Glu	11–15		
F-Iawata	72 Gly → Arg	11		
F-Sardinia	75 Ile → Thr	15		
F-Damman	79 Asp → Asn	6.9	13.1	
F-Victoria Jubilee	80 Asp → Tyr	7.0		
F-Hull	121 Glu → Lys	7–9		

is an unstable hemoglobin that presents as a Heinz-body hemolytic anemia during the first weeks of life.[299]

DEFECTS IN HEMOGLOBIN SYNTHESIS

In newborn infants, defects in hemoglobin synthesis create a greater variety of thalassemia syndromes than those that may occur at any other time of life. Newborns may demonstrate all varieties of α-thalassemia, β-thalassemia, γ-thalassemia, δ-thalassemia, or any combination of these.

Alpha-Thalassemia Syndromes in the Neonate. In the newborn period, hemolytic disease caused by thalassemia has invariably been associated with homozygous α-thalassemia. A large spectrum of α-thalassemia syndromes may be observed in the newborn period.

Silent Carrier (One-Gene Defect). Thus far, no observations have been made of this disorder in the neonatal period. This entity would be suspected only if a parent were known to be a silent carrier.

Alpha-Thalassemia Trait (Two-Gene Defect). Although the α-thalassemia syndromes have been described for more than 20 years, the heterozygous state (trait or two genes deleted in cis or trans) has been difficult to identify because of the mild hematologic changes that accompany this disorder. Older children and adults may exhibit a very mild anemia and microcytosis in the presence of a normal hemoglobin electrophoresis. The diagnosis is more easily made in the neonatal period than at any other time of life. This is because of two unique occurrences. First, microcytosis is observed in the cord blood of newborns with α-thalassemia trait. Because other causes of microcytosis are rare at this age, infants who are born with a low MCV are more likely to have α-thalassemia trait than any other disease. Second, α-thalassemia in newborns is associated with the presence of Bart's Hb (γ_4), which is easily identified.

Hemoglobin values in neonates with thalassemia trait are no different from those of normal neonates (range, 15.2 to 18.5 g/dL).[300] The MCVs are significantly lower (~94 μm^3) than those of normal-term infants (106.4 ± 5.7 μm^3). In addition, patients with the trait syndrome usually have a mean corpuscular hemoglobin (MCH) value less than 29.3 pg. The determination of MCV and MCH appears to be an adequate screening test. The presence of Bart's Hb is the confirmatory finding.

Hemoglobin H Disease. This disorder appears to be the result of the inheritance of a three-gene deletion, which causes sufficient α/β + γ chain imbalance to result in the presence of large quantities of Bart's Hb (γ_4) and some HbH (β_4) in the newborn period. After the first few months of life, the Bart's Hb disappears, and the only remaining abnormal hemoglobin is HbH.

Infants born with HbH diseases have higher levels of Bart's Hb in their cord blood than do normal infants or individuals with α-thalassemia trait; however, they have lower levels than do homozygous infants with hydrops fetalis. Unlike infants with α-thalassemia trait, infants with HbH disease are born with significant anemia. Microcytosis is present.[301] The hemolytic process may contribute to a somewhat increased incidence of neonatal jaundice.

Hydrops Fetalis. This four-gene deletion disease results in the death of the affected fetus. Because of the virtual absence of α chain synthesis, affected infants are born with Bart's Hb only (occasionally, however, some Hb Portland may be found). The peripheral blood smear demonstrates marked hypochromia, poikilocytosis, and target cells. This disorder must be distinguished from other causes of hydrops fetalis with severe anemia. A negative result on Coombs' test and the demonstration of intracellular crystals of Bart's Hb with supravital staining rapidly confirm the high probability of the homozygous state as the correct diagnosis. If death does not occur *in utero*, it occurs within minutes after birth. Although infants with hydrops fetalis have been reported to have cord hemoglobin values as high as 11 g/dL, the usual levels are much lower.[302] Oxygen delivery is severely impaired even when hemoglobin levels are greater because of the profound leftward shift of the oxyhemoglobin dissociation curve for Bart's Hb. There is a possible association between homozygous α-thalassemia and hypospadias.[303, 304] When this disorder is detected *in utero*, the fetus may be salvaged with intrauterine transfusion and maintained by a postdelivery transfusion program.[305, 306] Severe forms of α-thalassemia and hydrops fetalis can be prevented with prenatal testing and counseling.[307]

Beta-Thalassemias. In the β-thalassemia syndromes (both trait and homozygous states), the disorders become apparent only after 2 or 3 months of age. In β-thalassemia minor, hematologic findings at birth are entirely normal, with microcytosis being noted later in the first 6 months

of life. Similarly, in β-thalassemia major, no clinical findings are present initially; the first sign of any abnormality is the presence of nucleated red cells on smear or continued high HbF concentrations. Any disorder that significantly alters the survival of fetal red cells (e.g., intrauterine blood loss or blood group incompatibility) could make the β-thalassemia syndromes clinically obvious at an earlier age.

Erlandson and Hilgartner[308] recorded their observations of infants in whom thalassemia major was diagnosed during the first 3 months of life. In four infants in whom the disease was diagnosed between 1 and 2 months of age, the hemoglobin concentrations were abnormally low. Morphologic erythrocyte abnormalities were already present at 3 days of age in one infant who also was mildly anemic (Hb level, 12.7 g/dL). The earliest morphologic abnormalities were similar to those found in the heterozygous state; however, by 2 months of age, the presence of marked numbers of normoblasts, consistent with homozygous thalassemia, was noted in all infants. Splenomegaly was not present in the one infant who was examined at birth but was apparent in all infants between 1 and 3 months of age. The fetal hemoglobin levels were elevated at 1 to 2 months of age. It would seem then that at least some manifestations of thalassemia major may be present at birth.

Gamma-Thalassemias. Theoretically, a decrease in γ chain synthesis (γ-thalassemia) would produce symptoms *in utero*. Because there are multiple structural genes for γ chain synthesis, the severity of γ-thalassemia would depend on the extent to which these genes were involved. The condition would be lethal if no γ chains were formed; if only one or two genes were involved, only slight hypochromia or, at most, a mild anemia would ensue. If the diagnosis were not established in the neonatal period, it would be missed, because as β chain synthesis replaces γ chain synthesis, the red cell changes would disappear.[309]

Combinations of Thalassemia Syndromes. Kan and co-workers[310] described a full-term infant who had a hemolytic hypochromic anemia at birth associated with microcytosis and nucleated red cells on smear. Neither HbH nor Bart's Hb was detected. Studies of globin chain synthesis in peripheral blood revealed a deficiency in the synthesis of γ and β chains. As the infant matured, the peripheral smear morphology improved and became identical with that of the subject's father, who had β-thalassemia trait. Since then, several such cases have been reported (see Chapter 20).

Methemoglobinemia in Neonates Treated with Nitric Oxide

Methemoglobinemia is discussed in detail in Chapter 18. A new form of drug-induced MetHb has special relevance for oxygen transport in neonates. Pulmonary vasoconstriction is characteristic of persistent pulmonary hypertension of the newborn and is often seen in neonatal respiratory distress syndromes. Inhaled nitric oxide (NO) acts as a potent vasodilator on the pulmonary vasculature, improves oxygenation, and lowers pulmonary vascular resistance.[311–316] A potentially serious side effect of the administration of NO is the oxidation of Fe^{2+} of hemoglobin to form Fe^{3+} and MetHb. This is usually transient but has been reported to be as high as 40 percent.[317] Detection of MetHb formation is particularly problematic in neonates owing to the interference of HbF with MetHb determination. Multiwavelength Hb CO-oximeters can provide reliable estimates of MetHb in samples with high HbF, although their reliability differs in different models.[318–320] It is advisable to monitor MetHb levels in all neonates treated with NO.

Methemoglobinemia in Neonates with Diarrhea

Diarrhea in neonates can be associated with methemoglobinemia, in some cases requiring infusion of methylene blue. Patients are usually in the first 1 to 3 months of life. They often show failure to thrive, have weight on admission below the 10th percentile, and have been formula-fed.[321–323]

Hereditary Disorders of the Red Cell Membrane

Hereditary spherocytosis, hereditary elliptocytosis, hereditary stomatocytosis, and hereditary xerocytosis all may be manifest in the newborn period.[324] If a hemolytic anemia is detected during evaluation of hyperbilirubinemia, a precise diagnosis generally is not established in most patients until they are older. It should also be kept in mind that genetic defects in bilirubin metabolism may be associated with hereditary disorders of the red cell membrane, leading to marked neonatal hyperbilirubinemia.[325]

In only one third of patients is hereditary spherocytosis diagnosed during the first year of life. Neonates with hereditary spherocytosis have dehydrated erythrocytes with decreased membrane surface area and exhibit a sharp fall in Hb (near-normal at birth) and reticulocyte counts during the first 20 days of life, with 75 percent requiring transfusion.[326] The reticulocyte response to the anemia is also blunted in the first year of life.[326] Two cases have been reported of severe neonatal anemia caused by hereditary spherocytosis and the absence of the anion exchange protein band 3.[327, 328]

The classic morphologic abnormalities of patients with hereditary elliptocytosis may not be present during the first few weeks of life. Patients with the hemolytic form of hereditary elliptocytosis may display pyknocytes rather than elliptocytes early in life, and only after several months are the typical elliptocytes observed. These membrane disorders are described in detail in Chapter 16.

Dehydrated hereditary spherocytosis has been shown to be associated in some families with perinatal edema, which resolves in a few weeks after birth, and in some other families with pseudohyperkalemia. The MCV and MCH concentration in erythrocytes are both increased and the defect has been localized to 16q23-q24.[329, 330]

Red Cell Enzyme Deficiencies

Inherited disorders of red cell metabolism also may be anticipated to produce a hemolytic anemia early in life. The most common of these abnormalities are G6PD deficiency and pyruvate kinase deficiency.[331] These and other disorders of red cell metabolism are described in Chapters 16 and 17. G6PD deficiency may be associated with Gilbert's syndrome, leading to marked hyperbilirubinemia and jaundice.[332, 333]

Malaria

Although the pathophysiology of malaria-associated anemia is not fully understood,[334] it has been shown that congenital malaria and the presence of parasitemia at birth are strongly associated with neonatal anemia (Hb < 14 g/dL).[335–338]

IMPAIRED RED BLOOD CELL PRODUCTION

Diamond-Blackfan anemia (pure red cell anemia, erythrogenesis imperfecta, or chronic aregenerative anemia) is an uncommon condition characterized by a failure of erythropoiesis but normal production of white blood cells and platelets (see Chapter 8).[339] The disease may affect more than red cell production, because it is associated with pancytopenia, hypoplasia of the bone marrow, and reduced *in vitro* clonogenic potential.[340]

Two reviews of the subject suggest that as many as 25 percent of affected patients may be anemic at birth.[341, 342] Hemoglobin values as low as 9.4 g/dL, accompanied by reticulocytopenia, have been observed during the first days of life.[343] There is no correlation between the various kinds of gene mutations described in this disease and the clinical expression and severity.[344, 345] However, the severity of the disease is greater in patients who are seen at a young age and were born prematurely.[346]

Low birth weight occurs in approximately 10 percent of all affected patients, with about half of this group being small for gestational age. There appears to be a slight increase in the incidence of miscarriages, stillbirths, and complications of pregnancy among the mothers who have given birth to infants with this syndrome.

Described abnormalities include microcephaly, cleft palate, anomalies of the eye, web neck, and thumb deformity. Triphalangeal thumb, duplications of the thumb, and bifid thumb have been described in association with this syndrome.[347–349]

Another cause of impaired red cell production in the neonatal period is Pearson syndrome.[350] This syndrome is characterized by vacuolization of bone marrow precursors, sideroblastic anemia, and exocrine pancreatic dysfunction.[351] It may be associated with Leigh disease (subacute necrotizing encephalopathy)[352] or with Kearns-Sayre syndrome (bilateral ptosis and atypical retinitis pigmentosa).[353] A deletion in mitochondrial DNA has been found in Pearson syndrome.[354–356] A case of pyridoxine-refractory congenital sideroblastic anemia with autosomal recessive inheritance has also been described.[357] Neonatal anemia with macrocytosis has been described in some cases of cartilage-hair hypoplasia.[358]

Cases of congenital dyserythropoietic anemias (CDAs) resulting in severe fetal and/or neonatal anemia have been described.[204, 359] Association with Gilbert's syndrome increases neonatal hyperbilirubinemia in CDA type II.[360]

Impaired red cell production resulting in anemia during the neonatal period may also be observed as a result of congenital infections such as rubella, cytomegalovirus, adenovirus, and human parvovirus.[361–363] Congenital leukemia, Down syndrome, and osteoporosis may also produce anemia during the early days of life as a result of inadequate erythropoiesis.

A DIAGNOSTIC APPROACH TO THE ANEMIC NEWBORN

In view of the great number of entities that may be responsible for anemia in the newborn period, a disciplined approach to diagnosis is essential. A detailed family history and obstetric history should be obtained. The placenta should be examined whenever possible.

During the physical examination of the infant, particular attention should be devoted to detection of congenital anomalies, stigmata of intrauterine infection, internal hemorrhages, and the presence of hepatosplenomegaly.

Initial laboratory studies should include a complete blood count, red cell indices, reticulocyte count, direct Coombs' test, and examination of a well-prepared peripheral blood smear. Other useful simple procedures include a Heinz body preparation and the performance of a "wet prep" of the infant's erythrocytes.

One approach that relies on the reticulocyte count and cellular indices in arriving at a diagnosis is illustrated in Figure 2–11. This approach can be supplemented with specific diagnostic tests as indicated.

PHYSIOLOGIC ANEMIA OF PREMATURITY

The hemoglobin concentration of term infants normally decreases over the first weeks of life; this is known as the "physiologic anemia of infancy." Infants who are born prematurely but are otherwise healthy experience a more exaggerated decrease in hemoglobin concentration

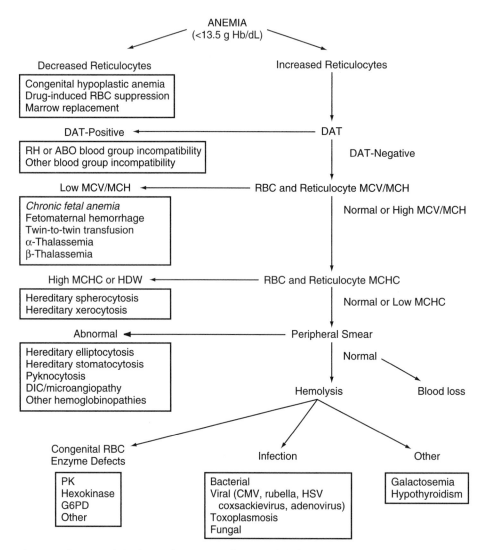

FIGURE 2–11. Diagnostic approach to anemia in the newborn. DAT = direct antiglobulin test; MCV/MCH = mean corpuscular volume/mean corpuscular hemoglobin; MCHC = mean corpuscular hemoglobin concentration; HDW = hemoglobin distribution width; DIC = disseminated intravascular coagulation; PK = pyruvate kinase; G6PD = glucose-6-phosphate dehydrogenase; CMV = cytomegalovirus; HSV = herpes simplex virus.

(see the next paragraph). This has been called the "physiologic anemia of prematurity."[364] The factors that influence the magnitude of this physiologic anemia include the nutritional status of the infant and a variety of complex adaptations to changes in oxygen availability.[365]

Cord hemoglobin values do not change significantly during the last trimester of pregnancy. After birth, the rapidity with which the hemoglobin level declines and the magnitude of the actual decrease vary directly with the degree of immaturity of the newborn. Although the nadir in hemoglobin concentration for normal full-term infants may be as low as 11.4 ± 0.9 g/dL by the age of 8 to 12 weeks, the average hemoglobin value observed by Schulman[364] in premature infants weighing less than 1500 g was 8.0 g/dL at the age of 4 to 8 weeks. These data are consistent with the normal data found by others.[366]

It is generally agreed that this fall in hemoglobin concentration results in greatest part from a decrease in the red cell mass rather than from a hemodilutional effect of an expanding plasma volume.[64] These changes occur at a time when the red cell survival of both term and premature infants is known to be shortened and when a striking decrease occurs in hematopoietic activity, as evidenced by a fall in reticulocyte count and a decrease in marrow erythroid elements.

Cord blood analysis generally demonstrates elevated levels of erythropoietin; these elevated levels are increased further in infants who experience transient hypoxemia at the time of delivery.[367, 368] One notable exception is seen in neonates with severe isoimmunization treated with intrauterine transfusion, who typically develop severe anemia postnatally. The anemia is due to a combination of continued immune-mediated hemolysis and suppressed erythropoiesis. Serum EPO in these neonates surged transiently at birth but did not reach "appropriate" levels until the hemoglobin level decreased to below 5 g/dL.[369] Otherwise, infants born anemic demonstrate a reticulocytosis. Increased erythropoiesis is generally seen in small-for-gestational-age infants who have suffered from intrauterine hypoxia.[370] The anemia of prematurity rarely occurs in association with cyanotic congenital heart disease or with respiratory insufficiency; this indicates that higher oxygen-carrying capacities can be maintained in infants in the first few weeks of life if the need arises. In premature infants, early neonatal anemia is an important predictor of mortality and neurologic sequelae.[371]

An important insight into the ability of hemoglobin levels to be adjusted adequately to a preterm infant's specific requirements may be noted if the hematologic statuses of infants who are born with widely varying hemoglobin concentrations are compared in the first few months of life. Differences in initial hemoglobin levels greatly affect the hemoglobin concentration in the weeks after birth. In infants with lower hemoglobin levels at birth minimum hemoglobin values are achieved more rapidly and the recovery phase occurs earlier compared with infants born with higher hemoglobin levels.[365] It is interesting, however, that the minimum hemoglobin levels achieved are similar in infants born with widely discrepant hemoglobin values; this suggests that the signal for return of active erythropoiesis is roughly equivalent among infants.

Until recently, it was not clear how systems of infants, particularly premature infants, could tolerate large declines in hemoglobin concentration while at the same time providing adequate supplies of oxygen to tissues. Adequate tissue oxygenation in the face of diminished oxygen-carrying capacity (lower hemoglobin concentration) can be accomplished only if oxygen demands are reduced or if one or more compensatory changes that are known to accompany anemia are observed. These responses include, in part, a higher cardiac output, an improved oxygen-unloading capacity, a redistribution of blood flow, and a greater oxygen extraction (a decrease in the oxygen tension in mixed central venous blood). Apparently, only some of these responses occur.

Cardiac output does not change significantly between the end of the first week of life and 3 months of age. Although the oxygen content of blood (milliliters of oxygen carried per 100 mL of blood) decreases to its lowest level in the first 2 to 3 months of life, this reflects nothing more than the overall decline in hemoglobin concentration. The oxygen-unloading capacity of blood—that is, the actual quantity of oxygen that is theoretically capable of being delivered to tissues—is constantly increasing from the moment of birth, even as the hemoglobin level falls.[372] This increase in oxygen unloading results from the gradual rightward shift in the oxyhemoglobin dissociation curve as the fetal hemoglobin levels decrease and the red cell 2,3-DPG level increases. The magnitude of this shift may have profound physiologic significance for both term and premature infants.

Recombinant Human Erythropoietin and the Anemia of Prematurity

In 1977, Stockman and associates[373] observed EPO concentrations within or below the normal adult range in infants with anemia of prematurity. Very low levels for the degree of anemia have subsequently been observed and reported by others.[374, 375] EPO levels in neonates of different birth weights vary over a wide range, but they seem to reach a nadir between days 7 and 50 independently of weight at birth; this is followed by the nadir in Hb concentration (between day 51 and 150).[376] These and other data indicate that the increase in EPO levels is insufficient for the degree of anemia when the neonates are compared with matched adults.[39, 377]

Investigation of *in vitro* erythroid colony growth has demonstrated normal numbers of both circulating BFU-Es[378] and bone marrow CFU-Es[379] in the anemia of prematurity. Both classes of erythroid progenitors show normal EPO dose-response curves. Taken together, the findings of low serum EPO concentrations, relative bone marrow erythroid hypoplasia, and a normal EPO dose-response curve suggest that inadequate EPO production is a major factor in the genesis of the anemia of prematurity.

The blunted EPO response to decreasing Hb levels[270] may be a consequence of the incomplete switch from liver to kidney as the major source of EPO production in premature infants and of the relative insensitivity to hypoxia of the liver-controlled EPO production.[374] An additional factor may be related to a different clearance and volume of distribution of EPO in neonates that results in lower EPO levels.[380, 381]The anemia of prematurity also is due to blood loss related to the shorter life span of neonatal erythrocytes and to the rapid growth observed in the first weeks of life, which is not accompanied by a parallel increase in red cell mass. Detailed reviews of the pathophysiology and therapy of the anemia of prematurity have been published.[228–230, 382, 383]

The use of recombinant human EPO (r-HuEPO) reduces the need for transfusions in premature infants weighing more than 1000 g, a group that rarely undergoes transfusions.[383] r-HuEPO may not be as effective in reducing transfusion requirements when it is used in infants weighing less than 1000 g or in neonates requiring artificial ventilation.[384–386] In a large, double-blind, placebo-controlled trial, r-HuEPO was shown to reduce the number of blood transfusions in preterm infants (weight at birth, 924 ±183 g).[387] Although the reduction in blood transfusions was statistically significant, the use of r-HuEPO resulted in only a small increase in the number of infants not undergoing transfusion (from 31 to 43 percent). This disappointing result could have been due to poor EPO responsiveness, the variability in the r-HuEPO dosages used, or inconsistency in providing supplemental iron for sustaining the enhanced erythropoiesis induced by r-HuEPO. A detailed cost analysis of the use of r-HuEPO in the anemia of prematurity has been published.[388] A meta-analysis study of 21 clinical trials with r-HuEPO in premature neonates showed an average reduction of 11 mL/kg in RBC transfusion in neonates weighing less than 1000 g.[389] However, the large variability in the published results does not allow the recommendation of r-HuEPO as a standard of care in these settings.[389] Early (first 2 weeks of life) use of r-HuEPO does not seem to reduce the number of transfusions in infants with birth weight less than 1250 g.[390] However, it lowers the number of transfusions in infants with birth weight less than 800 g and phlebotomy losses greater than 30 mL/kg.[390]

A potential advantage of the use of r-HuEPO in the anemia of prematurity is the associated right shift in the oxyhemoglobin dissociation curve, most likely due to the increased erythrocyte 2,3-DPG content.[391] The incidence of necrotizing enterocolitis is lower in very-low-birth-weight infants treated with r-HuEPO.[392], whereas neurodevelopmental outcomes are unaffected by r-HuEPO therapy.[393]

Studies in adult subjects have identified a functional iron deficiency in normal iron-replete subjects treated with r-HuEPO and oral iron.[394] Oral iron administration is insufficient for sustaining the increased marrow activity in the presence of r-HuEPO, and intravenous iron supplementation should always be considered for premature infants, possibly in association with vitamin E supplementation.

Studies in adult patients have indicated that autologous donation is not cost-effective when it is compared with allogeneic blood transfusion, mostly as a consequence of the high cost of collecting and discarding units that are not used.[395] However, reduction of allogeneic blood use by means of autologous blood donation (and the use of r-HuEPO) may be a prudent practice to follow, despite the associated additional cost.[396] Cost-benefit analysis does not indicate cost-effectiveness for the use of EPO in neonatal settings.[397] However, this conclusion is based on the high cost of the product (to reach a break-even point would require a 54 percent reduction in product cost) and on the way it is currently packaged: a 2000-U vial cannot be used more than once for the same patient, although it can be used for multiple patients on the same day. However, any vial-sharing practice should be carefully scrutinized, given the recent reports of *Serratia liquefaciens* sepsis resulting from multiple usage of single-use vials in adult dialysis centers.[398] Changes in r-HuEPO price and packaging could make r-HuEPO therapy more similar in cost to that of allogeneic blood transfusion. r-HuEPO is a remarkably safe drug. No significant side effects have been reported with its use, with the exception of the occurrence of seizures and blood pressure elevation when the circulating red cell mass is increased too rapidly. r-HuEPO has been shown to increase total bilirubin production in premature infants without inducing clinically significant jaundice.[399] Use of r-HuEPO in preterm infants does not affect the ratio of HbF to HbA.[400]

NEONATAL HYPERVISCOSITY

Neonates with hematocrits in excess of 65 percent are at some risk for *hyperviscosity syndrome*, which includes hypoglycemia, central nervous system injury,[401] and hypocalcemia with elevated plasma calcitonin gene–related peptide levels.[402] Infants with polycythemic hyperviscosity should undergo careful isovolumic partial plasma exchange transfusion, especially when abnormal results are obtained for cerebral blood flow velocity studies.[403] Although there is a good correlation between polycythemia and hyperviscosity, several infants with hyperviscosity syndrome have normal hematocrits and can be identified only with the use of viscosity measurements.[404] Several risk factors for neonatal polycythemia and hyperviscosity have been identified, such as maternal insulin-dependent diabetes,[405, 406] intrauterine growth retardation, perinatal asphyxia, twin-to-twin transfusion (recipient), delayed cord clamping, and Beckwith's syndrome.[407]

TRANSFUSIONS IN PREMATURE INFANTS

Red cell transfusion is discussed in Chapter 50; however, some of the problems unique to the neonatal setting are discussed in this section. For a more detailed discussion of issues relating to neonatal red cell transfusions, consult references 229, 230, and 408 through 410.

Decisions regarding the need for transfusion in low-birth-weight infants cannot be based on hemoglobin concentration or hematocrit alone. Wardrop and co-workers[411] demonstrated that "available oxygen" and not absolute hemoglobin level most closely correlates with the presence of symptoms and signs of hypoxemia such as tachycardia, tachypnea, easy fatigability, and poor feeding in low-birth-weight infants. Available oxygen is a reflection of the position of the oxyhemoglobin dissociation curve, the hemoglobin concentration, and the arterial oxygen saturation. Nomograms that illustrate the importance of these factors in making decisions regarding transfusion have been prepared.[412] These nomograms are based on assumptions regarding cardiac output and oxygen consumption that have been derived from serial measurements in low-birth-weight infants.[413] An example of the importance of the P_{50} and the arterial oxygen saturation in making decisions regarding the hemoglobin required for maintaining the central venous oxygen tension at 30 mm Hg is illustrated in Table 2–18.

As a general rule, hemoglobin values in otherwise healthy low-birth-weight infants should be maintained above 12 g/dL during the first 2 weeks of life. After that period, decisions regarding transfusion when available oxygen cannot be determined should be based on the infant's clinical condition. Factors to evaluate include the infant's weight gain, evidence of fatigue during feeding, tachycardia, tachypnea, and evidence of hypoxemia as reflected by an increase in blood lactic acid concentrations.[414] However, a study in premature infants has shown no relationship between Hct (values from 19 to 64 percent) and either heart or respiratory rates or occurrence of bradycardia.[415] Capillary whole blood lactate has been shown to have little value in transfusion decisions,[391, 416] although lactate plasma levels decrease after transfusion.[391]

Infants with cardiac or pulmonary disease that reduces arterial oxygen saturation may require hemoglobin concentrations of at least 16 to 17 g/dL for their oxygen requirements to be adequately met. No guidelines for neonatal transfusions have been clearly defined. It is common practice to transfuse neonates for the following reasons[417]:

1. Replacement of blood drawn for testing when the cumulative blood loss reaches 5 or 10 percent of the total blood volume.
2. Maintenance of hematocrit greater than 40 percent in patients with severe respiratory distress or symptomatic heart disease.
3. Maintenance of hematocrit greater than 30 percent in neonates with cardiopulmonary problems or growth failure.

It has been estimated that more than 300,000 red blood cell transfusions are given annually to 38,000 premature neonates in the United States.[417] Most infants who weigh more than 1000 g do not receive transfusions in this country.[418] There has been a significant reduction in the prevalence of transfusions owing to improved treatment and prevention of neonatal lung disease with surfactants, better ventilation, inhalation of NO, reduction in blood loss for analytical purposes, and less aggressive transfusion regimens. Neonatal transfusion practices in the United States have been studied in a national survey.[419, 420] The survey indicated that a large number of institutions in the United States still perform unnecessary major antiglobulin crossmatches for neonatal transfusions. This practice leads to a greater amount of blood being drawn and, thus, more transfusions. Standards issued by the American Association of Blood Banks (AABB) require testing for ABO group and Rh type, as well as red cell antibody screening before the first transfusion. If the red cell antibody screen is negative and group O red cells are used, no additional testing is required for subsequent red cell transfusions. If cells other than group O are transfused, the initial sample should also be tested for passively acquired anti-A or anti-B immunoglobulins.[421]

Infant do not usually produce red cell–specific antibodies. Production of antibodies against white cells has been described, but its clinical significance is unclear.[422, 423]

Traditionally, blood used for neonatal transfusion is less than 7 to 10 days old and is collected in anticoagulant citrate phosphate dextrose adenine (CPDA) rather than in additive solutions, even though there is no good scientific evidence to support this practice with small-volume (10 mL/kg) red cell transfusions.[419, 424, 425] When transfused in small volumes (15 mL/kg), up to 42-day-old red cells in additive solutions are equivalent to fresh red cells in CPDA.[426] Use of specifically assigned units less than 14 days old and of sterile connecting devices allows reduction of donor exposure and has no adverse effects.[427] The exposure to different donors can be drastically reduced by the multiple use of a single unit of blood for a patient over 35 to 42 days without affecting cost.[428–430]

Low-risk cytomegalovirus blood products (cytomegalovirus-negative or leukodepleted red cells) should be used only for neonates with birth weight less than 1200 g who are cytomegalovirus-negative or have unknown cytomegalovirus status.[431, 432] Universal leukodepletion is now applied to all red cells collected in the United States.[433]

Packed red cells should be adjusted to the desired hematocrit (60 to 79 percent) with normal saline or 5 percent albumin solution. However, a significant number of institutions still use fresh frozen plasma from the same donor or from a different donor for this purpose.[419] This practice is particularly widespread for exchange transfusions, in which red cells reconstituted in fresh frozen plasma from different donors are used—that is, each neonate is exposed to two different donors. In some settings, partial exchange transfusion may be preferable to simple transfusion.[434]

A significant factor in determining different blood uses in the neonatal setting is related to existing institutional practice. Comparison of blood utilization in two neonatal intensive care units (NICU) has revealed major differences in the percentage of patients receiving transfusions and the number of transfusions, which cannot be

TABLE 2–18. Hemoglobin Levels Required in Low-Birth-Weight Infants* to Maintain a Central Venous Oxygen Tension of 30 mm Hg

P_{50} (mm Hg)	Arterial Oxygen Saturation (%)			
	95	90	85	80
20	10.0	13.0	20.0	>25.0
23	7.3	9.0	11.0	15.5
25	6.2	7.3	8.8	11.0
27	5.3	6.3	7.3	8.9

*Assumes a cardiac output of 250 mL/kg per minute and an oxygen consumption of 6.5 mL/kg per minute.

accounted for by differences in disease severity.[435–437] Because no differences can be demonstrated in clinical outcome between NICUs with high-transfusion or low-transfusion rates, implementation of guidelines on blood drawing, use of arterial catheters, and transfusion should result in a reduction of transfusion rates and associated complications and costs.

REFERENCES

1. Wintrobe MM: Clinical Hematology, 5th ed. Philadelphia, Lea & Febiger, 1961, p 32.
2. Orkin SH: Diversification of haematopoietic stem cells to specific lineages. Nat Rev Genet 2000; 1:57–64.
3. Maximov AA: Relation of blood cells to connective tissue and endothelium. Physiol Rev 1924; 4:533.
4. Bloom W, Bartelmez GW: Hematopoiesis in young human embryos. Am J Anat 1940; 67:21.
5. Ehrlich P: De- und Regeneration roter Blutscheiben. Berhandl Gesellsch Charite Arzte 1880.
6. Migliaccio G, Migliaccio AR, et al: Human embryonic hemopoiesis. Kinetics of progenitors and precursors underlying the yolk sac→liver transformation. J Clin Invest 1986; 78:51.
7. Thomas DB, Yoffey JM: Human foetal haematopoiesis. II. Hepatic haematopoiesis in the human foetus. Br. J Haematol 1964; 10:193.
8. Tavian M, Coulombel L, et al: Aorta-associated CD34+ hematopoietic cells in the early human embryo. Blood 1996; 87:67.
9. Tavian M, Hallais MF, Peault B: Emergence of intraembryonic hematopoietic precursors in the pre-liver human embryo. Development 1999; 126:793.
10. Medvinsky AL, Dzierzak E: Definitive hematopoiesis is autonomously initiated by the AGM region. Cell 1996; 86:897.
11. Cumano A, Dieterlen-Lievre F, Godin I: Lymphoid potential, probed before circulation in mouse, is restricted to caudal intraembryonic splanchnopleura. Cell 1996; 86:907.
12. Fukuda A: Fetal hemopoiesis. II. Electron microscopic studies on human hepatic hemopoiesis. Virchows Arch B Zell Pathol 1974; 16:249.
13. Kimura N, Yamano Y, et al: Erythroid progenitors in human fetal liver. Nippon Ketsueki Gakkai Zasshi 1984; 47:1235.
14. Campagnoli C, Fisk NM, Overton T, et al: Circulating hematopoietic progenitor cells in first trimester fetal blood. Blood 2000; 95:1967–1972.
15. Linch DC, Knott LJ, et al: Studies of circulating hemopoietic progenitor cells in human fetal blood. Blood 1982; 59:976.
16. Zauli G, Vitale M, et al: In vitro growth of human fetal CD34+ cells in the presence of various combinations of recombinant cytokines under serum-free conditions. Br. J Haematol 1994; 86:461.
17. Lansdorp PM: Developmental changes in the function of hematopoietic stem cells. Exp Hematol 1995; 23:187.
18. Kelemen E, Calvo W, et al: Atlas of Human Hemopoietic Development. Berlin, Springer-Verlag, 1979.
19. Broxmeyer HE, Douglas GW, et al: Human umbilical cord blood as a potential source of transplantable hematopoietic stem/progenitor cells. Proc Natl Acad Sci USA 1989; 86:3828.
20. Liang DC, Ma SW, et al: Granulocyte/macrophage colony-forming units from cord blood of premature and full-term neonates: Its role in ontogeny of human hematopoiesis. Pediatr Res 1988; 24:701.
21. Forestier F, Daffos F, et al: Developmental hematopoiesis in normal human fetal blood. Blood 1991; 77:2360.
22. Murray NA, Roberts IAG: Circulating megakaryocytes and their progenitors (BFU-MK and CFU-MK) in term and pre-term neonates. Br. J Haematol 1995; 89:41.
23. Shields LE, Andrews RG: Gestational age changes in circulating CD34+ hematopoietic stem/progenitor cells in fetal cord blood. Am J Obstet Gynecol 1998; 178:931.
24. Valtieri M, Gabbianelli M, et al: Erythropoietin alone induces erythroid burst formation by human embryonic but not adult BFU-E in unicellular-serum-free culture. Blood 1989; 74:460.
25. Emerson S, Thomas S, et al: Developmental regulation of erythropoiesis by hematopoietic growth factors: Analysis of populations of BFU-E from bone marrow, peripheral blood, and fetal liver. Blood 1989; 74:49.
26. Gardner D, Liechty KW, Christensen RD: Effects of interleukin-6 on fetal hematopoietic progenitors. Blood 1990; 75:2150.
27. Holbrook ST, Ohls RK, et al: Effect of interleukin-9 on clonogenic maturation and cell-cycle status of fetal and adult hematopoietic progenitors. Blood 1991; 77:2129.
28. Schibler KR, Yang YC, Christensen RD: Effect of interleukin-11 on cycling status and clonogenic maturation of fetal and adult hematopoietic progenitors. Blood 1992; 80:900.
29. Schibler KR, Li Y, et al: Possible mechanisms accounting for the growth factor independence of hematopoietic progenitors from umbilical cord blood. Blood 1994; 84:3679.
30. Traycoff CM, Abboud MR, et al: Rapid exit from G0/G1 phases of cell cycle in response to stem cell factor confers on umbilical cord blood CD34+ cells an enhanced *ex vivo* expansion potential. Exp Hematol 1994; 22:1264.
31. Pettengell R, Luft T, et al: Direct comparison by limiting dilution analysis of long-term culture-initiating cells in human bone marrow, umbilical cord blood, and blood stem cells. Blood 1994; 84:3653.
32. Gluckman E, Broxmeyer HE, et al: Hematopoietic reconstitution in a patient with Fanconi's anemia by means of umbilical-cord blood from an HLA-identical sibling. N Engl J Med 1989; 321:1174.
33. Gale RP: Cord-blood-cell transplantation: A real sleeper. N Engl J Med 1995; 332:392.
34. Wagner JE, Kerman NA, et al: Transplantation of umbilical cord blood in 50 patients: Analysis of the registry data. Blood 1994; 84:395a.
35. Issaragrisil S, Visuthisakchai S, et al: Brief report: Transplantation of cord-blood stem cells into a patient with severe thalassemia. N Engl J Med 1995; 332:367.
36. Sirchia G, Rebulla P: Placental/umbilical cord blood transplantation. Haematologica 1999; 84:738–747.
37. Gluckman E, Locatelli F: Umbilical cord blood transplants. Curr Opin Hematol 2000; 7:353–357.
38. Hows JM: Status of umbilical cord blood transplantation in the year 2001. J Clin Pathol 2001; 54:428–434.
39. Halvorsen S: Plasma erythropoietin in cord blood during the first few hours of life. Acta Pediatr Scand 1963; 52:425.
40. Matoth Y, Zaizov R: Regulation of erythropoiesis in the fetal rat. In The Tel Aviv University Conference on Erythropoiesis, Petak Tikva, Israel. New York, Academic Press, 1970.
41. Jacobsen LO, Marks EK, et al: The effect of transfusion-induced polycythemia in the mother of the fetus. Blood 1959; 14:644.
42. Zanjani ED, Gidari AS, et al: Humoral regulation of erythropoiesis in the foetus. In Comline KS, Cross KW, et al: Foetal and Neonatal Physiology. London, Cambridge University Press, 1973, p 448.
43. Orkin SH: Transcription factors and hematopoietic development. J Biol Chem 1995; 270:4955.
44. Gregory T, Yu C, Ma A, et al: GATA-1 and erythropoietin cooperate to promote erythroid cell survival by regulating bcl-xL expression. Blood 1999; 94:87–96.
45. Simon MC, Pevny L, et al: Rescue of erythroid development in gene-targeted GATA-1-mouse embryonic stem cells. Nat Genet 1992; 1:92.
46. Perkins A, Sharpe AH, Orkin SH: Lethal beta-thalassemia in mice lacking the erythroid CACCC-transcription factor EKLF. Nature 1995; 375.
47. Nichols KE, Crispino JD, Poncz M, et al: Familial dyserythropoietic anaemia and thrombocytopenia due to an inherited mutation in GATA1. Nat Genet 2000; 24:266–270.
48. Ward AC, Touw I, Yoshimura A: The Jak-Stat pathway in normal and perturbed hematopoiesis. Blood 2000; 95:19–29.
49. Bromberg J, Darnell JEJ: The role of STATs in transcriptional control and their impact on cellular function. Oncogene 2000; 19:2468–2473.
50. Bromberg J, Darnell JEJ: The role of STATs in transcriptional control and their impact on cellular function. Oncogene 2000; 19:2468–2473.
51. Socolovsky M, Fallon AEJ, Wang S, et al: Fetal anemia and apoptosis of red cell progenitors in Stat5a$^{-/-}$5b$^{-/-}$ mice: A direct role for Stat5 in bcl-X$_L$ induction. Cell 1999; 98:181–191.
52. Socolovsky M, Nam H, Fleming MD, et al: Ineffective erythropoiesis in Stat5a$^{-/-}$5b$^{-/-}$ mice due to decreased survival of early erythroblasts. Blood 2001; 98:3261–3273.
53. Wagner KU, Claudio E, Rucker EB, et al: Conditional deletion of the BCl-x gene from erythroid cells results in hemolytic anemia and profound splenomegaly. Development 2000; 127:4949–4958.

54. Stamatoyannopoulos G, Rossenblum BB, et al: Hb F and Hb A production in erythroid cultures from human fetuses and neonates. Blood 1979; 54:440.

55. Orkin SH: Regulation of globin gene expression in erythroid cells. Eur J Biochem 1995; 231:271.

56. Lewis BA, Kim TK, Orkin SH: A downstream element in the human beta-globin promoter: Evidence of extended sequence-specific transcription factor IID contacts. Proc Natl Acad Sci USA 2000; 97:7172–7177.

57. Szelengi JG, Hollan SR: Studies on the structure of human embryonic haemoglobin. Acta Biochim Biophys Acad. Sci Hung 1969; 4:47.

58. Hecht F, Motulsky AG, et al: Predominance of hemoglobin Gower 1 in early human embryonic development. Science 1966; 152:91.

59. Kamuzora H, Lehmann H: Human embryonic haemoglobins including a comparison by homology of the human and ζ and a chains. Nature 1975; 256:511.

60. Ley T, Maloney K, et al: Globin gene expression in erythroid human fetal liver cells. J Clin Invest 1989; 83:1032.

61. He Z, Russell JE: Expression, purification, and characterization of human hemoglobins Gower-1 ($\zeta_2\epsilon_2$), Gower-2 ($\alpha_2\epsilon_2$), and Portland-2 ($\zeta_2\beta_2$) assembled in complex transgenic-knockout mice. Blood 2001; 97:1099–1105.

62. Seip M: The reticulocyte level and the erythrocyte production judged from reticulocyte studies in newborn infants during the first week of life. Acta Paediatr (Stockh) 1955; 44:355.

63. Garby L, Sjoli S, et al: Studies on erythrokinetics in infancy. III. Plasma disappearance and red cell uptake of intravenously injected radioiron. Acta Paediatr (Stockh) 1963; 52:537.

64. Bratteby LE: Studies on erythrokinetics in infancy. XI. The change in circulating red cell volume during the first five months of life. Acta Paediatr Scand 1968; 54:215.

65. Gairdner D, Marks J, et al: Blood formation in infancy. Normal erythropoiesis. Arch Dis Child 1952; 27:214.

66. Sturgeon P: Volumetric and microscopic pattern of bone marrow in normal infants and children. I. Volumetric pattern. Pediatrics 1951; 7:577.

67. Sturgeon P: Volumetric and microscopic pattern of bone marrow in normal infants and children. II. Cytologic pattern. Pediatrics 1951; 7:642.

68. Issaragrisil S: Correlation between hematopoietic progenitors and erythroblasts in cord blood. Am J Clin Pathol 1983; 80:865.

69. Man DL, Sites MD, et al: Erythropoietic stimulating activity during the first 90 days of life. Proc Soc Exp Biol Med 1965; 118:212.

70. Wranne L: Studies on erythrokinetics in infancy. Acta Paediatr Scand 1967; 56:381.

71. Perrine SP, Greene MF, Faller DV: Delay in the fetal globin switch in infants of diabetic mothers. N Engl J Med 1985; 327:569.

72. Little JA, Dempsey NJ, et al: Metabolic persistence of fetal hemoglobin. Blood 1995; 85:1712.

73. Bard H, Prosmanne J: Elevated levels of fetal hemoglobin synthesis in infants with chronic bronchopulmonary dysplasia. Pediatrics 1990; 86:193.

74. Bard H, Lachance C, et al: The reactivation of fetal hemoglobin synthesis during anemia of prematurity. Pediatr Res 1994; 36:253.

75. Pearson HA: Life span of the fetal red blood cell. J Pediatr 1967; 70:166.

76. Bratteby E, Garby L: Development of erythropoiesis: Infant erythrokinetics. In Nathan DG, Oski RA (eds): Hematology of Infancy and Child, 1st ed. Philadelphia, WB Saunders, 1974, p 56.

77. Landaw SA, Guancial RL: Shortened survival of fetal erythrocytes in the rat. Pediatr Res 1977; 11:1155.

78. Landaw SA: Decreased survival and altered membrane properties of red blood cells (RBC) in the newborn rat. Pediatr Res 1978; 12:395.

79. Meyburg J, Bohler T, Linderkamp O: Decreased mechanical stability of neonatal red cell membrane quantified by measurement of the elastic area compressibility modulus. Clin Hemorheol Microcirc 2000; 22:67–73.

80. Serrani RE, Alonso D, Corchs JL: States of stability/lysis in human fetal and adult red blood cells. Arch Int Physiol Biochim 1989; 97:309.

81. Sjölin S: The resistance of red cells in vitro. A study of the osmotic properties, the mechanical resistance and the behavior of red cells of fetuses, children and adults. Acta Paediatr 1954; 43:1.

82. Goldbloom RB, Fischer E, et al: Studies on the mechanical fragility of erythrocytes. I. Normal values for infants and children. Blood 1953; 8:165.

83. Colombel L, Tchernia G, Mohandas N: Human reticulocyte maturation and its relevance to erythropoietic stress. J Lab Clin Med 1979; 94:467.

84. Thatte HS, Schrier SL: Comparison of transferrin receptor B mediated endocytosis and drug-induced endocytosis in human neonatal and adult RBCs. Blood 1988; 72:1693.

85. Colin FC, Schrier SL: Myosin content and distribution in human neonatal erythrocytes are different from adult erythrocytes. Blood 1991; 78:3052.

86. Diagne I, Archambeaud MP, Diallo D, et al: Parametres erythocytaires et reserves en fer dans le sang du cordon. Arch Pediatr 1995; 2:208–214.

87. Zipursky A, Brown E, et al: The erythrocyte differential count in newborn infants. Am J Pediatr Hematol Oncol 1983; 5:45.

88. Maxwell DJ, Seshadri R, et al: Infantile pyknocytosis: A cause of intrauterine haemolysis in 2 siblings. Aust NZ J Obstet Gynaecol 1983; 23:182.

89. Holroyde CP, Oski FA, et al: The "pocked" erythrocyte. N Engl J Med 1969; 281:516.

90. Nathan DG, Gunn RB: Thalassemia: The consequences of unbalanced hemoglobin synthesis. Am J Med 1966; 41:815.

91. Pearson HA, Macintosh S, et al: Interference phase microscopic enumeration of pitted RBC and splenic function in sickle cell anemia. Pediatr Res 1978; 12:471.

92. Sills RH, Tamburlin JH, et al: Formation of intracellular vesicles in neonatal and adult erythrocytes: Evidence against the concept of neonatal hyposplenism. Pediatr Res 1988; 24:703.

93. Matovcik LM, Junga IG, Schrier SL: Drug-induced endocytosis of neonatal erythrocytes. Blood 1985; 65:1056.

94. Dervichian D, Fournet C, et al: Structure submicroscopique des globules rouges contenant des hémoglobines abnormales. Rev Hematol 1952; 7:567.

95. Haberman S, Blanton P, et al: Some observations on ABO antigen sites of the erythrocyte membranes of adults and newborn infants. J Immunol 1967; 98:150.

96. Kurantsin-Mills J, Lessin LS: Freeze-etching and biochemical analysis of human fetal erythrocyte membranes. Pediatr Res 1984; 18:1035.

97. Schekman R, Singer SJ: Clustering and endocytosis of membrane receptors can be induced in mature erythrocytes of neonatal but not adult humans. Proc Natl Acad Sci USA 1976; 73:4075.

98. Kehry M, Yguerabid J, et al: Fluidity in the membranes of adult and neonatal human erythrocytes. Science 1977; 195:486.

99. Polychronakos C, Ruggere MD, et al: The role of cell age in the difference in insulin binding between adult and cord erythrocytes. J Clin Endocrinol Metab 1982; 55:290.

100. Funakoshi T, Morikawa H, et al: Insulin-like growth factor (IGF) receptor in human fetal erythrocytes and fetal rat liver. Nippon Naibunpi Gakkai Zasshi 1989; 65:728.

101. Belussi G, Muccioli G, et al: Prolactin binding sites in human erythrocytes and lymphocytes. Life Sci 1987; 41:951.

102. Kearin M, Kelly JG: Digoxin "receptors" in neonates: An explanation of less sensitivity to digoxin than in adults. Clin Pharmacol Ther 1980; 28:346.

103. Koekebakker M, Barr RD: Acetylcholinesterase in the human erythron. I. Cytochemistry. Am J Hematol 1988; 28:252.

104. Miyazono Y, Hirono A, Miyamoto Y, et al: Erythrocyte enzyme activities in cord blood of extremely low-birth-weight infants. Am J Hematol 1999; 62:88–92.

105. Neerhout RC: Erythrocyte lipids in the neonate. Pediatr Res 1968; 2:172.

106. Younkin S, Oski FA, et al: Observations on the mechanism of the hydrogen peroxide hemolysis test and its reversal with phenols. Am J Clin Nutr 1971; 24:7.

107. Vengelen-Tyler V: Technical Manual, 13 ed. Bethesda, MD, American Association of Blood Banks, 1999.

108. Hollan SR, Szeleny JG, et al: Structural and functional differences between human foetal and adult erythrocytes. Haematology 1967; 4:409.

109. Serrani RE, Venera G, et al: Potassium influx in human neonatal red blood cells: Partition into its major components. Arch Int Physiol Biochim 1990; 98:27.

110. Moore TJ, Hall N: Kinetics of glucose transfer in adult and fetal human erythrocytes. Pediatr Res 1971; 5:536.

111. Schettini F, Bratta A, et al: Acid lysis of red blood cells in normal children. Acta Paediatr Scand 1971; 60:17.

112. Matsuo Y, Inoue F, et al: Changes of erythrocyte ouabain maximum binding after birth in neonates in relation to erythrocyte sodium and potassium concentrations. Early Hum Dev 1995; 43:59.

113. Brahm J, Wimberley PD: Chloride and bicarbonate transport in fetal red cells. J Physiol 1989; 419:141.

114. Linderkamp O, Hammer BJ, Miller R: Filterability of erythrocytes and whole blood in preterm and full-term neonates and adults. Pediatr Res 1986; 20:1269.

115. Colin FC, Gallois Y, et al: Impaired fetal erythrocyte's filterability: Relationship with cell size, membrane fluidity, and membrane lipid composition. Blood 1992; 79:2148.

116. Buonocore G, Berni S, et al: Characteristics and functional properties of red cells during the first days of life. Biol Neonate 1991; 60:137.

117. Gross RT, Schroeder EA, et al: Energy metabolism in the erythrocytes of premature infants compared to full-term newborn infants and adults. Blood 1963; 21:755.

118. Konrad PN, Valentine WN, et al: Enzymatic activities and glutathione content of erythrocytes in the newborn: Comparison with red cells of older normal subjects and those with comparable reticulocytosis. Acta Haematol 1972; 48:193.

119. Oski FA: Red cell metabolism in the newborn infant. V. Glycolytic intermediates and glycolytic enzymes. Pediatrics 1969; 44:84.

120. Witt I, Herdan M, et al: Vergleichende Untersuchungen von enzymaktivitäten in Reticulocyten-reichen und Reticulocyten-armen Fraktionen aus Neugeborenen- und Erwachsenenblut. Klin Wochenschr 1968; 46:149.

121. Lestas AN, Rodeck CH, White JM: Normal activities of glycolytic enzymes in the fetal erythrocytes. Br J Haematol 1982; 50:439–444.

122. Mohrenweiser HW, Fielek S, Wurzinger KH: Characteristics of enzymes of erythrocytes from newborn infant and adults: Activity, thermostability, and electrophoretic profile as a function of cell age. Am J Hematol 1981; 11:125–136.

123. Travis SF, Garvin JH: In vivo lability of red cell phosphofructokinase in term infants: The possible molecular basis of the relative phosphofructokinase deficiency in neonatal red cells. Pediatr Res 1977; 11:1159–1161.

124. Vora S, Piomelli S: A fetal isozyme of phosphofructokinase in newborn erythrocytes. Pediatr Res 1977; 11:483.

125. Holmes EW, Malone JI, Winegrad AI, et al: Hexokinase isoenzymes in human erythrocytes. Association of type II with fetal hemoglobin. Science 1967; 156:646–648.

126. Schröter W, Tillman W: Hexokinase isoenzymes in human erythrocytes of adults and newborns. Biochem Biophys Res Commun 1968; 31:92.

127. Chen SH, Anderson JE, et al: Lysozyme patterns in erythrocytes from human fetuses. Am J Hematol 1977; 2:23.

128. Witt I, Witz D: Reinigung und Charakterisierung von Phosphopyruvatz-Hydratase (= Enolase; EC 4.2.1.11) aus Neugeborenen- und Erwachsenen-Erythrozyten. Hoppe Seylers Z Physiol Chem 1970; 351:1232.

129. Oski FA, Smith CA: Effect of pH on glycolysis in the erythrocytes of the newborn infant. Proc Soc Pediatr Res 1972:106.

130. Witt I, Müller H, Künzer W: Vergleichende biochemische Untersuchunger an Erythrocyten aus Neugeborenen- und Erwachsenen-blut. Klin Wochenschr 1967; 45:262.

131. Bentley HP, Alford CA, Diseker M: Erythrocyte glucose consumption in the neonate. J Lab Clin Med 1970; 76:311–321.

132. Oski FA: Red cell metabolism in the premature infant. II. The pentose phosphate pathway. Pediatrics 1967; 39:689.

133. Zipursky A, LaRue T, et al: The in vitro metabolism of erythrocytes from newborn infants. Can J Biochem Physiol 1960; 38:727.

134. Schröter W, Winter P: Der 2,3-Diphosphoglyceratstoffwechsel in den Erythrocyten Neugeborener und Erwachsener. Klin Wochenschr 1967; 45:255.

135. Trueworthy R, Lowman JT: Intracellular control of 2,3-diphosphoglycerate concentration in fetal red cells. Proc Soc Pediatr Res 1971:86.

136. Lestas AN, Bellingham AJ, Nicolaides KH: Red cell glycolytic intermediates in normal, anemic and transfused human fetuses. Br J Haematol 1989; 73:387.

137. Jain SK: The neonatal erythrocyte and its oxidative susceptibility. Semin Hematol 1989; 26:286.

138. Shahal Y, Bauminger ER, et al: Oxidative stress in newborn erythrocytes. Pediatr Res 1991; 29:119.

139. Abbasi S, Ludomirski A, et al: Maternal and fetal plasma vitamin E to total lipid ratio and fetal RBC antioxidant function during gestational development. J Am Coll Nutr 1990; 9:314.

140. Glader BE, Conrad MD: Decreased glutathione peroxidase in neonatal erythrocytes: Lack of relation to hydrogen peroxide metabolism. Pediatr Res 1972; 6:900.

141. Lestas AN, Rodeck CH: Normal glutathione content and some related enzyme activities in the fetal erythrocytes. Br J Haematol 1984; 57:695.

142. Gros RT, Bracci R, et al: Hydrogen peroxide toxicity and detoxification in the erythrocytes of newborn infants. Blood 1967; 29:481.

143. Whaun JM, Oski FA: Relation of red blood cell glutathione peroxidase to neonatal jaundice. J Pediatr 1970; 76:555.

144. Schröter W: Drug susceptibility and the development of erythrocyte enzyme systems. In Leiden, Stenfert, Krose (eds): Nutricia Symposium: Metabolic Processes in the Fetus and Newborn Infant. 1971, p 73.

145. Papp A, Nemeth I, Karg E, et al: Glutathione status in retinopathy of prematurity. Free Radic Biol Med 1999; 27:738–743.

146. Aliakbar S, Brown PR, et al: Human erythrocyte superoxide dismutase in adults, neonates, and normal, hypoxaemic, anaemic and chromosomally abnormal fetuses. Clin Biochem 1993; 26:109.

147. Agostoni A, Gerli GC, et al: Superoxide dismutase, catalase, and glutathione peroxidase activities in maternal and cord blood erythrocytes. J Clin Chem Clin Biochem 1980; 18:771.

148. Bracci R, Martini G, et al: Changes in erythrocyte properties during the first hours of life: Electron spin resonance of reacting sulfhydryl groups. Pediatr Res 1988; 24:391.

149. Haga P, Lunde G: Selenium and vitamin E in cord blood from preterm and full-term infants. Acta Paediatr Scand 1978; 67:735.

150. Travis SF, Kumar SP, Paez PC, et al: Red cell metabolic alterations in postnatal life in term infants: Glycolytic enzymes and glucose-6-phosphate dehydrogenase. Pediatr Res 1980; 14:1349–1352.

151. Jansen G, Koenderman L, Rijksen G, et al: Characteristics of hexokinase, pyruvate kinase, and glucose-6-phosphate dehydrogenase during adult and neonatal reticulocyte maturation. Am J Hematol 1985; 20:203–215.

152. Vetrella M, Barthelmai W: Enzyme activities in the erythrocytes of human fetuses. I. Glucose-6-phosphate dehydrogenase, 6-phosphogluconic dehydrogenase and glutathione reductase. Z Kinderheilkd 1971; 110:99–103.

153. Schröter W, Bodemann H: Experimentally induced cation leaks of the red cell membrane. Biol Neonate 1970; 15:291.

154. Tillman W, Menke J, et al: The formation of Heinz bodies in ghosts of human erythrocytes of adults and newborn infants. Klin Wochenschr 1973; 51:201.

155. Kleihauer E, Bernau A: Heinzkörperbildung in Neugeboren-erythrozyten. 1. In-vitro-Studien über experimentelle Bedingungen und den Einfluss von Austauschtransfusionen. Acta Haematol 1970; 43:333.

156. Schröter W, Tillman W: Heinz body susceptibility of red cells and exchange transfusion. Acta Haematol 1973; 49:74.

157. Bracci R, Benedetti PA, et al: Hydrogen peroxide generation in the erythrocytes of newborn infants. Biol Neonate 1970; 15:135.

158. Lipschutz F, Lubin B, et al: Red cell oxygen consumption and hydrogen peroxide formation. Proc Soc Pediatr Res 1972:1051.

159. Oettinger L Jr, Mills WB: Simultaneous capillary and venous hemoglobin determinations in newborn infants. J Pediatr 1949; 35:362.

160. Moe PJ: Umbilical cord blood and capillary blood in the evaluation of anemia in erythroblastosis fetalis. Acta Paediatr Scand 1967; 56:391.

161. Linderkamp O, Versmold HT: Capillary-venous hematocrit differences in newborn infants. I. Relationship to blood volume, peripheral blood flow, and acid-base parameters. Eur J Pediatr 1977; 127:9.

162. Larsson BA, Tannfeldt G, Lagercrantz H, et al: Venipuncture is more effective and less painful than heel lancing for blood tests in neonates. Pediatrics 1998; 101:882–886.

163. Vertanen H, Fellman V, Brommels M, et al: An automatic incision device for obtaining blood samples from the heels of preterm

infants causes less damage than a conventional manual lancet. Arch Dis Child Fetal Neonatal Ed 2001; 84:F53–F55.

164. Lindh V, Wiklund U, Hakansson S: Heel lancing in term new-born infants: An evaluation of pain by frequency domain analysis of heart rate variability. Pain 1999; 80:143–148.

165. Eriksson M, Gradin M, Schollin J: Oral glucose and venepuncture reduce blood sampling pain in newborns. Early Hum Dev 1999; 55(3):211–218.

166. Abril Martin JC, Aguilar Rodriguez L, Albinana Cilveti J: Flatfoot and calcaneal deformity secondary to osteomyelitis after neonatal heel puncture. J Pediatr Orthop B 1999; 8:122–124.

167. Jain A, Rutter N: Does topical amethocaine gel reduce the pain of venepuncture in newborn infants? A randomised double blind controlled trial. Arch Dis Child Fetal Neonatal Ed 2000; 83:F207–F210.

168. Lindh V, Wiklund U, Hakansson S: Assessment of the effect of EMLA during venipuncture in the newborn by analysis of heart rate variability. Pain 2000; 86:247–254.

169. Brisman M, Ljung BM, Otterbom I, et al: Methaemoglobin formation after the use of EMLA cream in term neonates. Acta Paediatr 1998; 87:1191–1194.

170. Usher R, Shepard M, et al: The blood volume of the newborn infant and placental transfusion. Acta Paediatr Scand 1963; 52:497.

171. Yao AC, Lind J, et al: Placental transfusion in the premature infant with observation on clinical course and outcome. Acta Paediatr Scand 1969; 58:561.

172. Gunther M: The transfer of blood between baby and placenta in the minutes after birth. Lancet 1957; 1:1277.

173. Ogata ES, Kitterman JA, et al: The effect of time of cord clamping and maternal blood pressure on placental transfusion with cesarean section. Am J Obstet Gynecol 1977; 128:197.

174. Linderkamp O, Nelle M, et al: The effect of early and late cord clamping on blood viscosity and other hemorheological parameters in full-term neonates. Acta Paediatr 1992; 81:745.

175. Nelle M, Zilow EP: The effect of Leboyer delivery on blood viscosity and other hemorheological parameters in term neonates. Am J Obstet Gynecol 1993; 169:189.

176. Kinmond S, Aitchison TC, et al: Umbilical cord clamping and preterm infants: A randomized trial. Br Med J 1993; 306:172.

177. Usher RH, Saigal S, et al: Estimation of red blood cell volume in premature infants with and without respiratory distress syndrome. Biol Neonate 1975; 26:241.

178. Hofmeyr GJ, Gobetz L, et al: Periventricular/intraventricular hemorrhage following early and delayed umbilical cord clamping: A randomized controlled trial. Online J Curr. Clin Trials 1993; Dec 29:Doc. No. 110.

179. Rabe H, Wacker A, Hulskamp G, et al: A randomised controlled trial of delayed cord clamping in very low birth weight preterm infants. Eur J Pediatr 2000; 159:775–777.

180. Ibrahim HM, Krouskop RW, Lewis DF, et al: Placental transfusion: Umbilical cord clamping and preterm infants. J Perinatol 2000; 20:351–354.

181. Saigal S, Usher RH: Symptomatic neonatal plethora. Biol Neonate 1977; 32:62.

182. Saigal S, Wilson R, Usher R: Radiological findings in symptomatic neonatal plethora resulting from placental transfusion. Radiology 1977; 125:185.

183. Yao AC, Lind J: Effect of early and late cord clamping on the systolic time intervals of the newborn infant. Acta Paediatr Scand 1977; 66:489.

184. Erkkola R, Kero P, et al: Delayed cord clamping in cesarean section with general anesthesia. Am J Perinatol 1984; 1:165.

185. Mollison PL, Veall N, et al: Red cell and plasma volume in newborn infants. Arch Dis Child 1950; 25:242.

186. Jegier W, MacLaurin J, et al: Comparative study of blood volume estimation in the newborn infant using I 131-labeled human serum albumin (IHSA) and T-1824. Scand J Clin Lab Invest 1964; 16:125.

187. Usher R, Lind J: Blood volume of the newborn premature infant. Acta Paediatr Scand 1965; 54:419.

188. Sisson TRC, Lund CJ, et al: The blood volume of infants. I. The full-term infant in the first year of life. J Pediatr 1959; 55:163.

189. Cassady G: Plasma volume studies in low birth weight infants. Pediatrics 1966; 38:1020.

190. Russell SJM: Blood volume studies in healthy children. Arch Dis Child 1949; 24:88.

191. Brines JK, Gibson JG Jr, et al: Blood volume in normal infants and children. J Pediatr 1941; 18:447.

192. Brown E, Krouskop RW, et al: Blood volume and blood pressure in infants with respiratory distress. J Pediatr 1975; 87:1133.

193. Faxelius G, Raye J, et al: Red cell volume measurements and acute blood loss in high risk newborn infants. J Pediatr 1977; 90:273.

194. Shepherd AJ, Richardson CJ, et al: Nuchal cord as a cause of neonatal anemia. Am J Dis Child 1985; 139:71.

195. Forestier F, Daffos F, et al: Hematological values of 163 normal fetuses between 18 and 30 weeks of gestation. Pediatr Res 1986; 20:342.

196. Dialio DH, Sidibe S, et al: Prévalence de l'anémie du nouveau-né au Mali. Cah Sante 1994; 4:341.

197. Harthoorn-Lasthuizen EJ, Lindemans J, Langenhuijsen MMAC: Does iron-deficient erythropoiesis in pregnancy influence fetal iron supply? Acta Obstetr Gynecol Scand 2001; 80:392–396.

198. Abdel-Fattah SA, Carroll SG, Kyle PM, et al: The effect of fetal hydrops on the rate of fall of hemoglobin after fetal intravascular transfusion for red cell alloimmunization. Fetal Diagn Ther 2000; 15:262–266.

199. Boyd PA, Keeling JW: Fetal hydrops. J Med Genet 1992; 29:91.

200. Horn LC, Faber R, Meiner A, et al: Greenberg dysplasia: First reported case with additional non-skeletal malformations and without consanguinity. Prenat Diagn 2000; 20:1008–1011.

201. Saltzman DH, Frigoletto FD, et al: Sonographic evaluation of hydrops fetalis. Obstet Gynecol 1989; 74:106.

202. Ferreira P, Morais L, Costa R, et al: Hydrops fetalis associated with erythrocyte pyruvate kinase deficiency. Eur J Pediatr 2000; 159:481–482.

203. Oie BK, Hertel J, et al: Hydrops foetalis in 3 infants of a mother with acquired chronic pure red cell aplasia: Transitory red cell aplasia in 1 of the infants. Scand J Haematol 1984; 33:466.

204. Parez N, Dommergues M, Zupan V, et al: Severe congenital dyserythropoietic anaemia type I: Prenatal management, transfusion support and alpha-interferon therapy. Br J Haematol 2000; 110:420–423.

205. Rejjal AL, Nazer H: Resolution of cystic hygroma, hydrops fetalis, and fetal anemia. Am J Perinatol 1993; 10:455.

206. Hirata GI, Masaki DI, et al: Color flow mapping and Doppler velocimetry in the diagnosis and management of a placental chorioangioma associated with non-immune fetal hydrops. Obstet Gynecol 1993; 81:850.

207. Panero C, Azzi A, et al: Fetoneonatal hydrops from human parvovirus B19. Case report. J Perinat Med 1994; 22:257.

208. Yaegashi N, Niinuma T, Chisaka H, et al: The incidence of, and factors leading to, parvovirus B19-related hydrops fetalis following maternal infection; report of 10 cases and meta-analysis. J Infect 1998; 37:28–35.

209. Essary LR, Vnencak-Jones CL, Manning SS, et al: Frequency of parvovirus B19 infection in nonimmune hydrops fetalis and utility of three diagnostic methods. Hum Pathol 1998; 29:696–701.

210. Rodis JF, Borgida AF, Wilson M, et al: Management of parvovirus infection in pregnancy and outcomes of hydrops: A survey of members of the Society of Perinatal Obstetricians. Am J Obstet Gynecol 1998; 179:985–988.

211. Forestier F, Tissot JD, Vial Y, et al: Haematological parameters of parvovirus B19 infection in 13 fetuses with hydrops foetalis. Br J Haematol 1999; 104:925–927.

212. Bousquet F, Segondy M, Faure JM, et al: B19 parvovirus-induced fetal hydrops: Good outcome after intrauterine blood transfusion at 18 weeks of gestation. Fetal Diagn Ther 2000; 15:132–133.

213. Inoue T, Matsumura N, Fukuoka M, et al: Severe congenital cytomegalovirus infection with fetal hydrops in a cytomegalovirus-seropositive healthy woman. Eur J Obstet Gynecol Reprod Biol 2001; 95:184–186.

214. Brabin B: Fetal anemia in malarious areas: Its causes and significance. Ann Trop Paediatr 1992; 12:303.

215. Willert JR, Feusner J, Beckwith JB: Congenital mesoblastic nephroma: A rare cause of perinatal anemia. J Pediatr 1999; 134:248.

216. Norton ME: Nonimmune hydrops fetalis. Semin Perinatol 1994; 18:321.

217. Lallemand AV, Doco-Fenzy M, Gaillard DA: Investigation of nonimmune hydrops fetalis: Multidisciplinary studies are necessary for diagnosis—Review of 94 cases. Pediatr Dev Pathol 1999; 2:432–439.

218. Nakayama H, Kukita J, Hikino S, et al: Long-term outcome of 51 liveborn neonates with non-immune hydrops fetalis. Acta Paediatr 1999; 88:24–28.

219. Wafelman LS, Pollock BH, Kreutzer J, et al: Nonimmune hydrops fetalis: Fetal and neonatal outcome during 1983–1992. Biol Neonate 1999; 75:73–81.

220. Smets K, Van Aken S: Fetomaternal haemorrhage and prenatal intracranial bleeding: Two more causes of blueberry muffin baby. Eur J Pediatr 1998; 157:932–934.

221. Sohan K, Carroll S, Byrne D, et al: Parvovirus as a differential diagnosis of hydrops fetalis in the first trimester. Fetal Diagn Ther 2000; 15:234–236.

222. Miyagawa S, Takahashi R, et al: Angio-oedema in a neonate with IgG antibodies to parvovirus B19 following intrauterine parvovirus B19 infection. Br J Dermatol 2000; 143:428–430.

223. Lubin B: Neonatal anaemia secondary to blood loss. Clin Haematol 1978; 7:19.

224. Glader BE, Platt O: Haemolytic disorders of infancy. Clin Haematol 1978; 7:35.

225. Oski FA, Naiman JL: Hematologic Problems of the Newborn, 3rd ed. Philadelphia, WB Saunders, 1982, pp 56–86.

226. Blanchette VS, Zipursky A: Assessment of anemia in newborn infants. Clin Perinatol 1984; 11:489.

227. Dickerman JD: Anemia in the newborn infant. Pediatr Rev 1984; 6:131.

228. Halperin DS: Use of recombinant erythropoietin in treatment of the anemia of prematurity. Am J Pediatr Hematol-Oncol 1991; 13:351–363.

229. Dallman PR: Anemia of prematurity: The prospects for avoiding blood transfusions by treatment with recombinant human erythropoietin. AdvPediatr 1993; 40:385–403.

230. Gallagher PG, Ehrenkranz RA: Erythropoietin therapy for anemia of prematurity. Clin Perinatol 1993; 20:169–191.

231. Kannourakis G: The biology of erythropoietin and its role in the anemia of prematurity. J Paediatr Child Health 1994; 30:293.

232. Zipursky A, Hull A, et al: Foetal erythrocytes in the maternal circulation. Lancet 1959; 1:451.

233. Ganshirt-Ahlert D, Borjesson-Stoll R, et al: Detection of fetal trisomies 21 and 18 from maternal blood using triple gradient and magnetic cell sorting. Am J Reprod Immunol (Copenh) 1993; 30:194–201.

234. Geifman-Holtzman O, Blatman RN, Bianchi DW: Prenatal genetic diagnosis by isolation and analysis of fetal cells circulating in maternal blood. Semin Perinatol 1994; 18:366–375.

235. Bianchi DW: Fetal cells in the mother: From genetic diagnosis to diseases associated with fetal cell microchimerism. Eur J Obstet Gynecol Reprod Biol 2000; 92:103–108.

236. Samura O, Sohda S, Johnson KL, et al: Diagnosis of trisomy 21 in fetal nucleated erythrocytes from maternal blood by use of short tandem repeat sequences. Clin Chem 2001; 47:1622–1626.

237. Pertl B, Bianchi DW: Fetal DNA in maternal plasma: Emerging clinical applications. Obstet Gynecol 2001; 98:483–490.

238. Bianchi DW, LeShane ES, Cowan JM: Large amounts of cell-free fetal DNA are present in amniotic fluid. Clin Chem 2001; 47:1867–1869.

239. Pertl B, Sekizawa A, Samura O, et al: Detection of male and female fetal DNA in maternal plasma by multiplex fluorescent polymerase chain reaction amplification of short tandem repeats. Hum Genet 2000; 106:45–49.

240. Sebring ES, Polesky HF: Fetomaternal hemorrhage: Incidence, risk factors, time of occurrence, and clinical effects [See comments]. Transfusion 1990; 30:344–357.

241. de Almeida V, Bowman JM: Massive fetomaternal hemorrhage: Manitoba experience. Obstetr Gynecol 1994; 83:323.

242. Pearlman MD, Tintinalli JE, Lorenz RP: A prospective controlled study of outcome after trauma during pregnancy. Am J Obstet Gynecol 1990; 162:1502–1507; discussion 1507–1510.

243. Duleba AJ, Miller D, Taylor G: Expectant management of choriocarcinoma limited to placenta. Gynecol Oncol 1992; 44:277.

244. Kleihauer E, Hildegard B, et al: Demonstration von fetalem Hämoglobin in den Erythrocyten eines Blutausstrichs. Klin Wochenschr 1957; 35:637.

245. Boulos J, Andrini P, Haddad J, et al: Fetomaternal hemorrhage: A series of 9 cases. Arch Pediatr 1998; 5:1206–1210.

246. Dupre AR, Morrison JC, Martin JN Jr, et al: Clinical application of the Kleihauer-Betke test. J Reprod Med 1993; 38:621–624.

247. Patton WN, Nicholson GS, et al: Assessment of fetal-maternal hemorrhage in mothers with hereditary persistence of fetal hemoglobin. J Clin Pathol 1990; 43:728.

248. Bayliss KM, Kueck BD, et al: Detecting fetomaternal hemorrhage: A comparison of five methods. Transfusion 1991; 31:303.

249. Greenwalt TJ, Dumaswala UJ, Domino MM: The quantification of fetomaternal hemorrhage by an enzyme-linked antibody test with glutaraldehyde fixation. Vox Sang 1992; 63:268.

250. Garratty G, Arndt P: Applications of flow cytometry to transfusion science. Transfusion 1995; 35:157.

251. Benirschke K: Accurate recording of twin placenta. Obstetr Gynecol 1961; 18:334.

252. Strong SJ, Comey G: The Placenta in Twin Pregnancy. New York, Pergamon Press, 1967.

253. Seng YC, Rajadurai VS: Twin-twin transfusion syndrome: A five year review. Arch Dis Child Fetal Neonatal Ed 2000; 83:F168–F170.

254. Fries MH, Goldstein RB, et al: The role of velamentous cord insertion in the etiology of twin-twin transfusion syndrome. Obstet Gynecol 1993; 81:569.

255. Gonsoulin W, Moise KJ, et al: Outcome of twin-twin transfusion diagnosed before 28 weeks of gestation. Obstet Gynecol 1990; 75:214.

256. Hayakawa M, Oshiro M, Mimura S, et al: Twin-to-twin transfusion syndrome with hydrops: A retrospective analysis of ten cases. Am J Perinatol 1999; 16:263–267.

257. Blickstein I: The twin-twin transfusion syndrome. Obstet Gynecol 1990; 75:714.

258. Bruner JP, Rosemond RL: Twin-to-twin transfusion syndrome: A subset of the twin oligohydramnios-polyhydramnios sequence. Am J Obstet Gynecol 1993; 169:925.

259. Pinette MG, Pan Y, et al: Treatment of twin-twin transfusion syndrome. Obstet Gynecol 1993; 82:841.

260. Pochedly C, Musiker S: Twin-to-twin transfusion syndrome. Postgrad Med 1970; 47:172.

261. Su RM, Yu CH, Chang CH, et al: Prenatal diagnosis of twin-twin transfusion syndrome complicated with hydrops fetalis at 14 weeks of gestation. Int J Gynaecol Obstet 2001; 73:151–154.

262. Tan KL, Tan R, et al: The twin transfusion syndrome: Clinical observations on 35 affected pairs. Clin Pediatr 1979; 18:111.

263. Klebe JG, Ingomar CJ: The fetoplacental circulation during parturition illustrated by the interfetal transfusion syndrome. Pediatrics 1972; 49:112.

264. Kirkman HN, Riley HD Jr: Posthemorrhagic anemia and shock in the newborn. A review. Pediatrics 1959; 24:97.

265. Weiner AS: Diagnosis and treatment of anemia of the newborn caused by occult placental hemorrhage. Am J Obstet Gynecol 1948; 56:717.

266. Novak F: Posthemorrhagic shock in newborns during labor and after delivery. Acta Med Iugoslav 1953; 7:280.

267. Clayton EM, Pryor JA, et al: Fetal and maternal components of third-trimester obstetric hemorrhage. Obstet Gynecol 1964; 24:56.

268. Leonard S, Anthony B: Giant cephalohematoma of newborn. Am J Dis Child 1961; 101:170.

269. Robinson RJ, Rossiter MA: Massive subaponeurotic hemorrhage in babies of African origin. Arch Dis Child 1968; 43:684.

270. Packman DJ: Massive hemorrhage in the scalp of the newborn infant. Hemorrhagic caput succedaneum. Pediatrics 1962; 29:907.

271. Florentino-Pineda I, Ezhuthachan SG, et al: Subgalean hemorrhage in the newborn infant associated with silicone elastomer vacuum extractor. J Perinatol 1994; 14:95.

272. Rausen AR, Diamond LK: Enclosed hemorrhage and neonatal jaundice. Am J Dis Child 1961; 101:164.

273. Potter EL: Fetal and neonatal deaths: A statistical analysis of 2000 autopsies. JAMA 1940; 115:996.

274. Henderson JL: Hepatic hemorrhage in stillborn and newborn infants; clinical and pathological study of 47 cases. J Obstet Gynaecol Br Emp 1941; 48:377.

275. Erakalis AJ: Abdominal injury related to the trauma of birth. Pediatrics 1967; 39:421.

276. Philipsborn HF Jr, Traisman HS, et al: Rupture of the spleen: A complication of erythroblastosis fetalis. N Engl J Med 1955; 252:159.

277. Leape LL, Bordy MD: Neonatal rupture of the spleen. Report of a case successfully treated after spontaneous cessation of hemorrhage. Pediatrics 1971; 47:101.

278. Yerby M: Epilepsy and pregnancy: New issues for an old disorder. Neurol Clin 1993; 4:777.

279. Abzug AJ, Levin MJ: Neonatal adenovirus infection: Four patients and review of the literature. Pediatrics 1991; 87:890.

280. Hohlfeld P, Vial Y, et al: Cytomegalovirus fetal infection: Prenatal diagnosis. Obstet Gynecol 1991; 78:615.

281. Nader PR, Margolin F: Hemangioma causing gastrointestinal bleeding. Case report and review of the literature. Am J Dis Child 1966; 111:215.

282. Svane S: Foetal exsanguination from hemangioendothelioma of the skin. Acta Paediatr Scand 1966; 55:536.

283. Rumack CM, Guggenheim MA, et al: Neonatal intracranial hemorrhage and maternal use of aspirin. Obstet Gynecol 1981; 58 (Suppl):528.

284. Papile L, Burstein J, et al: Incidence and evolution of subependymal and intraventricular hemorrhage: Study of infants with birth weights less than 1500 grams. J Pediatr 1978; 92:529.

285. Nexo E, Christensen NC, Olesen H: Volume of blood removed for analytical purposes during hospitalization of low-birthweight infants. Clin Chem 1981; 27:759.

286. Obladen M, Sachsenweger M, Stahnke M: Blood sampling in very low birth weight infants receiving different levels of intensive care. Eur J Pediatr 1988; 147:399–404.

287. Madsen LP, Rasmussen MK, Bjerregaard LL, et al: Impact of blood sampling in very preterm infants. Scand J Clin Lab Invest 2000; 60:125–132.

288. Shulman RJ, Phillips S, et al: Volume of blood required to obtain central venous catheter blood cultures in infants and children. JPEN J Parent Ent Nutr 1993; 17:177.

289. Thorkelsson T, Hoath SB: Accurate micromethod of neonatal blood sampling from peripheral arterial catheters. J Perinatol 1995; 15:43.

290. Gleason E, Grossman S, Campbell C: Minimizing diagnostic blood loss in critically ill patients. Am J Crit Care 1992; 1:85.

291. Silver MJ, Yh L, et al: Reduction of blood loss from diagnostic sampling in critically ill patients using a blood-conserving arterial line system. Chest 1993; 104: 1711–1715.

292. Lin JC, Strauss RG, Kulhavy JC, et al: Phlebotomy overdraw in the neonatal intensive care nursery. Pediatrics 2000; 106:E19.

293. Necheles TF, Rai US, et al: The role of haemolysis in neonatal hyperbilirubinemia as reflected in carboxyhaemoglobin levels. Acta Paediatr Scand 1976; 65:361.

294. Minnich V, Cordonnier JK, et al: Alpha, beta and gamma hemoglobin polypeptide chains during the neonatal period with a description of a fetal form of hemoglobin D St. Louis. Blood 1962; 19:137.

295. Levine RL, Lincoln DR: Hemoglobin Hasharon in a premature infant with hemolytic anemia. Pediatr Res 1975; 9:7.

296. van Wijgerden JA: Clinical expression of sickle cell anemia in the newborn. South Med J 1983; 76:478.

297. Hegyi T, Delphin ES: Sickle cell anemia in the newborn. Pediatrics 1977; 60:213.

298. Veiga S, Varthianathan T: Massive intravascular sickling after exchange transfusion with sickle cell trait blood. Transfusion 1963; 3:387.

299. Lee-Potter JP, Deacon-Smith RA, et al: A new cause of hemolytic anemia in the newborn. J Clin Pathol 1975; 28:317.

300. Schmairer AH, Mauer HM, et al: Alpha thalassemia screening in neonates by mean corpuscular volume and mean corpuscular hemoglobin concentration. J Pediatr 1973; 83:794.

301. Koenig HM, Vedvidk TS, et al: Prenatal diagnosis of hemoglobin H disease. J Pediatr 1978; 92:278.

302. Thumasathit B, Nondasuta A, et al: Hydrops fetalis associated with Bart's hemoglobin in northern Thailand. J Pediatr 1968; 73:132.

303. Fung TY, Kin LT, Kong LC, et al: Homozygous alpha-thalassemia associated with hypospadias in three survivors. Am J Medical Genet 1999; 82:225–227.

304. Dame C, Albers N, Hasan C, et al: Homozygous alpha-thalassaemia and hypospadias—Common aetiology or incidental association? Long-term survival of Hb Bart's hydrops syndrome leads to new aspects for counselling of alpha-thalassaemic traits. Eur J Pediatrics 1999; 158:217–220.

305. Beaudry MA, Ferguson DJ, et al: Survival of a hydropic infant with homozygous alpha-thalassemia-I. J Pediatr 1986; 108:713.

306. Bianchi DW, Beyer EC, et al: Normal long-term survival with alpha-thalassemia. J Pediatr 1986; 108:716.

307. Tongsong T, Wanapirak C, Sirivatanapa P, et al: Prenatal eradication of Hb Bart's hydrops fetalis. J Reprod Med 2001; 46:18–22.

308. Erlandson ME, Hilgartner M: Hemolytic disease in the neonatal period. J Pediatr 1959; 54:566.

309. Stamatoyannopoulos G: Gamma-thalassemia. Lancet 1971; 2:192.

310. Kan YW, Forget BG, et al: Gamma-beta thalassemia: A cause of hemolytic disease of the newborn. N Engl J Med 1972; 286:129.

311. Abman SH, Griebel JL, et al: Acute effect of inhaled nitric oxide in children with severe hypoxemic respiratory failure. J Pediatr 1994; 124:881.

312. Journois D, Pouard P, et al: Inhaled nitric oxide as a therapy for pulmonary hypertension after operation for congenital heart defects. J Thorac Cardiovasc Surg 1994; 107:1129.

313. Winberg P, Lundell BP, Gustafsson LE: Effect of inhaled nitric oxide on raised pulmonary vascular resistance in children with congenital heart disease. Br Heart J 1994; 71:282.

314. Wessel DL, Adatia I, Van Marter LJ, et al: Improved oxygenation in a randomized trial of inhaled nitric oxide for persistent pulmonary hypertension of the newborn. Pediatrics 1997; 100:E7.

315. Roberts JD Jr, Fineman JR, Morin FC 3rd, et al: Inhaled nitric oxide and persistent pulmonary hypertension of the newborn: The Inhaled Nitric Oxide Study Group. N Engl J Med 1997; 336:605–610.

316. Banks BA, Seri I, Ischiropoulos H, et al: Changes in oxygenation with inhaled nitric oxide in severe bronchopulmonary dysplasia. Pediatrics 1999; 103:610–618.

317. Nakajima W, Ishida A, Arai H, et al: Methaemoglobinemia after inhalation of nitric oxide in infant with pulmonary hypertension. Lancet 1997; 350:1002–1003.

318. Speakman ED, Boyd JC, Bruns DE: Measurement of methemoglobin in neonatal samples containing fetal hemoglobin. Clin Chem 1995; 41:458.

319. Lynch PL, Bruns DE, Boyd JC, et al: Chiron 800 system CO-oximeter module overestimates methemoglobin concentrations in neonatal samples containing fetal hemoglobin. Clin Chem 1998; 44:1569–1570.

320. de Keijzer MH, Brandts R, Giesendorf BA: Comment on the overestimation of methemoglobin concentrations in neonatal samples with the Chiron 800 system CO-oximeter module. Clin Chem 1999; 45(8 Pt 1):1313–1314.

321. Lebby T, Roco JJ, Arcinue EL: Infantile methemoglobinemia associated with acute diarrheal illness. Am J Emerg Med 1993; 11:471–472.

322. Pollack ES, Pollack CV Jr: Incidence of subclinical methemoglobinemia in infants with diarrhea. Ann Emerg Med 1994; 24:652–656.

323. Hanukoglu A, Danon PN: Endogenous methemoglobinemia associated with diarrheal disease in infancy. J Pediatr Gastroenterol Nutr 1996; 23:1–7.

324. Ogburn PL Jr, Ramin KD, Danilenko-Dixon D, et al: In utero erythrocyte transfusion for fetal xerocytosis associated with severe anemia and non-immune hydrops fetalis. Am J Obstet Gynecol 2001; 185:238–239.

325. del Giudice EM, Perrotta S, Nobili B, et al: Coinheritance of Gilbert syndrome increases the risk for developing gallstones in patients with hereditary spherocytosis. Blood 1999; 94:2259–2262.

326. Delhommeau F, Cynober T, Schischmanoff PO, et al: Natural history of hereditary spherocytosis during the first year of life. Blood 2000; 95:393–397.

327. Ribeiro ML, Alloisio N, et al: Severe hereditary spherocytosis and distal renal tubular acidosis associated with the total absence of band 3. Blood 2000; 96:1602–1604.

328. Perrotta S, Nigro V, et al: Dominant hereditary spherocytosis due to band 3 Neapolis produces a life-threatening anemia at the homozygous state. Blood 1998; 92(Suppl):9a.

329. Grootenboer S, Schischmanoff PO, Cynober T, et al: A genetic syndrome associating dehydrated hereditary stomatocytosis, pseudohyperkalaemia and perinatal oedema. Br J Haematol 1998; 103:383–386.

330. Grootenboer S, Schischmanoff PO, Laurendeau I, et al: Pleiotropic syndrome of dehydrated hereditary stomatocytosis,

pseudohyperkalemia, and perinatal edema maps to 16q23-q24. Blood 2000; 96:2599–2605.

331. Zanella A, Bianchi P, Fermo E, et al: Molecular characterization of the PK-LR gene in sixteen pyruvate kinase-deficient patients. Br J Haematol 2001; 113:43–48.

332. Iolascon A, Faienza MF, Perrotta S, et al: Gilbert's syndrome and jaundice in glucose-6-phosphate dehydrogenase deficient neonates. Haematologica 1999; 84:99–102.

333. Iolascon A, Faienza MF, Giordani L, et al: Bilirubin levels in the acute hemolytic crisis of G6PD deficiency are related to Gilbert's syndrome. Eur J Haematol 1999; 62:307–310.

334. English M: Life-threatening severe malarial anaemia. Trans R Soc Trop Med Hyg 2000; 94:585–588.

335. Ndyomugyenyi R, Magnussen P: Chloroquine prophylaxis, iron/folic-acid supplementation or case management of malaria attacks in primigravidae in western Uganda: Effects on congenital malaria and infant haemoglobin concentrations. Ann Trop Med Parasitol 2000; 94:759–768; discussion 769–770.

336. Viraraghavan R, Jantausch B: Congenital malaria: Diagnosis and therapy. Clin Pediatr 2000; 39:66–67.

337. Brabin BJ, Premji Z, Verhoeff F: An analysis of anemia and child mortality. J Nutr 2001; 131(2S–2):636S–645S; discussion 646S–648S.

338. Brabin BJ, Hakimi M, Pelletier D: An analysis of anemia and pregnancy-related maternal mortality. J Nutr 2001; 131(2S–2):604S–614S; discussion 614S–615S.

339. Sieff CA, Nisbet-Brown E, Nathan DG: Congenital bone marrow failure syndromes. Br J Haematol 2000; 111:30–42.

340. Giri N, Kang E, Tisdale JF, et al: Clinical and laboratory evidence for a trilineage haematopoietic defect in patients with refractory Diamond-Blackfan anaemia. Br J Haematol 2000; 108:167–175.

341. Alter BP, Nathan DG: Red cell aplasia in children. Arch Dis Child 1979; 54:263.

342. Diamond LK, Wang WC, et al: Congenital hypoplastic anemia. Adv. Pediatr 1976; 22:349.

343. Diamond LK, Allen DM, et al: Congenital (erythroid) hypoplastic anemia. Am J Dis Child 1961; 102:149.

344. Willig TN, Draptchinskaia N, Dianzani I, et al: Mutations in ribosomal protein S19 gene and Diamond Blackfan anemia: Wide variations in phenotypic expression. Blood 1999; 94:4294–306.

345. Matsson H, Klar J, Draptchinskaia N, et al: Truncating ribosomal protein S19 mutations and variable clinical expression in Diamond-Blackfan anemia. Hum Genet 1999; 105:496–500.

346. Willig TN, Niemeyer CM, Leblanc T, et al: Identification of new prognosis factors from the clinical and epidemiologic analysis of a registry of 229 Diamond-Blackfan anemia patients. Pediatr Res 1999; 46:553–561.

347. Da Costa L, Willig TN, Fixler J, et al: Diamond-Blackfan anemia. Curr Opin Pediatrics 2001; 13:10–15.

348. Dianzani I, Garelli E, Ramenghi U: Diamond-Blackfan anaemia: An overview. Paediatr Drugs 2000; 2:345–355.

349. Willig TN, Gazda H, Sieff CA: Diamond-Blackfan anemia. Curr Opin Hematol 2000; 7:85–94.

350. Pearson HA, Lobel JS, et al: A new syndrome of refractory sideroblastic anemia with vacuolization of marrow precursors and exocrine pancreatic dysfunction. J Pediatr 1979; 95:976.

351. Mayes C, Sweeney C, Savage JM, et al: Pearson's syndrome: A multisystem disorder. Acta Paediatr 2001; 90:235–237.

352. Blatt J, Katerji A, et al: Pancytopenia and vacuolization of marrow precursors associated with necrotizing encephalopathy. Br. J Haematol 1994; 86:207.

353. Simonsz HJ, Barlocher K, Rotig A: Kearns-Sayre's syndrome developing in a boy who survived Pearson's syndrome caused by mitochondrial DNA deletion. Doc Ophthalmol 1992; 82:73.

354. Rotig A, Colonna M, et al: A 13-bp direct repeat in mitochondrial DNA promotes deletions in Pearson's syndrome. Lancet 1989; 1:250.

355. Lestienne P, Bataille N: Mitochondrial DNA alterations and genetic diseases: A review. Biomed Pharmacol 1994; 48:199.

356. Lacbawan F, Tifft CJ, Luban NL, et al: Clinical heterogeneity in mitochondrial DNA deletion disorders: A diagnostic challenge of Pearson syndrome. Am J Med Genet 2000; 95:266–268.

357. Jardine PE, Cotter PD, et al: Pyridoxine-refractory congenital sideroblastic anemia with evidence for autosomal inheritance: Exclusions of linkage to ALAS2 at Xp11.21 by polymorphism analysis. J Med Genet 1994; 31:213.

358. Mäkitie O, Rajantie J, Kaitila I: Anemia and macrocytosis C unrecognized features in cartilage-hair hypoplasia. Acta Paediatr 1992; 81:1026.

359. Shalev H, Tamary H, Shaft D, et al: Neonatal manifestations of congenital dyserythropoietic anaemia. J Pediatr 1997; 131:95–97.

360. Perrotta S, del Giudice EM, Carbone R, et al: Gilbert's syndrome accounts for the phenotypic variability of congenital dyserythropoietic anemia type II (CDA-II). J Pediatr 2000; 136:556–559.

361. Tugal O, Pallant B, et al: Transient erythroblastopenia of the newborn caused by human parvovirus. Am J Pediatr Hematol Oncol 1994; 16:352.

362. Heegaard ED, Hasle H, Skibsted L, et al: Congenital anemia caused by parvovirus B19 infection. Pediatr Infect Dis J 2000; 19:1216–1218.

363. von Kaisenberg CS, Jonat W: Fetal parvovirus B19 infection. Ultrasound Obstetr Gynecol 2001; 18:280–288.

364. Schulman J: The anemia of prematurity. J Pediatr 1959; 54:663.

365. Stockman JA: The anemia of prematurity and the decision when to transfuse. Adv Pediatr 1983; 30:191.

366. Melhorn DK, Gross S: Vitamin E-dependent anemia in the preterm infant. I. Effects of large doses of medicinal iron. J Pediatr 1971; 79:569.

367. Halvorsen S, Finne PH: Erythropoietin production in the human fetus and newborn. Ann NY Acad Sci 1968; 149:516.

368. Rollins MD, Maxwell AP, et al: Cord blood erythropoietin, pH, PaO$_2$ and hematocrit following caesarean section before labour. Biol Neonate 1993; 63:147.

369. Willard DD, Gidding SS, et al: Effect of intravascular, intrauterine transfusion on prenatal and postnatal hemolysis and erythropoiesis in severe fetal isoimmunization. J Pediatr 1990; 117:447.

370. Humbert JR, Abelson H, et al: Polycythemia in small for gestational age infants. J Pediatr 1969; 75:812.

371. Sann L, Bourgeois J, Stephant A, et al: Outcome of 249 premature infants, less than 29 weeks gestational age. Arch Pediatr 2001; 8:250–258.

372. Cook CD, Brodie HR, et al: Measurement of fetal hemoglobin in newborn infants. Correlation with gestational age and intrauterine hypoxia. Pediatrics 1957; 20:272.

373. Stockman JA, III, Garcia JF, et al: The anemia of prematurity. Factors governing the erythropoietin response. N Engl J Med 1977; 296:647.

374. Brown MS: Phibb RH, et al: Decreased response of plasma immunoreactive erythropoietin to "available oxygen" in anemia of prematurity. J Pediatr 1984; 105:793.

375. Stockman JAI, Graeber JE, et al: Anemia of prematurity. Determinants of erythropoietin response. J Pediatr 1984; 105:786.

376. Yamashita H, Kukita J, Ohga S: Serum erythropoietin levels in term and preterm infants during the first year of life. Am J Pediatr Hematol Oncol 1994; 16:213.

377. Emmerson AJB, Westwood NB, et al: Erythropoietin responsive progenitors in anemia of prematurity. Arch Dis Child 1991; 66:810.

378. Shannon KM, Naylor GS, et al: Circulating erythroid progenitors in the anemia of prematurity. N Engl J Med 1987; 317:728.

379. Rhondeau SM, Christensen RD, et al: Responsiveness to recombinant erythropoietin of marrow erythroid progenitors in infants with anemia of prematurity. J Pediatr 1988; 112:935.

380. Ruth V, Widness JA, et al: Postnatal changes in serum immunoreactive erythropoietin in relation to hypoxia before and after birth. J Pediatr 1990; 116:950.

381. Brown MS, Jones MA, et al: Single-dose pharmacokinetics of recombinant human erythropoietin in preterm infants after intravenous and subcutaneous administration. J Pediatr 1993; 122:655.

382. Attias D: Pathophysiology and treatment of the anemia of prematurity. J Pediatr Hematol Oncol 1995; 17:13.

383. Meyer M, Meyer JH, et al: Recombinant human erythropoietin in the treatment of the anemia of prematurity: Results of a double-blind, placebo-controlled study. Pediatrics 1994; 93:918.

384. Soubasi V, Kremenopoulos G, et al: In which neonates does early recombinant human erythropoietin treatment prevent anemia of prematurity? Results of a randomized, controlled study. Pediatr Res 1993; 34:675.

385. Brown MS, Keith JF III: Comparison between two and five doses a week of recombinant human erythropoietin for anemia of prematurity: A randomized trial. Pediatrics 1999; 104(2 Pt 1):210–215.

386. Reiter PD: Rosenberg AA, Valuck RJ: Factors associated with successful epoetin alfa therapy in premature infants. Ann Pharmacother 2000; 34:433–439.

387. Shannon KM, Keith JF, et al: Recombinant human erythropoietin stimulates erythropoiesis and reduces erythrocyte transfusions in very low birth weight preterm infants. Pediatrics 1995; 95:1.

388. Fain J, Hilsenrath P, et al: A cost analysis comparing erythropoietin and red cell transfusions in the treatment of anemia of prematurity. Transfusion 1995; 35:936.

389. Vamvakas EC, Strauss RG: Meta-analysis of controlled clinical trials studying the efficacy of rHuEPO in reducing blood transfusions in the anemia of prematurity. Transfusion 2001; 41:406–415.

390. Donato H, Vain N, Rendo P, et al: Effect of early versus late administration of human recombinant erythropoietin on transfusion requirements in premature infants: Results of a randomized, placebo-controlled, multicenter trial. Pediatrics 2000; 105:1066–1072.

391. Soubasi V, Kremenopoulos G, Tsantali C, et al: Use of erythropoietin and its effects on blood lactate and 2, 3-diphosphoglycerate in premature neonates. Biol Neonate 2000; 78:281–287.

392. Ledbetter DJ, Juul SE: Erythropoietin and the incidence of necrotizing enterocolitis in infants with very low birth weight. J Pediatr Surg 2000; 35:178–181; discussion 182.

393. Newton NR, Leonard CH, Piecuch RE, et al: Neurodevelopmental outcome of prematurely born children treated with recombinant human erythropoietin in infancy. J Perinatol 1999; 19(6 Pt 1):403–406.

394. Brugnara C, Colella GM, et al: Effects of subcutaneous recombinant human erythropoietin in normal subjects: Development of decreased reticulocyte hemoglobin content and iron-deficient erythropoiesis. J Lab Clin Med 1994; 123:660.

395. Etchason J, Petz L, et al: The cost effectiveness of preoperative autologous blood donations. N Engl J Med 1995; 332:719.

396. Rutherford CJ, Kaplan HS: Autologous blood donation—Can we bank on it? N Engl J Med 1995; 332:740.

397. Shireman TI, Hilsenrath P, et al: Recombinant human erythropoietin vs. transfusions in the treatment of anemia of prematurity. Arch Pediatr Adolesc Med 1994; 148:582.

398. Grohskopf LA, Roth VR, et al: *Serratia liquefaciens* bloodstream infections from contamination of epoetin alfa at a hemodialysis center. N Engl J Med 2001; 344:1491–1497.

399. Baxter LM, Vreman HJ, et al: Recombinant human erythropoietin (r-HuEPO) increases total bilirubin production in premature infants. Clin Pediatr 1995; 34:213.

400. Bechensteen AG, Refsum HE, et al: Effects of recombinant human erythropoietin on fetal and adult hemoglobin in preterm infants. Pediatr Res 1995; 38:729.

401. Black DB, Lubchenco LO, et al: Developmental and neurologic sequelae of neonatal hyperviscosity syndrome. Pediatrics 1982; 69:426.

402. Saggese G, Bertelloni S, et al: Elevated calcitonin gene-related peptide in polycythemic newborn infants. Acta Paediatr 1992; 81:966.

403. Bada HS, Korones SB, et al: Asymptomatic syndrome of polycythemic hyperviscosity: Effect of partial plasma exchange transfusion. J Pediatr 1992; 120:579.

404. Drew JH, Guaran RL, et al: Cord whole blood hyperviscosity: measurement, definition, incidence and clinical features. J Paediatr Child Health 1991; 26:363.

405. Mimouni F, Miodovnik M, et al: Neonatal polycythemia in infants of insulin-dependent diabetic mothers. Obstet Gynecol 1986; 68:370.

406. Piacquadio K, Hollingsworth DR, Murphy H: Effects of in-utero exposure to oral hypoglycemic drugs. Lancet 1991; 338:866.

407. Oh W: Neonatal polycythemia and hyperviscosity. Pediatr Clin North Am 1986; 33:523.

408. Sacher R, Luban NLC, Strauss RG: Current practice and guidelines for the transfusion of cellular blood components in the newborn. Transfus Med Rev 1989; 3:39.

409. Yu VY, Gan TE: Red cell transfusion in the preterm infant. J Paediatr Child Health 1994; 30:301.

410. Shannon K: Recombinant erythropoietin in anemia of prematurity: Five years later. Pediatrics 1993; 92:614.

411. Wardrop CA, Holland BM, et al: Non physiological anemia of prematurity. Arch Dis Child 1978; 53:855.

412. Schneider AJ, Stockman JA III, Oski FA: Transfusion nomogram: An application of physiology to clinical decisions regarding the use of blood. Crit Care Med 1981; 9:469.

413. Stockman JA III, Levin E, et al: O_2 consumption of premature infants in the first 10 weeks of life: Response to transfusion. Pediatr Res 1979; 13:442.

414. Izraeli S, Ben-Sira L, et al: Lactic acid as a predictor for erythrocyte transfusion in healthy preterm infants with anemia of prematurity. J Pediatr 1993; 122:629.

415. Keyes WG, Donohue PK, Spivak JL, et al: Assessing the need for transfusion of premature infants and role of hematocrit, clinical signs, and erythropoietin level. Pediatrics 1989; 84:412–417.

416. Frey B, Losa M: The value of capillary whole blood lactate for blood transfusion requirements in anaemia of prematurity. Intens Care Med 2001; 27:222–227.

417. Strauss RG: Transfusion therapy in neonates. Am J Dis Child 1991; 145:904.

418. Strauss RG: Erythropoietin and neonatal anemia. N Engl J Med 1994; 330:1227.

419. Levy GJ, Strauss RG, et al: National survey of neonatal transfusion practices: I. Red blood cell therapy. Pediatrics 1993; 91:523.

420. Strauss RG, Levy GJ, et al: National survey of neonatal transfusion practices: II. Blood component therapy. Pediatrics 1993; 91:530.

421. American Association of Blood Banks: Standards for Blood Banks and Transfusion Services, 20th ed. Bethesda, MD, American Association of Blood Banks, 2000.

422. Strauss RG, Cordle DG, Quijana J, et al: Comparing alloimmunization in preterm infants after transfusion of fresh unmodified versus stored leukocyte-reduced red blood cells. J Pediatr Hematol/Oncol 1999; 21:224–230.

423. Strauss RG, Johnson K, Cress G, et al: Alloimmunization in preterm infants after repeated transfusions of WBC-reduced RBCs from the same donor. Transfusion 2000; 40:1463–1468.

424. Luban NL, Strauss RG, Hume HA: Commentary on the safety of red cells preserved in extended-storage media for neonatal transfusions. Transfusion 1991; 31:229.

425. Patten E, Robbins M, et al: Use of red blood cells older than five days for neonatal transfusion. J Perinatol 1991; 11:37.

426. Strauss RG, Burmeister LF, Johnson K, et al: Feasibility and safety of AS-3 red blood cells for neonatal transfusions. J Pediatr 2000; 136:215–219.

427. Cook S, Gunter J, Wissel M, Effective use of a strategy using assigned red cell units to limit donor exposure for neonatal patients. Transfusion 1993; 33:379.

428. Liu EA, Mannino FL, Lane TA: Prospective randomized trial of the safety and efficacy of a limited donor exposure transfusion program for premature neonates. J Pediatr 1994; 125:92.

429. Strauss RG, Burmeister LF, Johnson K, et al: Randomized trial assessing the feasibility and safety of biologic parents as RBC donors for their preterm infants. Transfusion 2000; 40:450–456.

430. Hilsenrath P, Nemecek J, Widness JA, et al: Cost-effectiveness of a limited-donor blood program for neonatal red cell transfusions. Transfusion 1999; 39:938–943.

431. Strauss RG: Leukocyte-reduction to prevent transfusion-transmitted cytomegalovirus infections. Pediatr Transplant 1999; 3(Suppl 1):19–22.

432. Luban NL, Manno C: Lack of difference in CMV transmission via the transfusion of filtered irradiated and nonfiltered irradiated blood to newborn infants in an endemic area. Transfusion 2000; 40:387–389.

433. Thurer RL, Luban NL, AuBuchon JP, et al: Universal WBC reduction. Transfusion 2000; 40:751–752.

434. Naulaers G, Barten S, Vanhole C, et al: Management of severe neonatal anemia due to fetomaternal transfusion. Am J Perinatol 1999; 16:193–196.

435. Ringer SA, Richardson D, et al: Blood utilization in neonatal intensive care. Blood 1991; 78:353a.

436. Ringer SA, Richardson DK, Sacher RA, et al: Variations in transfusion practice in neonatal intensive care. Pediatrics 1998; 101:194–200.

437. Bednarek FJ, Weisberger S, Richardson DK, et al: Variations in blood transfusions among newborn intensive care units. SNAP II Study Group. J Pediatr 1998; 133:601–607.

3 | Immune Hemolytic Disease

Helen G. Liley

HISTORICAL ASPECTS

Whereas many serious complications of pregnancy were well known in antiquity, maternofetal blood group incompatibility is a young subject. Much of the understanding of the disease developed between the 1930s and 1970s, although since the late 1980s the molecular basis of both Rh and other blood group genotypes and phenotypes has been revealed. The lack of ancient recognition may seem surprising, considering the spectacular appearance of a hydropic fetus and placenta and the drastic effect of recurrent perinatal death on family size and structure. However, only about 1 pregnancy in 200 in occidental societies is vulnerable to complication by antibodies. Even without any effective treatment only about one half of the babies would die, giving a perinatal mortality of about 1 in 400. Against the high perinatal mortality prevailing in most countries up until the start of the last century, deaths from

hemolytic disease were of little statistical significance. Louyse Bourgeois, midwife to Marie de Medici, is credited with the first description (in 1609) of hemolytic disease of the fetus and newborn (HDN). She described twins: the first was hydropic and died shortly after birth; the second initially appeared well but rapidly became jaundiced, then opisthotonic, and subsequently died.

The physiologic connection between "congenital anemia," icterus gravis, and hydrops fetalis was not recognized until 1932, despite detailed descriptions of each condition by pathologists. Diamond and co-workers[1] deduced that these were variations on a common theme and coined the term *erythroblastosis fetalis* for the disease characterized by hemolytic anemia, intra- and extramedullary erythropoiesis, and hepatosplenomegaly. Darrow, who had lost a baby of her own to kernicterus, correctly speculated in 1938 that the disease was caused by maternal antibodies to fetal antigens developed as a result of transplacental fetomaternal hemorrhage.[2] However, because she was incorrect in her conclusion that the antibody was to fetal hemoglobin, much of the recognition for this remarkable insight was given to those who provided the evidence.

Landsteiner and Wiener's description in 1929 of the Rh blood groups had not matched the spectacular significance for transfusion practice of the discovery of the ABO system in 1900. A decade elapsed before Levine (a student of Landsteiner) and Stetson linked a woman's severe transfusion reaction to her husband's blood with her recent delivery of a hydropic stillborn infant.[3] She was found to have an antibody that agglutinated her husband's red blood cells (RBCs). Levine postulated that she had become sensitized to a RBC surface antigen that the fetus had inherited from its father.

In 1940, Landsteiner and Wiener[4] proposed the identity of the antigen by generating antibodies to rhesus monkey RBCs in guinea pigs and rabbits. The antisera agglutinated RBCs from 85 percent of whites. These subjects were designated *rhesus (Rh) positive*. The 15 percent whose RBCs were not agglutinated were *rhesus (Rh) negative*.

Levine and associates then used Landsteiner and Wiener's antiserum to show that Levine and Stetson's patient was Rh negative and her husband was Rh positive. Furthermore, her serum agglutinated the RBCs from Wiener and Landsteiner's Rh-positive individuals but not RBCs from their Rh-negative subjects.[5] Although the monkey RBC antigen and antibody (LW and anti-LW) are not the same as the human RhD antigen and antibody, their discovery was important. In subsequent years progress was rapid and dramatic. It included the recognition that immunoglobulin (Ig) G (7S antibody) crossed the placenta and the development of Coombs' test.[6] This test uses rabbit anti-IgG antibodies to agglutinate IgG-labeled RBCs and remains important in the detection and management of HDN to this day. Chown reported in 1954[7] that mothers could be sensitized by a transplacental hemorrhage of fetal blood, although until crossmatching for Rh groups became routine, transfusion for postpartum hemorrhage and other indications also contributed to the incidence of the disease. Chown's observation plus subsequent recognition that most sensitizing fetomaternal hemorrhages occurred at delivery, explaining why Rh HDN was mainly a disease of multipara, paved the way for development of immunoprophylaxis. Since the late 1960s, RhD immunoglobulin treatment has been available to treat Rh-negative mothers of Rh-positive infants at delivery to prevent effects on future pregnancies.

These discoveries all contributed to understanding of the delicate balance in the immunology of pregnancy; the maternal immune system generally remains in a state of armed neutrality toward the fetus and its foreign antigens, which remain shielded by the trophoblast. Meanwhile, the advantages of maternal immunologic memory are conferred on the fetus and newborn via active transplacental passage of antibodies, creating optimal conditions for the awakening of the newborn's own adaptive immune system. However, if a maternal antibody develops to a self-antigen or a fetal antigen, fetal disease can result. Thus, when an Rh-negative woman exposed to Rh-positive RBCs develops anti-D IgG, the antibody traverses the placenta and can bind fetal D-positive RBCs, leading to their destruction. The subsequent fetal hemolysis can lead to icterus gravis, kernicterus, and hydrops fetalis.

For many problems of pregnancy, obscurity of the pathophysiology until recently often led to management that, at best, was symptomatic. In contrast, with hemolytic disease the genetic predilection, molecular mechanism, and rationale for treatment were rapidly deduced, which led to remarkable success in preventing the disease and mitigating its effects. Indeed, the history of the prevention and management of Rh HDN includes a number of epic discoveries that have influenced the management of other diseases. These breakthroughs include exchange transfusion for neonatal treatment, development of screening programs for maternal blood group antibodies, strategies for inducing early delivery to optimize neonatal outcomes, the use of amniocentesis for fetal diagnosis, the first example of intrauterine fetal treatment, and the development of one of the earliest and most successful forms of immuno-prophylaxis using human antibodies. Subsequently, many of the successes of fetal and neonatal treatment of Rh HDN have been extrapolated to HDN due to other blood group antibodies and to other problems of pregnancy.

Advances in molecular biology and biochemistry allowed the identification of the Rh polypeptides in 1982 and the Rh genes in 1991. Until these discoveries, a controversy existed between two models to explain Rh genotype and phenotype relationships. Wiener and Wexler[8] proposed the existence of a single gene with multiple epitopic sites, whereas Fisher and Race[9] postulated that there were two closely linked genes encoding three pairs of Rh antigens: Dd, Cc, and Ee inherited in two sets of three (one set from each parent) (Table 3–1). Both models have been shown to be partly correct, although like many disorders that were once thought to have been genetically simple and phenotypically diverse, the diversity of Rh genotype/phenotype relationships is much greater than once envisaged.

THE Rh BLOOD GROUP SYSTEM

Biochemistry and Molecular Genetics

Although the incidence of Rh HDN has been declining and the incidence of HDN due to other alloantibodies has increased, the *Rh blood group system* remains the most common cause of HDN (particularly severe HDN), especially in whites, for which about one in seven conceptions involves an Rh-negative woman and an Rh-positive man. Individuals are classed as Rh positive or negative based on expression of the major D antigen on their RBCs; however, at least 44 other Rh antigens have been identified. Those most commonly recognized in clinical practice are the antigens designated D, C, c, E, and e. The Rh blood group system is the most complex blood group system in humans.[11]

After the landmark descriptions of the RhD protein in 1982,[12, 13] the non-D[14, 15] and D complementary DNAs (cDNAs) and genes were cloned in the early 1990s.[16, 17] In most individuals the Rh blood group loci are the products of two very similar genes, one of which encodes CD240CE, the polypeptide that carries the Cc/Ee epitopes in combinations (Ce, ce, cE, or CE); the other encodes CD240D, the D antigen polypeptide[18, 19] (Table 3–2). The two genes are separated by only 30 kb and are organized

TABLE 3–1. Incidence of Rh Allelic Combinations Expressed by Fisher-Race and Wiener Nomenclature

	Nomenclature			Frequency[10]		
	Fisher-Race	**Wiener**	**Expressed Alleles**	**Whites**	**Blacks**	**Asians***
RhD positive	CDe	R_1	*RHD RHCe*	0.42	0.17	0.70
	cDE	R_2	*RHD RHcE*	0.14	0.11	0.21
	cDe	R_0	*RHD RHce*	0.04	0.44	0.03
	CDE	R_z	*RHD RHCE*	0.00	0.00	0.01
TOTAL				**0.6**	**0.72**	**0.95**
RhD negative[†]	cde	r	*RHce*	0.37	0.26	0.03
	Cde	r'	*RHCe*	0.02	0.02	0.02
	cdE	r''	*RHcE*	0.01	<0.01	<0.01
	CdE	r^y	*RHCE*	<0.01	<0.01	<0.01
TOTAL				**0.4**	**0.28**	**0.05**
RATIO OF RHD-POSITIVE TO RHD-NEGATIVE PHENOTYPES				**0.84: 0.16**	**0.92: 0.08**	**0.99: <0.01**

*The predominant reasons for failure to express RHD vary by racial group. RHD deletions predominate in whites, but other variants such as partial deletions and RHD RHCE recombinations are more common in other populations.
†Rh negativity is more common in Indo-Asians.

TABLE 3–2. Incidence of Common Rh Haplotypes

			Allele Frequency in United States (%)			
Gene	**Allele**	**Translated Product**	**Whites**	**Blacks**	**Native Americans**	**Asians**
RHD	*RHD*	RhD polypeptide	61	97	99	99
	RHD silent	None	39	3	1	1
RHCE	*RHCe*	RhCe polypeptide	44	19	46	72
	RHcE	RhcE polypeptide	15	11	40	21
	RHce	Rhce polypeptide	41	70	8	6
	RHCE	RhCE polypeptide	0	0	6	1

From Huang CH: Blood Group Antigen Gene Mutation Database: Rh Blood Group System. HUGO Mutation Database Initiative, 2001. Available at http://www.bioc.aecom.yu.edu/bgmut/index.htm.

TABLE 3–3. Examples of Variant Rh Phenotypes for Which a Corresponding Genotype Has Been Described, Illustrating the Diversity of the *RHD* Genotype

Category	**Phenotype**	**Typical Mutations**
Partial D	D^{II} to D^{VII} and others	Variety of point mutations and *RHD-RHCE* hybrids
Weak D	Weak D (D^u) types 1–16	Variety of point mutations leading to amino acid substitutions in transmembrane or cytoplasmic domains
D negative (silent D or d)	D negative	Variety of mechanisms: *RHD* complete or partial deletion, *CE* hybrids, point mutations; some prevent transcription, but all prevent expression at the cell surface
CE variants	RN, E^{I-III}, VN, CX, C^W, etc.	Variety of hybrids and point mutations
CE silent	D.., D-- and various others	Mostly *RHD-RHCE* hybrids
Rh deficiency states (no D or CE expression)	D_{null} amorph	*RHCE* silent genes plus *RHD* deletion
	$D_{null\ reg}$, $D_{null\ mod}$	*RHAG* mutations that prevent expression

as a cluster in opposite orientation on chromosome bands 1p34–p36. The small *SMP1* gene (putatively a "small membrane protein" family member) lies between them. They share a very similar 10-exon structure and their intronic sequences are also highly conserved. Their sequence identity strongly suggests that they evolved by the fairly recent duplication of an ancestral gene. However,

worldwide, the Rh blood group system displays considerable polymorphism. A wide variety of both small and large mutations (including gene deletion and recombination to form hybrid *RHD-RHCE* products) and the effects of other modifying genes account for the diverse common and rare Rh phenotypes[19–21] (Table 3–3). Although some genotypic and phenotypic variants are confined to a single family, for others the incidence in various gene pools is much higher or unknown. This diversity mandates caution in the use of DNA-based clinical diagnostic approaches, especially when these approaches are applied to populations other than the ones in which they were piloted but may open the door for future individualization of prevention and therapy.[22]

The predicted product of the RhD messenger RNA is a 417-amino acid polypeptide with a molecular mass of 45,100. The D and Cc/Ee polypeptides have 94 percent identity and almost 96 percent similarity. Although E/e specificity appears to be conferred primarily by a single amino acid substitution (P226A) encoded by exon 5 of the *RHCE* gene, C/c specificity is associated with four amino acid differences: C16W encoded by exon 1 and I60L, S68N, and S103P all encoded by exon 2 of the *RHCE* gene[23] (Table 3–4). Of these, the S103P substitution is the most important in determining the antigenic reactivity.[23, 24]

It has been well established for decades that no d antigen exists. RhD negativity is defined as the absence of RhD antigen and its incidence is highest in the Basque population.[25] It has been suggested that peripatetic Basque traders and fishermen (or their ancestors) may have spread this genotype to other populations. In these European-descended populations in which Rh negativity is relatively common, most RhD-negative individuals lack the *RHD* gene altogether.[16, 17] This mutation appears to have arisen because two highly homologous sequences (1463 bp "rhesus boxes") flank the *RHD* gene and provide the opportunity for *RHD* deletion by unequal crossing over.[26] However, other mechanisms for D negativity appear more commonly in other populations such as those of African, Chinese, or Japanese ancestry.[27–30] These alternative mechanisms include partial deletion, recombination between *RHD* and *RHCE* genes, and point mutation. An Rh allele that comprises a pseudogene (*RHD ψ*) is prevalent among people of African ancestry.[29] An interaction with expression of Cc polypeptides has also been proposed, because of an observation that D-negative individuals who had intact *RHD* genes were CC or Cc, but not cc.[28] Rh-associated proteins (described later) may also be able to affect expression of RhD, conferring the D-negative phenotype.

The molecular basis of the D-positive phenotype is also intricate. Studies using site-directed mutagenesis or naturally occurring variants of *RHD* and monoclonal antibodies offer support for two models, one proposing that the D antigen may be composed of several epitopes,[31–34] some of which are missing in individuals who express partial D antigenicity. An alternative view is that most anti-D antigens bind a similar "footprint" in which the size and arrangement of residues differs slightly.[35] Of the 30 to 36 amino acid substitutions that usually differ between the D and the CE polypeptides, only about one quarter are in extracellular domains of the protein. Although transmembrane, cytoplasmic, and extracellular substitutions could all affect antigenicity by altering epitope conformation, all epitope-modifying variations recognized so far affect extracellular domains.[11, 20]

The RHD and RHCE gene products are unique among blood group antigens in being nonglycosylated, palmitoylated integral membrane proteins (Fig. 3–1). Their 12 predicted transmembrane domains are connected by relatively small extracellular and cytoplasmic domains. They are also unusual in that their expression is confined to erythroid cells, whereas most other blood group antigens are present in many tissues. They are found in hetero-oligomeric complexes, the structure and function of which is still under investigation. In these oligomers, Rh antigens are found in association with a glycosylated membrane component, which migrates diffusely on sodium dodecyl sulfate–polyacrylamide gel electrophoresis at approximately 45 to 75 kd. This 409-amino acid glycoprotein was formerly known as Rh50 glycoprotein, but is now designated Rh-associated glycoprotein (RhAG). It is 36 percent identical to RhD and RhCE and, putatively, has a similar configuration involving 12 helical membrane-spanning domains. Its gene has an exon-intron organization very similar to that of *RHD* and *CE*; however, it maps to chromosome bands 6p11–p21.1. Its expression is also confined to erythroid cells, although its regulation probably differs from that of *RHD* and *RHCE*.[36] Nonerythroid homologs (*RHBG* and *RHCG*) have been found in other tissues.[37] The Rh complex is thought to comprise a tetramer of one D subunit, one CE subunit, and two RhAG subunits in D-positive RBCs or a tetramer of two CE subunits and two RhAg subunits in D-negative RBCs (Fig. 3–2).

Cartron[11] and Cartron and Colin[18] have reviewed the *Rh deficiency states*. The rare individuals with the Rh deficiency syndrome (formerly known as Rh$_{null}$) lack expression of all or virtually all RhD, C/c, and E/e antigens. This recessive condition can result from mutations

TABLE 3–4. Differences between the Common *RH* Genotypes*

Gene (GenBank Accession No.)	cDNA Change (from *RHCe*)	Amino Acid Change
RHD (L08429)	150 C → T; 178 C → A; 201 A → G; 203 A → G; 307 C → T	L60I; N68S; P103S
RHCe	48G → C; 150C → T; 178C → A; 201A → G; 203A → G; 307C → T; 676G → C	W16C; L60I; N68S; P103S
RHCE	48G → C; 150C → T; 178C → A; 201A → G; 203A → G; 307C → T; 676G → C	W16C; L60I; N68S; P103S; A226P
RhcE (M34015)	676G → C	A226P

*RHCe is used as the reference.

From Huang CH: Blood Group Antigen Gene Mutation Database: Rh Blood Group System. HUGO Mutation Database Initiative, 2001. Available at http://www.bioc.aecom.yu.edu/bgmut/index.htm.

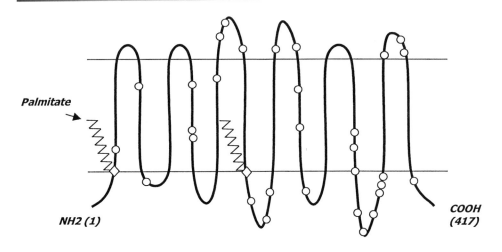

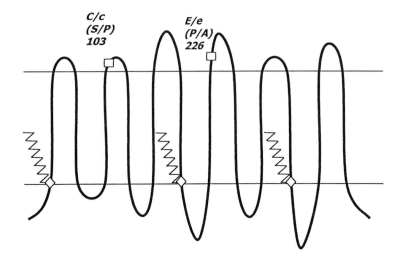

FIGURE 3–1. Diagram of the Rh peptides: RhD *(top)* and RhCE *(bottom)*, inserted in the cell membrane *(parallel horizontal lines)*. The amino acid sequence of both proteins predicts 12 transmembrane domains. Neither is glycosylated, but RhD has two sites of palmitoylation *(zigzag lines)* and RhCE has three. D-specific amino acids are marked with *open circles*. The predicted position of most is in transmembrane and cytoplasmic domains. E/e specificity appears to be conferred by a single amino acid substitution (P226A) encoded by exon 5 of the *RHCE* gene and C/c specificity by the S103P substitution encoded by exon 2. Four other amino acid differences are also associated with C/c polymorphism but do not appear to affect antigen characteristics: C16W encoded by exon 1 and I60L, S68N, and S103P all encoded by exon 2 of the *RhCE* gene.[23]

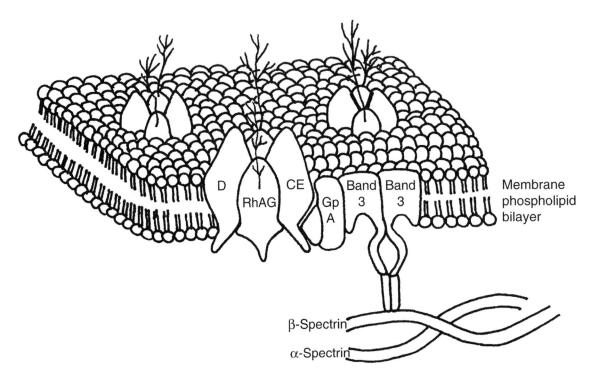

FIGURE 3–2. Diagram of the Rh complex and its interactions. The tetramer composed of two RhAg molecules and either two RhCE molecules (RhD negative) or one RhCE and one RhD (RhD positive) interacts with other membrane proteins and either directly or indirectly with the cytoskeleton. (Artist M. Swaminathan.)

in the *RHCE* gene, which appear to prevent cell surface expression of RhCE and reduce that of RhAG ("amorph type"). Homozygotes for mutations that prevent expression of RhAG have the more common "regulator type" or the Rh_{mod} phenotype. Despite normal transcription of Rh genes the proteins are not found at the cell surface.[38]

The *functional significance of the Rh complex* is indicated by the fact that Rh-deficient individuals have spherocytosis, stomatocytosis, and chronic hemolysis of varying severity. Their RBCs have altered ion transport and membrane composition and are partly or completely deficient in certain other membrane proteins including RhAG, CD47 (integrin associated protein), LW (Landsteiner-Wiener glycoprotein, ICAM-4), glycophorin B (which confers the Ss blood group), and Duffy Fy5 (Duffy antigen receptor for chemokines). These deficiencies suggest that Rh proteins form complexes with RhAG and other proteins and that the complexes fail to form if components are missing.[11, 20] There is also evidence for an interaction with the anion-exchange protein (band 3). However, many details of when, how, and why the Rh complexes form remain to be explained.

An important functional role for the Rh complex components is also suggested by their evolutionary conservation, particularly in regard to molecules similar to the *RHAG* gene family.[11, 37, 39] A likely function of the Rh complex was recently deduced because of sequence identity between Rh antigens and the yeast Mep proteins. This led to the discovery that RhAG and a second Rh related glycoprotein, RhGK (normally expressed in kidney cells) rescue Mep-deficient mutant cells grown on medium with low ammonium. These and related experiments indicate a probable role for Rh complexes in ammonium ion import and export across cell membranes.[40–42] However, the diversity of abnormalities in Rh-deficient RBCs raises the possibility of ancillary functions. There is also good evidence that the Rh complex is linked to the spectrin-based RBC membrane skeleton, and failure of this association may explain some of the dysfunction.[11]

In contrast to the common Rh-negative and very rare Rh deficiency states, *weak and partial D phenotypes* are fairly common (e.g., 0.2 to 1 percent of populations of European ancestry) and are caused by *RHD* coding region alterations that affect the number and antibody binding affinity of RhD sites per cell. The term "partial D" has been used to describe RBCs that react with some monoclonal anti-D antibodies and not others, whereas "weak D" has been used for RBCs with markedly reduced numbers of antigenic sites. However, it has been recognized that there is overlap in these phenotypes and the term "aberrant D" has been proposed for these plus the D_{el} phenotype[20, 43] (see Table 3–3).

The weak and partial D phenotypes can be significant in transfusion therapy and in pregnancy. For example, if blood donors with aberrant D are regarded as D negative, their blood can cause alloimmunization of D-negative recipients. On rare occasions, women with aberrant D can develop anti-D antibodies if they carry a D-positive child, or D negative women can develop antibodies if their babies have aberrant D. Some partial D phenotypes are also associated with distinct antigens.

The C antigen is most common in Southeast Asia, parts of South America, and the southern tip of Greenland, whereas the E antigen occurs most often in populations indigenous to parts of South America and Alaska.[25] The genetics underlying RhCc/Ee phenotypes also display more subtle variation than was once envisaged, and weak, partial, and variant antigen phenotypes have also been recognized. Internet databases are a good source of up-to-date information about the phenotype-genotype relationships for RhD and RhCE.[44, 45]

RhD ALLOIMMUNIZATION

HDN is a disease of the fetus caused by a maternal response to pregnancy. As such the pathogenesis can be considered in three stages: maternal alloimmunization, antibody transfer to the fetus, and fetal response.

Maternal Rh Sensitization

Maternal sensitization to Rh antigens can occur as a result of exposure to antigenically dissimilar fetal RBCs during pregnancy, as a result of therapeutic transfusion, or occasionally as a result of needle sharing.[46, 47] Transfusion has become a rare cause because compatibility testing for Rh antigens has been a routine practice for several decades. However, it accounts for a high proportion of sensitization to other blood group antigens. Furthermore, the need for emergency transfusion of Rh-positive blood to Rh-negative women is likely to remain an occasional cause of sensitization to RhD in locations where the Rh-negative phenotype is rare and Rh-negative blood is scarce.

Exposure to fetal antigens remains the most common cause of maternal antibodies to RhD. Although Chown first described maternal Rh immunization that occurred as a result of fetal transplacental hemorrhage (TPH), the test of Kleihauer and associates in 1957[48] was needed to show the incidence, size, and timing of these events and to show that most maternal Rh sensitization occurs this way.[49] The test, which depends on the resistance of fetal hemoglobin to acid elution (Fig. 3–3), can detect 1 fetal RBC in 200,000 adult RBCs, corresponding to a fraction of a milliliter in the circulating maternal blood volume. Bowman and colleagues[50] used this technique for two weekly tests in a group of 33 women and showed that 76 percent had had a TPH. The incidence increased as pregnancy progressed: 3 percent had a TPH in the first trimester, 12 percent in the second trimester, 45 percent in the third trimester, and 64 percent immediately after birth (Table 3–5). Subsequently, using flow cytometric techniques and DNA amplification of fetal sequences researchers have confirmed that fetal cells can be detected in maternal blood during all trimesters of most pregnancies.[51] Because the strategies for detection vary among studies and because of uncertainties about the persistence of various types of fetal cells in the maternal circulation, the volume and timing of this transplacental passage of fetal cells remain unclear. However, most of these "hemorrhages" are likely to be tiny.

Larger TPHs are uncommon; the amount of fetal blood exceeds 5 mL in less than 1 percent of gestations

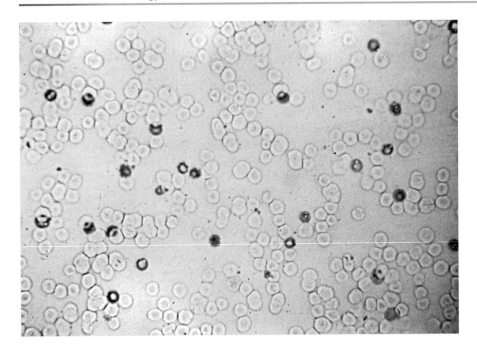

FIGURE 3–3. Acid elution technique of Kleihauer. Fetal RBCs stain with eosin and appear dark. Adult RBCs do not stain and appear as ghosts. This maternal blood smear contained 11.2 percent fetal RBCs, representing a transplacental hemorrhage of about 450 mL of blood. (From Bowman JM: Hemolytic disease of the newborn. In Conn HF, Conn RB (eds): Current Diagnosis 5. Philadelphia, WB Saunders, 1977, p 1103.)

TABLE 3–5. Prevalence of Fetal Transplacental Hemorrhage in 33 Women Delivering ABO-Compatible Babies

Gestation	No. with TPH (%)	No. without TPH (%)
First trimester	1 (3)	32 (97)
Second trimester	4 (12)	29 (88)
Third trimester	15 (45)	18 (55)
After delivery	21 (64)	12 (36)
At any time during pregnancy and delivery	25 (76)	8 (24)

TPH = transplacental hemorrhage.
From Bowman JM, Pollock JM, Penston LE: Feto-maternal transplacental hemorrhage during pregnancy and after delivery. Vox Sang 1986; 100:567. Copyright 1986 S. Karger AG, Basel, Switzerland.

and is greater than 30 mL in less than 0.25 percent.[50] However, certain obstetric situations increase the risk of significant TPH; these include antepartum hemorrhage, toxemia of pregnancy, external version,[52] cesarean section,[53, 54] and manual removal of the placenta.[55] Amniocentesis is risky in these patients, particularly if it is not carried out under ultrasound guidance (TPH occurred in 11.2 percent in one series).[56] Even with the use of ultrasound, TPH occurs in about 2.5 to 8.4 percent of patients after amniocentesis.[57, 58] Both spontaneous and therapeutic abortions are also associated with fetal TPH, and the Rh antigen is expressed early enough in gestation (by 30 to 45 days) for early pregnancy loss to present a risk.

All studies have focused on fetal cells in the maternal bloodstream, but the responses to submucosal, subcutaneous, or intramuscular antigen presentation differ from the responses to intravascular presentation. Therefore, deposition of fetal RBCs in these sites could be more immunogenic than with the intravascular route and could account for some of the propensity for Rh sensitization

after invasive procedures. If this is the case, techniques such as those developed to minimize exposure of the fetus to maternal blood in pregnant women who are human immunodeficiency virus positive[59] might be effective in reducing risk of blood group sensitization.

The Nature of Rh Sensitization

PRIMARY AND SECONDARY IMMUNE RESPONSES

In most subjects, the primary immune response develops slowly. In experimental Rh immunization of male volunteers, antibody responses are typically detected at 8 to 9 weeks, although they can occur at any time from 4 weeks to 6 months. Hemolytic anemia caused by anti-D has been detected as early as 10 days after a massive Rh-incompatible transfusion in a previously unsensitized patient.[60] A primary, often weak, IgM response will not affect the fetus even if it occurs before delivery in a sensitizing pregnancy, because IgM anti-D does not cross the placenta. However, IgG anti-D production usually ensues, especially if there is continued antigenic challenge, which accounts for fetuses with HDN in some women during their first Rh-positive pregnancy.

After a primary response has been invoked, subsequent exposure to Rh-positive RBCs produces a rapid increase in anti-D IgG, which can cross the placenta and affect the fetus. Repeated exposures can progressively increase the titer and change the characteristics (including IgG subclass distribution) of the Rh antibody, thus increasing the severity of Rh erythroblastosis in successive pregnancies.

DOSE OF Rh ANTIGEN NECESSARY TO PRODUCE Rh SENSITIZATION

Experiments using injection of Rh-positive blood into Rh-negative males show, not unexpectedly, that Rh sensitization depends on dose and repetition of exposure to the antigen. In one study, 50 percent of volunteers were immunized by 10 mL of Rh-positive blood. In other experiments, two thirds were immunized by five injections of 3.5 mL of Rh-positive RBCs, 80 percent by one injection of 0.5 mL of Rh-positive RBCs,[61] and 30 percent by repeated injections of 0.1 mL of RBCs.[62] About one third of subjects failed to be immunized after a 250-mL infusion, indicating that some subjects are anergic to RhD regardless of dose. Secondary immune responses may occur after exposure to much smaller amounts of RhD-positive RBCs (as little as 0.03 mL).

Studies during and immediately after pregnancy using the Kleihauer technique indicate that if the volume of TPH is always less than 0.1 mL of RBCs, the prevalence of Rh sensitization detectable up to 6 months after delivery is 3 percent,[62] whereas when volumes exceed 0.4 mL, the prevalence is 22 percent.[61] Nevertheless, because in 75 to 80 percent of pregnancies the amount of the TPH is always less than 0.1 mL, either small or undetectable TPHs or fetal cells deposited in other sites account for the majority of sensitizations.

INCIDENCE OF Rh SENSITIZATION

Rh sensitization has decreased markedly with the introduction of Rh immunoprophylaxis. In its absence, about 16 percent of Rh-negative women become sensitized in their first ABO-compatible Rh-positive pregnancy. Of these, about one half have detectable anti-D 6 months after delivery and in one half a rapid secondary response is seen in the next susceptible pregnancy, indicating that previous primary sensitization had occurred.[63] If sensitization does not occur, the risk in a second D-positive, ABO-compatible pregnancy is similar, and by the time an Rh-negative woman has completed her fifth ABO-compatible, Rh-positive pregnancy, the probability that she will be Rh sensitized is about 50 percent.

However, as parity increases and the number of women capable of an Rh immune response diminishes because they have already become immunized, the proportion of the remainder whose systems mount a primary immune response decreases because of a greater residual number of "nonresponders." About 25 to 30 percent of D-negative women are nonresponders, in that they do not become Rh sensitized, despite having many D-positive pregnancies; however, some may yet become Rh sensitized if they are exposed to a very large amount of Rh-positive blood. Immunologic tolerance can be induced by several different mechanisms and can depend on the context of antigen presentation to the immune system. It is not known which mechanisms of tolerance predominate in nonresponding Rh-negative women.

ABO incompatibility provides partial protection against Rh sensitization. Without anti-D immunoprophylaxis, the incidence of Rh sensitization 6 months after delivery of an ABO-incompatible, D-positive infant is 1.5 to 2 percent.[61] Bowman[63] suggested that this partial protection is due to rapid intravascular hemolysis of the ABO-incompatible, D-positive RBCs, with sequestration of D-positive cells in the stroma in the liver (an organ with poor antibody-forming potential) rather than in the spleen (the site of RBC sequestration when extravascular RBC

destruction occurs). However, it is not clear whether the immune system remains naïve with respect to the Rh antigens or tolerance is induced in these instances. Although ABO incompatibility provides substantial protection against the primary Rh immune response, it provides no protection against the secondary Rh immune response[64, 65] and should not influence management of an already affected pregnancy. Maternal HLA type does not have any consistent effect on risk of sensitization.[66, 67]

Other factors that influence the likelihood and severity of sensitization include fetal red cell phenotype, which affects the number and antigenicity of D antigen sites on fetal RBCs. For example, R1r (CDe/cde) cells, with only 9900 to 14,400 D antigen sites per cell are less immunogenic than R2r (cDE/cde) cells which have 14,000 to 16,000 sites.[68, 69] The possibility that Rh-negative women are exposed to RhD during their own fetal life has been considered. Scott and colleagues[69] performed a case-control study of sensitized Rh-negative primigravidas and showed not only that they had no excess of Rh-positive mothers but also that they did have evidence of TPH from their fetuses.[70] They also failed to find antibodies in 70 Rh-negative infants of Rh-positive mothers. These findings argue against the concept that sensitization is caused by exposure of the Rh-negative woman to Rh antigens via maternal-to-fetal hemorrhage while she herself was a fetus (the so-called "grandmother theory"). Nevertheless, convincing evidence of maternal-to-fetal hemorrhage has been found in other circumstances, and these events could explain the occasional presence of Rh antibodies in Rh-negative men who have never had a transfusion and occasional instances of Rh sensitization in women.

Rh sensitization during pregnancy, once considered to be rare, occurred in about 1.8 percent of susceptible pregnancies in one study.[71] The proportion of all occurrences of Rh sensitization that are attributable to antenatal sensitization now varies among studies, depending on the application of antenatal immunoprophylaxis.

The risk of Rh sensitization occurring after a threatened or spontaneous abortion is about 1.5 to 2 percent and increases the later in gestation that abortion occurs. The risk is greater after therapeutic abortion, being 4 to 5 percent.[72]

In summary, some general rules apply to Rh HDN. The probability of incompatible pregnancies is predictable from Hardy-Weinberg genetic principles, but the impact of HDN on a population will also depend on typical family size and on careful management of obstetric complications.[73] The risk should be low when good blood bank procedures, parsimonious approaches to blood transfusion, effective screening of pregnant women, and evidence-based administration of Rh immunoprophylaxis are applied. The disease should be uncommon or mild in a woman's first incompatible pregnancy, and 50 percent of the infants of heterozygous fathers and sensitized mothers should be safe. However, as pointed out by Kinnock and Liley,[64] the striking feature of pregnancies in severely isoimmunized women is their clinical variability. Because these women have often become sensitized despite the predictions of conventional wisdom, their care requires astute and conscientiousness management to ensure satisfactory outcomes.

Prevention of Rh Sensitization

The background to the prevention of Rh sensitization lies in the experiments of Von Dungern, at the beginning of the 20th century.[74] He showed that serum from rabbits that had previously been injected with ox cells prevented the development of antibodies to ox cells in a second group of rabbits. The partial protective effect of ABO incompatibility also suggested that antibody-mediated destruction of fetal RBCs could prevent maternal Rh sensitization. Finn et al[75] suggested a strategy of administering anti-D immunoprophylaxis, and it was put to the test almost simultaneously in New York[76] and Liverpool[77] and shortly thereafter in Winnipeg.[62] Because anti-RhD immunoglobulin was strikingly successful in preventing sensitization in males, clinical trials were then undertaken in which Rh-negative, unsensitized women were given anti-D intramuscularly after delivery of an Rh-positive infant.[78–80] The licensing of Rh immune globulin in 1968 profoundly influenced the prevalence of Rh sensitization. Despite its success, the exact mechanism of action of anti-D remains elusive.[81, 82]

The level of evidence for the use of postpartum anti-D immunoprophylaxis is high. A recent systematic review collated data from the six eligible trials involving more than 10,000 women that compared postpartum anti-D prophylaxis with no treatment or placebo. The conclusion was that anti-D prophylaxis strikingly lowered the incidence of RhD alloimmunization 6 months after birth (relative risk 0.04, 95 percent confidence interval 0.02 to 0.06) and in a subsequent pregnancy (relative risk 0.12, 95 percent confidence interval 0.07 to 0.23). These benefits were seen regardless of the ABO status of the mother and baby, when anti-D was given within 72 hours of birth. Higher doses (up to 200 µg) were more effective than lower doses (up to 50 µg) in preventing RhD alloimmunization in a subsequent pregnancy.[83] The usual dose after full-term delivery in the United States is 300 µg, although elsewhere lower doses are administered with almost equivalent effectiveness. Postpartum prophylaxis is recommended whenever a weak D- or D-positive infant is born to an unsensitized D-negative mother.[84]

After postnatal immunoprophylaxis, the risk of RhD alloimmunization during or immediately after a first pregnancy is about 1.5 percent. Administration of 100 µg (500 IU) of anti-D at 28 and 34 weeks' gestation to women in their first pregnancy can reduce this risk to about 0.2 percent, meaning that fewer women will have D antibodies in their next pregnancy.[85] Most current guidelines[84, 86–88] therefore recommend routine administration of Rh immunoglobulin to all D-negative pregnant women in the early and mid third trimester unless the father of the fetus is known and can be shown conclusively to be Rh negative. This combined antenatal and postnatal prophylaxis will prevent 96 percent of RhD isoimmunization.[84] The level of evidence is lower, but the current recommendation is to also offer prophylaxis to weak D-positive women. Additional or earlier doses (depending on the timing and circumstances) for those weak D-positive or D-negative women who are not already sensitized and who are likely to or do abort or who are undergoing amniocentesis, chorionic villus sampling, or other relevant procedures may further reduce the risk of sensitization. Small amounts of anti-D cross the placenta and cause a weakly positive antiglobulin test, but there are no apparent adverse effects on the infant.[89] It is important to note that results of maternal antibody screening tests done near term may be positive (albeit usually at low titer) after anti-D administration during pregnancy, but under the current guidelines these results should not preclude administration of postnatal anti-D.

About 1 in 400 woman will have a fetal-to-maternal TPH of greater than 30 mL of fetal blood at the time of delivery. Prevention of Rh sensitization in the presence of such a large dose of antigen requires prompt assessment (by the Kleihauer-Betke test or flow cytometry) and administration of a titrated dose of anti-D.[88] Pediatricians must be aware of this possibility and promptly notify their obstetric colleagues of any suspected anemia or blood loss in the newborn infant of an Rh-negative mother.

Certain knowledge of Rh negativity in the biologic father of the fetus can obviate the need for immunoprophylaxis. However, this information should be established with a very high degree of certainty because of the potential for severe consequences in a future pregnancy in case of error.[88]

Reports from numerous countries document the reduction in RhD HDN as a result of anti-D immunoglobulin. Nevertheless, there is no room for complacency, because 30 to 40 percent of the reduction in incidence of HDN over recent decades has been attributed to decreased family size, rather than to administration of anti-D.[90] Chavez and colleagues[91] noted that the incidence of Rh sensitization in the United States is three times the rate predicted if anti-D were always applied according to guidelines issued by the American College of Obstetricians and Gynecologists. The failure of the anti-D program to completely abolish RhD HDN can be partly attributed to noncompliance with guidelines. In addition, recommendations for additional doses during pregnancy have led to scarcity of anti-D.[92] These problems are even greater in poorer countries. Giving booster doses to donors, using carefully screened RhD-positive RBCs, has been a necessity as the number of suitable sensitized donors decreases, but this practice requires extreme care to protect both the donor and eventual recipients. The distribution of the Rh-negative phenotype may increase as a result of migration. As with use of any blood product, issues of safety cannot be disregarded.[93] All these forces threaten the supply of anti-D. Monoclonal preparations, which could, in principle, replace the current polyclonal anti-D, thereby resolving problems of availability and safety, have been under development in recent years. However, although monoclonal antibodies have significant diagnostic and research applications, they are not yet available for prophylaxis against sensitization.[94]

Overall, it is unlikely that the incidence of Rh HDN will ever return to the levels seen in previous generations, but it is also not likely to be abolished altogether.

Pathogenesis of Rh Hemolytic Disease

Erythropoiesis begins in the yolk sac by the third week of gestation, and Rh antigen is expressed by the sixth week. By 6 to 8 weeks' gestation, the liver replaces the yolk sac as the main site of RBC production. Normally, erythropoiesis then diminishes in the liver and takes place nearly entirely in the bone marrow by the late third trimester of pregnancy.[95] In the presence of fetal anemia due either to hemolysis or to blood loss, erythropoiesis can persist in the liver and spleen and may be extreme.

The fundamental cause of erythroblastosis is maternal D IgG coating of D-positive fetal RBCs, leading to their destruction. The subsequent fetal anemia stimulates erythropoiesis via the production of erythropoietin and other erythroid growth factors. When fetal marrow RBC production cannot keep up with RBC destruction, extramedullary erythropoiesis can be found in other organs including the liver and in more severe conditions also in the spleen, kidneys, skin, intestines, and adrenal glands. Hepatosplenomegaly is a hallmark of erythroblastosis fetalis.

In the presence of extramedullary erythropoiesis, immature nucleated RBCs, from normoblasts to early erythroblasts (Fig. 3–4), are poured into the circulation.

SEVERITY OF Rh HEMOLYTIC DISEASE

Degrees of Severity

For purposes of audit, research, and planning of treatment, degrees of severity of HDN have been used since the 1950s.

In general, fetuses and infants with *mild HDN* have had antibody-coated RBCs, yielding positive results on a direct antiglobulin (Coombs') test, but they have no anemia or anemia that is well-compensated for *in utero* and after birth and do not require exchange transfusion to prevent bilirubin toxicity. This group comprised about one half of affected fetuses (but now includes a higher proportion of infants as a result of effective intrauterine treatment). Nearly all survive and do well without invasive treatment.

Moderately affected fetuses are at risk of neural toxicity from bilirubin if they do not receive treatment. They are likely to have signs of anemia *in utero* and *ex utero* but are not severely acidotic or hydropic. Peripheral blood typically shows polychromasia, anisocytosis, and reticulocytosis, although these can be suppressed by intrauterine treatment. Maternal clearance copes with the products of hemolysis, and the fetus is usually born in good condition at or near term. This category comprises about one third of fetuses, but again now includes a higher proportion newborn infants as a result of fetal treatment. Moderately affected neonates do require vigilant neonatal management, including intensive phototherapy or exchange transfusion to manage jaundice.

Severely affected fetuses have hydrops or hydrops is impending, and they would die before, during, or after birth unless managed intensively. Untreated, one half develop hydrops between 18 and 34 weeks' gestation and the other one half between 34 and 40 weeks' gestation. Polyhydramnios usually occurs early in the course of or precedes the development of hydrops. Ascites and pleural and pericardial effusions develop. In infants with the most extreme conditions, compression hypoplasia of the lungs makes gas exchange after birth precarious.

When these categories of disease were first devised, severe fetal disease predicted severe neonatal disease. However, as effective fetal and neonatal interventions are introduced and worthless or outdated treatments are discarded, the predictions must be updated. For example, an anemic but not hydropic neonate who met previous criteria for exchange transfusion may now be managed effectively with intensive phototherapy and would therefore be regarded as having mild rather than moderate disease. Similarly, a fetus with early development of hydrops (severe fetal HDN) may respond well to one or more intrauterine transfusions and therefore be born with mild neonatal disease and yet still have severe late anemia that is as much a consequence of the effective intrauterine treatment as of the underlying disease. A suggested update to the working definitions that separates the criteria into epochs and includes a summary of implications for practice is given in Table 3–6.

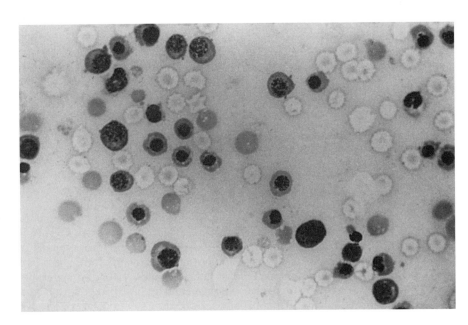

FIGURE 3–4. Cord blood of baby with severe Rh erythroblastosis fetalis who required multiple fetal transfusions and exchange transfusions. The smear was treated by Kleihauer's technique with Wright's staining. Note the adult donor ghost red blood cells (RBCs), dark fetal RBCs, and early fetal erythroid series from erythroblasts through to normoblasts. (From Bowman JM: The management of Rh-isoimmunization. Obstet Gynecol 1978; 52:1. Reprinted with permission from The American College of Obstetricians and Gynecologists.)

TABLE 3–6. Degrees of Severity of Rh Hemolytic Disease of the Fetus and Newborn[225]

Severity	Mild	Moderate	Severe
IN FETUS			
Historical proportion of Rh HDN before intrauterine therapy was available	~50%	25–30%	20–25%
Likely history in previous siblings	No exchange	Exchange unless *in utero* treatment	Death unless *in utero* treatment
Maternal anti-D titer	<1:64	>1:64	>1:64
Ultrasound abnormalities	None	Altered patterns of flow in fetal vessels, polyhydramnios	Hydrops, portal hypertension, ascites and other effusions
IN NEONATE			
Clinical condition at birth	Normal	Moderately ill	Hydrops
Hemoglobin cord	No anemia	Mild, or moderate anemia HgB >0.6 multiples of mean (MoM) for gestation	Severe, symptomatic anemia <0.6 MoM
Hemoglobin nadir	Transfusion not needed	At risk for symptomic anemia`	Risk of death unless transfusion
Bilirubin cord	<3.5 mg/dL (≈70 μmol/L)	>3.5 mg/dL (≈70 μmol/L)	>3.5 mg/dL (≈70 μmol/L)
Bilirubin peak	Term: <20 mg/dL (~380 μmol/L) Premature: Lower levels depending on prematurity	Term: >20 mg/dL (~380 μmol/L) Premature: lower levels depending on prematurity	Rate of RBC destruction depends on (low) hemoglobin B; peak bilirubin is variable, but toxicity increased
Phototherapy	If bilirubin increases faster than 0.4–0.5 mg/dL/hr; lower threshold for premature infants	If bilirubin increases faster than 0.4–0.5 mg/dL/hr; lower threshold for premature infants	Immediate, double, pending measurement of bilirubin increase
"Early" exchange	No	If rate of increase of bilirubin >0.8–1 mg/dL/hr; lower threshold for premature infants	Yes
"Late" exchange	If bilirubin > exchange level	If bilirubin ≥ exchange level	If bilirubin approaching exchange level
Heme oxygenase inhibition	Unnecessary—number needed to treat to avoid exchange will be high	In context of well-designed clinical trials	In clinical trial to avert late exchange; unlikely to allow avoidance of early exchange
Intravenous immunoglobulin	Unnecessary—number needed to treat to avoid exchange will be high	In context of well-designed clinical trials	In clinical trial to avert late exchange; unlikely to allow avoidance of early exchange
Phenobarbital	No	No	No clear benefit if optimal phototherapy
Erythropoietin for late anemia	No	In context of well-designed clinical trials	In context of well-designed clinical trials

Pathogenesis of Hydrops

Hydrops in HDN was originally attributed to fetal heart failure, but other factors probably play a role. Although heart failure does occur in some fetuses and in others if they live long enough (Fig. 3–5), a significant number of hydropic infants are not hypervolemic or in heart failure at birth.[96]

With severe hemolysis and progressively greater extramedullary erythropoiesis, the hepatic architecture and circulation are distorted by the islets of erythropoiesis. It has been suggested that this could result in portal and umbilical venous obstruction and portal hypertension. Impairment of umbilical venous return would exacerbate the fetal tissue hypoxia caused by anemia and explain the placental edema that is usually seen in severe hydrops. The placental edema, by increasing the placental barrier to gas exchange, could then impair oxygen delivery even more.

Hypoalbuminemia is a common feature, but the mechanism has not been explained. It could be caused by a greater volume of distribution for albumin or reversion to α-fetoprotein expression rather than failure of hepatic synthesis.

The theory that liver distortion and dysfunction are at least as important as heart failure in the pathogenesis of hydrops fetalis could explain why hydrops is not always accompanied by hypervolemia or even anemia.[96] Support for the suggestion that portal hypertension is present is provided by ultrasound assessment of waveforms in the portal venous system.[97]

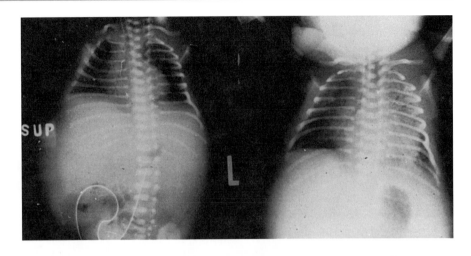

FIGURE 3–5. Radiograph of a hydropic newborn at birth and 6 hours later after exchange transfusion. Note the small size of the heart at the time of birth and the very marked increase in heart size and evidence of pulmonary congestion denoting heart failure 6 hours later. The fetus has extreme ascites. (From Bowman JM: Blood-group incompatibilities. In Iffy L, Kaminetzky HA (eds): Principles and Practice of Obstetrics and Perinatology. New York, John Wiley & Sons, 1981, p 1203. © Leslie Iffy, MD, Newark, NJ.)

The mechanisms that lead to hydrops, both in anemic fetuses and in nonanemic fetuses with "nonimmune" hydrops, remain poorly understood. Various inflammatory mediators could play a role but have not been examined. Genes that are regulated by hypoxia include those for vascular endothelial growth factor and other molecules involved in capillary morphogenesis. Depending on the pattern of expression, these molecules can markedly affect capillary permeability and could also play a role.

Factors Affecting the Severity of HDN

If a sensitized mother is pregnant with an Rh-incompatible fetus, a number of factors influence the severity of disease in the fetus. These factors include placental transfer of antibody, antibody characteristics, antigen characteristics, state of maturation of the fetal spleen, and resilience of fetal erythropoiesis.

TRANSFER OF ANTIBODY TO THE FETUS

All four IgG subclasses are transported across the placenta, via FcRn receptor–mediated endocytosis and then exocytosis.[98–100] The fetal-to-maternal ratio for total IgG is approximately 0.4 at 28 weeks' gestation and increases to 1.4 at term,[101] but fetal levels of IgG1 are close to maternal levels by 17 to 20 weeks' gestation.[102] The efficiency of placental transport of antibody may be an important factor in the severity of Rh HDN, and reduced IgG transport can result in unexpectedly mild disease.[103]

MECHANISM OF RED BLOOD CELL HEMOLYSIS

When anti-RBC antibodies bind complement and are present in high concentrations (as with transfusion reactions to ABO-incompatible blood in adults), RBC extravascular destruction occurs and may cause a clinically severe reaction including hemoglobinemia, shock, and disseminated intravascular coagulopathy. Products of RBC destruction are cleared predominantly by the liver.

When antibodies do not fix complement, as is typical with anti-D in the fetus and neonate, the mechanisms of hemolysis are more subtle but, in the end, equally destructive. Three Fc receptor–mediated pathways have been implicated in the destruction of opsonized RBCs:

direct phagocytosis, phagocytic damage leading to later lysis, and killer cell–mediated damage. When anti-D becomes concentrated on the membrane of RhD-positive RBCs, the RBCs adhere to macrophages and form rosettes. This occurs particularly in the red pulp of the spleen, where RBCs and macrophages come into close apposition. The phagocytic cell can then destroy the RBC or damage and deplete the membrane, causing loss of RBC deformability. If the RBC escapes being consumed by the macrophage, its membrane is damaged, and its osmotic fragility and likelihood of lysis are greater (Fig. 3–6).

Antibody-dependent cellular cytotoxicity (ADCC) probably also accounts for the destruction of some RBCs.[104] Large granular "K cells" (natural killer lymphocytes) or myeloid cells (polymorphonuclear leukocytes and monocytes) bind antibody-labeled cells and release lysosomal enzymes and perforin, causing lysis.

Hemolysis also requires a competent system of phagocytic cells in the fetus. The clinical manifestations of the disease suggest that maturation is sufficient as early as the mid-second trimester.

ANTIBODY SPECIFICITY AND SEVERITY OF HEMOLYTIC DISEASE

Antigen characteristics, including details of antibody distribution, density, and structure, all affect risk for HDN; and these have been reviewed by Hadley.[105] Antibodies with the potential to cause HDN generally recognize antigens restricted to erythroid cells (such as Rh antigens) rather than those with a wider tissue distribution (such as A and B antigens, found on many cell types). The antigens must be expressed in the fetus and neonate. Thus antibodies to Kell and Rh antigens, which are expressed early in fetal life, cause severe HDN, whereas antibodies to Lewis antigens, which are not synthesized in erythrocyte progenitors, never cause HDN. The circulating glycosphingolipids carrying the antigenic Le^a or Le^b epitopes generally only adsorb to the erythrocyte membrane during postnatal life. Lewis antibodies are also usually IgM. Lewis is the only human blood group system that has never been reported to cause HDN of any severity.

Antigen density is also an important factor. Within the Rh system, even in the presence of high maternal anti-D

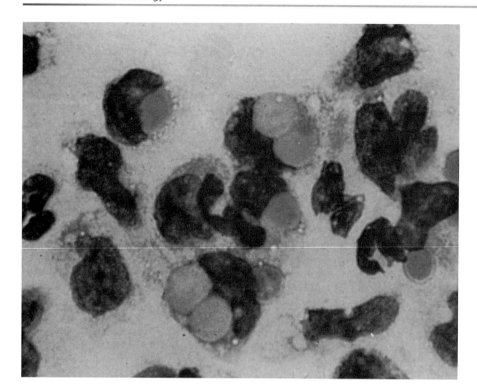

FIGURE 3–6. A Rebuck skin window preparation in which anti-D–sensitized erythrocytes have been ingested by macrophages. Note that neutrophil erythrophagocytosis is not seen. (From Zipursky A, Bowman JM: Isoimmune hemolytic disease. In Nathan DG, Oski FA (eds): Hematology of Infancy and Childhood, 4th ed. Philadelphia, WB Saunders, 1993, p 53.)

titers, fetuses with aberrant D phenotypes are unlikely to be severely affected. The density of several other antigens, including A and B and the Lutheran antigens,[106] is developmentally regulated, and antigen density on immature RBCs limits the severity of hemolysis.

Antigen structure may also play a role, with some antigens being more capable of promoting recognition of RBCs by phagocytic cells.

Antibody characteristics also play a role in determining the severity of HDN. IgG subclasses bind different classes of Fc receptors, although it has not yet been established conclusively which receptors are involved in RBC destruction *in vivo*. Fc receptor polymorphisms (analogous to an *FcRII* allele found in whites, which binds IgG2 very avidly and may play a role in ABO HDN) may yet be found to account for some of the heterogeneity of Rh HDN.[105]

Whereas anti-A and anti-B antibodies are predominantly IgG2, IgG1 and IgG3 anti-D antibodies tend to predominate in Rh-sensitized women.[107–110] They are often present in combination.

The capacity of RBC-bound IgG3 antibodies to bind to Fc receptors of monocytes is greater than that of IgG1 antibodies. Threshold levels of antibody binding for rosette formation *in vitro* were approximately 1000 IgG3 or 2000 IgG1 molecules per RBC.[111] Both can promote phagocytosis, but their relative potencies depend on circumstances. IgG3 usually causes more efficient lysis by monocytes than does IgG1.[112–114] Clearance of Rh-positive RBCs is caused by fewer molecules of IgG3 anti-D than of IgG1 anti-D.[115] However, the relationship of these factors to HDN is still unclear. Studies of maternal IgG subclasses do not indicate a clear relationship between subclass distribution and disease severity.[116]

HLA antibodies have been found in sera of some women who have infants with mild HDN despite high antibody levels. The HLA antibodies may block antibody-antigen interactions on the macrophage membrane.[105]

ANTIBODY DETECTION

ABO and RhD typing plus antibody screening is recommended at the first prenatal visit, including visits for elective abortion, in all pregnancies. A history of prior pregnancies and blood transfusions should also be taken. If the blood group is D-negative or weak D, another antibody screening is recommended at 24 to 28 weeks' gestation, before administration of anti-D immunoprophylaxis. If an alloantibody is detected at a low titer, screening is usually repeated at regular intervals to detect any increase. There are a variety of methods for assessing maternal antibodies, some that are better suited for screening methods and some that are more useful for predicting severity of disease.[105]

Manual Methods

Rh-positive RBCs suspended in isotonic *saline* are agglutinated only by IgM anti-D, because although IgG anti-D can bind to antigen, it cannot bridge the gap between RBCs suspended in saline. Therefore, a maternal serum sample containing only IgG anti-D does not agglutinate Rh-positive RBCs suspended in saline. Addition of *albumin* lowers the negative electrical potential of the RBC membrane, and IgG anti-D can then bridge the smaller gaps between the RBCs.[117] Because IgM anti-D also agglutinates Rh-positive RBCs suspended in albumin, if saline and albumin titers are similar, the albumin titer does not accurately assess IgG anti-D. Addition of dithiothreitol disrupts IgM sulfhydryl bonds and reveals the true IgG anti-D titer. Albumin methods have been surpassed but are described to clarify the earlier literature that refers to them.

Coombs' serum is an anti-human globulin produced by immunizing another species.[6] Rh-positive RBCs are incubated, with the serum being tested for the presence of anti-D. If anti-D is present in the serum, it adheres to the Rh-positive RBC membrane. The RBCs are then washed to remove nonadherent human protein and suspended in Coombs' serum. If the RBCs are coated with anti-D, they are agglutinated by the antibodies to human immunoglobulin (positive test result). The reciprocal of the highest dilution of maternal serum that produces agglutination is the *indirect antiglobulin titer*.

Incubation of RBCs with enzymes such as papain, trypsin, and bromelin reduces the electrical potential of the RBC membranes, allowing agglutination of Rh-positive cells by IgG anti-D even in saline. Enzyme screening methods are the most sensitive manual techniques available for detecting Rh sensitization, but they detect many antibodies that have no clinical significance.[118]

These manual methods have the advantages of sensitivity and flexibility, but the correlation between antibody titer and disease severity is poor.

Automated Analysis

Autoanalyzer methods have been developed and refined for more efficient and reproducible detection and quantitation of Rh and other antibodies.[119–121] Autoanalyzer techniques are very sensitive, and the finding of an Rh antibody detected only by an Autoanalyzer method and not by any manual method must be viewed with skepticism. In 85 percent of instances, if a maternal serum Rh antibody was identified by Autoanalyzer only and the identification was not confirmed by other methods, the mother may not be truly Rh immunized. Gel and solid-phase assays have also been developed.[122–125]

PREDICTION OF FETAL HEMOLYTIC DISEASE

Once sensitization is detected, subsequent investigative and treatment measures are inconvenient for the mother and have some risk for the fetus. To refine the estimation of risk, many or all the following may need to be considered.

Fetal blood type is determined by

- Paternal blood typing
- Fetal blood typing

Severity of disease is predicted by

- History indicating the severity of HDN in previous infants
- Maternal antibody titers
- Cell-mediated maternal antibody functional assays
- Amniotic fluid spectrophotometry
- Fetal ultrasound
- Percutaneous fetal blood sampling

Determination of Fetal Blood Type

PATERNAL BLOOD TYPING

In some instances paternal blood typing can indicate that the baby has no risk for HDN. This situation occurs if the father is Rh negative and the mother was sensitized not by his offspring but by those of a previous partner or by transfusion. If the father is predicted to be heterozygous, there is a chance that the fetus may be completely unaffected regardless of the maternal antibody titer. In predominantly white populations, about 56 percent of Rh-positive individuals are heterozygous. It is important not to place too much weight on heterozygosity when it is present. One half of the offspring of a heterozygous father should be Rh negative, but to come reliably ($P = 0.95$) within 20 percent of this ideal state, it can be deduced statistically that each mother would have to have about 30 pregnancies.[64]

Historically, paternal genotype was estimated by determination of the father's RhCE type, used in combination with information about distribution of Rh phenotypes in different racial groups. Molecular genetic techniques now allow more direct determination of genotype and correlation with phenotype.

FETAL BLOOD TYPING

Fetal Rh typing, either by traditional antigen typing or genotyping using DNA amplification techniques, is becoming increasingly feasible. It can be an important technique if paternity is uncertain or the father is heterozygous.

Molecular methods are now used routinely in many locations to detect fetal *RHD, RHCE, KEL, FY,* and *JK* genes in fetal DNA obtained by amniocentesis, or even from maternal blood [126–133] These tests have the potential to reduce the need for assessment throughout the pregnancy, including the need for other invasive tests, and to avert the need for anti-D administration during some pregnancies. Single cell preimplantation diagnosis has also been described.[134]

The genetic diversity of the Rh blood group system outlined in an earlier section of this chapter provides an important reminder to use caution in choosing primers that minimize false-positive and false-negative test results and to keep in mind the fact that genotype does not always obviously predict phenotype. The prevalence of *RHD-RHCE* hybrids and partially intact but functionally inert *RH* genes in certain populations can render useless tests designed for application in whites. Current recommendations include amplifying at least two diagnostic sites, preferably checking the correlation between parents' genotype and phenotype in parallel, and using the tests with a good understanding of the typical genotypes in the populations for which they were developed and to which they are being applied.[22, 127, 132, 135]

Bennett and associates[136] showed that RhD genotyping of amniotic and chorionic cells agrees with serologic and tissue typing. Thus, either chorionic villus sampling (CVS) or amniocentesis can be used for typing of the fetus. However, CVS is usually avoided because of the risk of exacerbating sensitization. Diagnosis using maternal blood samples has the advantages that their acquisition does not have any risk for the fetus and that there is no risk of increasing maternal exposure to fetal antigens and consequently elevating the mother's antibody titer.[132] Several types of fetal cells can be identified in maternal blood in early gestation and used for other diagnostic purposes. However, they may not present a reliable solution to early, noninvasive Rh typing of the fetus because of their rarity and the fact that in searching for evidence of a deletion of *RHD*, the need to have a good positive control value to identify false-negative results is critical. No ideal positive control value has yet been found. Lo[131, 137] has reported that analysis of fetal DNA in maternal serum or plasma can provide reliable results in the first trimester.

In most pregnancies, the initial invasive procedure to determine fetal blood type can wait until 18 to 20 weeks' gestation, because it is rare for fetuses to be severely affected before then, and intervention to treat the severely affected fetus is difficult. However, if there is a history of a previous fetus severely affected in the second trimester or ultrasound evidence of early fetal anemia, earlier diagnosis is warranted.

Prediction of Severity of Disease

The relative roles of a variety of methods for assessing the severity of hemolytic disease in the fetus are still evolving.[138]

PREGNANCY HISTORY

Although it is usually true that the severity of HDN remains the same or increases during subsequent affected pregnancies, the disease sometimes becomes less severe. If a previous baby was hydropic, a subsequent affected fetus has a 90 percent, but not a 100 percent, chance of developing hydrops. If hydrops is going to develop, it does so usually at the same gestation or earlier, but occasionally it develops later. In a first D-sensitized pregnancy, with no prior history of HDN, there is an 8 to 10 percent probability that hydrops will develop. If a mother has a prior history of having a fetus with hydrops and the father is heterozygous for the offending antigen, the fetus may be D negative and completely unaffected or D positive and very severely affected, creating a dilemma that requires resolution, usually by fetal typing.

MATERNAL ANTIBODY TITERS

Although antibody titrations carried out in the same laboratory by the same experienced personnel using the same methods and test cells are reproducible and do give the physician some indication of risk, their predictive value is inadequate to guide invasive fetal treatment. The autoanalyzer technique provides somewhat better prediction of the severity of HDN than manual methods, but the two approaches have not been compared rigorously. Hadley[105] has recommended that whereas many laboratories can and should undertake screening for alloantibodies, antibody quantitation is best limited to regional centers with proven reliability. Ideally, these laboratories will also have programs auditing the outcomes of

pregnancies in which antibodies have been detected. This will lead over time to the recognition of a critical titer, below which no cases of severe disease have occurred, allowing targeting of more extensive and invasive tests to those with titers above the threshold. However, the follow-up needed is laborious and prone to ascertainment bias and can threaten patient privacy. Generally, if the obstetric history is good, low titers (≤1:16 by manual methods or <5 IU/mL [1 µg/mL] by Autoanalyzer) that increase slowly or not at all are reassuring and indicate continued surveillance using antibody titers and ultrasound.

Although rising titers suggest increasing risk to the fetus, it has not been possible, even with Autoanalyzer methods, to establish a titer above which the fetus must be sensitized,[139, 140] and sometimes, antibody levels increase significantly (but presumably nonspecifically) despite the presence of a compatible and therefore unaffected fetus. Nevertheless, in the presence of very high or rising titers, fetal assessment becomes urgent.

MATERNAL ANTIBODY FUNCTIONAL ASSAYS

Various functional assays that measure the ability of maternal antibody to promote interactions between RBC and monocytes or K cells have been developed.[141] These assays include the monocyte monolayer assay,[109, 142] the ADCC assay using lymphocytes[143] or monocytes,[144] and monocyte chemiluminescence.[111]

Each assay has its proponents, and the advantages and limitations have been reviewed.[105, 145] Hadley and associates[122] compared monocyte chemiluminescence, K-cell lymphocyte ADCC, monocyte-macrophage ADCC, and a rosette assay using U937 cells. They found that monocyte chemiluminescence and monocyte ADCC functional assays predicted severity of disease better than rosette assay with U937 cells and K-lymphocyte ADCC. Similarly, Zupanska and colleagues[109] found that the results of a monocyte-based assay (monocyte monolayer assay) correlated better with the clinical severity of hemolytic disease than did the results of rosette assays using lymphocytes. A survey of nine European laboratories that carried out functional assays, testing sera from mothers delivering babies with varying degrees of HDN, revealed correct results as follows: ADCC (monocytes), 60 percent; ADCC (lymphocytes), 57 percent; chemiluminescence, 51 percent; and rosetting and phagocytosis with peripheral monocytes, 41 percent (with U937 cells or cultured macrophages, 32 percent).[147] However, a more recent report has cast doubt on the ability of the monocyte-macrophage assay to predict the severity of HDN.[148]

Overall, when taken in conjunction with ultrasonography, consideration of the outcomes of previous pregnancies, and antibody quantitation, bioassays are somewhat useful in helping to weigh the risks of invasive procedures in women with borderline levels of alloantibodies, because they seem to be better for predicting mild rather than severe disease. However, there is no consensus that bioassays reduce the number of amniocenteses and cordocenteses, and it is important to note that most published reports involve relatively small numbers of subjects. These tests should be carried out in reference laboratories that perform them regularly and validate them carefully.

Because they are measuring characteristics of the antibody, not the fetal antigen, bioassays are of no use in excluding an antigen-negative, unaffected fetus.

AMNIOTIC FLUID SPECTROPHOTOMETRY

Bevis[149] showed that bilirubin could be found in the amniotic fluid of infants with HDN, and in 1961, Liley[150] plotted fetal outcomes by gestation and results of amniotic fluid spectrophotometry, thus devising a test that still plays a role in managing fetal hemolytic disease. Liley used the ΔOD_{450} reading (the deviation from linearity at 450 nm due to the absorption spectrum of bilirubin) as a measurement of the amniotic fluid bilirubin level (Fig. 3–7). Readings in zone I indicate either no disease or no anemia at the time of testing but reflect a 10 percent chance that exchange transfusion will be needed. Readings in zone II indicate moderate disease that becomes more severe as readings approach the zone III boundary. Readings falling into very high zone II or zone III indicate severe disease. Hydrops is present or will develop within 7 to 10 days. When serial ΔOD_{450} measurements are taken, the overall accuracy of prediction of hemolytic disease with the amniotic fluid technique is 95 percent. Accuracy is higher in the third trimester than in the second trimester. Because the graphs were developed before intervention at earlier than 27 weeks' gestation was

contemplated, zone boundaries in the second trimester were not defined. The Liley zone boundaries have subsequently been modified by inclining them downward before 24 weeks' gestation because of the observation that ΔOD_{450} readings peak at 23 to 24 weeks' gestation in pregnancies unaffected by HDN.[151-154] The division lines for Queenan's chart are lower at all gestations than those of Liley's system. Although it has been suggested that Queenan's modification may result in overestimation of severity, leading to too many interventions,[156] others have concluded that a more conservative approach is appropriate now that safer and more effective intervention is available.[157] Direct fetal blood sampling has reduced but not abolished the need for assessment by amniocentesis. Because the skills and technology needed to perform amniocentesis are more widely available, it can be used to guide timing of referral to a center of excellence in management of the disease and to assess severity when factors such as fetal and placental position complicate fetal umbilical blood sampling.

Amniocentesis has risks, although good ultrasound guidance has improved the safety and reliability considerably. Among the other known risks, blood in the amniotic fluid can obscure the 450-nm peak, making the fluid worthless for predicting the severity of hemolytic disease and complicating the determination of fetal genotype. Ultrasound guidance has reduced this risk from about 10

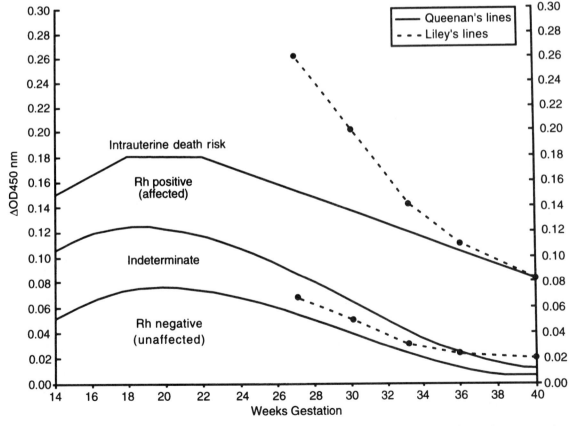

FIGURE 3–7. Superimposed Queenan and Liley charts of the deviation of absorbance at a wavelength of 450 nm (ΔOD_{450}) versus gestation. Liley's lines began at 27 weeks, and they were rectilinear when shown on a log-linear plot.[150] They were subsequently extrapolated back to 20 weeks.[151] Queenan's chart demonstrates that the lines should deflect downward in the early second trimester.[154] However, the division lines for Queenan's chart are lower at all gestations and may overestimate risk in some fetuses. Current practice is to use other indicators in addition to amniotic fluid results in determining the need and timing for intrauterine treatment. (From Scott F, Chan FY: Assessment of the clinical usefulness of the 'Queenan' chart versus the 'Liley' chart in predicting severity of rhesus iso-immunization. Prenat Diagn 1998; 18:1143–1148.)

percent to 2.5 percent. Increases in antibody titer occur after some amniocenteses, although the risk is reported to be lower than that after umbilical blood sampling.[56, 57]

ULTRASOUND ASSESSMENT

The development of obstetric ultrasonography in the late 1970s was a major advance in the management of maternal blood group alloimmunization. Ultrasound allows estimation of placental and hepatic size and determination of the presence or absence of polyhydramnios, edema, ascites, and other effusions. It has increased the safety of amniocentesis and intraperitoneal transfusion and is essential for umbilical blood sampling and intravascular fetal transfusions.

Although ultrasound was previously said to be of little use in assessing the severity of disease until hydrops had developed, assessment of flow velocities in major fetal vessels has now been shown by several groups to be very reliable for detecting significant fetal anemia.[97, 158–165] Middle cerebral artery velocimetry is the most extensively used assessment. As with any critical test, responsible practitioners should audit outcomes and refine their judgments according to them, but when skills to perform it are available, ultrasound has become the method of choice in monitoring women with blood group-sensitized pregnancies and in the planning and timing of invasive fetal sampling, fetal treatment, and delivery.

PERCUTANEOUS FETAL BLOOD SAMPLING

With the development of sophisticated ultrasound equipment and the availability of perinatologists skilled in its use, percutaneous fetal umbilical blood sampling became feasible in the mid-1980s[166] (Fig. 3–9). This procedure allows direct diagnosis of fetal blood type, anemia, and acidosis. It provides the "gold standard" for diagnosis of fetal anemia against which the accuracy of other assessment techniques can be measured. The procedure does carry with it a likelihood of fetal-to-maternal hemorrhage[167] and a small risk of mortality.[166] Generally, it should be reserved for use when ultrasound or amniocentesis indicates moderately severe or severe disease with a probable need for intrauterine treatment. It has a definite role at 18 to 24 weeks' gestation when the reliability of other assessment methods is less certain and is generally not indicated unless fetal treatment of severe anemia appears to be necessary for safe delivery. Fetal blood sampling may be possible as early as 18 weeks' gestation; it usually is feasible by 20 to 21 weeks' gestation. The preferred sampling site is an umbilical vessel (preferably the vein) at its insertion into the placenta. For this reason, the procedure is technically easier to perform if the placenta is implanted on the anterior uterine wall.

MANAGEMENT OF MATERNAL ALLOIMMUNIZATION

Suppression of Alloimmunization

Since the mid-1940s, efforts have been made to suppress the strength of already developed maternal immune responses against fetal RBC. Methods previously used and discarded include Rh hapten, Rh-positive RBC stroma, and promethazine hydrochloride. Administration of Rh immune globulin, of great value in preventing Rh sensitization, has been shown to be quite ineffective in suppressing an established antibody response, no matter how weak, once it has begun.[168, 169]

Two measures that may have greater potential to reduce maternal antibody levels and ameliorate hemolytic disease are (1) intensive plasma exchange[170, 171] and (2) the administration of nonspecific intravenous immune serum globulin (IVIG).[172–174] With intensive plasma exchange, alloantibody levels can be lowered by as much as 75 percent but tend to rebound, at times to levels higher than they were before.[175] Vascular access becomes difficult and IgG and albumin administration is needed. Plasma exchange is tedious, costly, and uncomfortable.[176] It may have a role in a mother with a fetus known to be susceptible to the antigen to which she is immunized, who has a prior history of hydrops at or before 24 to 26 weeks' gestation. However, the published evidence for its benefits remains insufficiently strong to recommend it for routine management.

The value of high-dose IVIG administration in the severely alloimmunized pregnant woman is also uncertain and its use should also be the subject of carefully designed clinical studies. The mechanism of action has not been defined, but it could include inhibition of antibody synthesis or competitive blockade of receptor-mediated transfer across the placenta or binding sites on fetal immune cells. If IVIG therapy is considered, it should be used in the same situation as intensive plasma exchange, beginning at 10 to 12 weeks' gestation. Ongoing assessment of fetal disease remains essential, because not all fetuses respond adequately. Because of its cost, inconvenience, and uncertain benefit, like plasmapheresis its use is reserved for fetal disease that is expected to be refractory to other therapy.[177]

Fetal Treatment

INDUCED EARLY DELIVERY

Premature delivery of fetuses with Rh HDN has been important in prevention of mortality since the late 1940s. With the introduction of amniotic fluid assessment in 1961, it became possible for the first time to predict which fetuses should be considered candidates for early delivery. Subsequent advances in perinatal and neonatal management of premature infants have had a major impact on survival. However, HDN is different from many other fetal conditions in that intrauterine treatment has been effective in prolonging many gestations. As the effectiveness of fetal treatment has improved, particularly after the introduction of intravascular intrauterine transfusions, the need for premature delivery of infants with HDN has diminished. If premature delivery is required, antenatal betamethasone therapy should be given to the mother according to consensus guidelines. Antenatal betamethasone therapy has not been put to the test in the subgroup of premature infants with HDN in a randomized trial, but it is probable that infants with HDN have as much or more to gain from use of this important preparation for extrauterine life than their gestation-matched peers with other fetal conditions. The risk-to-benefit ratio of repeated courses of antenatal steroids during the second and early third trimester is much more uncertain and is currently the subject of clinical trials.

INTRAUTERINE TRANSFUSIONS FOR FETAL HEMOLYTIC DISEASE

In 1961, induced early delivery could not be undertaken before 31 to 32 weeks' gestation without the risk of prohibitive mortality from prematurity and severe Rh disease. Eight percent of fetuses develop hydrops before 32 weeks' gestation. In 1963, the introduction of *intraperitoneal fetal transfusions (IPT)* by Liley[178] completely altered the prognosis for these most severely affected of all fetuses (Fig. 3–8).

Since the beginning of the 20th century, it was known that RBCs placed in the peritoneal cavity are absorbed and function normally. At one time, IPT was a favorite method for giving transfusions to children with thalassemia. It was abandoned in favor of vascular transfusions because of the severe discomfort that it caused. Absorption is via the subdiaphragmatic lymphatic lacunae, up the right lymphatic duct, and into the venous circulation. In the fetus, breathing movements are necessary for absorption to occur.[179] In the absence of hydrops, 10 to 12 percent of infused RBCs are absorbed daily. Ascites does not prevent absorption per se, although the rate of absorption in its presence is less predictable and the procedure is more risky. Placental damage and spontaneous labor after IPT are also significant risks.

Although IPT was a major advance in the management of severe erythroblastosis fetalis, *intravascular transfusion (IVT)* has proved to be even more successful for most fetuses. The earliest attempts at direct IVTs, either into a fetal or placental blood vessel approached via a hysterotomy incision, were attempted in the mid-1960s, but outcomes were poor because complications including premature labor almost invariably ensued.[180, 181]

In 1981, Rodeck and co-workers[182] reported direct fetal transfusions through a fetoscope. Intracardiac trans-

fusion has also been described,[183] but these methods were soon superseded by percutaneous transfusion into umbilical vessels.[184–188] Under ultrasound guidance and local anesthesia, the tip of a 22- or 20-gauge spinal needle is introduced into an umbilical blood vessel (preferably the vein, but occasionally the artery) at its insertion into the placenta or, if necessary, at another site (Fig. 3–9). Fetal blood sampling usually precedes and follows the transfusion, and confirmation that the needle tip remains in the correct position can be obtained throughout the procedure by observing altered echoes in the vessel via ultrasonography.

There are a number of advantages of IVT compared with IPT. IVT allows direct diagnostic sampling at the onset and completion of the procedure. For skilled practitioners the failure rate and procedure-related mortality are lower, especially in hydropic fetuses. It allows larger transfusions and administration of platelets if needed.[188, 189] It is effective in correcting anemia and its immediate physiologic consequences[190, 191] and in reversing hydrops.[187] Survival and neonatal condition were improved so rapidly by the introduction of IVT that, just as with IPT before it, its merits have been determined by comparison with historical control data rather than with prospective randomized studies. Comparison with historical control data may fail to take into account numerous other improvements in perinatal and neonatal care since the 1970s. However, babies with more severe disease respond to IVT, and they need less invasive and intensive neonatal care afterwards. Undoubtedly, if an intrauterine procedure is necessary and IVT is feasible, it is the procedure of choice. Because of the rarity of severe disease, follow-up studies are small, but they indicate that most survivors of both IPT and IVT have good prognoses for neurologic development and general health.[192–196] Umbilical and inguinal hernias are reported to occur often after IPT.[193]

Despite the great advantages of IVT, there remain some situations in which IPT is necessary and, therefore, the skill needed to perform it must be maintained. These include the fetus that is severely afflicted early in pregnancy, at a time when the cord vessels are too small for a successful venipuncture. A more common situation tends

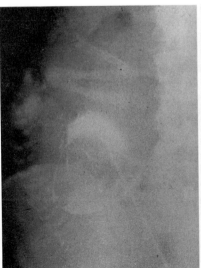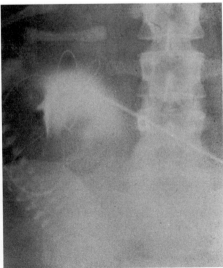

FIGURE 3–8. Hydrops fetalis at intraperitoneal fetal transfusion (IPT). Note the gross ascites at both the first and second IPTs. The fetus, hydropic at birth with a cord hemoglobin level of 9 g/100 mL (all donor RBCs) survived. (From Bowman JM: Maternal blood group immunization. In Creasy RK, Resnik R (eds): Maternal-Fetal Medicine: Principles and Practice, 2nd ed. Philadelphia, WB Saunders, 1989, p 636.)

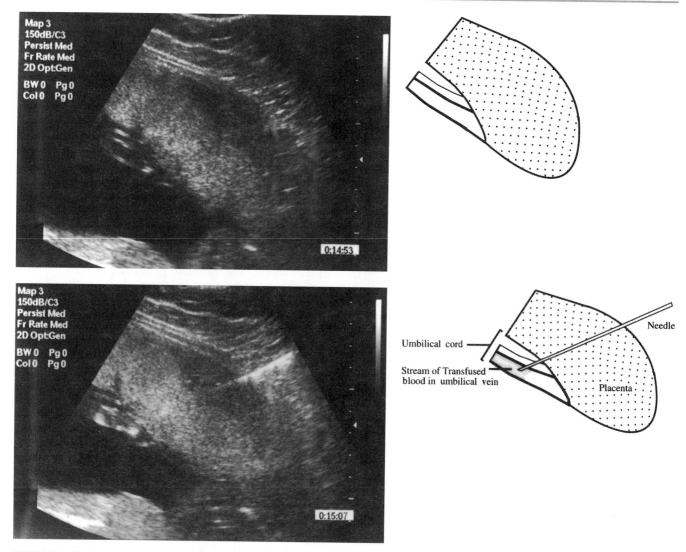

FIGURE 3–9. Real-time scan ultrasound view of the insertion of the umbilicus into an anterior placenta. The large umbilical vein is sonar lucent. The bottom panel shows a needle inserted (via the placenta) into the umbilical vein. The intravascular transfusion in progress is shown by the echogenicity of the transfused blood in the umbilical vein.

to occur late in pregnancy when fetal size and position may preclude access to the umbilical vessels. IPT may also be necessary to "top-up" an incomplete IVT if needle dislodgement or other immediate complications occur.

Although IVT and IPT can both expose the mother to fetal cells, raising her antibody titer and potentially worsening disease, the risk may be greater with IPT. As stated earlier, there is no benefit to giving anti-D antibody to these already sensitized mothers. In the future, other methods of immunomodulation might prove beneficial to improve the safety of this aspect of treatment.

It has been recommended that both IPT and IVT be performed in centers that perform at least 20 to 30 cordocenteses and 10 to 15 transfusions annually to maintain competence and to allow adequate surveillance of outcomes.[197, 198] Some perinatologists advocate the use of pancuronium before IVT to prevent fetal movement, but others use it selectively. Complications include fetal bradycardia, cord hematomas or bleeding, rupture of membranes, infection, and premature labor.

BLOOD FOR INTRAUTERINE TRANSFUSION

No general guidelines have been published recently for many aspects of intrauterine transfusions. Although there have undoubtedly been advances in equipment design and blood banking techniques, reports of their application to intrauterine transfusion have not been published in peer-reviewed literature. By extrapolation from results from neonatal transfusion therapy, it seems reasonable to propose that cytomegalovirus-negative packed RBCs with a packed cell volume of 0.85 to 0.88 should be used for intrauterine transfusion. Cells should be as fresh as is compatible with careful screening and crossmatch against maternal blood and should be leukocyte depleted and **irradiated.** The risk of graft-versus-host disease is very low but not zero.[199–201] The use of Kell antigen-negative blood is optimal, if it is available.

Treatment of the Neonate with Hemolytic Disease

GENERAL MEASURES

As a result of advances in antenatal assessment and treatment, the pediatrician often has the benefit of treating an infant with HDN whose condition is better and whose disease course is more predictable than those of infants with HDN in previous decades. Nevertheless, the management of the infant with severe hydrops fetalis remains difficult, and because the disease is now very uncommon, there is little opportunity for well-designed trials to test various approaches to management. Uncertainties include the role of antenatal drainage of pleural effusions and ascites, which resuscitation fluids and drugs to use, and when to perform top-up or exchange transfusion. Surfactant therapy may be necessary because of prematurity or surfactant inactivation.[202, 203] Top-up transfusion may be useful for stabilization[96, 204] because nearly all hydropic infants are severely anemic and some have low central venous pressures.

Even in the mildly affected infant careful assessment and anticipatory management are required. The fetus that has coped well in the intrauterine environment and has not needed or has responded well to intrauterine treatment can still have significant problems with the transition to independent extrauterine life. Problems attributable to HDN such as hyperinsulinemic hypoglycemia[205] may be compounded by the problems of prematurity. The baby should be assessed promptly at birth and any immediate resuscitation issues should be addressed. A complete physical examination may reveal hepatic and splenic enlargement and signs of anemia. Occasionally, stigmata resulting from accidents of intrauterine therapy are found.

Laboratory assessment should include a complete blood count, blood group assessment, assessment of relevant antibodies, and baseline measurement of bilirubin level, so that the rate of increase of bilirubin can be calculated. In severely affected infants, liver function, acid-base balance, and coagulation profile should also be assessed. In infants who have received multiple transfusions, assessment of iron status should be considered, especially if there is evidence of liver dysfunction.[206–208] Cord blood can be useful for these tests but may provide misleading results unless the sample is promptly obtained. Many blood banks will not accept cord blood for crossmatch.

In regard to general care, breast-feeding is strongly recommended and it should commence early in infants well enough to tolerate it. If the infant is mature and in good condition, he or she can be breast-fed while receiving phototherapy (if necessary) via a suitable fiberoptic blanket or spotlight. Although Rh antibodies are present in breast milk, particularly in colostrum, very little antibody is absorbed.[209] There is no evidence that forced fluid administration (beyond requirements for nutrition and compensation for any increased insensible losses) improves the outcome of the disease, and it is hazardous in premature infants and those in heart failure.

Folate is normally stored in the liver in late gestation, but reserves may be deficient in premature infants and depleted by ineffective erythropoiesis or by exchange transfusion, which replaces the infant's blood with adult blood that has a lower folate level.[210,211] Supplemental folic acid at a dose of 100 to 200 μg/day is recommended for several weeks. Vitamin B_{12} will usually be supplied in adequate amounts in breast milk (unless the mother has a deficiency), and supplemental iron is not only unnecessary but potentially hazardous.[206] Drugs that interfere with bilirubin binding to albumin or with bilirubin metabolism should be avoided.

The use of *phototherapy* and other measures for hyperbilirubinemia is discussed in Chapter 4 and has been reviewed elsewhere.[212, 213] The principles we now apply in deciding when to begin and end phototherapy are little more than traditional rules of thumb; but evidence to base guidelines on is unlikely to be seen in the near future. However, it also seems clear that phototherapy is effective in preventing many exchange transfusions in infants with hemolysis.[214, 215] Most guidelines still recommend lower thresholds for beginning phototherapy for HDN than for nonhemolytic jaundice, despite the improved condition of most of the infants with HDN whom we now treat. The use of phototherapy is not strongly supported by evidence, but its risks and resource implications are low compared with those of exchange transfusion.

Phototherapy can be discontinued when serum bilirubin levels decrease, or if the conjugated fraction of bilirubin increases significantly. As a rule, well term infants who have received intrauterine transfusions can be discharged at about 1 week of age. Conversely, the many weeks of specialized care needed by premature, very anemic prehydropic or hydropic infants may challenge the resources of the most highly developed tertiary-level neonatal intensive care unit.

The administration of IVIG to prevent the need for exchange transfusion in HDN has been the subject of limited investigation.[216–219] These small studies used different IVIG preparations and for different thresholds.[220] IVIG therapy deserves further investigation in selected infants, but there is not sufficient evidence to recommend it outside of carefully conducted clinical trials.

EXCHANGE TRANSFUSION

Exchange transfusion originated in the 1920s in a procedure done via the anterior fontanelle. Refinements to the technique of "exsanguination transfusion" were introduced by Wallerstein and Wiener in 1946.[146, 221] Generations of infants and pediatric residents should be very grateful for Diamond's decision to pioneer the use of umbilical catheters,[222] because Wiener's technique involved infusion of blood through a saphenous vein cutdown and drainage (after heparinization of the baby) via an incision in the radial artery at the wrist. A randomized controlled trial in 1952 confirmed that the technique could save lives and prevent kernicterus.[223]

During exchange transfusion, RBCs coated with antibody are replaced with RBCs negative for the antigen to which the mother is alloimmunized. Exchange transfusion corrects the anemia of the severely affected newborn, prevents hyperbilirubinemia by removing the infant's hemolyzing erythrocytes and suppressing erythropoiesis, removes some of the already formed bilirubin, and depletes any unbound anti-D antibody. Only modest amounts of the offending antibody are removed by exchange transfusion because the antibody (IgG) is widely distributed in extracellular fluid, both within and outside the vascular compartment.

Exchange transfusion produces a significant drop in neutrophil levels. Whether or not this has any functional significance is not known, but the initial neutropenia and subsequent "left shift" during the rebound from it can certainly complicate the diagnosis of sepsis in the hours and days after exchange. A similar decrease in platelets is generally well tolerated provided that the baby does not have thrombocytopenia or other coagulopathy before the exchange transfusion. Because a variety of coagulation defects increase the risk for intraventricular hemorrhage,[224] platelet therapy should be considered in sick and premature infants, unless whole blood is used for the exchange transfusion.

Indications for Exchange Transfusion

Exchange transfusion is generally performed early for severe anemia or later when phototherapy and other conservative measures fail to control the bilirubin level. However, the exact thresholds at which it should be applied are controversial and warrant the development of contemporary guidelines.[225] Traditional criteria for early exchange transfusion included cord hemoglobin level less than 13 to 15 g/dL (130–150 g/L) and cord serum bilirubin level greater than 60 to 130 μmol/L (3 to 7 mg/dL). However, Wennberg and colleagues[226] showed in 1978 that neither cord hematocrit nor bilirubin level had much value in predicting a postnatal increase in bilirubin level. They suggested using the criterion of rate of increase of bilirubin. Rates of increase of 8 to 13 μmol/L/hr, despite intensive phototherapy, indicate that exchange transfusion is likely to be needed. Improved antenatal treatment, phototherapy, and other supportive care have cast even these guidelines into doubt. Many neonatal intensive care units that have prompt blood bank support and the ability to perform exchange transfusion at short notice will delay exchange transfusion in babies who do not have symptomatic anemia until the risk of exchange transfusion is thought to approximate the risk of kernicterus. The decision process is clearly hampered by imprecise knowledge of where these risk boundaries lie, although Jackson[227] recently estimated the risk of serious complications of exchange transfusion to be less than 1 percent in previously well infants and about 12 percent in ill infants. In severely anemic hydropic babies, early exchange transfusion still seems warranted to improve oxygen transport. Peterec[225] has suggested working guidelines.

Free Bilirubin and Reserve Albumin Binding Studies

It appears that the level of free unconjugated bilirubin is the determining factor in the pathogenesis of bilirubin encephalopathy (kernicterus; see Chapter 4), but measurements of free bilirubin, although accessible, have not routinely influenced clinical practice.

Technique of Exchange Transfusion

The specific technical details of exchange transfusion are clearly set out elsewhere[228] and are only discussed briefly here. The safest location for catheter tips and whether it is better to use a single catheter "push-pull" technique or a double catheter continuous technique have not been conclusively determined. In practice, these decisions are often based on local tradition and on the number and type of catheters that can be easily inserted. The procedure should be conducted precisely and with meticulous attention to precautions against infection.

The blood should be ABO compatible and for anti-D HDN, Rh negative. If the mother is alloimmunized to an antigen other than D, the blood should be missing that antigen. It should be crossmatch compatible with the mother's serum. Ideally, the blood should also be negative for Kell antigen (to avoid sensitizing the infant) and hemoglobin S (to avoid problems with filtration). If the initial exchange transfusion is carried out using group O blood, any further exchange transfusions should use group O blood. Otherwise, brisk hemolysis and jaundice due to ABO incompatibility may become a further complication. Graft-versus-host disease occurs rarely after exchange transfusion, but blood should be irradiated if possible, especially for premature infants. The question of whether to use whole blood or packed RBCs partially reconstituted with plasma or saline plus or minus platelets has not been subjected to a rigorous study, but component therapy is widely used. Component therapy potentially exposes the infant to more donors and more risk of handling errors, but less risk of white blood cell–related complications. For very unusual antibodies or combinations of antibodies, RBCs may need to be transported over long distances. Occasionally, stored washed maternal RBCs must be used. In these circumstances, whole blood is unlikely to be available.

Depending on the local strategy for neonatal screening for metabolic and other diseases, it is strongly recommended that some of the blood from the first drawback be applied to a neonatal screening card. Otherwise, the diagnosis of some disorders such as galactosemia may be masked for some time to come. If any blood for serologic analysis or a DNA sample is needed for other diagnostic purposes such as congenital infection, it should also be collected at this time.

Aliquots of the infant's blood are removed and replaced with antigen-negative donor blood. In choosing a technique for transfusion, the practitioner should take into account the following considerations: the infant's tolerance of the metabolic, hemodynamic, and hematologic demands; the effectiveness of the procedure in treating anemia and preventing an increase in bilirubin level; and safe handling of the blood for transfusion. The size of aliquot should be chosen to take into account the tolerance of the infant and if a single catheter is used, its dead space. Principles of calculus make it clear that the largest aliquots the infant can tolerate will correct anemia most rapidly, but very rapid correction of anemia is not usually the prime objective. Allowing sufficient time for equilibration of bilirubin and antibody between vascular and extravascular compartments is another concern, but with very long procedures there is the risk of clotted catheters and degradation of the donor blood. Generally, between 1.5 and 2 infant blood volumes are exchanged (130 to 170 mL/kg of body weight) over 1 to 2 hours. A two–blood volume exchange transfusion removes approximately 90 percent of the affected RBCs of the infant, but the response is asymptotic rather than linear and 70 percent removal occurs after the first blood volume has been exchanged. Only about 25 to 30 percent of total bilirubin is removed because it is sequestered in extravascular and cellular compartments. A decrease of about 50 percent in the serum bilirubin level can be expected, but a rapid rebound to about 75 percent of the pre-exchange level typically is seen.

The administration of albumin, 1 g/kg of body weight, before the exchange transfusion, or the addition of albumin, 4 to 6 g, to blood used for exchange transfusion modestly increases the amount of bilirubin removed to about 35 percent of the total body bilirubin by drawing bilirubin into the vascular compartment. Caution is advised in administering albumin to the severely anemic infant, because it may precipitate heart failure.

Many previous guidelines suggested routine administration of calcium gluconate. However, contemporary anticoagulants affect the ionized calcium much less than the citrate-phosphate-dextrose used in years gone by. Furthermore, most neonatal units now have immediate access to blood gas analyzers that also measure ionized calcium, electrolytes, and glucose in tiny samples. Periodic measurement of ionized calcium, electrolytes, glucose, and blood gas are therefore a reasonable alternative (e.g., every 30 minutes or earlier if the infant manifests any instability).

Complications of Exchange Transfusion

Complications of exchange transfusion include all those of simple transfusion plus a variety of others related to the large size of the transfusion, to the catheters, and to the technique.[227, 228] As fewer procedures are being performed, experience with the procedure among neonatal and pediatric medical and nursing staff is declining. Furthermore, well infants who were previously given exchange transfusions are now managed conservatively, whereas the sickest and most premature infants still require exchange transfusion. Thus, paradoxically, at a time when most transfusion therapy has never been safer, exchange transfusion is likely to become more hazardous.

Necrotizing enterocolitis is a potentially life-threatening hazard. The occurrence of necrotizing enterocolitis may be related to the technique. In the absence of evidence-based guidelines, effort should be made to prevent wide pressure and volume variations during exchange transfusion. Blood injection and withdrawal should be carried out smoothly without undue haste. The use of blood products that are anti-T cryptantigen–negative, prolonging the interval until oral feeding is restarted and the use of prophylactic antibiotics might also influence risk of necrotizing enterocolitis, but there is no clear evidence for any of these practices in relation to exchange transfusion.

As was discussed earlier for intrauterine transfusions, the performance of exchange transfusions in neonatal intensive care units with experienced staff and with blood banks familiar with supplying neonates is likely to yield the best results for infants and the best hope of accumulating evidence to guide practice.

OTHER MATERNAL ALLOANTIBODIES CAUSING FETAL/NEONATAL HEMOLYTIC DISEASE

Alloantibodies Other Than A and B

Although reports from numerous geographic areas demonstrate the effectiveness of administration of anti-D IgG to prevent RhD alloimmunization, most find that Rh is still the blood group system causing most cases of HDN and anti-D is still the most common single antibody causing severe HDN. However, there are at least 26 blood group systems, and the molecules carrying these antigens are very diverse in structure, function and tendency to cause HDN. The molecules include transporters and channels (e.g., Diego, Kidd, and Rh), receptors for pathogens (Duffy, P, and others) and for adhesion to other cells (e.g., Landsteiner-Wiener), enzymes (ABO, H, Lewis, and Kell), structural proteins (GE), and complement receptors (CH/RG).[18]

As the incidence of RhD HDN has been decreasing, other blood group antibodies have assumed a greater importance. Bowman[229] found that in Manitoba (population, 1 million), the mean annual occurrence of D alloimmunization in pregnant women dropped from 194 in 1962 through 1967 to 23 in 1989 through 1994. In the same two periods, the mean annual occurrence of detected non-D alloimmunization in pregnant women, excluding ABO alloimmunization, increased from 14 to 108. This increase was partially the result of the increased screening of pregnant D-positive women. It also reflected a real increase in the occurrence of non-D alloimmunization because of the increased incidence of blood transfusion (transfused blood is generally only crossmatched for ABO and D). A summary of results from five studies from the 1960s to the 1990s is shown in Table 3–7.

The alloantibodies listed by Mollison and co-workers[235] and Bowman[236] as having been reported to cause HDN are listed in Table 3–8. Of the multitude of antibodies implicated as causes of HDN, fortunately most are rare or rarely cause severe disease (Table 3–9). Some are the subject of single case reports.

There are various reasons why the incidence and severity of HDN differ from one blood group antigen system to another. In some cases, it is because of the rarity of the offending antigen or the lack of it and the likelihood of incompatibility between parents being low. An example is the Colton blood group system, which comprises the high-incidence antigens Co_a and Co_3 found on aquaporin-1. Rare individuals lacking aquaporin can produce antibodies that lead to severe HDN.

In others, it is because of low levels of expression on the RBC surface. For this reason, maternal anti-I and anti-Lutheran antibodies, even when present at high titer usually do not cause HDN because of low cell surface

TABLE 3–7. Antibody Occurrence in Five Series[234]

Antibody*	Polesky (1967)[230]	Queenan et al. (1969)[231]	Pepperell et al. (1977)[232]	Filbey et al. (1995)[233]	Geifman-Holtzman et al. (1996)[234]
D	1864 (63.1)	304 (48. 3)	958 (65. 3)	159 (19. 0)	101 (18. 4)
E	80 (2.7)	34 (5. 3)	69 (4. 7)	51 (6. 1)	77 (14. 0)
C	448 (15.2)	34 (5. 3)	9 (0. 6)	36 (4. 3)	26 (4. 7)
C^w	4 (0.14)	—	—	10 (1. 2)	1 (0. 2)
c	68 (2.3)	12 (1. 9)	59 (4. 0)	38 (4. 5)	32 (5. 8)
E	2 (0.07)	3 (0. 4)	6 (0. 04)	1 (0. 1)	—
Kell	93 (3. 1)	30 (4. 7)	34 (2. 3)	48 (5. 7)	121 (22)
Duffy	17 (0.6)	12 (1. 9)	8 (0. 5)	26 (3. 1)	31 (5. 6)
MNS	45 (1.5)	20 (3. 1)	18 (1. 2)	35 (4. 2)	26 (4. 7)
Kidd	7 (0.2)	7 (1. 1)	2 (0. 14)	10 (1. 2)	8 (1. 5)
Lutheran	—	3 (0. 4)	—	13 (1.6)	7 (1. 3)
P$_1$	27 (0.9)	15 (2. 3)	129 (8. 8)	48 (5. 7)	1 (0. 2)
Le^a, Le^b	94 (3. 2)	51 (8. 1)	174 (11. 9)	241 (28. 8)	113 (20. 5)
I	13 (0.4)	15 (2. 3)	—	—	5 (0. 9)
Others	194 (6.6)	90 (14. 3)	1 (0. 07)	120 (14. 4)	1 (0. 2)
Total antibodies	2956	630	1467	836	550
Blood samples	43,000	18,378	72,138	110,765	37,506
Time period	1960–1966 (7 yr)	1960–1967 (8 yr)	1965–1975 (10 yr)	1980–1991 (12 yr)	1993–1995 (2.5 yr)
Place	Minnesota	New York	Australia	Sweden	Central New York
D†	43.3	16.5	1.3	1.4	2.6
E†	1.9	1.9	1.0	0.5	2.0
C†	1.6	0.7	0.8	0.3	0.7
Kell†	2.2	1.6	0.5	0.4	3.2
Le^a, Le^{b†}	2.2	2.8	2.4	2.2	3.2

*Values are given as number (%) of antibodies.
†Values are given as number of antibodies per 1000 samples.

TABLE 3–8. Non-ABO Alloantibodies Reported to Cause Hemolytic Disease[229, 235]

	Any HDN	Moderate or severe HDN
Within the Rh system	Anti-D, -c, -C, -C^w, -C^x, -e, -E, -E^w, -ce, -Ce^s, -Rh32, -Go^a, -Be^a, -Evans, -Rh17	Anti-D, -c, -C, -C^w, -C^x, -e, -E, -E^w, -ce, -Ce^s, -Rh32, -Go^a, -Be^a, -Evans, -Rh17
Outside the Rh system	Anti-LW, -K, -k, -Ku, -Kp^a, -Kp^b, -Js^a, -Js^b, -Fy^a, -Fy3, -Jk^a, -Jk^b, -M, -N, -S, -s, -U, -Vw, -M^v -Mit, -Mt^a, -Mur, -Hil, -Hut, -En^a, -PP$_1$P^k, -Lu^a, -Lu^b, -Lu9, -Di^a, -Di^b, -Yt^a, -Yt^b, -Do^a, -Co^a, -Wr^a	Anti-LW, -K, -k, -Kp^a -Jk^a, -Js^a, -Js^b, -Ku, -Fy^a, -M, -N, -S, -s, -U, -PP$_1$P^k, -Di^b, -Far,
Antibodies to low-incidence antigens	Anti-Bi, -By, -Fr^a, -Good, -Rd, -Re^a, -Zd	-Good, -Zd
Antibodies to high-incidence antigens	Anti-At^a, -Jr^a, -Lan, -Ge	-Lan

HDN = Hemolytic disease of the fetus and newborn.

expression of these antigens on fetal RBCs. Lutheran antigens are also widely distributed in endothelial cells.

Disease due to *anti-Kell antibodies* can be very severe. Maternal antibodies to KEL1 causing neonatal anemia were first described in 1945,[6] and the blood group system was named for Mrs. Kell, in whom the antibodies were found. Kell glycoprotein is an endopeptidase involved in endothelin activation,[237] and it is more properly regarded as a subunit of a larger protein because it is linked via disulfide bond to the XK protein. Redman and associates[238, 239] reviewed the Kell blood group and summarized the low- and high-incidence antigens, of which at least 23 have been described. The most immunogenic,

KEL1, is second to RhD in its immunizing potential and occurs in about 9 percent of whites and 2 percent of blacks. It results from a point mutation causing a Thr^{193} (KEL2) to Met^{193} (KEL1) substitution, which in turn leads to loss of a glycosylation site. The other Kell phenotypes are also generally due to single base substitutions, so genotyping is more straightforward than that in the Rh system. Skilled assessment of the fetus by ultrasound for signs of anemia is recommended.

Sensitization occurs most commonly via unmatched blood transfusion but can arise during pregnancy. Although the number of incompatible pregnancies is lower for Kell than for RhD, the proportion of anti-KEL1–affected fetuses

TABLE 3–9. Severity of Hemolytic Disease in Manitoba over 32 Years[*][229]

Alloantibody Specificity	No. of Patients	Affected Patients (%)	No Treatment Required (%)	Phototherapy and/or Exchange Transfusion Required (%)	Stillborn Hydropic or Hb <60 g/L (%)
D (19 yr)	566	257 (47)	51	30	19
E	633	162 (26)	89	11	—
c, cE	302	164 (54)	70	23	7
C, Ce, C^w, e	193	50 (36)	86	14	—
Kell	478	16 (3.3)	50	37	13
Kp^a	7	3 (43)	67	33	—
k	1	1 (100)	—	100	—
Fy^a	35	6 (17)	67	16	16
S	20	11 (55)	64	36	—

Hb = hemoglobin.
[*]From November 1, 1962, to October 31, 1994, except for anti-D (November 1, 1975, to October 31, 1994).

that are severely affected is reported to be as high as 40 to 50 percent.[153, 240]

Kell antibodies, which recognize antigens expressed in early erythroid progenitors and at an early stage of erythropoiesis in fetal liver, appear to be capable of suppressing erythropoiesis.[241] This is the putative reason for the tendency for hydrops early in pregnancy seen in anti-Kell HDN. It has also been proposed as the reason why amniotic fluid spectrophotometry is not as reliable as in Rh hemolytic disease, although not all studies agree on this point.[153, 242, 243] Paternal typing followed, where necessary, by fetal genotyping is recommended in pregnancies complicated by significant anti-Kell antibody titers.

Rarely, anti-C, -Ce, -C^W, -Kp^a, -k, -Fy^a, and -S and occasionally other antibodies (see Table 3–8) have caused hemolytic disease severe enough to require treatment after birth, but only one, anti-Fy^a, resulted in disease so severe that hydrops developed or that fetal transfusions were required in Bowman's Manitoba series.[244] Other blood group antibodies in these patients caused either no or mild clinical disease. Bowman also reported that 34 pregnant non-D-alloimmunized women referred from *outside* Manitoba (a highly selected group with very severely affected fetuses drawn from a much greater population base) showed the following distribution of antibodies that produced HDN so severe that intrauterine treatment was required: anti-K (18 fetuses), -c (9 fetuses), -cE (2 fetuses) -k^34 (1 fetus), -Jk^a (1 fetus), -Fy^a (1 fetus), -CC^W (1 fetus), and -E (1 fetus). There are rare instances of other alloantibodies, usually benign ones, causing severe hemolytic disease (e.g., anti-Kp^b and anti-M).[245, 246]

ABO Hemolytic Disease

ABO HDN behaves differently from HDN due either to anti-D or to other blood group antibodies. Anti-A and anti-B, which bind complement in adults, cause violent, life-threatening intravascular hemolysis after transfusion of ABO-incompatible blood. Fetal ABO HDN usually is much milder than HDN due to D, c, K, and E. Although kernicterus may develop if the baby with ABO HDN is left untreated, hydrops rarely occurs and anemia at birth is usually absent or moderate and late anemia is rare. There are rare reports of hydrops fetalis due to ABO

erythroblastosis.[247] It is possible that some of these involve other causes of increased ineffective erythropoiesis (such as RBC enzyme deficiency or α-thalassemia trait) or nonimmune hydrops superimposed upon ABO HDN. ABO antibodies are a more common cause of HDN (and of severe HDN) in Southeast Asia, Africa, and Latin America, for reasons that have yet to be determined.

Several reasons have been proposed for the mildness of ABO HDN, compared with HDN caused by other antibodies and with adult ABO hemolysis.[248] First, there are fewer A and B antigenic sites on the fetal RBC membrane,[249] and anti-A and anti-B do not bind complement on the fetal RBC membrane.[250] Second, anti-A and anti-B are often IgM, which does not cross the placenta, or IgG2, which plays a minor role in HDN.[251] Third, the small amounts of IgG anti-A and anti-B that do traverse the placenta have myriad antigenic sites both on tissues other than on RBCs and on secretions to which they may bind. Because there is very little antibody on the RBC, the cord blood direct antiglobin test result in ABO hemolytic disease is usually only weakly positive and may be negative unless a sensitive test is used. Capillary blood taken at 2 or 3 days of age often yields a negative direct antiglobin test result regardless of test sensitivity. In at least 25 percent of ABO-incompatible babies, cord blood RBCs give weakly positive results on the direct antiglobin test at delivery, and an excess of babies with blood types A and B of mothers with blood type O become severely jaundiced.[252, 253] The A- or B-incompatible infants of mothers with blood type A or B do not appear to be at increased risk for hemolysis or jaundice.[254]

Only a small fraction of A- or B-incompatible infants of O mothers develop clinical evidence of HDN (early and severe jaundice).[253, 255, 256] One study found that only 0.07 percent of more than 88,000 infants required exchange transfusion for anti-A or -B HDN.[255] Nevertheless, ABO HDN continues to account for a significant proportion of infants with troublesome jaundice, necessitating prolongation of hospital stay, readmission to the hospital, or home therapy. The same large study found that ABO incompatibility accounted for 5.5 percent of infants with jaundice.

Although anemia is rarely severe, mild hemolysis appears to be common. In a series of 1704 infants of blood group O mothers, the infants with blood group A or

B had significantly higher cord bilirubin and lower cord hemoglobin concentrations than the babies with blood group O.[257] Blood films tend to show polychromasia, reticulocytosis, and prominent spherocytosis, which can be difficult at times to differentiate from hereditary spherocytosis.

Control of hyperbilirubinemia is usually the major issue in infants with ABO HDN, and thresholds for phototherapy and exchange transfusion are generally regarded as similar to those for Rh HDN. The risk of symptomatic late anemia in ABO HDN is very low. The risk of recurrence of jaundice due to anti-A or -B in future incompatible siblings is high and mothers should be counseled accordingly.[258]

MANAGEMENT OF SPECIAL PROBLEMS

Syndrome of Hepatocellular Damage

Most infants with severe anemia and erythroblastosis, particularly those who are hydropic or prehydropic, show signs of obstructive jaundice. There is extreme hepatomegaly and evidence of biliary canalicular obstruction. These infants may develop extreme or prolonged jaundice but with one half or more of the total bilirubin being direct-acting conjugated bilirubin. The threshold for exchange transfusion in such infants is unclear and should be individualized. If hepatic damage is so severe that a symptomatic coagulopathy has ensued, exchange transfusion (with appropriate components) may be necessary to remove activated clotting factors and degradation products and to replenish clotting factor levels.

Infants Who Have Undergone Fetal Transfusions

Assessment of infants who have undergone IVT or IPT does not differ from that of other babies with HDN. Because these infants are often delivered with few residual Rh-positive hemolyzing RBCs, their postdelivery management may be simple. Nevertheless, some require multiple exchange transfusions. Compared to those who received IPTs, relatively few babies born after having IVTs require exchange transfusion. However, careful individual assessment is still required and delivery in or near a center that can perform exchange transfusion is still advisable.

Follow-up Care of the Infant with Hemolytic Disease

Whether or not the affected infant has required fetal transfusions or exchange transfusions, anemia in the first few weeks of life is commonly seen.[259] Hemoglobin levels should be checked at 10- to 14-day intervals until the infant is 8 to 12 weeks of age. The anemia is due to the gradual loss of transfused Rh-negative RBCs and to the failure of the infant's Rh-positive RBCs to replace them. This failure is initially due to hemolysis of any RBCs produced and to transient erythroblastopenia, which usually resolves spontaneously at about 6 to 8 weeks of age.

In the interim, if symptomatic anemia develops or if hemoglobin levels are falling rapidly toward symptomatic levels, a simple transfusion of 20 mL/kg of body weight of crossmatched, packed RBCs compatible with the infant's serum is administered. Iron supplementation is not indicated, but folic acid and, in some circumstances, vitamin B_{12} should be given.

Recently, recombinant erythropoietin has been used with some success in the treatment of the anemia of prematurity. Erythropoietin treatment for prevention of "late" anemia in infants with HDN has been tested in small trials.[260–262] A larger trial is needed to evaluate the role of erythropoietin in preventing late anemia of HDN.

CONCLUSIONS

Advances in prevention of Rh sensitization and the management of immune HDN in the past 30 years have been dramatic. Statistics from all over the developed world have indicated that the prevalence of Rh sensitization in pregnant women has been reduced by more than 90 percent. The number of exchange transfusions has also been decreased by more than 100-fold. In addition, the number of perinatal deaths due to HDN has plummeted. However, for those still affected by anti-D or other significant antibodies, the disease burden remains significant.

Despite a recent explosion in knowledge about antigen presentation and provocation of the immune response in general, little detail at the molecular and cellular level is known about maternal sensitization to RhD. A better understanding of these events, taken together with the recent elucidation of the molecular genetics of RhD and other blood groups, is likely to provide new tools for prevention, diagnosis, and treatment.

REFERENCES

1. Diamond L, Blackfan K, Baty J: Erythroblastosis fetalis and its association with universal edema of the fetus, icterus gravis neonatorum and anemia of the newborn. J Pediatr 1932; 1:269.
2. Darrow R: Icterus gravis (erythroblastosis neonatorum). An examination of etiologic considerations. Arch Pathol 1938; 25:378.
3. Levine P, Stetson R: An unusual case of intra-group agglutination. JAMA 1939; 113:126.
4. Landsteiner K, Wiener A: An agglutinable factor in human blood recognized by immune sera for rhesus blood. Proc Soc Exp Biol Med 1940; 43:223.
5. Levine P, Katzin E, Burnham L: Isoimmunization in pregnancy: Its possible bearing on the etiology of erythroblastosis foetalis. JAMA 1941; 116:825.
6. Coombs R, Mourant A, Race R: Detection of weak and 'incomplete' Rh agglutinins: A new test. Lancet 1945; 2:15.
7. Chown B: Anemia from bleeding of the fetus into the mother's circulation. Lancet 1954; 1:1213.
8. Wiener A, Wexler I: Heredity of the blood groups. New York, Grune & Stratton, 1958.
9. Race R: The Rh genotype and Fisher's theory. Blood 1948; 3:27.
10. Urbaniak SJ, Greiss MA: RhD haemolytic disease of the fetus and newborn. Blood Rev 2000; 14:44–61.
11. Cartron JP: RH blood group system and molecular basis of Rh-deficiency. Balliere's Clin Haematol 1999; 12:655.
12. Moore S, Woodrow CF, McClelland DB: Isolation of membrane components associated with human red cell antigens Rh(D), (c), (E) and Fy. Nature 1982; 295:529.
13. Gahmberg CG: Molecular identification of the human Rho(D) antigen. FEBS Lett 1982; 140:93.

14. Cherif-Zahar B, Bloy C, Le Van Kim C, et al: Molecular cloning and protein structure of a human blood group Rh polypeptide. Proc Natl Acad Sci USA 1990; 87:6243.

15. Avent ND, Ridgwell K, Tanner MJ, et al: cDNA cloning of a 30 kDa erythrocyte membrane protein associated with Rh (rhesus)-blood-group-antigen expression. Biochem J 1990; 271:821.

16. Le van Kim C, Mouro I, Cherif-Zahar B, et al: Molecular cloning and primary structure of the human blood group RhD polypeptide. Proc Natl Acad Sci USA 1992; 89:10925.

17. Arce MA, Thompson ES, Wagner S, et al: Molecular cloning of RhD cDNA derived from a gene present in RhD-positive, but not RhD-negative individuals. Blood 1993; 82:651.

18. Cartron JP, Colin Y: Structural and functional diversity of blood group antigens. Transfus Clin Biol 2001; 8:163.

19. Avent ND, Reid ME: The Rh blood group system: A review. Blood 2000; 95:375.

20. Avent ND: Molecular biology of the Rh blood group system. J Pediatr Hematol Oncol 2001; 23:394.

21. Okuda H, Suganuma H, Kamesaki T, et al: The analysis of nucleotide substitutions, gaps, and recombination events between *RHD* and *RHCE* genes through complete sequencing. Biochem Biophys Res Commun 2000; 274:670.

22. Flegel WA, Wagner FF, Muller TH, et al: Rh phenotype prediction by DNA typing and its application to practice. Transfus Med 1998; 8:281.

23. Mouro I, Colin Y, Cherif-Zahar B, et al: Molecular genetic basis of the human rhesus blood group system. Nat Genet 1993; 5:62.

24. Simsek S, de Jong CA, Cuijpers HT, et al: Sequence analysis of cDNA derived from reticulocyte mRNAs coding for Rh polypeptides and demonstration of E/e and C/c polymorphisms. Vox Sang 1994; 67:203.

25. Mourant A, Kopec A, Domaniewska-Sobczak K: The distribution of the human blood groups and other polymorphisms. London, Oxford University Press, 1976.

26. Wagner FF, Flegel WA: *RHD* gene deletion occurred in the rhesus box. Blood 2000; 95:3662.

27. Lan JC, Chen Q, Wu DL, et al: Genetic polymorphism of RhD-negative associated haplotypes in the Chinese. J Hum Genet 2000; 45:224.

28. Okuda H, Kawano M, Iwamoto S, et al: The RHD gene is highly detectable in RhD-negative Japanese donors. J Clin Invest 1997; 100:373.

29. Singleton BK, Green CA, Avent ND, et al: The presence of an *RHD* pseudogene containing a 37 base pair duplication and a nonsense mutation in Africans with the Rh D-negative blood group phenotype. Blood 2000; 95:12.

30. Avent ND, Martin PG, Armstrong-Fisher SS, et al: Evidence of genetic diversity underlying Rh D-, weak D (Du), and partial D phenotypes as determined by multiplex polymerase chain reaction analysis of the *RHD* gene. Blood 1997; 89:2568.

31. Cartron JP: A molecular approach to the structure, polymorphism and function of blood groups. Transfus Clin Biol 1996; 3:181.

32. Jones J, Scott ML, Voak D: Monoclonal anti-D specificity and Rh D structure: Criteria for selection of monoclonal anti-D reagents for routine typing of patients and donors. Transfus Med 1995; 5:171.

33. Avent ND, Jones JW, Liu W, et al: Molecular basis of the D variant phenotypes DNU and DII allows localization of critical amino acids required for expression of Rh D epitopes epD3, 4 and 9 to the sixth external domain of the Rh D protein. Br J Haematol 1997; 97:366.

34. Liu W, Smythe JS, Scott ML, et al: Site-directed mutagenesis of the human D antigen: Definition of D epitopes on the sixth external domain of the D protein expressed on K562 cells. Transfusion 1999; 39:17.

35. Chang TY, Siegel DL: Genetic and immunological properties of phage-displayed human anti-Rh(D) antibodies: Implications for Rh(D) epitope topology. Blood 1998; 91:3066.

36. Iwamoto S, Omi T, Yamasaki M, et al: Identification of 5′ flanking sequence of *RH50* gene and the core region for erythroid-specific expression. Biochem Biophys Res Commun 1998; 243:233.

37. Liu Z, Chen Y, Mo R, et al: Characterization of human RhCG and mouse Rhcg as novel nonerythroid Rh glycoprotein homologues predominantly expressed in kidney and testis. J Biol Chem 2000; 275:25641.

38. Huang CH, Cheng G, Liu Z, et al: Molecular basis for Rh_{null} syndrome: Identification of three new missense mutations in the Rh50 glycoprotein gene. Am J Hematol 1999; 62:25.

39. Matassi G, Cherif-Zahar B, Pesole G, et al: The members of the *RH* gene family (*RH50* and *RH30*) followed different evolutionary pathways. J Mol Evol 1999; 48:151.

40. Marini AM, Matassi G, Raynal V, et al: The human rhesus-associated RhAG protein and a kidney homologue promote ammonium transport in yeast. Nat Genet 2000; 26:341.

41. Marini AM, Vissers S, Urrestarazu A, et al: Cloning and expression of the *MEP1* gene encoding an ammonium transporter in *Saccharomyces cerevisiae*. EMBO J 1994; 13:3456.

42. Heitman J, Agre P: A new face of the rhesus antigen. Nat Genet 2000; 26:258.

43. Flegel WA, Wagner FF: Molecular genetics of RH. Vox Sang 2000; 78:109.

44. Huang CH: Blood Group Antigen Gene Mutation Database: Rh Blood Group System. HUGO Mutation Database Initiative, 2002. Available at http://www.bioc.aecom.yu.edu/bgmut/index.htm.

45. Flegel W, Wagner F: The Rhesus Site. Abteilung Blutgruppenserologie und Immunhämatologie, DRK-Blutspendedienst Baden-Württemberg, Institut Ulm, 2002. Available at http://www.uni-ulm.de/~wflegel/RH/.

46. Williamson I, Hofmeyr GJ, Crookes RL: Hemolytic disease of the newborn as an unusual consequence of drug abuse. A case report. J Reprod Med 1990; 35:46.

47. Vontver LA: RH sensitization associated with drug use [letter]. JAMA 1973; 226:469.

48. Kleihauer E, Braun H, Betke K: Demonstration von fetalem Haemoglobin in den Erythrozyten eines Blutausstriches. Klin Wochenschr 1957; 35:637.

49. Clarke CA: Prevention of RH haemolytic disease. A method based on the post-delivery injection of the mother with anti-D antibody. Vox Sang 1966; 11:641.

50. Bowman JM, Pollock JM, Penston LE: Fetomaternal transplacental hemorrhage during pregnancy and after delivery. Vox Sang 1986; 51:117.

51. Medearis AL, Hensleigh PA, Parks DR, et al: Detection of fetal erythrocytes in maternal blood post partum with the fluorescence-activated cell sorter. Am J Obstet Gynecol 1984; 148:290.

52. Lau TK, Lo KW, Chan LY, et al: Cell-free fetal deoxyribonucleic acid in maternal circulation as a marker of fetal-maternal hemorrhage in patients undergoing external cephalic version near term. Am J Obstet Gynecol 2000; 183:712.

53. Harrison KL, Baker JW: Fetal-maternal macrotransfusion—A study of 400 postpartum women. Aust NZ J Obstet Gynaecol 1978; 18:176.

54. Feldman N, Skoll A, Sibai B: The incidence of significant fetomaternal hemorrhage in patients undergoing cesarean section. Am J Obstet Gynecol 1990; 163:855.

55. Lloyd LK, Miya F, Hebertson RM, et al: Intrapartum fetomaternal bleeding in Rh-negative women. Obstet Gynecol 1980; 56:285.

56. Peddle LJ: Increase of antibody titer following amniocentesis. Am J Obstet Gynecol 1968; 100:567.

57. Bowman JM, Pollock JM: Transplacental fetal hemorrhage after amniocentesis. Obstet Gynecol 1985; 66:749.

58. Mennuti MT, Brummond W, Crombleholme WR, et al: Fetal-maternal bleeding associated with genetic amniocentesis. Obstet Gynecol 1980; 55:48.

59. Towers CV, Deveikis A, Asrat T, et al: A "bloodless cesarean section" and perinatal transmission of the human immunodeficiency virus. Am J Obstet Gynecol 1998; 179:708.

60. von Zabern I, Ehlers M, Grunwald U, et al: Release of mediators of systemic inflammatory response syndrome in the course of a severe delayed hemolytic transfusion reaction caused by anti-D. Transfusion 1998; 38:459.

61. Woodrow J: Rh immunization and its prevention. The immune response in the mother. In Jensen K, Killmann S (eds): Series Hematologica III. Copenhagen, Munksgaard, 1970, p 3.

62. Zipursky A, Israels LG: The pathogenesis and prevention of Rh immunization. Can Med Assoc J 1967; 97:1245.

63. Bowman JM: The prevention of Rh immunization. Transfus Med Rev 1988; 2:129.

64. Kinnock S, Liley AW: The epidemiology of severe haemolytic disease of the newborn. NZ Med J 1970; 71:76.

65. Bowman JM: Fetomaternal AB0 incompatibility and erythroblastosis fetalis. Vox Sang 1986; 50:104.

66. Hilden JO, Gottvall T, Lindblom B: HLA phenotypes and severe Rh(D) immunization. Tissue Antigens 1995; 46:313.

67. Kruskall MS, Yunis EJ, Watson A, et al: Major histocompatibility complex markers and red cell antibodies to the Rh(D) antigen. Absence of association. Transfusion 1990; 30:15.

68. Murray S: The effect of Rh genotypes on severity of Rh haemolytic disease of the newborn. Br J Haematol 1957; 3:143.

69. Rochna E, Hughes-Jones NC: The use of purified ^{125}I labelled anti gamma globulin in the determination of the number of D antigen sites on red cells of different phenotypes. Vox Sang 1965; 10:675.

70. Scott JR, Beer AE, Guy LR, et al: Pathogenesis of Rh immunization in primigravidas. Fetomaternal versus maternofetal bleeding. Obstet Gynecol 1977; 49:9.

71. Bowman JM, Chown B, Lewis M, et al: Rh isoimmunization during pregnancy: Antenatal prophylaxis. Can Med Assoc J 1978; 118:623.

72. Leong M, Duby S, Kinch RA: Fetal-maternal transfusion following early abortion. Obstet Gynecol 1979; 54:424.

73. Joseph KS, Kramer MS: The decline in Rh hemolytic disease: Should Rh prophylaxis get all the credit? Am J Public Health 1998; 88:209.

74. Von Dungern F: Beiträge zur Immunitätslehr. Munch Med Wochenschr 1900; 47:677.

75. Finn R, Clarke C, Donohow WT: Experimental studies on the prevention of Rh haemolytic disease. BMJ 1961; 1:1486.

76. Freda V, Gorman J, Pollack W: Successful prevention of experimental Rh sensitization in man with an anti-Rh gamma-2-globulin antibody preparation: A preliminary report. Transfusion 1964; 4:26.

77. Clarke C, Donohow WT, McConnell R: Further experimental studies in the prevention of Rh-haemolytic disease. BMJ 1963; 1:979.

78. Chown B, Duff A, James J, et al: Prevention of primary Rh immunization: First report of the Western Canadian Trial. Can Med Assoc J 1969; 100:1021.

79. Pollack W, Gorman JG, Freda VJ, et al: Results of clinical trials of RhoGAM in women. Transfusion 1968; 8:151.

80. Prevention of Rh-haemolytic disease: Results of the clinical trial. A combined study from centres in England and Baltimore. BMJ 1966; 2:907.

81. Ware RE, Zimmerman SA: Anti-D: Mechanisms of action. Semin Hematol 1998; 35:14.

82. Kumpel BM, Elson CJ: Mechanism of anti-D-mediated immune suppression—A paradox awaiting resolution? Trends Immunol 2001; 22:26.

83. Crowther C, Middleton P: Anti-D administration after childbirth for preventing rhesus alloimmunisation (Cochrane review). In The Cochrane Library, Issue 2. Oxford, UK, Update Software, 2002.

84. DiGuiseppi C: Screening for D (Rh) incompatibility. In Guide to Clinical Preventive Services Report of the US Preventive Services Task Force, Chapter 38. Bethesda, MD, National Library of Medicine, 1996.

85. Crowther CA, Keirse MJ: Anti-D administration in pregnancy for preventing rhesus alloimmunisation. In Cochrane Database of Systematic Reviews, CD000020. Oxford, UK, Update Software, 2000.

86. Prevention of Rh D Alloimmunization. ACOG Practice Bulletin 63. Washington, DC, American College of Obstetricians and Gynecologists, 1999.

87. Papers and abstracts. Consensus Conference on Anti-D Prophylaxis, Edinburgh, UK, April 8–9, 1997. Br J Obstet Gynaecol 1998; 105:iv.

88. Hartwell EA: Use of Rh immune globulin: ASCP practice parameter. Am J Clin Pathol 1998; 110:281.

89. Maayan-Metzger A, Schwartz T, Sulkes J, et al: Maternal anti-D prophylaxis during pregnancy does not cause neonatal haemolysis. Arch Dis Child Fetal Neonatal Ed 2001; 84:F60.

90. Adams MM, Marks JS, Gustafson J, et al: Rh hemolytic disease of the newborn: Using incidence observations to evaluate the use of RH immune globulin. Am J Public Health 1981; 71:1031.

91. Chavez G, Mulinare J, Edmonds LD: Epidemiology of RH hemolytic disease of the newborn in the United States. JAMA 1991; 24:3270.

92. Zavala C, Salamanca F: Mothers at risk of alloimmunization to the Rh(D) antigen and availability of gamma-globulin at the Mexican Institute of Social Security. Arch Med Res 1996; 27:373.

93. Kenny-Walsh E: Clinical outcomes after hepatitis C infection from contaminated anti-D immune globulin. Irish Hepatology Research Group. N Engl J Med 1999; 340:1228.

94. Scott ML, Voak D: Monoclonal antibodies to Rh D—Development and uses. Vox Sang 2000; 78:79.

95. Ohls R: Developmental erthropoiesis. In Polin R, Fox W (eds): Fetal and Neonatal Physiology, Vol. 2. Philadelphia, WB Saunders, 1998, p 1762.

96. Phibbs RH, Johnson P, Tooley WH: Cardiorespiratory status of erythroblastotic newborn infants. II. Blood volume, hematocrit, and serum albumin concentration in relation to hydrops fetalis. Pediatrics 1974; 53:13.

97. d'Ancona RL, Rahman F, Ozcan T, et al: The effect of intravascular blood transfusion on the flow velocity waveform of the portal venous system of the anemic fetus. Ultrasound Obstet Gynecol 1997; 10:333.

98. Pearse BM: Coated vesicles from human placenta carry ferritin, transferrin, and immunoglobulin G. Proc Natl Acad Sci USA 1982; 79:451.

99. Story CM, Mikulska JE, Simister NE: A major histocompatibility complex class I-like Fc receptor cloned from human placenta: Possible role in transfer of immunoglobulin G from mother to fetus. J Exp Med 1994; 180:2377.

100. Leach JL, Sedmak DD, Osborne JM, et al: Isolation from human placenta of the IgG transporter, FcRn, and localization to the syncytiotrophoblast: Implications for maternal-fetal antibody transport. J Immunol 1996; 157:3317.

101. Pitcher-Wilmott RW, Hindocha P, Wood CB: The placental transfer of IgG subclasses in human pregnancy. Clin Exp Immunol 1980; 41:303.

102. Malek A, Sager R, Kuhn P, et al: Evolution of maternofetal transport of immunoglobulins during human pregnancy. Am J Reprod Immunol 1996; 36:248.

103. Dooren MC, Engelfriet CP: Protection against Rh D-haemolytic disease of the newborn by a diminished transport of maternal IgG to the fetus. Vox Sang 1993; 65:59.

104. Urbaniak SJ: Lymphoid cell dependent (K-cell) lysis of human erythrocytes sensitized with rhesus alloantibodies. Br J Haematol 1976; 33:409.

105. Hadley AG: A comparison of in vitro tests for predicting the severity of haemolytic disease of the fetus and newborn. Vox Sang 1998; 74:375.

106. Novotny VM, Kanhai HH, Overbeeke MA, et al: Misleading results in the determination of haemolytic disease of the newborn using antibody titration and ADCC in a woman with anti-Lu[b]. Vox Sang 1992; 62:49.

107. Frankowska K, Gorska B: IgG subclasses of anti-Rh antibodies in pregnant women. Arch Immunol Ther Exp (Warsz) 1978; 26:1095.

108. Pollock JM, Bowman JM: Anti-Rh(D) IgG subclasses and severity of Rh hemolytic disease of the newborn. Vox Sang 1990; 59:176.

109. Zupanska B, Brojer E, Richards Y, et al: Serological and immunological characteristics of maternal anti-Rh(D) antibodies in predicting the severity of haemolytic disease of the newborn. Vox Sang 1989; 56:247.

110. Parinaud J, Blanc M, Grandjean H, et al: IgG subclasses and Gm allotypes of anti-D antibodies during pregnancy: Correlation with the gravity of the fetal disease. Am J Obstet Gynecol 1985; 151:1111.

111. Hadley AG, Kumpel BM, Merry AH: The chemiluminescent response of human monocytes to red cells sensitized with monoclonal anti-Rh(D) antibodies. Clin Lab Hematol 1988; 10:377.

112. Hadley AG, Wilkes A, Goodrick J, et al: The ability of the chemiluminescence test to predict clinical outcome and the necessity for amniocenteses in pregnancies at risk of haemolytic disease of the newborn. Br J Obstet Gynaecol 1998; 105:231.

113. Hadley AG, Kumpel BM, Leader K, et al: An in-vitro assessment of the functional activity of monoclonal anti-D. Clin Lab Haematol 1989; 11:47.

114. Kumpel BM, Hadley AG: Functional interactions of red cells sensitized by IgG1 and IgG3 human monoclonal anti-D with enzyme-modified human monocytes and FcR-bearing cell lines. Mol Immunol 1990; 27:247.

115. Thomsom A, Contreras M, Gorick B: Clearance of D-positive cells with monoclonal anti-D. Lancet 1990; 336:1147.

116. Hadley AG, Kumpel BM: The role of Rh antibodies in haemolytic disease of the newborn. Baillieres Clin Haematol 1993; 6:423.

117. Lewis M, Chown B: A short albumin method for the determination of isohemagglutinins, particularly incomplete Rh antibodies. J Lab Clin Med 1957; 50:494.

118. Filbey D, Garner SF, Hadley AG, et al: Quantitative and functional assessment of anti-RhD: A comparative study of non-invasive methods in antenatal prediction of Rh hemolytic disease. Acta Obstet Gynecol Scand 1996; 75:102.

119. Rosenfield RE, Haber GV: Detection and measurement of homologous human hemagglutinins. Presented at the Technicon Symposia, Tarrytown, NY, 1965.

120. Lalezari P: A polybrene method for the detection of red cell antibodies. Fed Proc 1967; 26:756.

121. Moore BPL: Automation in the blood transfusion laboratory: I. Antibody detection and quantitation in the Technicon AutoAnalyzer. Can Med Assoc J 1969; 100:381.

122. Hadley AG, Kumpel BM, Leader KA, et al: Correlation of serological, quantitative and cell-mediated functional assays of maternal alloantibodies with the severity of haemolytic disease of the newborn. Br J Haematol 1991; 77:221.

123. Hirvonen M, Tervonen S, Pirkola A, et al: An enzyme-linked immunosorbent assay for the quantitative determination of anti-D in plasma samples and immunoglobulin preparations. Vox Sang 1995; 69:341.

124. Lambin P, Ahaded A, Debbia M, et al: An enzyme-linked immunosorbent assay for the quantitation of IgG anti-D and IgG subclasses in the sera of alloimmunized patients. Transfusion 1998; 38:252.

125. Alie-Daram SJ, Fournie A, Dugoujon JM: Gel test assay for IgG subclass detection by GM typing: Application to hemolytic disease of the newborn. J Clin Lab Anal 2000; 14:1.

126. Hessner MJ, McFarland JG, Endean DJ: Genotyping of KEL1 and KEL2 of the human Kell blood group system by the polymerase chain reaction with sequence-specific primers. Transfusion 1996; 36:495.

127. Faas BH, Maaskant-Van Wijk PA, von dem Borne AE, et al: The applicability of different PCR-based methods for fetal RHD and K1 genotyping: A prospective study. Prenat Diagn 2000; 20:453.

128. Yankowitz J, Li S, Murray JC: Polymerase chain reaction determination of RhD blood type: An evaluation of accuracy. Obstet Gynecol 1995; 86:214.

129. Spence WC, Maddalena A, Demers DB, et al: Molecular analysis of the RhD genotype in fetuses at risk for RhD hemolytic disease. Obstet Gynecol 1995; 85:296.

130. Spence WC, Potter P, Maddalena A, et al: DNA-based prenatal determination of the *RhEe* genotype. Obstet Gynecol 1995; 86:670.

131. Lo YM, Hjelm NM, Fidler C, et al: Prenatal diagnosis of fetal RhD status by molecular analysis of maternal plasma. N Engl J Med 1998; 339:1734.

132. Avent ND: Antenatal genotyping of the blood groups of the fetus. Vox Sang 1998; 74:365.

133. Maaskant-van Wijk PA, Faas BH, de Ruijter JA, et al: Genotyping of RHD by multiplex polymerase chain reaction analysis of six RHD-specific exons. Transfusion 1998; 38:1015.

134. Van den Veyver IB, Chong SS, Cota J, et al: Single-cell analysis of the RhD blood type for use in preimplantation diagnosis in the prevention of severe hemolytic disease of the newborn. Am J Obstet Gynecol 1995; 172:533.

135. Allen RW, Ward S, Harris R: Prenatal genotyping for the RhD blood group antigen: Considerations in developing an accurate test. Genet Test 2000; 4:377.

136. Bennett PR, Kim CLV, Colin Y, et al: Prenatal determination of fetal RhD type by DNA amplification. N Engl J Med 1993; 329:607.

137. Lo YM: Fetal RhD genotyping from maternal plasma. Ann Med 1999; 31:308.

138. Oepkes D: Invasive versus non-invasive testing in red-cell alloimmunized pregnancies. Eur J Obstet Gynecol Reprod Biol 2000; 92:83.

139. Harrison KL, Baker JW, Popper EI, et al: Value of maternal anti-D concentration in predicting the outcome of Rh(D) haemolytic disease. Aust NZ J Obstet Gynaecol 1984; 24:6.

140. Bowell P, Wainscoat JS, Peto TE, et al: Maternal anti-D concentrations and outcome in rhesus haemolytic disease of the newborn. Br Med J (Clin Res Ed) 1982; 285:327.

141. Hadley AG: In vitro assays to predict the severity of hemolytic disease of the newborn. Transfus Med Rev 1995; 9:302.

142. Nance SJ, Nelson JM, Horenstein J, et al: Monocyte monolayer assay: An efficient noninvasive technique for predicting the severity of hemolytic disease of the newborn. Am J Clin Pathol 1989; 92:89.

143. Urbaniak SJ, Greiss MA, Crawford RJ, et al: Prediction of the outcome of rhesus haemolytic disease of the newborn: Additional information using an ADCC assay. Vox Sang 1984; 46:323.

144. Engelfriet CP, Brouwers HA, et al: Prognostic value of the ADCC with monocytes and maternal antibodies for haemolytic disease if the newborn (abstract). In Abstracts of the XXIst Congress of the International Society of Hematology and XIXth Congress of the International Society of Blood Transfusion, Sydney, Australia, 1986, p 162.

145. Zupanska B: Assays to predict the clinical significance of blood group antibodies. Curr Opin Hematol 1998; 5:412.

146. Wiener AS, Wexler LB: The use of heparin when performing exchange transfusions in newborn infants. J Lab Clin Med 1946; 31:1016.

147. Results of tests with different cellular bioassays in relation to severity of RhD haemolytic disease. Report from nine collaborating laboratories. Vox Sang 1991; 60:225.

148. Moise KJ Jr, Perkins JT, Sosler SD, et al: The predictive value of maternal serum testing for detection of fetal anemia in red blood cell alloimmunization. Am J Obstet Gynecol 1995; 172:1003.

149. Bevis DCA: Blood pigments in hemolytic disease of the newborn. J Obstet Gynaecol Br Emp 1956; 63:68.

150. Liley AW: Liquor amnii analysis in management of pregnancy complicated by rhesus immunization. Am J Obstet Gynecol 1961; 82:1359.

151. Management of Isoimmunization in Pregnancy. ACOG Educational Bulletin 90. Washington, DC, American College of Obstetricians and Gynecologists, 1986.

152. Nicolaides KH, Rodeck CH, Mibashan RS, et al: Have Liley charts outlived their usefulness? Am J Obstet Gynecol 1986; 155:90.

153. Bowman JM, Pollock JM, Manning FA, et al: Maternal Kell blood group alloimmunization. Obstet Gynecol 1992; 79:239.

154. Queenan JT, Tomai TP, Ural SH, et al: Deviation in amniotic fluid optical density at a wavelength of 450 nm in Rh-immunized pregnancies from 14 to 40 weeks' gestation: A proposal for clinical management. Am J Obstet Gynecol 1993; 168:1370.

155. Grannum PA, Copel JA: Prevention of Rh isoimmunization and treatment of the compromised fetus. Semin Perinatol 1988; 12:324.

156. Spinnato JA, Clark AL, Ralston KK, et al: Hemolytic disease of the fetus: A comparison of the Queenan and extended Liley methods. Obstet Gynecol 1998; 92:441.

157. Scott F, Chan FY: Assessment of the clinical usefulness of the 'Queenan' chart versus the 'Liley' chart in predicting severity of rhesus iso-immunization. Prenat Diagn 1998; 18:1143.

158. Detti L, Oz U, Guney I, et al: Doppler ultrasound velocimetry for timing the second intrauterine transfusion in fetuses with anemia from red cell alloimmunization. Am J Obstet Gynecol 2001; 185:1048.

159. Bahado-Singh RO, Oz AU, Hsu C, et al: Middle cerebral artery Doppler velocimetric deceleration angle as a predictor of fetal anemia in Rh-alloimmunized fetuses without hydrops. Am J Obstet Gynecol 2000; 183:746.

160. Bahado-Singh R, Oz U, Deren O, et al: Splenic artery Doppler peak systolic velocity predicts severe fetal anemia in rhesus disease. Am J Obstet Gynecol 2000; 182:1222.

161. Mari G, Deter RL, Carpenter RL, et al: Noninvasive diagnosis by Doppler ultrasonography of fetal anemia due to maternal red-cell alloimmunization. Collaborative Group for Doppler Assessment of the Blood Velocity in Anemic Fetuses. N Engl J Med 2000; 342:9.

162. Mari G, Rahman F, Olofsson P, et al: Increase of fetal hematocrit decreases the middle cerebral artery peak systolic velocity in pregnancies complicated by rhesus alloimmunization. J Matern Fetal Med 1997; 6:206.

163. Delle Chiaie L, Buck G, Grab D, et al: Prediction of fetal anemia with Doppler measurement of the middle cerebral artery peak systolic velocity in pregnancies complicated by maternal blood group

alloimmunization or parvovirus B19 infection. Ultrasound Obstet Gynecol 2001; 18:232.

164. Teixeira JM, Duncan K, Letsky E, et al: Middle cerebral artery peak systolic velocity in the prediction of fetal anemia. Ultrasound Obstet Gynecol 2000; 15:205.

165. Roberts AB, Mitchell JM, Lake Y, et al: Ultrasonographic surveillance in red blood cell alloimmunization. Am J Obstet Gynecol 2001; 184:1251.

166. Daffos F, Capella-Pavlovsky M, Forestier F: Fetal blood sampling during pregnancy with use of a needle guided by ultrasound: A study of 606 consecutive cases. Am J Obstet Gynecol 1985; 153:655.

167. Bowman JM, Pollock JM, Peterson LE, et al: Fetomaternal hemorrhage following funipuncture: Increase in severity of maternal red-cell alloimmunization. Obstet Gynecol 1994; 84:839.

168. de Silva M, Contreras M, Mollison PL: Failure of passively administered anti-Rh to prevent secondary Rh responses. Vox Sang 1985; 48:178.

169. Bowman JM, Pollock JM: Reversal of Rh alloimmunization. Fact or fancy? Vox Sang 1984; 47:209.

170. Graham-Pole J, Barr W, Willoughby ML: Continuous-flow plasmapheresis in management of severe rhesus disease. Br Med J 1977; 1:1185.

171. Angela E, Robinson E, Tovey LA: Intensive plasma exchange in the management of severe Rh disease. Br J Haematol 1980; 45:621.

172. Gottvall T, Selbing A: Alloimmunization during pregnancy treated with high dose intravenous immunoglobulin. Effects on fetal hemoglobin concentration and anti-D concentrations in the mother and fetus. Acta Obstet Gynecol Scand 1995; 74:777.

173. Berlin G, Selbing A, Ryden G: Rhesus haemolytic disease treated with high-dose intravenous immunoglobulin. Lancet 1985; 1:1153.

174. Margulies M, Voto LS, Mathet E: High-dose intravenous IgG for the treatment of severe rhesus alloimmunization. Vox Sang 1991; 61:181.

175. Barclay GR, Greiss MA, Urbaniak SJ: Adverse effect of plasma exchange on anti-D production in rhesus immunisation owing to removal of inhibitory factors. Br Med J 1980; 280:1569.

176. Huntley B: Red cell antigens. The fetus as a patient. Lancet 2001; 358:S58.

177. Porter TF, Silver RM, Jackson GM, et al: Intravenous immune globulin in the management of severe Rh D hemolytic disease. Obstet Gynecol Surv 1997; 52:193.

178. Liley AW: Intrauterine transfusion of foetus in haemolytic disease. BMJ 1963; 2:1107.

179. Menticoglou SM, Harman CR, Manning FA, et al: Intraperitoneal fetal transfusion: Paralysis inhibits red cell absorption. Fetal Ther 1987; 2:154.

180. Adamsons KJ, Freda VJ, James LS, et al: Prenatal treatment of erythroblastosis fetalis following hysterotomy. Pediatrics 1965; 35:848.

181. Asensio SH, Figueroa-Longo JG, Pelegrina IA: Intrauterine exchange transfusion. Am J Obstet Gynecol 1966; 95:1129.

182. Rodeck CH, Kemp JR, Holman CA, et al: Direct intravascular fetal blood transfusion by fetoscopy in severe rhesus isoimmunisation. Lancet 1981; 1:625.

183. Galligan BR, Cairns R, Schifano JV, et al: Preparation of packed red cells suitable for intravascular transfusion in utero. Transfusion 1989; 29:179.

184. de Crespigny LC, Robinson HP, Quinn M, et al: Ultrasound-guided fetal blood transfusion for severe rhesus isoimmunization. Obstet Gynecol 1985; 66:529.

185. Berkowitz RL, Chitkara U, Goldberg JD, et al: Intrauterine intravascular transfusions for severe red blood cell isoimmunization: Ultrasound-guided percutaneous approach. Am J Obstet Gynecol 1986; 155:574.

186. Nicolaides KH, Soothill PW, Rodeck CH, et al: Rh disease: Intravascular fetal blood transfusion by cordocentesis. Fetal Ther 1986; 1:185.

187. Grannum PA, Copel JA, Moya FR, et al: The reversal of hydrops fetalis by intravascular intrauterine transfusion in severe isoimmune fetal anemia. Am J Obstet Gynecol 1988; 158:914.

188. Harman CR, Bowman JM, Manning FA, et al: Intrauterine transfusion—intraperitoneal versus intravascular approach: A case-control comparison. Am J Obstet Gynecol 1990; 162:1053.

189. Bennebroek Gravenhorst J: Management of serious alloimmunization in pregnancy. Vox Sang 1988; 55:1.

190. Moise KJ Jr, Mari G, Fisher DJ, et al: Acute fetal hemodynamic alterations after intrauterine transfusion for treatment of severe red blood cell alloimmunization. Am J Obstet Gynecol 1990; 163:776.

191. Soothill PW, Lestas AN, Nicolaides KH, et al: 2,3-Diphosphoglycerate in normal, anaemic and transfused human fetuses. Clin Sci (Lond) 1988; 74:527.

192. Stewart G, Day RE, Del Priore C, et al: Developmental outcome after intravascular intrauterine transfusion for rhesus haemolytic disease. Arch Dis Child Fetal Neonatal Ed 1994; 70:F52.

193. White CA, Goplerud CP, Kisker CT, et al: Intrauterine fetal transfusion, 1965–1976, with an assessment of the surviving children. Am J Obstet Gynecol 1978; 130:933.

194. Janssens HM, de Haan MJ, van Kamp IL, et al: Outcome for children treated with fetal intravascular transfusions because of severe blood group antagonism. J Pediatr 1997; 131:373.

195. Hudon L, Moise KJ Jr, Hegemier SE, et al: Long-term neurodevelopmental outcome after intrauterine transfusion for the treatment of fetal hemolytic disease. Am J Obstet Gynecol 1998; 179:858.

196. Doyle LW, Kelly EA, Rickards AL, et al: Sensorineural outcome at 2 years for survivors of erythroblastosis treated with fetal intravascular transfusions. Obstet Gynecol 1993; 81:931.

197. Murphy KW, Whitfield CR: Rhesus disease in this decade. Contemp Rev Obstet Gynecol 1994; 6:61.

198. Anderson KC, Ness PM: Scientific Basis of Transfusion Medicine. Implications for Clinical Practice. Philadelphia, WB Saunders, 2000.

199. Naiman JL, Punnett HH, Lischner HW, et al: Possible graft-versus-host reaction after intrauterine transfusion for Rh erythroblastosis fetalis. N Engl J Med 1969; 281:697.

200. Harte G, Payton D, Carmody F, et al: Graft versus host disease following intrauterine and exchange transfusions for rhesus haemolytic disease. Aust NZ J Obstet Gynaecol 1997; 37:319.

201. Plecas DV, Chitkara U, Berkowitz GS, et al: Intrauterine intravascular transfusion for severe erythroblastosis fetalis: How much to transfuse? Obstet Gynecol 1990; 75:965.

202. Phibbs RH, Johnson P, Kitterman JA, et al: Cardiorespiratory status of erythroblastotic infants. 1. Relationship of gestational age, severity of hemolytic diseases, and birth asphyxia to idiopathic respiratory distress syndrome and survival. Pediatrics 1972; 49:5.

203. Amato M, Schurch S, Grunder R, et al: Influence of bilirubin on surface tension properties of lung surfactant. Arch Dis Child Fetal Neonatal Ed 1996; 75:F191.

204. Phibbs RH, Johnson P, Kitterman JA, et al: Cardiorespiratory status of erythroblastotic newborn infants: III. Intravascular pressures during the first hours of life. Pediatrics 1976; 58:484.

205. Barrett CT, Oliver TK Jr: Hypoglycemia and hyperinsulinism in infants with erythroblastosis fetalis. N Engl J Med 1968; 278:1260.

206. Abbas A, Nicolaides K: Fetal serum ferritin and cobalamin in red blood cell isoimmunisation. Fetal Diagn Ther 1995; 10:297.

207. Lasker MR, Eddleman K, Toor AH: Neonatal hepatitis and excessive hepatic iron deposition following intrauterine blood transfusion. Am J Perinatol 1995; 12:14.

208. Sreenan C, Idikio HA, Osiovich H: Successful chelation therapy in a case of neonatal iron overload following intravascular intrauterine transfusion. J Perinatol 2000; 20:509.

209. Bowman JM: Gastro-intestinal absorption of iso-hemagglutinin. Am J Dis Child 1963; 105:352.

210. Puruggan G, Leikin S, Gautier G: Folate metabolism in erythroid hyperplastic and hypoplastic states. Am J Dis Child 1971; 122:48.

211. Gallagher PG, Ehrenkranz RA: Nutritional anemias in infancy. Clin Perinatol 1995; 22:671.

212. Mills JF, Tudehope D: Fibreoptic phototherapy for neonatal jaundice (Cochrane review). In Cochrane Database of Systematic Reviews, CD002060. Oxford, UK, Update Software, 2001

213. Dennery PA, Seidman DS, Stevenson DK: Neonatal hyperbilirubinemia. N Engl J Med 2001; 344:581.

214. Valaes T, Koliopoulos C, Koltsidopoulos A: The impact of phototherapy in the management of neonatal hyperbilirubinemia: Comparison of historical cohorts. Acta Paediatr 1996; 85:273.

215. Hansen TW: Acute management of extreme neonatal jaundice—The potential benefits of intensified phototherapy and interruption of enterohepatic bilirubin circulation. Acta Paediatr 1997; 86:843.

216. Rubo J, Albrecht K, Lasch P, et al: High-dose intravenous immune globulin therapy for hyperbilirubinemia caused by Rh hemolytic disease. J Pediatr 1992; 121:93.

217. Rubo J, Wahn V: [High-dose immunoglobulin therapy of hyper-bilirubinemia in rhesus incompatibility]. Infusionsther Transfusionsmed 1993; 20:104.

218. Dagoglu T, Ovali F, Samanci N, et al: High-dose intravenous immunoglobulin therapy for rhesus haemolytic disease. J Int Med Res 1995; 23:264.

219. Alpay F, Sarici SU, Okutan V, et al: High-dose intravenous immunoglobulin therapy in neonatal immune haemolytic jaundice. Acta Paediatr 1999; 88:216.

220. Alcock GS, Liley HG: Immunoglobulin infusion for isoimmune hemolytic jaundice in neonates. (Cochrane Review). Cochrane Database Syst Rev 2002; CD 003313.

221. Alcode GS, Liley H: Immunoglobulin infusion for isoimmune haemolytic jaundice in neonates (Cochrane Review). Cochrane Database Syst Rev 2002; CD 003313.

222. Diamond L: Replacement transfusion as a treatment for erythroblastosis fetalis. Pediatrics 1948; 2:520.

223. Mollison PL, Walker W: Controlled trials of the treatment of haemolytic disease of the newborn. Lancet 1952; 262:429.

224. Setzer ES, Webb IB, Wassenaar JW, et al: Platelet dysfunction and coagulopathy in intraventricular hemorrhage in the premature infant. J Pediatr 1982; 100:599.

225. Peterec SM: Management of neonatal Rh disease. Clin Perinatol 1995; 22:561.

226. Wennberg RP, Depp R, Heinrichs WL: Indications for early exchange transfusion in patients with erythroblastosis fetalis. J Pediatr 1978; 92:789.

227. Jackson JC: Adverse events associated with exchange transfusion in healthy and ill newborns. Pediatrics 1997; 99:e7.

228. Edwards MC, Fletcher MA: Exchange transfusions. In Fletcher MA, MacDonald MG (eds): Atlas of Procedures in Neonatology. Philadelphia, JB Lippincott, 1993, p 363.

229. Bowman JM: Immune hemolytic disease. In Nathan DG, Orkin SH (eds): Nathan and Oski's Hematology of Infancy and Childhood, 5th ed. Philadelphia, WB Saunders, 1998.

230. Polesky HF: Blood group antibodies in prenatal sera. Minn Med 1967; 50:601.

231. Queenan JT, Smith BD, Haber JM, et al: Irregular antibodies in the obstetric patient. Obstet Gynecol 1969; 34:767.

232. Pepperell RJ, Barrie JV, Fliegner JR: Significance of red cell irregular antibodies in the obstetric patient. Med J Aust 1977; 2:453.

233. Filbey D, Hanson U, Wesstrom G: The prevalence of red cell antibodies in pregnancy correlated to the outcome of the newborn: A 12 year study in central Sweden. Acta Obstet Gynecol Scand 1995; 74:687.

234. Geifman-Holtzman O, Wojtowycz M, Kosmas E, et al: Female alloimmunization with antibodies known to cause hemolytic disease. Obstet Gynecol 1997; 89:272.

235. Mollison PL, Engelfriet CP, Contreras M: Hemolytic disease of the newborn. In Mollison PL (ed): Blood Transfusion in Clinical Medicine. Oxford, UK, Blackwell Scientific Publications, 1987, p 639.

236. Bowman JM: Treatment options for the fetus with alloimmune hemolytic disease. Transfus Med Rev 1990; 4:191.

237. Lee S, Lin M, Mele A, et al: Proteolytic processing of big endothelin-3 by the Kell blood group protein. Blood 1999; 94:1440.

238. Redman CM, Russo D, Lee S: Kell, Kx and the McLeod syndrome. Balliere's Clin Haematol 1999; 12:621.

239. Lee S, Russo D, Redman CM: The Kell blood group system: Kell and XK membrane proteins. Semin Hematol 2000; 113.

240. Caine ME, Mueller-Heubach E: Kell sensitization in pregnancy. Am J Obstet Gynecol 1986; 154:85.

241. Vaughan JI, Manning M, Warwick RM, et al: Inhibition of erythroid progenitor cells by anti-Kell antibodies in fetal alloimmune anemia. N Engl J Med 1998; 338:798.

242. Babinszki A, Lapinski RH, Berkowitz RL: Prognostic factors and management in pregnancies complicated with severe Kell alloimmunization: Experiences of the last 13 years. Am J Perinatol 1998; 15:695.

243. McKenna DS, Nagaraja HN, O'Shaughnessy R: Management of pregnancies complicated by anti-Kell isoimmunization. Obstet Gynecol 1999; 93:667.

244. Bowman JM: Immune hemolytic disease. In Nathan DG, Orkin SH (eds): Nathan and Oski's Hematology of Infancy and Childhood, 5th ed. Philadelphia, WB Saunders, 1998.

245. Dacus JV, Spinnato JA: Severe erythroblastosis fetalis secondary to anti-Kpb sensitization. Am J Obstet Gynecol 1984; 150:888.

246. Thompson DJ, Stults DZ, Daniel SJ: Anti-M antibody in pregnancy. Obstet Gynecol Surv 1989; 44:637.

247. McDonnell M, Hannam S, Devane SP: Hydrops fetalis due to ABO incompatibility. Arch Dis Child Fetal Neonatal Ed 1998; 78:F220.

248. Grundbacher FJ: The etiology of ABO hemolytic disease of the newborn. Transfusion 1980; 20:563.

249. Romano EL, Mollison PL, Linares J: Number of B sites generated on group O red cells from adults and newborn infants. Vox Sang 1978; 34:14.

250. Brouwers HA, Overbeeke MA, Huiskes E, et al: Complement is not activated in ABO-haemolytic disease of the newborn. Br J Haematol 1988; 68:363.

251. Ukita M, Takahashi A, Nunotani T, et al: IgG subclasses of anti-A and anti-B antibodies bound to the cord red cells in ABO incompatible pregnancies. Vox Sang 1989; 56:181.

252. Feng CS, Wan CP, Lau J, et al: Incidence of ABO haemolytic disease of the newborn in a group of Hong Kong babies with severe neonatal jaundice. J Paediatr Child Health 1990; 26:155.

253. Meberg A, Johansen KB: Screening for neonatal hyperbilirubinaemia and ABO alloimmunization at the time of testing for phenylketonuria and congenital hypothyreosis. Acta Paediatr 1998; 87:1269.

254. Ozolek JA, Watchko JF, Mimouni F: Prevalence and lack of clinical significance of blood group incompatibility in mothers with blood type A or B. J Pediatr 1994; 125:87.

255. Guaran RL, Drew JH, Watkins AM: Jaundice: Clinical practice in 88,000 liveborn infants. Aust NZ J Obstet Gynaecol 1992; 32:186.

256. Palmer DC, Drew JH: Jaundice: A 10 year review of 41,000 live born infants. Aust Paediatr J 1983; 19:86.

257. Desjardins L, Blajchman MA, Chintu C, et al: The spectrum of ABO hemolytic disease of the newborn infant. J Pediatr 1979; 95:447.

258. Katz MA, Kanto WP Jr, Korotkin JH: Recurrence rate of ABO hemolytic disease of the newborn. Obstet Gynecol 1982; 59:611.

259. al-Alaiyan S, al Omran A: Late hyporegenerative anemia in neonates with rhesus hemolytic disease. J Perinat Med 1999; 27:112.

260. Zuppa AA, Maragliano G, Scapillati ME, et al: Recombinant erythropoietin in the prevention of late anaemia in intrauterine transfused neonates with Rh-haemolytic disease. Fetal Diagn Ther 1999; 14:270.

261. Ovali F, Samanci N, Dagoglu T: Management of late anemia in rhesus hemolytic disease: use of recombinant human erythropoietin (a pilot study). Pediatr Res 1996; 39:831.

262. Ohls RK, Wirkus PE, Christensen RD: Recombinant erythropoietin as treatment for the late hyporegenerative anemia of Rh hemolytic disease. Pediatrics 1992; 90:678.

4 | Disorders of Bilirubin Metabolism

Peter F. Whitington ● Estella M. Alonso

Jaundice is among the most common clinical signs observed in the newborn; thus, an understanding of bilirubin metabolism is important for pediatricians. Bilirubin determination is a valuable tool in clinical evaluation because it represents an interface of the hematologic and hepatobiliary systems. Pediatricians should understand the normal metabolism of bilirubin and the clinical conditions in which its metabolism is altered if they are to effectively manage the large number of jaundiced infants encountered in their practices. This chapter discusses the chemistry, synthesis, transport, metabolism, and disposal of bilirubin, both in health and in disease.

CHEMISTRY OF BILIRUBIN AND ANALYTICAL CONSIDERATIONS

Structure and Physical Chemistry of Bilirubin

Bilirubin is a compound with a molecular weight of 584 composed of four substituted pyrrole rings linked by two outer methylene —CH= groups and one central methene (—CH2=) group[1] (Fig. 4–1). It is derived entirely from the protoporphyrin in hemoglobin and other iron-containing heme proteins.[1] The structure of bilirubin determines its physical characteristics.[2] The central carbon bridge is flexible, permitting the molecule in its diacidic form to twist so that intramolecular hydrogen bonds can form between the propionic acid carboxyl groups and the opposing pyrrole lactam systems. This causes the molecule to fold on itself and form a ridge-tile structure with both planes being apolar and either end having a hydrophilic domain. The diacid is, therefore, almost insoluble in water at physiologic pH (Fig. 4–2).[2–6] Its aqueous solubility is less than 0.005 mg/dL (86 nmol/L) at pH 7.4.[3] It is more water-soluble in the ionized form when the hydrogen bonds are partially broken. The apparent pK_a for bilirubin is 8.1.[7] When the hydrogen bonds are broken, the pK_a values of the carboxyl groups are 4.2 and 4.9, very similar to those of other carboxyl compounds.[8] The diacid is soluble in relatively polar

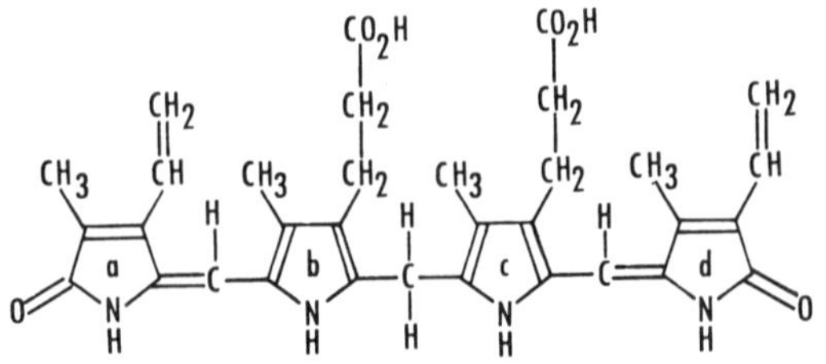

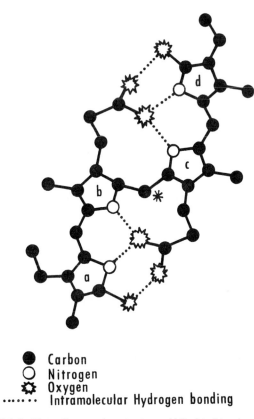

FIGURE 4–1. Standard chemical structure of bilirubin IXa.

● Carbon
○ Nitrogen
✿ Oxygen
······· Intramolecular Hydrogen bonding

FIGURE 4–2. Naturally occurring structure of bilirubin IXα, demonstrating intramolecular hydrogen bonding (·····) and rotation of a-b and c-d dipyrroles around the central methene carbon (*). (From Bonnett R, Davies JE, Hursthouse MB: The structure of bilirubin. Nature (Lond) 1976; 262:326. Reprinted with permission from *Nature.* Copyright © MacMillan Magazines Ltd.)

organic solvents such as chloroform and essentially insoluble in nonpolar solvents such as diethyl ether.[1, 3] It is insoluble in biologic membranes; rather it associates with the surface of membranes by interaction with the relatively polar ends of the ridge-tile molecule and the polar head groups of membrane phospholipids. It can move rapidly across the surface of membranes in a tumbling fashion and readily flip-flops through membranes to gain access to the inside of organelles such as endoplasmic reticulum. The movement of bilirubin from albumin through membranes displays first-order kinetics with a $t_{1/2}$ of 130 msec.[9]

Isomers of Bilirubin

The asymmetry of the molecule, which determines its peculiar physical chemistry, is caused by the specificity of heme oxygenase for cleaving heme (IX ferroprotoporphyrin) at the α-methylene linkage, which results in the production of only bilirubin IXα (see section on bilirubin synthesis).[10–13] Nonenzymatic cleavage of the β-, γ-, and δ- sites results in the production of trace amounts of the IXβ, γ, and δ bilirubin isomers.[14, 15] Acid-catalyzed cleavage of the central methene bridge of bilirubin IXα and scrambling of the dissimilar dipyrrole halves can result in the formation of three α-isomers: bilirubin III, IX, and XIIIα.[16] Trace quantities of all these isomers of bilirubin can be found in bile.[17] The isomers of bilirubin that are formed during phototherapy are discussed in the section dealing with that therapeutic technique.

Conjugated Bilirubin

The conjugation of bilirubin occurs at the C8 and C12 propionic acid carboxyl groups by the enzymatic formation of ester bonds, usually with a glycoside moiety. Glucuronide esters are the most common conjugates of bilirubin in man.[18, 19] Conjugation abolishes internal hydrogen bonding by consuming one or both of the carboxyl groups and by introducing a bulky glycoside moiety that prevents the bilirubin molecule from folding on itself. As a consequence, conjugated bilirubin is much more water-soluble than bilirubin.[20] It does not flip-flop through membranes as does bilirubin, but requires facilitated transport.[9]

Bilirubin Covalently Bound to Albumin

Some serum bilirubin is covalently bound to albumin and is known as *delta bilirubin* or *biliprotein*.[21, 22] This fraction may account for a significant proportion of the total bilirubin in patients with cholestatic jaundice, but is absent in patients with nonconjugated hyperbilirubinemia.[23, 24] This complex is formed in plasma by a nonenzymatic process that involves acyl migration of bilirubin from its glucuronide ester with the formation of an amide linkage between one propionic acid side chain and a lysine residue of plasma albumin.[25] Its plasma half-life is equal to that of the albumin to which it is bound, about 18 to 20 days.[26]

Measurement of Bilirubin in Serum

The diazo reaction is the basis for most clinical determinations of bilirubin. This reaction, which was discovered by Ehrlich in 1883 and fully described by van den Bergh in 1916, involves the hydrolysis of bilirubin at the central methene bridge and the subsequent reaction of one dipyrrole with the diazonium to form an azodipyrrole. The second dipyrrole combines with the complementary half of another previously hydrolyzed bilirubin molecule to form bilirubin, which can further react. In stepwise fashion, all available bilirubin is converted to azodipyrroles, which are red and have an absorption maximum at 530 to 540 nm.[1] The procedure calls for the dilution of serum with water and the addition of a diazotizing agent, usually diazosulfanilic acid. Some of the bilirubin, the *direct-reacting* fraction, reacts immediately. The remainder does not react until an "accelerator" is added, usually alcohol or caffeine, which causes a conformational change in albumin that displaces bilirubin. In the presence of an accelerator, all serum bilirubin reacts, yielding the *total bilirubin value*. The total bilirubin value minus the direct-reacting bilirubin value is the *indirect-reacting bilirubin value*.

The measurement of total bilirubin by the van den Bergh reaction is very reproducible, but the direct-reacting bilirubin measurement is not reproducible because of its dependence upon the conditions of the assay and on time.[27] The direct-reacting fraction comprises all bilirubin conjugates and biliprotein. A portion of nonconjugated bilirubin also reacts, which confounds the interpretation of results particularly in patients with high levels of nonconjugated bilirubin. The higher the total bilirubin concentration, even if it is all nonconjugated bilirubin, the higher the direct-reacting bilirubin value will be. Despite its problems, the direct bilirubin value is still a standard clinical measurement in many hospitals. Any value less than 1 mg/dL is considered normal (the test is highly inaccurate at low levels of conjugated bilirubin), and in samples with high total bilirubin concentrations, any value less than 20 percent of the total bilirubin should be considered normal. The presence of bilirubin covalently bound to albumin (delta bilirubin) presents another problem with interpretation[24]; the direct-reacting fraction remains high for a period equal to the life of circulating serum albumin even if the conjugated bilirubin concentration decreases to normal. Thus, after relief of extrahepatic bile duct obstruction, the direct-reacting bilirubin level can remain increased even in the absence of conjugated bilirubin.

The Kodak Ektachem system[28, 29] uses film technology to separate the various species of bilirubin before they react with the diazotizing agent. It allows independent and extremely accurate measurement of total bilirubin, nonconjugated bilirubin, and conjugated bilirubin concentrations. The quantity of delta bilirubin is calculated. This system precisely measures the level of conjugated bilirubin in the physiologic range (<0.3 mg/dL), and the conjugated bilirubin value is not affected by a high total bilirubin concentration. It does not, however, permit the separate measurement of bilirubin monoglucuronide and diglucuronide. At present only complex methodology using high-performance liquid chromatography of azodipyrroles is able to distinguish between mono- and diconjugated bilirubin.[22, 24, 30–32]

Cutaneous Bilirubinometry

The presence of jaundice correlates with an elevated serum bilirubin concentration. In the newborn with an elevated nonconjugated bilirubin level, icteric skin is generally perceptible at a serum bilirubin level of about 5 mg/dL. It has been noted that jaundice in a newborn progresses caudally.[33] It is apparent in the head and neck at bilirubin levels of 4 to 8 mg/dL, the upper trunk at 5 to 12 mg/dL, the lower trunk and legs at 11 to 18 mg/dL, and the palms and soles at greater than 15 mg/dL. In the older child and adult, scleral icterus can be seen with bilirubin levels as low as 2.0 mg/dL. Jaundice in the newborn has been quantitated by cutaneous bilirubinometry using reflectance spectroscopy.[34–38] The technique involves a probe that emits light at 465 nm wavelength perpendicularly to the plane of the skin; the amount reflected back into a photodiode array is then measured. The device is placed tightly over a blanched area of skin, usually over the sternum. Because bilirubin absorbs light at this wavelength, the amount of light returning to the photodiode is inversely proportional to the amount of bilirubin in the skin. Cutaneous bilirubinometry is an inaccurate means of measuring serum bilirubin because the relationship between skin reflectance and serum bilirubin is complex. However, in an individual infant, cutaneous bilirubinometry results correlate very closely with serum bilirubin level; thus, this technique can be used to record change over time.

BILIRUBIN SYNTHESIS, TRANSPORT, AND METABOLISM

Serum concentrations of both bilirubin and its conjugates are determined by the rates of entry of the pigments into the circulation and their rates of removal.[39, 40] For nonconjugated bilirubin, two major sources of entry must be considered: new synthesis from heme and reabsorption from the intestine after biliary excretion (Fig. 4–3). Virtually all of the circulating bilirubin in the normal adult is derived from new synthesis, whereas in the newborn the enteric pool contributes a significant proportion.[40, 41] Clearance of bilirubin depends entirely on the liver. The minute amount of conjugated bilirubin in serum of healthy individuals ($\approx$0.1 mg/dL) evidently comes from regurgitation from hepatocytes. In patients with cholestasis, conjugated bilirubin can account for almost all serum bilirubin. Clearance of conjugated bilirubin can be hepatic or renal.[20] In conditions of total hepatic excretory failure, such as total extrahepatic biliary atresia, renal clearance and other poorly understood disposal mechanisms maintain bilirubin concentrations usually below 20 mg/dL.

Bilirubin Synthesis

The normal adult makes 250 to 350 mg of bilirubin per day, averaging 4.4 mg/kg of body weight per day.[39] Approximately 70 to 80 percent of new bilirubin is derived from senescent circulating erythrocytes and is formed approximately 120 days after the original synthesis of the heme. The remainder is formed from degradation of heme from immature erythrocyte precursors and tissue hemeproteins—in particular hepatic cytochromes, catalase, and tryptophan pyrrolase.[42, 43] The synthesis of bilirubin from these sources follows original heme synthesis by only 1 to 5 days and is often referred to as *early-labeled bilirubin production*, as defined by studies in which isotopically labeled heme precursors are administered and bile pigment excretion is monitored over time.[43, 44] Although nearly every tissue is capable of degrading heme to bilirubin, the reticuloendothelial organs, especially the spleen and liver, are responsible for the majority of bilirubin synthesis.

The conversion of heme to bilirubin requires two closely linked enzymatic steps. The first step involves heme

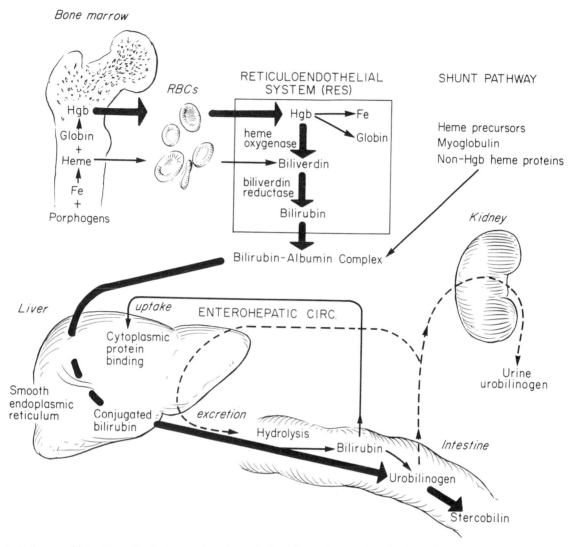

FIGURE 4–3. Pathways of bilirubin synthesis, transport, and metabolism. (From Gartner LM: Disorders of bilirubin metabolism. In Assali NS (ed): *Pathophysiology of Gestation*, Vol III. New York, Academic Press, 1972, p 457.)

oxygenase, which can be isolated from the microsomal fractions of macrophages in spleen, bone marrow, liver, hepatocytes, renal tubular epithelial cells, and the choroid plexus.[13, 45] It functions in combination with reduced nicotinamide adenosine phosphate (NADPH)-cytochrome *c* reductase to remove the α-meso bridge carbon, which is oxidized to carbon monoxide[46]; as a result, the cyclic tetrapyrrole heme is converted to the linear tetrapyrrole biliverdin and one molecule of ferrous iron is released.[45, 47, 48] Free hemoporphyrin is cleaved more rapidly than hemoglobin, so it seems that the iron-containing protoporphyrin IX molecule is first removed from the protein moiety before it reacts with heme oxygenase.[13] The process is stereospecific and yields only biliverdin IXα. Molecular oxygen and NADPH are required.

The heme oxygenase reaction is the rate-limiting step in bilirubin synthesis and can be upregulated three- to fivefold in response to hemolysis.[13] Substrate-mediated regulation occurs at the transcriptional level. Similarly, after splenectomy hepatic heme oxygenase activity increases two- to threefold in compensation. Fasting results in increased bilirubin production by temporarily

increasing the activity of heme oxygenase.[49, 50] This is thought to be one reason why patients with Gilbert syndrome exhibit increased serum bilirubin after fasting and may contribute to the jaundice observed in infants with pyloric stenosis.[51–53]

The carbon monoxide formed during heme degradation is excreted unchanged by the lung. Although there are other potential endogenous sources of small amounts of carbon monoxide (e.g., lipid peroxidation),[46, 54] quantitative estimation of its excretion offers a reasonably accurate assessment of the rate of heme degradation from all sources and, therefore, of bilirubin synthesis.[46, 54–62]

The second step of bilirubin synthesis involves biliverdin reductase, which is found in the cytosol of most cells. This enzyme catalyzes the conversion of biliverdin to bilirubin by reduction at the central methylene bridge, with NADPH as the hydrogen donor.[63–66] Biliverdin reductase is stereospecific for biliverdin IXα.[67] The three enzymes involved in bilirubin synthesis— heme oxygenase, cytochrome *c* reductase, and biliverdin reductase—may exist as a ternary complex located at the cytosol–endoplasmic reticulum interface in tissues involved in bilirubin synthesis.[47, 48, 66, 68, 69] Such a configuration may account for the rapidity with which bilirubin is synthesized. Exogenously administered heme first appears in bile as conjugated bilirubin within 2 minutes, while administered biliverdin appears in less than 1 minute.[12, 70, 71]

There seems to be little biologic advantage to converting biliverdin, a green, water-soluble, and apparently nontoxic pigment, to the water-insoluble and toxic bilirubin. One possible advantage is improved placental transport. Heme turnover occurs throughout gestation, and removal of the metabolic end-products is an important placental function. A specific transporter for bilirubin and passive diffusion are apparently important for bilirubin clearance. Biliverdin, with its increased water solubility, would not be cleared as well as bilirubin by the placenta.[72–74] Bilirubin formation may, therefore, have an advantage in mammals that is not shared by birds and reptiles, which do not reduce biliverdin to bilirubin. Postnatally, bilirubin synthesis may serve to protect the kidneys and other tissues. If it were filtered in large amounts by a kidney capable of concentrating the urine, biliverdin could "salt out," forming crystals and producing obstruction of renal tubules and collecting ducts.

Bilirubin is an antioxidant that is potentially capable of protecting tissues against peroxidative injury.[75–80] Bilirubin, with its extended system of conjugated double bonds and a reactive hydrogen atom, could function as an important scavenger for peroxyl radicals. Both bilirubin and biliverdin function as effective antioxidants at micromolar concentrations in multilamellar liposomes.[80] This antioxidant activity increases as the oxygen concentration in the system decreases, and at low oxygen tensions bilirubin is more effective than α-tocopherol at suppressing lipid peroxidation.[77] In primary rat hepatocyte culture, bilirubin in solution with albumin has a cytoprotective effect on cells exposed to inducers of free radical stress.[81] This cytoprotection was also demonstrated for human erythrocytes and was significant at physiologic levels of bilirubin (3.4 to 26 μmol/L). In addition, an *in vivo* study examining rat liver chemiluminescence demonstrated that induction of heme oxygenase by cobalt chloride increased the level of reactive oxygen species, reduced intrahepatic glutathione content, and markedly decreased the activity of the important antioxidant enzymes superoxide dismutase, catalase, and glutathione peroxidase. Pretreatment of the animals with bilirubin infusion prevented the heme oxygenase induction, attenuated the increase in chemiluminescence, and prevented a drop in hepatic glutathione.[82] Both of these studies strongly suggest that the antioxidant properties of bilirubin are important under physiologic and stress conditions. However, a protective effect has been difficult to demonstrate in human neonates. Increased bilirubin production may, indeed, increase tissue lipid peroxidation.[83] Further work in this area is needed to determine the teleologic role of bilirubin in protecting the newborn animal during its transition to an oxygen-rich environment. Some similar protection may also be conferred by bilirubin excreted in bile into the intestine, which is particularly well endowed with mechanisms for producing oxidative tissue injury.[84–89]

Bilirubin Transport in Plasma

Bilirubin in plasma is tightly bound to albumin.[90, 91] The primary binding site has a binding affinity of 10^8 mol^{-1}.[3, 92, 93] A second binding site of somewhat lower affinity also exists, and additional weaker binding sites have been postulated.[94, 95] One gram of albumin can bind 8.3 mg of bilirubin at the primary binding site; thus, a patient with an albumin concentration of 3.5 g/dL can potentially bind 29 mg/dL of plasma. The second binding site could double the theoretical capacity to 58 mg/dL. Diminished albumin concentrations, the presence of substances competing with bilirubin for the same sites, and alterations in the configuration of albumin that diminish the affinity of the binding sites can reduce the binding capacity and affinity. Conjugates of bilirubin are also bound to albumin in serum, with less than 1 percent existing in free form, but their binding affinity is much less than that for bilirubin.[92]

Studies in analbuminemic rats have demonstrated that plasma lipoproteins can serve as important carriers for bilirubin.[96–98] Serum bilirubin in analbuminemic rats is bound to a lipoprotein fraction, which effectively protects the animals from brain injury. Furthermore, exogenously administered bilirubin is transported to the liver, where uptake is undisturbed by the absence of albumin.[99] Interestingly, about 40 percent of bilirubin in hyperbilirubinemic Gunn rats, which have normal serum albumin, is bound to a similar protein fraction.[98] The key element of lipoproteins that permits bilirubin transport is apolipoprotein D on the surface of high-density lipoprotein particles.[100]

The binding capacity and affinity of albumin for bilirubin have been measured for both investigative and clinical purposes using a variety of techniques. These include competitive dye binding, spectral characteristics, binding of pigment to alternate artificial and natural ligands, fluorescence of bilirubin itself when bound, quenching of albumin fluorescence, and enzymatic measurement of free or unbound bilirubin. Although these techniques have been studied for almost 20 years, much uncertainty still remains about the interpretation of results relating to theories of binding and even greater uncertainty about the application of these techniques to clinical evaluation or prediction of toxicity. The concepts and methodology of determining binding capacity, constraints in interpreting results, and relationships of binding to bilirubin toxicity have been reviewed in detail elsewhere.[101–105]

Hepatic Uptake of Bilirubin

The liver is uniquely structured for the uptake of protein bound metabolites from plasma. Because the hepatocyte has no basement membrane, its plasma membrane is separated from the blood within the hepatic sinusoids only by vascular endothelial cells that contain fenestrae large enough to permit access of plasma proteins to the perihepatocytic space (space of Disse). Furthermore, the hepatic cord structure permits contact with plasma by a large portion of the surface of each hepatocyte. Hepatic uptake of albumin-bound bilirubin is efficient and under normal conditions works at far less than saturation kinetics.[106–108] Even under conditions of extremely high rates of bilirubin production, hepatic uptake is probably not limiting to bilirubin clearance.

Bilirubin enters the hepatocyte from plasma by a non–energy-dependent process. Whether it moves across the hepatocyte plasma membrane by simple diffusion (flip-flop) or is facilitated by a membrane transport protein is still being debated.[109, 110] A variety of candidate organic anion transport proteins (OATPs) have been isolated.[111] In the rat, a 55-kd organic anion binding protein has been determined to be important in bilirubin uptake. Its function can be inhibited by an antibody to the purified protein.[112] Uptake is not enhanced or reduced by the binding of bilirubin to albumin, leading to the conclusion that the membrane receptor has an *in vivo* affinity that allows it to readily extract bilirubin from albumin.[113] Recently it has been shown that the human *OATP2* gene product participates in the transport of bilirubin and sulfobromophthalein (BSP), but not other organic anions.[114] However, Zucker and Goessling[7] very clearly showed rapid transmembrane movement of bilirubin into lipid vesicles in the absence of carrier protein. The rate of flux is dependent on the dissociation of bilirubin from albumin and could easily account for bilirubin uptake *in vivo*.[7] Additional work is needed to clarify this issue.

After uptake, bilirubin briefly accumulates in the hepatocyte. Again, there is some controversy about intracellular binding and trafficking. It has been thought for years that protein binding is important to prevent reflux of bilirubin back to plasma. Two cytosolic proteins have significant bilirubin-binding capacity. The most important is *ligandin* or *Y protein*, a 47-kd basic protein that accounts for 10 percent of all liver cytoplasmic protein and is also found in kidney and small intestinal mucosa. It can efficiently bind bilirubin, as well as a number of other organic anions.[115–117] It also possesses an enzymatic activity, glutathione S-transferase.[118–120] The ligandin molecule consists of two subunits; one is required for binding of organic anions and both are required for its enzymatic activity. A second, smaller (12-kd) cytoplasmic protein designated as *Z protein* also binds bilirubin, although with less affinity than ligandin.[115, 121] Z protein is identical to fatty acid–binding protein of intestinal mucosa and liver.[122] Its major function appears to be the intracellular binding and trafficking of fatty acids, and its role in bilirubin metabolism is unclear. Recent concepts about the physical interaction of bilirubin with biologic membranes and the speed with which bilirubin can move across and through membranes have left the role of protein binding in question.[9, 123–127] It may be that cytosolic proteins co-contribute to intracellular bilirubin trafficking or represent a redundant system in this important process.

Considerable data indicate that bilirubin flux across the hepatocyte basolateral membrane is bidirectional.[128] It has been estimated that in normal people up to 40 percent of bilirubin taken up by hepatocytes refluxes unchanged back into plasma.[39] Ligandin appears not to be directly involved in bilirubin uptake, but it may help to limit the amount of reflux back into plasma. Although the binding affinity of ligandin for bilirubin is less than that of albumin, the total binding capacity of ligandin permits sufficient retention of bilirubin to make its overall uptake efficient. Induction of increased levels of ligandin, as occurs with the administration of phenobarbital and with thyroidectomy, increases the overall efficiency of bilirubin uptake. Reduced levels of ligandin correlate with reduced uptake in newborn monkeys.[129]

The current model of bilirubin uptake suggests that the rate-limiting event is its delivery to the sinusoidal membrane.[130] With increasing concentrations of bilirubin in plasma, the rate of bilirubin uptake by the liver increases, although the process may be saturable at the extreme. The normal low level of serum bilirubin results from inefficient delivery at low concentrations and reflux from hepatocytes. Chronic hemolytic states produce increased synthesis and delivery of bilirubin to the liver and increased uptake. An incremental increase in serum bilirubin is seen with any major increase in production because of relatively inefficient delivery and increased reflux.

Bilirubin Conjugation

The conjugation process that results in the formation of bilirubin mono- and diglucuronide accounts for the disposal of essentially all bilirubin.[18, 19] Small amounts are converted to a water-soluble substance by conjugation with substances other than glucuronic acid[18] and trivial amounts by other hepatic biotransformation reactions.[17, 131–136] Bilirubin uridine diphosphate (UDP)–glucuronyl transferase (BUGT) catalyzes the transfer of glucuronic acid from UDP–glucuronic acid (UDPGA) to form glucuronide esters at the C8 and C12 carboxyl groups of bilirubin.[137] UDPGA is derived from glucose and is synthesized from uridine diphosphoglucose by the soluble cytoplasmic enzyme uridine diphosphoglucose dehydrogenase. The products of the reaction are bilirubin monoglucuronine (BMG) and diglucuronine (BDG).[138–141] β-Glucuronidase within the endoplasmic reticulum may function to deconjugate BDG and BMG; the resulting bilirubin can either be reconjugated or be efflux from the endoplasmic reticulum.[142] The regulatory role this reaction plays is unknown.

Within the hepatocyte, bilirubin must be delivered to the endoplasmic reticulum, the site of conjugation. Ligandin may play a role in the intracellular trafficking of bilirubin, but growing evidence suggests that intracellular membranes primarily serve this function. Recent evidence suggests that the unique physical chemistry of bilirubin, which is neither water nor lipid soluble, causes it to adsorb to, rather than be solubilized in, the phospholipid bilayers of intracellular organelles.[9, 123, 124, 143, 144] Transfer of bilirubin molecules from donor lipid vesicles to acceptor vesicles occurs at very rapid rates (<20 msec).[144] Also, the rate of glucuronidation by microsomal vesicles *in vitro* is enhanced by delivery of bilirubin bound to phospholipid vesicles.[145] At present the relative contributions of ligandin and membrane-to-membrane transfer to the transport of bilirubin from the plasma membrane to the endoplasmic reticulum is not known.

Cloning of rat and human BUGT genes has resulted in major advances in the understanding of the function of this enzyme and the molecular genetics of disorders in which it is deficient (Crigler-Najjar syndrome, the Gunn rat; see section on disorders of hepatic bilirubin metabolism).[146–160]

BUGT is a member of a multigene family encoding for various UGTs with more or less homology and selective or overlapping substrate specificities.[149, 161–166] In the human there are multiple unique exons number 1 (13 reported to date), each with a unique promoter. These are differentially spliced to four common exons (numbers 2 through 5), which leads to generation of different mRNAs that encode for the many UGT isoforms. The members of the UGT family are synthesized as pre-proteins of about 530 amino acids. A signal peptide on the amino terminal end functions to localize the protein in the endoplasmic reticulum, after which it is cleaved from the UGT molecule. Latency experiments have demonstrated the functional moiety to be inside the endoplasmic reticulum.[167, 168] Sequencing data suggest that it is anchored in the membrane by a C-terminal hydrophobic domain and that most of the enzyme resides within the lumen of the endoplasmic reticulum.[137, 150, 151] The functional portion of the molecule resides in the lumen of the endoplasmic reticulum. The region encoded by exon 1 provides substrate specificity, while exons 2 to 5 provide for the binding site for UDPGA and the membrane-spanning domain and a cytoplasmic tail. The close association of all UGTs with the membrane environment is crucial for function.[169] Delipidation or treatment with detergents markedly reduces or eliminates enzyme activity.[167, 170–173] Although UGT is predominantly located in the liver, it has been detected also in kidney, stomach, small bowel, colon, and skin.[174–176]

Two isoforms of human BUGT have been identified (BUGT1 and BUGT2) that share a common functionally important 3′ region with phenol-UGT (functions in conjugating menthol), but each have a unique functionally important 5′ region.[164] Only UGT1A1 appears to be functionally relevant in bilirubin metabolism.[177] Two genetic defects in patients with Crigler-Najjar syndrome type 1—one a substitution producing a serine to phenylalanine change and the other a substitution producing a premature stop codon—are in the common region and result in defective bilirubin UGT and phenol UGT.[178–182] The bilirubin UGT complementary deoxyribonucleic acids (cDNAs) of several patients have been expressed in a BUGT-deficient cell line, and all resulted in the complete absence of active BUGT.[183] Two other affected individuals have been discovered to have defects in the unique 5′ region of BUGT-1. If both BUGT-1 and BUGT-2 function to conjugate bilirubin, these patients should not have been severely affected, but they were. Again, cDNAs were expressed in a BUGT-deficient cell line, demonstrating that only BUGT-1 is active *in vivo* in the conjugation of bilirubin.[177] BUGT appears to be relatively selective for bilirubin and BMG as substrates.[141, 184] Evidence suggests that the enzyme exists as a tetramer, with one subunit being required for the conjugation of bilirubin and all four for the further conjugation of BMG to BDG.[185, 186]

The total capacity of BUGT to form BMG has been estimated to be 100-fold greater than the normal load of bilirubin presented to the liver for disposal, and it does not, therefore, work at saturation for bilirubin.[187] BUGT catalyzes the formation of BMG at either the C8 or the C12 position without preference.[188, 189] The same active site catalyzes the formation of BDG from BMG.[189] The enzyme has more affinity for bilirubin ($K_m \approx 981$ μmol/L)

than for BMG ($K_m \approx 10$ μmol/L).[135, 190, 191] Its affinity for UDPGA is lower ($K_m \approx 200$ to 600 μmol/L), and it appears to function below saturation for UDPGA, which is present in liver tissue at a concentration of 0.6 to 1.2 mmol/L.[189, 191, 192] This may explain why bilirubin conjugation is sensitive to factors that affect UDPGA concentration in liver. Factors (e.g., ethanol intake) that shift the redox state of the hepatocyte toward NADH, a potent inhibitor of uridine diphosphoglucose dehydrogenase, reduce BUGT activity.[185, 186] Also, depletion of UDPGA resulting from administration of xenobiotics requiring glucuronidation can affect the conjugation of bilirubin.[190, 193] Reduced UDPGA formation probably contributes to hyperbilirubinemia in infants of diabetic mothers. As mentioned earlier, fasting decreases UDPGA concentration, which may contribute to fasting hyperbilirubinemia in Gilbert syndrome.[185, 186]

For conjugation to take place, bilirubin and UDPGA must gain access to the enzyme, which is located within the endoplasmic reticulum.[194, 195] Bilirubin probably gains access rapidly by its physical interaction with lipid bilayers and its ability to spontaneously flip through them.[123, 124, 127] A specific transport protein or bilirubin translocase has not been identified. A specific transporter for UDPGA has been identified and functionally characterized.[194–197] Another cytosolic sugar nucleotide, UDP-N-acetylglucosamine, greatly enhances conjugation, probably by allosteric interaction with BUGT that greatly increases its affinity for UDPGA.[172, 198–200] Uridine diphosphoxylose enhances BUGT activity by stimulating transport of UDPGA across the endoplasmic reticulum membrane.[201] Divalent cations may also play a role in the regulation of BUGT activity.[202]

Two patterns of UGT development have been demonstrated: a fetal pattern that results in adult levels of UGT activity at birth and an adult pattern in which adult activities are reached a few weeks after birth.[203–206] BUGT belongs to the group demonstrating the adult pattern of development.[207, 208] BUGT activity at 17 to 30 weeks of gestation is about 0.1 percent of adult levels, and at 30 to 40 weeks of gestation, it is about 1 percent of adult values. Adult values are reached by about 14 weeks after birth. This accelerated development appears to be turned on by birth itself. It follows premature birth without delay, and postmaturity delays its onset.[204, 207, 209] Ultimately, female rats have greater BUGT activity than do male rats,[210] and women have lower serum bilirubin concentrations than do men; these findings suggest that sex hormones influence development.

At least two additional carbohydrate conjugates of bilirubin, a glucoside and a xyloside, can also be found in small amounts in human bile.[18, 19] Other species, particularly the dog, produce much larger proportions of nonglucuronide conjugates and have a mixed glucuronide-glucoside diester as the predominant conjugate in bile.[211] Apparently only one transferase enzyme mediates the formation of all of these conjugates,[141] and there is some debate about why bilirubin is selectively conjugated with glucuronic acid in humans. One theory involves the limited entry of water-soluble UDP-glycosides into the smooth endoplasmic reticulum, which is postulated to involve a transport mechanism that is substrate-specific.[194, 195] Other potential substrates for the transferase enzyme are not transported into the smooth endoplasmic reticulum and are available to the transferase enzyme only in trace amounts as a result of nonspecific leakage. Opponents of this theory suggest that there are different enzyme affinities for the various UDP-glycosides,[192, 212, 213], but evidence to the contrary exists.[138] The increased proportion of nonglucuronide conjugates in the bile of fetuses can be explained by either theory—developmentally reduced specificity of either the transporter or BUGT. Differences in the lipid microenvironment in which BUGT functions is thought to have some effect on substrate specificity.[143, 214–218] Changes in microsomal microviscosity that occur in fetal and early postnatal development[219, 220] may explain the patterns of bilirubin conjugation with sugars other than glucuronic acid in the fetus and newborn.[221–224]

Although BMG is water-soluble and capable of being excreted into bile without further alteration by the hepatocyte, 80 percent of bilirubin is excreted in normal adults as BDG.[18, 19] In conditions associated with reduced transferase activity, such as Gilbert syndrome, and in the neonate, BMG is the predominant bile pigment.[18, 19, 225–227] A direct correlation exists between the relative amounts of BDG and BMG in bile and the level of BUGT activity.[228, 229] Because the glucuronide esters are formed sequentially, not simultaneously, and the affinity of BUGT for bilirubin is greater than that for BMG, BMG is the predominant product as the system approaches the maximum rate of conjugation (saturation kinetics). In severe hemolysis, a shift toward the excretion of BMG may occur.[230]

Bilirubin Excretion

Hepatic excretion into bile rapidly follows conjugation, so rapidly, in fact, that BDG cannot be recovered from the liver even after bilirubin loading. Further, it proceeds against a large concentration gradient, because biliary bilirubin concentrations are 40 times greater than those in serum and 100 times greater than those in liver cytoplasm.[231, 232] Excretion involves two steps, the movement of bilirubin conjugates from the endoplasmic reticulum to the canalicular membrane and their translocation across the membrane into canalicular bile.

Little is known about the movement of bilirubin conjugates within the hepatocyte. Obviously, some system directs the movement toward the canalicular domain because very little of the conjugate refluxes into serum. Evidence exists that vectoring is accomplished by way of a microtubule-dependent membrane translocation mechanism.[70, 71, 233, 234] Bilirubin excretion somewhat depends on the rates of bile salt and biliary lipid excretion, which depend on the hepatocyte microtubular system.[233–235] Xenobiotics that interfere with lipid excretion reduce bilirubin excretion as well.[236, 237] These findings have been interpreted to indicate either a primary dependence of bilirubin excretion on the microtubular system or its association with lipids destined for excretion.[238–242] Conjugated bilirubin adheres to biologic membranes with a similar avidity to bilirubin, but cannot flip through them.[9, 124] Microtubules may represent a membrane conduit along which conjugated bilirubin can slide at high speed from the site of conjugation to the site of excretion, a sort of wormhole for BMG and BDG to traverse the cytoplasmic universe. Binding to cytosolic proteins may also occur, but their role in intracellular transport is probably minimal because of their size-limited rate of diffusion.

The canalicular excretory process appears to depend in part on a carrier-mediated adenosine triphosphate (ATP)–dependent process that is shared by a variety of endogenous and exogenous organic anions.[243–252] There is evidence for a family of carriers with overlapping substrate specificity for organic anions. Bilirubin transport is stimulated by the bicarbonate ion.[253] Evidence that there are redundant pathways for BMG and BDG excretion is plentiful. None of the mutant animal species or patients with Dubin-Johnson syndrome are profoundly jaundiced.

Bilirubin excretion depends to a degree on bile formation; thus, significant reductions in bile salt excretion and bile flow reduce bilirubin excretory capacity,[254–256] but bilirubin is in no way responsible for bile formation. Even though relatively soluble, bilirubin conjugates do not remain monomeric in bile, but form dimers or highly aggregated multimers or enter mixed biliary micelles.[5, 257] Therefore, even at very high concentrations, bilirubin in bile exerts a minimal osmotic effect.

Excretion is considered to be the rate-limiting step of overall bilirubin clearance from plasma. In situations of markedly increased bilirubin production, the retention of bilirubin conjugates is a reflection of this normal physiologic limitation.[231] It is not unusual to observe moderate elevations of conjugated bilirubin (usually <2 mg/dL) during periods of brisk hemolysis (e.g., Rh incompatibility). This should not raise concerns that liver disease is present. Severe or chronic hemolysis can result in combined conjugated and nonconjugated hyperbilirubinemia. The nonconjugated fraction may result from inefficient uptake and retention by hepatocytes or from intracellular deconjugation. Microsomal β-glucuronidase is possibly responsible for this phenomenon as well as for the appearance of BMG as a small proportion of bile pigment.[142]

Enterohepatic Circulation of Bilirubin

Although hepatic excretion is often viewed as the final event in the disposal of bilirubin, events occurring within the intestine and enterohepatic circulation significantly influence serum bilirubin concentrations, particularly in the newborn.[41, 94, 258] Bilirubin conjugates are relatively unstable ester glucuronides and are readily hydrolyzed to nonconjugated bilirubin within the intestinal lumen. β-Glucuronidase is the enzyme responsible for enzymatic deconjugation of bilirubin ester glucuronides. Mucosal β-glucuronidase is plentiful in fetal intestinal mucosa and persists in the newborn, whereas the bacterial β-glucuronidase level increases with the establishment of the enteric microflora.[187] Nonenzymatic hydrolysis may also occur in the alkaline environment of the neonate's upper intestine. Once hydrolysis occurs, bilirubin can be reabsorbed across the intestinal mucosa, probably through passive mechanisms to return to the liver via the portal circulation.[259]

Bilirubin reaching the distal bowel is converted to a series of urobilinoids by a hydroxylation-reduction process performed by intestinal bacteria, primarily *Clostridium perfringens* and *Escherichia coli*.[260, 261] Urobilinoids include urobilins, urobilinogens, stercobilinogens, and stercobilin; each of these is produced at a further step in the reduction process.[262] Urobilinoid formation occurs in the distal intestinal tract, primarily in the colon, except when purulent infection of the upper intestine is present. Urobilinoids formed in the intestine are partially absorbed and enter an enterohepatic recirculation. A small portion is excreted in the urine, forming the basis of a clinical test for the differential diagnosis of cholestasis. Complete obstruction of the flow of bile, such as that seen in the presence of a common duct stone, results in complete absence of urobilinoids in urine because no bilirubin is being delivered to the intestine. Patients with cellular cholestasis, in contrast, usually have elevated urine urobilinogen concentrations. The bilirubin entering the intestine, even though the amounts are reduced, results in urobilinogen formation and absorption. However, because cholestasis exists, hepatic clearance is reduced and excess urobilinogen is excreted into the urine. This test is not reliable in the neonate because the intestinal microflora may not yet be established.

DEVELOPMENTAL ASPECTS OF BILIRUBIN METABOLISM AND TRANSPORT

Normal human newborns regularly develop elevated serum nonconjugated bilirubin concentrations during the first 1 to 2 weeks of life (Fig. 4–4). This pattern of hyperbilirubinemia is known as *physiologic jaundice of the newborn* and results from a complex interaction of several normal, developmentally determined disturbances in bilirubin metabolism and transport. Many of the mechanisms of bile formation are defective in the newborn of several species, resulting in developmentally impaired bile formation that resolves by 6 to 12 months in the human infant. This does not contribute to physiologic jaundice, and the serum concentration of conjugated bilirubin is not increased in human newborns. Physiologic jaundice results from the presentation of an increased load of bilirubin to an immature liver.[187] The increased load results from increased synthesis and an overactive enterohepatic recirculation of bilirubin.

Bilirubin synthesis is normally increased in neonates. The technique used most often for indirect estimation of heme degradation in the newborn, carbon monoxide production, indicates that heme degradation and bilirubin formation are increased significantly.[55, 57, 62, 258] The erythrocyte life span is diminished in the newborn (70 to 90 days in the neonate versus 120 days in the adult) and may be even briefer in the premature infant.[263, 264] In addition, in both mature and immature neonates, large pools of erythrocyte precursors that exist within the bone marrow, liver, and spleen may also contribute to excessive bilirubin production.

Direct measurement of bilirubin excretion in the bile of newborn rhesus monkeys has shown that the total load of bilirubin presented to the liver for excretion is at least five-

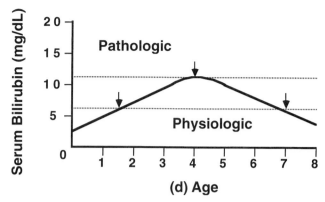

FIGURE 4–4. Defining pathologic jaundice. Infants whose total serum bilirubin falls above the curve cannot be considered to have physiologic jaundice and deserve evaluation. The arrows indicate three points that warrant particular consideration. The *left arrow* indicates early jaundice: infants who are visibly jaundiced (having a serum bilirubin level of about 7 mg/dL *[lower broken line]*) at or before 36 hours of age probably have increased bilirubin production and should be evaluated for hemolysis. The *middle arrow* indicates exaggerated hyperbilirubinemia: infants with serum bilirubin concentrations above 12 mg/dL *(upper broken line)* require diagnostic study to determine the cause as well as close monitoring to ensure that any further increase does not reach toxic levels (≈15 mg/dL in the healthy premature neonate and 20 mg/dl in the full-term neonate). These infants may have increased bilirubin production, reduced clearance, or increased enterohepatic circulation. The *right arrow* indicates prolonged jaundice: infants who are jaundiced for longer than 1 week probably have reduced clearance (hypothyroidism, hereditary hyperbilirubinemia) or increased enterohepatic circulation (breast-feeding). Any conjugated bilirubin level greater than 1 mg/dL or direct-reacting bilirubin level greater than 1 mg/dL or 10 percent of the total bilirubin level indicates hepatic dysfunction. (Adapted from Odell GB. Neonatal Hyperbilirubinemia. New York, Grune & Stratton, 1980, p 36.)

fold greater in the neonate during the first 6 weeks of life than it is in older monkeys.[187] Diversion of bile away from the intestine in newborn rhesus monkeys has shown that nearly the entire increased bilirubin load after the first week of life is derived from intestinal reabsorption. Enteric bilirubin absorption also has a key role in physiologic jaundice of the human neonate. Evidence of this is the observation that oral administration of nonabsorbable substances that bind bilirubin, such as agar and activated charcoal, results in a significant reduction in peak serum bilirubin concentrations.[41, 265–267] Increased bilirubin absorption in the newborn probably results from the deconjugation of conjugated bilirubin by the action of mucosal β-glucuronidase. Studies in animals suggest that the colon may also serve as an effective site for bilirubin absorption if sufficient nonconjugated bile pigment is present and bacterial flora are minimal, as it may be in the newborn. Meconium is another source of bilirubin to be absorbed[268]; the nonconjugated bilirubin in meconium is estimated to be 80 to 180 mg, or 5 to 10 times the normal amount of bilirubin produced in a day.[258] Nonconjugated bilirubin absorbed from the bowel becomes a portion of the total bilirubin load that the liver must handle. There is no evidence to suggest that increased enterohepatic recirculation of bilirubin is a major cause for the increased physiologic jaundice of premature infants. Reduced BUGT activity probably accounts for the increased jaundice in premature infants.[204, 207]

A somewhat limited capacity for bilirubin clearance also probably contributes to physiologic jaundice.[204, 207] A mature liver would handle the increased load with only slight elevation of serum bilirubin. In the full-term rhesus monkey, hepatic BUGT activity during the first 24 hours of life is approximately 5 percent of normal adult values, but it doubles by 24 hours of age. Peak serum bilirubin concentrations in the newborn monkey are reached at 24 hours and decline thereafter, coincident with the increase in transferase activity. Studies of autopsy material from aborted human fetuses, from infants, and from children have yielded similar information. Early in fetal development, there is a quantitative defect in bilirubin conjugation and a lack of specificity for conjugation with glucuronide. At 20 to 24 weeks of gestation, enzyme activity increases, and glucuronide monoconjugates appear in bile. At term, enzyme activity is 1 percent of adult activity, and BMG is the predominant bile pigment. Although this degree of reduced conjugating capacity is not sufficient by itself to cause retention of bilirubin, the simultaneous sixfold increase in bilirubin load is sufficient to produce the observed increase in serum bilirubin. As soon as BUGT activity increases sufficiently to accommodate the bilirubin load, the serum bilirubin concentration decreases. This occurs in the newborn monkey by 24 hours and in the human neonate by 72 to 96 hours.

Events that alter the BUGT activity have an effect on physiologic jaundice. Prepartum induction of BUGT activity by the administration of phenobarbital to the mother in the last 2 weeks of gestation can eliminate physiologic jaundice in the newborn monkey. Administration of phenobarbital to pregnant women similarly reduces the severity of physiologic jaundice.[269, 270] In premature infants, delayed maturation of BUGT results in exaggerated physiologic jaundice.[204, 207] In a rat model, this coincides with a reduction in the mass of endoplasmic reticulum.[209] Phenobarbital has little or no effect on serum bilirubin concentrations when it is administered to premature monkeys or to human premature neonates and is of little value in clinical management of the jaundiced premature infant.

A relatively stable but elevated serum nonconjugated bilirubin concentration of approximately 2 mg/dL often persists for a time after jaundice abates, normally until 12 to 14 days of life. In the premature infant, hyperbilirubinemia may persist for 4 or 5 weeks. The reasons for this are poorly understood, but evidence from the rhesus monkey indicates that it results from the simultaneous occurrence of defective hepatic uptake and a continued increased bilirubin load, primarily from enteric bilirubin absorption.[41, 187] Defective hepatic uptake may result from a developmental delay in production of ligandin, with increased reflux of bilirubin from hepatocytes under conditions of reduced BUGT activity[129, 271] or theoretically from a defect in the hepatocyte plasma membrane receptor for bilirubin. The uptake defect in the newborn is only relative, and an increased bilirubin load causes increased uptake, as it does in the adult. BUGT has no role in this prolongation of hyperbilirubinemia in full-term newborns because its activity matures earlier in life.

Fetal serum bilirubin is maintained at a low level (<2.0 mg/dL), exclusively by placental clearance, even though fetal hepatic bilirubin metabolism and excretion are established early in gestation. Placental transfer of nonconjugated bilirubin results from active transport and passive diffusion.[72–74] In the normal situation, there is a chemical gradient for bilirubin from fetus to mother, and bilirubin movement is favored by the higher albumin concentration in maternal plasma and the greater binding affinity of albumin relative to α-fetoprotein.[272, 273] In the rare circumstance that a mother has an elevated nonconjugated bilirubin concentration, the fetus may exhibit a similar elevation.[258] Even in situations of marked increased fetal bilirubin production (e.g., Rh isoimmune hemolysis), fetal serum bilirubin concentrations rarely exceed 5 to 7 mg/dL, which explains the usual absence of jaundice at birth in such babies. Immediately after cord clamping and elimination of placental clearance, serum bilirubin concentrations in these neonates rise rapidly, and clinical jaundice may be seen within 30 minutes after delivery. In contrast, fetal cholestatic liver diseases that cause retention of conjugated bilirubin are associated with jaundice at birth. The placenta is relatively impermeable to bilirubin conjugates because of their inability to flip through membranes. Cord serum direct-reacting bilirubin concentrations often exceed 7 mg/dL. The presence of delta bilirubin in cord blood indicates fetal cholestasis.[221, 274]

GENERAL CONCEPTS OF DISORDERED BILIRUBIN METABOLISM AND TRANSPORT IN THE NEWBORN

The processes that cause physiologic jaundice are present in virtually every neonate, so diseases that alter bilirubin metabolism must be diagnosed while superimposed on this background.[94, 105, 258] A difficult problem facing a clinician caring for a jaundiced newborn is distinguishing between simple physiologic jaundice and jaundice that is a manifestation of a pathologic process. In most infants a superimposed disease such as hemolysis will result in a serum bilirubin concentration above that expected in the normal newborn. Figure 4–4 provides guidelines regarding serum bilirubin and postpartum age that can help in making decisions about the need for further evaluation. Sometimes, however, knowledge of the serum bilirubin concentration alone is not adequate to distinguish between normal physiologic hyperbilirubinemia and pathologic conditions. The premature infant normally has a higher peak serum bilirubin concentration because of physiologic immaturity, but also more often exhibits hyperbilirubinemia as the result of pathologic conditions.[275] Thus, it is always wise to consider the possibility of a superimposed disease in premature infants with jaundice.

Elevated concentrations of conjugated or direct-reacting bilirubin always indicate a pathologic condition and must be evaluated (see section on conjugated hyperbilirubinemia). In some hospitals direct-reacting or conjugated fractions are not routinely determined when a serum bilirubin concentration is requested, particularly in a newborn. Occasional measurement of the direct-reacting or conjugated fraction during the course of jaundice should be standard practice. In addition, direct-reacting or conjugated bilirubin concentrations should always be determined before initiation of phototherapy, because the infant with hepatocellular disease may develop the "bronze baby syndrome" when exposed to therapeutic light.[276-280] This is more fully discussed in the section on management of neonatal hyperbilirubinemia.

SPECIFIC DISEASES ASSOCIATED WITH NONCONJUGATED HYPERBILIRUBINEMIA OF THE NEWBORN

Hemolytic Disorders and Increased Bilirubin Production

The specific conditions causing increased erythrocyte destruction have been discussed in detail in the preceding chapter. In nearly all newborn infants with hemolytic disease, a major manifestation in addition to anemia is jaundice. Even mildly increased rates of hemolysis that may not cause anemia can lead to substantial increases in serum bilirubin, reflecting the delicate balance in the newborn between bilirubin load and hepatic clearance.

Rh ISOIMMUNE HEMOLYSIS (ERYTHROBLASTOSIS FETALIS)

The most severe degrees of hyperbilirubinemia are seen in this disorder[281] (see Chapter 3). Affected infants develop jaundice within the first few hours of life, and serum bilirubin concentrations routinely exceed safe limits within 48 hours. The magnitude of the peak serum bilirubin concentration may be crudely predicted from cord hemoglobin and bilirubin concentrations and reticulocyte and nucleated red blood cell counts, as well as from amniotic fluid bilirubin concentrations measured as the optical density at 450 nm.[282] These parameters also give an indication of the possible need for exchange transfusion. Exceptions to these indications result from individual variations in infants' abilities to handle bilirubin loads.

Conjugated hyperbilirubinemia is occasionally observed in Rh erythroblastosis, particularly when intrauterine transfusions have effectively supported an infant with otherwise fatal intrauterine hemolysis.[230] This may be the result of exceeding the hepatic excretory capacity, but true cholestasis may also result from hepatic congestion from extramedullary erythropoiesis and heart failure or from tissue hypoxia caused by reduced hepatic blood flow and anemia.[283] The development of secondary complications, including bacterial sepsis, biliary obstruction, or hepatic failure, can also contribute to cholestasis in infants with erythroblastosis fetalis.[281]

Infants with severe hyperbilirubinemia in association with Rh erythroblastosis appear to have a greater risk for bilirubin encephalopathy (kernicterus) than do infants with an equally high serum bilirubin level in the absence of severe hemolysis.[284] Circulating heme pigments or other erythrocyte components may interfere with albumin binding of bilirubin,[285] and complications of severe hemolytic disease such as cerebral hypoxia, acidosis, and infection may interrupt the defenses against bilirubin entry into brain cells[105] (see section on bilirubin encephalopathy). Therapy should be initiated at lower serum bilirubin concentrations in infants with Rh hemolysis than in infants with nonhemolytic hyperbilirubinemia.

Phototherapy and exchange transfusions are the major modes of therapy for hyperbilirubinemia in Rh erythroblastosis (see section on treatment of hyperbilirubinemia). With severe disease, exchange transfusions may be performed as emergency procedures almost immediately after delivery, but this is for treatment of anemia and heart failure, not for hyperbilirubinemia.[281] Theoretically, removal of sensitized red cells before their destruction should reduce the degree of hyperbilirubinemia, but indications for exchange transfusion should be based upon the need for immediate resuscitative treatment or the results of specific serum bilirubin concentration determinations. It should be kept in mind that serum bilirubin concentrations can increase extremely rapidly and that therapy should be instituted in anticipation of the increase. Serum bilirubin concentrations should be determined at 4-hour intervals in infants with Rh erythroblastosis so the rate of increase can be determined.

ABO ISOIMMUNE HEMOLYSIS (ABO ERYTHROBLASTOSIS)

Hemolysis is generally milder and briefer in ABO hemolytic disease, and hyperbilirubinemia is less extreme although it occasionally may be severe.[286, 287] Even in the absence of overt anemia, neonates with ABO incompatibility with the mother and a positive result on Coombs' test should be observed carefully, and serum bilirubin concentrations should be determined at the first sign of jaundice.

OTHER HEMOLYTIC DISORDERS

Glucose-6-phosphate dehydrogenase (G6PD) deficiency of erythrocytes is the most common enzyme deficiency of the red cells found to be associated with hyperbilirubinemia.[288-294] American black neonates with a mild form of disease usually only exhibit normal physiologic jaundice, but they may have exaggerated hyperbilirubinemia even in the absence of overt hemolysis. The reasons are unknown. In the Mediterranean and Asian types of G6PD deficiency, severe hemolysis and jaundice may be seen.[292] Chemical exposure (e.g., to naphthalene vapors or high-dose synthetic vitamin K) and infection can incite brisk hemolysis and hyperbilirubinemia. Mild hemolysis in the third or fourth week of life often does not produce jaundice because hepatic mechanisms for disposal of bilirubin may have matured sufficiently by that time. Chronic brisk hemolysis may be associated with a mixed (conjugated and nonconjugated) hyperbilirubinemia after the hepatic uptake and conjugating mechanisms mature.

Structural abnormalities of the red cells, such as spherocytosis, elliptocytosis, and pyknocytosis, are rare causes of exaggerated neonatal hyperbilirubinemia and of chronic hyperbilirubinemia.[288]

Bacterial infection can increase the rate of erythrocyte destruction and jaundice. Congenital syphilis, rubella, and toxoplasmosis are infections that may be associated with increased hemolytic rates and hyperbilirubinemia. In each of these diseases, hepatocellular damage and conjugated hyperbilirubinemia may also be present. Sequestered blood in hematomas and ecchymoses sometimes contributes to exaggerated hyperbilirubinemia. A hematoma may only slowly release bilirubin as macrophages gradually enter the mass and convert the heme to bilirubin, but a diffuse and widespread area of subcutaneous blood is more rapidly converted to bile pigment. Red cell destruction may also be accelerated because of trapping in massive capillary and cavernous hemangiomas (so-called *Waring blender hemolysis*). If these involve the liver, a complex picture of anemia, heart failure, and mixed hyperbilirubinemia may be confused initially with severe isoimmune hemolytic disease.

Congenital erythropoietic porphyria is one of the rarest causes of hyperbilirubinemia related to hemolysis in the newborn period. Pink urine and neonatal onset of severe photosensitivity with formation of cutaneous bullae strongly suggest the diagnosis of congenital erythropoietic porphyria.[295] It is important to identify this rare disorder before institution of phototherapy because intense light will induce severe skin inflammation with bullae and may be fatal (see Chapter 13).

Hereditary Disorders of Hepatic Bilirubin Metabolism

GILBERT SYNDROME

Gilbert syndrome is a common disorder that is manifested by mild nonconjugated hyperbilirubinemia, usually presenting in adolescence and early adulthood.[296-298] In various studies, it has been identified in 3 to 6 percent of the population. It is clinically apparent and the male-to-female ratio is 4:1.[299] This disparity is probably related to intrinsically better bilirubin clearance in females. If the antimode for normal serum bilirubin is set at 1.4 mg/dL in males and 0.7 mg/dL in females (serum bilirubin values higher than these are considered abnormal), there is no male predominance.

A strong association has been established between a defect in the promoter region of the *BUGT1* gene and Gilbert syndrome.[159] Homozygous elongation of the TATAA element of the promoter from the normal A(TA)6TAA to A(TA)7TAA has been found in a large proportion of patients from Western Europe and the United States.[298, 300-304] This defect results in reduced gene expression.[305] Molecular diagnosis to detect this common defect is now commercially available.[306] There is, however, considerable genetic variation in the population of patients with clinically apparent Gilbert syndrome.[304, 307] Further elongation of the TATAA element to (TA)8 and a homozygous missense mutation (Tyr486Asp) have been identified in a relatively large proportion of Japanese patients but also in some patients of European descent.[308-315] It is not known for sure that all patients with clinically apparent Gilbert syndrome have a defect in the *BUGT1* gene, and it remains to be determined by molecular methods if Gilbert syndrome is one or a collection of disorders.

The exact pathophysiology of the disease remains unclear, and Gilbert syndrome seems to be a common manifestation of a variety of minor defects in the hepatic metabolism of organic anions. A universal defect appears to be a 50 percent or more reduction in hepatic BUGT activity.[159, 297, 316-321] Although in general conflict with current thinking regarding the dependence of serum bilirubin on transferase activity, the 50 percent reduction in transferase activity observed in patients with Gilbert syndrome is probably an important factor related to their jaundice. There is poor correlation between the activity of hepatic BUGT measured *in vitro* and bilirubin clearance capacity, however, administration of phenobarbital to these patients results in normalization of serum bilirubin activity.[322, 323] This probably reflects the inadequacy of the measurement of transferase activity because there is no other good explanation for these observations. In patients with Gilbert syndrome, reduced BUGT activity evidently places it nearer saturation kinetics, which results in an alteration of the pattern of bilirubin conjugates in bile with a predominance of BMG.[225-227] A significant proportion of these patients also have increased bilirubin production as a result of slightly increased red cell turnover, dyserythropoiesis, or increased hepatic heme turnover.[323-325] These are not overt, pathologic defects and are only detected in the presence of reduced bilirubin clearance. Indeed, the defect in Gilbert syndrome appears to be mainly in the liver as evidenced by the transference of the disease with a hepatic allograft into liver transplant recipients.[326] Several reports indicate that Gilbert syndrome can complicate hemolytic and dyserythropoietic disease and contribute to the degree of jaundice patients with these diseases exhibit.[327-331]

The heterogeneity of Gilbert syndrome is best indicated by variable defects in clearance of bilirubin, BSP, and indocyanine green that can be detected, indicating variable uptake and intracellular transport defects.[297] Clearance of an intravenous bilirubin load test or of radiolabeled bilirubin is abnormal in patients with Gilbert syndrome, who uniformly retain more than 15 percent after 4 hours (the normal amount retained is less than 5 percent).[227, 296, 332-335] Bile salt clearance is generally normal,[336, 337] but some subjects have shown abnormal patterns of bile acid conjugates and abnormal clearance of ursodeoxycholic acid.[338] Based on the clearance of various organic anions, patients with phenotypic Gilbert syndrome can be shown to have variable defects of anion clearance.[332, 334, 339, 340]

The serum bilirubin concentration of patients with Gilbert syndrome normally varies between 1 and 6 mg/dL, of which 95 percent is nonconjugated.[341] The bile from patients with Gilbert syndrome also contains an excess of BMG: 23 percent compared with 7 percent in normal individuals.[227, 317] Fasting and nicotinic acid infusion cause an increase in serum bilirubin levels of patients with Gilbert syndrome and may be helpful manipulations in establishing the diagnosis.[342-345] Fasting causes an approximately three- to fourfold increase in the serum bilirubin level from baseline, which may be related to reduced bilirubin clearance, increased bilirubin production, or both. Intravenous injection of 50 mg of nicotinic acid causes the serum bilirubin level to increase more than threefold in contrast to the less than twofold increase in the normal individual. Evidence suggests that normal individuals and patients with Gilbert syndrome experience equal degrees of increased bilirubin production after the injection of nicotinic acid, but the serum bilirubin level increases in inverse proportion to the clearance capacity, which is lower in patients with Gilbert syndrome.[346]

The diagnosis of Gilbert syndrome rests on a combination of biochemical findings, examination of the family, and exclusion of other causes of hyperbilirubinemia. A presumptive diagnosis can be made in the individual with (1) a mild increase in the serum nonconjugated bilirubin level (total, <6 mg/dL total; nonconjugated, >95 percent), (2) no evidence of hemolytic disease (normal complete blood count, blood smear, and reticulocyte count), (3) no evidence of liver disease (normal concentrations of aminotransferases, alkaline phosphatase, γ-glutamyl transpeptidase, and serum bile acid), and (4) no other contributing factors (e.g. breast-feeding or intestinal disease). Finding Gilbert syndrome in a parent or sibling provides important supporting evidence for the diagnosis. Follow-up over 1 to 2 years that demonstrates the same findings confirms the diagnosis. Invasive tests such as liver biopsy with measurement of BUGT activity are not necessary except in very unusual circumstances. No treatment is necessary. However, it has become increasing evident that the common gene defects that contribute to Gilbert syndrome can impair the metabolism of xenobiotics, particularly chemotherapeutic agents, and contribute to drug toxicity.[347–351] It may be that genetic testing for this common disease should be part of the strategy in formulating a course of treatment for cancer patients.

The importance of Gilbert syndrome in neonatal hyperbilirubinemia is unknown. It appears to contribute to the level of serum bilirubin achieved and the length of jaundice.[313,352–354] Certainly in the presence of isoimmune and other hemolytic diseases, patients with Gilbert syndrome exhibit greater than normal elevations of serum bilirubin.[327–329, 355] Exaggerated jaundice in association with pyloric stenosis has also been observed, which is consistent with the general effect of fasting in Gilbert syndrome.[53, 356–363] Finally, in the authors' experience, Gilbert syndrome has been diagnosed in several patients with apparent severe and prolonged breast milk–related jaundice.

CRIGLER-NAJJAR SYNDROME

Two genetically determined disorders with severe defects in hepatic BUGT activity have been described.[186, 364, 365] Both are associated with lifelong nonconjugated hyperbilirubinemia with onset in the newborn period. Early in the newborn period it may be extremely difficult to separate the two disorders from each other and from other causes of nonconjugated hyperbilirubinemia.

Crigler-Najjar Syndrome Type I

Crigler-Najjar syndrome type I is characterized by persistent nonconjugated hyperbilirubinemia. If the disease is untreated, bilirubin concentrations are almost always greater than 20 mg/dL and often exceed 30 mg/dL. Affected individuals have a marked defect in bilirubin clearance to less than 1 percent of normal; the half-life of circulating bilirubin exceeds 156 hours.[366] Bile contains only minute amounts of bilirubin, of which about half is nonconjugated bilirubin IXα.[225, 229, 367] Other bile pigments include photoisomers of bilirubin, trace xylose and glucose conjugates of bilirubin, and diazo-negative products of bilirubin oxidation.

The disease is caused by an autosomal recessive inherited complete absence of BUGT. Several gene defects have been identified (see section on conjugation of bilirubin), and the disease seems to have major genetic heterogeneity.[160, 169, 178–180, 318, 365, 368–370] Parents of affected patients have normal serum bilirubin levels, but they have transferase activity that is approximately 50 percent of normal. Compound heterozygotes for major *BUGT1* gene defects causing Crigler-Najjar syndrome type I have been identified. A recent report demonstrates how defects in the *BUGT1* gene can act in concert to produce severe hereditary jaundice. An adult with kernicterus was shown to be homozygous for the (TA)7 Gilbert syndrome defect in the promoter region and heterozygous for a major Crigler-Najjar syndrome defect.[371] At present, genetic diagnosis plays a limited role in diagnosis of Crigler-Najjar syndrome and remains a research tool, although it has been used in prenatal diagnosis.[369] To date no comprehensive analysis of the relationship between genotype and phenotype in Crigler-Najjar syndrome has been performed.

The homozygous jaundiced (jj) Gunn rat is the animal equivalent of Crigler-Najjar syndrome type I. This animal resulted from a spontaneous mutation in the *BUGT* gene in the Wistar rat strain. It is a true equivalent of the Crigler-Najjar syndrome type I in humans and has been used to study the molecular mechanism of human disease and approaches to treatment. Homozygous defective rats have life-long jaundice and a total absence of hepatic BUGT activity. Small amounts of bilirubin can be identified in the bile of jaundiced (jj) rats, mainly as BMG,[17] despite the absence of bilirubin-specific transferase activity. These rats also excrete BMG and BDG when infused with bilirubin dimethyl ester.[228, 372] Together, these observations suggested that the conjugation defect could result from an abnormal microsomal membrane environment for transferase that alters its interaction with its natural substrate, bilirubin. However, when this was examined, microsomal membrane vesicles from jaundiced (jj) Gunn rats were found not to be different from those of outbred Wistar rats with regard to several measures of membrane order.[373] More recently, isoforms of glucuronyl transferase have been isolated from the microsomal fraction from jaundiced (jj) and outbred (JJ) Wistar rats.[147, 148] These studies have shown that jaundiced (jj) rats have transferase isoforms that are recognized by anti-rat liver UGT and have electrophoretic mobility identical to that from congenic Wistar rats. However, isoform V, which is normally active in conjugation of bilirubin, has no activity in the jaundiced rats. Isoform I, which is normally active with *p*-nitrophenol as a substrate, is also partially defective. These data suggest that BUGT produced by the Gunn rat is defective, probably as the result of a single amino acid substitution, and that more than one transferase is affected, perhaps as the result of a repeated defective sequence in both proteins. A single base deletion has been identified that results in a frameshift mutation that removes 115 amino acid residues from the carboxy terminus of the enzyme.[374] The identification of this gene defect has improved the understanding of the function of the complex BUGT gene.

The principal sign to suggest Crigler-Najjar syndrome type I is persistence of severe hyperbilirubinemia beyond the end of the first week of life. A family history of similar illness or of consanguineous mating further strengthens the suspicion. Collection of duodenal bile with analysis of the bilirubin and its azodipyrroles after the van den Bergh reaction by high-performance liquid chromatography is the preferred method of diagnosis at present.[375] Neonatal liver biopsy with microassay for BUGT activity can be used to confirm the diagnosis but is rarely necessary. Trial therapy with phenobarbital fails to alter serum bilirubin concentrations, indicating a complete absence of inducible transferase activity, in contrast to the response in patients with the Crigler-Najjar syndrome type II (see later).

The major complication resulting from the Crigler-Najjar syndrome type I is bilirubin encephalopathy (kernicterus).[376-378] Before the advent of effective therapy, the majority of affected infants developed kernicterus in the newborn period. In recent years, many affected infants have survived without clinical evidence of bilirubin encephalopathy, probably reflecting generally improved perinatal management and treatment. No specific treatment is available for this disorder in the newborn period. The goal of therapy is to maintain serum bilirubin concentrations at less than 20 mg/dL. Exchange transfusions and phototherapy are used to carry the infant past the second or third week of life, followed by home use of phototherapy for periods of 8 to 14 hours/day.[376, 379, 380] The response to phototherapy in some of these children diminishes over time, as evidenced by gradually rising serum bilirubin concentrations from low levels of 12 to 15 mg/dL to levels higher than 25 mg/dL. Agar or other bilirubin binding agents can be administered by mouth to augment the effect of phototherapy, but they are of limited value.[381] Acute inhibition of bilirubin production may be accomplished with metalloporphyrins, which can be of therapeutic benefit.[382-384] Alternative pathways for bilirubin catabolism may function in the setting of defective conjugation.[17, 131-134, 136] One alternate pathway is dependent upon a specific cytochrome P-450 activity that can be induced by the administration of certain chemicals and may be auto-induced in the absence of BUGT activity.[131, 132, 136] Chlorpromazine in low doses is capable of inducing this activity and could be safely used in therapy of Crigler-Najjar syndrome type I, but it is not proven to be effective in any series of patients. Anesthesia, infections, and other physiologic stresses have been associated with acute development of kernicterus and should be either avoided or treated promptly. Despite improved medical therapy, every known patient has ultimately developed neurologic disease during late adolescence or early adulthood unless he or she has undergone liver transplantation.[376] The general strategy for treatment involves medical therapy until serum bilirubin levels

cannot be maintained in a safe range (<35 mg/dL in older children), at which time liver transplantation is performed. Transplantation may entail replacing the entire liver or providing an auxiliary liver graft to provide the necessary BUGT activity.[385-387] Hepatocyte transplantation as an approach to treating Crigler-Najjar syndrome has been explored in detail in the Gunn rat and has been used successfully in one human subject.[388] The major difficulty with this approach has been repopulating the liver with sufficient numbers of hepatocytes to provide sufficient BUGT activity to maintain a low serum bilirubin concentration. Over time, the infused cells are depleted, and the procedure must be repeated. The Gunn rat has also been the subject of experimental gene replacement therapy.[389, 390] It seems likely that a specific treatment for Crigler-Najjar syndrome other than liver transplantation is just over the horizon.[391]

Crigler-Najjar Syndrome Type II

Crigler-Najjar syndrome type II presents in the newborn period as neonatal jaundice followed by persistent elevated concentrations of serum nonconjugated bilirubin.[392] Serum bilirubin concentrations often exceed 20 mg/dL in the newborn, whereas in older children and adults, they usually range from 6 to 20 mg/dL. Crigler-Najjar syndrome type II may be differentiated from Crigler-Najjar syndrome type I by the lower serum bilirubin concentrations after the newborn period[392, 393] and the response to phenobarbital administration.[322, 394, 395] Duodenal bile contains more than trace amounts of bilirubin, most of which is BMG.[225, 375, 396]

Family studies suggested that this disorder may be inherited as an autosomal dominant trait with marked variability of penetrance.[397] One of the parents was often found to have nonconjugated hyperbilirubinemia and profound reduction of hepatic transferase activity, and more distant relations from the affected parent's side were also found to have the deficiency even though some of them did not have overt disease. Recent molecular genetic studies have shown homozygous defects in the *BUGT1* gene that do not completely ablate enzyme activity.[169, 181, 183, 318, 395] The defective cDNAs from two patients have been expressed in a BUGT-deficient cell line. In contrast to the complete inactivation in Crigler-Najjar syndrome type I, BUGT was only partially inactivated, with residual activity being about 4 percent of normal.[183] The major effect was a 10-fold decrease in the affinity of the expressed enzyme for bilirubin. These data suggest a recessively inherited defect involving a gene mutation at a site that alters, but does not completely inactivate, the bilirubin binding domain of BUGT. In another patient, the gene defect was in the hydrophobic, membrane-spanning domain, which could affect the stability of the enzyme in the microsomal environment.[169] Crigler-Najjar syndrome type II may, therefore, represent a common manifestation of several genetic defects.

Hepatic BUGT activity of patients with Crigler-Najjar syndrome type II is just barely detectable, so low that measurement of transferase activity cannot be used to reliably differentiate Crigler-Najjar syndrome type II from type I.[392, 398] Because only about 1 percent of normal enzyme activity is required for clearance of bilirubin, a very small shift in the low level of enzyme activity in Crigler-Najjar syndrome type II can effect a marked change in serum bilirubin concentration. Small differences in enzyme activity in affected individuals apparently account for the variability of expression of the disorder. Administration of phenobarbital produces a significant decline in serum bilirubin concentration, often to less than 4 mg/dL.[322, 394, 395] Continued administration of the drug maintains nearly normal serum bilirubin concentrations, but discontinuation results in a return to pretreatment levels in 1 to 4 weeks. This finding suggests that the drug has induced increased BUGT activity, but the presence of such activity has been difficult to prove by enzyme assay, again probably because of the intrinsic difficulties of measuring activity at such low levels. Because patients with Crigler-Najjar syndrome type I fail to respond to phenobarbital, its administration may be used in the differential diagnosis of severe nonhemolytic jaundice. Chronic phenobarbital administration is useful for maintaining cosmetically more acceptable skin color, but no patients with type II syndrome have ever been shown to develop kernicterus beyond the immediate neonatal period.

Acquired Nonconjugated Hyperbilirubinemia

JAUNDICE ASSOCIATED WITH BREAST-FEEDING

A significant number of breast-fed infants develop moderately severe nonconjugated hyperbilirubinemia, which in some cases persists through the first 3 or 4 months of life. Two separate periods of time must be considered when jaundice in the breast-fed infant is evaluated. During the first few days of life, breast-feeding is superimposed on the developmental factors that cause physiologic jaundice, which may cause it to be exaggerated. After the first week of life, physiologic jaundice should have abated, so breast-feeding is acting alone to cause jaundice, albeit acting in a less than mature environment.

The concept that breast-feeding exaggerates physiologic jaundice is based on the observation that serum bilirubin levels exceed 12 mg/dL more often in breast-fed infants than in bottle-fed infants.[399] Although this is evidently a commonly observed phenomenon, it has not been a universal finding in all studies.[400] The phenomenon may be related to inadequate caloric intake, which can increase bilirubin production[49, 51, 401, 402] and may reduce intestinal transit and enhance bilirubin absorption.[403, 404] In some hospital settings, breast-feeding mothers are not encouraged to nurse often enough to permit rapid and effective development of lactation. This may explain differences in the occurrence and intensity of jaundice in breast-fed infants among hospitals. No therapy is needed beyond ensuring adequate caloric intake.[405] If anything, attention should probably be given to ensuring the adequacy of breast-feeding and, if this cannot be accomplished, caloric supplementation should be provided.

Prolonged jaundice is seen in approximately 1 in every 100 otherwise normal breast-fed infants throughout the world; up to 40 percent have abnormally high serum nonconjugated bilirubin levels at 2 to 3 weeks of age.[406, 407] Bilirubin concentrations rise to peak levels that may exceed 20 mg/dL by the end of the second week of life.[408] With continued nursing, serum bilirubin concentrations typically decline gradually from their peak, reaching normal serum concentrations by 4 to 16 weeks of life. If one infant in a family has had breast milk–related jaundice, a recurrence rate of approximately 70 percent is to be anticipated in subsequently nursed infants.[408]

The mechanism by which breast milk causes infantile jaundice remains uncertain. Investigation has centered on the roles of two observed effects of breast milk on bilirubin metabolism: inhibition of BUGT and enhancement of bilirubin absorption from the intestine. These may act alone or in conjunction to produce the breast milk–related jaundice syndrome. To date, no factor in milk that inhibits BUGT has been identified as the cause for breast milk–related jaundice. It can be demonstrated in the laboratory that breast milk enhances the absorption of nonconjugated bilirubin from the intestine of the rat.[406] In this study there was a good correlation between the absorption of bilirubin and the degree of infantile jaundice. This effect, if expressed *in vivo* in the neonate, could increase the bilirubin load and produce jaundice. β-Glucuronidase activity in breast milk has been suggested to have a role in producing this syndrome.[409] Also, a β-glucuronidase inhibitor has been shown to be present in cow milk formula, which could inhibit mucosal enzyme activity and therefore inhibit the enterohepatic recirculation of bilirubin in the neonate.[410] Much more work is needed to determine the cause of this relatively common disorder.[411]

A clinical diagnosis of the breast milk–related jaundice syndrome may be established by the characteristic pattern of prolonged hyperbilirubinemia in a breast-feeding infant. The infant should be thriving, with good appetite, milk intake, and weight gain, and other definable causes of jaundice should be excluded. Mutations of the *BUGT* gene have been identified in this setting and should be considered in any infant whose symptoms do not fit the normal parameters of breast milk–related jaundice.[412] Any breast-fed baby with an elevated conjugated bilirubin level should be investigated for liver disease. Tragically, the authors have seen several infants with biliary atresia and conjugated hyperbilirubinemia whose condition was dismissed as breast milk–related jaundice. A specific test for breast milk–related jaundice entails interruption of nursing, which will result in a significant decline in serum bilirubin concentrations in 24 to 72 hours.[413, 414] Failure of serum bilirubin concentrations to decrease after 3 days of interruption indicates that the jaundice was probably not related to breast milk. Resumption of nursing usually results in no more than a 2 to 3 mg/dL increase in serum bilirubin level. Temporary interruption of nursing is not recommended for diagnostic purposes alone because it may lead to detrimental biologic and psychological effects and should be practiced only when the serum bilirubin concentration is at or close to the estimated toxic level. Kernicterus has been seen in otherwise healthy breast-feeding infants; thus, careful observation is warranted.[415]

INTESTINAL DISORDERS

Disorders that reduce intestinal clearance are associated with an increased incidence of pathologic jaundice.[53] Up to 50 percent of infants with pyloric stenosis have elevated serum bilirubin concentrations, and about 10 percent develop jaundice.[361] Pyloric stenosis has been shown to be associated with markedly suppressed levels of hepatic BUGT activity,[363] and it has been shown that jaundice with pyloric stenosis can be an early manifestation of mutations in the *BUGT* gene (Gilbert syndrome).[357, 360, 362] Infants with pyloric stenosis also have reduced indocyanine green clearance, indicating an abnormality in hepatic clearance of organic anions that would also include bilirubin.[359] The cause of a clearance defect is not understood, but it is consistent with Gilbert syndrome. Congenital intestinal obstruction usually presents with other signs, and the effect of obstruction on serum bilirubin concentrations is impossible to distinguish from the effects of general sickness and starvation. Hyperbilirubinemia is also occasionally associated with large bowel obstruction, as in Hirschsprung's disease.

DRUGS AND NONCONJUGATED HYPERBILIRUBINEMIA

Xenobiotics have a potential for broad-spectrum effects on bilirubin metabolism and transport. No drugs commonly used therapeutically for newborns are known to precipitate hemolytic disorders in otherwise normal infants, although some may affect infants with G6PD deficiency (see Chapter 17). Novobiocin, an antibiotic that is an inhibitor of BUGT, is the only drug ever demonstrated to produce nonconjugated hyperbilirubinemia in the newborn and has been withdrawn from clinical use for many years. All newly introduced drugs should be used in the newborn with great caution and with an eye to potential detrimental metabolic effects, including induction of jaundice.

ENDOCRINE DISORDERS

Congenital hypothyroidism is associated with prolonged nonconjugated hyperbilirubinemia in approximately 10 percent of cases. This probably results from the general depression of metabolism in the hypothyroid infant or from the dependence of the maturation of innumerable hepatic metabolic pathways on thyroxin. Infants of diabetic mothers likewise have an increased occurrence of exaggerated and prolonged nonconjugated hyperbilirubinemia. One explanation is deficient production of UDPGA that results in reduced conjugation. Early feeding may help to alleviate the severity and duration of the jaundice.

ETHNIC FACTORS IN NEONATAL JAUNDICE

Infants of Asian descent, including Chinese, Japanese, and Korean, and also Native American infants have peak serum bilirubin levels approximately twice those of white or black infants during the first 3 or 4 days of life.[416–420] The pattern of hyperbilirubinemia and its universality suggest a genetically determined delayed maturation of the basic mechanisms responsible for physiologic jaundice. An increase in the endogenous carbon monoxide production suggests hemolysis in some cases, but in the majority of infants of Asian descent, no hemolytic contribution can be demonstrated.[417, 418]

Experiences with exaggerated transient neonatal jaundice in more geographically localized areas have also been observed, the most intensively studied being on the island of Lesbos in Greece.[289, 419, 420]. Although the island has a high incidence of G6PD deficiency, only about 5 percent of jaundiced infants have the enzyme deficiency.[293] A local environmental factor may contribute, but whether infants of Greek origin when born outside of Greece are equally affected remains a subject of controversy.[420] Phenobarbital prophylaxis with treatment of both the pregnant mother and neonate will ameliorate the severity of jaundice and the frequent need for exchange transfusions to prevent kernicterus. Heme-oxygenase inhibition with tin-mesoporphyrin has also been shown to be effective in this situation.[294]

BILIRUBIN NEUROTOXICITY

Nonconjugated bilirubin can, under certain conditions, enter the central nervous system and injure neurons in specific areas of the brain, resulting in the condition known as *kernicterus*.[258, 421] The pathophysiology of bilirubin neurotoxicity has not been established despite years of major investigative effort. The word actually means "nuclear jaundice", which refers to the staining of dead neurons in the basal ganglia, hippocampal cortex, cerebellum, and subthalamic nuclei that fulfills the pathologist's definition of kernicterus.[421–424] The clinical definition includes progressive lethargy, muscular rigidity, opisthotonus, high-pitched cry, fever, and convulsions that develop in an infant at risk.[423] Fortunately, the full-blown clinical and pathologic syndrome of kernicterus is rarely encountered with modern nursery care. The focus of most recent clinical investigation is to assess the risk of jaundiced infants for developing neurotoxicity that is manifest in more subtle ways, such as learning deficits.[425–427] It seems that bilirubin neurotoxicity includes a spectrum of clinical illness and pathologic injury that ranges from full-blown kernicterus to minimally detectable learning deficits.

Pathogenesis of Kernicterus

In formulating our current understanding of neurotoxicity, the assumption has been that circulating bilirubin is the source of bilirubin deposited in the brain.[428] If that is the case, two key factors, albumin binding of bilirubin and the blood-brain barrier, must be considered in the pathophysiology of bilirubin neurotoxicity.[421, 429, 430] The protection conferred by albumin binding of bilirubin is clearly important in preventing neurotoxicity.[95, 431] It should be noted, however, that analbuminemic rats and humans do not suffer brain injury; thus, albumin is not crucial in protecting against the movement of bilirubin into the central nervous system. The adequacy of binding is determined by the concentrations of albumin and bilirubin and the binding affinity, which can be affected by substances that compete for bilirubin-binding sites. The theoretical binding capacity has been discussed in the section dealing with bilirubin transport in plasma. In theory, the plasma albumin of a newborn can fully bind bilirubin at concentrations well above those that are considered to be safe. The theoretical situation is confounded in the clinical setting by variable binding affinity caused by circulating chemicals, whether xenobiotics or endogenous metabolites.

The sick neonate may be exposed to many chemicals that have the potential for interfering with albumin binding of bilirubin. Competition for binding at the high-affinity site is the mechanism by which sulfisoxazole and other sulfonamide drugs enhance the risk for kernicterus. This has provided a useful model for the study of kernicterus in animals, particularly with regard to the manipulation of a single limb of the complex equation that determines the movement of bilirubin into the central nervous system.[422, 432–434] Drugs known to reduce the affinity of albumin binding should be avoided, and new drugs should be considered as possible inhibitors when they are evaluated clinically in the care of neonates.[435] Some cephalosporins have been shown to interfere with bilirubin binding to such a degree that their use should be avoided in infants at risk for kernicterus.[436, 437]

Elevated free fatty acids may have an effect on bilirubin binding, but the direction and the magnitude of the effect are not clear. Fatty acids bind to albumin in a region close to the high-affinity binding site for albumin. Various studies suggest that fatty acid binding to albumin interferes with or produces allosteric enhancement of bilirubin binding.[438–440] In the clinical setting, conditions that produce elevated serum free fatty acid concentrations have been associated with an increased risk of neurotoxicity, which is thought to be due to reduced binding affinity.[441] The major problem with this interpretation is the fact that conditions that increase fatty acid concentrations, such as fasting, cause many other changes that could affect binding or the blood-brain barrier. In infants without acute illness, moderate increases in the serum free fatty acid concentration that can result from the administration of intravenous lipid and heparin probably do not significantly alter the bilirubin binding capacity of neonates.

Conjugated bilirubin does not enter the central nervous system but does bind to albumin and possibly competes with bilirubin for albumin binding. Although in clinical practice it has been traditional to subtract the direct-reacting fraction of bilirubin from the total serum bilirubin concentration in estimation of the risk for bilirubin neurotoxicity, this method may not be completely accurate. Rather, conjugated bilirubin should be considered as an additional risk factor at any given level of nonconjugated bilirubin.

The blood-brain barrier is also important in preventing bilirubin neurotoxicity.[429–431, 442] Certain clinical phenomena appear to enhance the risk for development of kernicterus by interfering with the blood-brain barrier. These include prematurity, hypoxia, acidosis, hypoglycemia, hemolysis, and sepsis with or without meningitis.[275, 443–445] Useful animal models have been developed to investigate the mechanisms by which the blood-brain barrier is breached in various clinical settings and are providing valuable insights.[431, 446–452] Bacterial endotoxins and hypoxia appear to have particularly profound effects and increase the risk for kernicterus by damaging the endothelial lining cells of the cerebral capillaries or by altering the neuronal cell membranes to permit entry of bilirubin.[453]

Some clinical conditions affect both binding and the blood-brain barrier, placing the jaundiced infant in double jeopardy. Acidosis is one of these conditions. Lowered pH weakens the binding affinity and circulating organic acids compete with bilirubin for binding sites; at the same time clinical acidosis is often encountered in settings in which the blood-brain barrier is impaired.[454, 455]

Having gained entry into the neuron, bilirubin interferes with cellular function. In model systems, it can be shown to affect oxidative phosphorylation, cell respiration, protein synthesis, cell membrane transport, and glucose metabolism.[421, 456–462] Bilirubin can directly induce apoptosis in rat brain neurons.[463] Bilirubin has also been shown to disrupt the uptake and release of neurotransmitters, particularly glutamate.[464–466] The particular affinity of bilirubin for the basal ganglia, hippocampal cortex, cerebellum, and subthalamic nuclei is not understood.[467] Recent animal studies suggest that the clinical symptomatology of kernicterus may be produced by intravenous infusions of nonconjugated bilirubin in the absence of staining of the brain and normal brain histology. Acute manipulations of bilirubin binding and the blood-brain barrier can be monitored by changes in auditory evoked potentials in these animal models.[433, 468–470]

The assumption that circulating bilirubin is the culprit in neurotoxicity is now being questioned on the basis of recent experimental data. Brain tissues are clearly capable of synthesizing bilirubin. Both heme oxygenase and biliverdin reductase have been shown to be present in the brain and have a pattern of developmental expression that suggests functional importance.[64, 471–473] The ability of the brain to synthesize bilirubin appears to confer protection against oxidative injury.[82, 474] Mice that express heme oxygenase are clearly protected from acute ischemia.[475–477] Evident also is the fact that by producing CO heme oxygenase functions in the system of neurotransmitters.[478] Heme oxygenase colocalizes with NO-synthase, which suggests that it has a role in the complex system of gaseous neurotransmitters.[479] The ability to synthesize bilirubin locally may, however, be a double-edged sword for the brain. Although mice that overexpress heme oxygenase are protected from acute ischemia, they develop the equivalent of attention deficit disorder with attenuated exploratory behavior.[480] Increased bilirubin in brain tissue can incite peroxidative injury of membranes as it is oxidized.[83, 481] In the past, considerable attention has been paid to the risk of neurotoxicity in newborn babies with brisk hemolysis as a factor independent of the serum bilirubin concentration.[482, 483] It may be that increased circulating hemoproteins during hemolysis provides a source for increased endogenous brain bilirubin production and greater risk of neurotoxicity.

Clinical Manifestations of Bilirubin Neurotoxicity

The clinical manifestations correlating with bilirubin injury to brain range from complete absence of specific signs or symptoms to full-blown kernicterus. Approximately one half of infants demonstrating kernicterus die. Survivors of this clinical complex, as well as some infants who are essentially asymptomatic as newborns, demonstrate choreoathetoid cerebral palsy, high-frequency deafness, and, less commonly, mental retardation.[429, 483–488] Alterations in neurophysiologic studies such as auditory evoked potentials have been related to risk factors for bilirubin neurotoxicity.[489] Magnetic resonance imaging can also be an aid in diagnosis.[490, 491] Other epidemiologic studies have associated mild motor, cognitive, and behavioral disorders later in infancy and childhood with elevated neonatal serum bilirubin concentrations.[425, 492, 493] The importance of the effect of mild hyperbilirubinemia on neural development, however, remains to be determined.

Bilirubin is toxic to tissues other than brain. Infants found to have kernicterus at autopsy often have extraneural deposits of bilirubin, particularly in the intestinal mucosa, pancreas, and renal papillae.[494] Bilirubin nephropathy can be demonstrated in the jaundiced Gunn rat,[495] but the human clinical condition remains to be defined. However, the possibility of extraneural toxicity accounting for clinical disease cannot be ignored.

TREATMENT OF NEONATAL HYPERBILIRUBINEMIA AND PREVENTION OF BILIRUBIN NEUROTOXICITY

At the present time, the prevention of bilirubin injury to the brain is empirical and based upon "safe" serum bilirubin concentrations adjusted according to birth weight or gestational age and clinical status. Although earlier studies indicated the critical importance of serum bilirubin concentrations in excess of 20 mg/dL in the etiology of kernicterus, this value should not be considered as a "magic number" below which there is no danger. As previously discussed, many factors contribute to the risk for development of neurotoxicity, and kernicterus can occur in the sick neonate even at serum nonconjugated bilirubin concentrations as low as 5 mg/dL. Vigorous attention to the intensive care of small and sick neonates appears to be effective in preventing the development of kernicterus in high-risk infants if it is kept in mind that serum bilirubin represents a loaded gun that can be discharged by a variety of insults.[415, 496] The sicker the infant, the greater is the risk at any given bilirubin level. Although neonates are at the greatest risk for bilirubin neurotoxicity and advancing age provides some protection, older children and even adults can develop kernicterus if serum bilirubin levels reach critical levels.[371, 377, 497] Exchange transfusion and phototherapy are the two treatment modalities most commonly used to lower serum bilirubin concentrations or maintain them in a safe range. The technique and complications of exchange transfusions are discussed in Chapter 3.

Phototherapy

Phototherapy is effective for the treatment of neonatal jaundice from a variety of causes.[498–500] It has been adopted worldwide as the first-line treatment of nonconjugated hyperbilirubinemia.

Indications for Use. Phototherapy should be considered as the first-line therapy for all nonconjugated hyperbilirubinemia that needs to be treated. For example, in severe hyperbilirubinemia due to Rh hemolytic disease, it reduces the need for exchange transfusion, thereby reducing morbidity.[501] In such a case the benefit clearly outweighs the risk. On the other hand, phototherapy should not be used for patients with physiologic jaundice, in whom there is no risk of bilirubin-induced injury. Phototherapy is limited with regard to its ability to acutely reduce serum bilirubin in states with markedly increased production. It is most effective when used prophylactically in anticipation of the need for exchange transfusion.

Mechanism of Action. Phototherapy reduces serum bilirubin mainly by the mechanism of photoisomerization of bilirubin.[502–516] *Photoisomerization* is defined as a change in the configuration of the bilirubin molecule as a consequence of the absorption of light energy. This mechanism was first identified in Gunn rats, which lack the ability to conjugate bilirubin. When exposed to therapeutic light, these rats rapidly exhibit biliary excretion of bilirubin.[511, 517] A similar effect has been confirmed in jaundiced human infants and probably represents the major effect of therapeutic light.[516, 518]

Bilirubin absorbs light energy mainly in the blue-green range. The energy is dissipated in the complex system of conjugated and double bonds of the molecule, which results in configurational changes, including the production of a class of compounds collectively called *photobilirubin* (Fig. 4–5). The folding that makes nonconjugated bilirubin IXα insoluble in water is made possible by the flexibility of the central methene carbon bridge and the *Z configuration* (from *zusammen*, German for "together") of the 4- and 15-methylene carbon bridges. With the energy supplied by light, these relatively rigid bridges are converted to the *E configuration* (from *entgegen*, German for "opposite") with disruption of internal hydrogen bonds. The bilirubin molecule is unfolded, freeing the carboxyl groups to interact with the aqueous environment and making the compound much more soluble in water. Three configurational isomers are formed: 4*E*,15*Z*-photobilirubin; 4*Z*,15*E*-photobilirubin; and 4*E*,15*E*-photobilirubin. The first two are thermodynamically unstable and spontaneously revert to insoluble bilirubin in minutes; the 4*E*,15*E*-photobilirubin isomer is more stable but is formed only in small quantities.[510, 513, 514] The configurational isomers are rapidly formed during phototherapy and are easily excreted by the liver without conjugation.[509, 515, 519–521] Another phototherapy-induced isomer of bilirubin called *cyclobilirubin* or *lumirubin* is the product of intramolecular endovinyl cyclization of 4*E*,15*Z*-photobilirubin.[522] Although accounting for only a small percentage of photoisomers formed, it is perhaps the most important product of phototherapy because it is totally stable and cannot revert back to bilirubin.[516] Cyclobilirubin is excreted less

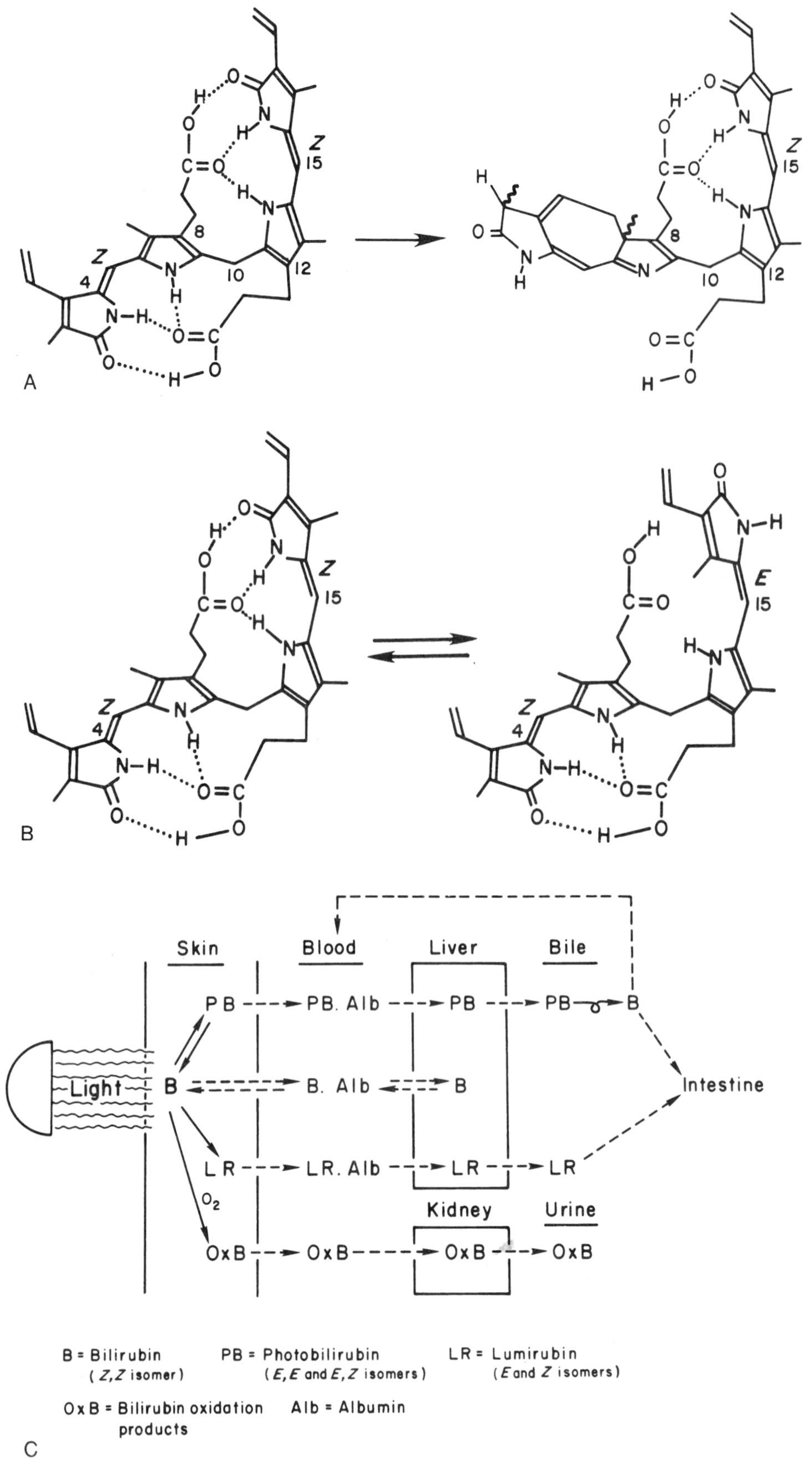

FIGURE 4–5. The mechanism of phototherapy. *A, Z-E* carbon double-bond configurational isomerization of bilirubin. *B,* Intramolecular cyclization of bilirubin in the presence of light to form lumirubin. *C,* General mechanism of phototherapy for neonatal jaundice. *Solid arrows* represent chemical reactions; *broken arrows* represent transport processes. Pigments may be bound to proteins in compartments other than blood. Some excretion of photoisomers in urine also occurs. (From McDonagh AF, Lightner DA: Like a shrivelled blood orange—bilirubin, jaundice, and phototherapy. Pediatrics 1985; 75:443. Copyright American Academy of Pediatrics 1985.)

rapidly in the Gunn rat during phototherapy than are the configurational isomers.[523] However, the clearance of cyclobilirubin formed during phototherapy in premature infants appears to be more rapid than that of the configurational isomers, with a mean half-life of 111 minutes compared with 15 hours for the isomers.[507] The extent to which formation of cyclobilirubin contributes to the clearance of bilirubin during phototherapy, therefore, remains unclear. Overall, photoisomerization is responsible for more than 80 percent of the effect of phototherapy.[514]

The efficiency of phototherapy is reduced because the configurational isomers in the intestine revert to bilirubin, which is readily absorbed.[381] Adequate caloric intake and frequent feeding increase the effectiveness of phototherapy, whereas partial or complete starvation decreases the level of reduction of serum bilirubin by phototherapy. The efficacy of phototherapy can be enhanced by the simultaneous oral administration of agents that bind bilirubin.[267, 381]

Photodegradation also occurs to a small degree.[514] When bilirubin in the skin absorbs light energy and is elevated from its triplet (ground) energy state to the singlet state, the energy can be transferred to molecular oxygen. This produces singlet oxygen, which is capable of oxidizing compounds containing double bonds. Free radicals, which are capable of a wide variety of oxidizing reactions, are also generated. Bilirubin, in addition to sensitizing these reactions, is oxidized by them. The products formed by these reactions include biliverdin, dipyrroles, and monopyrroles, all of which are water-soluble and can be excreted by the liver or kidney without conjugation. Evidence suggests that photodegradation is a minor mechanism of phototherapy, but significant amounts of water-soluble photodegradation products of bilirubin can be identified in the urine of infants receiving light therapy.[524] This class of reactions may account for up to 20 percent of the bilirubin excreted as a result of phototherapy.

In both mechanisms, bilirubin absorbs the energy of light to initiate the photodynamic reaction.[514] Only tissue bilirubin is subject to the photodynamic reaction, and light effectively penetrates only the outermost 2 mm of the skin.[525] It is imperative that as much skin as possible be exposed for the effect to be maximal. Newer methods of distributing light to greater areas of skin, such as fiberoptic blankets, are effective.[526] Because the maximum absorption bilirubin IXα is in the wavelength range of 425 to 475 nm, blue light has been considered to be the most effective for therapy.[527] Recent studies have shown that tissue and protein binding of bilirubin alters the absorption spectrum, and the maximum quantum yield for photoisomerization occurs at 520 nm wavelength (green light).[528–532] Light of longer wavelength would also be safer in theory, but this wavelength would not penetrate skin as well.[501, 529, 530, 533–536]

Complications. High-energy light has considerable potential to cause toxicity in the developing neonate.[503, 514, 537, 538] Phototherapy has been shown to result in a number of physiologic changes and pathologic alterations in the newborn undergoing treatment for jaundice. The potential for injury from light is compounded by the fact that nonconjugated bilirubin is a sensitizer of photodynamic reactions that result in the production of singlet oxygen. This, in turn, can result in the oxidation of a variety of compounds containing double bonds. Thus, cell membranes and other important organic compounds can be injured as a result of phototherapy. A few important complications of phototherapy have been recorded, but the full toxicity potential of this modality has yet to be determined.

Riboflavin, a vitamin that contains double bonds, can be oxidized during phototherapy. A deficiency state can develop with the use of prolonged phototherapy, which can be prevented by a daily riboflavin intake of 0.3 mg.[539, 540] Riboflavin is itself a sensitizer of photodynamic reactions and has been shown to accelerate the destruction of methionine, tryptophan, and histidine in amino acid solutions exposed to light. Likewise, oxidation of polyunsaturated, essential fatty acids is accelerated by exposure to light *in vitro*.[541] The binding of some fatty acids to albumin, however, increases the quantum yield of phototherapy for the production of bilirubin photoisomers.[542] The innumerable possible interactions of light energy, bilirubin, and organic compounds must be considered in assessing the safety of this therapy.

Some infants treated with phototherapy exhibit increased bilirubin excretion but no reduction of serum bilirubin, suggesting that light may increase the rate of hemolysis. *In vitro*, blue light causes increased loss of erythrocyte potassium and membrane adenosine triphosphatase (ATPase) activity, lysis of resealed erythrocyte membranes, and cross-linking of erythrocyte membrane polypeptides.[543–545] The Gunn rat treated with blue light exhibits increased osmotic fragility of erythrocytes,[546] but no apparent alteration in red cell survival.[547] However, the human fetal erythrocyte membrane is quite susceptible to oxidative stress. A variety of erythrocyte membrane enzymes are inactivated, and the O_2 dissociation curve of fetal blood is shifted by bilirubin sensitized photoreaction.[548] Finally, patients with inherited deficiency of G6PD of the Mediterranean type may develop significant hemolysis upon exposure to therapeutic light.[291]

The effect of phototherapy on the binding capacity of albumin for bilirubin has been investigated with conflicting results. *In vitro*, photo-oxidation of albumin can be demonstrated, but *in vivo*, there appears to be no reduction in the binding affinity or capacity of albumin during phototherapy.[549, 550] Therapeutic light does decrease the concentration of serum albumin in treated infants, presumably because of photo-oxidation, but this reduction is not clinically significant.[550] Administration of albumin increases the effectiveness of phototherapy in low-birth-weight infants.[551]

A number of potentially important alterations of physiology have been observed during phototherapy.[537] Retinal changes can result from prolonged exposure to intense light, but shielding the eyes from light, as is now common practice, prevents any long-term measurable optic injury.[552–555] Preterm infants demonstrate a reduced growth rate and an increased occurrence of hypocalcemia.[556, 557] These effects may be caused by the influence of light on hormone production directly or to the disruption of the circadian rhythm.[558, 559]

A dramatic alteration in intestinal physiology is caused by the large increase of nonconjugated bilirubin delivered to the intestine.[518] Clinically apparent diarrhea occurs in 10 percent of treated infants.[538] Diarrhea is probably due to intestinal secretion induced by bilirubin,[560, 561] which can be reversed by the administration of agar.[562] Transient lactase deficiency probably does not occur as previously thought.[563–565]

A specific, pathologic complication of phototherapy is the *bronze baby syndrome*. This rare disorder, which occurs in fewer than 1 in 1000 infants receiving phototherapy, is characterized by the development of brown-black discoloration of the serum, urine, and skin.[276–280, 566] It appears after many hours of exposure to light and has almost always been associated with the presence of mild or moderate conjugated hyperbilirubinemia before phototherapy. The development of this complication probably requires preexisting cholestatic liver disease in the infant; thus, it has been assumed that a pigment normally excreted into bile during phototherapy is retained. Based on chromatographic and spectroscopic data, the retained pigments are either polymers of photobilirubin[278] or photodegradation products of Cu(II)-porphyrin.[279, 566] It is not known at this time whether the bronze baby syndrome is simply a cosmetic defect or whether it is associated with a risk for secondary tissue damage. It is generally recommended that infants with cholestasis not be exposed to phototherapy lights and that light therapy be promptly discontinued in all infants who develop cholestasis or bronze coloration. Discontinuation of phototherapy is usually associated with prompt disappearance of the pigment from the serum, urine, and skin.

Metalloporphyrins

The metalloporphyrins are substituted heme compounds, in which other multivalent metals are chelated by protoporphyrin IX in the place of iron.[384] The discovery that metalloporphyrins can inhibit bilirubin formation has led to their potential use in chemotherapy of neonatal hyperbilirubinemia.[105, 384, 567–571] They interact with the prosthetic site of heme oxygenase and have variable effects on enzyme activity, some acting as competitive inhibitors and some as inducers of the enzyme.[567, 569]

The best studied metalloporphyrins have been Sn-protoporphyrin and Sn-mesoporphyrin. Studies in animals have shown impressive reduction of bilirubin production and serum bilirubin levels in a variety of experimental conditions. Normal physiologic jaundice in newborn rats can be prevented by the administration of Sn-protoporphyrin.[572] The compound also inhibits carbon monoxide excretion in adult mice[59] and reduces endogenous bilirubin production in adult rats.[573] It effectively reduces bilirubin production in normal human subjects.[574] It has not shown serious toxicity in animals, but there remain important questions about the potential for light-induced oxidative injury.[571, 575] Sn-protoporphyrin is a potent photosensitizer, accepting light energy with a maximum absorption at 400 nm wavelength, elevating electrons to the triplet excited state. As it gives up energy it elevates available oxygen to produce toxic singlet oxygen, which can injure cells and membranes, particularly the skin. This potential for toxicity must be studied in greater detail.

Sn-substituted porphyrins have been developed to the point that they have been used in clinical trials with good success. In an early study Greek infants with ABO incompatibility received Sn-protoporphyrin.[576] The group treated with higher doses had a significant reduction in serum bilirubin and a reduced need for phototherapy, but the effect was small. There were few toxic effects. Of 12 babies given both Sn-protoporphyrin and phototherapy, two developed mild skin sensitivity. Other studies in newborns have shown similar effect and lack of toxicity.[382, 577, 578] Sn-mesoporphyrin has also been used in a patient with Crigler-Najjar syndrome, in which it may have value in temporarily reducing serum bilirubin concentrations.[383]

At the present time, considerable interest remains in the metalloporphyrins and their application to the treatment of neonatal jaundice. Improved methods for targeting the drugs to improve efficacy and reduce toxicity may increase their clinical usefulness.[384, 579] It will probably be several years before they have general clinical application.

CONJUGATED HYPERBILIRUBINEMIA OF THE NEWBORN

Elevated serum concentrations of conjugated or direct bilirubin virtually always indicates the presence of liver dysfunction. Rarely, very brisk rates of bilirubin production and conjugation can overwhelm the excretory capacity of the liver and result in mild retention of conjugated bilirubin. This clinical situation is not likely to be confused with liver disease, but some systemic disease states, such as sepsis, can cause both hemolysis and hepatocyte dysfunction. The conditions of liver dysfunction to be considered here are the hereditary conjugated hyperbilirubinemias and cholestasis. The former is considered in some detail in this section. Only a conceptual overview of the latter is presented.

Hereditary Conjugated Hyperbilirubinemia

Two extremely rare hereditary disorders that affect the excretion of conjugated bilirubin by the hepatocyte have been described.[580, 581] These have the common characteristic of producing elevated serum concentrations of conjugated bilirubin, but they vary in other respects.

DUBIN-JOHNSON SYNDROME

This is the more common of the two hereditary conjugated hyperbilirubinemias. This benign condition is characterized by an excretory defect for several organic anions, including conjugated bilirubin.[581,582] Serum bilirubin varies from 1.5 to 6.0 mg/dL, over half of which is conjugated. Results of other routine liver function tests are normal, including serum bile salt concentrations. The liver is often grossly black in color, and histologically a dark pigment in hepatocyte lysosomes that is either derived from melanin or catecholamines is retained.[583] Oral cholecystography dye is not excreted normally, which results in failure to visualize the gallbladder. Techniques using the study of kinetics of excretion of scintigraphic dyes can now be used to confirm this diagnosis and differentiate it from Rotor syndrome.[582, 584]

The Dubin-Johnson defect involves the canalicular transport mechanism, specifically a genetic alteration of the canalicular multispecific organic anion–transporter gene (*MRP2/cMOAT*).[243, 248, 249, 585–588] The BSP clearance study demonstrates an excretory defect. BSP is normally taken up by the hepatocyte and conjugated with glutathione before excretion. The normal plasma disappearance curve reflects uptake only, because there is no regurgitation of conjugated BSP. The curve in a patient with Dubin-Johnson syndrome demonstrates normal early clearance, but reflux of conjugated BSP after 45 minutes causes a secondary increase in serum BSP concentration.[589] Further studies with BSP have demonstrated a normal storage capacity but a marked reduction in excretion.

Animal equivalents of Dubin-Johnson syndrome have permitted more careful investigation of organic anion transport defects. These are the Corriedale sheep and three rat strains—the Groningen yellow (GY) rat, the transport negative (TR⁻) rat, and the Eisai hyperbilirubinemic (EHBR) rat.[245, 250–252, 590] Most work has used rat models for obvious reasons. These rats are thought to have similar if not identical defects, and they are similar in most respects to the human disorder. Most studies have led to the conclusion that these rats, and by inference humans with Dubin-Johnson syndrome, have a genetic defect in a canalicular ATP-dependent organic anion transporter (see section on bilirubin excretion). This results in defective excretion of bilirubin conjugates (BMG and BDG). It should be emphasized that these rats and humans with Dubin-Johnson syndrome have normal concentrations of bilirubin in bile and that they depend almost exclusively on the liver for clearance of bilirubin. The defect is mild and results only in a steady-state condition that is different from the normal one.

A hallmark of Dubin-Johnson syndrome is a defect in the clearance of coproporphyrin that results in an abnormal ratio of isomers in the urine of affected patients. The total excretion of coproporphyrin is normal. However, more than 80 percent of coproporphyrin in the urine of these patients is coproporphyrin I, whereas in normal subjects 75 percent of coproporphyrin is coproporphyrin III.[591] The cause for this is unknown.

Dubin-Johnson syndrome is inherited as an autosomal recessive trait, and obligate heterozygotes have normal serum bilirubin concentrations. The diagnosis is established in the individual with a moderate degree of conjugated hyperbilirubinemia, without abnormal liver function tests and with abnormal urinary coproporphyrin I excretion. Liver biopsy will demonstrate hepatocyte pigment, but is not necessary for establishing the diagnosis. No therapy is needed.

ROTOR SYNDROME

This very rare autosomal recessive familial disorder involves the storage capacity and excretion of conjugated bilirubin and results in elevated levels of conjugated and nonconjugated bilirubin.[581] Results of other liver function tests are normal, and in contrast to the findings in Dubin-Johnson syndrome, the gallbladder is visualized with orally administered cholecystography dye and no abnormal hepatocyte pigment is present.[584, 592–594] The baseline serum bilirubin concentration varies from 2 to 7 mg/dL, but during illness can rise to 25 mg/dL. BSP clearance is delayed and does not show the secondary rise seen in Dubin-Johnson syndrome.[595] Urinary coproporphyrin excretion is two to five times normal, and compared with

that in normal subjects coproporphyrin I predominates (about 40 percent).[596] Obligate homozygotes also excrete abnormal amounts of coproporphyrin in the urine, whereas serum bilirubin levels are normal. No treatment is needed.

The lack of an animal model has limited the investigation of the pathophysiology of Rotor syndrome. Current understanding of the postconjugation processing of bilirubin suggests that it involves vesicular storage and transport (see section on bilirubin excretion). The defect in Rotor syndrome can be explained by a defective vesicular transport system, but proof of this is lacking.[581]

Acquired Conjugated Hyperbilirubinemia (Cholestasis)

Cholestasis is defined as a pathologic state of reduced bile formation or flow. The clinical definition of cholestasis, therefore, is any condition in which there is retention of substances normally excreted into bile.[597] The serum concentrations of conjugated bilirubin and bile salts are commonly measured. It should be noted that not all substances normally excreted into bile are retained to the same extent in various cholestatic disorders. In some conditions, the level of serum bile salts may be markedly elevated whereas the bilirubin level is only modestly elevated and vice versa. The histopathologic definition of cholestasis is the appearance of bile within the elements of the liver, usually associated with secondary cell injury.

Most cholestatic conditions can be classified as either obstructive or hepatocellular. Obstructive cholestasis results from impedance of bile hydraulics. In other words, there is an anatomic or functional obstruction of the biliary system. This obstruction can be at the level of the large or extrahepatic bile ducts (e.g., cholelithiasis). The distinguishing histopathologic feature of large duct obstruction is the presence of bile plugs in the interlobular bile ducts. Histologic evidence of secondary hepatocellular injury may be minimal to severe. Findings often involve central lobular hepatocytes and include hepatocyte cholestasis, ballooning, and necrosis. Within the liver, the biliary system ramifies, with 10 to 12 orders of branches, and the cross-sectional area increases by several orders of magnitude. Intrahepatic obstructive cholestasis requires the obstruction or obliteration of enough smaller bile ducts to alter bile flow. Sclerosing cholangitis in older patients typically involves one to four orders of bile ducts, so relatively few ducts need to be involved to produce cholestasis. In neonatal sclerosing cholangitis, the interlobular (terminal order) bile ducts are more often involved. In this situation, much more extensive involvement is needed to produce clinical cholestasis. Biliary atresia affects the extrahepatic bile ducts first, but it is often seen as an ascending obliterative cholangitis, which may explain the high failure rate of the Kasai operation. Diseases that are associated with ductal paucity manifest varying forms of cholestasis depending on the degree of paucity. The principal causes of obstructive cholestasis in children are presented in Table 4–1. Of these, biliary atresia accounts for more than 90 percent of cases.

TABLE 4–1. Major Causes of Cholestasis in Infancy

OBSTRUCTIVE CHOLESTASIS

Biliary atresia
Congenital bile duct anomalies (choledochal cyst)
Cholelithiasis
Primary sclerosing cholangitis
Infectious cholangitis
Cholangitis associated with Langerhans cell histiocytosis

CHOLESTASIS WITH DUCTAL PAUCITY

Alagille syndrome
Nonsyndromic ductal paucity
Ductopenic allograft rejection
Hepatocellular cholestasis
Hepatitis
α_1-Antitrypsin deficiency
Inborn errors of bile acid synthesis
Drug-induced cholestasis
Total parenteral nutrition-associated cholestasis
Progressive familial intrahepatic cholestasis

Hepatocellular cholestasis results from impairment of mechanisms of bile formation. This is sometimes called *hepatocanalicular cholestasis* in recognition of the canaliculus as the bile-forming apparatus of the hepatocyte and the fact that canalicular bile plugs are often observed in biopsy specimens. Several mechanisms that have been identified in experimental hepatocellular cholestasis are thought to be important in human cholestasis as well. These are presented in Table 4–2. Even though there is a lobular gradient for bile formation, with periportal hepatocytes most active in this regard, hepatocellular cholestasis implies defective function of most or all hepatocytes—a global defect must be in place to produce cholestasis. Whatever the primary defect, once cholestasis begins, amplification by several mechanisms occurs.

The typical histopathologic features of hepatocellular cholestasis include the presence of bile within hepatocytes and bile plugs in canalicular spaces. Histologic evidence of extensive secondary hepatocellular injury is often seen. In most clinical forms of hepatocellular cholestasis, the molecular mechanism is unknown. The principal causes of hepatocellular cholestasis in children are listed in Table 4–1. Idiopathic neonatal giant cell hepatitis accounts for the majority of cases, but in the last decade improved understanding of the causes of hepatocellular cholestasis in children has resulted in a reduction in the percentage of idiopathic cases.

TABLE 4–2. Molecular Mechanisms of Hepatocellular Cholestasis

PRIMARY HEPATOCYTE MEMBRANE INJURY

INHIBITION OF ACTIVE TRANSPORT PROCESSES

SUBCELLULAR ANATOMIC ALTERATIONS

AMPLIFICATION BY SEVERAL MECHANISMS

Cholesterol retention with altered membrane fluidity
Bile salt retention with secondary membrane injury
Formation of secondary "cholestatic" bile acids
Reduced bile salt pool and enterohepatic recirculation

The newborn's liver is relatively sensitive to the development of cholestasis in response to a wide variety of insults. Several of the critical mechanisms for bile salt uptake and bile formation are underdeveloped at birth, which probably accounts for the tendency of neonates to develop cholestasis. Indeed, "physiologic cholestasis," in which serum bile salt concentrations are elevated to a level equal to that in the adult with pathologic cholestasis, is evident in the infant during the first several months of life.[598, 599] A wide variety of insults, such as gram-negative sepsis, heart failure, metabolic disease, or exposure to toxic substances, are capable of further compromising the mechanisms for bile formation and can cause clinical cholestasis in the neonate.

To attempt a discussion of the diagnosis and management of the diseases causing neonatal cholestasis is outside the scope of this chapter. The reader is referred to recent reviews on the subject.[600, 601]

REFERENCES

1. With TK: Bile Pigments: Chemical, Biological, and Clinical Aspects. London, Academic Press, 1968.
2. Bonnett R, Davies JE, Hursthouse MB: Structure of bilirubin. Nature 1976; 262:327.
3. Brodersen R: Bilirubin. Solubility and interaction with albumin and phospholipid. J Biol Chem 1979; 254:2364.
4. Hutchinson DW, Johnson B, Knell AJ: Tautomerism and hydrogen bonding in bilirubin. Biochem J 1971; 123:483.
5. Ostrow JD, Celic L, Mukerjee P: Molecular and micellar associations in the pH-dependent stable and metastable dissolution of unconjugated bilirubin by bile salts. J Lipid Res 1988; 29:335.
6. Hahm JS, Ostrow JD, Mukerjee P, et al: Ionization and self-association of unconjugated bilirubin, determined by rapid solvent partition from chloroform, with further studies of bilirubin solubility. J Lipid Res 1992; 33:1123.
7. Zucker SD, Goessling W: Mechanism of hepatocellular uptake of albumin-bound bilirubin. Biochim Biophys Acta 2000; 1463:197.
8. Lightner DA, Holmes DL, McDonagh AF: On the acid dissociation constants of bilirubin and biliverdin. pK_a values from ^{13}C NMR spectroscopy. J Biol Chem 1996; 271:2397.
9. Zucker SD, Goessling W, Hoppin AG: Unconjugated bilirubin exhibits spontaneous diffusion through model lipid bilayers and native hepatocyte membranes. J Biol Chem 1999; 274:10852.
10. Schmid R, McDonagh AF: The enzymatic formation of bilirubin. Ann NY Acad Sci 1975; 244:533.
11. Brown SB, Thomas SE: The mechanism of haem degradation in vitro. Kinetic evidence for the formation of a haem-oxygen complex. Biochem J 1978; 176:327.
12. Brown SB, King RF: The mechanism of haem catabolism. Bilirubin formation in living rats by [^{18}O]oxygen labelling. Biochem J 1978; 170:297.
13. Tenhunen R, Marver HS, Schmid R: The enzymatic catabolism of hemoglobin: Stimulation of microsomal heme oxygenase by hemin. J Lab Clin Med 1970; 75:410.
14. Blanckaert N, Heirwegh KP, Compernolle F: Synthesis and separation by thin-layer chromatography of bilirubin-IX isomers. Their identification as tetrapyrroles and dipyrrolic ethyl anthranilate azo derivatives. Biochem J 1976; 155:405.
15. Bonnett R, McDonagh AF: The meso-reactivity of porphyrins and related compounds. VI. Oxidative cleavage of the haem system. The four isomeric biliverdins of the IX series. J Chem Soc 1973; 9:881.
16. McDonagh AF, Assisi F: The ready isomerization of bilirubin IX- in aqueous solution. Biochem J 1972; 129:797.
17. Blanckaert N, Fevery J, Heirwegh KP, et al: Characterization of the major diazo-positive pigments in bile of homozygous Gunn rats. Biochem J 1977; 164:237.
18. Fevery J, Van Damme B, Michiels R, et al: Bilirubin conjugates in bile of man and rat in the normal state and in liver disease. J Clin Invest 1972; 51:2482.

19. Fevery J, Blanckaert N, Heirwegh KP, et al: Bilirubin conjugates: Formation and detection. Prog Liver Dis 1976; 5:183.

20. Ullrich D, Tischler T, Sieg A, et al: Renal clearance of bilirubin conjugates in newborns of different gestational age. Eur J Pediatr 1993; 152:837.

21. Lauff JJ, Kasper ME, Wu TW, et al: Isolation and preliminary characterization of a fraction of bilirubin in serum that is firmly bound to protein. Clin Chem 1982; 28:629.

22. Lauff JJ, Kasper ME, Ambrose RT: Quantitative liquid-chromatographic estimation of bilirubin species in pathological serum. Clin Chem 1983; 29:800.

23. Weiss JS, Gautam A, Lauff JJ, et al: The clinical importance of a protein-bound fraction of serum bilirubin in patients with hyperbilirubinemia. N Engl J Med 1983; 309:147.

24. Blanckaert N, Servaes R, Leroy P: Measurement of bilirubin-protein conjugates in serum and application to human and rat sera. J Lab Clin Med 1986; 108:77.

25. Ding A, Ojingwa JC, McDonagh AF, et al: Evidence for covalent binding of acyl glucuronides to serum albumin via an imine mechanism as revealed by tandem mass spectrometry. Proc Natl Acad Sci USA 1993; 90:3797.

26. Reed RG, Davidson LK, Burrington CM, et al: Non-resolving jaundice: Bilirubin covalently attached to serum albumin circulates with the same metabolic half-life as albumin. Clin Chem 1988; 34:1992.

27. Killenberg PG, Stevens RD, Wildermann RF, et al: The laboratory method as a variable in the interpretation of serum bilirubin fractionation. Gastroenterology 1980; 78:1011.

28. Wu TW, Dappen GM, Powers DM, et al: The Kodak Ektachem clinical chemistry slide for measurement of bilirubin in newborns: Principles and performance. Clin Chem 1982; 28:2366.

29. Wu TW, Dappen GM, Spayd RW, et al: The Ektachem clinical chemistry slide for simultaneous determination of unconjugated and sugar-conjugated bilirubin. Clin Chem 1984; 30:1304.

30. Lauff JJ, Kasper ME, Ambrose RT: Separation of bilirubin species in serum and bile by high-performance reversed-phase liquid chromatography. J Chromatogr 1981; 226:391.

31. Muraca M, Blanckaert N: Liquid-chromatographic assay and identification of mono- and diester conjugates of bilirubin in normal serum. Clin Chem 1983; 29:1767.

32. Odell GB, Mogilevsky WS, Gourley GR: High-performance liquid chromatographic analysis of bile pigments as their native tetrapyrroles and as their dipyrrolic azosulfanilate derivatives. J Chromatogr 1990; 529:287.

33. Kramer LI: Advancement of dermal icterus in the jaundiced newborn. Am J Dis Child 1969; 118:454.

34. Ballowitz L, Avery ME: Spectral reflectance of the skin. Studies on infant and adult humans, Wistar and Gunn rats. Biol Neonate 1970; 15:348.

35. Schreiner RL, Hannemann RE, DeWitt DP, et al: Relationship of skin reflectance and serum bilirubin: Full term Caucasian infants. Hum Biol 1979; 51:31.

36. Amato M, Huppi P, Markus D: Assessment of neonatal jaundice in low birth weight infants comparing transcutaneous, capillary and arterial bilirubin levels. Eur J Pediatr 1990; 150:59.

37. Dai J, Parry DM, Krahn J: Transcutaneous bilirubinometry: Its role in the assessment of neonatal jaundice. Clin Biochem 1997; 30:1.

38. Maisels MJ, Kring E: Transcutaneous bilirubinometry decreases the need for serum bilirubin measurements and saves money. Pediatrics 1997; 99:599.

39. Berk PD, Howe RB, Bloomer JR, et al: Studies of bilirubin kinetics in normal adults. J Clin Invest 1969; 48:2176.

40. Berk PD, Martin JF, Blaschke TF, et al: Unconjugated hyperbilirubinemia. Physiologic evaluation and experimental approaches to therapy. Ann Intern Med 1975; 82:552.

41. Poland RL, Odell GB: Physiologic jaundice: The enterohepatic circulation of bilirubin. N Engl J Med 1971; 284:1.

42. Robinson SH: The origins of bilirubin. N Engl J Med 1968; 279:143.

43. Israels LG: The bilirubin shunt and shunt hyperbilirubinemia. Prog Liver Dis 1970; 3:1.

44. Robinson SH: Early labeled bilirubin. N Engl J Med 1968; 278:565.

45. Tenhunen R, Marver HS, Schmid R: Microsomal heme oxygenase. Characterization of the enzyme. J Biol Chem 1969; 244:6388.

46. Rodgers PA, Vreman HJ, Dennery PA, et al: Sources of carbon monoxide (CO) in biological systems and applications of CO detection technologies. Semin Perinatol 1994; 18:2.

47. Yoshinaga T, Sassa S, Kappas A: A comparative study of heme degradation by NADPH-cytochrome *c* reductase alone and by the complete heme oxygenase system. Distinctive aspects of heme degradation by NADPH-cytochrome *c* reductase. J Biol Chem 1982; 257:7794.

48. Yoshinaga T, Sassa S, Kappas A: The occurrence of molecular interactions among NADPH-cytochrome *c* reductase, heme oxygenase, and biliverdin reductase in heme degradation. J Biol Chem 1982; 257:7786.

49. Bloomer JR, Barrett PV, Rodkey FL, et al: Studies on the mechanism of fasting hyperbilirubinemia. Gastroenterology 1971; 61:479.

50. Bakken AF, Thaler MM, Schmid R: Metabolic regulation of heme catabolism and bilirubin production. I. Hormonal control of hepatic heme oxygenase activity. J Clin Invest 1972; 51:530.

51. Felsher BF, Redeker AG: Bilirubinemia and fasting. N Engl J Med 1970; 283:823.

52. Felsher BF, Carpio NM: Caloric intake and unconjugated hyperbilirubinemia. Gastroenterology 1975; 69:42.

53. Chaves-Carballo E, Harris LE, Lynn HB: Jaundice associated with pyloric stenosis and neonatal small-bowel obstructions. Clin Pediatr 1968; 7:198.

54. Berk PD, Rodkey FL, Blaschke TF, et al: Comparison of plasma bilirubin turnover and carbon monoxide production in man. J Lab Clin Med 1974; 83:29.

55. Bartoletti AL, Stevenson DK, Ostrander CR, et al: Pulmonary excretion of carbon monoxide in the human infant as an index of bilirubin production. I. Effects of gestational and postnatal age and some common neonatal abnormalities. J Pediatr 1979; 94:952.

56. Cohen RS, Ostrander CR, Cowan BE, et al: Pulmonary excretion rates of carbon monoxide using a modified technique: Differences between premature and full-term infants. Biol Neonate 1982; 41:289.

57. Maisels MJ, Pathak A, Nelson NM, et al: Endogenous production of carbon monoxide in normal and erythroblastotic newborn infants. J Clin Invest 1971; 50:1.

58. Maisels MJ, Pathak A, Nelson NM: The effect of exchange transfusion on endogenous carbon monoxide production in erythroblastotic infants. J Pediatr 1972; 81:705.

59. Milleville GS, Levitt MD, Engel RR: Tin protoporphyrin inhibits carbon monoxide production in adult mice. Pediatr Res 1985; 19:94.

60. Stevenson DK, Bartoletti AL, Ostrander CR, et al: Pulmonary excretion of carbon monoxide in the human infant as an index of bilirubin production. II. Infants of diabetic mothers. J Pediatr 1979; 94:956.

61. Stevenson DK, Bartoletti AL, Ostrander CR, et al: Pulmonary excretion of carbon monoxide in the human newborn infant as an index of bilirubin production: III. Measurement of pulmonary excretion of carbon monoxide after the first postnatal week in premature infants. Pediatrics 1979; 64:598.

62. Stevenson DK, Vreman HJ, Oh W, et al: Bilirubin production in healthy term infants as measured by carbon monoxide in breath. Clin Chem 1994; 40:1934.

63. Huang TJ, Trakshel GM, Maines MD: Detection of 10 variants of biliverdin reductase in rat liver by two-dimensional gel electrophoresis. J Biol Chem 1989; 264:7844.

64. Maines MD: Multiple forms of biliverdin reductase: Age-related change in pattern of expression in rat liver and brain. Mol Pharmacol 1990; 38:481.

65. Maines MD, Trakshel GM: Purification and characterization of human biliverdin reductase. Arch Biochem Biophys 1993; 300:320.

66. Pereira PJ, Macedo-Ribeiro S, Parraga A, et al: Structure of human biliverdin IXβ reductase, an early fetal bilirubin IXβ producing enzyme. Nat Struct Biol 2001; 8:215.

67. Frydman RB, Bari S, Tomaro ML, et al: The enzymatic and chemical reduction of extended biliverdins. Biochem Biophys Res Commun 1990; 171:465.

68. Salim M, Brown-Kipphut BA, Maines MD: Human biliverdin reductase is autophosphorylated, and phosphorylation is required for bilirubin formation. J Biol Chem 2001; 276:10929.

69. Tenhunen R, Ross ME, Marver HS, et al: Reduced nicotinamide-adenine dinucleotide phosphate dependent biliverdin reductase: Partial purification and characterization. Biochemistry 1970; 9:298.

70. Crawford JM, Ransil BJ, Potter CS, et al: Hepatic disposition and biliary excretion of bilirubin and bilirubin glucuronides in intact rats. Differential processing of pigments derived from intra- and extrahepatic sources. J Clin Invest 1987; 79:1172.

71. Crawford JM, Hauser SC, Gollan JL: Formation, hepatic metabolism, and transport of bile pigments: A status report. Semin Liver Dis 1988; 8:105.

72. Brandes JM, Berk PD, Urbach J, et al: Transport of bilirubin and glucose by the isolated perfused human placenta. Contrib Gynecol Obstet 1985; 13:147.

73. McDonagh AF, Palma LA, Schmid R: Reduction of biliverdin and placental transfer of bilirubin and biliverdin in the pregnant guinea pig. Biochem J 1981; 194:273.

74. Pascolo L, Fernetti C, Garcia-Mediavilla MV, et al: Mechanisms for the transport of unconjugated bilirubin in human trophoblastic BeWo cells. FEBS Lett 2001; 495:94.

75. Frei B, Stocker R, Ames BN: Antioxidant defenses and lipid peroxidation in human blood plasma. Proc Natl Acad Sci USA 1988; 85:9748.

76. Krinsky NI: Mechanism of action of biological antioxidants. Proc Soc Exp Biol Med 1992; 200:248.

77. Neuzil J, Stocker R: Free and albumin-bound bilirubin are efficient co-antioxidants for α-tocopherol, inhibiting plasma and low density lipoprotein lipid peroxidation. J Biol Chem 1994; 269:16712.

78. Stocker R, Yamamoto Y, McDonagh AF, et al: Bilirubin is an antioxidant of possible physiological importance. Science 1987; 235:1043.

79. Stocker R, Glazer AN, Ames BN: Antioxidant activity of albumin-bound bilirubin. Proc Natl Acad Sci USA 1987; 84:5918.

80. Stocker R, McDonagh AF, Glazer AN, et al: Antioxidant activities of bile pigments: Biliverdin and bilirubin. Methods Enzymol 1990; 186:301.

81. Wu TW, Carey D, Wu J, et al: The cytoprotective effects of bilirubin and biliverdin on rat hepatocytes and human erythrocytes and the impact of albumin. Biochem Cell Biol 1991; 69:828.

82. Llesuy SF, Tomaro ML: Heme oxygenase and oxidative stress. Evidence of involvement of bilirubin as physiological protector against oxidative damage. Biochim Biophys Acta 1994; 1223:9.

83. Olinescu R, Alexandrescu R, Hulea SA, et al: Tissue lipid peroxidation may be triggered by increased formation of bilirubin in vivo. Res Commun Chem Pathol Pharmacol 1994; 84:27.

84. Zimmerman BJ, Grisham MB, Granger DN: Mechanisms of oxidant-mediated microvascular injury following reperfusion of the ischemic intestine. Basic Life Sci 1988; 49:881.

85. Parks DA, Granger DN: Ischemia-reperfusion injury: A radical view. Hepatology 1988; 8:680.

86. Grisham MB, Granger DN: Neutrophil-mediated mucosal injury. Role of reactive oxygen metabolites. Dig Dis Sci 1988; 33(Suppl):6.

87. Granger DN: Role of xanthine oxidase and granulocytes in ischemia-reperfusion injury. Am J Physiol 1988; 255:H1269.

88. Crissinger KD: Animal models of necrotizing enterocolitis. J Pediatr Gastroenterol Nutr 1995; 20:17.

89. Crissinger KD: Regulation of hemodynamics and oxygenation in developing intestine: Insight into the pathogenesis of necrotizing enterocolitis. Acta Paediatr Suppl 1994; 396:8.

90. Tiribelli C, Ostrow JD: New concepts in bilirubin chemistry, transport and metabolism: Report of the International Bilirubin Workshop, April 6–8, 1989, Trieste, Italy. Hepatology 1990; 11:303.

91. Wennberg R: Bilirubin transport and toxicity. Mead Johnson Symp Perinat Dev Med 1982:25.

92. Jacobsen J, Brodersen R: Albumin-bilirubin binding mechanism. J Biol Chem 1983; 258:6319.

93. Jacobsen C, Jacobsen J: Dansylation of human serum albumin in the study of the primary binding sites of bilirubin and L-tryptophan. Biochem J 1979; 181:251.

94. Odell GB: Neonatal jaundice. Prog Liver Dis 1976; 5:457.

95. Brodersen R: Bilirubin transport in the newborn infant, reviewed with relation to kernicterus. J Pediatr 1980; 96:349.

96. Inoue M: Metabolism and transport of amphipathic molecules in analbuminemic rats and human subjects. Hepatology 1985; 5:892.

97. Inoue M, Hirata E, Morino Y, et al: The role of albumin in the hepatic transport of bilirubin: Studies in mutant analbuminemic rats. J Biochem 1985; 97:737.

98. Takahashi M, Sugiyama K, Shumiya S, et al: Penetration of bilirubin into the brain in albumin-deficient and jaundiced rats (AJR) and Nagase analbuminemic rats (NAR). J Biochem 1984; 96:1705.

99. Yamashita M, Adachi Y, Kambe A, et al: Serum binding and biliary excretion of bilirubin after bilirubin loading in Nagase analbuminemic rats and heterozygous (Jj) Gunn rats. J Lab Clin Med 1988; 112:443.

100. Goessling W, Zucker SD: Role of apolipoprotein D in the transport of bilirubin in plasma. Am J Physiol 2000; 279:G356.

101. Cashore WJ, Gartner LM, Oh W, et al: Clinical application of neonatal bilirubin-binding determinations: Current status. J Pediatr 1978; 93:827.

102. Ebbesen F: Bilirubin, reserve albumin for binding of bilirubin and pH in plasma during phototherapy (ordinary and double light) of term newborn infants. Acta Paediatr Scand 1981; 70:223.

103. Lee KS, Gartner LM, Vaisman SL: Measurement of bilirubin-albumin binding. I. Comparative analysis of four methods and four human serum albumin preparations. Pediatr Res 1978; 12:301.

104. Ryall RG, Peake MJ: Theoretical constraints in the measurement of serum bilirubin binding capacity. Clin Biochem 1982; 15:146.

105. Dennery PA, Seidman DS, Stevenson DK: Neonatal hyperbilirubinemia. N Engl J Med 2001; 344:581.

106. Paumgartner G, Reichen J: Kinetics of hepatic uptake of unconjugated bilirubin. Clin Sci Mol Med 1976; 51:169.

107. Sorrentino D, Berk PD: Mechanistic aspects of hepatic bilirubin uptake. Semin Liver Dis 1988; 8:119.

108. Sorrentino D, Potter BJ, Berk PD: From albumin to the cytoplasm: The hepatic uptake of organic anions. Prog Liver Dis 1990; 9:203.

109. Berk PD, Bradbury M, Zhou SL, et al: Characterization of membrane transport processes: Lessons from the study of BSP, bilirubin, and fatty acid uptake. Semin Liver Dis 1996; 16:107.

110. Ockner RK, Weisiger RA, Gollan JL: Hepatic uptake of albumin-bound substances: Albumin receptor concept. Am J Physiol 1983; 245:G13.

111. Weinman SA: Identifying the hepatic organic anion transporter: One of many? Hepatology 1994; 20:1642.

112. Stremmel W, Berk PD: Hepatocellular uptake of sulfobromophthalein and bilirubin is selectively inhibited by an antibody to the liver plasma membrane sulfobromophthalein/bilirubin binding protein. J Clin Invest 1986; 78:822.

113. Goeser T, Nakata R, Braly LF, et al: The rat hepatocyte plasma membrane organic anion binding protein is immunologically related to the mitochondrial F1 adenosine triphosphatase beta-subunit. J Clin Invest 1990; 86:220.

114. Cui Y, Konig J, Leier I, et al: Hepatic uptake of bilirubin and its conjugates by the human organic anion transporter SLC21A6. J Biol Chem 2001; 276:9626.

115. Fleischner GM, Arias IM: Structure and function of ligandin (Y protein, GSH transferase B) and Z protein in the liver: A progress report. Prog Liver Dis 1976; 5:172.

116. Torres AM, Kaplowitz N, Tiribelli C: Role of BSP/bilirubin binding protein and bilitranslocase in glutathione uptake in rat basolateral liver plasma membrane vesicles. Biochem Biophys Res Commun 1994; 200:1079.

117. Ookhtens M, Lyon I, Fernandez-Checa J, et al: Inhibition of glutathione efflux in the perfused rat liver and isolated hepatocytes by organic anions and bilirubin. Kinetics, sidedness, and molecular forms. J Clin Invest 1988; 82:608.

118. Kaplowitz N: Physiological significance of glutathione S-transferases. Am J Physiol 1980; 239:G439.

119. DeLeve LD, Kaplowitz N: Importance and regulation of hepatic glutathione. Semin Liver Dis 1990; 10:251.

120. Wolkoff AW, Weisiger RA, Jakoby WB: The multiple roles of the glutathione transferases (ligandins). Prog Liver Dis 1979; 6:213.

121. Theilmann L, Stollman YR, Arias IM, et al: Does Z-protein have a role in transport of bilirubin and bromosulfophthalein by isolated perfused rat liver? Hepatology 1984; 4:923.

122. Ockner RK, Manning JA, Kane JP: Fatty acid binding protein. Isolation from rat liver, characterization, and immunochemical quantification. J Biol Chem 1982; 257:7872.

123. Zucker SD, Storch J, Zeidel ML, et al: Mechanism of the spontaneous transfer of unconjugated bilirubin between small unilamellar phosphatidylcholine vesicles. Biochemistry 1992; 31:3184.

124. Zucker SD, Goessling W, Zeidel ML, et al: Membrane lipid composition and vesicle size modulate bilirubin intermembrane transfer. Evidence for membrane-directed trafficking of bilirubin in the hepatocyte. J Biol Chem 1994; 269:19262.

125. Zucker SD, Goessling W, Ransil BJ, et al: Influence of glutathione S-transferase B (ligandin) on the intermembrane transfer of bilirubin. Implications for the intracellular transport of nonsubstrate ligands in hepatocytes. J Clin Invest 1995; 96:1927.

126. Zucker SD, Goessling W, Gollan JL: Kinetics of bilirubin transfer between serum albumin and membrane vesicles. Insight into the mechanism of organic anion delivery to the hepatocyte plasma membrane. J Biol Chem 1995; 270:1074.

127. Zucker SD: Kinetic model of protein-mediated ligand transport: Influence of soluble binding proteins on the intermembrane diffusion of a fluorescent fatty acid. Biochemistry 2001; 40:977.

128. Farrell GC, Gollan JL, Schmid R: Efflux of bilirubin into plasma following hepatic degradation of exogenous heme. Proc Soc Exp Biol Med 1980; 163:504.

129. Levi AJ, Gatmaitan Z, Arias IM: Deficiency of hepatic organic anion-binding protein, impaired organic amnion uptake by liver and "physiologic" jaundice in newborn monkeys. N Engl J Med 1970; 283:1136.

130. Weisiger RA: Dissociation from albumin: A potentially rate-limiting step in the clearance of substances by the liver. Proc Natl Acad Sci USA 1985; 82:1563.

131. Kapitulnik J, Ostrow JD: Stimulation of bilirubin catabolism in jaundiced Gunn rats by an induced of microsomal mixed-function monooxygenases. Proc Natl Acad Sci USA 1978; 75:682.

132. Kapitulnik J, Gonzalez FJ: Marked endogenous activation of the CYP1A1 and CYP1A2 genes in the congenitally jaundiced Gunn rat. Mol Pharmacol 1993; 43:722.

133. Cardenas-Vazquez R, Yokosuka O, Billing BH: Enzymic oxidation of unconjugated bilirubin by rat liver. Biochem J 1986; 236:625.

134. Berry CS, Zarembo JE, Ostrow JD: Evidence for conversion of bilirubin to dihydroxyl derivatives in the Gunn rat. Biochem Biophys Res Commun 1972; 49:1366.

135. Cuypers HT, Ter Haar EM, Jansen PL: Microsomal conjugation and oxidation of bilirubin. Biochim Biophys Acta 1983; 758:135.

136. De Matteis F, Dawson SJ, Boobis AR, et al: Inducible bilirubin-degrading system of rat liver microsomes: Role of cytochrome P450IA1. Mol Pharmacol 1991; 40:686.

137. Burchell B, Coughtrie MW: UDP-glucuronosyltransferases. Pharmacol Ther 1989; 43:261.

138. Burchell B, Blanckaert N: Bilirubin mono- and di-glucuronide formation by purified rat liver microsomal bilirubin UDP-glucuronyltransferase. Biochem J 1984; 223:461.

139. Blanckaert N, Gollan J, Schmid R: Bilirubin diglucuronide synthesis by a UDP-glucuronic acid-dependent enzyme system in rat liver microsomes. Proc Natl Acad Sci USA 1979; 76:2037.

140. Chowdhury JR, Chowdhury NR, Wu G, et al: Bilirubin mono- and diglucuronide formation by human liver in vitro: Assay by high-pressure liquid chromatography. Hepatology 1981; 1:622.

141. Chowdhury NR, Arias IM, Lederstein M, et al: Substrates and products of purified rat liver bilirubin UDP-glucuronosyltransferase. Hepatology 1986; 6:123.

142. Whiting JF, Narciso JP, Chapman V, et al: Deconjugation of bilirubin-IXα glucuronides: A physiologic role of hepatic microsomal β-glucuronidase. J Biol Chem 1993; 268:23197.

143. Whitmer DI, Russell PE, Ziurys JC, et al: Hepatic microsomal glucuronidation of bilirubin is modulated by the lipid microenvironment of membrane-bound substrate. J Biol Chem 1986; 261:7170.

144. Whitmer DI, Russell PE, Gollan JL: Membrane-membrane interactions associated with rapid transfer of liposomal bilirubin to microsomal UDP-glucuronyltransferase. Relevance for hepatocellular transport and biotransformation of hydrophobic substrates. Biochem J 1987; 244:41.

145. Whitmer DI, Ziurys JC, Gollan JL: Hepatic microsomal glucuronidation of bilirubin in unilamellar liposomal membranes. Implications for intracellular transport of lipophilic substrates. J Biol Chem 1984; 259:11969.

146. Jackson MR, McCarthy LR, Harding D, et al: Cloning of a human liver microsomal UDP-glucuronosyltransferase cDNA. Biochem J 1987; 242:581.

147. Roy Chowdhury J, Roy Chowdhury N, Falany CN, et al: Isolation and characterization of multiple forms of rat liver UDP-glucuronate glucuronosyltransferase. Biochem J 1986; 233:827.

148. Roy Chowdhury N, Gross F, Moscioni AD, et al: Isolation of multiple normal and functionally defective forms of uridine diphosphate-glucuronosyltransferase from inbred Gunn rats. J Clin Invest 1987; 79:327.

149. Burchell B, Nebert DW, Nelson DR, et al: The UDP glucuronosyltransferase gene superfamily: Suggested nomenclature based on evolutionary divergence. DNA Cell Biol 1991; 10:487.

150. Burchell B, Jackson MR, Coarser RB, et al: The molecular biology of UDP-glucuronyltransferases. Biochem Soc Trans 1987; 15:581.

151. Burchell B, Coughtrie MW, Jackson MR, et al: Genetic deficiency of bilirubin glucuronidation in rats and humans. Mol Aspects Med 1987; 9:429.

152. Mackenzie PI: Rat liver UDP-glucuronosyltransferase. Sequence and expression of a cDNA encoding a phenobarbital-inducible form. J Biol Chem 1986; 261:6119.

153. Mackenzie PI, Rodbourn L: Organization of the rat UDP-glucuronosyltransferase, UDPGTr-2, gene and characterization of its promoter. J Biol Chem 1990; 265:11328.

154. Robertson KJ, Clarke D, Sutherland L, et al: Investigation of the molecular basis of the genetic deficiency of UDP-glucuronosyltransferase in Crigler-Najjar syndrome. J Inherit Metab Dis 1991; 14:563.

155. Clarke DJ, Keen JN, Burchell B: Isolation and characterisation of a new hepatic bilirubin UDP-glucuronosyltransferase. Absence from Gunn rat liver. FEBS Lett 1992; 299:183.

156. Clarke DJ, Moghrabi N, Monaghan G, et al: Genetic defects of the UDP-glucuronosyltransferase-1 (UGT1) gene that cause familial non-haemolytic unconjugated hyperbilirubinaemias. Clin Chim Acta 1997; 266:63.

157. Ritter JK, Crawford JM, Owens IS: Cloning of two human liver bilirubin UDP-glucuronosyltransferase cDNAs with expression in COS-1 cells. J Biol Chem 1991; 266:1043.

158. Bosma PJ, Chowdhury NR, Goldhoorn BG, et al: Sequence of exons and the flanking regions of human bilirubin-UDP-glucuronosyltransferase gene complex and identification of a genetic mutation in a patient with Crigler-Najjar syndrome, type I. Hepatology 1992; 15:941.

159. Bosma PJ, Chowdhury JR, Bakker C, et al: The genetic basis of the reduced expression of bilirubin UDP-glucuronosyltransferase 1 in Gilbert's syndrome. N Engl J Med 1995; 333:1171.

160. Aono S, Yamada Y, Keino H, et al: A new type of defect in the gene for bilirubin uridine 5′-diphosphate-glucuronosyltransferase in a patient with Crigler-Najjar syndrome type I. Pediatr Res 1994; 35:629.

161. Nagai F, Homma H, Tanase H, et al: Studies on the genetic linkage of bilirubin and androsterone UDP-glucuronyltransferases by cross-breeding of two mutant rat strains. Biochem J 1988; 252:897.

162. Mackenzie PI: Expression of chimeric cDNAs in cell culture defines a region of UDP glucuronosyltransferase involved in substrate selection. J Biol Chem 1990; 265:3432.

163. Mackenzie PI, Owens IS, Burchell B, et al: The UDP glycosyltransferase gene superfamily: Recommended nomenclature update based on evolutionary divergence. Pharmacogenetics 1997; 7:255.

164. Ritter JK, Chen F, Sheen YY, et al: Two human liver cDNAs encode UDP-glucuronosyltransferases with 2 log differences in activity toward parallel substrates including hyodeoxycholic acid and certain estrogen derivatives. Biochemistry 1992; 31:3409.

165. Owens IS, Ritter JK: The novel bilirubin/phenol UDP-glucuronosyltransferase UGT1 gene locus: Implications for multiple nonhemolytic familial hyperbilirubinemia phenotypes. Pharmacogenetics 1992; 2:93.

166. Owens IS, Ritter JK: Gene structure at the human UGT1 locus creates diversity in isozyme structure, substrate specificity, and regulation. Prog Nucleic Acid Res Mol Biol 1995; 51:305.

167. Vanstapel F, Blanckaert N: Topology and regulation of bilirubin UDP-glucuronyltransferase in sealed native microsomes from rat liver. Arch Biochem Biophys 1988; 263:216.

168. Vanstapel F, Hammaker L, Pua K, et al: Properties of membrane-bound bilirubin UDP-glucuronyltransferase in rough and smooth endoplasmic reticulum and in the nuclear envelope from rat liver. Biochem J 1989; 259:659.

169. Seppen J, Steenken E, Lindhout D, et al: A mutation which disrupts the hydrophobic core of the signal peptide of bilirubin UDP-glucuronosyltransferase, an endoplasmic reticulum membrane protein, causes Crigler-Najjar type II. FEBS Lett 1996; 390:294.

170. Jansen PL, Arias IM: Delipidation and reactivation of UDPglucuronosyltransferase from rat liver. Biochim Biophys Acta 1975; 391:23.

171. Erickson RH, Zakim D, Vessey DA: Preparation and properties of a phospholipid-free form of microsomal UDP-glucuronyltransferase. Biochemistry 1978; 17:3706.

172. Vessey DA, Goldenberg J, Zakim D: Kinetic properties of microsomal UDP-glucuronyltransferase. Evidence for cooperative kinetics and activation by UDP-N-acetylglucosamine. Biochim Biophys Acta 1973; 309:58.

173. Shepherd SR, Baird SJ, Hallinan T, et al: An investigation of the transverse topology of bilirubin UDP-glucuronosyltransferase in rat hepatic endoplasmic reticulum. Biochem J 1989; 259:617.

174. Chowdhury JR, Novikoff PM, Chowdhury NR, et al: Distribution of UDPglucuronosyltransferase in rat tissue. Proc Natl Acad Sci USA 1985; 82:2990.

175. Peters WH, Nagengast FM, van Tongeren JH: Glutathione S-transferase, cytochrome P450, and uridine 5′-diphosphate-glucuronosyltransferase in human small intestine and liver. Gastroenterology 1989; 96:783.

176. Sutherland L, Ebner T, Burchell B: The expression of UDP-glucuronosyltransferases of the UGT1 family in human liver and kidney and in response to drugs. Biochem Pharmacol 1993; 45:295.

177. Bosma PJ, Seppen J, Goldhoorn B, et al: Bilirubin UDP-glucuronosyltransferase 1 is the only relevant bilirubin glucuronidating isoform in man. J Biol Chem 1994; 269:17960.

178. Bosma PJ, Chowdhury JR, Huang TJ, et al: Mechanisms of inherited deficiencies of multiple UDP-glucuronosyltransferase isoforms in two patients with Crigler-Najjar syndrome, type I. FASEB J 1992; 6:2859.

179. Ritter JK, Yeatman MT, Ferreira P, et al: Identification of a genetic alteration in the code for bilirubin UDP-glucuronosyltransferase in the UGT1 gene complex of a Crigler-Najjar type I patient. J Clin Invest 1992; 90:150.

180. Erps LT, Ritter JK, Hersh JH, et al: Identification of two single base substitutions in the UGT1 gene locus which abolish bilirubin uridine diphosphate glucuronosyltransferase activity in vitro. J Clin Invest 1994; 93:564.

181. Moghrabi N, Clarke DJ, Boxer M, et al: Identification of an A-to-G missense mutation in exon 2 of the UGT1 gene complex that causes Crigler-Najjar syndrome type 2. Genomics 1993; 18:171.

182. Moghrabi N, Clarke DJ, Burchell B, et al: Cosegregation of intragenic markers with a novel mutation that causes Crigler-Najjar syndrome type I: Implication in carrier detection and prenatal diagnosis. Am J Hum Genet 1993; 53:722.

183. Seppen J, Bosma PJ, Goldhoorn BG, et al: Discrimination between Crigler-Najjar type I and II by expression of mutant bilirubin uridine diphosphate-glucuronosyltransferase. J Clin Invest 1994; 94:2385.

184. Burchell B, Brierley CH, Rance D: Specificity of human UDP-glucuronosyltransferases and xenobiotic glucuronidation. Life Sci 1995; 57:1819.

185. Jansen PL, Bosma PJ, Chowdhury JR: Molecular biology of bilirubin metabolism. Prog Liver Dis 1995; 13:125.

186. Jansen PL, Oude Elferink RP: Hereditary hyperbilirubinemias: A molecular and mechanistic approach. Semin Liver Dis 1988; 8:168.

187. Gartner LM, Lee KS, Vaisman S, et al: Development of bilirubin transport and metabolism in the newborn rhesus monkey. J Pediatr 1977; 90:513.

188. Crawford JM, Ransil BJ, Narciso JP, et al: Hepatic microsomal bilirubin UDP-glucuronosyltransferase. The kinetics of bilirubin mono- and diglucuronide synthesis. J Biol Chem 1992; 267:16943.

189. Vanstapel F, Blanckaert N: On the binding of bilirubin and its structural analogues to hepatic microsomal bilirubin UDPglucuronyltransferase. Biochemistry 1987; 26:6074.

190. Hjelle JJ: Hepatic UDP-glucuronic acid regulation during acetaminophen biotransformation in rats. J Pharmacol Exp Ther 1986; 237:750.

191. Peters WH, Jansen PL: Microsomal UDP-glucuronyltransferase-catalyzed bilirubin diglucuronide formation in human liver. J Hepatol 1986; 2:182.

192. Mackenzie PI: The effect of N-linked glycosylation on the substrate preferences of UDP glucuronosyltransferases. Biochem Biophys Res Commun 1990; 166:1293.

193. Kamisako T, Adachi Y, Yamamoto T: Effect of UDP-glucuronic acid depletion by salicylamide on biliary bilirubin excretion in the rat. J Pharmacol Exp Ther 1990; 254:380.

194. Hauser SC, Ziurys JC, Gollan JL: A membrane transporter mediates access of uridine 5′-diphosphoglucuronic acid from the cytosol into the endoplasmic reticulum of rat hepatocytes: Implications for glucuronidation reactions. Biochim Biophys Acta 1988; 967:149.

195. Bossuyt X, Blanckaert N: Carrier-mediated transport of intact UDP-glucuronic acid into the lumen of endoplasmic-reticulum-derived vesicles from rat liver. Biochem J 1994; 302:261.

196. Berg CL, Radominska A, Lester R, et al: Membrane translocation and regulation of uridine diphosphate-glucuronic acid uptake in rat liver microsomal vesicles. Gastroenterology 1995; 108:183.

197. Bossuyt X, Blanckaert N: Carrier-mediated transport of uridine diphosphoglucuronic acid across the endoplasmic reticulum membrane is a prerequisite for UDP-glucuronosyltransferase activity in rat liver. Biochem J 1997; 323:645.

198. Bossuyt X, Blanckaert N: Functional characterization of carrier-mediated transport of uridine diphosphate N-acetylglucosamine across the endoplasmic reticulum membrane. Eur J Biochem 1994; 223:981.

199. Bossuyt X, Blanckaert N: Mechanism of stimulation of microsomal UDP-glucuronosyltransferase by UDP-N-acetylglucosamine. Biochem J 1995; 305:321.

200. Hauser SC, Ransil BJ, Ziurys JC, et al: Interaction of uridine 5′-diphosphoglucuronic acid with microsomal UDP-glucuronosyltransferase in primate liver: The facilitating role of uridine 5′-diphospho-N-acetylglucosamine. Biochim Biophys Acta 1988; 967:141.

201. Bossuyt X, Blanckaert N: Uridine diphosphoxylose enhances hepatic microsomal UDP-glucuronosyltransferase activity by stimulating transport of UDP-glucuronic acid across the endoplasmic reticulum membrane. Biochem J 1996; 315:189.

202. Zakim D, Goldenberg J, Vessey DA: Effects of metals on the properties of hepatic microsomal uridine diphosphate glucuronyltransferase. Biochemistry 1973; 12:4068.

203. Goldstein RB, Vessey DA, Zakim D, et al: Perinatal developmental changes in hepatic UDP-glucuronyltransferase. Biochem J 1980; 186:841.

204. Campbell MT, Wishart GJ: The effect of premature and delayed birth on the development of UDP-glucuronosyltransferase activities towards bilirubin, morphine and testosterone in the rat. Biochem J 1980; 186:617.

205. Leakey JE, Hume R, Burchell B: Development of multiple activities of UDP-glucuronyltransferase in human liver. Biochem J 1987; 243:859.

206. Burchell B, Coughtrie M, Jackson M, et al: Development of human liver UDP-glucuronosyltransferases. Dev Pharmacol Ther 1989; 13:70.

207. Kawade N, Onishi S: The prenatal and postnatal development of UDP-glucuronyltransferase activity towards bilirubin and the effect of premature birth on this activity in the human liver. Biochem J 1981; 196:257.

208. Coughtrie MW, Burchell B, Leakey JE, et al: The inadequacy of perinatal glucuronidation: Immunoblot analysis of the developmental expression of individual UDP-glucuronosyltransferase isoenzymes in rat and human liver microsomes. Mol Pharmacol 1988; 34:729.

209. Cukier JO, Whitington PF, Odell GB: Bilirubin, UDP-glucuronyl transferase of liver in postmature rats. A functional and morphologic comparison. Lab Invest 1981; 44:368.

210. Muraca M, Fevery J: Influence of sex and sex steroids on bilirubin uridine diphosphate-glucuronosyltransferase activity of rat liver. Gastroenterology 1984; 87:308.

211. Heirwegh KP, Fevery J, Michiels R, et al: Separation by thin-layer chromatography and structure elucidation of bilirubin conjugates isolated from dog bile. Biochem J 1975; 145:185.

212. Sommerer U, Gordon ER, Goresky CA: Microsomal specificity underlying the differing hepatic formation of bilirubin glucuronide and glucose conjugates by rat and dog. Hepatology 1988; 8:116.

213. Senafi SB, Clarke DJ, Burchell B: Investigation of the substrate specificity of a cloned expressed human bilirubin UDP-glucuronosyltransferase: UDP-sugar specificity and involvement in steroid and xenobiotic glucuronidation. Biochem J 1994; 303:233.

214. Eletr S, Zakim D, Vessey DA: A spin-label study of the role of phospholipids in the regulation of membrane-bound microsomal enzymes. J Mol Biol 1973; 78:351.

215. Hochman Y, Kelley M, Zakim D: Modulation of the number of ligand binding sites of UDP-glucuronyltransferase by the gel to liquid-crystal phase transition of phosphatidylcholines. J Biol Chem 1983; 258:6509.

216. Hochman Y, Zakim D: Evidence that UDP-glucuronyltransferase in liver microsomes at 37 °C is in a gel phase lipid environment. J Biol Chem 1983; 258:11758.

217. Magdalou J, Hochman Y, Zakim D: Factors modulating the catalytic specificity of a pure form of UDP-glucuronyltransferase. J Biol Chem 1982; 257:13624.

218. Zakim D, Vessey DA: The effect of a temperature-induced phase change within membrane lipids on the regulatory properties of microsomal uridine diphosphate glucuronyltransferase. J Biol Chem 1975; 250:342.

219. Kapitulnik J, Tshershedsky M, Barenholz Y: Fluidity of the rat liver microsomal membrane: Increase at birth. Science 1979; 206:843.

220. Kapitulnik J, Weil E, Rabinowitz R, et al: Fetal and adult human liver differ markedly in the fluidity and lipid composition of their microsomal membranes. Hepatology 1987; 7:55.

221. Rosenthal P, Blanckaert N, Kabra PM, et al: Formation of bilirubin conjugates in human newborns. Pediatr Res 1986; 20:947.

222. Vaisman SL, Lee KS, Gartner LM: Xylose, glucose, and glucuronic acid conjugation of bilirubin in the newborn rat. Pediatr Res 1976; 10:967.

223. Blumenthal SG, Ikeda RM, Ruebner BH: Bile pigments in humans and in nonhuman primates during the perinatal period: Composition of meconium and gallbladder bile of newborns and adults. Pediatr Res 1976; 10:664.

224. Blumenthal SG, Stucker T, Rasmussen RD, et al: Changes in bilirubins in human prenatal development. Biochem J 1980; 186:693.

225. Fevery J, Blanckaert N, Heirwegh KP, et al: Unconjugated bilirubin and an increased proportion of bilirubin monoconjugates in the bile of patients with Gilbert's syndrome and Crigler-Najjar disease. J Clin Invest 1977; 60:970.

226. Fevery J, Blanckaert N, Leroy P, et al: Analysis of bilirubins in biological fluids by extraction and thin-layer chromatography of the intact tetrapyrroles: Application to bile of patients with Gilbert's syndrome, hemolysis, or cholelithiasis. Hepatology 1983; 3:177.

227. Goresky CA, Gordon ER, Shaffer EA, et al: Definition of a conjugation dysfunction in Gilbert's syndrome: Studies of the handling of bilirubin loads and of the pattern of bilirubin conjugates secreted in bile. Clin Sci Mol Med 1978; 55:63.

228. Gourley GR, Arend R, Mogilevsky WS, et al: Bilirubin conjugate excretion and bilirubin uridine diphosphoglucuronyltransferase activity in nonjaundiced homozygous and heterozygous Gunn rats. J Lab Clin Med 1986; 108:436.

229. Adachi Y, Yamashita M, Nanno T, et al: Proportion of conjugated bilirubin in bile in relation to hepatic bilirubin UDP-glucuronyltransferase activity. Clin Biochem 1990; 23:131.

230. Muraca M, Rubaltelli FF, Blanckaert N, et al: Unconjugated and conjugated bilirubin pigments during perinatal development. II. Studies on serum of healthy newborns and of neonates with erythroblastosis fetalis. Biol Neonate 1990; 57:1.

231. Gartner LM, Lane DL, Cornelius CE: Bilirubin transport by liver in adult *Macaca mulatta*. Am J Physiol 1971; 220:1528.

232. Wolkoff AW, Ketley JN, Waggoner JG, et al: Hepatic accumulation and intracellular binding of conjugated bilirubin. J Clin Invest 1978; 61:142.

233. Crawford JM, Berken CA, Gollan JL: Role of the hepatocyte microtubular system in the excretion of bile salts and biliary lipid: Implications for intracellular vesicular transport. J Lipid Res 1988; 29:144.

234. Crawford JM, Gollan JL: Hepatocyte cotransport of taurocholate and bilirubin glucuronides: Role of microtubules. Am J Physiol 1988; 255:G121.

235. Verkade HJ, Havinga R, Gerding A, et al: Mechanism of bile acid-induced biliary lipid secretion in the rat: Effect of conjugated bilirubin. Am J Physiol 1993; 264:G462.

236. Apstein MD: Inhibition of biliary phospholipid and cholesterol secretion by bilirubin in the Sprague-Dawley and Gunn rat. Gastroenterology 1984; 87:634.

237. Roman ID, Monte MJ, Gonzalez-Buitrago JM, et al: Inhibition of hepatocytary vesicular transport by cyclosporin A in the rat: Relationship with cholestasis and hyperbilirubinemia. Hepatology 1990; 12:83.

238. Crawford JM, Crawford AR, Strahs DC: Microtubule-dependent transport of bile salts through hepatocytes: Cholic vs. taurocholic acid. Hepatology 1993; 18:903.

239. Crawford JM, Crawford JJ: Push me-pull you: The challenge of endocytic sorting. Hepatology 1993; 17:342.

240. Crawford JM, Strahs DC, Crawford AR, et al: Role of bile salt hydrophobicity in hepatic microtubule-dependent bile salt secretion. J Lipid Res 1994; 35:1738.

241. Dubin M, Maurice M, Feldmann G, et al: Influence of colchicine and phalloidin on bile secretion and hepatic ultrastructure in the rat. Possible interaction between microtubules and microfilaments. Gastroenterology 1980; 79:646.

242. Gregory DH, Vlahcevic ZR, Prugh MF, et al: Mechanism of secretion of biliary lipids: Role of a microtubular system in hepatocellular transport of biliary lipids in the rat. Gastroenterology 1978; 74:93.

243. Kajihara S, Hisatomi A, Mizuta T, et al: A splice mutation in the human canalicular multispecific organic anion transporter gene causes Dubin-Johnson syndrome. Biochem Biophys Res Commun 1998; 253:454.

244. Kitamura T, Jansen P, Hardenbrook C, et al: Defective ATP-dependent bile canalicular transport of organic anions in mutant (TR-) rats with conjugated hyperbilirubinemia. Proc Natl Acad Sci USA 1990; 87:3557.

245. Nishida T, Hardenbrook C, Gatmaitan Z, et al: ATP-dependent organic anion transport system in normal and TR- rat liver canalicular membranes. Am J Physiol 1992; 262:G629.

246. Paulusma CC, Oude Elferink RP: The canalicular multispecific organic anion transporter and conjugated hyperbilirubinemia in rat and man. J Mol Med 1997; 75:420.

247. Paulusma CC, Kool M, Bosma PJ, et al: A mutation in the human canalicular multispecific organic anion transporter gene causes the Dubin-Johnson syndrome. Hepatology 1997; 25:1539.

248. Toh S, Wada M, Uchiumi T, et al: Genomic structure of the canalicular multispecific organic anion-transporter gene (MRP2/cMOAT) and mutations in the ATP-binding-cassette region in Dubin-Johnson syndrome. Am J Hum Genet 1999; 64:739.

249. Wada M, Toh S, Taniguchi K, et al: Mutations in the canalicular multispecific organic anion transporter (cMOAT) gene, a novel ABC transporter, in patients with hyperbilirubinemia II/Dubin-Johnson syndrome. Hum Mol Genet 1998; 7:203.

250. Jansen PL, Peters WH, Meijer DK: Hepatobiliary excretion of organic anions in double-mutant rats with a combination of defective canalicular transport and uridine 5′-diphosphate-glucuronyltransferase deficiency. Gastroenterology 1987; 93:1094.

251. Nishida T, Gatmaitan Z, Roy-Chowdhry J, et al: Two distinct mechanisms for bilirubin glucuronide transport by rat bile canalicular membrane vesicles. Demonstration of defective ATP-dependent transport in rats (TR-) with inherited conjugated hyperbilirubinemia. J Clin Invest 1992; 90:2130.

252. Sathirakul K, Suzuki H, Yasuda K, et al: Kinetic analysis of hepatobiliary transport of organic anions in Eisai hyperbilirubinemic mutant rats. J Pharmacol Exp Ther 1993; 265:1301.

253. Adachi Y, Kobayashi H, Kurumi Y, et al: Bilirubin diglucuronide transport by rat liver canalicular membrane vesicles: Stimulation by bicarbonate ion. Hepatology 1991; 14:1251.

254. Ricci GL, Cornelis M, Fevery J, et al: Maximal hepatic bilirubin transport in the rat during somatostatin-induced cholestasis and taurocholate-choleresis. J Lab Clin Med 1983; 101:835.

255. Ricci GL, Michiels R, Fevery J, et al: Enhancement by secretin of the apparently maximal hepatic transport of bilirubin in the rat. Hepatology 1984; 4:651.

256. Sieg A, Stiehl A, Heirwegh KP, et al: Similarities in maximal biliary bilirubin output in the normal rat after administration of unconjugated bilirubin or bilirubin diglucuronide. Hepatology 1989; 10:14.

257. Carey MC, Koretsky AP: Self-association of unconjugated bilirubin-IXα in aqueous solution at pH 10.0 and physical-chemical interactions with bile salt monomers and micelles. Biochem J 1979; 179:675.

258. Odell GB: Neonatal Hyperbilirubinemia. New York, Grune & Stratton, 1980.

259. Lester R, Schmid R: Intestinal absorption of bile pigments. II. Bilirubin absorption in man. N Engl J Med 1963; 269:178.

260. Dhar GJ: Enterohepatic circulation and plasma transport of uro-bilinogen. In Berk PD, Berlin NI (eds): Chemistry and Physiology of Bile Pigments. Bethesda, MD, US Department of Health, Education and Welfare, 1977, p 526.

261. Watson CJ: The urobilinoids: Milestones in their history and some recent developments. In Berk PD, Berlin NI (eds): Chemistry and Physiology of Bile Pigments. Bethesda, MD, US Department of Health, Education and Welfare, 1977, p 469.

262. Watson CJ: Composition of the urobilinin in urine, bile and feces and the significance of variations in health and disease. J Lab Clin Med 1959; 1:54.

263. Pearson H: Life-span of the fetal red blood cell. J Pediatr 1967; 70:166.

264. West MF: Erythrocyte survival in newborn infants as measured by chromium and its relation to postnatal serum bilirubin level. J Pediatr 1961; 54:194.

265. Poland RL, Odell GB: The binding of bilirubin to agar. Proc Soc Exp Biol Med 1974; 146:1114.

266. Ustrom RA, Eisenklam E: The enterohepatic shunting off bilirubin in the newborn infant. I. Use of oral activated charcoal to reduce normal serum bilirubin values 1964; J Pediatr 65:27.

267. Maurer HM, Shumway CN, Draper DA, et al: Controlled trial comparing agar, intermittent phototherapy, and continuous phototherapy for reducing neonatal hyperbilirubinemia. J Pediatr 1973; 82:73.

268. Weisman LE, Merenstein GB, Digirol M, et al: The effect of early meconium evacuation on early-onset hyperbilirubinemia. Am J Dis Child 1983; 137:666.

269. Maurer HM, Wolff JA, Finster M, et al: Reduction in concentration of total serum-bilirubin in offspring of women treated with pheno-barbitone during pregnancy. Lancet 1968; 2:122.

270. Vaisman SL, Gartner LM: Pharmacologic treatment of neonatal hyperbilirubinemia. Clin Perinatol 1975; 2:37.

271. Levi AJ, Gatmaitan Z, Arias IM: Deficiency of hepatic organic anion-binding protein as a possible cause of non-haemolytic unconjugated hyperbilirubinaemia in the newborn. Lancet 1969; 2:139.

272. Ruoslahti E, Estes T, Seppala M: Binding of bilirubin by bovine and human α-fetoprotein. Biochim Biophys Acta 1979; 578:511.

273. Hsia JC, Er SS, Tan CT, et al: α-Fetoprotein binding specificity for arachidonate, bilirubin, docosahexaenoate, and palmitate. A spin label study. J Biol Chem 1980; 255:4224.

274. Ostrea EM, Jr., Ongtengco EA, Tolia VA, et al: The occurrence and significance of the bilirubin species, including delta bilirubin, in jaundiced infants. J Pediatr Gastroenterol Nutr 1988; 7:511.

275. Ackerman BD, Dyer GY, Leydorf MM: Hyperbilirubinemia and kernicterus in small premature infants. Pediatrics 1970; 45:918.

276. Clark CF, Torii S, Hamamoto Y, et al: The "bronze baby" syndrome: Postmortem data. J Pediatr 1976; 88:461.

277. Kopelman AE, Brown RS, Odell GB: The "bronze" baby syndrome: A complication of phototherapy. J Pediatr 1972; 81:466.

278. Onishi S, Itoh S, Isobe K, et al: Mechanism of development of bronze baby syndrome in neonates treated with phototherapy. Pediatrics 1982; 69:273.

279. Rubaltelli FF, Jori G, Reddi E: Bronze baby syndrome: A new porphyrin-related disorder. Pediatr Res 1983; 17:327.

280. Tan KL, Jacob E: The bronze baby syndrome. Acta Paediatr Scand 1982; 71:409.

281. Grannum PA, Copel JA: Prevention of Rh isoimmunization and treatment of the compromised fetus. Semin Perinatol 1988; 12:324.

282. Gottvall T, Hilden JO, Selbing A: Evaluation of standard parameters to predict exchange transfusions in the erythroblastotic newborn. Acta Obstet Gynecol Scand 1994; 73:300.

283. Barss VA, Doubilet PM, St John-Sutton M, et al: Cardiac output in a fetus with erythroblastosis fetalis: Assessment using pulsed Doppler. Obstet Gynecol 1987; 70:442.

284. Maisels MJ: Bilirubin; on understanding and influencing its metabolism in the newborn infant. Pediatr Clin North Am 1972; 19:447.

285. Kirk JJ, Ritter DA, Kenny JD: The effect of hematin on bilirubin binding in bilirubin-enriched neonatal cord serum. Biol Neonate 1984; 45:53.

286. Levine DH, Meyer HB: Newborn screening for ABO hemolytic disease. Clin Pediatr (Phila) 1985; 24:391.

287. Sivan Y, Merlob P, Nutman J, et al: Direct hyperbilirubinemia complicating ABO hemolytic disease of the newborn. Clin Pediatr (Phila) 1983; 22:537.

288. Oski FA: The erythrocyte and its disorders. In Nathan DG, Oski FA (eds): Hematology of Infancy and Childhood. Philadelphia, WB Saunders, 1992, p 26.

289. Drew JH, Smith MB, Kitchen WH: Glucose-6-phosphate dehydrogenase deficiency in immigrant Greek infants. J Pediatr 1977; 90:659.

290. Kaplan M, Hammerman C: Severe neonatal hyperbilirubinemia. A potential complication of glucose-6-phosphate dehydrogenase deficiency. Clin Perinatol 1998; 25:575.

291. Kopelman AE, Ey JL, Lee H: Phototherapy in newborn infants with glucose-6-phosphate dehydrogenase deficiency. J Pediatr 1978; 93:497.

292. Meloni T, Cutillo S, Testa U, et al: Neonatal jaundice and severity of glucose-6-phosphate dehydrogenase deficiency in Sardinian babies. Early Hum Dev 1987; 15:317.

293. Valaes T, Karaklis A, Stravrakakis D, et al: Incidence and mechanism of neonatal jaundice related to glucose-6-phosphate dehydrogenase deficiency. Pediatr Res 1969; 3:448.

294. Valaes T, Drummond GS, Kappas A: Control of hyperbilirubinemia in glucose-6-phosphate dehydrogenase-deficient newborns using an inhibitor of bilirubin production, Sn-mesoporphyrin. Pediatrics 1998; 101:E1.

295. Eriksen L, Hofstad F, Seip M: Congenital erythropoietic porphyria. The effect of light shielding. Acta Paediatr Scand 1973; 62:385.

296. Berk PD, Bloomer JR, Howe RB, et al: Constitutional hepatic dysfunction (Gilbert's syndrome). A new definition based on kinetic studies with unconjugated radiobilirubin. Am J Med 1970; 49:296.

297. Fevery J: Pathogenesis of Gilbert's syndrome. Eur J Clin Invest 1981; 11:417.

298. Bosma P, Chowdhury JR, Jansen PH: Genetic inheritance of Gilbert's syndrome. Lancet 1995; 346:314.

299. Owens D, Evans J: Population studies on Gilbert's syndrome. J Med Genet 1975; 12:152.

300. Kavazarakis E, Tsezou A, Tzetis M, et al: Gilbert syndrome: Analysis of the promoter region of the uridine diphosphate-glucuronosyltransferase 1 gene in the Greek population. Eur J Pediatr 2000; 159:873.

301. Te Morsche RH, Zusterzeel PL, Raijmakers MT, et al: Polymorphism in the promoter region of the bilirubin UDP-glucuronosyltransferase (Gilbert's syndrome) in healthy Dutch subjects. Hepatology 2001; 33:765.

302. Biondi ML, Turri O, Dilillo D, et al: Contribution of the TATA-box genotype (Gilbert syndrome) to serum bilirubin concentrations in the Italian population. Clin Chem 1999; 45:897.

303. Borlak J, Thum T, Landt O, et al: Molecular diagnosis of a familial nonhemolytic hyperbilirubinemia (Gilbert's syndrome) in healthy subjects. Hepatology 2000; 32:792.

304. Burchell B, Hume R: Molecular genetic basis of Gilbert's syndrome. J Gastroenterol Hepatol 1999; 14:960.

305. Raijmakers MT, Jansen PL, Steegers EA, et al: Association of human liver bilirubin UDP-glucuronyltransferase activity with a polymorphism in the promoter region of the UGT1A1 gene. J Hepatol 2000; 33:348.

306. Pirulli D, Giordano M, Puzzer D, et al: Rapid method for detection of extra (TA) in the promoter of the bilirubin-UDP-glucuronosyl transferase 1 gene associated with Gilbert syndrome. Clin Chem 2000; 46:129.

307. Monaghan G, Ryan M, Seddon R, et al: Genetic variation in bilirubin UPD-glucuronosyltransferase gene promoter and Gilbert's syndrome. Lancet 1996; 347:578.

308. Aono S, Adachi Y, Uyama E, et al: Analysis of genes for bilirubin UDP-glucuronosyltransferase in Gilbert's syndrome. Lancet 1995; 345:958.

309. Maruo Y, Sato H, Yamano T, et al: Gilbert syndrome caused by a homozygous missense mutation (Tyr486Asp) of bilirubin UDP-glucuronosyltransferase gene. J Pediatr 1998; 132:1045.

310. Soeda Y, Yamamoto K, Adachi Y, et al: Predicted homozygous missense mutation in Gilbert's syndrome. Lancet 1995; 346.

311. Tsezou A, Tzetis M, Kitsiou S, et al: A Caucasian boy with Gilbert's syndrome heterozygous for the (TA)(8) allele. Haematologica 2000; 85:319.

312. Iolascon A, Faienza MF, Centra M, et al: (TA)8 allele in the UGT1A1 gene promoter of a Caucasian with Gilbert's syndrome. Haematologica 1999; 84:106.

313. Akaba K, Kimura T, Sasaki A, et al: Neonatal hyperbilirubinemia and a common mutation of the bilirubin uridine diphosphate-glucuronosyltransferase gene in Japanese. J Hum Genet 1999; 44:22.

314. Ando Y, Chida M, Nakayama K, et al: The UGT1A1*28 allele is relatively rare in a Japanese population. Pharmacogenetics 1998; 8:357.

315. Koiwai O, Nishizawa M, Hasada K, et al: Gilbert's syndrome is caused by a heterozygous missense mutation in the gene for bilirubin UDP-glucuronosyltransferase. Hum Mol Genet 1995; 4:1183.

316. Black M, Billing BH: Hepatic bilirubin UDP-glucuronyl transferase activity in liver disease and Gilbert's syndrome. N Engl J Med 1969; 280:1266.

317. Felsher BF, Craig JR, Carpio N: Hepatic bilirubin glucuronidation in Gilbert's syndrome. J Lab Clin Med 1973; 81:829.

318. Sampietro M, Iolascon A: Molecular pathology of Crigler-Najjar type I and II and Gilbert's syndromes. Haematologica 1999; 84:150.

319. Ullrich D, Sieg A, Blume R, et al: Normal pathways for glucuronidation, sulphation and oxidation of paracetamol in Gilbert's syndrome. Eur J Clin Invest 1987; 17:237.

320. Auclair C, Hakim J, Boivin P, et al: Bilirubin and paranitrophenol glucuronyl transferase activities of the liver in patients with Gilbert's syndrome. An attempt at a biochemical breakdown of the Gilbert's syndrome. Enzyme 1976; 21:97.

321. Debinski HS, Lee CS, Dhillon AP, et al: UDP-glucuronosyltransferase in Gilbert's syndrome. Pathology 1996; 28:238.

322. Black M, Fevery J, Parker D, et al: Effect of phenobarbitone on plasma (14C)bilirubin clearance in patients with unconjugated hyperbilirubinaemia. Clin Sci Mol Med 1974; 46:1.

323. Metreau JM, Yvart J, Dhumeaux D, et al: Role of bilirubin overproduction in revealing Gilbert's syndrome: Is dyserythropoiesis an important factor? Gut 1978; 19:838.

324. Berk PD, Blaschke TF: Detection of Gilbert's syndrome in patients with hemolysis. A method using radioactive chromium. Ann Intern Med 1972; 77:527.

325. Powell LW, Billing BH, Williams HS: An assessment of red cell survival in idiopathic unconjugated hyperbilirubinaemia (Gilbert's syndrome) by the use of radioactive diisopropylfluorophosphate and chromium. Australas Ann Med 1967; 16:221.

326. Te HS, Schiano TD, Das S, et al: Donor liver uridine diphosphate (UDP)-glucuronosyltransferase-1A1 deficiency causing Gilbert's syndrome in liver transplant recipients. Transplantation 2000; 69:1882.

327. Iolascon A, Faienza MF, Perrotta S, et al: Gilbert's syndrome and jaundice in glucose-6-phosphate dehydrogenase deficient neonates. Haematologica 1999; 84:99.

328. Kaplan M: Gilbert's syndrome and jaundice in glucose-6-phosphate dehydrogenase deficient neonates. Haematologica 2000; 85.

329. Kaplan M, Hammerman C, Renbaum P, et al: Gilbert's syndrome and hyperbilirubinaemia in ABO-incompatible neonates. Lancet 2000; 356:652.

330. Perrotta S, del Giudice EM, Carbone R, et al: Gilbert's syndrome accounts for the phenotypic variability of congenital dyserythropoietic anemia type II (CDA-II). J Pediatr 2000; 136:556.

331. Sharma S, Vukelja SJ, Kadakia S: Gilbert's syndrome co-existing with and masking hereditary spherocytosis. Ann Hematol 1997; 74:287.

332. Berk PD, Blaschke TF, Waggoner JG: Defective bromosulphthalein clearance in patients with constitutional hepatic dysfunction (Gilbert's syndrome). Gastroenterology 1972; 63:472.

333. Okolicsanyi L, Ghidini O, Orlando R, et al: An evaluation of bilirubin kinetics with respect to the diagnosis of Gilbert's syndrome. Clin Sci Mol Med 1978; 54:539.

334. Martin JF, Vierling JM, Wolkoff AW, et al: Abnormal hepatic transport of indocyanine green in Gilbert's syndrome. Gastroenterology 1976; 70:385.

335. Persico M, Persico E, Bakker CT, et al: Hepatic uptake of organic anions affects the plasma bilirubin level in subjects with Gilbert's syndrome mutations in UGT1A1. Hepatology 2001; 33:627.

336. Roda A, Roda E, Sama C, et al: Serum primary bile acids in Gilbert's syndrome. Gastroenterology 1982; 82:77.

337. Vierling JM, Berk PD, Hofmann AF, et al: Normal fasting-state levels of serum cholyl-conjugated bile acids in Gilbert's syndrome: An aid to the diagnosis. Hepatology 1982; 2:340.

338. Ohkubo H, Okuda K, Iida S, et al: Ursodeoxycholic acid oral tolerance test in patients with constitutional hyperbilirubinemias and effect of phenobarbital. Gastroenterology 1981; 81:126.

339. Nambu M, Namihisa T: Hepatic transport and metabolism of various organic anions in patients with congenital non-hemolytic hyperbilirubinemia, including constitutional indocyanine green excretory defect. J Gastroenterol 1994; 29:228.

340. Ohkubo H, Okuda K, Iida S: A constitutional unconjugated hyperbilirubinemia combined with indocyanine green intolerance: A new functional disorder? Hepatology 1981; 1:319.

341. Sieg A, Stiehl A, Raedsch R, et al: Gilbert's syndrome: Diagnosis by typical serum bilirubin pattern. Clin Chim Acta 1986; 154:41.

342. Olsson R, Lindstedt G: Evaluation of tests for Gilbert's syndrome. Acta Med Scand 1980; 207:425.

343. Thomsen HF, Hardt F, Juhl E: Diagnosis of Gilbert's syndrome. Reliability of the caloric restriction and phenobarbital stimulation tests. Scand J Gastroenterol 1981; 16:699.

344. Owens D, Sherlock S: Diagnosis of Gilbert's syndrome: Role of reduced caloric intake test. Br Med J 1973; 3:559.

345. Rollinghoff W, Paumgartner G, Preisig R: Nicotinic acid test in the diagnosis of Gilbert's syndrome: Correlation with bilirubin clearance. Gut 1981; 22:663.

346. Gentile S, Tiribelli C, Persico M, et al: Dose dependence of nicotinic acid-induced hyperbilirubinemia and its dissociation from hemolysis in Gilbert's syndrome. J Lab Clin Med 1986; 107:166.

347. Iyer L, King CD, Whitington PF, et al: Genetic predisposition to the metabolism of irinotecan (CPT-11). Role of uridine diphosphate glucuronosyltransferase isoform 1A1 in the glucuronidation of its active metabolite (SN-38) in human liver microsomes. J Clin Invest 1998; 101:847.

348. Owens IS, Ritter JK, Yeatman MT, et al: The novel UGT1 gene complex links bilirubin, xenobiotics, and therapeutic drug metabolism by encoding UDP-glucuronosyltransferase isozymes with a common carboxyl terminus. J Pharmacokinet Biopharm 1996; 24:491.

349. Wasserman E, Myara A, Lokiec F, et al: Severe CPT-11 toxicity in patients with Gilbert's syndrome: Two case reports. Ann Oncol 1997; 8:1049.

350. Bourdeaut F, Matei L, Labrune P, et al: Gilbert syndrome revealed during chemotherapy. Med Pediatr Oncol 2001; 36:400.

351. Burchell B, Soars M, Monaghan G, et al: Drug-mediated toxicity caused by genetic deficiency of UDP-glucuronosyltransferases. Toxicol Lett 2000; 113:333.

352. Bancroft JD, Kreamer B, Gourley GR: Gilbert syndrome accelerates development of neonatal jaundice. J Pediatr 1998; 132:656.

353. Monaghan G, McLellan A, McGeehan A, et al: Gilbert's syndrome is a contributory factor in prolonged unconjugated hyperbilirubinemia of the newborn. J Pediatr 1999; 134:441.

354. Maruo Y, Nishizawa K, Sato H, et al: Association of neonatal hyperbilirubinemia with bilirubin UDP-glucuronosyltransferase polymorphism. Pediatrics 1999; 103:1224.

355. Lake AM, Truman JT, Bode HH, et al: Marked hyperbilirubinemia with Gilbert syndrome and immunohemolytic anemia. J Pediatr 1978; 93:812.

356. Garrow E, Hertzler J: Hypertrophic pyloric stenosis with jaundice. A case report of one family. J Pediatr Surg 1966; 1:284.

357. Labrune P, Myara A, Huguet P, et al: Jaundice with hypertrophic pyloric stenosis: A possible early manifestation of Gilbert syndrome. J Pediatr 1989; 115:93.

358. Levine G, Favara BE, Mierau G, et al: Jaundice, liver ultrastructure, and congenital pyloric stenosis. A study in infants. Arch Pathol 1973; 95:267.

359. Roth B, Statz A, Heinisch HM, et al: Elimination of indocyanine green by the liver of infants with hypertrophic pyloric stenosis and the icteropyloric syndrome. J Pediatr 1981; 99:240.

360. Roth B, Statz A, Heinisch HM: Jaundice with hypertrophic pyloric stenosis: A possible manifestation of Gilbert syndrome. J Pediatr 1990; 116:1003.

361. Scharli A, Sieber WK, Kiesewetter WB: Hypertrophic pyloric stenosis at the Children's Hospital of Pittsburgh from 1912 to 1967. A critical review of current problems and complications. J Pediatr Surg 1969; 4:108.

362. Trioche P, Chalas J, Francoual J, et al: Jaundice with hypertrophic pyloric stenosis as an early manifestation of Gilbert syndrome. Arch Dis Child 1999; 81:301.

363. Woolley MM, Felsher BF, Asch J, et al: Jaundice, hypertrophic pyloric stenosis, and hepatic glucuronyl transferase. J Pediatr Surg 1974; 9:359.

364. Jansen PL: Diagnosis and management of Crigler-Najjar syndrome. Eur J Pediatr 1999; 158 (Suppl 2):89.

365. Kadakol A, Ghosh SS, Sappal BS, et al: Genetic lesions of bilirubin uridine-diphosphoglucuronate glucuronosyltransferase (UGT1A1) causing Crigler-Najjar and Gilbert syndromes: Correlation of genotype to phenotype. Hum Mutat 2000; 16:297.

366. Schmid R, Hammaker L: Metabolism and disposition of C^{14}-bilirubin in congenital nonhemolytic jaundice. J Clin Invest 1963; 42:1720.

367. Kotal P, Van der Veere CN, Sinaasappel M, et al: Intestinal excretion of unconjugated bilirubin in man and rats with inherited unconjugated hyperbilirubinemia. Pediatr Res 1997; 42:195.

368. Labrune P, Myara A, Hadchouel M, et al: Genetic heterogeneity of Crigler-Najjar syndrome type I: A study of 14 cases. Hum Genet 1994; 94:693.

369. Ciotti M, Obaray R, Martin MG, et al: Genetic defects at the UGT1 locus associated with Crigler-Najjar type I disease, including a prenatal diagnosis. Am J Med Genet 1997; 68:173.

370. Ritter JK, Yeatman MT, Kaiser C, et al: A phenylalanine codon deletion at the UGT1 gene complex locus of a Crigler-Najjar type I patient generates a pH-sensitive bilirubin UDP-glucuronosyltransferase. J Biol Chem 1993; 268:23573.

371. Chalasani N, Chowdhury NR, Chowdhury JR, et al: Kernicterus in an adult who is heterozygous for Crigler-Najjar syndrome and homozygous for Gilbert-type genetic defect. Gastroenterology 1997; 112:2099.

372. Odell GB, Cukier JO, Gourley GR: The presence of a microsomal UDP-glucuronyl transferase for bilirubin in homozygous jaundiced Gunn rats and in the Crigler-Najjar syndrome. Hepatology 1981; 1:307.

373. Whitington PF, Black DD, Struve W, et al: Evidence against an abnormal hepatic microsomal lipid matrix as the primary genetic defect in the jaundiced Gunn rat. Biochim Biophys Acta 1985; 812:774.

374. Iyanagi T, Watanabe T, Uchiyama Y: The 3-methylcholanthrene-inducible UDP-glucuronosyltransferase deficiency in the hyperbilirubinemic rat (Gunn rat) is caused by a −1 frameshift mutation. J Biol Chem 1989; 264:21302.

375. Sinaasappel M, Jansen PL: The differential diagnosis of Crigler-Najjar disease, types 1 and 2, by bile pigment analysis. Gastroenterology 1991; 100:783.

376. van der Veere CN, Sinaasappel M, McDonagh AF, et al: Current therapy for Crigler-Najjar syndrome type 1: Report of a world registry. Hepatology 1996; 24:311.

377. Ihara H, Hashizume N, Shimizu N, et al: Threshold concentration of unbound bilirubin to induce neurological deficits in a patient with type I Crigler-Najjar syndrome. Ann Clin Biochem 1999; 36:347.

378. Labrune PH, Myara A, Francoual J, et al: Cerebellar symptoms as the presenting manifestations of bilirubin encephalopathy in children with Crigler-Najjar type I disease. Pediatrics 1992; 89:768.

379. Arrowsmith WA, Payne RB, Littlewood JM: Comparison of treatments for congenital nonobstructive nonhaemolytic hyperbilirubinaemia. Arch Dis Child 1975; 50:197.

380. Gorodischer R, Levy G, Krasner J, et al: Congenital nonobstructive, nonhemolytic jaundice. Effect of phototherapy. N Engl J Med 1970; 282:375.

381. Odell GB, Gutcher GR, Whitington PF, et al: Enteral administration of agar as an effective adjunct to phototherapy of neonatal hyperbilirubinemia. Pediatr Res 1983; 17:810.

382. Kappas A, Drummond GS, Henschke C, et al: Direct comparison of Sn-mesoporphyrin, an inhibitor of bilirubin production, and phototherapy in controlling hyperbilirubinemia in term and near-term newborns. Pediatrics 1995; 95:468.

383. Galbraith RA, Drummond GS, Kappas A: Suppression of bilirubin production in the Crigler-Najjar type I syndrome: Studies with the heme oxygenase inhibitor tin-mesoporphyrin. Pediatrics 1992; 89:175.

384. Drummond GS, Valaes T, Kappas A: Control of bilirubin production by synthetic heme analogs: Pharmacologic and toxicologic considerations. J Perinatol 1996; 16:S72.

385. Whitington PF, Emond JC, Heffron T, et al: Orthotopic auxiliary liver transplantation for Crigler-Najjar syndrome type 1. Lancet 1993; 342:779.

386. Rela M, Muiesan P, Vilca-Melendez H, et al: Auxiliary partial orthotopic liver transplantation for Crigler-Najjar syndrome type I. Ann Surg 1999; 229:565.

387. Kaufman SS, Wood RP, Shaw BW, Jr., et al: Orthotopic liver transplantation for type I Crigler-Najjar syndrome. Hepatology 1986; 6:1259.

388. Fox IJ, Chowdhury JR, Kaufman SS, et al: Treatment of the Crigler-Najjar syndrome type I with hepatocyte transplantation. N Engl J Med 1998; 338:1422.

389. Kren BT, Parashar B, Bandyopadhyay P, et al: Correction of the UDP-glucuronosyltransferase gene defect in the Gunn rat model of Crigler-Najjar syndrome type I with a chimeric oligonucleotide. Proc Natl Acad Sci USA 1999; 96:10349.

390. Sauter BV, Parashar B, Chowdhury NR, et al: A replication-deficient rSV40 mediates liver-directed gene transfer and a long-term amelioration of jaundice in Gunn rats. Gastroenterology 2000; 119:1348.

391. Green RM, Gollan JL: Crigler-Najjar disease type I: Therapeutic approaches to genetic liver diseases into the next century. Gastroenterology 1997; 112:649.

392. Arias IM, Gartner LM, Cohen M, et al: Chronic nonhemolytic unconjugated hyperbilirubinemia with glucuronyl transferase deficiency. Clinical, biochemical, pharmacologic and genetic evidence for heterogeneity. Am J Med 1969; 47:395.

393. Gollan JL, Huang SN, Billing B, et al: Prolonged survival in three brothers with severe type 2 Crigler-Najjar syndrome. Ultrastructural and metabolic studies. Gastroenterology 1975; 68:1543.

394. Crigler JF, Gold NI: Effect of sodium phenobarbital on bilirubin metabolism in an infant with congenital, nonhemolytic, unconjugated hyperbilirubinemia, and kernicterus. J Clin Invest 1969; 48:42.

395. Ciotti M, Werlin SL, Owens IS: Delayed response to phenobarbital treatment of a Crigler-Najjar type II patient with partially inactivating missense mutations in the bilirubin UDP-glucuronosyltransferase gene. J Pediatr Gastroenterol Nutr 1999; 28:210.

396. Gordon ER, Shaffer EA, Sass-Kortasak A: Bilirubin secretion and conjugation in the Crigler-Najjar syndrome type II. Gastroenterology 1976; 70:761.

397. Hunter JO, Thompson RP, Dunn PM, et al: Inheritance of type 2 Crigler-Najjar hyperbilirubinaemia. Gut 1973; 14:46.

398. Duhamel G, Blanckaert N, Metreau JM, et al: An unusual case of Crigler-Najjar disease in the adult. Classification into types I and II revisited. J Hepatol 1985; 1:47.

399. Lascari AD: "Early" breast-feeding jaundice: Clinical significance. J Pediatr 1986; 108:156.

400. Dahms BB, Krauss AN, Gartner LM, et al: Breast feeding and serum bilirubin values during the first 4 days of life. J Pediatr 1973; 83:1049.

401. Gartner U, Goeser T, Wolkoff AW: Effect of fasting on the uptake of bilirubin and sulfobromophthalein by the isolated perfused rat liver. Gastroenterology 1997; 113:1707.

402. Whitmer DI, Gollan JL: Mechanisms and significance of fasting and dietary hyperbilirubinemia. Semin Liver Dis 1983; 3:42.

403. Kotal P, Vitek L, Fevery J: Fasting-related hyperbilirubinemia in rats: The effect of decreased intestinal motility. Gastroenterology 1996; 111:217.

404. De Carvalho M, Robertson S, Klaus M: Fecal bilirubin excretion and serum bilirubin concentrations in breast-fed and bottle-fed infants. J Pediatr 1985; 107:786.

405. Auerbach KG, Gartner LM: Breastfeeding and human milk: Their association with jaundice in the neonate. Clin Perinatol 1987; 14:89.

406. Alonso EM, Whitington PF, Whitington SH, et al: Enterohepatic circulation of nonconjugated bilirubin in rats fed with human milk. J Pediatr 1991; 118:425.

407. Winfield CR, MacFaul R: Clinical study of prolonged jaundice in breast- and bottle-fed babies. Arch Dis Child 1978; 53:506.

408. Gartner LM, Arias IM: Studies of prolonged neonatal jaundice in the breast-fed infant. J Pediatr 1966; 68:54.

409. Gourley GR, Arend RA: β-Glucuronidase and hyperbilirubinaemia in breast-fed and formula-fed babies. Lancet 1986; 1:644.

410. Gourley GR, Kreamer BL, Cohnen M: Inhibition of β-glucuronidase by casein hydrolysate formula. J Pediatr Gastroenterol Nutr 1997; 25:267.

411. Gartner LM, Herschel M: Jaundice and breastfeeding. Pediatr Clin North Am 2001; 48:389.

412. Maruo Y, Nishizawa K, Sato H, et al: Prolonged unconjugated hyperbilirubinemia associated with breast milk and mutations of the bilirubin uridine diphosphate-glucuronosyltransferase gene. Pediatrics 2000; 106:E59.

413. Martinez JC, Maisels MJ, Otheguy L, et al: Hyperbilirubinemia in the breast-fed newborn: A controlled trial of four interventions. Pediatrics 1993; 91:470.

414. Amato M, Howald H, von Muralt G: Interruption of breast-feeding versus phototherapy as treatment of hyperbilirubinemia in full-term infants. Helv Paediatr Acta 1985; 40:127.

415. Maisels MJ, Newman TB: Kernicterus in otherwise healthy, breast-fed term newborns. Pediatrics 1995; 96:730.

416. Lu TC, Wei H, Blackwell RQ: Increased incidence of severe hyperbilirubinemia among newborn Chinese infants with G-6-P D deficiency. Pediatrics 1966; 37:994.

417. Horiguchi T, Bauer C: Ethnic differences in neonatal jaundice: Comparison of Japanese and Caucasian newborn infants. Am J Obstet Gynecol 1975; 121:71.

418. Johnson JD, Angelus P, Aldrich M, et al: Exaggerated jaundice in Navajo neonates. The role of bilirubin production. Am J Dis Child 1986; 140:889.

419. Drew JH, Kitchen WH: Jaundice in infants of Greek parentage: The unknown factor may be environmental. J Pediatr 1976; 89:248.

420. Drew JH, Barrie J, Horacek I, et al: Factors influencing jaundice in immigrant Greek infants. Arch Dis Child 1978; 53:49.

421. Odell GB: Bilirubin encephalopathy. In McCandless DW (ed): Cerebral Energy Metabolism and Metabolic Encephalopathy. New York, Plenum Press, 1985, p 229.

422. Rose AL, Wisniewski H: Acute bilirubin encephalopathy induced with sulfadimethoxine in Gunn rats. J Neuropathol Exp Neurol 1979; 38:152.

423. Sherwood AJ, Smith JF: Bilirubin encephalopathy. Neuropathol Appl Neurobiol 1983; 9:271.

424. Hansen TW: Bilirubin in the brain. Distribution and effects on neurophysiological and neurochemical processes. Clin Pediatr 1994; 33:452.

425. Rubin RA, Balow B, Fisch RO: Neonatal serum bilirubin levels related to cognitive development at ages 4 through 7 years. J Pediatr 1979; 94:601.

426. Scheidt PC, Graubard BI, Nelson KB, et al: Intelligence at six years in relation to neonatal bilirubin levels: Follow-up of the National Institute of Child Health and Human Development Clinical Trial of Phototherapy. Pediatrics 1991; 87:797.

427. Odell GB, Storey GN, Rosenberg LA: Studies in kernicterus. 3. The saturation of serum proteins with bilirubin during neonatal life and its relationship to brain damage at five years. J Pediatr 1970; 76:12.

428. Brodersen R, Stern L: Deposition of bilirubin acid in the central nervous system—A hypothesis for the development of kernicterus. Acta Paediatr Scand 1990; 79:12.

429. Cashore WJ: Kernicterus and bilirubin encephalopathy. Semin Liver Dis 1988; 8:163.

430. Wennberg RP: The blood-brain barrier and bilirubin encephalopathy. Cell Mol Neurobiol 2000; 20:97.

431. Wennberg RP, Hance AJ: Experimental bilirubin encephalopathy: Importance of total bilirubin, protein binding, and blood-brain barrier. Pediatr Res 1986; 20:789.

432. Brann BS, Stonestreet BS, Oh W, et al: The in vivo effect of bilirubin and sulfisoxazole on cerebral oxygen, glucose, and lactate metabolism in newborn piglets. Pediatr Res 1987; 22:135.

433. Shapiro SM: Acute brainstem auditory evoked potential abnormalities in jaundiced Gunn rats given sulfonamide. Pediatr Res 1988; 23:306.

434. Silver S, Sohmer H, Kapitulnik J: Postnatal development of somatosensory evoked potential in jaundiced Gunn rats and effects of sulfadimethoxine administration. Pediatr Res 1996; 40:209.

435. Walker PC: Neonatal bilirubin toxicity. A review of kernicterus and the implications of drug-induced bilirubin displacement. Clin Pharmacokinet 1987; 13:26.

436. Martin E, Fanconi S, Kalin P, et al: Ceftriaxone-bilirubin-albumin interactions in the neonate: An in vivo study. Eur J Pediatr 1993; 152:530.

437. Nerli B, Pico G: Identification of the cephalosporin human serum albumin binding sites. Pharmacol Toxicol 1993; 73:297.

438. Jacobsen J, Theissen H, Brodersen R: Effect of fatty acids on the binding of bilirubin to albumin. Biochem J 1972; 126:7.

439. Starinsky R, Shafrir E: Displacement of albumin-bound bilirubin by free fatty acids. Implications for neonatal hyperbilirubinemia. Clin Chim Acta 1970; 29:311.

440. Soltys BJ, Hsia C: Human serum albumin. I. On the relationship of fatty acid and bilirubin binding sites and the nature of fatty acid allosteric effects—A monoanionic spin label study. J Biol Chem 1978; 253:3023.

441. Ostrea EM, Bassel M, Fleury CA, et al: Influence of free fatty acids and glucose infusion on serum bilirubin and bilirubin binding to albumin: Clinical implications. J Pediatr 1983; 102:426.

442. Perlman M, Frank JW: Bilirubin beyond the blood-brain barrier. Pediatrics 1988; 81:304.

443. Cashore WJ, Oh W: Unbound bilirubin and kernicterus in low-birth-weight infants. Pediatrics 1982; 69:481.

444. Gartner LM, Snyder RN, Chabon RS, et al: Kernicterus: High incidence in premature infants with low serum bilirubin concentrations. Pediatrics 1970; 45:906.

445. Pearlman MA, Gartner LM, Lee K, et al: The association of kernicterus with bacterial infection in the newborn. Pediatrics 1980; 65:26.

446. Burgess GH, Oh W, Bratlid D, et al: The effects of brain blood flow on brain bilirubin deposition in newborn piglets. Pediatr Res 1985; 19:691.

447. Bratlid D, Cashore WJ, Oh W: Effect of serum hyperosmolality on opening of blood-brain barrier for bilirubin in rat brain. Pediatrics 1983; 71:909.

448. Burgess GH, Stonestreet BS, Cashore WJ, et al: Brain bilirubin deposition and brain blood flow during acute urea-induced hyperosmolality in newborn piglets. Pediatr Res 1985; 19:537.

449. Hansen TW, Sagvolden T, Bratlid D: Open-field behavior of rats previously subjected to short-term hyperbilirubinemia with or without blood-brain barrier manipulations. Brain Res 1987; 424:26.

450. Ives NK, Bolas NM, Gardiner RM: The effects of bilirubin on brain energy metabolism during hyperosmolar opening of the blood-brain barrier: An in vivo study using ^{31}P nuclear magnetic resonance spectroscopy. Pediatr Res 1989; 26:356.

451. Ives NK, Gardiner RM: Blood-brain barrier permeability to bilirubin in the rat studied using intracarotid bolus injection and in situ brain perfusion techniques. Pediatr Res 1990; 27:436.

452. Levine RL, Fredericks WR, Rapoport SI: Clearance of bilirubin from rat brain after reversible osmotic opening of the blood-brain barrier. Pediatr Res 1985; 19:1040.

453. Allen JW, Tommarello S, Carcillo J, et al: Effects of endotoxemia and sepsis on bilirubin oxidation by rat brain mitochondrial membranes. Biol Neonate 1998; 73:340.

454. Meisel P, Jahrig D, Beyersdorff E, et al: Bilirubin binding and acid-base equilibrium in newborn infants with low birthweight. Acta Paediatr Scand 1988; 77:496.

455. Ebbesen F, Knudsen A: The possible risk of bilirubin encephalopathy as predicted by plasma parameters in neonates with previous severe asphyxia. Eur J Pediatr 1992; 151:910.

456. Amit Y, Chan G, Fedunec S, et al: Bilirubin toxicity in a neuroblastoma cell line N-115: I. Effects on Na$^+$K$^+$ ATPase, [^{3}H]-thymidine uptake, L-[^{35}S]-methionine incorporation, and mitochondrial function. Pediatr Res 1989; 25:364.

457. Amit Y, Poznansky MJ, Schiff D: Bilirubin toxicity in a neuroblastoma cell line N-115: II. Delayed effects and recovery. Pediatr Res 1989; 25:369.

458. Amit Y, Brenner T: Age-dependent sensitivity of cultured rat glial cells to bilirubin toxicity. Exp Neurol 1993; 121:248.

459. Cowger ML: Mechanism of bilirubin toxicity on tissue culture cells: Factors that affect toxicity, reversibility by albumin, and comparison with other respiratory poisons and surfactants. Biochem Med 1971; 5:1.

460. Noir BA, Boveris A, Garaza Pereira AM, et al: Bilirubin: A multi-site inhibitor of mitochondrial respiration. FEBS Lett 1972; 27:270.

461. Weil ML, Menkes JH: Bilirubin interaction with ganglioside: Possible mechanism in kernicterus. Pediatr Res 1975; 9:791.

462. Gurba PE, Zand R: Bilirubin binding to myelin basic protein, histones and its inhibition in vitro of cerebellar protein synthesis. Biochem Biophys Res Commun 1974; 58:1142.

463. Grojean S, Koziel V, Vert P, et al: Bilirubin induces apoptosis via activation of NMDA receptors in developing rat brain neurons. Exp Neurol 2000; 166:334.

464. McDonald JW, Shapiro SM, Silverstein FS, et al: Role of glutamate receptor-mediated excitotoxicity in bilirubin-induced brain injury in the Gunn rat model. Exp Neurol 1998; 150:21.

465. Ochoa EL, Wennberg RP, An Y, et al: Interactions of bilirubin with isolated presynaptic nerve terminals: Functional effects on the uptake and release of neurotransmitters. Cell Mol Neurobiol 1993; 13:69.

466. Grojean S, Lievre V, Koziel V, et al: Bilirubin exerts additional toxic effects in hypoxic cultured neurons from the developing rat brain by the recruitment of glutamate neurotoxicity. Pediatr Res 2001; 49:507.

467. Johnston MV, Hoon AH, Jr. Possible mechanisms in infants for selective basal ganglia damage from asphyxia, kernicterus, or mitochondrial encephalopathies. J Child Neurol 2000; 15:588.

468. Ahlfors CE, Bennett SH, Shoemaker CT, et al: Changes in the auditory brainstem response associated with intravenous infusion of unconjugated bilirubin into infant rhesus monkeys. Pediatr Res 1986; 20:511.

469. Jirka JH, Duckrow RB, Kendig JW, et al: Effect of bilirubin on brainstem auditory evoked potentials in the asphyxiated rat. Pediatr Res 1985; 19:556.

470. Shapiro SM, Hecox KE: Development of brainstem auditory evoked potentials in heterozygous and homozygous jaundiced Gunn rats. Brain Res 1988; 469:147.

471. Ewing JF, Maines MD: Immunohistochemical localization of biliverdin reductase in rat brain: Age related expression of protein and transcript. Brain Res 1995; 672:29.

472. Maines MD: The heme oxygenase system and its functions in the brain. Cell Mol Biol 2000; 46:573.

473. Sun Y, Rotenberg MO, Maines MD: Developmental expression of heme oxygenase isozymes in rat brain. Two HO-2 mRNAs are detected. J Biol Chem 1990; 265:8212.

474. Dennery PA, McDonagh AF, Spitz DR, et al: Hyperbilirubinemia results in reduced oxidative injury in neonatal Gunn rats exposed to hyperoxia. Free Radic Biol Med 1995; 19:395.

475. Panahian N, Yoshiura M, Maines MD: Overexpression of heme oxygenase-1 is neuroprotective in a model of permanent middle cerebral artery occlusion in transgenic mice. J Neurochem 1999; 72:1187.

476. Panahian N, Huang T, Maines MD: Enhanced neuronal expression of the oxidoreductase—biliverdin reductase—after permanent focal cerebral ischemia. Brain Res 1999; 850:1.

477. Chen K, Gunter K, Maines MD: Neurons overexpressing heme oxygenase-1 resist oxidative stress-mediated cell death. J Neurochem 2000; 75:304.

478. Maines MD: The heme oxygenase system: A regulator of second messenger gases. Annu Rev Pharmacol Toxicol 1997; 37:517.

479. Vincent SR, Das S, Maines MD: Brain heme oxygenase isoenzymes and nitric oxide synthase are co-localized in select neurons. Neuroscience 1994; 63:223.

480. Maines MD, Polevoda B, Coban T, et al: Neuronal overexpression of heme oxygenase-1 correlates with an attenuated exploratory behavior and causes an increase in neuronal NADPH diaphorase staining. J Neurochem 1998; 70:2057.

481. Hansen TW, Allen JW: Oxidation of bilirubin by brain mitochondrial membranes—Dependence on cell type and postnatal age. Biochem Mol Med 1997; 60:155.

482. Brown AK: Erythrocyte metabolism and hemolysis in the newborn. Pediatr Clin North Am 1966; 13:879.

483. Hyman CB, Keaster J, Hanson V, et al: CNS abnormalities after neonatal hemolytic disease or hyperbilirubinemia. A prospective study of 405 patients. Am J Dis Child 1969; 117:395.

484. Ackerman BD: What should kernicterus mean as a clinical diagnosis? Pediatrics 1970; 46:156.

485. Elhassani SB, Feingold M: Kernicterus. Am J Dis Child 1986; 140:247.

486. Gourley GR: Bilirubin metabolism and kernicterus. Adv Pediatr 1997 1997; 44:173.

487. Roth P, Polin RA: Controversial topics in kernicterus. Clin Perinatol 1988; 15:965.

488. Turkel SB, Miller CA, Guttenberg ME, et al: A clinical pathologic reappraisal of kernicterus. Pediatrics 1982; 69:267.

489. Hung KL: Auditory brainstem responses in patients with neonatal hyperbilirubinemia and bilirubin encephalopathy. Brain Dev 1989; 11:297.

490. Martich-Kriss V, Kollias SS, Ball WS, Jr. MR findings in kernicterus. AJNR Am J Neuroradiol 1995; 16:819.

491. Yokochi K: Magnetic resonance imaging in children with kernicterus. Acta Paediatr 1995; 84:937.

492. Boggs TR, Jr., Hardy JB, Frazier TM: Correlation of neonatal serum total bilirubin concentrations and developmental status at age eight months. A preliminary report from the collaborative project. J Pediatr 1967; 71:553.

493. Naeye RL: Amniotic fluid infections, neonatal hyperbilirubinemia, and psychomotor impairment. Pediatrics 1978; 62:497.

494. Bernstein J, Landing BJ: Extraneural lesions associated with neonatal hyperbilirubinemia and kernicterus. Am J Pathol 1961; 40:371.

495. Odell GB, Natzschka JC, Storey GN: Bilirubin nephropathy in the Gunn strain of rat. Am J Physiol 1967; 212:931.

496. Newman TB, Maisels MJ: Less aggressive treatment of neonatal jaundice and reports of kernicterus: Lessons about practice guidelines. Pediatrics 2000; 105:242.

497. Waser M, Kleihues P, Frick P: Kernicterus in an adult. Ann Neurol 1986; 19:595.

498. Ennever JF: Phototherapy in a new light. Pediatr Clin North Am 1986; 33:603.

499. Ennever JF: Phototherapy for neonatal jaundice. Photochem Photobiol 1988; 47:871.

500. Tan KL: Phototherapy for neonatal jaundice. Acta Paediatr 1996; 85:277.

501. Ebbesen F: Superiority of intensive phototherapy—blue double light—in rhesus haemolytic disease. Eur J Pediatr 1979; 130:279.

502. Agati G, Fusi F, Pratesi S, et al: Bilirubin photoisomerization products in serum and urine from a Crigler-Najjar type I patient treated by phototherapy. J Photochem Photobiol B 1998; 47:181.

503. Cohen AN, Ostrow JD: New concepts in phototherapy: Photoisomerization of bilirubin IX alpha and potential toxic effects of light. Pediatrics 1980; 65:740.

504. Costarino AT, Ennever JF, Baumgart S, et al: Bilirubin photoisomerization in premature neonates under low- and high-dose phototherapy. Pediatrics 1985; 75:519.

505. Ennever JF, Knox I, Denne SC, et al: Phototherapy for neonatal jaundice: In vivo clearance of bilirubin photoproducts. Pediatr Res 1985; 19:205.

506. Ennever JF, Knox I, Speck WT: Differences in bilirubin isomer composition in infants treated with green and white light phototherapy. J Pediatr 1986; 109:119.

507. Ennever JF, Costarino AT, Polin RA, et al: Rapid clearance of a structural isomer of bilirubin during phototherapy. J Clin Invest 1987; 79:1674.

508. Knox I, Ennever JF, Speck WT: Urinary excretion of an isomer of bilirubin during phototherapy. Pediatr Res 1985; 19:198.

509. Lamola AA, Blumberg WE, McClead R, et al: Photoisomerized bilirubin in blood from infants receiving phototherapy. Proc Natl Acad Sci USA 1981; 78:1882.

510. Lightner DA, Wooldridge TA, McDonagh AF: Configurational isomerization of bilirubin and the mechanism of jaundice phototherapy. Biochem Biophys Res Commun 1979; 86:235.

511. McDonagh AF, Ramonas LM: Jaundice phototherapy: Micro flow-cell photometry reveals rapid biliary response of Gunn rats to light. Science 1978; 201:829.

512. McDonagh AF: Phototherapy: A new twist to bilirubin. J Pediatr 1981; 99:909.

513. McDonagh AF, Lightner DA: 'Like a shrivelled blood orange'—Bilirubin, jaundice, and phototherapy. Pediatrics 1985; 75:443.

514. McDonagh AF, Lightner DA: Phototherapy and the photobiology of bilirubin. Semin Liver Dis 1988; 8:272.

515. Onishi S, Isobe K, Itoh S, et al: Demonstration of a geometric isomer of bilirubin-IX alpha in the serum of a hyperbilirubinaemic newborn infant and the mechanism of jaundice phototherapy. Biochem J 1980; 190:533.

516. Onishi S, Isobe K, Itoh S, et al: Metabolism of bilirubin and its photoisomers in newborn infants during phototherapy. J Biochem (Tokyo) 1986; 100:789.

517. Ostrow JD: Photocatabolism of labeled bilirubin in the congenitally jaundiced (Gunn) rat. J Clin Invest 1971; 50:707.

518. Lund HT, Jacobsen J: Influence of phototherapy on unconjugated bilirubin in duodenal bile of newborn infants with hyperbilirubinemia. Acta Paediatr Scand 1972; 61:693.

519. Lightner DA, Wooldridge TA, McDonagh AF: Photobilirubin: An early bilirubin photoproduct detected by absorbance difference spectroscopy. Proc Natl Acad Sci USA 1979; 76:29.

520. Isobe K, Onishi S: Kinetics of the photochemical interconversion among geometric photoisomers of bilirubin. Biochem J 1981; 193:1029.

521. Pellegrino JM, Roma MG, Mottino AD, et al: Hepatic handling of photoirradiated bilirubin. A study in isolated perfused Wistar rat liver. Biochim Biophys Acta 1991; 1074:25.

522. Onishi S, Miura I, Isobe K, et al: Structure and thermal interconversion of cyclobilirubin IX alpha. Biochem J 1984; 218:667.

523. Onishi S, Ogino T, Yokoyama T, et al: Biliary and urinary excretion rates and serum concentration changes of four bilirubin photoproducts in Gunn rats during total darkness and low or high illumination. Biochem J 1984; 221:717.

524. Lightner DA, Linnane WP, Ahlfors CE: Bilirubin photooxidation products in the urine of jaundiced neonates receiving phototherapy. Pediatr Res 1984; 18:696.

525. Vogl TP: Phototherapy of neonatal hyperbilirubinemia: Bilirubin in unexposed areas of the skin. J Pediatr 1974; 85:707.

526. Tan KL: Efficacy of bidirectional fiber-optic phototherapy for neonatal hyperbilirubinemia. Pediatrics 1997; 99:13.

527. Gutcher GR, Yen WM, Odell GB: The in vitro and in vivo photoreactivity of bilirubin: I. Laser-defined wavelength dependence. Pediatr Res 1983; 17:120.

528. Amato M, Inaebnit D: Clinical usefulness of high intensity green light phototherapy in the treatment of neonatal jaundice. Eur J Pediatr 1991; 150:274.

529. Ennever JF, Sobel M, McDonagh AF, et al: Phototherapy for neonatal jaundice: In vitro comparison of light sources. Pediatr Res 1984; 18:667.

530. Romagnoli C, Marrocco G, de Carolis MP, et al: Phototherapy for hyperbilirubinemia in preterm infants: Green versus blue or white light. J Pediatr 1988; 112:476.

531. Vecchi C, Donzelli GP, Migliorini MG, et al: Green light in phototherapy. Pediatr Res 1983; 17:461.

532. McDonagh AF, Agati G, Fusi F, et al: Quantum yields for laser photocyclization of bilirubin in the presence of human serum albumin. Dependence of quantum yield on excitation wavelength. Photochem Photobiol 1989; 50:305.

533. Ennever JF, McDonagh AF, Speck WT: Phototherapy for neonatal jaundice: Optimal wavelengths of light. J Pediatr 1983; 103:295.

534. Agati G, Fusi F, Pratesi R, et al: Wavelength-dependent quantum yield for Z-E isomerization of bilirubin complexed with human serum albumin. Photochem Photobiol 1992; 55:185.

535. Agati G, Fusi F, Donzelli GP, et al: Quantum yield and skin filtering effects on the formation rate of lumirubin. J Photochem Photobiol B 1993; 18:197.

536. Seidman DS, Moise J, Ergaz Z, et al: A new blue light-emitting phototherapy device: A prospective randomized controlled study. J Pediatr 2000; 136:771.

537. Wu PY, Hodgman JE, Kirkpatrick BV, et al: Metabolic aspects of phototherapy. Pediatrics 1985; 75:427.

538. John E: Complications of phototherapy in neonatal hyperbilirubinaemia. Aust Paediatr J 1975; 11:53.

539. Tan KL, Chow MT, Karim SM: Effect of phototherapy on neonatal riboflavin status. J Pediatr 1978; 93:494.

540. Gromisch DS, Lopez R, Cole HS, et al: Light (phototherapy)–induced riboflavin deficiency in the neonate. J Pediatr 1977; 90:118.

541. Ostrea EM, Fleury CA, Balun JE, et al: Accelerated degradation of essential fatty acids as a complication of phototherapy. J Pediatr 1983; 102:617.

542. Malhotra V, Greenberg JW, Dunn LL, et al: Fatty acid enhancement of the quantum yield for the formation of lumirubin from bilirubin bound to human albumin. Pediatr Res 1987; 21:530.

543. Odell GB, Brown RS, Kopelman AE: The photodynamic action of bilirubin on erythrocytes. J Pediatr 1972; 81:473.

544. Ostrea EM, Jr., Cepeda EE, Fleury CA, et al: Red cell membrane lipid peroxidation and hemolysis secondary to phototherapy. Acta Paediatr Scand 1985; 74:378.

545. Girotti AW: Bilirubin-photosensitized cross-linking of polypeptides in the isolated membrane of the human erythrocyte. J Biol Chem 1978; 253:7186.

546. Cukier JO, Maglalang AC, Odell GB: Increased osmotic fragility of erythrocytes in chronically jaundiced rats after phototherapy. Acta Paediatr Scand 1979; 68:903.

547. Howe RB, Hadland CR, Engel RR: Effect of phototherapy on serum bilirubin levels and red blood cell survival in congenitally jaundiced Gunn rats. J Lab Clin Med 1978; 92:221.

548. Ostrea EM, Jr., Odell GB: Photosensitized shift in the O_2 dissociation curve of fetal blood. Acta Paediatr Scand 1974; 63:341.

549. Cashore WJ, Karotkin EH, Stern L, et al: The lack of effect of phototherapy on serum bilirubin-binding capacity in newborn infants. J Pediatr 1975; 87:977.

550. Ebbesen F, Jacobsen J: Bilirubin-albumin binding affinity and serum albumin concentration during intensive phototherapy (blue double light) in jaundiced newborn infants. Eur J Pediatr 1980; 134:261.

551. Ebbesen F, Brodersen R: Albumin administration combined with phototherapy in treatment of hyperbilirubinaemia in low-birth-weight infants. Acta Paediatr Scand 1981; 70:649.

552. Sisson TR, Glauser SC, Glauser EM, et al: Retinal changes produced by phototherapy. J Pediatr 1970; 77:221.

553. Dobson V, Riggs LA, Siqueland ER: Electroretinographic determination of dark adaptation functions of children exposed to phototherapy as infants. J Pediatr 1974; 85:25.

554. Dobson V, Cowett RM, Riggs LA: Long-term effect of phototherapy on visual function. J Pediatr 1975; 86:555.

555. Valkeakari T, Anttolainen I, Aurekoski H, et al: Follow-up study of phototreated fullterm newborns. Acta Paediatr Scand 1981; 70:21.

556. Romagnoli C, Polidori G, Cataldi L, et al: Phototherapy-induced hypocalcemia. J Pediatr 1979; 94:815.

557. Wu PY, Lim RC, Hodgman JE, et al: Effect of phototherapy in preterm infants on growth in the neonatal period. J Pediatr 1974; 85:563.

558. Hakanson DO, Bergstrom WH: Phototherapy-induced hypocalcemia in newborn rats: Prevention by melatonin. Science 1981; 214:807.

559. Lemaitre BJ, Toubas PL, Dreux C, et al: Increased gonadotropin levels in newborn premature females treated by phototherapy. J Steroid Biochem 1979; 10:335.

560. Whitington PF, Olsen WA, Odell GB: The effect of bilirubin on the function of hamster small intestine. Pediatr Res 1981; 15:1009.

561. Guandalini S, Fasano A, Albini F, et al: Unconjugated bilirubin and the bile from light exposed Gunn rats inhibit intestinal water and electrolyte absorption. Gut 1988; 29:366.

562. Li BU, Whitington PF, Odell GB: The reversal of bilirubin-induced intestinal secretion by agar. Pediatr Res 1984; 18:79.

563. Whitington PF: Effect of jaundice phototherapy on intestinal mucosal bilirubin concentration and lactase activity in the congenitally jaundiced Gunn rat. Pediatr Res 1981; 15:345.

564. Bakken AF: Temporary intestinal lactase deficiency in light-treated jaundiced infants. Acta Paediatr Scand 1977; 66:91.

565. Dinari G, Cohen MI, McNamara H, et al: The effect of phototherapy on intestinal mucosal enzyme activity in the Gunn rat. Biol Neonate 1980; 38:179.

566. Jori G, Reddi E, Rubaltelli FF: Bronze baby syndrome: An animal model. Pediatr Res 1990; 27:22.

567. Kappas A, Drummond GS, Simionatto CS, et al: Control of heme oxygenase and plasma levels of bilirubin by a synthetic heme analogue, tin-protoporphyrin. Hepatology 1984; 4:336.

568. Drummond GS, Kappas A: Prevention of neonatal hyperbilirubinemia by tin protoporphyrin IX, a potent competitive inhibitor of heme oxidation. Proc Natl Acad Sci USA 1981; 78:6466.

569. Maines MD, Kappas A: Studies on the mechanism of induction of haem oxygenase by cobalt and other metal ions. Biochem J 1976; 154:125.

570. Kappas A, Drummond GS: Control of heme metabolism with synthetic metalloporphyrins. J Clin Invest 1986; 77:335.

571. McDonagh AF: Purple versus yellow: Preventing neonatal jaundice with tin-porphyrins. J Pediatr 1988; 113:777.

572. Drummond GS, Kappas A: Chemoprevention of neonatal jaundice: Potency of tin-protoporphyrin in an animal model. Science 1982; 217:1250.

573. Whitington PF, Moscioni AD, Gartner LM: The effect of tin (IV)-protoporphyrin-IX on bilirubin production and excretion in the rat. Pediatr Res 1987; 21:487.

574. Berglund L, Angelin B, Blomstrand R, et al: Sn-protoporphyrin lowers serum bilirubin levels, decreases biliary bilirubin output, enhances biliary heme excretion and potently inhibits hepatic heme oxygenase activity in normal human subjects. Hepatology 1988; 8:625.

575. McDonagh AF, Palma LA: Tin-protoporphyrin: A potent photosensitizer of bilirubin destruction. Photochem Photobiol 1985; 42:261.

576. Kappas A, Drummond GS, Manola T, et al: Sn-protoporphyrin use in the management of hyperbilirubinemia in term newborns with direct Coombs-positive ABO incompatibility. Pediatrics 1988; 81:485.

577. Valaes T, Petmezaki S, Henschke C, et al: Control of jaundice in preterm newborns by an inhibitor of bilirubin production: Studies with tin-mesoporphyrin. Pediatrics 1994; 93:1.

578. Martinez JC, Garcia HO, Otheguy LE, et al: Control of severe hyperbilirubinemia in full-term newborns with the inhibitor of bilirubin production Sn-mesoporphyrin. Pediatrics 1999; 103:1.

579. Landaw SA, Drummond GS, Kappas A: Targeting of heme oxygenase inhibitors to the spleen markedly increases their ability to diminish bilirubin production. Pediatrics 1989; 84:1091.

580. Wolkoff AW: Inheritable disorders manifested by conjugated hyperbilirubinemia. Semin Liver Dis 1983; 3:65.

581. Zimniak P: Dubin-Johnson and Rotor syndromes: Molecular basis and pathogenesis. Semin Liver Dis 1993; 13:248.

582. Pinos T, Constansa JM, Palacin A, et al: A new diagnostic approach to the Dubin-Johnson syndrome. Am J Gastroenterol 1990; 85:91.

583. Swartz HM, Sarna T, Varma RR: On the natural and excretion of the hepatic pigment in the Dubin-Johnson syndrome. Gastroenterology 1979; 76:958.

584. Bar-Meir S, Baron J, Seligson U, et al: ^{99m}Tc-HIDA cholescintigraphy in Dubin-Johnson and Rotor syndromes. Radiology 1982; 142:743.

585. Kartenbeck J, Leuschner U, Mayer R, et al: Absence of the canalicular isoform of the MRP gene-encoded conjugate export pump from the hepatocytes in Dubin-Johnson syndrome. Hepatology 1996; 23:1061.

586. Keitel V, Kartenbeck J, Nies AT, et al: Impaired protein maturation of the conjugate export pump multidrug resistance protein 2 as a consequence of a deletion mutation in Dubin-Johnson syndrome. Hepatology 2000; 32:1317.

587. Kagawa T, Sato M, Hosoi K, et al: Absence of R1066X mutation in six Japanese patients with Dubin-Johnson syndrome. Biochem Mol Biol Int 1999; 47:639.

588. Tsujii H, Konig J, Rost D, et al: Exon-intron organization of the human multidrug-resistance protein 2 (MRP2) gene mutated in Dubin-Johnson syndrome. Gastroenterology 1999; 117:653.

589. Erlinger S, Dhumeaux D, Desjeux JF, et al: Hepatic handling of unconjugated dyes in the Dubin-Johnson syndrome. Gastroenterology 1973; 64:106.

590. Kitamura T, Alroy J, Gatmaitan Z, et al: Defective biliary excretion of epinephrine metabolites in mutant (TR-) rats: Relation to the pathogenesis of black liver in the Dubin-Johnson syndrome and Corriedale sheep with an analogous excretory defect. Hepatology 1992; 15:1154.

591. Koskelo P, Toivonen I, Adlercreutz H: Urinary coproporphyrin isomer distribution in the Dubin-Johnson syndrome. Clin Chem 1967; 13:1006.

592. Fretzayas AM, Garoufi AI, Moutsouris CX, et al: Cholescintigraphy in the diagnosis of Rotor syndrome. J Nucl Med 1994; 35:1048.

593. Fretzayas AM, Stavrinadis CS, Koukoutsakis PM, et al: Diagnostic approach of Rotor syndrome with cholescintigraphy. Clin Nucl Med 1997; 22:635.

594. Tutus A, Silov G, Kula M: Cholescintigraphy in the diagnosis of Rotor syndrome. Clin Nucl Med 1997; 22:306.

595. Wolpert E, Pascasio FM, Wolkoff AW, et al: Abnormal sulfobromophthalein metabolism in Rotor's syndrome and obligate heterozygotes. N Engl J Med 1977; 296:1099.

596. Shimizu Y, Naruto H, Ida S, et al: Urinary coproporphyrin isomers in Rotor's syndrome: A study in eight families. Hepatology 1981; 1:173.

597. Phillips MJ, Suchy FJ: Mechanisms and morphology of cholestasis. In Suchy FJ, Sokol RJ, Balistreri WF (eds): Liver Disease in Children. Philadelphia, Lippincott, Williams & Wilkins, 2001, p 23.

598. Suchy FJ, Balistreri WF, Heubi JE, et al: Physiologic cholestasis: Elevation of the primary serum bile acid concentrations in normal infants. Gastroenterology 1981; 80:1037.

599. Karpen SJ, Suchy FJ: Structural and functional development of the liver. In Suchy FJ, Sokol RJ, Balistreri WF (eds): Liver Disease in Children. Philadelphia, Lippincott, Williams & Wilkins, 2001, p 3.

600. Emerick KM, Whitington PF: Molecular basis of neonatal cholestasis. Pediatr Clin North Am 2002; 49:221.

601. Suchy FJ: Approach to the infant with cholestasis. In Suchy FJ, Sokol RJ, Balistreri WF (eds): Liver Disease in Children. Philadelphia, Lippincott, Williams & Wilkins, 2001, p 187.

5 | Developmental Hemostasis: Relevance to Newborns and Infants

Paul Monagle[*] ● Maureen Andrew[†]

---

[*]Dr. Monagle is supported by a research fellowship from the Murdoch Children's Research Institute.

[†]Dr. Maureen Andrew (1952–2001) died suddenly during the preparation of this chapter. Dr. Andrew was one of the most influential pediatric researchers/clinicians of our time. A past president of the Society for Pediatric Research, she worked actively in research until her death, introducing the concept of developmental hemostasis, and leading the field of thromboembolic disease in children with an evidence-based approach. As founder of the 1–800-NO-CLOTS service, she directly helped thousands of babies as a source of clinical expertise. Dr. Andrew trained numerous pediatricians in the art of pediatric hematology. She will be remembered by many, including the editors of this textbook, as a brilliant scientist, a caring doctor, a thoughtful mentor, and, for those of us lucky enough to know her well, as a warm and wonderful friend.—*PM*

Over the past century, the discovery of individual components of the hemostatic system and their interactions has been accompanied by the realization that hemostasis is a dynamic, evolving process that is age dependent and begins *in utero*. Recent studies have provided reference ranges that delineate the age-dependent features of hemostasis and facilitate the evaluation of infants with hemostatic disorders. Although evolving, the hemostatic system in healthy fetuses and infants must be considered physiologic. However, the susceptibility of the young to complications associated with disturbed hemostasis differs significantly from that of adults. For example, the prevalence of thromboembolic complications in hospitalized sick newborns is relatively rare compared with that in adults. In contrast, hemorrhagic complications are not uncommon in sick newborns and most often are due to events such as vitamin K (VK) deficiency and asphyxia.

The first week of life is a time when serious hemorrhagic and thrombotic complications occur from either hereditary or, more commonly, acquired pathologic disorders. The evaluation of newborns for hemorrhagic or thrombotic complications presents unique problems that are not encountered in older children and adults. For example, physiologic levels of many coagulation proteins in newborns are low, and this makes the diagnosis of some inherited and acquired hemostatic problems difficult to establish. Because the hemostatic system is dynamic, multiple reference ranges to reflect the gestational age (GA) and postnatal age of infants are necessary.[1-3] The index of suspicion for severe congenital deficiencies of the components of hemostasis must be increased in newborns, because most severe deficiencies present in the neonatal period.

After confirming the presence of a hemostatic problem, the clinician is faced with the challenge of providing a safe and effective form of therapy. Just as for adults, the efficacy and safety of therapeutic interventions for infants must be tested in randomized, controlled trials, whenever feasible, and alternative study designs can be useful in dealing with rare or consistently life-threatening events. Guidelines for the classification of study design, and therefore the strength of the findings, have been established.[4] In this chapter, conclusions from studies with strong designs are given greater weight than conclusions from studies with weaker designs. When clinical data from studies in newborn infants are not available, extrapolations are made from data for adults in combination with results from *in vitro* studies and newborn animal models. An understanding of developmental hemostasis in the broadest sense optimizes the prevention, diagnosis, and treatment of hemostatic problems during childhood and undoubtedly provides new insights into the pathophysiology of hemorrhagic and thrombotic complications for all age groups. In this chapter, platelet function, coagulation, and fibrinolysis are reviewed in the context of developmental hemostasis.

DEVELOPMENTAL HEMOSTASIS

Platelets

GENERAL INFORMATION

Platelets from cord blood have been extensively studied and compared with platelets from adults. Flow cytometry has facilitated the study of platelets directly from newborns because of the small sample volume required for extensive platelet function studies. Because platelets from cord blood and from newborns may have some differences in function, they are discussed separately in this chapter. Differences in sample timing, method of collection, concentrations and compositions of platelet agonists, and laboratory testing probably contribute to apparently conflicting reports on cord blood platelet function.

MEGAKARYOCYTE AND PLATELET PRECURSORS

Increased numbers of all megakaryocyte precursors are found in cord blood of preterm babies compared with that of term infants. Term infants, with no evidence of platelet consumption, have increased circulating megakaryocyte progenitor numbers at birth correlated with platelet numbers compared with those of adults.[5] Cord blood megakaryocyte progenitors are exquisitely sensitive to exogenous cytokines. The magnitude of their proliferative and maturational responses to cytokines is related to developmental age.[6] Reticulated platelets are newly synthesized platelets with increased ribonucleic acid content. Reticulated platelet counts are reported to be similar to adult levels in healthy neonates older than 30 weeks' gestation and increased in neonates younger than 30 weeks' gestation,[7] although another study reports reduced reticulated platelet counts in neonates of all GAs compared with adults.[8] The median level in term babies (0.000145 µg/mL; range 0.000052–0.000237 µg/mL) is similar to that observed in preterm babies (0.000132 µg/mL; 0.000032–0.000318 µg/mL).[9] There is no information on developmental differences of megakaryocyte and platelet precursors during childhood.

PLATELET NUMBER, SIZE, AND SURVIVAL

Platelet counts and mean platelet volumes in newborns are similar to those in adults, with values of 150,000 to 450,000 × 10^9/L and 7 to 9 fL, respectively.[10–18] Platelet counts in fetuses between 18 and 30 weeks' gestation also fall within the adult range, with the average value being 250 × 10^9/L.[19] Platelet survival has not been measured in healthy infants. However, the survival of ^{111}In oxine-labeled platelets is similar in adult and newborn rabbits,[15, 20] and in humans the platelet survival times are the longest in the least thrombocytopenic infants.[21] Together, these studies suggest that platelet survivals in newborns probably do not differ significantly from those in adults (i.e., 7 to 10 days).

PLATELET STRUCTURE

Cord platelets have been examined for the presence of secretory granules and defects in release mechanisms. Electron microscopy studies have demonstrated normal numbers of granules; however, serotonin and adenosine diphosphate (ADP), which are stored in dense granules, are present at concentrations that are less than 50 percent of adult values. Flow cytometry studies in whole blood without added agonist show that there are no significant differences between newborns and adults in platelet binding of monoclonal antibodies for glycoprotein (GP) Ib or P-selectin; however, GP IIb/IIIa is significantly reduced.[22, 23]

PLATELET ADHESION

When the endothelial lining of blood vessels is damaged or removed, platelets adhere to subendothelial layers, undergo changes in shape, and spread over the damaged surface. This process requires that *von Willebrand's factor (VWF)*, a plasma factor, binds to a specific component of the platelet membrane, GP Ib, forming a bridge between the subendothelial surface and platelet.[24] Platelet adhesion at birth has not been assessed with sensitive and reproducible assays; this may explain the conflicting *in vitro* results given in the literature.[25, 26] GP Ib is present on fetal platelet membranes in adult quantities.[27] Both the plasma concentrations of VWF and the proportion of high-molecular-weight multimers (and therefore more active forms) of VWF are increased in newborns.[28, 29] The cord multimeric pattern of VWF appears similar to that of the forms released by endothelial cells. This similarity may be explained by the recent finding that newborn plasma has little if any detectable VWF cleaving protease.[30] The quantitative and qualitative differences in VWF at birth are probably responsible for the enhanced agglutination of cord platelets to low concentrations of ristocetin[28, 29, 31] and contribute to the short bleeding time in newborns.[25, 32–36]

PLATELET AGGREGATION

After activation of platelets, GP IIb and IIIa come together on platelet surfaces to form 1:1 complexes that are binding sites for fibrinogen and, to a lesser extent, VWF and fibronectin. Platelet-to-platelet adherence or aggregation is mediated by fibrinogen bound to GP IIb/IIIa. GP IIb/IIIa complexes are expressed on platelet membranes early in gestation,[27] and fibrinogen is present in adult amounts by the time of viability.[1–3] The capacity of cord platelets to aggregate after exposure to a variety of agonists has been variable, with some observations being more consistent than others. Recently differences between cord blood of premature and full-term infants have been described, with reduced aggregation in preterm infants.[37]

Epinephrine-induced aggregation of cord platelets is consistently decreased compared with that of adult platelets because of the decreased availability of α-adrenergic receptors.[25, 26, 31, 33–36, 38–45] This phenomenon is transient and is due to either delayed maturation of these receptors or occupation by catecholamines released during birth. Ristocetin-induced agglutination of cord platelets is consistently increased compared with that of adult platelets, probably because of quantitative and qualitative increases in the level of VWF.[1–3] Aggregation of cord platelets induced by ADP, collagen, thrombin, and arachidonic acid varies and may be moderately decreased in relation to or similar to that of adult platelets.[38, 40, 41, 46–48] There is reduced thromboxane A[2] production in neonates despite normal receptor binding, suggesting a postreceptor signal transduction problem.[49]

Decreased aggregation of cord platelets implies either a storage pool deficiency or an abnormality in secretion. The modestly decreased aggregation with some platelet agonists was initially thought to be due to a physiologic storage pool deficiency.[26, 26, 50] However, differences from adult platelets are small, and after incubation of newborn platelets with radiolabeled adenine, normal specific radioactivities of platelet adenosine triphosphate (ATP) and ADP are measured.[26] The absence of a classic storage pool deficiency was further supported by normal studies of newborn platelet granules with electron microscopy.[31, 51]

An aspirin-like defect does not occur in platelets from newborns because mixing studies of newborn and aspirin-treated platelets reveal normal platelet aggregation, production of arachidonic acid, and products of both the lipoxygenase and cyclooxygenase pathway.[26, 46, 51–55] Thus, neither a classic storage pool deficiency nor an aspirin-like platelet defect adequately explains the functional deficit of newborn platelets. Clots from adults and newborns exhibit similar platelet-mediated clot retraction.[56]

PLATELET ACTIVATION AND SECRETION

Studies of activation pathways leading to release have not identified specific abnormalities in cord platelets. Inositol phosphate production and protein phosphorylation are normal, as is production of arachidonic acid and its metabolites.[48] In fact, cord platelets release more arachidonic acid than adult platelets in response to stimulation by thrombin.[38] This increased release may be due to the greater reactivity of platelet membranes induced by low levels of vitamin E.[53, 57] The number of agonist receptors, with the exception of the α-adrenergic receptor discussed previously, does not appear to be decreased. Despite a poor response to collagen stimulation, cord platelets have normal numbers of the collagen receptor GP Ia/IIa present on platelet membranes.[27] Coupling of agonist receptors to phospholipases may be the site of this transient activation defect in response to collagen.[58]

STUDIES OF PLATELETS FROM NEWBORNS

A few studies have assessed aggregation of platelets from newborns obtained during the first few days of life; other studies have evaluated platelets of older neonates.[42, 45] In one study, abnormal platelet aggregation in response to

ADP (decreased primary wave and absent secondary wave) was observed in cord platelet–rich plasma.[42] However, improved platelet aggregation was seen in newborn platelets (blood drawn 2 hours after birth), with normalization of platelet aggregation at 48 hours.[45] Studies using whole-blood flow cytometry show that, compared with adult platelets, neonatal platelets are hyporeactive to thrombin, a combination of ADP and epinephrine, and a thromboxane A[2] analog (Fig. 5–1).[38, 39, 43, 59] The clinical significance of these observations remains unknown.

BLEEDING TIME

Measurement of the bleeding time is currently the best *in vivo* test of platelet interaction with the vessel wall.[32] Automated devices modified for newborns and children are available and have been standardized.[33] Bleeding times in infants during the first week of life are significantly shorter than those in adults.[25, 32–36] Several mechanisms contribute to this enhanced platelet/vessel wall interaction, including higher plasma concentrations of VWF,[1–3] enhanced function of VWF due to a disproportional increase in the high-molecular-weight multimeric forms,[28, 29] active multimers, large red cells,[60] and high hematocrits.[61] The significance of mild platelet aggregation defects in cord platelets is uncertain when bleeding times in newborns are shorter than those in adults.

The PFA–100 system provides an *in vitro* method of assessing primary platelet-related hemostasis by measuring the time (closure time) taken for a platelet plug to occlude a microscopic aperture cut into a membrane coated with collagen and either adrenaline or ADP. The PFA–100 system is ideal for neonates because of the small volume required and the rapidity of testing. Normal ranges for the clotting times of children are similar to those for adults.[62] Platelets from newborns have shorter clotting times, which are not influenced by red cells or white cells.[63] The sensitivity of the PFA–100 system for identifying von Willebrand disease (VWD) is reported to be 86 percent and the specificity more than 98 percent.[64] For platelet function defects the sensitivity is 86 percent and specificity is 82 percent,[65] although some authors question the reliability of the technique in this setting.[66] The ease of the PFA–100 system and the associated difficulties in performing skin bleeding times have reduced the clinical utility of skin bleeding times. Further studies are required to determine the optimal method of assessing primary hemostasis in newborns and children.

ACTIVATION DURING THE BIRTH PROCESS

There is strong evidence that platelets are activated during the birth process. Cord plasma levels of thromboxane B[2], β-thromboglobulin, and platelet factor 4 are increased,[53, 67, 68] the granular content of cord platelets is decreased, and epinephrine receptor availability is reduced, perhaps as a result of occupation.[67, 69] The mechanisms of activation are probably multifactorial and include thermal changes, hypoxia, acidosis, adrenergic stimulation, and the thrombogenic effects of amniotic fluid. Activation of the coagulation system may provide an

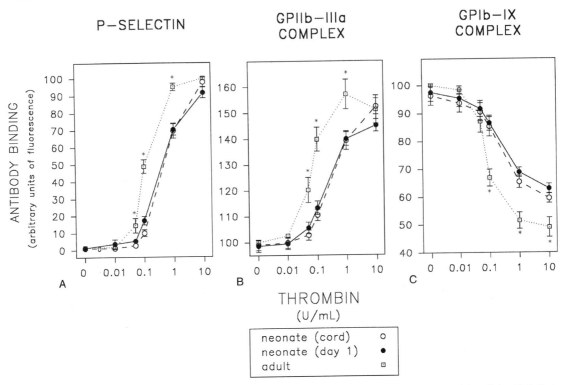

FIGURE 5–1. Effect of thrombin on the surface expression of P-selectin *(A)*, the glycoprotein (GP) IIb/IIIa complex *(B)*, and the GP Ib/factor IX complex *(C)* on neonatal and adult platelets in whole blood. Results were similar for cord and neonatal day 1 values. Expression of P-selectin and GP IIb/IIIa complexes was decreased in newborns, whereas GP Ib/factor IX expression was relatively preserved in newborns compared with adults after stimulation with thrombin. Data are expressed as mean ± SEM; *n* = 20. Asterisks indicate *P* > .05 for both cord blood and day 1 neonatal platelets compared with adult platelets. (From Rajasekhar D, Kestin AS, Bednarek FJ, et al: Neonatal platelets are less reactive than adult platelets to physiological agonists in whole blood. Thromb Haemost 1994; 72:957–963.)

explanation for the paradox that one-stage coagulation times are prolonged in the newborn but that various measures of whole-blood clotting duration are shortened relative to those in the adult.[25, 70, 71]

Blood Vessel Wall: Age and Anticoagulant Properties

In the 1980s, it was established that the endothelium fulfills a complex role in hemostasis, preventing thrombotic complications under physiologic conditions and promoting fibrin formation when injured. One of the anticoagulant properties of endothelial cell surfaces is mediated by lipoxygenase and cyclooxygenase metabolites of unsaturated fatty acids. Prostacyclin (prostaglandin [PG] I_2) production by cord vessels exceeds that by vessels in adults.[72] A second endothelial cell-mediated antithrombotic property is the promotion of antithrombin (AT) neutralization of thrombin by cell surface proteoglycans. Structurally, there is evidence that vessel wall glycosaminoglycans of the young differ from those of adults.[73, 74] In a rabbit venous model, increased amounts of glycosaminoglycans are seen in inferior vena cavae from rabbit pups compared with those in adults. Similarly, in the rabbit arterial model, increased glycosaminoglycan-mediated AT activity in seen in rabbit pups compared with that in adult rabbits.[75, 76]

Nitric oxide, or endothelium-derived relaxing factor, is a labile humoral agent that modulates vascular tone in the fetal and postnatal lung and contributes to the normal decline in pulmonary vascular resistance at birth. Like prostacyclin, nitric oxide is a potent inhibitor of platelet activation and adhesion to the damaged vessel wall.[77] Cord plasma can generate less thrombin in the presence of human umbilical endothelial cells than it can against a plastic surface. This is related to the cell surface promotion of AT inhibition of thrombin.[78]

THE COAGULATION SYSTEM

General Information

Our understanding of the physiology of hemostasis in newborns and infants is deficient compared with our knowledge of this subject in adults. The reasons for this deficit are several: in newborns and infants, multiple reference ranges are required because these patients have rapidly evolving systems[1–3, 79]; blood sampling in the young is technically difficult; only small blood samples can be obtained; microtechniques are required[80]; and greater variability in plasma concentrations of coagulation proteins necessitates the use of large patient numbers to establish normative data.

Coagulation proteins do not cross the placental barrier but are independently synthesized by the fetus.[19, 81-92] Plasma concentrations of most coagulation proteins are measurable by a 10 weeks' gestation, and they continue to increase gradually in parallel with the GA. Samples obtained during fetoscopy provide the best assessment of normal values for fetuses, and by extrapolation, for very premature infants (Tables 5–1 and 5–2). True reference ranges for extremely premature infants are not available because the majority of these infants have postnatal complications. Tables 5–3 to 5–6 provide reference ranges for coagulation proteins, inhibitors of coagulation, and components of the fibrinolytic system for premature (30 to 36 weeks' gestation) and full-term infants on day 1 of life as well as longitudinally, over the first 6 months of life.[1] Tables 5–7 to 5–9 provide similar data for older children.

Screening Tests

The variable results for coagulation screening tests reflect the use of cord blood samples rather than samples from infants or differing ethnic populations or the use of different reagents.[93, 94] Variation in prothrombin time (PT) results can be minimized by reporting the PT as an *international normalized ratio (INR)*.[95] The INR is calculated as

TABLE 5–1. Coagulation Screening Tests and Coagulation Factor Levels in Fetuses, Full-Term Infants, and Adults

Parameter	Fetuses (Weeks' Gestation)			Newborn (n = 60)	Adult (n = 40)
	19–23 (n = 20)	24–29 (n = 22)	30–38 (n = 22)		
PT (sec)	32.5 (19–45)	32.2 (19–44)[†]	22.6 (16–30)[†]	16.7 (12.0–23.5)[*]	13.5 (11.4–14.0)
PT (INR)	6.4 (1.7–11.1)	6.2 (2.1–10.6)[†]	3.0 (1.5–5.0)[*]	1.7 (0.9–2.7)[*]	1.1 (0.8–1.2)
APTT (sec)	168.8 (83–250)	154.0 (87–210)[†]	104.8 (76–128)[†]	44.3 (*35–52)[*]	33.0 (25–39)
TCT (sec)	34.2 (24–44)[*]	26.2 (24–28)	21.4 (17.0–23.3)	20.4 (15.2–25.0)[†]	14.0 (12–16)
Factor I von Clauss (g/L)	0.85 (0.57–1.50)	1.12 (0.65–1.65)	1.35 (1.25–1.65)	1.68 (0.95–2.45)[†]	3.0 (1.78–4.50)
Factor I Ag (g/L)	1.08 (0.75–1.50)	1.93 (1.56–2.40)	1.94 (1.30–2.40)	2.65 (1.68–3.60)[†]	3.5 (2.50–5.20)
Factor IIc (%)	16.9 (10–24)	19.9 (11–30)[*]	27.9 (15–50)[†]	43.5 (27–64)[†]	98.7 (70–125)
Factor VIIc (%)	27.4 (17–37)	33.8 (18–48)[*]	45.9 (31–62)	52.5 (28–78)[†]	101.3 (68–130)
Factor IXc (%)	10.1 (6–14)	9.9 (5–15)	12.3 (5–24)[†]	31.8 (15–50)[†]	104.8 (70–142)
Factor Xc (%)	20.5 (14–29)	24.9 (16–35)	28.0 (16–36)[†]	39.6 (21–65)[†]	99.2 (75–125)
Factor Vc (%)	32.1 (21–44)	36.8 (25–50)	48.9 (23–70)[†]	89.9 (50–140)	99.8 (65–140)
Factor VIIIc (%)	34.5 (18–50)	35.5 (20–52)	50.1 (27–78)[†]	94.3 (38–150)	101.8 (55–170)
Factor XIc (%)	13.2 (8–19)	12.1 (6–22)	14.8 (6–26)[†]	37.2 (13–62)[†]	100.2 (70–135)
Factor XIIc (%)	14.9 (6–25)	22.7 (6–40)	25.8 (11–50)[†]	69.8 (25–105)[†]	101.4 (65–144)
PK (%)	12.8 (8–19)	15.4 (8–26)	18.1 (8–28)[†]	35.4 (21–53)[†]	99.8 (65–135)
HMWK (%)	15.4 (10–22)	19.3 (10–26)	23.6 (12–34)[†]	38.9 (28–53)[†]	98.8 (68–135)

All values are given as a mean followed in parentheses by the lower and upper boundaries including 95% of the population.

n = number of subjects; PT = prothrombin time; INR = international normalized ratio; APTT = activated partial thromboplastin time; TCT = thrombin clotting time; Ag = antigen; PK = prekallikrein, HMWK = high-molecular-weight kininogen.

[*]P < .05.

[†]P < .01.

From Reverdiau-Moalic P, Delahousse B, Body G, et al: Evolution of blood coagulation activators and inhibitors in the healthy human fetus. Blood 1996; 88:900–906.

TABLE 5–2. Blood Coagulation Inhibitor Levels in Fetuses, Full-Term Infants, and Adults

Parameter	Fetuses (Weeks' Gestation)			Newborns (n = 60)	Adults (n = 40)
	19–23 (n = 20)	24–29 (n = 22)	30–38 (n = 22)		
AT (%)	20.2 (12–31)[*]	30.0 (20–39)	37.1 (24–55)[†]	59.4 (42–80)[†]	99.8 (65–130)
HCII (%)	10.3 (6–16)	12.9 (5.5–20)	21.1 (11–33)[†]	52.1 (19–99)[†]	101.4 (70–128)
TFPI (%)[‡]	21.0 (16.0–29.2)	20.6 (13.4–33.2)	20.7 (10.4–31.5)[†]	38.1 (22.7–55.8)[†]	73.0 (50.9–90.1)
PC Ag (%)	9.5 (6–14)	12.1 (8–16)	15.9 (8–30)[†]	32.5 (21–47)[†]	100.8 (68–125)
PC Act (%)	9.6 (7–13)	10.4 (8–13)	14.1 (8–18)[†]	28.2 (14–42)[†]	98.8 (68–125)
Total PS (%)	15.1 (11–21)	17.4 (14–25)	21.0 (15–30)[†]	38.5 (22–55)[†]	99.6 (72–118)
Free PS (%)	21.7 (13–32)	27.9 (19–40)	27.0 (18–40)[†]	49.3 (33–67)[†]	98.7 (72–128)
Free PS/Total PS	0.82 (0.75–0.92)	0.83 (0.76–0.95)	0.79 (0.70–0.89)[†]	0.64 (0.59–0.98)[†]	0.41 (0.38–0.43)
C4b-BP (%)	1.8 (0–6)	6.1 (0–12.5)	9.3 (5–14)	18.6 (3–40)[†]	100.3 (70–124)

All Values are given as a mean followed in parentheses by the lower and upper boundaries including 95% of the population.

AT = antithrombin; HCII = heparin cofactor II; TFPI = tissue factor pathway inhibitor; PC = protein C; ACT = activity; PS = protein S .

[*]P < .05.

[†]P < .01.

[‡]Twenty samples were assayed for each group but only 10 for 19- to 23-week-old fetuses.

From Reverdiau-Moalic P, Delahousse B, Body G, et al: Evolution of blood coagulation activators and inhibitors in the healthy human fetus. Blood 1996; 88:900–906.

TABLE 5–3. Reference Values for Coagulation Tests in Healthy Premature Infants (30 to 36 Weeks' Gestation) during the First 6 Months of Life

Coagulation Tests	Day 1	Day 5	Day 30	Day 90	Day 180	Adult
PT (sec)	13.0 (10.6–16.2)*	12.5 (10.0–15.3)*	11.8 (10.0–13.6)*	12.3 (10.0–14.6)	12.5 (10.0–15.0)*	12.4 (10.8–13.9)
INR	1.0 (0.61–1.70)	0.91 (0.53–1.48)	0.79 (0.53–1.11)	0.88 (0.53–1.32)	0.91 (0.53–1.48)	0.89 (0.64–1.17)
APTT (sec)	53.6 (27.5–79.4)†	50.5 (26.9–74.1)	44.7 (26.9–62.5)	39.5 (28.3–50.7)	37.5 (27.2–53.3)	33.5 (26.6–40.3)
TCT (sec)	24.8 (19.2–30.4)	24.1 (18.8–29.4)*	24.4 (18.8–29.9)	25.1 (19.4–30.8)	25.2 (18.9–31.5)	25.0 (19.7–30.3)
Fibrinogen (g/L)	2.43 (1.50–3.73)*, †	2.80 (1.60–4.18)*, †	2.54 (1.50–4.14)	2.46 (1.50–3.52)	2.28 (1.50–3.60)	2.78 (1.56–4.00)
Factor II (U/mL)	0.45 (0.20–0.77)	0.57 (0.29–0.85)†	0.57 (0.36–0.95)	0.68 (0.30–1.06)	0.87 (0.51–1.23)	1.08 (0.70–1.46)
Factor V (U/mL)	0.88 (0.41–1.44)*, †	1.00 (0.46–1.54)*	1.02 (0.48–1.56)*	0.99 (0.59–1.39)	1.02 (0.58–1.46)*	1.06 (0.62–1.50)
Factor VII (U/mL)	0.67 (0.21–1.13)	0.84 (0.30–1.38)	0.83 (0.21–1.45)	0.87 (0.31–1.43)	0.99 (0.47–1.51)*	1.05 (0.67–1.43)
Factor VIII (U/mL)	1.11 (0.50–2.13)	1.15 (0.53–2.05)*, †	1.11 (0.50–1.99)	1.06 (0.58–1.88)*, †	0.99 (0.50–1.87)*, †	0.99 (0.50–1.49)
VWF (U/mL)	1.36 (0.78–2.10)	1.33 (0.72–2.19)	1.36 (0.66–2.16)	1.12 (0.75–1.84)*, †	0.98 (0.54–1.58)*	0.92 (0.50–1.58)
Factor IX (U/mL)	0.35 (0.19–0.65)†	0.42 (0.14–0.74)†	0.44 (0.13–0.80)	0.59 (0.25–0.93)	0.81 (0.50–1.20)	1.09 (0.55–1.63)
Factor X (U/mL)	0.41 (0.11–0.71)	0.51 (0.19–0.83)	0.56 (0.20–0.92)	0.67 (0.35–0.99)	0.77 (0.35–1.19)	1.06 (0.70–1.52)
Factor XI (U/mL)	0.30 (0.08–0.52)†	0.41 (0.13–0.69)†	0.43 (0.15–0.71)†	0.59 (0.25–0.93)*	0.78 (0.46–1.10)	0.97 (0.67–1.27)
Factor XII (U/mL)	0.38 (0.10–0.66)†	0.39 (0.09–0.69)†	0.43 (0.11–0.75)	0.61 (0.15–1.07)	0.82 (0.22–1.42)	1.08 (0.52–1.64)
PK (U/mL)	0.33 (0.09–0.57)	0.45 (0.25–0.75)	0.59 (0.31–0.87)	0.79 (0.37–1.21)	0.78 (0.40–1.16)	1.12 (0.62–1.62)
HK (U/mL)	0.49 (0.09–0.89)	0.62 (0.24–1.00)†	0.64 (0.16–1.12)†	0.78 (0.32–1.24)	0.83 (0.41–1.25)*	0.92 (0.50–1.36)
Factor XIIIa (U/mL)	0.70 (0.32–1.08)	1.01 (0.57–1.45)*	0.99 (0.51–1.47)*	1.13 (0.71–1.55)*	1.13 (0.65–1.61)*	1.05 (0.55–1.55)
Factor XIIIb (U/mL)	0.81 (0.35–1.27)	1.10 (0.68–1.58)*	1.07 (0.57–1.57)*	1.21 (0.75–1.67)	1.15 (0.67–1.63)	0.97 (0.57–1.37)

All factors except fibrinogen are expressed as units per milliliter (U/mL), where pooled plasma contains 1.0 U/mL. All values are given as a mean followed by the lower and upper boundary encompassing 95% of the population. Between 40 and 96 samples were assayed for each value for the newborn. Some measurements were skewed owing to a disproportionate number of high values.

Factor VIII = factor VIII procoagulant; VWF = von Willebrand factor.

*Values indistinguishable from those of adults.

†Measurements are skewed owing to a disproportionate number of high values.

From Andrew M, Paes B, Milner R, et al: Development of the human coagulation system in the healthy premature infant. Blood 1988; 72:1651–1657.

the patient PT/control PT ratio to the power of the *international sensitivity index (ISI)*.[1–3] The ISI corrects for the large variation in sensitivity of thromboplastin reagents to plasma concentrations of coagulation proteins. The thrombin clotting time measured in the absence of calcium is prolonged because of the presence of the "fetal" form of fibrinogen at birth.[1–3] For Tables 5–3 and 5–4, the thrombin clotting time was measured in the presence of calcium, so that abnormal values caused by the presence of heparin, as well as low levels of fibrinogen, could be detected.

Coagulant Proteins

The VK-dependent factors are the most extensively studied group of factors in infants. This attention reflects the importance of hemolytic disease of the newborn, an acquired bleeding disorder caused by pathologically low levels of the VK-dependent proteins.[96–98] Physiologically low levels of factors II, VII, IX, and X in

Tables 5–3 and 5–4 are similar to those in other reports[1–3, 10, 99–108] and were measured in infants who received VK prophylaxis at birth. The levels of both the VK-dependent factors and the four contact factors (factor XI, factor XII, prekallikrein, and high-molecular-weight kininogen) gradually increase to values approaching those in the adult by 6 months of life.[1–3, 10] The prolonged activated partial thromboplastin time (APTT) seen during the first months of life is in large part due to the low levels of the contact factors.[109]

Plasma levels of fibrinogen, factors V, VIII, and XIII, and VWF are not decreased at birth (Tables 5–3 and 5–4).[1–3, 10, 99–108] Fibrinogen levels continue to increase after birth; this is important to recognize when an elevated fibrinogen level is used as a marker of sepsis.[110] Plasma levels of factor VIII are skewed toward the high measurements, necessitating an adjustment of the lower limit of normal (Tables 5–3 and 5–4). Fewer than 1 percent of values for factor VIII are less than 0.40 unit/mL, and all values are greater than 0.30 unit/mL. Levels of both VWF

TABLE 5–4. Reference Values for Coagulation Tests in Healthy Full-Term Infants during the First 6 Months of Life

Coagulation Tests	Day 1	Day 5	Day 30	Day 90	Day 180	Adult
PT (sec)	13.0 (10.1–15.9)*	12.4 (10.0–15.3)*	11.8 (10.0–14.3)*	11.9 (10.0–14.2)*	12.3 (10.7–13.9)*	12.4 (10.8–13.9)
INR	1.00 (0.53–1.62)	0.89 (0.53–1.48)	0.79 (0.53–1.26)	0.81 (0.53–1.26)	0.88 (0.61–1.17)	0.89 (0.64–1.17)
APTT (sec)	42.9 (31.3–54.5)	42.6 (25.4–59.8)	40.4 (32.0–55.2)	37.1 (29.0–50.1)*	35.5 (28.1–42.9)	33.5 (26.6–40.3)*
TCT (sec)	23.5 (19.0–28.3)*	23.1 (18.0–29.2)	24.3 (19.4–29.2)*	25.1 (20.5–29.7)*	25.5 (19.8–31.2)	25.0 (19.7–30.3)*
Fibrinogen (g/L)	2.83 (1.67–3.99)*	3.12 (1.62–4.62)*	2.70 (1.62–3.78)*	2.43 (1.50–3.79)*	2.51 (1.50–3.87)	2.78 (1.56–4.00)*
Factor II (U/mL)	0.48 (0.26–0.70)	0.63 (0.33–0.93)	0.68 (0.34–1.02)	0.75 (0.45–1.05)	0.88 (0.60–1.16)	1.08 (0.70–1.46)
Factor V (U/mL)	0.72 (0.34–1.08)	0.95 (0.45–1.45)	0.98 (0.62–1.34)	0.90 (0.48–1.32)	0.91 (0.55–1.27)	1.06 (0.62–1.50)
Factor VII (U/mL)	0.66 (0.28–1.04)	0.89 (0.35–1.43)	0.90 (0.42–1.38)	0.91 (0.39–1.43)	0.87 (0.47–1.27)	1.05 (0.67–1.43)
Factor VIII (U/mL)	1.00 (0.50–1.78)*	0.88 (0.50–1.54)*	0.91 (0.50–1.57)*	0.79 (0.50–1.25)*	0.73 (0.50–1.09)	0.99 (0.50–1.49)
VWF (U/mL)	1.53 (0.50–2.87)	1.40 (0.50–2.54)	1.28 (0.50–2.46)	1.18 (0.50–2.06)	1.07 (0.50–1.97)	0.92 (0.50–1.58)
Factor IX (U/mL)	0.53 (0.15–0.91)	0.53 (0.15–0.91)	0.51 (0.21–0.81)	0.67 (0.21–1.13)	0.86 (0.36–1.36)	1.09 (0.55–1.63)
Factor X (U/mL)	0.40 (0.12–0.68)	0.49 (0.19–0.79)	0.59 (0.31–0.87)	0.71 (0.35–1.07)	0.78 (0.38–1.18)	1.06 (0.70–1.52)
Factor XI (U/mL)	0.38 (0.10–0.66)	0.55 (0.23–0.87)	0.53 (0.27–0.79)	0.69 (0.41–0.97)	0.86 (0.49–1.34)	0.97 (0.67–1.27)
Factor XII (U/mL)	0.53 (0.13–0.93)	0.47 (0.11–0.83)	0.49 (0.17–0.81)	0.67 (0.25–1.09)	0.77 (0.39–1.15)	1.08 (0.52–1.64)
PK (U/mL)	0.37 (0.18–0.69)	0.48 (0.20–0.76)	0.57 (0.23–0.91)	0.73 (0.41–1.05)	0.86 (0.56–1.16)	1.12 (0.62–1.62)
HMWK (U/mL)	0.54 (0.06–1.02)	0.74 (0.16–1.32)	0.77 (0.33–1.21)	0.82 (0.30–1.46)*	0.82 (0.36–1.28)*	0.92 (0.50–1.36)
Factor XIIIa (U/mL)	0.79 (0.27–1.31)	0.94 (0.44–1.44)*	0.93 (0.39–1.47)*	1.04 (0.36–1.72)*	1.04 (0.46–1.62)*	1.05 (0.55–1.55)
Factor XIIIb (U/mL)	0.76 (0.30–1.22)	1.06 (0.32–1.80)	1.11 (0.39–1.73)*	1.16 (0.48–1.84)*	1.10 (0.50–1.70)*	0.97 (0.57–1.37)

All factors except fibrinogen are expressed as units per milliliter (U/mL), where pooled plasma contains 1.0 U/mL. All values are expressed as mean followed by the lower and upper boundary encompassing 95% of the population. Between 40 and 77 samples were assayed for each value for the newborn. Some measurements were skewed owing to a disproportionate number of high values.

*Values indistinguishable from those of adults.
From Andrew M, Paes B, Milner R, et al: Development of the human coagulation system in the full-term infant. Blood 1987; 70:165–172.

TABLE 5–5. Reference Values for the Inhibitors of Coagulation in Infants during the first 6 Months of Life

Inhibitor Levels	Day 1	Day 5	Day 30	Day 90	Day 180	Adult
Healthy Full-Term Infants						
AT (U/mL)	0.63 (0.39–0.87)	0.67 (0.41–0.93)	0.78 (0.48–1.08)	0.97 (0.73–1.21)*	1.04 (0.84–1.24)*	1.05 (0.79–1.31)
α_2M (U/mL)	1.39 (0.95–1.83)	1.48 (0.98–1.98)	1.50 (1.06–1.94)	1.76 (1.26–2.26)	1.91 (1.49–2.33)	0.86 (0.52–1.20)
C_1E-INH (U/mL)	0.72 (0.36–1.08)	0.90 (0.60–1.20)*	0.89 (0.47–1.31)	1.15 (0.71–1.59)	1.41 (0.89–1.93)	1.01 (0.71–1.31)
α_1AT (U/mL)	0.93 (0.49–1.37)*	0.89 (0.49–1.29)*	0.62 (0.36–0.88)	0.72 (0.42–1.02)	0.77 (0.47–1.07)	0.93 (0.55–1.31)
HCII (U/mL)	0.43 (0.10–0.93)	0.48 (0.00–0.96)	0.47 (0.10–0.87)	0.72 (0.10–1.46)	1.20 (0.50–1.90)	0.96 (0.66–1.26)
Protein C (U/mL)	0.35 (0.17–0.53)	0.42 (0.20–0.64)	0.43 (0.21–0.65)	0.54 (0.28–0.80)	0.59 (0.37–0.81)	0.96 (0.64–1.28)
Protein S (U/mL)	0.36 (0.12–0.60)	0.50 (0.22–0.78)	0.63 (0.33–0.93)	0.86 (0.54–1.18)*	0.87 (0.55–1.19)*	0.92 (0.60–1.24)
Healthy Premature Infants (30–36 Weeks' Gestation)						
AT (U/mL)	0.38 (0.14–0.62)†	0.56 (0.30–0.82)	0.59 (0.37–0.81)†	0.83 (0.45–1.21)†	0.90 (0.52–1.28)†	1.05 (0.79–1.31)
α_2 M (U/mL)	1.10 (0.56–1.82)†	1.25 (0.71–1.77)	1.38 (0.72–2.04)	1.80 (1.20–2.66)	2.09 (1.10–3.21)	0.86 (0.52–1.20)
C_1E-NH (U/mL)	0.65 (0.31–0.99)	0.83 (0.45–1.21)	0.74 (0.40–1.24)†	1.14 (0.60–1.68)*	1.40 (0.96–2.04)	1.01 (0.71–1.31)
α_1AT (U/mL)	0.90 (0.36–1.44)*	0.94 (0.42–1.46)*	0.76 (0.38–1.12)†	0.81 (0.49–1.13)*,†	0.82 (0.48–1.16)*	0.93 (0.55–1.31)
HCII (U/mL)	0.32 (0.10–0.60)†	0.34 (0.10–0.69)	0.43 (0.15–0.71)	0.61 (0.20–1.11)	0.89 (0.45–1.40)*,†	0.96 (0.66–1.26)
Protein C (U/mL)	0.28 (0.12–0.44)†	0.31 (0.11–0.51)	0.37 (0.15–0.59)†	0.45 (0.23–0.67)†	0.57 (0.31–0.83)	0.96 (0.64–1.28)
Protein S (U/mL)	0.26 (0.14–0.38)†	0.37 (0.13–0.61)	0.56 (0.22–0.90)	0.76 (0.40–1.12)†	0.82 (0.44–1.20)	0.92 (0.60–1.24)

All values are expressed in units per milliliter (U/mL), where pooled plasma contains 1.0 U/mL. All values are given as a mean followed by the lower and upper boundary encompassing 95% of the population. Between 40 and 75 samples were assayed for each value for the newborn. Some measurements were skewed owing to a disproportionate number of high values. The lower limits exclude the lower 2.5% of the population.

AT = antithrombin; α_2M = α_2-macroglobulin; C_1-INH = C_1-esterase inhibitor; α_1-AT = α_1-antitrypsin.
*Values indistinguishable from those of adults.
†Values different from those of full-term infants.
From Andrew M, Paes B, Johnston M: Development of the hemostatic system in the neonate and young infant. Am J Pediatr Hematol Oncol 1990; 12:95–104.

and high-molecular-weight multimers are increased at birth and for the first 3 months of life.[1, 2]

Regulation of Thrombin

Thrombin regulation, a key step in hemostasis, is both delayed and decreased in plasma from newborns com-pared with plasma from adults and is similar to that in plasma samples from adults receiving therapeutic doses of warfarin or heparin (Fig. 5–2).[111] The amount of thrombin generated is directly proportional to the prothrombin concentration,[36] whereas the rate of thrombin generation reflects the concentration of other procoagulants. Thrombin generation in plasma from newborns is further

TABLE 5–6. Reference Values for the Components of the Fibrinolytic System during the First 6 Months of Life

Fibrinolytic System	Day 1	Day 5	Day 30	Day 90	Day 180M (B)	AdultM (B)
			Healthy Full-Term Infants			
Plasminogen (U/mL)	1.95 (1.25–2.65)	2.17 (1.41–2.93)	1.98 (1.26–2.70)	2.48 (1.74–3.22)	3.01 (2.21–3.81)	3.36 (2.48–4.24)
TPA (ng/mL)	9.6 (5.0–18.9)	5.6 (4.0–10.0)*	4.1 (1.0–6.0)*	2.1 (1.0–5.0)*	2.8 (1.0–6.0)*	4.9 (1.4–8.4)
α_2AP (U/mL)	0.85 (0.55–1.15)	1.00 (0.70–1.30)*	1.00 (0.76–1.24)*	1.08 (0.76–1.40)*	1.11 (0.83–1.39)*	1.02 (0.68–1.36)
PAI-1 (U/mL)	6.4 (2.0–15.1)	2.3 (0.0–8.1)*	3.4 (0.0–8,8)*	7.2 (1.0–15.3)	8.1 (6.0–13.0)	3.6 (0.0–11.0)
			Healthy Premature Infants (30–36 Weeks' Gestation)			
Plasminogen (U/mL)	1.70 (1.12–2.48)†	1.91 (1.21–2.61)†	1.81 (1.09–2.53)	2.38 (1.58–3.18)	2.75 (1.91–3.59)†	3.36 (2.48–4.24)
TPA (ng/mL)	8.48 (3.00–16.70)	3.97 (2.00–6.93)*	4.13 (2.00–7.79)*	3.31 (2.00–5.07)*	3.48 (2.00–5.85)*	4.96 (1.46–8.46)
α_2AP (U/mL)	0.78 (0.40–1.16)	0.81 (0.49–1.13)†	0.89 (0.55–1.23)†	1.06 (0.64–1.48)*	1.15 (0.77–1.53)	1.02 (0.68–1.36)
PAI-1 (U/mL)	5.4 (0.0–12.2)*†	2.5 (0.0–7.1)*	4.3 (0.0–10.9)*	4.8 (1.0–11.8)*†	4.9 (1.0–10.2)*†	3.6 (0.0–11.0)

Plasminogen units are those recommended by the Committee on Thrombolytic Agents. Values for TPA are given as nanograms per milliliter (ng/mL). For α_2AP, values are expressed as units per milliliter (U/mL), where pooled plasma contains 1.0 U/mL. Values for PAI-1 are given as units per milliliter (U/mL) where 1 unit of PAI-1 activity is defined as the amount of PAI-1 that inhibits the one international unit of human single chain TPA.

TPA = tissue plasminogen activator; α_2AP = α_2–antiplasmin; PAI–1 = plasminogen activator inhibitor 1.

*Values indistinguishable from those of adults.

†Values different from those of full-term infants.

From Andrew M, Paes B, Johnston M: Development of the hemostatic system in the neonate and young infant. Am J Pediatr Hematol Oncol 1990; 12:95–104.

TABLE 5–7. Reference Values for Coagulation Tests in Healthy Children Aged 1 to 16 Years Compared with Adults

Coagulation Tests	1–5 Years	6–10 Years	11–16 Years	Adult
PT (sec)	11 (10.6–11.4)	11.1 (10.1–12.1)	11.2 (10.2–12.0)	12 (11.0–14.0)
PT (INR)	1.0 (0.96–1.04)	1.01 (0.91–1.11)	1.02 (0.93–1.10)	1.10 (1.0–1.3)
APTT (sec)	30 (24–36)	31 (26–36)	32 (26–37)	33 (27–40)
Fibrinogen (g/L)	2.76 (1.70–4.05)	2.79 (1.57–4.0)	3.0 (1.54–4.48)	2.78 (1.56–4.0)
Bleeding time (min)	6 (2.5–10)*	7 (2.5–13)*	5 (3–8)*	4 (1–7)
Factor II (U/mL)	0.94 (0.71–1.16)*	0.88 (0.67–1.07)	0.83 (0.61–1.04)*	1.08 (0.70–1.46)
Factor V (U/mL)	1.03 (0.79–1.27)	0.90 (0.63–1.16)*	0.77 (0.55–0.99)*	1.06 (0.62–1.50)
Factor VII (U/mL)	0.82 (0.55–1.16)	0.85 (0.52–1.20)	0.83 (0.58–1.15)*	1.05 (0.67–1.43)
Factor VIII (U/mL)	0.90 (0.59–1.42)	0.95 (0.58–1.32)	0.92 (0.53–1.31)	0.99 (0.50–1.49)
VWF (U/mL)	0.82 (0.60–1.20)	0.95 (0.44–1.44)	1.00 (0.46–1.53)	0.92 (0.50–1.58)
Factor IX (U/mL)	0.73 (0.47–1.04)	0.75 (0.63–0.89)*	0.82 (0.59–1.22)*	1.09 (0.55–1.63)
Factor X (U/mL)	0.88 (0.58–1.16)	0.75 (0.55–1.01)*	0.79 (0.50–1.17)*	1.06 (0.70–1.52)
Factor XI (U/mL)	0.97 (0.56–1.50)	0.86 (0.52–1.20)	0.74 (0.50–0.97)	0.97 (0.67–1.27)
Factor XII (U/mL)	0.93 (0.64–1.29)	0.92 (0.60–1.40)	0.81 (0.34–1.37)*	1.08 (0.52–1.64)
PK (U/mL)	0.95 (0.65–1.30)	0.99 (0.66–1.31)	0.99 (0.53–1.45)	1.12 (0.62–1.62)
HMWK (U/mL)	0.98 (0.64–1.32)	0.93 (0.60–1.30)	0.91 (0.63–1.19)	0.92 (0.50–1.36)
Factor XIIIa (U/mL)	1.08 (0.72–1.43)	1.09 (0.65–1.51)*	0.99 (0.57–1.40)	1.05 (0.55–1.55)
Factor XIIIb (U/mL)	1.13 (0.69–1.56)	1.16 (0.77–1.54)*	1.02 (0.60–1.43)	0.97 (0.57–1.37)

All factors except fibrinogen are expressed as units per milliliter (U/mL), where pooled plasma contains 1.0 U/mL. All data are expressed as the mean followed by the upper and lower boundary encompassing 95% of the population. Between 20 and 50 samples were assayed for each value for each age group. Some measurements were skewed owing to a disproportionate number of high values. The lower limit, which excludes the lower 2.5% of the population, has been given.

*Values significantly different from those of adults.

From Andrew M, Vegh P, Johnston M, et al: Maturation of the hemostatic system during childhood. Blood 1992; 80:1998–2005.

decreased in the presence of endothelial cell surfaces, but not to the same extent as that in plasma from adults.[78]

DIRECT INHIBITORS OF THROMBIN

Thrombin is directly inhibited by AT, heparin cofactor II, and α_2-macroglobulin. α_2-Macroglobulin is a more important inhibitor of thrombin in plasmas from newborns than it is in plasmas from adults.[112] α_2-Macroglobulin compensates, in part, for the low levels of AT in newborns, even in the presence of endothelial cell

surfaces (Fig. 5–3).[112, 113] In addition, a circulating physiologic anticoagulant in cord blood has properties similar to those of the glycosaminoglycans dermatan sulfate.[74] The fetal proteoglycan is present in plasma in concentrations of 0.29 µg/mL, has a molecular weight of 150,000, and catalyzes thrombin inhibition by means of the natural inhibitor heparin cofactor II.[67, 69] The fetal anticoagulant also is present in plasma from pregnant women and is produced by the placenta.[114] The length of time that the fetal anticoagulant circulates in newborns is not known; however, it is still present during the first week

TABLE 5–8. Reference Values for the Inhibitors of Coagulation in Healthy Children Aged 1 to 16 Years Compared with Adults

Inhibitors	1–5 Years	6–10 Years	11–16 Years	Adult
AT (U/mL)	1.11 (0.82–1.39)	1.11 (0.90–1.31)	1.05 (0.77–1.32)	1.0 (0.74–1.26)
α_2M (U/mL)	1.69 (1.14–2.23)*	1.69 (1.28–2.09)*	1.56 (0.98–2.12)*	0.86 (0.52–1.20)
C_1E-INH (U/mL)	1.35 (0.85–1.83)*	1.14 (0.88–1.54)	1.03 (0.68–1.50)	1.0 (0.71–1.31)
α_1AT (U/mL)	0.93 (0.39–1.47)	1.00 (0.69–1.30)	1.01 (0.65–1.37)	0.93 (0.55–1.30)
HCII (U/mL)	0.88 (0.48–1.28)*	0.86 (0.40–1.32)*	0.91 (0.53–1.29)*	1.08 (0.66–1.26)
Protein C (U/mL)	0.66 (0.40–0.92)*	0.69 (0.45–0.93)*	0.83 (0.55–1.11)*	0.96 (0.64–1.28)
Protein S				
Total (U/mL)	0.86 (0.54–1.18)	0.78 (0.41–1.14)	0.72 (0.52–0.92)	0.81 (0.60–1.13)
Free (U/mL)	0.45 (0.21–0.69)	0.42 (0.22–0.62)	0.38 (0.26–0.55)	0.45 (0.27–0.61)

All values are expressed in units per milliliter (U/mL), where for all factors pooled plasma contains 1.0 U/mL, with the exception of free protein S which contains a mean of 0.4 U/mL. All values are given as a mean, followed by the lower and upper boundary encompassing 95% of the population. Between 20 and 30 samples were assayed for each value for each age group. Some measurements were skewed owing to a disproportionate number of high values.

*Values significantly different from those of adults.

From Andrew M, Vegh P, Johnston M, et al: Maturation of the hemostatic system during childhood. Blood 1992; 80:1998–2005.

TABLE 5–9. Reference Values for the Fibrinolytic System in Healthy Children Aged 1 to 16 Years Compared with Adults

Fibrinolytic System	1–5 Years	6–10 Years	11–16 Years	Adult
Plasminogen (U/mL)	0.98 (0.78–1.18)	0.92 (0.75–1.08)	0.86 (0.68–1.03)*	0.99 (0.77–1.22)
TPA (ng/mL)	2.15 (1.0–4.5)*	2.42 (1.0–5.0)*	2.16 (1.0–4.0)*	4.90 (1.40–8.40)
α_2AP (U/mL)	1.05 (0.93–1.17)	0.99 (0.89–1.10)	0.98 (0.78–1.18)	1.02 (0.68–1.36)
PAI-1 (U/mL)	5.42 (1.0–10.0)	6.79 (2.0–12.0)*	6.07 (2.0–10.0)	3.60 (0–11.0)

Plasminogen units are those recommended by the Committee on Thrombolytic Agents. Values for TPA are given as nanograms/milliliter (ng/mL). For α_2AP, values are expressed as units per milliliter (U/mL), where pooled plasma contains 1.0 U/mL. Values for PAI-1 are given as units per milliliter (U/mL) where 1 unit of PAI-1 activity is defined as the amount of PAI-1 that inhibits 1 IU of human single-chain TPA. All values are given as mean followed by the lower and upper boundary encompassing 95% of the population.

*Values significantly different from those of adults.

From Andrew M, Vegh P, Johnston M, et al: Maturation of the hemostatic system during childhood. Blood 1992; 80:1998–2005.

of life in sick premature infants with respiratory distress syndrome (RDS). Despite these differences, the rate of inhibition of thrombin is still slower in newborns than it is in adults.[112]

PROTEIN C/PROTEIN S SYSTEM

A second mechanism for inhibiting thrombin coagulant activity is the *protein C/protein S system*. When thrombin binds to the endothelial cell surface receptor thrombomodulin, it no longer cleaves fibrinogen or factors V and VIII, nor does it activate platelets. However, it can change the VK-dependent inhibitor protein C to its activated form, which, in the presence of protein S, inactivates factors Va and VIIIa by proteolytic degradation. At birth, plasma concentrations of protein C are very low, and they remain decreased during the first 6 months of life.[1–3] The single-chain form of protein C in neonatal plasma is increased twofold compared with the double-chain form, which is prominent in adults. Animal data suggest that glycosylation in fetal protein C is increased compared with that in adults. Despite these changes there is no evidence that protein C is functionally different in newborns.[115, 116] Although total amounts of protein S are decreased at birth, functional activity is similar to that in the adult because protein S is completely present in the free, active form owing to the absence of C4 binding protein.[117, 118] Further, the interaction of protein S with acti-

vated protein C in plasma from newborns may be regulated by the increased levels of α_2-macroglobulin.[119] Plasma concentrations of thrombomodulin are increased in early childhood and decrease to adult values by the late teenage years; however, the influence of age on endothelial cell expression of thrombomodulin has not been determined.[120–124] Whether the overall activity of the protein C/protein S system varies with age is unknown.

TISSUE FACTOR PATHWAY INHIBITOR

Tissue factor pathway inhibitor (TFPI) effects a third mechanism regulating the generation of thrombin. A TFPI/factor Xa complex binds to factor VIIa/tissue factor in a factor Xa calcium-dependent reaction that results in the inhibition of factor VIIa. After the generation of small amounts of thrombin, TFPI prevents further generation of thrombin via tissue factor/factor VIIa. Total TFPI levels in newborns are reported to be similar to levels in older children or adults. The free TFPI level is reported to be significantly lower in newborns.[125]

REGULATION OF THROMBIN BY FIBRIN

The capacity of fibrin clots from newborns to bind thrombin has been assessed through the measurement of fibrinopeptide A (FPA) production.[126] Clots from cord blood plasma generate significantly less FPA than do clots

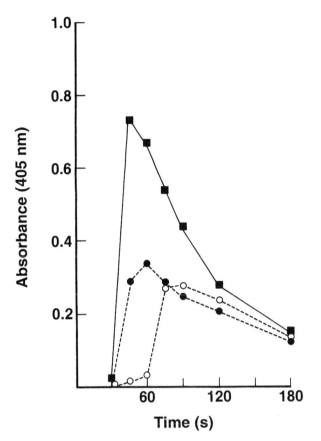

FIGURE 5–2. Thrombin generation after activation in the partial thromboplastin system was significantly decreased in plasma from full-term infants on day 1 of life *(solid circles)* and in that from premature infants on day 1 of life *(open circles)* compared with that from adults *(solid squares)*. The amount of thrombin generated was determined on the basis of its ability to cleave a chromogenic substrate, which results in a change in the absorbance reading at 405 nm.

from adult blood plasma[126] because of the decreased plasma concentrations of prothrombin in cord blood plasma.[126] This observation suggests that thrombi in newborns may not have the same propensity to propagate as do thrombi in adult patients.

Physiologic Mechanisms

Potential mechanisms explaining the physiologically different plasma concentrations of coagulation proteins at birth include decreased production, accelerated clearance, and activation at birth.

PRODUCTION

Messenger ribonucleic acid (mRNA) levels have been measured for factors VII, VIII, IX, and X, fibrinogen, AT, and protein C in hepatocytes from 5- to 10-week-old human embryos, fetuses, and adults.[127] Embryonic-fetal transcripts and adult mRNAs were similar in size, and the nucleotide sequences of mRNA for factors IX and X were identical.[128] However, the expression of mRNA was variable, with adult values existing for some coagulation proteins but decreased expression for others (Fig. 5–4). Similar concentrations of prothrombin mRNA were

found in the livers of newborn and adult rabbits[129]; another study reported lower prothrombin mRNA concentrations in sheep.[127]

CLEARANCE

Fibrinogen, whether of fetal or adult origin, is cleared more rapidly in newborn lambs than it is in sheep.[130] Similarly, clearance of fibrinogen is accelerated in premature infants with or without RDS.[131] Antithrombin survival times are shorter in healthy infants who require exchange transfusion than they are in adults.[132] An increased basal metabolic rate in the young probably contributes to the accelerated clearance of proteins.[133] Although activation of the coagulation system occurs at birth,[82, 83, 134] it does not account for low concentrations of some coagulation proteins.[135–137]

ACTIVATION

Activation of coagulation *in vivo*, with the generation of thrombin, can be quantitated by specific activation peptides. Increased plasma concentrations of FPA and thrombin/AT complexes in cord plasma suggest that coagulation is activated at birth.[67, 69, 112, 138] However, this process seems to be well controlled and self-limited. Indeed, activation of coagulation during the birth process does not result in significant consumption of circulating plasma coagulation proteins nor clinical morbidity.[82, 83]

THE FIBRINOLYTIC SYSTEM

Age and Components of the Fibrinolytic System

Although plasmin is generated and inhibited similarly in infants and adults, important differences do exist.[1] In newborns, plasminogen levels are only 50 percent of adult values, α_2-antiplasmin levels are 80 percent of adult values, and plasma concentrations of plasminogen activator inhibitor (PAI) 1 and tissue plasminogen activator (TPA) are significantly greater than adult levels.[1–3, 10, 99–107, 139–141] Increased levels of TPA and PAI–1 found on day 1 of life contrast markedly with values from cord blood, in which concentrations of these two proteins are significantly lower than they are in adults.[139–141] The discrepancy between newborn and cord plasma concentrations of TPA and PAI–1 can be explained by the enhanced release of TPA and PAI–1 from the endothelium shortly after birth. PAI–2 levels are detectable in cord blood but are significantly lower than they are in pregnant women.[142] Plasminogen, like fibrinogen, has a fetal form. Fetal plasminogen exists in two glycoforms that have increased amounts of mannose and sialic acid.[143] The enzymatic activity of "fetal plasmin" and its binding to cellular receptors for fetal plasminogen are decreased.

Influence of Age on Endogenous Regulation of Fibrinolysis

Short whole-blood clotting times, short euglobulin lysis times, and increased plasma concentrations of the

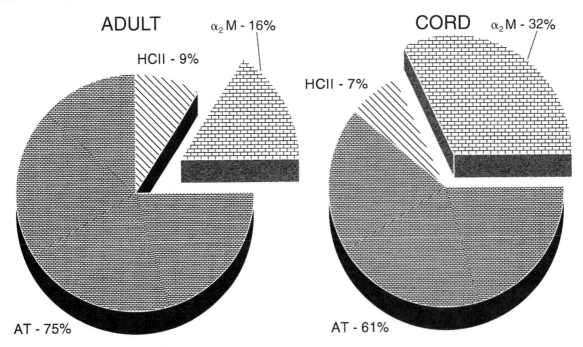

FIGURE 5–3. Percentage of ^{125}I-labeled thrombin complexed with inhibitors in pooled plasma from adults and newborns. In adult plasma, antithrombin (AT) inhibits 75 percent of the complexed thrombin, whereas α_2-macroglobulin (α_2M) and heparin cofactor II (HCII) inhibit only 16 and 9 percent, respectively. In newborn plasma, α_2M inhibits 32 percent of the complexed thrombin, whereas AT and HCII inhibit 61 and 7 percent, respectively.

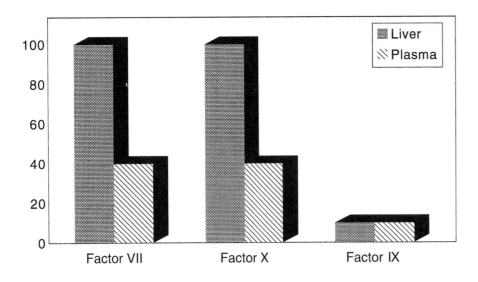

FIGURE 5–4. Concentrations of coagulation factors VII, IX, and X at 7 to 8 weeks' gestation in liver and plasma. Values are expressed as a percentage of adult levels. Interpretation: Liver and plasma values are similar for factor IX but are discordant for factors VII and X, indicating that multiple regulation mechanisms influence the ontogenic biologic availability of coagulation proteins.

Bβ15–42 fibrin-related peptides all suggest that the fibrinolytic system is activated at birth.[2, 140] At the same time, the capacity of the fetal fibrinolytic system to generate plasmin in response to stimulation by a thrombolytic agent is decreased compared with that of adults[144]; this reflects low levels of plasminogen.[2, 140]

HEMORRHAGIC DISORDERS

Although acquired disorders are more commonly seen, severe forms of congenital factor deficiencies often present first in early infancy and should be seriously considered in otherwise healthy infants who are seen with bleeding.[10, 100–105, 145]

Clinical Presentation

The clinical presentation of bleeding disorders is different in newborns than it is in children and adults. Bleeding may appear as oozing from the umbilicus, bleeding into the scalp, large cephalohematomas, bleeding after circumcision, bleeding from peripheral sites from which blood samples have been obtained, and bleeding into the skin. A small but important proportion of infants are seen with an intracranial hemorrhage (ICH) as the first manifestation of their bleeding tendency.[146–152] Sick infants can bleed from mucous membranes, the bladder, and sites of invasive procedures. Joint bleeding is rare. The most common causes of bleeding in healthy infants are thrombocytopenia resulting from transplacental passage of a maternal antiplatelet antibody or sepsis, VK deficiency, and congenital coagulation factor deficiencies.

Laboratory Evaluation

In addition to a workup for sepsis, the laboratory evaluation of infants with bleeding complications should include determination of PT, APTT, thrombin clotting time, fibrinogen level, and platelet count, and possibly screening for primary hemostasis with the PFA–100 or a similar system. Abnormalities in test results usually prompt additional tests, such as specific factor assays and paracoagulation tests. For a male child in whom hemophilia A or B is suspected, specific factor assays should be performed regardless of the APTT value. Screening tests are not prolonged in the presence of deficiencies of factor XIII and α_2-antiplasmin. These must be measured directly if deficiencies are suspected.

Management

The appropriate management of an infant with a hemorrhagic disorder depends on the correct identification of the hemostatic defect. This information allows replacement therapy with specific factor concentrates, fresh frozen plasma (FFP), stored plasma, platelet concentrates, or cryoprecipitate.

QUANTITATIVE PLATELET DISORDERS

General Information

Healthy infants have the same platelet counts as adults do,[10, 16] whereas premature infants have platelet counts that are slightly lower but still within the normal adult range (150×10^9 to 450×10^9/L).[10–12] The definition of thrombocytopenia in newborns is the same as that in adults: a platelet count less than 150×10^9/L. Studies of fetuses between 18 and 30 weeks' gestation show a stable platelet count of approximately 250×10^9/L.[19] Consequently, platelet counts less than 150×10^9/L are abnormal and indicate the need for investigation and, sometimes, treatment. Mean volumes of platelets in newborns are similar to those of adults, with values less than 10 fL (range, 7 to 9 fL).[14–16] Postnatally, mean platelet volumes increase slightly over the first 2 weeks of life, concomitantly with an increase in platelet count.[17, 18]

Epidemiology

Thrombocytopenia is the most common hemostatic abnormality in newborns admitted to neonatal intensive care units.[11, 13–15, 153] A single prospective cohort study[15] and five retrospective reviews[14, 154–157] have provided the most reliable information on the occurrence, natural history, mechanisms, and clinical impact of thrombocytopenia in newborns. There is general agreement that thrombocytopenia indicates the presence of an underlying pathologic process; however, the clinical relevance of mild thrombocytopenia remains to be proved. Approximately

22 percent of infants admitted into neonatal intensive care units of tertiary hospitals develop thrombocytopenia.[15] For some infants, the thrombocytopenia is trivial, with platelet counts being between 100 and 150×10^9/L. However, for 50 percent of affected infants, platelet counts decrease to less than 100×10^9/L, and for 20 percent of infants platelet counts are less than 50×10^9/L.[15] The natural history of thrombocytopenia in sick newborns is remarkably consistent[15]: it is present by day 2 of life in 75 percent of infants, reaches a nadir by day 4 in 75 percent of infants, and recovers to more than 150×10^9/L by day 10 of life in 86 percent of infants.[15, 156]

Pathogenesis

Thrombocytopenia can be caused by decreased platelet production, increased platelet destruction, platelet pooling in an enlarged spleen, or a combination of these mechanisms. Characterization of mechanisms responsible for thrombocytopenia is important because these mechanisms have practical implications in assessing the risk of bleeding and its management. Increased platelet destruction is the mechanism responsible for thrombocytopenia in most infants,[15, 20] whereas splenic sequestration contributes to thrombocytopenia in some infants.[20]

At autopsy, thrombocytopenic infants have megakaryocyte numbers similar to those of nonthrombocytopenic infants.[15] The strongest evidence of platelet consumption comes from uniformly short survival times of radiolabeled platelets in thrombocytopenic infants.[15, 20, 34] Hypersplenism also is present in some infants.[20]

Increased Platelet Destruction

Thrombocytopenia due to increased platelet destruction can be considered as a nonimmune or an immune event. Common nonimmune causes of thrombocytopenia include sepsis with or without disseminated intravascular coagulation (DIC) and exchange transfusion.[15] Exchange transfusions and intrauterine transfusions cause thrombocytopenia by a dilutional effect that depends on the amount of blood transfused.[156, 158] After an exchange transfusion, platelet counts increase within 3 days and reach preexchange levels by about 7 days.[100]

IMMUNE THROMBOCYTOPENIA

Immune thrombocytopenia is defined as an increased rate of platelet clearance caused by platelet-associated immunoglobulin G (IgG) or complement. Idiopathic thrombocytopenic purpura is not diagnosed by elevated platelet-associated IgG levels, but they are associated with a variety of thrombocytopenic disorders. For reasons that are not clear, 50 percent of infants with platelet counts less than 100×10^9/L have increased amounts of platelet-associated IgG on their platelets.[157, 159] Specific disorders associated with platelet-associated IgG are neonatal sepsis,[159] preeclampsia,[160] maternal idiopathic thrombocytopenic purpura, and neonatal alloimmune thrombocytopenia.

DISEASE STATES ASSOCIATED WITH PLATELET CONSUMPTION

Neonatal thrombocytopenia is associated with many pathologic states (Table 5–10).[11–13, 100] Acute asphyxia is a consistent cause of DIC and thrombocytopenia.[21] Chronic hypoxia is associated with placental dysfunction and intrauterine growth retardation and also with significant thrombocytopenia.[159] Both viral (rubella, herpesvirus, echovirus, *Toxoplasma*, cytomegalovirus, and human immunodeficiency virus) and bacterial infections cause severe thrombocytopenia.[161] Mechanisms responsible for bacterial sepsis–induced thrombocytopenia are multifactorial and include consumption resulting from DIC, endothelial damage, platelet aggregation caused by binding of bacterial products to platelet membranes, immune-mediated thrombocytopenia, and decreased production due to marrow infection.[162] Mechanisms responsible for thrombocytopenia caused by viruses include loss of sialic acid from platelet membranes due to viral neur-

TABLE 5–10. Etiology of Thrombocytopenia

INCREASED DESTRUCTION
Immune-Mediated
Maternal idiopathic thrombocytopenic purpura
Maternal systemic lupus erythematosus
Maternal hyperthyroidism
Maternal drugs
Maternal preeclampsia
Neonatal alloimmune thrombocytopenia

Non-Immune-Mediated (Probably Related to DIC)
Asphyxia
Perinatal aspiration
Necrotizing enterocolitis
Hemangiomas
Neonatal thrombosis
Respiratory distress syndrome

Unknown
Hyperbilirubinemia
Phototherapy
Polycythemia
Rh hemolytic disease
Congenital thrombotic thrombocytopenic purpura
Total parenteral nutrition
Inborn errors of metabolism
Wiskott-Aldrich syndrome
Multiple congenital anomalies

HYPERSPLENISM
DECREASED PRODUCTION OF PLATELETS
Bone Marrow Replacement Disorders
Congenital leukemia
Congenital leukemoid reactions
Neuroblastoma
Histiocytosis
Osteopetrosis

Bone Marrow Aplasia
Thrombocyopenia with absence of the radius
Amegakaryocytic thrombocytopenia
Fanconi anemia
Other marrow hypoplastic or aplastic disorders

DIC = disseminated intravascular coagulation.

aminidase, intravascular platelet aggregation, and degeneration of megakaryocytes. Congenital rubella causes thrombocytopenia in three quarters of infants with platelet counts ranging from 20 to 60×10^9/L for the first 4 to 8 weeks of life. For premature infants, thrombocytopenia often complicates other disorders such as RDS, persistent pulmonary hypertension, necrotizing enterocolitis, conditions associated with preeclampsia, and hyperbilirubinemia treated with phototherapy.[158] Activation of coagulation with platelet consumption occurs in RDS, and mechanical ventilation may be an independent factor contributing to thrombocytopenia.[163] Persistent pulmonary hypertension in newborns may be due in part to intrapulmonary platelet aggregation and the release of platelet-derived vasoactive substances such as thromboxane A_2.[164] These infants are frequently thrombocytopenic and, at autopsy, have pulmonary microthrombi. Necrotizing enterocolitis is characterized by bloody stools, vomiting of bile-stained gastric residue, and abdominal distention. Approximately half of the affected infants are thrombocytopenic, with about 20 percent having laboratory evidence of DIC. Both hyperbilirubinemia and phototherapy are associated with mild thrombocytopenia in newborn humans and shortened platelet survival in rabbits.[20] When platelets are exposed to a broad-spectrum blue fluorescent light *in vitro,* aggregation is decreased and microscopic alterations in granules and external membranes occur.

GIANT HEMANGIOMAS

Giant hemangiomas, or Kasabach-Merritt syndrome (see Chapter 45),[165–168] cause a local consumptive coagulopathy characterized by hypofibrinogenemia, elevated levels of fibrinogen-fibrin degradation products, microangiopathic fragmentation of red cells, and thrombocytopenia.[169] The thrombocytopenia is usually severe, with platelet counts of less than 50×10^9/L.[170] Approximately 50 percent of affected infants experience systemic bleeding during the first month of life.[170]

DRUG-INDUCED THROMBOCYTOPENIA

Transplacental passage of drugs and drug-dependent antibodies can result in both maternal and neonatal thrombocytopenia.[26] However, these causes are rare, and the evidence for them is weak.[171–175] Agents implicated are quinine, hydralazine, tolbutamide, and thiazide diuretics. Heparin has been identified as a cause of thrombocytopenia. If heparin-induced thrombocytopenia is suspected, heparin therapy should be discontinued immediately and alternative forms of anticoagulation therapy considered if necessary (see Chapter 40).

OTHER ASSOCIATIONS

Thrombocytopenia is loosely associated with thromboembolic complications and polycythemia in infants with hematocrits greater than 0.70. However, thrombocytopenia may also indicate the presence of other concurrent disease processes. Infants with a familial form of hemolytic-uremic syndrome or thrombotic thrombocytopenic purpura have a schistocytic hemolytic anemia in association with transient neurologic or renal abnormalities.[176]

Decreased Platelet Production

Thrombocytopenia due to decreased platelet production is rare, accounting for less than 5 percent of thrombocytopenic infants (Table 5–10).[11–13, 100] Causes in neonates include congenital leukemia, congenital leukemoid reactions with Down syndrome, neuroblastoma, histiocytosis, some viral infections, osteopetrosis, and disorders causing bone marrow failure.

APLASTIC DISORDERS
(see Chapter 7)

Aplastic disorders include thrombocytopenia absent radius syndrome and amegakaryocytic thrombocytopenia (Chapter 7).[177, 178] Infants with aplastic disorders have the greatest risk of serious bleeding in the form of ICH in the first months of life. Neither splenectomy nor steroids are beneficial for infants with this syndrome.[177, 178] Platelet transfusions are highly effective but should be reserved for symptomatic infants because prophylactic platelet transfusions could result in refractoriness due to alloimmunization.[178] By several months of age, increased numbers of megakaryocytes usually appear in the bone marrow, and platelet counts increase.[177, 178] A functional platelet defect may be present in some children with thrombocytopenia absent radius syndrome.[179] Isolated amegakaryocytic thrombocytopenia with normal radii and other rare reports of inherited forms of thrombocytopenia may present with bleeding during the newborn period[180] and develop into complete aplastic anemia.

Hypersplenism

Decreased recovery of ^{111}In oxine-labeled platelets (fewer than 40 to 50 percent) indicates that increased splenic sequestration is a cause of thrombocytopenia.[20] Thrombocytopenia resulting from hypersplenism is usually mild, with platelet counts ranging from 50×10^9 to 100×10^9/L.

Clinical Impact of Neonatal Thrombocytopenia

Clinically important bleeding is less likely to occur in patients with consumptive disorders than in patients with a regenerative thrombocytopenia. The bleeding risk is increased in patients who have both thrombocytopenia and a platelet function defect. The choice of a platelet count at which one should intervene, although a simplistic response, provides a guideline for therapy. A platelet count less than 50×10^9/L places some otherwise healthy full-term newborns at risk for serious ICH.[181] The importance of "moderate" thrombocytopenia (platelet counts between 50×10^9 and 100×10^9/L) in sick premature infants has been a subject of controversy. A randomized, controlled trial assessed the potential benefits of platelet concentrate transfusions in 154 premature thrombocytopenic infants during the first 72 hours of life.[182]

Treated infants received platelet concentrates to maintain platelet counts greater than 150×10^9/L. No beneficial effect on the incidence or extension of ICH was shown in this study, which was designed to detect an effect of 25 percent or greater.[182] However, infants who had received transfusions had shortened bleeding times and required significantly less blood product support.

Treatment

The management of thrombocytopenic infants depends in part on the underlying disorder. If an infant is bleeding, a trial of platelet concentrates (10 to 20 mL/kg) is indicated. The increased platelet count usually shortens the bleeding time and is frequently clinically effective.[35] Autoimmune and alloimmune thrombocytopenias do not respond to random donor platelet concentrates and require specific forms of therapy.

Autoimmune and Alloimmune Thrombocytopenia

Immune thrombocytopenia should always be suspected in otherwise healthy infants with isolated severe thrombocytopenia. The differentiation of autoimmune thrombocytopenia from alloimmune thrombocytopenia in neonates is critical because the management and severity of these disorders are quite different. Chapter 44 discusses these two forms of immune thrombocytopenia in detail.

Thrombocytosis

Elevated platelet counts are frequently observed in premature infants at approximately 4 to 6 weeks after birth.[183] There are no clinical manifestations of neonatal thrombocytosis, and therapeutic intervention is not indicated.

QUALITATIVE PLATELET DISORDERS

Despite the physiologic hyporeactivity of neonatal platelets in response to exposure to some agents, healthy infants do not have an increased risk of bleeding. Pathologic impairment of platelet function may occur, to a variable extent, as a result of the use of certain drugs or the presence of pathologic states in either mothers or infants. In mothers, these causative factors include the use of some drugs,[183] diabetes,[184–187] dietary abnormalities,[188–194] smoking,[195–197] and ethanol abuse[198]; in infants, they include the use of some drugs, perinatal aspiration syndrome,[156, 158, 199–201] hyperbilirubinemia,[202, 203] phototherapy,[203, 204] renal failure,[205] and hepatic failure.

Aspirin

Salicylate crosses the placenta and can be detected in fetuses after maternal ingestion.[171–174, 206–210] Clearance of salicylate is slower in newborns than it is in adults, and thus infants have a potential risk for bleeding for a longer period of time.[172] However, *in vitro* studies have not demonstrated an additive effect of aspirin on platelets of newborns,[53, 208] and evidence linking maternal aspirin ingestion to clinically important bleeding in newborns is weak.[174, 211–214] There is little reason to have serious concerns about maternal ingestion of aspirin, but it is reasonable to advise mothers not to ingest aspirin unless specifically indicated by their physician.

Indomethacin

Indomethacin is an antiplatelet agent used for nonsurgical closure of a patent ductus arteriosus in premature infants.[215–217] Indomethacin, like salicylate, has a longer half-life in newborns than in adults (21 to 24 hours and 2 to 3 hours, respectively).[218] This is probably due to underdevelopment of hepatic drug metabolism or renal excretory function or to altered protein binding.[219, 220] Indomethacin inhibits platelet function in newborns, as shown by prolongation of bleeding times.[36, 221, 222] Randomized, controlled trials have provided conflicting conclusions on the effect of indomethacin on intraventricular hemorrhage in premature infants.[223]

Maternal Diabetes

The reactivity of platelets from diabetic mothers and their infants is increased, with enhanced thromboxane B_2 production, enhanced platelet aggregation,[186, 224] and a lower threshold to many aggregating agents.[225] The enhanced platelet function in diabetes is associated with increased synthesis of a PGE-like material that crosses the placenta and can affect the fetus.[226] The evidence linking enhanced platelet reactivity to thromboembolic complications in newborns is weak.[227, 228]

Diet

Alterations in the diet of mothers or infants during the postnatal period can affect newborn platelet function. Increases in the ratio of polyunsaturated fatty acids to saturated fatty acids in the diet of mothers who breast-feed their infants result in increases in the concentration of linoleic acid and enhance thromboxane B_2 production.[188] Infants receiving a diet deficient in essential fatty acids may have arachidonic acid depletion and platelet dysfunction.[190, 191, 229] Vitamin E functions as an antioxidant and as an inhibitor of platelet aggregation/release in humans.[192–194, 230, 231] Instances of vitamin E–deficient infants with increased platelet aggregation that reversed after vitamin E supplementation have been reported.[194, 232]

Amniotic Fluid

Amniotic fluid contains procoagulant activity that enhances the generation of thromboxane A_2 by platelets.[158, 199–201] Infants who develop a perinatal aspiration syndrome have pulmonary hypertension characterized by platelet thrombi in the pulmonary microcirculation. The exact mechanism or mechanisms leading to persistent pulmonary hypertension in these infants is unknown; however, alterations in PG synthesis,[194, 233] as well as in thrombocytopenia, hypoxia, and acidosis, have been suggested.[14, 158, 199–201]

Nitric Oxide

Nitric oxide prevents adhesion of platelets to endothelial cells and inhibits ADP-induced aggregation of cord platelets in a manner similar to that in adults.[234–237]

CONGENITAL FACTOR DEFICIENCIES

For most hemostatic components, both severe and mild forms of deficiency can occur, with severe deficiencies often characterized by significant bleeding in newborns. Chapters 41 and 42 discuss congenital factor deficiencies in detail.

General Information

INHERITANCE

Deficiencies of factors II, FV, FVII, FXI, and FXII, prekallikrein, and high-molecular-weight kininogen are rare, autosomally inherited disorders, with consanguinity present in many families. Deficiencies of factor XII, prekallikrein, and high-molecular-weight kininogen do not result in hemorrhagic complications and thus are not considered further. Deficiencies of factors VIII and IX are sex-linked and are the most common congenital bleeding disorders in newborns. Rarely, combined deficiencies of factors II, VII, IX, and or of factors V and VIII present in the neonatal period.[238, 239] Tests are available to diagnose most congenital factor deficiencies prenatally so that either termination of pregnancy or management of affected infants can be planned (see Chapters 41 and 42).

CLINICAL PRESENTATION

The majority of newborns with congenital coagulation factor deficiencies do not present with bleeding in the perinatal period unless a hemostatic challenge is present. On the other hand, unexplained bleeding in an otherwise healthy newborn should be carefully investigated because it may reflect the presentation of a congenital coagulation factor deficiency. With few exceptions, only severe forms of congenital coagulation factor deficiencies are manifested by bleeding in newborns. The most common sites of bleeding include the penis (i.e., after circumcision), umbilical cord, central nervous system (ICH), scalp, and heel (i.e., after peripheral heel sticks).

ICH is rare in full-term newborns and usually occurs either spontaneously or after a insults such as birth asphyxia or trauma, VK deficiency, and several congenital factor deficiencies. Other risk factors include small birth weight, young GA, and race.[240–248] In a review of 75 cases of factor VII deficiency, 12 (16 percent) patients had an ICH. ICH occurred in the first week of life in 5 of these 12 patients, and in the first year of life in 9 of them. The risk of ICH in children with severe hemophilia A or B ranges from 2 to 8 percent. The location of the ICH is most commonly the subarachnoid area, but subdural and parenchymal bleeding also occur. Some infants require surgical intervention, and many have long-term neurologic deficits.[240–246, 248–250]

Full-term infants with unexplained ICH should be carefully evaluated for congenital or acquired hemostatic defects.[146, 240–248] Unfortunately, the diagnosis of ICH may be delayed because of the nonspecific nature of the early clinical presentation, which includes lethargy, apnea, vomiting, and irritability. Further delays can occur when secondary coagulopathies such as DIC occur[251–254] and when plasma concentrations of the coagulation protein in question are physiologically low in newborns. The more extreme clinical presentation of ICH is usually recognized early and is characterized by seizures, meningismus, and a tense fontanelle.

Although severe deficiency of factor VIII is the most common cause of ICH from a coagulation factor deficiency,[255] severe congenital deficiencies of fibrinogen and factors II, V, VII, VIII, IX, X, XI, and XIII can also cause ICH at birth. The incidence of ICH in newborns is unknown and probably is changing, reflecting improvements in perinatal care. The widespread use of ultrasound, a safe modality for the monitoring of fetuses at risk, has resulted in the detection of ICH *in utero. In utero* factor replacement has also been accomplished in several infants.[89] Although less common than ICH, subgaleal bleeding with concurrent shock and DIC may be the initial presentation of a congenital factor deficiency.[256]

DIAGNOSIS

Unexpected congenital factor deficiencies are usually diagnosed by abnormal results for coagulation screening tests (APTT, PT, and fibrinogen) and subsequent specific coagulation protein assays. In newborns, the diagnosis of many congenital factor deficiencies based upon plasma concentrations can be difficult because plasma concentrations of several coagulation proteins are physiologically decreased at birth.[2, 3] Mild-to-moderate congenital deficiencies of prothrombin and factors V, VIII, IX, X, and XI

result in plasma concentrations that may overlap with neonatal physiologic values. In contrast, plasma concentrations resulting from either mild-to-moderate factor VII deficiency or severe deficiency of factors V, VII, VIII, IX, X, and XIII can be easily distinguished from physiologic values (see Table 5–1). Prenatal diagnosis of most congenital factor deficiencies is performed by amniocentesis or chorionic villus biopsy. The prenatal diagnosis of congenital deficiencies of specific coagulation proteins is largely confined to severe hemophilia A and B although deficiencies of factors V, VII, and XIII and VWF have also been diagnosed prenatally.[89, 257, 258] Prenatal diagnosis of VWF deficiency is only indicated for type 3 or severe VWD. Early diagnosis permits either termination of the pregnancy or early intervention when indicated (see Chapters 41 and 42).[1–3, 89, 257–259]

TREATMENT

In the presence of active bleeding or a planned hemostatic challenge, the fundamental principle of management is to increase the plasma concentration of the deficient coagulation protein to a minimal hemostatic level. The minimal hemostatic level of a particular coagulation protein varies; it depends on the protein and the nature of the hemostatic challenge (Tables 5–11 and 5–12) There are a variety of plasma products available for use (Tables 5–13 and 5–14).

Specific Coagulation Factor Deficiencies

FIBRINOGEN DEFICIENCY

Fibrinogen deficiency is rare. Bleeding due to afibrinogenemia has been reported in newborns after circumcision or as umbilical stump bleeding and soft tissue hemorrhage, with some cases being fatal. Replacement

TABLE 5–11. Properties of Coagulation Proteins

Factor	Chromosome	Molecular Weight	Plasma Concentration (μg/mL)	Half-life (hrs)	Minimal Hemostatic Level	Replacement Therapy
Factor I	4q26-q28	330,000	3000	120	0.5–1.0 g/L	FFP/cryoprecipitate, fibrinogen concentrate
Factor II	11p11-q12	72,000	100	72	0.15–0.40 U/mL	FFP/PPC
Factor V	1q21-q25	330,000	10	12–36	0.10–0.25 U/mL	FFP
Factor VII	13q34	50,000	0.5	4–6	0.05–0.10 U/mL	Factor VII concentrate, PCC/FF
Factor VIII	Xq28	330,000	0.1	12–15	0.30–0.50 U/mL	Factor VIII concentrate
Factor IX	Xq27	56,000	5	18–30	0.20–0.50 U/mL	Factor IX concentrate, PCC
Factor X	13q34	58,800	10	65	0.10–0.20 U/mL	PCC/FFP
Factor XI	4q32-q35	160,000	5	65	0.10–0.30 U/mL	Factor XI concentrate, FFP
Factor XIII	a: 6p24p25 b: 1q31-q32	320,000	60	72–240	0.10–0.50 U/mL	Factor XIII concentrate, cryoprecipitate, FFP
VWF	12pter-p12	309,000	5–10	12	0.30–0.50 U/mL	Factor VIII-VWF concentrate, cryoprecipitate

a = a subunit of factor XIII; b = b subunit of factor XIII; FFP = fresh frozen plasma; PCC = prothrombin complex concentrate.
Adapted from Andrew M, Brooker LA: Blood component therapy in neonatal hemostatic disorders. Transfus Med Rev 1995; 9:231–250.

TABLE 5–12. Factor VIII and Factor IX Replacement Therapy in Children with Severe Hemophilia A and B

Type of Bleeding	Minimum Hemostatic Level	Hemophilia A (Factor VIII)	Hemophilia B (Factor IX)
Joint	30%–50%	20–40 U/kg qd usually 2 days	30–40 U/kg qd usually 2 days
Muscle	40%–50%	20–40 U/kg qd	40–60 U/kg qd
Oral mucosa	50%	25 U/kg	50 U/kg
Epistaxis	Initially 80%–100%, then 30% until resolution	40–50 U/kg, then 30–40 U/kg qd	80–100 U/kg, then 70–80 U/kg qd
Gastrointestinal	Initially 100%, then 30% until resolution	40–50 U/kg, then 30–40 U/kg qd	80–100 U/kg qd, then 70–80 U/kg qd
Hematuria	Initially 100%, then 30% until resolution	40–50 U/kg, then 30–40 U/kg qd	80–100 U/kg, then 70–80 U/kg qd
CNS	Initially 100%, then 50%–100% for 10–14 days	50 U/kg, then 25 U/kg q12h or continuous infusion	100 U/kg, then 50 U/kg q24h or continuous infusion*
Surgery	Initially 100%, then 50% until wound healing begins, then 30% until wound healing is complete	50 U/kg, then dose q12h or by continuous infusion	100 U/kg, then dose q24h or by continuous infusion*

CNS = central nervous system.
*Continuous infusion of high-purity product may be possible.
Adapted from DiMichele D, Neufeld EJ: Hemophilia. A new approach to an old disease. Hematol Oncol Clin North Am 1998; 12:1315–1344.

therapy consisted of the use of whole blood, cryoprecipitate, FFP, and fibrinogen concentrates. One fibrinogen concentrate (Haemocomplettan HS, Centeon/Aventis Behring) is available in Europe and North America. One infant, who was seen with bleeding from the umbilicus after circumcision, was treated with Gelfoam and thrombin.[260–263]

FACTOR II DEFICIENCY

Deficiency of prothrombin is very rare. Bleeding complications due to prothrombin deficiency were reported in two newborns and consisted of gastrointestinal bleeding and ICH.[264, 265] Reviews of adult patients have reported bleeding after invasive events such as circumcision and venipunctures or as soft tissue hematomas; umbilical cord bleeding or hemarthrosis was not reported.[261]

Although FFP can be used as initial therapy, factor II concentrate or prothrombin complex concentrate (PCC) is the preferred replacement product.

FACTOR V DEFICIENCY

Bleeding due to severe factor V deficiency has been reported in newborns. The clinical presentations include ICH, subdural hematoma, bleeding from the umbilical stump, gastric hemorrhage, and soft tissue hemorrhage.[266, 267] Antenatal intraventricular hemorrhage was reported in two newborns.[268] Replacement therapy included whole blood, FFP, and the application of pressure on local sites of bleeding. One infant with ICH died at 6 days of age.[89] Although thrombotic complications occur in some patients with factor V deficiency, they have not been reported in newborns.[266–270]

FACTOR VII DEFICIENCY

Severe factor VII deficiency (factor VII level < 1 percent) usually causes significant bleeding equivalent to that seen in patients with severe hemophilia. Patients with factor VII

levels greater than 5 percent generally have mild hemorrhagic episodes. The most commonly reported bleeding complication in newborns with congenital factor VII deficiency is ICH.[71–73, 271, 272] In a review of 75 patients with factor VII deficiency, ICH was observed in 12 (16 percent) patients. In 5 (41 percent) of these 12 patients, ICH occurred in the first week of life with fatal outcome.[74] Congenital factor VII deficiency may occur in infants with Dubin-Johnson syndrome[21, 77, 273] or Gilbert syndrome.[20] Bleeding episodes due to factor VII deficiency can be treated with FFP, PCC, or purified factor VIIa concentrates (Tables 5–13 and 5–14).[271–277]

In 1988, Daffos and associates[89] used fetal blood sampling to diagnose factor VII deficiency at 24 weeks' gestation, and the fetus underwent *in utero* transfusion with 200 units of factor VII concentrate at 37 weeks. The baby was born without hemorrhagic complications and did not bleed as a newborn. Although FFP or PCC can be used as initial therapy, factor VII concentrate is the replacement product of choice.

FACTOR VIII DEFICIENCY

The severity of factor VIII deficiency is determined by the plasma concentration of factor VIII, with a level of less than 1 percent being severe, 1 to 5 percent being moderate, and 5 to 50 percent being mild.[278] Severe factor VIII deficiency is the most common congenital disorder of the neonatal period. In addition, a small number of neonates with moderate and mild hemophilia are seen after a hemostatic challenge.[148, 152, 279–283] Large cohort studies have revealed that approximately 10 percent of children with hemophilia have clinical symptoms in the neonatal period.[255] An additional 40 percent are seen by 1 year of age; by 1.5 years, more than 70 percent have had a major bleeding event.[255] In less severe factor VIII deficiency, a major hemorrhage occurs in only 2.5 percent of patients by the end of the neonatal period.[255]

In approximately 50 percent of factor VIII–deficient children who have bleeding in the neonatal period, it

TABLE 5–13. Common Factor Concentrates Available in Europe and/or North America in 2001

Name	Manufacturer	Availability	
		Europe	North America
FACTOR VIII			
High-purity			
Hemofil M	Baxter	Yes	Yes
Monoclate-P	Centeon (Aventis Behring)	Yes	Yes
Recombinant			
Bioclate	Centeon (Aventis Behring)	Yes	Yes
Helixate	Centeon (Aventis Behring)	Yes	Yes
Kogenate	Bayer	Yes	Yes
Kogenate SF	Bayer	Yes	No
Recombinate	Baxter	Yes	Yes
FACTOR IX			
High-purity			
AlphaNine SD	Alpha	Yes	Yes
Berinin HS	Centeon (Aventis Behring)	Yes	No
Immunine	Baxter	Yes	No
Mononine	Centeon (Aventis Behring)	Yes	Yes
Recombinant			
BeneFIX	Genetic Institute★	Yes	Yes
FIBRINOGEN			
Haemocomplettan HS	Centeon (Aventis Behring)	Yes	Yes
FACTOR VII			
Factor VII	BioProducts Laboratory LFB France Baxter	Yes	Yes
Recombinant			
NovoSeven	NovoNordisk	Yes	Yes
FACTOR XI			
Factor XI	BioProducts Laboratory	Yes	Yes
Hemoleven	LFB France	Yes	No
FACTOR XIII			
Fibrogammin HS	Centeon (Aventis Behring)	Yes	Yes
FACTOR XIII			
	BioProducts Laboratory	Yes	No

★Distributed in Europe by Baxter.

TABLE 5–14. Factor VIII-von Willebrand Factor Concentrates

Name	Manufacturer	Availability		Method of Purification	Method of Viral Inactivation
		Europe	North America		
Alphanate	Alpha	Yes	Yes	Affinity chromatography	Solvent detergent + dry heat at 80°C for 72 hr
Haemate HS	Centeon (Aventis Behring)	Yes	No	Multiple precipitation	Pasteurization at 60°C for 10 hr
Humate P	Centeon (Aventis Behring)	No	Yes	Multiple precipitation	Pasteurization at 60°C for 10 hr
Immunate	Baxter	Yes	No	Anion exchange chromatography	Vapor heat at 60°C for 10 hr

occurred after circumcision. Almost 20 percent had intracranial bleeding.[148, 152, 251, 252, 279–293] Death may occur from neonatal bleeding.[148, 251, 252, 290] In contrast to older infants and children, bleeding into joints is extremely rare in neonates.[294] Severe factor VIII deficiency can, on rare occasions, occur in female infants with clinical presentation in the neonatal period. Three female infants were reported to have bleeding from puncture sites and into the skin at birth. The levels of factor VIII were less than 0.01 unit/mL in two of these infants and 0.04 unit/mL in the third.[295, 296] Factor VIII deficiency was diagnosed in all three girls later in life, and they did not receive any form of replacement therapy at birth.

Management of bleeding due to factor VIII deficiency is discussed in detail in Chapter 41.

FACTOR IX DEFICIENCY

The severity of factor IX deficiency is identical to that of factor VIII deficiency. Diagnosis of milder forms of factor IX deficiency is complicated by physiologic levels of factor IX that can be as low as 0.15 unit/mL, and, in the rare infant, by the potential for concurrent VK deficiency. Bleeding after circumcision and ICH is described in detail in Chapter 41.[148, 152, 279, 291, 297, 298]

VON WILLEBRAND DISEASE

Although VWD is the most common congenital bleeding disorder, patients with the disease are rarely seen in the neonatal period. Plasma concentrations of VWF are increased, as is the proportion of high-molecular-weight multimers.[28, 29] Only three newborns with bleeding caused by VWD have been identified.[299–301] One infant with type IIA VWD was seen with umbilical bleeding and later with life-threatening epistaxis.[302] Two infants with type IIB VWD were seen with bleeding at blood sampling sites and in soft tissue.[299] Platelet counts were less than 50 × 10⁹/L, and the bleeding time and APTT were prolonged. The VWF multimeric structure was characterized by the absence of the high-molecular-weight forms, and the patients' platelets aggregated at much lower ristocetin concentrations than did control subjects' platelets.[299] One infant was seen on day 7 of life with an intracerebral and subdural hemorrhage.[301] The factor VIII level was 0.03 unit/mL, and the VWF/antigen and VWF/ristocetin cofactors were undetectable. This infant was treated with a factor VIII concentrate of intermediate purity at a dose of 60 units/kg twice per day for 10 days, followed by once-per-day dosing for 10 days. The bleeding stopped, and the infant's neurologic status was normal.[301]

Management of VWD is discussed in detail in Chapter 41.

FACTOR X DEFICIENCY

Five newborns with bleeding due to severe factor X deficiency have been identified.[303–307] Four of the five infants had ICH; two subsequently died, and one remained in a coma.[303] ICH was diagnosed *in utero* in one of these four infants and, despite prophylactic administration of PCC in the first months of life, the infant died as a result of ICH.[305]

Other sites of bleeding were umbilical, gastrointestinal, and intra-abdominal.[303, 304, 306] Replacement therapy included whole blood, FFP, and PCC (see Chapter 42).

FACTOR XI DEFICIENCY

Deficiency of factor XI is rare. It is different from other coagulation protein deficiencies in that bleeding symptoms do not necessarily correlate with plasma concentrations of factor XI nor do all patients bleed. Bleeding complications due to severe factor XI deficiency were reported in two newborns. One bled after circumcision at the age of 3 days and had a factor XI level of 0.07 unit/mL. In another newborn factor XI deficiency was diagnosed prenatally with bilateral subdural hemorrhage.[308–310] Either FFP or cryoprecipitate can be used for the treatment of factor XI–deficient patients if factor XI concentrate is not available.

FACTOR XIII DEFICIENCY

Severe factor XIII deficiency typically manifests at birth with bleeding from the umbilical stump or ICH.[149, 311–320] Other clinical presentations of homozygous factor XIII deficiency include delayed wound healing, abnormal scar formation, and recurrent soft tissue hemorrhage with a tendency to form hemorrhagic cysts. ICH occurs even in the absence of a trauma in approximately one third of all affected patients. Newborns with heterozygous factor XIII deficiency are not clinically affected.

FFP, cryoprecipitate, or factor XIII concentrates can be used for the treatment of factor XIII–deficient patients. Newborns with factor XIII deficiency should receive a prophylactic regimen of factor XIII because of the high incidence of ICH. Plasma concentrations of factor XIII greater than 1 percent are effective, and the very long half-life of factor XIII permits once-per-month therapy. Therefore, prophylactic replacement therapy consists of either small doses of FFP (2 to 3 mL/kg) administered every 4 to 6 weeks, cryoprecipitate at a dose of 1 bag/10 to 20 kg of weight every 3 to 6 weeks, or preferably factor XIII concentrate at a dose of 10 to 20 U/kg every 4 to 6 weeks depending on the clinical situation and the preinfusion plasma concentration of factor XIII (Tables 5–11 and 5–13).[149, 311–322]

FAMILIAL MULTIPLE FACTOR DEFICIENCIES

Congenital deficiencies of two or more coagulation proteins have been reported for 16 different combinations of coagulation factors.[323] Bleeding in the neonatal period has only been reported for two infants with combined factor deficiencies. One infant had deficiencies of FII, FVII, FIX, and FX and was seen with spontaneous bruising and umbilical stump bleeding; the bruising and bleeding continued until 3 months after birth, when the infant was treated with FFP.[239] A second infant who had deficiencies of FV and FVIII was seen with serious bleeding (undescribed) in the first week of life.[238] FFP was administered, but no improvement was seen. Administration of FFP is usually the initial therapy. Subsequent treatment varies, depending on the specific factors affected.

ACQUIRED HEMOSTATIC DISORDERS

Disseminated Intravascular Coagulation

GENERAL INFORMATION

The term *disseminated intravascular coagulation* was first used to describe the pathologic feature of diffuse fibrin deposition in the microvasculature.[323–325] Subsequently, a relationship between the clinicopathologic findings and the decrease in the concentration of coagulation factors due to consumption was noted for both adults and infants.[326–330] Most recently, the definition of the term has been extended to include evidence of endogenous thrombin and plasmin generation on the basis of sensitive biochemical markers such as F1.2, thrombin/AT complex, and D-dimer. The following discussion focuses particularly on DIC in newborns.

ETIOLOGY

DIC is not a disorder in itself but a process that results from a variety of underlying diseases in newborns.[110, 330–341] Adverse events related to the fetal-placental unit may result in asphyxia and shock and thereby contribute to the release of tissue thromboplastin at the time of birth. Some of the common pathologic disorders related to prematurity, such as RDS, can be associated with DIC. A variety of other disorders such as viral or bacterial infections, hypothermia, and meconium or amniotic fluid aspiration syndromes may initiate DIC.[323–325, 342]

CLINICAL PRESENTATION

The clinical spectrum of DIC is changing, reflecting the ever-improving perinatal care of sick infants. The intensity and duration of activation of the hemostatic system, the degree of blood flow impairment, and the functioning of the liver all influence the clinical severity of DIC.[341] In the past, infants who had clinical manifestations of hemorrhagic or thrombotic complications from DIC often died.[323–325] Now the majority of infants with DIC survive, and for some DIC is of little clinical significance.[342]

DIAGNOSIS

Historically, the laboratory diagnosis of DIC was characterized by prolonged PT, prolonged APTT, depletion of certain coagulation factors (fibrinogen, factor V, and factor VIII), increased levels of fibrin degradation products, thrombocytopenia, and microangiopathic hemolytic anemia.[110, 330–341] Physiologic concentrations of fibrinogen and factors V and VIII are similar in newborns and adults; thus, pathologic decreases, as in DIC, are readily identified. The availability of sensitive markers for endogenous thrombin and plasmin generation has complicated the diagnosis of DIC in newborns. For example, plasma concentrations of thrombin/AT complexes are increased in healthy infants, probably as a reflection of activation of the coagulation system during birth.[67, 69, 112, 138] Positive results for these sensitive paracoagulation tests do not indicate the presence of DIC or the need for intervention.

In practice, no single laboratory test can be used to confirm or exclude DIC.

TREATMENT

DIC is a secondary disease. The cornerstone of treatment of DIC in all patients remains the successful treatment of the underlying disease. Treatment of the secondary hemostatic disorder may be helpful, but it has to be considered as an adjuvant therapy. Because decreased concentrations of platelets and coagulation factors may cause serious bleeding, replacement therapy with platelet concentrates and plasma in the form of FPP or cryoprecipitate may be beneficial in infants with clinical symptoms. Transfusion of factor concentrates is generally not recommended because of contamination with activated coagulation factors, which could, at least theoretically, augment the already activated coagulation system. Clinically practical goals for the treatment of infants who are bleeding from DIC are to maintain a platelet count greater than 50×10^9/L, fibrinogen concentrations greater than 1.0 g/L, and PT and APTT near normal values for age. Replacement of natural inhibitors of coagulation including AT and protein C may be an appropriate therapy in patients with DIC. However, because large clinical trials of replacement therapies are lacking, a general recommendation to use them cannot be supported.[343] Another attractive therapy option in patients with DIC is to inhibit the activation of the coagulation system by using heparin. However, heparin may increase the risk of bleeding, and there are no trials showing that it is helpful. The use of heparin is usually limited to patients with large vessel thrombosis.[344–346]

Several uncontrolled and two randomized clinical trials in newborns with DIC have been published.[338, 341, 347–358] Gobel et al[358] randomly assigned 36 infants to receive either unfractionated heparin or placebo, whereas Gross et al[354] randomly assigned 33 newborns to receive either exchange transfusion, administration of FFP and platelets, or no specific therapy. Although no beneficial effect of therapy was shown, results of both trials were not conclusive because the sample sizes were insufficient to detect a 50 percent reduction in mortality.[338, 341, 343–352, 354–358] No large trials of the use of fractionated heparin preparations have been reported.

Liver Disease

GENERAL INFORMATION

The coagulopathies of liver disease in newborns are similar to those of adults and reflect the failure of hepatic synthetic functions superimposed upon a physiologic immaturity, activation of the coagulation and fibrinolytic systems, poor clearance of activated coagulation factors, and the loss of hemostatic proteins into ascitic fluid.[359] The secondary effects of liver disease on platelet number and function also occur in newborns.[360–362] Thrombocytopenia is due to the impairment of platelet production, perhaps as a result of the direct invasion of megakaryocytes by the virus, splenic sequestration, and accelerated clearance.[363–366]

Only 28 reports in the literature have dealt with coagulopathies of liver disease in newborns, and all of these are case series.[367–376] Common causes of hepatic dysfunction in newborns include viral hepatitis, hypoxia, total parenteral nutrition, shock, and fetal hydrops.

The laboratory abnormalities induced by acute liver disease include prolongation of the PT and low plasma concentrations of several coagulation proteins, including fibrinogen.[377, 378] Chronic liver failure with cirrhosis is also characterized by a coagulopathy[379–381] and mild thrombocytopenia due to splenic sequestration.[382, 383] Secondary VK deficiency may occur owing to impaired absorption from the small intestine, particularly in intra- and extrahepatic biliary atresia.[384] Patients with clinical bleeding may benefit temporarily from replacement of coagulation proteins with FFP, cryoprecipitate, or exchange transfusion. However, without recovery of hepatic function, replacement therapy is futile. VK should be administered to infants in whom cholestatic liver disease is suspected.

Periventricular-Intraventricular Hemorrhage

The characteristic form of ICH in premature newborns is *periventricular-intraventricular hemorrhage (PIVH)*, which is characterized by bleeding from the fragile microvasculature of the subependymal germinal matrix that may extend into the lateral ventricles and/or brain parenchyma.[385–387] Approximately 20 to 40 percent of premature infants born before 32 weeks' gestation or with a birth weight less than 1500 g develop an ICH.[388] Most PIVH occurs in the first 24 hours, with almost all developing by 72 hours of life.[245, 387, 389–391] In more than half of the affected newborns PIVH is clinically silent.[386, 390–395] The use of ultrasonography allows accurate bedside diagnosis and follow-up of PIVH.[386, 387, 389 391–395] Four severity grades of PIVH have been defined using ultrasonography. Grade I is defined as bleeding in the subependymal matrix, grade II involves intraventricular bleeding, grade III indicates intraventricular bleeding and dilation, and grade IV includes intraventricular bleeding with extension into the parenchyma. The incidence of PIVH in premature infants is decreasing; this decrease is probably a reflection of improvements in neonatal care.

EVOLUTION OF PERIVENTRICULAR-INTRAVENTRICULAR HEMORRHAGE

Germinal matrix hemorrhages rupture into the adjacent ventricle in approximately 80 percent of infants and may incite an arachnoiditis that obstructs cerebrospinal fluid flow. The consequences of PIVH include destruction of the germinal matrix with cyst formation, progressive posthemorrhagic ventricular dilation, and periventricular hemorrhagic infarction. Periventricular hemorrhagic infarction occurs in 15 to 20 percent of infants with PIVH and is located in the periventricular white matter.[396–404] The hemorrhagic infarction is frequently asymmetric, is associated with an extensive PIVH, and occurs late, with peak incidence on day 4 of life.[401, 402, 405, 406]

ETIOLOGY OF PERIVENTRICULAR-INTRAVENTRICULAR HEMORRHAGE

The pathophysiologic mechanism of PIVH in premature infants is incompletely understood and is probably multifactorial.[407–412] Abnormalities of cerebral blood flow resulting in ischemia and subsequent reperfusion of brain tissue are the most likely causes.[413–417] Other potential contributing mechanisms include the fragility of the germinal matrix capillaries, oxidative damage to the endothelium, and concurrent impairment of the coagulation system including decreased plasma concentrations of some coagulant proteins, thrombocytopenia, and enhanced local fibrinolytic activity.[35, 405, 418] Factors such as vaginal delivery, labor, intrapartum asphyxia, RDS, increased mean, diastolic, and systolic blood pressure, and decreased superior vena cava flow due to an immature myocardium have been associated with PIVH in premature newborns.[35, 145, 419–421]

THERAPEUTIC MODALITIES

A variety of therapeutic modalities directed at decreasing the frequency and severity of PIVH have been tested.[422] In general, therapeutic interventions have included the use of agents that affect cerebral blood flow (phenobarbital before and after birth, indomethacin, and pancuronium bromide), drugs that affect cell membranes (ethamsylate and vitamin E), and products that enhance hemostasis (ethamsylate, VK, FFP, tranexamic acid, and platelet concentrates). Only the studies testing interventions to alter hemostasis are discussed in this section.[423]

Trials of Coagulation Factor Replacement before the 1980s

The immature physiologic state of hemostasis in premature infants and the association of pathologic alterations of hemostasis with PIVH form the rationale for intervention studies to enhance hemostasis. Six clinical trials with coagulation factor replacement were conducted between 1968 and 1981.[145, 350, 352, 424–426] The results of these early trials cannot be extrapolated to current practice because of significant improvements in neonatal intensive care management and the availability of ultrasound for diagnosing PIVH. Since 1980, a number of drugs or blood products that enhance specific aspects of hemostasis have been tested in infants at risk for PIVH (Table 5–15).

Antenatal Administration of Vitamin K

Beginning antenatally, VK was administered to mothers to increase plasma activities of VK-dependent coagulation proteins in premature infants. Of the three clinical trials conducted to test this hypothesis, two reported a benefit and one did not.[213, 214, 427] A placebo control group was not present in any study. Despite randomization, there were imbalances in the two positive studies between treatment and control groups that may have conferred a positive bias for the use of VK. Both positive studies reported an effect on coagulation tests that might reflect the administration of VK. The negative study did not identify a positive effect on the infant's coagulation system. For all of

TABLE 5–15. Periventricular/Intraventricular Hemorrhage Prevention Studies

Study	Number	Weight (kg)	Dose 1 (mg/kg)	Dose 2 (mg/kg)	PIVH
VITAMIN K					
Pomerance et al (1987)[213]	53	1.5	10	10 × 2	↓
Morales et al (1988)[214]	100	1.5	10	10 for 5 days	↓
Kazzi et al (1989)[427]	98	2.5	10	20/day	↔
Thorp et al (1994)[638]	164	1.3	10	10 × 1	↔
BLOOD PRODUCTS					
Beverley et al (1985)[351] (FFP)	73	1.5	10 mL	10 mL × 2	↓
Shirahata et al (1990)[428] (factor XIII C)	21	–	100 U	None	↓
Andrew et al (1991)[626] (platelet C)	154	1.5	10 mL	10 mL × 1–3	↔
TRANSEXAMIC ACID					
Hensey et al (1984)[430]	105	1.25	25 (IV)	25 × 20	↔
ETHAMSYLATE					
Morgan et al (1981)[639]	73	1.5	12.5	12.5 × 16	↓
Benson et al (1986)[440]	330	1.5	12.5	12.5 × 16	↓
INDOMETHACIN					
Krueger (1987)[640]	32	1.5	0.2	None	↓
Hanigan et al (1988)[442]	111	1.3	0.4	0.4 × 3	↓
Ment et al (1988)[443]	36	1.25	0.1	0.1 × 3	↓
Bandstra et al (1988)[641]	199	1.3	0.2	0.1 × 2	↓
Bada et al (1989)[642]	141	1.5	0.2	0.1 × 2	↓
Mahony et al (1985)[643]	104	1.3	0.2	0.1 × 2	↓
Ment et al (1985)[441]	48	1.25	0.6	0.1 × 8	↓
Rennie et al (1986)[444]	50	1.75	0.2	0.2 × 2	↔
Vincer et al (1987)[644]	30	1.5	0.2	0.2 × 2	↔
Brangenburg et al (1997)[634]	103	1.3	50–200 IU/kg		↔

PIVH = Periventricular intraventricular hemorrhage; FFP = fresh frozen plasma; FXIII C = factor XIII concentrate; platelet C = platelet concentrate; IV = intravenous.

these reasons, antenatal VK administration for the prevention of PIVH cannot be recommended at this time. This statement does not contradict the well-substantiated need for postnatal VK supplementation.

Trials of Replacement with Blood Products since 1980

Blood products have been tested in randomized, controlled trials in infants with PIVH. FFP was tested in one randomized, controlled trial conducted in 1985. Treated newborns received 10 mL/kg of FFP on admission and at 24 hours of age.[351] Of the treated newborns, 5 of 36 developed ICH, whereas 15 of 37 control newborns did—a significant difference. However, without a placebo control group, it is possible that the beneficial effect observed was the result of "stabilizing the circulation" rather than of improving hemostasis. In a second study of a blood product, factor XIII concentrates were given to premature infants to prevent ICH through enhancement of fibrin cross-linking.[428] Although this study reported a significant effect, the analysis was performed on a small subset of infants that was not balanced. Furthermore, there is no strong biologic rationale to support the probable benefit of factor XIII concentrates because plasma concentrations of factor XIII at birth are well within the adult range. In a third study of a blood product, platelet concentrates were administered to thrombocytopenic infants because of the close association of PIVH and thrombocytope-

nia.[182] In this study 154 premature infants who were thrombocytopenic during the first 72 hours of life were randomly assigned to either a control or a treated group. Treated infants received platelet concentrates to maintain platelet counts greater than 150×10^9/L. No beneficial effect on the incidence or extension of ICH was shown in this study, which was designed to detect an effect of 25 percent or greater. Antithrombin replacement has also been reported, but no significant benefit was seen.[429]

Inhibition of Fibrinolysis

Tranexamic acid, an inhibitor of fibrinolysis, was tested in infants with ICH because of increased fibrinolytic activity at birth.[430] Tranexamic acid has been shown to reduce the incidence of recurrent subarachnoid hemorrhage in adults[431, 432] and to prevent bleeding after oral surgery in high-risk patients.[433, 434] In this study, 105 infants were randomly assigned to receive tranexamic acid or placebo on day 1 of life and for 4 subsequent days. No significant effect was demonstrated.

Stabilization of Capillary Membranes

The microvasculature of the germinal matrix is fragile and thereby susceptible to rupture. Ethamsylate is a drug that may stabilize capillary membranes and increase platelet adhesiveness. In addition, ethamsylate is an inhibitor of PG synthesis and may have effects on the cerebral vasculature. Ethamsylate reduces capillary bleeding during selected surgical interventions in humans (e.g., ear, nose, and throat surgery)[435–437] and decreases the incidence of PIVH in the beagle puppy model.[438] Two randomized, controlled trials and one controlled trial have reported a reduction in PIVH with ethamsylate.[439, 440] However, before ethamsylate can be generally recommended, neurodevelopmental follow-up is needed because of the possibility that treatment could cause brain ischemia.[422]

Cerebral Blood Flow Regulation

Cerebral blood flow is regulated in part by PGs such as prostacyclin and thromboxane A_2. Prostacyclin is a potent vasodilator that inhibits platelet aggregation, and thromboxane A_2 is a potent vasoconstrictor that promotes platelet aggregation. In the beagle puppy model, indomethacin, a drug that blocks the enzyme cyclooxygenase, significantly decreased the incidence of ICH. Indomethacin reduced plasma concentrations of 6-keto-$PGF_{1\alpha}$ and thromboxane B_2, the stable metabolites of prostacyclin and thromboxane A_2.[438] Four randomized, controlled trials have been conducted with indomethacin, three of which demonstrated a beneficial effect[441–443] and one of which did not detect a change.[444]

Recommendations

Several confounding variables may have contributed to the differing results of the trials discussed. Of particular importance is the declining incidence of PIVH, which is probably a reflection of improvements in perinatal care. Ongoing clinical studies are necessary for testing potentially beneficial therapeutic agents within the context of improving clinical care. At this time, no firm recommendations can be made for any of the intervention modalities discussed because of a lack of consistent results and neurodevelopmental follow-up.[223]

Respiratory Distress Syndrome

Respiratory distress syndrome, an acute lung disorder that primarily affects premature infants, is characterized by diffuse atelectasis, hyaline membrane formation, permeability edema, and right-to-left shunting of pulmonary blood flow.[154, 445] Increased pulmonary surface tension secondary to surfactant deficiency is an important mechanism that contributes to RDS.

POTENTIAL ROLE OF COAGULATION

One of the pathologic characteristics of RDS is fibrin deposition in both intra-alveolar and intravascular sites.[154, 445] This observation has led several investigators to look for evidence of activation of coagulation in infants with RDS. Early studies reported decreased plasma concentrations of some coagulation proteins and inhibitors. However, these tests were neither sensitive nor specific for activation of coagulation with thrombin generation. The sensitive paracoagulation markers F1.2, thrombin/AT complex, and D-dimer have been measured in newborns with a spectrum of mild to severe RDS. A direct correlation among increasing thrombin generation, decreased

AT levels, and the severity of RDS was observed. Furthermore, there is evidence to support that fibrin deposition within the lung probably contributes to the severity of lung disease.[446–449] In a piglet model of neonatal acute lung injury, increasing plasma concentrations of AT by infusion of AT concentrates decreased the severity of the lung disease.[450]

INTERVENTION TRIALS INFLUENCING HEMOSTASIS

The possible role of coagulation in acute neonatal lung disease has provided the rationale for five intervention studies with the aim of decreasing fibrin deposition through the use of anticoagulants, thrombolytic therapy, and AT concentrates (Table 5–16). In 1966, the value of urokinase-activated human plasmin was tested in a randomized, placebo-controlled, double-blind study of 60 infants with severe RDS; the study revealed that the plasmin effected a substantial increase in survival rate without toxicity.[56] In a second double-blind randomized study, 500 premature infants were treated with plasminogen or placebo intravenously within 60 minutes of birth. There was a substantial decrease in severe clinical respiratory distress, in the number of deaths caused by hyaline membrane disease, and in the total mortality in the plasminogen-treated infants compared with the control subjects.[451] In a third trial, the effect of heparin on the development of RDS as well as its effect on the incidence of ICH was tested.[452] High-risk, low-birth-weight infants were randomly assigned to receive heparin or placebo (saline), with nurses blinded to treatment. Of the 81 infants included, 39 were in the heparin group and 42 were in the placebo group. In the primary analyses, there was no difference in the number of deaths, the incidence of RDS, or bleeding. However, on a subanalysis in which 7 moribund infants treated with heparin and 3 moribund infants treated with saline were excluded, the investigators suggested that there was a positive effect on mortality with heparin treatment.[452] The fourth study was an open, randomized, controlled clinical trial that assessed the role of AT concentrates in 103 infants.[453] There was no difference in duration of ventilation, incidence of ICH, or mortality.[453] Finally, Schmidt et al[454] randomly assigned 122 infants with mean GA of 28 weeks to receive AT (100 IU/kg at birth followed by 50 IU/kg every 6 hours for 48 hours) or placebo. The group receiving AT had more deaths and significantly longer requirements for mechanical ventilation and supplemental oxygen. Future clinical trials are needed to assess the benefits of antithrombotic or thrombolytic therapy in RDS.

Vitamin K Deficiency

HISTORICAL VIEW

Hemolytic disease of the newborn (HDN), as first described by Townsend in 1894, consisted of hemorrhaging from multiple sites in otherwise healthy infants in the absence of trauma, asphyxia, or infection on days 1 through 5 of life.[96] This report was followed by recognition that blood from newborns takes longer to clot than does adult blood.[10] Subsequently, a causal link between HDN

TABLE 5–16. Clinical Trials Assessing the Potential Benefits of Anticoagulant or Thrombolytic Therapy in Neonates with Respiratory Distress Syndrome

Study	No. of Subjects	Outcome		
		Death (%)	RDS (%)	ICH (%)
Markarian et al (1971)[635]				
Heparin	39	17(44%)*	26 (68.8%)*	40% mild† 10% severe
Placebo	42	16 (38%)	22 (53.3%)	0% mild 61% severe
Ambrus et al (1966)[56]				
UK-plasmin	32	9 (28%)‡	—	7 (22%)*
Placebo	28	17 (61%)	—	6 (21%)
Ambrus et al (1977)[451]				
Plasminogen concentrate	251	6 (2%)‡	35 (14%) mild* 19 (7%) severe‡	1 (0.4%)*
Placebo	249	20 (8%)	22 (9%) mild 31 (12%) severe	1 (0.4%)
Muntean and Rosseger (1989)[453]				
AT concentrate	45	9 (20%)*	23 (51%)*	—
Control	53	8 (15%)	28 (53%)	—
Schmidt et al (1998)[454]			(MDMV)	
AT	61	11.5%	7.1	—
Placebo	61	4.9%	4.8	—

RDS = respiratory distress syndrome; ICH = intracranial hemorrhage; UK = urokinase; AT = antithrombin I; MDMV = mean days mechanical ventilation.
*Not significantly different from placebo/control group.
†Patients in whom ICH was diagnosed at autopsy.
‡Significantly different from placebo/control group.
Reproduced with permission.[628]

and abnormal blood clotting was made.[10, 79, 455, 456] Initial treatment of infants with HDN consisted of intravenous, intramuscular, or subcutaneous injection of blood or serum. At this very early time, the difficulty of separating treatment response from spontaneous improvements was recognized. Later, a randomized, controlled trial showed that the injection of intramuscular blood was not helpful in preventing the abnormalities in blood coagulation that occurred during the first week of life.[79] The link between VK deficiency and spontaneous hemorrhaging was first recognized in chicks in 1929.[457] The association between VK deficiency and HDN quickly followed, as subsequently did the treatment of infants with HDN.[10, 97, 98, 458]

The next historical step was the recognition of the link between decreased prothrombin activity and increased PTs on days 2 to 4 of life in the absence of prophylactic VK. Prothrombin activity was observed to return to normal by days 5 to 7 of life (Fig. 5–5).[10, 459–462] These observations led to the hypothesis that VK administered prophylactically could prevent HDN.[325, 459, 460, 463–468] There was uniform agreement that the prophylactic administration of VK to mothers or infants prevented the decrease in prothrombin activity during the first 3 to 4 days of life.[10, 458, 459, 464] On the basis of these studies, VK prophylaxis was widely recommended. Subsequently, the scientific basis for this policy became less clear for several reasons. First, plasma concentrations of other coagulation proteins besides prothrombin were shown to be low in newborns. Second, there was increasing recognition that bleeding in neonates was often not due to VK deficiency.[10, 455, 456, 469, 470] Third, administration of high amounts (50 to 70 mg) of a water-soluble form of VK, resulted in a hemolytic anemia with kernicterus in some infants.[10, 471, 472] Fourth, many clinicians suggested that

VK prophylaxis was not needed for all healthy full-term infants.[470, 473–475] Consequently, VK prophylaxis was suspended in some countries, and this resulted in a recurrence of HDN.[10, 460, 476–487] Subsequently, numerous reports advocating or refuting the need for VK prophylaxis were seen. Over time, publications confirming and refuting the link between prophylactic VK and cancer have been published.[79, 105, 470, 488–494] At this time, the authors believe that the available evidence overwhelmingly supports the prophylactic administration of VK to all infants.

The following section critically analyzes the studies supporting or refuting the benefits and risks of prophylactic treatment for VK deficiency. In this discussion, the term *vitamin K–deficiency bleeding (VKDB)* is used instead of HDN, because neonatal bleeding often is not due to VK deficiency and because VKDB may occur after the neonatal period.

CLINICAL PRESENTATION

Infants are at greater risk for hemorrhagic complications from VK deficiency than are similarly affected adults because their plasma concentrations of VK-dependent factors are physiologically decreased.[1–3, 10, 487, 495] The clinical presentation of VKDB can be classified as classic, early, or late on the basis of the timing and type of complications (Table 5–17).[10, 477, 496–499] *Classic VKDB* presents on days 2 to 7 of life in breast-fed, healthy, full-term infants.[10, 481, 495, 498–501] Causes include poor placental transfer of VK,[502–505] marginal VK content in breast milk (less than 20 μg/L), inadequate milk intake, and a sterile gut.[10] VKDB rarely occurs in formula-fed infants because commercially available formulas are supplemented with VK (≈830 mg/L).[506, 507] How often classic VKDB occurs in

Prothrombin Activity %

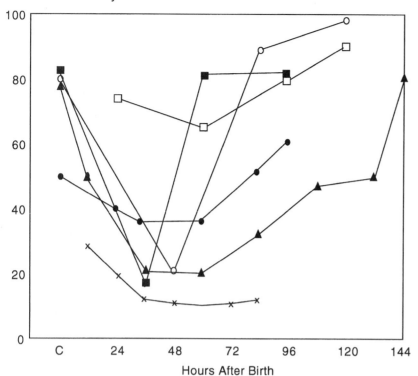

FIGURE 5–5. The plasma prothrombin activity in the neonatal period from various studies is shown.[10, 97, 459, 462] A consistent decrease in plasma prothrombin activity is demonstrated on days 2 and 3 of life; this is followed by increase in activity.[10] The infants did not receive vitamin K.

Hours After Birth

the absence of VK prophylaxis depends on the population studied, the supplemental formula, and the number of mothers breast-feeding. In the absence of prophylactic VK, the occurrence of VKDB ranges from 0.25 to 1.7 percent.[10, 508] *Early VKDB* presents in the first 24 hours of life and is linked to maternal use of specific medications that interfere with VK stores or function.[509–511] *Late VKDB* presents between weeks 2 and 8 of life and is linked to disorders that compromise the supply of VK.[512, 513]

LABORATORY DIAGNOSIS

Laboratory tests used to detect VK deficiency include screening tests, factor assays, determination of decarboxylated forms of VK-dependent factors and protein induced by VK antagonists (PIVKA), and direct measurements of VK. The results of these tests must always be compared with values for age-matched, healthy, non–VK-deficient infants in order to distinguish physiologic and pathologic deficiencies.[514, 515] PIVKA can be measured directly[33, 102, 145, 516–519] or as a discrepancy between coagulant activity and protein concentration measured immunologically or with a clotting assay using venom from *Echis carinatus*.[518] Recently, PIVKA II was demonstrated to be reliable in the postmortem period for determining VK deficiency.[520] Other tests have also been used to screen for VK deficiency.[521, 522]

FORMS OF VITAMIN K

VK exists in three forms: VK_1 (phytonadione), which is present in leafy green vegetables; VK_2 (menaquinone), which is synthesized by intestinal bacterial flora; and VK_3 (menadione), which is a synthetic, water-soluble form. VK_3 is rarely used in newborns because at high doses it

causes hemolytic anemia, which results in jaundice and potential morbidity.[10, 471, 472] Stores of VK in newborns are low, as shown by low levels of VK in cord blood and the livers of aborted fetuses.[224, 504, 523, 524] Studies measuring placental transport of VK show that only about 10 percent of maternally administered VK reaches the fetus.[525]

PROPHYLACTIC VITAMIN K

Most of the controversy concerning the prophylactic use of VK can be explained by the design of the trials and the subsequent interpretation of their results. The strongest form of evidence comes from randomized, controlled trials. Two randomized, controlled trials have assessed the benefits of VK prophylaxis, using clinical bleeding as the outcome measure (Table 5–18).[508, 526] In the first study, 3338 full-term infants were randomly assigned to receive either placebo, 100 μg of menadione, or 5 mg of menadione intramuscularly.[508] The risk of ICH and of minor bleeding was significantly greater in the placebo group than in both of the treatment groups. These clinical results were supported by prolonged PTs in infants with hemorrhagic complications and by the correction of PT values after VK administration. In a second study 470 male infants who were undergoing circumcision were randomly assigned to receive VK or nothing.[526] Infants who received prophylactic VK had significantly less bleeding than those who did not.[526] A subsequent smaller, nonblinded trial conducted by the same group produced similar results.[527]

A second level of support for the use of prophylactic VK comes from numerous studies in which laboratory evidence of VK deficiency was compared in infants who

TABLE 5–17. Forms of Vitamin K–Deficiency Bleeding in Infancy

Parameter	Early Form	Classic Form	Late Form
Age	<24 hr	2–7 days	0.5–6 mo
Causes and risk factors	Medications during pregnancy	Breast-feeding	Marginal VK content in breast milk resulting from low VK intake and absorption
	Anticonvulsants	Inadequate VK intake	Cystic fibrosis
	Oral anticoagulants (rifampin, isoniazid)		Diarrhea
	Antibiotics (rarely, idiopathic or hereditary)		α_1AT deficiency
			Hepatitis
			Celiac disease
Localization in order of occurrence	ICH	ICH	ICH (>50%)
	GI	GI	GI
	Umbilicus	Umbilicus	Skin
	Intra-abdominal	ENT region	ENT region
	Cephalhematoma	Injection sites	Injection sites
		Circumcision	Urogenital tract
			Intrathoracic
Occurrence without VK prophylaxis	Very rare	1.5% (1/10,000 births)	4–10/10,000 births[*]
Prophylaxis	Discontinue or replace offending medications	Adequate VK supply	Adequate VK supply
	Maternal VK prophylaxis	Early and adequate breast-feeding	Adequate breast-feeding
		Formula	Formula
		VK prophylaxis	VK prophylaxis[†]

VK = vitamin K; GI = gastrointestinal bleeding; ENT = ear, nose, and throat region; α_1AT = α_1-antitrypsin.
[*]More common in Southeast Asia.
[†]Single intramuscular injection is better than a single oral dose; repeated small doses are closer to physiologic conditions.

TABLE 5–18. Prophylactic Vitamin K: Randomized, Controlled Trials

Study	All Bleeding[*]			Significant Bleeding[†]		Coagulation Studies[‡]	
	n	*n*	%	*n*	%	*n*	Abnormal
Sutherland and Glueck (1967)[508]							
Vitamin K	2195		5.5	7	0.3	76	1
Control	1143		7.5	19	1.7[§]	60	18
Vietti et al (1960)[526]							
Vitamin K	240	6	2.5	1	0.4	22	1
Control	230	32	13.9	14	6.0[§]	25	11

[*]Sutherland and Glueck: bleeding from any site; Vietti et al: any bleeding after circumcision.
[†]Sutherland and Glueck: in a significant site (central nervous system, adrenal) causing anemia, resuturing a circumcision; Vietti et al: bleeding requiring resuturing of a circumcision.
[‡]Prothrombin time in both studies
[§]$P < .01$.

received VK at birth and in infants who did not receive VK (Table 5–19). These studies consistently indicate that biochemical evidence of VK deficiency is detected less often in infants who received VK prophylaxis than in those who did not. A third level of support for prophylactic VK comes from cohort studies reporting biochemical indices of VK deficiency at birth[224, 504, 505, 524]; large population–based studies in which VK prophylaxis was never instituted; and studies in which VK prophylaxis was instituted and then withdrawn.[10, 460, 477, 478, 495, 501] In general, VKDB rarely occurred when VK prophylaxis was used but was observed when prophylactic VK therapy was withdrawn. Evidence also comes from numerous studies reporting beneficial effects (either clinically or biochemically) after the administration of VK to mothers.[10, 463–465, 472, 528] The weakest supporting data come from comparisons of the incidence of VKDB in countries that do not provide prophylactic VK with that in countries that do administer VK prophylaxis.[10, 477] Finally, numerous cases of infants with VKDB who for a variety of reasons did not receive VK at birth have been reported.[190, 483, 484, 529]

TABLE 5–19. Evidence Supporting the Benefits of Vitamin K Prophylaxis: Laboratory Surrogate Outcomes

Reference	No. of Subjects	Coagulation Test		Comments
Ogata et al (1988)[645]		*PIVKA-II (day 7)★*		
Control	23	15 (65%)		
VK	11	0 (0%)		Affected infants responded to VK
Widdershoven et al (1986)[33]		*PIVKA-II*		*Days 1–4* *Days 29–35*
Control	12	5 (42%)		378 707
VK	13	0 (0%)		32,711[†] 698
Motohara et al (1987)[646]		*PIVKA-II (1 mo)*		
Control (breastfed)	5090	26 (0.51%)[†]		Affected infants responded to VK
VK (breastfed)	3206	6 (0.19%)		
Von Kries et al (1987)[647]		*PIVKA-II*		
Control	95	47 (48%)		Factor II 40% of adult level in 36% of control babies and 0% of treated babies
VK	95	0[†] (0%)		
Garrow et al (1986)[522]		*Thrombotest*		
Control	24	15.2[†]		—
VK	24	39.1		
O'Connor and Addiego (1986)[648]		*Factor II/Echis II*		
Control	15	0.68		Similar results with oral VK
VK	15	0.96[†]		
Motohara et al (1985)[479]		*PIVKA-II (day 3)*		
Control	51	61.5%[†]		Affected infants responded to VK
VK	51	18.5%		
Aballi and de Lamerens (1978)[10]		*Factor II (%)*		
		Before	*After*	
Control	57	23	20	Four hour response to VK prophylaxis
VK	58	20	53[†]	
Keenan et al (1971)[649]		*PT (sec)*		
Control	61	22		Affected infants responded to VK
VK	13	14[†]		
Wefring et al (1962)[650]		*Thrombotest (<10%)*		
Control	28	16 (57%)		Affected infants responded to VK
VK	83	2 (2%)		
Vietti et al (1961)[526]★		*PT (sec)*		
Control	50	14 (28%)		Bleeding seen in 0/39 (0%) circumcised male infants in the control group and in 4/15 (27%) in the VK group
VK	85	1 (1.1%)		
Lehmann (1944)[495]★		*PI (<30%)*		
Control	90	55.5%		Death from bleeding occurred in 34 of 17,741, compared with 6 of 13,250 treated infants
VK	122	0.8%[†]		
Bruchsaler (1941)[458]		*PI*		
		Day 1	*Day 4*	—
Control	30	58.3	55.4	
VK	30	59.0	81.0	
Astrowe and Palmerton (1941)[651]		*PT (sec)*		
		Birth	*Day 3*	
Control	28	38.4	51.8	—
VK	18	46.0	34.0★	

PI = prothrombin index; PIVKA-II = protein induced by VK antagonists.

★Control groups did not receive VK prophylaxis. The VK groups received prophylactic VK K in differing amounts, by differing routes, and, in some cases, by formula supplementation.

†Statistically significant differences ($P < .05$) between control and VK groups.

Studies reported to refute the benefits of prophylactic VK use are also ranked by the strength of their study designs (Table 5–20). No randomized, controlled trials had large enough sample sizes to show that prophylactic VK does not prevent bleeding. Some small studies reported no clinical benefit from prophylactic VK. However, the strength of the conclusions from these studies is consider- ably reduced because of small sample sizes, sequential rather than concurrent controls, and the absence of infor- mation on feeding practices.[470] Some investigators stud- ied cord blood only and did not demonstrate biochemical evidence of VK deficiency. In other studies, mothers rather than infants received VK prophylaxis, which intro- duced the confounding variable of placental transport and delivery of VK to fetuses. Some of the latter studies did show a benefit of maternal VK prophylaxis on biochemical outcomes.

In 1990 a cohort study with the aim of determining perinatal risk factors for childhood cancer reported an association between drugs administered in the peripartum period (maternal pethidine or neonatal VK) and childhood cancer with an odds ratio of 2.6.[491] A subsequent case-control study by the same authors found no association between maternal pethidine and childhood cancer; however, they again reported an increased risk of childhood cancer after neonatal intramuscular VK administration (odds ratio 1.97).[530] A further case-control study of seven cases, one ecological study, and one meta-analysis have shown that there is no association between VK administration and childhood cancer.[531] The current con-

sensus is that the risk of increased childhood cancer is probably minimal, if any, and the benefits of VK prophylaxis in terms of reduced bleeding are substantial.

Prophylactic Vitamin K Administration

The recommendations for VK prophylaxis in many countries are reasonably similar.[525] Daily requirements of VK are approximately 1 to 5 µg/kg of body weight for newborns.[525] Most groups recommend a single dose of 0.5 to 1 mg intramuscularly or an oral dose of 2 to 4 mg at birth, with subsequent dosing for breast-fed infants. Oral VK prophylaxis is preferred to parenteral prophylaxis; studies have shown that oral administration of VK is as effective, less expensive, and less traumatic than intramuscular administration in preventing the classic presentation of VK deficiency.[525] However, orally administered VK_1 or

TABLE 5–20. Studies Refuting the Benefits of Prophylactic Vitamin K in Neonates

Reference	No. of Subjects	CoagulationTest			Comments
Sanford et al (1942)[79]		*PT (%)*			
		Day 1		*Day 3*	
Control	55	80		20*	No apparent difference in bleeding
Vitamin K	40	82		75	
Potter (1945)[470]		*Mortality*			
Control	6630	90 (1.4%)†			Death from all causes, not HDN; sequential study.
VK	6004	89 (1.5%)			
Muller et al (1977)[488]		*Prothrombin*			—
		ACT	*Ag*	*Echis*	
Cord blood	43	51	53	54	
Gobel et al (1977)[105]		*Factor II (%)*			
Control	15	20.8*			VK given as early feedings
VK	15	22.6			
Mori et al (1977)[490]		*Factor II (%)*			
		Day 1		*Day 2*	
Control	29	30.5		30.4	VK group had at least 10% increase in VK-dependent factors
VK	31	30.3		33.2	
Malia et al (1980)[475]					
Cord blood	24	Similar values for activity and immunologic measurements for factors II, VII, IX, and X			—
Corrigan and Kryc (1980)[627]	40	*Factor II Activity: Ag Ratio*			
Cord blood	40	0.90			Similar results for premature infants and adults
Pietersma-de Bruyn (1990)[652]		*Factor II (ACT) (%)*	*Factor II (%) (ANT)*	*Factor X (%) (ACT)*	
Formula VK	8	58†	53†	74†	1 wk after birth
Breast milk	10	54	50	49	
Greer et al (1991)[653]		*Plasma phylloquinone*			
Formula VK	11	5.19 ng/mL*			No apparent VK deficiency
Breast milk	23	<0.25 ng/mL			
Anai et al (1993)[654]		*Normotest (%)*			Maternal VK (oral)
Control	186	53.4 ± 9.9*			
VK	74	59.6 ± 10.1			
Dickson et al (1994)[655]		*PT (sec)*	*APTT(sec)*	*Factor II (%) (ACT)*	*Factor II (%) (ANT)*	Maternal VK (intramuscular) or placebo
Control	16	17.0	53.4	35.7	39.8	
VK	17	14.6	59.5	38.8	43.2	

HDN = hemolytic disease of the newborn.
*Statistically significant differences between control and VK groups, *P* <.05.
†Not significant.

VK_3 is not as effective as intramuscularly injected VK in the prevention of late VK deficiency (Table 5–21). In a 1990 randomized, controlled trial in Thailand,[532] infants were given a single 2-mg dose of VK orally, 5 mg orally, or 1 mg intramuscularly. Although the mean levels of VK_1 were not significantly different in the treated infants given the various dosage forms, a trend toward the manifestation of higher levels was observed in intramuscularly treated infants. Strategies for preventing late VK deficiency include repeat administration of oral VK in Germany[486] and Japan[533] or continuous low-dose VK supplementation in the Netherlands.[486]

In addition to general prophylaxis at birth, patients in certain risk groups require additional VK prophylaxis (e.g., infants with α_1-antitrypsin deficiency, chronic diarrhea, cystic fibrosis, or celiac disease). Pregnant women receiving oral anticonvulsant therapy should receive about 5 mg of VK_1 daily during the third trimester for the prevention of overt VK deficiency in their infants at birth.

New Developments in Vitamin K Prophylaxis

A new mixed micelle oral VK_1 preparation that is readily absorbed has been tested in children.[525] Whether this preparation will negate the need for repeated dosing if the oral route is chosen requires further testing.

TREATMENT

An infant suspected of having VK deficiency should be treated immediately with VK while laboratory confirmation is awaited. All infants with VKDB should be given VK either subcutaneously or intravenously, depending on the clinical problem. VK should not be given intramuscularly to infants with VKDN, because large hematomas may form at the site of the injection. The absorption of subcutaneously administered VK is rapid, and its effect occurs only slightly slower than that of systemically administered VK. Intravenous VK should be given slowly because it may induce an anaphylactoid reaction. Infants with major bleeding because of VK deficiency should also be treated with plasma products to rapidly increase levels of VK-dependent proteins. Plasma is the product of choice for the treatment of a non–life-threatening hemorrhagic event, whereas the use of PCCs should be considered for the management of life-threatening bleeding.

Extracorporeal Membrane Oxygenation

The use of extracorporeal membrane oxygenation (ECMO) began in the 1960s. Since then, thousands of infants have been treated; the survival rate of those treated is approximately 60 percent. ECMO permits the transfer of oxygen into blood across a semipermeable membrane and is currently used for infants with life-threatening severe respiratory insufficiency. The underlying respiratory disorders include meconium aspiration syndrome, severe RDS, congenital diaphragmatic hernia, persistent pulmonary hypertension, and sepsis. Despite the widespread use of ECMO, few controlled trials assessing its efficacy have been published.[534–537] Clearly, more definitive trials are needed to validate the use of ECMO. The follow-up studies of infants who were treated with ECMO and survived are encouraging, with a majority of infants having normal developmental follow-up.

Hemorrhage, particularly ICH, is one of the most serious complications of this technique. The incidence of ICH is 25 to 50 percent in treated newborns and ICH is associated with increased mortality and long-term neurologic morbidity rates.[538] Similar to that found with cardiopulmonary bypass, the increased risk of bleeding during ECMO is due mostly to the use of heparin in combination with hemostatic defects, which include significant decreased plasma concentrations of coagulation proteins and platelet dysfunction.[539] Other recognized factors

TABLE 5–21. Oral Vitamin K Is Not as Effective as Intramuscular Vitamin K in the Prevention of Late Vitamin K Deficiency

Country	Vitamin K	No. of Patients	Rate per 100,000	95% CI
United Kingdom (1991)[486]	Nil	9	4.4	2.0–8.4
	Oral: 1–2 mg	7	1.5	0.6–3.2
	IM: 1mg	0	0	0.0–0.4
Sweden (1991)[656]	Oral: 1–2 mg	16	6	3.7–9.8
	IM: 1mg	0	0	0.0–5.6
Switzerland (1986)[657]	Oral: 1–3 mg	7	6.4	2.5–13.1
	IM: 1mg	0	0	0.0–5.3
Germany (1992)[533]	Nil	10	7.2	3.5–13.3
	Oral: 1–2 mg	2	1.4	0.2–5.2
	IM (SC): 1 mg	1	0.25	0.01–1.32
Japan (1992)[658]	Nil	20.4*	10.5†	7.0–15.0
	MK–4 (2 mg: 1–3×)	29.5*	2.8†	2.0–3.78
United States (1995)[659]	Oral: 2 mg	23,228	1.4–6.4	—
Germany (1995)[513]	Nil	89	5.13	2.81–29.58
	Oral: 2 mg	10	1.21	0.97–11.52
	IM: 1 mg	2	0.36	—

CI = confidence interval; IM = intramuscular injection; SC = subcutaneous injection; MK–4 = menaquinone–4.

*Estimated number of cases.

†Including patients with strictly idiopathic disease and patients with recognized associated disease (almost all with ICH) but no patients with VK deficiency detected by mass screening; if clear information on VK prophylaxis was not available, patients were included in the VK prophylaxis group.

associated with an increased risk of ICH during ECMO include prolonged hypoxia, ischemia, general anesthesia, acidosis, sepsis, and treatment with epinephrine.[538–545]

Data to date suggest that thrombin generation is impaired due to a consumptive coagulopathy and that a hyperfibrinolytic state exists along with impairment of platelet number and function.[546, 547] Heparin is used in full systemic doses, with a bolus of 100 to 150 U/kg followed by a continuous systemic infusion at 20 to 70 U/kg/hr. The laboratory goal is to maintain the activated clotting time at two- to threefold baseline values (240 to 280 seconds). Although anticoagulation is required for ECMO, the optimal use of heparin has never been tested in clinical trials. Whether lower doses of heparin or the potentially safer anticoagulant drugs, such as low-molecular-weight heparins, have a role in ECMO remains to be determined.

THROMBOTIC DISORDERS

Congenital Prethrombotic Disorders

Patients with single-gene defects for recognized inherited prethrombotic disorders rarely are seen with their first thromboembolic complication during childhood unless another pathologic event unmasks the problem. In contrast, patients who are homozygotes or double heterozygotes for a congenital prethrombotic disorder usually are seen as newborns or young children. The following discussion is limited to the unique aspects of these inherited deficiencies in newborns. Chapter 42 discusses congenital prethrombotic disorders in detail.

Homozygous Prothrombotic Disorders

GENERAL INFORMATION

Although rare, the most commonly reported homozygous prothrombotic disorder presenting during the newborn period is protein C deficiency. Homozygous protein S deficiency is even less common.[47, 548–569] All patients seen in the newborn period had undetectable levels of protein C (or protein S), whereas children with delayed presentation had detectable levels ranging between 0.05 and 0.20 unit/mL.

CLINICAL PRESENTATION

The classic clinical presentation of homozygous protein C/protein S deficiency consists of cerebral or ophthalmic damage (or both) that occurred *in utero*, purpura fulminans within hours or days of birth, and, on rare occasions, large vessel thrombosis. Purpura fulminans is an acute, lethal syndrome of DIC characterized by rapidly progressive hemorrhagic necrosis of the skin due to dermal vascular thrombosis.[278, 570, 571] The skin lesions start as small, ecchymotic sites that increase in a radial fashion, become purplish black with bullae, and then turn necrotic and gangrenous.[278, 571] The lesions occur mainly on the extremities but can occur on the buttocks, abdomen, scrotum, and scalp. They also occur at pressure points, at sites of previous punctures, and at previously affected sites.

Affected infants also have severe DIC with hemorrhagic complications.

DIAGNOSIS

The diagnosis of homozygous protein C/protein S deficiency in infants is based on the appropriate clinical picture, a protein C/protein S level that is usually undetectable, a heterozygous state in the parents, and, ideally, identification of the molecular defect. The presence of very low levels of protein C/protein S in the absence of clinical manifestations and of a family history cannot be considered diagnostic because physiologic plasma levels can be as low as 0.12 unit/mL. The homozygous forms of AT (or heparin cofactor II) deficiency have not been confirmed in newborns, but one would anticipate that affected infants would have with severe life-threatening thromboembolic complications. Molecular diagnosis is available for identified families (see Chapter 43).

INITIAL TREATMENT

The diagnosis of homozygous protein C/protein S deficiency is usually unanticipated and is made at the time of the clinical presentation. Although numerous forms of initial therapy have been used, 10 to 20 mL/kg of FFP every 6 to 12 hours is usually the form of therapy that is most readily available.[572] Plasma levels of protein C achieved with these doses of FFP vary from 15 to 32 percent at 30 minutes after the infusion and from 4 to 10 percent at 12 hours.[559] Plasma levels of protein S (which was entirely bound to C4b) were 23 percent at 2 hours and 14 percent at 24 hours, with an approximate half-life of 36 hours.[573] Doses of protein C concentrate have ranged from 20 to 60 units/kg. In one study, a dose of 60 units/kg resulted in peak protein C levels greater than 0.60 unit/mL.[574] Replacement therapy should be continued until all of the clinical lesions resolve, which is usually at 6 to 8 weeks. In addition to the clinical course, plasma D-dimer concentrations may be useful for monitoring the effectiveness of protein C replacement.[575]

LONG-TERM THERAPY

The modalities used for the long-term management of infants with homozygous protein C/protein S deficiency included oral anticoagulation therapy, replacement therapy with either FFP or protein C concentrate, and liver transplantation.[569] When oral anticoagulation therapy is initiated, replacement therapy should be continued until the INR is at a therapeutic value so that skin necrosis can be avoided. The therapeutic range for the INR can be individualized to some extent but is usually between 2.5 and 4.5. The risks of oral anticoagulation therapy include bleeding with high INR values and recurrent purpuric lesions with low INR values. Frequent monitoring of INR values is required if these complications are to be avoided. Bone development also should be monitored because the long-term effects of warfarin use on bones of young infants is unknown.

Heterozygous Prothrombotic Disorders

GENERAL INFORMATION

Thromboembolic events rarely occur in infants. When they do occur, a secondary, acquired insult is usually present. The few case reports in the literature described a diversity of clinical presentations that usually reflected the site of the thrombus. Purpura fulminans did not occur in any case. Although most infants died, many were left with residual complications resulting from the location of the thrombus, including the venous (systemic and central nervous system) and arterial systems (aorta and coronary arteries).[576–582]

TREATMENT

Treatments consisted of supportive therapy alone, anticoagulation with heparin, thrombolytic therapy, and replacement with specific factor concentrates.[583–585] Removal or treatment of the secondary acquired insult is important. For AT deficiency, AT concentrates were administered to four infants as either boluses or as continuous infusions. Boluses of 52 and 104 units/kg of AT concentrate increased AT levels from 0.10 unit/mL to 0.75 and 1.48 units/mL, respectively, at 1 hour.[585] At 24 hours, levels of AT had decreased to approximately 0.20 unit/mL.[585] A continuous infusion of AT concentrate at a rate of 2.1 units/kg/hr maintained a plasma level of 0.40 to 0.50 unit/mL.[585]

ACQUIRED PROTHROMBOTIC DISORDERS

General Information

Reviews of the literature[106, 586, 587] and an international registry of neonatal thrombotic disease[588] have provided valuable information on the epidemiology of venous and arterial thrombotic disease in newborns. Symptomatic secondary thromboembolic complications occur more frequently in sick newborns than in children of any other age, with an incidence of approximately 2.4 per 1000 hospital admissions to the neonatal intensive care unit.[588] Intravascular catheters are responsible for more than 80 percent of venous and 90 percent of arterial thrombotic complications.[588] Catheters are responsible for many of the factors that initiate thrombus formation (e.g., the presence of a foreign surface, endothelial cell damage, impairment of flow, and infusion of noxious substances).[588] Renal vein thrombosis (RVT) is the most common form of non–catheter-related thrombosis.[588] Other risk factors include increased blood viscosity, poor deformability of physiologically large red cells, polycythemia, dehydration, and activation of the coagulation and fibrinolytic systems caused by a variety of medical problems. The following section discusses the epidemiology, diagnosis, and treatment of thromboembolic complications in newborns.

Venous Catheter-Related Thrombosis

The use of umbilical venous catheters and other forms of central venous catheters is associated with a significant risk of thrombosis.[588–590] According to autopsy studies, 20 to 65 percent of infants who die with an umbilical venous catheter in place have an associated thrombus. A database search of the literature from 1966 to 1995 identified 60 references to catheter-related thrombosis in infants. Of these, 44 were case reports or small case series. The appropriate placement of umbilical venous catheters is critical to the prevention of serious organ impairment, such as portal vein thrombosis and hepatic necrosis. Long-term sequelae of umbilical venous catheters have not been rigorously studied but include portal vein thrombosis with portal hypertension, splenomegaly, gastric and esophageal varices, and hypertension. Until recently, pulmonary embolism was rarely diagnosed in sick newborns because its clinical signs were easily confused with those of RDS. The use of ventilation lung scintigraphy in newborns has facilitated the diagnosis of pulmonary embolism.[591]

Arterial Catheter-Related Thrombosis

GENERAL INFORMATION

Seriously ill infants require indwelling arterial catheters, which present a risk of thrombosis, regardless of the vessel and type of catheter chosen.[386, 453, 592–595] Catheter-related thrombosis not only occludes catheters with loss of patency but also may obstruct major arterial vessels. In a retrospective examination of approximately 4000 infants who underwent umbilical artery catheterization, 1 percent had severe symptomatic vessel obstruction. Asymptomatic catheter-related thrombi occur more frequently, as evidenced by postmortem (3 to 59 percent of cases) and angiographic studies (10 to 90 percent of cases).

DIAGNOSIS

Contrast angiography is considered the reference test for diagnosis of arterial thrombosis. Noninvasive techniques such as Doppler ultrasound offer advantages, but their sensitivity and specificity are unknown. A review of 20 neonates with aortic thromboses treated in one institution revealed that ultrasound failed to identify thrombi in 4 patients, 3 of whom had complete aortic obstruction.[596]

SEQUELAE

The sequelae of catheter-related thrombosis can be immediate or long term. Acute symptoms reflect the location of the catheter and include renal hypertension, intestinal necrosis, and peripheral gangrene.[586] The long-term side effects of symptomatic and asymptomatic thrombosis of major vessels have not been studied but are probably significant.[586]

PROPHYLAXIS WITH HEPARIN

A low-dose continuous heparin infusion (3 to 5 units/hr) is commonly used to maintain catheter patency. The effectiveness of heparin was assessed in seven studies focusing on three outcomes: patency, local thrombus, and

ICH (Table 5–22).[592–595, 597, 598] Patency, which is probably linked to the presence of local thrombus, is prolonged by the use of low-dose heparin.[593–595, 597, 598] Local thromboses were assessed by ultrasound in two randomized studies. The sample sizes were too small to allow the forming of any meaningful conclusions.[592, 593] The evidence linking heparin to ICH in newborns is similarly weak.[595, 599] One study had a sample size of only 15 per arm,[595] and another case-control study had a broad odds ratio that ranged from 1.4 to 11.0.[599] Thus, the magnitude of risk for ICH is uncertain.[599] Heparin is used in at least three quarters of American nurseries.[586]

Renal Vein Thrombosis

GENERAL INFORMATION

Renal vein thrombosis occurs primarily in newborns and young infants. Approximately 80 percent present within the first month and usually within the first week of life. Some infants develop RVT *in utero*. The incidence among male and female infants is similar, and the left and right sides are affected equally. Bilateral RVT occurs in 24 percent of pediatric patients.

CLINICAL PRESENTATION AND ETIOLOGY

Presenting symptoms and clinical findings are different in neonates and older patients and are influenced by the extent and rapidity of thrombus formation. Neonates usually have a flank mass, hematuria, proteinuria, thrombocytopenia, and nonfunction of the involved kidney. Clinical findings suggesting acute inferior vena caval thrombosis include cold, cyanotic, and edematous lower extremities. Renal vein thromboses result from pathologic states characterized by reduced renal blood flow, increased blood viscosity, hyperosmolality, or hypercoagulability.

COAGULATION ABNORMALITIES

The most common coagulation abnormality is thrombocytopenia, which is usually mild, with average values of $100,000 \times 10^9$/L. Coagulation may be prolonged, and levels of fibrinogen-fibrin degradation products increased. Children with RVT are often evaluated for a congenital prothrombotic disorder, although the significance of thrombophilic markers in this disease is unknown.[578]

DIAGNOSIS AND TREATMENT

The diagnosis of RVT has changed from an autopsy finding to an antemortem diagnosis that requires confirmation with an objective test. Ultrasound is the radiographic test of choice owing to ease of testing and sensitivity to an enlarged kidney. Treatment options include supportive care, anticoagulation, and thrombolytic therapy. In the 1990s, there has been uniform agreement that aggressive supportive care is indicated. However, the use of anticoagulants and thrombolytic agents is controversial. One approach is to use supportive care for unilateral RVT in the absence of uremia and extension into the inferior vena cava. Heparin therapy should be considered for unilateral RVT that does extend into the inferior vena cava or for bilateral RVT owing to the risk of pulmonary embolism and complete renal failure. Thrombolytic therapy should be considered in the presence of bilateral RVT and renal failure. Thrombectomy, although a common therapeutic choice in the past, is rarely indicated.

TABLE 5–22. Umbilical Artery Catheterization

Outcome					
Reference	Level	Intervention	No. of Patients	Bleeding	Event(B or TE)
Jackson et al (1987)[592]	II	HB–PU	61	*	13 TE
		PVC	64	*	23 TE
Horgan et al (1987)[593]	II	Heparin	59	*	16 TE
		No heparin	52	*	18 TE
Rajani et al (1979)[594]	I	Heparin	32	*	4 B†
		Saline	30	*	19 B
David et al (1981)[598]	II	Heparin	26	0‡	3 B†
		No heparin	26	0‡	15 B
Bosque and Weaver (1986)[597]	II	Heparin (continuous)	18	*	0 B†
		Heparin (intermittent)	19	*	8 B
Horgan et al (1987)[593]	II	Heparin	59	*	2 B†
		No heparin	52	*	10 B
Ankola and Atakent (1993)[595]	II	Heparin	15	4 ICH	2 B†
		No heparin	15	5 ICH	11 B
Chang et al (1997)[636]	II	Heparin	55	19 ICH	—
		No heparin	58	17 ICH	—

HB-PU = heparin-bonded polyurethane; PVC = polyvinyl chloride; TE = thromboembolic event; B = blocked.
*Not reported.
†$P < .05$.
‡No hemorrhage.
From Michelson AD, Bovill E, Andrew M: Antithrombotic therapy in children. Chest 1995; 108:506S–522S.

OUTCOME

Renal vein thrombosis has changed from a frequently lethal complication to one that more than 85 percent of children survive. Unfortunately, no recent studies have assessed the long-term morbidity, such as hypertension and renal atrophy.

Spontaneous Venous and Arterial Thrombosis

Spontaneous venous thrombosis occurs in adrenal veins, the inferior vena cava, the portal vein, the hepatic veins, and the venous system of the brain.[586, 587] Spontaneous occlusion of arterial vessels in the absence of a catheter is unusual, but it can occur in ill infants. As in catheter-related thrombosis, the clinical presentation reflects the vessel that is occluded. Complete occlusion of a vessel can lead to gangrene and loss of the affected limb or to ischemic organ damage.[586, 587] The presence of systemic hypertension in newborns is frequently related to renal artery thrombosis, even in the absence of a catheter.

Heparin Therapy in Newborns

The lack of consensus for prophylaxis and treatment of thromboembolic complications in newborns reflects the lack of controlled trials in this area. Recommendations for adult patients provide useful guidelines but probably do not reflect the optimal therapy for newborns. Current therapeutic options include supportive care alone, anticoagulant therapy, thrombolytic therapy, and thrombectomy. For most infants who develop thrombotic complications, the cause of thrombosis is a catheter-related thrombus that does not produce clinical symptoms. In most nurseries, catheters are not routinely checked for associated thrombosis; thus, by exclusion, most infants with clinically silent thrombi receive supportive care alone.

AGE-DEPENDENT FEATURES

Heparin's anticoagulant activities are mediated by catalysis of AT inhibition of thrombin and, secondarily, of other serine proteases. Although dosing for heparin therapy in newborns differs from that in adults, optimal dosing cannot be predicted. Several observations suggest that the heparin requirements of neonates are decreased compared with those of adults. First, the capacity of plasma from healthy newborns to generate thrombin is both delayed and decreased compared with that of adult plasma and is similar to that of plasma from adults receiving therapeutic amounts of heparin.[36, 111] Second, at heparin concentrations in the therapeutic range, the capacity of plasma from healthy newborns to generate thrombin is barely measurable.[600] Third, the amount of clot-bound thrombin is decreased in newborns because low plasma concentrations of prothrombin probably reduce heparin requirements.[126] Observations suggesting that heparin requirements are increased in neonates compared with adults include the following: (1) the clearance of heparin is accelerated in newborns[601, 602]; (2) plasma concentrations of AT are decreased to levels frequently less than 0.40 in premature infants, which may limit heparin's antithrombotic activities[1–3]; and (3) studies in a newborn piglet model of venous thrombosis have shown that low AT levels limit the anticoagulant and antithrombotic effectiveness of heparin.[585, 603]

INDICATIONS, THERAPEUTIC RANGE, AND DOSE

Indications for heparin therapy in newborns remain unclear. Although the benefits of heparin therapy in newborns are probably similar to those in adults, the relative risk that major bleeding will occur with its use may be increased. Infants with thromboses that are extending or infants whose organ or limb viability is threatened by a thrombosis may benefit from heparin therapy.

Therapeutic ranges reflect the optimal risk/benefit ratio of anticoagulant therapy with regard to recurrent thrombotic events and bleeding complications. In the absence of clinical trials in newborns, one approach is to use heparin in doses that achieve the lower therapeutic range for adults (see Chapter 45). Close monitoring of the thrombus with objective tests such as ultrasound is recommended.

Average doses of heparin required in newborns to achieve adult therapeutic APTT values are bolus doses of 75 to 100 units/kg and average maintenance doses of 28 units/kg/hr. The duration of heparin therapy required for the treatment of thromboembolic complications is uncertain. One approach is to treat the infant for 10 to 14 days with heparin alone. If there is subsequent extension of the thrombus in the absence of anticoagulation therapy, treatment with oral anticoagulants should be considered. In general, the use of oral anticoagulants should be avoided whenever possible in newborns because of the risk of bleeding and difficulties in monitoring. There are clear exceptions to this approach, such as the infant with homozygous protein C/protein S deficiency or recurrent thrombotic events.

ADVERSE EFFECTS

There are two clinically important adverse effects of heparin therapy: ICH and heparin-induced thrombocytopenia.[604, 605] In the absence of an alternative cause, thrombocytopenic patients should be evaluated for heparin-induced thrombocytopenia and treated with alternative therapy.

The use of low-molecular-weight heparins offers significant therapeutic advantages over use of heparin for newborns.[586, 606] Potential advantages include predictable bioavailability, the need for minimal monitoring, ease of administration, decreased bleeding, and equal or increased efficacy. Low-molecular-weight heparins are particularly useful in patients who are susceptible to bleeding complications, such as sick premature infants.

Oral Anticoagulant Therapy in Newborns

AGE-DEPENDENT FEATURES

Chapter 45 discusses oral anticoagulation therapy in children in detail; thus, only specific issues related to newborns are discussed in this section. Oral anticoagulants function by reducing plasma concentrations of the VK-dependent proteins. At birth, levels of the VK-dependent proteins are similar to those found in adults receiving therapeutic amounts of oral anticoagulants for deep venous thrombosis/PE embolism.[1–3, 600, 607–609] In addition, stores of VK are low, and a small number of newborns have evidence of functional VK deficiency.[514] These features significantly increase the sensitivity of newborns to oral anticoagulants and potentially their risk of bleeding. Oral anticoagulant therapy should be avoided when possible during the first month of life.[514, 610] Unfortunately, a small number of infants require extended anticoagulation therapy, and heparin cannot be used for extended periods of time because of the risk of osteopenia. The use of low-molecular-weight heparin is an option that should be considered; however, studies of its use in newborns are limited.[586]

INDICATIONS, THERAPEUTIC RANGE, AND DOSE

The optimal therapeutic INR range is unknown for newborns and almost certainly differs from that for adults. Recommendations for oral anticoagulation therapy in adults can be used as a guideline for determining the lowest effective dose, which to some extent can be individualized. Maintenance doses for therapeutic amounts of oral anticoagulants are age-dependent, with infants requiring the highest doses (0.32 mg/kg).

ADVERSE EFFECTS

Close monitoring of oral anticoagulation in newborns is required if both hemorrhagic and recurrent thrombotic complications are to be prevented. Unfortunately, these infants have poor venous access as well as complicated medical problems.[611–619] Weekly or biweekly measurements of the INR and frequent dose adjustments are required (see Chapter 45).[620] Doses are affected by diet, medication, and intercurrent illnesses.

Breast-fed infants are very sensitive to oral anticoagulants because of the low concentrations of VK in breast milk.[10, 170, 224, 506, 524, 621] Daily supplementation of breast-fed infants with small amounts of commercial formulas reduces their sensitivity to oral anticoagulants and the risk of sudden increases in INR values. In contrast to breast-fed infants, infants receiving commercial formulas or total parenteral nutrition are resistant to oral anticoagulants because of VK supplementation.[506, 622] Reducing or removing VK supplementation in infants receiving total parenteral nutrition significantly reduces the dose requirements. Most infants requiring oral anticoagulants also require other medications on an intermittent and long-term basis. The effects of dosage changes and the introduction of new medications must be closely supervised.

Antiplatelet Agents in Newborns

Antiplatelet agents are rarely used in newborns for antithrombotic therapy. The hyporeactivity of neonatal platelets and the paradoxically short bleeding time suggest that optimal use of antiplatelet agents differs in newborns and in adults. Aspirin is the most commonly used antiplatelet agent. The use of empirical low doses of 1 to 5 mg/kg/day has been proposed as adjuvant therapy for patients with Blalock-Taussig shunts, some endovascular stents, and some cerebrovascular events.[623, 624]

Thrombolytic Therapy in Newborns

AGE-DEPENDENT FEATURES

The activities of thrombolytic agents depend on the endogenous concentrations of plasminogen, which are physiologically decreased at birth.[144] Low plasminogen levels result in impairment of the capacity to generate plasmin[140] and a decrease in the capacity to thrombolyse fibrin clots.[144] Increasing plasma concentrations of plasminogen with purified plasminogen has resulted in fibrin clot lyses that were greater than those occurring in adult plasma, probably owing to the decreased levels of α_2-antiplasmin in the plasma of newborns. If an infant's condition does not respond to thrombolytic therapy, replacement of plasminogen should be considered.

INDICATIONS, THERAPEUTIC RANGE, AND DOSE

Infants who develop serious thrombotic complications, as defined by organ or limb impairment, may benefit from thrombolytic therapy. The clinical objective is removal of the clot as quickly and safely as possible. The surgical removal of a clot in a major vessel can be curative; however, it is technically difficult and poses a considerable life-threatening risk to infants, who often are premature. In the absence of contraindications, the use of thrombolytic agents in these infants is a preferred approach. Doses, monitoring, and adverse effects are discussed in Chapter 45.

REFERENCES

1. Andrew M, Paes B, Milner R, et al: Development of the human coagulation system in the full-term infant. Blood 1987; 70:165–172.
2. Andrew M, Paes B, Johnston M: Development of the hemostatic system in the neonate and young infant. Am J Pediatr Hematol Oncol 1990; 12:95–104.
3. Andrew M, Paes B, Milner R, et al: Development of the human coagulation system in the healthy premature infant. Blood 1988; 72:1651–1657.
4. Cook DJ, Guyatt GH, Laupacis A, et al: Rules of evidence and clinical recommendations on the use of antithrombotic agents. Chest 1992; 102(4 Suppl):305S–311S.
5. Deutsch VR, Olson TA, Nagler A, et al: The response of cord blood megakaryocyte progenitors to IL–3, IL–6 and aplastic canine serum varies with gestational age. Br J Haematol 1995; 89:8–16.
6. Murray NA, Roberts IA: Circulating megakaryocytes and their progenitors (BFU-MK and CFU-MK) in term and pre-term neonates. Br J Haematol 1995; 89:41–46.
7. Peterec SM, Brennan SA, Rinder HM, et al: Reticulated platelet values in normal and thrombocytopenic neonates. J Pediatr 1996; 129:269–274.
8. Joseph MA, Adams D, Maragos J, et al: Flow cytometry of neonatal platelet RNA. J Pediatr Hematol Oncol 1996; 18:277–281.
9. Murray NA, Watts TL, Roberts IA: Endogenous thrombopoietin levels and effect of recombinant human thrombopoietin on megakaryocyte precursors in term and preterm babies. Pediatr Res 1998; 43:148–151.
10. Aballi AJ, de Lamerens S: Coagulation changes in the neonatal period and in early infancy. Pediatr Clin North Am 1962; 9:785–817.

11. Andrew M, Kelton J: Neonatal thrombocytopenia. Clin Perinatol 1984; 11:359–391.
12. Pearson HA, McIntosh S: Neonatal thrombocytopenia. Clin Haematol 1978; 7:111–122.
13. Gill FM: Thrombocytopenia in the newborn. Semin Perinatol 1983; 7:201–212.
14. Mehta P, Vasa R, Neumann L, et al: Thrombocytopenia in the high-risk infant. J Pediatr 1980; 97:791–794.
15. Castle V, Andrew M, Kelton J, et al: Frequency and mechanism of neonatal thrombocytopenia. J Pediatr 1986; 108(5 Pt 1):749–755.
16. Beverley DW, Inwood MJ, Chance GW, et al: 'Normal' haemostasis parameters: A study in a well-defined inborn population of preterm infants. Early Hum Dev 1984; 9:249–257.
17. Kipper SL, Sieger L: Whole blood platelet volumes in newborn infants. J Pediatr 1982; 101:763–766.
18. Arad ID, Alpan G, Sznajderman SD, et al: The mean platelet volume (MPV) in the neonatal period. Am J Perinatol 1986; 3:1–3.
19. Forestier F, Daffos F, Galacteros F, et al: Hematological values of 163 normal fetuses between 18 and 30 weeks of gestation. Pediatr Res 1986; 20:342–346.
20. Castle V, Coates G, Kelton JG, et al: ^{111}In-oxine platelet survivals in thrombocytopenic infants. Blood 1987; 70:652–656.
21. Castle V, Coates G, Mitchell LG, et al: The effect of hypoxia on platelet survival and site of sequestration in the newborn rabbit. Thromb Haemost 1988; 59:45–48.
22. Rajasekhar D, Kestin AS, Bednarek FJ, et al: Neonatal platelets are less reactive than adult platelets to physiological agonists in whole blood. Thromb Haemost 1994; 72:957–963.
23. Hurtaud-Roux MF, Hezard N, Lefranc V, et al: Quantification of the major integrins and P-selectin in neonatal platelets by flow cytometry [abstract]. Thromb Haemost 2001; Suppl:P284.
24. Jenkins CS, Phillips DR, Clemetson KJ, et al: Platelet membrane glycoproteins implicated in ristocetin-induced aggregation. Studies of the proteins on platelets from patients with Bernard-Soulier syndrome and von Willebrand's disease. J Clin Invest 1976; 57:112–124.
25. Mull MM, Hathaway WE: Altered platelet function in newborns. Pediatr Res 1970; 4:229–237.
26. Whaun JM, Smith GR, Sochor VA: Effect of prenatal drug administration on maternal and neonatal platelet aggregation and PF4 release. Haemostasis 1980; 9:226–237.
27. Gruel Y, Boizard B, Daffos F, et al: Determination of platelet antigens and glycoproteins in the human fetus. Blood 1986; 68:488–492.
28. Katz JA, Moake JL, McPherson PD, et al: Relationship between human development and disappearance of unusually large von Willebrand factor multimers from plasma. Blood 1989; 73:1851–1858.
29. Weinstein MJ, Blanchard R, Moake JL, et al: Fetal and neonatal von Willebrand factor (VWF) is unusually large and similar to the VWF in patients with thrombotic thrombocytopenic purpura. Br J Haematol 1989; 72:68–72.
30. Takahashi Y, Kawaguchi C, Hanesaka Y, et al: Plasma von Willebrand factor-cleaving protease is low in newborns [abstract]. Thromb Haemost 2001; Suppl:P285.
31. Ts'ao CH, Green D, Schultz K: Function and ultrastructure of platelets of neonates: Enhanced ristocetin aggregation of neonatal platelets. Br J Haematol 1976; 32:225–233.
32. Harker LA, Slichter SJ: The bleeding time as a screening test for evaluation of platelet function. N Engl J Med 1972; 287:155–159.
33. Widdershoven J, Kollee L, van Munster P, et al: Biochemical vitamin K deficiency in early infancy: Diagnostic limitation of conventional coagulation tests. Helvetica Paediatrica Acta 1986; 41:195–201.
34. Feusner JH: Normal and abnormal bleeding times in neonates and young children utilizing a fully standardized template technic. Am J Clin Pathol 1980; 74:73–77.
35. Andrew M, Castle V, Saigal S, et al: Clinical impact of neonatal thrombocytopenia. J Pediatr 1987; 110:457–464.
36. Andrew M, Schmidt B, Mitchell L, et al: Thrombin generation in newborn plasma is critically dependent on the concentration of prothrombin. Thromb Haemost 1990; 63:27–30.
37. Ucar T, Gurman C, Kemahli S: Platelet functions in preterm and term newborns [abstract]. Thromb Haemost 2001; Suppl:CD3398.
38. Stuart MJ, Dusse J, Clark DA, et al: Differences in thromboxane production between neonatal and adult platelets in response to arachidonic acid and epinephrine. Pediatr Res 1984; 18:823–826.

39. Corby DG, O'Barr TP: Decreased alpha-adrenergic receptors in newborn platelets: Cause of abnormal response to epinephrine. Dev Pharmacol Ther 1981; 2:215–225.
40. Barradas MA, Mikhailidis DP, Imoedemhe DA, et al: An investigation of maternal and neonatal platelet function. Biol Res Pregnancy Perinatol 1986; 7:60–65.
41. Gader AM, Bahakim H, Jabbar FA, et al: Dose-response aggregometry in maternal/neonatal platelets. Thromb Haemost 1988; 60:314–318.
42. Hicsonmez G, Prozorova-Zamani V: Platelet aggregation in neonates with hyperbilirubinaemia. Scand J Haematol 1980; 24:67–70.
43. Alebouyeh M, Lusher JM, Ameri MR, et al: The effect of 5-hydroxytryptamine and epinephrine on newborn platelets. Eur J Pediatr 1978; 128:163–168.
44. Sadowitz PD, Walenga RW, Clark D, et al: Decreased plasma arachidonic acid binding capacity in neonates. Biol Neonate 1987; 51:305–311.
45. Landolfi R, De Cristofaro R, Ciabattoni G, et al: Placental-derived PGI$_2$ inhibits cord blood platelet function. Haematologica 1988; 73:207–210.
46. Ahlsten G, Ewald U, Tuvemo T: Arachidonic acid-induced aggregation of platelets from human cord blood compared with platelets from adults. Biol Neonate 1985; 47:199–204.
47. Andrews NP, Broughton PF, Heptinstall S: Blood platelet behaviour in mothers and neonates. Thromb Haemost 1985; 53:428–432.
48. Israels SJ, Daniels M, McMillan EM: Deficient collagen-induced activation in the newborn platelet. Pediatr Res 1990; 27(4 Pt 1):337–343.
49. Israels SJ, Gowen B, Gerrard JM: Contractile activity of neonatal platelets. Pediatr Res 1987; 21:293–295.
50. Corby DG, Zuck TF: Newborn platelet dysfunction: A storage pool and release defect. Thromb Haemost 1976; 36:200–207.
51. Kosztolanyi G, Jobst K, Kellermayer M, et al: ADP induced surface charge changes of adult and newborn platelets. Br J Haematol 1980; 46:257–262.
52. Stuart MJ: The neonatal platelet: Evaluation of platelet malonyl dialdehyde formation as an indicator of prostaglandin synthesis. Br J Haematol 1978; 39:83–90.
53. Stuart MJ, Dusse J: In vitro comparison of the efficacy of cyclooxygenase inhibitors on the adult versus neonatal platelet. Biol Neonate 1985; 47:265–269.
54. Walenga RW, Sunderji S, Stuart MJ: Formation of hydroxyeicosatetraenoic acids (HETE) in blood from adults versus neonates: Reduced production of 12-HETE in cord blood. Pediatr Res 1988; 24:563–567.
55. Weiss HJ, Aledort LM, Kochwa S: The effect of salicylates on the hemostatic properties of platelets in man. J Clin Invest 1968; 47:2169–2180.
56. Ambrus CM, Weintraub DH, Ambrus JL: Studies on hyaine membrane disease.3. Therapeutic trial of urokinase-activated human plasmin. Pediatrics 1966; 38:231–243.
57. Stuart MJ, Oski FA: Vitamin E and platelet function. Am J Pediatr Hematol Oncol 1979; 1:77–82.
58. Corby DG, O'Barr TP: Neonatal platelet function: A membrane-related phenomenon? Haemostasis 1981; 10:177–185.
59. Jones CR, McCabe R, Hamilton CA, et al: Maternal and fetal platelet responses and adrenoceptor binding characteristics. Thromb Haemost 1985; 53:95–98.
60. Aarts PA, Bolhuis PA, Sakariassen KS, et al: Red blood cell size is important for adherence of blood platelets to artery subendothelium. Blood 1983; 62:214–217.
61. Fernandez F, Gaudable C, Sie P, et al: Low hematocrit and prolonged bleeding time in uraemic patients: Effect of red cell transfusions. Br J Haematol 1985; 59:139–148.
62. Carcao MD, Blanchette VS, Dean JA, et al: The platelet function analyzer (PFA-100): A novel in vitro system for evaluation of primary haemostasis in children. Br J Haematol 1998; 101:70–73.
63. Sudi K, Kostenberger M, et al: Shorter PFA-100 closure time in neonates than in adults is not caused by high red or white blood cell counts but depends on platelets and von Willebrand factor [abstract]. Thromb Haemost 2001; Suppl:P280.
64. Slavec B, Benedik DM: The platelet function analyzer (PFA-100): A novel system for evaluation of primary haemostasis [abstract]. Thromb Haemost 2001; Suppl:CD3310.

65. Harrison P, Robinson M, Liesner R, et al: Performance of the PFA–100R as a potential screening tool for platelet dysfunction [abstract]. Thromb Haemost 2001; Suppl:P376.

66. Burgess CA, Credland P, Khair K, et al: An evaluation of the usefulness of the PFA–100 device in 60 consecutive paediatric patients referred for investigation of potential haemostatic disorders [abstract]. Thromb Haemost 2001; Suppl:P378.

67. Suarez CR, Menendez CE, Walenga JM, et al: Neonatal and maternal hemostasis: Value of molecular markers in the assessment of hemostatic status. Semin Thromb Hemost 1984; 10:280–284.

68. Kaplan KL, Owen J: Plasma levels of beta-thromboglobulin and platelet factor 4 as indices of platelet activation in vivo. Blood 1981; 57:199–202.

69. Suarez CR, Gonzalez J, Menendez C, et al: Neonatal and maternal platelets: Activation at time of birth. Am J Hematol 1988; 29:18–21.

70. Blifeld C, Courtney JT, Gross JR: Assessment of neonatal platelet function using a viscoelastic technique. Ann Clin Lab Sci 1986; 16:373–379.

71. Saleem A, Blifeld C, Saleh SA, et al: Viscoelastic measurement of clot formation: A new test of platelet function. Ann Clin Lab Sci 1983; 13:115–124.

72. Jacqz EM, Barrow SE, Dollery CT: Prostacyclin concentrations in cord blood and in the newborn. Pediatrics 1985; 76:954–957.

73. Kumar V, Berenson GS, Ruiz H, et al: Acid mucopolysaccharides of human aorta.1. Variations with maturation. J Atheroscler Res 1967; 7:573–581.

74. Andrew M, Mitchell L, Berry L, et al: An anticoagulant dermatan sulfate proteoglycan circulates in the pregnant woman and her fetus. J Clin Invest 1992; 89:321–326.

75. Nitschmann E, Berry L, Bridge S, et al: Morphological and biochemical features affecting the antithrombotic properties of the aorta in adult rabbits and rabbit pups. Thromb Haemost 1998; 79:1034–1040.

76. Nitschmann E, Berry L, Bridge S, et al: Morphologic and biochemical features affecting the antithrombotic properties of the inferior vena cava of rabbit pups and adult rabbits. Pediatr Res 1998; 43:62–67.

77. Abman SH: Pathogenesis and treatment of neonatal and postnatal pulmonary hypertension. Curr Opin Pediatr 1994; 6:239–247.

78. Xu L, Delorme M, Berry L, et al: Thrombin generation in newborn and adult plasma in the presence of an endothelial surface [abstract]. Thromb Haemost 1991; 65:1230.

79. Sanford HN, Gasteyer TH, Wyat L: The substances involved in the coagulation of the blood of the newborn [abstract]. Am J Dis Child 1932; 43:58.

80. Johnston M, Zipursky A: Microtechnology for the study of the blood coagulation system in newborn infants. Can J Med Tech 1980; 42:159–164.

81. Cade JF, Hirsh J, Martin M: Placental barrier to coagulation factors: Its relevance to the coagulation defect at birth and to haemorrhage in the newborn. BMJ 1969; 2:281–283.

82. Kisker CT, Robillard JE, Clarke WR: Development of blood coagulation—A fetal lamb model. Pediatr Res 1981; 15:1045–1050.

83. Andrew M, O'Brodovich H, Mitchell L: Fetal lamb coagulation system during normal birth. Am J Hematol 1988; 28:116–118.

84. Holmberg L, Henriksson P, Ekelund H, et al: Coagulation in the human fetus. Comparison with term newborn infants. J Pediatr 1974; 85:860–864.

85. Jensen AH, Josso F, Zamet P, et al: Evolution of blood clotting factors in premature infants during the first 10 days of life: A study of 96 cases with comparison between clinical status and blood clotting factor levels. Pediatr Res 1973; 7:638–644.

86. Mibashan RS, Rodeck CH, Thumpston JK, et al: Plasma assay of fetal factors VIIIC and IX for prenatal diagnosis of haemophilia. Lancet 1979; 1:1309–1311.

87. Forestier F, Cox WL, Daffos F, et al: The assessment of fetal blood samples. Am J Obstet Gynecol 1988; 158:1184–1188.

88. Forestier F, Daffos F, Rainaut M, et al: Vitamin K dependent proteins in fetal hemostasis at mid trimester of pregnancy. Thromb Haemost 1985; 53:401–403.

89. Forestier F, Daffos F, Sole Y, et al: Prenatal diagnosis of hemophilia by fetal blood sampling under ultrasound guidance. Haemostasis 1986; 16:346–351.

90. Toulon P, Rainaut M, Aiach M, et al: Antithrombin III (ATIII) and heparin cofactor II (HCII) in normal human fetuses (21st–27th week) [letter]. Thromb Haemost 1986; 56:237.

91. Barnard DR, Simmons MA, Hathaway WE: Coagulation studies in extremely premature infants. Pediatr Res 1979; 13:1330–1335.

92. Nossel HL, Lanzkowsky P, Levy S, et al: A study of coagulation factor levels in women during labour and in their newborn infants. Thromb Diath Haemorrh 1966; 16:185–197.

93. Hirsh J, Ofosu F, Cairns J: Advances in antithrombotic therapy. In Hoffbrand AV (ed): Recent Advances in Hematology. London, Churchill Livingstone, 1985, pp 333–367.

94. Koepke JA: Partial thromboplastin time test—Proposed performance guidelines. ICSH Panel on the PTT. Thromb Haemost 1986; 55:143–144.

95. Hirsh J: Oral anticoagulant drugs [see comments]. N Engl J Med 1991; 324:1865–1875.

96. Townsend CW: The haemorrhagic disease of the newborn. Arch Pediatr 1894; 11:559.

97. Dam H, Tage-Hansen E, Plum P: K-avitaminose hos spaede born som aarag til hemorrhagisk diathese. Ugesk Laeger 1939; 101:896.

98. Brinkhous KM, Smith HP, Warner ED: Plasma prothrombin level in normal infancy and in hemorrhagic disease of the newborn. Am J Med Sci 1937; 193:475.

99. Bleyer WA, Hakami N, Shepard TH: The development of hemostasis in the human fetus and newborn infant [abstract]. J Pediatr 1971; 79:838–853.

100. Hathaway WE, Bonnar J: Bleeding disorders in the newborn infant. In Oliver TK Jr (ed): Perinatal Coagulation. Monographs in Neonatology. New York, Grune and Stratton, 1978, pp 115–169.

101. Gross S, Melhorn D: Exchange transfusion with citrated whole blood for disseminated intravascular coagulation. J Pediatr 1971; 78:415–419.

102. Buchanan GR: Coagulation disorders in the neonate. Pediatr Clin North Am 1986; 33:203–220.

103. Montgomery RR, Marlar RA, Gill JC: Newborn haemostasis. Clin Haematol 1985; 14:443–460.

104. Gibson B: Neonatal haemostasis. Arch Dis Child 1989; 64:503–506.

105. Gobel U, von Voss H, Petrich C, et al:. Etiopathology and classification of acquired coagulation disorders in the newborn infant. Klin Wochenschr 1979; 57:81–86.

106. McDonald MM, Hathaway WE: Neonatal hemorrhage and thrombosis. Semin Perinatol 1983; 7:213–225.

107. Stothers J, Boulton F, Wild R, et al: Letter: Neonatal coagulation. Lancet 1975; 1:408–409.

108. Bahakim H, Gader AGMA, Galil A, et al: Coagulation parameters in maternal and cord blood at delivery. Ann Saud Med 1990; 10:149–155.

109. Andrew M, Karpatkin M: A simple screening test for evaluating prolonged partial thromboplastin times in newborn infants. J Pediatr 1982; 101:610–612.

110. Zipursky A, Jaber HM: The haematology of bacterial infection in newborn infants. Clin Haematol 1978; 7:175–193.

111. Schmidt B, Ofosu FA, Mitchell L, et al: Anticoagulant effects of heparin in neonatal plasma. Pediatr Res 1989; 25:405–408.

112. Schmidt B, Mitchell L, Ofosu FA, et al: Alpha–2-macroglobulin is an important progressive inhibitor of thrombin in neonatal and infant plasma. Thromb Haemost 1989; 62:1074–1077.

113. Levine JJ, Udall JN, Evernden BA, et al: Elevated levels of α-macroglobulin-protease complexes in infants. Biol Neonate 1987; 51:149.

114. Delorme MA, Xu L, Berry L, et al: Anticoagulant dermatan sulfate proteoglycan (decorin) in the term human placenta. Thromb Res 1998; 90:147–153.

115. Greffe BS, Marlar RA, Manco-Johnson MJ: Neonatal protein C: Molecular composition and distribution in normal term infants. Thromb Res 1989; 56:91–98.

116. Manco-Johnson MJ, Spedale S, Peters M, et al: Identification of a unique form of protein C in the ovine fetus: Developmentally linked transition to the adult form. Pediatr Res 1995; 37:365–372.

117. Moalic P, Gruel Y, Body G, et al: Levels and plasma distribution of free and C4b-BP-bound protein S in human fetuses and full-term newborns. Thromb Res 1988; 49:471–480.

118. Schwarz HP, Muntean W, Watzke H, et al: Low total protein S antigen but high protein S activity due to decreased C4b-binding protein in neonates. Blood 1988; 71:562–565.

119. Cvirn G, Gallistl S, Kostenberger M, et al: Efficacy of the anticoagulant action of protein S is regulated by the alpha 2

macroglobulin level in cord and adult plasma. Thromb Haemost 2001; Suppl:P282.

120. Knofler R, Hofmann S, Weissbach G, et al: Molecular markers of the endothelium, the coagulation and the fibrinolytic systems in healthy newborns [abstract]. Semin Thromb Hemost 1998; 24:453–461.

121. Yurdakok M, Yigit S, Aliefendioglu D, et al: Plasma thrombomodulin levels in early respiratory distress syndrome. Turk J Pediatr 1998; 40:85–88.

122. Distefano G, Romeo MG, Betta P, et al: Thrombomodulin serum levels in ventilated preterm babies with respiratory distress syndrome. Eur J Pediatr 1998; 157:327–330.

123. Yurdakok M, Yigit S: Plasma thrombomodulin, plasminogen activator and plasminogen activator inhibitor levels in preterm infants with or without respiratory distress syndrome [letter; comment]. Acta Paediatr 1997; 86:1022–1023.

124. Nako Y, Ohki Y, Harigaya A, et al: Plasma thrombomodulin level in very low birthweight infants at birth. Acta Paediatr 1997; 86:1105–1109.

125. Van Dreden P, Auvrignon A, Leverger G, et al: Tissue factor pathway inhibitor in infants and children. Thromb Haemost 2001; Suppl:P2134.

126. Patel P, Weitz J, Brooker LA, et al: Decreased thrombin activity of fibrin clots prepared in cord plasma compared with adult plasma [abstract]. Pediatr Res 1996; 39:826–830.

127. Kisker CT, Perlman S, Bohlken D, et al: Measurement of prothrombin mRNA during gestation and early neonatal development. J Lab Clin Med 1988; 112:407–412.

128. Hassan HJ, Leonardi A, Chelucci C, et al: Blood coagulation factors in human embryonic-fetal development: Preferential expression of the FVII/tissue factor pathway. Blood 1990; 76:1158–1164.

129. Karpatkin M, Blei F, Hurlet A, et al: Prothrombin expression in the adult and fetal rabbit liver. Pediatr Res 1991; 30:266–269.

130. Andrew M, Mitchell L, Berry LR, et al: Fibrinogen has a rapid turnover in the healthy newborn lamb. Pediatr Res 1988; 23:249–252.

131. Karitzky D, Kleine N, Pringsheim W, et al: Fibrinogen turnover in the premature infant with and without idiopathic respiratory distress syndrome. Acta Paediatr Scand 1971; 60:465–470.

132. Schmidt B, Wais U, Pringsheim W, et al: Plasma elimination of antithrombin III (heparin cofactor activity) is accelerated in term newborn infants. Eur J Pediatr 1984; 141:225–227.

133. Esmon NL, Owen WG, Esmon CT: Isolation of a membrane-bound cofactor for thrombin-catalyzed activation of protein C. J Biol Chem 1982; 257:859–864.

134. Andrew M, O'Brodovich H, Mitchell L: Fetal lamb coagulation system during birth asphyxia. Am J Hematol 1988; 28:201–203.

135. Witt I, Muller H, Kunzer W: Evidence for the existence of foetal fibrinogen. Thromb Diath Haemorrh 1969; 22:101–109.

136. Hamulyak K, Nieuwenhuizen W, Devilee PP, et al: Reevaluation of some properties of fibrinogen, purified from cord blood of normal newborns. Thromb Res 1983; 32:301–310.

137. Galanakis DK, Mosesson MW: Evaluation of the role of in vivo proteolysis (fibrinogenolysis) in prolonging the thrombin time of human umbilical cord fibrinogen. Blood 1976; 48:109–118.

138. Yuen PM, Yin JA, Lao TT: Fibrinopeptide A levels in maternal and newborn plasma. Eur J Obstet Gynecol Reprod Biol 1989; 30:239–244.

139. Corrigan JJ Jr: Neonatal thrombosis and the thrombolytic system: Pathophysiology and therapy. Am J Pediatr Hematol Oncol 1988; 10:83–91.

140. Corrigan JJ Jr, Sleeth JJ, Jeter M, et al: Newborn's fibrinolytic mechanism: Components and plasmin generation. Am J Hematol 1989; 32:273–278.

141. Kolindewala JK, Das BK, Dube RK, et al: Blood fibrinolytic activity in neonates: Effect of period of gestation, birth weight, anoxia and sepsis. Indian Pediatr 1987; 24:1029–1033.

142. Lecander I, Astedt B: Specific plasminogen activator inhibitor of placental type PAI 2 occurring in amniotic fluid and cord blood. J Lab Clin Med 1987; 110:602–605.

143. Edelberg JM, Enghild JJ, Pizzo SV, et al: Neonatal plasminogen displays altered cell surface binding and activation kinetics. Correlation with increased glycosylation of the protein. J Clin Invest 1990; 86:107–112.

144. Andrew M, Brooker L, Leaker M, et al: Fibrin clot lysis by thrombolytic agents is impaired in newborns due to a low plasminogen concentration. Thromb Haemost 1992; 68:325–330.

145. Gray OP, Ackerman A, Fraser AJ: Intracranial haemorrhage and clotting defects in low-birth-weight infants. Lancet 1968; 1:545–548.

146. Girolami A, De Marco L, Dal Bo ZR, et al: Rarer quantitative and qualitative abnormalities of coagulation. Clin Haematol 1985; 14:385–411.

147. Silverstein A: Intracranial bleeding in hemophilia. Arch Neurol 1960; 94:12–26.

148. Yoffe G, Buchanan GR: Intracranial hemorrhage in newborn and young infants with hemophilia. J Pediatr 1988; 113:333–336.

149. Abbondanzo SL, Gootenberg JE, Lofts RS, et al: Intracranial hemorrhage in congenital deficiency of factor XIII. Am J Pediatr Hematol Oncol 1988; 10:65–68.

150. Struwe F: Intracranial hemorrhage and occlusive hydrocephalus in hereditary bleeding disorders. Dev Med Child Neurol 1970; 12:165–169.

151. Mariani G, Mazzucconi MG: Factor VII congenital deficiency. Clinical picture and classification of the variants. Haemostasis 1983; 13:169–177.

152. Baehner RL, Strauss HS: Hemophilia in the first year of life. N Engl J Med 1966; 275:524–528.

153. Pearson HA, Shulman NR, Marder VJ, et al: Isoimmune neonatal thrombocytopenic purpura. Clinical and therapeutic considerations. Blood 2001; 23:154–177.

154. Gajl-Paczalska K: Plasma protein composition of hyaline membrane in the newborn as studies by immunofluorescence. Arch Dis Child 1964; 39:226–231.

155. Lupton BA, Hill A, Whitfield MF, et al: Reduced platelet count as a risk factor for intraventricular hemorrhage. Am J Dis Child 1988; 142:1222–1224.

156. Austin N, Darlow BA: Transfusion-associated fall in platelet count in very low birthweight infants. Aust Paediatr J 1988; 24:354–356.

157. Samuels P, Main EK, Tomaski A, et al: Abnormalities in platelet antiglobulin tests in preeclamptic mothers and their neonates. Am J Obstet Gynecol 1987; 157:109–113.

158. Stuart M, Wu J, Sunderji S, et al: Effect of amniotic fluid on platelet thromboxane production. J Pediatr 1987; 110:289–292.

159. Tate DY, Carlton GT, Johnson D, et al: Immune thrombocytopenia in severe neonatal infections. J Pediatr 1981; 98:449–453.

160. Podolsak B: Thrombopoiesis in newborn infants after exchange blood transfusion. Z Kinderheilkd 1973; 114:13–26.

161. Patrick CH, Lazarchick J: The effect of bacteremia on automated platelet measurements in neonates. Am J Clin Pathol 1990; 93:391–394.

162. Weinblatt ME, Scimeca PG, James-Herry AG, et al: Thrombocytopenia in an infant with AIDS. Am J Dis Child 1987; 141:15.

163. Ballin A, Koren G, Kohelet D, et al: Reduction of platelet counts induced by mechanical ventilation in newborn infants. J Pediatr 1987; 111:445–449.

164. Horgan MJ, Carrasco NJ, Risemberg H: The relationship of thrombocytopenia to the onset of persistent pulmonary hypertension of the newborn in the meconium aspiration syndrome. NY State J Med 1985; 85:245–247.

165. Shim WK: Hemangiomas of infancy complicated by thrombocytopenia. Am J Surg 1968; 116:896–906.

166. Fost NC, Esterly NB: Successful treatment of juvenile hemangiomas with prednisone. J Pediatr 1968; 72:351–357.

167. Johnson DH, Vinson AM, Wirth FH, et al: Management of hepatic hemangioendotheliomas of infancy by transarterial embolization: A report of two cases. Pediatrics 1984; 73:546–549.

168. Orchard PJ, Smith CM III, Woods WG, et al: Treatment of haemangioendotheliomas with alpha interferon. Lancet 1989; 2:565–567.

169. Larsen EC, Zinkham WH, Eggleston JC, et al: Kasabach-Merritt syndrome: Therapeutic considerations. Pediatrics 1987; 79:971–980.

170. Andrew M: The hemostatic system in the infant. In Nathan D, Oski F (eds): Hematology of Infancy and Childhood, 4th ed. Philadelphia, WB Saunders, 1992, pp 115–154.

171. Corby DG, Schulman I: The effects of antenatal drug administration on aggregation of platelets of newborn infants. J Pediatr 1971; 79:307–313.

172. Levy G, Garrettson LK: Kinetics of salicylate elimination by newborn infants of mothers who ingested aspirin before delivery. Pediatrics 1974; 53:201–210.

173. Ylikorkala O, Makila UM, Kaapa P, et al: Maternal ingestion of acetylsalicylic acid inhibits fetal and neonatal prostacyclin and thromboxane in humans. Am J Obstet Gynecol 1986; 155:345–349.

174. Haslam RR, Ekert H, Gillam GL: Hemorrhage in a neonate possibly due to maternal ingestion of salicylate. J Pediatr 1974; 84:556–557.

175. Cariou R, Tobelem G, Bellucci S, et al: Effect of lupus anticoagulant on antithrombogenic properties of endothelial cells—Inhibition of thrombomodulin-dependent protein C activation. Thromb Haemost 1988; 60:54–58.

176. Murphy WG, Moore JC, Kelton JG: Calcium-dependent cysteine protease activity in the sera of patients with thrombotic thrombocytopenic purpura. Blood 1987; 70:1683–1687.

177. Hall JG, Levin J, Kuhn JP, et al: Thrombocytopenia with absent radius (TAR). Medicine (Baltimore) 1969; 48:411–439.

178. Hedberg VA, Lipton JM: Thrombocytopenia with absent radii. A review of 100 cases. Am J Pediatr Hematol Oncol 1988; 10:51–64.

179. Homans AC, Cohen JL, Mazur EM: Defective megakaryocytopoiesis in the syndrome of thrombocytopenia with absent radii. Br J Haematol 1988; 70:205–210.

180. Lecompte T: Hereditary thrombocytopenias. Curr Stud Hematol Blood Transfus 1988;:162–173.

181. Hegde UM: Immune thrombocytopenia in pregnancy and the newborn. Br J Obstet Gynaecol 1985; 92:657–659.

182. Andrew M, Vegh P, Caco C, et al: A randomized, controlled trial of platelet transfusions in thrombocytopenic premature infants. J Pediatr 1993; 123:285–291.

183. Chan KW, Kaikov Y, Wadsworth LD: Thrombocytosis in childhood: A survey of 94 patients. Pediatrics 1989; 84:1064–1067.

184. Ostermann H, van de Loo J: Factors of the hemostatic system in diabetic patients. A survey of controlled studies. Haemostasis 1986; 16:386–416.

185. Stuart MJ, Elrad H, Graeber JE, et al: Increased synthesis of prostaglandin endoperoxides and platelet hyperfunction in infants of mothers with diabetes mellitus. J Lab Clin Med 1979; 94:12–26.

186. Kaapa P, Knip M, Viinikka L, et al: Increased platelet thromboxane B_2 production in newborn infants of diabetic mothers. Prostaglandins Leukot Med 1986; 21:299–304.

187. Stuart MJ, Sunderji SG, Allen JB: Decreased prostacyclin production in the infant of the diabetic mother. J Lab Clin Med 1981; 98:412–416.

188. Kaapa P, Uhari M, Nikkari T, et al: Dietary fatty acids and platelet thromboxane production in puerperal women and their offspring. Am J Obstet Gynecol 1986; 155:146–149.

189. Friedman Z, Lamberth EL Jr, Stahlman MT, et al: Platelet dysfunction in the neonate with essential fatty acid deficiency. J Pediatr 1977; 90:439–443.

190. Friedman Z, Danon A, Stahlman MT, et al: Rapid onset of essential fatty acid deficiency in the newborn. Pediatrics 1976; 58:640–649.

191. Friedman Z, Seyberth H, Lamberth EL, et al: Decreased prostaglandin E turnover in infants with essential fatty acid deficiency. Pediatr Res 1978; 12:711–714.

192. Machlin LJ, Filipski R, Willis AL, et al: Influence of vitamin E on platelet aggregation and thrombocythemia in the rat. Proc Soc Exp Biol Med 1975; 149:275–277.

193. Stuart MJ: Vitamin E deficiency: Its effect on platelet-vascular interaction in various pathologic states. Ann NY Acad Sci 1972; 277.

194. Lake AM, Stuart MJ, Oski FA: Vitamin E deficiency and enhanced platelet function: Reversal following E supplementation. J Pediatr 1977; 90:722–725.

195. Ahlsten G, Ewald U, Kindahl H, et al: Aggregation of and thromboxane B_2 synthesis in platelets from newborn infants of smoking and non-smoking mothers. Prostaglandins Leukot Med 1985; 19:167–176.

196. Ahlsten G, Ewald U, Tuvemo T: Maternal smoking reduces prostacyclin formation in human umbilical arteries. A study on strictly selected pregnancies. Acta Obstet Gynecol Scand 1986; 65:645–649.

197. Davis RB, Leuschen MP, Boyd D, et al: Evaluation of platelet function in pregnancy. Comparative studies in non-smokers and smokers. Thromb Res 1987; 46:175–186.

198. Ylikorkala O, Halmesmaki E, Viinikka L: Effect of ethanol on thromboxane and prostacyclin synthesis by fetal platelets and umbilical artery. Life Sci 1987; 41:371–376.

199. Segall ML, Goetzman BW, Schick JB: Thrombocytopenia and pulmonary hypertension in the perinatal aspiration syndromes. J Pediatr 1980; 96:727–730.

200. Levin DL, Weinberg AG, Perkin RM: Pulmonary microthrombi syndrome in newborn infants with unresponsive persistent pulmonary hypertension. J Pediatr 1983; 102:299–303.

201. Suzuki S, Wake N, Yoshiaki K: New neonatal problems of blood coagulation and fibrinolysis. II. Thromboplastic effect of amniotic fluid and its relation to lung maturity. J Perinat Med 1976; 4:221–226.

202. Kaapa P: Immunoreactive thromboxane B_2 and 6-keto-prostaglandin $F_{1\alpha}$ in neonatal hyperbilirubinemia. Prostaglandins Leukot Med 1985; 17:97–105.

203. Maurer HM, Haggins JC, Still WJ: Platelet injury during phototherapy. Am J Hematol 1976; 1:89–96.

204. Karim MA, Clelland IA, Chapman IV, et al: β-Thromboglobulin levels in plasma of jaundiced neonates exposed to phototherapy. J Perinat Med 1981; 9:141–144.

205. Remuzzi G: Bleeding in renal failure. Lancet 1988; 1:1205–1208.

206. Bleyer WA, Breckenridge RT: Studies on the detection of adverse drug reactions in the newborn. II. The effects of prenatal aspirin on newborn hemostasis. JAMA 1970; 213:2049–2053.

207. Rumack CM, Guggenheim MA, Rumack BH, et al: Neonatal intracranial hemorrhage and maternal use of aspirin. Obstet Gynecol 1981; 58(5 Suppl):52S–56S.

208. Ts'ao CH: Comparable inhibition of aggregation of PRP of neonates and adults by aspirin. Haemostasis 1977; 6:118–126.

209. Palmisano PA, Cassady G: Salicylate exposure in the perinate. JAMA 1969; 209:556–558.

210. Casteels-Van Daele M, Jaeken J, Eggermont E, et al: More on the effects of antenatally administered aspirin on aggregation of platelets of neonates. J Pediatr 1972; 80:685–686.

211. Territo M, Finklestein J, Oh W, et al: Management of autoimmune thrombocytopenia in pregnancy and in the neonate. Obstet Gynecol 1973; 41:579–584.

212. Peters M, Jansen E, ten Cate JW, et al: Neonatal antithrombin III. Br J Haematol 1984; 58:579–587.

213. Pomerance JJ, Teal JG, Gogolok JF, et al: Maternally administered antenatal vitamin K_1: Effect on neonatal prothrombin activity, partial thromboplastin time, and intraventricular hemorrhage. Obstet Gynecol 1987; 70:235–241.

214. Morales WJ, Angel JL, O'Brien WF, et al: The use of antenatal vitamin K in the prevention of early neonatal intraventricular hemorrhage. Am J Obstet Gynecol 1988; 159:774–779.

215. Heymann MA, Rudolph AM, Silverman NH: Closure of the ductus arteriosus in premature infants by inhibition of prostaglandin synthesis. N Engl J Med 1976; 295:530–533.

216. Friedman WF, Hirschklau MJ, Printz MP, et al: Pharmacologic closure of patent ductus arteriosus in the premature infant. N Engl J Med 1976; 295:526–529.

217. Gersony WM, Peckham GJ, Ellison RC, et al: Effects of indomethacin in premature infants with patent ductus arteriosus: Results of a national collaborative study. J Pediatr 1983; 102:895–906.

218. Friedman Z, Whitman V, Maisels MJ, et al: Indomethacin disposition and indomethacin-induced platelet dysfunction in premature infants. J Clin Pharmacol 1978; 18(5–6):272–279.

219. Guignard JP, Torrado A, Da Cunha O, et al: Glomerular filtration rate in the first three weeks of life. J Pediatr 1975; 87:268–272.

220. Brown AK, Zeulzer WW, Brunett HH: Studies on the neonatal development of the glucoronide system. J Clin Invest 1958; 37:332.

221. Setzer ES, Webb IB, Wassenaar JW, et al: Platelet dysfunction and coagulopathy in intraventricular hemorrhage in the premature infant. J Pediatr 1982; 100:599–605.

222. Corazza MS, Davis RF, Merritt TA, et al: Prolonged bleeding time in preterm infants receiving indomethacin for patent ductus arteriosus. J Pediatr 1984; 105:292–296.

223. Ment LR, Ehrenkranz RA, Duncan CC: Intraventricular hemorrhage of the preterm neonate: Prevention studies. Semin Perinatol 1988; 12:359–372.

224. Shearer MJ, Rahim S, Barkhan P, et al: Plasma vitamin K₁ in mothers and their newborn babies. Lancet 1982; 2:460–463.

225. Sagel J, Colwell JA, Crook L, et al: Increased platelet aggregation in early diabetus mellitus. Ann Intern Med 1975; 82:733–738.

226. Halushka PV, Lurie D, Colwell JA: Increased synthesis of prostaglandin-E-like material by platelets from patients with diabetes mellitus. N Engl J Med 1977; 297:1306–1310.

227. Oppenheimer EH, Esterly JR: Thrombosis in the newborn: Comparison between infants of diabetic and nondiabetic mothers. J Pediatr 1965; 67:549–556.

228. Cowett RM, Schwartz R: The infant of the diabetic mother. Pediatr Clin North Am 1982; 29:1213–1231.

229. Dixon RH, Rosse WF: Platelet antibody in autoimmune thrombocytopenia. Br J Haematol 1975; 31:129–134.

230. Cox AC, Rao GH, Gerrard JM, et al: The influence of vitamin E quinone on platelet structure, function, and biochemistry. Blood 1980; 55:907–914.

231. Steiner M, Anastasi J: Vitamin E—An inhibitor of the platelet thromboxane production. J Pediatr 1987; 110:289–290.

232. Khurshid M, Lee TJ, Peake IR, et al: Vitamin E deficiency and platelet functional defect in a jaundiced infant. BMJ 1975; 4:19–21.

233. Kaapa P: Platelet thromboxane B₂ production in neonatal pulmonary hypertension. Arch Dis Child 1987; 62:195–196.

234. Varela AF, Runge A, Ignarro LJ, et al: Nitric oxide and prostacyclin inhibit fetal platelet aggregation: A response similar to that observed in adults. Am J Obstet Gynecol 1992; 167:1599–1604.

235. Radomski MW, Palmer RM, Moncada S: Endogenous nitric oxide inhibits human platelet adhesion to vascular endothelium. Lancet 1987; 2:1057–1058.

236. Golino P, Cappelli-Bigazzi M, Ambrosio G, et al: Endothelium-derived relaxing factor modulates platelet aggregation in an in vivo model of recurrent platelet activation. Circ Res 1992; 71:1447–1456.

237. Bodzenta-Lukaszyk A, Gabryelewicz A, Lukaszyk A, et al: Nitric oxide synthase inhibition and platelet function. Thromb Res 1994; 75:667–672.

238. Mazzone D, Fichera A, Pratico G, et al: Combined congenital deficiency of factor V and factor VIII. Acta Haematol 1982; 68:337–338.

239. McMillan CW, Roberts HR: Congenital combined deficiency of coagulation factors II, VII, IX and X. Report of a case. N Engl J Med 1966; 274:1313–1315.

240. Scher MS, Wright FS, Lockman LA, et al: Intraventricular hemorrhage in the full-term neonate. Arch Neurol 1982; 39:769–772.

241. Jackson JC, Blumhagen JD: Congenital hydrocephalus due to prenatal intracranial hemorrhage. Pediatrics 1983; 72:344–346.

242. Serfontein GL, Rom S, Stein S: Posterior fossa subdural hemorrhage in the newborn. Pediatrics 1980; 65:40–43.

243. Gunn TR, Mok PM, Becroft DM: Subdural hemorrhage in utero. Pediatrics 1985; 76:605–610.

244. Cartwright GW, Culbertson K, Schreiner RL, et al: Changes in clinical presentation of term infants with intracranial hemorrhage. Dev Med Child Neurol 1979; 21:730–737.

245. Palma PA, Miner ME, Morriss FH Jr, et al: Intraventricular hemorrhage in the neonate born at term. Am J Dis Child 1979; 133:941–944.

246. Chaplin ER Jr, Goldstein GW, Norman D: Neonatal seizures, intracerebral hematoma, and subarachnoid hemorrhage in full-term infants. Pediatrics 1979; 63:812–815.

247. Guekos-Thoeni U, Boltshauser E, Willi UV: Intraventricular haemorrhage in full-term neonates. Dev Med Child Neurol 1982; 24:704–705.

248. Mackay RJ, de Crespigny LC, Murton LJ, et al: Intraventricular haemorrhage in term neonates: Diagnosis by ultrasound. Aust Paediatr J 1982; 18:205–207.

249. Hayden CK Jr, Shattuck KE, Richardson CJ, et al: Subependymal germinal matrix hemorrhage in full-term neonates. Pediatrics 1985; 75:714–718.

250. Guekos-Thoeni U, Boltshauser E, Willi UV: Intraventricular haemorrhage in full-term neonates. Dev Med Child Neurol 1982; 24:704–705.

251. Bray GL, Luban NL: Hemophilia presenting with intracranial hemorrhage. An approach to the infant with intracranial bleeding and coagulopathy. Am J Dis Child 1987; 141:1215–1217.

252. Schmidt B, Zipursky A: Disseminated intravascular coagulation masking neonatal hemophilia. J Pediatr 1986; 109:886–888.

253. Baugh RF, Deemar KA, Zimmermann JJ: Heparinase in the activated clotting time assay: Monitoring heparin-independent alterations in coagulation function. Anesth Analg 1992; 74:201–205.

254. Karpatkin S, Strick N, Karpatkin MB, et al: Cumulative experience in the detection of antiplatelet antibody in 234 patients with idiopathic thrombocytopenic purpura, systemic lupus erythematosus and other clinical disorders. Am J Med 1972; 52:776–785.

255. Smith PS: Congenital coagulation protein deficiencies in the perinatal period. Semin Perinatol 1990; 14:384–392.

256. Rohyans JA, Miser AW, Miser JS: Subgaleal hemorrhage in infants with hemophilia: Report of two cases and review of the literature. Pediatrics 1982; 70:306–307.

257. Killick CJ, Barton CJ, Aslam S, et al: Prenatal diagnosis in factor XIII—A deficiency. Arch Dis Child Fetal Neonatal Ed 1999; 80:F238-F239.

258. Antonarakis SE, Copeland KL, Carpenter RJ, et al: Prenatal diagnosis of haemophilia A by factor VIII gene analysis. Lancet 1985; 1:1407–1409.

259. Peake IR, Bowen D, Bignell P, et al: Family studies and prenatal diagnosis in severe von Willebrand disease by polymerase chain reaction amplification of a variable number tandem repeat region of the von Willebrand factor gene. Blood 1990; 76:555–561.

260. Manios SG, Schenck W, Kunzer W: Congenital fibrinogen deficiency. Acta Paediatr Scand 1968; 57:145–150.

261. Lewis JH, Spero JA, Ragni MV, et al: Transfusion support for congenital clotting deficiencies other than haemophilia. Clin Haematol 1984; 13:119–135.

262. Zenny JC, Chevrot A, Sultan Y, et al: [Intra-osseus hemorrhagic lesions in congenital afibrinogenemia. A new case (author's transl)]. J Radiol 1981; 62:263–266.

263. Fried K, Kaufman S: Congenital afibrinogenemia in 10 offspring of uncle-niece marriages. Clin Genet 1980; 17:223–227.

264. Gill FM, Shapiro SS, Schwartz E: Severe congenital hypoprothrombinemia. J Pediatr 1978; 93:264–266.

265. Viola L, Chiaretti A, Lazzareschi I, et al: [Intracranial hemorrhage in congenital factor II deficiency]. Pediatr Med Chir 1995; 17:593–594.

266. Ehrenforth S, Klarmann D, Zabel B, et al: Severe factor V deficiency presenting as subdural haematoma in the newborn. Eur J Pediatr 1998; 157:1032.

267. Kashyap R, Saxena R, Choudhry VP: Rare inherited coagulation disorders in India. Haematologia (Budap) 1996; 28:13–19.

268. Seeler RA: Parahemophilia. Factor V deficiency. Med Clin North Am 1972; 56:119–125.

269. Roberts H, Lefkowitz J: Inherited disorders of prothrombin conversion. In Colman R, Hirsh J, Marder V, et al (eds): Philadelphia, JB Lippincott, 1994, pp 200–218.

270. Salooja N, Martin P, Khair K, et al: Severe factor V deficiency and neonatal intracranial haemorrhage: A case report. Haemophilia 2000; 6:44–46.

271. Matthay KK, Koerper MA, Ablin AR: Intracranial hemorrhage in congenital factor V deficiency. J Pediatr 1979; 94:413–415.

272. Schubert B, Schindera F: Congenital factor VII deficiency in a newborn [abstract]. Hamophilie-Symposion, 1988.

273. Levanon M, Rimon S, Shani M, et al: Active and inactive factor VII in Dubin-Johnson syndrome with factor VII deficiency, hereditary factor VII deficiency and on Coumadin administration. Br J Haematol 1972; 23:669.

274. Seligsohn U, Shani M, Ramot B: Gilbert syndrome and factor-VII deficiency. Lancet 1970; 1:1398.

275. Rabiner S, Winick M, Smith C: Congenital deficiency of factor VII associated with hemorrhagic disease of the newborn. Pediatrics 1960; 25:101–105.

276. Ragni M, Lewis J, Spero J, et al: Factor VII deficiency. Am J Hematol 1986; 10:79–88.

277. Seligsohn U, Shani M, Ramot B, et al: Dubin-Johnson syndrome in Israel. II. Association with factor-VII deficiency. Q J Med 1970; 39:569–584.

278. Adcock DM, Brozna J, Marlar RA: Proposed classification and pathologic mechanisms of purpura fulminans and skin necrosis. Semin Thromb Hemost 1990; 16:333–340.

279. Schulman I: Pediatric aspects of the mild hemophilias. Med Clin North Am 1962; 46:93–105.
280. Kozinn P, Ritz N, Moss A, et al: Massive hemorrhage—Scalps of newborn infants. Am J Dis Child 1964; 108:413–417.
281. Kozinn P, Ritz N, Horowitz A: Scalp hemorrhage as an emergency in the newborn. JAMA 1965; 194:179–180.
282. McCarthy JW, Coble LL: Intracranial hemorrhage and subsequent communicating hydrocephalus in a neonate with classical hemophilia. Pediatrics 1973; 51:122–124.
283. Umetsu M, Chiba Y, Horino K, Chiba S, Nakao T: Cytomegalovirus-mononucleosis in a newborn infant. Arch Dis Child 1975; 50:396–397.
284. Volpe JJ, Manica JP, Land VJ, et al: Neonatal subdural hematoma associated with severe hemophilia A. J Pediatr 1976; 88:1023–1025.
285. Cohen DL: Neonatal subgaleal hemorrhage in hemophilia. J Pediatr 1978; 93:1022–1023.
286. Eyster ME, Gill FM, Blatt PM, et al: Central nervous system bleeding in hemophiliacs. Blood 1978; 51:1179–1188.
287. Koch JA: Haemophilia in the newborn. A case report and literature review. S Afr Med J 1978; 53:721–722.
288. Pettersson H, McClure P, Fitz C: Intracranial hemorrhage in hemophilic children. CT follow-up. Acta Radiol Diagn (Stockh) 1984; 25:161–164.
289. Bisset RA, Gupta SC, Zammit-Maempel I: Radiographic and ultrasound appearances of an intra-mural haematoma of the pylorus. Clin Radiol 1988; 39:316–318.
290. Kletzel M, Miller CH, Becton DL, et al: Postdelivery head bleeding in hemophilic neonates. Causes and management. Am J Dis Child 1989; 143:1107–1110.
291. Ljung R, Petrini P, Nilsson IM: Diagnostic symptoms of severe and moderate haemophilia A and B. A survey of 140 cases. Acta Paediatr Scand 1990; 79:196–200.
292. Oski F: Blood coagulation and its disorders in the newborn. In Oski F, Naiman J (eds): Hematologic Problems in the Newborn, 2nd ed. Philadelphia, WB Saunders, 1982, pp 137–174.
293. Hartmann J, Diamond L: Hemophilia and related hemorrhagic disorders. Practitioner 1957; 178:179–190.
294. Rosendaal FR, Smit C, Briet E: Hemophilia treatment in historical perspective: A review of medical and social developments. Ann Hematol 1991; 62:5–15.
295. Stormorken H, Hessel B, Lunde J, et al: Severe factor VIII deficiency in a chromosomally normal female. Thromb Res 1986; 44:113–117.
296. Mannucci PM, Coppola R, Lombardi R, et al: Direct proof of extreme lyonization as a cause of low factor VIII levels in females. Thromb Haemost 1978; 39:544–545.
297. Stowell KM, Figueiredo MS, Brownlee GG, et al: Haemophilia B Liverpool: A new British family with mild haemophilia B associated with a –6 G to A mutation in the factor IX promoter. Br J Haematol 1993; 85:188–190.
298. Trotter CW, Hasegawa DK: Hemophilia B. Case study and intervention plan. JOGN Nurs 1983; 12:82–85.
299. Donner M, Holmberg L, Nilsson IM: Type IIB von Willebrand's disease with probable autosomal recessive inheritance and presenting as thrombocytopenia in infancy. Br J Haematol 1987; 66:349–354.
300. Bignell P, Standen GR, Bowen DJ, et al: Rapid neonatal diagnosis of von Willebrand's disease by use of the polymerase chain reaction. Lancet 1990; 336:638–639.
301. Gazengel C, Fischer AM, Schlegel N, et al: Treatment of type III von Willebrand's disease with solvent/detergent-treated factor VIII concentrates. Nouv Rev Fr Hematol 1988; 30:225–227.
302. Pasi KJ, Williams MD, Enayat MS, et al: Clinical and laboratory evaluation of the treatment of von Willebrand's disease patients with heat-treated factor VIII concentrate (BPL 8Y). Br J Haematol 1990; 75:228–233.
303. Girolami A, Molaro G, Calligaris A, et al: Severe congenital factor X deficiency in 5-month-old child. Thromb Diath Haemorrh 1970; 24:175–184.
304. Machin SJ, Winter MR, Davies SC, et al: Factor X deficiency in the neonatal period. Arch Dis Child 1980; 55:406–408.
305. de Sousa C, Clark T, Bradshaw A: Antenatally diagnosed subdural haemorrhage in congenital factor X deficiency. Arch Dis Child 1988; 63(10 Spec No):1168–1170.
306. Sandler E, Gross S: Prevention of recurrent intracranial hemorrhage in a factor X deficient infant. Am J Pediatr Hematol Oncol 1992; 14:163–165.
307. Ruane BJ, McCord FB: Factor X deficiency—A rare cause of scrotal haemorrhage. Ir Med J 1990; 83:163.
308. Edson JR, White JG, Krivit W: The enigma of severe factor XI deficiency without hemmorrhagic symptoms. Distinction from Hageman factor and "Fletcher factor" deficiency; family study; and problems of diagnosis. Thromb Diath Haemorrh 1967; 18:342–348.
309. Kitchens CS: Factor XI: A review of its biochemistry and deficiency. Semin Thromb Hemost 1991; 17:55–72.
310. Barozzino T, Sgro M, Toi A, et al: Fetal bilateral subdural haemorrhages. Prenatal diagnosis and spontaneous resolution by time of delivery. Prenat Diagn 1998; 18:496–503.
311. Barry A, Delage M: Congenital deficiency of fibrin stabilizing factor: Observation of a new case. N Engl J Med 1965; 272:943–946.
312. Fisher S, Rikover M, Naor S: Factor 13 deficiency with severe hemorrhagic diathesis. Blood 1966; 28:34–39.
313. Britten AF: Congenital deficiency of factor 13 (fibrin-stabilizing factor): Report of a case and review of the literature. Am J Med 1967; 43:751–761.
314. Ozsoylu S, Altay C, Hicsonmez G: Congenital factor 13 deficiency. Observation of two new cases in the newborn period. Am J Dis Child 1971; 122:541–543.
315. Francis J, Todd P: Congenital factor XIII deficiency in a neonate. BMJ 1978; 2:1532.
316. Merchant RH, Agarwal BR, Currimbhoy Z, et al: Congenital factor XIII deficiency. Indian Pediatr 1992; 29:831–836.
317. Seitz R, Duckert F, Lopaciuk S, et al:: ETRO Working Party on Factor XIII questionnaire on congenital factor XIII deficiency in Europe: Status and perspectives. Study Group. Semin Thromb Hemost 1996; 22:415–418.
318. Blanckaert D, Oueidat I, Chelala J, et al: [Congenital deficiency of fibrin stabilizing factor (factor XIII)]. Pediatrie 1993; 48:451–453.
319. Daly HM, Haddon ME: Clinical experience with a pasteurised human plasma concentrate in factor XIII deficiency. Thromb Haemost 1988; 59:171–174.
320. Landman J, Creter D, Homburg R, et al: Neonatal factor XIII deficiency. Clin Pediatr (Phila) 1985; 24:352–353.
321. Duckert F, Jung E, Shmerling D: Hitherto undescribed congenital haemorrhage diathesis probably due to fibrin stabilizing factor deficiency. Throm Diath Haemorrh 1960; 5:179–180.
322. Solves P, Altes A, Ginovart G, et al: Late hemorrhagic disease of the newborn as a cause of intracerebral bleeding. Ann Hematol 1997; 75:65–66.
323. Mammen E, Murano G, Bick RL: Combined congenital clotting factor abnormalities. Semin Thromb Hemost 1983; 9:55–56.
324. Boyd JF: Disseminated fibrin thromboembolism among neonates dying within 48 hours of birth. Arch Dis Child 1967; 42:401–409.
325. Boyd JF: Disseminated fibrin thrombo-embolism in stillbirths: A histological picture similar to one form of maternal hypofibrinogenaemia. J Obstet Gynaecol Br Commonw 1966; 73:629–639.
326. Lascari AD, Wallace PD: Disseminated intravascular coagulation in newborns. Survey and appraisal as exemplified in two case histories. Clin Pediatr (Phila) 1971; 10:11–17.
327. Dube B, Bhargava V, Dube RK, et al: Disseminated intravascular coagulation in neonatal period. Indian Pediatr 1986; 23:925–931.
328. Phillips LL: Alterations in the blood clotting system in disseminated intravascular coagulation. Am J Cardiol 1967; 20:174–184.
329. Rodriguez-Erdmann F: Bleeding due to increased intravascular blood coagulation. Hemorrhagic syndrome caused by consumption of blood clotting factors (consumption coagulates). N Engl J Med 1965; 273:1310.
330. Hathaway WE, Mull MM, Pechet GS: Disseminated intravascular coagulation in the newborn. Pediatrics 1969; 43:233–240.
331. Abildgaard CF: Recognition and treatment of intravascular coagulation. J Pediatr 1969; 74:163–176.
332. Watkins MN, Swan S, Caprini JA, et al: Coagulation changes in the newborn with respiratory failure. Thromb Res 1980; 17:153–175.
333. Markarian M, Lindley A, Jackson JJ, et al: Coagulation factors in pregnant women and premature infants with and without the respiratory distress syndrome. Thromb Diath Haemorrh 1967; 17:585–594.

334. Appleyard WJ, Cottom DG: Effect of asphyxia on Thrombotest values in low birthweight infants. Arch Dis Child 1970; 45:705–707.

335. Anderson JM, Brown JK, Cockburn F: On the role of disseminated intravascular coagulation in the pathology of birth asphyxia. Dev Med Child Neurol 1974; 16:581–591.

336. Chessells JM, Wigglesworth JS: Coagulation studies in severe birth asphyxia. Arch Dis Child 1971; 46:253–256.

337. Chessells JM, Wigglesworth JS: Haemostatic failure in babies with rhesus isoimmunization. Arch Dis Child 1971; 46:38–45.

338. Chessells JM, Wigglesworth JS: Coagulation studies in preterm infants with respiratory distress and intracranial haemorrhage. Arch Dis Child 1972; 47:564–570.

339. Altstatt LB, Dennis LH, Sundell H, et al: Disseminated intravascular coagulation and hyaline membrane disease. Biol Neonate 1971; 19:227–240.

340. Edson JR, Blaese RM, White JG, et al: Defibrination syndrome in an infant born after abruptio placentae. J Pediatr 1968; 72:342–346.

341. Corrigan JJ Jr: Activation of coagulation and disseminated intravascular coagulation in the newborn. Am J Pediatr Hematol Oncol 1979; 1:245–249.

342. Schmidt BK, Vegh P, Andrew M, et al: Coagulation screening tests in high risk neonates: A prospective cohort study. Arch Dis Child 1992; 67(10 Spec No):1196–1197.

343. Rintala E, Kauppila M, Seppala OP, et al: Protein C substitution in sepsis-associated purpura fulminans. Crit Care Med 2000; 28:2373–2378.

344. Haneberg B, Gutteberg TJ, Moe PJ, et al: Heparin for infants and children with meningococcal septicemia. NIPH Ann 1983; 6:43–47.

345. Blum D, Fondu P, Denolin-Reubens R, et al: Early heparin therapy in 60 children with acute meningococcemia: Relationship between clinical manifestations and coagulation abnormalities. Acta Chir Belg 1973; 4:288–297.

346. Hathaway WE: Heparin therapy in acute meningococcemia. J Pediatr 1991; 82:900–901.

347. Dudley DK, Dalton ME: Single fetal death in twin gestation. Semin Perinatol 1986; 10:65.

348. Chuansumrit A, Manco-Johnson MJ, Hathaway WE: Heparin cofactor II in adults and infants with thrombosis and DIC. Am J Hematol 1989; 31:109.

349. Schmidt BK, Muraji T, Zipursky A: Low antithrombin III in neonatal shock: DIC or non-specific protein depletion? Eur J Pediatr 1986; 145:500.

350. Turner T, Prowse CV, Prescott RJ, et al: A clinical trial on the early detection and correction of haemostatic defects in selected high-risk neonates. Br J Haematol 1981; 47:65–75.

351. Beverley DW, Pitts-Tucker TJ, Congdon PJ, et al: Prevention of intraventricular haemorrhage by fresh frozen plasma. Arch Dis Child 1985; 60:710–713.

352. Hambleton G, Appleyard WJ: Controlled trial of fresh frozen plasma in asphyxiated low birthweight infants. Arch Dis Child 1973; 48:31–35.

353. Snydor MS, Weaver RL, Johnson CA: Effects of fresh frozen plasma infusions on coagulation screening tests in sick neonates (abstract). Pediatr Res 1977; 11:542.

354. Gross SJ, Filston HC, Anderson JC: Controlled study of treatment for disseminated intravascular coagulation in the neonate. J Pediatr 1982; 100:445–448.

355. Ettingshausen CE, Veldmann A, Beeg T, et al: Replacement therapy with protein C concentrate in infants and adolescents with meningococcal sepsis and purpura fulminans. Semin Thromb Hemost 1999; 25:537–541.

356. Hunter J: Heparin therapy in meningoccal septicaemia. Arch Dis Child 1973; 48:233–235.

357. Johnson CA, Snyder MS, Weaver RL: Effects of fresh frozen plasma infusions on coagulation screening tests in neonates. Arch Dis Child 1982; 57:950–952.

358. Gobel U, von Voss H, Jurgens H, et al: Efficiency of heparin in the treatment of newborn infants with respiratory distress syndrome and disseminated intravascular coagulation. Eur J Pediatr 1980; 133:47–49.

359. Kelly DA, Summerfield JA: Hemostasis in liver disease. Semin Liver Dis 1987; 7:182–191.

360. von Breedin K: Hamorrhagische diathesen bei lebererkrankungen unter besonderer berucksichtigung der thrombocytenfunction. Acta Haematol 1962; 27:1–2.

361. Rubin MH, Weston MJ, Bullock G, et al: Abnormal platelet function and ultrastructure in fulminant hepatic failure. Q J Med 1977; 46:339–352.

362. Weston MJ, Langley PG, Rubin MH, et al: Platelet function in fulminant hepatic failure and effect of charcoal haemoperfusion. Gut 1977; 18:897–902.

363. Osborn JE, Shahidi NT: Thrombocytopenia in murine cytomegalovirus infection. J Lab Clin Med 1973; 81:53–63.

364. Chesney PJ, Taher A, Gilbert EM, et al: Intranuclear inclusions in megakaryocytes in congenital cytomegalovirus infection. J Pediatr 1978; 92:957–958.

365. Zinkham WH, Medearis DN Jr, Osborn JE: Blood and bone-marrow findings in congenital rubella. J Pediatr 1967; 71:512–524.

366. Lafer CZ, Morrison AN: Thrombocytopenic purpura progressing to transient hypoplastic anemia in a newborn with rubella syndrome. Pediatrics 1966; 38:499–501.

367. Bortolotti F, Vajro P, Barbera C, et al: Hepatitis C in childhood: Epidemiological and clinical aspects. Bone Marrow Transplant 1993; 12 Suppl 1:21–23.

368. Kulhanjian J: Fever, hepatitis and coagulopathy in a newborn infant. Pediatr Infect Dis J 1992; 11:1069, 1072.

369. Telfer MC: Clinical spectrum of viral infections in hemophilic patients. Hematol Oncol Clin North Am 1992; 6:1047–1056.

370. van Saene HK, Stoutenbeek CP, Faber-Nijholt R, et al: Selective decontamination of the digestive tract contributes to the control of disseminated intravascular coagulation in severe liver impairment. J Pediatr Gastroenterol Nutr 1992; 14:436–442.

371. Horowitz IN, Galvis AG, Gomperts ED: Arterial thrombosis and protein S deficiency. J Pediatr 1992; 121:934–937.

372. Meili EO: Treatment of hemophilia. Schweiz Med Wochenschr Suppl 1991; 43:82–89.

373. Dresse MF, David M, Hume H, et al: Successful treatment of Kasabach-Merritt syndrome with prednisone and epsilon-aminocaproic acid. Pediatr Hematol Oncol 1991; 8:329–334.

374. Noseda G, Roy C, Phan P, et al: [Acute hepatic insufficiency disclosing congenital syphilis]. Arch Fr Pediatr 1990; 47:445–446.

375. Rathgeber J, Rath W, Wieding JU: [Anesthesiologic and intensive care aspects of severe pre-eclampsia with HELLP syndrome]. Anasth Intensivther Notfallmed 1990; 25:206–211.

376. Kurzel RB: Can acetaminophen excess result in maternal and fetal toxicity? South Med J 1990; 83:953–955.

377. Dupuy JM, Frommel D, Alagille D: Severe viral hepatitis type B in infancy. Lancet 1975; 1:191–194.

378. Mindrum G, Glueck H: Plasma prothrombin time in liver disease: Its clinical and prognostic significance. Ann Intern Med 1959; 50:1370–1371.

379. Hope PL, Hall MA, Millward-Sadler GH, et al: Alpha–1-antitrypsin deficiency presenting as a bleeding diathesis in the newborn. Arch Dis Child 1982; 57:68–70.

380. Olivera JE, Elcarte R, Erice B, et al: [Galactosemia of early diagnosis with psychomotor retardation]. An Esp Pediatr 1986; 25:267–270.

381. Di Battista C, Rossi L, Marcelli P, et al: [Hereditary tyrosinemia in an acute form: A case report (author's transl)]. Pediatr Med Chir 1981; 3:101–104.

382. Aster RH: Pooling of platelets in the spleen: Role in the pathogenesis of "hypersplenic" thrombocytopenia. J Clin Invest 1966; 45:645–657.

383. Stein SF, Harker LA: Kinetic and functional studies of platelets, fibrinogen, and plasminogen in patients with hepatic cirrhosis. J Lab Clin Med 1982; 99:217–230.

384. Blanchard RA, Furie BC, Jorgensen M, Kruger SF, Furie B: Acquired vitamin K-dependent carboxylation deficiency in liver disease. N Engl J Med 1981; 305:242–248.

385. Wesstrom G: Umbilical artery catheterization in newborns. V. A clinical follow-up study. Acta Paediatr Scand 1980; 69:371–376.

386. Bejar R, Curbelo V, Coen RW, et al: Diagnosis and follow-up of intraventricular and intracerebral hemorrhages by ultrasound studies of infant's brain through the fontanelles and sutures. Pediatrics 1980; 66:661–673.

387. Mack LA, Wright K, Hirsch JH, et al: Intracranial hemorrhage in premature infants: Accuracy in sonographic evaluation. AJR Am J Roentgenol 1981; 137:245–250.

388. Antoniuk S, da Silva RV: [Periventricular and intraventricular hemorrhage in the premature infants]. Rev Neurol 2000; 31:238–243.

389. Pape KE, Bennett-Britton S, Szymonowicz W, et al: Diagnostic accuracy of neonatal brain imaging: A postmortem correlation of computed tomography and ultrasound scans. J Pediatr 1983; 102:275–280.

390. Graziani LJ, Pasto M, Stanley C, et al: Cranial ultrasound and clinical studies in preterm infants. J Pediatr 1985; 106:269–276.

391. Sinha SK, Davies JM, Sims DG, et al: Relation between periventricular haemorrhage and ischaemic brain lesions diagnosed by ultrasound in very pre-term infants. Lancet 1985; 2:1154–1156.

392. Dubowitz LM, Levene MI, Morante A, et al: Neurologic signs in neonatal intraventricular hemorrhage: A correlation with real-time ultrasound. J Pediatr 1981; 99:127–133.

393. Perlman JM, Nelson JS, McAlister WH, et al: Intracerebellar hemorrhage in a premature newborn: Diagnosis by real-time ultrasound and correlation with autopsy findings. Pediatrics 1983; 71:159–162.

394. Dolfin T, Skidmore MB, Fong KW, et al: Incidence, severity, and timing of subependymal and intraventricular hemorrhages in preterm infants born in a perinatal unit as detected by serial real-time ultrasound. Pediatrics 1983; 71:541–546.

395. Trounce JQ, Fagan D, Levene MI: Intraventricular haemorrhage and periventricular leucomalacia: Ultrasound and autopsy correlation. Arch Dis Child 1986; 61:1203–1207.

396. Papile LA, Burstein J, Burstein R, et al: Incidence and evolution of subependymal and intraventricular hemorrhage: A study of infants with birth weights less than 1,500 gm. J Pediatr 1978; 92:529–534.

397. Tsiantos A, Victorin L, Relier JP, et al: Intracranial hemorrhage in the prematurely born infant. Timing of clots and evaluation of clinical signs and symptoms. J Pediatr 1974; 85:854–859.

398. Shinnar S, Molteni RA, Gammon K, et al: Intraventricular hemorrhage in the premature infant. N Engl J Med 1982; 306:1464–1468.

399. Ahmann PA, Lazzara A, Dykes FD, et al: Intraventricular hemorrhage in the high-risk preterm infant: Incidence and outcome. Ann Neurol 1980; 7:118–124.

400. Levene MI, de Vries L: Extension of neonatal intraventricular haemorrhage. Arch Dis Child 1984; 59:631–636.

401. Guzzetta F, Shackelford GD, Volpe S, et al: Periventricular intraparenchymal echodensities in the premature newborn: Critical determinant of neurologic outcome. Pediatrics 1986; 78:995–1006.

402. Gould SJ, Howard S, Hope PL, et al: Periventricular intraparenchymal cerebral haemorrhage in preterm infants: The role of venous infarction. J Pathol 1987; 151:197–202.

403. Rushton DI, Preston PR, Durbin GM: Structure and evolution of echo dense lesions in the neonatal brain. A combined ultrasound and necropsy study. Arch Dis Child 1985; 60:798–808.

404. Takashima S, Mito T, Ando Y: Pathogenesis of periventricular white matter hemorrhages in preterm infants. Brain Dev 1986; 8:25–30.

405. Szymonowicz W, Yu VY: Timing and evolution of periventricular haemorrhage in infants weighing 1250 g or less at birth. Arch Dis Child 1984; 59:7–12.

406. Menkes JH: Intracranial hemorrhage: Pathogenesis and pathology. In Taeusch HW, Ballard RA, Avery ME (eds): Diseases of the Newborn. Philadelphia, WB Saunders, 1991, pp 422–425.

407. Goddard-Finegold J: Periventricular, intraventricular hemorrhages in the premature newborn. Update on pathologic features, pathogenesis and possible means of prevention. Arch Neurol 1984; 41:766–771.

408. Burstein J, Papile L, Burstein R: Subependymal germinal matrix and intraventricular hemorrhage in premature infants: Diagnosis by CT. Am J Roentgenol 1977; 128:971.

409. Volpe JJ: Neonatal intraventricular hemorrhage. N Engl J Med 1981; 304:886–891.

410. Ment LR, Duncan CC, Ehrenkranz RA: Intraventricular hemorrhage of the preterm neonate. Semin Perinatol 1987; 11:132–141.

411. Hambleton G, Wigglesworth JS: Origin of intraventricular haemorrhage in the preterm infant. Arch Dis Child 1976; 51:651–659.

412. Szymonowicz W, Yu VYH, Wilson FE: Antecedents of periventricular hemorrhage in infants weighing 1250 g or less at birth. Arch Dis Child 1984; 59:13.

413. Lipscomb AP, Thorburn RJ, Reynolds EOR: Pneumothorax and cerebral haemorrhage in preterm infants. Lancet 1981; 1:414.

414. Clark CE, Clyman RI, Roth RS, et al: Risk factor analysis of intraventricular haemorrhage in low-birth-weight infants. J Pediatr 1981; 99:625.

415. Kosmetatos N, Dinter C, Williams ML, et al: Intracranial haemorrhage in the premature: Its predictive features and outcome. Am J Dis Child 1980; 13:855.

416. Cooke RWI: Factors associated with periventricular haemorrhage in very low birthweight infants. Arch Dis Child 1981; 56:425.

417. Dykes FD, Lazzara A, Ahmann P, et al: Intraventricular haemorrhage: A prospective evaluation of etiopathogenesis. Pediatrics 1980; 66:42.

418. Ackerman A, Fraser AJ: Intracranial haemorrhage and clotting defects in low-birth-weight infants. Lancet 1968; 1:545.

419. Vohr B, Ment LR: Intraventricular hemorrhage in the preterm infant. Early Hum Dev 1996; 44:1–16.

420. Gronlund JU, Korvenranta H, Kero P, et al: Elevated arterial blood pressure is associated with peri-intraventricular haemorrhage. Eur J Pediatr 1994; 153:836–841.

421. Kluckow M, Evans N: Low superior vena cava flow and intraventricular haemorrhage in preterm infants. Arch Dis Child Fetal Neonatal Ed 2000; 82:F188-F194.

422. Horbar J: Prevention of periventricular-intraventricular hemorrhage. In Sinclair J, Bracken MB (eds): Effective Care of the Newborn Infant. Oxford, UK, Oxford University Press, 1992, pp 562–589.

423. Shankaran S, Papil LA, Wright LL, et al: The effect of antenatal phenobarbital therapy on neonatal intracranial hemorrhage in preterm infants. N Engl J Med 1997; 337:466–471.

424. Thomas DB, Burnard ED: Prevention of intraventricular haemorrhage in babies receiving artificial ventilation. Med J Aust 1973; 1:933–936.

425. Waltl H, Kurz R, Mitterstieler G, Fodisch JH, et al: Intracranial hemorrhage in low birth weight infants and prophylactic administration of coagulation factor concentrates. Lancet 1973; 1:1284–1288.

426. Gupta JM, Starr H, Fincher P, et al: Intraventricular haemorrhage in the newborn. Med J Aust 1976; 2:338–340.

427. Kazzi NJ, Ilagan NB, Liang KC, et al: Maternal administration of vitamin K does not improve the coagulation profile of preterm infants. Pediatrics 1989; 84:1045–1050.

428. Shirahata A, Nakamura T, Shimono M, et al: Blood coagulation findings and the efficacy of factor XIII concentrate in premature infants with intracranial hemorrhages. Thromb Res 1990; 57:755–763.

429. Brandenberg R, Bodensohn M, Burger U: Antithrombin III substitution in preterm infants: Effects on intracranial hemorrhage and coagultion parameters. Biol Neonate 1997; 72:76–83.

430. Hensey OJ, Morgan ME, Cooke RW: Tranexamic acid in the prevention of periventricular haemorrhage. Arch Dis Child 1984; 59:719–721.

431. Fodstad H, Forssell A, Liliequist B, et al: Antifibrinolysis with tranexamic acid in aneurysmal subarachnoid hemorrhage: A consecutive controlled clinical trial. Neurosurgery 1981; 8:158–165.

432. Bartlett JR: Subarachnoid haemorrhage. Br Med J (Clin Res Ed) 1981; 283:1347–1348.

433. Sindet-Pedersen S, Stenbjerg S: Effect of local antifibrinolytic treatment with tranexamic acid in hemophiliacs undergoing oral surgery. J Oral Maxillofac Surg 1986; 44:703–707.

434. Sindet-Pedersen S, Ramstrom G, Bernvil S, et al: Hemostatic effect of tranexamic acid mouthwash in anticoagulant-treated patients undergoing oral surgery. N Engl J Med 1989; 320:840–843.

435. Paptheodossiou N: A double blind clinical trial on dicynone in tonsillectomy. Med Hyg 1973; 31:1818–1819.

436. Symes DM, Offen DN, Lyttle JA, et al: The effect of dicynene on blood loss during and after transurethral resection of the prostate. Br J Urol 1975; 47:203–207.

437. Harrison RF, Cambell S: A double-blind trial of ethamsylate in the treatment of primary and intrauterine-device menorrhagia. Lancet 1976; 2:283–285.

438. Ment L, Stewart W, Scott D, et al: Beagle puppy model of intraventricular hemorrhage: Randomized indomethacin prevention trial. Neurology 1983; 33:179–184.

439. Cooke RW, Morgan ME: Prophylactic ethamsylate for periventricular haemorrhage. Arch Dis Child 1984; 59:82–83.

440. Benson JW, Drayton MR, Hayward C, et al: Multicentre trial of ethamsylate for prevention of periventricular haemorrhage in very low birthweight infants. Lancet 1986; 2:1297–1300.

441. Ment LR, Duncan CC, Ehrenkranz RA, et al: Randomized indomethacin trial for prevention of intraventricular hemorrhage in very low birth weight infants. J Pediatr 1985; 107:937–943.

442. Hanigan WC, Kennedy G, Roemisch F, et al: Administration of indomethacin for the prevention of periventricular-intraventricular hemorrhage in high-risk neonates. J Pediatr 1988; 112:941–947.

443. Ment LR, Duncan CC, Ehrenkranz RA, et al: Randomized low-dose indomethacin trial for prevention of intraventricular hemorrhage in very low birth weight neonates. J Pediatr 1988; 112:948–955.

444. Rennie JM, Doyle J, Cooke RW: Early administration of indomethacin to preterm infants. Arch Dis Child 1986; 61:233–238.

445. Bachofen M, Weibel ER: Structural alterations of lung parenchyma in the adult respiratory distress syndrome. Clin Chest Med 1982; 3:35–56.

446. Seeger W, Stohr G, Wolf H: Alteration of surfactant function due to protein leakage: Special interaction with fibrin monomer. J Appl Physiol 1985; 58:326–338.

447. Saldeen T: Fibrin-derived peptides and pulmonary injury. Ann NY Acad Sci 1982; 384:319–331.

448. Fukuda Y, Ishizaki M, Masuda Y, et al: The role of intraalveolar fibrosis in the process of pulmonary structural remodeling in patients with diffuse alveolar damage. Am J Pathol 1987; 126:171–182.

449. Damiano VV, Cherian PV, Frankel FR, et al: Intraluminal fibrosis induced unilaterally by lobar instillation of $CdCl_2$ into the rat lung. Am J Pathol 1990; 137:883–894.

450. Schmidt B, Davis P, La Pointe H, et al: Thrombin inhibitors reduce intrapulmonary accumulation of fibrinogen and procoagulant activity of bronchoalveolar lavage fluid during acute lung injury induced by pulmonary overdistention in newborn piglets. Pediatr Res 1996; 39:798–804.

451. Ambrus CM, Choi TS, Cunnanan E, et al: Prevention of hyaline membrane disease with plasminogen. A cooperative study. JAMA 1977; 237:1837–1841.

452. Markarian M, Githens JH, Rosenblut E, et al: Hypercoagulability in premature infants with special reference to the respiratory distress syndrome and hemorrhage. I. Coagulation studies. Biol Neonate 1971; 17:84–97.

453. Muntean W, Rosseger H: Antithrombin III concentrate in preterm infants with IRDS: An open, controlled, randomized clinical trial. Thromb Haemost 1989; 62:288 (abst). (Abstract)

454. Schmidt B, Gillie P, Mitchell L, et al: A placebo-controlled randomized trial of antithrombin therapy in neonatal respiratory distress syndrome. Am J Respir Crit Care Med 1998; 158:470–476.

455. Kugelmass IN: The management of hemorrhagic problems in infancy and childhood. JAMA 1932; 99:895.

456. Clifford SH: Hemorrhagic disease of the newborn. A critical consideration. J Pediatr 1941; 18:333.

457. Dam CPH: Cholesterinstoffwechsel in Huhnereiern und Huhnchen. Biochemischeschr Z 1929; 215:475–492.

458. Bruchsaler FS: Vitamin K and the prenatal and postnatal prevention of hemorrhagic disease in newborn infants. J Pediatr 1941; 18:317.

459. Nygaard KK: Prophylactic and curative effect of vitamin K in hemorrhagic disease of the newborn (hypothrombinemia hemorrhagica neonatorum). A preliminary report. Acta Obstet Gynecol Scand 1939; 19:361.

460. Waddell WW, Guerry D: The role of vitamin K in the etiology, prevention, and treatment of hemorrhage in the newborn infant. Part II. J Pediatr 1939; 15:802.

461. Dam H, Glavind J, Larsen EH, et al: Investigations into the cause of the physiological hypoprothrombinemia in new-born children. IV. The vitamin K content of woman's milk and cow's milk. Acta Med Scand 1942; 112:211.

462. Quick AJ, Grossman AM: Prothrombin concentration in newborns. Proc Soc Exp Biol Med 1939; 41:227.

463. Fitzgerald JE, Webster A: Effect of vitamin K administered to patients in labor. Am J Obstet Gynecol 1940; 40:413.

464. Hellman LM, Shettles LB: The prophylactic use of vitamin K in obstetrics. South Med J 1942; 35:289.

465. Mull JW, Bill AH, et al: Effect on the newborn of vitamin K administered to mothers in labor. J Lab Clin Med 1941; 26:1305.

466. Sanford HN, Morrison HJ, Wyat L, et al: The substances involved in the coagulation of the blood of the newborn. III. The effect of with-holding protein and fat from the diet. Am J Dis Child 1932; 43:571.

467. Gellis SS, Lyon RA: The influence of the diet of the newborn infant on the prothrombin index. J Pediatr 1941; 19:495.

468. Motohara K, Matsukane I, Endo F, et al: Relationship of milk intake and vitamin K supplementation to vitamin K status in newborns. Pediatrics 1989; 84:90–93.

469. Aballi AJ, Lopez Banus V, et al: The coagulation defect of fulltern infants. Pediatr Internaz 1959; 9:315.

470. Potter EL: The effect on infant mortality of vitamin K administered during labor. Am J Obstet Gynecol 1945; 50:235.

471. Committee on Nutrition, American Academy of Pediatrics: Vitamin K compounds and water-soluble analogues: Use in therapy and prophylaxis in pediatrics. Pediatrics 1961; 28:501–507.

472. Lucey JF, Dolan RG: Hyperbilirubinemia of newborn infants associated with the parenteral administration of a vitamin K analogue to the mothers. Pediatrics 1959; 23:553.

473. Parks J, Sweet LK: Does the antenatal use of vitamin K prevent hemorrhage in the newborn infant? Am J Obstet Gynecol 1942; 44:432.

474. Waddell WW Jr, Whitehead BW: Neonatal mortality rates in infants receiving prophylactic doses of vitamin K. South Med J 1945; 38:349.

475. Malia RG, Preston FE, Mitchell VE: Evidence against vitamin K deficiency in normal neonates. Thromb Haemost 1980; 44:159–160.

476. Dyggve H: The prophylactic use of vitamin K in obstetrics. South Med J 1942; 35:289.

477. MacElfresh ME: Coagulation during the neonatal period. Am J Med Sci 1961; 242:77.

478. Lawson RB: Treatment of hypoprothrombinemia (hemorrhagic disease) of the newborn infant. J Pediatr 1941; 18:224.

479. Motohara K, Endo F, Matsuda I: Effect of vitamin K administration on acarboxy prothrombin (PIVKA-II) levels in newborns. Lancet 1985; 2:242–244.

480. Lane PA, Hathaway WE: Vitamin K in infancy. J Pediatr 1985; 106:351–359.

481. Rose SJ: Neonatal haemorrhage and vitamin K. Acta Haematol 1985; 74:121.

482. O'Connor ME, Livingstone DS, Hannah J, et al: Vitamin K deficiency and breast-feeding. Am J Dis Child 1983; 137:601–602.

483. Behrmann BA, Chan WK, Finer NN: Resurgence of hemorrhagic disease of the newborn: A report of three cases. CMAJ 1985; 133:884–885.

484. Binder L: Hemorrhagic disease of the newborn: An unusual etiology of neonatal bleeding. Ann Emerg Med 1986; 15:935–938.

485. Tulchinsky T, Patton M, Randolph L, et al: Mandating vitamin K prophylaxis for newborns in New York State. Am J Public Health 1993; 83:1166–1168.

486. McNinch A, Tripp J: Haemorrhagic disease of the newborn in the British Isles: Two year prospective study. BMJ 1991; 303:1105–1109.

487. Von Kries R, Shearer MJ, Gobel U: Vitamin K in infancy. Eur J Pediatr 1988; 147:106–112.

488. Muller AD, Van Doorm JM, Hemker HC: Heparin-like inhibitor of blood coagulation in normal newborn. Nature 1977; 267:616–617.

489. Kryc JJ, Corrigan JJ: Idiopathic thrombocytopenic purpura during pregnancy. A pediatric viewpoint. Am J Pediatr Hematol Oncol 1983; 5:21–25.

490. Mori PG, Bisogni S, Odini S, et al: Vitamin K deficiency in the newborn [letter]. Lancet 1977; 2:188.

491. Golding J, Paterson M, Kinlen L: Factors associated with childhood cancer in a national cohort study. Br J Cancer 1990; 62:304–308.

492. Golding J, Greenwood R: Intramuscular vitamin K and childhood cancer: Two British studies. In Sutor AH, Hathaway WE (eds): Vitamin K in Infancy. Stuttgart, Schattauer, 1995, pp 283–289.

493. Ekelund H, Finnstrom O, Gunnarskog J, et al: Administration of vitamin K to newborn infants and childhood cancer. BMJ 1993; 307:89–91.

494. Klebanoff M, Read J, Mills J, et al: The risk of childhood cancer after neonatal exposure to vitamin K. N Engl J Med 1993; 329:905–908.

495. Lehmann J: Vitamin K as a prophylactic in 13,000 infants. Lancet 1944; i:493.

496. Fetus and Newborn Committee, Canadian Pediatric Society. The use of vitamin K in the perinatal period. CMAJ 1988; 139:127–130.

497. Hathaway WE: ICTH Subcommittee on Neonatal Hemostasis. Thromb Haemostas 1986; 55:145.

498. Hathaway WE: New insights on vitamin K. Hematol Oncol Clin North Am 1987; 1:367–379.

499. Shapiro AD, Jacobson LJ, Aramon ME, et al: Vitamin K deficiency in the newborn infant: Prevalence and perinatal risk factors. J Pediatr 1986; 109:675–680.

500. Hall MA, Pairaudeau P: The routine use of vitamin K in the newborn. Midwifery 1987; 3:170.

501. Hanawa Y, Maki M, Murata B, et al: The second nation-wide survey in Japan of vitamin K deficiency in infants. Eur J Pediatr 1988; 147:472–477.

502. Mandelbrot L, Guillaumont M, Forestier F, et al: Placental transfer of vitamin K_1 and its implications in fetal haemostasis. Thromb Haemost 1988; 60:39–43.

503. Hamulyak K, de Boer-van den Berg MAG: The placental transport of [^{3}H]vitamin K_1 in rats. Br J Haematol 1987; 65:335–338.

504. Hiraike H, Kimura M, Itokawa Y: Determination of K vitamins (phylloquinone and menaquinones) in umbilical cord plasma by a platinum-reduction column. J Chromotog 1988; 430:143–148.

505. Hiraike H, Kimura M, Itokawa Y: Distribution of K vitamins (phylloquinone and menaquinones) in human placenta and maternal and umbilical cord plasma. Am J Obstet Gynecol 1988; 158:564–569.

506. Haroon Y, Shearer MJ, Rahim S, et al: The content of phylloquinone (vitamin K_1) in human milk, cow's milk and infant formula foods determined by high-performance liquid chromatography. J Nutr 1982; 112:1105–1117.

507. Von Kries R, Becker A, Gobel U: Vitamin K in the newborn: Influence of nutritional factors on acarboxy-prothrombin detectability and factor II and VII clotting activity. Eur J Pediatr 1987; 146:123–127.

508. Sutherland JM, Glueck HI: Hemorrhagic disease of the newborn; breast feeding as a necessary factor in the pathogenesis. Am J Dis Child 1967; 113:524–533.

509. Srinivasan G, Seeler RA, Tiruvury A, et al: Maternal anticonvulsant therapy and hemorrhagic disease of the newborn. Obstet Gynecol 1982; 59:250–252.

510. Mountain KR, Hirsh J, Gallius AS: Neonatal coagulation defect due to anticonvulsant drug treatment in pregnancy. Lancet 1970; 1:265–268.

511. Laosombat V: Hemorrhagic disease of the newborn after maternal anticonvulsant therapy: A case report and literature review. J Med Assoc Thailand 1988; 71:643–648.

512. Martin-Bouyer G, Linh PD, Tuan LC: Epidemic of haemorrhagic disease in Vietnamese infants caused by warfarin-contaminated talcs. Lancet 1983; 1:230–233.

513. Sutor AH, Dagres N, Niederhoff H: Late form of vitamin K deficiency bleeding in Germany. Klin Padiatr 1995; 207:89–97.

514. Bovill EG, Soll R, Lynch M, et al: Vitamin K_1 metabolism and the production of des-carboxy prothrombin and protein C in the term and premature neonate. Blood 1993; 81:77–83.

515. Pietersma-de Bruyer AL, van Haard PM, et al: Vitamin K_1 levels and coagulation factors in healthy term newborns untill 4 weeks after birth. Haemostasis 1990; 20:8–14.

516. Motohara K, Kuroki Y, Kan H, et al: Detection of vitamin K deficiency by use of an enzyme-linked immunosorbent assay for circulating abnormal prothrombin. Pediatr Res 1985; 19:354.

517. Widdershoven J, Lambert W, Motohara K, et al: Plasma concentrations of vitamin K_1 and PIVKA-II in bottle-fed and breast-fed infants with and without vitamin K prophylaxis at birth. Eur J Pediatr 1988; 148:139–142.

518. Fujimura Y, Okubo Y, Sakai T, et al: Studies on precursor proteins PIVKA-II, -IX, and -X in the plasma of patients with 'hemorrhagic disease of the newborn.' Haemostasis 1984; 14:211–217.

519. Kotohara K, Endo F: Effect of vitamin K administration of acarboxy prothrombin (PIVKA-II) levels in newborns. Lancet 1985; 2:243.

520. Brookfield C, Rutty GN, Wooley A, et al: The PIVKA II test: The first reliable coagulation test for autopsy investigations? Thromb Haemost 2001; Suppl:CD3174.

521. Shirahata A, Nojiri T, Takaragi S, et al: Normotest screenings and prophylactic oral administration for idiopathic vitamin K deficiency in infancy [abstract]. Acta Haematol (Jpn) 1982; 45:867–875.

522. Garrow D, Chisolm M, Radford M: Vitamin K and Thrombotest values in fullterm infants. Arch Dis Child 1986; 61:349–351.

523. Herman J, Jumbelic MI, Anconer RJ, et al: In utero cerebral haemorrhage in alloimmune thrombocytopenia. Am J Pediatr Hematol Oncol 1986; 8:312–317.

524. Greer FR, Mummah-Schendel LL, Marshall S, et al: Vitamin K_1 (phylloquinone) and vitamin K_2 (menaquinone) status in newborns during the first week of life. Pediatrics 1988; 81:137–140.

525. Von Kries R, Hanawa Y: Neonatal vitamin K prophylaxis. Report of Scientific and Standardization Committee on Perinatal Hemostasis. Thromb Haemost 1993; 69:293–295.

526. Vietti TJ, Murphy TP, James JA, et al: Observation on the prophylactic use of vitamin K in the newborn. J Pediatr 1960; 56:343–346.

527. Vietti TJ, Stephens JC, Bennett KR: Vitamin K–1 prophylaxis in the newborn. JAMA 1961; 176:791.

528. Fresh JW, Adams H, Morgan FM: Vitamin K-blood clotting studies during pregnancy and prothrombin and proconvertin levels in the newborn. Obstet Gynecol 1959; 13:37–40.

529. Chaou W-T, Chou M-L, Eitzman DV: Intracranial hemorrhage and vitamin K deficiency in early infancy. J Pediatr 1984; 105:880–884.

530. Golding J, Greenwood R, Birmingham K, et al: Childhood cancer, intramuscular vitamin K, and pethidine given during labour. BMJ 1992; 305:341–346.

531. Brousson MA, Klein MC: Controversies surrounding the administration of vitamin K to newborns: A review. CMAJ 1996; 154:307–315.

532. Hathaway W, Isarangkura P, Mahasandana C, et al: Comparison of oral and parenteral vitamin K prophylaxis for prevention of late hemorrhagic disease of the newborn. J Pediatr 1991; 119:461–464.

533. Von Kries R, Gobel U: Vitamin K prophylaxis and vitamin K deficiency bleeding (VKDB) in early infancy. Acta Paediatr 1992; 81:655–657.

534. Zreik H, Bengur R, Meliones J, et al: Superior vena cava obstruction after extracorporeal membrane oxygenation. J Pediatr 1995; 127:314–316.

535. Sutor AH, Weibach G, Schreiber R, et al: Thrombosen im Kindesalter. Hemostaseologie (Germany) 1992; 12:82–93.

536. Bartlett RH, Roloff D, Cornell R, et al: Extracorporeal circulation in neonatal respiratory failure: A prospective randomized study. Pediatrics 1985; 76:479–487.

537. Rosenberger WF, Lachin JM: The use of response-adaptive designs in clinical trials. Control Clin Trials 1993; 14:471–484.

538. Canady AI, Fessler RD, Klein MD: Ultrasound abnormalities in term infants on ECMO. Pediatr Neurosurg 1993; 19:202–205.

539. Cheung PY, Sawicki G, Salas E, et al: The mechanisms of platelet dysfunction during extracorporeal membrane oxygenation in critically ill neonates [see comments]. Crit Care Med 2000; 28:2584–2590.

540. Chan AKC, Leaker M, Burrows FA, et al: Coagulation and fibrinolytic profile of paediatric patients undergoing cardiopulmonary bypass. Thromb Haemost 1997; 77:270–277.

541. Watson JW, Brown DM, Lally KP, et al: Complications of extracorporeal membrane oxygenation in neonates. South Med J 1990; 83:1262–1265.

542. Zavadil DP, Stammers AH, Willett LD, et al: Hematological abnormalities in neonatal patients treated with extracorporeal membrane oxygenation (ECMO). J Extra Corpor Technol 1998; 30:83–90.

543. Jarjour I, Ahdab-Barmada M: Cerebrovascular lesions in infants and children dying after extracorporeal membrane oxygenation. Pediatr Neurol 1994; 10:13–19.

544. McManus M, Kevy S, Bower LK, et al: Coagulation factor deficiencies during initiation of extracorporeal membrane oxygenation. J Pediatr 1995; 126:900–904.

545. Hardart GE, Fackler JC: Predictors of intracranial hemorrhage during neonatal extracorporeal membrane oxygenation. J Pediatr 1999; 134:156–159.

546. Robinson T, Kickler T, Walker L, et al: Effect of extracorporeal membrane oxygenation on platelets in newborns. Crit Care Med 1993; 21:1029–1034.

547. Plotz F, van Oeveren W, Bartlett RH, et al: Blood activation during neonatal extracorporeal life support. J Thorac Cardiovasc Surg 1993; 105:823–832.

548. Ozkutlu S, Saraclar M, Atalay S, et al: Two-dimensional echocardiographic diagnosis of tricuspid valve noninfective endocarditis due to protein C deficiency (lesion mimicking tricuspid valve myxoma). Jpn Heart J 1991; 32:139–145.

549. Pescatore P, Horellou HM, Conard J, et al: Problems of oral anticoagulation in an adult with homozygous protein C deficiency and late onset of thrombosis [see comments]. Thromb Haemost 1993; 69:311–315.

550. Marlar RA, Sills RH, Groncy PK, et al: Protein C survival during replacement therapy in homozygous protein C deficiency. Am J Hematol 1992; 41:24–31.

551. Deguchi K, Tsukada T, Iwasaki E, et al et al: Late-onset homozygous protein C deficiency manifesting cerebral infarction as the first symptom at age 27. Intern Med 1992; 31:922–925.

552. Yamamoto K, Matsushita T, Sugiura I, et al: Homozygous protein C deficiency: Identification of a novel missense mutation that causes impaired secretion of the mutant protein C [see comments]. J Lab Clin Med 1992; 119:682–689.

553. Auberger K: Evaluation of a new protein-C concentrate and comparison of protein-C assays in a child with congenital protein-C deficiency. Ann Hematol 1992; 64:146–151.

554. Grundy CB, Melissari E, Lindo V, et al: Late-onset homozygous protein C deficiency [letter] [see comments]. Lancet 1991; 338:575–576.

555. Marlar RA, Neumann A: Neonatal purpura fulminans due to homozygous protein C or protein S deficiencies. Semin Thromb Hemost 1990; 16:299–309.

556. Tripodi A, Franchi F, Krachmalnicoff A, et al: Asymptomatic homozygous protein C deficiency. Acta Haematol 1990; 83:152–155.

557. Petrini P, Segnestam K, Ekelund H, et al: Homozygous protein C deficiency in two siblings. Pediatr Hematol Oncol 1990; 7:165–175.

558. Marlar RA, Adcock DM, Madden RM: Hereditary dysfunctional protein C molecules (type II): Assay characterization and proposed classification. Thromb Haemost 1990; 63:375–379.

559. Marlar RA, Montgomery RR, Broekmans AW: Report on the diagnosis and treatment of homozygous protein C deficiency. Report of the Working Party on Homozygous Protein C Deficiency of the ICTH-Subcommittee on Protein C and Protein S. Thromb Haemost 1989; 61:529–531.

560. Ben Tal O, Zivelin A, Seligsohn U: The relative frequency of hereditary thrombotic disorders among 107 patients with thrombophilia in Israel. Thromb Haemost 1989; 61:50–54.

561. Burrows RF, Kelton J: Low fetal risks in pregnancies associated with idiopathic thrombocytopenic purpura do not justify obstetrical interventions. Am J Obstet Gynecol 1990; 163:1147–1150.

562. Manco-Johnson MJ, Marlar RA, Jacobson LJ, et al: Severe protein C deficiency in newborn infants. J Pediatr 1988; 113:359–363.

563. Vukovich T, Auberger K, Weil J, et al: Replacement therapy for a homozygous protein C deficiency-state using a concentrate of human protein C and S. Br J Haematol 1988; 70:435–440.

564. Gladson CL, Groncy P, Griffin JH: Coumarin necrosis, neonatal purpura fulminans, and protein C deficiency. Arch Dermatol 1987; 123:1701a–1706a.

565. Casella JF, Lewis JH, Bontempo FA, et al: Successful treatment of homozygous protein C deficiency by hepatic transplantation. [published erratum appears in Lancet 1988; 1:1238] Lancet 1988; 1:435–438.

566. Peters C, Casella JF, Marlar RA, et al: Homozygous protein C deficiency: Observations on the nature of the molecular abnormality and the effectiveness of warfarin therapy. Pediatrics 1988; 81:272–276.

567. Miletich J, Sherman L, Broze G Jr: Absence of thrombosis in subjects with heterozygous protein C deficiency. N Engl J Med 1987; 317:991–996.

568. Rappaport ES, Speights VO, Helbert B, et al: Protein C deficiency. South Med J 1987; 80:240–242.

569. Marlar RA, Montgomery RR, Broekmans AW: Diagnosis and treatment of homozygous protein C deficiency. Report of the Working Party on Homozygous Protein C Deficiency of the Subcommittee on Protein C and Protein S, International Committee on Thrombosis and Haemostasis. J Pediatr 1989; 114(4 Pt 1):528–534.

570. Auletta MJ, Headington JT: Purpura fulminans. A cutaneous manifestation of severe protein C deficiency [see comments]. Arch Dermatol 1988; 124:1387–1391.

571. Adcock DM, Hicks MJ: Dermatopathology of skin necrosis associated with purpura fulminans. Semin Thromb Hemost 1990; 16:283–292.

572. Estelles A, Garcia-Plaza I, Dasi A, et al: Severe inherited "homozygous" protein C deficiency in a newborn infant. Thromb Haemost 1984; 52:53–56.

573. Mahasandana C, Suvatte V, Chuansumrit A, et al: Homozygous protein S deficiency in an infant with purpura fulminans. J Pediatr 1990; 117:750–753.

574. Dreyfus M, Magny JF, Bridey F, et al: Treatment of homozygous protein C deficiency and neonatal purpura fulminans with a purified protein C concentrate. N Engl J Med 1991; 325:1565–1568.

575. Reverdiau-Moalic P, Gruel Y, Delahousse B, et al: Comparative study of the fibrinolytic system in human fetuses and in pregnant women. Thromb Res 1991; 61:489–499.

576. Dahlback B, Hildebrand B: Inherited resistance to activated protein C is corrected by anticoagulant cofactor activity found to be a property of factor V. Proc Natl Acad Sci USA 1994; 91:1396–1400.

577. Svensson PJ, Dahlback B: Resistance to activated protein C as a basis for venous thrombosis. N Engl J Med 1994; 330:517–522.

578. Rogers PC, Silva MP, Carter JE, et al: Renal vein thrombosis and response to therapy in a newborn due to protein C deficiency. Eur J Pediatr 1989; 149:124–125.

579. Lobato-Mendizabal E, Ruiz-Arguelles GJ, Toquero-Franco O: [Effect of danazol on heterozygous protein C coagulation deficiency exacerbated by *Salmonella typhi* sepsis]. Bol Med Hosp Infant Mex 1989; 46:343–345.

580. Simioni P, de Ronde H, Prandoni P, et al: Ischemic stroke in young patients with activated protein C resistance. A report of three cases belonging to three different kindreds. Stroke 1995; 26:885–890.

581. Cucuianu M, Blaga S, Pop S, et al: Homozygous or compound heterozygous qualitative antithrombin III deficiency. Nouv Rev Fr Hematol 1994; 35:335–337.

582. Glueck CJ, Glueck HI, Greenfield D, et al: Protein C and S deficiency, thrombophilia, and hypofibrinolysis: Pathophysiologic causes of Legg-Perthes disease. Pediatr Res 1994; 35(4 Pt 1):383–388.

583. Schander K, Niessen M, Rehm A, et al: Diagnose und Therapie eines kongenitalen Antithrombin III Manglels in der neonatalen Periode. Blut 1980; 40:68.

584. Soutar R, Marzinotto V, Andrew M: Overtight nappy precipitating thrombosis in antithrombin III deficiency. Arch Dis Child 1993; 69:599–600.

585. Shiozaki A, Arai T, Izumi R, et al: Congenital antithrombin III deficient neonate treated with antithrombin III concentrates. Thromb Res 1993; 70:211–216.

586. Schmidt B, Andrew M: Neonatal thrombotic disease: Prevention, diagnosis, and treatment. J Pediatr 1988; 113:407–410.

587. Schmidt B, Zipursky A: Thrombotic disease in newborn infants. Clin Perinatol 1984; 11:461–488.

588. Schmidt B, Andrew M: Neonatal thrombosis: Report of a prospective Canadian and international registry. Pediatrics 1995; 96(5 Pt 1):939–943.

589. David M, Andrew M: Venous thromboembolic complications in children. J Pediatr 1993; 123:337–346.

590. Andrew M, David M, Adams M, et al: Venous thromboembolic complications (VTE) in children: First analyses of the Canadian Registry of VTE. Blood 1994; 83:1251–1257.

591. O'Brodovich H, Coates J: Quantitative ventilation perfusion lung scans in infants and children: Utility of a submicronic radiolabelled aerosol to assess ventilation. J Pediatr 1984; 105:377–383.

592. Jackson JC, Truog WE, Watchko JF, et al: Efficacy of thromboresistant umbilical artery catheters in reducing aortic thrombosis and related complications. J Pediatr 1987; 110:102–105.

593. Horgan MJ, Bartoletti A, Polansky S, et al: Effect of heparin infusates in umbilical arterial catheters on frequency of thrombotic complications. J Pediatr 1987; 111:774–778.

594. Rajani K, Goetzman BW, Wennberg RP, et al: Effect of heparinization of fluids infused through an umbilical artery catheter on

catheter patency and frequency of complications. Pediatrics 1979; 63:552–556.

595. Ankola PA, Atakent YS: Effect of adding heparin in very low concentration to the infusate to prolong the patency of umbilical artery catheters. Am J Perinatol 1993; 10:229–232.

596. Vailas GN, Brouillette RT, Scott JP, et al: Neonatal aortic thrombosis: Recent experience. J Pediatr 1986; 109:101–108.

597. Bosque E, Weaver L: Continuous versus intermittent heparin infusion of umbilical artery catheters in the newborn infant. J Pediatr 1986; 108:141–143.

598. David RJ, Merten DF, Anderson JC, et al: Prevention of umbilical artery catheter clots with heparinized infusates. Dev Pharmacol Ther 1981; 2:117–126.

599. Lesko SM, Mitchell AA, Epstein MF, et al: Heparin use as a risk factor for intraventricular hemorrhage in low-birth-weight infants. N Engl J Med 1986; 314:1156–1160.

600. Andrew M, Mitchell L, Vegh P, et al: Thrombin regulation in children differs from adults in the absence and presence of heparin. Thromb Haemost 1994; 72:836–842.

601. Andrew M, Ofosu F, Schmidt B, et al: Heparin clearance and ex vivo recovery in newborn piglets and adult pigs. Thromb Res 1988; 52:517–527.

602. McDonald MM, Jacobson LJ, Hay WW Jr, et al: Heparin clearance in the newborn. Pediatr Res 1981; 15:1015–1018.

603. Schmidt B, Buchanan MR, Ofosu F, et al: Antithrombotic properties of heparin in a neonatal piglet model of thrombin-induced thrombosis. Thromb Haemost 1988; 60:289–292.

604. Murdoch IA, Beattie RM, Silver DM: Heparin-induced thrombocytopenia in children. Acta Paediatr 1993; 82:495–497.

605. Spadone D: Heparin induced thrombocytopenia in the newborn. J Vasc Surg 1996; 15:306–312.

606. Hirsh J, Levine MN: Low molecular weight heparin. Blood 1992; 79:1–17.

607. Hathaway W, Corrigan J: Report of Scientific and Standardization Subcommittee on Neonatal Hemostasis. Normal coagulation data for fetuses and newborn infants. Thromb Haemost 1991; 65:323–325.

608. Corrigan J: Normal hemostasis in fetus and newborn. In Polin R, Fox W (eds): Fetal and Neonatal Physiology. Philadelphia, WB Saunders, 1992, pp 1368–1371.

609. Hathaway WE, Bonnar J: Hemostatic disorders of the pregnant woman and newborn infant. New York: Elsevier, 1987.

610. Schmidt B, Andrew M: Report of Scientific and Standardization Subcommittee on Neonatal Hemostasis Diagnosis and Treatment of Neonatal Thrombosis. Thromb Haemost 1992; 67:381–382.

611. el Makhlouf A, Friedli B, Oberhansli I, et al: Prosthetic heart valve replacement in children. Results and follow-up of 273 patients. J Thorac Cardiovasc Surg 1987; 93:80–85.

612. Sade RM, Crawford FA Jr, Fyfe DA, et al: Valve prostheses in children: A reassessment of anticoagulation. J Thorac Cardiovasc Surg 1988; 95:553–561.

613. Rao S, Solymar L, Mardini M, et al: Anticoagulant therapy in children with prosthetic valves. Ann Thorac Surg 1989; 47:589–592.

614. Serra AJ, McNicholas KW, Olivier HF Jr, et al: The choice of anticoagulation in pediatric patients with the St. Jude Medical valve prostheses. J Cardiovasc Surg (Torino) 1987; 28:588–591.

615. McGrath LB, Gonzalez-Lavin L, Eldredge WJ, et al: Thromboembolic and other events following valve replacement in a pediatric population treated with antiplatelet agents. Ann Thorac Surg 1987; 43:285–287.

616. Spevak PJ, Freed MD, Castaneda AR, et al: Valve replacement in children less than 5 years of age. J Am Coll Cardiol 1986; 8:901–908.

617. Harada Y, Imai Y, Kurosawa H, et al: Ten-year follow-up after valve replacement with the St. Jude Medical prosthesis in children. J Thorac Cardiovasc Surg 1990; 100:175–180.

618. Stewart S, Cianciotta D, Alexson C, et al: The long-term risk of warfarin sodium therapy and the incidence of thromboembolism in children after prosthetic cardiac valve replacement. J Thorac Cardiovasc Surg 1987; 93:551–554.

619. Woods A, Vargas J, Berri G, et al: Antithrombotic therapy in children and adolescents. Thromb Res 1986; 42:289–301.

620. Andrew M, Marzinotto V, Brooker LA, et al: Oral anticoagulation therapy in pediatric patients: A prospective study. Thromb Haemost 1994; 71:265–269.

621. Von Kries R, Shearer MJ, McCarthy PT, et al: Vitamin K$_1$ content of maternal milk: Influence of the stage of lactation, lipid composition, and vitamin K$_1$ supplements given to the mother. Pediatr Res 1987; 22:513–517.

622. Von Kries R, Stannigel H, Gobel U: Anticoagulant therapy by continuous heparin-antithrombin III infusion in newborns with disseminated intravascular coagulation. Eur J Pediatr 1985; 144:191–194.

623. Hathaway WE: Use of antiplatelet agents in pediatric hypercoagulable states. Am J Dis Child 1984; 138:301–304.

624. Barnard DR, Simmons M, Hathaway W: Coagulation studies in extremely premature infants. Pediatr Res 1979; 13:1330–1335.

625. Beverley DW, Chance GW, Inwood MJ, et al: Intraventricular haemorrhage and haemostasis defects. Arch Dis Child 1984; 59:444–448.

626. Andrew M, Caco C, Vegh P, et al: Benefits of platelet transfusions in premature infants: A randomized controlled trial. Thromb Haemost 1991; 65:721.

627. Corrigan J, Kryc JJ: Factor II (prothrombin) levels in cord blood. Correlation of coagulant activity with immunoreactive protein. J Pediatr 1980; 97:979–983.

628. Andrew M: Developmental hemostasis: Relevance to newborns and infants. In Nathan DG, Orkin SH (eds): Nathan and Oski's Hematology of Infancy and Childhood, 5th ed. Philadelphia, WB Saunders, 1998, pp 114–157.

629. Monagle P, Andrew M, Halton J, et al: Homozygous protein C deficiency: Description of a new mutation and successful treatment with low molecular weight heparin. Thromb Haemost 1998; 79:756–761.

630. Reverdiau-Moalic P, Delahousse B, et al: Evolution of blood coagulation activators and inhibitors in the healthy human fetus. Blood 1996; 88:900–906.

631. Andrew M, Vegh P, Johnston M, et al: Maturation of the hemostatic system during childhood. Blood 1992; 80:1998–2005.

632. Andrew M, Brooker LA: Blood component therapy in neonatal hemostatic disorders. Transfus Med Rev 1995; 9:231–250.

633. DiMichele D, Neufeld EJ: Hemophilia. A new approach to an old disease. Hematol Oncol Clin North Am 1998; 12:1315–1344.

634. Brangenberg R, Bodensohn M, Burger U: Antithrombin III substitution in preterm infants; effects on intracranial hemorrhage and coagulation parameters. Biol Neonate 1997; 72:76–83.

635. Markarian M, Githens JH, Rosenblut E, et al: Hypercoagulability in premature infants with special reference to the respiratory distress syndrome and hemorrhage. I. Coagulation studies. Biol Neonate 1971; 17:84–97.

636. Chang GY, Lueder FL, DiMichele DM, et al: Heparin and the risk of intraventricular hemorrhage in premature infants. J Pediatr 1997; 131:362–366.

637. Michelson AD, Bovill E, Andrew M: Antithrombotic therapy in children. Chest 1995; 108:506S–522S.

638. Thorp JA, Parriott J, Ferrette-Smith D, et al: Antepartum vitamin K and phenobarbital for preventing intraventricular hemorrhage in the premature newborn: a randomized double-blind, placebo-controlled trial. Obstet Gynecol 1994; 83:70–76.

639. Morgan ME, Benson JW, Cooke RW: Ethamsylate reduces the incidence of periventricular haemorrhage in very low birth-weight babies. Lancet 1981; 2:830–831.

640. Krueger E, Mellander M, Bratton D, et al: Prevention of symptomatic patent ductus arteriosus with a single dose of indomethacin. J Pediatr 1987; 111:749–754.

641. Bandstra ES, Montalvo BM, Goldberg RN, et al: Prophylactic indomethacin for prevention of intraventricular hemorrhage in premature infants. Pediatrics 1988; 82:533–542.

642. Bada HS, Green RS, Pourcyrous M, et al: Indomethacin reduces the risk of severe intraventricular hemorrhage. J Pediatr 1989; 115:631–637.

643. Mahony L, Caldwell RL, Girod DA, et al: Indomethacin therapy on the first day of life in infants with very low birth weight. J Pediatr 1985; 106:801–805.

644. Vincer M, Allen A, Evans J et al: Early intravenous indomethacin prolongs respiratory support in very low birth weight infants. Acta Paediatr Scand 1987; 76:894–897.

645. Ogata T, Motohara K, Endo F, et al: Vitamin K effect in low birth weight infants. Pediatrics 1988; 81:423–427.

646. Motohara K, Endo F, Matsuda I: Screening for late neonatal vitamin K deficiency by acarboxyprothrombin in dried blood spots. Arch Dis Child 1987; 62:370–375.

647. von Kries R, Kreppel S, Becker A, et al: Acarboxyprothrombin concentration after oral prophylactic vitamin K. Arch Dis Child 1987; 62:938–940.

648. O'Connor ME, Addiego JE Jr: Use of oral vitamin K1 to prevent hemorrhagic disease of the newborn infant. J Pediatr 1986; 108:616–619.

649. Keenan WJ, Jewett T, Glueck HI: Role of feeding and vitamin K in hypoprothrombinemia of the newborn. Am J Dis Child 1971; 121:271–277.

650. Wefring KW: Hemorrhage in the newborn and vitamin K prophylaxis. J Pediatr 1962; 61:686.

651. Astrowe PS, Palmerton ES: Clinical studies with vitamin K in newborn infants. J Pediatr 1941; 18:507.

652. Pietersma-de Bruyn AL, van Haard PM, Beunis MH, et al: Vitamin K1 levels and coagulation factors in healthy term newborns till 4 weeks after birth. Haemostasis 1990; 20:8–14.

653. Greer FR, Marshall S, Cherry J, et al: Vitamin K status of lactating mothers, human milk, and breast-feeding infants. Pediatrics 1991; 88:751–756.

654. Anai T, Hirota Y, Yoshimatsu J, et al: Can prenatal vitamin K1 (phylloquinone) supplementation replace prophylaxis at birth? Obstet Gynecol 1993; 81:251–254.

655. Dickson RC, Stubbs T, Lazarchick J: Antenatal vitamin K therapy of the low-birth-weight infant. Am J Obstet Gynecol 1994; 170:85–89.

656. Ekelund H: Late haemorrhagic disease in Sweden 1987-1989. Acta Paediatr Scand 1991; 80:966–968.

657. Tonz O, Schubinger G: Neonatale vitamin K prophylaxe and vitamin K mangelblutungen in der Schweiz 1986-1988. Schweiz Med Wochenschr 1988; 118:1747–1752.

658. Hanawa Y: Vitamin K deficiency in infancy: the Japanese experience. Acta Paediatr Jpn 1992; 34:107–116.

659. Clark F, James E: Twenty-seven years of experience with oral vitamin K1 therapy in neonates. J Pediatr 1995; 127:301–304.

III Bone Marrow Failure

6 | The Anatomy and Physiology of Hematopoiesis

Steven C. Clark ● David G. Nathan ● Colin A. Sieff

A review of the anatomy and physiology of normal hematopoiesis is presented in this chapter to provide a basis of understanding of the marrow failure syndromes described at length in the Chapters 7 and 8. We briefly discuss the phylogeny of hematopoiesis and describe marrow anatomy and the egress of recognizable hematopoietic cells from the marrow into the peripheral blood. A more detailed analysis of the cellular bases of erythrocyte, granulocyte-macrophage, and megakaryocyte development follows, including discussions of the pluripotent stem cell, the more committed but still undifferentiated progenitor cells, and the differentiated precursors of the mature formed elements of the blood. Much of this chapter is devoted to the interactions of growth factors and the cells that produce them in the up-regulation of hematopoiesis. The mechanisms of down-regulation of hematopoiesis by cell interactions and cytokines are touched upon here, but they are less well understood despite the fact that they are likely to influence the pathophysiology of aplastic anemia and other marrow failure syndromes.

HISTORY*

That "blood is life" was acknowledged by Empedocles in the fifth century BC. The theory that the vasculature contains blood, phlegm, black bile, and yellow bile, all revealed when freshly let blood is permitted to separate, is attributed to Polibus, the son-in-law of Hippocrates. Servetus recognized the systemic and lesser circulations in the 16th century. He was burned at the stake, in part because he did not accept the dogma that blood must pass through the intraventricular cardiac septum. (Grant disapproval and, more recently, approval without funding have been substituted for immolation. The effects are not entirely dissimilar.)

In view of the present growth of knowledge of hematology, it is remarkable to realize that the concept of the circulation of the blood was finally established by Harvey only a little more than 300 years ago. With this finding the clinical application of blood transfusion began, of which Pepys wrote "it gave rise to many pretty wishes as of the blood of a Quaker to be let into an Archbishop and such like."

In the mid-17th century, Swammerdam observed red blood corpuscles in the microscope, and Malpighi discovered the capillary circulation in the lung and in the omentum. However, it was not until the 19th century that the source of blood cell production began to be successfully explored. Houston suggested that red cells were derived from leukocytes in the lymphoid system. Zimmerman believed that erythrocytes were derived from platelets, an opinion shared by Hayem. Addison, perhaps not surprisingly, attributed red cell production to the adrenal glands, and Reikert finally suggested that red cells might be produced in the embryonic liver. In fact, it was not until 1868 that Neumann demonstrated that red cells arise from precursors in the marrow. This discovery began the modern understanding of the physiology of hematopoiesis.

PHYLOGENY

Much can be learned about the physiology of hematopoiesis from study of the evolution of oxygen transport, a subject reviewed by Lehmann and Huntsman.[1]

One of the major advantages of mammalian life over that of invertebrates is the capacity to package large amounts of hemoglobin within cells. This permits the delivery of oxygen to tissues without the enormous increase in oncotic pressure that would be induced by a similar concentration of high-molecular-weight hemoglobin free in the plasma. The renewal rate of red cells is a function of metabolic rate or basal heat production. This is illustrated dramatically in studies of the animal kingdom, ranging from the turtle to the pygmy shrew, and by comparisons of red cell renewal in marmots during periods at ambient and cold temperatures,[2] in rats,[3] and in frogs.[4]

The production of blood cells in bone marrow is a late development in phylogeny. Red cells are found in the coelomic cavity of the worm and are produced in the kidneys of the goldfish. The influence of oxygen demand on the production of red cells[5] is illustrated by the effects of hyperoxia on bled rats[6] and the behavior of the European eel, one of the few vertebrate forms that ordinarily lacks erythrocytes in its juvenile state. When the adult eel struggles against the current up the rivers of Europe, hemoglobin-containing nucleated cells appear in its plasma. This influence of oxygen demand on respiratory pigment production is also illustrated in non–red cell-producing organisms such as *Daphnia*, the English water flea, a creature that produces high-molecular-weight hemoglobin in its ovaries when it is exposed to low oxygen tension in stagnant ponds. The discovery of transcription factors that function as oxygen sensors provides a potential

---

*For an entertaining review from which this précis was in part drawn, see Robb-Smith AHT: The growth of knowledge of functions of the blood. In MacFarlane RG, Robb-Smith AHT (eds): Functions of the Blood. Oxford, Blackwell Scientific Publications, 1961. For more details, see also Wintrobe MM: Blood Pure and Simple. New York, McGraw-Hill Book Company, 1980.

molecular explanation for these regulatory mechanisms.[7-9]

MARROW ANATOMY

The relative red (active) marrow space of a child is much greater than that of an adult, presumably because the high requirements for red cell production during neonatal life demand the resources of the entire production potential of the marrow. During postnatal life the demands for red cell production ebb, and much of the marrow space is slowly and progressively filled with fat (Fig. 6–1). In certain disease states that are usually associated with anemia, such as myeloid metaplasia, hematopoiesis may return to its former sites in the liver, spleen, and lymph nodes and may also be found in the adrenal glands, cartilage, adipose tissue, thoracic paravertebral gutters, and even in the kidneys.

The microenvironment of the marrow cavity is a vast network of vascular channels or sinusoids in which float fronds of hematopoietic cells, including fat cells. This complex area of cell biology and anatomy has been the subject of several reviews.[10-13] The cells are found in the intrasinusoidal fronds. The vascular and hematopoietic compartments are joined by reticular fibroblastoid cells that form the adventitial surfaces of the vascular sinuses and extend cytoplasmic processes to create a lattice on which blood cells are found. The lattice itself is illustrated by reticulin stains of marrow sections (Fig. 6–2). The conformation of the meshwork of reticulin and the location of hematopoietic cells in the network of vascular sinuses are best illustrated by scanning electron microscopy (Fig.

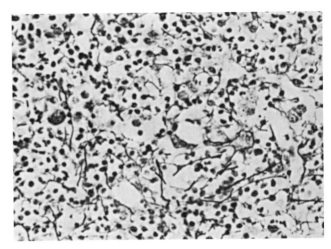

FIGURE 6–2. Bone marrow biopsy of a patient with mild myelofibrosis showing a slight increase in the number of reticulin fibers in a delicate discontinuous fiber network. (Gomori stain ×350.) (From Lennert K, Nagai K, Schwarze EW: Patho-anatomical features of the bone marrow. Clin Hematol 1975; 4:335.)

6–3). The fibroblastoid network provides two major functions: (1) an adhesive framework onto which the developing cells are bound and (2) the production by these cells of essential hematopoietic colony-stimulating factors (discussed later).[14] Cell-cell adhesion may be mediated by binding of the hematopoietic very late antigen (VLA) 4 integrin to stromal fibronectin or vascular cell adhesion molecule 1 (VCAM-1).[15-18] In addition, cytokine receptors such as c-kit can bind to the membrane-bound form of stem cell factor (SCF), also called Steel factor (SF)[19] and the extracellular matrix proteins secreted by stromal cells may actually provide a binding site for some growth factors or for hematopoietic cells.[20-22] In addition,

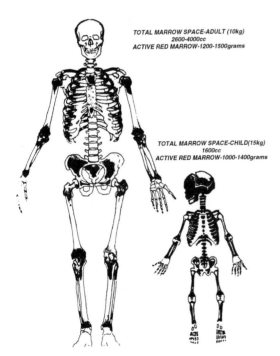

FIGURE 6–1. Comparison of active red marrow–bearing areas in the child and the adult. Note the almost identical amount of active red marrow in the child and adult despite a fivefold discrepancy in body weight. (From MacFarlane RC, Robb-Smith AHT (eds): Functions of the Blood. Oxford, Blackwell Scientific Publications, 1961, p 357.)

TOTAL MARROW SPACE-ADULT (10kg)
2600-4000cc
ACTIVE RED MARROW-1200-1500grams

TOTAL MARROW SPACE-CHILD(15kg)
1600cc
ACTIVE RED MARROW-1000-1400grams

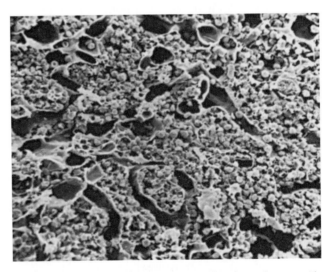

FIGURE 6–3. Scanning electron micrograph of rat femoral marrow. The hematopoietic cells are grouped between the interlacing network of vascular sinuses. Many cells are dislodged when the marrow is transected, and separate spaces are present where cells had been. (From Lichtman MA, Chamberlain JK, et al: Factors thought to contribute to the regulation of egress of cells from marrow. In Silber K, LoBue L, et al (eds): The Year in Hematology, 1978. New York, Plenum Medical Book Company, 1978, pp 243–279.)

data show that a family of small molecules called chemokines may have a role in stromal function. Specifically, stroma-derived factor 1 (SDF-1) is a potent attractant for hematopoietic cells (both mature leukocytes and progenitor cells that express its receptor CXCR4).[23] Gene disruption studies in mice of both ligand and receptor are embryonic lethal, with defects in B lymphopoiesis and myelopoiesis.[24, 25] These defects may relate to a critical role for CXCR4 in bone marrow engraftment in nonobese diabetic/severe combined immunodeficient (NOD/SCID) mice[26]; SDF-1 has been shown to activate the integrins VLA-4, VLA-5, and lymphocyte function antigen (LFA) 1) on CD34[+] cells.[27] Last, there is evidence that SDF-1 may also play a role in the egress of progenitor cells from bone marrow to blood during stem cell mobilization.[28, 29]

A schema of the marrow circulation is shown in Figure 6–4. The central and radial arteries ramify in the cortical capillaries, which in turn join the marrow sinusoids and drain into the central sinus. Cells that egress from the marrow sinusoids then join the venous circulation through the comitant veins. The inner, or luminal, surface of the vascular sinusoids is lined with endothelial cells, the cytoplasmic extensions of which overlap, or interdigitate, with one another. The escape of developing hematopoietic cells into the sinus for transport to the general circulation occurs through gaps that develop in this endothelial lining and even through endothelial cell cytoplasmic pores.

The location of the different hematopoietic cells is not random. Clumps of megakaryocytes are found adjacent to marrow sinuses. They shed platelets, the fragments of their cytoplasm, directly into the lumen. This reduces the requirement for movement of bulky mature megakaryocytes, a mobility characteristic of the granuloid- and erythroid-differentiated precursors as they approach the point at which they egress from the marrow. A schema that illustrates the transfer of hematopoietic cells into the sinus is shown in Figure 6–5. Disruption of the function

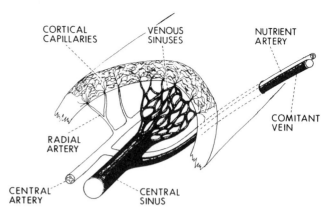

FIGURE 6–4. A schematic representation of the circulation of the marrow. The nutrient artery, central arteries, and radial arteries feed the cortical capillaries. The cortical capillaries anastomose with the marrow sinuses, which drain into the large central sinus. The central sinus enters the comitant vein by which the marrow effluent enters the systemic venous circulation. An interesting feature of the circulation of marrow is the transit of nearly all arterial blood through cortical capillaries before it enters the marrow sinuses. Not shown are the arterial communications from muscular arteries that feed the periosteum and penetrate the cortex to anastomose with intracortical vessels. (From Lichtman MA, Chamberlain JK, et al: Factors thought to contribute to the regulation of egress of cells from marrow. In Silber K, LoBue L, et al (eds): The Year in Hematology, 1978. New York, Plenum Medical book Company, 1978, pp 243–279.)

of microenvironmental cells inhibits long-term murine marrow cultures.[30] Such disruptions may be responsible for aplastic anemia in certain patients.

HEMATOPOIETIC CELLS

Stem Cells

The concept that sustained hematopoiesis derives from pluripotent stem cells was first suggested by Jacobson and co-workers,[31] who showed that mice can be protected from the lethal effects of whole-body irradiation by exte-

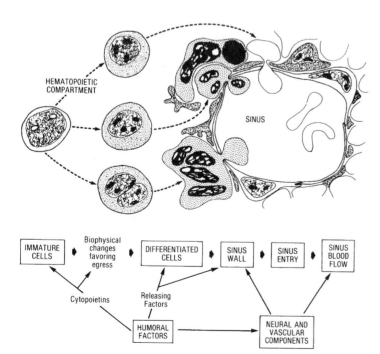

FIGURE 6–5. A schematic diagram of the factors that may be involved in controlling the release of marrow cells. The central relationship between the hematopoietic compartment and the marrow sinus is depicted. The drawing highlights the similarity of the egress process for the three major hematopoietic cells: reticulocytes in the top pathway, granulocytes and monocytes in the center pathway, and platelets in the lower pathway. Immature cells undergo biophysical changes under the influence of cytopoietins that favor egress. In the case of the reticulocyte, enucleation precedes egress. This is shown by the solid black inclusion in the perisinal macrophage representing nucleophagocytosis antecedent to digestion of the erythroblast nucleus. The cytoplasmic protrusion of the megakaryocyte presumably detaches itself from the cell and will further fragment into platelets in the circulation. (From Lichtman MA, Chamberlain JK et al: Factors thought to contribute to the regulation of egress of cell from marrow. In Silber R, LoBue J, et al (eds): The Year in Hematology, 1978. New York, Plenum Medical Book Company, 1978, pp 243–279.)

riorization and shielding of the spleen. This protective effect was shown to be cell-mediated by the observation that the injection of spleen cells could initiate recovery and reestablish hematopoiesis in irradiated animals.[32] The clonal nature of hematopoiesis and the concept that a single pluripotent stem cell exhibits the capacity to repopulate the entire hematopoietic system was first demonstrated experimentally by Till and McCulloch,[33] who also used the mouse as an experimental system. They demonstrated that colonies of hematopoietic cells could be observed in the spleen of the irradiated transplant recipients within 10 days after the transplant. These colonies contained precursors to erythrocytes, granulocytes and macrophages, and megakaryocytes. Subsequent experiments using karyotypically marked donor cells confirmed the clonal origin of the differentiated cells in the colony, proving that a single pluripotent stem cell had given rise to these differentiated cells.[34] It was also shown that each colony contained a number of stem cells that could again form a colony of differentiated progeny in a second irradiated recipient, demonstrating their self-renewal capacity. This is true only of spleen colonies that are present on days 12 through 14 (spleen colony-forming unit [$CFU-S_{12}$]). Colonies observed on days 7 to 8 after marrow infusion are transient, disappear by day 12, and are neither multipotential nor self-maintaining.[35] Under steady-state conditions no more than 10 percent of the CFU-S become committed to differentiation during any given 3-hour period. The demonstration of a stem cell that can differentiate to form progenitor cells for erythropoiesis, granulopoiesis, and megakaryopoiesis is completely consistent with subsequent observations in disease states such as chronic myelogenous leukemia[36, 37] and polycythemia vera,[38, 39] in which a clonal origin of abnormal erythroid, granulocytic, and megakaryocytic precursor cells and lymphocytes can be demonstrated (see Chapter 34).

The demonstration of a pluripotent stem cell in adult bone marrow led to a systematic search for the ontogenic origins of hematopoietic stem cells (HSCs). Experiments performed by Moore and Metcalf [40, 41] clearly demonstrated the presence of cells capable of repopulating the adult marrow in the yolk sac and the murine fetal liver. Subsequent work has confirmed and extended these observations,[42] although data show that HSCs may arise simultaneously in yolk sac and the intraembryonic aorta/gonad/mesonephros region.[43] A difficulty here is that primordial germ cells also arise or migrate through this region and have been shown to have the potential to generate HSCs.[44] A point of interest that arises is whether the stem cells observed in yolk sac, fetal liver, and adult marrow and spleen are functionally equivalent in every respect. One experimental finding that suggests functional differences between CFU-S at different stages of development of the mouse was made by Micklem and Ross.[45] Their experimental approach was to transfer spleen cells sequentially from a repopulated recipient to an irradiated recipient. Experiments of this type had previously shown that the capacity for transfer of CFU-S from adult marrow or spleen was finite, and in fact only three serial transfers could be accomplished.[46] Micklem and Ross showed that cells transplanted from the yolk sac to the spleen of an

irradiated recipient could be serially transplanted as many as seven times before further proliferative capacity was lost. CFU-S derived from fetal livers were capable of five to six serial transfers.

Studies of Hellman and co-workers[47] have provided a model of the stem cell compartment in which there is a continuum of cells with decreasing capacities for self-renewal, increasing likelihood for differentiation, and increasing proliferative activity. Cells progress in a unidirectional fashion in this continuum. It is the most primitive cells with the greatest self-renewal capacity that reconstitute long-term hematopoiesis after transfer into irradiated recipient mice. These cells, termed *long-term reconstituting hematopoietic stem cells* (LTR-HSCs), were shown to be separable from $CFU-S_{12}$ in a limiting dilution assay designed to detect and enumerate "cobblestone areas."[48] This assay is derived from the original "Dexter" technique for long-term culture of murine marrow in which CFU-S, granulocyte-macrophage colony-forming units (CFU-GM), and erythroid burst-forming units (BFU-E) flourish for many months on and within an adherent stromal monolayer.[49] The areas of active hematopoiesis have a cobblestone appearance. In the limiting dilution assay, different concentrations of bone marrow cells are plated onto a series of microwells that contain a preestablished stromal monolayer, and at 5 weeks the cobblestone areas that comprise proliferating blast cells within the stromal cell layer are counted.[48] In cell separation experiments, their numbers correlate with a cell fraction that is characterized by low mitochondrial mass per cell (minimal retention of the supravital fluorochrome rhodamine 123); this cell fraction is enriched for marrow repopulating cells but depleted of $CFU-S_{12}$.[48, 50] An even more impressive separation of pre-CFU-S from $CFU-S_{12}$ was obtained by counter-current elutriation.[51] Intermediate and rapidly sedimenting cells contained more than 99 percent $CFU-S_{12}$ as well as the cells responsible for short-term reconstitution. In contrast, long-term reconstituting cells (>60 days) came from a slowly sedimenting fraction that contained only 0.25 percent $CFU-S_{12}$.

In summary, LTR-HSCs are cells capable of long-term reconstitution of myelopoiesis and lymphopoiesis. More mature progenitor cells, represented by $CFU-S_{12}$, give rise to spleen colonies 12 to 14 days after injection into irradiated recipients, exhibit less self-renewal and proliferative capacity, and are generally limited to myeloid differentiation. The most mature compartment, represented by cells that give rise to spleen colonies 6 to 8 days after transplantation ($CFU-S_8$), has limited self-renewal and proliferative capacities. The relationship between the *in vivo* LTR-HSC assay and *in vitro* assays that measure blast cell colonies capable of forming additional colonies after replating,[52] high proliferative potential colony-forming cells (HPP-CFCs) that form large monocyte colonies (up to 5×10^4 cells),[53] or cells that survive in long term cultures[54] is at this point unresolved.

The stem cell model of hemopoiesis has parallels in other organ systems. The fact that rapidly self-renewing epithelial tissues such as skin and intestine have stem cells that continually replenish the cells lost by differentiation is well described, and it is likely that most epithelial tissues, for example, liver and pancreas, also contain stem cells that function after organ damage. However, the recent demonstration of the existence of neural stem cells[55, 56] has raised the possibility that many organ systems might retain a population of self-renewing stem cells. Muscle satellite cells also appear to fulfill this role. These organ- or tissue-specific stem cells arise during early fetal development from embryonic stem cells of the inner cell mass of the blastocyst that are totipotent and give rise to all body cell types.

Much more surprising are the demonstrations of stem cell "plasticity," in which organ-specific stem cells have been reported to differentiate into cells of other lineages, either *in vitro* or after transplantation *in vivo*. The first reports of (murine) bone marrow–derived cells differentiating into brain and muscle[57, 58] and cultured neural cells differentiating into blood[59] have now been followed by a spate of studies documenting bone marrow stroma into brain,[60] bone marrow into liver[61] and other ectodermal tissues[62], neural cells into cardiac muscle, and muscle cells into blood.[63, 64] Recent intriguing data show that "multipotent adult progenitor cells" derived from bone marrow stroma can apparently differentiate into multiple lineages (including hematopoietic),[64a] and that ES cells can be induced to differentiate into dopamine-secreting neurons[64b] (reviewed in reference 64c) (Fig. 6–6). Because of their challenge to the dogma that commitment of embryonic totipotential stem cells to organ-specific stem cells during embryogenesis is irreversible as well as their important potential therapeutic applications, these results have caused much excitement. It is therefore important to examine rigorously claims of unexpected heterologous differentiation outcomes, by noting whether differentiation is complete with production of functional cells or whether a few phenotypic markers only characterize the new cell population. Second, did the demonstration of plasticity involve purification of the stem cells from which the unexpected outcome was observed without extensive *in vitro* culture. And third, what is the rate of occurrence within the purified stem cell population? The interested reader may consult several excellent recent reviews.[65–67] Even data obtained with highly purified stem cells can be difficult to interpret. Purified "side population" cells from muscle were shown to be capable of hematopoietic reconstitution.[63, 64] The analysis of Ly-5.1/Ly-5.2 chimeric transplantation experiments from Ogawa's group[68] shows that after transplantation the percentage of Ly-5.1 (donor) progenitors cultured from muscle correlated with the percentage of those cultured from bone marrow, indicating their bone marrow origin; furthermore, secondary transplantation studies showed that the muscle-derived cells capable of long-term reconstitution were also of bone marrow origin. These results are important because they clearly demonstrate the hematopoietic origin of the muscle stem cells. However, the existence of a bipotent bone marrow–derived stem cell capable of both hematopoietic and muscle differentiation is still open to question.

Purified HSCs have been shown to differentiate into muscle,[63] although the rate may be low, and into functional hepatocytes after transplantation into a mouse model of fatal hereditary tyrosinemia type I.[69] Recently, single HSCs recovered from the bone marrow 48 hours after transplantation with highly enriched PKH26 (a

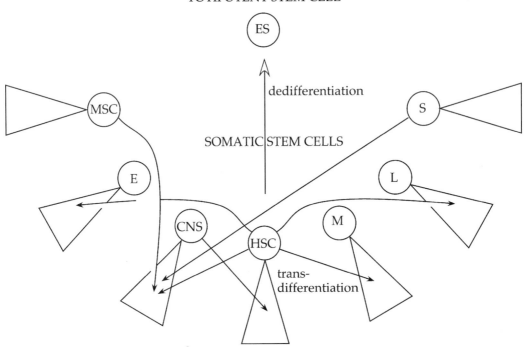

FIGURE 6–6. Lineage plasticity of stem cells. Data suggest that organ-specific stem cells are capable of contributing to tissues of diverse organs. Thus hematopoietic stem cells (HSC) have been reported to contribute to muscle (M), hepatocytes (L), epithelial cells of gut and skin (E), and brain (CNS), whereas CNS- and muscle-derived stem cells are reported to differentiate into blood (see text for discussion). Bone marrow mesenchymal cells (MSC) and skin cells (S) can differentiate into neural (CNS) cells and, perhaps less surprising, into other mesodermal-derived tissues (chondrocytes, osteoblasts, adipocytes, myoblasts, and endothelial cells). Whether dedifferentiation into a totipotent stem cell analogous to the embryonic stem cell (ES) or transdifferentiation underlies these phenomena is uncertain.

fluorescent membrane label)-labeled stem cells were shown to be capable of long-term reconstitution of hematopoiesis and also of contributing to several ectodermal and endodermal derived lineages.[62] After transplantation of human bone marrow[70, 71] or mobilized blood[72] stem cells, a small proportion of hepatocytes and both skin and gut epithelial cells were shown to be of donor origin, based on fluorescence Y-chromosome analysis in female recipients of male grafts. Although these data suggest that plasticity can be extended to human stem cells, the lack of purification of the transplanted cells as well as certain technical limitations invites a cautious interpretation.[73] The exciting possibility that useful cells of other lineages may be generated from HSCs awaits further experimentation.

Considerations of stem cell heterogeneity are of clinical relevance, because any manipulations of human bone marrow before allogeneic or autologous transplantation requires preservation of the most primitive stem cell compartment. Morphologically, stem cells appear to be medium-sized mononuclear cells with a very high nuclear-to-cytoplasmic ratio, basophilic cytoplasm devoid of granules, and prominent nucleoli.

A cell with the characteristics of a self-renewing multipotential stem cell has not been clearly defined in humans for obvious reasons. However, the presence of stem cells capable of long-term hematopoietic reconstitution (i.e., LTR-HSCs) is inferred from the success of bone marrow transplantation, using bone marrow or blood as a source of cells in humans[74, 75] and blood as a source of reconstituting cells in canine models.[76] However, these transplantation experiments do not prove that the LTR-HSCs present in the marrow and blood of human and canine species are capable of self-renewal. More differentiated stem cells could have established the hematopoietic graft. Rigid proof of the presence of self-renewing stem cells requires the use of a secondary transfer assay, in which the primary transplanted cells themselves are used for reconstitution of second irradiated hosts. Colonies morphologically similar to CFU-S have been observed after careful examination of spleens from bone marrow transplant recipients who died early in the engraftment process, which then allowed analysis of their spleens at times similar to days 8 to 14 after transplants in the mouse.[77] Obviously, however, cells from such colonies cannot be used to attempt reconstitution of secondary hosts.

The growth of LTR-HSCs in the marrow may require a microenvironmental "niche".[78, 79] Thus, isogeneic marrow infusions are not successful unless the recipient is irradiated or treated with sufficient doses of cytotoxic drugs to create an adequate number of niches. Therefore, reports of failure of engraftment after transplants using identical twin donors in aplastic anemia do not necessarily suggest an immunologic basis for the disease but could just as well imply persistence of nonfunctional pluripotent progenitors in the aplastic marrow niches. These abnormal cells must be destroyed, if present, to allow implantation of transfused normal progenitors.

Many assays have been proposed as "surrogate" stem cell assays, but until homogeneous populations can be evaluated in both *in vitro* and *in vivo* assays it will be impossible to determine the precise cell type measured by these methods. Fauser and Messner and others[37, 80-82] demonstrated colonies in semisolid media that contain granulocytes, erythrocytes, monocytes, and megakaryocytes (CFU-GEMM) in methylcellulose cultures of human bone marrow. A unique type of *in vitro* blast cell colony that comprises small numbers of blast cells with higher self-renewal capacity (secondary colonies on replating) than CFU-GEMM has been described.[52] Evidence for the presence of pluripotent HSCs is also derived from the Dexter technique for liquid culture of human marrow in which myeloid progenitors (mostly CFU-GM) are sustained for about 2 months on and within an adherent stromal monolayer.[83, 84] The progenitors can be detected by replating into methylcellulose with several growth factors at 5 to 8 weeks, thereby demonstrating that unipotent and multipotent cells are generated in this culture system. Eaves and colleagues[85] have adapted this long-term culture technique to a limiting dilution assay in which long-term culture-initiating cells (LTC-ICs) can be quantitated after culture at different concentrations on a stromal layer for 5 weeks followed by replating in methylcellulose to score for the number of wells that do not contain colonies. The analogous cobblestone area–forming cell assay has also been adapted to human cells.[86] Another method that measures the enormous proliferative capacity of primitive progenitor cells is the HPP-CFC assay that gives rise to macroscopically (>5 mm) visible *in vitro* colonies.[53, 87] In an effort to establish a more direct measure of the ability of human stem cells to reconstitute hematopoiesis, Kamel-Reid and Dick developed an *in vivo* assay.[88] In this method human cells are injected into immunodeficient NOD/SCID mice, and 5 to 8 weeks later the animals are killed and tested for the presence of human cells in blood and progenitors in bone marrow. By limiting dilution these SCID-reconstituting cells (SRC) can be quantitated. A tentative relationship of the cells measured in these different assays to the stem cell is shown in Figure 6–7.

Application of these assays and analysis of HCSs, in general, has been hindered by the low rate of occurrence of the cell type in the hematopoietic cell population and the lack of reagents to identify stem cells. However, it is now possible to purify murine stem cells by several methods. Murine HSCs can be highly purified by density gradient centrifugation combined with labeling with antibodies, lectins, or intracellular dyes (alone or in combination) followed by separation using fluorescence-activated cell sorting (FACS), immunopanning, or immunomagnetic beads. Immunologic reagents that define murine stem cell populations include Thy-1, Sca-1, and Qa-m7. Weissman and co-workers[89] used FACS in combination with negative expression of T-cell, B-cell, granulocyte, and monocyte lineage (lin)–specific markers; low expression of Thy-1; and expression of the stem cell antigen (Sca-1). As few as 30 lin^-, Thy-1^{lo}, Sca-1^+ cells can ensure survival at 30 days for 50 percent of lethally irradiated syngeneic recipients. This cell fraction is highly enriched for CFU-S_{12}, but its content of long-term repopulating cells (pre-CFU-S, discussed earlier) is uncertain. Bertoncello and co-workers[90] used antibodies to the Qa-m7 antigen and immunomagnetic bead separation to purify HPP-CFCs. These cells are considered by some to

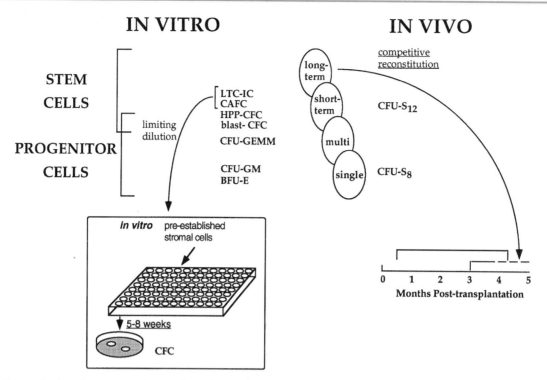

FIGURE 6–7. Schematic view of some general properties and assays for the heterogeneous cells that comprise the stem cell and progenitor cell compartments. Cells capable of permanently reconstituting *in vivo* hematopoiesis are separable from cells that give rise to day 12 spleen colony-forming units (CFU-S$_{12}$), but the precise developmental stage of *in vitro* long-term culture initiating cells (LTC-IC), cobblestone area–forming cells (CAFC), high proliferative potential colony-forming cells (HPP-CFC), and blast CFC is not established. In the progenitor compartment, mixed colonies of almost all lineage combinations have been described. CFU-GEMM = granulocyte-erythrocyte-monocyte-megakaryocyte colony-forming unit; CFU-GM = granulocyte-macrophage colony-forming unit; BFU-E, burst-forming unit-erythroid.

be the equivalent of the reconstituting stem cell. In these studies, up to 30 percent of the final cell population were HPP-CFCs. Visser and co-workers[91] used combinations of density gradient centrifugation and labeling with wheat germ agglutinin and rhodamine 123 dye to purify stem cells capable of 30-day radioprotection after transplantation into lethally irradiated syngeneic murine recipients. Differences in physical properties and expression of the antigens CD34 and CD33 have been used to enrich for human stem cells. Although most colony-forming cells (CFCs) express both the CD34 and CD33 antigens, cells that give rise to CFCs in long-term bone marrow cultures (i.e., pre-CFCs) can be separated by their expression of CD34, lack of expression of CD33, and intermediate forward light–scattering properties.[92] A G$_0$ CD34$^+$cell population has been isolated by exploiting the resistance of these cells to 5-fluorouracil in the presence of SCF and interleukin (IL)-3.[93] The G$_0$ cells are also c-kit, IL-6 receptor (IL-6R), and interleukin-1 receptor (IL-1R) positive; do not form progenitor-derived colonies upon direct culture in methylcellulose; but, after 5 weeks in culture on stromal cells, do form primary colonies in methylcellulose, 40 percent of which are replatable. Furthermore, 89 percent of the cells (normalized for the maximum number of positive wells) score positive in an LTC-IC assay, and in long-term culture myeloid and lymphoid cells can be derived. These data are unconfirmed but suggest that this cell population may represent a primitive resting multipotent HSC, possibly the LTR-HSC. The importance of CD34$^+$ marrow cells is emphasized by *in vivo* simian studies. Similar to its expression in human

bone marrow, the CD34 antigen is expressed by a minority of baboon cells, and infusion of these cells isolated by immunoabsorption chromatography and FACS can reconstitute lymphohematopoiesis in lethally irradiated baboons.[94] The cloning of the murine CD34 complementary DNA (cDNA) has cast some doubt on expression of CD34 by LTR-HSCs, at least in the mouse. A monoclonal antibody raised to a murine CD34-GST fusion protein was use to separate purified Sca-1$^+$, c-kit$^+$, and lin$^-$ bone marrow cells into CD34$^{lo/-}$,CD34^{lo}, and CD34$^+$ fractions. Interestingly, long-term multilineage reconstitution was observed after transplantation of the CD34$^{lo/-}$ cells, whereas the CD34$^+$ fraction gave early but unsustained multilineage reconstitution.[95] It is possible that murine and primate LTR-HSCs differ in their expression of CD34; however, the human and primate transplants have not used very highly purified cells, and so it is also possible that CD34$^{lo/-}$ cells could account for the long-term engraftment. These data are supported by experiments demonstrating that a tiny subset of murine bone marrow cells that exclude the Hoechst 33342 dye (called the side population) contains all the LTR-HSC activity, but is CD34$^-$.[96] Primate and human studies have also raised the possibility that HSCs do not express CD34.[97] When primitive human lin$^-$ cells are separated into CD34$^+$ and CD34$^-$ fractions, the capacity to reconstitute hemopoiesis in immunodeficient mice (cells called SRCs) is found in both cell fractions.[98] A resolution to this controversy may come from the recent demonstration that resting murine HSCs are CD34$^-$, while HSC activated with 5-fluorouracil or cytokines such as granulocyte colony-stimulating factor (G-CSF) express the CD34 antigen.[99, 100] The most interesting finding is that when activated CD34+ HSCs are transplanted, they can lose CD34 expression after return of the recipients to the resting steady state and still retain the capacity to reconstitute secondary recipients, demonstrating that CD34 expression is reversible.[100]

Progenitor Cells

The pluripotent stem cells of the marrow slowly self-replicate while occasionally (and stochastically) differentiating into a stage of either lymphoid or myeloid commitment. The first step of myeloid commitment produces a progenitor capable of self-renewal and stochastic differentiation into all of the progenitors of the blood cells other than lymphoid cells. This is the myeloid stem cell. This cell, in turn, slowly self-replicates or stochastically enters a more committed progenitor stage such as that of the progenitors responsible for phagocytopoiesis or eosinophilopoiesis or the progenitors responsible for erythropoiesis, basophilopoiesis, and megakaryocytopoiesis.

ERYTHROID COLONY-FORMING CELLS

The compartment of erythroid progenitors is invisible to the light microscope. These committed progenitors of a single lineage are derived from the stochastic differentiation of bi- or multipotential progenitors[101] that are, in turn, derived from a tiny population of totipotential stem cells (Fig. 6–8). In humans, the most primitive single lineage-committed erythroid progenitor is the erythroid burst-forming unit (BFU-E). BFU-E are so named because, in response to the combination of erythropoietin (EPO) and either SCF, IL-3, or granulocye-macrophage colony-stimulating factor (GM-CSF) *in vitro* in semisolid (methylcellulose) cultures, the progenitor divides several times when still motile, thereby forming subpopulations of erythroid colony-forming units (CFU-E).[102] Then, each of the latter forms a large colony of proerythroblasts that go on to form more mature erythroblasts and even reticulocytes. The burstlike morphology of the colony is responsible for the name of the progenitor. The entire process requires about 2 weeks *in vitro*. Bone marrow also contains the more mature CFU-E that, under the influence of EPO, form small colonies of erythroblasts in 7 days.

GRANULOCYTE AND MACROPHAGE COLONY-FORMING CELLS

The first colony assays relevant to the study of the production of granulocytes and monocytes in the mouse were described in 1965 by Pluznik and Sachs[103] and in 1966 by Bradley and Metcalf.[104] Analogous assays have been developed in the human system.[105] These groups demonstrated that individual cells derived from mouse spleen or bone marrow could give rise to colonies of up to several thousand differentiated granulocytes and macrophages in a soft agar medium. A period of 7 to 8 days was required for full maturation of these colonies (12 to 14 days is required in humans). Appropriate studies were performed to demonstrate the single cell origin of the colonies. These studies also demonstrated that a single progenitor cell, which was termed the *colony-forming unit in culture* (CFU-C), was capable of differentiation into both granulocytes and macrophages, thus the designation CFU-GM. Unit gravity sedimentation and other separation methods have been used to demonstrate that CFU-GM represents a cell population distinguishable from the pluripotent stem cell population.[106] The use of long-term liquid bone marrow cultures has been particularly helpful in defining humoral and cell-cell interactions that induce myeloid differentiation.[107] CFU-GM give rise to the more mature granulocyte colony-forming units (CFU-G) and macrophage colony-forming units (CFU-M).[103, 104] In addition, CFU-GM can be distinguished from the eosinophil progenitor (CFU-Eo), each arising independently from the myeloid stem cell. A progenitor more mature than the CFU-GM, which differentiates to smaller clusters of mature myeloid cells earlier in culture than does CFU-GM, has been described.[53, 105, 108, 109] This is analogous to the erythroid system, in which the BFU-E differentiates to a more mature progenitor, the CFU-E. A pre–CFU-GM similar to the most immature BFU-E with a slower sedimentation rate and lower cycling index than the CFU-GM has been described in humans.[110–112] Thus, the myeloid progenitor population, like the erythroid, represents a continuum with respect to proliferative potential.

MEGAKARYOCYTE COLONY-FORMING CELLS

Figure 6–8 provides an accepted, if idealized, schema of lineage-restricted megakaryocyte progenitor development. Evidence strongly suggests that the initial phase of differentiation into erythrocyte, basophil, and megakaryocyte (e/b/meg) commitment involves a single progenitor capable of giving rise to colonies of differentiated cells, all of which express a nuclear transcription factor known as GATA-1.[113, 114] Further evidence of a close developmental relationship between erythroid and megakaryocytic lineages comes from the *in vitro* cultures of progenitor-derived colonies in human erythroid leukemia cell lines. Studies of the erythroid colonies produced *in vitro* after culture of low-density marrow cells in the presence of EPO reveal that a small but readily demonstrable fraction of the erythroid colonies are interspersed with megakaryocytes. Finally, human erythroid leukemia cells which express an erythroid phenotype constitutively, become even more strikingly erythroid when incubated with δ-aminolevulinic acid but express a megakaryocyte phenotype when they are exposed to low doses of phorbol myristate acetate.[115]

When the e/b/meg progenitor finally differentiates to a stage called megakaryocyte-burst-forming units (BFU-meg), a restricted commitment to megakaryocyte differentiation is achieved. This is entirely analogous to the events previously described with respect to phagocyte and erythroid development. When driven by the appropriate growth factors (those that comprise megakaryocyte colony-stimulating activity [meg-CSA]), BFU-meg divide in culture for several days before they begin to differentiate into colonies that although few in number are relatively large and have a burstlike morphology. *In vivo*, BFU-meg mature to megakaryocyte colony-forming units

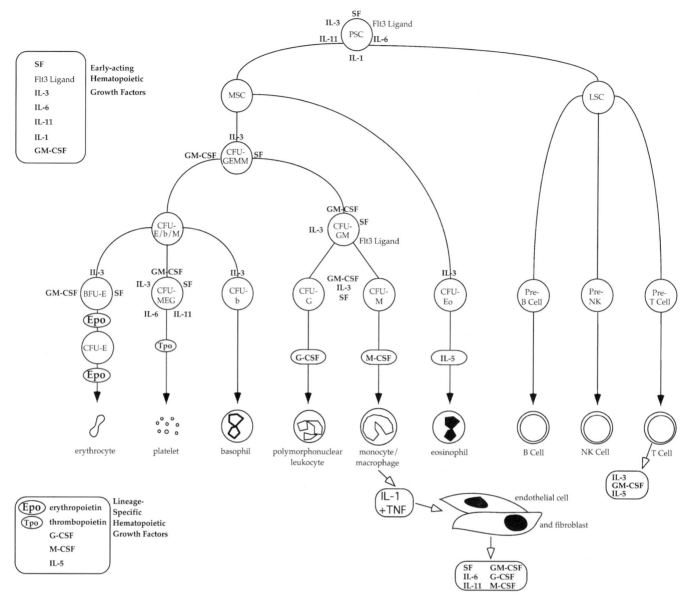

FIGURE 6–8. Major cytokine sources and actions. Cells of the bone marrow microenvironment such as macrophages (ma), endothelial cells (ec), and reticular fibroblastoid cells (fb) produce macrophage colony-stimulating factor (M-CSF), granulocyte-macrophage colony-stimulating factor (GM-CSF), granulocyte colony-stimulating factor (G-CSF), interleukin (IL) 6, and probably Steel factor (SF: cellular sources not yet precisely determined) after induction with endotoxin (ma) or IL-1/tumor necrosis factor (TNF) (ec, fb). T-cells produce IL-3, GM-CSF, and IL-5 in response to antigenic and IL-1 stimulation. These cytokines have overlapping actions during hematopoietic differentiation, as indicated, and for all lineages optimal development requires a combination of early- and late-acting factors. PSC = pluripotent stem cells; MSC = myeloid stem cells; CFU-E/b/M = erythrocyte, basophil, and megakaryocyte colony-forming unit; CFU-E = erythroid colony-forming unit; CFU-G = granulocyte colony-forming unit; CFU-M = macrophage colony-forming unit; CFU-Eo = eosinophil colony forming unit; NK = natural killer.

(CFU-meg). When suitably stimulated by the growth factors in meg-CSA and by thrombopoietin (TPO), CFU-meg, which are found more often in human marrow than are BFU-meg, form relatively small single colonies. CFU-meg express HLA-DR and CD34 antigens whereas it is said that BFU-meg express only CD34.[116] This, of course, may be a matter of detection. Of great interest is the fact that at least one transcription factor, NF-E2, has been shown to regulate platelet production.[117] Mice rendered NF-E2 deficient die from bleeding due to absence of platelets. The thrombocytopenia is due to a block late in megakaryocyte maturation. Interestingly, these animals do not show an increase in thrombopoietin levels, suggesting

that the megakaryocyte mass rather than the platelet count regulates TPO production.

Precursors and Mature Cells

The erythroid precursor or erythroblast pool represents about one third of the marrow cell population in the normal child older than age 3 or in the adult. Proerythroblasts are the earliest recognizable forms. These divide and mature through various stages, which involve nuclear condensation and extrusion and hemoglobin accumulation. On average, each erythroblast can form about eight reticulocytes. Measurement of the total marrow proerythrob-

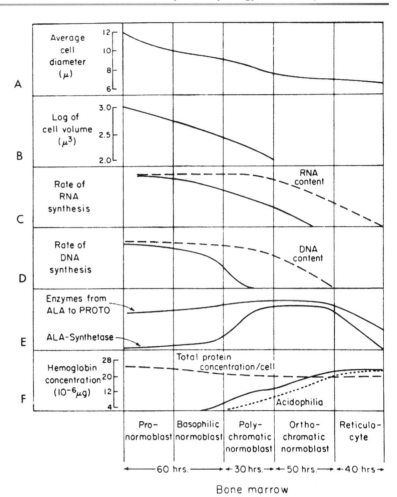

FIGURE 6–9. Erythroid maturation: alterations in cell size, rates of DNA and RNA synthesis, enzymes involved in heme synthesis, and hemoglobin concentration. Substances listed in the left-hand column are represented by corresponding *solid black lines.* Unless specified, graphs represent relative values. ALA = δ-aminolevulinic acid; PROTO = protoporphyrin. Considerable protein synthesis takes place during the earliest phase. After this, the nucleolus disappears but mitochondria remain. As the concentration of DNA decreases and the concentration of RNA starts to fall, hemoglobin begins to appear, rapidly increasing in amount. (From Granick S, Levere RD: Heme synthesis in erythroid cells. In Moore CV, Brown EB (eds): Progress in Hematology, Vol. IV. New York, Grune & Stratton, 1964, p 1. By permission of Grune & Stratton.)

last content[118] and daily reticulocyte production shows that under normal conditions replicating proerythroblasts largely maintain the reticulocyte pool being renewed from the progenitor compartment at a rate of about 10 percent per day.[119]

ERYTHROID DEVELOPMENT

Up to this point we have discussed the nondescript progenitors of erythropoiesis without reference to their physical appearance or to the appearance of their differentiated daughter cells. The best evidence to date suggests that hematopoietic progenitors or stem cells look like lymphoblasts,[120–122] and studies of peripheral blood have shown that BFU-E reside in the nonadherent "null" lymphocyte population.[123]

The pathway of erythroid *precursor* differentiation between the development of proerythroblasts and the mature red cell is known as the *erythron* and includes the functioning differentiated precursor cells observed in bone marrow aspirates and biopsies. The morphology of erythroid precursor maturation is well described in several texts and is not to be repeated here. The salient features of the morphologic changes during cell development are related to biochemical and kinetic alterations that were reviewed by Granick and Levere[124] and are shown in Figure 6–9. The residence times spent in each morphologic compartment are shown at the bottom of the figure,

but the average transit time from proerythroblast to emergence of the reticulocyte into the circulation is approximately 5 days.[125] In acute anemia, the transit time may decrease to as little as 1 or 2 days by means of skipped divisions.[126] The red cells that emerge are macrocytic and may bear surface i antigen and other fetal characteristics because the abbreviated time in the marrow compartment does not permit complete conversion of i antigen to I antigen or acquisition of certain other adult characteristics.[127] The cells also contain excessive burdens of the rubbish that normally accumulates during cell assembly,[128] because less time is available for the cleansing action of cell proteases and nucleases.[129] Thus, stress erythropoiesis is associated with circulating Pappenheimer bodies (iron granules), basophilic stippling (ribosomes), Heinz bodies (hemoglobin inclusions), and Howell-Jolly bodies (nuclear remnants).

The kinetics of erythropoiesis can be monitored by the use of radioactive iron and surface scanning. The various ferrokinetic patterns in human diseases are shown in Figure 6–10. The total distribution of erythroid marrow can be determined by scintigraphy using indium-111 chloride (^{111}InCl) bound to transferrin, as shown in Figure 6–11. Both iron-59 (^{59}Fe) kinetics and ^{111}InCl scintigraphy can be useful in the diagnosis of marrow failure, but these techniques are rarely necessary. The initial uptake of ^{59}Fe in marrow is found primarily in proerythroblasts and early basophilic erythroblasts.[130] The same is

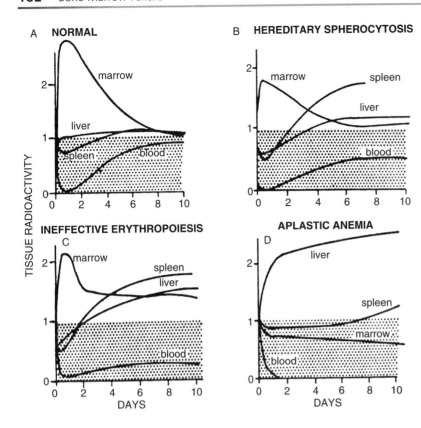

A **NORMAL**

B **HEREDITARY SPHEROCYTOSIS**

C **INEFFECTIVE ERYTHROPOIESIS**

D **APLASTIC ANEMIA**

FIGURE 6–10. Pattern of radioactivity in blood and over sacrum (marrow), liver, and spleen during a ferrokinetic study. Representative data from patients with three different disorders and one normal individual are presented. (From Finch CA: Ferrokinetics in man. Medicine 1970; 49:17. Copyright 1970, Williams & Wilkins, Baltimore.)

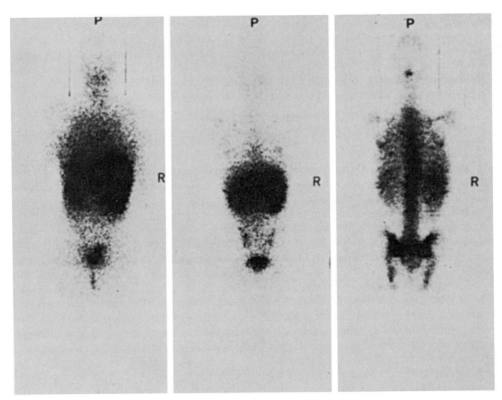

FIGURE 6–11. Spectrum of scintigraphic patterns in patients with idiopathic aplastic anemia. On the *left* is a scintigram of a patient with renal but no marrow activity before transplantation. In the *middle* is a scintigram of a patient with activity in the kidneys and borderline uptake within the marrow. On the *right* is a normal bone marrow scan in a patient after transplantation. Liver activity is seen in all three patterns, and splenic activity is seen in none. (From McNeil BJ, Rappeport JM, et al: Indium chloride scintigraphy: an index of severity in patients with aplastic anaemia. Br J Haematol 1976; 34:599.)

true of ^{111}In if it is bound to transferrin prior to injection.[131] Otherwise, ^{111}In labels marrow reticulum cells.

NEUTROPHIL PRODUCTION

A model that describes the production and kinetics of neutrophils in human is shown in Figure 6–12. It is highly compartmentalized. The relatively tiny peripheral blood pool is divided into two components in equilibrium; the circulatory pool (CGP) and the marginating pool (MGP). These pools provide entrance into the tissues. The level of circulating cells is buffered by an immense narrow reserve of identifiable precursors, some of which are in the mitotic compartment and others in a maturing storage compartment. The transit times within each compartment are relatively long, so that a huge reserve remains available. The responses of these compartments to various diseases are detailed in Chapter 22. The kinetics of proliferation of recognizable cell precursors have been studied using labeled precursors of DNA. The so-called labeling indices from which measurements of cell cycle times can be made have served as important approaches to the study of the pharmacology and toxicity of chemotherapy (see Chapter 31).

The final stages of granulocyte production, their release from the marrow, is also multifaceted.[132] At least four factors may influence granulocyte egress: (1) the organization and localization of the cells in relation to vascular channels; (2) the development of nuclear and cytoplasmic changes that increase cell deformability; (3) a hypothetical hormone called cell-releasing factor; and, finally, (4) the regulation of blood flow through vascular channels in the marrow.

MEGAKARYOCYTE DEVELOPMENT

As shown in Figure 6–13, a morphologically detectable process of megakaryocyte formation begins with the development of an acetylcholinesterase-positive cell (in the mouse) that is probably analogous to a megakaryoblast and remains capable of division in response to appropriate growth factors that must include the regulatory protein, TPO (see later discussion of hematopoietic growth factors [HGFs]). Further differentiation of the acetylcholinesterase-positive cell into the mature megakaryocyte involves a unique process of cytoplasmic enlargement and nuclear endoreduplication, events that are also influenced by HGFs.

Levine and co-workers[133] and Williams and Levine[134] have provided some valuable cytologic characteristics of the megakaryocytic maturation process (Table 6–1 and Fig. 6–14). The progressive differentiation of megakaryocytes involves the curious endoreduplication phenomenon in which two episodes of chromosomal reduplication proceed apparently at the level of the late progenitor to produce the earliest recognizable megakaryoblast, an 8N cell.[135–137] The process of reduplication of chromosomes continues at the megakaryoblast level to produce 16N and 32N megakaryoblasts. The modal ploidy of the population is 16N. The endowment of DNA within each megakaryocyte is strongly correlated with the cytoplasmic volume of the cell and with the size of individual fragments that emerge from the extruded cytoplasm,[138, 139] but newly formed platelets are remodeled in the circulation to achieve a reasonably uniform size distribution. The spleen probably contributes significantly to the remodeling.

The process of endoreduplication of DNA ceases at the mature megakaryocyte stage. This is why sensitivity to cytotoxic agents is characteristic of early megakaryocyte precursors rather than of more mature precursors and why S-phase–specific cytotoxic agents destroy recognizable megakaryocytes if most of the megakaryocytes are relatively immature,[140, 141] which is seen in marrow recovering from a previous insult or after an episode of thrombolytic thrombocytopenia.

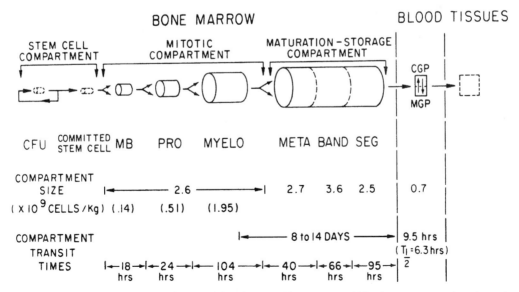

FIGURE 6–12. Model of the production and kinetics of neutrophils in humans. The marrow and blood compartments have been drawn to show their relative sizes. The compartment transit times, as derived from DF^{32}P studies, are shown on the next to the last line. Values derived from titrated thymidine studies are shown on the last line. CGP = circulatory pool; MGP = marginating pool; MB = myeloblast; PRO = promyelocyte; MYELO = myelocyte; META = metamyelocyte; BAND = band neutrophil; SEG = segmented neutrophil. (From Wintrobe MM, Lee RG, et al: Clinical Hematology. Philadelphia, Lea & Febiger, 1975, p 244.)

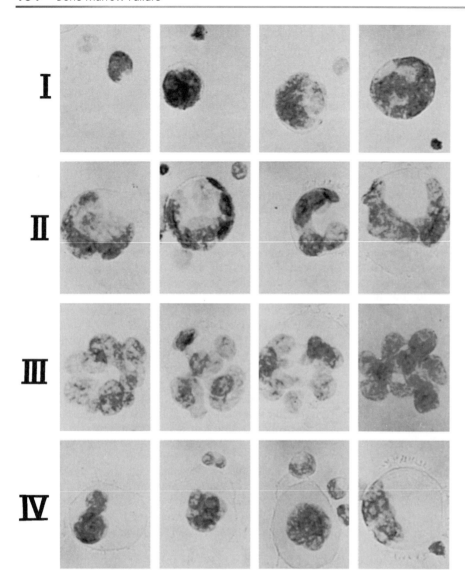

FIGURE 6–13. Photomicrographs of maturation stages of Feulgen-stained guinea pig megakaryocytes (magnification ×760). Each row illustrates representative nuclear configurations of maturation stages I, II, III, and IV, respectively. (From Levine RF: The significance of megakaryocyte size. Blood 1982; 60:1122.)

Thus, increased platelet production seems to be derived from megakaryocytes with high ploidy,[142–144] whereas the megakaryocyte pool is replenished by division of cells with lower ploidy.[145, 146] In addition to its effects on platelet production, TPO appears to be largely responsible for endoreduplication and thus for increased megakaryocyte ploidy[146–148] and for the general process of megakaryocyte morphogenesis.[149] In experimental thrombocytopenia, thrombopenic plasma contains increased amounts of TPO,[150–153] because platelets specif-

TABLE 6–1. Cytologic Characteristics of Megakaryocyte Maturation Stages

Stage	Nuclear Morphology	Cytoplasmic Staining (Wright-Giemsa)	Approximate Size Range	Demarcation Membranes	Granules	Suggested Name
I	Compact (lobed)	Basophilic	6–24 µm	Present by electron microscopy	Few present by electron microscopy	Megakaryoblast
II	Horseshoe	Pink center	14–30 µm	Proliferating to center of cell	Starting to increase	Promegakaryocyte
III	Multilobed	Increasingly more pink than blue	15–56 µm	Extensive but asymmetric	Great numbers	Granular megakaryocyte
IV	Compact highly lobulated	Wholly eosinophilic	20–50 µm	Evenly distributed	Organized into "platelet field"	Mature megakaryocyte

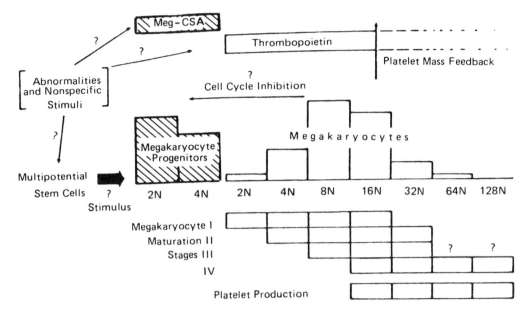

FIGURE 6–14. Thrombopoiesis. Shown horizontally in the *center* is the progression from uncommitted multipotential stem cells, through the proliferating progenitors detected in the *in vitro* clonogenic assays, to the spectrum of maturing megakaryocytes. The relative DNA levels of megakaryocytes and their precursors are given as ploidy values (N), where 2N is a diploid cell. The megakaryocytes are also presented vertically in terms of their maturation stages, ending in platelet shedding; a detailed classification of these stages in given in Table 6–1 and Figure 6–13. The columns show the maturation stages at particular ploidy ranges. Thus, 4N megakaryocytes are found at maturation stages I and II. The *top row* shows a postulated two-level regulatory process with megakaryocyte colony-stimulating activity (Meg-CSA) primarily influencing proliferation of progenitors and thrombopoietin required for megakaryocyte ploidy amplification and possibly for maturation. It is not certain that these regulators are completely exclusive in their target cell specificities as shown. Furthermore, no clear distinction is currently possible between the specific or nonspecific control of the two factors. Thrombopoietin production is sensitive to variations in platelet mass, as indicated in the figure; it is assumed that this feedback mechanism operates on the source of thrombopoietin. The progenitors might be controlled by cell cycle inhibition, perhaps as a consequence of normal numbers of megakaryocytes. (From Williams N, Levine RF: The origin, development and regulation of megakaryocytes. Br J Haematol 1982; 52:173)

ically bind TPO and remove it from the circulation.[154] When platelet levels fall, plasma levels of "free" TPO increase.[154] TPO mRNA levels in some murine tissues are also inversely correlated with circulating platelet count.[155] Increased levels of circulating TPO also increase megakaryocyte ploidy.[156]

BONE MARROW EXAMINATION AND MEGAKARYOCYTOPOIESIS

Despite the fact that the morphology of megakaryocyte development is fairly well established, bone marrow examinations can be of limited value in the various platelet disorders. Bone marrow smears and biopsy specimens provide insufficient data about thrombopoiesis because the final stage of platelet production, extrusion of cytoplasm into the sinusoid and shedding of platelets (to be described later), is not recognized by these techniques; only the relative numbers of megakaryocytes and their size and ploidy can be identified by routine morphologic methods. It is not surprising that such information is only loosely correlated with platelet production. Furthermore, sampling errors can be responsible for serious misinterpretations. This is a particular hazard in aspirates of neonatal marrow, in which megakaryocytes may be hard to detect whether platelet production is normal or not. Furthermore, megakaryocytes are not evenly distributed in marrow smears. They are more readily found around the edges of the particles, and they may be mistaken for broken cells by the untrained observer. Megakaryocyte nuclei are often found lying free in marrow smears, where they may be erroneously scored as tumor cells. Biopsy sections provide more accurate assessments of megakaryocyte number and distribution than smears, although the latter are usually sufficient (except in neonates) if examined carefully. Biopsies should not be attempted merely to define megakaryocytes in neonates; clinical judgment is a safer tool in these patients.

Examinations of routine marrow smears and biopsies, although instructive, are limited by their two-dimensional views and the thickness of the sections. Megakaryocytes have a peculiar predilection to lie next to the endothelial cell lining of the fronds of developing marrow cells, perhaps because thrombopoietin is produced by these cells. In general, megakaryocytes are too large to squeeze through the sinusoidal meshwork so they merely push their cytoplasms through the fenestrations. The protruding cytoplasms form demarcation lines and then shatter into platelets, which are swept into the blood. The megakaryocyte nuclei rarely make the transfenestration journey into the sinusoids and then into the blood. If they do, they may be mistakenly interpreted by the unwary microscopist as tumor cells in the blood. Intact or partial megakaryocytes are regularly observed in the blood of patients with marrow-invasive diseases such as certain leukemias, metastatic cancers, granulomatous disorders, and fibrosis.

HEMATOPOIETIC GROWTH FACTORS

Since the pioneering work in the early 1960s by Bradley and Metcalf[104] and Pluznik and Sachs,[103] it has been recognized that normal and leukemic blood progenitor cells can be propagated in culture in the presence of soluble protein growth factors. These factors were originally termed *colony-stimulating factors* (CSFs), based on their ability to support the formation of colonies of blood cells by bone marrow cells plated in semisolid medium.[157, 158] During the 1970s and 1980s, it was recognized that many types of CSFs exist, based on the different types of blood cells found in the colonies that grow in the presence of the different factors, leading to the hypothesis that the growth and differentiation of different lineages of blood cells are controlled, at least in part, by exposure of progenitor cells to CSFs having different lineage specificities.[157–159] With the molecular cloning of the genes for many of these factors and their receptors during the 1980s and 1990s it became possible to study in detail the structure, function, and biology of the recombinant CSFs as well as the molecular biology of their respective genes.[158–163] This analysis, along with similar work on the regulation of cells in the immune system, led to the realization that there are a large number of interacting regulatory molecules, now generally known as cytokines or lymphohematopoietic cytokines, that together control the hematopoietic and immune systems and to integrate the responses of these systems with those of many other physiologic systems.[161, 164–167] These "control" molecules regulate the growth, development, differentiation, activation, and trafficking of cells within the hematopoietic and immune systems. With the elucidation of the sequence of most of the human genome in the final years of the 1990s, even more cytokine and growth factor genes have been discovered, providing both new insights into how all these systems have evolved with common themes and also further challenges to cell biologists in their attempts to understand the functions and interactions of all of the different molecules.

The cytokine gene families that contain at least one member that functions within the hematopoietic or immune systems include the lymphohematopoietic cytokines (including many interleukins and CSFs[157, 158, 163]), the receptor tyrosine kinase ligands (CSF-1,[168] stem cell factor [SCF] [also known as Steel factor[169]], and the ligand for the Flk2/Flt3 receptor [FL]),[170] the IL-1 gene family,[171] the chemokines,[172] the tumor necrosis factors,[173] the interferons,[174] the IL-10 gene family,[175] the transforming growth factor β (TGF-β) gene family,[176] and the IL-17 gene family.[177] We will briefly describe these families and the molecules among the family members selected as HGFs for further discussion. Three other ligand/receptor pairs that are important in development and may play a role in stem cell renewal are discussed later in the section on stem cells; they are Delta and Jagged/Notch, Sonic Hedgehog/Smoothened, and Wnt/Frizzled.

Lymphohematopoietic Cytokines

For our purposes, the lymphohematopoietic cytokines are defined as the protein ligands for the members of the hematopoietin receptor gene family, also known as the cytokine receptor class I gene family.[178] This gene family is characterized by an extracellular domain with pairs of conserved cysteine residues and the distinctive amino acid sequence element Trp-Ser-Xaa-Trp-Ser (WSXWS).[179] These receptors all signal at least partly through the JAK-STAT pathway[180, 181] This rather large family of hematopoietins now includes many interleukins[182] (IL-2, IL-3, IL-4, IL-5, IL-6, IL-7, IL-9, IL-11, IL-12, IL-13, IL-15, IL-21, and IL-23)[163, 183, 184] GM-CSF,[158, 185] G-CSF,[186] EPO,[187] TPO,[188] thymic stromal thymopoietin,[189–191] leukemia inhibitory factor (LIF),[192] oncostatin M (OSM), cardiotropin-1 (CT-1), and ciliary neurotrophic factor (CNTF).[193] The hematopoietin receptors on the cell surface signal as multimers, either homo- or heteromeric, and the family can be further divided into subfamilies based on the molecular composition of their receptor complexes. The lymphohematopoietic cytokines with homodimeric receptors include EPO, TPO, and G-CSF.[163] A second subgroup comprising GM-CSF, IL-3, and IL-5 in the human system have receptor complexes that share a common subunit known as the β_c chain that forms heterodimers with unique cytokine α subunits to give selectivity for the respective cytokines.[163] A third group including IL-6, IL-11, LIF, OSM,[194] CNTF, and CT-1 all share a common receptor signaling chain known as gp130, with unique chains that provide ligand specificity.[193] A fourth group largely involved in lymphocyte development and activation, including IL-2, IL-4, IL-7, IL-9, IL-15, and IL-21[195] share a hematopoietin receptor component known as the γ_c chain, originally identified as a component of the IL-2 receptor.[167] A fifth group, comprising IL-7 and thymic stromal thymopoietin share the IL-7Rα chain,[196] and the last group, IL-12 and IL-23, heterodimeric cytokines with a common subunit (p40) shared by each cytokine, also share the IL-12Rβ1 component.[184] The cytokines from the first two groups (EPO, TPO, G-CSF, GM-CSF, IL-3, and IL-5) all have predominant activities on the growth and differentiation of various myeloid cell populations and are traditionally included among the HGFs. Among the gp130 family of cytokines, IL-6 and IL-11 have multiple activities in different biologic systems but also, at least *in vitro*, play important roles in regulating myeloid cell growth and development, and therefore we also consider them HGFs.[197] Although IL-4, IL-9, IL-12, and LIF display some activities as growth factors for myeloid cells, they all also have prominent activities in other systems and will not be considered further here.[163] The other interleukins, CNTF,[198] and CT-1 (the latter two of which act primarily outside the hematopoietic and immune systems) act predominantly on the growth, development, and activation of various lymphocyte populations, and, although these activities are extremely important in controlling the immune system and possibly indirectly the hematopoietic system, we will leave them aside for simplicity and concentrate on the activities of the previously mentioned lymphohematopoietic HGFs.

Receptor Tyrosine Kinase Ligands

Three HGFs, macrophage CSF (M-CSF, also known as CSF-1[168]), SCF,[170, 199] and FL,[200] have been identified.

These signal through related receptors which themselves have tyrosine kinase activity.[170] The receptors for these HGFs are all evolutionarily related as are the ligands themselves, and each plays an important role in controlling blood cell production.[201, 202]

Interleukin 1 Gene Family

The IL-1[203, 204] gene family has grown substantially in the last few years and now includes at least six IL-1s (IL-1α through IL-1ξ), the IL-1 receptor antagonist (IL-1RA), and IL-18.[171, 205] IL-1α, IL-1β, and IL-18 all have a potent ability to induce cytokine production. IL-18 in combination with IL-12 in particular induces interferon (IFN)-γ,[206] but the two IL-1s have also been shown to synergize with other HGFs in support of early blood cell proliferation and, therefore, will be considered further here.[207] The functions of the other novel members of the IL-1 gene family are still unknown.

Chemokines

The chemokines represent a large family of generally small proteins (usually 8 to 12 kD) readily identifiable by sequence homology, including twin characteristic cysteine residues near the amino termini, which separate the family into CC chemokines if the cysteines are adjacent or CXC if they are separated by one residue.[172] Currently, there are more than 50 members of the gene family that have demonstrated important roles in cell trafficking in many systems. The receptor gene family for this cytokine family comprises about 20 members of the G protein—coupled receptor family. However, their biologic function is not limited to chemotaxis because several have been shown to effect gene transcription, apoptosis, and cell proliferation. IL-8 is a prominent CXC chemokine, which regulates neutrophil trafficking and therefore has a prominent effect in inflammatory responses.[172] However, two chemokines, SDF-1[208] and macrophage inflammatory protein 1α (MIP-1α,)[209] have been reported to inhibit the cycling of very early stem cells and therefore may be important molecules in halting cycling stem cells and returning them to their normal, quiescent state. SDF-1 is clearly very interesting and important in the hematopoietic system as a chemotactic factor for very primitive stem cells, providing possible mechanisms for the homing of cells both as hematopoiesis moves from the fetal liver to the bone marrow and during transplantation of cells in adults.[210]

Tumor Necrosis Factors

The tumor necrosis factor (TNF) gene family[173] now includes TNFα, lymphotoxin α and β, CD27 ligand, CD30 ligand, CD40 ligand, Fas ligand, TNF-related apoptosis-inducing ligand (TRAIL), and TNF-related activation-induced cytokine (Trance).[167] Many of these molecules are involved in regulating activation and death of various cells including T lymphocytes. TNFα itself has many biologic activities, particularly in inflammation. However, it is mentioned here because of its potent and important role in promotion of dendritic cell differentiation and activation.[211, 212]

Interferons

The type I interferons (13 species of IFN-α, IFN-β, and IFN-ω) are closely linked on human chromosome 9. The type II interferon (IFN-γ) demonstrates little if any sequence homology with the type I interferons, but the receptors for all of these cytokines are members of cytokine receptor class 2, which is related to but distinct from cytokine receptor class 1 (hemopoietin receptors), because they lack the distinctive WSXWS sequence.[213] In addition to their antiviral activities, both type I and type II interferons have many other regulatory activities with many cell types including T cells. In the human system, type I interferons play a prominent role in polarizing T helper cells toward the type 1 (Th1) phenotype.[167] However, none of these molecules appear to have prominent roles in directly controlling blood cell production and will not be considered further here.[174]

Interleukin 10 Gene Family

IL-10, an immunosuppressive cytokine[214, 215] at human chromosome 1q32, is pleiotropic in activity and also has some effects on megakaryocytes and stem cells.[163] The receptor for IL-10 is composed of members of the interferon receptor gene family (cytokine receptor class 2).[216] More recently, three related genes that are closely linked to IL-10 on chromosome 1 have been identified. They have been designated *IL-19*,[217] *IL-20*,[175] and *mda-7*.[218] A fifth member of the gene family, now designated *IL-22* (also known as *IL-TIF*),[219] has been localized to human chromosome 12q15, along with a related gene known as *AK155*, which is expressed in *Herpesvirus saimiri*–transformed T cells. All of these family members have been discovered recently, and their biologic function remains to be elucidated. It will be interesting to see if the receptors for each of these are also members of the cytokine receptor class 2 family. Because the IL-10 family appears to be largely involved with lymphocyte activation and development, none of these cytokines will be considered further here.

Transforming Growth Factor β Gene Family

The TGF-β gene family is a large family of genes, which includes TGF-β1, TGF-β2, and TGF-β3, the bone morphogenetic proteins (BMPs) 2 through 16, the growth and differentiation factor (GDF) genes 1 through 10, activin, and inhibin. Like those for many of the other cytokines, the receptors for the TGF-β family members are multimers composed of two different members of the serine/threonine kinase receptor gene family.[176] Receptors of different ligand specificities are generated by combining these gene products in different combinations. TGF-β1 itself is a very important regulator of cell cycling in many cell systems including the hematopoietic system and will be considered here further as a negative regulator of hematopoiesis.[220, 221] The BMPs and GDFs have been implicated in many developmental systems. Interestingly, BMP-4 has been shown to be essential in *Xenopus* for the embryonic development of HSCs, and it seems possible that this molecule might play a role in mammals as well in blood cell development during embryogenesis if not in adult hematopoiesis, an area worth investigating.[222] However, for our purposes, we include only TGF-β1 itself as a HGF.

Interleukin 17 Gene Family

IL-17 was originally identified as a T cell–derived inflammatory mediator capable of inducing cytokine expression by many cells including stomal fibroblasts.[177] Two related cytokines designated IL-17B and IL-17C[223] have been identified. They are interestingly scattered throughout the genome and also have some ability to induce cytokine expression by various cells. Another member of the gene family, designated IL-17e, has recently been reported. It is also an apparently proinflammatory cytokine because it is capable of inducing IL-8 expression.[224] The various IL-17s and the currently known IL-17 receptors are unrelated to any of the other cytokines or receptors, hence their splitting out as a separate cytokine gene family. Several reports have linked administration of IL-17 to animals with increased granulopoiesis and have suggested a role for this molecule in hematopoiesis, but this role seems to result from its activity in promoting expression of other cytokine genes. Therefore, IL-17 will not be considered further as an HGF.[225]

In summary, the cytokines that have been selected here for further consideration of their biologic function as important HGFs are the CSFs (G-CSF, GM-CSF, and M-CSF [also known as CSF-1]),[162] certain interleukins (IL-1,[207] IL-3,[159, 226] IL-5,[161, 227] IL-6,[228] and IL-11[229–231]), other positive HGFs (EPO,[187, 232, 233] TPO,[150] SCF[169] (also known as kit ligand [KL] or Steel factor [SF]), FL [234, 235] and the negative regulator of hematopoiesis, TGF-β1.[208]

Types of Hematopoietic Growth Factors

The HGFs that have been selected for discussion can be separated into five groups based on their biologic function. These include (1) lineage-specific factors, including G-CSF, M-CSF, EPO, TPO, and IL-5; (2) multilineage factors including IL-3 and GM-CSF; (3) stem cell factors including SCF and FL; (4) "synergistic" factors including IL-1, IL-6 and IL-11; and (5) the negative regulator of hematopoiesis, TGF-β1.

LINEAGE-SPECIFIC HEMATOPOIETIC GROWTH FACTORS: G-CSF, M-CSF, IL-5, TPO, AND EPO

Early on, it was recognized that different CSFs could selectively support the growth of specific types of hematopoietic colonies.[157] Thus, when human bone marrow cells are cultured in semisolid medium in the presence of G-CSF, 7 to 8 days later colonies emerge which consist largely of mature neutrophilic granulocytes and their precursors.[157, 186] This led to the model that G-CSF, to a large degree, interacts with relatively late hematopoietic progenitors that have already committed to the neutrophil lineage (CFU-G) and serves to support their growth and final maturation into functional neutrophils.[186] Similar analysis has revealed that the other major hematopoietic cell lineages have analogous, lineage-specific late-acting

factors and that these molecules often serve as important, if not primary, regulators of their respective pathways. Thus, M-CSF supports monocyte/macrophage colony growth and is important in supporting the growth and maturation of monocyte progenitors (CFU-M),[168] IL-5 supports eosinophilic granulocyte colony-formation and therefore supports the growth and maturation of eosinophil progenitors (CFU-Eo) and activates eosinophils,[227, 236] EPO is necessary for the growth and maturation of both earlier (BFU-E) and later (CFU-E) progenitors of the erythroid lineage,[187] and TPO directly supports the growth and maturation of megakaryocyte progenitors (CFU-meg) and the subsequent production of functional platelets.[150, 188]

Although the regulation of the respective blood cell pathways by the lineage-specific HGFs is likely to be their major function, in no case is this lineage specificity absolutely maintained. G-CSF has been found to influence the migration and proliferation of endothelial cells, cells that express high-affinity receptors for this cytokine.[237] IL-5 serves as a growth factor for activated B-cells, particularly in the mouse, and affects the type of immunoglobulin secreted by mature B cells.[238] EPO[239] and TPO[240] have been noted to interact with megakaryocyte and erythroid progenitors, respectively. M-CSF appears to be important in trophoblast development.[168] Finally, populations of early HSCs have been found to express receptors for many cytokines; typically, these cells do not respond to single factors but require combinations of factors to trigger them into cycle.[241, 242] "Lineage-specific" factors that have been reported to act in various combinations to trigger cycling of early "stem" cells include G-CSF,[243] M-CSF,[244] and TPO,[245] demonstrating that the molecules are not strictly lineage-specific even within the hematopoietic system. Mice deficient in either the TPO receptor (mpl) or G-CSF have deficient levels of all progenitor cells, consistent with the idea that these factors indeed are involved in expansion of early lineage cells.[162] However, when administered in vivo each of these molecules largely influences the growth and development of the expected lineage and the designation of lineage specificity seems warranted.

MULTILINEAGE HEMATOPOIETIC GROWTH FACTORS: IL-3 AND GM-CSF

Initial analysis of human bone marrow cell cultures grown in the presence of GM-CSF revealed that a variety of different colony types develop over a period of 10 to 14 days.[246] Mature blood cells that could be readily identified included neutrophils, monocytes/macrophages, and eosinophils. This led to the designation of the molecule as a "granulocyte-macrophage" colony-stimulating factor. Compared with G-CSF, it took longer for colonies with identifiable neutrophils to be produced but the ultimate variety of cell types was greater. This led to a model in which GM-CSF acts on progenitors committed to produce either neutrophils or monocytes (CFU-GM), which is a precursor to the G-CSF–responsive CFU-G and the M-CSF–responsive CFU-M.[157, 246] These later progenitors apparently retain responsiveness to GM-CSF as well, because mature monocytes and neutrophils can be observed in cultures supported by GM-CSF alone. That this model is not strictly correct was shown when recombinant GM-CSF was introduced into human bone marrow cultures in the presence of EPO, and it was found that this combination of factors effectively supported the development of erythroid colonies (murine GM-CSF is somewhat less effective in this regard).[157, 247, 248] Thus, despite its name, GM-CSF generally interacts with intermediate multilineage progenitors that yield neutrophils, eosinophils, monocytes, erythroid cells, and megakaryocytes (CFU-GEMM). These activities were similar to those ascribed to IL-3 in the murine system.[249] When human IL-3 was identified, its abilities to support multilineage colony formation were found to be similar to those of human GM-CSF, indicating that it interacts with slightly different but strongly overlapping subsets of progenitors.[250, 251] Compared with GM-CSF, IL-3 is somewhat more effective in supporting multilineage, erythroid and megakaryocyte colony formation, and GM-CSF is slightly more effective with granulocyte and monocyte/macrophage colony formation.[250, 251] In serum-free conditions, the ability of IL-3 to support final neutrophil and monocyte maturation is significantly depressed, indicating that the later-acting factors, G-CSF or GM-CSF in the case of neutrophils or M-CSF or GM-CSF in the case of monocytes, are necessary for final end cell production.[252]

In addition to acting slightly earlier than GM-CSF, IL-3 is clearly distinguished by its ability to support the growth and maturation of mast cells and basophils.[253, 254] In the mouse, this was one of the first recognized activities of IL-3[249] and when IL-3 was first administered to primates, basophilia was one of the most prominent findings.[254, 255] Thus, IL-3 appears to be capable of supporting the growth and development of basophil and mast cell progenitors. In the human system, both IL-3 and GM-CSF can support the development and differentiation of dendritic cells of either myeloid or lymphoid origin, especially in combination with SCF, FL, and TNF.[256–258]

IL-4 in mice and humans has also been reported to support multilineage colony formation, including colonies that contain cells from the erythroid, megakaryocytic, neutrophilic, and monocytic lineages.[259–261] IL-4 in the mouse supports mast cell growth and therefore shares many activities with IL-3.[238] However, IL-4 plays very important roles in the development and maturation of T cells and B cells,[238, 261, 262] particularly in the polarization of cytokine production by helper T cells toward the type 2 (Th2) response.[263] Therefore, on balance, it is likely to be more important in controlling immune cell development and function and will not be discussed further here. IL-9 has been shown to enhance erythroid colony formation in the presence of EPO in both the murine and human systems[264] and appears to play a role in T- and B-cell development as well.[265] IL-9 has also been shown to have some effects on the growth and activation of mast cells and may play a role in the pathologic course of asthma.[266]

EARLY-ACTING HEMATOPOIETIC GROWTH FACTORS: SCF AND FL

SCF[169, 170, 199] and FL,[200, 235, 267] both receptor tyrosine kinase ligands, interact with a variety of hematopoietic progenitor cells, perhaps most importantly with very early stem cell populations. SCF also play an important role in melanocyte growth and development, which is reflected in the coat color effects of mutations in SCF or its receptor, c-kit.[169] Genetic analysis of mice clearly showed that mice defective in either SCF (Steel strain *[Sl]* mice) or in c-kit (dominant white spotting strain *[W]* mice) have serious hematopoietic defects, including macrocytic anemia, mast cell deficiencies, and deficiencies in the stem cell compartment.[169] These early studies had already indicated the critical importance of SCF in the survival and development of stem cells. Mutations in the human c-kit gene lead to a similar phenotype in melanocyte development in humans known as the piebald mutation; however, these patients do not have any hematologic problems, probably because severe mutations in this locus are likely to be lethal.[268] *In vitro*, the activities of SCF are generally most evident when it is combined with other HGFs; its proliferative activity with hematopoietic cells in culture as a single factor is minimal.[169] In fact, culture of murine bone marrow cells in SCF alone ultimately yields largely mast cells.[269] However, SCF acts synergistically to enhance the activities of most of the other HGFs in culture and is particularly effective when combined with HGFs such as IL-3, IL-1, or IL-11 at promoting the expansion of "blast"-like cells that retain considerable potential for yielding multilineage colonies in secondary culture.[270–272] These colonies, when replated under conditions that support B lymphocyte development or when transplanted into animals also yield B and T lymphocytes, indicating that SCF-responsive cells include primitive stem cells with both lymphoid and myeloid potential.[273, 274] SCF has also been implicated in combination with IL-2 or IL-7 in early stages of T-cell development in the thymus,[275] with IL-7 in pre-B–cell growth,[276] and with IL-7 in enhancing natural killer (NK) cell responsiveness to IL-2.[169] However, that none of these lineages are dramatically affected in *W* or *Sl* mice indicates that SCF-independent mechanisms can compensate in these systems.

SCF,[277] M-CSF,[278] and FL[202] are all expressed both as membrane-bound and soluble forms. In the case of SCF, expression of membrane-bound forms of the molecule in the marrow microenvironment provides a nice model for how this growth factor might act locally. Indeed, cell lines that express membrane-associated SCF only are much more effective in supporting long-term hematopoiesis *in vitro* than cell lines that produce only soluble forms of the molecule.[277] This interaction of membrane-associated SCF with c-kit provides one mechanism for the adherence of hematopoietic cells to stroma; binding of human megakaryocytes to fibroblasts can be blocked by antibodies to c-kit.[279] Finally, membrane-associated forms of SCF in which the cytoplasmic domain is essentially missing result in male but not female sterility, suggesting that the cytoplasmic domain may have an as yet undetermined important biologic function.[169, 280]

As shown by the early genetic studies and confirmed through analysis of the recombinant protein, SCF is not specific for the hematopoietic system. It is also an important growth factor for melanocytes and primordial germ cells, and it appears to play a role in development of the nervous system, perhaps as a neuronal guidance factor, although it has been difficult to demonstrate neurologic defects in *W* or *Sl* mice.[169]

The Flt3 receptor tyrosine kinase was originally identified as a novel receptor present in HSCs; with human marrow, the expression is largely limited to the CD34+ cell population.[228, 281, 282] FL alone yields low numbers of CFU-GM colonies from human bone marrow but acts synergistically with other cytokines including IL-3, GM-CSF, EPO, and SCF to yield enhanced colony formation, both in terms of size and numbers of colonies.[234, 235, 283] The synergy observed between FL and the other HGFs is comparable to that observed with SCF in similar systems with the exception that FL has little effect on BFU-E.[267] Multifactor combinations with SCF have been used for expansion of CFCs in long-term cultures; FL has effects comparable to those of SCF when combined with IL-1, IL-3, IL-6, and EPO in 4-week cultures.[284, 285] Like SCF, FL in combination with other cytokines such as GM-CSF, supports dendritic cell development from CD34+ bone marrow cells.[256] In contrast to SCF, FL does not support the growth and development of mast cells.[234, 235] Despite this overlap in bioactivities, mice in which the Flt3 receptor tyrosine kinase has been disrupted appear to have normal hematopoiesis with the only detectable defects observed within the B-lymphocyte lineage.[286] However, mice with disruptions in both the c-*kit* and Flt3 receptor tyrosine kinase genes display more severe hematologic complications than mice with a mutation in either single gene, suggesting that the two pathways can to some degree compensate for one another.[286] The importance of FL in B-cell growth has also been shown with cultures of primitive B-cell progenitors (CD43+B220lo) in combination with either IL-7 or SCF.[287] Altogether, these findings argue for an important role for FL in hematopoiesis.

SYNERGISTIC FACTORS: IL-1, IL-6, AND IL-11

Early in the 1980s, factors were identified that had the ability to enhance hematopoietic colony formation supported by other HGFs, particularly with early progenitor cells. One factor, designated hematopoietin 1 was subsequently purified and discovered to be IL-1.[244] In this fashion, IL-1 was recognized as having little ability on its own to stimulate hematopoietic colony formation but is able to act in synergy with other HGFs, notably IL-3, in increasing both the rate of occurrence of colony formation and the numbers of cells per colony. Subsequent to the discovery of the synergistic activity of IL-1, numerous other cytokines with similar activity have been found including IL-6,[288] IL-11,[289] LIF,[290] and IL-12.[291] Of these, IL-6, IL-11, and LIF all signal through a common signal transducing molecule, the gp130 component of the IL-6 receptor.[292] Because these molecules are likely to behave similarly in most systems and because IL-6 and IL-11 have been the most thoroughly studied, we limit our discussion to these two members of this family. IL-12, which signals through a distinct but perhaps similar pathway to gp130,[293] has interesting effects in combinations with other cytokines[291] but appears to be more important in regulating the development and activities of T and NK cells[294, 295] and will therefore not be discussed further.

The effects of IL-1 on hematopoiesis are highly complicated because this cytokine is a potent inducer of secondary cytokine production often by accessory cells in the culture.[296] The induction of other growth factors, notably IL-6, G-CSF, GM-CSF, and IL-11, is likely to contribute to the activity of IL-1 as a synergistic factor in hematopoietic colony formation. Nevertheless, combinations of IL-1 with other factors in cultures of highly purified hematopoietic cells typically yield synergistic effects, suggesting that at least some of the effects are direct.[297, 298] However, even with highly purified hematopoietic progenitor cell populations, the effects of IL-1 can be indirect. For example, Rodriguez and associates[299] have reported that IL-1 can prevent apoptotic death of CD34+/lin− human bone marrow cells, but the effect is largely abrogated by antibodies to GM-CSF, suggesting that some progenitor cells in the population can produce their own GM-CSF. Thus, the survival effect of IL-1 in some systems may also be indirectly mediated by induction of GM-CSF expression in CD34+/lin− bone marrow cells themselves.

IL-6 is an extremely pleiotropic cytokine with important effects on the growth and differentiation of T and B cells, on the induction of the hepatic acute phase response, and enhancement of proliferation of hematopoietic progenitor cells.[228] IL-6 signaling, mediated by two members of the hematopoietin receptor gene family, IL-6R[300] and gp130,[301] was the first example of signaling through a commonly shared receptor subunit, gp130, which now is known to be involved in the signaling of LIF, IL-11, OSM, CNTF, and CT-1.[292, 302] Because most cells express gp130, the expression of other receptor components such as IL-6R or IL-11R generally determines whether or not a cell will respond to one of these family members; cells that express receptors for multiple members of this cytokine subgroup generally exhibit identical or nearly identical responses to each member whose receptor component is expressed by the cell.[193, 292, 303]

The HGF activity of IL-6 was recognized when the cDNA for this cytokine was cloned by functional expression cloning from a human T-cell line that produced a weak colony-stimulating activity that supported modest CFU-GM colony formation with murine bone marrow target cells.[304] More detailed analysis in the murine system and subsequently the human system led to the realization that IL-6 has little if any ability to support colony formation on its own but can enhance colony formation supported by other HGFs, particularly IL-3 and SCF.[271, 288] This effect was most prominent using bone marrow cells from mice isolated 2 days after treatment with 5-fluorouracil, a drug that enriches for primitive progenitors by selectively killing later, actively cycling cells in the bone marrow.[241] Bone marrow cells treated in this fashion generally yield significant numbers of colonies only when plated in the presence of multiple HGFs. In this system, IL-6 was found to enhance colony formation supported by IL-3 or SCF. These early cells are typically quiescent in the G$_0$ phase of the growth cycle, and combined effects of cytokines, such as IL-3 and IL-6, are required to push them into active cycling.[241] Similar effects have been observed with cultures of purified early human hematopoietic progenitor cells.[305]

IL-11 was originally identified as having stimulatory activity for a murine hybridoma cell line,[306] but characterization in various hematopoietic cell culture system soon revealed a much broader spectrum of biologic effects.[229, 307] Evaluation of various properties of IL-11 led to the realization that the IL-11 receptor complex uses the IL-6 gp130 signal transducing system. These two HGFs appear to have somewhat overlapping biologic activities.[308] In general, IL-6 has proved to have more effects on T and B cells than IL-11[228, 307] and similar effects in the hepatic acute phase response[309] and on osteoclast formation,[310] but IL-11 is somewhat more potent in megakaryocytopoiesis.[311] Like those of IL-6, the effects of IL-11 in hematopoietic cultures are largely observed only in combination with other factors. IL-11 in combination with SCF or FL is very effective in supporting the growth of primitive hematopoietic progenitors.[283] In the murine system, the early targets of IL-11 in combination with SCF include primitive stem cells that in secondary cultures yield hematopoietic cells and B lymphocytes and when transplanted into irradiated hosts yield T lymphocytes.[273] In combination with FL, IL-11, when plated with highly purified Sca$^+$/lin$^-$ bone marrow cells in single cell per well cultures, yielded colonies in 25 percent of the wells (75 of 300), and 23 percent of the colonies consisted of immature blastlike cells, a higher proportion than with any of the other factor combinations tested.[283] Similarly, IL-11 in combination with FL or SCF supports the expansion of CD34$^+$ bone marrow cells *in vitro*.[284, 305, 312]

Early after its discovery, IL-11 was shown to have important effects on the growth and development of megakaryocyte progenitors.[306, 307, 311] Again, in this system, IL-11 had little effect on colony formation on its own but was found to act in synergy with IL-3, SCF, or TPO in supporting CFU-meg colony formation.[313] When combined with IL-3, IL-11 increases the number as well as the size of the megakaryocyte colonies.[311] In human cell cultures, these effects are observed preferentially with earlier (BFU-meg) rather than later (CFU-meg) progenitor cell populations.[314] With more mature cells, IL-11 acts by itself in increasing the average ploidy of the megakaryocyes.[311] These effects of IL-11 on megakaryocytopoiesis have also been seen *in vivo*; administration of IL-11 to normal mice,[315] primates,[231] or humans[316] results in a significant increase in levels of circulating platelets. After myelosuppressive chemotherapy, administration of IL-11 results in a decrease in the number of patients needing platelet transfusions.[317] Finally, although TPO levels are likely to control the daily levels of platelets in circulation, circulating levels of IL-11 have been found to increase in patients undergoing intensive myelosuppressive therapy,[317] suggesting that IL-11 may contribute to hematopoietic recovery after severe damage to the bone marrow.

IL-11 has also shown biologic effects in other systems as well. Within the erythroid lineage, IL-11 interacts with SCF and EPO in supporting the formation of macroscopic erythroid bursts.[318] IL-11 appears to affect monocyte/macrophage development; secondary replating of blast colonies in IL-11 alone yields monocyte/macrophage colonies.[289] IL-11 has been found to significantly inhibit production of inflammatory cytokines, including produc-

tion of TNF by cultured macrophages.[319, 320] This effect is likely to be a significant component of the anti-inflammatory properties of IL-11 that have been observed.[321] Other cell types that are affected by IL-11 include epithelial cells which, at least *in vivo*, can be protected from radiation by treatment with IL-11,[322] and adipocyte progenitors, which are blocked from differentiation by exposure to IL-11.[323]

NEGATIVE REGULATOR OF HEMATOPOIESIS: TRANSFORMING GROWTH FACTOR β

TGF-β has long been recognized as a negative regulator in many cell systems, causing cycling cells to leave the active phase of the cell cycle.[176] In the normal hematopoietic system, the majority of early stem cells are quiescent and out of the cell cycle; that is, they are in the G_0 state.[197, 324] This is believed to be important for the long-term maintenance of the stem cells in the hematopoietic system over the life-time of the animal and therefore, the control of cell cycling of the stem cell is likely to be an important regulatory component of the system. A variety of cytokines have been reported to reversibly inhibit cycling of early hematopoietic cells including the chemokines SDF-1[208] and MIP-1α[209] and TGF-β, perhaps the most potent of all.[325–327] Interestingly, when individual early cells were plated in wells, either antibody to TGF-β1 or an antisense oligonucleotide to the mRNA for this factor could trigger the release of the cells from quiescence in the presence of appropriate combinations of early-acting cytokines which, by themselves, failed to trigger the cycling of the cells.[326, 327] This demonstrated that at least some early HSCs rely on continuous autocrine production of TGF-β1 to maintain them in a quiescent state and that this loop, again at least in some cells, is not interrupted by exposure to combinations of currently studied cytokines. It will be of interest to see if similar autocrine loops by TGF-β1 regulate stem cells in other biologic systems and to determine the physiologic mechanism that results in shutting off the loop and allowing stem cells to begin cycling.

MOLECULAR BIOLOGY OF THE HGFs

Cloning Hematopoietic Growth Factor Genes

Over the past 20 years, the cDNAs and genes for the HGFs and many other cytokines and their receptors have been cloned.[167] This work provided a powerful array of tools for analysis of the molecular and cellular biology of hematopoiesis beginning with molecular clones for analysis of the expression of the HGF and HGF receptor (HGFR) genes as well as recombinant proteins for evaluation of the biologic activities of the various factors *in vivo* and *in vitro* (Table 6–2).

Although each cloning project is an important story in its own right, today, the more important information is what has been learned with the various molecular tools. We therefore refer the interested reader to the literature to learn the details of how cDNAs encoding each HGF were isolated. Essentially, the cloning efforts have followed five

TABLE 6–2. Human Hematopoietic Growth Factors

Factor	Synonym	Chromosome	Protein (kD)	Source	Biologic Activities	
					Progenitors	Mature Cells
SCF	Stem cell factor Steel factor Kit ligand	12q2-24	15-20 (×2) soluble and membrane forms	Stromal F, Vasc Endo	Synergistic: IL-3, IL-11, IL-6 on blast CFC; Synergistic: IL-3, GM-CSF, G-CSF, EPO, TPO on committed CFC	Mast cell growth
Flk2/Flt3 ligand				Spleen, lung	Synergistic: SCF, IL-3, IL-11 on blast CFC; Synergistic: IL-3, GM-CSF, G-CSF on committed CFC; Synergistic: IL-7, SCF on B cell progenitors	
IL-3	MultiCSF	5g23-31	15.14	T, mast	All CFC	eo, b, mo
GM-CSF	CSFα	5q23-31	14.4	T, Endo, F, M0	All CFC	n, mo, eo
G-CSF	CSFβ	17q11.2-21	18.6	M0, Endo, F	CFU-G	n
IL-5		5q31	13.2 (2)	T, mast	CFU-eo	eo
M-CSF	CSF-1	1p13-21	26 (×2)	F, Endo, F	CFU-M	m
EPO		7q11-22	18.4	Kidney	BFU-E, CFU-E,	eb
TPO		3q27-28	35	Liver, kidney, F, Endo	CFU-meg	meg
IL-1α		2q13	17	M0, F, Endo, Epi, K, SM	Synergistic: SCF, IL-3, on blast CFU	Activates cytokine production
IL-1β		2q13	17	M0, F, Endo, Epi, K, SM	Synergistic: SCF, IL-3, on blast CFU	
IL-6		7p15	20.8	M0, T, B, F, Endo, K	Synergistic: SCF, IL-3 on blast CFC; IL-3, SF on CFU-meg	
IL-11		19q13.3-13.4	22	Stromal F		meg

eo = eosinophil; n = polymorphonuclear neutrophil; mo = monocyte; b = basophil; eb = erythroblast; meg = megakaryocyte; mast = mast cell; Endo = endothelial cell; Epi = epithelial cell; F = fibroblast; T = T cell; B = B cell; K = kidney; SM = smooth muscle; CFC = colony-forming cell; CFU = colony-forming unit; CFU-G = granulocyte CFU; CFU-M = monocyte/macrophage CFU; BFU-E = erythroid burst-forming unit; CFU-E = erythroid CFU; CFU-Eo = eosinophil CFU; CFU-meg = megakaryocyte CFU; IL = interleukin; GM-CSF = granulocyte-macrophage colony-stimulating factor; G-CSF = granulocyte CSF; M-CSF = monocyte CSF; multiCSF = multipotential colony-stimulating factor EPO = erythropoietin; SCF = stem cell factor; TPO = thrombopoietin.

different strategies. The first to be used successfully was hybridization selection in which pools of candidate cDNAs are placed on nitrocellulose filters to test the ability to selectively enrich for messenger RNAs (mRNAs) that can be translated by microinjection into *Xenopus laevis* oocytes to yield the desired HGF biologic activity. This tedious strategy was successfully used to identify several cytokine genes in the early 1980s, including the gene for IL-6.[328] A second approach, which has been highly successful, is based on the purification to homogeneity of the protein to be molecularly cloned. By determination of amino acid sequences of peptides from the purified protein, it is possible to synthesize small (generally 13- to 25 mer) DNA probes based on the genetic code that can be used directly to screen cDNA libraries for the desired clone. This methodology has been used by various laboratories to isolate the cDNAs for G-CSF,[329, 330] M-CSF,[331] EPO,[332] SCF,[333, 334] and TPO.[156, 335] In a third approach, begun in the early 1980s, several laboratories developed methods for screening pools of cDNA clones for the ability to direct the expression of functionally active proteins after DNA transfection in mammalian COS cells. By testing the medium conditioned by the transfected COS cells for the bioactivity, it was possible to identify the desired cDNA clone. This methodology was effective in the identification of cDNA clones for GM-CSF,[336] IL-3,[337] IL-5,[238] and IL-11.[306] In a fourth approach, several HGFs have been identified through the use of their receptors when receptors with unknown ligands had been identified. This approach was used by various groups to identify cDNAs encoding SCF,[338] FL,[234, 235] and, TPO.[335, 339, 340] Finally, during the current genomic era when most of the sequences of the human and mouse genomes are available from the National Center for Biotechnology Information (NCBI) (at http://www.ncbi.nlm.nih.gov/LocusLink/index.htm), many cytokine genes have been identified through sequence homology either experimentally by nucleic acid cross-hybridization as in the case of several new members of the IL-1 gene family[341] or *in silico* using statistical methods as was the case for IL-17B and C.[223]

Genomic Analysis of the Cytokine and Cytokine Receptor Genes

During the 1980s and most of the 1990s, the tedious isolation of cDNA clones led to the isolation of each of the individual HGF genes and provided important molecular tools for probing their structure and organization in the genomes. However, in the last few years, the availability of the sequence of most of the human and mouse genomes has greatly sped up this analysis and led to the identification, through sequence similarities, of many more cytokine genes and receptors, thus providing a much more complete picture of how the genome is organized and more insights into the evolution of the individual factors. From the analysis of the human genome, several common themes and relationships have emerged about the different types of cytokine/growth factor and receptor genes. First, as we have already noted, most of the cytokines and their receptors exist as members of distinct evolutionarily related gene families; examples of single cytokine or growth factor genes with no relatives are rare.

Similarly, the receptors also fall into gene families. Thus, a relatively small number of primordial growth factor/cytokine genes were duplicated many times, forming families of genes whose roles evolved into regulatory functions for many different systems. As has have been discussed, cytokines that signal through the gp130 receptor component are important regulators in many different systems including embryonic development, the central nervous system, the myocardium, the hematopoietic system, and the immune systems.[193] That different physiologic systems share cytokines and receptor components from common gene families gives us more assurance that lessons learned from the relatively accessible hematopoietic system will at least provide guidance as we begin to dissect other systems. Interestingly, in most cases, each of the individual cytokines of a particular gene family uses members of a single receptor gene family. For example, all of the chemokines use G protein–coupled receptors as their signaling/recognition molecules[172] whereas all members of the TGF-β gene family use different combinations of the serine/threonine kinase receptors as their recognition and signaling molecules.[176] All of these receptor/ligand pairs must have evolved in concert as they were selected to control different cellular processes.

Despite the obvious gene duplications that have occurred in all these gene families, there is no absolute rule for how the genes are arranged today. In some cases, the related genes are still closely linked in tandem in the genome as is the case for the IL-3 and GM-CSF genes on chromosome 5 at 5q31.1 (Fig. 6–15). In this case, another duo of related genes, IL-4 and IL-13, are very closely linked to one another but slightly more separated from the IL-3/GM-CSF cluster. Similarly, in the case of the IL-10 gene family, several of the members are closely linked at 1q32 (IL-10, IL-19, IL-20, and MDA-7) whereas IL-22 and AK155 are linked at 12q15 (MDA and AK195),[218] another example for which genes have either been split out of a tandem array on one chromosome during recombination or individual genes have migrated from the original site of the primordial gene and subsequently undergone further gene duplication and separate evolution events.

Detailed sequence analysis of many of the chromosome regions surrounding these gene clusters has been very illuminating. In the interesting region of chromosome 5, 5q31, a segment of roughly 5 megabase pairs has been identified. This segment contains approximately 115 genes, 5 of which were previously known to be related to lymphohematopoietic cytokine genes, including the IL-3/GM-CSF cluster, the IL-4/IL-13 gene cluster, and, slightly more distal from the centromere, the IL-9 gene (Fig. 6–15). In addition, the sequence analysis identified a previously unknown IL-13–related gene of unknown function designated LOC153844, closely linked to IL-4 with the same orientation as both IL-4 and IL-13. Similar observations in other regions has led to a plethora of new cytokine genes of unknown function for evaluation by cell biologists. Also in this region, most likely by serendipity, is the gene for an unknown CXC chemokine SCYB14 (Fig. 6–15), consistent with the fact that the roughly 50 chemokine genes are scattered throughout the genome.[172] Finally, the sequence analysis has revealed the existence of

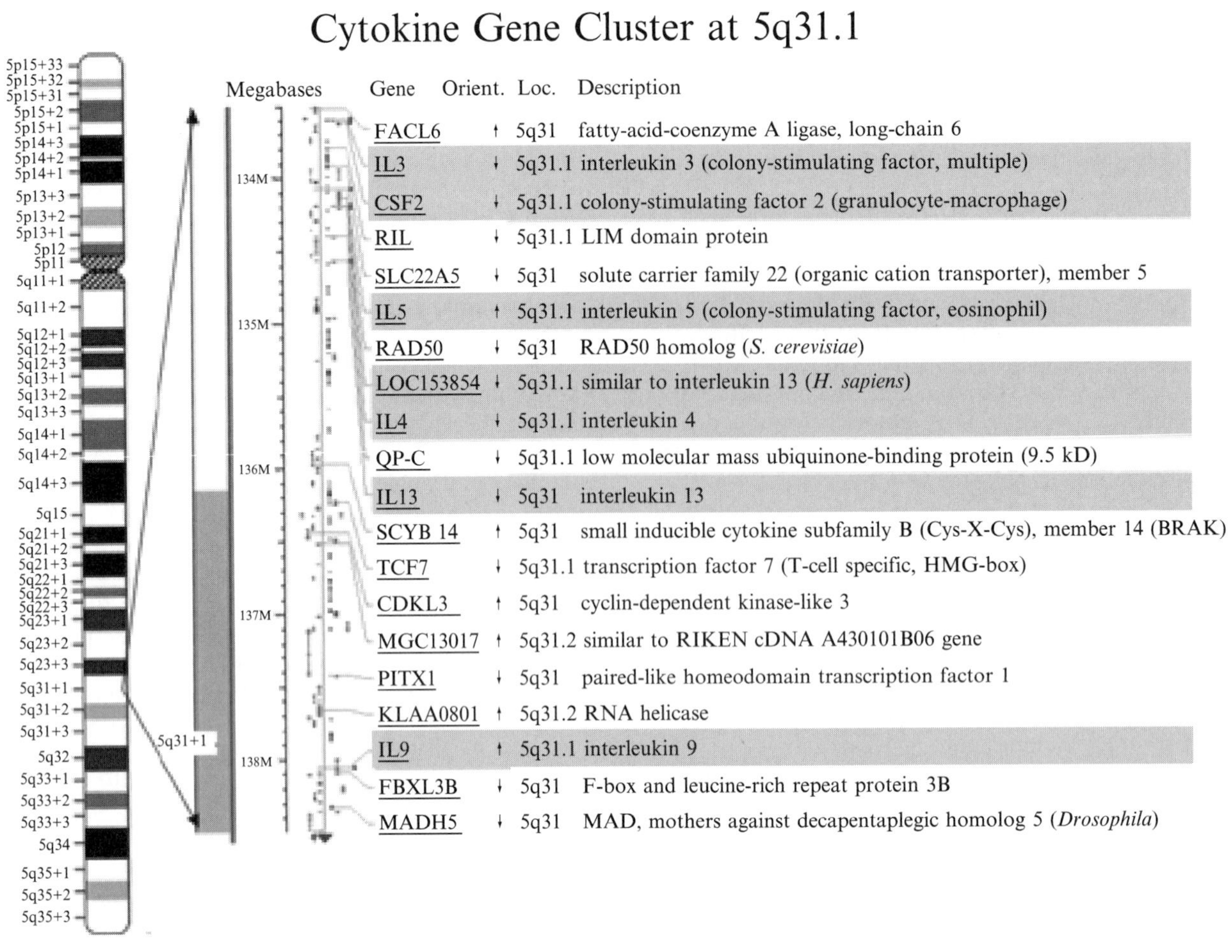

Cytokine Gene Cluster at 5q31.1

Megabases	Gene	Orient.	Loc.	Description
	FACL6	↑	5q31	fatty-acid-coenzyme A ligase, long-chain 6
134M	IL3	↓	5q31.1	interleukin 3 (colony-stimulating factor, multiple)
	CSF2	↓	5q31.1	colony-stimulating factor 2 (granulocyte-macrophage)
	RIL	↓	5q31.1	LIM domain protein
	SLC22A5	↓	5q31	solute carrier family 22 (organic cation transporter), member 5
135M	IL5	↑	5q31.1	interleukin 5 (colony-stimulating factor, eosinophil)
	RAD50	↓	5q31	RAD50 homolog (S. cerevisiae)
	LOC153854	↓	5q31.1	similar to interleukin 13 (H. sapiens)
	IL4	↓	5q31.1	interleukin 4
	QP-C	↓	5q31.1	low molecular mass ubiquinone-binding protein (9.5 kD)
136M	IL13	↓	5q31	interleukin 13
	SCYB 14	↓	5q31	small inducible cytokine subfamily B (Cys-X-Cys), member 14 (BRAK)
	TCF7	↓	5q31.1	transcription factor 7 (T-cell specific, HMG-box)
	CDKL3	↑	5q31	cyclin-dependent kinase-like 3
137M	MGC13017	↑	5q31.2	similar to RIKEN cDNA A430101B06 gene
	PITX1	↓	5q31	paired-like homeodomain transcription factor 1
	KLAA0801	↑	5q31.2	RNA helicase
138M	IL9	↑	5q31.1	interleukin 9
	FBXL3B	↓	5q31	F-box and leucine-rich repeat protein 3B
	MADH5	↓	5q31	MAD, mothers against decapentaplegic homolog 5 (Drosophila)

FIGURE 6–15. Cytokine gene cluster at 5q31.1. The region from chromosome 5, comprising 5 Mb of DNA sequence, is expanded as shown. Structures of the individual genes with GenBank notations, descriptions, and gene orientations are indicated. The region contains approximately 115 genes, 21 of which are illustrated. The data were collected and assembled from the NCBI database.

many pseudogenes. For example, sequence analysis of the type 1 interferon gene cluster on chromosome 9 revealed the existence of multiple residual inactivated interferon genes, presumably through negative selective pressure as their function was no longer needed.[167]

Structures of the Hematopoietic Growth Factor Proteins

The availability of the cDNAs for the individual cytokines facilitated rapid determination of their primary amino acid sequences, allowed their expression in quantities large enough for direct radiographic determination of their crystal structures and, more broadly, helped in prediction of structures based on those of proteins related even distantly by sequence. One of the clear results of this structural analysis of the different cytokines was the realization that, despite generally low conservation of amino acid sequences, many of the lymphohematopoietic cytokines are distantly related in evolution. Most of the lymphohematopoietic cytokines are believed to assume a tightly packed, antiparallel four α-helix bundled structure with either short or long helical bundles.[163, 167] Lymphohematopoietins having the short

helical bundle structure include IL-2, IL-3, IL-4, IL-5, IL-7, IL-9, IL-13, IL-15, and GM-CSF; cytokines having the long helical structures include the gp130 signaling proteins IL-6, IL-11, LIF, and OSM and the homodimeric receptor signaling proteins EPO, TPO, and G-CSF.[150, 163, 342] With the exception of IL-12, which is a covalently linked heterodimer of two chains, designated p40 and p35,[295] all of these are believed to act as monomers. Because IL-23 is composed of the IL-12p40 with a novel p19 subunit, distantly related to p35, it seems likely that p19 will also have the long helical structure.[184]

Sequence and structural information suggest that cytokines with the long helical bundle structure are all distantly related in evolution. Members of the IL-6 subfamily, including IL-6, IL-11, and G-CSF show rather modest sequence similarity but display common gene organization and certain structural features that suggest evolutionary relatedness.[166, 342, 343] Sequence alignments of IL-6 and G-CSF show conservation of cysteine residues.[344] Interestingly, a cytokine identified in the chicken, myelomonocytic growth factor,[345] displays sequence similarities with G-CSF and IL-6, which suggests that all three are derived from a common ancestral gene. EPO shows some structural features similar to those of growth hormone and G-CSF but at a very low level.[342] In contrast, the amino-terminal half of TPO shows strong sequence similarity with EPO whereas the carboxy-terminal half is unrelated to any known protein.[346–348] The four-helical bundle structure of EPO is clearly related to the amino-terminal, helically structured portion of TPO, whereas the additional domain of TPO, which is heavily glycosylated, may increase the serum half-life of the molecule. Both of these family members are believed to act as monomers.

The ligands for the receptor tyrosine kinase gene family members, SCF, FL, and M-CSF, share many common structural similarities.[169, 202, 349] All three contain transmembrane domains and are initially synthesized as homodimeric integral membrane proteins. Although the membrane-bound forms are functional, dimeric soluble forms are released from the cell by proteolysis and also display biologic activity. The extracellular domains display low but significant sequence similarity, including conservation of the positions of the cysteine residues involved in disulfide bridge formation.[202] Modeling of these extracellular domains indicates that they, too, are likely to form four α-helical bundle structures tethered to the membrane through variable spacer domains with dimerization through a cysteine located in the spacer domain.[163, 201, 202]

Hematopoietic Growth Factor Gene Structures and Gene Disruptions

HEMATOPOIETIN RECEPTOR LIGANDS

G-CSF. The G-CSF gene, which has been localized to chromosome 17 at 17 q11-q12,[350] consists of five exons spread over approximately 2.3 kb.[351] At the 5′ end of the second intron, there are two donor splice sites separated by 9 bp; alternate splicing at these two different sites results in two forms of G-CSF differing by the insertion of three amino acids corresponding to the nine nucleotides present when the more distal splice donor is used.[351] However, no functional difference has been found between the two different forms of G-CSF and it is not clear if differential splicing in the G-CSF gene serves a purpose. The chromosomal localization of the G-CSF gene initially led to speculation that it might be involved in the breakpoints of the t(15;17) translocation characteristic of acute promyelocytic leukemia. However, this proved not to be the case because the gene maps proximal to the breakpoint and is not rearranged in the malignant clone that gives rise to this disorder.[351]

The combination of technology for regenerating mice from cultured embryonic stem cells and the ability to selectively disrupt genes in cultured mammalian cells has led to new methodology for studying gene function *in vivo* (mutants related to HGFs are summarized in Table 6–3).[352] Using this approach, Lieschke and associates[353] were able to generate mice with both copies of the G-CSF gene disrupted. These animals develop normally but, as adults display 70 to 80 percent reduction in the levels of circulating neutrophils; a 50 percent reduction in the numbers of progenitors in all lineages, and impaired resistance to challenge infections with *Listeria monocyto-*

genes. These findings, which are in agreement with earlier observations by Hammond and colleagues[354] in dogs that had developed cross-reacting antibodies to canine G-CSF, demonstrate the central role for G-CSF in controlling neutrophil levels. However, the decline in all populations of progenitors is consistent with a role for G-CSF before commitment to the neutrophil lineage, perhaps at the early stem cell stage as suggested by the synergy of G-CSF and SCF in generating blast cell colonies.[355, 356]

EPO and TPO. The *EPO* gene, which spans roughly 3000 bp and consists of five exons and four introns has been mapped to chromosome 7q22.[357, 358] The *TPO* gene has been localized to chromosome 3q27.[346–348] At the amino acid level, the first 153 residues (of a total of 353) show 23 percent identity to *EPO* (50 percent with conservative amino acid changes) whereas the remaining 181 residues of the carboxy-terminal domain of *TPO* are unrelated to any known proteins.[346] Even more compelling, the intron/exon junctions of the five protein-coding exons of *TPO* exactly match, in phase with the intron/exon boundaries of the five exons of the *EPO* gene.[346] Thus, the *TPO* and *EPO* genes have clearly evolved from a common ancestor and at some point the extra protein-coding region found in the final coding exon of the *TPO* gene was either removed (in the case of the *EPO* gene) or added (in the case of the *TPO* gene) after the early duplication event. Analogous to the situation with IL-6 and G-CSF noted earlier, it may be interesting to analyze the corresponding gene structures in lower vertebrates to better understand how these important genes have evolved.

Although disruption of the *TPO* gene has not been reported, mice in which the c-*mpl* gene has been deleted have been described.[359] Although these animals develop normally and do not display significant abnormalities in bleeding times, they do have only 15 to 20 percent normal levels of circulating platelets. This result implies that TPO is very important for maintaining circulating levels of platelets but that other cytokines might have some capacity to generate platelets at low levels. Interestingly, through elegant study of various combinations of receptor gene disruptions, Gainsford and associates[360, 361] have shown that known cytokines with megakaryocyte-stimulating activity in culture, including IL-3, IL-6, IL-11, and LIF, play no role in basal platelet production in the mouse with *mpl* gene disruption.

In the case of *EPO*, gene disruption results in embryonic lethality owing to failure of fetal liver erythropoiesis[362]; furthermore, immunization of sheep or rabbits with human EPO results in the development of cross-reacting antibodies that causes life-threatening anemia in the animals.* Thus, in the absence of functioning EPO, no other growth factors can sufficiently substitute for maintenance of homeostasis.

IL-6–gp130 Complex Ligands: IL-6 and IL-11. The genes for IL-6 and IL-11 have been localized to chromosomes 7p21 and 19q13.3-q13.4,[363, 364] respectively. Both genes consist of five exons and four introns. The gene for G-CSF, which has been mapped to chromosome

---

*Sklut P, Foster B: unpublished results.

TABLE 6–3. Genetic Defects in Receptors or Signaling Proteins

		Human Mutations	
Gene	Mutation	Phenotype	Reference
IL2R$_{\gamma c}$	Deletion	X-linked severe combined immunodeficiency (SCID)	1089
JAK 3	Deletion	SCID	1090
GCSFR	C-terminal deletion	Fragment in Kostmann disease with AML	521
EPOR	C-terminal deletion	Benign erythrocytosis	594

			Nonhuman Mutations	
Species	Gene	Name	Phenotype	Reference
Mouse	*C-kit*	White-spotting	Macrocytic anemia, mast cell deficiency, lack of pigmentation, sterile	643, 644, 678
	Steel factor	Steel	Macrocytic anemia, mast cell deficiency, lack of pigmentation, sterile	643, 644, 678
	CSF1	Microphthalmia	Osteopetrosis due to decreased osteoclast function	385
	HCP	Moth-eaten	Immunodeficiency, autoimmune disease, and increased sensitivity to EPO	596
Drosophila	*JAK* homologue	Hopscotch	Tum^L allele is a gain-of-function mutation that causes leukemia	1091, 1092

	Targeted Disruption in Murine Embryonic Stem Cells	
Gene	Phenotype	Reference
IL6	Decreased CFU-S and stem cell function	367
GMCSF	Hematopoiesis normal; progressive accumulation of pulmonary surfactant	380, 381
GCSF	Neutrophils 25% normal; impaired response to *Listeria monocytogenes* infection	353
Epo	Embryonic lethal—failure of definitive erythropoiesis	362
EpoR	Embryonic lethal—failure of definitive erythropoiesis	362
TpoR (c-*mpL*)	Platelets 15–20% normal	359
IL3Rβ	Normal hematopoiesis	827
IL3/5/GMRβ$_c$	Similar to GM-CSF$^{-/-}$ mice; also low eosinophils and impaired eosinophil response to *Nippostrongylus brasiliensis*	827
Vav	Not required for hematopoiesis	1093

17q11-q12, has a similar structure and is almost certainly distantly related in evolution.[365]

Animals that have been engineered to lack the IL-6 gene develop normally but display significant deficiencies in various immune and inflammatory responses.[366] Interestingly, the hepatic acute phase response in these animals is severely compromised after tissue damage but only moderately in response to lipopolysaccharide (LPS). The effects of disruption of the IL-6 gene on normal hematopoiesis are relatively minor: a slight decrease in peripheral blood leukocyte counts, 10 percent reduction in bone marrow cellularity, and 50 percent reduction in CFU-S$_{d12}$ and a four- to fivefold reduction of pre-CFU-S.[367] This relatively minor effect on hematopoiesis of disruption of the IL-6 gene points out the difficulty in evaluating the relative importance of cytokines *in vivo* through *in vitro* culture systems: IL-6 in cultures of mouse bone marrow cells is one of the most potent synergistic factors for all lineages yet gene disruption experiments suggest that it is either highly redundant with other cytokines or its role in regulating normal hematopoiesis is relatively minor.[162]

Although numerous investigators have tried without success to generate mice with disruption of the IL-11 gene, Nandurkar and associates[368] have been successful in generating mice with the IL-11Rα gene for the purpose of investigating the biologic activity of the cytokine. Interestingly, the resulting female mice are infertile because of defective decidualization, revealing an important role for IL-11 in female reproduction and possibly explaining the difficulty in generating an IL-11 gene disruption.[369] Evaluation of hematopoiesis in the receptor-deleted animals revealed no significant defects in normal blood or progenitor cell levels in any lineage, nor did the animals show impaired recovery when challenged with 5-fluorouracil or phenylhydrazine, indicating that IL-11 is not essential for hematopoiesis in normal or stressed mouse.

GM-CSFR Complex Ligands: IL-3, GM-CSF, and IL-5. The genes for each of these proteins comprise approximately 3000 bp divided among four (GM-CSF[370, 371] and IL-5,[238, 372]) or five (IL-3[371, 373]) exons with somewhat similar structures. All of these genes have been localized to the long arm of chromosome 5 at 5q31.1[374] a region commonly disrupted or deleted in patients with various malignant myeloid neoplasms.[375] This region also contains the genes for other important cytokines including IL-4, IL-9, IL-12p40 and IL-13.[374–376] Despite this close clustering of important genes involved in various aspects of regulating the hematopoietic system, analysis of the defects in chromosome 5 from 135 patients has revealed that a minimal critical region at 5q31, deleted in every patient, does not contain any of **these cytokine genes, suggesting that they are not generall**y involved in these malignancies.[375] Detailed mapping of the region has demonstrated that several of these genes are very closely linked: the GM-CSF and IL-3 genes are tandemly arrayed within 9 kb of one another,[377] and the IL-4 and IL-13 genes are separated by only 12.5 kb.[374] This clustering of molecules with similar structures and functions, including sharing receptor components in the case of GM-CSF, IL-3, and IL-5[378, 379] provides further strong support for the evolutionary relatedness of their respective genes.

Mice with homozygous disruption of the GM-CSF gene develop normally and do not display any defects in the levels of circulating granulocytes or monocytes nor in the levels of CFU-GM progenitors in marrow or spleen.[380, 381] However, these animals exhibit alveolar proteinosis with surfactant accumulation in the lungs based on defective alveolar macrophage function. Thus, GM-CSF plays an irreplaceable role in the function/ development of certain macrophage populations, but any function of this cytokine in controlling basal or stimulated production of granulocytes or monocytes can be replaced by other factors.

To evaluate the role of the entire IL-3–GM-CSF–IL-5 complex, Nishinakamura and associates[382] engineered a mouse lacking the βc receptor component shared by all three cytokines as well as a disruption in the IL-3 gene. Mice lacking the βc receptor show a pulmonary alveolar proteinosis-like disease and reduced numbers of peripheral eosinophils, which are explained by the lack of GM-CSF and IL-5 function, respectively. Combination with IL-3 gene disruption caused no further abnormalities in hematopoiesis, demonstrating that the entire IL-3/GM-CSF/IL-5 axis is dispensable for hematopoiesis both in normal and stressed mice.

RECEPTOR TYROSINE KINASE LIGANDS: M-CSF, STEM CELL FACTOR, AND FLT3 LIGAND

With the isolation of the genes encoding SCF and the FL, it has become clear that, like their receptor genes, the M-CSF, SCF, and FL genes are all evolutionarily related.[201, 202] The first of these to be identified was the gene for M-CSF, which is a large gene (spanning more than 20 kb[383]) containing nine exons that has been localized to chromosome 1p13-p21.[384] The gene for SCF has a similar exon structure and has been localized to chromosome 12q22-q24.[349] The amino acid sequence identity shared by the external domains of these proteins is 16 percent (32 percent similarity with conservative changes[201]), and the disulfide structures have been preserved. The more recently cloned gene for FL also shows a similar gene structure with locations of introns reasonably well preserved with those of M-CSF and SCF. However, if the sizes of exons are used as a measure of relatedness, the corresponding exons of the latter two factors are more similar, suggesting that they might be more closely related to one another than to FL.[202]

The gene for M-CSF is defective in the spontaneous mutant, osteopetrosis *(op/op)*.[385] Female *op/op* mice are infertile, confirming the role of M-CSF in the biologic activity of the pregnant uterus.[386] They also have a severe deficiency of the ability to develop osteoclasts derived from the monocytic lineage, resulting in the development of osteopetrosis and the failure to develop teeth.[387] However, the animals do develop some macrophages populations, indicating that M-CSF is important in many but not all macrophage-related lineages. The observation that some of the defects in the *op/op* mouse are corrected as the animals mature has led to speculation that alternative splicing of the mutant M-CSF transcript can lead to production of some functional M-CSF.[388] This raises the necessity of genetically engineering mice with substantial deletions in this gene to see if there is some redundancy in HGF function or if *op* is not a true null mutation.

Naturally occurring mutations in the SCF locus (*Sl* mice) or in the receptor for SCF, c-*kit* (*W* mice) result in profound effects on many stages of hematopoiesis, most notably in the stem cell, erythroid, and mast cell compartments.[169] These studies have clearly demonstrated the central role of SCF in controlling hematopoietic cell function. Interestingly, disruption of the Flt3 receptor gene, has relatively minor effects on hematopoiesis, the most notable being somewhat depressed levels of B-lymphocyte precursors.[286] However, mice with both the c-*kit* and Flt3 receptor tyrosine kinase genes disrupted display more severe hematologic complications than mice with either single mutation,[286] suggesting that the two factors do, at some level, complement one another *in vivo.*

Hematopoietic Growth Factor Genes: Regulation of Expression

Many different cell types, including T and B cells, monocytes/macrophages, fibroblasts, epithelial cells, endothelial cells, elaborate various HGFs, especially after stimulation.[159–161, 186] Indeed, Metcalf and associates[389] have reported that conditioned media from murine organ cultures of lung, muscle, thymus, bone shaft, and heart all contain readily detectable levels of many different HGFs and cytokines. However, serum levels of HGFs under steady-state conditions are very low but elevate rapidly after systemic administration of agents such as LPS.[389] Thus, it seems likely that normal hematopoiesis is maintained by low-level expression of HGFs locally in the microenvironment of the bone marrow, spleen, and thymus whereas systemic circulation of HGFs becomes more important after infection.[390] Because HGF production is closely regulated in most cell types, it may be that binding of hematopoietic cells to stromal cells also activates stromal HGF production, analogous to the induction of IL-6 expression by binding of myeloma cells to stromal fibroblasts.[391] Indeed, Gupta and associates[392] have shown that coculture of primitive CD34[+] cells with bone marrow stromal cell layers results in a four- to fivefold increase in levels of both IL-6 and G-CSF.

Activation of HGF gene expression by various stimuli has been reported for many different cell types.[159–161, 186] This activation accelerates blood cell production in times of stress, such as a response to infection, marrow damage, or severe bleeding. Among the many types of HGF-producing cells, the most prominent include T and B lymphocytes, monocytes/macrophages, and mesodermal cells, including fibroblasts, endothelial cells, and epithelial cells. Expression of some of the HGF genes, notably IL-3 and IL-5, is restricted largely to activated T cells.[238, 393, 394] Activated T cells also produce GM-CSF,[395] M-CSF,[396] and IL-6[397] but these HGFs are produced by many other cells as well, including monocytes/macrophages and the various mesodermally derived cells. G-CSF[186] is expressed by monocytes/macrophages and the various mesodermally derived cells whereas the expression of IL-11 is even further restricted because it does not appear to be made by T cells nor by monocyte/macrophages.[230, 307, 398] EPO expression is highly regulated by oxygen tension and is expressed during fetal development in the liver and in adults largely in the kidney.[232, 233] TPO appears to be made constitutively in liver and kidney and at lower but inducible levels in the bone marrow.[150] SCF[169] and FL[234, 235] are broadly expressed in many mesodermal cell types, but thus far little is known about the regulation of their expression.

The expression of the HGFs and other cytokines is often triggered in cells by exposure to other cytokines or growth factors, leading to the concept that there are complicated interacting networks of cytokines that control and coordinate many physiologic responses.[164, 165] Finally, the circulating levels of blood cells are known to be directly controlled by production of the HGFs (e.g., EPO in the case of red cells),[232, 233] and therefore the control of expression of these genes is probably critically important for maintaining the appropriate numbers of cells. In this section, we review the expression and regulation of expression of the different cytokine genes in different cell types.

REGULATION OF mRNA PRODUCTION

The activation of HGF gene expression is generally reflected by increases in the levels of the respective mRNAs, which often provide reasonable surrogates for measuring cytokine levels. This is achieved either by enhancing the rate of transcription of the gene or by increasing the half-life of decay of the mRNA or by both mechanisms as in the case of IL-11 expression in stromal cells.[398] Activators of gene expression, whether they are cytokines such as IL-1[203] or TNF[399] or bacterial products such as LPS,[203] interact with specific cellular receptors. This interaction results in activation of signal transduction cascades that generally involve phosphorylation and dephosphorylation of specific intracellular proteins, calcium fluxes, and translocations of cytoplasmic proteins into the nucleus of the cell.[400] Transcriptional activation begins with opening up of the chromatin structure and demethylation of critical CpG sites in the cytokine promoter so that it can become accessible to RNA polymerase II.[401] The initiation of transcription begins with the activation and translocation into the nucleus of positive transcription factors, which interact with regulatory elements (see, for example, references 393, 402, and 403) that have been identified in the promoters or enhancers of

the different cytokine genes.[404] These sequences, which act as targets or "receptors" for the different transcription factors and transcription factor complexes appear in different combinations in many of the different HGF promotors. These combinations probably provide the basis for the unique regulation of each gene in each specific cell type. Prominent among the many transcription factors that interact with their regulatory sequences in the cytokine gene promotors are members of the NF-κB,[405] NF-AT,[406] AP-1,[407] ETS,[408] and GATA[409] families of regulatory proteins. The NF-κB family members have been implicated in the activation of many cytokine genes, particularly those associated with inflammatory responses whereas several members of the NF-AT gene family are prominent in controlling the expression of genes in activated T cells.

Stabilization of mRNAs inside cells is also a prominent regulatory mechanism for activation of gene expression.[410, 411] In many cell types, cytokine genes are continually transcribed, but the resulting RNAs are rapidly degraded under steady-state conditions; in such cells, cytokine mRNA levels can be increased rapidly simply by inhibition of their degradation. This mechanism was first demonstrated for GM-CSF when Shaw and Kamen[410] found that a conserved sequence element, AUUUA, in the 3'-untranslated region of the mRNA decreased its stability, probably through interaction with specific proteins.[412] This destabilizer sequence as well as a second different element based on a stem-loop structure of the mRNA sequence is found in the mRNAs for cytokine and transcription factor genes and is often important for regulating the levels of those particular mRNAs.[413] The mechanism of increasing the mRNA half-life through interactions mediated by the destabilizer sequence is still poorly understood[414]; however it is clear, for example, that stimulation of fibroblasts with IL-1 results both in activation of specific positive transcription factors and in activation of a pathway that blocks AUUUA-mediated mRNA degradation.[415] Perhaps not surprisingly, it has also been shown that multiple pathways are involved that can distinguish, for example, between Fos and various cytokine mRNAs in different cell types.[414, 415] Thus, regulation of gene expression through mRNA stabilization is gene and cell type specific, analogous to the regulation through transcriptional activation.

EXPRESSION OF HEMATOPOIETIC GROWTH FACTORS BY ACTIVATED T CELLS: IL-3, IL-5, GM-CSF, IL-6, AND M-CSF

Activation of T cells in response to antigens represents one of the key regulatory steps in control of the immune system.[416] As part of this process, a variety of T-cell genes become transcriptionally active along with the genes for many cytokines, including GM-CSF,[371, 395] IL-3,[238, 371, 393, 394] IL-5,[238, 393, 417], IL-6,[397] and M-CSF.[396] Among these, expression of IL-3 and IL-5 is largely limited to activated T cells (but also to mast cells activated through the immunoglobulin [Ig] E receptor), at least in the mouse,[238, 393, 417] whereas the expression of GM-CSF, IL-6, and M-CSF has been observed after activation of many different cell types. IL-6 expression has been commonly observed in murine T cells and T-cell clones, but with human cultures IL-6 expression by mitogen-stimulated T cells requires monocytes; the monocytes could be replaced by phorbol ester.[397] Hempel and co-workers[418] have found that IL-10 interacts directly with T cells to inhibit IL-6 production, suggesting that IL-6 production may be controlled by important components of the cytokine network. M-CSF, although not classically thought to be a T cell–derived HGF, has been shown to be expressed by normal T-cell populations in response to combined triggering of CD2 and CD28.[396]

Antigen recognition by the T-cell receptor in combination with a co-stimulatory signal such as that provided by CD28 interacting with the B7 co-stimulatory molecules rapidly switches on intercellular signaling events, including protein phosphorylation, calcium mobilization, and inositol phospholipid hydrolysis.[419] Signal transduction resulting in cytokine gene activation by the T-cell receptor can largely be bypassed by exposure of the cells to phorbol esters such as phorbol-12-myristate 13 acetate (PMA) which activate protein kinase C and calcium ionophores (ionomycin) that mobilize calcium ions into the cell.[416, 420] Thus, triggering of the T-cell receptor results in protein kinase C activation and calcium mobilization that ultimately leads to activation of transcription of various cytokine genes. This activation can be blocked by treatment with cyclosporine or FK506 (tacrolimus).[416, 421] These findings have led to the study of cytokine gene expression in T cell lines or clones after stimulation with phytohemagglutinin to mimic T-cell receptor cross-linking, PMA to induce protein kinase C activation/translocation, and ionomycin to induce calcium mobilization and in the presence of cyclosporine or FK506 as a check for physiologic relevance although such powerful stimulation is likely to override many of the more subtle mechanisms regulating T-cell expression of cytokines.

In situ hybridization studies with purified human cell subsets suggest that CD4, CD8, and NK cells all express GM-CSF and IL-3; however, only a small fraction of T cells produce IL-3 or GM-CSF in response to PMA and the calcium ionophore ionomycin.[395] These studies indicated that only 1 and 10 percent of the activated T cells express IL-3 and GM-CSF, respectively, but this level could be increased substantially with the addition of IL-2 to the cultures. IL-3 expression is also limited to the CD28+ subset of human T cells.[422] Expression of the IL-5 gene, like that of the IL-3 gene is largely restricted to activated T cells and mast cells (at least in the mouse).[423]

To turn to a possibly more physiologic situation, it has long been recognized that different subsets of CD4+ helper T cells become polarized in the types of cytokines that they produce when activated; type 1 (Th1) prominently secretes IL-2 and IFN-γ and type 2 (Th2) produces IL-4, IL-5, IL-6, IL-10, and IL-13.[424] GM-CSF and IL-3 are actively produced by both helper cell subtypes. CD8+ cells can also be polarized along the same lines. In addition, T-cell clones expressing different combinations of cytokines have been identified, which define yet other types, including type 3 (production of high levels of TGF-β) and Tr1 (production of high levels of IL-10 and IFN-γ, low levels of IL-2, and no IL-4).[425] Thus, the patterns of cytokine expression are not

as simple as originally thought, and it may turn out that there are no discrete subsets, but different clones of cells may fall on a continuum between the two extremes.[167] Naive peripheral T cells are multipotent in their ability to synthesize the various cytokines, and upon activation they acquire a more restricted pattern of expression. In the type 1 direction, these patterns are best influenced by IL-12[295] and in the type 2 direction by either IL-4[426] or IL-13.[427] These are examples of how the different members of the cytokine family interact in a network to further control responses, both hematopoietic and within the immune system, through complicated interactions with T cells.

EXPRESSION OF HEMATOPOIETIC GROWTH FACTORS BY MONOCYTES/MACROPHAGES, DENDRITIC CELLS, AND MYELOID LEUKEMIAS: G-CSF, M-CSF, GM-CSF, IL-6, AND SCF

Monocytes/macrophages and related cells including dendritic cells, Kupffer cells in the liver, and Langerhans cells in the skin are key cells that serve many important functions in regulating the immune system.[428] Among the functions performed by these cells is the production of many cytokines, including TNF,[429] IL-1,[204] G-CSF,[186] M-CSF,[429] GM-CSF,[159] IL-6,[228] and IL-12,[428] in response to various stimuli including LPS,[428, 429] IL-1,[164] IL-3,[430] GM-CSF,[431] and M-CSF.[432] Other cytokines including IL-4,[433] IL-10[434] and IL-11[319] down-regulate monocyte production of many of these cytokines. Several of the newer cytokines, including IL-18,[206] various members of the IL-17 gene family[435] and IL-23[184] are likely to play important roles in control of cytokine production by monocytes and macrophages.

All of these interactions are key components of the interactions between T cells and monocytes in determining the nature and direction of the immune response. Different regulators have been found to induce different subsets of these cytokines. For example, LPS has been shown to induce expression of IL-1, IL-6, TNF, IL-1RA, GM-CSF, and G-CSF.[430] In contrast, IL-3 and GM-CSF failed to induce the expression of either GM-CSF or G-CSF but were found to induce M-CSF expression. M-CSF has been shown to induce peritoneal macrophages to activate expression of GM-CSF and IL-6 at the transcriptional level, but additional signals are necessary to induce the release of the functional cytokine proteins from the cells.[436] Murine bone marrow–derived macrophages have been reported to constitutively express the mRNA for M-CSF and SCF, and the level of expression can be enhanced by treating the cultures with pokeweed mitogen.[437]

The different HGF genes in monocytes can be up-regulated by a variety of different mechanisms. In the case of IL-6, LPS and *Mycobacterium tuberculosis* activate gene expression at the transcriptional level through activation of the transcription factors NF-IL6 and NF-κB.[438] In contrast, activation of IL-1 and IL-6 expression by *Salmonella typhimurium* porins is largely mediated by mRNA stabilization.[439] Cytokine activation of monocyte IL-6 expression also occurs by various mechanisms, often involving interactions between NF-κB and NF-IL6.[440]

However, LIF treatment of monocytes induces transcriptional activation of the IL-6 gene, and this is largely mediated by NF-κB and not by NF-IL6.[441] IL-2, IL-3, and GM-CSF have all been shown to induce monocyte expression of IL-6 and this expression is inhibited post-transcriptionally by treatment with IL-4.[430, 433] LPS-activated expression of IL-6 is potently inhibited at the transcriptional level by IL-10.[442] Activation of IL-6 expression by the combination of TNF and IFN-γ in the human THP-1 monocytic cell line involves requires activation of NF-κB. Perhaps surprisingly, treatment of monocytes with the anti-inflammatory cytokine TGF-β also activates IL-6 expression.[443] In the case of G-CSF, expression can be activated by treatment of monocytes with either IL-1 or LPS (IFN-γ potentiates the LPS response[444]), and IL-4 given simultaneously can block this induction, an effect that is not mediated by mRNA stability but rather at the transcriptional level.[445] However, the IFN-γ enhancement effect appears to be largely at the level of mRNA stability; the mRNA half-life with LPS treatment alone is roughly 20 minutes, but after exposure to IFN-γ, the half-life increased to 120 minutes.[444] M-CSF gene expression can be activated in HL-60 cells, an event mediated by NF-κB.[446] These interactions between monocytes and T cells and the cytokines they produce, although complicated, are clearly important in determining the direction and extent of the resulting immune responses and are likely to play a key role in control of the cytokine network.

Dendritic cells, which have been characterized as potent antigen-presenting cells, are also an important source of HGFs and other cytokines.[447] With the availability of cytokines such as FL, GM-CSF, IL-3, and IL-4, it has become much easier to generate significant numbers of dendritic cells for further studies from both myeloid and lymphoid sources.[257, 448] Originally believed to be largely of myeloid cell origin, it is now recognized that some are probably derived from myeloid cells whereas others have their origins in the lymphoid lineages.[449] Interestingly, different types of dendritic cells matured under different conditions can polarize cytokine production by maturing T-helper cells[450] and therefore probably play key roles in determining the outcomes of immune responses. Murine bone marrow–derived immature dendritic cells (CD86⁻) produce high levels of IL-1α and IL-1β, TNF-α, and TGF-β1 but upon maturation (CD86+) in the presence of CD40 ligand, the levels of TGF-β dropped whereas levels of IL-6, IL-12p40, IL-15, IL-18, and TNF-α increased as did the ability of the cells to prime naïve T cells.[450] With the availability of new cytokines for expanding both myeloid and dendritic cells in culture, it will be very interesting to further elucidate how these important cells interact with T cells through the cytokine network in up- and down-regulation of immune responses.

The growth factor responsiveness of primary leukemias and leukemic cell lines in culture raises the possibility that leukemogenesis might involve the disruption of the normal pathways of growth factor control of hematopoietic cell development.[451, 452] However, analysis of many primary samples from patients with acute myeloid leukemia has revealed that in culture, most require exogenous growth factors, although occasionally the cells spontaneously produce G-CSF or GM-CSF.[451, 453, 454] In some of these cases, GM-CSF production is actually regulated through a paracrine loop in which the leukemic cells make and secrete IL-1 which in turn stimulates endogenous GM-CSF.[455] Thus, despite the commonly observed defects in chromosome 5[375] surrounding the genes for IL-3 and GM-CSF, activation of the expression does not appear to be a primary event in leukemogenesis but as a secondary event may contribute to the severity of the leukemia.[454] Frank overexpression of IL-3 genes by acute lymphocytic leukemic cells have been reported in a few patients, in whom the IL-3 gene became activated through translocation into an immunoglobulin locus.[456, 457] At least one of these patients had eosinophilia, presumably due to increased levels of IL-3.[457] Both IL-3[458] and IL-11[459] have been reported to be autocrine growth factors for different megakaryoblastic leukemia cell lines, but it is not clear if this represents a property of the original leukemic cells or if selection of the cells in culture might have resulted in the activation of expression of these genes. The IL-3 promoter in megakaryoblastic leukemic cell lines uses many of the same transcription factors that it uses in activated T cells.[460] Finally, juvenile chronic myeloblastic leukemia was suspected as the cause of autocrine expression of the GM-CSF gene, but more recent evidence indicates that it appears to be due to hyper-responsiveness to this HGF.[461, 462]

EXPRESSION OF HEMATOPOIETIC GROWTH FACTORS BY FIBROBLASTS, ENDOTHELIAL CELLS, AND EPITHELIAL CELLS: G-CSF, M-CSF, SCF, FL, GM-CSF, IL-6, AND IL-11

Different populations of fibroblasts, endothelial cells, and epithelial cells can be stimulated to produce cytokines by treatment with LPS,[463] phorbol esters,[371] or other cytokines including IL-1,[203] TNF,[464] and platelet-derived growth factor.[465] In many tissues, this is likely to be an integral part of the host response to infection: cytokine production at the site of infection should result in local activation of host defense effector cells and in the systemic recruitment of more effector cells until the infection is resolved.[389] In bone marrow, thymus, and spleen, these cell populations are probably critical components of the local microenvironment, which is involved in the normal proliferation, development, and differentiation of cells of the hematopoietic and lymphopoietic systems. The control of production of the various HGFs in the steady state is still poorly understood.[389]

Fibroblasts and endothelial cells are important sources of many of the HGFs, including G-CSF,[186] M-CSF,[168] GM-CSF,[371] IL-6,[466] IL-11,[307] SCF,[169] and FL.[234, 235] This expression is regulated both transcriptionally and post-transcriptionally by exposure to LPS, phorbol esters, or cytokines such as IL-1, TNF, and IFN-γ.[186, 467, 468] SCF expression has been reported to be constitutive in human stromal bone marrow cultures, in endothelial cells, and in bone marrow–derived fibroblasts and is not responsive to IL-1.[469]

Although it is not clear that stromal fibroblasts from bone marrow are any more or less capable of cytokine production than fibroblasts from other tissues, because of their proximity to stem and progenitor cells they have long been studied for their ability to express HGFs. Many of these cells constitutively express the tyrosine kinase receptor ligands M-CSF and SLF.[469, 470] IL-1 stimulation induces expression of G-CSF, GM-CSF, IL-6, and IL-11[398, 471, 472] and further up-regulates the M-CSF gene, a gene also further activated by IL-6.[464] Much of this induction is mediated via mRNA stability. In the case of G-CSF, despite the presence of an IL-1 response element in the promoter region,[473] most of the effect on marrow-derived stromal fibroblasts appears to be related to mRNA stability.[472] IL-6, GM-CSF, and IL-11 all behave similarly.[464] In the case of IL-11, several stromal cell lines have been found to express low constitutive levels of the cytokine, and IL-1 induction results in enhanced mRNA stability. The constitutive expression and the activation of IL-11 expression by phorbol esters in the same cells is mediated through binding of a JunD–AP-1 complex to an AP-1 site in the promoter region. Expression of many cytokines, including GM-CSF and IL-6 but not M-CSF, by lung fibroblasts is down-regulated by glucocorticoid hormones such as dexamethasone and is mediated by mRNA destablization.[474]

After myeloablation, circulating levels of many HGFs increase dramatically. In some instances this might result from mechanisms that sense low levels of the various blood cells. However, Hachiya and associates[475] have found that, in culture, TNF and IL-1 synergize with irradiation to up-regulate the expression of GM-CSF through both mRNA stabilization and activation of gene transcription. These observations raise the possibility that the myeloablative agents themselves may directly induce or enhance HGF production *in vivo* after various cancer therapy regimens.

IL-6 is expressed constitutively by thymic epithelial cells but is strongly further up-regulated by IL-1, LPS, or TNF.[476] IL-6 expression is also activated in normal bone marrow fibroblasts by binding to multiple myeloma cells, cells that generally require IL-6 for growth. This effect is at least partly transcriptionally regulated through NF-κB.[477] TNF and IL-1 induction of human fibroblasts is also at least in part mediated by NFκB.[478] In bone marrow fibroblasts and in osteoblasts, IL-6 gene expression is down-regulated by the estrogen receptor; an effect mediated through interactions in the nucleus of the estrogen receptor with NF-κB and NF-IL6.[479] These effects of estrogen on IL-6 expression provide a possible explanation for the relationship between IL-6 and bone loss osteoporosis related to estrogen deficiency.[480]

Endothelial cells are another important source of HGFs. Human endothelial cells produce G-CSF, GM-CSF, and M-CSF in response to inflammatory cytokines such as IL-1 and TNF.[481, 482] In contrast to that for G-CSF and GM-CSF, SCF mRNA is expressed constitutively by human umbilical vein endothelial cells.[483] The levels of SCF mRNA are further increased in response to inflammatory mediators such as IL-1 and LPS. This induction results predominantly from mRNA stabilization by approximately threefold. Increased expression of GM-CSF mRNA in human umbilical vein endothelial cells is also at least partly mediated by mRNA stabilization.[484]

The induction of SCF mRNA in endothelial cells may contribute to the elevated plasma levels of this factor in patients with sepsis and patients with inflammatory diseases.[483] Finally, vascular endothelial cells express M-CSF in response to minimally modified low-density lipoprotein though transcriptional activation mediated by NF-κB; however, it is not clear how this might contribute to the biologic activity of the macrophage-derived foam cell in the atherosclerotic lesion.[485]

REGULATION OF ERYTHROPOIETIN EXPRESSION BY HYPOXIA

EPO has long been recognized as the physiologic regulator of red cell production.[232, 233, 486] It is produced in the kidney and in the fetal liver in response to hypoxia or exposure to cobalt(II) chloride; the mechanism of the switch of production from predominantly fetal liver to predominantly kidney in adults is largely unknown.[487] Using a transgenic approach, Semenza and associates[488] showed that *EPO* gene constructs containing 0.7 kb of 3′-flanking sequence and 0.4 kb of 5′-flanking sequence were inducible in the liver but not the kidneys of hypoxic mice; addition of 5.6 kb of additional 5′-flanking sequence suppressed the relatively high basal levels of improper expression, and, finally, the further addition of 8 kb of 5′-flanking sequence resulted in proper, kidney-specific *EPO* gene expression.[488, 489] These studies mapped important negative regulatory elements between 0.4 and 6 kb upstream of the EPO gene and kidney-specific regulatory elements to an area between 6 and 14 kb 5′ to the gene, indicating a complicated mechanism for regulation of its expression.

Given the complexity and large size of the EPO gene with its regulatory regions and the lack of kidney-derived cell lines, the study of the regulation of *EPO* expression has largely focused on two liver-derived cell lines, Hep G2 and Hep 3B, in which expression is inducible by hypoxia or cobalt chloride.[232, 233] These studies have provided important basic information about the regulation of EPO gene expression in response to oxygen deprivation, but it should be remembered that this does not include the mechanism for kidney-specific expression in adults. Many proteins that react with molecular oxygen do so through a heme moiety as is best studied in the case of oxygen binding to hemoglobin. In hemoglobin, the oxygen binds reversibly to the ferrous iron atom in the center of the heme porphyrin. Upon oxygen binding, the conformation of the hemoglobin molecule changes. Cobalt or nickel can substitute for ferrous iron, but the poor binding of oxygen to cobalt and the lack of binding to nickel lock the hemoglobin molecule in the "deoxy" state.[232, 233] Finally, carbon monoxide competes with oxygen for binding to the ferrous iron atom. In Hep 3B cells, hypoxia, cobalt, and nickel significantly stimulate EPO production while carbon monoxide inhibits hypoxia- but not cobalt-induced *EPO* expression.[7] These results have been formulated into a model in which primary regulation of *EPO* gene expression is mediated by a heme protein–based oxygen sensor. Binding of oxygen in equilibrium to this putative sensor would shift its conformation between an oxygenated (off) state and a deoxy (on) state; the deoxy form would activate a series of events leading to *EPO* gene transcription.[232, 233] In this model, cobalt substitution for ferrous iron would result in a failure to bind oxygen (deoxy state), thereby resulting in activation of *EPO* expression and, because carbon monoxide does not bind cobalt, it would not be expected to interfere with cobalt activation of *EPO* expression. However, cobalt should interfere with hypoxia-induced expression by binding ferrous iron and locking the putative heme protein in the "oxy" state. Further support for this model comes from the observation that inhibition of heme synthesis causes a fivefold reduction in hypoxia-induced *EPO* production.[232]

Downstream events from the oxygen sensor involved in activation of *EPO* gene expression require *de novo* protein synthesis, including the production of specific transcription factors.[490] One of these, a heterodimeric (subunits of 120 and 93 kD) basic helix-loop-helix transcription factor complex designated hypoxia-inducible factor 1 (HIF-1) has been purified and molecularly cloned.[8, 491, 492] HIF-1 is induced in a variety of cell types in response to hypoxia or cobalt, indicating that, although it is important in activation of *EPO* expression, it is also important in the activation of other hypoxia-inducible genes.[8, 492] HIF-1 has been shown to bind to an enhancer sequence located approximately 130 bp downstream from the poly(A) addition signal of the *EPO* gene. This enhancer segment has been shown to render other promoter-reporter gene constructs hypoxia-responsive with typical inductions in the range of 4 to 15-fold, significantly less than the 50- to 100-fold induction observed with the chromosomal *EPO* gene in Hep 3B cells.[488]

In addition to HIF-1 and its role on the 3′ *EPO* gene enhancer, other studies have identified a 53-bp sequence from the *EPO* promoter that confers oxygen-sensitivity (6- to 10-fold inducibility) to a luciferase reporter gene.[493] Combination of the enhancer and promoter sequences results in cooperative (50-fold) inducibility of transcription in response to hypoxia, approaching that observed *in vivo*. Because these sequence elements included the consensus hexanucleotide nuclear hormone receptor response elements, various orphan members of this gene family were examined for binding to the *EPO* promoter and enhancer and for their presence in transcription complexes isolated from Hep 3B nuclear extracts. One of these, hepatic nuclear factor 4 (HNF-4), was found to be present in these extracts and to play a critical role in hypoxia-induced activation of *EPO* gene expression in Hep 3B cells.[9] Together, HIF-1 and HNF-4, which are activated in response to hypoxia, have provided considerable insight into the transcriptional regulation of the *EPO* gene, but, thus far the kidney restriction of expression in adults has not been accounted for.

REGULATION OF THROMBOPOIETIN GENE EXPRESSION

The cloning and expression of the gene for TPO[150] have provided new insight into the regulation of levels of platelets.[170] Gene disruption studies of *c-mpl*, the receptor for TPO, in mice have shown that in the absence of the function of this pathway, mice have only 15 percent of the normal levels of circulating platelets.[359] Thus, whereas redundancy among the growth factors, perhaps including SCF, IL-3, IL-6 and IL-11, can partially compensate for dysfunctional *c-mpl* signaling, TPO, like EPO in the erythrocyte lineage, appears to be the major regulator of circulating platelet levels.[150] However, in contrast to the control of *EPO* production, *TPO* gene expression does not seem to be transcriptionally regulated nor significantly influenced by platelet levels.[494] In adult mice, the major sources of *TPO* mRNA are the liver and kidney; in both organs, the gene is constitutively expressed and is not significantly up-regulated during thrombocytopenia. However, circulating levels of TPO increase rapidly during thrombocytopenia and decline as platelet counts return to normal.[154, 495] The observation that platelets themselves can remove TPO from thrombocytopenic plasma *in vitro* has led to the model that TPO is constantly produced and released into the circulation but, in normal circumstances, is rapidly removed by the circulating platelets.[154, 495] During thrombocytopenia, because of the platelet shortage TPO is not removed as fast as it is made, resulting in elevated levels and stimulation of platelet production. This mechanism is similar to one proposed some years ago by Stanley and associates[496] for the regulation of circulating M-CSF levels directly through consumption by the monocytes themselves.

HEMATOPOIETIC GROWTH FACTOR RECEPTORS

Types of Hematopoietic Growth Factor Receptors

Analysis of the actions of the HGFs on purified murine or human stem and progenitor cells (see later) has shown that there is considerable overlap in the action of the HGFs. Some insight into the apparent overlap in the biologic activities of many cytokines has come from analysis of their structural homologies and from the recent cloning of many of their receptors. These receptors are all type 1 membrane glycoproteins with extracellular N termini and single transmembrane domains, and fall into two major classes. Receptors such as c-kit, c-fms (the M-CSF receptor), and Flt3 are characterized by a cytoplasmic tyrosine kinase domain, whereas most of the other receptors lack cytoplasmic tyrosine kinase activity and can be divided into four subclasses (Table 6–4). Most of the HGFRs (class 1) fall into a superfamily with structural features based on two linked fibronectin (FBN) type III domains (Fig. 6–16). Analogous FBN domains are found in the interferon (class 2) receptors, and the class 1 and 2 structures probably evolved from a common primitive adhesion molecule.[497] Although the TNF family of receptors (class 3) are characterized by an extracellular fourfold repeat of approximately 40 amino acids that contains six conserved cysteine residues (Cys repeat),[166] the IL-1Rs (class 4) feature extracellular Ig-like repeats. Although the later discussion is focused mainly on the HGFRs, the tyrosine kinase receptors activate many of the same signaling cascades.[498, 499]

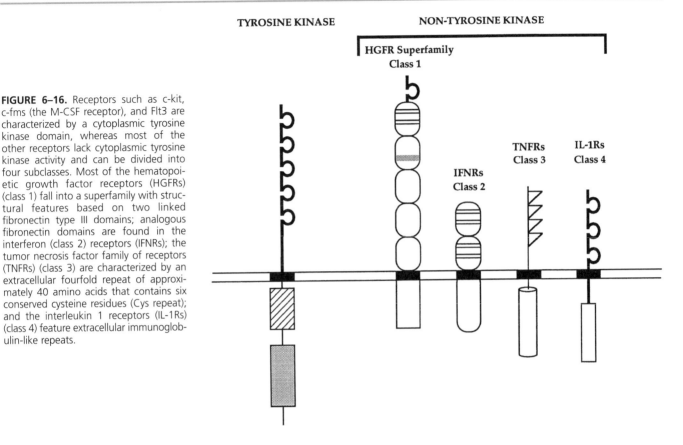

FIGURE 6–16. Receptors such as c-kit, c-fms (the M-CSF receptor), and Flt3 are characterized by a cytoplasmic tyrosine kinase domain, whereas most of the other receptors lack cytoplasmic tyrosine kinase activity and can be divided into four subclasses. Most of the hematopoietic growth factor receptors (HGFRs) (class 1) fall into a superfamily with structural features based on two linked fibronectin type III domains; analogous fibronectin domains are found in the interferon (class 2) receptors (IFNRs); the tumor necrosis factor family of receptors (TNFRs) (class 3) are characterized by an extracellular fourfold repeat of approximately 40 amino acids that contains six conserved cysteine residues (Cys repeat); and the interleukin 1 receptors (IL-1Rs) (class 4) feature extracellular immunoglobulin-like repeats.

TABLE 6–4. Hematopoietic Growth Factor Receptor Classes

Type	Receptor	Cytokine
Tyrosine kinase (Ig repeats)	c-*kit*, M-CSFR (c-fms), Flt3	Four α-helix bundle
Non–tyrosine kinase		
Class 1: HGFRs (FBN III domains)		Four α-helix bundle
Shared β$_c$	IL-3R, GM-CSFR, IL-5R	
Shared gp130	IL-6R, LIFR, IL-11R, IL-12R, OSMR	
Shared γ$_c$	IL-2R, IL-4R, IL-7R, IL-9R, IL-15R	
Single chain	G-CSFR, EPOR, TPOR (c-mp1)	
Class 2 (FBN III domains)	IFNα/βR, IFNγR	
Class 3 (Cys repeats)	TNFR I, TNFR II, FAS, CD40	β-Jellyroll wedge
Class 4 (Ig repeats)	IL-1R I and II	β-Trefoil fold

R = receptor; HGF = hematopoietic growth factor; LIF = leukemia inhibitory factor; OSM = oncostatin M; FBN = fibronectin; IFN = interferon; TNF = tumor necrosis factor.

Structure and Binding Properties

Prototypes for the class 1 structure are the (non-hematopoietic) prolactin and growth hormone receptors.[500–502] All these polypeptides show no apparent homology to other known receptors, and share a number of features (Fig. 6–17). The major homology lies in the extracellular domain, which is characterized by four conserved cysteine residues in the amino-terminal FBN III repeat and a Trp-Ser-X-Trp-Ser (WSXWS) motif in the linked carboxy-terminal FBN III repeat that forms a hydrophobic hinge between the two domains. In addition, the IL-6 family of receptors comprise members that each have an amino-terminal immunoglobulin-like domain as well as extra FBN III repeats. The cytoplasmic regions of

the receptor family show much less homology, although membrane proximal domains rich in prolines (box 1, within 20 amino acids of the membrane) and acidic residues (box 2), separated by a positionally conserved tryptophan, have been defined. Mutations within the box 1/2 domains have inactivated the mitogenic function of the receptors that have been examined,[503] whereas mutations of the conserved tryptophan inactivate some but not other receptors.[504] An additional interesting feature of many of the HGFRs is that receptor subunits are shared. GM-CSF, IL-3, and IL-5 all have receptors with unique α chains that bind their respective ligands with low affinity. They share a common β chain that converts ligand binding from low to high affinity in each case and is thought to be critical for

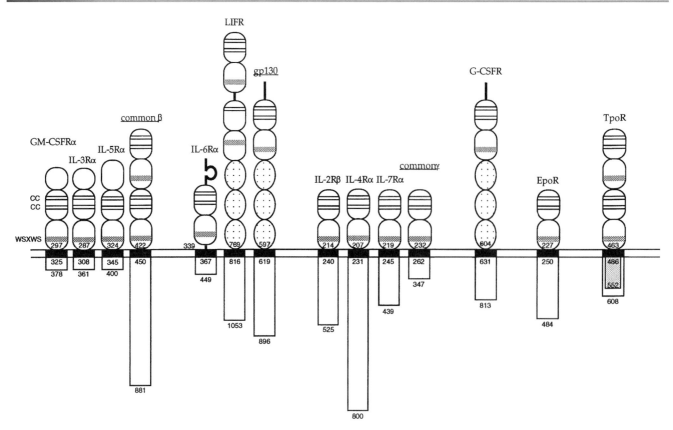

FIGURE 6–17. HGFR receptor family. Diagram of some of the HGFRs that have been cloned. The extracellular domains are all characterized by one or two regions that contain four conserved cysteines and a tryptophan-serine-x-tryptophan-serine (WSXWS) motif, like the prolactin receptor. Unique features are the following: IL-6 contains an immunoglobulin-like domain *(open circle)*; G-CSF contains a fibronectin type III-like region *(cross-hatched)*. The intracellular domains show less homology. An additional interesting feature of many of the HGFRs is that receptor subunits are shared (in particular the IL-3R, IL-6R, and IL-2R groups). In contrast, lineage-restricted receptors such as the erythropoietin receptor (EpoR), granulocyte colony-stimulating factor receptor (G-CSFR), and thrombopoietin receptor (TpoR) appear not to require an additional subunit for ligand binding or signal transduction. LIFR = leukemia inhibitory factor receptor.

signal transduction.[505] A similar arrangement is evident with the IL-6, LIF, OSM, IL-11, and CNTF receptors, all of which share a common β chain, namely gp130. An additional subunit, the low-affinity LIF receptor (LIFR), is shared by LIF, OSM, and CNTF. IL-6 and CNTF also use ligand-specific α receptor components, and gp130 is thought to form homodimers when IL-6 binds the IL-6Rα and heterodimers with LIFR in the presence of LIF, OSM, or CNTF. The finding of shared subunits explains to a certain extent why the actions of GM-CSF and IL-3 overlap on many cells, and why IL-6, LIF, and IL-11 all share pleiotropic actions on HSCs and hepatic cells. The fact that IL-12 is a heterodimer of two polypeptides that are similar to IL-6 and the IL-6Rα provides an explanation for its biologic activities, at least on stem cells, because it falls into the IL-6 group.[344] The γ chain of the IL-2R (called common γ) is now known to be shared by the IL-4,[506, 507] IL-7,[508] IL-9,[509] and IL-15[510] receptors. Other members of the HGFR superfamily that act on lineage-restricted cells such as the EPO receptor (EPOR), the G-CSF receptor (G-CSFR), and the TPO receptor appear not to require an additional subunit for ligand binding or signal transduction.

The binding properties of receptors for the murine and human HGFs have been characterized using iodinated, purified natural or recombinant ligands.[157, 511] Distribution of receptors within the hematopoietic system is restricted to undifferentiated and maturing cells of the appropriate target cell lineages. Because lineage-committed progenitor cells respond to more than one factor, overlap in receptor expression occurs, as noted earlier. A major challenge is to determine whether the overlap represents functional redundancy or indicates subtle and complex control mechanisms that dictate the degree and perhaps localization of the hematopoietic response under different physiologic circumstances.[512] The number of IL-3, GM-CSF, G-CSF, and EPORs per cell is strikingly low 1000 sites/cell), whereas those for M-CSF are about 1 log unit higher. In all cases, affinity of a receptor for its ligand is high, with dissociation constants usually in the picomolar range. Stimulation of target cells can occur at concentrations of factor orders of magnitude lower than the equilibrium constant at which 50 percent of receptors are occupied, and therefore it is apparent that low receptor occupancy is sufficient to produce biologic effects.

Receptor Function

SELECTION VERSUS INSTRUCTION

A major issue is whether HGFs act merely by supporting the survival (i.e., the prevention of apoptosis), proliferation, and differentiation of intrinsically programmed hematopoietic progenitor cells or whether they can recruit or direct differentiation along a particular pathway. If lineage-restricted receptors are important in directing the differentiation of multipotent cells to a particular lineage rather than acting merely as permissive factors, one might expect their expression on earlier multipotent cells or at least induction of expression very early in the sequence of commitment to that lineage. In the case of EPO for example, binding to the EPOR would then lead to expression of other "downstream" erythroid lineage-specific proteins. Data on the expression of different receptors by the most primitive HSCs from adults are very incomplete. The c-kit receptor appears certainly to be expressed on stem cells, but whether receptors for other early-acting factors such as the IL-3 or IL-6 groups are expressed at this stage is still uncertain. CD34 cells, a mixture of stem and progenitor cells, express IL-6, IL-3, GM-CSF, and a small number of EPORs,[513] whereas noncycling or "G_0" cells that survive 5-fluorouracil treatment and are enriched for LTC-IC express c-kit, IL-6Rα, gp130, and IL-1R, but interestingly not IL-3Rα or βc.[93] Some studies at the single cell level suggest that multilineage receptor gene expression is not observed,[514, 515] whereas other data suggest that some CD34+lin− cells (≈50 percent) can promiscuously express genes of both erythroid (EPOR and β-globin) and myeloid (myeloperoxidase) programs.[516] An alternate model, for which there is both murine[517] and human[513] evidence, suggests that the early-acting synergistic HGFs such as IL-6 up-modulate IL-3R expression, IL-3 in turn up-modulates GM-CSFR and EPOR expression, and GM-CSF also up-modulates EPOR expression. Although these data on normal marrow cells do not show modulation of upstream HGFRs by downstream factors, some data suggest that in cell lines, any mitogenic stimulus, including EPO, can up-modulate IL-3R expression.[518]

LINEAGE-SPECIFIC FACTORS AND THE INDUCTION OF DIFFERENTIATION

Do lineage-specific receptors direct differentiation or do intracellular proteins specific for lineage-restricted cells have that function? With respect to receptor-driven events, a proximal cytoplasmic domain of the G-CSFR is essential for proliferation whereas a more distal domain is important for induction of acute-phase plasma protein expression when the receptor is transfected into hepatoma cell lines[519] or granulocyte-specific proteins when it is introduced into murine IL-3–dependent FDC-P1 cells.[520] Support for a role for the G-CSFR in granulocyte differentiation comes from sequence analysis of the receptor in two patients with severe congenital neutropenia (Kostmann disease) who developed acute myeloid leukemia.[521] Two different point mutations in the G-CSFR gene resulted in truncations of the carboxy-terminal cytoplasmic region of the receptor and co-expression of both mutant and wild-type genes. The mutation was present in the neutropenic phase in one of the patients, suggesting that the mutation was not acquired along with the leukemia. Functional analysis by transfection of mutant or wild-type genes into murine 32D.C10 cells showed that the mutation acted as a "dominant negative" and prevented differentiation in response to G-CSF. Other evidence for an inductive role of receptors comes from murine long-term bone marrow cultures infected with a retroviral c-*fms* vector that yielded a pre-B line with an Ig heavy chain gene rearrangement. This line grew in IL-7 or M-CSF, but interestingly, the switch to M-CSF led to macrophage maturation, suggesting that signals from this receptor can determine differentiation in these bipotent cells.[522] Last, transduction and stable expression of the EPOR in IL-3–dependent Ba/F3 cells results in cells that produce globin mRNA upon stimulation with EPO but not with IL-3,[523] and a chimeric receptor that comprises the extracellular domain of GM-Rα and the cytoplasmic domain of the EPOR can induce increased glycophorin A expression in Ba/F3 cells, in contrast to the GM-Rα/βc control.[524] All of these experiments suggest that elements of the cytoplasmic domains of these receptors can direct both proliferation and differentiation.

Although it is intuitively easy to accept that the cytoplasmic domain of a receptor drives a specific response to its ligand, data for hybrid receptors appear to show just the opposite. These experiments show that the pattern of tyrosine phosphorylation induced by ligand binding is dictated more by the extracellular domain of the hybrid receptor than by the intracellular domain.[525–527] Although the pattern of tyrosine phosphorylation does not correlate with any specific differentiation response, these experiments are perhaps most easily explained by postulating that the extracellular domain of these receptors can interact with other proteins that dictate the phosphorylation response.

The view of lineage specific receptors such as the G-CSFR or EPOR dictating differentiation signals has also been challenged by the introduction of the *Bcl-2* gene into murine multipotent IL-3–dependent FDCP-Mix cells.[528] Parental FDCP-Mix cells continue to proliferate as blasts in IL-3 and differentiate into myeloid or erythroid cells if the concentration of IL-3 is reduced and GM-CSF, G-CSF, or EPO is added; upon withdrawal of IL-3, the cells die by apoptosis. The FDCP-Mix (*Bcl-2*) cells, however, show a delay in apoptosis in the absence of IL-3, and, remarkably, differentiate into granulocytes, monocytes, or erythroblasts in the absence of added growth factors. The horse serum used in these experiments was, however, able to modulate the differentiation outcome, which suggests that some factors present in serum do influence differentiation in this system.

Thus, it is reasonable to conclude that the major role of HGFRs is the survival, amplification, and, particularly in the case of the lineage-specific receptors, the completion of an intrinsic differentiation program of committed progenitor cells.

SIGNAL TRANSDUCTION

HGF–Induced Tyrosine Phosphorylation. More support for the notion that HGFRs merely amplify populations of intrinsically programmed differentiating hematopoietic cells comes from a wealth of data showing that several signaling proteins and pathways are common to many different receptor types. A paradigm common to receptors both with and without endogenous tyrosine kinase activity is that ligand binding induces homodimerization or heterodimerization of receptor subunits, and this is followed rapidly by transient tyrosine phosphorylation of the cytoplasmic domain of the receptor itself, of cytoplasmic tyrosine kinases, and of other cytoplasmic proteins involved in generating different signaling cascades (Fig. 6–18). In the case of the receptors with intrinsic tyrosine kinases, ligand-induced activation of their catalytic function leads to trans- or autophosphorylation of dimerized receptor subunits, but receptors that lack a tyrosine kinase domain must recruit cytoplasmic tyrosine kinases. Data demonstrate that the family of Janus kinases (JAKs) may fulfill this role, but other nonreceptor kinases have been identified and may also be important. It is thought that tyrosine phosphorylation within the receptor cytoplasmic domain creates docking sites for substrates characterized by the presence of Src homology 2 (SH2) domains. These SH2 domains recognize phosphotyrosine in the context of specific short sequences of amino acids.[529]

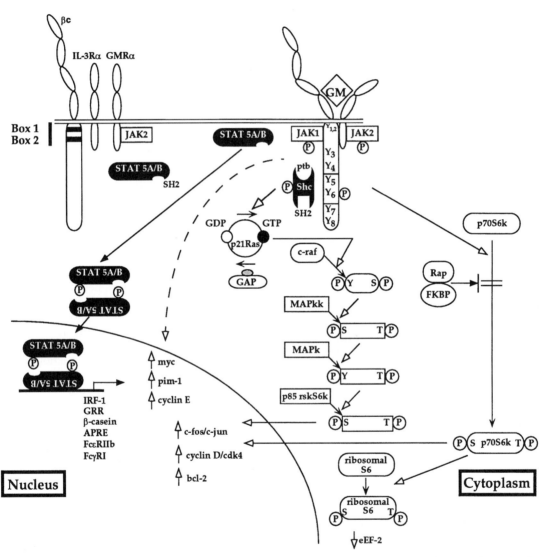

FIGURE 6–18. Signal transduction through the GM-CSF/IL-3 receptor. The figure illustrates that ligand binding (indicated by GM) induces the formation of GMRα/βc heterodimers. This is followed by recruitment of signaling molecules, many of which are shared by other receptors (see Table 6–5). Essential to a proliferative response are the Box 1 and Box 2 proximal cytoplasmic regions of βc and the proximal cytoplasmic domain of GMRα. Janus kinases JAK1 and JAK2 and other nonreceptor tyrosine kinases become phosphorylated, as does βc itself on Y750 (Y6 in the diagram). At least four major pathways are activated: c-*myc* and pim-1 induction by the proximal domain, essential for a proliferative response; JAK-mediated activation of STAT5A and STAT5B, which translocate to the nucleus and activate transcription of genes with specific recognition sequences in their promoters; Shc phosphorylation and binding to βc, followed by Ras activation and phosphorylation of c-raf, mitogen-activated protein kinase kinase (MAPkk), mitogen-activated protein kinase (MAPk), and p85S6k(rsk) and induction of c-Fos/c-Jun and probably bcl-2, important for cell proliferation and survival; and activation of p70S6k, also correlated with the cell proliferation and inhibited by rapamycin (Rap) bound to FK506-binding protein (FKBP). GAP = GTPase-activating proteins; GDP = guanosine diphosphatase; GTP = guanosine triphosphatase; IRF-1 = interferon regulatory factor 1; GRR = interferon-γ response region; APRE = acute phase response element; GMR = GM-CSF receptor; eEF-2 = eukaryotic elongation factor-2.

There are four known members of the JAK family: JAK1, JAK2, JAK3, and Tyk2.[530–532] All are 130- to 134-kD related proteins that have a carboxy-terminal kinase domain immediately downstream of a pseudokinase domain (Fig. 6–19); three of them (JAK1, JAK2, and Tyk2) were first cloned by cDNA rescue of mutagenized cells that failed to respond to IFN-α or to IFN-γ. Thus, both the *TYK2* and *JAK1* genes could functionally reconstitute the cellular response to IFN-α in mutant cells that lack the Tyk2 or JAK1 proteins, respectively.[533, 534]

Although it first appeared that HGFs activated JAK proteins in a rather promiscuous manner, some patterns have emerged (Table 6–5). Thus, receptors that comprise single chains such as the EPOR, G-CSFR, and TPO receptor associate with JAK2 (or to a lesser extent JAK1) in either a constitutive or ligand-dependent manner. Ligand binding and consequent clustering of receptor molecules leads to JAK2 aggregation and transphosphorylation at the lysine-glutamic acid-tyrosine-tyrosine (KEYY) site in the kinase activation loop (Fig. 6–19). For example, EPO induces the rapid tyrosine phosphorylation of JAK2.[535] *In vitro* experiments show that JAK2 phosphorylation leads to activation of its kinase function, which, taken together with evidence of association of JAK2 with the EPOR, suggests that JAK2 may act as the "master" protein tyrosine kinase that mediates the biologic response to EPO. Support for this theory comes from observations that a kinase-negative JAK2 acts as a dominant negative suppressor of the proliferative response to EPO,[536] and that the box1/box2 proximal cytoplasmic domain of the EPOR is the region that both binds JAK2 and is essential for receptor function.[535] However, a number of other substrates are phosphorylated in response to EPO,[537–539] including nonreceptor kinases such as c-fes,[540] the p85 subunit of phosphatidylinositol 3-OH kinase and Vav, substrates such as phospholipase C-γ1 and the adaptor molecule Shc, and the tyrosine phosphatases

hematopoietic cell phosphatase (HCP or PTP-1C) and Syp (also known as PTP-1D or SH-PTP2).

The other receptors that comprise more than one chain appear to associate with and activate several JAKs (see Table 6–5).[541] The β common component of the IL-3/GM-CSF receptor is tyrosine phosphorylated after IL-3 or GM-CSF stimulation.[542, 543] The tyrosine kinase that is responsible for ligand-induced receptor phosphorylation could be JAK2[544] or JAK1,[545] but the role of other recruited nonreceptor kinases such as lyn,[546] fyn,[547] or c-fes[548] has not been clearly defined. Truncation mutants of βc show that the proximal cytoplasmic domain (amino acids 449 to 517) can induce JAK2 tyrosine phosphorylation and kinase activation,[549] and this truncated receptor also retains the capacity to induce c-*myc* and pim-1 and to induce proliferation in serum-replete but not in serum-free conditions.[542, 550–552] Both gp130 and LIFR can associate with and activate JAK1, JAK2, and Tyk2, but the pattern of such JAK family activation is distinct in different cell types.[553]

HGF–Induced Activation of STAT Proteins. The paradigm of the response to interferon has provided another major insight into a subsequent step in JAK family signal transduction. The kinase activities of Tyk2 and JAK1 that are activated after IFN-α binding lead to phosphorylation of 91/84-kD and 113-kD cytoplasmic proteins now referred to as STAT1α/STAT1β, and STAT2, respectively, where STAT stands for signal transducer and activator of transcription. STAT proteins are characterized by conserved carboxy-terminal SH2 domains and less conserved SH3 domains (Fig. 6–19). Tyrosine-phosphorylated STAT1α/β and STAT 2 form heterodimers through their SH2 domains, bind to a 48-kD protein, translocate to the nucleus, and activate gene expression by binding to an interferon-stimulated response element.[554–556] STAT1α is also tyrosine phosphorylated (at Y_{701}) after IFN-γ binds to the IFN-γR, and

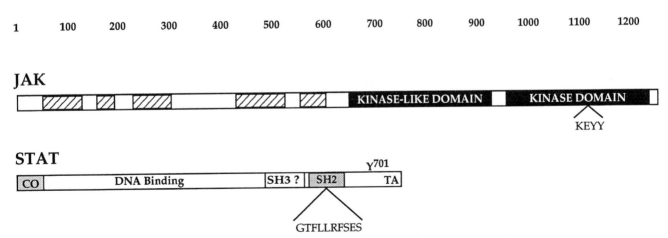

FIGURE 6–19. Structure of JAK and STAT proteins. The JAKs contain a carboxy-terminal tyrosine kinase domain and, immediately amino-terminal, a kinase-like domain of unknown function. Blocks that are homologous among family members are indicated as *black boxes*. The STAT proteins contain an SH2 domain that contains the completely conserved GTFLLRFSS sequence; mutation of the arginine residue eliminates function. The SH2 domain is critical for recruitment to receptors and for STAT dimerization. The SH3-like domain is less conserved and is not known to bind to proline-containing proteins. The DNA binding domain is highly conserved, and after STAT dimerization binds similar symmetrical dyad sequences (e.g., STAT5: TTCC(A→T)GGAA). DNA binding is totally dependent on phosphorylation of a critical tyrosine (Y^{701} in STAT1). The carboxy terminus is required for transcriptional activation (TA). STAT1β lacks this sequence and acts as a dominant negative. The amino terminus is conserved (CO) and is essential for function. (Reviewed by Ihle.[1123]) (Data from Nemunaitis J, Singer JW, Buckner CD, et al: Use of recombinant human granulocyte-macrophage colony-stimulating factor in graft failure after bone marrow transplantation. Blood 1990; 76:345.)

TABLE 6–5. JAK/STAT and Non Receptor Protein Tyrosine Kinases Activated by Hematopoietic Growth Factor Receptors

Receptor	JAK Family	JAK Activated STATS	Other Non-Receptor PTKs
c-kit	JAK2[1094]		PI3K[1095–1097]
IFNRα/β	JAK1[534,557,1098]	Tyk2[533], STAT1[1099], STAT2[1099], STAT3[556]	
IFNRγ	JAK1[534,557,1098], JAK2[534,557,1098]	STAT1[1100]	
IL-3Rα (→β$_c$)	**JAK1**[544], **JAK2**[544]	STAT5[566, 567], STAT6[1101]	Lyn[546,547], Fyn[547], Fes[548], Tec[1102]
GM-CSFRα (→β$_c$)	JAK1[545,549], **JAK2**[545,549]	STAT5[566,567]	**Fes**[548]
IL-6Rα (→gp130)	**JAK1**[559], **JAK2**[559], **Tyk2**[559]	STAT1[560,561,1103], STAT3[559]	**Hck**[1104], **Btk**[1105], **Tec**[1105]
IL-2Rα (→β, γ$_c$)	**JAK1**[1106,1107]	STAT3[1108], STAT5[1109,1110] STAT6(IL-4[1101])	**Lck**[1111], **Fyn**[547], Lyn[547,1112], **Syk**[1113]
EPOR	**JAK2**[535]	STAT5[567,1114,1115]	**Fes**[540]
G-CSFR	**JAK1**[1116], **JAK2**[1117–1119]	STAT3[1117]	**Lyn**[1120], **Syk**[1120], c-rel[1121]

Non-receptor tyrosine kinases that associate with receptors are indicated in bold, and references are in superscript. Adapted from a detailed review by Taniguchi T: Cytokine signaling through nonreceptor protein tyrosine kinases. Science 1995; 268:251. Copyright 1995, American Association for the Advancement of Science.

this event is associated with tyrosine phosphorylation of JAK1 and JAK2.[557, 558] STAT1α homodimerizes, translocates to the nucleus, and binds to the IFN-γ activated sequence (GAS), thereby transcriptionally activating genes that contain this sequence in their promoters.

It was therefore no surprise that the JAK proteins activated by HGFRs also lead to phosphorylation and DNA binding of STAT proteins, and four additional members of the STAT family have recently been cloned, STAT3, STAT4, STAT5, and STAT6 (see Table 6–5). Thus, it has been shown that ligand-induced activation of gp130, the signal-transducing component of the IL-6, LIF, IL-11, OSM, and CNTF family of receptors, leads to tyrosine phosphorylation of the JAK-Tyk family and activation of DNA binding of acute-phase response factor, an 89-kD phosphoprotein antigenically related to STAT1α.[553, 559] The gene for p89 has been cloned (STAT3).[560] Because of its relatedness to STAT1 and STAT2, STAT4 was cloned by low-stringency screening of a cDNA library[561] and by degenerate polymerase chain reaction.[562] Unlike the other STAT proteins, which are ubiquitously expressed, STAT4 expression is restricted to spermatogonia and to thymic and myeloid cells. STAT4 mRNA levels appear to decline when 32Dcl1 cells differentiate in either G-CSF or EPO.[562] IL-12 has been shown to activate STAT4.[563] IL-3 and GM-CSF have been shown to activate a DNA binding protein of 80 kD that, like STAT1α, recognizes the IFN-γ response region located in the promoter of the Fcγ receptor gene.[564] An ovine DNA-binding activity induced by prolactin called mammary gland factor was cloned and is now named STAT5.[565] STAT5 is activated by EPO and growth hormone,[566] and the murine homolog has been shown to be activated by IL-3, GM-CSF, and IL-5.[567] This 92-kD protein exists as two highly related proteins, STAT 5A and STAT 5B (96 percent identical) that are encoded by different genes. STAT6 is most closely related to STAT5 and is induced by IL-4.[568]

Do the JAK or STAT proteins account for the specificity of signaling through different receptors? The JAK family appears to be rather promiscuous in that any JAK appears capable of phosphorylating any STAT in coexpression studies in COS cells. However, studies of factor-dependent cells do show that there is some specificity in receptor recruitment of JAK and STAT proteins (see

Table 6–5).[1122] Taking this information together with the ability of STAT proteins to form homodimers and heterodimers with different affinities to GAS-like promoter elements might begin to explain the specific responses associated with distinct receptors.

HGF Signaling through the Ras Pathway. Attention has focused on Ras as a "turnstile" through which signals from many receptors are routed.[569, 570] Ras guanosine triphosphatase (GTP) can associate with and activate Raf-1 and mitogen-activated protein kinase (MAPK).[571] Ras is a 21-kD membrane-associated protein that cycles between the active GTP-bound and inactive guanosine diphosphate (GDP)-bound forms in response to extracellular signals from various HGFRs, including c-kit, IL-3, and GM-CSF receptors, T-cell receptor, IL-2R, and EPOR.[572–575] Activation of Ras is mediated by guanine nucleotide–releasing factors (GRFs) that catalyze the release of bound GDP and its exchange for GTP, whereas deactivation occurs by GTPase-activating proteins (GAPs) such as p120^{GAP} and neurofibromin that accelerate the intrinsic activity of Ras, leading to hydrolysis of GTP to GDP. The mammalian prototype for GRF-mediated Ras activation is the epidermal growth factor (EGF) receptor, the cytoplasmic domain of which bears intrinsic tyrosine kinase activity. After ligand-mediated dimerization the EGF receptor is activated through auto- or transphosphorylation of tyrosine 1068. An adaptor protein, GRB2, binds to this phosphotyrosine through its SH2 domain. This, in turn, leads to the formation of a ternary complex of EGF receptor, GRB2, and a GRF called SOS, which is analogous to the *Drosophila* son of sevenless (SOS) protein.[569, 570] SOS contains a proline-rich region that recognizes two SH3 domains of GRB2, and the complex then activates membrane-bound Ras GDP to Ras GTP. The proto-oncogene *vav* also has Ras GDP/GTP nucleotide exchange activity[576] and is activated through tyrosine phosphorylation after cross-linking of the T cell antigen receptor–CD3 complex. With respect to the HGFRs, IL-2–mediated activation of the IL-2R leads to IL-2R β chain tyrosine phosphorylation and association of the receptor with Shc, another adaptor protein that is characterized by both an SH2 domain and a second phosphotyrosine binding domain.[577, 578] Shc itself becomes phosphorylated on tyrosine, and this in turn leads to recruitment of GRB2 and SOS.[579] The IL-3/GM-CSF-mediated signaling cascade involves phosphorylation of the β subunit itself as well as of Shc, with subsequent increased levels of Ras GTP and activation of Raf-1, MAPK kinase, and MAPK, followed by induction of c-*fos* and c-*jun*. Interestingly, this activity was mapped to the cytoplasmic domain of $β_c$ between amino acids 626 and 763, whereas a more proximal domain (amino acids 449 to 517) retains the capacity to induce c-*myc* and pim-1.[551] The phosphotyrosine binding domain of Shc has been shown to bind to tyrosine 577 of $β_c$ after JAK2-mediated phosphorylation of $β_c$.[580] The carboxy-terminal domain of $β_c$, including the region that activates Ras appeared not to be important for the proliferative response in experiments with receptor-transduced cell lines that were cultured in serum.[542, 550] However, serum can activate Ras independently of the receptor, and in serum-free cultures Ras activation is important for both proliferative and survival (prevention of apoptosis) functions.[552, 581] In the case of the EPOR, ligand-induced phosphorylation of Shc and the association of Shc with the EPOR has also been demonstrated; phosphorylated Shc associates with GRB2, and Ras and the MAPK pathway is activated.[582–586] In summary, these three examples show that Ras is activated by a number of HGFRs and that the Ras-Raf-MAPK pathway may be important for proliferation and survival of hematopoietic cells.

The Ras pathway may also be important in certain leukemias. Neurofibromin, encoded by the *NF1* gene, is mutated in patients with autosomal dominant neurofibromatosis type 1 (NF-1). *NF1* shows sequence homology with yeast and mammalian *GAP* genes. Children with neurofibromatosis have an increased risk for juvenile chronic myeloid leukemia, monosomy 7 syndrome, and acute myeloblastic leukemia.[587, 588] An important finding is that leukemic cells from children with NF-1 and myelodysplastic syndrome show loss of the normal *NF1* allele, thus implicating *NF1* as a tumor suppressor gene.[588] $NF1^{GAP}$ activity is significantly lower in cell lysates prepared from patients with NF-1-associated leukemia than that in normal bone marrow or non–NF-1-associated leukemic lysates.[589] Bone marrow mononuclear cells from patients with juvenile chronic myeloid leukemia show an increase in CFU-GM in response to GM-CSF, but not IL-3. Interestingly, fetal liver cells from mice that are rendered null for the *NF1* gene show similar hypersensitivity to GM-CSF, indicating that $NF1^{GAP}$ may play a crucial and specific role in the response of myeloid cells to GM-CSF.[589, 590] $NF1^{-/-}$ mice die *in utero* around day 13.5 to 14.5 from complex cardiac defects, but transplantation of day 11.5 to 13.5 fetal liver cells into lethally irradiated recipients produces a myeloproliferative syndrome similar to the human disease.[590] BCR-ABL is a chimeric oncogenic protein that shows dysregulated tyrosine kinase activity and is implicated in the pathogenesis of Philadelphia chromosome–positive chronic myeloid leukemia. A phosphorylated tyrosine (Y^{177}) in the *BCR* first exon binds to the SH2 domain of GRB2 and activates Ras.[591] Mutation of the Y^{177} *BCR-ABL* to phenylalanine abolishes GRB2 binding and abrogates both BCR-ABL-induced Ras activation and transformation of primary bone marrow cultures.[591] In summary, Ras dysregulation may contribute to the increased proliferation that characterizes these two chronic leukemias.

Phosphatases and Receptor Signaling. The carboxy-terminal domain of the EPOR has a negative regulatory role.[592] It is likely that this effect is mediated by a phosphatase that dephosphorylates kinase-associated tyrosine(s) in this region, as has been shown for the IL-3R.[593] There is a fascinating report of a Finnish family with dominantly inherited benign erythrocytosis.[594] The proband, an Olympic cross-country skier, has a mutation in the EPOR that introduces a premature stop codon and generates a receptor lacking the carboxy-terminal 70 amino acids. This mutation co-segregates with the disease phenotype in this large family. Data show that the non-transmembrane protein tyrosine phosphatase SH-PTP1 (also called HCP and PTP-1C) associates via its SH2 domain with tyrosine-phosphorylated EPOR.[595] Mutational analysis mapped the binding site most probably to Y_{429}, and this tyrosine is deleted with the carboxy-terminal truncation of the EPOR in the Finnish family with benign erythrocytosis. Factor-dependent cells that express a $Y_{429,431}F$ mutant EPOR show increased sensitivity to EPO, as do cultured erythroid progenitors from patients with benign erythrocytosis.[595] CFU-E from mice that lack or have impaired SH-PTP1 activity (motheaten or motheaten viable) show a similar increased sensitivity to EPO.[596, 597] Therefore, a strong case can be made for postulating that EPO-induced activation and subsequent tyrosine phosphorylation of the EPOR leads to recruitment of SH-PTP1, which then plays a major role in terminating the EPO signal, possibly through dephosphorylation of JAK2[595] or other tyrosine kinases. Another nonreceptor protein tyrosine phosphatase called SH-PTP2, Syp, or PTP-1B has 50 to 60 percent identity with SH-PTP1 in both SH2 and catalytic domains. Despite this similarity SH-PTP2 appears to be a positive regulator of some growth factor pathways.[598]

Other Inhibitors of HGF Signaling. Two new families of negative regulators have been discovered, the suppressors of cytokine signaling (SOCS) and protein inhibitors of activated STAT (PIAS) proteins. SOCS-1 was discovered by three groups, contains an SH2 domain, and has sequence and structural similarities to an immediate early gene called CIS (cytokine-inducible SH2-containing protein).[498, 499, 516, 599] It is one of an eight-member gene family (SOCS1 through SOCS7 and CIS) that are characterized by a central SH2 domain and a carboxy-terminal conserved motif called a SOCS box. Unlike the constitutively expressed phosphatases, SOCS expression is induced by many cytokines including IL-3, EPO, TPO, IL-6, and LIF, and the proteins are expressed in hematopoietic and other tissues.[600] SOCS-1, expressed predominantly in the thymus, interacts directly with the phosphorylated activation loop of (activated) JAKs, and its amino-terminus is thought to inhibit adenosine triphosphate binding to the activation cleft.[498, 499, 601] Subsequently, the SOCS box is hypothesized to target the SOCS-signaling complex to the proteosome for degradation by recruiting components of the proteosome machinery including elongins B and C and Cullin 2.[602, 603] SOCS-3 has been shown to inhibit signaling by a different mechanism—binding directly to activated receptors and to JAKs without inhibiting JAK activity,[604] whereas CIS can bind to phosphorylated tyrosines on the EPOR and thereby inhibit STAT5 signaling.[516]

SOCS knockout mice have provided insight into the important physiologic roles of some of these proteins. SOCS-1$^{-/-}$ mice die before weaning with fatty degeneration of liver, reduced thymic size, lack of T and B cells, and monocytic infiltration of organs,[605, 606] This phenotype is similar to mice with elevated IFN-γ, and indeed SOCS-1$^{-/-}$ mice have increased IFN-γ levels; rescue of the animals can be achieved by using antibodies to IFN-γ or by crossing mice with IFN-γ$^{-/-}$ mice.[514, 607] SOCS-2$^{-/-}$ mice are normal at birth but then become significantly larger than wild-type mice, with thickening of the dermis due to excess collagen deposition.[608] Therefore, SOCS-2 appears to play an important role in postnatal growth, possibly through the growth hormone/insulin-like growth factor-1 axis. SOCS-3$^{-/-}$ mice are hematopoietically most interesting in that they die at embryonic days 12 to 14 from massive erythrocytosis.[609] Progenitor cells appear to be hyperresponsive to IL-3 and EPO. Thus, SOCS-3 plays a crucial role in inhibiting fetal erythropoiesis. Although CIS-deleted mice show no abnormalities, overexpression of CIS induces a phenotype similar to STAT5a$^{-/-}$ or STAT5b$^{-/-}$ animals.[610–613]

PIAS1 is a member of a family of related proteins that share a putative zinc-binding and highly acidic domains.[614] It appears to be constitutively expressed and binds to activated STAT1 dimers, inhibiting their DNA-binding activity.[615] STAT1 dimers are methylated on a conserved arginine, and methylation appears to be important for PIAS1 binding. PIAS3 is also constitutively expressed and inhibits STAT3-mediated gene transcription in IL-6–stimulated M1 cells.[616]

HEMATOPOIETIC GROWTH FACTORS AND THE CELL CYCLE

To induce cell division, the HGF signaling cascade must eventually activate the cell cycle machinery, which is composed of cyclins, cyclin-dependent kinases (cdks), and other regulatory proteins. Data show that HGFs induce cell proliferation by acting during the G_1 phase of the cell cycle on a family of G_1 or D-type cyclins.[617] Unlike the A-, B-, and E-type cyclins, which periodically oscillate during the cell cycle and regulate the functions of p34^{cdc2} (cyclin B) and p33^{cdk2} (cyclins A and E), the D-type cyclins (D1, D2, and D3) are synthesized in G_1 as delayed early response genes in response to growth factors (Fig. 6–20). Cyclin D1 associates only with p34^{cdk4}, whereas cyclins D2 and D3 can associate with both p33^{cdk2} and p34^{cdk4}. Overexpression of cyclin E leads to a reduction in the duration of the G_1 interval,[618] whereas interference with cyclin D1 function by either antibodies or antisense oligonucleotides can prevent entry into S phase.[619] D-type cyclins contain an amino-terminal LXCXE motif that binds to the retinoblastoma gene product pRb. This motif is shared by the oncoproteins SV40 large T antigen, adenovirus E1A, and papillomavirus E7 that also bind to pRb. The generally accepted view of cyclin function is that the cyclin D–p34^{cdk4} complex initiates pRb phosphorylation in mid-G_1, after which cyclin E-p33^{cdk2} becomes active and phosphorylates pRb on additional sites. Hypophosphorylated pRb binds to the transcription factor E2F, whereas hyperphosphorylation of pRb and its consequent dissociation from E2F allows E2F to promote the expression of target genes, some of which are expressed in S phase.[620] Further insight into the relationships between cyclins, HGFs, and proliferation versus differentiation comes from cyclin D overexpression studies in murine myeloid IL-3–dependent 32Dcl3 cells.[621] The parental cells, which normally express cyclins D2 and D3 but not D1, self-renew in IL-3 but growth arrest and differentiate into granulocytes if switched to G-CSF. p34^{cdk4}, D2, and D3 cyclin levels correlate with the concentration of IL-3, whereas TGFβ1, which induces cell cycle arrest in mid-G_1, blocks IL-3–induced expression of p34^{cdk4} but not of cyclin D2 or D3.[622] In parallel, cyclin D2–associated kinase activity of pRb is induced by IL-3 in vitro and inhibited by TGF-β1 both in vitro and in vivo.[622] Cells that overexpress cyclins D2 and D3 (but not D1) show shortening of the G_1 interval, compensatory lengthening of the S phase, and inability to differentiate in G-CSF.[621, 623] Cells that express a mutant D2 that cannot bind to or hyperphosphorylate pRb are not blocked in differentiation, while the introduction of a kinase-defective mutant p34^{cdk4} into D2 overexpressors restores the G-CSF differentiation response.[621] Thus these data suggest that pRb (and/or related proteins) may play an important role in the regulation of differentiation, consistent with the observations that targeted disruption of the *Rb-1* gene results in death *in utero* with defects in neural development and erythroid differentiation.[624–626] Lethality is probably due to profound anemia, similar to that in the GATA-1[627] and c-*myb*[628] knockouts, which develops during hepatic hematopoiesis. The control and mutant animals contain equivalent numbers of hepatic CFU-E at day 12.5, but those derived from mutant animals are defective in their differentiation capacity and generate fewer erythrocytes.

Several lines of evidence suggest a role for cyclins in oncogenesis. The proliferating cell nuclear antigen and p21 proteins normally associate with cyclin–cyclin-dependent kinase complexes. In cells transformed with DNA tumor viruses, p34^{cdk4} dissociates from cyclin D, proliferating cell nuclear antigen, and p21, and associates instead with a novel 16-kD polypeptide.[629] Cyclin D1 has been implicated in oncogenesis as the putative oncogene *(PRAD1)* that is rearranged in parathyroid tumors, is translocated (as the *bcl-1* oncogene) to an immunoglobulin gene enhancer in some B-cell lymphomas and leukemias, and is amplified in other carcinomas (breast, head, and neck).[630–634]

BIOLOGY OF HEMATOPOIESIS

Stem Cells

The formed elements of the blood in vertebrates, including humans, continuously undergo replacement to maintain a constant number of red cells, white cells, and platelets. The number of cells of each type is maintained in a very narrow range in the physiologically normal adult

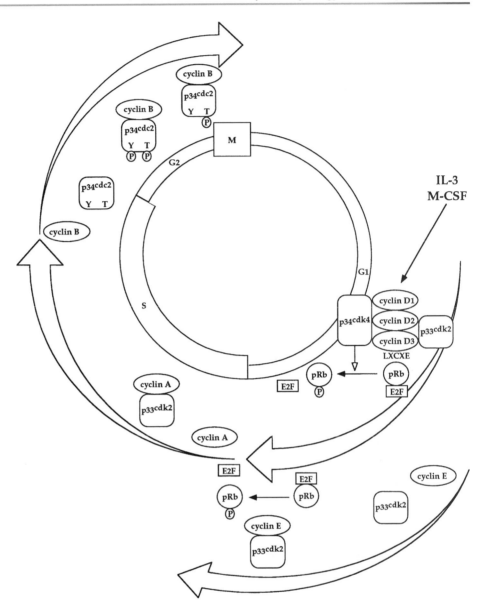

FIGURE 6–20. The cell cycle. The *inner part* of the figure shows the phases of the cell cycle. The *arrows* illustrate the approximate times and oscillating nature of the cyclin regulatory proteins. A, B, and E cyclins appear to oscillate as part of the intrinsic machinery of the cell cycle clock, and as levels increase, they bind to the kinases p33^{cdk2} and p34^{cdc2}. These kinases are activated through complex phosphorylation-dephosphorylation reactions mediated by other kinases and phosphatases (not shown). The G$_1$ or D cyclins are synthesized in response to HGF stimulation such as IL-3 or CSF-1 and bind to p34^{cdk4} (D1, D2, or D3 cyclins) or p33^{cdk2} (D2 and D3 cyclins). These cyclins bear an LXCXE motif that can hyperphosphorylate the retinoblastoma protein (pRb), dissociating it from the transcription factor E2F, which induces genes normally expressed in S phase. Cyclin E-p33^{cdk2} can also mediate this function. (From Sieff CA: Hematopoietic cell proliferation and differentiation. Curr Opin Hematol 1994; 1:310. Copyright 1994, Rapid Science Publishers.)

individual—approximately 5000 granulocytes, 5×10^6 red blood cells, and 150,000 to 300,000 platelets/mL or μL of whole blood (see Appendix for normal values in infancy and childhood). In this section we examine the normal regulatory mechanisms that maintain a balanced production of new blood cells. These regulatory systems are far from completely understood, but present evidence strongly supports the following basic principles, schematically depicted in Figure 6–8:

1. A single pluripotent stem cell is capable of giving rise to many committed progenitor cells. These committed progenitors are destined to form differentiated recognizable precursors of the specific types of blood cells.
2. The pluripotent stem cell is capable of self-renewal. The committed progenitor cells are limited in proliferative potential and are not capable of indefinite self-renewal. In addition to their limited proliferative potential, committed progenitors also "die by differentiation,"[635] and their numbers depend on influx from the pluripotent stem cell pool.

3. The proliferative potential and differentiation of stem cells and committed progenitors may be influenced by adventitial cells or factors derived from them. Thymus-derived lymphocytes appear to contribute to the induction of spleen colony formation in irradiated recipients.[636–639] The hematopoietic role of thymus-derived cells is further supported by experiments demonstrating the defective restorative capacity of bone marrow from congenitally athymic[640] or neonatally thymectomized[641] mice or rigorously T cell–depleted human bone marrow.[642]
4. Committed progenitor cells are capable of response to humoral or marrow stroma–derived regulators, some produced in reaction to the circulating levels of a particular differentiated cell type. In this response, they proliferate and differentiate to form the recognizable blood cells. Under this type of control, amplification of production occurs at the committed progenitor cell level. Most of the regulatory molecules are produced by hematopoietic accessory cells in close proximity to progenitor cells. These

molecules are produced as part of an incompletely understood complex regulatory network operating at close range and may involve accessory cell-progenitor cell interactions. For most hematopoietic lineages studied, there appear to be at least two humoral regulators that work sequentially. The immature progenitor of a particular lineage has a greater requirement for a regulator that acts on all or many immature progenitors than do its more mature counterparts. As differentiation proceeds, sensitivity to the late-acting factor increases. This variable degree of response to late-acting regulators that are present at high concentrations during hematopoietic stress (e.g., EPO in anemia) may protect the highly proliferative but numerically limited immature progenitor compartment from exhaustion or death by differentiation under these stress conditions.

5. Hematopoietic differentiation requires an appropriate microenvironment. In normal humans, this environment is confined to the bone marrow, whereas in the mouse the microenvironment includes both the spleen and bone marrow. The existence of the *Sl* strains of mutant mice[643, 644] that exhibit a deficiency in the hematopoietic microenvironment (see discussion later in this chapter) suggests that the interactions between hematopoietic progenitors and the bone marrow microenvironment involve very specific molecular mechanisms, and data have shown that this is, in fact, so.[645] Progenitors may exist outside the marrow but do not normally differentiate in these extramedullary sites. A number of early hematopoietic cells including the pluripotent stem cells and certain committed progenitor cells have been demonstrated in the circulation of normal individuals and/or experimental animals.[76, 80, 646, 647] The capacity of HSCs to negotiate nonhematopoietic tissues through the circulation is especially significant in relation to bone marrow transplantation, which is carried out by infusion of bone marrow or blood cells from the donor into the circulation of the recipient.[74] For example, blockade of hepatic asialoglycoprotein receptors enhances stem cell engraftment in murine spleen and marrow.[648] There is also convincing evidence that murine stem cells (CFU-S) and progenitors (CFU-GM) express "homing" or adhesive lectin receptors that bind to the mannose or galactose presented on stromal cells. For example, homing of transplanted mouse progenitors can be blocked by synthetic neoglycoproteins with these specificities, suggesting that stromal cells are likely to express these sugars.[649]

What controls the decision of CFU-S to undergo either self-replication or commitment to one of the many alternative differentiation pathways? In 1964 Till and coworkers,[635] in their seminal article, proposed that control of this process was "lax" and that any CFU-S could give rise to "colonies with widely differing characteristics." Careful analysis of CFU-S colonies revealed that while most colonies contained new CFU-S (self-replication), "their distribution among colonies was quite heterogenous with many colonies containing few CFCs and few containing very many." Twenty years later, Suda and colleagues[101] analyzed the differentiation of murine hematopoietic colonies derived from paired progenitors (i.e., CFU-blast progenitors allowed to undergo one division) in culture and showed similar diversity in the colonies derived from each member of more than 25 percent of the pairs. These observations lend further support for lax control or a "stochastic" mechanism of stem cell differentiation and indicate that control of differentiation, as well as amplification, must occur at the committed progenitor cell level.

If only 10 to 20 percent of stem cells are in cycle in the resting state, what is their role with regard to self-renewal versus differentiation, and what is the role of the noncycling stem cells? The hypothesis that a series of stem cells may contribute clones successively to maintain hematopoiesis throughout the life span of an individual was first advanced by Kay.[650] Support for this hypothesis comes from transplant studies of recipients of small numbers of bone marrow cells[651, 652] and from experiments in which mixtures of fetal liver cells from different inbred mouse strains were introduced into *W*-mutant fetuses. *W* mutants exhibit a genetically determined deficiency of HSCs (as well as germ and follicle cells) (see later). Long-term monitoring showed clonal dominance followed by a decline in cells of particular genotypes.[652]

The use of retrovirus-mediated gene transfer to mark HSCs at first lent support to this hypothesis. Analysis of the viral integration patterns at intervals after transplantation has documented concurrent contributions of small numbers of stem cells to hematopoiesis, with changing patterns over time.[653, 654] These conclusions are not supported by the work of Harrison and associates,[655] who measured variances at successive intervals in recipients of marrow mixtures from two congenic donors. The high correlations observed in this study suggest that the transplanted stem cells continuously produce descendants. However, if 10 to 20 (or more) clones are contributing to hematopoiesis simultaneously, then even with clonal succession one might expect variances between two alloenzymes at sequential samplings to be minimized. Furthermore, a longer-term analysis of viral integration patterns in multiple lineage progeny of stem cells transplanted into mice show that integration patterns are unstable initially but then stabilize and maintain a consistent pattern over many months.[656] Although this consistency does not appear to support the clonal succession hypothesis, the contributory role of unmarked stem cells in these experiments cannot be assessed. Furthermore, it is not possible to determine whether the immediate progeny of the transplanted (and retrovirally marked) stem cells might not all still have self-renewal capacity and subsequently contribute to hematopoiesis successively. Such clones would carry the same integration marker. Long-term analysis of female Safari cats (heterozygous for two glucose 6-phosphodiesterase isoforms) that received transplants of small numbers (1 to 2×10^7/kg) of autologous marrow cells showed extensive variation in glucose 6-phosphodiesterase phenotype over a 4-year period.[657] A computer model of the data was consistent with a stochastic model in which stem cells did not replicate more often than once every 3 weeks, which challenges many of the current strategies for inserting foreign genes into HSCs. A problem with the transplant approach discussed earlier is that the preparation required for successful transplantation may perturb hematopoiesis and complicate interpretation of the results. A resolution to the problem came from studies in which a nontoxic dose of bromodeoxyuridine in drinking water was fed to mice.[658, 659] Bromodeoxyuridine is incorporated into DNA by proliferating cells, and measurement of incorporation rates into primitive stem cell populations over time can be used as a monitor of proliferative history. Under steady-state conditions approximately 5 percent of LTR-HSCs were in cycle and another 20 percent in the G_1 phase, with approximately 8 percent entering the cell cycle per day. By 6 days, 1 month, and 6 months 50, 90, and 99 percent, respectively, of the stem cell pool had incorporated the label.[659] Because the size of the stem cell pool remains constant, these data indicate that 50 percent of dividing LTR-HSCs must self-renew; this could be accomplished by asymmetric division or by symmetric division in which half the cells give rise to LTR-HSCs and the other half to differentiating cells.

TRANSCRIPTION FACTORS AND STEM CELLS

Although the factors that control the decision of stem cells to undergo either self-renewal or commitment to differentiate down one of the alternate lineage pathways are poorly understood, nuclear transcription factors have been characterized that play a role in stem or early progenitor cell proliferation and lineage commitment.[660] The tal-1/SCL, rbtn2/LMO2, and GATA families of transcription factors are important for this role. In particular, tal-1/SCL, a basic helix-loop-helix transcription factor, is expressed in biphenotypic (lymphoid/myeloid) and T-cell leukemias[661, 662] and in both early hematopoietic progenitors and more mature erythroid, mast, megakaryocyte, and endothelial cells.[663, 664] Targeted disruption of the *tal-1/SCL* gene leads to death *in utero* from absence of blood formation, and lack of *in vitro* myeloid colony formation suggests a role for this factor very early during hematopoiesis at the pluripotent or myeloid-erythroid stem cell level.[665, 666] Another transcription factor implicated in T-cell acute lymphocytic leukemia is the LIM domain nuclear protein rhombotin 2 (rbtn2/LMO2).[667, 668] Mice that lack this factor die *in utero* and have the same bloodless phenotype as the tal-1/SCL$^{-/-}$ animals.[669] Interestingly, although rbtn2/LMO2 does not show sequence specific DNA binding, immunoprecipitates in erythroid cells show that rbtn2/LMO2 exists in a complex with tal-1/SCL,[670, 671] suggesting a physiologic interaction *in vivo*. GATA-2 is expressed in the regions of the *Xenopus* and zebrafish embryos that are fated to become hematopoietic and is highly expressed in progenitor cells.[664, 672–674] Overexpression of GATA-2 in chicken erythroid progenitors leads to proliferation at the expense of differentiation.[675] Targeted disruption of the *GATA-2* gene by homologous recombination in embryonic stem cells leads to reduced primitive hematopoiesis in the yolk sac and embryonic death by days 10 to 11.[676] Definitive hematopoiesis in liver and bone marrow is profoundly reduced with loss of virtually all lineages, and *in vitro* differentiation data show a marked deficiency of SCF-responsive definitive erythroid and mast cell colonies and reduced macrophage colonies, suggesting that GATA-2 serves as a regulator of genes that control HGF responsiveness or proliferation of stem and/or early progenitor cells. These data contrast with the later time of embryonic death (day 15) from anemia during the mid fetal liver stage in mice with targeted disruption of c-*myb*,[628] *Rb*,[624, 625, 677] and severe forms of *W* and *Sl* mutations (see later).[678] Similarly, loss of function of the *AML-1* gene, which encodes one of the α subunits of the heterodimeric core binding factor (CBF), results in fetal death by day 12.5 due to failure of production of all definitive hematopoietic lineages.[679] CBF recognition sequences are present in the IL-3, GM-CSF, M-CSFR, and T-cell antigen receptor promoters. The *AML-1* gene is often rearranged in acute myeloid leukemia and childhood acute lymphocytic leukemia and is expressed in myeloid and lymphoid cells.[668]

Homeobox (HOX) genes encode transcription factors involved in the establishment of body pattern and tissue identity during development.[680] The human genes occur in four clusters, *HOXA, HOXB, HOXC,* and *HOXD,* on chromosomes 7, 17, 12, and 2, respectively. *HOXA* and *HOXB* genes are expressed in CD34$^+$ cells and are downregulated as these cells mature. Intriguingly, murine bone marrow cells engineered to overexpress *HOXB4* by retrovirus-mediated gene transfer show a dramatic up-regulation in stem cell activity both *in vitro* and *in vivo*.[681] Serial transplantation studies showed a greatly enhanced ability of *HOXB4*-transduced bone marrow cells to regenerate the most primitive hematopoietic stem cell compartment, resulting in 50-fold higher numbers of transplantable totipotent HSCs in primary and secondary recipients, compared with serially passaged control (neo-transduced) cells. This *in vivo* expansion of *HOXB4*-transduced HSCs was not accompanied by identifiable anomalies in the blood of these mice, suggesting that *HOXB4* is an important regulator of very early but not late hematopoietic cell proliferation. Data show that ectopic expression of *HOXB4* in yolk sac and embryonic stem cells confirms long-term engraftment capacity in primary and secondary recipients.[682, 683]

GROWTH FACTORS AND STEM CELLS

HGFs also appear to influence at least some classes of stem cells. Analysis of the actions of HGFs on "purified" murine or human stem and progenitor cells has led to several major conclusions that should be interpreted in the light that, to date, even the most highly purified "stem cell" fractions are still heterogeneous with respect to content of LTR-HSCs, HSCs with short-term reconstituting potential, and lineage-committed progenitors. HGFs such as SCF and perhaps IL-3, GM-CSF, and G-CSF can independently support the survival of murine and/or human stem cell populations.[305, 684–686] However, of all these HGFs only SCF has been shown to enhance the survival of murine LTR-HSCs, and no single HGF or combination of HGFs has unequivocally shown the capacity to induce significant self-renewal of LTR-HSCs.[687, 688] However, SCF and SCF plus G-CSF have been shown to increase the murine

HSC content approximately threefold as determined by competitive reconstitution measured 4 months after transplantation.[689, 690] IL-6–deficient mice show a reduction in CFU-S and failure of IL-6$^{-/-}$ bone marrow cells to contribute to long-term hematopoiesis after serial transfer.[367] In addition to its effect on megakaryocyte and platelet formation TPO is also vital for stem cell production. Mice that lack the receptor for TPO, c-*mpl*, show reduced numbers of blast colonies and CFU-S and fail to compete effectively with normal stem cells for reconstitution of hematopoiesis in irradiated recipients, even when they are transplanted at a 10-fold excess.[691] Furthermore, both murine and human repopulating activity segregates with primitive cells that express c-mpl.[692] In the human system information on HSC self-renewal is not available because no human assay measures this property. Combinations of HGFs are necessary to induce or shorten the time to cell cycling of the most immature stem and progenitor cells. Examples are SCF plus IL-3 or either of these two factors plus IL-6, IL-11, IL-12, LIF, or G-CSF.[241]

Analysis of mutations that affect the function of stem cells and the hematopoietic microenvironment through HGF interactions have provided important insights. Two murine mutations have been characterized in some detail, the *Sl* and *W* mutations.[643, 644, 678] Genetically affected mice that are defective at these loci have a severe macrocytic anemia associated with increased radiation sensitivity, lack of pigmentation, and sterility. Although phenotypically similar, these mutations map to different chromosomes (*W*—chromosome 5, *Sl*—chromosome 10) and have distinct hematologic characteristics. Best characterized at the molecular level, the *W* mutation results in a functional deficiency of HSCs and particularly erythroid progenitors. Transplantation of normal bone marrow into homozygous *W* recipients completely corrects the hematopoietic abnormalities, whereas transplantation of *W* bone marrow into normal mice fails to reconstitute hematopoiesis.[644, 693] The *W* gene is allelic with the c-*kit* proto-oncogene,[694, 695] which, as discussed earlier, is known to be a member of a tyrosine kinase receptor family,[696] as is c-fms, the receptor for M-CSF. Several variants of the W mutation have been shown to be phenotypic expressions of specific mutations of the c-*kit* gene, and the severity of the phenotypic changes associated with specific alleles correlates with the degree of functional impairment of kinase activity.[697]

In contrast, the Steel mutation affects the function of the cells of the microenvironment. *Sl/Sl^d* bone marrow cells are capable of reconstituting hematopoiesis in irradiated normal mice, whereas transplantation of normal bone marrow into *Sl/Sl^d* animals fails to cure the defect.[698] A deeper insight into the molecular nature of this defect was provided by the purification of a factor that is active on mast cells and on mouse bone marrow (enriched for primitive stem cells but depleted of mature progenitors) after 5-fluorouracil treatment.[699, 700] This "stem cell factor" or "mast cell growth factor" was purified, and its cDNA was cloned. Labeling studies with the purified recombinant protein demonstrate that it is the ligand for c-*kit*.[333, 338, 701, 702] Furthermore, administration of the factor to *Sl/Sl^d* mice corrects their macrocytic anemia and repairs their mast cell deficiency. The SCF gene maps to the *Steel* locus on chromosome 10.[703] Confirmation for the hypothesis that SCF is encoded by the Steel gene comes from Southern analysis of stromal lines from normal and *Sl/Sl* embryos (lethal).[334] Although multiple bands are present in the *Eco*RI-digested normal DNA hybridized with the SCF probe, there is no hybridization with the *Sl/Sl* DNA. Moreover, less severe mutations at the *Sl* locus such as *Sl^d* are associated with smaller deletions at the *Sl* locus. The gene encodes a protein that exists in both transmembrane and secreted forms.[333, 704, 705] Thus, it is intriguing to speculate on a stromal cell-stem cell interaction role for SCF, whose biologic properties are characterized by lack of colony stimulating activity alone but marked synergy with many CSFs specific for different cell lineages.

Recently, other growth factor pathways that are important during embryogenesis and that have been subverted in certain cancers have also been implicated in stem cell self-renewal. Notch receptors (four members: Notch1, Notch2, Notch3, and Notch4) are expressed on the surface of a variety of hematopoietic cells as proteolytically cleaved dimers comprising an EGF repeat–rich extracellular domain and a transmembrane/intracellular domain that contains two motifs (RAM and ANK) that can bind to a transcriptional repressor CBF1/RBPJκ.[706] After ligand binding (three ligands: Delta, Jagged1, or Jagged2) the transmembrane/intracellular domain is cleaved to release the active intracellular domain of Notch (ICN), which translocates to the nucleus, binds to CBF1/RPBJk, and transactivates genes such as hairy and Enhancer of split homolog 1 (HES-1), a basic-helix-loop-helix protein that suppresses transcription of N-box (CACNAG) target genes. Human Notch1 was first identified as a gene called TAN-1 that is involved in some T-cell leukemias by generating an intracellular activated form of Notch1 (ICN1).[707] Remarkably, overexpression of ICN1 in murine stem cells leads to immortalization of cytokine-dependent cell lines that can generate lymphoid or myeloid progeny *in vitro* and *in vivo*, suggesting a role for Notch1 in stem cell self-renewal.[708] Addition of soluble Jagged1 to cultures of human purified stem and progenitor cells also increased NOD/SCID repopulating activity.[709] A second signaling pathway that may be involved in stem cell self-renewal involves the Sonic hedgehog (Shh) protein. Shh activates the Smoothened receptor (Smo) by binding to its inhibitor Patched. Smo initiates signaling that regulates transcription factors of the Gli family, which modify expression of genes that encode BMP-4 and its inhibitor Noggin. Shh has recently been shown to induce expansion of human NOD/SCID repopulating cells, possibly through regulation of BMP-2.[709a] Finally, Wnt signaling may also be involved in stem cell self-renewal. Wnt signals through the receptors Frizzled and lipoprotein receptor-related protein to activate a cytoplasmic protein called Dishevelled, which in turn stabilizes β-catenin, a transcriptional co-activator that associates with the Tcf/LEF family of transcription factors.[710] Without Wnt signaling β-catenin is normally destabilized by a cytoplasmic complex that comprises Axin, adenomatous polyposis coli, and glycogen synthase kinase-3β. Overexpression of activated β-catenin in highly purified murine HSCs appears able to expand the pool of transplantable cells.[711]

Two models have been proposed to explain the mechanisms that influence the choice of stem cells between self-renewal and commitment. A *stochastic model* was proposed by Till and colleagues.[635] In this model, self-renewal or differentiation is considered to occur in a random or stochastic manner, only dictated by a certain probability. Because no extrinsic source of stem cells exists, under steady-state conditions the overall probability of stem cell division resulting in self-renewal must be 0.5; probabilities less than or greater than this value would lead to progressive stem cell depletion (aplasia) or expansion (leukemia), respectively. The commitment of stem cells could occur symmetrically, where, overall, half the stem cells divide to produce progeny, both of which enter a differentiation pathway, whereas half the stem cells generate progeny that are both stem cells. Alternatively asymmetric division would give rise to one stem cell and one cell committed to differentiate. Analysis of single cells from blast cell colonies has shown that hematopoietic cells can divide asymmetrically; these micromanipulated single cells give rise to colonies that comprise almost all possible lineage combinations.[101] Single cell analysis of purified human CD34+CD45RA[lo]CD71[lo] provides evidence for quiescent survival, self-renewal, and asymmetric division.[712] These data provide strong support for a stochastic mechanism to explain both commitment and restriction of differentiation potential. Differentiation of single blast cells into mature cells occurs in these methycellulose cultures in the absence of an intact microenvironment. A source of HGFs is obligatory, however, as is the case for all colonies grown in semisolid media. It is important to recognize that although these random events occur with a given probability, it must be possible for that probability to be altered. For example, during the regeneration of hematopoietic tissues after injury by irradiation or cytotoxic drugs, the probability of generating stem cells must increase. How this probability is altered is one of the outstanding unanswered questions in hematopoiesis.

A contrasting model, proposed by Curry and Trentin,[713] postulates that the *hematopoietic microenvironment is inductive* and is based on the observation that domains of a given lineage exist within single spleen colonies. Erythroid hematopoietic inductive microenvironments are thought to be more predominant in murine spleen, whereas granulocytic inductive microenvironments predominate in bone marrow. Transfer experiments showed that granulocytic cells predominate in the junctional region of bone marrow fragments implanted in spleen.[714] A major drawback of this model comes from an analysis of progenitors within these colonies. Correlations are not observed between mature cells and their respective committed progenitors.[715] The preponderance of differentiating cells of one or another type within colonies thus appears to result from events that affect maturation rather than lineage commitment. The nature of these events has not been established, but possibilities include the release of short-range lineage-specific factors by stromal cells, or perhaps the display of such growth factor molecules on the surface of their cell membranes. The Dexter culture system also lends powerful support to an essential role of stromal cells for stem cell survival, because the concentration of stem cells is highest within the adherent stromal

layer itself. This and other observations related to the morphologic characterization of the focal development of hematopoietic islands attached to adherent cells has led to the postulate that HSCs reside within stromal cell "niches" that play a vital role in supporting stem cell survival, perhaps by intimate cell contact.[78]

Whether a stochastic mechanism or one influenced by environmental cues dictates the outcome of the stem cell decision to commit to one or other hematopoietic lineage is also uncertain. Experiments suggest that cross-antagonism among lineage-specific transcription factors may provide a mechanistic explanation for lineage specification. Forced expression of the erythroid-specific factor GATA-1 in myelomonocytic cells perturbs their ability to differentiate,[716] and evidence is accumulating that this is due to direct physical interaction and cross-antagonism of PU.1, the myeloid transcription factor, and GATA-1. GATA-1 inhibits PU.1 by preventing it from interacting with its cofactor c-Jun, whereas PU.1 prevents GATA-1 from binding to DNA.[717–720] Another example is the antagonism between FOG-1 and C/EBP-β in an eosinophilic cell line, in that enforced expression of FOG-1 blocks C/EBP-β–mediated eosinophil differentiation.[721] It is therefore possible that lineage-specific transcription factors not only have potent inductive effects but also exert blocking effects on alternate lineage choices. The observation that forced expression of C/EBP-β in pancreatic cells promoted their differentiation into a hepatic phenotype raises the intriguing possibility that this mechanism underlies stem cell plasticity as well.[722, 723]

In summary, it appears likely that two types of extrinsic control can affect stem cell regulation: at one level is control by stromal cells, perhaps primarily on stem cell survival but also on their response to humoral factors; at a second level are the humoral growth factors, which appear to affect stem cells but probably have a greater effect on the amplification of committed maturing progenitors and precursors. Responses to these growth factors are dictated by the combinations of transcription factors expressed in the developing cells, but how those combinations are regulated remains a major question.

Erythropoiesis

It is well established that the level of oxyhemoglobin and the rate of delivery of oxygen to the tissues is the fundamental stimulus of erythropoiesis.[5] In species that package hemoglobin in erythrocytes, EPO mediates the response to oxygen demand and does so by interacting with specific receptors[724] that are found on the surface of committed erythroid progenitor cells[725–727] and erythroblasts.[728] As discussed earlier, insight into the mechanism by which hypoxia induces a transcriptional increase in the expression of the EPO gene has come from the identification of the hypoxia-inducible transcription factors HIF-1α and HIF-1β.[491, 729]

It is believed that BFU-E do not ordinarily give rise to erythroblasts *in vivo* except under conditions of extreme anemic stress. Instead, they mature to single erythroid CFUs or CFU-E, which divide *in vivo*, and under the influence of lower concentrations of EPO form single, relatively small colonies of proerythroblasts at about 1 week *in vitro*. Many (at least half) CFU-E will form erythroid colonies *in vitro* in response to EPO alone. They do not require the additional presence of either GM-CSF or IL-3, having differentiated beyond this requirement.[730] All proerythroblasts can differentiate in the presence of EPO alone. In the steady state, the number of human CFU-E exceeds the number of BFU-E by a factor of 10. CFU-E are larger than BFU-E and because a larger fraction of CFU-E are in the S phase of DNA synthesis than the fraction of BFU-E, the former exhibit a higher rate of "suicide" in response to exposure to tritiated thymidine. The membranes of mature BFU-E and CFU-E are CD34$^+$ and HLA-DR$^+$, and various negative and positive selection methods may be used to purify them from sources such as bone marrow and human fetal liver.[120, 731] They have the appearance of lymphoblasts.

The bone marrow of an adult mouse contains about 500 CFU-E/10^5 nucleated cells. In response to anemic stress, as in hemorrhage or hemolysis, nearly the entire burden of accelerated reticulocyte production is born by the rapid EPO-dependent influx into the proerythroblast pool from the progenitor compartment.[119, 130] This produces an expanded proerythroblast pool. Little or no increase in the mitotic rate of recognizable erythroid precursors occurs.[119] Instead, the late BFU-E and CFU-E proliferate in response to the engagement of their EPO receptors by the hormone and also differentiate to proerythroblasts and beyond. In normal murine marrow, the CFU-E occurrence of about 500/10^5 nucleated cells increases to 1000 to 2000 CFU-E/10^5 nucleated cells after experimental hemorrhage or hemolysis. In contrast, hypertransfused mice exhibit a reduced number of CFU-E/10^5 nucleated marrow cells (values between 10 and 20 percent of normal have been reported).

During stress erythropoiesis induced by anemia, the orderly progression from immature BFU-E through CFU-E to proerythroblasts is interrupted as high EPO levels appear to permit or induce differentiation of immature progenitors to proerythroblasts. In the rhesus monkey, this premature terminal differentiation may account for the marked increase in fetal hemoglobin content and F cells seen in simian stress erythropoiesis.[732] The ability of human progenitors to generate erythroblasts capable of synthesizing large quantities of fetal hemoglobin is less pronounced.[733] Thus, the accumulation of F cells in peripheral blood in response to anemia is relatively small.[734] Such red cells are usually macrocytic and carry the i antigen as well, but these two characteristics may relate to a short transit time through the marrow in response to EPO rather than to an intrinsic characteristic of fetal hemoglobin–containing cells themselves (see later). F cells are also present in very small numbers in the blood of normal individuals, but these cells are not macrocytic and do not bear i antigen. F cell progenitors can be detected easily in the bone marrow of patients with various dyspoieses[735, 736] and even in marrow from normal individuals.[737]

TRANSCRIPTION FACTORS AND ERYTHROPOIESIS

As discussed earlier, targeted disruption of the *tal-1/SCL*, *rbtn2/LMO2*, and *GATA-2* genes lead to embryonic lethality due to failure of blood production, probably at the level of HSCs. *GATA-1* expression is limited to multipotent progenitors and erythroid, megakaryocyte, mast, and eosinophil lineages.[113, 738, 739] Analysis of chimeric mice injected at the blastocyst stage with GATA-1$^{-/-}$ embryonic stem cells shows a failure of a contribution of the GATA-1$^{-/-}$ cells to erythrocytes but development into other hematopoietic lineages, as well as other tissues.[627, 740] Differentiation assays *in vitro* show proerythroblast arrest and apoptosis of these cells.[741–743] A transcriptional cofactor of GATA-1, Friend of GATA-1 (FOG-1) was discovered and found to be essential for erythropoiesis and megakaryopoiesis.[744, 745] Evidence that this interaction is essential *in vivo* comes from studies of a family with severe dyserythropoietic anemia and thrombocytopenia. Affected family members have a mutation in GATA-1 that disrupts its interaction with FOG-1 without affecting DNA-binding affinity.[746]

GROWTH FACTORS AND ERYTHROPOIESIS

The regulation of the proliferation and maturation of erythroid progenitors depends on interaction with a number of growth factors. The availability of pure recombinant growth factors, the enrichment of target progenitor cells, and the use of defined "serum-free" culture conditions have provided insights into the role of these factors during hematopoiesis.

EPO is essential for the terminal maturation of erythroid cells. Its major effect appears to be at the level of the CFU-E during adult erythropoiesis, and recombinant preparations[730] are as effective as the natural hormone.[747, 748] These progenitors do not require "burst-promoting activity"[749, 750] in the form of IL-3 or GM-CSF, and their dependence on EPO is exemplified by the observation that they will not survive *in vitro* in the absence of EPO. Because the majority of CFU-E are in cycle, their survival in the presence of EPO is probably tightly linked to their proliferation and differentiation to mature erythrocytes. EPO also acts on a subset of presumptive mature BFU-E, which also require EPO for survival and terminal maturation. A second subset of BFU-E, presumably less mature, survive EPO deprivation if burst-promoting activity is present, either as IL-3 or GM-CSF (IL-3 > GM-CSF). When EPO is added to these cultures on day 3, these BFU-E form typical colonies. Similar results are obtained in serum-deprived methylcellulose cultures in which the usual 30 percent fetal calf serum is substituted by bovine serum albumin–adsorbed cholesterol, iron-saturated transferrin, and insulin.[751] Under serum-deprived culture conditions the combination of IL-3 and GM-CSF results in more BFU-E than seen with either factor alone when EPO is added on day 3.[751] Although EPO is crucial for the terminal differentiation of erythroid progenitors, data show that mice with homozygous null mutations of the *EPO* or *EPOR* genes form BFU-E and CFU-E normally, but they fail to differentiate into mature erythrocytes.[362] Both the *EPO*$^{-/-}$ and *EPOR*$^{-/-}$ mutations are embryonic lethal owing to failure of definitive (fetal liver) erythropoiesis. However, yolk sac erythropoiesis is only partially impaired, indicating the existence of a population of EPO-independent primary erythropoietic precursors. SCF has marked synergistic effects on BFU-E cultured in the presence of EPO,[169], [752–754] although alone it has no colony-forming ability. SCF is crucial for the normal development of CFU-E, because mice that lack SCF (*Sl* mutants) or its receptor c-*kit* (*W* mutants) are severely anemic and show a reduction in fetal liver CFU-E.[755] Studies of cell lines that express both c-kit and EPOR (HCD57 cells) or are transduced with cDNAs for these two receptors (32D cells) showed that SCF supports the proliferation of these cells only if the EPOR is also present.[756] Further studies showed that SCF induces tyrosine phosphorylation of the EPOR and that c-kit associates with the cytoplasmic domain of the tyrosine phosphorylated EPOR. Whether such an interaction between c-kit and the EPOR occurs during normal erythropoiesis is not known. Further insight into the molecular mechanism by which EPO prevents apoptosis in erythroid cells comes from studies of STAT5A$^{-/-}$5B$^{-/-}$ mice. During fetal development the embryos are severely anemic; the erythroid progenitors in fetal liver are reduced in number and show increased apoptosis.[757] This result was explained by the finding that STAT5 mediates the early induction of the anti-apoptotic gene *Bcl-X$_L$* through direct binding to its promoter. Interestingly, although adult animals were thought to be hematologically normal, about one half have chronic anemia with splenomegaly, owing to an increase in early erythroid precursors. Erythropoiesis is ineffective because of an increase in apoptosis in these early normoblasts that show reduced levels of *Bcl-X$_L$*.[758]

Progenitors obtained from human fetal liver and cultured in serum-free conditions differ in their requirements for burst-promoting activity and EPO.[759, 760] Although adult BFU-E require IL-3 or GM-CSF and EPO for the development of maximal BFU-E colony number and size, embryonic BFU-E require only EPO for maximal BFU-E cloning efficiency; the addition of IL-3 or GM-CSF increases BFU-E size but not number. These results suggest that EPORs are expressed at an earlier stage of erythroid maturation in fetal cells and that during ontogeny expression of the EPOR becomes restricted to a subset of mature BFU-E and CFU-E. However, cord blood progenitors, in contrast to their adult counterparts, form "spontaneous" CFU-GM in the absence of HGFs, and this can be abrogated by the addition of antibodies to GM-CSF and IL-3. Interestingly, GM-CSF and IL-3 transcripts were detected by reverse transcription–polymerase chain reaction in cord blood CD34$^+$ cells and in the spontaneous colonies, suggesting that the progenitor cells or their immediate progeny may produce these two factors.[761] This provides an alternative explanation for the burst-promoting activity independence of primitive erythroid progenitors. During fetal development, the EPOR may be expressed by even more immature myeloid-erythroid progenitors such as CFU-Mix. Neonates with severe Rh hemolytic disease and very high EPO levels are born with neutropenia and thrombocytopenia.[762] Furthermore, premature infants who received recombinant EPO in a clinical trial developed neutropenia. *In vitro*, high concentrations of EPO reduce the number of CFU-GM colonies and decrease the number of granulocytes per colony, with newborn cells being more sensitive to this effect than progenitors from adults.[763] These results do not appear to result from "crowding" in the culture dishes, because cord blood cells were plated at 10^4 cells/mL. In summary, the data are consistent with the hypothesis that the fetal EPOR is expressed on bi-potent progenitor cells and can influence the subsequent maturation of these cells.

Factors distinct from the classical CSFs may positively regulate erythropoiesis, either directly or indirectly. Limiting dilution studies of highly purified CFU-E in serum-free culture show that insulin and insulin-like growth factor I act directly on these cells.[764] The presence of EPO is essential in these studies, which contrast with earlier murine studies of unfractionated cells in which CFU-E respond to insulin-like growth factor 1 or insulin in the absence of EPO.[765] Another factor that enhances both BFU-E and CFU-E colony formation is activin. This protein dimer, also known as follicle-stimulating hormone-releasing protein, appears to have a lineage-specific effect on erythropoiesis that is indirect, because removal of monocytes or T lymphocytes abrogates its effect.[766] It is interesting that activin has been identified as the factor produced by vegetal cells during blastogenesis that induces animal ectodermal cells to form primary mesoderm.[767] Hepatocyte growth factor has also been shown to have synergistic effects on CFU-GEMM and BFU-E in EPO containing cultures.[768]

NEGATIVE REGULATION OF ERYTHROPOIESIS

Observations that subsets of lymphocytes with an immunologic suppressor phenotype isolated from normal subjects can inhibit erythroid activity *in vitro*[769–771] correlate with reports of patients with a variety of disorders in whom anemia or granulocytopenia is associated with an expansion of certain T-lymphocyte populations.[772–776] In the rare disorder T lymphocytosis with cytopenia,[777] *in vitro* suppression of erythropoiesis has been correlated with the expansion of a T-lymphocyte population that may be the counterpart of the hematopoietic suppressor cells isolated from normal blood. The phenotype of these cells has been described in detail.[777, 778] The cell is a large granular lymphocyte that is both E rosette-positive and CD8 (classic suppressor phenotype)-positive. Suppressor T cells may also be involved in some patients who have aplastic anemia[779, 780] or neutropenia[781] without an underlying immunologic disorder or an overt T-cell proliferation. Exactly how such suppressor T cells interact with hematopoietic progenitors and what surface antigens are "seen" by the suppressors are under investigation. There is evidence to support the concept that suppression of erythroid colony expression *in vitro* is regulated by T cells and may be genetically restricted.[778, 782] Cell-cell interactions in immunologic systems have been well characterized with regard to surface determinants that allow for cellular recognition. That certain phenotypes of T cells "recognize" distinct classes of histocompatibility antigens on immunologic cell surfaces has been well described.[783] Thus, the observation that hematopoietic progenitors have a unique distribution of class II histocompatibility antigens on their cell surface[784–787] suggests a role for these antigens in the cell-cell interactions that regulate hematopoietic differentiation.

T cells may also inhibit erythropoiesis in a non-HLA restricted fashion by the production of inhibitory cytokines. Some lymphokines may inhibit erythropoiesis *in vitro* by a complex lymphokine cascade. Activation of T cells by the T-cell antigen receptor CD3 results in cell surface expression of the IL-2α chain (p55) and the acquisition of IL-2 responsiveness.[788] IL-2 inhibits BFU-E in the presence of these IL-2R[+] cells, possibly by inducing their release of IFN-γ. CD2 can serve as an alternative pathway of T-cell activation, and may do so through binding to its ligand LFA-3 on antigen-presenting cells. Blockade of CD2 with monoclonal antibody leads to abrogation of IL-2/IFN-γ–mediated BFU-E suppression.[789] These data are difficult to reconcile with the observation that IL-2 incubation of PMA/calcium ionophore–activated CD4[+] T cells leads to marked expansion of IL-3 and GM-CSF mRNA[+] cells by *in situ* hybridization.[395] Most, but not all, CD4[+] T cells express CD28 as well, and there is evidence to suggest that IL-3 production is restricted to CD28[+] T cells.[422] It thus appears paradoxical that both potent stimulating and inhibitory lymphokines can be produced by activating T cells through the same pathway.

Tumor necrosis factor also suppresses erythropoiesis *in vitro*.[790, 791] The injection of peritoneal macrophages into Friend murine leukemia virus–infected animal results in rapid, but transient, resolution of the massive erythroid hyperplasia associated with this disease. This may be due to elaboration by macrophages of IL-1α, which does not suppress erythropoiesis itself, but acts by the induction of TNF. This effect is reversed by EPO.[792]

Myelopoiesis

PHAGOCYTE DEVELOPMENT

Although a clonogenic assay of granulocyte progenitors was developed almost a decade before the erythroid clonogenic assay, the various factors responsible for granulocyte-macrophage development remain incompletely understood. Excellent reviews of early work in this field have been provided by Metcalf[108] and Moore.[105]

It is now accepted that CFU-GM is derived from the pluripotent progenitor and, under the influence of SCF, IL-3, GM-CSF, G-CSF, or M-CSF ultimately gives rise to mature granulocytes and monocytes. Monocytes irreversibly leave the circulation[793, 794] and differentiate further into fixed-tissue macrophages, a category comprising the alveolar macrophages,[795] hepatic Kupffer cells,[796] dermal Langerhans cells,[797] osteoclasts,[798] peritoneal and pleural macrophages, and perhaps brain microglial cells.[799] The enormous diversity of this system and the high turnover rate of granulocytes, as well as the necessity to maintain splenic, marginated, and bone marrow granulocyte pools to meet sudden demands caused by infection, has led to the evolution of an extremely complex regulatory network. Indeed, although many of the factors that allow release of granulocytes from storage pools are distinct from CSF,[132] GM-CSF can inhibit granulocyte motility[800] and be an activator of granulocyte superoxide anion generation.[801] This complexity *in vivo* does not per-

mit studies analogous to those in which erythropoiesis is influenced by hypertransfusion or hemorrhage,[802, 803] and megakaryocytopoiesis is stimulated by induced thrombocytopenia.[804] Thus, investigators have relied heavily upon *in vitro* progenitor assays to study the regulation of myelopoiesis.

TRANSCRIPTION FACTORS AND MYELOPOIESIS

A family of transcription factors important for commitment to myeloid and lymphoid lineages and for regulation of myeloid-specific promoters such as those of the myeloperoxidase and neutrophil elastase genes are factors that were first identified on the basis of their ability to bind to the polyomavirus enhancer-binding protein 2/core binding factor (PEBP2/CBF). Two α subunits (CBFα1 and CBFα2 [the human homologue is known as AML-1]) bind DNA with low affinity, and affinity is strengthened in the presence of the non–DNA-binding β subunit (CBFβ). As noted earlier AML-1[−/−] mice die *in utero* by day 12.5 due to failure of production of all definitive hematopoietic lineages.[679] The CCAAT/enhancer binding protein (C/EBP) family of transcription factors bind to DNA through a basic region-leucine zipper domain (bZIP). There are several family members (C/EBPα, C/EBPβ [NF-IL-6], C/EBPγ, C/EBPδ, C/EBPζ, and C/EBPε) that are differentially expressed during myelopoiesis, with an increase (C/EBPβ) or an increase followed by either a partial (C/EBPδ) or a marked (C/EBPα) reduction in the level of expression during maturation of 32D.cl3 cells to terminally differentiated granulocytes.[805] C/EBPα has been implicated in the regulation of hepatocyte and adipocyte differentiation (levels are low in undifferentiated dividing cells but high in quiescent terminally differentiated cells) and also in myeloid CSF receptor promoter function; AML-1 can act synergistically with C/EBPα to activate the M-CSFR promoter.[806] Mice with disruption of the *C/EBP-α* gene show arrested myelopoiesis at the myeloblast stage due to failure of expression of G-CSF and IL-6 receptors.[807, 808] Mice that lack C/EBPβ produce monocytes that are defective in bactericidal and tumoricidal function, and their macrophages and fibroblasts, but interestingly not their endothelial cells, fail to produce G-CSF in response to LPS.[809] C/EBPε is produced primarily in myeloid lineages. Knockout mice are viable and fertile but die at 50 to 75 days from opportunistic infections with *Pseudomonas aeruginosa*.[810] Nullizygous animals fail to produce normal neutrophils and eosinophils. Functional abnormalities include diminished release of hydrogen peroxide in response to PMA stimulation, because of a failure to produce secondary and tertiary granules, which are important reservoirs of membrane-bound components of the reduced nicotinamide adenine dinucleotide phosphate (NADPH) oxidase apparatus. Additional components of secondary and tertiary granules, lactoferrin and gelatinase B, are absent because of failure of transcriptional activation of C/EBPε.[810, 811] Interestingly, similar abnormalities characterize the rare neutrophil-specific granule deficiency,[812] and, indeed, mutations in C/EBPε have recently been found in these patients.[813–815] The PU.1(Spi-1) transcription factor is a member of the Ets family and is expressed principally in monocytes/macrophages and B lymphocytes and also in erythroid cells and granulocytes.[816, 817] Potential target genes include the integrin CD11b, M-CSFR, GM-CSFRα, G-CSFR, and the Igλ light chain.[818–822] Mice that lack PU.1 die *in utero* with absence of monocytes, granulocytes, and T and B lymphocytes; anemia is variable and thus does not explain the prenatal mortality.[823]

GROWTH FACTORS AND MYELOPOIESIS

Murine IL-3 stimulates a broad spectrum of myeloid progenitor cells, including pluripotent stem cells, granulocyte or macrophage CFCs or units (CFU-GM, CFU-G, and CFU-M), BFU-E, CFU-Eo, CFU-meg, and mast cells. As its name implies, GM-CSF was initially shown to act only as a stimulus for the proliferation and development of CFU-GM. However, murine studies with purified or recombinant factor have shown that it also stimulates the initial proliferation of other progenitors such as BFU-E as well (see earlier).[248, 824] The actions of other murine factors, G-CSF and M-CSF, are more restricted; they predominantly stimulate granulocyte and monocyte colony-forming units (CFU-G and CFU-M), respectively.[825, 826]

With the possible exception of GM-CSF, the activities of the human CSFs are similar to those of the corresponding murine factors. Both IL-3 and GM-CSF affect a similar broad spectrum of human progenitor cells. This includes CFU-GEMM, CFU-GM, CFU-G, CFU-M, CFU-Eo, and CFU-meg. In full serum cultures, IL-3 and GM-CSF alone stimulate the formation of colonies derived from CFU-GM, CFU-G, CFU-M, CFU-Eo, and CFU-meg. Data from serum-free cultures suggest that in the presence of IL-3 or GM-CSF alone, myeloid colony formation is much reduced and that optimal CFU-G or CFU-M proliferation requires the addition of G-CSF or M-CSF, respectively, to the cultures.[252, 751] Even in serum-replete conditions, IL-3 acts additively or synergistically with G-CSF to induce more granulocyte colony formation than is observed with either factor alone.[251]

Insight into the *in vivo* role of GM-CSF comes from studies in which the GM-CSF gene was disrupted by homologous recombination in embryonic stem cells.[381] Mice that carried two null alleles of the GM-CSF gene showed normal basal hematopoiesis but developed progressive accumulation of surfactant lipids and proteins in the alveolar space, the defining characteristic of idiopathic human pulmonary alveolar proteinosis. Extensive lymphoid hyperplasia associated with lung airways and blood vessels was also found. Surfactant proteins and lipids are synthesized by type II pneumocytes and cleared from the alveolar space by type II cells and by alveolar macrophages. The lungs from the animals with null mutations showed normal surfactant synthetic capacity and no accumulation in type II pneumocytes. In contrast, the alveolar macrophages showed a marked increase of surfactant protein and lipid, suggesting strongly that these cells cannot process surfactant as a result of the lack of GM-CSF. Mice that were generated with null mutations of the common chain of the GM-CSF/IL-3/IL-5 receptor (β_c) show similar pulmonary pathologic changes and also show low basal numbers of eosinophils and absence of

blood and lung eosinophilia in response to infection with the parasite *Nippostrongylus brasiliensis*.[827] The G-CSF gene has also been disrupted by homologous recombination in embryonic stem cells.[353] G-CSF$^{-/-}$ mice have a chronic neutropenia (20 to 30 percent of normal levels of neutrophils) and reduced numbers of bone marrow myeloid precursors and progenitors. The animals also had a markedly impaired capacity to increase neutrophil and monocyte counts after infection with *L. monocytogenes*.

In addition to their effects on progenitor differentiation, the CSFs also induce a variety of functional changes in mature cells. GM-CSF inhibits polymorphonuclear neutrophil migration under agarose,[800] induces antibody-dependent cytotoxicity for human target cells,[801] and increases neutrophil phagocytic activity.[246] Some of these functional changes may be related to GM-CSF–induced increase in the cell surface expression of a family of antigens that function as cell adhesion molecules.[828] The increase in antigen expression is rapid and is associated with increased aggregation of neutrophils; both are maximal at the migration inhibitory concentration of 500 pmol/L, and granulocyte-granulocyte adhesion can be inhibited by an antigen-specific monoclonal antibody. GM-CSF also acts as a potent stimulus of eosinophil antibody-dependent cytotoxicity, superoxide production, and phagocytosis.[829] G-CSF acts as a potent stimulus of neutrophil superoxide production, antibody-dependent cytotoxicity, and phagocytosis,[830] whereas M-CSF activates mature macrophages[831] and enhances macrophage cytotoxicity.

It is apparent then that the actions of the CSFs on mature cells parallels their spectrum of activity on immature progenitors. Murine IL-3, in contrast to human IL-3, does activate neutrophil function. The explanation for this difference lies in the observation that murine IL-3 neutrophils express the IL-3 receptor,[832] whereas it is undetectable on the surface of human neutrophils.

Megakaryocytopoiesis

The cloning of TPO has greatly clarified our understanding of the regulation of megakaryocytopoiesis.[150] Before the discovery of TPO, several factors,[833] including IL-3,[834] IL-6,[835] IL-11,[836] SCF,[837, 838] and even EPO[839–841] were shown to stimulate megakaryocytopoiesis and thrombopoiesis *in vitro* and *in vivo*. IL-11 has even entered clinical trials.[317] IL-3, IL-6, and IL-11 engage heterodimeric receptors of the β common (IL-3R) and gp130 families (IL-6R and IL-11R). SCF engages a receptor the intracellular domain of which expresses tyrosine kinase activity upon ligand binding. As already emphasized in this chapter, ligand engagements of these receptor families are known to induce early multipotent progenitors to proliferate and even differentiate toward lineage-specific progenitors, and SCF, IL-3, and IL-11 participate in the induction of the proliferation and differentiation of lineage-specific progenitors. Hence, all of the just-mentioned HGFs, except EPO, can contribute collectively to what is known biologically as megakaryocyte colony-stimulating activity (meg-CSA).[840] EPO is probably not a functional component of meg-CSA. It induces only slight megakaryocyte differentiation and only at high concentrations.[842] It probably does so because the developing erythroid progenitor passes through a stage of trilineage restriction that includes erythroid, megakaryocytic, and basophil potential,[113] and because, as previously mentioned, EPO and TPO share structural homology.

Meg-CSA is therefore a "soup" of growth factors that transduce three of the four classes of receptors that drive hematopoietic differentiation.[833] Three of these include the familiar β common, tyrosine kinase, and gp130 families. All of these receptors, when engaged, drive early progenitor proliferation and partial differentiation to more mature progenitors, but the final steps of lineage-committed mature progenitor development into recognizable marrow precursors require a lineage-specific growth factor—G-CSF for the granulocyte, M-CSF for the macrophage, IL-5 for the eosinophil, and EPO for the erythrocyte.

The discovery of TPO provides the final step of understanding of megakaryocytopoiesis because this factor, and probably none other, actually induces lineage-restricted megakaryocyte progenitor proliferation, differentiation of those committed progenitors to megakaryoblasts, and, finally, differentiation of megakaryoblasts to the megakaryocytes that in turn produce platelets (Fig. 6–14). However, this in no way implies that other meg-CSA components may not be useful in the therapy of hypoplastic thrombocytopenias. As is emphasized later, circulating TPO levels are high in those conditions just as EPO levels are elevated in the erythroid hypoplasias. Administration of high doses of EPO is usually of little benefit in the latter conditions. TPO may be just as unsuccessful in certain megakaryocyte hypoplasias because those conditions are often associated with severe depletion of lineage-specific or multipotent progenitors. One or more of the growth factors that comprise meg-CSA, such as IL-11, may be more useful in such circumstances. Clinical trials now in progress will decide that issue.

THROMBOPOIETIN

In 1993, Methia and co-workers[843] performed what proved to be a critically important experiment. They demonstrated that exposure of CD34+ progenitor cells in culture to oligonucleotides that were antisense to c-*mpl*, a proto-oncogene, inhibited the ability of these cells to form megakaryocyte, but not other hematopoietic, colonies. This experiment, conceived in the laboratory of Francoise Wendling, had its roots in Wendling's 1986 description of *mpl*, an oncogenic viral complex that produces a murine myeloproliferative and, ultimately, leukemic disease.[844] Four years later, Wendling's group cloned the virus and demonstrated that a gene transduced by the virus might be a cytokine receptor and was responsible for the transforming function.[845] Two years later, another French group, including one member of Wendling's laboratory, cloned the human homologue of *mpl* and demonstrated that it is a member of the HGFR superfamily. The physiologic ligand for this receptor was, as yet, unknown.[846, 847]

Wendling's 1993 experiment strongly suggested that the unknown ligand might be the long-sought TPO, and in 1994 several laboratories cloned or purified and sequenced the all-important growth factor[151, 335, 339, 848] and important physiologic studies of TPO were launched, particularly by Kaushansky.[150] As previously mentioned, the *TPO* gene is localized on the long arm of chromosome 3. It contains five exons, the boundaries of which line up precisely with those of the *EPO* gene. The gene enjoys widespread tissue expression, including liver, kidney, smooth muscle, endothelial cells, and fibroblasts. Thus, TPO is produced at the site of hematopoiesis. Therefore, although its activity is increased in the blood during episodes of thrombopenia, it does not necessarily function as a hormone because it is produced directly at the site of thrombopoiesis. In this sense, it differs from EPO, which is not produced at all in marrow stroma. It is likely that the level of production of TPO is quite constant in all tissues. The blood levels may increase in thrombopenic states merely because circulating platelets and tissue megakaryocytes sop up the growth factor and carry it out of the circulation.[154, 849] This theory has received support from observations in mice with disruption of the murine transcription factor gene called *NF-E2*[117]; although these animals are thrombocytopenic, they have an increase in megakaryocyte mass and no increase in serum TPO levels.★

As reviewed by Kaushansky,[150] the TPO molecule is considerably longer than the other HGF polypeptides. Its 5′ half has 23 percent sequence homology to EPO, while the 3′ half has no structural homology to any cytokine and may be removed by a proteolytic mechanism. Indeed, removal of this half does not ablate physiologic function. The resemblance of the 5′ domain of the molecule to EPO may explain the synergy of TPO and EPO in megakaryocyte colony formation and platelet production.[150, 833] It is well recognized that splenectomized individuals with persistent anemia usually have significant thrombocytosis, and many individuals with red cell aplasia and high EPO levels also have thrombocytosis and megakaryocytosis.

The function of TPO has been studied carefully *in vivo* and *in vitro*. Although some of the *in vitro* experiments can be criticized because it is very difficult to achieve conditions in which only one factor at a time is studied, the model of megakaryocytosis discussed in the introduction to this section has been loosely confirmed.[150] Lineage-specific CD34+ megakaryocyte progenitors have receptors for SCF, IL-3, IL-11, and TPO, the four major classes of hematopoietic cytokine receptors. Maximal megakaryocyte colony formation probably requires signaling by all four receptors, but TPO is absolutely required for the final stages of megakaryocyte maturation, including maximal ploidy and cytoplasmic volume, and, therefore, platelet production.

Early therapeutic trials of TPO in mice have shown that TPO is species specific. Treatment of mice with murine TPO induces massive thrombocytosis, whereas human TPO is much less active in these animals. More importantly, TPO is active in reducing the platelet nadir in mice and primates rendered thrombopenic by chemotherapy or radiation. Whether it will be superior to IL-11 in this regard will probably depend upon the extent of the progenitor depletion that occurs in human diseases. For

---

★(Shivdasani R, Orkin S, de Sauvage F: unpublished observations.

example, repeated doses of chemotherapy in patients with cancer may reduce the progenitor pool so much that drugs that induce proliferation of progenitors such as IL-3 or IL-11 may be more effective than TPO or be required in addition to TPO for maximal restoration of megakaryocyte development.

CIRCULATING PLATELETS

The differential diagnosis of thrombocytopenia depends first on evaluation of platelet morphologic characteristics. In conditions in which megakaryocytopoiesis is accelerated, circulating platelet volume (and usually diameter) is increased. The reasons for this shift in volume are disputed. Some claim that young platelets are larger than old platelets.[850] Others suggest that large megakaryocytes give rise to large platelets.[851] Neither explanation satisfies all experimental and clinical conditions, but, in general, thrombocytopenia secondary to increased destruction of platelets is associated with platelets of large volume, and thrombocytopenia related to decreased production of platelets is associated with platelets of normal size. There are major exceptions to this rule. Patients with hyposplenism tend to have large platelets in their blood, whether thrombopoiesis is increased or not, and patients with primary abnormalities of platelet function, such as Wiskott-Aldrich syndrome or Bernard-Soulier syndrome, have platelet sizes that have no relationship to platelet production. TPO increases platelet production by increasing both the number and size of individual megakaryocytes. Although TPO is probably solely responsible for the later stages of recognizable megakaryocyte differentiation and proliferation of megakaryocyte progenitors, its function depends, at least in part, on the additional stimulation of megakaryocyte progenitors (and probably early megakaryocytes as well) with other growth factors, including IL-3, IL-11, and SCF. As discussed earlier, the latter contribute, in combination, to what is known as "meg-CSA."

DOWN-REGULATION OF MEGAKARYOCYTES

There is great uncertainty about possible down-regulation of megakaryocytes. Platelet factor 4 seems to down-regulate colony formation *in vitro*,[852] which, if active *in vivo*, would provide an interesting feedback loop. TGF-β is also a potent inhibitor *in vitro*.[853] NK cells, which are thought by some to be general suppressors of hematopoiesis *in vitro*, actually enhance megakaryocyte colony formation *in vitro*.[852] In addition, an antibody to NK cells, when it is given intraperitoneally in massive doses to mice, abolishes the formation of colonies of megakaryocytes that can be grown in culture from murine marrow, suggesting that NK cells may actually play a stimulatory role *in vivo*.[854] These are interesting studies that are, however, subject to varying interpretations.

MEGAKARYOCYTE PROGENITORS IN DISEASE

A number of attempts have been made to relate diseases associated with elevated or depressed platelet counts to the number or the growth characteristics of megakaryocyte progenitors.[855] Most attempts have been relatively nonproductive, and very few have been carried out for childhood platelet disorders. Of particular interest is thrombocytosis, a generally benign condition in childhood.[856] Of greater importance is essential thrombocythemia. Megakaryocyte progenitors in the latter condition have growth characteristics similar to those of the expanded numbers of erythroid progenitors in polycythemia vera. The latter develop into erythroid colonies without additions of EPO to the culture medium. The trace of EPO in the serum is sufficient to drive the sensitive receptor system in these progenitors. In a similar fashion, the numerous CFU-meg in essential thrombocythemia develop into megakaryocyte colonies in the absence of stimulation by aplastic anemia serum.[857] They are "TPO independent" and many produce endogenous TPO.

CONCLUSION

It is obvious that the literature on megakaryocytopoiesis is becoming understandable. The general rules are similar to those that pertain in erythropoiesis and phagocytopoiesis, and the specific details have been greatly clarified by the discovery of TPO.

CLINICAL USE OF HEMATOPOIETIC GROWTH FACTORS

Correction or amelioration of marrow failure syndromes by administration of HGFs has been and continues to be the major practical goal of research in hematopoiesis. The goal could not be achieved, however, until recombinant DNA technology provided sufficient amounts of the hormones to permit interpretable investigations.

Animal Studies

IL-3

The discovery, cloning, and expression of the gene for murine multipotential CSF (multi-CSF) or IL-3 presented the first opportunity to evaluate HGFs in an unambiguous fashion.[858, 859] Sublethally irradiated mice were infused for 7 days with recombinant multi-CSF or with control protein.[860] The spleens of the multi-CSF–treated marrow recipients were much larger than those of the controls, were more cellular, and contained more progenitors. The increase in progenitor cells affected erythroid and myeloid lineages. In contrast, bone marrow cellularity was unaffected and progenitor content was reduced. Metcalf and colleagues[861] injected mice with purified bacterially synthesized IL-3 by the intraperitoneal route and obtained similar results. In addition, 10-fold increases in blood eosinophil and 2- to 3-fold increases in neutrophil and monocyte levels were observed. The intraperitoneal injections also resulted in 6- to 15-fold increase in peritoneal phagocytes with an increase in macrophage phagocytic activity.

These experiments clearly demonstrate that murine IL-3 influences the replication and growth potential of primitive hematopoietic progenitors and strongly suggest that whatever effect such hormones have on blood counts are related to their influences on progenitor function rather than to their effects on peripheral blood cell kinetics. They also suggest that the function of mature cells can be altered *in vivo*, an effect that would be expected to decrease rather than increase numbers of circulating phagocytes.

GM-CSF

The first indications that the human hematopoietic growth factor, GM-CSF, could broadly stimulate hematopoiesis *in vivo* resulted from studies of the infusion of COS cell–produced GM-CSF into cynomolgus macaques.[862] Recombinant (r) human (h) GM-CSF acts on simian progenitors. The disappearance curve of intravenously injected metabolically labeled factor is complex and suggests a multicompartment turnover model, but the overall initial half-time of 15 to 20 minutes clearly demonstrated that infusion of the hormone at a concentration sufficient to maintain a functional blood level could be achieved.[862] The effects of such infusions into normal *Macaca fasicularis* were striking. Large increments in all classes of leukocytes, including eosinophils and lymphocytes as well as reticulocytes, were observed during the hormone infusion. When the hormone treatment was terminated, the blood counts rapidly fell toward normal. A particularly striking reticulocytosis was observed in an animal with an acquired retroviral infection that was associated with secondary pancytopenia and an elevated EPO level. This "preclinical" trial in a severely ill monkey encouraged the conclusion that GM-CSF might play an important therapeutic role in various cytopenias such as those observed in viral infections, including acquired immunodeficiency syndrome (AIDS), or in autologous or allogeneic marrow transplantation.

The potential role of human recombinant GM-CSF in marrow transplantation was evaluated by the infusion of autologous marrow into rhesus monkeys (*Macaca mulatta*) 2 hours after lethal total body irradiation.[863] Recombinant hGM-CSF was administered at a daily dose of 50 units/min/kg continuously from 10 to 19 days before radiation or from 9 to 17 days beginning 2 or 3 days after irradiation. Both dosage schedules produced the same final results, although the blood counts of the animals that received the hormone before radiation were much higher at the onset of radiation than those who received the hormone only after radiation. In five separate studies, granulocytes recovered to a level greater than $1,000/mm^3$ in 9 days rather than the minimum of 17 days observed in two untreated controls. In four of the five experiments, platelets recovered more rapidly as well.

G-CSF

Human G-CSF has also been evaluated in simian preclinical trials. Cynomolgus monkeys treated with two daily subcutaneous injections of purified G-CSF for 14 to 28 days showed a dose-related increase in polymorphonuclear neutrophils, the plateau being reached after 1 week.[864] At the intermediate dose of 10 µg/kg/day, total white blood cell counts of 40,000 to 50,000/µL were observed. Neutrophil function was also enhanced. In addition, results were achieved in two cyclophosphamide-treated animals that received G-CSF either from 6 days before until 21 days after the cyclophosphamide treatment or for 14 days from day 3 after cyclophosphamide. In both monkeys, the neutrophil count increased dramatically by days 6 to 7 after cyclophosphamide administration, reaching levels of 50,000/µL by the 10th day. The control animal remained pancytopenic for 3 to 4 weeks after treatment.

THROMBOPOIETIN

rhTPO or its polyethylene glycol (PEG)-derivatized 163-residue amino terminus megakaryocyte growth and development factor (PEG-MGDF) stimulates megakaryocyte proliferation and endoreduplication *in vitro* and is a potent inducer of megakaryocytopoiesis and platelet production *in vivo* in mice and nonhuman primates.[335, 339, 340, 865–867]

Human Clinical Studies

Several recombinant HGFs are currently being evaluated in a variety of clinical settings. Largely because of availability, initial studies focused on GM-CSF and G-CSF in both transient and long-standing bone marrow failure syndromes and EPO in the anemia of chronic renal failure. Other HGFs, such as M-CSF, SCF, IL-1, IL-11, and TPO are being evaluated. The availability of recombinant growth factors that stimulate myeloid progenitors raised several possibilities. First, they might shorten or prevent the hypoplasia that follows chemotherapy and make more intensive myeloablative chemotherapy regimens possible. However, because GM-CSF and IL-3 receptors are expressed by several nonhematopoietic cell types, malignancies of these cell lineages might also respond to growth factor therapy.

MALIGNANT DISEASE

G-CSF. In the first phase I/II clinical studies in patients with malignant disease, administration of G-CSF by bolus or continuous intravenous infusion before chemotherapy led to a dose-related increase in polymorphonuclear neutrophils.[868, 869] Rapid increases in neutrophil counts were observed, with maximal counts of 80 to 100×10^9/L at doses of 10 to 30 µg/kg/day. A transient depression in neutrophil counts was noted to precede this increase in one study.[870] In another study, rhG-CSF was given for 14 days after alternate cycles of intensive chemotherapy.[871] The period of neutropenia was reduced by a median of 80 percent (52 to 100 percent) in the chemotherapy/G-CSF cycles, with a return to normal neutrophil counts within 2 weeks after chemotherapy. Infective episodes were observed during the cycles with chemotherapy that did not include G-CSF, whereas no infective episode occurred in those that did. G-CSF treatment after chemotherapy results in a significant reduction in the number of days per patient in which the neutrophil count is less than 1.0×10^9/L.[868] Antibiotic use to treat fever and neutropenia is also reduced, and all the patients could receive their next course of chemotherapy on schedule (versus 29 percent of patients who did not receive G-CSF). The mature neutrophils produced in response to G-CSF have normal mobility and bactericidal capacity.[872] A double-blind, randomized, placebo-controlled U.S. multicenter trial in which patients with lung carcinoma who received up to 6 cycles of cyclophosphamide, doxorubicin, and etoposide were given G-CSF or placebo from days 4 to 17 of each cycle. The results showed a reduction in the median duration of severe neutropenia ($<0.5 \times 10^9$/L) from 6 to 3 days in the G-CSF arm and a 50 percent reduction of febrile neutropenia, hospitalizations, confirmed infections, and antibiotic use with G-CSF.[873] This study and other reports[874, 875] have led the American Society of Clinical Oncology to recommend the primary use of G-CSF in patients with an expected rate of neutropenia that exceeds 40 percent.[876] The use of G-CSF has allowed dose intensification in patients with lung carcinoma, with the suggestion that overall survival may be improved.[877, 878] However, larger randomized clinical trials are needed to answer this question more conclusively. Patients in the placebo arm of the U.S. multicenter trial[873] who developed fever in the first treatment cycle were subsequently treated with G-CSF, and this reduced the duration of severe neutropenia from 6 to 3 days and the duration of neutropenic fever from 100 percent in cycle 1 to 23 percent in cycle 2. Thus, the prophylactic use of G-CSF in chemotherapy-induced neutropenia is supported. However, the literature does not support the use of G-CSF or GM-CSF after afebrile[879] or febrile neutropenia has developed,[880, 881] with the exception of one study.[882] Although the number of days of neutropenia may be fewer, it has been difficult to show an effect on clinically significant endpoints such as shortened duration of hospitalization, which was seen in only one of the studies.[881]

The effect of G-CSF on progenitor cells is interesting. After administration of melphalan and GCF, the absolute number of *circulating* progenitor cells of the granulocyte-macrophage, erythroid, mixed, and megakaryocyte lineages show a dose-related increase up to 100-fold after 4 days of treatment with rhG-CSF,[883] confirming earlier animal studies.[884, 885] The relative proportions of the early and late granulocyte progenitors and of early progenitors of different lineages remain unchanged; however, the number of CFU-E, normally undetectable in blood, is markedly increased. In most patients there was a slight reduction in the occurrence of *bone marrow* progenitors, although this is difficult to interpret in view of the possibility of variable blood cell contamination of bone marrow samples. The mechanism for this increase in all progenitors in the blood is unclear; G-CSF has been shown to affect immature blast CFCs, and it is possible that stem cells are stimulated *in vivo* to produce increased progenitors of all classes; alternatively, G-CSF may indirectly stimulate progenitors by induction of HGF production or by release into the circulation of bone marrow progenitor cells.

GM-CSF. rhGM-CSF has been administered in phase I/II studies to several adult groups of patients with advanced malignancy, both before and after chemotherapy.[886–888] Glycosylated GM-CSF produced in either mammalian (Chinese hamster ovary) cells or yeast and *Escherichia coli*–derived nonglycosylated GM-CSF have been evaluated with comparable results. A rapid, dose-related increase in polymorphonuclear neutrophils, monocytes, and eosinophils is observed in patients treated before chemotherapy. Neutrophils peak at approximately 20 to 30×10^9/L at doses from 4 to 32 µg/kg/day and GM-CSF is well tolerated at doses up to this level. A capillary leak syndrome and venous thrombi are observed at higher doses (64 µg/kg/day).[886] Phase III randomized trials in patients with lymphoma or breast cancer have confirmed that GM-CSF given after chemotherapy is associated with shorter periods of neutropenia and higher leukocyte nadirs.[889–891] However, one of these studies included only the patients able to tolerate treatment and was not significant on an intention-to-treat basis. Furthermore, another study of GM-CSF after chemotherapy showed decreased neutropenia after the first treatment cycle only,[892] whereas another two studies showed no improvement in neutrophil counts.[893, 894] In one of these studies[893] patients with small cell lung cancer were given chemotherapy and radiation; compared with the placebo control group, patients in the GM-CSF arm suffered more infections, deaths from toxicity. and longer hospital stays, and therefore the American Society for Clinical Oncology panel has cautioned against the use of CSFs in combined chemotherapy/radiation regimens.[876, 895]

Similar encouraging results have been obtained in children with solid tumors undergoing intensive chemotherapy.[896–898] Significantly shorter durations of severe neutropenia and thrombocytopenia were observed in a study of 25 children in whom yeast-derived GM-CSF was given at 60 to 1500 µg/m^2/day for 14 days after chemotherapy.[896]

Like G-CSF, GM-CSF also produced an increase in blood progenitor cells of both erythroid and myeloid lineages. Before chemotherapy, an 18-fold increase in blood CFU-GM and an 8-fold increase in BFU-E was noted; after chemotherapy, GM-CSF produced a much greater increase of progenitors (60-fold) when given during the recovery period.[899]

IL-3. A phase I/II study of the effect of rhIL-3 in patients with nonhematopoietic malignancies with normal marrow function, as well as lymphomas and bone marrow failure, was reported.[900] Doses that ranged from 30 to 500 µg/m^2 were given for 15 days by daily subcutaneous injection. In the patients with normal hematopoiesis a dose-dependent increase (1.4- to 3.0-fold) in neutrophils was observed, with the major increase during the second week. This contrasts with the rapid neutrophil response that has been the experience with GM-CSF or G-CSF. Platelets and eosinophils also increased in a dose-dependent fashion up to the dose of 250 µg/m^2/day (1.3- to 1.9-fold), and increases in basophil and lymphocytes were noted. Increases in reticulocytes that did not appear to be dose-related were also observed in 70 percent of the patients. Similar results were observed in the patients with bone marrow failure, but stimulation of malignant B cells was seen in two patients with lymphoma. Examination of the bone marrow showed increases in cycling of CFU-GEMM, BFU-E, and CFU-GM, with increased bone marrow cellularity.[901] There was also an increase in blood CFU-GEMM and CFU-GM, but a reduction in BFU-E.

In conclusion, results from this initial human IL-3 study indicate that IL-3 can induce a multilineage hematopoietic response.

TPO. Because of TPO's potent *in vitro* activity and its role as the factor essential for terminal megakaryocytic differentiation, analogous to EPO for the erythroid lineage, clinical studies designed to assess its affect on platelet production have been reported. Both rhTPO and PEG-MGDF are safe and show no organ toxicity, and in normal volunteers a single bolus of 3 µg/kg/day of PEG-MGDF doubles the blood platelet concentration by day 12 with a return to baseline by day 28.[867] A stimulatory effect on platelet production was observed when TPO or PEG-MGDF was administered after chemotherapy to more than 100 cancer patients, with a decrease in the time for platelet counts to return to normal and elevated platelet nadirs.[902–904]

Other HGFs. Partially purified urinary M-CSF has been evaluated in patients with different malignancies who received myelotoxic chemotherapy. After treatment, patients received M-CSF for 5 days, and a modest increase in neutrophils was observed. Monocytes and other hematopoietic lineages were unaffected.[905] IL-11 has been shown to ameliorate the thrombocytopenia associated with chemotherapy for breast cancer[317, 906] and has been approved by the Food and Drug Administration for secondary prophylaxis of thrombocytopenia after chemotherapy. IL-1, given at 0.03, 0.1, or 0.3 µg/kg/day for 5 days, was used in 43 adults with advanced neoplasms, before or after carboplatin chemotherapy.[907] A third of the patients (5 of 15) given one of the higher two doses after chemotherapy had minimal thrombocytopenia (platelets >90,000/µL versus median 19,000/µL. without IL-1).

BONE MARROW TRANSPLANTATION

GM-CSF, G-CSF, and M-CSF have been evaluated in clinical autotransplantation trials.

GM-CSF. Patients with nonhematopoietic malignancies were treated with high-dose combination chemotherapy, autologous bone marrow transplantation, and rhGM-CSF given by continuous intravenous infusion for 14 days beginning 3 hours after bone marrow infusion. There was a dose-related increase in the neutrophil count at day 14 (1411 cells/µL at 2 to 8 µg/kg/day, 2575 cells/µL at 16 µg/kg/day, and 3120 cells/µL at 32 µg/kg/day, compared with 863/µL in 24 historical control subjects).[908] Although not statistically significant, there was an improved neutrophil count in patients who had not received previous chemotherapy compared with those who had (1832 versus 833/µL). A lower morbidity and mortality were also noted among the patients who received the GM-CSF; bacteremia occurred in 16 percent of treated patients compared with 35 percent of control subjects able to be evaluated. Comparable results were reported in a study of patients with lymphoid malignancies who received rhGM-CSF as a 2-hour infusion daily for 14 days after chemotherapy, radiotherapy, and autologous bone marrow transplantation.[909] Neutrophil and platelet counts recovered more rapidly, there were fewer days with fever, and the extent of hospitalization was reduced in comparison with a historical control group. In the only reported pediatric study, nine patients received 5 to 10 µg/kg/day of GM-CSF after bone marrow transplantation. Neutrophil recovery was accelerated, although there was no difference in the incidence of fever infection or length of hospitalization compared with historical control subjects.[910]

The response to GM-CSF after myelosuppression may depend on the infusion of sufficient progenitor cells. In an autotransplantation study of patients with acute lymphoblastic leukemia, bone marrows were purged with 4-hydroperoxycyclophosphamide and anti-T- or anti-B-cell lineage-specific antibodies before transplantation.[911] In 30 percent of the patients who received >64 µg/m²/day an absolute neutrophil count of more than 1000/µL by day 21 was achieved, whereas the absolute neutrophil count in none of patients who showed no response reached this level by day 27 after transplant. The responder group required only one third as many platelet transfusions, and there was a trend for fewer red cell transfusions, higher ratio of myeloid cells to erythroid cells in the bone marrow, and an earlier day of discharge in the responder group as well. Although bone marrow cell dose did not differ among the two groups, the number of CFU-GM progenitors infused per kilogram was significantly higher in the responder group compared with the nonresponder group (17.5 [12 to 27] × 10³/kg versus 2 [0 to 7.2] × 10³/kg). It is possible that this increased number of progenitors accounts for the more rapid recovery rather than the rhGM-CSF infusion because the responder group all showed a rapid decrease in absolute neutrophil count within 48 to 72 hours of discontinuation of GM-CSF. This result is consistent with a stimulatory effect on bone marrow. One can conclude that GM-CSF is effective in this context provided that sufficient progenitor cells are present.

G-CSF. rhG-CSF was evaluated in patients with hematopoietic and nonhematopoietic malignancies after intensive chemotherapy and reinfusion of cryopreserved autologous bone marrow.[912] The rhG-CSF was given by continuous intravenous infusion from 24 hours after marrow infusion for a maximum of 28 days, beginning at 20 µg/kg/day; the dose was reducing after the neutrophil count persistently exceeded 1 × 10⁹/L. The mean time to recovery of neutrophil count (>0.5 × 10⁹/L) occurred by day 11, 9 days earlier than in historical control subjects. This led to significantly fewer days of parental antibiotic therapy, but there was no effect on red cell or platelet counts. Although the rate of recovery from neutropenia was faster than that reported for rhGM-CSF, the latter studies were phase I dose escalation evaluations, and many patients did not receive an optimal dose of GM-CSF. One study compared G-CSF with GM-CSF in exactly the same analogous bone marrow transplant protocol. The G-CSF group contained more patients with breast carcinoma who had received previous chemotherapy, and this group did not show a dose-related increase in neutrophil count after a 14-day continuous intravenous infusion at doses of 16, 32, and 64 μg/kg/day. Overall, however, recovery of total leukocyte count was slightly more rapid in the G-CSF group compared with the GM-CSF group. G-CSF administration resulted in two leukocyte count peaks. The first at day 10 comprised lymphocytes, while the second at day 14 comprised mostly granulocytes; in contrast, GM-CSF produced a single peak at the end of the period of infusion. A major difference was observed with respect to neutrophil migration to an inflammatory site during CSF infusion after hematopoietic reconstitution.[913] Neutrophils did not migrate to skin chambers filled with autologous serum during GM-CSF treatment, a defect not encountered during the administration of G-CSF. There was, however, a similar reduction in the incidence of bacteremia with both GM-CSF and G-CSF (18 and 19 percent, respectively) in comparison with the historical control subjects (35 percent).

In conclusion, if neutrophil count recovery is the goal after bone marrow transplantation, then G-CSF appears to be the factor of choice. It preserves neutrophil function and is well tolerated. The inability to hasten platelet count recovery is still the major challenge.

TPO. PEG-MGDF was evaluated in a controlled trial of 50 breast cancer patients who received chemotherapy with autologous bone marrow; the time during which platelets numbered less than 20,000/μL was reduced (P <0.6), and the time to recovery of normal platelet counts was significantly shortened. However, when mobilized blood progenitor support was given rather than bone marrow, the more rapid recovery made it difficult to demonstrate an effect of PEG-MGDF on duration of thrombocytopenia or platelet transfusion requirements.[867]

M-CSF. Human urinary M-CSF has been evaluated in a phase II study of patients with different malignancies who received cyclophosphamide, total-body irradiation, and either allogeneic or autologous bone marrow.[914] Human urinary CSF was given for 14 days by a 2-hour intravenous infusion daily starting at day 1, day 4, or day 14. In patients who received CSF early, there was a significant reduction in the time to a neutrophil count to reach greater than 1×10^9/L compared with a control group (16.7 versus 25.4 days). However, the time to recovery of the control group is somewhat delayed in comparison with other reports (17 to 21 days).

MYELODYSPLASIA

GM-CSF. Despite the theoretical risks of treating patients with myeloid stem cell clonal diseases with the CSFs, the factors have been evaluated in patients with refractory anemia, refractory anemia with an excess of blasts, refractory anemia with an excess of blasts in transformation, and chronic myelomonocytic leukemia.[915–917] In an early study, GM-CSF was given by continuous infusion for 14 days and repeated after a 2-week rest period.[915] Five of the eight patients had received chemotherapy up to 4 weeks before study. Doses of 30 to 500 μg/m² were used. Blood leukocytes rose 5- to 70-fold and neutrophils rose 5- to 373-fold, and an absolute

increase in monocytes, eosinophils, and lymphocytes was also observed. Three of the eight patients also had a 2- to 10-fold increase in platelet count and improvement in erythropoiesis, and two of the three no longer required transfusions. Marrow cellularity increased, and there was a reduction in the proportion of blasts, although there was a transient and dose-related increase in the absolute number of circulating blasts. No patient developed overt leukemia during the period of follow-up (up to 32 weeks). There was no cytogenetic evidence for a reduction in the number of abnormal clones, and it is likely that the stimulatory effect on hematopoiesis affects both normal and abnormal cells. A dose-related increase in neutrophils, monocytes, eosinophils, and lymphocytes was also noted in a study of 11 patients with myelodysplasia. However, four patients who had more than 14 percent blasts in the bone marrow showed an increase in blasts after therapy, whereas an additional three patients showed an increase in blasts in the blood; five patients developed acute leukemia either during or within 4 weeks after treatment.[917] Unlike the earlier report, none of these patients had received previous chemotherapy.

G-CSF. A small number of patients have been treated with G-CSF.[918, 918] Neutrophil count responses were seen in five patients with myelodysplasia who received 50 to 1600 μg/m²/day by a 30-minute infusion daily for 6 days. At the higher doses (400 μg/m²/day), the increase was sustained and associated with an increase in bone marrow cellularity. No reticulocyte or platelet count increases were observed, and no patient's condition progressed to an acute phase. Similar results were reported in a study of 12 patients given G-CSF by daily subcutaneous injection, with dose escalation from 0.1 to 3 μg/kg/day over an 8-week period.[919] Although 10 of the 12 patients showed elevations in neutrophil counts (5- to 40-fold), an increase in reticulocyte count occurred in five patients with a reduction in requirements for transfusions in two patients. There was no response in other cell lineages and no progression to acute leukemia.

Other HGFs and Combinations of HGFs. Approximately 20 percent of patients show an increase in platelet counts during treatment with IL-3,[920, 921] and a similar proportion show an increase in hematocrit or a reduced requirement for transfusions with EPO administration.[922] This erythroid cell response can be increased to about 40 percent if EPO treatment is combined with either G-CSF[923, 924] or GM-CSF.[925]

APLASTIC ANEMIA

GM-CSF. Establishing a role for the CSFs in aplastic anemia will challenge investigators. Severe aplastic anemia is a heterogeneous disease that may result from either absent or defective stem cells, from microenvironmental defects, or from immunologically mediated suppression. Mortality is high and therapeutic options are limited to bone marrow transplantation if an appropriate donor is available or to immunosuppression (see Chapters 7 and 8). Whereas bone marrow transplantation can be curative, treatment with antithymocyte globulin is sometimes effective but generally is not curative. Other modalities such as cyclosporine and androgens may be partially effective in some patients. For these reasons rhGM-CSF has been evaluated in a number of phase I/II studies. Administration of rhGM-CSF by bolus or continuous IV infusion for 7 or 14 days resulted in increased granulocyte, monocyte, and reticulocyte counts in six of eight patients.[916] In another small study rhGM-CSF was given to cohorts of patients in escalating doses from 4 to 64 μg/kg/day by continuous intravenous infusion for 14 days. Although a dose-related effect was not observed, 10 of 11 patients able to be evaluated had partial or complete responses indicated by increases in neutrophil, monocyte, and eosinophil counts, with increases in bone marrow cellularity also. Importantly, the greatest increments occurred in patients with higher pretreatment neutrophil counts and more cellular marrows. Only 10 to 20 percent of patients show an increase in hemoglobin concentration and platelet count, and in all patients counts return to baseline after cessation of treatment.[926, 927] In the first report of rhGM-CSF treatment in childhood, three quarters of the patients able to be evaluated responded with a significant increase in neutrophil count during the 28-day induction period.[928] Although neutrophil counts returned to baseline after cessation of treatment in all the patients with severe aplastic anemia who responded, in one patient with moderate aplasia a trilineage response was maintained for longer than 1 year with no therapy. One cannot extrapolate from such a small experience, but the data underscore the point that responses are more likely in patients with less severe disease.

Thus, in summary, it appears as though rhGM-CSF treatment has a palliative effect in aplastic anemia, with greater neutrophil count responses seen in patients with less severe disease. Patients with the most severe disease respond poorly.[929] No infections were observed during the study period in several reports, whereas infections were observed in others. Longer-term prospective comparative studies are necessary to investigate morbidity.

G-CSF. Neutrophil count responses have also been reported in a study of 20 children given 400 μg/m²/day G-CSF for 14 days.[930] In 12 patients neutrophil counts were doubled, but other lineages were unaffected. In another pediatric study high doses of G-CSF (400 to 2000 μg/m²/day) induced neutrophil count responses in 6 of 10 patients with very severe aplastic anemia.[931] Long-term treatment may be associated with multilineage cell responses when given alone[932] or in combination with cyclosporine.[933]

IL-3, IL-6, and EPO. Hematopoietic responses have been reported in a small phase I study of nine patients with aplastic anemia given IL-3 250 to 500 μg/m² (in five neutrophil counts were doubled, in four an increase in reticulocyte counts but no reduction in requirements for transfusion was seen, and in one platelet counts increased from 1 to 31×10^9/L).[900] An increase in platelet count was reported in one of six patients entered in a phase I study of IL-6, although a dose-related decrease in neutrophil, monocyte, and lymphocyte counts was observed, and a proportion (approximately one third) of patients given EPO show a reduced requirement for transfusion and/or an increase in Hb.[934] Also promising preliminary results, including trilineage cell responses, have been reported in a small number of patients with refractory aplastic anemia

treated with low doses of GM-CSF plus EPO[935] or G-CSF plus EPO.[936] The effects of EPO are unexpected because endogenous levels are very high in aplastic anemia.

HUMAN IMMUNODEFICIENCY VIRUS INFECTION

GM-CSF. Human immunodeficiency virus (HIV) infection is associated with several hematologic abnormalities including neutropenia, anemia, and thrombocytopenia. Anemia and neutropenia can be exacerbated by treatment with azidothymidine, and rhGM-CSF has been evaluated in an effort to enhance immunologic and hematopoietic function and improve tolerance to therapeutic agents. In the first report of the use of rhGM-CSF in humans, cohorts of AIDS patients were treated with increasing doses of factor given by 14-day continuous intravenous infusion.[937] This resulted in a rapid, dose-related increase in neutrophil, band cell, and eosinophil counts, with a slight increase in monocyte count. A follow-up study with subcutaneous administration showed that these effects could be sustained for up to 6 months without evidence of tachyphylaxis.[938]

A concern with the use of GM-CSF in AIDS is possible enhancement of HIV replication. In one study of azidothymidine given on an alternate-week schedule with GM-CSF, some patients showed increased viral p24 levels during therapy with GM-CSF. There is evidence, however, that GM-CSF may in fact augment azidothymidine levels in monocytes, which suggests that the combination of azidothymidine and GM-CSF might be advantageous.[939] This is not the case with newer nucleoside analogs such as dideoxycytidine and dideoxyinosine.[940] Two clinical studies have documented an increase in HIV p24 antigen while patients were receiving GM-CSF,[941, 942] and therefore GM-CSF has been replaced by G-CSF for the treatment of neutropenia.

G-CSF. In a pilot study at the National Institutes of Health G-CSF was evaluated in 19 pediatric patients with AIDS who developed neutropenia while receiving azidothymidine. The neutrophil count increased from a median of 1×10^9/L to 2.9×10^9/L at doses from 1 to 20 μg/kg/day, and in 17 of the 19 patients continued azidothymidine therapy was well tolerated.[943] Of note was the development of thrombocytopenia in some patients; two patients developed G-CSF–dependent disseminated intravascular coagulation; and one patient developed an increase in myeloblasts that disappeared after G-CSF treatment was stopped.[940]

EPO. EPO has been used in 12 anemic pediatric patients to determine if tolerance to azidothymidine could be improved.[940] EPO administration was well tolerated, and at doses from 150 to 400 units/kg subcutaneously or intravenously three times per week azidothymidine therapy could be maintained in all patients with a marked (four patients) or moderate (four patients) reduction in the requirement for transfusion.

TPO. PEG-MGDF has been evaluated in six thrombocytopenic patients with HIV infection in a randomized placebo-controlled study.[944] Platelet counts increased 10-fold within 14 days and were sustained for the 16 weeks of the study, returning to previous levels within 2 weeks of cessation of treatment. There was no evidence of increased viral load or anti–PEG-MGDF antibodies. Megakaryocytic apoptosis, which was abnormal before treatment, was shifted into the normal range by TPO treatment, suggesting that the mechanism of action involves increased effectiveness of the platelets that are produced.

BONE MARROW FAILURE SYNDROMES

The use of HGFs in the treatment of inherited bone marrow failure syndromes has been reviewed in detail.[945]

Fanconi Anemia. GM-CSF has been studied in seven patients with Fanconi anemia,[946] and, IL-3 and G-CSF are being evaluated in clinical trials.[945] Results show that all three HGFs can improve the neutrophil count in most pancytopenic patients, but platelet and hemoglobin levels are unaffected.

Diamond-Blackfan Anemia. Although there is no evidence that Diamond-Blackfan anemia is due to deficiency of EPO,[947] IL-3, or GM-CSF,[753] or an abnormality of c-*kit* or its ligand SCF,[948, 949] it is possible that pharmacologic doses of these factors might stimulate erythropoiesis. Niemeyer et al[950] observed no reticulocyte count or hemoglobin responses in nine patients treated with rhEPO doses as high as 2000 units/kg/day. In contrast, three of six patients treated with IL-3 (60 to 125 $\mu g/m^2$/day subcutaneously for 4 to 6 weeks) had increases in reticulocyte counts, and two of the patients who responded did not require transfusions for 1.5 to 2 years after no therapy.[951] In another IL-3 study[952] 4 of 18 patients treated with 0.5 to 10 $\mu g/kg$ subcutaneously responded. Two of the patients who responded developed deep vein thromboses necessitating discontinuation of treatment, whereas in the other two patients responses were sustained, one of these received maintenance treatment with IL-3 for 31 months and one received no treatment for 12 months after 30 months of therapy. In another study of 13 patients no responses were observed.[953] Thus, 6 patients have had significant erythroid cell responses to IL-3 of a total of 37 (14 percent), a rate similar to that reported by the European working group for Diamond-Blackfan anemia (3 of 25).[954]

Amegakaryocytic Thrombocytopenia. Amegakaryocytic thrombocytopenia is a rare disease that presents in infancy or early childhood with thrombocytopenia, often with anemia, and with development of pancytopenia. Bone marrow megakaryocytes are absent or extremely scarce. A phase I/II IL-3 dose escalation study without or with sequential GM-CSF in five children with amegakaryocytic thrombocytopenia showed that IL-3 (but not IL-3/GM-CSF) induced platelet count increases in two patients and decreased bruising, bleeding, and transfusion requirement in the other three.[834] In the two patients with initial platelet count increases, a reversal was seen after several months of IL-3 maintenance treatment (125 to 250 $\mu g/m^2$/day), whereas another patient no longer needed platelet transfusions after 4 months of IL-3 treatment and had a trilineage cell response that was sustained for almost 2 years. Five patients have been treated with PIXY321 (IL-3/GM-CSF fusion protein), and in two the platelet count increased.[945]

Severe Congenital Neutropenia (Kostmann Disease). Severe congenital neutropenia (SCN) (Kostmann disease) (see also Chapter 8) is a disorder of myelopoiesis characterized by impaired neutrophil differentiation and absolute neutrophil counts less than 200/μL. In contrast, monocyte and eosinophil counts are normal or increased. The bone marrow shows maturation arrest at the promyelocyte stage, and these cells are often atypical, with abnormal nuclei and vacuolated cytoplasm. The pathophysiology is uncertain. Reduced production of or abnormal G-CSF is a possibility, but unlikely in view of data showing that serum from these patients contains normal or elevated levels of G-CSF, as determined by Western blot and bioassay.[955] A progenitor defect is a more likely cause, because *in vitro* cultures show normal CFU-M and CFU-Eo but impaired differentiation of CFU-G in the presence of either GM-CSF or G-CSF. Another possibility is that the GM-CSF or G-CSF receptor is abnormal. The number and affinity of G-CSFRs is normal in patients with SCN,[956] and a single-strand conformational polymorphism analysis of the cytoplasmic domain of the receptor showed no evidence for structural abnormality in six patients.[957] However, other investigations show mutations in the C-terminal "differentiation" domain of the G-CSFR in two patients.[521] Recently, the majority of patients with SCN were shown to have mutations in the neutrophil elastase gene *ELA-2*.[957a,957b]

The responses of these patients to administration of exogenous G-CSF and GM-CSF are of great interest. One study compared the effects of GM-CSF and G-CSF in a small number of patients, and G-CSF alone was evaluated in other studies.[958–960] In these investigations *G-CSF produced a remarkable increase in neutrophil count in all patients*. The dose necessary to maintain a neutrophil count greater than 1000/μL varied and ranged from 3 to 15 $\mu g/kg$/day. The monocyte count was also increased. In contrast, rhGM-CSF produced an increase in neutrophil count in only one patient, whereas the others showed an increase in eosinophil and monocyte counts. Although the period on study was short, no new episodes of severe bacterial infection occurred during either GM-CSF or G-CSF treatment; this contrasts with the recurrent bacterial and fungal infections that occurred before treatment. In a multicenter phase III study of G-CSF in 120 patients with severe chronic neutropenic disorders including SCN, Shwachman-Diamond syndrome, and myelokathexis, complete responses were seen in 108 patients (absolute neutrophil count > 1.5×10^9/L), partial responses in 4 patients, and failure to respond in 8 patients.[961]

Somatic mutations of a single allele of the G-CSFR that result in loss of the C-terminal differentiation domain of the receptor were described in several patients with SCN and shown to act as a dominant negative in transduced cells.[962, 963] These patients may eventually develop myelodysplastic syndrome (MDS) or acute myeloblastic leukemia (AML) or both.[521] Data from the SCN International Registry[964] for 506 patients with SCN, cyclic neutropenia, and idiopathic neutropenia who were treated in phase I, II, and III clinical G-CSF trials showed that 23 of 249 patients with SCN/Shwachman-Diamond syndrome (neutropenia and pancreatic insufficiency) patients developed MDS/AML, compared with none of the 97 patients with cyclic neutropenia or 160 patients with idiopathic neutropenia. The observation that patients with SCN but not with cyclic or idiopathic neutropenia who are receiving G-CSF develop MDS/AML is consistent with reports of AML in patients with SCN before the introduction of G-CSF treatment[965, 966] and show that SCN is a preleukemic disease. Additional cytogenetic changes (translocations and monosomy 7) and oncogene *(ras)* mutations are common in the patients that develop MDS/AML.[967] The G-CSFR mutation is present in myeloid cells only and was not present in first-degree relatives of affected patients, including a sibling with SCN,[968] demonstrating that the mutation is acquired.

In summary, treatment with G-CSF has had a major positive impact on the lives of the majority of patients with SCN. Continued treatment has increased the risk of emergence of leukemic clones in this preleukemic disease, and patients need to be monitored regularly for their appearance.

Cyclic Neutropenia. Cyclic neutropenia (see also Chapter 22) is a rare hematopoietic stem cell disease due to mutations in neutrophil elastase. It is characterized by regular 21-day cyclic fluctuations in numbers of neutrophils, monocytes, eosinophils, lymphocytes, platelets, and reticulocytes. Patients typically have recurrent episodes of fever, malaise, mucosal ulceration, and, occasionally, life-threatening infection during periods of neutropenia. Six patients were treated with intravenous or subcutaneous rhG-CSF for 3 to 15 months at doses ranging from 3 to 10 µg/kg/day.[969] The median neutrophil count increased from 0.7×10^9/L to 9.8×10^9/L. In five of the patients, cycling of blood counts continued, but the length of cycles decreased from 21 to 14 days. The number of days of severe neutropenia (<200/µL) was reduced from a mean of 12.7/mo to less than 1/mo and, importantly, the nadir counts increased; neutrophil turnover increased almost fourfold, and migration to a skin window was normal. Average counts of other cells did not increase. One patient with disease of adult onset had a qualitatively different response with an increase in neutrophil count and disappearance of the cyclic fluctuations in the count. Therapy reduced the occurrence of oropharyngeal inflammation, fever, and infections, demonstrating that treatment with rhG-CSF is effective management for such patients. These results have been confirmed in other studies and rhG-CSF is well tolerated.[970–972] GM-CSF was not effective in two patients but eliminated severe neutropenia when given at a low dose (0.3 µg/kg/day).[973–975]

Chronic Idiopathic Neutropenia. This disorder of myelopoiesis is characterized by maturation arrest of neutrophil precursors in the bone marrow and neutrophil counts of less than 1.5×10^9/L; and other cell lineages are not affected. Patients have mucosal ulcers, periodontal disease, and recurrent infections. The pathophysiology is uncertain; *in vitro* bone marrow culture shows normal numbers of myeloid progenitors, and antineutrophil antibodies are absent. A single patient who received 1 to 3 µg/kg/day of rhG-CSF by subcutaneous injection showed normalization of the absolute neutrophil count with healing of chronic oral ulceration, reduction of episodes of recurrent infection, and minimal side effects.[976] Cycling of neutrophil, monocyte, and platelet counts was induced with a 40-day periodicity; this contrasts with the normal 21-day cycle and out-of-phase fluctuation of neutrophil and monocyte counts seen in cyclic neutropenia.

ANEMIA OF CHRONIC RENAL FAILURE

EPO. Anemia is a major complication of end-stage renal failure and is due primarily to a reduction in EPO production. Other mechanisms that may be involved are shortened red cell survival, iron deficiency, hypersplenism, possible circulating inhibitors of erythropoiesis, and aluminum-induced microcytosis. Several phase I, II, and III studies have documented that rhEPO can induce a dose-dependent increase in effective erythropoiesis.[977–979]

In a phase III study patients received 150 or 300 units of rhEPO three times per week after hemodialysis; a target hematocrit of 35 percent was reached by 8 to 12 weeks.[978, 979] The majority of patients required a dose of 50 to 125 units/kg intravenously three times per week after dialysis to maintain a hematocrit of approximately 35 percent. The increase in erythropoiesis required to normalize the hemoglobin concentration requires mobilization of a considerable amount of iron; patients whose conditions improve rapidly, in particular, can develop absolute or relative iron deficiency. If iron is not given, the response to rhEPO becomes blunted; the standard corrective measure is intravenous administration of iron dextran or oral iron supplementation. Regular measurements of ferritin and transferrin saturation are necessary to ensure that iron stores are adequate.

EPO has been well tolerated, has resulted in elimination of patients' dependence on transfusions, and has not led to antibody formation. Hypertension, occasionally with encephalopathy, has been observed, particularly with rapid increases in hematocrit that lead to an increase in peripheral vascular resistance; induction with doses not greater than 150 units/kg is recommended to produce a gradual increase in hemoglobin levels. Some patients require either initiation of antihypertensive medication or an adjustment of dose.

The effect of rhEPO in most studies appears to be restricted to the erythroid lineage. However, data from a phase III study of 303 patients show a significant increase in mean platelet count (224 to 241×10^9/L at 6 months), which is not biologically meaningful. There is also a slight increase in blood urea nitrogen, creatinine, and serum potassium levels. The bone marrow progenitors from patients with end-stage renal failure were studied before and 2 weeks after rhEPO treatment. The concentration of BFU-E, CFU-E, and CFU-meg increased after therapy. Surprisingly, an increment in CFU-GM also occurred, and the number of progenitors of all classes in the cell cycle almost doubled.[980]

Subjective improvement in appetite, energy, sleep pattern, and libido are also noted. A Canadian double-blind, placebo-controlled study of rhEPO treatment has provided objective evidence of benefit.

Extending this treatment to patients who do not yet require dialysis has met with similar success.[981] An issue that has yet to be resolved is financial; rhEPO is not inexpensive, and the National Kidney Foundation in the United States has issued guidelines for the use of rhEP in which all patients with a hematocrit of less than 30 percent will be eligible. rhEPO is more effective when administered by the subcutaneous route; this will be more convenient for patients and also will allow a dose reduction.[982, 983] In patients who have not yet undergone dialysis, 100 units/kg subcutaneously provided a response similar to that seen with 150 units/kg given intravenously.[982] The bioavailability of subcutaneous EPO is seven times greater than that of intravenously administered drug, and a large controlled study showed that the mean EPO dose to maintain a stable hematocrit was 32 percent lower by the subcutaneous than the intravenous route.[984]

Similar results have been obtained in several rhEPO studies in children (reviewed by Müller-Wiefel and associates[985]). Anemia was corrected by 3 to 4 months in 24 children with preterminal chronic renal failure (CRF) treated with rhEPO and iron treatment, which was adjusted by careful monitoring of iron status. Hypertension is the most common side effect.[986–989] Interestingly, although the growth failure of children with terminal CRF is unaffected by rhEPO treatment, mean growth velocity in 22 children with preterminal CRF increased from −2.29 to −0.56 within the first 6 months of treatment.[985] Other possible benefits include reports of delay in progression of renal dysfunction in children with preterminal CRF, and improvement in cognitive function.

Other Indications for rEPO Therapy. Several small clinical trials have evaluated the use of rhEPO in the anemia of prematurity.[990–996] These studies have been reviewed by Mentzer and Shannon,[997] and although study differences in patient population, transfusion criteria, rhEPO dose, and iron therapy make comparisons difficult, rhEPO treatment is safe and stimulates a reticulocyte count response. An effect on hematocrit was observed only in the studies in which doses greater than 500 units/kg/wk were used,[990, 992, 994, 995] and there appears to be a modest effect on transfusion requirement. Increasing the dose from 750 to 1500 units/kg/wk was not supported by a large European study of 184 very low-birth-weight infants.[998]

Preliminary data suggest that rhEPO may be useful in the treatment of patients with the anemia of chronic disease associated with rheumatoid arthritis[999] and the anemia that complicates azidothymidine treatment in patients with AIDS (see earlier).

In simian studies, hemoglobin F levels can be increased by administration of EPO.[1000] If similar changes occur in humans, EPO may have a role in the management of sickle cell disease and thalassemia. Several small studies in sickle cell disease have shown that an F reticulocytosis can occur in some patients, whereas other patients show an increase in hemoglobin without a sustained F reticulocyte response, a finding that is of some concern because blood viscosity might be increased.[1001] Data also suggest that hydroxyurea in combination with EPO can augment the F reticulocyte response, although the contribution of EPO is still uncertain.[1002, 1003] In patients with thalassemia who require transfusions or those who have not received transfusions, variable responses to EPO alone have also been reported,[1004–1007] with some patients showing an increase in hemoglobin and F cells. The only report to show a consistent increase in fetal hemoglobin was a study of 10 tha-

lassemic patients who had not received transfusions and were given received rhEPO (400 to 800 units/kg three times per week) as well as iron and hydroxyurea 4 days/wk. The hemoglobin level increased significantly in 8 of the 10 patients with concomitant increases in the fetal hemoglobin level to 5 to 20 percent above baseline.[1007]

Finally, EPO can be used to increase the number of units of blood that can be obtained preoperatively for autologous blood donation.[1008]

OSTEOPETROSIS

M-CSF. An interesting series of studies showed that osteopetrotic *op/op* mice do not produce M-CSF,[1009, 1010] that the *op* locus maps to the same region of chromosome 3 as the M-CSF gene, and that fibroblasts from the mice have a single base insertional mutation in the M-CSF gene that results in a premature stop codon.[385] Based on the observations that osteopetrosis in *op/op* mice can be corrected by M-CSF treatment[1011–1013] a phase I/II study was designed to evaluate the administration of escalating doses of M-CSF in children with severe infantile osteopetrosis.[1014] Preliminary results showed that one patient had a partial response; in particular, growth velocity was maintained, and relatively normal bone trabecular formation was observed on biopsy after 2 months of treatment. However, biochemical evidence of bone resorption was not seen.

Osteoclastic superoxide production and bone resorption can be stimulated by IFN-γ in osteopetrotic *mi/mi* mice,[1015] and this cytokine has been evaluated in a phase I/II study in 14 patients with osteopetrosis.[1016] An increase in leukocyte superoxide production, a decrease in trabecular bone volume, and an increase in hemoglobin level and platelet counts after 6 months of treatment were seen.

STEM AND PROGENITOR CELL MOBILIZATION

As noted earlier, the effect of G-CSF on progenitor cells is interesting. After administration of melphalan and G-CSF, the absolute numbers of *circulating* progenitor cells of the granulocyte-macrophage, erythroid, mixed, and megakaryocyte lineages show a dose-related increase up to 100-fold after 4 days of treatment with rhG-CSF,[883] confirming earlier animal studies.[884, 885] Like G-CSF, GM-CSF also produced an increase in blood progenitor cells of both erythroid and myeloid lineages. Before chemotherapy, an 18-fold increase in blood CFU-GM and an 8-fold increase in BFU-E was noted; after chemotherapy, GM-CSF produced a much greater increase of progenitors (60-fold) when given during the recovery period.[899]

These early studies set the stage for attempts to administer high-dose chemotherapy followed by mobilized blood progenitor cell rescue in a number of chemosensitive tumors such as lymphoma, breast cancer, and multiple myeloma. Time to engraftment is critically related to the number of CD34$^+$ cells infused, and a number of studies indicate that a dose greater than or equal to 5×10^6 CD34$^+$ cells/kg results in prompt neutrophil and platelet engraftment.[1017–1020] G-CSF is the usual HGF used to mobilize progenitors, and multiple apheresis procedures (≥4) are commonly required to achieve this dose of CD34[+] cells. Strategies to increase the yield and thereby reduce the number of apheresis procedures include the combination of G-CSF with chemotherapy, SCF,[1020–1023] TPO,[1024, 1025] a high-affinity IL-3 receptor agonist,[1026] or FL in animal studies.[1027–1031] Two studies suggested that SCF in combination with G-CSF can decrease the number of required apheresis procedures,[1020, 1032] which might be expected to have several advantages, including reduction of apheresis-associated morbidity, less delay in administration of chemotherapy, and decreased cost.

EX VIVO EXPANSION OF STEM AND PROGENITOR CELLS

The recognition that HGFs play a major role in the proliferation and differentiation of immature cells has led to intense interest in *ex vivo* expansion of stem and progenitor cells for clinical use. Because the rapidity, degree, and longevity of engraftment depends on the number and quality of transplanted stem cells, the ability to expand these critical cells might have great clinical potential in graft engineering, tumor purging, and gene therapy. Current efforts to achieve the goal of *ex vivo* culture and amplification of HSCs have mainly involved the use of different cytokine combinations. However, there is little evidence to support the notion that the true LTR-HSCs can be induced to divide and self-renew in such conditions, raising the concern that even if cell division is induced, the dividing cells may differentiate and eventually die. Several factors such as SCF, FL, IL-3, TPO, IL-6, IL-11, G-CSF, and GM-CSF appear to act on very primitive hematopoietic cells including stem cells. Despite intensive investigation only murine studies have demonstrated that cytokines can indeed increase self-renewal among the most immature HSCs capable of self-renewal and long-term hematopoietic reconstitution.[1033, 1034] In human studies the lack of a suitable stem cell assay has made it difficult to investigate the regulatory mechanisms of HSC self-renewal. Very high concentrations of a combination of SCF, FL, and IL-3 can lead to significant expansion of primitive human hematopoietic cells that initiate long-term cultures (LTC-IC),[1035] but the relationship of this cell to the LTR-HSC is uncertain. Data using a xenogeneic assay in which human cells are injected into immunodeficient NOD/SCID mice suggest that the SRC assay detects a cell more primitive than the LTC-IC.[88, 1036–1038] Reports suggest that it may be possible to maintain or increase SRC numbers in serum-free cultures supplemented with a cytokine combination that comprised SCF, FL, IL-3, IL-6, and G-CSF.[1039, 1040] However, our data[1041] show that incubation of cord blood CD34[+] cells in a similar combination of cytokines (SCF, FL, and IL-3) results in rapid loss of SRC activity over 3 days. These data emphasize the need for new approaches to investigate and induce HSC self-renewal and for caution in the clinical use of these *ex vivo* expanded cells.

Ex vivo expanded progenitors were first used clinically by Brugger and associates[1042] who cultured CD34+ mobilized blood progenitors in the combination of SCF,

IL-1, IL-3, IL-6, and EPO and showed rapid short-term engraftment of autografts given to patients with breast cancer after high-dose chemotherapy. However, it was not possible to assess the contribution of these unmarked cells to long-term reconstitution. When expanded progenitors were used in a similar protocol in patients with hematopoietic malignancies who received myeloablation therapy, short-term but not long-term engraftment was observed, with no sustained neutrophil engraftment and no evidence of platelet reconstitution.[1043]

In addition to attempts to expand the stem cell population and perhaps partly because this aim has been rather difficult to achieve, there is considerable interest in amplifying "post-progenitor" cells, that is, myeloid and platelet precursors, for therapeutic use. Although a number of different HGF combinations can generate impressive amplification, clinically effective use of these cells has yet to be achieved.[1044] However, recent studies suggest that the time to recovery of neutrophils may be reduced.[1045–1047]

GENE TRANSFER INTO HEMATOPOIETIC STEM CELLS

Retrovirus-mediated gene transfer into long-lived pluripotent HSCs could provide permanent correction of hematopoietic gene dysfunction in a variety of genetic diseases. However, the results of clinical gene therapy trials are disappointing, because of the low efficiency of gene transfer into HSCs and/or poor expression in the differentiated progeny of these cells.[1048–1051] Major problems of human retrovirus–mediated gene transfer include poor HSC expression of amphotropic receptors for the retroviral envelope gene[1052, 1053] and the quiescent state of the majority of HSCs, which does not favor the integration of retroviral vectors, because cell division is thought to be required.[1054] Difficulties in assaying human HSCs have compounded these problems, and protocols for clinical trials based on results from *in vitro* clonogenic assays of human progenitors, and, in particular, the LTC-IC assay, have not correlated with clinical outcome.

One approach to the amphotropic receptor problem has been the development of new vectors such as Moloney murine leukemia virus–based retrovirus or lentivirus pseudotyped with the vesicular stomatitis virus G protein.[1055–1057] Vesicular stomatitis virus G protein pseudotyped retroviruses, like conventional retroviruses, can stably integrate into the host genome, but have a much broader host range than conventional retroviruses and are more stable, thus permitting concentration by ultracentrifugation to more than 10^9 infectious particles/mL.[1058, 1059] These vectors can efficiently infect mammalian and nonmammalian cells that are resistant to infection by conventional Moloney-based retroviruses.

The problem of stem cell quiescence is usually approached by using HGFs *ex vivo* to stimulate murine[1060] or human[1061–1063] stem and progenitor cells into cycle, and this paradigm has driven much research in animal models and clinical trials. The human studies are based on investigations showing that stimulation with combinations of HGFs such as IL-3, IL-6, and SCF can increase the efficiency of gene transfer into LTC-IC in clinically applicable supernatant infection procedures in the absence of stroma.[1064, 1065] Although stromal support has been shown to increase the efficiency of gene transfer and may be necessary for optimal stem cell survival,[1065–1067] stromal cell–based gene transfer methods are impractical. Stromal components such as fibronectin have been shown to improve gene transfer efficiency, possibly by colocalization of virus and target cell on the 30- to 35-kD carboxy-terminal fragment of fibronectin.[1068] Despite these laboratory advances, HSC gene transfer efficiency in primate[1069, 1070] and human[1048–1051] clinical studies has been disappointingly low. Although strategies using combinations of HGFs have increased the efficiency of gene transfer into *in vitro* clonogenic progenitors, there is little evidence that cytokines increase the occurrence of gene transfer into long-term repopulating stem cells as measured in blood cells obtained from patients. Indeed, it is possible that stimulation with HGFs may irreversibly alter HSC properties, and there is now strong evidence that sustained HSC self-renewal may not be possible.[1071–1073] Instead, the potential of HSCs to self-renew is finite, determined by replicative history.[1074, 1075]

An alternative approach may eventually become feasible. Recently Daley, Jaenisch, and colleagues reported that nuclei from Rag2$^{-/-}$ tail cells could be transferred into enucleated oocytes, and embryonic stem cell lines derived from the resulting blastocysts.[1076] The *Rag2* mutation was then corrected by homologous recombination. Insertion of *HOXB4* into the corrected embryonic stem cells allowed their expansion into transplantable HSCs.[680, 1076] These cells were able to partially correct the defect in immunoglobulin production in Rag2$^{-/-}$ recipients after bone marrow transplantation.

EX VIVO RESPONSE OF SCID-RECONSTITUTING CELLS TO HEMATOPOIETIC GROWTH FACTORS

In a system that is modeled closely on human bone marrow transplantation and the long-term repopulation assay in mice, Kamel-Reid and Dick[88] injected 10^7 human bone marrow cells into irradiated bg/nu/xid mice. By molecular analysis, low levels (0.1 to 1 percent) of DNA from bone marrow and spleen were positive with a human probe, and these organs also contained human progenitor cells. Improved results with this technique have come from increasing the cell dose, regular intraperitoneal injection of SCF, IL-3/GM-CSF fusion protein (PIXY321), and EPO,[1077] and use of the NOD/SCID strain, which in addition to the T- and B-cell defects present in SCID mice has defects of innate immunity in NK cells, macrophages, and complement.[1078–1080] Cell fractionation and gene marking studies provide some evidence that the NOD SRC is more primitive than the LTC-IC.[1038, 1081] Although SRCs may still be a heterogeneous population of cells that includes long-term repopulating HSC, this assay provides a better measure of stem cell properties than the LTC-IC assay, especially with regard to the multipotent (i.e., myeloid and lymphoid) and self-renewal properties of HSCs. Recent reports suggest that it may be possible to maintain or increase numbers of SRCs in serum-free cultures supplemented with a cytokine combination that comprised SCF, FL, IL-3, IL-6, and G-CSF.[1039, 1040] These findings appear to conflict with our

data that numbers and quality of SRCs decline rapidly in culture.[1041] However, Conneally and associates[1039] report that after culture the number of CFCs and LTC-ICs generated per SRC is lower than before culture, despite correction for the observed twofold increase in the number of SRCs. Data from Bhatia and colleagues[1040] suggests a decline in the quality of SRCs as well. They calculate a fourfold increase in SRCs after 4 days in culture; however, despite this increase, the level of engraftment of 500 CD34$^+$CD38$^-$ cells was low (<1 percent), similar to the level obtained with fourfold fewer day 0 cells.[1081] This is consistent with their further observation that by day 9 no SRC activity was detectable at all. Thus, in summary it is still uncertain whether human HSCs can be maintained, expanded, or induced to cycle *ex vivo*, and these obstacles still present major challenges to successful gene therapy.

TOXICITY OF COLONY-STIMULATING FACTOR TREATMENT

The CSFs tested in all these clinical trials have, in general, been well tolerated. Both GM-CSF and G-CSF induce a *transient leukopenia* in the first 30 minutes after administration by intravenous bolus injection. GM-CSF rapidly induces surface expression of the leukocyte adhesion protein CD11b (MO1) *in vitro*, and this is accompanied by an increase in neutrophil aggregation.[828] CD11a (LFA-1) and CD11c (gp150 or gp95), two other members of this family of cell surface adhesion glycoproteins that have distinct α-chains but share a common β-chain (CD18) with CD11b, are unaffected by GM-CSF. These results have been corroborated by *in vivo* studies of patients with sarcoma who received 32 or 64 µg/kg/day GM-CSF. A marked increase of CD11b was noted that was evident by 30 minutes and persisted for 12 to 24 hours after treatment.[899] Radionuclide-labeled leukocytes are sequestered in the lungs after GM-CSF treatment,[870] probably owing to the aggregability and adhesiveness induced by increased CD11b expression. Breathlessness and hypoxia have been observed in some patients, particularly after short-duration intravenous administration. CD11b is not modulated by G-CSF, and the reason for the transient leukopenia after treatment with G-CSF is at present unclear.

Both GM-CSF and G-CSF have been associated with *bone pain* coincident with or shortly after administration. Occasional increases in leukocyte alkaline phosphatase and/or lactate dehydrogenase levels have been noted. In contrast, GM-CSF has also induced *flulike symptoms,* including fever, flushing malaise, myalgia, arthralgia, anorexia, and headache. Mild elevations of *transaminase levels* and *rash* are also reported. These effects are usually mild, are alleviated by antipyretics, and disappear with continued administration. More serious toxic effects have been observed at higher dose levels of GM-CSF (>32 µg/kg/day intravenously or >15 µg/kg/day subcutaneously). A capillary leak syndrome has been seen with weight gain due to fluid retention, manifested as pericardial or pleural effusions, ascites, or edema.[886, 908] Phlebitis was noted in initial studies when the GM-CSF was infused into small veins; large-vessel thrombosis has occurred with infusion of high doses into central veins.[886]

Antibodies to Recombinant Factors. rhGM-CSF that is produced in mammalian cells (Chinese hamster ovary cells) is variably glycosylated on both O-linked and N-linked sites. Production in *E. coli* results in nonglycosylated GM-CSF, and the yeast product is glycosylated at N-linked sites. All three products appear to be equally efficacious, but antibodies have been reported in 4 of 13 patients given the yeast-derived product in phase I/II studies.[1082] The IgG antibodies developed by 7 days after the start of the infusion in all 4 patients, 3 of whom had received a bolus test dose. These antibodies were non-neutralizing as judged by a bone marrow colony-forming assay, and they were directed at sites on the protein backbone of the GM-CSF molecule that are normally protected by O-linked glycosylation but which are exposed in the yeast and *E. coli*–derived products. Transient antibodies to TPO have been reported in one patient with cancer.[1083] However, the development of antibodies in both patients and volunteers given PEG-MGDF led to termination of further clinical development of this TPO formulation, because transient decreases in platelet count were noted.[867, 1084–1086] Antibodies to EPO can also develop in patients with the anemia of chronic renal failure who are receiving treatment with EPO.[1087]

No dose limiting toxic effects have been observed with G-CSF. However, one patients with pathogenic neutrophil infiltration (acute febrile neutrophilic dermatosis or Sweet syndrome) has been reported.[1088] One patient with SCN developed cutaneous necrotizing vasculitis (leukoclastic vasculitis) while receiving G-CSF treatment.[955, 959] As noted earlier, there is also concern that G-CSF will induce or accelerate the development of AML or MDS with monosomy 7 in aplastic anemia and SCN, which is perhaps more likely in those patients with G-CSF receptor mutations that can transduce a proliferative but not a differentiation signal.

Fever is the most common side effect associated with administration of human urinary M-CSF.[905, 914] Malaise and headache and slight depression of blood pressure have also been observed.

CONCLUSION

Advances in molecular and cell biology have led to an unraveling of some of the most challenging and confusing aspects of the study of hematopoiesis. Therapeutic benefits are rapidly emerging from these discoveries. The field of hematopoiesis, once a jumble of unknown factors and activities, has come of age, providing direct benefits to countless patients.

REFERENCES

1. Lehmann H, Huntsman RG: Why are red cells the shape they are? The evolution of the human red cell. In: MacFarlane RG, Robb-Smith AHT (eds): Function of the Blood. Oxford, Blackwell Scientific Publications, 1961, p 73.
2. Brace KC: Life span of the marmot erythrocyte. Blood 1953; 8:648.
3. Everett NB, Caffrey RW: Rate of red cell formation in rats at 24° C and 5° C. Anat Rec 1962; 143:339.
4. Cline MJ, Waldmann TA: Effect of temperature on erythropoiesis. Am J Physiol 1962; 203:401.
5. Grant WC, Root WS: Fundamental stimulus for erythropoiesis. Physiol Rev 1952; 32:449.
6. Necas E, Neuwirt J: Response of erythropoiesis to blood loss in hyperbaric air. Am J Physiol 1969; 216:800.
7. Goldberg MA, Dunning SP, Bunn HF: Regulation of the erythropoietin gene: Evidence that the oxygen sensor is a heme protein. Science 1988; 242:1412.
8. Wang GL, Jiang BH, Rue EA, et al: Hypoxia-inducible factor 1 is a basic-helix-loop-helix-PAS heterodimer regulated by cellular O_2 tension. Proc Natl Acad Sci USA 1995; 92:5510.
9. Galson DL, Tsuchiya T, Tendler DS, et al: The orphan receptor hepatic nuclear factor 4 functions as a transcriptional activator for tissue-specific and hypoxia-specific erythropoietin gene expression and is antagonized by ear3/coup-tf1. Mol Cell Biol 1995; 15:2135.
10. Clark BR, Keating A: Biology of bone marrow stroma [review]. Ann NY Acad Sci 1995; 770:70.
11. Muller-Sieburg CE, Deryugina E: The stromal cells? guide to the stem cell universe [review]. Stem Cells 1995; 13:477.
12. Wolf NS: The haemopoietic microenvironment. Clin Haematol 1979; 8:469.
13. Lichtman MA, Chamberlain JK, Santillo PA: Factors thought to contribute to the regulation of egress of cells from marrow. In: Silber R, LoBue J, Gordon AS (eds): The Year in Hematology. New York, Plenum Medical Book Company, 1978, p 243.
14. Bagby GC: Production of multilineage growth factors by hematopoietic stromal cells: An intracellular regulatory network involving mononuclear phagocytes and interleukin-1. Blood Cells 1987; 13:147.
15. Simmons PJ, Masinovsky B, Longenecker BM, et al: Vascular cell adhesion molecule-1 expressed by bone marrow stromal cells mediates the binding of hematopoietic progenitor cells. Blood 1992; 80:388.
16. Miyake K, Weissman IL, Greenberger JS, et al: Evidence for the role of the integrin VLA-4 in lympho-hemopoiesis. J Exp Med 1991; 173:599.
17. Teixido J, Hemler ME, Greenberger JS, et al: Role of β1 and β2 integrins in the adhesion of CD34^{hi} stem cells to bone marrow stroma. J Clin Invest 1996; 90:358.
18. Williams DA, Rios M, Stephens C, et al: Fibronectin and VLA-4 in hematopoietic stem cell-microenvironment interactions. Nature 1991; 352:438.
19. Kodama H, Nose M, Niida S, et al: Involvement of the c-kit receptor in the adhesion of hematopoietic stem cells to stromal cells. Exp Hematol 1994; 22:979.
20. Gordon MY, Riley GP, Watt SM, et al: Compartmentalization of a haemopoietic growth factor. Nature 1987; 326:403.
21. Dexter TM, Coutinho LH, et al: Stromal cells in haemopoiesis [review]. Ciba Found Symp 1990; 148:76x.
22. Baumheter S, Singer MS, Henzel W, et al: Binding of L-selectin to the vascular sialomucin CD34. Science 1993; 262:436.
23. Aiuti A, Webb IJ, Bleul C, et al: The chemokine SDF-1 is a chemoattractant for human CD34$^+$ hematopoietic progenitor cells and provides a new mechanism to explain the mobilization of CD34$^+$ progenitors to peripheral blood. J Exp Med 1997; 185:111.
24. Ma Q, Jones D, Borghesani PR, et al: Impaired B-lymphopoiesis, myelopoiesis, and derailed cerebellar neuron migration in CXCR4- and SDF-1-deficient mice. Proc Natl Acad Sci USA 1998; 95:9448.
25. Nagasawa T, Hirota S, Tachibana K, et al: Defects of B-cell lymphopoiesis and bone-marrow myelopoiesis in mice lacking the CXC chemokine PBSF/SDF-1. Nature 1996; 382:635.
26. Peled A, Petit I, Kollet O, et al: Dependence of human stem cell engraftment and repopulation of NOD/SCID mice on CXCR4. Science 1999; 283:845.
27. Peled A, Kollet O, Ponomaryov T, et al: The chemokine SDF-1 activates the integrins LFA-1, VLA-4, and VLA-5 on immature human CD34$^+$ cells: Role in transendothelial/stromal migration and engraftment of NOD/SCID mice. Blood 2000; 95:3289.
28. Hattori K, Heissig B, Tashiro K, et al: Plasma elevation of stromal cell-derived factor-1 induces mobilization of mature and immature hematopoietic progenitor and stem cells. Blood 2001; 97:3354.
29. Sweeney EA, Lortat-Jacob H, Priestley GV, et al: Sulfated polysaccharides increase plasma levels of SDF-1 in monkeys and mice: Involvement in mobilization of stem/progenitor cells. Blood 2002; 99:44.

30. Zuckerman KS, Rhodes RK, Goodrum DD, et al: Inhibition of collagen deposition in the extracellular matrix prevents the establishment of a stroma supportive of hematopoiesis in long-term murine bone marrow cultures. J Clin Invest 1985; 75:970.

31. Jacobson LO, Marks EK, Gaston EO, et al: Role of the spleen in radiation injury. Proc Soc Exp Biol Med 1949; 70:7440.

32. Ford CE, Hamerton JL, Barnes DWH, et al: Cytological identification of radiation-chimaeras. Nature 1956; 177:452.

33. Till JE, McCulloch EA: A direct measurement of the radiation sensitivity of normal mouse bone marrow cells. Radiat Res 1961; 14:213.

34. Becker AJ, McCulloch EA, et al: Cytological demonstration of the clonal nature of spleen colonies. J Cell Physiol 1967; 69:65.

35. Magli MC, Iscove NN, Odartchenko N: Transient nature of early haematopoietic spleen colonies. Nature 1982; 295:527.

36. Whang J, Frei E, et al: The distribution of the Philadelphia chromosome in patients with chronic myelogenous leukemia. Blood 1963; 22:644.

37. Fauser AA, Kanz L, et al: T cells and probably B cells arise from the malignant clone in chronic myelogenous leukemia. J Clin Invest 1985; 75:1080.

38. Raskind HS, Jacobson R, et al: Evidence for involvement of B lymphoid cells in polycythemia vera and essential thrombocythemia. J Clin Invest 1985; 75:1388.

39. Adamson JW, Fialkow PJ, et al: Polycythemia vera: Stem cell and probably clonal origin of the disease. N Engl J Med 1975; 295:913.

40. Metcalf D, Moore MAS: Haematopoietic cells. Amsterdam, North-Holland, 1971.

41. Moore MAS, Metcalf D: Ontogeny of the haemopoietic system: Yolk sac origin of *in vivo* and *in vitro* colony forming cells in the developing mouse embryo. Br J Haematol 1970; 18:279.

42. Huang H, Auerbach R: Identification and characterization of hematopoietic stem cells from the yolk sac of the early mouse embryo. Proc Natl Acad Sci USA 1993; 90:10110.

43. Godin I, Dieterlen-Lievre F, Cumano A: Emergence of multipotent hemopoietic cells in the yolk sac and paraaortic splanchnopleura in mouse embryos, beginning at 8.5 days postcoitus. Proc Natl Acad Sci USA 1995; 92:773.

44. Rich IN: Primordial germ cells are capable of producing cells of the hematopoietic system in vitro. Blood 1995; 86:463.

45. Micklem HS, Ross E: Heterogeneity and aging of hematopoietic stem cells. Ann Immunol 1978; 129:367.

46. Siminovitch L, Till JE, et al: Decline in colony-forming ability of marrow cells subjected to serial transplantation into irradiated mice. J Cell Comp Physiol 1964; 64:23.

47. Hellman S, Botnick LE, Hannon EC, et al: Proliferative capacity of murine hematopoietic stem cells. Proc Natl Acad Sci USA 1978; 75:490.

48. Ploemacher RE, van der Sluijs JP, Voerman SA, et al: An in vitro limiting-dilution assay of long-term repopulating hematopoietic stem cells in the mouse. Blood 1989; 74:2755.

49. Dexter TM: Cell interactions in vivo. Clin Haematol 1979; 8:453.

50. Ploemacher RE, Brons RHC: Separation of CFU-S from primitive cells responsible for reconstitution of the bone marrow hemopoietic stem cell compartment following irradiation: Evidence for a pre-CFU-S cell. Exp Hematol 1989; 17:263.

51. Jones RJ, Wagner JE, Celano P, et al: Separation of pluripotent haematopoietic stem cells from spleen colony-forming cells. Nature 1990; 347:188.

52. Nakahata T, Ogawa M: Identification in culture of a new class of hematopoietic colony forming units with extreme capability to self-renew and generate multipotential colonies. Proc Natl Acad Sci USA 1982; 79:3943.

53. Bradley TK, Hodgson GS: Detection of primitive macrophage progenitor cells in mouse bone marrow. Blood 1979; 54:1446.

54. Harrison DE, Lerner CP, Spooncer E: Erythropoietic repopulating ability of stem cells from long-term marrow cultures. Blood 1987; 69:1021.

55. Morrison SJ, White PM, Zock C, et al: Prospective identification, isolation by flow cytometry, and in vivo self-renewal of multipotent mammalian neural crest stem cells. Cell 1999; 96:737.

56. Uchida N, Buck DW, He D, et al: Direct isolation of human central nervous system stem cells. Proc Natl Acad Sci USA 2000; 97:14720.

57. Eglitis MA, Mezey E: Hematopoietic cells differentiate into both microglia and macroglia in the brains of adult mice. Proc Natl Acad Sci USA 1997; 94:4080.

58. Ferrari G, Cusella-De Angelis G, Coletta M, et al: Muscle regeneration by bone marrow-derived myogenic progenitors. Science 1998; 279:1528.

59. Bjornson CR, Rietze RL, Reynolds BA, et al: Turning brain into blood: A hematopoietic fate adopted by adult neural stem cells in vivo. Science 1999; 283:534.

60. Kopen GC, Prockop DJ, Phinney DG: Marrow stromal cells migrate throughout forebrain and cerebellum, and they differentiate into astrocytes after injection into neonatal mouse brains. Proc Natl Acad Sci USA 1999; 96:10711.

61. Petersen BE, Bowen WC, Patrene KD, et al: Bone marrow as a potential source of hepatic oval cells. Science 1999; 284:1168.

62. Krause DS, Theise ND, Collector MI, et al: Multi-organ, multi-lineage engraftment by a single bone marrow-derived stem cell. Cell 2001; 105:369.

63. Gussoni E, Soneoka Y, Strickland CD, et al: Dystrophin expression in the *mdx* mouse restored by stem cell transplantation. Nature 1999; 401:390.

64. Jackson KA, Mi T, Goodell MA: Hematopoietic potential of stem cells isolated from murine skeletal muscle. Proc Natl Acad Sci USA 1999; 96:14482.

65. Anderson DJ, Gage FH, Weissman IL: Can stem cells cross lineage boundaries? Nat Med 2001; 7:393.

66. Morrison SJ: Stem cell potential: Can anything make anything? Curr Biol 2001; 11:R7.

67. Gage FH: Mammalian neural stem cells. Science 2000; 287:1433.

68. Kawada H, Ogawa M: Bone marrow origin of hematopoietic progenitors and stem cells in murine muscle. Blood 2001; 98:2008.

69. Lagasse E, Connors H, Al-Dhalimy M, et al: Purified hematopoietic stem cells can differentiate into hepatocytes in vivo. Nat Med 2000; 6:1229.

70. Theise ND, Nimmakayalu M, Gardner R, et al: Liver from bone marrow in humans. Hepatology 2000; 32:11.

71. Alison MR, Poulsom R, Jeffery R, et al: Hepatocytes from non-hepatic adult stem cells. Nature 2000; 406:257.

72. Korbling M, Katz RL, Khanna A, et al: Hepatocytes and epithelial cells of donor origin in recipients of peripheral-blood stem cells. N Engl J Med 2002; 346:738.

73. Abkowitz JL: Can human hematopoietic stem cells become skin, gut, or liver cells? N Engl J Med 2002; 346:770.

74. Thomas ED, Storb R, et al: Bone marrow transplantation. N Engl J Med 1975; 292:832.

75. To LB, Juttner CA: Peripheral blood stem cell autographing: A new therapeutic option for AML? Br J Haematol 1987; 66:285.

76. Calvo W, Fleidner TM, et al: Regeneration of blood-forming organs after autologous leukocyte transfusion in lethally irradiated dogs. II. Distribution and cellularity of bone marrow in irradiated and transfused animals. Blood 1976; 47:593.

77. Antin JH, Weinberg DS, Rappeport JM: Evidence that pluripotent stem cells form splenic colonies in humans after marrow transplantation. Transplantation 1985; 39:102.

78. Schofield R: The relationship between the spleen colony-forming cell and the haemopoietic stem cell. Blood Cells 1978; 4:7.

79. Schofield R: The pluripotent stem cell. Clin Haematol 1979; 8:221.

80. Fauser AA, Messner HA: Granuloerythropoietic colonies in human bone marrow, peripheral blood, and cord blood. Blood 1978; 52:1243.

81. Fauser AA, Messner HA: Identification of megakaryocytes, macrophages and eosinophils in colonies of human bone marrow containing neutrophilic granulocytes and erythroblasts. Blood 1979; 53:1023.

82. Leary AG, Ogawa M, et al: Single cell origin of multilineage colonies in culture. J Clin Invest 1984; 74:2193.

83. Coulombel L, Kalousek DK, Eaves CJ, et al: Long-term marrow culture reveals chromosomally normal hematopoietic progenitor cells in patients with Philadelphia chromosome positive chronic myelogenous leukemia. N Engl J Med 1983; 308:1493.

84. Greenberg HM, Newberger PE, et al: Generation of physiologically normal human peripheral blood granulocytes in continuous bone marrow cultures. Blood 1981; 58:724.

85. Sutherland HJ, Lansdorp PM, Henkelman DH, et al: Functional characterization of individual human hematopoietic stem cells cultured at limiting dilution on supportive marrow stromal layers. Proc Natl Acad Sci USA 1990; 87:3584.

86. Breems DA, Blokland EAW, Neben S, et al: Frequency analysis of human primitive haematopoietic stem cell subsets using a cobblestone area forming cell assay. Leukemia 1994; 8:1095.

87. McNiece IK, Stewart FM, Deacon DM, et al: Detection of human CFC with a high proliferative potential. Blood 1989; 74:609.
88. Kamel-Reid S, Dick JE: Engraftment of immune-deficient mice with human hematopoietic stem cells. Science 1988; 242:1706.
89. Spangrude GJ, Heimfeld S, Weissman IL: Purification and characterization of mouse hematopoietic stem cells. Science 1988; 241:58.
90. Bertoncello I, Bradley TR, Hodgson GS: The concentration and resolution of primitive hemopoietic cells from normal mouse bone marrow by negative selection using monoclonal antibodies and Dynabead monodisperse magnetic microspheres. Exp Hematol 1989; 17:171.
91. Visser JWM, Bauman JGJ, Mulder AH, et al: Isolation of murine pluripotent hemopoietic stem cells. J Exp Med 1984; 59:1576.
92. Andrews RG, Singer JW, Bernstein ID: Precursors of colony-forming cells in humans can be distinguished from colony-forming cells by expression of the CD33 and CD34 antigens and light scatter properties. J Exp Med 1989; 169:1721.
93. Berardi AC, Wang A, Levine JD, et al: Functional isolation and characterization of human hematopoietic stem cells. Science 1995; 267:104.
94. Berenson RJ, Andrews RG, Bensinger WI, et al: Antigen CD 34+ marrow cells engraft lethally irradiated baboons. J Clin Invest 1988; 81:951.
95. Osawa M, Hanada K, Hamada H, et al: Long-term lymphohematopoietic reconstitution by a single CD34-low/negative hematopoietic stem cell. Science 1996; 273:242.
96. Goodell MA, Brose K, Paradis G, et al: Isolation and functional properties of murine hematopoietic stem cells that are replicating in vivo. J Exp Med 1996; 183:1797.
97. Goodell MA, Rosenzweig M, Kim H, et al: Dye efflux studies suggest that hematopoietic stem cells expressing low or undetectable levels of CD34 antigen exist in multiple species. Nat Med 1997; 3:1337.
98. Bhatia M, Bonnet D, Murdoch B, et al: A newly discovered class of human hematopoietic cells with SCID-repopulating activity. Nat Med 1998; 4:1038.
99. Tajima F, Sato T, Laver JH, et al: CD34 expression by murine hematopoietic stem cells mobilized by granulocyte colony-stimulating factor. Blood 2000; 96:1989.
100. Sato T, Laver JH, Ogawa M: Reversible expression of CD34 by murine hematopoietic stem cells. Blood 1999; 94:2548.
101. Suda T, Suda J, Ogawa M: Disparate differentiation in mouse hemopoietic colonies derived from paired progenitors. Proc Natl Acad Sci USA 1984; 81:2520.
102. Axelrad AA, McLeod DL, et al. Properties of cells that produce erythocytic colonies in vitro. In: Robinson WA (ed): Hemopoiesis in Culture. Washington, DC, DHEW Publication NIH-74–205, 1974, p 226.
103. Pluznik DH, Sachs L: The cloning of normal "mast" cells in tissue cultures. J Cell Comp Physiol 1965; 66:319.
104. Bradley TR, Metcalf D: The growth of mouse bone marrow cells in vitro. Aust J Exp Biol Med Sci 1966; 44:287.
105. Moore MAS: Humoral regulation of granulopoiesis. Clin Haematol 1979; 8:263.
106. Haskill JS, Moore MAS: Two-dimensional cell separation: A comparison of embryonic and adult haematopoietic stem cells. Nature 1970; 266:853.
107. Dexter TM, Allen TD, Lajtha LG: Conditions controlling the proliferation of haemopoietic stem cells in vitro. J Cell Physiol 1977; 91:335.
108. Metcalf D: Detection and analysis of human granulocyte-monocyte precursors using semi-solid cultures. Clin Haematol 1979; 8:263.
109. Haskill JS, McNeil TA, et al: Density distribution analysis of in vivo and in vitro colony-forming cells in bone marrow. J Cell Physiol 1970; 75:167.
110. Jacobsen N, Broxmeyer HE, et al: Diversity of human granulopoietic precursor cells: Separation of cells that form colonies in diffusion chambers (CFU-d) from populations of colony-forming cells in vitro (CFU-c) by velocity sedimentation. Blood 1978; 52:221.
111. Jacobsen N, Broxmeyer HE, et al: Colony-forming units in diffusion chambers (CFU-d) and colony-forming units in agar culture (CFU-c) obtained from normal human bone marrow: A possible parent-progeny relationship. Cell Tissue Kinet 1979; 12:213.
112. Moore MAS, Broxmeyer HE, et al: Continuous human bone marrow culture: Ia antigen characterization of probable pluripotent stem cells. Blood 1980; 55:682.
113. Martin DIK, Zon LI, Mutter G, et al: Expression of an erythroid transcription factor in megakaryocytic and mast cell lineages. Nature 1990; 344:444.
114. Orkin SH: GATA-binding transcription factors in hematopoietic cells. Blood 1992; 80:575.
115. Long MW, Heffner CH, et al: Regulation of megakaryocyte phenotype in human erythroleukemia cells. J Clin Invest 1990; 85:1072.
116. Briddell RA, Brandt JE, Straneva JE, et al: Characterization of the human burst-forming unit-megakaryocyte. Blood 1989; 74:145.
117. Shivdasani RA, Rosenblatt MF, Zucker-Franklin D, et al: Transcription factor NF-E2 is required for platelet formation independent of the actions of thrombopoietin/MGDF in megakaryocyte development. Cell 1995; 81:695.
118. Duebelbeiss KA, Dancey JR, et al: Marrow erythroid and neutrophil cellularity in the dog. J Clin Invest 1975; 55:825.
119. Alpen EL, Cranmore D: Cellular kinetics and iron utilization in bone marrow as observed by Fe-59 radioautography. Ann NY Acad Sci 1959; 77:753.
120. Emerson SG, Sieff CA, Wang EA, et al: Purification of fetal hematopoietic progenitors and demonstration of recombinant multipotential colony-stimulating activity. J Clin Invest 1985; 76:1286.
121. Duke KA, Van Nuord MJ, et al: Identification of cells in primate bone marrow resembling the hematopoietic stem cell in the mouse. Blood 1973; 42:195.
122. Rosse C: Small lymphocyte and transitional cell populations of the bone marrow: Their role in the mediation of immune and hemopoietic progenitor cell functions. Int Rev Cytol 1976; 45:155.
123. Nathan DG, Chess L, Hillman DG, et al: Human erythroid burst-forming unit: T-cell requirement for proliferation in vitro. J Exp Med 1978; 147:324.
124. Granick S, Levere RD: Heme synthesis in erythroid cells. Progr Hematol 1964; 4:1.
125. Finch CA: Ferrokinetics in man. Medicine (Baltimore) 1970; 49:17.
126. Lord BI: Kinetics of the recognizable erythrocyte precursor cells. Clin Haematol 1979; 9:355.
127. Hillman RS, Giblett ER: Red cell membrane alteration associated with "marrow stress." J Clin Invest 1965; 44:1730.
128. Nathan DG: Rubbish in the cell [editorial]. N Engl J Med 1969; 281:558.
129. Etlinger JD, Goldberg AL: Control of protein degradation in reticulocyte extracts by hemin. J Biol Chem 1980; 255:4563.
130. Alpen EL, Cranmore D: Observations on the regulation of erythropoiesis and on cellular dynamics by Fe-59 autoradiography. In Stohlman F Jr (ed): The Kinetics of Cellular Proliferation. New York, Grune & Stratton, 1959, p 290.
131. McNeil BJ, Rappeport JM, et al: Indium chloride scintigraphy: An index of severity in patients with aplastic anaemia. Br J Haematol 1976; 34:599.
132. Lichtman MA, Chamberlain JK, Weed RI, et al: The regulation of the release of granulocytes from normal marrow. In Greenwalt TJ, Jamieson GA (eds): The Granulocyte: Function and Clinical Utilization. New York, Alan R. Liss, 1977, p 53.
133. Levine RF, Hazzard KC, et al: The significance of megakaryocyte size. Blood 1982; 60:1122.
134. Williams N, Levine RF: The origin, development and regulation of megakaryocytes. Br J Haematol 1982; 52:173.
135. Odell TT Jr, Jackson CW, et al: Megakaryocytopoiesis in rats with special reference to polyploidy. Blood 1970; 35:775.
136. Odell TT Jr, Jackson CW: Polyploidy and maturation of rat megakaryocytes. Blood 1968; 32:102.
137. deLaval M, Paulus JM: Megakaryocytes, uninucleate polyploidy or plurinucleate cells. In Paulus JM (ed): Platelet Kinetics. Amsterdam, North Holland, 1971, p 90.
138. Jackson CW: Cholinesterase as a possible marker for early cells of the megakaryocytic series. Blood 1973; 42:413.
139. Nakeff A, Floech DP: Separation of megakaryocytes from mouse bone marrow by density gradient centrifugation. Blood 1976; 48:133.

140. Feinendegen LE, Odartchenko N, et al: Kinetics of megakaryocyte proliferation. Proc Soc Exp Biol Med 1962; 111:177.

141. Ebbe S, Howard D, et al: Effects of vincristine on normal and stimulated megakaryopoiesis in the rat. Br J Haematol 1975; 29:593.

142. Odell TT Jr, Murphy JR: Effects of degree of thrombocytopenia on thrombocytopoietic response. Blood 1974; 44:147.

143. Levine RF: Culture *in vitro* of isolated guinea pig megakaryocytes in the rat. Blood 1977; 50:713.

144. Long MW, Henry RL: Thrombocytosis-induced suppression of small acetylcholinesterase-positive cells in bone marrow of rats. Blood 1979; 54:1338.

145. Mayer M, Schaefer J, et al: Identification of young megakaryocytes by immunofluorescence and cytophotometry. Blood 1978; 37:265.

146. Williams N, Eger RR, Jackson HM, et al: Two-factor requirement for murine megakaryocyte colony formation. J Cell Physiol 1982; 110:101.

147. Levin J, Levin FC, et al: The effects of thrombopoietin on megakaryocyte-CFC, megakaryocytes, and thrombopoiesis: With studies of ploidy and platelet size. Blood 1982; 60:989.

148. Long MW, Williams N, Ebbe S: Immature megakaryocytes in the mouse: Physical characteristics, cell cycle status, and *in vitro* responsiveness to thrombopoietic stimulating factor. Blood 1982; 59:569.

149. Leven RM, Yee MK: Megakaryocytes morphogenesis stimulated *in vitro* by whole and partially fractionated thrombocytopenic plasma: A model system for the study of platelet formation. Blood 1987; 69:1046.

150. Kaushansky K: Thrombopoietin: The primary regulator of platelet production [review]. Blood 1995; 86:419.

151. Kato T, Ogami K, Shimada Y, et al: Purification and characterization of thrombopoietin. J Biochem (Tokyo) 1995; 118:229.

152. Wendling F, Maraskovsky E, Debili N, et al: c-Mpl ligand is a humoral regulator of megakaryocytopoiesis. Nature 1994; 369:571.

153. Hunt P, Hokom M, Dwyer E, et al: Megakaryocyte growth and development factor (MGDF) is a potent, physiological regulator of platelet production in normal and myelocompromised animals [abstract]. Blood 1994; 84(Suppl 1): 390a.

154. Kuter DJ, Rosenberg RD: The reciprocal relationship of thrombopoietin (c-Mpl ligand) to changes in the platelet mass during busulfan-induced thrombocytopenia in the rabbit. Blood 1995; 85:2720.

155. McCarty JM, Sprugel KH, Fox NE, et al: Murine thrombopoietin mRNA levels are modulated by platelet count. Blood 1995; 86:3668.

156. Kaushansky K, Lok S, Holly RD, et al: Promotion of megakaryocyte progenitor expansion and differentiation by the c-Mpl ligand thrombopoietin. Nature 1994; 369:568.

157. Metcalf D. The Molecular Control of Blood Cells. Cambridge, MA, Harvard University Press, 1988.

158. Metcalf D: Hemopoietic regulators and leukemia development: A personal retrospective. Adv Cancer Res 1994; 63:41.

159. Clark SC, Kamen R: The human hematopoietic colony-stimulating factors. Science 1987; 236:1229.

160. Metcalf D: The colony stimulating factors. Cancer 1990; 65:2185.

161. Moore MAS: Haemopoietic growth factor interactions: In vitro and in vivo preclinical evaluation. Cancer Surv 1990; 9:7.

162. Metcalf D: Cell-cell signalling in the regulation of blood cell formation and function. Immunol Cell Biol 1998; 76:441.

163. Alexander WS: Cytokines in hematopoiesis. Int Rev Immunol 1998; 16:651.

164. Wong GG, Clark SC: Multiple actions of interleukin-6 within a cytokine network. Immunol Today 1988; 9:137.

165. Bazan JF: Neuropoietic cytokines in the hematopoietic fold. Neuron 1991; 7:197.

166. Bazan JF: Emerging families of cytokines and receptors. Curr Biol. 1993; 3:603.

167. Kelso A: Cytokines: Principles and prospects. Immunol Cell Biol 1998; 76:300.

168. Roth P, Stanley ER: The biology of CSF-1 and its receptor. Curr Top Microbiol Immunol 1992; 181:141.

169. Galli SJ, Zsebo KM, Geissler EN: The kit ligand, stem cell factor. Adv Immunol 1994; 55:1.

170. Lyman SD, Jacobsen SE: C-kit ligand and flt3 ligand: Stem/progenitor cell factors with overlapping yet distinct activities. Blood 1998; 91:1101.

171. Sims JE, Nicklin MJ, Bazan JF, et al: A new nomenclature for IL-1-family genes. Trends Immunol 2001; 22:536.

172. Rollins BJ: Chemokines. Blood 1997; 90:909.

173. Shalaby MR, Pennica D, Palladino MA Jr: An overview of the history and biologic properties of tumor necrosis factors. Springer Semin Immunopathol 1986; 9:33.

174. Pestka S, Langer JA, Zoon KC, et al: Interferons and their actions. Annu Rev Biochem 1987; 56:727.

175. Blumberg H, Conklin D, Xu WF, et al: Interleukin 20: Discovery, receptor identification, and role in epidermal function. Cell 2001; 104:9.

176. Massague J: TGF-beta signal transduction. Annu Rev Biochem 1998; 67:753.

177. Fossiez F, Bancherau J, Murray R, et al: Interleukin-17. Int Rev Immunol 1998; 16:541.

178. Miyazaki T, Maruyama M, Yamada G, et al: The integrity of the conserved 'ws motif' common to IL-2 and other cytokine receptors is essential for ligand binding and signal transduction. EMBO J 1991; 10:3191.

179. Nicola NA: Guidebook to Cytokines and Their Receptors. Oxford, UK, Oxford University Press, 1994.

180. Darnell JE: STATS and gene regulation. Science 1997; 277:1630.

181. Ihle JN: Cytokine receptor signalling. Nature 1995; 377:591.

182. Strober W, James SP: The interleukins. Pediatr Res 1988; 24:549.

183. Vosshenrich CA, Di Santo JP: Cytokines: IL-21 joins the gamma(c)-dependent network? Curr Biol 2001; 11:R175.

184. Oppmann B, Lesley R, Blom B, et al: Novel p19 protein engages IL-12p40 to form a cytokine, IL-23, with biological activities similar as well as distinct from IL-12. Immunity 2000; 13:715.

185. Clark SC: Biological activities of human granulocyte-macrophage colony-stimulating factor. Int J Cell Cloning 1988; 6:365.

186. Demetri GD, Griffin JD: Granulocyte colony-stimulating factor and its receptor. Blood 1991; 78:2791.

187. Goldwasser E, Beru N, Smith D: Erythropoietin. Immunol Ser 1990; 49:257.

188. Alexander WS: Thrombopoietin. Growth Factors 1999; 17:13.

189. Quentmeier H, Drexler HG, Fleckenstein D, et al: Cloning of human thymic stromal lymphopoietin (TSLP) and signaling mechanisms leading to proliferation. Leukemia 2001; 15:1286.

190. Reche PA, Soumelis V, Gorman DM, et al: Human thymic stromal lymphopoietin preferentially stimulates myeloid cells. J Immunol 2001; 167:336.

191. Sims JE, Williams DE, Morrissey PJ, et al: Molecular cloning and biological characterization of a novel murine lymphoid growth factor. J Exp Med 2000; 192:671.

192. Metcalf D: Murine hematopoietic stem cells committed to macrophage/dendritic cell formation: Stimulation by Flk2-ligand with enhancement by regulators using the gp130 receptor chain. Proc Natl Acad Sci USA 1997; 94:11552.

193. Taga T, Kishimoto T: Gp130 and the interleukin-6 family of cytokines. Annu Rev Immunol 1997; 15:797.

194. Loy JK, Davidson TJ, Berry KK, et al: Oncostatin M: Development of a pleiotropic cytokine. Toxicol Pathol 1999; 27:151.

195. Asao H, Okuyama C, Kumaki S, et al: Cutting edge: The common γ-chain is an indispensable subunit of the IL-21 receptor complex. J Immunol 2001; 167:1.

196. Pandey A, Ozaki K, Baumann H, et al: Cloning of a receptor subunit required for signaling by thymic stromal lymphopoietin. Nature Immunol 2000; 1:59.

197. Ogawa M, Matsunaga T: Humoral regulation of hematopoietic stem cells. Ann NY Acad Sci 1999; 872:17.

198. Marz P, Otten U, Rose-John S: Neural activities of IL-6-type cytokines often depend on soluble cytokine receptors. Eur J Neurosci 1999; 11:2995.

199. Ashman LK: The biology of stem cell factor and its receptor c-kit. Int J Biochem Cell Biol 1999; 31:1037.

200. Lyman SD: Biologic effects and potential clinical applications of Flt3 ligand. Curr Opin Hematol 1998; 5:192.

201. Bazan JF: Genetic and structural homology of stem cell factor and macrophage colony-stimulating factor. Cell 1991; 65:9.

202. Lyman SD, Stocking K, Davison B, et al: Structural analysis of human and murine flt3 ligand genomic loci. Oncogene 1995; 11:1165.

203. Dinarello CA: The interleukin-1 family: 10 years of discovery. FASEB J 1994; 8:1314.

204. Dinarello CA: The biological properties of interleukin-1. Eur Cytokine Netw 1994; 5:517.

205. Nakanishi K, Yoshimoto T, Tsutsui H, et al: Interleukin-18 is a unique cytokine that stimulates both Th1 and Th2 responses depending on its cytokine milieu. Cytokine Growth Factor Rev 2001; 12:53.

206. Dinarello CA: IL-18: A TH1-inducing, proinflammatory cytokine and new member of the IL-1 family. J Allergy Clin Immunol 1999; 103:11.

207. Zhou YQ, Stanley ER, Clark SC, et al: Interleukin-3 and interleukin-1α allow earlier bone marrow progenitors to respond to human colony-stimulating factor 1. Blood 1988; 72:1870.

208. Cashman J, Clark-Lewis I, Eaves A, et al: Stromal-derived factor 1 inhibits the cycling of very primitive human hematopoietic cells in vitro and in NOD/SCID mice. Blood 2002; 99:792.

209. Mayani H, Little MT, Dragowska W, et al: Differential effects of the hematopoietic inhibitors MIP-1α, TGF-β, and TNF-α on cytokine-induced proliferation of subpopulations of CD34+ cells purified from cord blood and fetal liver. Exp Hematol 1995; 23:422.

210. Jo D-Y, Rafii S, Hamada T, et al: Chemotaxis of primitive hematopoietic cells in response to stromal cell-derived factor-1. J Clin Invest 2000; 105:101.

211. Palucka KA, Taquet N, Sanchez-Chapuis F, et al: Dendritic cells as the terminal stage of monocyte differentiation. J Immunol 1998; 160:4587.

212. Pasparakis M, Alexopoulou L, Episkopou V, et al: Immune and inflammatory responses in TNF α-deficient mice: A critical requirement for TNF α in the formation of primary B cell follicles, follicular dendritic cell networks and germinal centers, and in the maturation of the humoral immune response. J Exp Med 1996; 184:1397.

213. Pestka S: The interferon receptors. Semin Oncol 1997; 24(3 Suppl 9): S9.

214. Moore KW, de Waal Malefyt R, Coffman RL, et al: Interleukin-10 and the interleukin-10 receptor. Annu Rev Immunol 2001; 19:683.

215. Akdis CA, Blaser K: Mechanisms of interleukin-10-mediated immune suppression. Immunology 2001; 103:131.

216. Donnelly RP, Dickensheets H, Finbloom DS: The interleukin-10 signal transduction pathway and regulation of gene expression in mononuclear phagocytes. J Interferon Cytokine Res 1999; 19:563.

217. Gallagher G, Dickensheets H, Eskdale J, et al: Cloning, expression and initial characterization of interleukin-19 (IL-19), a novel homologue of human interleukin-10 (IL-10). Genes Immun 2000; 1:442.

218. Dumoutier L, Leemans C, Lejeune D, et al: Cutting edge: STAT activation by IL-19, IL-20 and mda-7 through IL-20 receptor complexes of two types. J Immunol 2001; 167:3545.

219. Dumoutier L, Van Roost E, Ameye G, et al: IL-TIF/IL-22: Genomic organization and mapping of the human and mouse genes. Genes Immun 2000; 1:488.

220. Fortunel NO, Hatzfeld A, Hatzfeld J: Transforming growth factor β: Pleiotropic role in the regulation of hematopoiesis. Blood 2000; 96:3722.

221. Cashman JD, Clark-Lewis I, Eaves AC, et al: Differentiation stage-specific regulation of primitive human hematopoietic progenitor cycling by exogenous and endogenous inhibitors in an in vivo model. Blood 1999; 94:3722.

222. Zhang C, Evans T: BMP-like signals are required after the mid-blastula transition for blood cell development. Dev Genet 1996; 18:267.

223. Li H, Chen J, Huang A, et al: Cloning and characterization of IL-17B and IL-17C, two new members of the IL-17 cytokine family. Proc Natl Acad Sci USA 2000; 97:773.

224. Lee J, Ho WH, Maruoka M, et al: IL-17E, a novel proinflammatory ligand for the IL-17 receptor homolog IL-17Rh1. J Biol Chem 2001; 276:1660.

225. Cai XY, Gommoll CP Jr, Justice L, et al: Regulation of granulocyte colony-stimulating factor gene expression by interleukin-17. Immunol Lett 1998; 62:51.

226. Yang YC, Clark SC: Interleukin-3: Molecular biology and biologic activities. Hematol Oncol Clin North Am 1989; 3:441.

227. Sanderson CJ: Interleukin-5, eosinophils, and disease. Blood 1992; 79:3101.

228. Akira S, Taga T, Kishimoto T: Interleukin-6 in biology and medicine. Adv Immunol 1993; 54:1.

229. Du XX, Williams DA: Interleukin-11: A multifunctional growth factor derived from the hematopoietic microenvironment. Blood 1994; 83:2023.

230. Yang YC: Interleukin 11: An overview. Stem Cells 1993; 11:474.

231. Goldman SJ: Preclinical biology of interleukin 11: A multifunctional hematopoietic cytokine with potent thrombopoietic activity. Stem Cells 1995; 13:462.

232. Blanchard KL, Fandrey J, Goldberg MA, et al: Regulation of the erythropoietin gene. Stem Cells 1993; 11(Suppl 1):1.

233. Porter DL, Goldberg MA: Regulation of erythropoietin production. Exp Hematol 1993; 21:399.

234. Lyman SD, James L, Vanden Bos T, et al: Molecular cloning of a ligand for the flt3/flk-2 tyrosine kinase receptor: A proliferative factor for primitive hematopoietic cells. Cell 1993; 75:1157.

235. Hannum C, Culpepper J, Campbell D, et al: Ligand for FLT3/FLK2 receptor tyrosine kinase regulates growth of haematopoietic stem cells and is encoded by variant RNAs. Nature 1994; 368:643.

236. Lopez AF, Sanderson CJ, Gamble JR, et al: Recombinant human interleukin-5 (IL-5) is a selective activator of human eosinophil function. J Exp Med 1988; 167:219.

237. Bussolino F, Wang JM, Defilippi P, et al: Granulocyte- and granulocyte-macrophage-colony stimulating factors induce human endothelial cells to migrate and proliferate. Nature 1989; 337:471.

238. Yokota T, Arai N, de Vries J, et al: Molecular biology of interleukin 4 and interleukin 5 genes and biology of their products that stimulate B cells, T cells and hemopoietic cells. Immunol Rev 1988; 102:137.

239. Berridge MV, Fraser JK, Carter JM, et al: Effects of recombinant human erythropoietin on megakaryocytes and on platelet production in the rat. Blood 1988; 72:970.

240. Kobayashi M, Laver JH, Kato T, et al: Recombinant human thrombopoietin (Mpl ligand) enhances proliferation of erythroid progenitors. Blood 1995; 86:2494.

241. Ogawa M: Differentiation and proliferation of hematopoietic stem cells. Blood 1993; 81:2844.

242. McKinstry WJ, Li CL, Rasko JE, et al: Cytokine receptor expression on hematopoietic stem and progenitor cells. Blood 1997; 89:65.

243. Ikebuchi K, Clark SC, Ihle JW, et al: Granulocyte colony-stimulating factor enhances interleukin-3-dependent proliferation of multipotential hemopoietic progenitors. Proc Natl Acad Sci USA 1988; 85:3445.

244. Stanley ER, Bartocci A, Patinkin D, et al: Regulation of very primitive, multipotent, hemopoietic cells by hemopoietin-1. Cell 1986; 45:667.

245. Zeigler FC, de Sauvage F, Widmer HR, et al: In vitro megakaryocytopoietic and thrombopoietic activity of c-mpl ligand (tpo) on purified murine hematopoietic stem cells. Blood 1994; 84:4045.

246. Metcalf D, Begley CG, Johnson GR, et al: Biologic properties in vitro of a recombinant human granulocyte-macrophage colony-stimulating factor. Blood 1986; 67:37.

247. Metcalf D: Lineage commitment of hemopoietic progenitor cells in developing blast cell colonies: Influence of colony-stimulating factors. Proc Natl Acad Sci USA 1991; 88:11310.

248. Sieff CA, Emerson SG, Donahue RE, et al: Human recombinant granulocyte-macrophage colony-stimulating factor: A multilineage hematopoietin. Science 1985; 230:1171.

249. Ihle JN, Keller J, Oroszalan S, et al: Biologic properties of homogeneous interleukin 3. I. Demonstration of WEHI-3 growth factor activity, mast cell growth factor activity, P cell-stimulating activity, and histamine-producing cell-stimulating activity. J Immunol 1983; 131:282.

250. Leary AG, Yang Y-C, Clark SC, et al: Recombinant gibbon interleukin 3 supports formation of human multilineage colonies and blast cell colonies in culture: Comparison with recombinant human granulocyte-macrophage colony-stimulating factor. Blood 1987; 70:1343.

251. Sieff CA, Niemeyer CM, Nathan DG, et al: Stimulation of human hematopoietic colony formation by recombinant gibbon multi-colony-stimulating factor or interleukin 3. J Clin Invest 1987; 80:818.

252. Sonoda Y, Yang Y-C, Wong GG, et al: Analysis in serum-free culture of the targets of recombinant human hemopoietic growth factors: Interleukin 3 and granulocyte-macrophage colony-stimulating factor are specific for early developmental stages. Proc Natl Acad Sci USA 1988; 85:4360.

253. Ottmann OG, Abboud M, Welte K, et al: Stimulation of human hematopoietic progenitor cell proliferation and differentiation by recombinant human interleukin 3. Comparison and interactions with recombinant human granulocyte-macrophage and granulocyte colony-stimulating factors. Exp Hematol 1989; 17:191.

254. Mayer P, Valent P, Schmidt G, et al: The in vivo effects of recombinant human interleukin-3: Demonstration of basophil differentiation factor, histamine-producing activity, and priming of GM-CSF-responsive progenitors in nonhuman primates. Blood 1989; 74:613.

255. Donahue RE, Seehra J, Metzger M, et al: Human interleukin-3 and GM-SCF act synergistically in stimulating hematopoiesis in primates. Science 1988; 241:1820.

256. Szabolcs P, Moore MA, Young JW: Expansion of immunostimulatory dendritic cells among the myeloid progeny of human CD34+ bone marrow precursors cultured with c-kit ligand, granulocyte-macrophage colony-stimulating factor, and TNF-α. J Immunol 1995; 154:5851.

257. Kelly KA, Lucas K, Hochrein H, et al: Development of dendritic cells in culture from human and murine thymic precursor cells. Cell Mol Biol 2001; 47:43.

258. McKenna HJ: Role of hematopoietic growth factors/flt3 ligand in expansion and regulation of dendritic cells. Curr Opin Hematol 2001; 8:149.

259. Keller U, Aman MJ, Derigs G, et al: Human interleukin-4 enhances stromal cell-dependent hematopoiesis: Costimulation with stem cell factor. Blood 1994; 84:2189.

260. Sonoda Y, Okuda T, Yokota S, et al: Actions of human interleukin-4/B-cell stimulatory factor-1 on proliferation and differentiation of enriched hematopoietic progenitor cells in culture. Blood 1990; 75:1615.

261. Kishi K, Ihle JN, Urdal DL, et al: Murine B-cell stimulatory factor-1 (BSF-1/interleukin-4 (IL-4) is a multilineage colony-stimulating factor that acts directly on primitive hemopoietic progenitors. J Cell Physiol 1989; 139:463.

262. Paul WE: Interleukin-4: A prototypic immunoregulatory lymphokine. Blood 1991; 77:1859.

263. Mosmann TR, Coffman RL: Th1 and Th2 cells: Different patterns of lymphokine secretion lead to different functional properties. Annu Rev Immunol 1989; 7:145.

264. Donahue RE, Yang Y-C, Clark SC: Human P40 T-cell growth factor (interleukin-9) supports erythroid colony formation. Blood 1993; 75:2271.

265. Renauld JC, Houssiau F, Louahed J, et al: Interleukin-9. Adv Immunol 1993; 54:79.

266. Demoulin JB, Renauld JC: Interleukin 9 and its receptor: An overview of structure and function. Int Rev Immunol 1998; 16:345.

267. Lyman SD, James L, Johnson L, et al: Cloning of the human homologue of the murine flt3 ligand: A growth factor for early hematopoietic progenitor cells. Blood 1994; 83:2795.

268. Spritz RA, Giebel LB, Holmes SA: Dominant negative and loss of function mutations of the c-kit (mast/stem cell growth factor receptor) proto-oncogene in human piebaldism [see comments]. Am J Hum Genet 1992; 50:261.

269. Alexander WS, Lyman SD, Wagner EF: Expression of functional c-kit receptors rescues the genetic defect of w mutant mast cells. EMBO J 1991; 10:3683.

270. Tsuji K, Lyman SD, Sudo T, et al: Enhancement of murine hematopoiesis by synergistic interactions between Steel factor (ligand for c-kit), interleukin-11, and other early acting factors in culture. Blood 1992; 79:2855.

271. Tsuji K, Zsebo KM, Ogawa M: Enhancement of murine blast cell colony formation in culture by recombinant rat stem cell factor, ligand for c-kit. Blood 1991; 78:1223.

272. Metcalf D, Nicola NA: Direct proliferative actions of stem cell factor on murine bone marrow cells *in vitro*: Effects of combination with colony-stimulating factors. Proc Natl Acad Sci USA 1991; 88:6239.

273. Hirayama F, Ogawa M: Negative regulation of early T lymphopoiesis by interleukin-3 and interleukin-1α. Blood 1995; 86:4527.

274. Hirayama F, Shih JP, Awgulewitsch A, et al: Clonal proliferation of murine lymphohemopoietic progenitors in culture. Proc Natl Acad Sci USA 1992; 89:5907.

275. Williams DE, de Vries P, Namen AE, et al: The Steel factor. Dev Biol 1992; 151:368.

276. McNiece IK, Langley KE, Zsebo KM: The role of recombinant stem cell factor in early B cell development. Synergistic interaction with IL-7. J Immunol 1991; 146:3785.

277. Toksoz D, Zsebo KM, Smith KA, et al: Support of human hematopoiesis in long-term bone marrow cultures by murine stromal cells selectively expressing the membrane-bound and secreted forms of the human homolog of the Steel gene product, stem cell factor. Proc Natl Acad Sci USA 1992; 89:7350.

278. Cerretti DP, Wignall J, Anderson D, et al: Human macrophage-colony stimulating factor: Alternative RNA and protein processing from a single gene. Mol Immunol 1988; 25:761.

279. Avraham H, Scadden D, Chi S, et al: Interaction of human bone marrow fibroblasts with megakaryocytes: Role of the c-kit ligand. Blood 1992; 80:1679.

280. Brannan CI, Lyman SD, Williams DE, et al: Steel-Dickie mutation encodes a c-Kit ligand lacking transmembrane and cytoplasmic domains. Proc Natl Acad Sci USA 1991; 88:4671.

281. Matthews W, Jordan C, Wiegand G, et al: A receptor tyrosine kinase specific to hematopoietic stem and progenitor cell-enriched populations. Cell 1991; 65:1143.

282. Small D, Levenstein M, Kim E, et al: STK-1, the human homolog of Flk-2/Flt-3, is selectively expressed in CD34+ human bone marrow cells and is involved in the proliferation of early progenitor/stem cells. Proc Natl Acad Sci USA 1994; 91:459.

283. Hirayama F, Lyman SD, Clark SC, et al: The flt3 ligand supports proliferation of lymphohematopoietic progenitors and early B-lymphoid progenitors. Blood 1995; 85:1762.

284. McKenna HJ, de Vries P, Brasel K, et al: Effect of flt3 ligand on the ex vivo expansion of human CD34+ hematopoietic progenitor cells. Blood 1995; 86:3413.

285. Hudak S, Hunte B, Culpepper J, et al: FLT3/FLK2 ligand promotes the growth of murine stem cells and the expansion of colony-forming cells and spleen colony-forming units. Blood 1995; 85:2747.

286. Mackarehtschian K, Hardin JD, Moore KA, et al: Targeted disruption of the flk2/flt3 gene leads to deficiencies in primitive hematopoietic progenitors. Immunity 1995; 3:147.

287. Hunte BE, Hudak S, Campbell D, et al: Flk2/flt3 ligand is a potent cofactor for the growth of primitive B cell progenitors. J Immunol 1996; 156:489.

288. Ikebuchi K, Wong GG, Clark SC, et al: Interleukin-6 enhancement of interleukin-3-dependent proliferation of multipotential hemopoietic progenitors. Proc Natl Acad Sci USA 1987; 84:9035.

289. Musashi M, Yang Y-C, Paul SR, et al: Direct and synergistic effects of interleukin 11 on murine hemopoiesis in culture. Proc Natl Acad Sci USA 1991; 88:765.

290. Leary AG, Wong GG, Clark SC, et al: Leukemia inhibitory factor/differentiation-inhibiting activity/human interleukin for DA cells augments proliferation of human hemopoietic stem cells. Blood 1990; 75:1960.

291. Hirayama F, Katayama N, Neben S, et al: Synergistic interaction between interleukin-12 and Steel factor in support of proliferation of murine lymphohematopoietic progenitors in culture. Blood 1994; 83:92.

292. Zhang XG, Gu JJ, Lu ZY, et al: Ciliary neurotropic factor, interleukin 11, leukemia inhibitory factor, and oncostatin M are growth factors for human myeloma cell lines using the interleukin 6 signal transducer gp130. J Exp Med 1994; 179:1337.

293. Chua AO, Chizzonite R, Desai BB, et al: Expression cloning of a human IL-12 receptor component. a new member of the cytokine receptor superfamily with strong homology to gp130. J Immunol 1994; 153:128.

294. Trinchieri G: Interleukin-12: A proinflammatory cytokine with immunoregulatory functions that bridge innate resistance and antigen-specific adaptive immunity. Annu Rev Immunol 1995; 13:251.

295. Trinchieri G: Interleukin-12: A cytokine at the interface of inflammation and immunity. Adv Immunol 1998; 70:63.

296. Leary AG, Ikebuchi K, Hirai Y, et al: Synergism between interleukin-6 and interleukin-3 in supporting proliferation of human hematopoietic stem cells: Comparison with interleukin-1α. Blood 1988; 71:1759.

297. Srour EF, Brandt JE, Leemhuis T, et al: Relationship between cytokine-dependent cell cycle progression and MHC class II antigen expression by human CD34+HLA-DR− bone marrow cells. J Immunol 1992; 148:815.

298. Jacobsen SE, Ruscetti FW, Okkenhaug C, et al: Distinct and direct synergistic effects of IL-1 and IL-6 on proliferation and differentiation of primitive murine hematopoietic progenitor cells in vitro. Exp Hematol 1994; 22:1064.

299. Rodriguez C, Lacasse C, Hoang T: Interleukin-1β suppresses apoptosis in CD34 positive bone marrow cells through activation of the type i IL-1 receptor. J Cell Physiol 1996; 166:387.

300. Yamasaki K, Taga T, Hirata Y, et al: Cloning and expression of the human interleukin-6 (BSF-2/IFN β2) receptor. Science 1988; 241:825.

301. Hibi M, Murakami M, Saito M, et al: Molecular cloning and expression of an IL-6 signal transducer, gp130. Cell 1990; 63:1149.

302. Pennica D, Shaw KJ, Swanson TA, et al: Cardiotrophin-1. Biological activities and binding to the leukemia inhibitory factor receptor/gp130 signaling complex. J Biol Chem 1995; 270:10915.

303. Nishimoto N, Ogata A, Shima Y, et al: Oncostatin M, leukemia inhibitory factor, and interleukin 6 induce the proliferation of human plasmacytoma cells via the common signal transducer, gp130. J Exp Med 1994; 179:1343.

304. Wong GG, Witek-Giannotti JS, Temple PA, et al: Stimulation of murine hemopoietic colony formation by human IL-6. J Immunol 1988; 140:3040.

305. Leary AG, Zeng HQ, Clark SC, et al: Growth factor requirements for survival in G_0 and entry into the cell cycle of primitive human hematopoietic progenitors. Proc Natl Acad Sci USA 1992; 89:4013.

306. Paul SR, Bennett F, Calvetti JA, et al: Molecular cloning of a cDNA encoding interleukin-11, a novel stromal cell-derived lymphopoietic and hematopoietic cytokine. Proc Natl Acad Sci USA 1990; 87:7512.

307. Turner KJ, Clark SC: Interleukin-11: Biological and clinical perspectives. In Mertelsmann R, Herrmann F (eds): Hematopoietic Growth Factors in Clinical Applications, vol 2. New York, Marcel Dekker, 1995, p 315.

308. Yin T, Taga T, Tsang MLS, et al: Interleukin (IL)-6 signal transducer, gp130, is involved in IL-11 mediated signal transduction. Blood 1992; 80(Suppl 1):151a.

309. Baumann H, Schendel P: Interleukin-11 regulates the hepatic expression of the same plasma protein genes as interleukin-6. J Biol Chem 1991; 266:20424.

310. Suda T, Udagawa N, Nakamura I, et al: Modulation of osteoclast differentiation by local factors. Bone 1995; 17:87S.

311. Burstein SA, Mei R-L, Henthorn J, et al: Leukemia inhibitory factor and interleukin-11 promote the maturation of murine and human megakaryocytes in vitro. J Cell Physiol 1992; 153:305.

312. van de Ven C, Ishizawa L, Law P, et al: IL-11 in combination with SLF and G-CSF or GM-CSF significantly increases expansion of isolated CD34+ cell population from cord blood vs. adult bone marrow. Exp Hematol 1995; 23:1289.

313. Broudy V, Lin N, Kaushansky K: Thrombopoietin (c-mpl ligand) acts synergistically with erythropoietin, stem cell factor, and interleukin-11 to enhance murine megakaryocyte colony growth and increases megakaryocyte ploidy in vitro. Blood 1995; 85:1719.

314. Bruno E, Briddell RA, Cooper RJ, et al: Effects of recombinant interleukin 11 on human megakaryocyte progenitor cells. Exp Hematol 1991; 19:378.

315. Neben TY, Loebelenz J, Hayes L, et al: Recombinant human interleukin 11 stimulates megakaryocytopoiesis and increases peripheral plateletes in normal and splenectomized mice. Blood 1993; 81:901.

316. Gordon MS, Nemunaitis J, Hoffman R, et al: A phase 1 trial of recombinant human interleukin-6 in patients with myelodysplastic syndromes and thrombocytopenia. Blood 1995; 85:3066.

317. Tepler I, Elias L, Smith JW II, et al: A randomized placebo-controlled trial of recombinant human interleukin-11 in cancer patients with severe thrombocytopenia due to chemotherapy. Blood 1996; 87:3607.

318. Quesniaux VF, Clark SC, Turner K, et al: Interleukin-11 stimulates multiple phases of erythropoiesis in vitro. Blood 1992; 80:1218.

319. Trepicchio WL, Bozza M, Pedneault G, et al: Recombinant human interleukin-11 attenuation of the inflammatory response through down-regulation of proinflammatory cytokine release and nitric oxide production. J Immunol 1996; 157: 3627.

320. Schwertschlag US, Trepicchio WL, Dykstra KH, et al: Hematopoietic, immunomodulatory and epithelial effects of interleukin-11. Leukemia 1999; 13:1307.

321. Keith JCJr, Albert L, Sonis ST, et al: IL-11, a pleiotropic cytokine: Exciting new effects of IL-11 on gastrointestinal mucosal biology. Stem Cells 1994; 12(Suppl 1):79.

322. Potten CS: Interleukin-11 protects the clonogenic stem cells in murine small-intestinal crypts from impairment of their reproductive capacity by radiation. Int J Cancer 1995; 62:356.

323. Ohsumi J, Miyadai K, Kawashima I, et al: Regulation of lipoprotein lipase synthesis in 3T3-L1 adipocytes by interleukin-11/adipogenesis inhibitory factor. Biochem Mol Biol Int 1994; 32:705.

324. Hatzfeld J, Li ML, Brown EL, et al: Release of early human hematopoietic progenitors from quiescence by antisense transforming growth factor β1 or Rb oligonucleotides. J Exp Med 1991; 174:925.

325. Eaves AC, Eaves CJ: Maintenance and proliferation control of primitive hemopoietic progenitors in long-term cultures of human marrow cells. Blood Cells 1988; 14:355.

326. Cardoso AA, Li ML, Batard P, et al: Release from quiescence of CD34+ CD38− human umbilical cord blood cells reveals their potentiality to engraft adults. Proc Natl Acad Sci USA 1993; 90:8707.

327. Li ML, Cardoso AA, Sansilvestri P, et al: Additive effects of Steel factor and antisense TGF-β1 oligodeoxynucleotide on CD34+ hematopoietic progenitor cells. Leukemia 1994; 8:441.

328. Zilberstein A, Ruggieri R, Korn JH, et al: Structure and expression of cDNA and genes for human interferon-β-2, a distinct species inducible by growth-stimulatory cytokines. EMBO J 1986; 5:2529.

329. Nagata S, Tsuchiya M, Asano S, et al: Molecular cloning and expression of cDNA for human granulocyte colony-stimulating factor. Nature 1986; 319:415.

330. Souza LM, Boone TC, Gabrilove JL, et al: Recombinant human granulocyte colony-stimulating factor: Effects on normal and leukemic myeloid cells. Science 1986; 232:61.

331. Kawasaki ES, Ladner MB, Wang AM, et al: Molecular cloning of a complementary DNA encoding human macrophage-specific colony-stimulating factor (CSF-1). Science 1985; 230:291.

332. Jacobs K, Shoemaker B, Rudersdorf R, et al: Isolation and characterization of genomic and cDNA clones of human erythropoietin. Nature 1985; 313:806.

333. Anderson DM, Lyman SD, Baird A, et al: Molecular cloning of mast cell growth factor, a hematopoietin that is active in both membrane bound and soluble forms. Cell 1990; 63:235.

334. Zsebo KM, Williams DA, Geissler EN, et al: Stem cell factor (SFC) is encoded at the *Sl* locus of the mouse and is the ligand for the c-kit tyrosine kinase receptor. Cell 1990; 63:213.

335. Bartley TD, Bogenberger J, Hunt P, et al: Identification and cloning of a megakaryocyte growth and development factor that is a ligand for the cytokine receptor Mpl. Cell 1994; 77:1117.

336. Wong GG, Witek JS, Temple PA, et al: Human GM-CSF: Molecular cloning of the complementary DNA and purification of the natural and recombinant proteins. Science 1985; 228:810.

337. Yang Y-C, Ciarletta AB, Temple PA, et al: Human IL-3 (multi-CSF): Identification by expression cloning of a novel hematopoietic growth factor related to murine IL-3. Cell 1986; 47:3.

338. Huang E, Nocka K, Beier DR, et al: The hematopoietic growth factor KL is encoded at the *Sl* locus and is the ligand of the c-kit receptor, the gene product of the *W* locus. Cell 1990; 63:225.

339. Lok S, Kaushansky K, Holly RD, et al: Cloning and expression of murine thrombopoietin cDNA and stimulation of platelet production in vivo. Nature 1994; 369:565.

340. de Sauvage FJ, Hass PE, Spencer SD, et al: Stimulation of megakaryocytopoiesis and thrombopoiesis by the c-Mpl ligand. Nature 1994; 369:533.

341. Smith DE, Renshaw BR, Ketchem RR, et al: Four new members expand the interleukin-1 superfamily. J Biol Chem 2000; 275:1169.

342. Boulay JL, Paul WE: Hematopoietin sub-family classification based on size, gene organization and sequence homology. Curr Biol 1993; 3:573.

343. Bazan JF: Haemopoietic receptors and helical cytokines. Immunol Today 1990; 11:350.

344. Merberg DM, Wolf SF, Clark SC: Sequence similarity between NKSF and the IL-6/G-CSF family. Immunol Today 1992; 13:77.

345. Leutz A, Damm K, Sterneck E, et al: Molecular cloning of the chicken myelomonocytic growth factor (CMGF) reveals relationship to interleukin 6 and granulocyte colony stimulating factor. EMBO J 1989; 8:175.

346. Sohma Y, Akahori H, Seki N, et al: Molecular cloning and chromosomal localization of the human thrombopoietin gene. FEBS Lett 1994; 353:57.

347. Foster DC, Sprecher CA, Grant FJ, et al: Human thrombopoietin: Gene structure, CDNA sequence, expression, and chromosomal localization. Proc Natl Acad Sci USA 1994; 91:13023.

348. Gurney A, Kuang W, Xie M, et al: Genomic structure, chromosomal localization, and conserved alternative splice forms of thrombopoietin. Blood 1995; 85:981.

349. Anderson DM, Williams DE, Tushinski R, et al: Alternate splicing of mRNAs encoding human mast cell growth factor and localization of the gene to chromosome 12q22-q24. Cell Growth Differ 1991; 2:373.

350. Simmers RN, Webber LM, Shannon MF, et al: Localization of the G-CSF gene on chromosome 17 proximal to the breakpoint in the t(15;17) in acute promyelocytic leukemia. Blood 1987; 70:330.

351. Nagata S, Tsuchiya M, Asano S, et al: The chromosomal gene structure and two mRNAs for human granulocyte colony-stimulating factor. EMBO J 1986; 5:575.

352. Thomas KR, Capecchi MR: Site-directed mutagenesis by gene targeting in mouse embryo-derived stem cells. Cell 1987; 51:503.

353. Lieschke GJ, Grail D, Hodgson G, et al: Mice lacking granulocyte colony-stimulating factor have chronic neuropenia, granulocyte and macrophage progenitor cell deficiency, and impaired neutrophil mobilization. Blood 1994; 84:1737.

354. Hammond WP, Csiba E, Canin A, et al: Chronic neutropenia. A new canine model induced by human granulocyte colony-stimulating factor. J Clin Invest 1991; 87:704.

355. Metcalf D: The molecular control of hematopoiesis: Progress and problems with gene manipulation. Stem Cells 1998; 16:314.

356. Ogawa M, Matsunaga T: Humoral regulation of hematopoietic stem cells. Ann NY Acad Sci 1999; 872:17.

357. Shoemaker CB, Mitsock LD: Murine erythropoietin gene: Cloning, expression, and human gene homology. Mol Cell Biol 1986; 6:849.

358. Law ML, Cai G-Y, Lin F-K: Chromosomal assignment of the human erythropoietin gene and its DNA polymorphism. Proc Natl Acad Sci USA 1986; 83:6920.

359. Gurney AL, Carver-Moore K, de Sauvage FJ, et al: Thrombocytopenia in c-mpl-deficient mice. Science 1994; 265:1445.

360. Gainsford T, Roberts AW, Kimura S, et al: Cytokine production and function in c-*mpl*-deficient mice: No physiologic role for interleukin-3 in residual megakaryocyte and platelet production. Blood 1998; 91:2745.

361. Gainsford T, Nandurkar H, Metcalf D, et al: The residual megakaryocyte and platelet production in c-*mpl*-deficient mice is not dependent on the actions of interleukin-6, interleukin-11, or leukemia inhibitory factor. Blood 2000; 95:528.

362. Wu H, Liu X, Jaenisch R, et al: Generation of committed erythroid BFU-E and CFU-E progenitors does not require erythropoietin or the erythropoietin receptor. Cell 1995; 83:59.

363. Sutherland GR, Baker E, Callen DF, et al: Interleukin 4 is at 5q31 and interleukin 6 is at 7p15. Hum Genet 1988; 79:335.

364. McKinley D, Wu Q, Yang-Feng T, et al: Genomic sequence and chromosomal location of human interleukin-11 gene (IL-11). Genomics 1992; 13:814.

365. Manavalan P, Swope DL, Withy RM: Sequence and structural relationships in the cytokine family. J Protein Chem 1992; 11:321.

366. Kopf M, Baumann H, Freer G, et al: Impaired immune and acute-phase responses in interleukin-6-deficient mice. Nature 1994; 368:339.

367. Bernad A, Kopf M, Kulbacki R, et al: Interleukin-6 is required in vivo for the regulation of stem cells and committed progenitors of the hematopoietic system. Immunity 1994; 1:725.

368. Nandurkar HH, Robb L, Begley CG: The role of IL-11 in hematopoiesis as revealed by a targeted mutation of its receptor. Stem Cells 1998; 16 (Suppl 2):53.

369. Robb L, Li R, Hartley L, et al: Infertility in female mice lacking the receptor for interleukin 11 is due to a defective uterine response to implantation. Nat Med 1998; 4:303.

370. Miyatake S, Otsuka T, Yokota T, et al: Structure of the chromosomal gene for granulocyte-macrophage colony stimulating factor: Comparison of the mouse and human genes. EMBO J 1985; 4:2561.

371. Nimer SD, Uchida H: Regulation of granulocyte-macrophage colony-stimulating factor and interleukin 3 expression. Stem Cells 1995; 13:324.

372. Campbell HD, Tucker WQJ, Hort Y, et al: Molecular cloning, nucleotide sequence, and expression of the gene encoding human eosinophil differentiation factor (interleukin 5). Proc Natl Acad Sci USA 1987; 84:6629.

373. Yang Y-C, Clark SC: Molecular cloning of a primate cDNA and the human gene for IL-3. Lymphokines 1988; 15:375.

374. Dolganov G, Bort S, Lovett M, et al: Coexpression of the interleukin-13 and interleukin-4 genes correlates with their physical linkage in the cytokine gene cluster on human chromosome 5q23-31. Blood 1996; 87:3316.

375. Le Beau MM, Espinosa III R, Neuman WL, et al: Cytogenetic and molecular delineation of the smallest commonly deleted region of chromosome 5 in malignant myeloid diseases. Proc Natl Acad Sci USA 1993; 90:5484.

376. Sieburth D, Jabs EW, Warrington JA, et al: Assignment of genes encoding a unique cytokine (IL12) composed of two unrelated subunits to chromosomes 3 and 5. Genomics 1992; 14:59.

377. Yang Y-C, Kovacic S, Kriz R, et al: The human genes for GM-CSF and IL 3 are closely linked in tandem on chromosome 5. Blood 1988; 71:958.

378. Tavernier J, Devos R, Cornelis S, et al: A human high affinity interleukin-5 receptor (IL5R) is composed of an IL5-specific α chain and a β chain shared with the receptor for GM-CSF. Cell 1991; 66:1175.

379. Kitamura T, Sato N, Arai K, et al: Expression cloning of the human IL-3 receptor cDNA reveals a shared beta subunit for the human IL-3 and GM-CSF receptors. Cell 1991; 66:1165.

380. Stanley E, Lieschke GJ, Grail D, et al: Granulocyte/macrophage colony-stimulating factor-deficient mice show no major perturbation of hematopoiesis but develop a characteristic pulmonary pathology. Proc Natl Acad Sci USA 1994; 91:5592.

381. Dranoff G, Crawford AD, Sadelain M, et al: Involvement of granulocyte-macrophage colony-stimulating factor in pulmonary homeostasis. Science 1994; 264:713.

382. Nishinakamura R, Miyajima A, Mee PJ, et al: Hematopoiesis in mice lacking the entire granulocyte-macrophage colony-stimulating factor/interleukin-3/interleukin-5 functions. Blood 1996; 88:2458.

383. Ladner MB, Martin GA, Noble JA, et al: Human CSF-1: Gene structure and alternative splicing of mRNA precursors. EMBO J 1987; 6:2693.

384. Morris SW, Valentine MS, Shapiro DW, et al: Reassignment of the human *CSF1* gene to chromosome 1P13-p21. Blood 1991; 78:2013.

385. Yoshida H, Hayashi S-I, Kunisada T, et al: The murine mutation osteopetrosis is in the coding region of the macrophage colony stimulating factor gene. Nature 1990; 345:442.

386. Pollard JW, Hunt JS, Wiktor-Jedrzejczak W, et al: A pregnancy defect in the osteopetrotic *(op/op)* mouse demonstrates the requirement for CSF-1 in female fertility. Dev Biol 1991; 148:273.

387. Wiktor-Jedrzejczak W, Ratajczak MZ, Ptasznik A, et al: CSF-1 deficiency in the *op/op* mouse has differential effects on macrophage populations and differentiation stages. Exp Hematol 1992; 20:1004.

388. Hume DA, Favot P: Is the osteopetrotic *(op/op* mutant) mouse completely deficient in expression of macrophage colony-stimulating factor? J Interferon Cytokine Res 1995; 15:279.

389. Metcalf D, Willson TA, Hilton DJ, et al: Production of hematopoietic regulatory factors in cultures of adult and fetal mouse organs: Measurement by specific bioassays. Leukemia 1995; 9:1556.

390. Quesenberry PJ, Crittenden RB, Lowry P, et al: In vitro and in vivo studies of stromal niches. Blood Cells 1994; 20:97.

391. Lokhorst HM, Lamme T, de Smet M, et al: Primary tumor cells of myeloma patients induce interleukin-6 secretion in long-term bone marrow cultures. Blood 1994; 84:2269.

392. Gupta P, Blazar BR, Gupta K, et al: Human CD34+ bone marrow cells regulate stromal production of interleukin-6 and granulocyte colony-stimulating factor and increase the colony-stimulating activity of stroma. Blood 1998; 91:3724.

393. Arai KI, Lee F, Miyajima A, et al: Cytokines: Coordinators of immune and inflammatory responses. Annu Rev Biochem 1990; 59:783.

394. Niemeyer CM, Sieff CA, Mathey-Prevot B, et al: Expression of human interleukin-3 (multi-CSF) is restricted to human lymphocytes and T-cell tumor lines. Blood 1989; 73:945.

395. Wimperis JZ, Niemeyer CM, Sieff CA, et al: Granulocyte-macrophage colony-stimulating factor and interleukin 3 mRNAs are produced by a small fraction of blood mononuclear cells. Blood 1989; 74:1525.

396. Cerdan C, Razanajaona D, Martin Y, et al: Contributions of the CD2 and CD28 T lymphocyte activation pathways to the regulation of the expression of the colony-stimulating factor (CSF-1) gene. J Immunol 1992; 149:373.

397. Horii Y, Muraguchi A, Suematsu S, et al: Regulation of BSF-2/IL-6 production by human mononuclear cells. Macrophage-dependent synthesis of BSF-2/IL-6 by T cells. J Immunol 1988; 141:1529.

398. Yang L, Yang YC: Regulation of interleukin (IL)-11 gene expression in IL-1 induced primate bone marrow stromal cells. J Biol Chem 1994; 269:32732.

399. Yamato K, El-Hajjaoui Z, Kuo JF, et al: Granulocyte-macrophage colony-stimulating factor: Signals for its mRNA accumulation. Blood 1989; 74:1314.

400. Tjian R, Maniatis T: Transcriptional activation: A complex puzzle with few easy pieces. Cell 1994; 77:5.

401. Fitzpatrick DR, Kelso A: Independent regulation of cytokine genes in T cells: The paradox in the paradigm. Transplantation 1998; 65:1.

402. Nimer SD, Uchida H: Regulation of granulocyte-macrophage colony-stimulating factor and interleukin 3 expression. Stem Cells 1995; 13:324.

403. Jones NC, Rigby PW, Ziff EB: Trans-acting protein factors and the regulation of eukaryotic transcription: Lessons from studies on DNA tumor viruses. Genes Dev 1988; 2:267.

404. Mitchell PJ, Tjian R: Transcriptional regulation in mammalian cells by sequence-specific DNA binding proteins. Science 1989; 245:371.

405. Akira S, Kishimoto T: NF-IL6 and NF-κB in cytokine gene regulation. Adv Immunol 1997; 65:1.

406. Rao A, Luo C, Hogan PG: Transcription factors of the nfat family: Regulation and function. Annu Rev Immunol 1997; 15:707.

407. Foletta VC, Segal DH, Cohen DR: Transcriptional regulation in the immune system: All roads lead to AP-1. J Leukoc Biol 1998; 63:139.

408. Wang CY, Bassuk AG, Boise LH, et al: Activation of the granulocyte-macrophage colony-stimulating factor promoter in T cells requires cooperative binding of elf-1 and AP-1 transcription factors. Mol Cell Biol 1994; 14:1153.

409. Weiss MJ, Orkin SH: GATA transcription factors: Key regulators of hematopoiesis. Exp Hematol 1995; 23:99.

410. Shaw G, Kamen R: A conserved AU sequence from the 3′ untranslated region of GM-CSF mRNA mediates selective mRNA degradation. Cell 1986; 46:659.

411. Sachs AB: Messenger RNA degradation in eukaryotes. Cell 1993; 74:413.

412. Nakamaki T, Imamura J, Brewer G, et al: Characterization of adenosine-uridine-rich RNA binding factors. J Cell Physiol 1995; 165:484.

413. Brown CY, Lagnado CA, Goodall GJ: A cytokine mRNA-destabilizing element that is structurally and functionally distinct from A+U-rich elements. Proc Natl Acad Sci USA 1996; 93:13721.

414. Curatola AM, Nadal MS, Schneider RJ: Rapid degradation of AU-rich element (ARE) mRNAs is activated by ribosome transit and blocked by secondary structure at any position 5′ to the ARE. Mol Cell Biol 1995; 15:6331.

415. Falkenburg JH, Harrington MA, de Paus RA, et al: Differential transcriptional and posttranscriptional regulation of gene expression of the colony-stimulating factors by interleukin-1 and fetal bovine serum in murine fibroblasts. Blood 1991; 78:658.

416. Fraser JD, Straus D, Weiss A: Signal transduction events leading to T-cell lymphokine gene expression. Immunol Today 1993; 14:357.

417. Prieschl EE, Gouilleux-Gruart V, Walker C, et al: A nuclear factor of activated T cell-like transcription factor in mast cells is involved in IL-5 gene regulation after IgE plus antigen stimulation. J Immunol 1995; 154:6112.

418. Hempel L, Korholz D, Bonig H, et al: Interleukin-10 directly inhibits the interleukin-6 production in T-cells. Scand J Immunol 1995; 41:462.

419. Blair PJ, Riley JL, Carroll RG, et al: CD28 co-receptor signal transduction in T-cell activation. Biochem Soc Trans 1997; 25:651.

420. Miyatake S, Shlomai J, Arai K, et al: Characterization of the mouse granulocyte-macrophage colony-stimulating factor (GM-CSF) gene promoter: Nuclear factors that interact with an element shared by three lymphokine genes—Those for GM-CSF, interleukin-4 (IL-4), and IL-5. Mol Cell Biol 1991; 11:5894.

421. Rao A: NF-ATp: A transcription factor required for the co-ordinate induction of several cytokine genes. Immunol Today 1994; 15:274.

422. Guba SC, Stella G, Turka LA, et al: Regulation of interleukin 3 gene induction in normal human T cells. J Clin Invest 1989; 84:1701.

423. Lee HJ, Masuda ES, Arai N, et al: Definition of cis-regulatory elements of the mouse interleukin-5 gene promoter. Involvement of nuclear factor of activated T cell-related factors in interleukin-5 expression. J Biol Chem 1995; 270:17541.

424. Mosmann TR, Coffman RL: TH1 and TH2 cells: Different patterns of lymphokine secretion lead to different functional properties. Annu Rev Immunol 1989; 7:145.

425. Groux H, O'Garra A, Bigler M, et al: A CD4+ T-cell subset inhibits antigen-specific T-cell responses and prevents colitis. Nature 1997; 389:737.

426. Pearce EJ, Reiner SL: Induction of Th2 responses in infectious diseases. Curr Opin Immunol 1995; 7:497.

427. Finkelman FD, Wynn TA, Donaldson DD, et al: The role of IL-13 in helminth-induced inflammation and protective immunity against nematode infections. Curr Opin Immunol 1999; 11:420.

428. Trinchieri G: Interleukin-12: A cytokine produced by antigen-presenting cells with immunoregulatory functions in the generation of T-helper cells type 1 and cytotoxic lymphocytes. Blood 1994; 84:4008.

429. Dinarello CA: Interleukin-1 and its biologically related cytokines. Adv Immunol 1989; 44:153.

430. Cluitmans FH, Esendam BH, Landegent JE, et al: Regulatory effects of T cell lymphokines on cytokine gene expression in monocytes. Lymphokine Cytokine Res 1993; 12:457.

431. Horiguchi J, Warren MK, Kufe D: Expression of the macrophage-specific colony-stimulating factor in human monocytes treated with granulocyte-macrophage colony-stimulating factor. Blood 1987; 69:1259.

432. Warren MK, Ralph P: Macrophage growth factor CSF-1 stimulates human monocyte production of interferon, tumor necrosis factor, and colony stimulating activity. J Immunol 1986; 137:2281.

433. Cluitmans FH, Esendam BH, Landegent JE, et al: IL-4 down-regulates IL-2-, IL-3-, and GM-CSF-induced cytokine gene expression in peripheral blood monocytes. Ann Hematol 1994; 68:293.

434. Fiorentino DF, Zlotnik A, Mosmann TR, et al: IL-10 inhibits cytokine production by activated macrophages. J Immunol 1991; 147:3815.

435. Chabaud M, Durand JM, Buchs N, et al: Human interleukin-17: A T cell-derived proinflammatory cytokine produced by the rheumatoid synovium. Arthritis Rheum 1999; 42:963.

436. Evans R, Kamdar SJ, Fuller JA, et al: The potential role of the macrophage colony-stimulating factor, CSF-1, in inflammatory responses: Characterization of macrophage cytokine gene expression. J Leukoc Biol 1995; 58:99.

437. Temeles DS, McGrath HE, Kittler EL, et al: Cytokine expression from bone marrow derived macrophages. Exp Hematol 1993; 21:388.

438. Zhang Y, Broser M, Rom W: Activation of the interleukin 6 gene by Mycobacterium tuberculosis or lipopolysaccharide is mediated by nuclear factors NF IL 6 and NF-κB. Proc Natl Acad Sci USA 1995; 92:3632.

439. Galdiero M, Cipollaro de L, Donnarumma G, et al: Interleukin-1 and interleukin-6 gene expression in human monocytes stimulated with Salmonella typhimurium porins. Immunology 1995; 86:612.

440. Matsusaka T, Fujikawa K, Nishio Y, et al: Transcription factors NF-IL6 and NF-κB synergistically activate transcription of the inflammatory cytokines, interleukin 6 and interleukin 8. Proc Natl Acad Sci USA 1993; 90:10193.

441. Gruss HJ, Brach MA, Herrmann F: Involvement of nuclear factor-κB in induction of the interleukin-6 gene by leukemia inhibitory factor. Blood 1992; 80:2563.

442. Wang P, Wu P, Siegel MI, et al: IL-10 inhibits transcription of cytokine genes in human peripheral blood mononuclear cells. J Immunol 1994; 153:811.

443. Moller A, Schwarz A, Neuner P, et al: Regulation of monocyte and keratinocyte interleukin 6 production by transforming growth factor β. Exp Dermatol 1994; 3:314.

444. de Wit H, Dokter WH, Esselink MT, et al: Interferon-γ enhances the LPS-induced G-CSF gene expression in human adherent monocytes, which is regulated at transcriptional and posttranscriptional levels. Exp Hematol 1993; 21:785.

445. Vellenga E, Dokter W, de Wolf JT, et al: Interleukin-4 prevents the induction of G-CSF mRNA in human adherent monocytes in response to endotoxin and IL-1 stimulation. Br J Haematol 1991; 79:22.

446. Yamada H, Iwase S, Mohri M, et al: Involvement of a nuclear factor-κB-like protein in induction of the macrophage colony-stimulating factor gene by tumor necrosis factor. Blood 1991; 78:1988.

447. Steinman RM: The dendritic cell system and its role in immunogenicity. Annu Rev Immunol 1991; 9:271.

448. Zhou LJ, Tedder TF: A distinct pattern of cytokine gene expression by human CD83+ blood dendritic cells. Blood 1995; 86:3295.

449. Galy A, Travis M, Cen D, et al: Human T, B, natural killer, and dendritic cells arise from a common bone marrow progenitor cell subset. Immunity 1995; 3:459.

450. Morelli AE, Zahorchak AF, Larregina AT, et al: Cytokine production by mouse myeloid dendritic cells in relation to differentiation and terminal maturation induced by lipopolysaccharide or CD40 ligation. Blood 2001; 98:1512.

451. Demetri GD, Griffin JD: Hemopoietins and leukemia [review]. Hematol Oncol Clin North Am 1989; 3:535.

452. Clark SC: Hematopoietic growth factors and the myeloid leukemias. In Brugge J, Curran T, Harlow E, McCormick F (eds): Origins of Human Cancer. A Comprehensive Review. Cold Spring Harbor, NY, Cold Spring Harbor Laboratory Press, 1991, p 453.

453. Vellenga E, Young DC, Wagner K, et al: The effects of GM-CSF and G-CSF in promoting growth of clonogenic cells in acute myeloblastic leukemia. Blood 1987; 69:1771.

454. Rogers SY, Bradbury D, Kozlowski R, et al: Evidence for internal autocrine regulation of growth in acute myeloblastic leukemia cells. Exp Hematol 1994; 22:593.

455. Griffin JD, Rambaldi A, Vellenga E, et al: Secretion of interleukin-1 by acute myeloblastic leukemia cells in vitro induces endothelial cells to secrete colony stimulating factors. Blood 1987; 70:1218.

456. Kishimoto H, Matsunaga T, Yamamoto T, et al: Leukemic erythroderma with elevated plasma IL-3 and hyperhistaminemia: In situ expression of IL-3 mRNA in leukemic cells. J Dermatol Sci 1995; 10:224.

457. Meeker TC, Hardy D, Willman C, et al: Activation of the interleukin-3 gene by chromosome translocation in acute lymphocytic leukemia with eosinophilia. Blood 1990; 76:285.

458. Chen YZ, Gu XF, Caen JP, et al: Interleukin-3 is an autocrine growth factor of human megakaryoblasts, the DAMI and MEG-01 cells. Br J Haematol 1994; 88:481.

459. Kobayashi S, Teramura M, Sugawara I, et al: Interleukin-11 acts as an autocrine growth factor for human megakaryoblastic cell lines. Blood 1993; 81:889.

460. Nimer S, Zhang J, Avraham H, et al: Transcriptional regulation of interleukin-3 expression in megakaryocytes. Blood 1996; 88:66.

461. Hess JL, Zutter MM, Castleberry RP, et al: Juvenile chronic myelogenous leukemia. Am J Clin Pathol 1996; 105:238.

462. Zecca M, Rosti V, Pinto L, et al: Juvenile chronic myelogenous leukemia: In vitro characterization before and after allogeneic bone marrow transplantation. Med Pediatr Oncol 1995; 24:166.

463. Watari K, Ozawa K, Tajika K, et al: Production of human granulocyte colony stimulating factor by various kinds of stromal cells in vitro detected by enzyme immunoassay and in situ hybridization. Stem Cells 1994; 12:416.

464. Mantovani L, Henschler R, Brach MA, et al: Regulation of gene expression of macrophage-colony stimulating factor in human fibroblasts by the acute phase response mediators interleukin (IL)-1β, tumor necrosis factor-α, and IL-6. FEBS Lett 1991; 280:97.

465. Walther Z, May LT, Sehgal PB: Transcriptional regulation of the interferon-β 2/B cell differentiation factor BSF-2/hepatocyte-stimulating factor gene in human fibroblasts by other cytokines. J Immunol 1988; 140:974.

466. Sironi M, Sciacca FL, Matteucci C, et al: Regulation of endothelial and mesothelial cell function by interleukin-13: Selective induction of vascular cell adhesion molecule-1 and amplification of interleukin-6 production. Blood 1994; 84:1913.

467. Hirano T, Akira S, Taga T, et al: Biological and clinical aspects of interleukin 6. Immunol Today 1990; 11:443.

468. Van Snick J: Interleukin-6: An overview. Annu Rev Immunol 1990; 8:253.

469. Heinrich MC, Dooley DC, Freed AC, et al: Constitutive expression of Steel factor gene by human stromal cells. Blood 1993; 82:771.

470. Cerretti DP, Wignall J, Anderson D, et al: Membrane bound forms of human macrophage colony stimulating factor (M-CSF, CSF-1). Prog Clin Biol Res 1990; 352:63.

471. Yang Y-C, Tsai S, Wong GG, et al: Interleukin-1 regulation of hematopoietic growth factor production by human stromal fibroblasts. J Cell Physiol 1988; 134:292.

472. Lilly M, Vo K, Le T, et al: Bryostatin 1 acts synergistically with interleukin-1α to induce secretion of G-CSF and other cytokines from marrow stromal cells. Exp Hematol 1996; 24:613.

473. Shannon MF, Coles LS, Fielke RK, et al: Three essential promoter elements mediate tumour necrosis factor and interleukin-1 activation of the granulocyte-colony stimulating factor gene. Growth Factors 1992; 7:181.

474. Tobler A, Meier R, Seitz M, et al: Glucocorticoids downregulate gene expression of GM-CSF, NAP-1/IL-8, and IL-6, but not of M-CSF in human fibroblasts. Blood 1992; 79:45.

475. Hachiya M, Koeffler HP, Suzuki G, et al: Tumor necrosis factor and interleukin-1 synergize with irradiation in expression of GM-CSF gene in human fibroblasts. Leukemia 1995; 9:1276.

476. Cohen-Kaminsky S, Delattre RM, Devergne O, et al: Synergistic induction of interleukin-6 production and gene expression in human thymic epithelial cells by LPS and cytokines. Cell Immunol 1991; 138:79.

477. Chauhan D, Uchiyama H, Akbarali Y, et al: Multiple myeloma cell adhesion-induced interleukin-6 expression in bone marrow stromal cells involves activation of NF-κB. Blood 1996; 87:1104.

478. Zhang YH, Lin JX, Vilcek J: Interleukin-6 induction by tumor necrosis factor and interleukin-1 in human fibroblasts involves activation of a nuclear factor binding to a κB-like sequence. Mol Cell Biol 1990; 10:3818.

479. Stein B, Yang MX: Repression of the interleukin-6 promoter by estrogen receptor is mediated by NF-κB and C/EBP β. Mol Cell Biol 1995; 15:4971.

480. Poli V, Balena R, Fattori E, et al: Interleukin-6 deficient mice are protected from bone loss caused by estrogen depletion. EMBO J 1994; 13:1189.

481. Seelentag WK, Mermod J-J, Montesano R, et al: Additive effects of interleukin 1 and tumor necrosis factor α on the accumulation of the three granulocyte and macrophage colony-stimulating factor mRNAs in human endothelial cells. EMBO J 1987; 6:2261.

482. Zsebo KM, Yuschenkoff VN, Schiffer S, et al: Vascular endothelial cells and granulopoiesis: Interleukin-1 stimulates release of G-CSF and GM-CSF. Blood 1988; 71:99.

483. Koenig A, Yakisan E, Reuter M, et al: Differential regulation of stem cell factor mRNA expression in human endothelial cells by bacterial pathogens: An in vitro model of inflammation. Blood 1994; 83:2836.

484. Bagby GC, Shaw G, Heinrich MC, et al: Interleukin-1 stimulation stabilizes GM-CSF mRNA in human vascular endothelial cells: Preliminary studies on the role of the 3′ AU rich motif. Prog Clin Biol Res 1990; 352:233.

485. Rajavashisth TB, Yamada H, Mishra NK: Transcriptional activation of the macrophage-colony stimulating factor gene by minimally modified LDL. Involvement of nuclear factor-κB. Arterioscler Thromb Vasc Biol 1995; 15:1591.

486. Jelkmann W: Erythropoietin: Structure, control of production, and function. Physiol Rev 1992; 72:449.

487. Eckardt KU, Ratcliffe PJ, Tan CC, et al: Age-dependent expression of the erythropoietin gene in rat liver and kidneys. J Clin Invest 1992; 89:753.

488. Semenza GL, Koury ST, Nejfelt MK, et al: Cell-type-specific and hypoxia-inducible expression of the human erythropoietin gene in transgenic mice. Proc Natl Acad Sci USA 1991; 88:8725.

489. Semenza GL, Nejfelt MK, Chi SM, et al: Hypoxia-inducible nuclear factors bind to an enhancer element located 3′ to the human erythropoietin gene. Proc Natl Acad Sci USA 1991; 88:5680.

490. Semenza GL: Regulation of erythropoietin production. New insights into molecular mechanisms of oxygen homeostasis. Hematol Oncol Clin North Am 1994; 8:863.

491. Wang GL, Semenza GL: Purification and characterization of hypoxia-inducible factor 1. J Biol Chem 1995; 270:1230.

492. Semenza GL: HIF-1: Mediator of physiological and pathophysiological responses to hypoxia. J Appl Physiol 2000; 88:1474.

493. Blanchard KL, Acquaviva AM, Galson DL, et al: Hypoxic induction of the human erythropoietin gene: Cooperation between the promoter and enhancer, each of which contains steroid receptor response elements. Mol Cell Biol 1992; 12:5373.

494. Stoffel R, Wiestner A, Skoda RC: Thrombopoietin in thrombocytopenic mice: Evidence against regulation at the mRNA level and for a direct regulatory role of platelets. Blood 1996; 87:567.

495. Chang M, Suen Y, Buzby G, et al: Differential mechanisms in the regulation of endogenous levels of thrombopoietin and interleukin-11 during thrombocytopenia: Insight into the regulation of platelet production. Blood 1996; 88:3354.

496. Bartocci A, Mastrogiannis DS, Migliorati G, et al: Macrophages specifically regulate the concentration of their own growth factor in the circulation. Proc Natl Acad Sci USA 1987; 84:6179.

497. Bazan JF: Structural design and molecular evolution of a cytokine receptor superfamily. Proc Natl Acad Sci USA 1990; 87:6934.

498. Endo TA, Masuhara M, Yokouchi M, et al: A new protein containing an SH2 domain that inhibits JAK kinases. Nature 1997; 387:921.

499. Naka T, Narazaki M, Hirata M, et al: Structure and function of a new STAT-induced STAT inhibitor. Nature 1997; 387:924.

500. Boutin J-M, Jolicoeur C, Okamura H, et al: Cloning and expression of the rat prolactin receptor, a member of the growth hormone/prolactin receptor gene family. Cell 1988; 53:69.

501. Edery M, Jolicoeur C, Levi-Meyrueis C, et al: Identification and sequence analysis of a second form of prolactin receptor by molecular cloning of complementary DNA from rabbit mammary gland. Proc Natl Acad Sci USA 1989; 86:2112.

502. Leung DW, Spencer SA, Cachianes G, et al: Growth hormone receptor and serum binding protein: Purification, cloning and expression. Nature 1987; 330:537.

503. Hatakeyama M, Mori H, Doi T, et al: A restricted cytoplasmic region of IL-2 receptor β chain is essential for growth signal transduction but not for ligand binding and internalization. Cell 1989; 59:837.

504. Miura O, Cleveland JL, Ihle JN: Inactivation of erythropoietin receptor function by point mutations in a region having homology with other cytokine receptors. Mol Cell Biol 1993; 13:1788.

505. Miyajima A, Mui ALF, Ogorochi T, et al: Receptors for granulocyte-macrophage colony-stimulating factor, interleukin-3, and interleukin-5. Blood 1993; 82:1960.

506. Kondo M, Takeshita T, Ishii N, et al: Sharing of the interleukin-2 (IL-2) receptor γ chain between receptors for IL-2 and IL-4. Science 1993; 262:1874.

507. Russell S, Keegan AD, Harada N, et al: Interleukin-2 receptor γ chain: A functional component of the interleukin-4 receptor. Science 1993; 262:1880.

508. Noguchi M, Nakamura Y, Russell SM, et al: Interleukin-2 receptor γ chain: A functional component of the interleukin-7 receptor. Science 1993; 262:1877.

509. Kimura Y, Takeshita T, Kondo M, et al: Sharing of the IL-2 receptor γ chain with the functional IL-9 receptor complex. Int Immunol 1995; 7:115.

510. Giri JG, Ahdieh M, Eisenman J, et al: Utilization of the β and γ chains of the IL-2 receptor by the novel cytokine IL-15. EMBO J 1994; 13:2822.

511. Nicola NA: Hemopoietic cell growth factors and their receptors. Annu Rev Biochem 1989; 58:45.

512. Metcalf D: Hemopoetic regulators—Redundancy or subtlety? Blood 1993; 82:3515.

513. Testa U, Pelosi E, Gabbianelli M, et al: Cascade transactivation of growth factor receptors in early human hematopoiesis. Blood 1993; 81:1442.

514. Alexander WS, Starr R, Fenner JE, et al: SOCS1 is a critical inhibitor of interferon γ signaling and prevents the potentially fatal neonatal actions of this cytokine. Cell 1999; 98:597.

515. Brady G, Billia F, Knox J, et al: Analysis of gene expression in a complex differentiation hierarchy by global amplification of cDNA from single cells [published erratum appears in Curr Biol 1995; 5:1201]. Curr Biol 1995; 5:909.

516. Yoshimura A, Ohkubo T, Kiguchi T, et al: A novel cytokine-inducible gene CIS encodes an SH2-containing protein that binds to tyrosine-phosphorylated interleukin 3 and erythropoietin receptors. EMBO J 1995; 14:2816.

517. Jacobsen SEW, Ruscetti FW, Dubois CM, et al: Induction of colony-stimulating factor receptor expression on hematopoietic progenitor cells: Proposed mechanism for growth factor synergism. Blood 1992; 80:678.

518. Liboi E, Jubinsky P, Andrews NC, et al: Enhanced expression of interleukin-3 and granulocyte-macrophage colony-stimulating factor receptor subunits in murine hematopoietic cells stimulated with hematopoietic growth factors. Blood 1992; 80:1183.

519. Ziegler SF, Bird TA, Morella KK, et al: Distinct regions of the human granulocyte-colony-stimulating factor receptor cytoplasmic domain are required for proliferation and gene induction. Mol Cell Biol 1993; 13:2384.

520. Fukunaga R, Ishizaka-Ikeda E, Nagata S: Growth and differentiation signals mediated by different regions in the cytoplasmic domain of granulocyte colony-stimulating factor receptor. Cell 1993; 74:1079.

521. Dong F, Brynes RK, Tidow N, et al: Mutations in the gene for the granulocyte colony-stimulating-factor receptor in patients with acute myeloid leukemia preceded by severe congenital neutropenia. N Engl J Med 1995; 333:487.

522. Borzillo GV, Ashmun RA, Sherr CJ: Macrophage lineage switching of murine early pre-B lymphoid cells expressing transduced *fms* genes. Mol Cell Biol 1990; 10:2703.

523. Liboi E, Carroll M, D'Andrea AD, et al: Erythropoietin receptor signals both proliferation and erythroid-specific differentiation. Proc Natl Acad Sci USA 1993; 90:11351.

524. Jubinsky PT, Nathan DG, Wilson DJ, et al: A low-affinity human granulocyte-macrophage colony-stimulating factor/murine erythropoietin hybrid receptor functions in murine cell lines. Blood 1993; 81:587.

525. Sakamaki K, Wang H-M, Miyajima I, et al: Ligand-dependent activation of chimeric receptors with the cytoplasmic domain of the interleukin-3 receptor β subunit (βIL3). J Biol Chem 1993; 268:15833.

526. Chiba T, Nagata Y, Machide M, et al: Tyrosine kinase activation through the extracellular domains of cytokine receptors. Nature 1993; 362:646.

527. Chiba T, Nagata Y, Kishi A, et al: Induction of erythroid-specific gene expression in lymphoid cells. Proc Natl Acad Sci USA 1993; 90:11593.

528. Fairbairn LJ, Cowling GJ, Reipert BM, et al: Suppression of apoptosis allows differentiation and development of a multipotent hemopoietic cell line in the absence of added growth factors. Cell 1993; 74:823.

529. Songyang Z, Shoelson SE, Chaudhuri M, et al: SH2 domains recognize specific phospopeptide sequences. Cell 1993; 72:767.

530. Ihle JN, Witthuhn BA, Quelle FW, et al: Signaling through the hematopoietic cytokine receptors. Annu Rev Immunol 1995; 13:369.

531. Schindler CW: Series introduction. JAK-STAT signaling in human disease. J Clin Invest 2002; 109:1133.

532. Aaronson DS, Horvath CM: A road map for those who know JAK-STAT. Science 2002; 296:1653.

533. Velazquez L, Fellous M, Stark GR, et al: A protein tyrosine kinase in the interferon α/β signaling pathway. Cell 1992; 70:313.

534. Müller M, Briscoe J, Laxton C, et al: The protein tyrosine kinase JAK1 complements defects in interferon-α/β and -γ signal transduction. Nature 1993; 366:129.

535. Witthuhn BA, Quelle FW, Silvennoinen O, et al: JAK2 associates with the erythropoietin receptor and is tyrosine phosphorylated and activated following stimulation with erythropoietin. Cell 1993; 74:227.

536. Zhuang H, Patel SV, He T, et al: Inhibition of erythropoietin-induced mitogenesis by a kinase-deficient form of Jak2. J Biol Chem 1994; 269:21411.

537. Linnekin D, Evans GA, D'Andrea A, et al: Association of the erythropoietin receptor with protein tyrosine kinase activity. Proc Natl Acad Sci USA 1992; 89:6237.

538. Miura O, D'Andrea A, Kabat D, et al: Induction of tyrosine phosphorylation by the erythropoietin receptor correlates with mitogenesis. Mol Cell Biol 1991; 11:4895.

539. Yoshimura A, Lodish HF: In vitro phosphorylation of the erythropoietin receptor and an associated protein, pp130. Mol Cell Biol 1992; 12:706.

540. Hanazono Y, Chib S, Sasaki K, et al: Erythropoietin induces tyrosine phosphorylation and kinase activity of the c-*fps*/*fes* proto-oncogene product in human erythropoietin-responsive cells. Blood 1993; 81:3193.

541. Ihle JN: Cytokine receptor signaling. Nature 1995; 377:591.

542. Sakamaki K, Miyajima I, Kitamura T, et al: Critical cytoplasmic domains of the common β subunit of the human GM-CSF, IL-3 and IL-5 receptors for growth signal transduction and tyrosine phosphorylation. EMBO J 1992; 11:3541.

543. Duronio V, Clark-Lewis I, Federsppiel B, et al: Tyrosine phosphorylation of receptor β subunits and common substrates in response to interleukin-3 and granulocyte-macrophage colony-stimulating factor. J Biol Chem 1992; 267:21856.

544. Silvennoinen O, Witthuhn BA, Quelle FW, et al: Structure of the murine JAK2 protein tyrosine kinase and its role in IL-3 signal transduction. Proc Natl Acad Sci USA 1993; 90:8429.

545. Shikama Y, Barber DL, D'Andrea A, et al: A constitutively activated chimeric cytokine receptor confers factor-dependent growth in hematopoietic cell lines. Blood 1996; 88:455.

546. Torigoe T, O'Connor R, Santoli D, et al: Interleukin-3 regulates the activity of the LYN protein-tyrosine kinase in myeloid-committed leukemic cell lines. Blood 1992; 80:617.

547. Kobayashi N, Kono T, Hatakeyama M, et al: Functional coupling of the src-family protein tyrosine kinases p59^{fyn} and p53/56^{lyn} with the interleukin 2 receptor: Implications for redundancy and pleiotopism in cytokine signal transduction. Proc Natl Acad Sci USA 1993; 90:4201.

548. Hanazono Y, Chiba S, Sasaki K, et al: c-*fps*/*fes* protein-tyrosine is implicated in a signaling pathway triggered by granulocyte-macrophage colony-stimulating factor and interleukin-3. EMBO J 1993; 12:1641.

549. Quelle FW, Sato N, Witthuhn BA, et al: JAK2 associates with the β$_c$ chain of the receptor for granulocyte-macrophage colony-stimulating factor, and its activation requires the membrane-proximal region. Mol Cell Biol 1994; 14:4335.

550. Weiss M, Yokoyama C, Shikama Y, et al: Human granulocyte-macrophage colony-stimulating factor receptor signal transduction requires the proximal cytoplasmic domains of the α and β subunits. Blood 1993; 82:3298.

551. Sato N, Sakamaki K, Terada N, et al: Signal transduction by the high-affinity GM-CSF receptor: Two distinct cytoplasmic regions of the common β subunit responsible for different signaling. EMBO J 1993; 12:4181.

552. Kinoshita T, Yokota T, Arai K-I, et al: Suppression of apoptotic death in hematopoietic cells by signalling through the IL-3/GM-CSF receptors. EMBO J 1995; 14:266.

553. Stahl N, Boulton TG, Farruggella T, et al: Association and activation of Jak-Tyk kinases by CNTF-LIF-OSM-IL-6β receptor components. Science 1994; 263:92.

554. Fu X-Y: A transcription factor with SH2 and SH3 domains is directly activated by an interferon α-induced cytoplasmic protein tyrosine kinase(s). Cell 1992; 70:323.

555. Fu X-Y, Schindler C, Improta T, et al: The proteins of ISGF-3, the interferon α-induced transcriptional activator, define a gene family involved in signal transduction. Proc Natl Acad Sci USA 1992; 89:7840.

556. Darnell Jr. JE, Kerr IM, Stark GR: Jak-STAT pathways and transcriptional activation in response to IFNs and other extracellular signaling proteins. Science 1994; 264:1415.

557. Watling D, Guschin D, Müller M, et al: Complementation by the protein tyrosine kinase JAK2 of a mutant cell line defective in the interferon-γ signal transduction pathway. Nature 1993; 366:166.

558. Shuai K, Stark GR, Kerr IM, et al: A single phosphotyrosine residue of STAT91 required for gene activation by interferon γ. Science 1993; 261:1744.

559. Lütticken C, Wegenka UM, Yuan J, et al: Association of transcription factor APRF and protein kinase Jak1 with the interleukin-6 signal transducer gp130. Science 1994; 263:89.

560. Zhong Z, Wen Z, Darnell Jr. JE: STAT3: A STAT family member activated by tyrosine phosphoryation in response to epidermal growth factor and interleukin-6. Science 1994; 264:95.

561. Zhong Z, Wen Z, Darnell JE Jr: Stat3 and Stat4: Members of the family of signal transducers and activators of transcription. Proc Natl Acad Sci USA 1994; 91:4806.

562. Yamamoto K, Quelle FW, Thierfelder WE, et al: Stat4, a novel γ interferon activation site-binding protein expressed in early myeloid differentiation. Mol Cell Biol 1994; 14:4342.

563. Jacobson NG, Szabo SJ, Weber-Nordt RM, et al: Interleukin 12 signaling in T helper type 1 (Th1) cells involves tyrosine phosphorylation of signal transducer and activator of transcription (Stat)3 and Stat4. J Exp Med 1995; 181:1755.

564. Larner AC, David M, Feldman GM, et al: Tyrosine phosphorylation of DNA binding proteins by multiple cytokines. Science 1993; 261:1730.

565. Wakao H, Gouilleux F, Groner B: Mammary gland factor (MGF) is a novel member of the cytokine regulated transcription factor gene family and confers the prolactin response. EMBO J 1994; 13:2182.

566. Gouilleux F, Pallard C, Dusanter-Fourt I, et al: Prolactin, growth hormone, erythropoietin and granulocyte-macrophage colony stimulating factor induce MGF-Stat5 DNA binding activity. EMBO J 1995; 14:2005.

567. Mui ALF, Wakao H, O'Farrell A-M, et al: Interleukin-3, granulocyte-macrophage colony stimulating factor and interleukin-5 transduce signals through two STAT5 homologs. EMBO J 1995; 14:1166.

568. Hou J, Schindler U, Henzel WJ, et al: An interleukin-4-induced transcription factor: IL-4 Stat. Science 1994; 265:1701.

569. McCormick F: How receptors turn Ras on. Nature 1993; 363:15.

570. Feig L: The many roads that lead to Ras. Science 1993; 260:767.

571. Moodie SA, Willumsen BM, Weber MJ, et al: Complexes of Ras-GTP with Raf-1 and mitogen-activated protein kinase kinase. Science 1993; 260:1658.

572. Satoh T, Nakafuku M, Miyajima A, et al: Involvement of *ras* p21 protein in signal-transduction pathways from interleukin 2, interleukin 3, and granulocyte/macrophage colony-stimulating factor, but not from interleukin 4. Proc Natl Acad Sci USA 1991; 88:3314.

573. Duronio V, Welham MJ, Abraham S, et al: p21^{ras} activation via hemopoietin receptors and c-Kit requires tyrosine kinase activity but not phosphorylation of p21^{ras} GTPase-activating protein. Proc Natl Acad Sci USA 1992; 89:1587.

574. Torti M, Marti KB, Altschuler D, et al: Erythropoietin induces p21^{ras} activation and p120GAP tyrosine phosphorylation in human erythroleukemia cells. J Biol Chem 1992; 267:8293.

575. Downward J, Graves JD, Warne PH, et al: Stimulation of p21^{ras} upon T-cell activation. Nature 1990; 346:719.

576. Gulbins E, Coggeshall KM, Baier G, et al: Tyrosine kinase-stimulated guanine nucleotide exchange activity of Vav in T cell activation. Science 1993; 260:822.

577. Kavanaugh WM, Williams LT: An alternative to SH2 domains for binding tyrosine-phosphorylated proteins. Science 1994; 266:1862.

578. van der Geer P, Pawson T: The PTB domain: A new protein module implicated in signal transduction. Trends Biochem Sci 1996; 20:277.

579. Ravichandran KS, Burakoff SJ: The adapter protein Shc interacts with the interleukin-2 (IL-2) receptor upon upon IL-2 stimulation. J Biol Chem 1994; 269:1599.

580. Pratt JC, Weiss M, Sieff CA, et al: Evidence for a physical association between the Shc-PTB domain and the β$_c$ chain of the granulocyte-macrophage colony stimulating receptor. J Biol Chem 1996; 271:12137.

581. Inhorn RC, Carlesso N, Durstin M, et al: Identification of a viability domain in the granulocyte/macrophage colony-stimulating factor receptor β-chain involving tyrosine-750. Med.Sci. 1995; 92:8665.

582. Damen JE, Liu L, Cutler RL, et al: Erythropoietin stimulates the tyrosine phosphorylation of Shc and its association with Grb2 and a 145-Kd tyrosine phosphorylated protein. Blood 1993; 82:2296.

583. Cutler RL, Liu L, Damen JE, et al: Multiple cytokines induce the tyrosine phosphorylation of Shc and its association with Grb2 in hemopoietic cells. J Biol Chem 1993; 268:21463.

584. Komatsu N, Adamson JW, Yamamoto K, et al: Erythropoietin rapidly induces tyrosine phosphorylation in the human erythropoietin-dependent cell line, UT-7. Blood 1992; 80:53.

585. Carroll MP, Spivak JL, McMahon M, et al: Erythropoietin induces Raf-1 activation and Raf-1 is required for erythropoietin-mediated proliferation. J Biol Chem 1991; 266:14964.

586. Miura Y, Miura O, Ihle JN, et al: Activation of the mitogen-activated protein kinase pathway by the erythropoietin receptor. J Biol Chem 1994; 269:29962.

587. Bader JL: Neurofibromatosis and cancer. Ann NY Acad Sci 1986; 486:57.

588. Shannon KM, O'Connell P, Martin GA, et al: Loss of the normal NF1 allele from the bone marrow of children with type 1 neurofibromatosis and malignant myeloid disorders. N Engl J Med 1994; 330:597.

589. Bollag G, Clapp DW, Shih S, et al: Loss of NF1 results in activation of the Ras signaling pathway and leads to aberrant growth in haematopoietic cells. Nat Genet 1996; 12:144.

590. Largaespada DA, Brannan CI, Jenkins NA, et al: NF1 deficiency causes Ras-mediated granulocyte/macrophage colony stimulating factor hypersensitivity and chronic myeloid leukaemia. Nat Genet 1996; 12:137.

591. Pendergast AM, Quilliam LA, Cripe LD, et al: BCR-ABL-induced oncogenesis is mediated by direct interaction with the SH2 domain of the GRB-2 adaptor protein. Cell 1993; 75:175.

592. D'Andrea AD, Yoshimura A, Youssoufian H, et al: The cytoplasmic region of the erythropoietin receptor contains nonoverlapping positive and negative growth-regulatory domains. Mol Cell Biol 1991; 11:1980.

593. Yi T, Mui ALF, Krystal G, et al: Hematopoietic cell phosphatase associates with the interleukin-3 (IL-3) receptor β chain and down-regulates IL-3-induced tyrosine phosphorylation and mitogenesis. Mol Cell Biol 1993; 13:7577.

594. de la Chapelle A, Traskelin A-L, Juvonen E: Truncated erythropoietin receptor causes dominantly inherited benign human erythrocytosis. Proc Natl Acad Sci USA 1993; 90:4495.

595. Klingmüller U, Lorenz U, Cantley LC, et al: Specific recruitment of SH-PTP1 to the erythropoietin receptor causes inactivation of JAK2 and termination of proliferative signals. Cell 1995; 80:729.

596. Van Zant G, Shultz L: Hematologic abnormalities of the immunodeficient mouse mutant, viable motheaten (me^v). Exp Hematol 1989; 17:81.

597. Schultz LD, Schweitzer PA, Rajan TV, et al: Mutations at the murine motheaten locus are within the hematopoietic cell protein-tyrosine phosphatase (Hcph) gene. Cell 1993; 73:1445.

598. Sun H, Tonks NK: The coordinated action of protein tyrosine phophatases and kinases in cell signaling. Trends Biochem Sci 1994; 19:480.

599. Starr R, Willson TA, Viney EM, et al: A family of cytokine-inducible inhibitors of signalling. Nature 1997; 387:917.

600. Greenhalgh CJ, Hilton DJ: Negative regulation of cytokine signaling. J Leukoc Biol 2001; 70:348.

601. Nicholson SE, Willson TA, Farley A, et al: Mutational analyses of the SOCS proteins suggest a dual domain requirement but distinct mechanisms for inhibition of LIF and IL-6 signal transduction. EMBO J 1999; 18:375.

602. Kamura T, Sato S, Haque D, et al: The elongin BC complex interacts with the conserved SOCS-box motif present in members of the SOCS, ras, WD-40 repeat, and ankyrin repeat families. Genes Dev 1998; 12:3872.

603. Zhang JG, Farley A, Nicholson SE, et al: The conserved SOCS box motif in suppressors of cytokine signaling binds to elongins B and C and may couple bound proteins to proteasomal degradation. Proc Natl Acad Sci USA 1999; 96:2071.

604. Sasaki A, Yasukawa H, Shouda T, et al: CIS3/SOCS-3 suppresses erythropoietin (EPO) signaling by binding the EPO receptor and JAK2. J Biol Chem 2000; 275:29338.

605. Starr R, Metcalf D, Elefanty AG, et al: Liver degeneration and lymphoid deficiencies in mice lacking suppressor of cytokine signaling-1. Proc Natl Acad Sci USA 1998; 95:14395.

606. Naka T, Matsumoto T, Narazaki M, et al: Accelerated apoptosis of lymphocytes by augmented induction of Bax in SSI-1 (STAT-induced STAT inhibitor-1) deficient mice. Proc Natl Acad Sci USA 1998; 95:15577.

607. Marine JC, Topham DJ, McKay C, et al: SOCS1 deficiency causes a lymphocyte-dependent perinatal lethality. Cell 1999; 98:609.

608. Metcalf D, Greenhalgh CJ, Viney E, et al: Gigantism in mice lacking suppressor of cytokine signalling-2. Nature 2000; 405:1069.

609. Marine JC, McKay C, Wang D, et al: SOCS3 is essential in the regulation of fetal liver erythropoiesis. Cell 1999; 98:617.

610. Matsumoto A, Seki Y, Kubo M, et al: Suppression of STAT5 functions in liver, mammary glands, and T cells in cytokine-inducible SH2-containing protein 1 transgenic mice. Mol Cell Biol 1999; 19:6396.

611. Liu X, Robinson GW, Wagner KU, et al: Stat5a is mandatory for adult mammary gland development and lactogenesis. Genes Dev 1997; 11:179.

612. Teglund S, McKay C, Schuetz E, et al: Stat5a and Stat5b proteins have essential and nonessential, or redundant, roles in cytokine responses. Cell 1998; 93:841.

613. Udy GB, Towers RP, Snell RG, et al: Requirement of STAT5b for sexual dimorphism of body growth rates and liver gene expression. Proc Natl Acad Sci USA 1997; 94:7239.

614. Liu B, Liao J, Rao X, et al: Inhibition of Stat1-mediated gene activation by PIAS1. Proc Natl Acad Sci USA 1998; 95:10626.

615. Mowen KA, Tang J, Zhu W, et al: Arginine methylation of STAT1 modulates IFNα/β-induced transcription. Cell 2001; 104:731.

616. Chung CD, Liao J, Liu B, et al: Specific inhibition of Stat3 signal transduction by PIAS3. Science 1997; 278:1803.

617. Sherr CJ: Mammalian G_1 cyclins. Cell 1993; 73:1059.

618. Ohtsubo M, Roberts JM: Cyclin-dependent regulation of G_1 in mammalian fibroblasts. Science 1993; 259:1908.

619. Baldin V, Lukas J, Marcote MJ, et al: Cyclin D1 is a nuclear protein required for cell cycle progression in G_1. Genes Dev 1993; 7:812.

620. Nevins JR: E2F: A link between the Rb tumor suppressor protein and viral oncoproteins. Science 1992; 258:424.

621. Kato J-Y, Sherr CJ: Inhibition of granulocyte differentiation by G_1 cyclins D2 and D3 but not D1. Proc Natl Acad Sci USA 1993; 90:11513.

622. Kurtzberg J, Laughlin M, Graham ML, et al: Placental blood as a source of hematopoietic stem cells for transplantation into unrelated recipients. N Engl J Med 1996; 335:157.

623. Ando K, Ajchenbaum-Cymbelista F, Griffin JD: Regulation of G_1/S transition by cyclins D2 and D3 in hematopoietic cells. Proc Natl Acad Sci USA 1993; 90:9571.

624. Lee EYHP, Chang C-Y, Hu N, et al: Mice deficient for Rb are nonviable and show defects in neurogeneisis and haematopoiesis. Nature 1992; 359:288.

625. Clarke AR, Maandag ER, van Roon M, et al: Requirement for a functional Rb-1 gene in murine development. Nature 1992; 359:328.

626. Jacks T, Fazeli A, Schmitt EM, et al: Effects of an RB mutation in the mouse. Nature 1992; 359:295.

627. Pevny L, Simon MC, Robertson E, et al: Erythroid differentiation in chimaeric mice blocked by a targeted mutation in the gene for transcription factor GATA-1. Nature 1991; 349:257.

628. Mucenski ML, McLain K, Kier AB, et al: A functional c-myb gene is required for normal murine fetal hepatic hematopoiesis. Cell 1991; 65:677.

629. Xiong Y, Zhang H, Beach D: Subunit rearrangement of the cyclin-dependent kinases is associated with cellular transformation. Genes Dev 1993; 7:1572.

630. Motokura T, Bloom T, Kim HG, et al: A novel cyclin encoded by a bcl1-linked candidate oncogene. Nature 1991; 350:512.

631. Rosenberg CL, Wong E, Petty EM, et al: PRAD1, a candidate BCL1 oncogene: Mapping and expression in centrocytic lymphoma. Proc Natl Acad Sci USA 1991; 88:9638.

632. Schuuring E, Verhoeven E, Mooi WJ, et al: Identification and cloning of two overexpressed genes, U21B31/PRAD1 and EMS1, within the amplified chromosome 11q13 region in human carcinomas. Oncogene 1992; 7:355.

633. Buckley MF, Sweeney KJ, Hamilton JA, et al: Expression and amplification of cyclin genes in human breast cancer. Oncogene 1993; 8:2127.

634. Callender T, el-Naggar AK, Lee MS, et al: PRAD-1 (CCND1)/cyclin D1 oncogene amplification in primary head and neck squamous cell carcinoma. Cancer 1994; 74:152.

635. Till JE, McCulloch EA, Siminovich L: A stochastic model of stem cell proliferation based on growth of spleen colony-forming cells. Proc Natl Acad Sci USA 1964; 51:29.

636. Petrov RV, Khaitov RM, et al: Factors controlling stem cell recirculation. III. Effect of thymus on the migration and differentiation of hematopoietic stem cells. Blood 1977; 29:40.

637. Lord BI, Schofield R: The influence of thymus cells in hemopoiesis: Stimulation of hemopoietic stem cells in a syngeneic, in vivo situation. Blood 1973; 42:395.

638. Trainin N, Resnitzky R: Influence of neonatal thymectomy on cloning capacity of bone marrow cells in mice. Nature 1963; 221:1154.

639. Prichard LL, Shinpock SG, et al: Augmentation of marrow growth by thymocytes separated by discontinuous albumin density-gradient centrifugation. Exp Hematol 1975; 3:94.

640. Zipori D, Trainin N: Defective capacity of bone marrow from nude mice to restore lethally irradiated recipients. Blood 1973; 42:671.

641. Zipori D, Trainin N: Impaired radioprotective capacity and reduced proliferative rate of bone marrow from neonatally thymectomized mice. Exp Hematol 1975; 3:1.

642. Martin PJ, Hansen JA, Buckner CD, et al: Effects of in vitro depletion of T cells in HLA-identical allogeneic marrow grafts. Blood 1985; 66:664.

643. Pinkerton PH, Bannerman RM: The hereditary anemias of mice. Hematol Rev 1968; 1:119.

644. Bernstein SE, Russell ES, Keighley G: Two hereditary mouse anemias (*Sl/Sl^d* and *W/W^v*) deficient in response to erythropoietin. Ann NY Acad Sci 1968; 149:475.

645. Witte ON: *Steel* locus defines new multipotent growth factor. Cell 1990; 63:5.

646. Barr RD, Wang-Peng J, et al: Hematopoietic stem cells in human peripheral blood. Science 1975; 109:284.

647. Clarke BJ, Housman D: Characterization of an erythroid precursor cell of high proliferative capacity in normal human peripheral blood. Proc Natl Acad Sci USA 1977; 74:1105.

648. Samlowski WE, Daynes RA: Bone marrow engraftment is enhanced by competitive inhibition of the hepatic asialoglycoprotein. Proc Natl Acad Sci USA 1985; 82:2508.

649. Tavassoli M, Hardy C: Molecular basis of homing of intravenously transplanted stem cells to the marrow. Blood 1990; 76:1059.

650. Kay HEM: Hypothesis: How many cell-generations? Lancet 1965; 2:418.

651. Micklem HS, Ansell JD, Wayman JER, et al: The clonal organization of hematopoiesis in the mouse. Prog Immunol 1983; 5:633.

652. Mintz B, Anthony K, Litwin S: Monoclonal derivation of mouse myeloid and lymphoid lineages from totipotent hematopoietic stem cells experimentally transplanted in fetal hosts. Proc Natl Acad Sci USA 1984; 81:7835.

653. Lemischka IR, Raulet DH, Mulligan RC: Developmental potential and dynamic behavior of hematopoietic stem cells. Cell 1986; 45:917.

654. Capel B, Hawley R, Covarrusias L, et al: Clonal contributions of small numbers of retrovirally marked hematopoietic stem cells engrafted in unirradiated neonatal *W/W^v* mice. Proc Natl Acad Sci USA 1989; 86:4564.

655. Harrison DE, Astle CM, Lerner C: Number and continuous proliferative pattern of transplanted primitive immunohematopoietic stem cells. Proc Natl Acad Sci USA 1988; 85:822.

656. Jordan CT, Lemischka IR: Clonal and systemic analysis of long-term hematopoiesis in the mouse. Genes Dev 1990; 4:220.

657. Abkowitz JL, Catlin SN, Guttorp P: Evidence that hematopoiesis may be a stochastic process *in vivo*. Nat Med 1996; 2:190.

658. Bradford GB, Williams B, Rossi R, et al: Quiescence, cycling, and turnover in the primitive hematopoietic stem cell compartment. Exp Hematol 1997; 25:445.

659. Cheshier SH, Morrison SJ, Liao X, et al: In vivo proliferation and cell cycle kinetics of long-term self-renewing hematopoietic stem cells. Proc Natl Acad Sci USA 1999; 96:3120.

660. Shivdasani RA, Orkin SH: The transcriptional control of hematopoiesis. Blood 1996; 87:4025.

661. Begley CG, Aplan PD, Davey MP, et al: Chromosomal translocation in a human leukemic stem-cell line disrupts the T-cell antigen receptor δ-chain diversity region and results in a previously unreported fusion transcript. Proc Natl Acad Sci USA 1989; 86:2031.

662. Finger LR, Kagan J, Christopher G, et al: Involvement of the *TCL5* gene on human chromosome 1 in T-cell leukemia and melanoma. Proc Natl Acad Sci USA 1989; 86:5039.

663. Begley CG, Aplan PD, Denning SM, et al: The gene *SCL* is expressed during early hematopoiesis and encodes a differentiation-related DNA-binding motif. Proc Natl Acad Sci USA 1989; 86:10128.

664. Mouthon MA, Bernard O, Mitjavila MT, et al: Expression of tal-1 and GATA-binding proteins during human hematopoiesis. Blood 1993; 81:647.

665. Shivdasani RA, Mayer EL, Orkin SH: Absence of blood formation in mice lacking the T-cell leukaemia oncoprotein tal-1/SCL. Nature 1995; 373:432.

666. Robb L, Lyons I, Li R, et al: Absence of yolk sac hematopoiesis from mice with a targeted disruption of the *scl* gene. Proc Natl Acad Sci USA 1995; 92:7075.

667. Boehm T, Foroni L, Kaneko Y, et al: The rhombotin family of cysteine-rich LIM-domain oncogenes: Distinct members are involved in T-cell translocations to human chromosomes 11p15 and 11p13. Proc Natl Acad Sci USA 1991; 88:4367.

668. Rabbitts TH: Chromosomal translocations in human cancer. Nature 1994; 372:143.

669. Warren AJ, Colledge WH, Carlton MBL, et al: The oncogenic cysteine-rich LIM domain protein rbtn2 is essential for erythroid development. Cell 1994; 78:45.

670. Valge-Archer VE, Osada H, Warren AJ, et al: The LIM protein RBTN2 and the basic helix-loop-helix protein TAL1 are present in a complex in erythroid cells. Proc Natl Acad Sci USA 1994; 91:8617.

671. Wadman I, Li J, Bash RO, et al: Specific in vivo association between the bHLH and LIM proteins implicated in human T cell leukemia. EMBO J 1994; 13:4831.

672. Dorfman DM, Wilson DB, Bruns GA, et al: Human transcription factor GATA-2. Evidence for regulation of preproendothelin-1 gene expression in endothelial cells. J Biol Chem 1992; 267:1279.

673. Leonard M, Brice M, Engel JD, et al: Dynamics of GATA transcription factor expression during erythroid differentiation. Blood 1993; 82:1071.

674. Visvader J, Adams JM: Megakaryocytic differentiation induced in 416B myeloid cells by GATA-2 and GATA-3 transgenes or 5-azacytidine is tightly coupled to GATA-1 expression. Blood 1993; 82:1493.

675. Briegel K, Lim KC, Plank C, et al: Ectopic expression of a conditional GATA-2/estrogen receptor chimera arrests erythroid differentiation in a hormone-dependent manner. Genes Dev 1993; 7:1097.

676. Tsai FY, Keller G, Kuo FC, et al: An early haematopoietic defect in mice lacking the transcription factor GATA-2. Nature 1994; 371:221.

677. Sposi NM, Zon LI, Carè A, et al: Cell cycle-dependent initiation and lineage-dependent abrogation of GATA-1 expression in pure differentiating hematopoietic progenitors. Proc Natl Acad Sci USA 1992; 89:6353.

678. Russell ES: Hereditary anemias of the mouse: A review for geneticists. Adv Genet 1979; 20:357.

679. Okuda T, van Deursen J, Hiebert SW, et al: AML1, the target of multiple chromosomal translocations in human leukemia, is essential for normal fetal liver hematopoiesis. Cell 1996; 84:321.

680. Boncinelli E, Simeone A, Acampora D, et al: *HOX* gene activation by retinoic acid. Trends Genet 1991; 7:329.

681. Sauvageau G, Thorsteinsdottir U, Eaves CJ, et al: Overexpression of HOXB4 in hematopoietic cells causes the selective expansion of more primitive populations in vitro and in vivo. Genes Dev 1995; 9:1753.

682. Kyba M, Perlingeiro RC, Daley GQ: HoxB4 confers definitive lymphoid-myeloid engraftment potential on embryonic stem cell and yolk sac hematopoietic progenitors. Cell 2002; 109:29.

683. Stegmaier K, Pendse S, Barker GF, et al: Frequent loss of heterozygosity at the *TEL* gene locus in acute lymphoblastic leukemia of childhood. Blood 1995; 86:38.

684. Bodine DM, Crosier PS, Clark SC: Effects of hematopoietic growth factors on the survival of primitive stem cells in liquid suspension culture. Blood 1991; 78:914.

685. Itoh Y, Ikebuchi K, Hirashima K: Interleukin-3 and granulocyte colony-stimulating factor as survival factors in murine hemopoietic stem cells in vitro. Int J Hematol. 1992; 55:139.

686. Katayama N, Clark SC, Ogawa M: Growth factor requirement for survival in cell cycle dormancy of primitive murine lymphohematopoietic progenitors. Blood 1993; 81:610.

687. Neben S, Donaldson D, Sieff C, et al: Synergistic effects of interleukin-11 with other growth factors on the expansion of murine hematopoietic progenitors and maintenance of stem cells in liquid culture. Exp Hematol 1994; 22:353.

688. Li CL, Johnson GR: Stem cell factor enhances the survival but not the self-renewal of murine hematopoietic long-term repopulating cells. Blood 1994; 84:408.

689. Bodine DM, Seidel NE, Zsebo KM, et al: In vivo administration of stem cell factor to mice increases the absolute number of pluripotent hematopoietic stem cells. Blood 1993; 82:445.

690. Bodine DM, Orlic D, Birkett NC, et al: Stem cell factor increases CFU-S number in vitro in synergy with interleukin-6, and in vivo in *SL/SL*^d mice as a single factor. Blood 1992; 79:913.

691. Kimura S, Roberts AW, Metcalf D, et al: Hematopoietic stem cell deficiencies in mice lacking c-Mpl, the receptor for thrombopoietin. Proc Natl Acad Sci USA 1998; 95:1195.

692. Solar GP, Kerr WG, Zeigler FC, et al: Role of c-mpl in early hematopoiesis. Blood 1998; 92:4.

693. McCulloch EA, Siminovich L, et al: Spleen colony formation of anemic mice of genotype WW^v. Science 1964; 144:844.

694. Chabot B, Stephenson DA, Chapman VM, et al: The proto-oncogenic c-*kit* encoding a transmembrane tyrosine kinase receptor maps to the mouse W locus. Nature 1988; 335:88.

695. Geissler EN, Ryan MA, Housman DE: The dominant-white spotting (W) locus of the mouse encodes the c-*kit* proto-oncogene. Cell 1988; 55:185.

696. Yarden Y, Kuang W-J, Yang-Feng T, et al: Human proto-oncogene c-*kit*: A new cell surface receptor tyrosine kinase for an unidentified ligand. EMBO J 1987; 6:3341.

697. Reith AD, Rottapel R, Giddens E, et al: *W* mutant mice with mild or severe developmental defects contain distinct point mutations in the kinase domain of the c-kit receptor. Genes Dev 1990; 4:390.

698. McCulloch EA, Siminovitch L, Till JE, et al: The cellular basis of the genetically determined hemopoietic defect in anemic mice of genotype Sl/Sl^d. Blood 1965; 26:399.

699. Williams DE, Eisenman J, Baird A, et al: Identification of a ligand for the c-*kit* proto-oncogene. Cell 1990; 63:167.

700. Zsebo KM, Wypych J, McNiece IK, et al: Identification, purification, and biological characterization of hematopoietic stem cell factor from buffalo rat liver-conditioned medium. Cell 1990; 63:195.

701. Martin FH, Suggs SV, Langley KE, et al: Primary structure and functional expression of rat and human stem cell factor DNAs. Cell 1990; 63:203.

702. Nocka K, Buck J, Levi E, et al: Candidate ligand for the c-kit transmembrane kinase receptor: KL, a fibroblast-derived growth factor stimulates mast cells and erythroid progenitors. EMBO J 1990; 9:3287.

703. Copeland NG, Gilbert DJ, Cho BC, et al: Mast cell growth factor maps near the steel locus on mouse chromosome 10 and is deleted in a number of steel alleles. Cell 1990; 63:175.

704. Flanagan JG, Leder P: The *kit* ligand: A cell surface molecule altered in steel mutant fibroblasts. Cell 1990; 63:185.

705. Flanagan JG, Chan DC, Leder P: Transmembrane form of the *kit* ligand growth factor is determined by alternative splicing and is missing in the *Sl*^d Mutant. Cell 1991; 64:1025.

706. Kojika S, Griffin JD: Notch receptors and hematopoiesis. Exp Hematol 2001; 29:1041.

707. Ellisen LW, Bird J, West DC, et al: TAN-1, the human homolog of the *Drosophila* notch gene, is broken by chromosomal translocations in T lymphoblastic neoplasms. Cell 1991; 66:649.

708. Varnum-Finney B, Xu L, Brashem-Stein C, et al: Pluripotent, cytokine-dependent, hematopoietic stem cells are immortalized by constitutive Notch1 signaling. Nat Med 2000; 6:1278.

709. Karanu FN, Murdoch B, Gallacher L, et al: The notch ligand jagged-1 represents a novel growth factor of human hematopoietic stem cells. J Exp Med 2000; 192:1365.

709a. Bhardwaj G, Murdoch B, Wu D, et al: Sonic hedgehog induces the proliferation of primitive human hematopoietic cells via BMP regulation. Nat Immunol 2001; 2:172.

710. Taipale J, Beachy PA: The Hedgehog and Wnt signalling pathways in cancer. Nature 2001; 411:349.

711. Reya T, Morrison SJ, Clarke MF, et al: Stem cells, cancer, and cancer stem cells. Nature 2001; 414:105.

712. Lansdorp PM, Dragowska W: Maintenance of hematopoiesis in serum-free bone marrow cultures involves sequential recruitment of quiescent progenitors. Exp Hematol 1993; 21:1321.

713. Curry JL, Trentin JJ: Hemopoietic spleen colony studies. I. Growth and differentiation. Dev Biol 1967; 15:395.

714. Trentin JJ: Influence of hematopoietic organ stroma (hematopoietic inductive microenvironments) on stem cell differentiation. In:

Gordon AS (ed): Regulation of Hematopoiesis. New York, Appleton-Century-Crofts, 1970, p 161.

715. Gregory CJ, McCulloch EA, Till JE: Repressed growth of C57BL marrow in hybrid hosts reversed by antisera directed against non-H-2 alloantigens. Transplantation 1972; 13:138.

716. Kulessa H, Frampton J, Graf T: GATA-1 reprograms avian myelomonocytic cell lines into eosinophils, thromboblasts, and erythroblasts. Genes Dev 1995; 9:1250.

717. Nerlov C, Querfurth E, Kulessa H, et al: GATA-1 interacts with the myeloid PU.1 transcription factor and represses PU.1-dependent transcription. Blood 2000; 95:2543.

718. Rekhtman N, Radparvar F, Evans T, et al: Direct interaction of hematopoietic transcription factors PU.1 and GATA-1: Functional antagonism in erythroid cells. Genes Dev 1999; 13:1398.

719. Zhang P, Behre G, Pan J, et al: Negative cross-talk between hematopoietic regulators: GATA proteins repress PU.1. Proc Natl Acad Sci USA 1999; 96:8705.

720. Zhang P, Zhang X, Iwama A, et al: PU.1 inhibits GATA-1 function and erythroid differentiation by blocking GATA-1 DNA binding. Blood 2000; 96:2641.

721. Querfurth E, Schuster M, Kulessa H, et al: Antagonism between C/EBPβ and FOG in eosinophil lineage commitment of multipotent hematopoietic progenitors. Genes Dev 2000; 14:2515.

722. Shen CN, Slack JM, Tosh D: Molecular basis of transdifferentiation of pancreas to liver. Nat Cell Biol 2000; 2:879.

723. Cantor AB, Orkin SH: Hematopoietic development: A balancing act. Curr Opin Genet Dev 2001; 11:513.

724. D'Andrea AD, Lodish HF, Wong GG: Expression cloning of the murine erythropoietin receptor. Cell 1989; 57:277.

725. Krantz SB, Goldwasser E: Specific binding of erythropoietin in spleen cells infected with the anemia strain of Friend virus. Proc Natl Acad Sci USA 1984; 81:7574.

726. Sawyer ST, Krantz SB, Sawada K: Receptors for erythropoietin in mouse and human erythroid cells and placenta. Blood 1989; 74:103.

727. Sawada K, Krantz SB, Sawyer ST, et al: Quantitation of specific binding of erythropoietin to human erythroid colony-forming cells. J Cell Physiol 1988; 137:337.

728. Akahane K, Tojo A, Fukamachi H, et al: Binding of iodinated erythropoietin to rat bone marrow cells under normal and anemic conditions. Exp Hematol 1989; 17:177.

729. Wang GL, Jiang B, Rue EA, et al: Hypoxia-inducible factor 1 is a basic-helix-loop-PAS heterodimer regulated by cellular O_2 tension. Proc Natl Acad Sci USA 1995; 92:5510.

730. Sieff CA, Emerson SG, Mufson A, et al: Dependence of highly enriched human bone marrow progenitors on hemopoietic growth factors and their response to recombinant erythropoietin. J Clin Invest 1986; 77:74.

731. Lansdorp PM, Dragowska W: Long-term erythropoiesis from constant numbers of CD34⁺ cells in serum-free cultures initiated with highly purified progenitor cells from human bone marrow. J Exp Med 1992; 175:1501.

732. Macklis RM, Javid J, et al: Synthesis of hemoglobin F in adult simian erythroid progenitor-derived colonies. J Clin Invest 1982; 70:752.

733. Friedman AD, Linch DC, et al: Determination of the hemoglobin F program in human progenitor-derived erythroid cells. J Clin Invest 1985; 75:1359.

734. Dover GJ, Boyer SH, et al: Production of erythrocytes that contains fetal hemoglobin in anemia: Transient in vivo changes. J Clin Invest 1979; 63:173.

735. Kidoguchi K, Ogawa M, et al: Augmentation of fetal hemoglobin (HbF) synthesis in culture by human erythropoietic precursors in the marrow and peripheral blood: Studies in sickle cell anemia and non-hemoglobinopathic adults. Blood 1978; 52:115.

736. Clarke BJ, Nathan DG, et al: Hemoglobin synthesis in human BFU-E and CFU-E-derived erythroid colonies. Blood 1979; 54:805.

737. Papayannopoulou T, Brice M, et al: Hemoglobin F synthesis in vitro: Evidence for control at the level of primitive erythroid stem cells. Proc Natl Acad Sci USA 1977; 74:2923.

738. Romeo P-H, Prandini M-H, Joulin V, et al: Megakaryocytic and erythrocytic lineages share specific transcription factors. Nature 1990; 344:447.

739. Zon LI, Yamaguchi Y, Yee K, et al: Expression of mRNA for the GATA-binding proteins in human eosinophils and basophils: Potential role in gene transcription. Blood 1993; 81:3234.

740. Simon MC, Pevny L, Wiles MV, et al: Rescue of erythroid development in gene targeted GATA-1 mouse embryonic stem cells. Nat Genet 1992; 1:92.

741. Weiss MJ, Keller G, Orkin SH: Novel insights into erythroid development revealed through in vitro differentiation of GATA-1-embryonic stem cells. Genes Dev 1994; 8:1184.

742. Pevny L, Lin C-S, D-Agati V, et al: Development of hematopoietic cells lacking transcription factor GATA-1. Development 1995; 121:163.

743. Weiss MJ, Orkin SH: Transcription factor GATA-1 permits survival and maturation of erythroid precursors by preventing apoptosis. Proc Natl Acad Sci USA 1995; 92:9623.

744. Tsang AP, Visvader JE, Turner CA, et al: FOG, a multitype zinc finger protein, acts as a cofactor for transcription factor GATA-1 in erythroid and megakaryocytic differentiation. Cell 1997; 90:109.

745. Tsang AP, Fujiwara Y, Hom DB, et al: Failure of megakaryopoiesis and arrested erythropoiesis in mice lacking the GATA-1 transcriptional cofactor FOG. Genes Dev 1998; 12:1176.

746. Nichols KE, Crispino JD, Poncz M, et al: Familial dyserythropoietic anaemia and thrombocytopenia due to an inherited mutation in *Gata1*. Nat Genet 2000; 24:266.

747. Eaves CJ, Eaves AC: Erythropoietin (Ep) dose-response curves for three classes of erythroid progenitors in normal human marrow and in patients with polycythemia vera. Blood 1978; 52:1196.

748. Eaves AC, Eaves CJ: Erythropoiesis in culture. Clin Haematol 1984; 13:371.

749. Iscove NN: Erythropoietin-independent stimulation of early erythropoiesis in adult bone marrow cultures by conditioned media from lectin stimulated mouse spleen cells. In Golde DW, Cline MJ, Metcalf D, et al (eds): Hematopoietic Cell Differentiation. New York, Academic Press, 1978, p 37.

750. Li CL, Johnson GR: Stimulation of multipotential erythroid and other murine haematopoietic progenitor cells by adherent cell lines in the absence of detectable multi-CSF (IL-3). Nature 1985; 316:633.

751. Sieff CA, Ekern SC, Nathan DG, et al: Combinations of recombinant colony stimulating factors are required for optimal hematopoietic differentiation in serum-deprived culture. Blood 1989; 73:688.

752. Abkowitz JL, Sabo KM, Nakamoto B, et al: Diamond-Blackfan anemia: In vitro response of erythroid progenitors to the ligand for c-kit. Blood 1991; 78:2198.

753. Bagnara GP, Zauli G, Vitale L, et al: In vitro growth and regulation of bone marrow enriched CD34+ hematopoietic progenitors in Diamond-Blackfan anemia. Blood 1991; 78:2203.

754. Olivieri NF, Grunberger T, Ben-David Y, et al: Diamond-Blackfan anemia: Heterogenous response of hematopoietic progenitor cells in vitro to the protein product of the *Steel* locus. Blood 1991; 78:2211.

755. Nocka K, Majumder S, Chabot B, et al: Expression of c-*kit* gene products in known cellular targets of *W* mutations in normal and *W* mutant mice—Evidence for an impaired c-kit kinase in mutant mice. Genes Dev 1989; 3:816.

756. Wu H, Klingmüller U, Besmer P, et al: Interaction of the erythropoietin and stem-cell-factor receptors. Nature 1995; 377:242.

757. Socolovsky M, Fallon AE, Wang S, et al: Fetal anemia and apoptosis of red cell progenitors in Stat5a$^{-/-}$5b$^{-/-}$ mice: A direct role for Stat5 in Bcl-X$_L$ induction. Cell 1999; 98:181.

758. Socolovsky M, Nam H, Fleming MD, et al: Ineffective erythropoiesis in Stat5a$^{-/-}$5b$^{-/-}$ mice due to decreased survival of early erythroblasts. Blood 2001; 98:3261.

759. Migliaccio AR, Migliaccio G: Human embryonic hemopoiesis: Control mechanisms underlying progenitor differentiation *in vitro*. Dev Biol 1988; 125:127.

760. Valtieri M, Gabbianelli M, Pelosi E, et al: Erythropoietin alone induces erythroid burst formation by human embryonic but not adult BFU-E in unicellular serum-free culture. Blood 1989; 74:460.

761. Schibler KR, Li Y, Ohls RK, et al: Possible mechanisms accounting for the growth factor independence of hematopoietic progenitors from umbilical cord blood. Blood 1994; 84:3679.

762. Koenig JM, Christensen RD: Neutropenia and thrombocytopenia in infants with Rh hemolytic disease. J Pediatr 1989; 114:625.

763. Christensen RD, Koenig JM, Viskochil DH, et al: Down-modulation of neutrophil production by erythropoietin in human hematopoietic clones. Blood 1989; 74:817.

764. Sawada K, Krantz SB, Dessypris EN, et al: Human colony-forming units-erythroid do not require accessory cells, but do require direct interaction with insulin-like growth factor I and/or insulin for erythroid development. J Clin Invest 1989; 83:1701.

765. Kurtz A, Jelkmann W: Insulin stimulates erythroid colony formation independently of erythropoietin. Br J Haematol 1983; 53:311.

766. Yu J, Shao L, Vaughan J, et al: Characterization of the potentiation effect of activin on human erythroid colony formation in vitro. Blood 1989; 73:952.

767. Smith JC, Price BM, van Nimmen K, et al: Identification of a potent *Xenopus* mesoderm-inducing factor as a homologue of activin A. Nature 1990; 345:729.

768. Galimi F, Bagnara GP, Bonsi L, et al: Hepatocyte growth factor induces proliferation and differentiation of multipotent and erythroid hemopoietic progenitors. J Cell Biol 1994; 127:1743.

769. Mangan KF, Chikkappa G, Sieler LZ, et al: Regulation of human blood erythroid burst-forming unit (BFU-E) proliferation by T lymphocyte subpopulations defined by Fc receptors and monoclonal antibodies. Blood 1982; 59:990.

770. Torok-Storb BJ, Martin PJ, Hansen JA: Regulation of in vitro erythropoiesis by normal T cells: Evidence for two T cell subsets with opposing functions. Blood 1981; 58:171.

771. Lipton JM, Smith BR, et al: Suppression of in vitro erythropoiesis by a subset of large granular lymphocytes. Blood 1984; 64:337a.

772. Hoffman R, Kopel SD, Hsu SD: T cell chronic lymphocytic leukemia: Presence in bone marrow and peripheral blood of cells that suppress erythropoiesis in vitro. Blood 1978; 52:255.

773. Bagby GC Jr: T lymphocytes involved in inhibition of granulopoiesis in two neutropenic patients are of the cytotoxic/suppressor (T3+T8+) subset. J Clin Invest 1981; 68:1597.

774. Abdou JI, NaPombejara C, Balentine L, et al: Suppressor cell-mediated neutropenia in Felty's syndrome. J Clin Invest 1978; 61:738.

775. Sugimoto M, Wakabayashi Y, Shiokawa Y, et al: Effect of peripheral blood lymphocytes from systemic lupus erythematosus patients on human bone marrow granulocyte precursor cells (colony-forming units in culture). Stem Cells 1982; 2:164.

776. Bom-van Noorloos AA, Pegels JG, van Oers RHJ, et al: Proliferation of T-gamma cells with killer-cell activity in two patients with neutropenia and recurrent infections. N Engl J Med 1980; 302:933.

777. Linch DC, Cawley JC, MacDonald SM, et al: Acquired pure red cell aplasia associated with an increase of T cells bearing receptors for the Fc of IgG. Acta Haematol 1981; 65:270.

778. Lipton JM, Nadler LM, Canellos GP, et al: Evidence for genetic restriction in the suppression of erythropoiesis by a unique subset of T lymphocytes in man. J Clin Invest 1983; 72:694.

779. Torok-Storb BJ, Sieff C, Storb R, et al: In vitro tests for distinguishing possible immune-mediated aplastic anemia from transfusion-induced sensitization. Blood 1980; 55:211.

780. Bacigalupo A, Podesta M, Mingari MC, et al: Immunosuppression of hematopoiesis in aplastic anemia: Activity of T lymphocytes. J Immunol 1980; 125:1449.

781. Smith BR, Lipton JM, et al: Multiparameter flow cytometric characterization of a unique T-lymphocyte subclass associated with granulocytopenia and pure red cell aplasia. Blood 1984; 64:343a.

782. Torok-Storb BJ, Hansen JA: Modulation of in vitro BFU-E growth by normal Ia-positive T cells is restricted by HLA-DR. Nature 1982; 298:473.

783. Krensky AM, Reiss CS, Mier JW, et al: Long-term human cytolytic T-cell lines allospecific for HLA-DR6 antigen are OKT4+. Proc Natl Acad Sci USA 1982; 79:2365.

784. Falkenburg JHF, Jansen J, van der Vaart-Duinkerken N, et al: Polymorphic and monomorphic HLA-DR determinants on human hematopoietic progenitor cells. Blood 1984; 63:1125.

785. Sieff C, Bicknell D, Caine G, et al: Changes in cell surface antigen expression during hemopoietic differentiation. Blood 1982; 60:703.

786. Greaves MF, Katz FE, Myers CD, et al: Selective expression of cell surface antigens on human haemopoietic progenitor cells. In Palek J (ed): Hematopoietic Stem Cell Physiology. New York, Alan R. Liss, 1985, p 301.

787. Sparrow RL, Williams N: The pattern of HLA-DR and HLA-DQ antigen expression on clonable subpopulations of human myeloid progenitor cells. Blood 1986; 67:379.

788. Burdach SEG, Levitt LJ: Receptor-specific inhibition of bone marrow erythropoiesis by recombinant DNA-derived interleukin-2. Blood 1987; 69:1368.

789. Burdach S, Shatsky M, Wagenhorst B, et al: The T-cell CD2 determinant mediates inhibition of erythropoiesis by the lymphokine cascade. Blood 1988; 72:770.

790. Roodman DC, Bird A, Hutzler D, et al: Tumor necrosis factor α and hematopoietic progenitors: Effects of tumor necrosis factor on the growth of erythroid progenitors CFU-E and BFU-E and the hematopoietic cell lines K562, HL60, and HEL cells. Exp Hematol 1987; 15:928.

791. Broxmeyer HE, Williams DE, Lu L, et al: The suppressive influences of human tumor necrosis factor on bone marrow hematopoietic progenitor cells from normal donors and patients with leukemia: Synergism of tumor necrosis factor and interferon-γ. J Immunol 1986; 136:4487.

792. Furmanski P, Johnson CS: Macrophage control of normal and leukemic erythropoiesis: Identification of the macrophage-derived erythroid suppressing activity as interleukin-1 and the mediator of its in vivo action as tumor necrosis factor. Blood 1990; 75:2328.

793. Van Furth R, Raeburn JA, et al: Characteristics of human mononuclear phagocytes. Blood 1979; 54:485.

794. Meuret G: Human monocytopoiesis. Exp Hematol 1974; 2:238.

795. Thomas ED, Ramberg RE, et al: Direct evidence for a bone marrow origin of the alveolar macrophage in man. Science 1976; 192:1016.

796. Gale RP, Sparkes RS, et al: Bone marrow origin of hepatic macrophages (Kupffer cells) in humans. Science 1978; 201:937.

797. Katz SI, Tamaki K, et al: Epidermal Langerhans cells are derived from cells originating in bone marrow. Nature 1979; 282:324.

798. Ash P, Loutit JF, et al: Osteoclasts derived from haematopoietic stem cells. Nature 1980; 283:669.

799. Carr I: The biology of macrophages. Clin Invest Med 1978; 1:59.

800. Gasson JC, Weisbart RH, Kaufman SE, et al: Purified human granulocyte-macrophage colony-stimulating factor: Direct action on neutrophils. Science 1984; 226:1339.

801. Weisbart RH, Golde DW, Clark SC, et al: Human granulocyte-macrophage colony-stimulating factor is a neutrophil activator. Nature 1985; 314:361.

802. Iscove NN: The role of erythropoietin in regulation of population size and cell cycling of early and late erythroid precursors in mouse bone marrow. Cell Tissue Kinet 1977; 10:373.

803. Udupa KB, Reissman KR: In vivo erythropoietin requirements of regenerating erythroid progenitors (BFU-e), CFU-e in bone marrow of mice. Blood 1979; 53:1164.

804. Odell TT Jr, McDonlad TP: Stimulation of platelet production by serum of platelet-depleted rats. Proc Soc Exp Biol Med 1961; 108:428.

805. Scott LM, Civin CI, Rorth P, et al: A novel temporal expression pattern of three C/EBP family members in differentiating myelomonocytic cells. Blood 1992; 80:1725.

806. Zhang DE, Hetherington CJ, Meyers S, et al: CCAAT enhancer-binding protein (C/EBP) and AML1 (CBFα2) synergistically activate the macrophage colony-stimulating factor receptor promoter. Mol Cell Biol 1996; 16:1231.

807. Zhang DE, Zhang P, Wang ND, et al: Absence of granulocyte colony-stimulating factor signaling and neutrophil development in CCAAT enhancer binding protein α-deficient mice. Proc Natl Acad Sci USA 1997; 94:569.

808. Zhang P, Iwama A, Datta MW, et al: Upregulation of interleukin 6 and granulocyte colony-stimulating factor receptors by transcription factor CCAAT enhancer binding protein α (C/EBPα) is critical for granulopoiesis. J Exp Med 1998; 188:1173.

809. Tanaka T, Akira S, Yoshida K, et al: Targeted disruption of the NF-IL6 gene discloses its essential role in bacteria killing and tumor cytotoxicity by macrophages. Cell 1995; 80:353.

810. Yamanaka R, Barlow C, Lekstrom-Himes J, et al: Impaired granulopoiesis, myelodysplasia, and early lethality in CCAAT/enhancer binding protein ε-deficient mice. Proc Natl Acad Sci USA 1997; 94:13187.

811. Lekstrom-Himes J, Xanthopoulos KG: CCAAT/enhancer binding protein ε is critical for effective neutrophil-mediated response to inflammatory challenge. Blood 1999; 93:3096.

812. Gallin JI: Neutrophil specific granule deficiency. Annu Rev Med 1985; 36:263.

813. Lekstrom-Himes JA, Dorman SE, Kopar P, et al: Neutrophil-specific granule deficiency results from a novel mutation with loss of function of the transcription factor CCAAT/enhancer binding protein ε. J Exp Med 1999; 189:1847.

814. Gombart AF, Shiohara M, Kwok SH, et al: Neutrophil-specific granule deficiency: homozygous recessive inheritance of a frameshift mutation in the gene encoding transcription factor CCAAT/enhancer binding protein-ε. Blood 2001; 97:2561.

815. Lekstrom-Himes JA: The role of C/EBP(ε) in the terminal stages of granulocyte differentiation. Stem Cells 2001; 19:125.

816. Goebl MK: The PU.1 transcription factor is the product of the putative oncogene Spi-1. Cell 1990; 61:1165.

817. Klemsz MJ, McKercher SR, Celada A, et al: The macrophage and B cell-specific factor PU.1 is related to the ets oncogene. Cell 1990; 61:113.

818. Pahl HL, Scheibe RJ, Zhang D-E, et al: The proto-oncogene PU.1 regulates expression of the myeloid-specific CD11b promotor. J Biol Chem 1993; 268:5014.

819. Pongubala JMR, Van Beveren C, Nagulapalli S, et al: Effect of PU.1 phosphorylation on interaction with NF-EM5 and transcriptional activation. Science 1993; 259:1622.

820. Shin MK, Koshland ME: Ets-related protein PU.1 regulates expression of the immunoglobulin J-chain gene through a novel Ets-binding element. Genes Dev 1993; 7:2006.

821. Zhang DE, Fujioka K, Hetherington CJ, et al: Identification of a region which directs the monocytic activity of the colony-stimulating factor 1 (macrophage colony-stimulating factor) receptor promoter and binds PEBP2/CBF (AML1). Mol Cell Biol 1994; 14:8085.

822. Hohaus S, Petrovick MS, Voso MT, et al: PU.1 (Spi-1) and C/EBPα regulate /expression of the granulocyte-macrophage colony-stimulating factor receptor α gene. Mol Cell Biol 1995; 15:5830.

823. Scott EW, Simon MC, Anastasi J, et al: Requirement of transcription factor PU.1 in the development of multiple hematopoietic lineages. Science 1994; 265:1573.

824. Metcalf D, Johnson GR, Burgess AW: Direct stimulation by purified GM-CSF of the proliferation of multipotential and erythroid precursor cells. Blood 1980; 55:138.

825. Metcalf D, Nicola NA: Proliferative effects of purified granulocyte colony-stimulating factor (G-CSF) on normal mouse hemopoietic cells. J Cell Physiol 1983; 116:198.

826. Metcalf D, Stanley ER: Haematological effects in mice of partially purified colony stimulating factor (CSF) prepared from human urine. Br J Haematol 1971; 21:481.

827. Nishinakamura R, Nakayama N, Hirabayashi Y, et al: Mice deficient for the IL-3/GM-CSF/IL-5 β_c receptor exhibit lung pathology and impaired immune response while β_{IL3} receptor-deficient mice are normal. Immunity 1995; 2:211.

828. Arnaout MA, Wang EA, Clark SC, et al: Human recombinant granulocyte macrophage colony-stimulating factor increases cell to cell adhesion and surface expression of adhesion promoting surface glycoproteins on mature granulocytes. J Clin Invest 1986; 78:597.

829. Lopez AF, To LB, Yang Y-C, et al: Stimulation of proliferation, differentiation, and function of human cells by primate interleukin 3. Proc Natl Acad Sci USA 1987; 84:2761.

830. Lopez AF, Nicola NA, Burgess AW, et al: Activation of granulocyte cytotoxic function by purified mouse colony stimulating factors. J Immunol 1983; 131:2983.

831. Hamilton JA, Stanley ER, Burgess AW, et al: Stimulation of macrophage plasminogen activator activity by colony-stimulating factors. J Cell Physiol 1980; 103:435.

832. Nicola NA, Metcalf D: Binding of iodinated multipotential colony-stimulating factor (interleukin-3) to murine bone marrow cells. J Cell Physiol 1986; 128:180.

833. Debili N, Masse JM, Katz A, et al: Effects of the recombinant hematopoietic growth factors interleukin-3, interleukin-6, stem cell factor, and leukemia inhibitory factor on the megakaryocytic differentiation of CD34⁺ cells. Blood 1993; 82:84.

834. Guinan EC, Lee YS, Lopez KD, et al: Effects of interleukin-3 and granulocyte-macrophage colony-stimulating factor on thrombopoiesis in congenital amegakaryocytic thrombocytopenia. Blood 1993; 81:1691.

835. Hill RJ, Warren MK, Stenberg P, et al: Stimulation of megakaryocytopoiesis in mice by human recombinant interleukin-6. Blood 1991; 77:42.

836. Neben S, Turner K: The biology of interleukin 11 [review]. Stem Cells 1993; 11(Suppl 2):156.

837. Broudy VC, Lin NL, Kaushansky K: Thrombopoietin (c-mpl ligand) acts synergistically with erythropoietin, stem cell factor, and

interleukin-11 to enhance murine megakaryocyte colony growth and increases megakaryocyte ploidy in vitro. Blood 1995; 85:1719.

838. Briddell RA, Bruno E, Cooper RJ, et al: Effect of c-kit ligand on in vitro human megakaryocytopoiesis. Blood 1991; 78:2854.

839. Ishibashi T, Koziol JA, Burstein SA: Human recombinant erythropoietin promotes differentiation of murine megakaryocytes in vitro. J Clin Invest 1987; 79:286.

840. McDonald TP, Sullivan PS: Megakaryocytic and erythrocytic cell lines share a common precursor cell. Exp Hematol 1993; 21:1316.

841. Longmore GD, Pharr P, Neumann D, et al: Both megakaryocytopoiesis and erythropoiesis are induced in mice infected with a retrovirus expressing an oncogenic erythropoietin receptor. Blood 1993; 82:2386.

842. McDonald TP, Cottrell MB, Clift RE, et al: High doses of recombinant erythropoietin stimulate platelet production in mice. Exp Hematol 1987; 15:719.

843. Methia N, Louache F, Vainchenker W, et al: Oligodeoxynucleotides antisense to the proto-oncogene c-*mpl* specifically inhibit in vitro megakaryocytopoiesis. Blood 1993; 82:1395.

844. Wendling F, Varlet P, Charon M, et al: A retrovirus complex including an acute myeloproliferative leukemia virus immortalizes hematopoietic progenitors. Virology 1986; 149:242.

845. Souyri M, Vigon I, Penciolelli JF, et al: A putative truncated cytokine receptor gene transduced by the myeloproliferative leukemia virus immortalizes hematopoietic progenitors. Cell 1990; 63:1137.

846. Vigon I, Mornon J-P, Cocault L, et al: Molcular cloning and characterization of *MPL*, the human homolog of the v-*mpl* oncogene: Identification of a member of the hematopoietic growth factor receptor superfamily. Proc Natl Acad Sci USA 1992; 89:5640.

847. Cosman D: The hematopoietin receptor superfamily [review]. Cytokine 1993; 5:95.

848. Kuter DJ, Beeler DL, Rosenberg RD: The purification of megapoietin: A physiological regulator of megakaryocyte growth and platelet production. Proc Natl Acad Sci USA 1994; 91:11104.

849. Emmons RV, Reid DM, Cohen RL, et al: Human thrombopoietin levels are high when thrombocytopenia is due to megakaryocyte deficiency and low when due to increased platelet destruction. Blood 1996; 87:4068.

850. Karpatkin S: Heterogeneity of human platelets. I. Metabolic and kinetic evidence suggestive of young and old platelets. J Clin Invest 1969; 48:1073.

851. Paulus JM, Breton-Gorius J, et al: Megakaryocyte ultrastructure and ploidy in human macrothrombocytosis. In: Baldini MG, Ebbe S (eds): Platelets, Production, Function, Transfusion and Storage. New York, Grune & Stratton, 1974, p 131.

852. Gewirtz AM, Calabretta B, Rucinksi B, et al: Inhibition of human megakaryocytopoiesis in vitro by platelet factor 4 (PF4) and a synthetic COOH-terminal PF4 peptide. J Clin Invest 1989; 83:1477.

853. Ishibashi T, Miller SL, Burstein SA: Type β transforming growth factor is a potent inhibitor of murine megakaryocytopoiesis in vitro. Blood 1987; 69:1737.

854. Pantel K, Nakeff A: Differential effect of natural killer cells on modulating CFU-meg and BFU-E proliferation in situ. Exp Hematol 1989; 17:1017.

855. Hoffman R: Regulation of megakaryocytopoiesis [review]. Blood 1989; 74:1196.

856. Chan KW, Kaikov Y, et al: Thrombocytosis in childhood: a survey of 94 patients. Pediatrics 1989; 84:1064.

857. Mazur EM, Cohen JL, et al: Growth characteristics of circulating hematopoietic progenitor cells from patients with essential thrombocythemia. Blood 1988; 71:1544.

858. Fung MC, Hapel AJ, Yuner S, et al: Molecular cloning for cDNA for murine interleukin-3. Nature 1984; 307:233.

859. Yokota T, Lee T, Rennick D, et al: Isolation and characterization of a mouse cDNA clone that expresses mast-cell growth factor activity in monkey cells. Proc Natl Acad Sci USA 1984; 81:1070.

860. Kindler V, Thorens B, De Kossodo S, et al: Stimulation of hematopoiesis *in vivo* by recombinant bacterial murine interleukin 3. Proc Natl Acad Sci USA 1986; 83:1001.

861. Metcalf D, Begley CG, Johnson GR, et al: Effects of purified bacterially synthesize murine multi-CSF (IL-3) on hematopoiesis in normal adult mice. Blood 1986; 68:46.

862. Donahue RE, Wang EA, Stone DK, et al: Stimulation of hematopoiesis in primates by continuous infusion of recombinant human GM-CSF. Nature 1986; 321:872.

863. Nienhuis AW, Donahue RE, Karlsson S, et al: Recombinant human granulocyte-macrophage colony stimulating factor (GM-CSF) shortens the period of neutropenia after autologous bone marrow transplantation in a primate model. J Clin Invest 1987; 80:573.

864. Welte K, Bonilla MA, Gillio AP, et al: Recombinant human granulocyte-colony-stimulating factor: Effects on hematopoiesis in normal and cyclophosphamide treated primates. J Exp Med 1987; 165:941.

865. Harker LA, Marzec UM, Hunt P, et al: Dose-response effects of pegylated human megakaryocyte growth and development factor on platelet production and function in nonhuman primates. Blood 1996; 88:511.

866. Harker LA, Marzec UM, Kelly AB, et al: Prevention of thrombocytopenia and neutropenia in a nonhuman primate model of marrow suppressive chemotherapy by combining pegylated recombinant human megakaryocyte growth and development factor and recombinant human granulocyte colony-stimulating factor. Blood 1997; 89:155.

867. Harker LA: Physiology and clinical applications of platelet growth factors. Curr Opin Hematol 1999; 6:127.

868. Gabrilove J, Jakubowski A, Scher H, et al: Effect of granulocyte colony-stimulating factor on neutropenia and associated morbidity due to chemotherapy for transitional-cell carcinoma of the urothelium. N Engl J Med 1988; 318:1414.

869. Morstyn G, Campbell L, Souza LM, et al: Effect of granulocyte colony stimulating factor on neutropenia induced by cytotoxic chemotherapy. Lancet 1988; I: 667.

870. Devereaux S, Linch DC, Campos-Costa D, et al: Transient leucopenia induced by granulocyte-macrophage colony-stimulating factor. Lancet 1987; 2:1523.

871. Bronchud MH, Scarffe JH, Thatcher N, et al: PhaseI/II study of recombinant human granulocyte colony-stimulating factor in patients receiving intensive chemotherapy for small cell lung cancer. Br.J Cancer 1987; 56:809.

872. Kodo H, Tajika K, Takahashi S, et al: Acceleration of neutrophilic granulocyte recovery after bone-marrow transplantation by the administration of recombinant human granulocyte colony-stimulating factor. Lancet 1988; 2:38.

873. Crawford J, Ozer H, Stoller R, et al: Reduction by granulocyte colony-stimulating factor of fever and neutropenia induced by chemotherapy in patients with small-cell lung cancer. N Engl J Med 1991; 325:164.

874. Pettengell R, Gurney H, Radford JA, et al: Granulocyte colony-stimulating factor to prevent dose-limiting neutropenia in non-Hodgkin's lymphoma: A randomized controlled trial. Blood 1992; 80:1430.

875. Zinzani PL, Pavone E, Storti S, et al: Randomized trial with or without granulocyte colony-stimulating factor as adjunct to induction VNCOP-B treatment of elderly high-grade non-Hodgkin's lymphoma. Blood 1997; 89:3974.

876. American Society of Clinical Oncology: Update of recommendations for the use of hematopoietic colony-stimulating factors: Evidence-based clinical practice guidelines. J Clin Oncol 1996; 14:1957.

877. Negoro S, Masuda N, Furuse K, et al: Dose-intensive chemotherapy in extensive-stage small-cell lung cancer. Cancer Chemother Pharmacol 1997; 40(Suppl):S70.

878. Woll PJ, Hodgetts J, Lomax L, et al: Can cytotoxic dose-intensity be increased by using granulocyte colony-stimulating factor? A randomized controlled trial of lenograstim in small-cell lung cancer. J Clin Oncol 1995; 13:652.

879. Hartmann LC, Tschetter LK, Habermann TM, et al: Granulocyte colony-stimulating factor in severe chemotherapy-induced afebrile neutropenia. N Engl J Med 1997; 336:1776.

880. Maher DW, Lieschke GJ, Green M, et al: Filgrastim in patients with chemotherapy-induced febrile neutropenia. A double-blind, placebo-controlled trial. Ann Intern Med 1994; 121:492.

881. Mayordomo JI, Rivera F, Diaz-Puente MT, et al: Improving treatment of chemotherapy-induced neutropenic fever by administration of colony-stimulating factors. J Natl Cancer Inst 1995; 87:803.

882. Aviles A, Guzman R, Garcia EL, et al: Results of a randomized trial of granulocyte colony-stimulating factor in patients with infection and severe granulocytopenia. Anticancer Drugs 1996; 7:392.

883. Duhrsen U, Villeval J-L, Boyd J, et al: Effects of recombinant human granulocyte colony-stimulating factor on hematopoietic progenitor cells in cancer patients. Blood 1988; 72:2074.

884. Tamura M, Hattori K, Nomura H, et al: Induction of neutrophilic granulocytes in mice by administration of purified human native granulocyte colony-stimulating factor (G-CSF). Biochem Biophys Res Commun 1987; 142:454.

885. Shimamura M, Kobayashi Y, Yuo A, et al: Effect of human recombinant granulocyte colony-stimulating factor on hematopoietic injury in mice induced by 5-fluorouracil. Blood 1987; 69:353.

886. Antman KS, Griffin JD, Elias A, et al: Effect of recombinant human granulocyte-macrophage colony-stimulating factor on chemotherapy-induced myelosuppression. N Engl J Med 1988; 319:593.

887. Herrmann F, Schulz G, Lindemann A, et al: Hematopoietic responses in patients with advanced malignancy treated with recombinant human granulocyte-macrophage colony-stimulating factor. J Clin Oncol 1989; 7:159.

888. Steward WP, Scarffe JH, Austin R, et al: Recombinant human granulocyte macrophage colony stimulating factor (rhGM-CSF) given as daily short infusions—A phase I dose-toxicity study. Br. J Cancer 1989; 59:142.

889. Kaplan LD, Kahn JO, Crowe S, et al: Clinical and virologic effects of recombinant human granulocyte-macrophage colony-stimulating factor in patients receiving chemotherapy for human immunodeficiency virus-associated non-Hodgkin's lymphoma: results of a randomized trial. J Clin Oncol 1991; 9:929.

890. Jones SE, Schottstaedt MW, Duncan LA, et al: Randomized double-blind prospective trial to evaluate the effects of sargramostim versus placebo in a moderate-dose fluorouracil, doxorubicin, and cyclophosphamide adjuvant chemotherapy program for stage II and III breast cancer. J Clin Oncol 1996; 14:2976.

891. Gerhartz HH, Engelhard M, Meusers P, et al: Randomized, double-blind, placebo-controlled, phase III study of recombinant human granulocyte-macrophage colony-stimulating factor as adjunct to induction treatment of high-grade malignant non-Hodgkin's lymphomas. Blood 1993; 82:2329.

892. Yau JC, Neidhart JA, Triozzi P, et al: Randomized placebo-controlled trial of granulocyte-macrophage colony-stimulating-factor support for dose-intensive cyclophosphamide, etoposide, and cisplatin. Am J Hematol 1996; 51:289.

893. Bunn PA Jr, Crowley J, Kelly K, et al: Chemoradiotherapy with or without granulocyte-macrophage colony-stimulating factor in the treatment of limited-stage small-cell lung cancer: A prospective phase III randomized study of the Southwest Oncology Group [published erratum appears in J Clin Oncol 1995;13:2860]. J Clin Oncol 1995; 13:1632.

894. Bajorin DF, Nichols CR, Schmoll HJ, et al: Recombinant human granulocyte-macrophage colony-stimulating factor as an adjunct to conventional-dose ifosfamide-based chemotherapy for patients with advanced or relapsed germ cell tumors: A randomized trial. J Clin Oncol 1995; 13:79.

895. American Society of Clinical Oncology. Recommendations for the use of hematopoietic colony-stimulating factors: Evidence-based, clinical practice guidelines. J Clin Oncol 1994; 12:2471.

896. Furman WL: Cytokine support following cytotoxic chemotherapy in children. Int Pediat Hematol Oncol 1995; 2:163.

897. Saarinen UM, Hovi L, Riikonen P, et al: Recombinant human granulocyte-macrophage colony-stimulating factor in children with chemotherapy-induced neutropenia. Med Pediatr Oncol 1992; 20:489.

898. Burdach S: Molecular regulation of hematopoietic cytokines: implications and indications for clinical use in pediatric oncology [review]. Med Pediatr Oncol Suppl 1992; 2:10.

899. Socinski MA, Cannistra SA, Elias A, et al: Granulocyte-macrophage colony stimulating factor expands the circulating haemopoietic progenitor cell compartment in man. Lancet 1988; 1:1194.

900. Ganser A, Lindemann A, Seipelt G, et al: Effects of recombinant human interleukin-3 in patients with normal hematopoiesis and in patients with bone marrow failure. Blood 1990; 76:666.

901. Ottmann OG, Ganser A, Seipelt G, et al: Effects of recombinant human interleukin-3 on human hematopoietic progenitor and precursor cells in vivo. Blood 1990; 76:1494.

902. O'Malley CJ, Rasko JE, Basser RL, et al: Administration of pegylated recombinant human megakaryocyte growth and development factor

to humans stimulates the production of functional platelets that show no evidence of in vivo activation. Blood 1996; 88:3288.

903. Vadhan-Raj S, Murray LJ, Bueso-Ramos C, et al: Stimulation of megakaryocyte and platelet production by a single dose of recombinant human thrombopoietin in patients with cancer. Ann Intern Med 1997; 126:673.

904. Fanucchi M, Glaspy J, Crawford J, et al: Effects of polyethylene glycol-conjugated recombinant human megakaryocyte growth and development factor on platelet counts after chemotherapy for lung cancer. N Engl J Med 1997; 336:404.

905. Motoyoshi K, Takaku F, Maekawa T, et al: Protective effect of partially purified human urinary colony-stimulating factor on granulocytopenia after antitumor chemotherapy. Exp Hematol 1986; 14:1069.

906. Gordon MS, Battiato L, Hoffman R, et al: Subcutaneously (SC) administered recombinant human interleukin-11 (neumega rhIL-11 growth factor; rhIL-11) prevents thrombocyteopenia following chemotherapy (CT) with cyclophosphamide (C) and doxorubicin (A) in women with breast cancer. Blood 1993; 82:318a.

907. Smith JW, Longo DL, Alvord WG, et al: The effects of treatment with interleukin-1α in platelet recovery after high-dose carboplatin. N Engl J Med 1993; 328:756.

908. Brandt SJ, Peters WP, Atwater SK, et al: Effect of recombinant human granulocyte-macrophage colony-stimulating factor of hematopoietic reconstitution after high-dose chemotherapy and autologous bone marrow transplantation. N Engl J Med 1988; 318:869.

909. Nemunaitis J, Singer JW, Buckner CD, et al: Use of recombinant human granulocyte-macrophage colony-stimulating factor in graft failure after bone marrow transplantation. Blood 1990; 76:345.

910. Tapp H, Vowels M: Prophylactic use of GM-CSF in pediatric marrow transplantation. Transplant Proc. 1992; 24:2267.

911. Blazar BR, Kersey JH, McGlave PB, et al: In vivo administration of recombinant human granulocyte/macrophage colony-stimulating factor in acute lymphoblastic leukemia patients receiving purged autografts. Blood 1989; 73:849.

912. Sheridan WP, Morstyn G, Wolf M, et al: Granulocyte colony-stimulating factor and neutrophil recovery after high-dose chemotherapy and autologous bone marrow transplantation. Lancet 1989; 2:891.

913. Peters WP, Stuart A, Affronti ML, et al: Neutrophil migration is defective during recombinant human granulocyte-macrophage colony-stimulating factor infusion after autologous bone marrow transplantation in humans. Blood 1988; 72:1310.

914. Masaoka T, Motoyoshi K, Takaku F, et al: Administration of human urinary colony stimulating factor after bone marrow transplantation. Bone Marrow Transplant 1988; 3:121.

915. Vadhan-raj S, Keating M, LeMaistre A, et al: Effects of recombinant human granulocyte-macrophage colony-stimulating factor in patients with myelodysplastic syndromes. N Engl J Med 1987; 317:1545.

916. Antin JH, Smith BR, Holmes W, et al: Phase I/II study of recombinant human granulocyte-macrophage colony-stimulating factor in aplastic anemia and myelodysplastic syndrome. Blood 1988; 72:705.

917. Ganser A, Volkers B, Greher J, et al: Recombinant human granulocyte-macrophage colony-stimulating factor in patients with myelodysplastic syndromes—A phase I/II trial. Blood 1989; 73:31.

918. Kobayashi Y, Okabe T, Ozawa K, et al: Treatment of myelodysplastic syndromes with recombinant human granulocyte colony-stimulating factor: A preliminary report. Am J Med 1989; 86:178.

919. Negrin RS, Haeuber D, Nagler A, et al: Treatment of myelodysplastic syndromes with recombinant human granulocyte colony-stimulating factor: A phase I/II trial. Ann Intern Med 1989; 110:976.

920. Ganser A, Ottmann OG, Seipelt G, et al: Effect of long-term treatment with recombinant human interleukin-3 in patients with myelodysplastic syndromes. Leukemia 1993; 7:696.

921. Nimer SD, Paquette RL, Ireland P, et al: A phase I/II study of interleukin-3 in patients with aplastic anemia and myelodysplasia. Exp Hematol 1994; 22:875.

922. Hellstrom-Lindberg E: Efficacy of erythropoietin in the myelodysplastic syndromes: A meta-analysis of 205 patients from 17 studies. Br J Haematol 1995; 89:67.

923. Hellstrom-Lindberg E, Negrin R, Stein R, et al: Erythroid response to treatment with G-CSF plus erythropoietin for the anaemia of patients with myelodysplastic syndromes: Proposal for a predictive model. Br J Haematol 1997; 99:344.

924. Hellstrom-Lindberg E, Ahlgren T, Beguin Y, et al: Treatment of anemia in myelodysplastic syndromes with granulocyte colony-stimulating factor plus erythropoietin: Results from a randomized phase II study and long-term follow-up of 71 patients. Blood 1998; 92:68.

925. Economopoulos T, Mellou S, Papageorgiou E, et al: Treatment of anemia in low risk myelodysplastic syndromes with granulocyte-macrophage colony-stimulating factor plus recombinant human erythropoietin. Leukemia 1999; 13:1009.

926. Champlin RE, Nimer SD, Ireland P, et al: Treatment of refractory aplastic anemia with recombinant human granulocyte-macrophage-colony-stimulating factor. Blood 1989; 73:694.

927. Vadhan-raj S, Buescher S, Broxmeyer HE, et al: Stimulation of myelopoiesis in patients with aplastic anemia by recombinanat human granulocyte-macrophage colony-stimulating factor. N Engl J Med 1988; 319:1628.

928. Guinan EC, Sieff CA, Oette DH, et al: A phase I/II trial of recombinant granulocyte-macrophage colony-stimulating factor for children with aplastic anemia. Blood 1990; 76:1077.

929. Nissen C, Tichelli A, Gratwohl A, et al: Failure of recombinant human granulocyte-macrophage colony-stimulating factor therapy in aplastic anemia patients with very severe neutropenia. Blood 1988; 72:2045.

930. Kojima S, Fukuda M, Miyajima Y, et al: Treatment of aplastic anemia in children with recombinant human granulocyte colony-stimulating factor. Blood 1991; 77:937.

931. Kojima S, Matsuyama T: Stimulation of granulopoiesis by high-dose recombinant human granulocyte colony-stimulating factor in children with aplastic anemia and very severe neutropenia. Blood 1994; 83:1474.

932. Sonoda Y, Yashige H, Fujii H, et al: Bilineage response in refractory aplastic anemia patients following long-term administration of recombinant human granulocyte colony-stimulating factor. Eur J Haematol 1992; 48:41.

933. Gluckman E, Esperou-Bourdeau H: Recent treatments of aplastic anemia. The International Group on SAA. Nouv Rev Fr Hematol 1991; 33:507.

934. Kojima S: Cytokine treatment of aplastic anemia. Int J Pediatr Hematol Oncol 1995; 2:135.

935. Kurzrock R, Talpaz M, Gutterman JU: Very low doses of GM-CSF administered alone with erythropoietin in aplastic anemia. Am J Med 1992; 93:41.

936. Hirashima K, Bessho M, Jinnai I, et al: Successful treatment of aplastic anemia and refractory anemia by combination therapy with recombinant human granulocyte colony-stimulating factor and erythropoietin. Exp Hematol 1993; 21:1080a.

937. Groopman JE, Mitsuyasu RT, DeLeo MJ, et al: Effects of recombinant human granulocyte-macrophage colony-stimulating factor on myelopoiesis in the acquired immunodeficiency syndrome. N Engl J Med 1987; 317:593.

938. Groopman JE, Molina J-M, Scadden DT: Hematopoietic growth factors: Biology and clinical applications. N Engl J Med 1989; 321:1449.

939. Perno CF, Yarchoan R, Conney DA, et al: Replication of human immunodeficiency virus in monocytes: Granulocyte/macrophage colony-stimulating factor (GM-CSF) potentiates viral production yet enhances the antiviral effect mediated by 3′-azido-2′3′-dideoxythymidine (AZT) and other dideoxynucleoside congeners of thymidine. J Exp Med 1989; 169:933.

940. Mueller BU: Role of cytokines in children with HIV infection. Int J Pediatr Hematol Oncol 1995; 2:151.

941. Pluda JM, Yarchoan R, Smith PD, et al: Subcutaneous recombinant granulocyte-macrophage colony-stimulating factor used as a single agent and in an alternating regimen with azidothymidine in leukopenic patients with severe human immunodeficiency virus infection. Blood 1990; 76:463.

942. Kaplan LD, Kahn JO, Crowe S, et al: Clinical and virologic effects of recombinant human granulocyte-macrophage colony-stimulating factor in patients receiving chemotherapy for human immunodeficiency virus-associated non-Hodgkin's lymphoma: Results of a randomized trial. J Clin Oncol 1991; 9:929.

943. Mueller BU, Jacobsen F, Butler KM, et al: Combination treatment with azidothymidine and granulocyte colony-stimulating factor in children with human immunodeficiency virus infection. J Pediatr 1992; 121:797.

944. Cole JL, Marzec UM, Gunthel CJ, et al: Ineffective platelet production in thrombocytopenic human immunodeficiency virus-infected patients. Blood 1998; 91:3239.

945. Gillio AP, Guinan EC: Cytokine treatment of inherited bone marrow failure syndromes. Int J Pediatr Hematol Oncol 1992; 2:123.

946. Guinan EC, Lopez KD, Huhn RD, et al: Evaluation of granulocyte-macrophage colony-stimulating factor for treatment of pancytopenia in children with Fanconi anemia. J Pediatr 1994; 124:144.

947. Hammond D, Keighley G: The erythrocyte-stimulating factor in serum and urine in congenital hypoplastic anemia. Am J Dis Child 1960; 100:466.

948. Abkowitz JL, Broudy VC, Bennett LG, et al: Absence of abnormalities of c-*kit* or its ligand in two patients with Diamond-Blackfan anemia. Blood 1992; 79:25.

949. Sieff CA, Yokoyama CT, Zsebo KM, et al: The production of Steel factor mRNA in Diamond-Blackfan anaemia long-term cultures and interactions of Steel factor with erythropoietin and interleukin-3. Br J Haematol 1992; 82:640.

950. Niemeyer CM, Baumgarten E, Holldack J, et al: Treatment trial with recombinant human erythropoietin in children with congenital hypoplastic anemia. Contrib Nephrol 1991; 88:276.

951. Dunbar CE, Smith DA, Kimball J, et al: Treatment of Diamond-Blackfan anaemia with haematopoietic growth factors, granulocyte-macrophage colony stimulating factor and interleukin 3: sustained remissions following IL-3. Br J Haematol 1991; 79:316.

952. Gillio AP, Faulkner LB, Alter BP, et al: Treatment of Diamond-Blackfan anemia with recombinant human interleukin-3. Blood 1993; 82:744.

953. Olivieri NF, Feig SA, Valentino L, et al: Failure of recombinant human interleukin-3 therapy to induce erythropoiesis in patients with refractory Diamond-Blackfan anemia. Blood 1994; 83:2444.

954. Bastion Y, Bordigoni P, Debre M, et al: Sustained response after recombinant interleukin-3 in Diamond Blackfan anemia [letter; comment]. Blood 1994; 83:617.

955. Pietsch T, Buhrer C, Mempel K, et al: Blood mononuclear cells from patients with severe congenital neutropenia are capable of producing granulocyte colony-stimulating factor. Blood 1991; 77:1234.

956. Kyas U, Pietsch T, Welte K: Expression of receptors for granulocyte colony-stimulating factor on neutrophils from patients with severe congenital neutropenia and cyclic neutropenia. Blood 1992; 79:1144.

957. Guba SC, Sartor CA, Hutchinson R, et al: Granulocyte colony-stimulating factor (G-CSF) production and G-CSF receptor structure in patients with congenital neutropenia. Blood 1994; 83:1486.

957a. Dale DC, Person RE, Bolyard AA, et al: Mutations in the gene encoding neutrophil elastase in congenital and cyclic neutropenia. Blood 2000; 96:2317.

957b. Aprikyan AA, Dale DC: Mutations in the neurophil elastase gene in cyclic and congenital neutropenia. Curr Opin Immunol 2001; 13:535.

958. Bonilla MA, Gillio AP, Ruggiero M, et al: Effects of recombinant human granulocyte colony-stimulating factor on neutropenia in patients with congenital agranulocytosis. N Engl J Med 1989; 320:1574.

959. Welte K, Zeidler C, Reiter A, et al: Differential effects of granulocyte-macrophage colony-stimulating factor and granulocyte-stimulating factor in children with severe congenital neutropenia. Blood 1990; 75:1056.

960. Boxer LA, Hutchinson R, Emerson S: Recombinant human granulocyte-colony-stimulating factor in the treatment of patients with neutropenia. Clin Immunol Immunopathol 1992; 62:539.

961. Dale DC, Bonilla MA, Davis MW, et al: A randomized controlled phase III trial of recombinant human granulocyte colony-stimulating factor (filgrastim) for treatment of severe chronic neutropenia. Blood 1993; 81:2496.

962. Dong F, van Buitenen C, Pouwels K, et al: Distinct cytoplasmic regions of the human G-CSF receptor involved in induction of proliferation and maturation. Mol Cell Biol 1993; 13:7774.

963. Dong F, Hoefsloot LH, Schelen AM, et al: Identification of a nonsense mutation in the granulocyte-colony-stimulating factor receptor in severe congenital neutropenia. Proc Natl Acad Sci USA 1994; 91:4480.

964. Welte K, Boxer LA: Severe chronic neutropenia: Pathophysiology and therapy. Semin Hematol 1997; 34:267.

965. Gilman PA, Jackson DP, Guild HG: Congenital agranulocytosis: Prolonged survival and terminal acute leukemia. Blood 1970; 36:576.

966. Rosen RB, Kang SJ: Congenital agranulocytosis terminating in acute myelomonocytic leukemia. J Pediatr 1979; 94:406.

967. Kalra R, Dale D, Freedman M, et al: Monosomy 7 and activating RAS mutations accompany malignant transformation in patients with congenital neutropenia. Blood 1995; 86:4579.

968. Tidow N, Pilz C, Teichmann B, et al: Clinical relevance of point mutations in the cytoplasmic domain of the granulocyte colony-stimulating factor receptor gene in patients with severe congenital neutropenia [see comments]. Blood 1997; 89:2369.

969. Hammond IV WP, Price TH, Souza LM, et al: Treatment of cyclic neutropenia with granulocyte colony-stimulating factor. N Engl J Med 1989; 320:1306.

970. Sugimoto K, Togawal A, Miyazono K: Treatment of childhood-onset cyclic neutropenia with recombinant human granulocyte colony stimulating factor. Eur J Haematol. 1990; 45:110.

971. Hanada T, Ono I, Nagasawa T: Childhood cyclic neutropenia treated with granulocyte colony-stimulating factor. Br J Haematol 1990; 75:135.

972. Dale D, Bolyard A, Hammond W: Cyclic neutropenia: Natural history and effects of long-term treatment with recombinant human granulocyte colony-stimulating factor. Cancer Invest 1993; 11:219.

973. Wright D, Oette D, Malech H: Treatment of cyclic neutropenia with recombinant human granulocyte-macrophage colony-stimulating factor (rhGM-CSF). Blood 1989; 74:231a.

974. Freund M, Luft S, Schober C, et al: Differential effect of GM-CSF and G-CSF in cyclic neutropenia. Lancet 1990; 336:313.

975. Kurzrock R, Talpaz M, Gutterman J: Treatment of cyclic neutropenia with very low-doses of GM-CSF. Am J Med 1991; 91:317.

976. Jakubowski AA, Souza L, Kelly F, et al: Effects of human granulocyte colony-stimulating factor in a patient with idiopathic neutropenia. N Engl J Med 1989; 320:38.

977. Winearls CG, Oliver DO, Pippard MJ, et al: Effect of human erythropoietin derived from recombinant DNA on the anemia of patients maintained by chronic haemodialysis. Lancet 1986; 11:1175.

978. Eschbach JW, Abdulhadi MH, Browne JK, et al: Recombinant human erythropoietin in anemic patients with end-stage renal disease. Ann Intern Med. 1989; 111:992.

979. Adamson JW: The promise of recombinant human erythropoietin. Semin Hematol 1989; 26(Suppl. 2):5.

980. Dessypris EN, Graber SE, Krantz SB, et al: Effects of recombinant erythropoietin on the concentration and cycling status of human marrow hematopoietic progenitor cells in vivo. Blood 1988; 72:2060.

981. Laupacis A: Changes in quality of life and functional capacity in hemodialysis patients treated with recombinant human erythropoietin. Semin Nephrol 1990; 10(Suppl 1):11.

982. Eschbach JW, Kelly MR, Haley NR, et al: Treatment of the anemia of progressive renal failure with recombinant human erythropoietin. N Engl J Med 1989; 321:158.

983. Bommer J, Ritz E, Weinrich T, et al: Subcutaneous erythropoietin. Lancet 1988; 2:406.

984. Kaufman JS, Reda DJ, Fye CL, et al: Subcutaneous compared with intravenous epoetin in patients receiving hemodialysis. Department of Veterans Affairs Cooperative Study Group on Erythropoietin in Hemodialysis Patients. N Engl J Med 1998; 339:578.

985. Müller-Wiefel DE, Amon O: Erythropoietin treatment of anemia associated with chronic renal failure in children. Int J Pediatr Hematol Oncol 1995; 2:87.

986. Offner G, Hoyer PF, Latta K, et al: One year's experience with recombinant erythropoietin in children undergoing continuous ambulatory or cycling peritoneal dialysis. Pediatr Nephrol 1990; 4:498.

987. Scigalla P, Bonzel KE, Bulla M, et al: Therapy of renal anemia with recombinant human erythropoietin in children with end-stage renal disease. Contrib Nephrol 1989; 76:227; discuss.

988. Scharer K, Klare B, Braun A, et al: Treatment of renal anemia by subcutaneous erythropoietin in children with preterminal chronic renal failure. Acta Pediatr 1993; 82:953.

989. Onkingco JRC, Ruley EJ, Turner ME: Use of low-dose subcutaneous recombinant human erythropoietin in end-stage renal disease: Experience with children receiving continuous cycling peritoneal dialysis. Am J Kidney Dis 1991; 18:446.

990. Ohls R, Christensen R: Recombinant erythropoietin compared with erythrocyte transfusion in the treatment of anemia of prematurity. J Pediatr 1991; 119:781.

991. Soubasi V, Kremenopoulos G, Diamandi E, et al: In which neonates does early recombinant human erythropoietin treatment prevent anemia of prematurity? Results of a randomized, controlled study. Pediatr Res 1993; 34:675.

992. Messer J, Haddad J, Donato L, et al: Early treatment of premature infants with recombinant human erythropoietin [see comments]. Pediatrics 1993; 92:519.

993. Bechensteen AG, Haga P, Halvorsen S, et al: Erythropoietin, protein, and iron supplementation and the prevention of anaemia of prematurity. Arch Dis Child 1993; 69:19.

994. Shannon KM, Mentzer WC, Abels RI, et al: Enhancement of erythropoiesis by recombinant human erythropoietin in low birth weight infants: a pilot study. J Pediatr 1992; 120:586.

995. Carnielli V, Montini G, Da Riol R, et al: Effect of high doses of human recombinant erythropoietin on the need for blood transfusions in preterm infants [see comments]. J Pediatr 1992; 121:98.

996. Halperin D, Felix M, Wacker P, et al: Recombinant human erythropoietin in the treatment of infants with anemia of prematurity. Eur J Pediatr 1992; 151:661.

997. Mentzer WC, Shannon KM: The use of recombinant human erythropoietin in preterm infants. Int J Pediatr Hematol Oncol 1995; 2:97.

998. Maier RF, Obladen M, Kattner E, et al: High-versus low-dose erythropoietin in extremely low birth weight infants. The European Multicenter rhEPO Study Group. J Pediatr 1998; 132:866.

999. Means RT, Olsen NJ, Krantz SB, et al: Treatment of the anemia of rheumatoid arthritis with recombinant human erythropoietin: Clinical and in vitro studies. Arthritis Rheum 1989; 32:638.

1000. Umemura T, al-Khatti A, Donahue RE, et al: Effects of interleukin-3 and erythropoietin on in vitro erythropoiesis and F cell formation in primates. Blood 1989; 74:1561.

1001. al-Khatti A, Umemura T, Clow J, et al: Erythropoietin stimulates F-reticulocyte formation in sickle cell anemia. Trans Assoc Am Physicians 1988; 101:54.

1002. Goldberg MA, Brugnara C, Dover GJ, et al: Treatment of sickle cell anemia with hydroxyurea and erythropoietin. N Engl J Med 1990; 323:366.

1003. Rodgers GP, Dover GJ, Uyesaka N, et al: Augmentation by erythropoietin of the fetal-hemoglobin response to hydroxyurea in sickle cell disease [see comments]. N Engl J Med 1993; 328:73.

1004. Rachmilewitz EA, Goldfarb A, Dover G: Administration of erythropoietin to patients with β-thalassemia intermedia: A preliminary trial. Blood 1991; 78:1145.

1005. Olivieri NF, Freedman MH, Perrine SP, et al: Trial of recombinant human erythropoietin: Three patients with thalassemia intermedia [letter]. Blood 1992; 80:3258.

1006. Aker M, Dover G, Schrier S, et al: Sustained increase in the hemoglobin, hematocrit and RBC following long term administration of recombinant human erythropoietin to patients with batal thalassemia intermedia [abstract]. Blood 1993; 82.

1007. Loukopoulos D, Voskaridou E, Cozma C, et al: Effective stimulation of erythropoiesis in thalassemia intermedia with recombinant human erythropoietin and hydroxyurea. Blood 1993; 82:357a.

1008. Goodnough LT, Rudnick S, Price TH, et al: Increased preoperative collection of autologous blood with recombinant human erythropoietin therapy. N Engl J Med 1989; 321:1163.

1009. Felix R, Cecchini MG, Hofstetter W, et al: Impairment of macrophage colony-stimulating factor production and lack of resident bone marrow macrophages in the osteopetrotic op/op mouse. J Bone Miner Res 1990; 5:781.

1010. Wiktor-Jedrzejczak W, Bartocci A, Ferrante AW Jr, et al: Total absence of colony-stimulating factor 1 in the macrophage-deficient osteopetrotic (op/op) mouse [published erratum appears in Proc Natl Acad Sci USA 1991; 88:5937]. Proc Natl Acad Sci USA 1990; 87:4828.

1011. Felix R, Cecchini MG, Fleisch H: Macrophage colony stimulating factor restores in vivo bone resorption in the op/op osteopetrotic mouse. Endocrinology 1990; 127:2592.

1012. Wiktor-Jedrzejczak W, Urbanowska E, Aukerman SL, et al: Correction by CSF-1 of defects in the osteopetrotic *op/op* mouse suggests local, developmental, and humoral requirements for this growth factor. Exp Hematol 1991; 19:1049.

1013. Kodama H, Yamasaki A, Nose M, et al: Congenital osteoclast deficiency in osteopetrotic *(op/op)* mice is cured by injections of macrophage colony-stimulating factor. J Exp Med 1991; 173:269.

1014. Key Jr. LL, Rodriguiz RM, Wang WC: Cytokines and bone resorption in osteopetrosis. Int J Pediatr Hematol Oncol 1995; 2:143.

1015. Rodriguiz RM, Key LL Jr, Ries WL: Combination macrophage-colony stimulating factor and interferon-γ administration ameliorates the osteopetrotic condition in microphthalmic *(mi/mi)* mice. Pediatr Res 1993; 33:384.

1016. Key LL, Ries WL, Rodriguiz RM, et al: Recombinant human interferon γ therapy of osteopetrosis. J Pediatr 1992; 121:119.

1017. Bensinger W, Appelbaum F, Rowley S, et al: Factors that influence collection and engraftment of autologous peripheral-blood stem cells. J Clin Oncol 1995; 13:2547.

1018. Weaver CH, Hazelton B, Birch R, et al: An analysis of engraftment kinetics as a function of the CD34 content of peripheral blood progenitor cell collections in 692 patients after the administration of myeloablative chemotherapy. Blood 1995; 86:3961.

1019. Pecora AL, Preti RA, Gleim GW, et al: CD34+CD33− cells influence days to engraftment and transfusion requirements in autologous blood stem-cell recipients. J Clin Oncol 1998; 16:2093.

1020. Glaspy JA, Shpall EJ, LeMaistre CF, et al: Peripheral blood progenitor cell mobilization using stem cell factor in combination with filgrastim in breast cancer patients. Blood 1997; 90:2939.

1021. Moskowitz CH, Stiff P, Gordon MS, et al: Recombinant methionyl human stem cell factor and filgrastim for peripheral blood progenitor cell mobilization and transplantation in non-Hodgkin's lymphoma patients—Results of a phase I/II trial. Blood 1997; 89:3136.

1022. Weaver A, Ryder D, Crowther D, et al: Increased numbers of long-term culture-initiating cells in the apheresis product of patients randomized to receive increasing doses of stem cell factor administered in combination with chemotherapy and a standard dose of granulocyte colony-stimulating factor. Blood 1996; 88:3323.

1023. Begley CG, Basser R, Mansfield R, et al: Enhanced levels and enhanced clonogenic capacity of blood progenitor cells following administration of stem cell factor plus granulocyte colony-stimulating factor to humans. Blood 1997; 90:3378.

1024. Basser RL, Rasko JE, Clarke K, et al: Randomized, blinded, placebo-controlled phase I trial of pegylated recombinant human megakaryocyte growth and development factor with filgrastim after dose-intensive chemotherapy in patients with advanced cancer [published erratum appears in Blood 1997; 90:2513]. Blood 1997; 89:3118.

1025. Rasko JE, Basser RL, Boyd J, et al: Multilineage mobilization of peripheral blood progenitor cells in humans following administration of PEG-rHuMGDF. Br J Haematol 1997; 97:871.

1026. Fleming WH, Lankford-Turner P, Turner CW, et al: Administration of daniplestim and granulocyte colony-stimulating factor for the mobilization of hematopoietic progenitor cells in nonhuman primates. Biol Blood Marrow Transplant 1999; 5:8.

1027. Pless M, Wodnar-Filipowicz A, John L, et al: Synergy of growth factors during mobilization of peripheral blood precursor cells with recombinant human Flt3-ligand and granulocyte colony-stimulating factor in rabbits. Exp Hematol 1999; 27:155.

1028. Brasel K, McKenna HJ, Charrier K, et al: Flt3 ligand synergizes with granulocyte-macrophage colony-stimulating factor or granulocyte colony-stimulating factor to mobilize hematopoietic progenitor cells into the peripheral blood of mice. Blood 1997; 90:3781.

1029. Papayannopoulou T, Nakamoto B, Andrews RG, et al: In vivo effects of Flt3/Flk2 ligand on mobilization of hematopoietic progenitors in primates and potent synergistic enhancement with granulocyte colony-stimulating factor. Blood 1997; 90:620.

1030. Molineux G, McCrea C, Yan XQ, et al: Flt-3 ligand synergizes with granulocyte colony-stimulating factor to increase neutrophil numbers and to mobilize peripheral blood stem cells with long-term repopulating potential. Blood 1997; 89:3998.

1031. Sudo Y, Shimazaki C, Ashihara E, et al: Synergistic effect of FLT-3 ligand on the granulocyte colony-stimulating factor-induced

mobilization of hematopoietic stem cells and progenitor cells into blood in mice. Blood 1997; 89:3186.

1032. Shpall EJ: The utilization of cytokines in stem cell mobilization strategies. Bone Marrow Transplant 1999; 23(Suppl 2):S13.

1033. Bodine DM, Seidel NE, Orlic D: Bone marrow collected 14 days after in vivo administration of granulocyte colony-stimulating factor and stem cell factor to mice has 10-fold more repopulating ability than untreated marrow. Blood 1996; 88:89.

1034. Miller CL, Eaves CJ: Expansion in vitro of adult murine hematopoietic stem cells with transplantable lympho-myeloid reconstituting ability. Proc Natl Acad Sci USA 1997; 94:13648.

1035. Zandstra PW, Conneally E, Petzer AL, et al: Cytokine manipulation of primitive human hematopoietic cell self-renewal. Proc Natl Acad Sci USA 1997; 94:4698.

1036. Vormoor J, Lapidot T, Pflumio F, et al: Immature human cord blood progenitors engraft and proliferate to high levels in severe combined immunodeficient mice. Blood 1994; 83:2489.

1037. Gan OI, Murdoch B, Larochelle A, et al: Differential maintenance of primitive human SCID-repopulating cells, clonogenic progenitors, and long-term culture-initiating cells after incubation on human bone marrow stromal cells. Blood 1997; 90:641.

1038. Larochelle A, Vormoor J, Hanenberg H, et al: Identification of primitive human hematopoietic cells capable of repopulating NOD/SCID mouse bone marrow: implications for gene therapy. Nat Med 1996; 2:1329.

1039. Conneally E, Cashman J, Petzer A, et al: Expansion in vitro of transplantable human cord blood stem cells demonstrated using a quantitative assay of their lympho-myeloid repopulating activity in nonobese diabetic-scid/scid mice. Proc Natl Acad Sci USA 1997; 94:9836.

1040. Bhatia M, Bonnet D, Kapp U, et al: Quantitative analysis reveals expansion of human hematopoietic repopulating cells after short-term ex vivo culture. J Exp Med 1997; 186:619.

1041. Rebel VI, Tanaka M, Lee JS, et al: One-day ex vivo culture allows effective gene transfer into human nonobese diabetic/severe combined immune-deficient repopulating cells using high-titer vesicular stomatitis virus G protein pseudotyped retrovirus. Blood 1999; 93:2217.

1042. Brugger W, Heimfeld S, Berenson RJ, et al: Reconstitution of hematopoiesis after high-dose chemotherapy by autologous progenitor cells generated ex vivo. N Engl J Med 1995; 333:283.

1043. Holyoake TL, Alcorn MJ, Richmond L, et al: CD34 positive PBPC expanded ex vivo may not provide durable engraftment following myeloablative chemoradiotherapy regimens. Bone Marrow Transplant 1997; 19:1095.

1044. Scheding S, Kratz-Albers K, Meister B, et al: Ex vivo expansion of hematopoietic progenitor cells for clinical use. Semin Hematol 1998; 35:232.

1045. Reiffers J, Cailliot C, Dazey B, et al: Abrogation of post-myeloablative chemotherapy neutropenia by ex-vivo expanded autologous CD34-positive cells. Lancet 1999; 354:1092.

1046. McNiece I, Jones R, Bearman SI, et al: Ex vivo expanded peripheral blood progenitor cells provide rapid neutrophil recovery after high-dose chemotherapy in patients with breast cancer. Blood 2000; 96:3001.

1047. Paquette RL, Dergham ST, Karpf E, et al: Ex vivo expanded unselected peripheral blood: Progenitor cells reduce posttransplantation neutropenia, thrombocytopenia, and anemia in patients with breast cancer. Blood 2000; 96:2385.

1048. Dunbar CE, Cottler-Fox M, O'Shaughnessy JA, et al: Retrovirally marked CD34-enriched peripheral blood and bone marrow cells contribute to long-term engraftment after autologous transplantation. Blood 1995; 85:3048.

1049. Bordignon C, Notarangelo LD, Nobili N, et al: Gene therapy in peripheral blood lymphocytes and bone marrow for ADA− immunodeficient patients. Science 1995; 270:470.

1050. Blaese RM, Culver KW, Miller AD, et al: T lymphocyte-directed gene therapy for ADA-SCID: Initial trial results after 4 years. Science 1995; 270:475.

1051. Kohn DB, Weinberg KI, Nolta JA, et al: Engraftment of gene-modified umbilical cord blood cells in neonates with adenosine deaminase deficiency. Nat Med 1995; 1:1017.

1052. Kavanaugh MP, Miller DG, Zhang W, et al: Cell-surface receptors for gibbon ape leukemia virus and amphotropic murine retrovirus are inducible sodium-dependent phosphate symporters. Proc Natl Acad Sci USA 1994; 91:7071.

1053. Orlic D, Girard LJ, Jordan CT, et al: The level of mRNA encoding the amphotropic retrovirus receptor in mouse and human hematopoietic stem cells is low and correlates with the efficiency of retrovirus transduction. Proc Natl Acad Sci USA 1996; 93:11097.

1054. Miller DG, Adam MA, Miller AD: Gene transfer by retrovirus vectors occurs only in cells that are actively replicating at the time of infection [published erratum appears in Mol Cell Biol 1992; 12:433]. Mol Cell Biol 1990; 10:4239.

1055. Emi N, Friedmann T, Yee JK: Pseudotype formation of murine leukemia virus with the G protein of vesicular stomatitis virus. J Virol 1991; 65:1202.

1056. Naldini L, Blomer U, Gallay P, et al: In vivo gene delivery and stable transduction of nondividing cells by a lentiviral vector. Science 1996; 272:263.

1057. Miyoshi H, Smith KA, Mosier DE, et al: Transduction of human CD34+ cells that mediate long-term engraftment of NOD/SCID mice by HIV vectors. Science 1999; 283:682.

1058. Burns JC, Friedmann T, Driever W, et al: Vesicular stomatitis virus G glycoprotein pseudotyped retroviral vectors: concentration to very high titer and efficient gene transfer into mammalian and nonmammalian cells. Proc Natl Acad Sci USA 1993; 90:8033.

1059. Friedmann T, Yee JK: Pseudotyped retroviral vectors for studies of human gene therapy [review]. Nat Med 1995; 1:275.

1060. Bodine DM, Karlsson S, Nienhuis AW: Combination of interleukins 3 and 6 preserves stem cell function in culture and enhances retrovirus-mediated gene transfer into hematopoietic stem cells. Proc Natl Acad Sci USA 1989; 86:8897.

1061. Laneuville P, Chang W, Kamel-Reid S, et al: High-efficiency gene transfer and expression in normal human hematopoietic cells with retrovirus vectors. Blood 1988; 71:811.

1062. Dick JE, Kamel-Reid S, Murdoch B, et al: Gene transfer into normal human hematopoietic cells using in vitro and in vivo assays. Blood 1991; 78:624.

1063. Hughes PF, Eaves CJ, Hogge DE, et al: High-efficiency gene transfer to human hematopoietic cells maintained in long-term marrow culture. Blood. 1989; 74:1915.

1064. Hughes PFD, Thacker JD, Hogge D, et al: Retroviral gene transfer to primitive normal and leukemic hematopoietic cells using clinically applicable procedures. J Clin Invest 1992; 89:1817.

1065. Xu LC, Kluepfel-Stahl S, Blanco M, et al: Growth factors and stromal support generate very efficient retroviral transduction of peripheral blood CD34+ cells from Gaucher patients. Blood 1995; 86:141.

1066. Moore KA, Deisseroth AB, Reading CL, et al: Stromal support enhances cell-free retroviral vector transduction of human bone marrow long-term culture-initiating cells. Blood 1992; 79:1393.

1067. Nolta JA, Smogorzewska EM, Kohn DB: Analysis of optimal conditions for retroviral-mediated transduction of primitive human hematopoietic cells. Blood 1995; 86:101.

1068. Moritz T, Dutt P, Xiao X, et al: Fibronectin improves transduction of reconstituting hematopoietic stem cells by retroviral vectors: Evidence of direct viral binding to chymotryptic carboxy-terminal fragments. Blood 1996; 88:855.

1069. van Beusechem VW, Kukler A, Heidt PJ, et al: Long-term expression of human adenosine deaminase in rhesus monkeys transplanted with retrovirus-infected bone-marrow cells. Proc Natl Acad Sci USA 1992; 89:7640.

1070. Bodine DM, Moritz T, Donahue RE, et al: Long-term in vivo expression of a murine adenosine deaminase gene in rhesus monkey hematopoietic cells of multiple lineages after retroviral mediated gene transfer into CD34+ bone marrow cells. Blood 1993; 82:1975.

1071. Harrison DE, Stone M, Astle CM: Effects of transplantation on the primitive immunohematopoietic stem cell. J Exp Med 1990; 172:431.

1072. Spangrude GJ, Brooks DM, Tumas DB: Long-term repopulation of irradiated mice with limiting numbers of purified hematopoietic stem cells: In vivo expansion of stem cell phenotype but not function. Blood 1995; 85:1006.

1073. Van Zant G, de Haan G, Rich IN: Alternatives to stem cell renewal from a developmental viewpoint. Exp Hematol 1997; 25:187.

1074. Morrison SJ, Wandycz AM, Akashi K, et al: The aging of hematopoietic stem cells. Nat Med 1996; 2:1011.

1075. Van Zant G, Holland BP, Eldridge PW, et al: Genotype-restricted growth and aging patterns in hematopoietic stem cell populations of allophenic mice. J Exp Med 1990; 171:1547.

1076. Rideout WM, Hochedlinger K, Kyba M, et al: Correction of a genetic defect by nuclear transplantation and combined cell and gene therapy. Cell 2002; 109:17.

1077. Lapidot T, Pflumio F, Doedens M, et al: Cytokine stimulation of multilineage hematopoiesis from immature human cells engrafted in SCID mice. Science 1992; 255:1137.

1078. Hesselton RM, Greiner DL, Mordes JP, et al: High levels of human peripheral blood mononuclear cell engraftment and enhanced susceptibility to human immunodeficiency virus type 1 infection in NOD/LtSz-scid/scid mice. J Infect Dis 1995; 172:974.

1079. Greiner DL, Shultz LD, Yates J, et al: Improved engraftment of human spleen cells in NOD/LtSz-scid/scid mice as compared with C.B-17-scid/scid mice. Am J Pathol 1995; 146:888.

1080. Shultz LD, Schweitzer PA, Christianson SW, et al: Multiple defects in innate and adaptive immunologic function in NOD/LtSz-scid mice. J Immunol 1995; 154:180.

1081. Bhatia M, Wang JCY, Kapp U, et al: Purification of primitive human hematopoietic cells capable of repopulating immune-deficient mice. Proc Natl Acad Sci USA 1997; 94:5320.

1082. Gribben JG, Devereux S, Thomas NSB, et al: Development of antibodies to unprotected glycosylation sites on recombinant human GM-CSF. Lancet 1990; 335:434.

1083. Vadhan-Raj S, Verschraegen CF, Bueso-Ramos C, et al: Recombinant human thrombopoietin attenuates carboplatin-induced severe thrombocytopenia and the need for platelet transfusions in patients with gynecologic cancer. Ann Intern Med 2000; 132:364.

1084. Crawford J, Glaspy J, Belani C, et al: A randomized, placebo-controlled, blinded, dose-scheduling trial of pegylated recombinant human megakaryocyte growth and development factor (PEG-rHuMGDF) with filgastrim support in small non-lung cancer (NSCLC) patients treated with paclitaxel and carboplatin during multiple cycles of chemotherapy. Proc Am Soc Clin Oncol 1998; 17:73a.

1085. Li J, Yang C, Xia Y, et al: Thrombocytopenia caused by the development of antibodies to thrombopoietin. Blood 2001; 98:3241.

1086. Yang C, Xia Y, Li J, et al: The appearance of anti-thrombopoietin antibody and circulating thrombopoietin-IgG complexes in a patient developing thrombocytopenia after the injection of PEG-rHuMGDF. Blood 1999; 94 (Suppl 1):681a.

1087. Casadevall N, Nataf J, Viron B, et al: Pure red-cell aplasia and antierythropoietin antibodies in patients treated with recombinant erythropoietin. N Engl J Med 2002; 346:469.

1088. Glaspy JA, Baldwin GC, Robertson PA, et al: Therapy for neutropenia in hairy cell leukemia with recombinant human granulocyte colony-stimulating factor. Ann Intern Med 1988; 109:789.

1089. Leonard WJ, Noguchi M, Russell SM, et al: The molecular basis of X-linked severe combined immunodeficiency: The role of the interleukin-2 receptor γ chain as a common γ chain, $γ_c$ [review]. Immunol Rev 1994; 138:61.

1090. Macchi P, Villa A, Gilliani S, et al: Mutations of Jak-3 gene in patients with autosomal severe combined immune deficiency (SCID). Nature 1995; 377:65.

1091. Luo H, Hanratty WP, Dearolf CR: An amino acid substitution in the *Drosophilia* hopTum-1 Jak kinase causes leukemia-like hematopoietic defects. EMBO J 1995; 14:1412.

1092. Harrison DA, Binari R, Nahreini TS, et al: Activation of a *Drosophila* Janus kinase (JAK) causes hematopoietic neoplasia and developmental defects. EMBO J 1995; 14:2857.

1093. Zmuidzinas A, Fischer KD, Lira SA, et al: The *vav* proto-oncogene is required early in embryogenesis but not for hematopoietic development in vitro. EMBO J 1995; 14:1.

1094. Brizzi MF, Zini MG, Aronica MG, et al: Convergence of signaling by interleukin-3, granulocyte-macrophage colony-stimulating factor, and mast cell growth factor on JAK2 tyrosine kinase. J Biol Chem 1994; 269:31680.

1095. Lev S, Givol D, Yarden Y: A specific combination of substrates is involved in signal transduction by the kit-encoded receptor. EMBO J 1991; 10:647.

1096. Rottapel R, Reedijk M, Williams DE, et al: The Steel/W transduction pathway: kit autophosphorylation and its association with a unique subset of cytoplasmic signaling proteins is induced by the Steel factor. Mol Cell Biol 1991; 11:3043.

1097. Herbst R, Lammers R, Schlessinger J, et al: Substrate phosphorylation specificity of the human c-kit receptor tyrosine kinase. J Biol Chem 1991; 266:19908.

1098. Hunter T: Cytokine connections. Nature 1993; 366:114.

1099. Leung S, Qureshi SA, Kerr IM, et al: Role of STAT2 in the α interferon signaling pathway. Mol Cell Biol 1995; 15:1312.

1100. Greenlund AC, Farrar MA, Viviano BL, et al: Ligand-induced IFN γ receptor tyrosine phosphorylation couples the receptor to its signal transduction system (p91). EMBO J 1995; 13:1591.

1101. Quelle FW, Shimoda K, Thierfelder W, et al: Cloning of murine Stat6 and human Stat6, Stat proteins that are tyrosine phosphorylated in responses to IL-4 and IL-3 but are not required for mitogenesis. Mol Cell Biol 1995; 15:3336.

1102. Mano H, Yamashita Y, Sato K, et al: Tec protein-tyrosine kinase is involved in interleukin-3 signaling pathway. Blood 1995; 85:343.

1103. Akira S, Nishio Y, Inoue M, et al: Molecular cloning of APRF, a novel IFN-stimulated gene factor 3 p91-related transcription factor involved in the gp130-mediated signaling pathway. Cell 1994; 77:63.

1104. Ernst M, Gearing DP, Dunn AR: Functional and biochemical association of Hck with the LIF/IL-6 receptor signal transducing subunit gp130 in embryonic stem cells. EMBO J 1994; 13:1574.

1105. Matsuda T, Takahashi-Tezuka M, Fukada T, et al: Association and activation of Btk and Tec tyrosine kinases by gp130, a signal transducer of the interleukin-6 family of cytokines. Blood 1995; 85:627.

1106. Miyazaki T, Kawahara A, Fujii H, et al: Functional activation of Jak1 and Jak3 by selective association with IL-2 receptor subunits. Science 1994; 266:1045.

1107. Johnston JA, Kawamura M, Kirken RA, et al: Phosphorylation and activation of the Jak-3 Janus kinase in response to interleukin-2. Nature 1994; 370:151.

1108. Nielsen M, Svejgaard A, Skov S, et al: Interleukin-2 induces tyrosine phosphorylation and nuclear translocation of stat3 in human T lymphocytes. Eur J Immunol 1994; 24:3082.

1109. Fujii H, Nakagawa Y, Schindler U, et al: Activation of Stat5 by interleukin 2 requires a carboxyl-terminal region of the interleukin 2 receptor β chain but is not essential for the proliferative signal transmission. Proc Natl Acad Sci USA 1995; 92:5482.

1110. Beadling C, Guschin D, Witthuhn BA, et al: Activation of JAK kinases and STAT proteins by interleukin-2 and interferon α, but not the T cell antigen receptor, in human T lymphocytes. EMBO J 1994; 13:5605.

1111. Hatakeyama M, Kono T, Kobayashi N, et al: Interaction of the IL-2 receptor with the src-family kinase p56lck: Identification of novel intermolecular association. Science 1991; 252:1523.

1112. Torigoe T, Saragovi HU, Reed JC: Interleukin 2 regulates the activity of the lyn protein-tyrosine kinase in a B-cell line. Proc Natl Acad Sci USA 1992; 89:2674.

1113. Minami Y, Nakagawa Y, Kawahara A, et al: Protein tyrosine kinase Syk is associated with and activated by the IL-2 receptor: Possible link with the c-myc induction pathway. Immunity 1995; 2:89.

1114. Gouilleux F, Wakao H, Mundt M, et al: Prolactin induces phosphorylation of Tyr694 of Stat5 (MGF), a prerequisite for DNA binding and induction of transcription. EMBO J 1994; 13:4361.

1115. Wakao H, Harada N, Kitamura T, et al: Interleukin 2 and erythropoietin activate STAT5/MGF via distinct pathways. EMBO J 1995; 14:2527.

1116. Nicholson SE, Oates AC, Harpur AG, et al: Tyrosine kinase KAK1 is associated with the granulocyte-colony-stimulating factor receptor and both become tyrosine-phosphorylated after receptor activation. Proc Natl Acad Sci USA 1994; 91:2985.

1117. Tian SS, Lamb P, Seidel HM, et al: Rapid activation of the STAT3 transcription factor by granulocyte colony-stimulating factor. Blood 1994; 84:1760.

1118. Nicholson SE, Novak U, Ziegler SF, et al: Distinct regions of the granulocyte colony-stimulating factor receptor are required for tyrosine phosphorylation of the signaling molecules JAK2, Stat3, and p42, p44MAPK. Blood 1995; 86:3698.

1119. Dong F, van Paassen M, van Buitenen C, et al: A point mutation in the granulocyte colony-stimulating factor receptor (G-CSF-R) gene in a case of acute myeloid leukemia results in the overexpression of a novel G-CSF-R isoform. Blood 1995; 85:902.

1120. Corey SJ, Burkhardt AL, Bolen JB, et al: Granulocyte colony-stimulating factor receptor signaling involves the formation of a three-component complex with Lyn and Syk protein-tyrosine kinases. Proc Natl Acad Sci USA 1994; 91:4683.

1121. Avalos BR, Hunter MG, Parker JM, et al: Point mutations in the conserved box 1 region inactivate the human granulocyte colony-stimulating factor receptor for growth signal transduction and tyrosine phosphorylation of p75^{c-rel}. Blood 1995; 85:3117.

1122. Taniguchi T: Cytokine signaling through nonreceptor protein tyrosine kinases. Science 1995; 268:251.

1123. Ihle JN: STATs: Signal transducers and activators of transcription. Cell 1996; 84:331.

7 | Acquired Aplastic Anemia

Akiko Shimamura • Eva C. Guinan

Bone marrow failure is characterized by a reduction in the effective production of mature erythrocytes, granulocytes, and platelets by the bone marrow that leads to peripheral blood pancytopenia. In some conditions, only one or two cell lines may be affected. Decreased production of *mature cells* may result from a reduction in the number or function of their *progenitors*. This results in a paucity of differentiated *precursors* in the marrow. Examples of such disorders include aplastic anemia (presumably involving the pluripotent hematopoietic progenitors) and Diamond-Blackfan anemia (involving the committed erythroid progenitors). In some disorders, derangement of the development of the differentiated precursors may occur, as in many neutropenias. The number of differentiated precursors may be paradoxically increased in the marrow, whereas the number of their mature products is diminished in the blood; this

state is referred to as *ineffective hematopoiesis*. It may be difficult to differentiate between primary progenitor abnormalities, environmental toxins, or nutritional insufficiency.

This chapter presents a review of the disorders associated with cytopenias due to bone marrow failure or ineffective hematopoiesis. Detailed discussion of neutropenias is found in Chapter 20. Disorders seen most often in the pediatric age group are emphasized.

OVERVIEW

In aplastic anemia, peripheral blood pancytopenia results from reduced or no production of blood cells in the bone marrow. The disorder may be acquired, inherited (genetic, but not necessarily expressed at birth), or congenital (present at birth) or any combination of these variants.

The causes are many, and natural histories are diverse. Isolated single-cell deficiencies may also be acquired or inherited, and they may remain single cytopenias or be precursors to complete aplasia. Classifications of the aplastic anemias and the single cytopenias are presented in Tables 7–1 and 7–2.[1] Several reviews provide more detailed information than can be presented here[2, 3]; references to many earlier publications can be found in the 5th edition of this book.[4]

The severity of aplastic anemia was classified by Camitta and co-workers[5] in an effort to make possible the comparison of diverse groups of patients and different therapeutic approaches. For the diagnosis of *severe aplastic anemia* the patient must have at least two of the following anomalies: a granulocyte count less than 500/μL, a platelet count less than 20,000/μL, and an absolute reticulocyte count less than or equal to 40×10^9/L. In addition, the bone marrow biopsy must contain less than 25 percent of the normal cellularity. Very severe aplastic anemia is further defined by a granulocyte count less than 200/μL.[6] *Mild* or *moderate aplastic anemia*, sometimes called "hypoplastic anemia," is distinguished from the severe form by the presence of mild or moderate cytopenias and more variable, but still deficient, bone marrow cellularity. These distinctions are more than semantic; they are critical for the prediction of outcome and the choice of therapy.

Aplastic anemia was first described in 1888 by Ehrlich[7] in a young pregnant woman (see later) who had an explosive fatal illness characterized by severe anemia, bleeding into skin and retinae, and high fever. At autopsy, the bone marrow was found to have been completely replaced by fat. The term *aplastic anemia* was apparently introduced by Vaquez and Aubertin[8] in discussions of the Society of the Hospital of Paris in 1904. The word *aplasia* is derived from the Greek verb, πλαθω, meaning "to create, give shape," and thus emphasizes the functional abnormality in blood cell production.

There are many large reported series of adult and pediatric patients with "acquired aplastic anemia," but studies in the older literature are difficult to interpret because of the absence of strict diagnostic criteria. Patients are now included in the group with acquired disease only if the bone marrow is hypocellular and if no evidence for inherited disease is apparent (see later). Making the distinction between acquired and inherited disease may present a clinical challenge, and the biologic separation may be subtle because acquired aplastic anemia may represent the outcome of an environmental insult in an individual of appropriate genetic background.

TABLE 7–1. Classification of the Aplastic Anemias

ACQUIRED

Secondary
Radiation
Drugs and chemicals
   Direct toxicity: chemotherapy, benzene
   Idiosyncratic: chloramphenicol, anti-inflammatory drugs, antiepileptic drugs, carbonic anhydrase inhibitors
Viruses
   Epstein-Barr virus
   Hepatitis (non-A, non-B, non-C, non-E, or non-G)
   Human immunodeficiency virus
Immune diseases
   Eosinophilic fasciitis
   Hypoimmunoglobulinemia
Thymoma
Pregnancy
Paroxysmal nocturnal hemoglobinuria
Myelodysplasia

Idiopathic

INHERITED

Fanconi anemia
Dyskeratosis congenita
Shwachman-Diamond syndrome
Reticular dysgenesis
Amegakaryocytic thrombocytopenia
Familial aplastic anemias
Nonhematologic syndromes (e.g., Down, Dubowitz and Seckel syndromes)

Modified from Alter BP, Potter NU, Li FP: Classification and aetiology of the aplastic anaemias. Clin Haematol 1978; 7:431.

EPIDEMIOLOGY

Epidemiologic studies performed in Europe have shown that the annual incidence of aplastic anemia is 2 per million per year.[9] In comparison, the incidence of acute leukemia is about 50 per million per year. Higher figures for the incidence of aplastic anemia have been obtained for smaller studies in the United States and earlier surveys in Europe, but these figures may have been inflated by the inclusion of patients with the more common syndrome

TABLE 7–2. Classification of the Single Cytopenias

Pure Red Cell Aplasia	Neutropenia	Thrombocytopenia
ACQUIRED		
Idiopathic	Idiopathic	Idiopathic
Drugs, toxins	Drugs, toxins	Drugs, toxins
Immune		
Thymoma		
Transient erythroblastopenia of childhood		
INHERITED		
Diamond-Blackfan anemia	Kostmann syndrome	Amegakaryocytic thrombocytopenia
	Shwachman-Diamond syndrome	Thrombocytopenia with absent radii
	Reticular dysgenesis	

Modified from Alter BP, Potter NU, Li FP: Classification and aetiology of the aplastic anaemias. Clin Hematol 1978; 7:431.

myelodysplasia. Aplastic anemia is more common in Asia (4 to 7 per million per year)[3] than in the West. Geographic variance in prevalence is apparently due to environmental, not genetic, factors. For example, in Thailand, significant risk factors include low socioeconomic status, exposure to solvents (in Bangkok), and rice farming (in the countryside). Because of its efficacy and low cost, chloramphenicol has been widely used in much of Asia, but reductions in its use have not been accompanied by reductions in the incidence of aplastic anemia in Japan[10, 11] or elsewhere,[12, 13] and no association was observed in case-control studies in Thailand.[14] Although one case-control study showed a relationship to exposures to chemicals or to viruses through blood transfusions, hepatitis, and occupation,[15] a more recent case-control study failed to confirm any association between household pesticide use and aplastic anemia in Thailand.[16]

The peak age of presentation of aplastic anemia is 15 to 25 years or older than 60 years (Fig. 7–1). The male-to-female ratio for acquired aplastic anemia is approximately 1:1.

Genetic associations are suggested by the correlation of aplastic anemia with certain human leukocyte antigen (HLA) types such as HLA-DR2.[17] In Japanese patients the class II haplotype DRB*1501 has been correlated with cyclosporine-responsive and cyclosporine-dependent disease.[18] There may be genetic abnormalities in DNA repair, drug metabolism, and immune response to viruses that are yet to be defined. Some of these possibilities are described in the following section. Families with higher-than-expected rates of aplastic anemia may represent kindreds with undiagnosed Fanconi anemia.

CAUSAL FACTORS

The actual cause of aplastic anemia in an individual patient is virtually impossible to determine. When no related factors are ascertained, the disease is classified as "idiopathic." Many patients have been exposed to several potential myelosuppressive agents, and the number of possible associations depends in part on the intensity of the investigation. A drug or toxin is often implicated if the exposure is to a previously implicated agent and is appropriately extensive or temporally proximate; sometimes a drug history is given significance only because all other factors are excluded. Therefore, the course, management, and outcome are related more to the severity of the hematopoietic depression than to the cause and are generally similar for disease with apparent cause and idiopathic disease.

Drugs

The incidence of drug- and chemical-related aplastic anemia varies over time and from place to place. Many drugs and toxins have been implicated by inferential and circumstantial evidence; the magnitude of the risk is usually unknown (Table 7–3). The presence of an agent on this list suggests caution regarding its use, but no drug on this list should be proscribed if there are strong clinical indications for its use. From a public health perspective, even drugs associated with an increased risk of marrow failure do not cause aplastic anemia in large numbers of patients.[9]

Note that even confirmed associations do not substantiate causality. Antibiotics felt to be causative may have been administered for the viral infection that led to the aplastic anemia or for symptoms from already established neutropenia in a patient with undiagnosed aplastic anemia. Bleeding may be precipitated in patients with undiagnosed thrombocytopenia who receive nonsteroidal anti-inflammatory drugs. To give an example of known errors in associations: among six patients who were reported to have sniffed glue and who developed aplasia, five had sickle cell anemia and aplastic crises now known to be due to parvovirus infection.[19]

The incidence of drug-related aplasia in pediatric patients is low, mainly because many of the drugs felt to be related to aplasia are not used in childhood. Exceptions include antiepileptic drugs, carbonic anhydrase inhibitors, nonsteroidal anti-inflammatory medications, and some antibiotics.

Drug-related aplasia may occur in several ways. Drugs may exert direct cytotoxic or suppressive effects on the bone marrow. Myelosuppressive drugs, such as those used in cancer chemotherapy, cause predictable and dose-related marrow suppression. Benzene, too, has been regu-

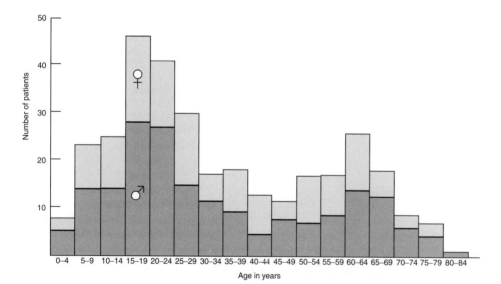

FIGURE 7–1. Age distribution at diagnosis of more than 300 patients seen with severe aplastic anemia at the Clinical Center of the National Institutes of Health between 1978 and 1998. (From Young NS: Acquired aplastic anemia. In NS Y (ed.): Bone Marrow Failure Syndromes. Philadelphia, WB Saunders, 2000, pp 1–46).

TABLE 7–3. Classification of Drugs and Chemicals Associated with Aplastic Anemia*

AGENTS THAT REGULARLY PRODUCE MARROW DEPRESSION

Antibiotics: daunorubicin, doxorubicin hydrochloride (Adriamycin), chloramphenicol
Antimetabolites: antifolic compounds, nucleotide analogs
Antimitotics: vincristine, vinblastine, colchicine
Benzene and chemicals containing benzene: carbon tetrachloride, chlorophenols, kerosene, Stoddard's solvent
Cytotoxic cancer chemotherapy alkylating drugs: busulphan, melphalan, cyclophosphamide

AGENTS POSSIBLY ASSOCIATED, WITH LOW PROBABILITY RELATIVE TO USE

Chloramphenicol
Insecticides: chlordane, chlorophenothane (DDT), γ-benzene hexachloride (lindane), parathion
Anticonvulsants: carbamazepine, hydantoins, phenacemide
Nonsteroidal anti-inflammatory agents: indomethacin, ibuprofen, oxyphenylbutazone, phenylbutazone, sulindac
Antihistamines: cimetidine, chlorpheniramine, ranitidine
Antiprotozoal drugs: quinacrine, chloroquine
Sulfonamides: some antibiotics, antidiabetics (chlorpropamide, tolbutamide), antithyroidal drugs (methimazole, methylthiouracil, propylthiouracil), carbonic anhydrase inhibitors (acetazolamide, methazolamide)
Penicillamine
Metals: gold, arsenic, bismuth, mercury

AGENTS MORE RARELY ASSOCIATED

Allopurinol (may potentiate marrow suppression by cytotoxic drugs)
Antibiotics: flucytosine, mebendazole, methicillin, sulfonamides, streptomycin, tetracycline, trimethoprim/sulfamethoxazole
Carbimazole
Guanidine
Lithium
Methyldopa
Potassium perchlorate
Quinidine
Sedatives and tranquilizers: chlordiazepoxide, chlorpromazine, meprobamate, methyprylon, piperacetazine, prochlorperazine
Thiocyanate

*Agents are listed because they have been cited in the literature; inclusion in this list does not imply acceptance by the authors of a causal relationship.
Modified from Young NS, Alter BP: Aplastic Anemia: Acquired and Inherited. Philadelphia, W.B. Saunders Co., 1994, p 104.

larly shown to suppress the bone marrow in animals in a dose-linked manner, and most individuals exposed to sufficient amounts of benzene will probably have some type of marrow damage. In practice, most drug-related aplastic anemia is "idiosyncratic"; that is, it occurs unpredictably in only rare individuals who receive the medication, sometimes weeks to months after its administration is discontinued. Patients in this last category may possess a genetic propensity for this phenomenon. In the case of agents that can cause both dose-related and idiosyncratic aplastic anemia, the mechanisms may be different because both forms have not been reported in the same patient.

CHLORAMPHENICOL

Chloramphenicol is the drug that was most often associated with idiosyncratic aplastic anemia in the past. A genetic predisposition for idiosyncratic aplasia may exist; however, its mechanism remains unknown despite extensive investigation.

This antibiotic was considered to be the most common cause of aplastic anemia at the peak of its use, which began in 1949.[20] It contains a nitrobenzene ring and thus resembles amidopyrine, a drug known to cause agranulocytosis.[21, 22] Chloramphenicol is the prime example of a drug that causes both dose-related marrow suppression and idiosyncratic aplastic anemia.[23]

The signs of dose-related toxicity appear more rapidly in patients with hepatic or renal disease because the drug

must be inactivated by conjugation with glucuronide in the liver and excreted in the urine. High doses and high plasma levels correlate with the characteristic reversible erythroid depression. *In vitro*, chloramphenicol inhibits the growth of both colony-forming units–granulocyte macrophage (CFU-GMs) and colony-forming units-erythroid (CFU-Es)[24–28] and also may inhibit the hematopoietic microenvironment.[26, 29]

OTHER DRUGS

Nonsteroidal anti-inflammatory drugs, which are used more extensively in adults than in children, are associated with aplasia.[9] Nonsteroidal anti-inflammatory drugs associated by occasional case reports with aplastic anemia include aspirin,[30] indomethacin,[31–34] and ibuprofen.[35] In several large studies an increased risk of aplastic anemia was found with use of phenylbutazone[36, 37] and even higher probabilities of disease were identified for some of the other nonsteroidal anti-inflammatory drugs.[9] Cimetidine is another drug associated with a risk of cytopenia of 2 per 100,000 patients.[38, 39] Sulfa-containing compounds, which appear as risk factors in most case-control studies of drugs and aplastic anemia, are used in a wide variety of clinical circumstances.[40–49] Other drugs commonly used in the pediatric population that are implicated in aplastic anemia include anticonvulsants (hydantoins[50–52] and carbamazepine[53–57]) and carbonic anhydrase inhibitors[58] (acetazolamide[59, 60] and methazolamide[61, 62]). Many of the drugs listed in Table 7–3 also have been associated with agranulocytosis. In general, only a minority of cases of aplastic anemia can be associated with a drug. Making the distinction between aplasia caused by medication versus that arising from the underlying disorder (or occult viral infection) requiring treatment can be difficult.

Chemicals and Toxins

BENZENE

Benzene is a particularly dangerous environmental contaminant.[63, 64] It is found in organic solvents, coal tar derivatives, and petroleum products.[65–68] Fatal aplastic anemia or leukemia or both have been reported years later in factory workers who were exposed to benzene. Benzene is concentrated in bone marrow fat,[69] forms water-soluble intermediates,[70–72] and damages DNA.[73–75] It decreases the numbers of progenitors and damages stroma as well. The risk of cytopenia is probably related to cumulative exposure.

OTHER AROMATIC HYDROCARBONS

Toxicity thought to be due to other organic solvents may in some instances be caused by benzene contaminants. Stoddard's solvent contains benzene. Neither pure toluene nor xylene is a marrow toxin. Aplastic anemia has been linked by many case reports to insecticides, particularly γ-benzene hexachloride (lindane) in children.[76] Aromatic hydrocarbons are present in insecticides and herbicides and may comprise the solvents for these agents. Some organophosphate insecticides have been shown to inhibit *in vitro* hematopoietic colony formation, as has lindane.[77]

IONIZING RADIATION

Marrow aplasia may occur as an acute toxic sequela of irradiation due to nuclear bomb explosion, radioactive fallout, reactor accidents, and accidental exposure in medicine and industry. Bone marrow cells may be affected by high-energy γ-rays as well as by ingested or absorbed lower-energy α particles. The radiation injures the actively replicating pool of precursor and progenitor cells and also stem cells, in which DNA damage may have a more severe effect. Nonetheless, radiation-related marrow aplasia is seen rarely. Even in a restricted episode, such as the Chernobyl reactor accident in 1986, most immediate deaths were due to skin burns and damage to gastrointestinal and pulmonary systems.

Chronic radiation-induced aplasia is dose related. Patients who were irradiated for ankylosing spondylitis had an increased risk of aplastic anemia, and American radiologists have been reported to have an increased death rate from aplasia (for both groups, the pathologic distinction between aplasia and myelodysplasia was not made). The incidence of late aplasia in persons exposed to radiation from an atomic bomb was not increased nor was it increased in patients receiving radiation therapy for malignancies. Knospe and Crosby[78] suggested that irradiation exposure greater than 4.4 Gy was required for the development of aplasia; they also postulated that low doses might damage only stem cells, whereas high doses would also damage the supportive hematopoietic stromal microenvironment.

Infectious Agents

Patients with bacterial or viral illnesses often develop mild pancytopenia during or after the infection (see Chapter 49). Patients with bacterial or viral infections often receive antibiotics and other medications, and it is often not clear whether an ensuing aplastic anemia was caused by the infection, by the drug, or by the combination of the two, or even whether the infectious illness was the result, and not the cause, of the pancytopenia (Table 7–4). However, several viruses do have specific hematopoietic effects (Fig. 7–2).[79]

HEPATITIS

Although hepatitis is often associated with mild depression of blood cell counts, aplasia is a rare sequela, estimated to occur in fewer than 0.07 percent of the total number of pediatric patients with hepatitis[80] and in fewer than 2 percent of those with non-A, non-B hepatitis.[81] Nonetheless, as an identifiable clinical event, a prior episode of hepatitis was recognized in 2 to 5 percent of patients with aplastic anemia in a Western series.[82] The prevalence of prior hepatitis is about twofold this proportion in the Far East.[83] Among children with aplastic anemia in Taiwan, 24 percent had a history of recent acute hepatitis.[84] The antecedent hepatitis may be subclinical, because about 50 percent of patients may have elevated hepatic transaminase levels before their first transfusion. In a report of 32 patients who had liver transplantation for hepatic failure after non-A, non-B hepatitis, however, 28 percent developed aplastic anemia.[85] Aplasia has been reported after both hepatitis A and B virus infections,[86, 87] but in almost all of these patients the hepatitis/aplasia syndrome was not linked with hepatitis virus A, B, C, E, or G.[88, 89]

Aplastic anemia associated with hepatitis is particularly severe. More than 200 patients with aplastic anemia

TABLE 7–4. Causes of Pancytopenia

HYPOCELLULAR BONE MARROW

Acquired aplastic anemia
Inherited bone marrow failure syndrome (Fanconi anemia, amegakaryocytic thrombocytopenia, dyskeratosis congenita)
Hypoplastic myelodysplastic syndrome
Virus-associated aplastic anemia

CELLULAR BONE MARROW

Primary Bone Marrow Disease
Myelodysplasia
Paroxysmal nocturnal hemoglobinuria

Secondary to Systemic Disease
Systemic lupus erythematosus, Sjögren syndrome
Hypersplenism
Vitamin B_{12} or folate deficiency
Infection
Storage disease (Gaucher, Niemann-Pick)
Alcoholism
Sarcoidosis

INFILTRATIVE BONE MARROW DISORDERS

Acute myelogenous leukemia
Hemophagocytic lymphohistiocytosis
Metastatic solid tumors
Osteopetrosis
Myelofibrosis

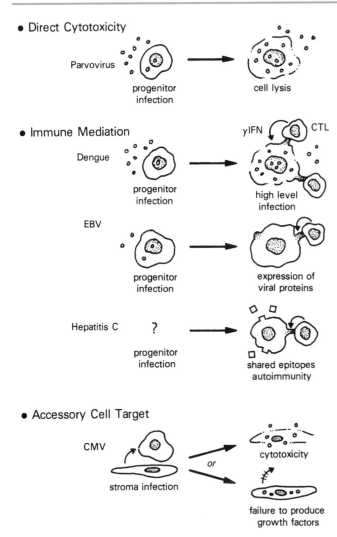

FIGURE 7–2. Potential models of virus-induced bone marrow failure. EBV = Epstein-Barr virus; CMV = cytomegalovirus; CLT = cytotoxic lymphocyte; HGF = hematopoietic growth factor; HSC = hematopoietic stem cell. (With permission from Young NS, Alter BP: Bone marrow failure. In Handin RI, Lux SE, Stossel TP (eds): Blood: Principles and Practice of Hematology. New York, Lippincott-Ravin, 1994. Illustrator, Joy D. Marlowe, M.A., A.M.I.)

and hepatitis have been reported, with two thirds of those affected being male and three quarters being younger than 20 years of age. In one series, more than 90 percent died within a year, and the mean survival was only 11 weeks,[90] although this study was done before modern treatment advances and it is unclear whether hepatitis still predicts a poor prognosis. Successful treatments with bone marrow transplantation, antithymocyte globulin, and androgens have been reported.

FLAVIVIRUSES

Flaviviruses cause arbovirus hemorrhagic fevers, dengue, and other hematodepressive syndromes. Dengue virus can propagate in bone marrow cultures without direct cytotoxicity, and dengue virus antigens induce lymphocyte activation and the release of marrow-suppressive cytokines.[91]

EPSTEIN-BARR VIRUS

Herpesviruses such as Epstein-Barr virus (EBV) are large, complex DNA viruses.[92] EBV causes infectious mononu-

cleosis, which has pancytopenic complications in fewer than 1 percent of patients. More than 12 such patients have been reported and in one half of these the outcome was fatal. EBV was demonstrated by immunologic and molecular methods in the bone marrow of six patients with aplastic anemia.[93] Only two had a history of typical mononucleosis, although all six had serologic evidence, suggesting that EBV may be an unrecognized cause of aplastic anemia. The target of EBV is B cells, although T cells also may be infected. Because EBV is a common infection, ascertainment of the cause of aplasia can be difficult.

CYTOMEGALOVIRUS AND HUMAN HERPESVIRUS 6

Infection with cytomegalovirus may lead to graft failure in immunosuppressed bone marrow transplant recipients.[94] Cytomegalovirus can infect marrow stromal cells *in vitro* and can inhibit their ability to produce growth factors[95]; direct progenitor cell infection by some cytomegalovirus strains also has been documented.[95, 96] Herpesvirus 6 is the cause of erythema subitum[97] and, like cytomegalovirus, may be found in the marrow of patients with graft failure after transplantation,[98] as well as in hematopoietic progenitors infected *in vitro*.[99] As with other viruses, both of these are ubiquitous infections, making causality difficult to ascertain.

HUMAN IMMUNODEFICIENCY VIRUS

Patients with acquired immunodeficiency virus (AIDS) often have cytopenias,[100] but their marrow is much more commonly cellular and dysplastic than empty. Colony formation by marrow from patients may be diminished.[101–104] The action of human immunodeficiency virus-1 (HIV-1), a lentivirus, on hematopoietic cells remains a subject of controversy. HIV-1 infection of CD34+ cells has been difficult to detect *in vivo* from patient material[103, 105] or after tissue culture infection of normal cells.[103, 106] The virus apparently directly infects megakaryocytes, which bear the CD4 receptor present on T cells.[107] The virus also may affect stroma functions, at least *in vitro*.[108, 109] HIV-1 can act indirectly on hematopoiesis through inhibitory lymphokine production: the envelope glycoprotein can stimulate macrophages to produce tumor necrosis factor, which in turn inhibits hematopoietic colony formation.[110] Hematologic suppression can also be due to opportunistic infections, neoplasms, or marrow suppression from the drugs used to treat AIDS and its complications.

OTHER VIRUSES

Blood cell count abnormalities, which are rarely severe, may be observed during the course of rubella, measles, mumps, varicella, and influenza A.[111]

Pregnancy

The first reported patient with aplastic anemia was a pregnant woman.[7] Although this finding is uncommon in pediatrics, it may occur within the context of the practice of pediatric hematology. More than 60 cases of aplastic anemia have now been reported as being first diagnosed during pregnancy, and more than 30 cases of the disease were diagnosed before pregnancy.[112] Among patients without known preceding aplasia, 25 percent died within the first 2 months after termination of pregnancy or delivery, and 50 percent eventually died from aplastic anemia. Although therapeutic pregnancy termination is often recommended, improvement was seen in only one of seven patients after termination. Among those with preexisting aplastic anemia, only seven died subsequent to delivery. Most fatal complications in both groups were due to bleeding. Red cell and platelet transfusion support can permit successful pregnancies, although clinical deterioration is possible. Increased levels of estrogens, which are seen during pregnancy, may have a role in the associated aplastic anemia. Animal studies suggest that high doses of estrogens may be responsible for bone marrow suppression.[113]

Paroxysmal Nocturnal Hemoglobinuria

Paroxysmal nocturnal hemoglobinuria (PNH) is a disease characterized by variable combinations of mild to severe intravascular hemolysis, large venous thromboses, and aplastic anemia.[114] It is uncommon in adults and even rarer in children (see Chapter 14). There is a clear association of PNH with aplastic anemia: 20 to 30 percent of patients with PNH first have pancytopenia and marrow hypoplasia, and 5 to 10 percent of patients with aplastic anemia develop PNH as they recover. According to flow cytometry results, a significant proportion of patients with newly diagnosed aplastic anemia manifest the PNH defect.[115]

PNH is characterized by an inability to inactivate complement on the erythrocyte cell surface, which results in increased sensitivity to complement. Deficits were subsequently identified in a family of membrane proteins, all of which were anchored to the cell membrane via glycosylphosphatidylinositol (GPI). GPI binds covalently to specific carboxyl terminal protein sequences and attaches them to cell membrane phosphatidylinositol residues. The genetic defect in PNH was localized to the X-linked *PIG-A* (phosphatidylinositol glycan class A) gene whose product functions in the transfer of *N*-acetylglucosamine to phosphatidylinositol as an early step in GPI anchor formation. The PNH defect can be detected by flow cytometry for the absence of GPI-anchored cell surface proteins.

The etiology of marrow aplasia in PNH remains unclear. Although SCID mice infused with bone marrow from patients with PNH show preferential engraftment with the PNH clones,[116] studies of hematopoiesis in patients with PNH have not detected any selective proliferative advantage of the *PIG-A*(−) hematopoietic clones.[117] A subsequent study comparing *in vitro* proliferation of *PIG-A*(−) and *PIG-A*(+) CD34 cells from patients with PNH found a selective growth deficiency in the *PIG-A*(+) cell population rather than an advantage for the *PIG-A* mutant cells: Fas receptor expression was elevated on the wild type compared with the GPI-deficient cells, suggesting increased resistance to apoptosis as one potential mechanism to explain these findings.[118] No proliferative advantage of PNH hematopoietic clones was observed in mice mosaic for the *PIG-A* gene.[119, 120] To evaluate the hypothesis that autoreactive T cells might preferentially eliminate *PIG-A*(+) hematopoietic stem cells while sparing the PNH clones, the sensitivity of normal versus PNH EBV-transformed B-cell lines to autologous

EBV-specific T-cell lines was examined.[121] The PNH cells were no less sensitive to T-cell–mediated cytotoxicity than the non-PNH cells; thus the GPI-linked cell surface molecules are not required for killing by T cells. An abnormal distribution of expanded T-cell clones detected by size analysis of the complementarity-determining region 3 (CDR3) in the beta variable region mRNA of the T-cell receptor has been noted in PNH patients,[122] although the targets of such T-cell populations remain to be ascertained.

Immunologic Diseases

In 10 percent of patients *eosinophilic fasciitis,* a rare collagen vascular syndrome, has been associated with aplastic anemia.[123] This condition is usually limited to adults. Thymoma associated with hematopoietic failure generally but not exclusively presents as pure red cell aplasia.[124] Some adults with this condition had also received drugs such as chloramphenicol or sulfonamides, and the aplasia could have been due to the drugs alone or to the combination. An iatrogenic aplasia can be induced by the transfusion of competent lymphocytes into immunodeficient hosts. In these patients, marrow failure arises from transfusional graft-versus-host disease.[125]

PATHOPHYSIOLOGY

The purported mechanisms for failure of hematopoiesis are predicated on our current knowledge of normal hematopoiesis (see Chapter 6). Disease could result from decreased numbers or defective function of the cellular or soluble components required for blood cell production or from combinations of these factors.

Figure 7–3 depicts two models for bone marrow damage. In type I, irradiation, drugs, chemicals, or an underlying cellular abnormality leads to DNA damage. In type II aplasia, viruses, or drugs or toxins incite an immune system reaction that in turn leads to cytotoxicity within the hematopoietic compartment. Recovery would occur if the stem cells could, in fact, repopulate adequately. With damage of both type I and type II, cell death among target cells occurs, probably by apoptotic mechanisms, and all proliferating cells are probably affected.

Hematopoietic Stem Cells and Clonality

Virtually all patients with aplastic anemia have greatly decreased numbers of committed progenitor cells in blood and marrow, assayed as myeloid colony-forming cells (CFU-GMs), erythroid colony-forming cells (CFU-Es) and burst-forming units–erythroid, megakaryocytic progenitors (CFU-megs), and multipotent colony-forming cells (CFU-granulocyte-erythroid-monocyte-macrophage). Until recently, true stem cells have not been assayable in humans; however, the *long-term culture–initiating cell* appears to be a surrogate test for this most primitive cell. These cells are severely reduced in number in both the marrow and blood in all patients with aplastic anemia.[126, 127] Hematopoietic cells can also be assessed phenotypically for the presence of the CD34 antigen, which defines a compartment of about 1 percent of marrow cells that includes progenitors and possibly activated stem cells.[128–131] Almost all patients with aplas-

PATHOPHYSIOLOGY OF APLASTIC ANEMIA

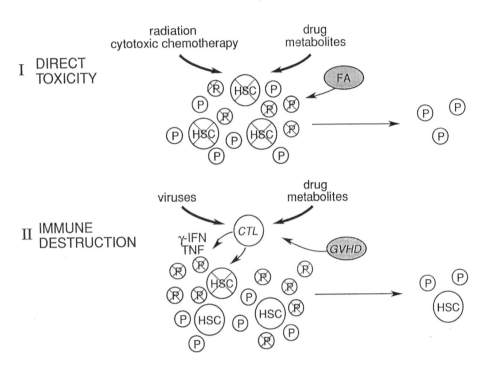

FIGURE 7–3. Two mechanisms of stem cell compartment damage. Type I involves DNA damaged by radiation and radiometric agents such as busulfan, as well as by other drugs (e.g., chloramphenicol). Fanconi anemia is an example of inheritance of the inability to repair DNA damage. Type II is at the level of the more mature cell and involves the cell membrane or metabolism; such damage can be caused by many drugs, viruses, and immune mechanisms. P = progenitor; HSC = hematopoietic stem cell; FA = Fanconi anemia; IFN = interferon; TNF = tumor necrosis factor; CTL = cytotoxic T lymphocyte; GVHD = Graft versus host disease.

tic anemic show not only severe reduction in the numbers of CD34+ cells but also poor plating efficiency for colony formation from purified CD34+ cells.[132, 133]

Several lines of evidence point to primary abnormalities in the hematopoietic stem cell as a potential etiology for aplastic anemia. Multiple studies have noted that simple infusion of stem cells from an identical twin donor without prior conditioning was sufficient to treat the aplasia in around 50 percent of patients.[134–137] These results strongly support a pathogenic stem cell defect and argue against permanent disorders of the bone marrow environment, including immunologic mechanisms, as the cause of stem cell destruction. The requirement for conditioning in a portion of patients with aplastic anemia before identical twin stem cell transplantation may reflect the required ablation of these abnormal clones to allow normal hematopoiesis in these patients. The persistence of low numbers of stem cells, even with hematologic recovery after immunosuppressive therapy, and the fact that blood cell parameters, such as macrocytosis, do not return to normal in many patients, again suggest an underlying stem cell abnormality. A primary stem cell defect probably also contributes to the observation of clonal hematopoiesis in aplastic anemia[138] as well as to the relative occurrence of relapse and late development of other hematologic diseases such as PNH, myelodysplasia, and acute leukemia (see later).

Immune Destruction

Several lines of data suggest that immune phenomena may be relevant in aplastic anemia.[139] In some syngeneic (twin) bone marrow transplant recipients, simple infusion of stem cells is not sufficient to reconstitute hematopoiesis. The requirement for prior conditioning of the host may reflect some operational immunologic process, although it is also consistent with the presence of an underlying clonal abnor-

mality that requires ablation.[140] Histocompatibility studies conducted in Europe, Asia, and America have indicated an increased representation of HLA-DR2 among patients with aplastic anemia, consistent with a genetically determined immune susceptibility to disease.[17, 140, 141] Evidence for specific immune mechanisms is reviewed below.

LYMPHOCYTES

Autologous recovery has been reported after either mismatched or matched transplants in patients prepared with antilymphocyte sera or cyclophosphamide.[142–144] Aplasia often responds to treatment with antilymphocyte globulin (ALG)/antithymocyte globulin (ATG) and/or cyclosporine without transplant. The antilymphocyte preparations contain heterogeneous mixtures of antibodies to many cells, including lymphocytes, and are clearly immunosuppressive as well as generally cytotoxic. They lead to rapid lymphopenia during and immediately after treatment, and reduced levels of activated lymphocytes persist for months. Cyclosporine exerts inhibitory T-cell effects and inhibits transcription of genes for cytokines including interleukin (IL)-2 and γ-interferon.[145] It has many other toxic effects on several tissues, including brain and kidney. The attribution of immune dysregulation as a cause of aplastic anemia based on therapy must be tempered with caution because ATG and cyclosporine exert many effects in addition to immunosuppression. The diverse antibodies in ATG react with a wide range of antigens, including signal transduction and adhesion molecules.[146] The active component(s) of ATG in aplastic anemia have not been isolated. Of note, therapies with mixtures of monoclonal antibodies specific for human T cells have not been very effective in clinical trials to date.[147] Furthermore, ATG can increase colony growth in normal, myelodysplasia, and aplastic anemia CD34+ bone marrow cells in culture[148] ATG treatment also reduces the expression of Fas antigen on aplastic anemia bone marrow CD34+ cells.[149] Cyclosporine is thought to be more specifically immunosuppressive than ATG and thus its efficacy further implicates T-cell participation in the pathophysiology of aplastic anemia. Nonetheless, cyclosporine therapy also has a broad range of additional effects. Effective treatment of myelodysplasia with cyclosporine has recently been reported and may suggest that cyclosporine exerts additional effects on the bone marrow,[150] although the possibility of an immune mechanism underlying myelodysplasia is also under investigation.[151]

A role for immune dysregulation in aplastic anemia in some patients is supported by several studies of T-cell characteristics in aplastic anemia. Lymphocytes with IgG receptors, Tγ+ cells, were reported in aplastic but not in normal bone marrow.[152] Later, these cells were characterized phenotypically as activated cytotoxic lymphocytes: *CD8+* T cells expressing the antigens HLA-DR and the receptor for IL-2; activated cytotoxic T cells circulate,[153] but they may be present in the marrow when they are not detected in the blood.[154] Cell clones of this phenotype have been isolated from patients, and *in vitro* they overproduce inhibitory cytokines and inhibit hematopoiesis.[155–157] Altered T-helper and T-cytotoxic cell profiles have been identified in patients with aplastic anemia.[158–160] Identification of a T-cell clone with HLA-DRB1 0405–restricted cytotoxicity for hematopoietic cells has been reported in one patient with aplastic anemia.[161] Studies of V_β T-cell receptors have not found any general restriction of T-cell clonality or of dominant lymphocyte clones.[162] A skewed distribution of the complementary-determining region 3 (CDR3) of the V_β region of the T-cell receptor, suggestive of clonal predominance, has been described in a small group of cyclosporine-dependent patients.[163] Analysis of the CDR3 region of CD4 cells derived from five patients with aplastic anemia and an HLA-DR2 haplotype showed a high frequency of clones bearing identical CDR3 DNA sequences that were not found in normal control subjects.[164] Of note, most of these reports studied T-cell characteristics of patients who had received treatment for aplastic anemia. Studies characterizing T cells of patients with aplastic anemia before therapy would be crucial for distinguishing possible confounding effects of therapy or transfusion. Furthermore, it remains to be determined whether such immunologic abnormalities are a general feature of all patients with aplastic anemia or are characteristic of a subset of such patients. Although genetically restricted suppression of erythropoiesis by a unique subset of T lymphocytes has been demonstrated in patients with pure red cell aplasia,[165] the coordinated identification and isolation of pathogenic T cells, demonstration of hematopoietic suppression by these T cells, and identification of antigen(s) recognized by such T cells have yet to be accomplished in a patient with aplastic anemia. This subject remains a critical area of active investigation.

LYMPHOKINES

Whether overproduction or dysregulated production of inhibitory cytokines represents a primary etiology or a secondary effect of an underlying bone marrow abnormality remains unclear. γ-Interferon, a soluble inhibitor produced by T cells was found to be produced at high levels in cultures from patients with aplastic anemia.[153, 166, 167] γ-Interferon is expressed in the marrow of most patients with aplastic anemia but not in marrow from normal subjects or from patients with other hematologic diseases who have undergone frequent transfusions.[168, 169] Other inhibitory cytokines, such as *tumor necrosis factor*[170] and *macrophage inflammatory protein–1*,[171, 172] also are overexpressed in aplastic marrow. Both interferon and tumor necrosis factor directly and synergistically inhibit hematopoiesis *in vitro*.[173] In long-term bone marrow cultures, constitutive low-level expression of γ-interferon markedly reduces the output of both committed progenitor cells and long-term cultureinitiating cells, the stem cell surrogates.[174] Both interferon and tumor necrosis factor increase the potential for programmed cell death within the CD34+ compartment by increasing Fas antigen expression on target cells.[175] (Fas antigen is a cell surface molecule in the tumor necrosis factor receptor family; its activation signals apoptosis.)

Microenvironment

In theory, aplastic anemia could be due to a microenvironment that fails to support hematopoiesis: a lesion of "soil" rather than "seed."[78] The anemia in the Sl/Sl^d murine strain, which is missing stem cell factor, the ligand for the c-*kit* receptor, is an example of such a defect.[176] Although defects in some stromal cell function have occasionally been measured in patients, these defects do not appear to be the cause of aplastic anemia in most patients. After marrow transplantation, most stromal cell elements remain of host origin,[177] yet these cells adequately support the donor's stem cells. In the laboratory, aplastic marrow usually provides normal adherent cell function in long-term or Dexter flask–type cultures; however, a patient's marrow is a poor source of clonogenic cells when grown on normal stroma, consistent with the defect in stem and progenitor cell numbers described earlier.[178] Some investigators have reported low fibroblast colony formation in aplastic anemia,[179] but this assay may not reflect stromal cell function.

Hematopoietic growth factor production and plasma levels are usually increased rather than decreased in patients with aplastic anemia.[180] Circulating levels of erythropoietin, granulocyte colony-stimulating factor (G-CSF) and granulocyte-macrophage colony-stimulating factor (GM-CSF), thrombopoietin, and flt-3 ligand are elevated in patients with aplastic anemia. Stem cell factor levels have been reported to be low to normal. Levels of IL-1, produced by monocytes, are low in aplastic anemia. Therapeutic trials with these factors have yielded divergent and incomplete responses,[181] casting doubt on the pathophysiologic significance of deficiency of these factors.

CLINICAL EVALUATION

The evaluation and diagnostic workup of the patient with presumed acquired aplastic anemia should be focused on eliminating alternative diagnoses for which curative therapies are available or for which the therapies for aplastic anemia would be inappropriate (Table 7–5).

TABLE 7–5. Clinical Evaluation

Test	Rationale
COMPLETE BLOOD COUNT AND DIFFERENTIAL	
Morphology	Malignant vs. benign
	Vitamin B_{12} deficiency
	Storage disease
Reticulocyte count	Defines severity
	Differentiates production vs. destruction
BONE MARROW BIOPSY	
Morphology	Malignant vs. benign
	Storage disease
	Hemophagocytosis
	Congenital disorder
Cytogenetics	Myelodysplasia
Culture	Infectious agent (e.g., tuberculosis, virus)
Other	DNA/antigen-based viral tests
PERIPHERAL BLOOD CHEMISTRY	
AST, ALT, GGT, bilirubin, alkaline phosphatase, LDH	Hepatitis
BUN, creatinine, electrolytes	Chronic renal failure
Serologic testing	Hepatitis, Epstein-Barr virus, other virus
Ham test/FACS	Paroxysmal nocturnal hemoglobinuria
Diepoxybutane chromosomal breakage	Fanconi anemia
Autoimmune disease evaluation	Evidence of collagen vascular disease
Histocompatibility testing	Establish potential donor pool

AST = aspartate aminotransferase; ALT = alanine aminotransferase; GGT = γ-glutamyl transferase; LDH = lactate dehydrogenase; BUN = blood urea nitrogen; FACS = fluorescence-activated cell sorting.
Modified from Guinan EC: Clinical aspects of aplastic anemia. Hematol Oncol Clin North Am 1997; 11:1028.

History

The chief presenting symptoms relate to low blood cell counts. Bleeding, such as gum oozing, nosebleeds, easy bruising with minimal trauma, or heavy menses, may be seen. Chronic anemia may present with fatigue, decreased activity, or exercise intolerance, although the gradual onset of severe anemia can be surprisingly well compensated for in young children. Serious infection is not a frequent presenting symptom early in the course of aplastic anemia. Many patients feel well with few symptoms on initial presentation. A careful family history for blood disorders or leukemias/solid tumors that might suggest an inherited bone marrow syndrome should be obtained. A developmental history can provide helpful information to screen for potential congenital, metabolic, or storage diseases. A detailed history of medications, environment, and infections, particularly for 1 to 12 months before presentation, should be obtained.

Physical Examination

Clinical appearance is related to the severity and duration of the underlying pancytopenia. Hemorrhagic manifestations from thrombocytopenia occur early and include petechiae (particularly on the border of the hard and soft palate), ecchymoses, epistaxis, and bleeding from mucous membranes. Neutropenia causes oral ulcerations, bacterial infections, and fever; these signs are rarely present early. Evidence of erythropoietic failure characterized by pallor, fatigue, and tachycardia is often seen late because the life span of the erythrocyte (120 days) far exceeds that of platelets (10 days) or white cells (variable, but measured in hours for granulo-

cytes). Mucous membranes and nailbeds may be pale. Lymphadenopathy, splenomegaly, and severe weight loss are uncommon and may suggest other underlying disorders. Short stature, congenital anomalies (particularly of the thumbs and forearms), areas of hyper- or hypopigmentation, or dystrophic nails should alert the examiner to possible inherited bone marrow failure disorders.

Laboratory Studies

Evaluation should include a complete blood count, reticulocyte count, Coombs' test to rule out autoimmune destruction, and biochemical profile including renal and hepatic evaluation.

A careful evaluation of the peripheral blood smear may suggest infection or dietary deficiency. Blood cell counts are often uniformly depressed. The blood smear shows a paucity of platelets and leukocytes, but in very acute disease essentially normal red cell morphology is seen. Automated counting indicates that the anemia is often macrocytic, although sometimes it is normocytic, and that the red cell distribution width, a numeric measure of anisocytosis, is usually normal. Platelet size is not increased, as it is in most patients with immune thrombocytopenias. The absolute reticulocyte count is decreased. Numbers of granulocytes are clearly diminished, as may be those of monocytes and lymphocytes.[182, 183] Increases in fetal hemoglobin (HbF) and red cell i antigen are manifestations of the fetal-like erythropoiesis seen in "stress" hematopoiesis[184] but occur irregularly in patients with aplastic anemia, have no prognostic value, and can persist in patients who have recovered.

Blood chemistry panels to evaluate hepatic and renal function should be obtained. Blood tests to rule out

Fanconi anemia and PNH are important because these diagnoses would entail alternative treatments. Patients with stigmata of collagen vascular disease should be appropriately evaluated. Early HLA typing of the patient and family members is helpful in guiding future therapies.

Bone marrow must be examined by both aspiration and biopsy so that cellularity can be evaluated both qualitatively and quantitatively. The bone marrow in aplastic anemia is hypocellular, with empty spicules, fat, reticulum cells, plasma cells, and mast cells (Fig. 7–4). Some dyserythropoiesis, with megaloblastosis and nuclear-cytoplasmic asynchrony, may be seen. Aspirates alone may appear hypocellular owing to dilution with peripheral blood, or they may look hypercellular because of areas of focal residual hematopoiesis. Biopsies provide larger, more reliable specimens for assessment of cellularity. Biopsies also provide critical information about bone marrow architecture such as fibrosis or granulomas. Bone marrow aspirates should also be sent for cytogenetic analysis and possibly for fluorescence *in situ* hybridization to identify abnormalities associated with myelodysplasia or malignancy. Bone marrow may also be sent for culture or DNA-based antigen detection of infectious agents such as viruses.

It is imperative that test results be obtained in an expeditious fashion to minimize the need for any blood transfusions before potential bone marrow transplantation. The outcome for patients undergoing allogeneic stem cell transplantation for aplastic anemia is generally better if they have had no or few transfusions (see later).

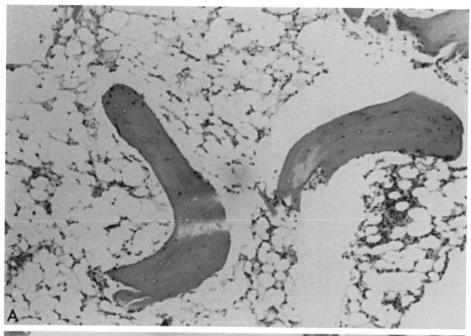

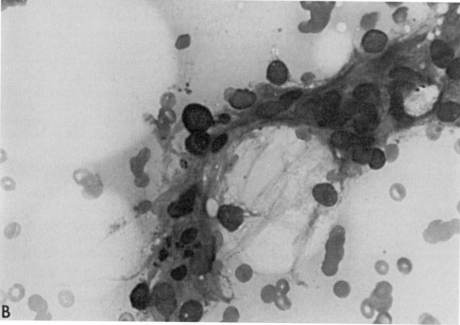

FIGURE 7–4. Bone marrow examination in severe aplastic anemia. *A,* Note hypercellularity in biopsy. *B,* Residual cells seen in aspirate are lymphocytes, stromal cells, plasma cells, and mast cells. (Courtesy of Dr. Gail Wolfe, Boston, MA.)

MANAGEMENT AND OUTCOME

Prognosis

Outcome depends on the types of treatments offered, the causes of the aplasias, and the eras and countries being analyzed. In a large series conducted before 1957, Wolff[185] found a survival rate of only 3 percent. In other series ending no later than 1965, complete recoveries were reported in 10 to 35 percent of patients. In a series of 40 pediatric patients seen before 1958, Diamond and Shahidi[186] found that only two patients recovered, one of whom later had a recurrence. The series summarized here may not have been rigorous with regard to the exclusion of patients with less than severe disease.[187]

SPONTANEOUS RECOVERY

Spontaneous recovery has been reported anecdotally, although most patients probably had moderate rather than severe aplastic anemia. Good supportive care (see later) may contribute to this recovery; in one series, 14 of 33 children recovered,[188] and children with moderate aplastic anemia have been found to have an excellent prognosis even without specific treatment.[189] A study in which 21 patients were randomly assigned to receive immunosuppressive therapy or only supportive care found no improvement in the control group after 3 months.[190] Spontaneous recovery is sufficiently rare in patients with severe aplastic anemia; thus, all current treatment modalities should be used.

Supportive Care

Blood product support should be used sparingly to avoid sensitization, and blood product donors should never be from the patient's family for the same reason. Complete red cell phenotyping should be done because erythrocyte antibodies may develop in patients who receive long-term blood product support. All blood products should be filtered and irradiated. In addition, any exposure to potentially hazardous drugs or toxins should be eliminated.

BLEEDING

The use of platelet (and red cell) support has probably had the greatest impact on survival of patients with aplastic anemia and has changed the cause of death from bleeding to infection. Platelets can be provided from several individual units of blood or, preferably, by platelet pheresis from a single donor (which reduces antigenic exposure).

The main role of prophylactic platelet support is reduction of the risk of intracranial hemorrhage, which is a rare but devastating event. The general threshold platelet count has long been 20,000 cells/μL; however, this figure and the entire practice of prophylactic administration of platelet transfusions have recently been questioned.[191–193] Platelet transfusions for outpatients with stable chronic severe aplastic anemia at platelet counts less than 5,000 to 10,000/μL were found to be feasible and safe in a recent study.[194] Chronic transfusions of platelets are not used as often for aplastic anemia as they are for leukemia. They are usually given when symptoms of bleeding are seen or if the patient has an increased risk of bleeding (e.g., toddlers learning to walk, patients with hypertension who are receiving cyclosporine, or patients with fever and infection).

Other measures to reduce bleeding include maintenance of good dental hygiene, use of a soft toothbrush, use of stool softeners, avoidance of trauma, and avoidance of vasoconstrictive drugs. Drugs that may interfere with platelet function, such as aspirin or nonsteroidal anti-inflammatory drugs, should be avoided in thrombocytopenia. Antifibrinolytic agents such as aminocaproic acid and tranexamic acid may decrease bleeding, particularly from the gums and nasal mucosa.

INFECTIONS

There are few reported studies of infection in aplastic anemia.[195, 196] Severe granulocytopenia may last for years. However, the immune systems of granulocytopenic patients remain intact; this is in contrast to the situation of patients with malignancies who receive chemotherapy and who experience simultaneous neutropenia and immunosuppression. Neutropenia (and perhaps monocytopenia) increases the risk of bacterial infection in aplastic anemia. Because neutropenia precludes the development of an inflammatory response, identification of an infected locus is often difficult. The bacterial organisms may be gram-negative bacilli such as *Escherichia coli*, *Klebsiella pneumoniae*, and *Pseudomonas aeruginosa* or gram-positive cocci, including *Staphylococcus aureus* and *Staphylococcus epidermidis* and streptococci. Immunosuppression in preparation for bone marrow transplantation or as the primary therapy for the aplastic anemia may lead to unusual bacterial, fungal, viral, and protozoan infections. Recommendations for specific antibiotics and other anti-infection agents are beyond the scope of this chapter. Moreover, regimens are changing rapidly as new generations of treatments are developed.

Prophylactic antibiotics have no role in the "well" patient with aplastic anemia. Patients undergoing immunosuppressive therapy should receive prophylaxis for *Pneumocystis carinii*. If fever and neutropenia are present, complete evaluation and cultures of all possible sites should be followed by the administration of broad-spectrum parenteral antibiotics. Fungal infections occur often in patients who have received repeated or extended courses of antibiotics; candidiasis and especially aspergillosis, which lead to sinusitis, lung disease, or disseminated infection, are distressingly common causes of death in patients with aplastic anemia.[195] Antecedent or concurrent administration of steroids increases this risk. Aggressive amphotericin B treatment is indicated in the patient with a persistent fever that is unresponsive to antibiotics or in the appropriate clinical setting.

ANEMIA

Red cells should be provided as needed. Hemoglobin should be maintained at a level consistent with normal activities if routine transfusions are to be used. Children can tolerate chronic anemia once adaptation has occurred, and this anemia should be permitted for a child in whom a hemoglobin level greater than 6 g/dL can be sustained without transfusions (i.e., a child who is not bleeding). Long-term use of transfusions leads to iron overload, with accumulation in critical organs. Permanent damage to heart, liver, and endocrine glands can be prevented by iron chelation therapy.[197] However, use of this therapy may be difficult in thrombocytopenic patients, who may not tolerate subcutaneous infusions.

Treatment

BONE MARROW TRANSPLANTATION

The general topic of bone marrow transplantation (BMT) is addressed in Chapter 8. The discussion below is limited to the role of BMT in treatment of aplastic anemia.

The earliest transplants for aplastic anemia involved identical twins. Subsequent definition of the human histocompatibility gene complex, development of immunosuppressive regimens, and improved support of patients with severe pancytopenia led to more general application of this form of therapy. Stem cell transplant between identical twins in the absence of any conditioning regimen was curative in approximately 50 percent of patients.[134–137] A recent study showed that the highest long-term survival of patients with identical twin transplants was achieved by following an algorithm of initial transplant without conditioning followed by a subsequent transplant with conditioning for any patients with engraftment failure after the first transplant. None of the patients in whom the first transplant failed died before receiving a second transplant, and they showed mortality similar to that of patients who received conditioning up front.[137] The European Group for Blood and Marrow Transplantation recently reported actuarial 5-year survival among patients receiving syngeneic twin transplants performed between 1976 and 1998 to be 91 percent.

Outcomes for patients who received HLA-matched allogeneic BMT have been reported by large registries, which combine the results of many contributing centers or in single-center studies by the largest referral centers[198–206] (Table 7–6). Survival rates after HLA-identical sibling transplant have improved over time, in large part due to improvements in prevention of graft-versus-host disease (GVHD).[204] Recent data reported to the International Bone Marrow Transplant Registry described 1699 patients who received HLA-identical sibling transplants for aplastic anemia between 1991 and 1997 (Fig. 7–5). The 5-year probabilities of survival (95 percent confidence intervals) were 75 ± 3 percent for patients up to 20 years of age, 68 ± 4 percent for patients between 21 and 39 years of age, and 35 ± 18 percent for patients older than 40 years of age. Survival data from single centers, while showing more variability, overlap with the 95 percent confidence intervals reported by the Registry[199] (Fig. 7–6). Patient age, duration of aplasia before transplant, prior transfusion history, and clinical status all affected survival rates. Survival was not affected by severity of aplasia.

Graft failure rates have been significantly higher after HLA-identical sibling transplants for aplastic anemia compared with those for such transplants performed to treat leukemia. Possible explanations include persistence of host immunocompetent cells capable of reacting to the donor cells, immune reactions against both host and donor hematopoietic precursors as suggested by results of identical twin transplants, persistent viral infections affecting the donor marrow, defects in the bone marrow microenvironment of some transplant recipients, or failure to eradicate an underlying abnormal stem cell clone. Risk factors for graft failure include older patient age, exposure to large numbers of blood transfusions leading to increased risk of

TABLE 7–6. Allogenic Bone Marrow Transplantation for Aplastic Anemia

Study	Years of Study	No. of Subjects	Age in Years (Median)	Rejection/ Failure (%)	Chronic Graft-versus- Host Disease (%)	Actual Survival (%)
Gluckman et al[200]	1980–1989	107	5–46 (19)	3	35	68 ± 10 (at 5 yr)
Champlin et al[201]	1984–1984	290	0.7–41 (19)	17	12	78 ± 10 (5 yr)
May et al[202]	1984–1991	24	4–53	29	0	79 ± 8
Storb et al[203]	1988–1993	39	2–52 (25)	5	34	92 (3 yr)*
Passweg et al[204]	1988–1992	471	1–51 (20)	16	32	66 ± 6 (5 yr)
Reiter et al[205]	1982–1996	20	17–37 (25)	0	53	95 (15 yr)

*In an update, a total of 55 patients treated by the same regimen were reported to have 89 percent survival at 8 years.[206]
From Young NS: Acquired aplastic anemia. In Young NS (ed): Bone Marrow Failure Syndromes. Phildadelphia, WB Saunders, 2000, p 19.

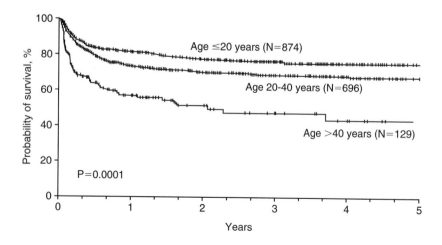

FIGURE 7–5. Effect of patient age on transplant outcome. Probability of survival by age after HLA-identical sibling bone marrow transplants for aplastic anemia come between 1991 and 1997 and reported to the International Bone Marrow Transplant Registry. (From Horwitz MM: Current status of allogeneic bone marrow transplantation in acquired aplastic anemia. Semin Hematol 2000; 37:37.)

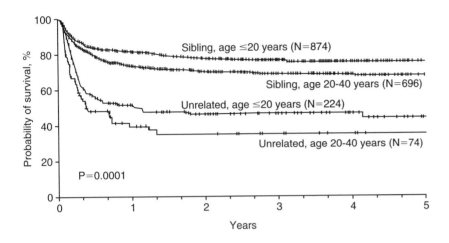

FIGURE 7–6. Effect of donor marrow on transplant outcome. Probability of survival by age after HLA-identical sibling and unrelated donor bone marrow transplants for aplastic anemia come between 1991 and 1997 and reported to the International Bone Marrow Transplant Registry. (From Horwitz MM: Current status of allogeneic bone marrow transplantation in acquired aplastic anemia. Semin Hematol 2000; 37:38.)

allosensitization, and disease duration. The detrimental role of transfusions may have decreased through the routine use of leukocyte-free products, as well as by the strict avoidance of the use of family members as donors.[207] The increased intensity of pretransplant conditioning regimens has been accompanied by significant decreases in graft rejection.[6, 208] The rate of successful second transplants in response to graft rejection has also improved.[208]

The International Bone Marrow Transplant Registry studied the efficacy of 1305 HLA-identical sibling bone marrow transplants performed between 1976 and 1992 and found that improvements in GVHD prophylaxis accounted for much of the improvements in 5-year survival. Although the proportion of patients who developed severe GVHD has declined, mortality from severe GVDH has not improved substantially over time.[209] The severity of GVHD increases with age. Children have a much lower rate of GVHD than do adults; this lower rate translates into improved survival for those younger than 20 or 30 years of age (see Chapter 8).

The above discussion refers to transplants from HLA-matched sibling donors. However, 75 percent of transplant patients do not have such a donor. Alternative donors include phenotypically but not genotypically matched relatives, partially matched (mismatched) relatives, and histocompatible but unrelated volunteers. Success has been reported in the occasional instance in which a family member is a phenotypic match as a result of, for example, haplotype sharing between parents.[210] The reader is referred to Chapter 8 for a detailed discussion of alternative donor bone marrow transplants. The European Group for Blood and Marrow Transplantation results for patients receiving transplants between 1976 and 1998 show an actuarial 5-year survival of 66 percent for patients who received HLA-identical sibling donor transplants and 37 percent for those who received alternative donor transplants.[211]

Immunosuppression

ANTITHYMOCYTE GLOBULIN

ALG and ATG (the sera produced by immunization of horses or rabbits with human thoracic duct lymphocytes or thymocytes) are highly cytotoxic reagents with activity against all blood and marrow cells, including progenitors. These reagents were initially used to decrease the rate of rejection of HLA-matched bone marrow. ALG and cyclophosphamide were also used to permit at least temporary engraftment of mismatched marrow in patients with aplastic anemia who do not have a matched donor.[142–144, 212, 213] Autologous recoveries occurred in some of these patients; these recoveries encouraged several groups to examine the use of ATG or ALG with and without haploidentical marrow.

Table 7–7 summarizes the data from several randomized studies.[214–221] Patients treated with ALG had a superior response rate and 3-year survival compared with control subjects. The addition of other agents to ALG therapy can further enhance the therapeutic effect.

ATG or ALG/antilymphocyte sera is often given to a total dose of 100 to 160 mg/kg divided over 4 to 10 days. Immediate allergic reactions to ALG are rare and can be predicted by skin testing followed by desensitization in those who are allergic.[222] The patient begins to make antibodies to horse protein about 1 week after first exposure; at this point, equine antibodies are rapidly cleared from the circulation. This clearance reduces the effective dose and enhances immune complex formation. *Serum sickness* due to immune complex deposition occurs in almost all patients who are treated for 10 days or longer. It manifests about 11 days after initiation of treatment as fever, a serpiginous rash at the volar-dorsal border of the hands and feet, arthralgia, myalgia, lassitude, and changes in urine sediment. Bronchospasm or liver chemistry abnormalities may also occur. Shorter courses of ATG treatment are less often associated with serum sickness and are advised. Corticosteroids are usually given (prednisone, 1 mg/kg) to reduce the symptoms from serum sickness. ATG binds to determinants on all cell types in blood and marrow and reduces platelet and granulocyte counts in addition to the lymphocyte counts and may lead to a positive Coombs' test. Thrombocytopenia may require intensive blood product support.[223]

Responses usually occur within the first 3 months, if at all, and some degree of blood cell count improvement by 3 months correlates with survival.[224] The earliest response to therapy may be heralded by the appearance of a few granulocytes and nucleated red cells in the circulation. Red cell size distribution histograms show a macrocytic shoulder.[225] Reticulocytes appear, the number of transfusions

TABLE 7–7. Immunosuppressive Therapy for Aplastic Anemia

Study Design	Disease Severity	% Response	Survival	Reference
IS ATG EFFECTIVE TREATMENT?				
ALG vs. control	Moderate-severe	53/0*	0.62/0.41 (3 yr)	Champlin et al (1983)[190]
CAN ATG BE REPLACED BY CSA?				
ATG vs. CsA	Severe	16/12 (3 mo)	0.64/0.70 (1 yr)	Gluckman et al (1982)[214]
ATG/CsA vs. CsA	Nonsevere	74/46* (6 mo)	0.93/0.91 (1 yr)	Marsh et al (1999)[215]
ATG/CsA vs. CsA/G-CSF	Severe	55/23* (4 mo)	0.82/0.71 (1 yr)	Raghavachar et al (1999)[216]
ARE THERE AGENTS THAT SYNERGIZE WITH ATG?				
ATG vs. ATG/oxymetholone	Severe	40/56* (4 mo)	0.71/0.73 (2 yr)	Camitta et al (1983)[217]
ATG vs. ATG/CsA	Severe	31/58* (3 mo)	0.55/0.80 (2 yr)	Frickhofen et al (1991)[218]
DO GROWTH FACTORS IMPROVE RESULTS OF IMMUNOSUPPRESSIVE PROTOCOLS?				
ATG vs. ATG/GM-CSF	Severe	64/18 (3 mo)	—	Gordon-Smith et al (1991)[219]
ATG/CsA vs. ATG/CsA/G-CSF	Severe	45/83* (4 mo)	0.82/0.81 (2 yr)	Gluckman et al (1999)[220]
ATG/CsA/danazol vs. ATG/CsA/danazol/G-CSF	Moderate-severe	77/55* (6 mo)	0.93/0.91 (4 yr)	Kojima et al (2000)[221]

ATG = antithymocyte globulin; ALG = antilymphocyte globulin; CsA = cyclosporine; G-CSF = granulocyte colony-stimulating factor; GM-CSF = granulocyte-macrophage colony-stimulating factor.

Modified from Frickhofen N, Rosenfeld SJ: Immunosuppressive treatment of aplastic anemia with antithymocyte globulin and cyclosporin. Semin Hematol 2000; 37:58.

declines, and the hemoglobin level increases slowly. The white cell count rises next. The last cell line to return is often the platelets, whose numbers may remain low for months or even years. The recovering red cells are not normal; in addition to macrocytosis, the HbF level is increased and fetal membrane antigens may remain.[226] Long-term survivors (except those with successful transplants) often have residual abnormalities, such as thrombocytopenia, red cell macrocytosis, and elevated HbF levels.[227] Clearly we do not understand either the mechanism of action of this poorly characterized drug, the ultimate course of patients with ATG-induced remissions, or the basis of their partial recovery.

CYCLOSPORINE

Cyclosporine (formerly cyclosporin A) is a fungal cyclic undecapeptide and an effective immunosuppressive agent.[228] Among its many effects, cyclosporine can inhibit T cells, preventing production of IL-2 and γ-interferon but not of CSFs.[145] Reports suggested that about one half of patients in whom ATG or ALG treatment had failed subsequently experienced remission with cyclosporine.[229, 230] Although one initial trial comparing treatment with ATG or cyclosporine found equivalent responses in the two groups, subsequent studies have shown significantly lower response rates and higher rates of disease progression with cyclosporine (Table 7–7).

Oral cyclosporine should be administered twice daily to maintain blood trough levels between 100 and 250 ng/mL as measured by radioimmunoassay. Hematologic responses can take weeks to months, and an initial trial period of 3 to 6 months is generally recommended.

Toxic effects from cyclosporine use are not insignificant and include hypertension, hypertensive encephalopa-thy, azotemia, hirsutism, gingival hypertrophy, coarsening of facial features, tremor, immunodeficiency, increase in serum creatinine levels, transient or irreversible nephrotoxicity, hepatotoxicity, and *P. carinii* pneumonia.[228] As with ATG, *in vitro* tests of the effect of cyclosporine on progenitor cells do not predict responses.[231]

COMBINATION IMMUNOSUPPRESSIVE THERAPY

Because androgens are effective in treating some patients with aplastic anemia (see later), the effect of combining androgen treatment with ATG was examined in several trials. Champlin et al[232] reported no difference in response rate or survival in patients with moderate to severe aplastic anemia. Studies by Kaltwasser et al[233] and the European Bone Marrow Transplant Severe Aplastic Anaemia Working Party (EBMT)[234] found significantly higher response rates after ALG plus androgens (73 and 56 percent) than those after ALG alone (31 and 40 percent).

The combination of ATG with cyclosporine is based on the clinical efficacy of each agent individually and on their separate and potentially complementary modes of action. Recent trials indicate that their combination induces hematologic responses more effectively than does either drug alone (Table 7–7). Importantly, intensive immunosuppressive therapy (IST) has greatly improved the results of treatment in two groups with aplastic anemia that is notoriously refractory to ALG or ATG alone: patients with very severe disease and children. In the National Institutes of Health (NIH) Clinical Center trial,[235] survival curves of those older and younger than 35 years of age were superimposable; also, there was no significant difference when the division was made at 20 years. A large ongoing study at the NIH, enrolling both children and adults, has found a response rate of 67 percent at 43 months and a 5-year actuarial survival rate of 70 percent (86 percent for responders and 16 percent for nonresponders).[236] The Gruppo Italiano Trapianto di Midollo Osseo (GITMO)/EBMT study of 100 patients with severe aplastic anemia including children (median age 16 years) treated with ALG, cyclosporine, prednisolone, and G-CSF found trilineage hematopoietic response in 77 percent after one or more courses of ALG. Three trials in children have confirmed the efficacy of the combination of ATG and cyclosporine in the pediatric population.[221, 237, 238]

ATG is typically given over a 4-day course followed by a 6- to 12-month course of cyclosporine. Cyclosporine should be tapered gradually with close monitoring of the blood cell counts before each decrease in dosage. A slow drop in the blood cell counts can often be treated with either an increase in cyclosporine dosage or a reinitiation of the full dose. Some patients require continuous cyclosporine treatment, and these patients should receive the lowest effective dose. A review of ongoing trials by the German multicenter group and the NIH revealed that 29 and 14 percent of patients who had an initial response, respectively, required continuous treatment.[236] The reoccurrence of frank pancytopenia generally requires a second course of ATG followed by a full dose of cyclosporine. Patients treated with immunosuppressive therapy often continue to have subnormal counts, although levels are functionally adequate.

RELAPSE

Relapse is common after immunosuppressive therapy. The EBMT reported an actuarial risk of relapse at 35 percent at 14 years. Relapses were observed as long as 10 years after treatment. Disease severity, age, sex, and etiology did not predict relapse. A short interval to response after initiation of therapy and a long interval from diagnosis to treatment correlated with an increased risk of relapse.[239] A review of ongoing unpublished trials from the German multicenter group and the NIH shows an actuarial risk of relapse of 40 percent at 8.7 years or 43 percent at 5 years, respectively.[236] The NIH study shows an apparent plateau at 64 percent between 7 and 10 years. Relapse has not significantly compromised survival in those patients whose aplasia continues to respond to additional courses of immunosuppression.

Tichelli et al[240] studied the efficacy of repeated treatment with ALG for patients with severe aplastic anemia whose anemia either failed to respond to an initial course of ALG or who experienced hematologic relapse. Transfusion independence was achieved in 63 percent and survival probability was 52± 8 percent at 10 years. No differences were noted between patients retreated for nonresponse versus those treated for relapse. No increases in acute toxicity were noted with additional courses of ALG, although serum sickness tended to occur earlier after repeat ALG administration.

COMPLICATIONS OF IMMUNOSUPPRESSIVE THERAPY

Patients treated for aplastic anemia with IST have an increased risk of developing clonal hematopoietic disorders.[241, 242] In an analysis of 860 patients treated with immunosuppression, 42 malignant conditions were reported including 19 cases of PNH, 11 cases of myelodysplasia, 15 cases of acute leukemia, 7 solid tumors, and 1 case of non-Hodgkin's lymphoma.[243] Of 748 patients treated with transplantation, 9 malignancies were reported: 2 patients with acute leukemias and 7 patients with solid tumors. The cumulative incidence of development of a malignant tumor at 10 years was 18.8 percent after immunosuppression and 3.1 percent after transplantation. A recent series of 122 NIH patients treated with immunosuppression showed a 33 percent actuarial risk of developing a clonal hematopoietic disorder at 10 years.[3] These data suggest that a clonal transformation of stem cells may underlie aplastic anemia. Prolonged survival as a result of ATG/ALG/cyclosporine treatment may permit the expected clonal evolution.

An intriguing report from Ball et al[244] noted significant telomere shortening in the leukocytes of patients with aplastic anemia. Of five patients reported to have mean telomere lengths less than 5 kb, three had acquired cytogenetic abnormalities, suggesting that compromise in the telomere's probable role in stabilizing chromosome ends may contribute to the increased incidence of myelodysplasias and acute leukemias. Brummendorf et al[245] reported relatively normal telomere lengths in patients whose disease responded to immunosuppression, whereas untreated patients or patients with unresponsive disease showed significant telomere shortening.[245] Whether telomere shortening represents a primary versus a secondary event in the genesis of aplastic anemia remains to be ascertained.

Transplantation versus Immunosuppression

The decision to treat with immunosuppression rather than HLA-identical sibling stem cell transplant for the 25 percent of patients for whom a suitable donor is available is based on a consideration of risks and benefits that vary depending on patient age and neutrophil count. Toxicities associated with the conditioning regimens, GVHD, and graft rejection are the major problems with stem cell transplantation, but this treatment offers the potential for long-term cure. Immunosuppression is associated with lower acute toxicities but may cause chronic end-organ damage and often yields incomplete hematologic recovery and late complications such as relapse and clonal hematologic disorders. Studies comparing BMT and immunosuppression in children have generally significantly favored stem cell transplant[246–253] (Table 7–8). Kojima et al[254] recently reported a prospective study of 100 children younger than 17 years of age with aplastic anemia between 1984 and 1998. Of these, 37 patients received an allogeneic bone marrow transplant and 63 patients received immunosuppression; 11 patients initially treated with IST received subsequent salvage treatment with an unrelated donor bone marrow transplant. The projected 10-year survival was 55 ± 8 percent with IST and 97 ± 3 percent with BMT. Failure-free survival at 10 years was 40 ± 8 percent for the IST group and 97 ± 3 percent for the BMT group. Seven patients in the IST group developed myelodysplasia with monosomy 7 and the estimated 10-year cumulative incidence of myelodysplasia was 20 ± 7 percent.

A recent report from the EBMT analyzed 1765 patients with aplastic anemia who received initial treatment with

TABLE 7–8. Studies Comparing Bone Marrow Transplantation to Immunosuppressive Therapy

Study	Population Age (yr)	BMT (No. of Patients)	Survival % (2–15 yr)	IST (No. of Patients)	Survival % (2–15 yr)	P
Speck et al (1981)[246]	All ages	18	44	32	69	NS
Bayever et al (1984)[247]	1–25	35	72	22	45	NS
Bacigalupo et al (1988)[6]	1–50	218	63	291	61	NS
Halperin et al (1989)[248]	Children	14	79	12	25	?
Locasciulli et al (1990)[249]	Children	171	63	133	48	0.002
Speck et al (1990)[250]	All ages	34	50	111	71	NS
Paquette et al (1995)[251]	Adults	55	72	155	45	NS
Lawlor et al (1997)[252]	Children	9	75	18	92	NS
Doney et al (1997)[253]	All ages	168	69	227	38	<0.001
Fuhrer et al (1998)[237]	Children	26	84	86	87	NS
Kojima, 2000[254]	Children	37	97	63	55	<0.0001

BMT = bone marrow transplantation; IST = immunosuppressive therapy.

Modified from Bacigalupo A, Brand R, Oneto R, et al: Treatment of acquired severe aplastic anemia: Bone marrow transplantation compared with immunosuppressive therapy—The European Group for Blood and Marrow Transplantation Experience. Semin Hematol 2000; 37:75.

either an HLA-identical sibling bone marrow transplant or IST.[198] Analysis was performed on an "intent-to-treat" basis. Patients were aged 1 to 50 years and treated between 1974 and 1996; 583 patients received HLA-identical sibling BMT and 1182 patients received IST. A comparison of immunosuppression versus bone marrow transplant in patients stratified by age and neutrophil count showed superior failure-free survival with BMT for children regardless of their neutrophil count. The advantage of BMT increased with increasing follow-up time, most likely because of the ongoing risks of late relapse and development of myelodysplasia and leukemia in the IST group. Children have a lower mortality with stem cell transplant and a longer post-treatment life expectancy, placing them at higher risk for IST-related late complications than adults. Thus, the current recommendation is to treat young patients (≤10 years) with HLA-identical sibling stem cell transplant when a suitable donor is available. Patients with severe disease who are younger than 40 years of age also do better with BMT. Patients older than 40 to 50 years of age generally do better with IST.

Note that many patients in these studies of long-term outcomes were treated before the development of current immunosuppressive regimens containing both ATG and cyclosporine. Any differential long-term effects of these more intensive immunosuppressive regimens remain to be ascertained.

Hematopoietic Growth Factors

Although patients with aplastic anemia do not have a deficiency of most hematopoietic growth factors (see earlier), it was hypothesized that pharmacologic levels might stimulate hematopoiesis of one or more cell lines.[181] Trials of GM-CSF, G-CSF, IL-3, IL-1, IL-6, and stem cell factor in patients with aplastic anemia have been published. The total number of patients treated in these protocols is not large, and because of their experimental nature, only a minority of participants have been children. These studies do not support the use of growth factors as primary treatment for aplastic anemia. To date, no consistent benefit in terms of response rate or survival after the adjunctive use of growth factors in immunosuppressive regimens has been

observed, including one recent prospective pediatric study.[221] Responses to a single growth factor or to a combination of growth factors have been reported in a few patients with refractory disease.

Toxicities of recombinant human growth factors vary. G-CSF is associated with flulike symptoms, bone pain, and splenomegaly. GM-CSF is generally well tolerated except at very high doses. Symptoms of "cytokine flu"—fever, rash, hives, headache, and myalgia—are common but do respond to acetaminophen or resolve with the passage of time. Bone pain may be a symptom of increased marrow activity, although this is more commonly seen with G-CSF. At higher doses, the severity of symptoms increases, and there may be evidence of visceral engorgement and fluid retention. The toxic effects of IL-3 are similar, usually including fever, chills, and headache. Hypotension is the dose-limiting toxicity of IL-1. Anaphylactic responses have been associated with the use of stem cell factor, also known as mast cell factor.

The potential risk of promoting or stimulating the development of abnormal hematopoietic clones, leading to a further increased risk of myelodysplasia or leukemia after prolonged treatment with growth factors remains a concern in patients with aplastic anemia. Although myelodysplasia and leukemia developing in such patients have been reported,[255] it is not clear whether these represent an effect of growth factor treatment or the natural history of their disease.

Androgens

Androgens no longer have a primary role in the management of aplastic anemia, unless the first-line therapies discussed earlier are unavailable or unsuccessful. As described earlier, androgens have been used as adjuncts to immunosuppression.

The mechanism of action of androgens has been reviewed extensively by Gardner and Besa.[256] Androgens increase erythropoietin production[257] and stimulate erythroid stem cells.[258] Hemoglobin levels increase in normal males at puberty and in patients treated with androgens for arthritis and breast cancer or in old age. Shahidi and Diamond[259] were the first to report success with testosterone, and large confirmatory series were published from

France[260] and Mexico.[261] However, later critical evaluations revealed no evidence to support the use of androgens. Despite the use of androgens, greater than 75 percent mortality has been reported in children[187] and adults.[262] Androgen-treated patients often did not do as well as those who were not treated with these hormones.[263, 264] The older publications often failed to distinguish patients with moderate disease from those with severe disease. Camitta and co-workers[265, 266] performed a prospective, multicenter analysis beginning in 1974 and concluded that androgens (whether oral or intramuscular) were no more effective than supportive care alone for severe aplastic anemia.

Improvement is usually greatest in the hematocrit, although increases in the granulocyte and platelet counts may also be seen. Response may take weeks to months, and trials of at least 3 months are recommended before declaring a patient's disease as unresponsive. The major side effect of androgens is liver toxicity. Cholestatic jaundice and hepatomegaly are usually reversible. Peliosis hepatis (blood lakes) has been reported.[267] Hepatic tumors are a serious risk, although the pathologic picture is usually that of a benign adenoma; such tumors may resolve when use of the androgen is discontinued. Other side effects include masculinization with hirsutism, baldness, deepening of the voice, and enlargement of the genitalia. Acne, flushing of the skin, nausea, and sodium and fluid retention also occur. The appetite is stimulated, and there is weight gain with increased muscular development. There may be an increase in the rate of skeletal maturation, with eventual premature fusion and ultimate short stature. However, treatment for up to 1 year may not be long enough for this problem to develop.[268] All patients who receive androgens should be monitored with frequent liver function testing, annual liver ultrasound examinations, and annual bone age determinations.

Corticosteroids

Modest doses of methylprednisolone are often given during ATG or ALG treatment to lessen the side effects of serum sickness. As a single agent, corticosteroids at very high doses can lead to responses in some patients.[269, 270] Treatment with high-dose steroids is associated with substantial toxicities, including hypertension, hyperglycemia, fluid retention, potassium wasting, psychosis, aseptic necroses of femoral and humeral heads, and increased susceptibility to fungal infections. Given the higher response rate and lower toxicity profile of ATG, high-dose steroids are not recommended as first-line therapy for aplastic anemia.

Splenectomy

Splenectomies were performed until recently, perhaps for want of something better to offer to patients. A review in 1957 indicated improvements in 20 of 35 patients.[271] More recently, the operation has been performed to facilitate supportive care.[272] Unless clear indications of hypersplenism significantly impeding platelet and red cell transfusion support are seen, the operation does not seem warranted.

Other Therapies

The aim of new therapeutic regimens is to improve rates of hematologic response and minimize acute and long-term complications of therapy.[147] The present status of new agents is summarized below.

CYCLOPHOSPHAMIDE

Administration of high doses of cyclophosphamide is an effective immunosuppressive therapy and is not myeloablative in normal hosts. Historically, a few patients who received high-dose cyclophosphamide as preparation for marrow transplant rejected their grafts and had autologous recovery. An early study of treatment with this drug without transplant indicated a complete response in 7 of 10 patients treated with 45 mg/kg/day for 4 days.[273] Based on these results, a phase III prospective randomized trial compared high-dose cyclophosphamide plus cyclosporin with ATG plus cyclosporine as first-line therapy.[274] The trial was terminated prematurely due to invasive fungal infections and three early deaths in the cyclophosphamide group (none in the ATG group). Responses at 6 months follow-up were seen in 6 of 13 (46 percent) patients treated with cyclophosphamide versus 9 of 12 (75 percent) patients treated with ATG.

RECOMBINANT HUMANIZED ANTI-INTERLEUKIN-2 RECEPTOR ANTIBODY

The high-affinity IL-2 receptor is present only on activated T cells and is required for T-cell activation and proliferation.[275] An anti-IL-2 receptor monoclonal antibody, daclizumab, has been approved for use in the prevention of renal transplant rejection. The use of this agent for the treatment of aplastic anemia is currently under investigation in phase II trials. It is usually administered together with cyclosporine and prednisone.

MYCOPHENOLATE MOFETIL

Mycophenolate mofetil (CellCept) is the prodrug of mycophenolic acid. It inhibits B- and T-cell proliferation through noncompetitive reversible inhibition of inosine monophosphate dehydrogenase, which is involved in the salvage pathway for guanine nucleotide synthesis.[276] It has antifungal, antibacterial, antiviral, and immunosuppressive activity. Mycophenolate mofetil has been approved for prevention of renal transplant rejection. Although generally well tolerated, side effects of mycophenolate mofetil include leukopenia and thrombocytopenia. Studies on use of mycophenolate mofetil in aplastic anemia are currently ongoing.

FK506 AND RAPAMYCIN

FK506 (tacrolimus, Prograf) has been effective in preventing organ transplant rejection, often in combination with other immunosuppressive agents. FK506 and cyclosporine are calcineurin inhibitors that decrease IL-2 production.[277] FK506 and cyclosporine also share similar toxicity profiles. Given the similarities in action, it is not clear whether FK506 offers any advantage over cyclosporine, although their toxicity profiles are subtly different.

Rapamycin (Rapamune, sirolimus) inactivates the serine/threonine protein kinase p70 and is a potent inhibitor of IL-2-dependent T-cell proliferation.[278, 279] Although rapamycin is an effective drug for the prevention of solid organ transplant rejection, its myelosuppressive side effects may render it potentially less useful for the treatment of aplastic anemia.

REFERENCES

1. Alter BP, Potter NU, Li FP: Classification and aetiology of the aplastic anaemias. Clin Hematol 1978; 7:431–465.
2. Young N: Introduction: Acquired aplastic anemia. Semin Hematol 2000; 37;2.
3. Young N: Acquired aplastic anemia. In: Young NS (ed): Bone Marrow Failure Syndromes. Philadelphia: WB Saunders, 2000, pp 1–46.
4. Alter BP, Young N: The Bone Marrow Failure Syndromes. In: Nathan DG, Oski SH (eds): Nathan and Oski's Hematology of Infancy and Childhood, 5th ed. Philadelphia, WB Saunders, 1998, pp 237–335.
5. Camitta BM, Thomas ED, Nathan DG, et al: Severe aplastic anemia: A prospective study of the effect of early marrow transplantation on acute mortality. Blood 1976; 48:63–70.
6. Bacigalupo A, Hows J, Gluckman E, et al: Bone marrow transplantation (BMT) versus immunosuppression for the treatment of severe aplastic anaemia (SAA): A report of the EBMT SAA working party. Br J Haematol 1988; 70:177–182.
7. Ehrlich P: Uber einen Fall von Anamie mit Bemerkungen uber regenerative Veranderungen des Knochenmarks. Charité-Ann 1888; 13:300.
8. Vaquez M, Aubertin C: L'anemie pernicieuse d'apres les conceptions actuelles. Bull Mem Soc Med Hop Paris 1904; 21:288.
9. Kaufman D, Kelly J, et al. The Drug Etiology of Agranulocytosis and Aplastic Anemia. New York, Oxford University Press, 1991, p 259.
10. Shimizu H, Kuroishi T, Tominaga S, et al: Production amount of chloramphenicol and mortality rate of aplastic anemia in Japan. Nippon Ketsueki Gakkai Zasshi [Acta Haematol Jpn] 1979; 42:689–696.
11. Mizuno S, Aoki K, Ohno Y, et al: Time series analysis of age-sex specific death rates from aplastic anemia and the trend in production amount of chloramphenicol. Nagoya J Med Sci 1982; 44:103–115.
12. Szklo M, Sensenbrenner L, Markowitz J, et al: Incidence of aplastic anemia in metropolitan Baltimore: A population-based study. Blood 1985; 66:115–119.
13. Bottiger LE, Furhoff AK, Holmberg L: Drug-induced blood dyscrasias. A ten-year material from the Swedish Adverse Drug Reaction Committee. Acta Med Scand 1979; 205:457–461.
14. Issaragrisil S, Kaufman DW, Anderson T, et al: Low drug attributability of aplastic anemia in Thailand. The Aplastic Anemia Study Group. Blood 1997; 89:4034–4039.
15. Linet MS, Markowitz JA, Sensenbrenner LL, et al: A case-control study of aplastic anemia. Leuk Res 1989; 13:3–11.
16. Kaufman D, Issaragrisil S, Anderson T, et al: Use of household pesticides and the risk of aplastic anaemia in Thailand. J. Epidemiol 1997; 26:643–650.
17. Nimer SD, Ireland P, Meshkinpour A, et al: An increased HLA DR2 frequency is seen in aplastic anemia patients. Blood 1994; 84:923–927.
18. Nakao S, Takamatsu H, Chuhjo T, et al: Identification of a specific HLA class II haplotype strongly associated with susceptibility to cyclosporine-dependent aplastic anemia. Blood 1994; 84:4257–4261.
19. Powars D: Aplastic anemia secondary to glue sniffing. N Engl J Med 1965; 273:700.
20. Scott J, Cartwright G, Wintrobe M: Acquired aplastic anemia: An analysis of thirty-nine cases and review of the pertinent literature. Medicine (Baltimore) 1958; 36:119.
21. Smadel J, Jackson E: Chloromycetin, an antibiotic with chemotherapeutic activity in experimental and viral infections. Science 1944; 106:41B.
22. Smadel J: Chloramphenicol (chloromycetin) in the treatment of infectious diseases. Am J Med 1949; 7:671.
23. Yunis A: Mechanisms underlying marrow toxicity from chloramphenicol and thiamphenicol. In: Silber R, LoBue J, Gordon A (eds): The Year in Hematology. New York: Plenum, 1978, p 143.
24. Ratzan RJ, Moore MA, Yunis AA: Effect of chloramphenicol and thiamphenicol on the in vitro colony-forming cell. Blood 1974; 43:363–369.
25. Bostrom B, Smith K, Ramsay NK: Stimulation of human committed bone marrow stem cells (CFU-GM) by chloramphenicol. Exp Hematol 1986; 14:156–161.
26. Sawada H, Tezuka H, Kamamoto T, et al: Effects of chloramphenicol on hemopoietic cells and their microenvironment in vitro. Acta Haematol 1985; 48:1323.
27. Hara H, Kohsaki M, Noguchi K, et al: Effect of chloramphenicol on colony formation from erythrocytic precursors. Am J Hematol 1978; 5:123–130.
28. Firkin FC, Sumner MA, Bradley TR: The influence of chloramphenicol on the bone marrow haemopoietic stem cell compartment. Exp Hematol 1974; 2:264–268.
29. Nara N, Bessho M, Hirashima K, et al: Effects of chloramphenicol on hematopoietic inductive microenvironment. Exp Hematol 1982; 10:20–25.
30. Wijnja L, Snijder JA, Nieweg HO: Acetylsalicylic acid as a cause of pancytopenia from bone-marrow damage. Lancet 1966; 2:768–770.
31. Menkes E, Kutas GJ: Fatal aplastic anemia following indomethacin ingestion. Can Med Assoc J 1977; 117:118.
32. Shearer CA: Indomethacin and aplastic anemia. Can Med Assoc J 1978; 118:18.
33. Canada AT Jr, Burka ER: Aplastic anemia after indomethacin. N Engl J Med 1968; 278:743–744.
34. Fredrick GR: Indomethacin and aplastic anemia [letter]. N Engl J Med 1968; 279:1290.
35. Gryfe CI: Letter: Agranulocytosis and aplastic anemia possibly due to ibuprofen. Can Med Assoc J 1976; 114:877.
36. McCarthy D, Chalmers T: Hematological complications of phenylbutazone therapy: Review of the literature and report of two cases. Can Med Assoc J 1964; 90:1061.
37. Gaisfort W: Fatality after oxyphenbutazone in Still's disease. BMJ 1962; 2:1517.
38. Chang HK, Morrison SL: Bone-marrow suppression associated with cimetidine. Ann Intern Med 1979; 91:580.
39. Tonkonow B, Hoffman R: Aplastic anemia and cimetidine. Arch Intern Med 1980; 140:1123–1124.
40. Kutscher AH, Lane SL, Segall R: The clinical toxicity of antibiotics and sulfonamides: A comparative review of the literature based on 104,672 cases treated systemically. J Allergy 1954; 25:135.
41. Holsinger DR, Hanlon DG, Welch JS: Fatal aplastic anemia following sulfamethoxypyridazine therapy. Mayo Clin Proc 1958; 33:679.
42. Tulloch AL: Pancytopenia in an infant associated with sulfamethoxazole-trimethoprim therapy. J Pediatr 1976; 88:499–500.
43. Levine B, Rosenberg DV: Aplastic anemia during the treatment of hyperthyroidism with tapazole. Ann Intern Med 1954; 41:844.
44. Edell SL, Bartuska DG: Aplastic anemia secondary to methimazole—Case report and review of hematologic side effects. J Am Med Womens Assoc 1975; 30:412–413.
45. Aksoy M, Erdem S: Aplastic anaemia after propylthiouracil. Lancet 1968; 1:1379.
46. Jost F: Blood dyscrasias associated with tolbutamide therapy. BMJ 1959; 169:1468.
47. Chapman I CW: Pancytopenia associated with tolbutamide therapy. JAMA 1963; 186:595.
48. White LLR: Fatal marrow aplasia during chlorpropamide therapy [letter]. Br Med J 1962; 1:691.
49. Recker RR, Hynes HE: Pure red blood cell aplasia associated with chlorpropamide therapy. Patient summary and review of the literature. Arch Intern Med 1969; 123:445–447.
50. Sparbert M: Diagnostically confusing complications of diphenylhydantoin therapy. Ann Intern Med 1963; 59:914.
51. Witkind EWM: Aplasia of the bone marrow during mesantoin therapy. Report of a fatal case. JAMA 1951; 147:757.
52. Isaacson S, Gold JA, Ginsberg V: Fatal aplastic anemia after therapy with nuvarone (3-methyl-5-phenylhydantoin). JAMA 1956; 160:1311.
53. Donaldson GW, Graham JG: Aplastic anaemia following the administration of tegretol. Br J Clin Pract 1965; 19:699–702.

54. Dyer NH, Hughes DT, Jenkins GC: Aplastic anaemia after carbamazepine. Br Med J 1966; 5479:108.

55. Pisciotta AV: Hematologic toxicity of carbamazepine. Adv Neurol 1975; 11:355–368.

56. Gayford JJ, Redpath TH: The side-effects of carbamazepine. Proc R Soc Med 1969; 62:615–616.

57. Pellock JM: Carbamazepine side effects in children and adults. Epilepsia 1987; 28:S64–70.

58. Wisch N, Fischbein FI, Siegel R, et al: Aplastic anemia resulting from the use of carbonic anhydrase inhibitors. Am J Ophthalmol 1973; 75:130–132.

59. Underwood LC: Fatal bone marrow depression after the treatment with acetazolamide (Diamox). JAMA 1956; 161:1477.

60. Lubeck MJ: Aplastic anemia following acetazolamide therapy. Am J Ophthalmol 1970; 69:684–685.

61. Gangitano JL, Foster SH, Contro RM: Nonfatal methazolamide-induced aplastic anemia. Am J Ophthalmol 1978; 86:138–139.

62. Werblin TP, Pollack IP, Liss RA: Aplastic anemia and agranulocytosis in patients using methazolamide for glaucoma. JAMA 1979; 241:2817–2818.

63. Smith M: Overview of benzene-induced aplastic anaemia. Eur J Haematol 1996; 57(Suppl):107–110.

64. Ross D: Metabolic basis of benzene toxicity. Eur J Haematol 1996; 57(Suppl):111–118.

65. Young N: Drugs and chemicals as agents of bone marrow failure. In: Testa N, Gale RC (eds): Hematopoiesis: Long-Term effects of Chemotherapy and Radiation, Vol. 131. New York, Marcel Dekker, 1988.

66. Snyder R, Kocsis JJ: Current concepts of chronic benzene toxicity. CRC Crit Rev Toxicol 1975; 3:265–288.

67. Fishbein L: An overview of environmental and toxicological aspects of aromatic hydrocarbons. I. Benzene. Sci Total Environ 1984; 40:189–218.

68. Brief RS, Lynch J, Bernath T, et al: Benzene in the workplace. Am Ind Hyg Assoc J 1980; 41:616–623.

69. Sato A, Nakajima T, Fujiwara Y, et al: Pharmacokinetics of benzene and toluene. Int Arch Arbeitsmed 1974; 33:169–182.

70. Kalf G, Post G, Snyder R: Solvent toxicology: Recent advances in the toxicology of benzene, the glycol ethers, and carbon tetrachloride. Annu Rev Pharmacol Toxicol 1987; 27:399.

71. Sawahata T, Rickert D, Greenlee W: Metabolism of benzene and its metabolites in bone marrow. In: Irons RD (ed): Toxicology of the Blood and Bone Marrow, Vol. 141. New York, Raven Press, 1985.

72. Greenlee WF, Sun JD, Bus JS: A proposed mechanism of benzene toxicity: Formation of reactive intermediates from polyphenol metabolites. Toxicol Appl Pharmacol 1981; 59:187–195.

73. Lee E, Garner C, Johnson J: A proposed role played by benzene itself in the induction of acute cytopenia: Inhibition of DNA synthesis. Res Commun Chem Pathol Pharmacol 1988; 60:27.

74. Kissling M, Speck B: Further studies on experimental benzene induced aplastic anemia. Blut 1972; 25:97–103.

75. Pellack-Walker P, Blumer JL: DNA damage in L5178YS cells following exposure to benzene metabolites. Mol Pharmacol 1986; 30:42–47.

76. Brahams D: Lindane exposure and aplastic anaemia. Lancet 1994; 343:1092.

77. Parent-Massin D, Thouvenot D, Rio B, et al: Lindane haematotoxicity confirmed by in vitro tests on human and rat progenitors. Hum Exp Toxicol 1994; 13:103–106.

78. Knospe WH, Crosby WH: Aplastic anaemia: A disorder of the bone-marrow sinusoidal microcirculation rather than stem-cell failure? Lancet 1971; 1:20–22.

79. Kurtzman G, Young N: Viruses and bone marrow failure. Baillieres Clin Haematol 1989; 2:51–67.

80. Pikis A, Kavaliotis J, Manios S: Incidence of aplastic anemia in viral hepatitis in children. Scand J Infect Dis 1988; 20:109–110.

81. Perrillo RP, Pohl DA, Roodman ST, et al: Acute non-A, non-B hepatitis with serum sickness-like syndrome and aplastic anemia. JAMA 1981; 245:494–496.

82. Bottiger LE, Westerholm B: Aplastic anaemia. 3. Aplastic anaemia and infectious hepatitis. Acta Med Scand 1972; 192:323–326.

83. Young NS, Issaragrasil S, Chieh CW, et al: Aplastic anaemia in the Orient. Br J Haematol 1986; 62:1–6.

84. Liang DC, Lin KH, Lin DT, et al: Post-hepatitic aplastic anaemia in children in Taiwan, a hepatitis prevalent area. Br J Haematol 1990; 74:487–491.

85. Tzakis AG, Arditi M, Whitington PF, et al: Aplastic anemia complicating orthotopic liver transplantation for non-A, non-B hepatitis. N Engl J Med 1988; 319:393–396.

86. Smith D, Gribble TJ, Yeager AS, et al: Spontaneous resolution of severe aplastic anemia associated with viral hepatitis A in a 6-year-old child. Am J Hematol 1978; 5:247–252.

87. Kindmark CO, Sjolin J, Nordlinder H, et al: Aplastic anaemia in a case of hepatitis B with a high titer of hepatitis B antigen. Acta Med Scand 1984; 215:89–92.

88. Hibbs JR, Frickhofen N, Rosenfeld SJ, et al: Aplastic anemia and viral hepatitis. Non-A, Non-B, Non-C? JAMA 1992; 267:2051–2054.

89. Brown KE, Tisdale J, Barrett AJ, et al: Hepatitis-associated aplastic anemia. N Engl J Med 1997; 336:1059–1064.

90. Hagler L, Pastore RA, Bergin JJ, et al: Aplastic anemia following viral hepatitis: Report of two fatal cases and literature review. Medicine (Baltimore) 1975; 54:139–164.

91. Nakao S, Lai CJ, Young NS: Dengue virus, a flavivirus, propagates in human bone marrow progenitors and hematopoietic cell lines. Blood 1989; 74:1235–1240.

92. Tosato G, Taga K, et al: Epstein-Barr virus as an agent for haematological disease. Baillieres Clin Haematol 1995; 8:165–199.

93. Baranski B, Armstrong G, Truman JT, et al: Epstein-Barr virus in the bone marrow of patients with aplastic anemia. Ann Intern Med 1988; 109:695–704.

94. Sing GK, Ruscetti FW: The role of human cytomegalovirus in haematological diseases. Baillieres Clin Haematol 1995; 8:149–163.

95. Simmons P, Kaushansky K, Torok-Storb B: Mechanisms of cytomegalovirus-mediated myelosuppression: Perturbation of stromal cell function versus direct infection of myeloid cells. Proc Natl Acad Sci USA 1990; 87:1386–1390.

96. Maciejewski JP, Bruening EE, Donahue RE, et al: Infection of hematopoietic progenitor cells by human cytomegalovirus. Blood 1992; 80:170–178.

97. Carrigan DR, Knox KK: Human herpesvirus 6 (HHV-6) isolation from bone marrow: HHV-6-associated bone marrow suppression in bone marrow transplant patients. Blood 1994; 84:3307–3310.

98. Lusso P, Gallo RC: Human herpesvirus 6. Baillieres Clin Haematol 1995; 8:201–223.

99. Knox KK, Carrigan DR: In vitro suppression of bone marrow progenitor cell differentiation by human herpesvirus 6 infection. J Infect Dis 1992; 165:925–929.

100. Davis BR, Zauli G: Effect of human immunodeficiency virus infection on haematopoiesis. Baillieres Clin Haematol 1995; 8:113–130.

101. Stella CC, Ganser A, Hoelzer D: Defective in vitro growth of the hemopoietic progenitor cells in the acquired immunodeficiency syndrome. J Clin Invest 1987; 80:286–293.

102. Bagnara GP, Zauli G, Giovannini M, et al: Early loss of circulating hemopoietic progenitors in HIV-1-infected subjects. Exp Hematol 1990; 18:426–430.

103. De Luca A, Teofili L, Antinori A, et al: Haemopoietic CD34+ progenitor cells are not infected by HIV-1 in vivo but show impaired clonogenesis. Br J Haematol 1993; 85:20–24.

104. Zauli G, Re MC, Davis B, et al: Impaired in vitro growth of purified (CD34+) hematopoietic progenitors in human immunodeficiency virus-1 seropositive thrombocytopenic individuals. Blood 1992; 79:2680–2687.

105. von Laer D, Hufert FT, Fenner TE, et al: CD34+ hematopoietic progenitor cells are not a major reservoir of the human immunodeficiency virus. Blood 1990; 76:1281–1286.

106. Molina JM, Scadden DT, Sakaguchi M, et al: Lack of evidence for infection of or effect on growth of hematopoietic progenitor cells after in vivo or in vitro exposure to human immunodeficiency virus. Blood 1990; 76:2476–2482.

107. Zucker-Franklin D, Seremetis S, Zheng ZY: Internalization of human immunodeficiency virus type I and other retroviruses by megakaryocytes and platelets. Blood 1990; 75:1920–1923.

108. Cen D, Zauli G, Szarnicki R, et al: Effect of different human immunodeficiency virus type-1 (HIV-1) isolates on long-term bone marrow haemopoiesis. Br J Haematol 1993; 85:596–602.

109. Schwartz GN, Kessler SW, Rothwell SW, et al: Inhibitory effects of HIV-1-infected stromal cell layers on the production of myeloid progenitor cells in human long-term bone marrow cultures. Exp Hematol 1994; 22:1288–1296.

110. Maciejewski JP, Weichold FF, Young NS: HIV-1 suppression of hematopoiesis in vitro mediated by envelope glycoprotein and TNF-α. J Immunol 1994; 153:4303–4310.

111. Young N, Alter B: Aplastic Anemia: Acquired and Inherited. Philadelphia, WB Saunders, 1994.

112. Alter B, Frissora C, et al: Fanconi's anemia and pregnancy. Br J Haematol 1991; 77:410.

113. Dukes P, Goldwasser E: Inhibition of erythropoiesis by estrogens. Endocrinology 1961; 69:21.

114. Yeh ET, Rosse WF: Paroxysmal nocturnal hemoglobinuria and the glycosylphosphatidylinositol anchor. J Clin Invest 1994; 93:2305–2310.

115. Schrezenmeier H, Hertenstein B, Wagner B, et al: A pathogenetic link between aplastic anemia and paroxysmal nocturnal hemoglobinuria is suggested by a high frequency of aplastic anemia patients with a deficiency of phosphatidylinositol glycan anchored proteins. Exp Hematol 1995; 23:81–87.

116. Iwamoto N, Kawaguchi T, Horikawa K, et al: Preferential hematopoiesis by paroxysmal nocturnal hemoglobinuria clone engrafted in SCID mice. Blood 1996; 87:4944–4948.

117. Maciejewski J, Sloand E, Sato T, et al: Impaired hematopoiesis in paroxysmal nocturnal hemoglobinuria/aplastic anemia is not associated with a selective proliferative defect in the glycosylphosphatidylinostol-anchored protein-deficient clone. Blood 1997; 89:1173–1181.

118. Chen R, Nagarajan S, Prince GM, et al: Impaired growth and elevated fas receptor expression in *PIGA*(+) stem cells in primary paroxysmal nocturnal hemoglobinuria. J Clin Invest 2000; 106:689–696.

119. Murakami Y, Kinoshita T, Maeda Y, et al: Different roles of glycosylphosphatidylinositol in various hematopoietic cells as revealed by a mouse model of paroxysmal nocturnal hemoglobinuria. Blood 1999; 94:2963–2970.

120. Tremml G, Dominguez C, Rosti V, et al: Increased sensitivity to complement and a decreased red blood cell life span in mice mosaic for a nonfunctional *Piga* gene. Blood 1999; 94:2945–2954.

121. Karadimitris A, Notaro R, Koehne G, et al: PNH cells are as sensitive to T-cell-mediated lysis as their normal counterparts: Implications for the pathogenesis of paroxysmal nocturnal haemoglobinuria. Br J Haematol 2000; 111:1158–1163.

122. Karadimitris A, Manavalan JS, Thaler HT, et al: Abnormal T-cell repertoire is consistent with immune process underlying the pathogenesis of paroxysmal nocturnal hemoglobinuria. Blood 2000; 96:2613–2620.

123. Hoffman R, Dainiak N, Sibrack L, et al. Antibody-mediated aplastic anemia and diffuse fasciitis. N Engl J Med 1979; 300:718–721.

124. Talerman A, Amigo A: Thymoma associated with aregenerative and aplastic anemia in a five-year-old child. Cancer 1968; 21:1212–1218.

125. Ferrara JL, Deeg HJ: Graft-versus-host disease. N Engl J Med 1991; 324:667–674.

126. Schrezenmeier H, Gerok M, Heimpel H: Assessment of frequency of hematopoietic stem cells in aplastic anemia by limiting dilution type long term marrow culture. Exp Hematol 1992; 20:806.

127. Maciejewski JP, Selleri C, Sato T, et al: A severe and consistent deficit in marrow and circulating primitive hematopoietic cells (long-term culture-initiating cells) in acquired aplastic anemia. Blood 1996; 88:1983–1991.

128. Sutherland HJ, Eaves CJ, Eaves AC, et al: Characterization and partial purification of human marrow cells capable of initiating long-term hematopoiesis in vitro. Blood 1989; 74:1563–1570.

129. Bhatia M, Wang JC, Kapp U, et al: Purification of primitive human hematopoietic cells capable of repopulating immune-deficient mice. Proc Natl Acad Sci USA 1997; 94:5320–5325.

130. Berenson RJ, Andrews RG, Bensinger WI, et al: Antigen CD34+ marrow cells engraft lethally irradiated baboons. J Clin Invest 1988; 81:951–955.

131. Civin CI, Trischmann T, Kadan NS, et al: Highly purified CD34-positive cells reconstitute hematopoiesis. J. Clin Oncol 1996; 14:2224–2233.

132. Maciejewski JP, Anderson S, Katevas P, et al: Phenotypic and functional analysis of bone marrow progenitor cell compartment in bone marrow failure. Br J Haematol 1994; 87:227–234.

133. Scopes J, Bagnara M, Gordon-Smith EC, et al: Haemopoietic progenitor cells are reduced in aplastic anaemia. Br J Haematol 1994; 86:427–430.

134. Lu DP: Syngeneic bone marrow transplantation for treatment of aplastic anaemia: Report of a case and review of the literature. Exp Hematol 1981; 9:257–263.

135. Champlin RE, Feig SA, Sparkes RS, et al: Bone marrow transplantation from identical twins in the treatment of aplastic anaemia: Implication for the pathogenesis of the disease. Br J Haematol 1984; 56:455–463.

136. Storb R: Bone marrow transplantation for aplastic anemia. Cell Transplant 1993; 2:365–379.

137. Hinterberger W, Rowlings PA, Hinterberger-Fischer M, et al: Results of transplanting bone marrow from genetically identical twins into patients with aplastic anemia. Ann Intern Med 1997; 126:116–122.

138. Young NS: The problem of clonality in aplastic anemia: Dr Dameshek's riddle, restated. Blood 1992; 79:1385–1392.

139. Young NS: Hematopoietic cell destruction by immune mechanisms in acquired aplastic anemia. Semin Hematol 2000; 37:3–14.

140. Hinterberger W, Raghavachar A, et al: Bone marrow transplantation from genotypically identical twins with aplastic anemia. In: Raghavachar A, Schrenzenmeier H, Frickhofen N (eds): Aplastic Anemia: Current Perspectives on the Pathogenesis and Treatment. Vienna, Blackwell-MZV, 1993, p 102.

141. Nakao S, Yamaguchi M, Saito M, et al: HLA-DR2 predicts a favorable response to cyclosporine therapy in patients with bone marrow failure. Am J Hematol 1992; 40:239–240.

142. Mathe G, Amiel JL, Schwarzenberg L, et al: Bone marrow graft in man after conditioning by antilymphocytic serum. BMJ 1970; 2:131–136.

143. Thomas ED, Storb R, Giblett ER, et al: Recovery from aplastic anemia following attempted marrow transplantation. Exp Hematol 1976; 4:97–102.

144. Territo MC: Autologous bone marrow repopulation following high dose cyclophosphamide and allogeneic marrow transplantation in aplastic anaemia. Br J Haematol 1977; 36:305–312.

145. Bickel M, Tsuda H, Amstad P, et al: Differential regulation of colony-stimulating factors and interleukin 2 production by cyclosporin A. Proc Natl Acad Sci USA 1987; 84:3274–3277.

146. Rebellato LM, Gross U, Verbanac KM, et al: A comprehensive definition of the major antibody specificities in polyclonal rabbit antithymocyte globulin. Transplantation 1994; 57:685–694.

147. Tisdale JF, Dunn DE, Maciejewski J: Cyclophosphamide and other new agents for the treatment of severe aplastic anemia. Semin Hematol 2000; 37:102–109.

148. Killick SB, Marsh JC, Gordon-Smith EC, et al: Effects of antithymocyte globulin on bone marrow CD34+ cells in aplastic anaemia and myelodysplasia. Br J Haematol 2000; 108:582–591.

149. Killick SB, Cox CV, Marsh JC, et al: Mechanisms of bone marrow progenitor cell apoptosis in aplastic anaemia and the effect of anti-thymocyte globulin: Examination of the role of the Fas-Fas-L interaction. Br J Haematol 2000; 111:1164–1169.

150. Jonasova A, Neuwirtova R, Cermak J, et al: Cyclosporin A therapy in hypoplastic MDS patients and certain refractory anaemias without hypoplastic bone marrow. Br J Haematol 1998; 100:304–309.

151. Young NS, Barrett AJ: Immune mediation of pancytopenia in myelodysplastic syndromes: Pathophysiology and treatment. In: Bennett JM (ed): The Myelodysplastic Syndromes: Pathobiology and Clinical Management, vol 27. New York, Marcel Dekker, 2002.

152. Koller U, Hinterberger W, Gschwandtler L, et al: Identification of activated T cells and the suppressor/inducer subset in patients suffering from severe aplastic anemia. Blut 1989; 58:21–26.

153. Zoumbos NC, Gascon P, Djeu JY, et al: Circulating activated suppressor T lymphocytes in aplastic anemia. N Engl J Med 1985; 312:257–265.

154. Maciejewski JP, Hibbs JR, Anderson S, et al: Bone marrow and peripheral blood lymphocyte phenotype in patients with bone marrow failure. Exp Hematol 1994; 22:1102–1110.

155. Herrmann F, Griffin JD, Meuer SG, et al: Establishment of an interleukin 2-dependent T cell line derived from a patient with severe aplastic anemia, which inhibits in vitro hematopoiesis. J Immunol 1986; 136:1629–1634.

156. Tong J, Bacigalupo A, Piaggio G, et al: In vitro response of T cells from aplastic anemia patients to antilymphocyte globulin and phytohemagglutinin: Colony-stimulating activity and lymphokine production. Exp Hematol 1991; 19:312–316.

157. Nakao S, Takamatsu H, Yachie A, et al: Establishment of a CD4+ T cell clone recognizing autologous hematopoietic progenitor cells from a patient with immune-mediated aplastic anemia. Exp Hematol 1995; 23:433–438.

158. Zoumbos NC, Ferris WO, Hsu SM, et al: Analysis of lymphocyte subsets in patients with aplastic anaemia. Br J Haematol 1984; 58:95–105.

159. Ruiz-Arguelles GJ, Katzmann JA, Greipp PR, et al: Lymphocyte subsets in patients with aplastic anemia. Am J Hematol 1984; 16:267–275.

160. Tsuda H, Yamasaki H: Type I and type II T-cell profiles in aplastic anemia and refractory anemia. Am J Hematol 2000; 64:271–274.

161. Nakao S, Takami A, Takamatsu H, et al: Isolation of a T-cell clone showing HLA-DRB1*0405-restricted cytotoxicity for hematopoietic cells in a patient with aplastic anemia. Blood 1997; 89:3691–3699.

162. Manz CY, Dietrich PY, Schnuriger V, et al: T-cell receptor beta chain variability in bone marrow and peripheral blood in severe acquired aplastic anemia. Blood Cells Mol Dis 1997; 23:110–122.

163. Zeng W, Nakao S, Takamatsu H, et al: Characterization of T-cell repertoire of the bone marrow in immune-mediated aplastic anemia: Evidence for the involvement of antigen-driven T-cell response in cyclosporine-dependent aplastic anemia. Blood 1999; 93:3008–3016.

164. Zeng W, Maciejewski J, Chen G, et al: Limited heterogeneity of T cell receptor BV usage in aplastic anemia. J Clin Invest 2001; 108:156–158.

165. Lipton JM, Nadler LM, Canellos GP, et al: Evidence for genetic restriction in the suppression of erythropoiesis by a unique subset of T lymphocytes in man. J Clin Invest 1983; 72:694–706.

166. Laver J, Castro-Malaspina H, Kernan NA, et al: In vitro interferon-γ production by cultured T-cells in severe aplastic anaemia: Correlation with granulomonopoietic inhibition in patients who respond to anti-thymocyte globulin. Br J Haematol 1988; 69:545–550.

167. Zoumbos NC, Gascon P, Djeu JY, et al: Interferon is a mediator of hematopoietic suppression in aplastic anemia in vitro and possibly in vivo. Proc Natl Acad Sci USA 1985; 82:188–192.

168. Nakao S, Yamaguchi M, Shiobara S, et al: Interferon-γ gene expression in unstimulated bone marrow mononuclear cells predicts a good response to cyclosporine therapy in aplastic anemia. Blood 1992; 79:2532–2535.

169. Nistico A, Young NS: γ-Interferon gene expression in the bone marrow of patients with aplastic anemia. Ann Intern Med 1994; 120:463–469.

170. Schultz JC, Shahidi NT: Detection of tumor necrosis factor-α in bone marrow plasma and peripheral blood plasma from patients with aplastic anemia. Am J Hematol 1994; 45:32–38.

171. Holmberg LA, Seidel K, Leisenring W, et al: Aplastic anemia: Analysis of stromal cell function in long-term marrow cultures. Blood 1994; 84:3685–3690.

172. Maciejewski JP, Liu JM, Green SW, et al: Expression of stem cell inhibitor (SCI) gene in patients with bone marrow failure. Exp Hematol 1992; 20:1112–1117.

173. Selleri C, Sato T, Anderson S, Young NS: Interferon-γ and tumor necrosis factor-α suppress both early and late stages of hematopoiesis and induce programmed cell death. J Cell Physiol 1995; 165:538–546.

174. Selleri C, Maciejewski JP, Sato T, et al: Interferon-γ constitutively expressed in the stromal microenvironment of human marrow cultures mediates potent hematopoietic inhibition. Blood 1996; 87:4149–4157.

175. Maciejewski J, Selleri C, Anderson S, et al: Fas antigen expression on CD34+ human marrow cells is induced by interferon γ and tumor necrosis factor α and potentiates cytokine-mediated hematopoietic suppression in vitro. Blood 1995; 85:3183–3190.

176. Bussel A, Dumont J, Schenmetzler C, et al: Long-term complete autologous reconstitution following cyclophosphamide and allogeneic marrow infusion in a case of severe aplastic anemia. Nouv Rev Fr Hematol 1985; 27:15–18.

177. Athanasou NA, Quinn J, Brenner MK, et al: Origin of marrow stromal cells and haemopoietic chimaerism following bone marrow transplantation determined by in situ hybridisation. Br J Cancer 1990; 61:385–389.

178. Marsh JC, Chang J, Testa NG, et al: In vitro assessment of marrow stem cell and stromal cell function in aplastic anaemia. Br J Haematol 1991; 78:258–267.

179. Juneja HS, Lee S, Gardner FH: Human long-term bone marrow cultures in aplastic anemia. Int J Cell Cloning 1989; 7:129–135.

180. Koijima S: Hematopoietic growth factors and marrow stroma in aplastic anemia. Int J Hematol 1998; 68:19–28.

181. Marsh JC: Hematopoietic growth factors in the pathogenesis and for the treatment of aplastic anemia. Semin Hematol 2000; 37:81–90.

182. Twomey JJ, Douglass CC, Sharkey O Jr. The monocytopenia of aplastic anemia. Blood 1973; 41:187–195.

183. Elfenbein GJ, Kallman CH, Tutschka PJ, et al: The immune system in 40 aplastic anemia patients receiving conventional therapy. Blood 1979; 53:652–665.

184. Alter BP: Fetal erythropoiesis in stress hematopoiesis. Exp Hematol 1979; 7:200–209.

185. Wolff J: Anemia caused by infections and toxins, idiopathic aplastic anemia and anemia caused by renal disease. Pediatr Clin North Am 1957; 4:469.

186. Diamond LK, Shahidi NT: Treatment of aplastic anemia in children. Semin Hematol 1967; 4:278–288.

187. Li FP, Alter BP, Nathan DG: The mortality of acquired aplastic anemia in children. Blood 1972; 40:153–162.

188. Heyn RM, Ertel IJ, Tubergen DG: Course of acquired aplastic anemia in children treated with supportive care. JAMA 1969; 208:1372–1378.

189. Khatib Z, Wilimas J, Wang W: Outcome of moderate aplastic anemia in children. Am J Pediatr Hematol Oncol 1994; 16:80–85.

190. Champlin R, Ho W, Gale RP: Antithymocyte globulin treatment in patients with aplastic anemia: A prospective randomized trial. N Engl J Med 1983; 308:113–118.

191. Herman JH, Kamel HT: Platelet transfusion. Current techniques, remaining problems, and future prospects. Am J Pediatr Hematol Oncol 1987; 9:272–286.

192. Heyman MR, Schiffer CA: Platelet transfusion therapy for the cancer patient. Semin Oncol 1990; 17:198–209.

193. Patten E: Controversies in transfusion medicine. Prophylactic platelet transfusion revisited after 25 years: Con. Transfusion 1992; 32:381–385.

194. Sagmeister M, Oec L, Gmur J: A restrictive platelet transfusion policy allowing long-term support of outpatients with severe aplastic anemia. Blood 1999; 93:3124–3126.

195. Weinberger M, Elattar I, Marshall D, et al: Patterns of infection in patients with aplastic anemia and the emergence of *Aspergillus* as a major cause of death. Medicine (Baltimore) 1992; 71:24–43.

196. Keidan AJ, Tsatalas C, Cohen J, et al: Infective complications of aplastic anaemia. Br J Haematol 1986; 63:503–508.

197. Brittenham GM, Griffith PM, Nienhuis AW, et al: Efficacy of deferoxamine in preventing complications of iron overload in patients with thalassemia major. N Engl J Med 1994; 331:567–573.

198. Bacigalupo A, Brand R, Oneto R, et al: Treatment of acquired severe aplastic anemia: Bone marrow transplantation compared with immunosuppressive therapy—The European Group for Blood and Marrow Transplantation Experience. Semin Hematol 2000; 37:69–80.

199. Horowitz MM: Current status of allogeneic bone marrow transplantation in acquired aplastic anemia. Semin Hematol 2000; 37:30–42.

200. Gluckman E, Socie G, Devergie A, et al: Bone marrow transplantation in 107 patients with severe aplastic anemia using cyclophosphamide and thoraco-abdominal irradiation for conditioning: Long-term follow-up. Blood 1991; 78:2451–2455.

201. Champlin RE, Ho WG, Nimer SD, et al: Bone marrow transplantation for severe aplastic anemia. Effect of a preparative regimen of cyclophosphamide-low-dose total-lymphoid irradiation and post-transplant cyclosporine-methotrexate therapy. Transplantation 1990; 49:720–724.

202. May WS, Sensenbrenner LL, Burns WH, et al: BMT for severe aplastic anemia using cyclosporine. Bone Marrow Transplant 1993; 11:459–464.

203. Storb R, Etzioni R, Anasetti C, et al: Cyclophosphamide combined with antithymocyte globulin in preparation for allogeneic marrow

transplants in patients with aplastic anemia. Blood 1994; 84:941–949.

204. Passweg JR, Socie G, Hinterberger W, et al: Bone marrow transplantation for severe aplastic anemia: Has outcome improved? Blood 1997; 90:858–864.

205. Reiter E, Keil F, Brugger S, et al: Excellent long-term survival after allogeneic marrow transplantation in patients with severe aplastic anemia. Bone Marrow Transplant 1997; 19:1191–1196.

206. Storb R, Leisenring W, Anasetti C, et al: Long-term follow-up of allogeneic marrow transplants in patients with aplastic anemia conditioned by cyclophosphamide combined with antithymocyte globulin. Blood 1997; 89:3890–3891.

207. Bordin JO, Heddle NM, Blajchman MA: Biologic effects of leukocytes present in transfused cellular blood products. Blood 1994; 84:1703–1721.

208. Stucki A, Leisenring W, Sandmaier BM, et al: Decreased rejection and improved survival of first and second marrow transplants for severe aplastic anemia (a 26-year retrospective analysis). Blood 1998; 92:2742–2749.

209. Deeg HJ, Leisenring W, Storb R, et al: Long-term outcome after marrow transplantation for severe aplastic anemia. Blood 1998; 91:3637–3645.

210. Vowels MR, Lam Po Tang R, et al: Bone marrow transplantation in children using closely matched related and unrelated donors. Bone Marrow Transplant 1991; 8:87–92.

211. Bacigalupo A, Oneto R, Bruno B, et al: Current results of bone marrow transplantation in patients with acquired severe aplastic anemia. Report of the European Group for Blood and Marrow transplantation. On behalf of the Working Party on Severe Aplastic Anemia of the European Group for Blood and Marrow Transplantation. Acta Haematol 2000; 103:19–25.

212. Jeannet M, Speck B, Rubinstein A, et al: Autologous marrow reconstitutions in severe aplastic anaemia after ALG pretreatment and HL-A semi-incompatible bone marrow cell transfusion. Acta Haematol 1976; 55:129–139.

213. Silingardi V, Torelli U: Recovery from aplastic anemia after treatment with antilymphocyte globulin. Arch Intern Med 1979; 139:582–583.

214. Gluckman E, Esperou-Bourdeau H, Baruchel A, et al: Multicenter randomized study comparing cyclosporine-A alone and antithymocyte globulin with prednisone for treatment of severe aplastic anemia. Blood 1992; 79:2540–2546.

215. Marsh J, Schrezenmeier H, Marin P, et al: Prospective randomized multicenter study comparing cyclosporin alone versus the combination of antithymocyte globulin and cyclosporin for treatment of patients with nonsevere aplastic anemia: A report from the European Blood and Marrow Transplant (EBMT) Severe Aplastic Anaemia Working Party. Blood 1999; 93:2191–2195.

216. Raghavachar A, Kolbe K, Hoffken K, et al: Standard immunosuppression is superior to cyclosporine/filgrastim in severe aplastic anemia: The German multicenter study. Bone Marrow Transplant 1999; 23:S31.

217. Camitta B, O'Reilly RJ, Sensenbrenner L, et al: Antithoracic duct lymphocyte globulin therapy of severe aplastic anemia. Blood 1983; 62:883–888.

218. Frickhofen N, Kaltwasser JP, Schrezenmeier H, et al: Treatment of aplastic anemia with antilymphocyte globulin and methylprednisolone with or without cyclosporine. The German Aplastic Anemia Study Group. N Engl J Med 1991; 324:1297–304.

219. Gordon-Smith EC, Yandle A, Milne A, et al: Randomised placebo controlled study of RH-GM-CSF following ALG in the treatment of aplastic anaemia. Bone Marrow Transplant 1991; 7:78–80.

220. Gluckman E, Rokicka-Milewska R, Gordon-Smith E, et al: Results of randomized study of glycosylated rHuG-CSF lenograstim in severe aplastic anemia. Blood 1999; 92:376a.

221. Kojima S, Hibi S, Kosaka Y, et al: Immunosuppressive therapy using antithymocyte globulin, cyclosporine, and danazol with or without human granulocyte colony-stimulating factor in children with acquired aplastic anemia. Blood 2000; 96:2049–2054.

222. Bielory L, Wright R, Nienhuis AW, et al: Antithymocyte globulin hypersensitivity in bone marrow failure patients. JAMA 1988; 260:3164–3167.

223. Greco B, Bielory L, Stephany D, et al: Antithymocyte globulin reacts with many normal human cell types. Blood 1983; 62:1047–1054.

224. Young N, Griffith P, Brittain E, et al: A multicenter trial of antithymocyte globulin in aplastic anemia and related diseases. Blood 1988; 72:1861–1869.

225. Bessman JD, Gardner FH: Persistence of abnormal RBC and platelet phenotype during recovery from aplastic anemia. Arch Intern Med 1985; 145:293–296.

226. Alter BP, Rappeport JM, Huisman TH, et al: Fetal erythropoiesis following bone marrow transplantation. Blood 1976; 48:843–853.

227. Freedman MH, Saunders EF, Hilton J, et al: Residual abnormalities in acquired aplastic anemia of childhood. JAMA 1974; 228:201–202.

228. Kahan BD: Cyclosporine. N Engl J Med 1989; 321:1725–1738.

229. Leonard EM, Raefsky E, Griffith P, et al: Cyclosporine therapy of aplastic anaemia, congenital and acquired red cell aplasia. Br J Haematol 1989; 72:278–284.

230. Hinterberger-Fischer M, Hocker P, et al: Oral cyclosporin-A is effective treatment for untreated and also for previously immunosuppressed patients with severe bone marrow failure. Eur J Haematol 1989; 43:136–142.

231. Bacigalupo A, Frassoni F, Podesta M, et al: Cyclosporin A (CyA) does not enhance CFU-c growth in patients with severe aplastic anaemia. Scand J Haematol 1985; 34:133–136.

232. Champlin RE, Ho WG, Feig SA, et al: Do androgens enhance the response to antithymocyte globulin in patients with aplastic anemia? A prospective randomized trial. Blood 1985; 66:184–188.

233. Kaltwasser JP, Dix U, Schalk KP, et al: Effect of androgens on the response to antithymocyte globulin in patients with aplastic anaemia. Eur J Haematol 1988; 40:111–118.

234. Bacigalupo A, Chaple M, Hows J, et al: Treatment of aplastic anaemia (AA) with antilymphocyte globulin (ALG) and methylprednisolone (MPred) with or without androgens: A randomized trial from the EBMT SAA working party. Br J Haematol 1993; 83:145–151.

235. Rosenfeld SJ, Kimball J, Vining D, et al: Intensive immunosuppression with antithymocyte globulin and cyclosporine as treatment for severe acquired aplastic anemia. Blood 1995; 85:3058–3065.

236. Frickhofen N, Rosenfeld SJ: Immunosuppressive treatment of aplastic anemia with antithymocyte globulin and cyclosporine. Semin Hematol 2000; 37:56–68.

237. Fuhrer M, Burdach S, Ebell W, et al: Relapse and clonal disease in children with aplastic anemia (AA) after immunosuppressive therapy (IST): The SAA 94 experience. German/Austrian Pediatric Aplastic Anemia Working Group. Klin Padiatr 1998; 210:173–179.

238. Matloub YH, Bostrom B, Golembe B, et al: Antithymocyte globulin, cyclosporine, and prednisone for the treatment of severe aplastic anemia in children. A pilot study. Am J Pediatr Hematol Oncol 1994; 16:104–106.

239. Schrezenmeier H, Marin P, Raghavachar A, et al: Relapse of aplastic anaemia after immunosuppressive treatment: A report from the European Bone Marrow Transplantation Group SAA Working Party. Br J Haematol 1993; 85:371–377.

240. Tichelli A, Passweg J, Nissen C, et al: Repeated treatment with horse antilymphocyte globulin for severe aplastic anaemia. Br J Haematol 1998; 100:393–400.

241. Tooze JA, Marsh JC, Gordon-Smith EC: Clonal evolution of aplastic anaemia to myelodysplasia/acute myeloid leukaemia and paroxysmal nocturnal haemoglobinuria. Leuk Lymphoma 1999; 33:231–241.

242. Socie G, Rosenfeld S, Frickhofen N, et al: Late clonal diseases of treated aplastic anemia. Semin Hematol 2000; 37:91–101.

243. Socie G, Henry-Amar M, Bacigalupo A, et al: Malignant tumors occurring after treatment of aplastic anemia. European Bone Marrow Transplantation-Severe Aplastic Anaemia Working Party. N Engl J Med 1993; 329:1152–1157.

244. Ball SE, Gibson FM, Rizzo S, et al: Progressive telomere shortening in aplastic anemia. Blood 1998; 91:3582–3592.

245. Brummendorf TH, Maciejewski JP, Mak J, et al: Telomere length in leukocyte subpopulations of patients with aplastic anemia. Blood 2001; 97:895–900.

246. Speck B, Gratwohl A, Nissen C, et al: Treatment of severe aplastic anaemia with antilymphocyte globulin or bone-marrow transplantation. BMJ (Clin Res Ed) 1981; 282:860–863.

247. Bayever E, Champlin R, Ho W, et al: Comparison between bone marrow transplantation and antithymocyte globulin in treatment of

young patients with severe aplastic anemia. J Pediatr 1984; 105:920–925.

248. Halperin DS, Grisaru D, Freedman MH, et al: Severe acquired aplastic anemia in children: 11-year experience with bone marrow transplantation and immunosuppressive therapy. Am J Pediatr Hematol Oncol 1989; 11:304–309.

249. Locasciulli A, van't Veer L, Bacigalupo A, et al: Treatment with marrow transplantation or immunosuppression of childhood acquired severe aplastic anemia: A report from the EBMT SAA Working Party. Bone Marrow Transplant 1990; 6:211–217.

250. Speck B, Tichelli A, Grathwohl A, et al: Treatment of severe aplastic anemia: A 12-year follow-up of patients after bone marrow transplantation or after therapy with antilymphocyte globulin. In: Shahidi T (ed): Aplastic Anemia and Other Bone Marrow Failure Syndromes. New York, Springer-Verlag, 1990, p 96.

251. Paquette RL, Tebyani N, Frane M, et al: Long-term outcome of aplastic anemia in adults treated with antithymocyte globulin: Comparison with bone marrow transplantation. Blood 1995; 85:283–290.

252. Lawlor ER, Anderson RA, Davis JH, et al: Immunosuppressive therapy: A potential alternative to bone marrow transplantation as initial therapy for acquired severe aplastic anemia in childhood? J Pediatr Hematol Oncol 1997; 19:115–123.

253. Doney K, Leisenring W, Storb R, et al: Primary treatment of acquired aplastic anemia: Outcomes with bone marrow transplantation and immunosuppressive therapy. Seattle Bone Marrow Transplant Team. Ann Intern Med 1997; 126:107–115.

254. Kojima S, Horibe K, Inaba J, et al: Long-term outcome of acquired aplastic anaemia in children: Comparison between immunosuppressive therapy and bone marrow transplantation. Br J Haematol 2000; 111:321–328.

255. Ohara A, Kojima S, Hamajima N, et al: Myelodysplastic syndrome and acute myelogenous leukemia as a late clonal complication in children with acquired aplastic anemia. Blood 1997; 90:1009–1013.

256. Gardner FH, Besa EC: Physiologic mechanisms and the hematopoietic effects of the androstanes and their derivatives. Curr Top Hematol 1983; 4:123–195.

257. Alexanian R: Erythropoietin and erythropoiesis in anemic man following androgens. Blood 1969; 33:564–572.

258. Singer JW, Adamson JW: Steroids and hematopoiesis. II: The effect of steroids on in vitro erythroid colony growth: Evidence for different target cells for different classes of steroids. J Cell Physiol 1976; 88:135–143.

259. Shahidi N, Diamond L: Testosterone-induced remission in aplastic anemia of both acquired and congenital types. Further observations in 24 cases. N Engl J Med 1961; 264:953.

260. Najean Y, Pecking A: Prognostic factors in acquired aplastic anemia. A study of 352 cases. Am J Med 1979; 67:564–571.

261. Sanchez-Medal L, Gomez-Leal A, Duarte L, et al: Anabolic androgenic steroids in the treatment of acquired aplastic anemia. Blood 1969; 34:283–300.

262. Davis S, Rubin AD: Treatment and prognosis in aplastic anaemia. Lancet 1972; 1:871–873.

263. Lynch RE, Williams DM, Reading JC, et al: The prognosis in aplastic anemia. Blood 1975; 45:517–528.

264. Williams DM, Lynch RE, Cartwright GE: Prognostic factors in aplastic anemia. Clin Haematol 1978; 7:467–474.

265. Camitta BM, Storb R, Thomas ED: Aplastic anemia (first of two parts): Pathogenesis, diagnosis, treatment, and prognosis. N Engl J Med 1982; 306:645–652.

266. Camitta BM, Storb R, Thomas ED: Aplastic anemia (second of two parts): Pathogenesis, diagnosis, treatment, and prognosis. N Engl J Med 1982; 306:712–718.

267. McGiven AR: Peliosis hepatis: Case report and review of pathogenesis. J Pathol 1970; 101:283–285.

268. Bourliere B, Najean Y: Influence of long-term androgen therapy on growth: An analysis of 18 cases of aplastic anemia in children. Am J Dis Child 1987; 141:718–719.

269. Marmont A, Bacigalupo A, et al: Treatment of severe aplastic anemia with high-dose methylprednisolone and antilyphocyte globulin. In: Young N, Levine A, Humphries R (eds): Aplastic Anemia: Stem Cell Biology and Advances in Treatment. New York, Alan R. Liss, 1984, p 271.

270. Gluckman E, Devergie A, Poros A, et al: Results of immunosuppression in 170 cases of severe aplastic anaemia. Report of the European Group of Bone Marrow Transplant (EGBMT). Br J Haematol 1982; 51:541–550.

271. Heaton L, Crosby W, Cohen A: Splenectomy in the treatment of hypoplasia of the bone marrow. With a report of twelve cases. Ann Surg 1957; 146:637.

272. Speck B, Gratwohl A, Nissen C, et al: Treatment of severe aplastic anemia. Exp Hematol 1986; 14:126–132.

273. Brodsky RA, Sensenbrenner LL, Jones RJ: Complete remission in severe aplastic anemia after high-dose cyclophosphamide without bone marrow transplantation. Blood 1996; 87:491–494.

274. Tisdale JF, Dunn DE, Geller N, et al: High-dose cyclophosphamide in severe aplastic anaemia: A randomised trial. Lancet 2000; 356:1554–1559.

275. Taniguchi T, Minami Y: The IL-2/IL-2 receptor system: A current overview. Cell 1993; 73:5–8.

276. Sievers TM, Rossi SJ, Ghobrial RM, et al: Mycophenolate mofetil. Pharmacotherapy 1997; 17:1178–1197.

277. Cai W, Hu L, Foulkes JG: Transcription-modulating drugs: Mechanism and selectivity. Curr Opin Biotechnol 1996; 7:608–615.

278. Kelly PA, Gruber SA, Behbod F, et al: Sirolimus, a new, potent immunosuppressive agent. Pharmacotherapy 1997; 17:1148–1156.

279. Sehgal SN: Rapamune (RAPA, rapamycin, sirolimus): Mechanism of action immunosuppressive effect results from blockade of signal transduction and inhibition of cell cycle progression. Clin Biochem 1998; 31:335–340.

8 | Inherited Bone Marrow Failure Syndromes

Blanche P. Alter

The term *constitutional aplastic anemia* was defined by O'Gorman Hughes as "chronic bone marrow failure associated with other features, such as congenital anomalies, a familial incidence, or thrombocytopenia at birth."[1] Although these disorders are "inherited bone marrow failure syndromes," the hematologic components are often not evident at birth. The subdivisions in the older literature are confusing and no longer relevant:

Type I, Fanconi anemia (FA), aplastic anemia with physical abnormalities, is now diagnosed if clastogen-induced chromosome breaks are present, and physical abnormalities may be absent.

Type II, the Estren-Dameshek disorder, familial aplastic anemia without physical anomalies, is a subset of FA.

Type III, amegakaryocytic thrombocytopenia, is now more stringently defined.

All of the specific disorders, both included and ignored by the terminology above, are referred to by their eponyms, until more specific information becomes available.

One hypothesis regarding "acquired" aplastic anemia is that it occurs in rare individuals (homozygotes or heterozygotes) who are genetically predisposed to marrow damage. In this section we will describe homozygotes for autosomal recessive bone marrow failure genes, heterozygotes for autosomal dominant genes, and hemizygotes for X-linked genes, who can be identified by their phenotype, and in some cases by specific laboratory tests including mutation analyses. Carriers are identified from their position in a family and by mutation testing. The phenotypes of patients with genes for aplastic anemia vary widely, and the categories may inadvertently include patients with congenital (i.e., present at birth) but not necessarily inherited phenocopies. Detailed references not provided here can be found in previous editions of this book,[2] as well as a monograph by Young and Alter.[3]

The incidence of these inherited conditions is difficult to ascertain. Among 134 children with aplastic anemia seen at the Children's Hospital Medical Center in Boston from 1958 to 1977, inherited diseases were diagnosed in 40 from birth to age 17.[4] Of these, 26 had FA, 10 had familial aplasia without physical or cytogenetic evidence for FA, and 4 developed pancytopenia after amegakaryocytic thrombocytopenia. In a similar interval at the Prince of Wales Hospital in Australia (1964 to 1984) 12 of 34 children had inherited syndromes, including 8 with FA.[5] We estimate that at least 25 percent of childhood aplastic anemia occurs in the presence of known marrow failure genes. Whether the remainder also have inherited dysfunction remains to be determined. Thus, the presence of the genetic syndromes must be determined in all patients with aplastic anemia, because treatment and prognoses for inherited and acquired disorders differ.

PANCYTOPENIAS

Fanconi Anemia

DESCRIPTION

In 1927, Fanconi[6] described three brothers who had pancytopenia as well as physical abnormalities; he called their macrocytic anemia "perniziosiforme." Uehlinger[7] soon described a similar patient with abnormalities of the thumb and kidney. According to Fanconi,[8] Naegeli suggested in 1931 that the term *Fanconi anemia* be used for familial aplastic anemia and congenital physical anomalies. Patients are included if they have characteristic chromosome breaks following clastogenic stress; physical anomalies and aplastic anemia are not required. Useful reviews of FA can be found in several sources.[3, 9–11]

More then 1200 cases have now been reported in varying detail, and many of the older case s are reviewed elsewhere.[2, 3, 9] Table 8–1 summarizes these patients according to the decade of the report; the ages at diagnosis are shown in Figure 8–1. The male-to-female ratio of occurrence is 1.2:1. Earlier diagnoses were made when aplastic anemia (or leukemia or cancer) developed; more recent diagnoses are also made with positive chromosome breakage studies in siblings of affected individuals or in patients with "characteristic" physical anomalies without aplastic anemia. The median age at diagnosis in male patients was 6.5 years of age and in female patients was 8 years of age, with ranges from birth to 48 years. All ethnic and racial groups from more than 60 countries have been represented, including whites, blacks, Asians, Native Americans, and Indians.

There are two extremes in the FA patient groups. In 4 percent of patients, FA was diagnosed between birth and 1 year of age, and at least half of these had hematologic signs at diagnosis. Thus, FA cannot be excluded from the differential diagnosis of aplastic anemia during infancy. In 9 percent FA was diagnosed at age 16 or older. This is only the tip of the iceberg, because the diagnosis of FA must be actively sought in adult patients with normal physical examinations or only subtle abnormalities (see later). FA is undoubtedly more common than it was thought to be before the development of specific chromosome testing.

Physical Examination. Until recently, patients were recognized only by the presence of some of the characteristic physical findings summarized in Tables 8–2 and 8–3. A higher proportion of patients with FA diagnosed in infancy had major characteristic anomalies, such as those involving thumbs and radii, kidneys, head, eyes, and ears, as well as gastrointestinal areas. Conversely, those with FA diagnosed in older years had fewer of those anomalies. Short stature and skin pigmentary problems are only apparent with increasing age and thus did not distinguish the two age extremes.

The patient shown in Figure 8–2 has the "classic" anomalies of FA: short stature, abnormal thumbs, microcephaly, café au lait and hypopigmented spots, and a characteristic facial appearance including a broad nasal base, epicanthal folds, and micrognathia.[12] FA and thrombocytopenia absent radii (TAR) (see later) can be distinguished: in FA, if the radii are affected, the thumbs are always abnormal; in TAR, where radii are absent, thumbs are always present. The list of anomalies in Table 8–3 includes both common and very rare findings, in approximate order of incidence. Involvement of the skin is seen most often, followed by poor growth, anomalies of the upper arms, and structural renal abnormalities. VATERL syndrome has been mistakenly diagnosed in some patients because of the specific types of anomalies (*v*ertebral defects, *a*nal atresia, *t*racheo*e*sophageal fistula, *r*enal defects, and radial *l*imb defects).[13] The malformations described in the 1993 International Fanconi Anemia Registry (IFAR) report are similar to those outlined here.[14]

The IFAR used a stepwise multivariate analysis to identify eight variables that differentiate patients with chromosome breakage (*FA homozygotes*) and those who do not have breakage (*non-FA*).[15] One point is given for microphthalmia, birthmarks, genitourinary anomalies, growth retardation, absence of radius or thumb, and thrombocytopenia, and a point is subtracted for learning disabilities and other skeletal abnormalities. Higher scores indicate an increased probability of FA. This scoring system, of course, does not detect the large group of patients with FA who do not have anomalies and only provides a probability determination for those who do have such findings.

The proportion of FA homozygotes with normal appearances is underestimated by literature review. Two such families were first described by Estren and Dameshek in 1947.[16] Subsequently, Li and Potter[17] reported that a cousin of one of the original families had typical FA, with chromosome breaks. The results of chromosome breakage studies in patients with the "Estren-Dameshek" disorder are indistinguishable from those in patients with classical FA with anomalies. Thus, patients without anomalies represent just one end of the spectrum of FA. Literature reports of patients identified because they had affected

TABLE 8–1. Fanconi Anemia Literature by Decade of First Report

	1927–1960	1961–1970	1971–1980	1981–1990	1991–2000	All Patients
No. of patients	118	119	262	316	391	1206
Male/female	68/50	74/44	151/108	163/153	205/179	661/534
Ratio	1.36	1.68	1.40	1.07	1.15	1.24
Male Age at Diagnosis (yrs)						
Mean	7.5	7.8	7.6	8.2	8.6	8.1
Median	6	7	6	6.5	6	6.5
Range	0.5–30	0.6–21	0–28	0–29	0–48	0–48
Female Age at Diagnosis (yrs)						
Mean	7.6	9.4	8.0	8.9	9.6	9.0
Median	7	8	7.8	8	7.8	8
Range	1–14	0–35	0–48	0–39	0–45	0–48
No. males ≤1 yr	1	1	9	8	8	27 (4%)
No. females ≤1 yr	2	1	3	5	5	16 (3%)
No. males ≥16 yrs	5	5	14	15	18	57 (9%)
No. females ≥16 yrs	0	5	10	17	15	47 (9%)
No. reported deceased	64	47	112	126	106	455
% reported deceased	54	39	43	40	27	38
Projected median survival (yrs)	13	17	16	19	30	20

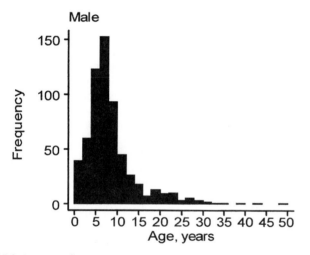
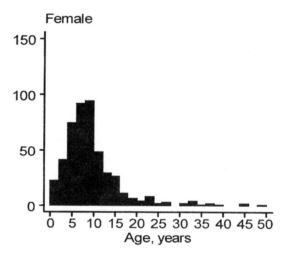

FIGURE 8–1. Age at diagnosis in approximately1200 published reports of patients with Fanconi anemia. *Left panel,* Males. *Right panel,* Females. (See text for definition of "diagnosis.")

siblings indicate that at least 25 percent do not have anomalies.[18, 19] Our own review (see Table 8–2) identified 25 percent of patients who fit into this category, whereas 11 percent were short and had skin findings. Almost 40 percent of the 370 patients analyzed in the IFAR were reported to be physically "normal."[14] These findings emphasize the importance of a careful search for genetic dysfunction in patients with marrow failure.

Inheritance and Environment. FA is an autosomal recessive disorder, despite the slight excess of occurrence in males reported in the literature (see Table 8–1). The

IFAR reported a male-to-female ratio of occurrence of 1.06. In a large single study,[20] 30 percent of families had two affected children, with consanguinity in 10 percent. Our survey identified at least 90 families with consanguinity, 325 with affected siblings, and 10 with affected cousins. At least 30 mothers of patients with FA had miscarriages; some of these fetuses had significant physical anomalies and are presumed to be homozygotes. Segregation analysis of the 86 patients reported by Schroeder et al[20] and 88 patients in the IFAR confirmed the monogenic autosomal recessive inheritance pattern.[21]

TABLE 8–2. Physical Abnormalities in Fanconi Anemia*

				Age at Diagnosis of Abnormality	
Abnormality	All Patients	Male	Female	≤1 yr	≥16 yrs
No. of patients (%)	1206	631	534	43 (4%)	104 (9%)
Skin pigment and/or café au lait	55%	57%	55%	37%	61%
Short stature	51%	54%	53%	47%	57%
Upper limbs	43%	46%	43%	63%	39%
Abnormal gonads, male	—	32%	—	37%	44%
Abnormal gonads, female	—	—	3%	50%	6%
Head	26%	27%	28%	37%	18%
Eyes	23%	25%	23%	33%	24%
Renal	21%	24%	19%	42%	19%
Birth weight ≤ 2500 g	11%	11%	12%	47%	8%
Developmental disability	11%	12%	12%	5%	8%
Ears, hearing	9%	11%	8%	23%	11%
Legs	8%	9%	7%	16%	7%
Cardiopulmonary	6%	5%	8%	16%	5%
Gastrointestinal	5%	4%	5%	28%	6%
No anomalies	25%	21%	26%	16%	23%
Short stature and/or skin only	11%	13%	10%	5%	19%

*Data represent percentage of patients with the abnormality.

The occurrence of heterozygotes is 1 in 300 persons in the United States and in Europe[20, 22] and approximately 1 per 100 Ashkenazi Jews and South African Afrikaans, owing to separate founder effects.[20, 23, 24] In some families, siblings had physical abnormalities without hematologic disease.[25–28] Anomalies have been seen in parents, consistent with a heterozygote phenotype.[29] In one family one brother had typical short stature, horseshoe kidney, and aplastic anemia; another brother had aplastic anemia followed by paroxysmal nocturnal hemoglobinuria (PNH), and a cousin died of aplastic anemia.[30] The brother with PNH was later proved to have FA by chromosome breakage studies and died from lung cancer at age 67.* All of the variations may reflect incomplete expression of the homozygous state or may occur in heterozygotes; testing for chromosome breakage would be helpful. The varied expression might also be the result of allelic but different gene defects or nonallelic mutations, or it may be related to different environmental influences.

In patients with characteristic malformations or with affected siblings FA can be diagnosed by chromosome studies in the *preanemic phase*.[3, 9] These patients should avoid use of drugs that are implicated in the occurrence of acquired aplastic anemia. Follow-up may permit definition of the reason for development of aplastic anemia or malignancy in patients with FA and may provide more accurate figures on the proportions of FA homozygotes who "escape" such complications.

The environment may explain aplasia in some patients. In one family with FA, one sister died of aplastic anemia at age 16 (she had a history of treating skin infections with topical coal tar).[31] The other two, with confirmed diagnosis of FA by chromosome breakage, had only mild pancytopenia for more than 20 years. One died at age 38 (with myelodysplastic syndrome as well as precancerous skin and cervical findings), whereas the other is in her 40s and remains hematologically well, although oral leukoplakia has developed (see later for discussion of the complications seen in older patients). Thus, the same FA genes in different external or internal (other gene) environments resulted in different phenotypes.

Aplastic anemia in FA homozygotes developed after several environmental events, such as viral illnesses, hepatitis, or primary tuberculosis.[32–35] Several patients received chloramphenicol before the onset of aplasia.[36–40] These examples also suggest that the environment may have a role. Several sets of siblings developed aplastic anemia at the same age, indicating a genetic component,[20, 34, 41, 42] and thus the relative roles of environment and genes may vary.

LABORATORY FINDINGS

Patients often have mild or moderate thrombocytopenia or leukopenia before pancytopenia, but severe aplasia eventually develops in most of these patients. Even in a patient with FA who has normal blood counts (preanemic or treatment-responsive), erythrocytes are often macrocytic. Examination of the blood smear shows large red cells with mild poikilocytosis and anisocytosis, as well as decreased numbers of platelets and leukocytes (Fig. 8–3). In FA the red cells may be larger than those seen in acquired aplastic anemia, and the fetal hemoglobin (HbF) level may be higher. When aplastic, the bone marrow in

*Dacie J, Gordon-Smith EC: personal communication.

TABLE 8–3. Specific Types of Anomalies in Fanconi Anemia*

SKIN

Generalized hyperpigmentation on trunk, neck, and intertriginous areas; café au lait spots; hypopigmented areas

BODY

Short stature; delicate features; small size; underweight

UPPER LIMBS

Thumbs: absent or hypoplastic; supernumerary or bifid, or duplicated; rudimentary; short, low set, attached by a thread, triphalangeal, tubular, stiff, hyperextensible
Radii: absent or hypoplastic (only with abnormal thumbs); absent or weak pulse
Hands: clinodactyly; hypoplastic thenar eminence; six fingers; absent first metacarpal; enlarged, abnormal fingers; short fingers, transverse crease
Ulnae: dysplastic

GONADS

Males: hypogenitalia; undescended testes; hypospadias; abnormal genitalia; absent testis; atrophic testes; azoospermia; phimosis; abnormal urethra; micropenis; delayed development
Females: hypogenitalia; bicornuate uterus; abnormal genitalia; aplasia of uterus and vagina; atresia of uterus, vagina, and ovary

OTHER SKELETAL ANOMALIES

Head and face: microcephaly; hydrocephalus; micrognathia; peculiar face; bird face; flat head; frontal bossing; scaphocephaly; sloped forehead; choanal atresia
Neck: Sprengel deformity; short, low hair line; webbed
Spine: spina bifida (thoracic, lumbar, cervical, occult sacral); scoliosis; abnormal ribs; sacrococcygeal sinus; Klippel-Feil syndrome; vertebral anomalies; extra vertebrae

EYES

Small eyes; strabismus; epicanthal folds; hypertelorism; ptosis; slanting; cataracts; astigmatism; blindness; epiphora; nystagmus; proptosis; small iris

EARS

Deafness (usually conductive); abnormal shape; atresia; dysplasia; low set, large, or small; infections; abnormal middle ear; absent drum; dimples; rotated; canal stenosis

KIDNEYS

Ectopic or pelvic; abnormal, horseshoe, hypoplastic, or dysplastic; absent; hydronephrosis or hydroureter; infections; duplicated; rotated; reflux; hyperplasia; no function; abnormal artery

GASTROINTESTINAL SYSTEM

High arched palate; atresia (esophagus, duodenum, jejunum); imperforate anus, tracheoesophageal fistula; Meckel diverticulum; umbilical hernia; hypoplastic uvula; abnormal biliary ducts; megacolon; abdominal diastasis; Budd-Chiari syndrome;

LOWER LIMBS

Feet: toe syndactyly; abnormal toes; flat feet; short toes; clubfeet; six toes; supernumerary toe
Legs: congenital hip dislocation; Perthes' disease; coxa vara; abnormal femur; thigh osteoma; abnormal legs

CARDIOPULMONARY SYSTEM

Patent ductus arteriosus; ventricular septal defect; abnormal heart; peripheral pulmonic stenosis; aortic stenosis; coarctation; absent lung lobes; vascular malformation; aortic atheromas; atrial septal defect; tetralogy of Fallot; pseudotruncus; hypoplastic aorta; abnormal pulmonary drainage; double aortic arch; cardiac myopathy

OTHER ANOMALIES

Slow development; hyperreflexia; Bell palsy; central nervous system arterial malformation; stenosis of the internal carotid artery; small pituitary gland; absent corpus callosum

*Abnormalities are listed in approximate order of frequency within each category.

patients with FA is hypocellular and fatty, with few hematopoietic elements and a relative increase in the numbers of lymphocytes, reticulum cells, mast cells, and plasma cells, identical to the marrow in patients with acquired aplasia. Areas of hypercellular marrow disappear as the aplasia progresses.[8]

Patients with FA have "stress erythropoiesis," producing erythrocytes with fetal characteristics, as also seen in patients during recovery from acquired aplastic anemia or after bone marrow transplantation (BMT).[43, 44] This "fetal-like" erythropoiesis, present in preanemic and anemic patients with FA or in patients whose FA is in

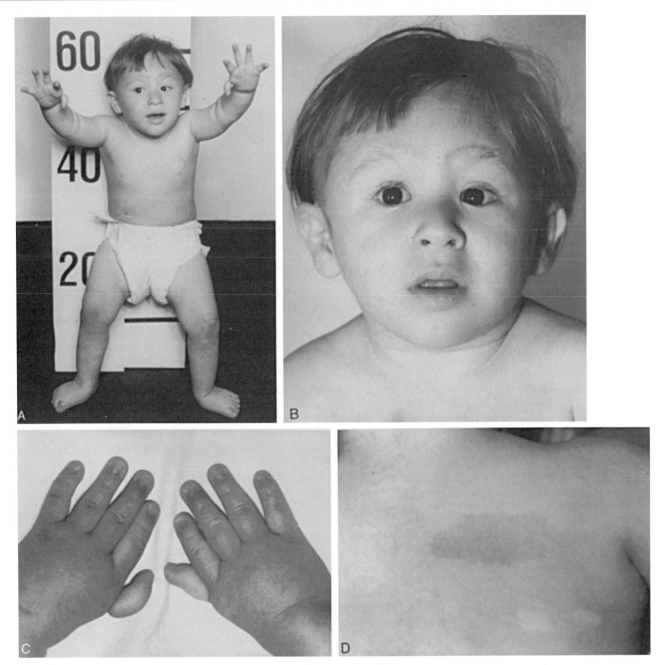

FIGURE 8–2. Three-year-old male with Fanconi anemia, who exhibits several classic phenotypic features. *A*, Front view. *B*, Face. *C*, Hands. *D*, Back right shoulder. The features to be noted include short stature, dislocated hips, microcephaly, broad nasal base, epicanthal folds, micrognathia, thumbs attached by threads, and café au lait spots with hypopigmented areas beneath.

remission, includes macrocytosis and increased levels of HbF (by alkali denaturation and Kleihauer-Betke acid elution) and i antigen. These features also identify nonanemic siblings with FA. The HbF is distributed unevenly, not clonally, and there is no single-cell concordance of the fetal-like features.[45] The level of HbF or degree of macrocytosis does not provide prognostic information. Serum erythropoietin levels are increased in patients with FA and are much higher than expected for the degree of anemia compared with levels in patients

with hemolytic anemias.[3] One group reported that the serum α-fetoprotein level was constitutively elevated in patients with FA,[46] although this has not been our experience.

We previously developed a classification scheme for FA,[47] using hematologic information. Group 1 includes patients with severe aplastic anemia, who are transfusion-dependent and are receiving no treatment, whereas Group 2 includes patients with similar disease except that they are receiving androgens but not responding to them.

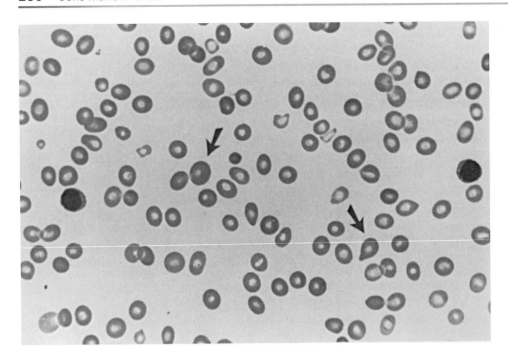

FIGURE 8–3. Peripheral blood from a patient with Fanconi anemia. Note anisocytosis, macrocytes *(arrows)*, thrombocytopenia, and neutropenia. (Courtesy of Dr. Gail Wolfe; with permission from Alter BP: The bone marrow failure syndromes. In Nathan DG, Oski FA (eds): Hematology of Infancy and Childhood, 3rd ed. Philadelphia, WB Saunders, 1987, p 159).

Groups 3 to 6 patients are not transfusion-dependent. Group 3 patients have severe aplasia, which is responding to androgens. Group 4 patients are developing aplasia and are in need of treatment. Group 5 includes patients who have stable disease with mild cytopenias, macrocytosis, or an increased HbF level, whereas Group 6 patients have normal blood counts and no signs of stress erythropoiesis. This classification may permit better interpretation of laboratory information, such as hematopoietic cultures, or other research data of potential relevance.

The red cell survival time is slightly shorter than normal, although hemolysis is not a major component. Ferrokinetics indicate ineffective erythropoiesis as well as relative marrow failure. Dyserythropoiesis has been noted, with fragmentation and multinuclearity. Marrow imaging with ^{99m}Tc sulfur colloid showed paradoxical and irregular tracer distribution in FA that was distinct from the uniform reduction seen in acquired aplastic anemia.[48] This may relate to the varied and irregular development of aplasia in patients with FA. The levels of several red cell enzymes were variably decreased, increased, or normal, reflecting the heterogeneity of red cell ages in the disease.[49–52]

The small size of patients with FA was ascribed to *growth hormone deficiency* in 22 of 28 patients whose growth hormone (GH) was measured.[3, 9, 53–56] Treatment with GH was reported to increase growth in 12 of 15 patients; hematologic improvement did not occur in any. In some families GH deficiency and FA segregated independently. The IFAR recently reported that 44 percent of the patients with FA studied (perhaps self-selected for short stature?) had GH deficiency, while 36 percent were hypothyroid.[57] One of the three patients treated with GH died from acute myelogenous leukemia. The role of recombinant GH in growth and hematopoiesis requires evaluation, and a potential association between GH therapy and leukemia needs careful consideration.[58–60]

The diagnostic laboratory test is chromosome breakage, using metaphase preparations of phytohemagglutinin-stimulated cultured peripheral blood lymphocytes. A high proportion of cells from patients with FA have breaks, gaps, rearrangements, exchanges, and endoreduplications (Fig. 8–4). Although the breakage rate is increased in baseline cultures,[3, 9] it is more dramatically increased when clastogenic agents such as diepoxybutane (DEB) or mitomycin C (MMC) are used (see later). Breakage is uncommon when direct preparations of bone marrow are examined, because cells with significant abnormalities may divide slowly or may not survive *in vivo*. Cultured skin fibroblasts also have abnormal chromosomes. The "spontaneous" aberrations seen in culture may be artifacts, induced by unknown factors in the medium; because marrow cells are not cultured, these abnormalities would not be evident. No apparent relationship exists between hematologic status or clinical course and chromosome findings. Some patients with FA may not have "spontaneous" breaks although breakage results with the use of DEB or MMC are positive. Similar spontaneous but not induced chromosomal changes are seen in Bloom syndrome and ataxia telangiectasia.[61] However, cells from patients with Bloom syndrome show increased sister chromatid exchange after treatment with bromodeoxyuridine, whereas cells from patients with FA do not.[62]

Another approach to the diagnosis of FA involves flow cytometry rather than counting chromosomal aberrations. FA cells grow slowly, owing to the prolongation of the G_2 phase of the cell cycle.[3, 9] Cells treated with alkylating agents fail to divide, but undergo DNA replication and accumulate in the G_2 phase, where they are detected because of the increased amount of DNA they contain.[63–67]

According to the IFAR, FA homozygotes have a mean of 8.96 breaks per cell after culture of blood lymphocytes with DEB, compared with a mean of 0.06 in

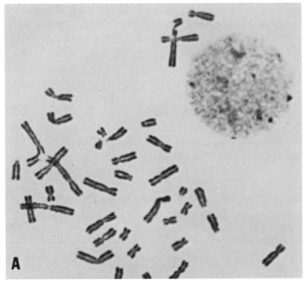

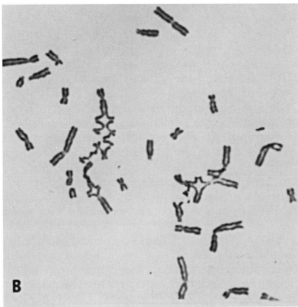

FIGURE 8–4. Cytogenetic findings in peripheral blood lymphocytes in Fanconi anemia. *A,* Spontaneous chromatid breakage. *B,* Multiple breakage following culture with diepoxybutane. (From Auerbach AD, Adler B, Changati RSK: Prenatal and postnatal diagnosis and carrier detection of Fanconi anemia by a cytogenetic method. Pediatrics 1981; 67:128. Copyright American Academy of Pediatrics 1981).

normal subjects.[68] Ten percent of patients in the IFAR had clonal rather than uniform breakage, with breaks in 10 to 40 percent of their cells[69]; others have also observed clonality.[70] Recent reports indicate that clonality is found in approximately 15 percent of patients[71,72] (see later for discussion of somatic mosaicism). The number of breaks seen in cells with breaks remains very high, and fibroblasts show uniform breakage. However, patients remain who have some of the phenotypic features of FA but whose chromosome breakage is not increased with DEB or MMC[10]; do these patients indeed have an extremely clonal variant of FA, or do they have gene mutations that are FA-like?

FA cells are sensitive to simian virus 40 (SV40) viral transformation,[73] ionizing radiation,[74] and alkylating agents.[75] The variety of chemicals includes DEB, nitrogen mustard, MMC, cyclophosphamide, and platinum compounds.[75–80]

Prenatal diagnosis can be done by chorionic villus sampling at 9 to 12 weeks' gestation, amniocentesis at approximately 16 weeks' gestation, or fetal blood sampling by cordocentesis.[68, 81–85] In one series, 10 of 58 chorionic villus and 10 of 64 amniocentesis samples had increased DEB-induced breaks.[86] There was one false-negative diagnosis by chorionic villus sampling, with no confirmatory amniocentesis sample. For the positive samples, the cultured cells grew more slowly. Only one third of the affected patients had physical anomalies, supporting the suggestion that many homozygotes may lack malformations. Increased breakage was reported in two fetuses not known to be at risk for FA.[84, 87] Prenatal diagnosis can now be performed by direct analysis of DNA for known mutations in families in which the genetic defect is known[88] (see later).

Laboratory evaluation of patients in whom FA is suspected should include complete blood counts, red cell size analysis, and HbF measurement. Skeletal radiography and renal ultrasonography can be done if physical anomalies are present or after the diagnosis has been confirmed. The specific test is chromosome breakage, both spontaneous and after clastogenic stress. These tests have identified FA in patients with physical anomalies who were not anemic[89–91] (see Fig. 8–2) and have been used to diagnose FA in patients with aplastic anemia without malformations.[81, 92] Patients with malformations who *may not* have FA also can be identified, and the possibility of their having FA may be excluded. Fanconi "anemia" is redefined to include patients who have the characteristic chromosomal response to clastogenic stress, may have normal physical examinations, and may not have hematologic disease.

FANCONI ANEMIA HETEROZYGOTES

Congenital malformations, particularly anomalies of the genitourinary system and those of the hand, are found more often in relatives of patients with FA (possible heterozygotes).[29] Some parents had physical abnormalities such as short stature without hematologic disease.[36, 93, 94] Petridou and Barrett[94] noted that obligate heterozygotes had increased levels of HbF, decreased natural killer cell counts, and poor responses to mitogens. FA heterozygotes may also be detected as a group by chromosome breakage analysis, but for individuals there is an overlap with the normal range.

PATHOPHYSIOLOGY

The underlying defect in FA is unknown, and the relationship between birth defects, hematopoietic failure, malignancies, and chromosome breakage is elusive. Development of hematopoiesis and the areas generally affected in FA occurs at 25 to 34 days' gestation, and a common toxic insult has been implicated.[42] The FA genotype presumably increases susceptibility to agents that may cause aplastic anemia in "normal" individuals. The oncogenic compounds that damage DNA *in vitro* may also be toxic *in vivo*. This section will provide a brief review of this topic; more details from the older literature can be found elsewhere.[3,11]

Clastogenic agents that cause chromosome breakage include radiation and bifunctional cross-linkers such as MMC, nitrogen mustard, DEB, and cyclophosphamide. Monofunctional agents are not toxic, which suggests that interstrand cross-links cannot be repaired. Table 8–4 lists several of the biochemical defects described in FA; more details can be found elsewhere.[95] The variable and sometimes contradictory results might now be ascribed to the fact that different cell lines were used in each study, and the complementation group and specific mutation of some of these lines have now been identified (see later).

One theory proposes that FA cells are damaged by accumulated oxygen free radicals, which are produced by mutagens such as high oxygen tension, γ-radiation, near-ultraviolet radiation, clastogens, and drugs that generate the reactive hydroxyl radical $HO^{\bullet}$.[125,126] Red cell levels of superoxide dismutase (SOD) were low,[3] whereas the white cell SOD concentrations were normal. Normal levels of red cell SOD, catalase, and glutathione peroxidase were also reported, although the concentration of glutathione transferase was increased. Normal levels of SOD were found in FA fibroblasts, which had increased Mn-SOD, catalase, and glutathione peroxidase concentrations; thus the suggestion was made that oxidant effects may be restricted to the hematopoietic system. The addition of SOD or catalase to FA lymphocyte cultures decreased the numbers of breaks. Other investigators found that SOD, catalase, or cysteine decreased MMC-induced breaks, but in similar proportions in normal and in FA fibroblasts. Culture of lymphocytes in the presence of increased oxygen tension resulted in an increase in the number of spontaneous breaks in some FA cells and not in normal cells and in all FA cells after addition of MMC. SOD increased the survival of FA fibroblasts cultured with MMC. Low oxygen tension or antioxidants were used to improve growth and decrease spontaneous and induced chromosome breaks in FA cells. A handful of patients with FA were treated with intravenous SOD, which resulted in only transient decreases in the number of spontaneous chromosome breaks and, in one patient, in an increase in marrow progenitors.[127,128]

FA cells grow slowly and have a prolonged G_2 phase (see earlier). They are susceptible to transformation by SV40 or adenovirus 12 and express SV40 T antigen.[3] Sister chromatid exchange is generally not increased in FA cells, either spontaneously or after treatment with mutagens. FA cells were found to be hypomutable by *in vitro* cross-linkers, and mutations in FA were primarily deletions, rather than point mutations, as are seen in normal cells.[113,129]

FA cells appear to have a defect in cell cycle regulation. Cell cycle arrest is increased when cells are treated with chemical cross-linkers. G_2 arrest can be corrected by overexpression of one of the cyclin family of proteins, SPHAR, and by caffeine, which activates cyclin-dependent kinase cdc2 and overrides a G_2 checkpoint.[115,130,131] FA cells also demonstrate increased homologous recombination and defective nonhomologous end joining.[132–134]

Hematopoietic Defect. The hematopoietic defect in FA is evident at the progenitor cell level. Colonies from bone marrow colony-forming units–granulocyte-macrophage (CFU-GM), colony-forming units–erythroid (CFU-E), burst-forming units–erythroid (BFU-E), and blood BFU-E, were all decreased in patients with aplastic FA, as they were as in a very small number who did not have aplasia.[47,119,121–123] Only one patient had a level of progenitor cells that was even close to normal.[135] Prospective studies of nonanemic patients with FA may be helpful in prediction of outcome; our results suggest a correlation between erythroid progenitor-derived colonies and clinical status.[47,121] Erythroid colony growth was improved with hematopoietic growth factors, such as stem cell factor (SCF), or with low oxygen,[121] although the effect of SCF was not found in all studies.[136] Although long-term marrow culture stromal layers were formed using bone marrow from patients with FA, Stark et al[122] found that the stroma did not generate CFU-GMs, although Butturini and Gale did find myelopoiesis in long-term marrow cultures.[137] Most of the culture data, however, as well as cures with BMT (see later), suggest a defect in the pluripotent stem cell in FA aplasia. In addition, Segal et al[138] inhibited *in vitro* hematopoiesis in normal cells treated with an antisense oligonucleotide to the *FAC* gene.[138] Although the DNA repair defect is present in all cells, hematopoietic failure happens to be what usually brings the patient to medical attention.

The level of tumor necrosis factor-α (TNF-α) was increased in plasma from FA patients, whereas that of interferon-γ was not.[139] Production of interleukin (IL)–6 was decreased by FA lymphoblasts or fibroblasts,[140–144] although some cell lines did produce increased levels of some cytokines.[144] Addition of IL-6

TABLE 8–4. Cellular Abnormalities in Fanconi Anemia

Feature	References
Spontaneous chromosome breaks	96–102
Sensitivity to cross-linking agents	75–80
Prolongation of G_2 phase of cell cycle	63, 103
SENSITIVITY TO OXYGEN:	
Poor growth at ambient O_2	104
Overproduction of O_2 radicals	105
Deficient O_2 radical defense	106
Deficiency in superoxide dismutase	107, 108
Sensitivity to ionizing radiation during G_2	109
Overproduction of TNF-α	110
DIRECT DEFECTS IN DNA REPAIR:	
Accumulation of DNA adducts	111
Defective repair of DNA cross-links	112
Hypermutability (by deletion)	113
Increased apoptosis	114–116
Abnormal induction of p53	115, 117
INTRINSIC STEM CELL DEFECT:	
Decreased colony growth in vitro	47, 118–123
Decreased gonadal stem cell survival	124

Adapted from D'Andrea AD, Grompe M: Molecular biology of Fanconi anemia: Implications for diagnosis and therapy. Blood 1997; 90:1725.

corrected MMC cytotoxicity.[140] TNF-α was overproduced by lymphoblasts from patients in four complementation groups, the addition of IL-6 decreased the overproduction of TNF-α, and antibodies to TNF-α decreased sensitivity to MMC.[110] SCF production was normal[141] or low,[143, 144] as was that of IL-1,[141] whereas granulocyte-macrophage colony-stimulating factor (GM-CSF) and granulocyte colony-stimulating factor (G-CSF) production was low, variable,[141, 143, 144] or even high.[142] The complementation groups were not known, and thus the cytokine heterogeneity may have a genetic basis.

One study suggested that tumor suppressor p53 was not mutated in 13 patients with FA,[145] although neither p53 expression nor apoptosis—perhaps related events— was induced by radiation.[117] MMC-induced apoptosis was normal in FA, suggesting that apoptosis is not involved in MMC hypersensitivity.[146]

Molecular Studies and Genes for Fanconi Anemia. Co-culture of FA cells with other FA, normal human, or Chinese hamster ovary cells corrected the sensitivity of FA cells to DNA cross-linkers by diffusible factors in some studies but not others.[147] Consistent correction was found in hybrid cells of different complementation groups.[148, 149] Duckworth-Rysiecki et al[150] defined complementation groups A and B, and Digweed et al[151] noted that the reported biochemical variations might be ascribed to such groupings, with those for group A being more severe. These types of complementation analyses have led to identification of eight different complementation groups—A through G, with D containing D1 and D2.[152–154] Table 8–5 provides a summary of the current state of knowledge about the FA (and other bone marrow failure syndrome) genes.

Gene cloning in FA was first described by the Buchwald laboratory. This group cloned the gene for FA complementation group C (*FANCC*) by functional complementation using an Epstein-Barr virus shuttle vector.[155] The complementary DNA has 4566 base pairs, codes for a 558-amino acid protein, and is located at 9q22.3.[156] Normal *FANCC* corrected MMC sensitivity in cells mutant from complementation group C[155]; an antisense oligonucleotide to *FANCC* inhibited growth of normal hematopoietic progenitors[138]; and the hematopoietic growth defect from progenitors of group C patients was corrected with a recombinant adenovirus-associated virus vector.[157]

FANCC is mutated in approximately 10 to 15 percent of patients with FA.[158, 159] A founder mutation common only to Ashkenazi Jews is IVS4 +4 A→T,[160] which is associated with a severe phenotype with multiple birth defects.[158] The occurrence of carriers in Ashkenazi Jews is almost 1 percent, and this mutation was not found in non-Jewish control subjects.[24, 161] However, the same mutation has been reported in Japanese patients with FA who have a mild phenotype, and thus phenotype cannot be inferred from genotype alone.[162] A milder phenotype is also seen in patients with FA of European ancestry who have other *FANCC* mutations, such as 322delG, Q13X, R185X, and D195V.[158, 163]

Six of the FA genes (Table 8–5 and Fig. 8–5) have now been cloned by functional complementation: *FANCA*, *FANCC*, *FANCD2*, *FANCE*, *FANCF*, and *FANCG*,[155, 164–168] and *FANCA* and *FANCD2* were also identified with positional cloning.[165, 169] Only *FANCG* has homology to a previously known gene, *XRCC9*.[170] *FANCB* and *FANCD1*, which complements in group D but is not

TABLE 8–5. Bone Marrow Failure Genes

Disease	Gene	Locus	Genomic DNA	cDNA	Exons	Protein	Amino Acids	Mutations	% of Patients	Genetics
FA	*FANCA*	16q24.3	80	5.5	43	163	1455	≈100	≈70	AR
	FANCB	N/A	—	—	—	—	—	—	Rare	AR
	FANCC	9q22.3	—	4.6	14	63	558	10	≈10	AR
	FANCD1	N/A	—	—	—	—	—	—	Rare	AR
	FANCD2	3p25.3	75	5	44	162	1451	5	Rare	AR
	FANCE	6p21.3	15	2.5	10	60	536	3	≈10	AR
	FANCF	11p15	3	1.3	1	42	374	6	Rare	AR
	FANCG	9p13	6	2.5	14	70	622	18	≈10	AR
DBA	*RPS19*	19q13.3	11	0.4	6	16	145	≈50	25	AD
	?	8p	—	—	—	—	—	—	35	
	Other	N/A	—	—	—	—	—	—	40	
DC	*DKC1*	Xq28	15	2.6	15	57	514	28	60 (males)	XLR
	DKC2 (hTR)	3q26	1704	1704	1	0	0	3	N/A	AD
	DKC3	N/A	—	—	—	—	—	—	N/A	AR
SD	?	7centromere	—	—	—	—	—	—	100	AR
SCN	*ELA2*	19p13.3	5.3	0.9	5	25	240	17	>90	AD
Amega	*mpl*	1p34	17	3.7	12	71	635	16	≈100	AR
TAR	N/A	—	—	—	—	—	—	—		AR

Information from references in text and GenBank. Thanks to Hans Joenje, Indirjeet Dokal, and David Dale for unpublished information.

cDNA = complementary DNA; FA = Fanconi anemia; AR = autosomal recessive; N/A = not available; DBA = Diamond-Blackfan anemia; AD = autosomal dominant; DC = dyskeratosis congenita; XLR = X-linked recessive; SD = Shwachman-Diamond syndrome; SCN = severe congenital neutropenia; Amega = amegakaryocytic thrombocytopenia; TAR = thrombocytopenia absent radii.

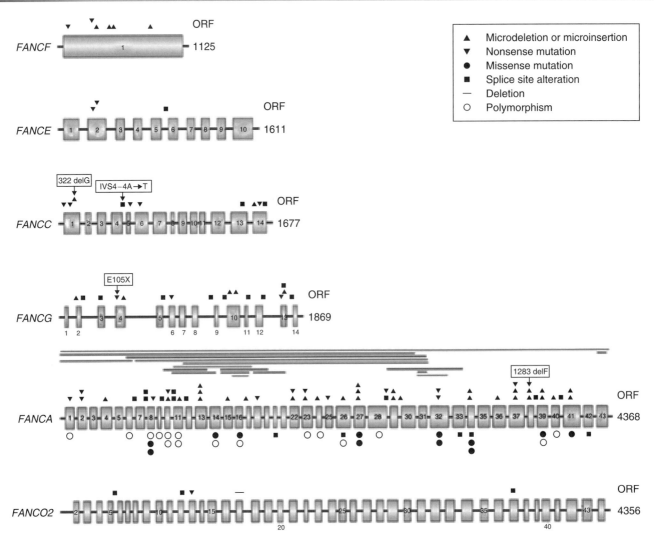

FIGURE 8–5. Mutations in *FANCA, FANCC, FANCD2, FANCE, FANCF,* and *FANCG* as of 2001. Figure shows open reading frames and exons, not to scale. (From Joenje H, Patel KJ: The emerging genetic and molecular basis of Fanconi anaemia. Nat Rev Genet 2:446, 2001.)

FANCD2, remain to be identified. An excellent review article summarizes the details of the FA genes.[171]

A model of the FA protein pathway is presented in Figure 8–6.[171] The similarity of FA patient phenotypes despite their genetic heterogeneity suggested that the FA gene products might interact in a common pathway, either as a complex or in sequence. In fact, the current model incorporates both concepts. The FANCA, FANCC, FANCE, FANCF, and FANCG proteins participate in a large nuclear complex,[167, 172–178] which functions as a ubiquitin ligase for FANCD2.[179] The addition of the 76-amino acid peptide ubiquitin appears to target FANCD2 to nuclear foci that develop during repair of DNA damage. These foci also contain other DNA-damage response proteins, such as BRA1, RAD51, and NBS.[179–181] Because individuals with mutations in other proteins in these foci, such as BRCA1, do not have FA phenotypes, this pathway cannot be the only function for FA proteins.[182, 183] In addition, data are not yet available to determine whether FA homozygotes or heterozygotes have an increased risk for breast cancer. There are also no large systematic investigations of the role of FA proteins in sporadic cancers of the types seen in patients with FA (see later).

FA in a member of the category "caretaker gene diseases" (reviewed in reference 171). These include single-gene diseases such as ataxia telangiectasia mutant in (*ATM*), which is involved in DNA-damage response, and Bloom syndrome, mutant in (*BLM*), involved in DNA unwinding. Other multiple gene syndromes in this category are xeroderma pigmentosum, with seven mutant genes involved in nucleotide excision/transcription-coupled repair; hereditary nonpolyposis colorectal cancer, in which there are five mutant genes relevant to mismatch repair; and hereditary breast/ovarian cancer, with mutations in *BRCA1* and *BRCA2*, involved in DNA-damage response and repair.

The *FANCA* gene is the most common, reported in approximately 70 percent of patients, and also the largest. Most mutations are private, with more than 100 reported to date (see Table 8–5). Except for a founder effect in South African Afrikaners,[184] molecular diagnostics are very complicated in patients with the *FANCA* mutation. There is also a common German mutation in *FANCG*.[185]

Correlation of genotype and phenotype is complicated, and phenotype probably correlates better with the type of mutation (absent versus partial gene product). There was a large study in which 169 patients had mutation analysis

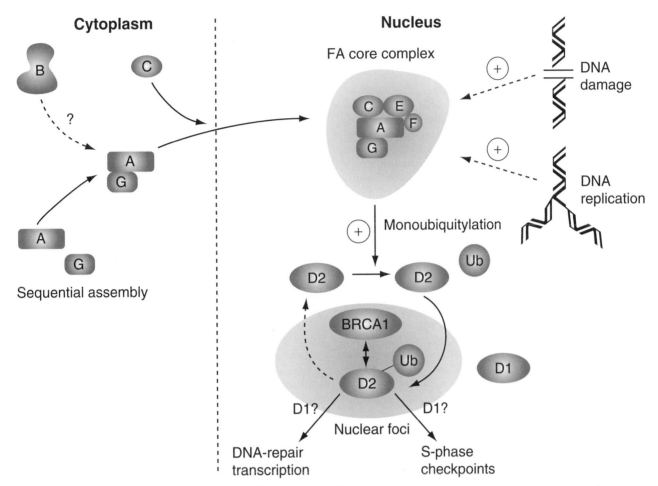

Cytoplasm

Nucleus

FA core complex

?

A
G

A
G

Sequential assembly

DNA damage

DNA replication

C E
A F
G

Monoubiquitylation

D2

D2

Ub

BRCA1

Ub

D2

D1

D1?

D1?

Nuclear foci

DNA-repair transcription

S-phase checkpoints

FIGURE 8–6. A model of the Fanconi anemia pathway. FA proteins assemble into a core complex in the cytoplasm and nucleus. In the presence of the complete complex, FANCD2 is monoubiquitinated during DNA damage repair or replication. Ubiquitinated FANCD2 is targeted to nuclear foci that form in response to DNA damage and that contain BRCA1. (From Joenje H, Patel KJ: The emerging genetic and molecular basis of Fanconi anaemia. Nat Rev Genet 2:446, 2001.)

and an additional 76 patients had complementation assignments by cell fusion or Western blotting.[186] Patients with the *FANCG* mutation had more severe cytopenia and increased leukemia, and somatic abnormalities were more common in patients with *FANCD*, *FANCE*, and *FANCF* mutations. However, patients who were homozygous for null mutations developed anemia sooner and had a higher incidence of leukemia. As mentioned above, patients with the *FANCC* IVS4 + 4A→T mutation developed aplastic anemia sooner and had more somatic abnormalities than those with 322delG mutations in the same gene.

Knockout mouse models for FA have been made for *FANCC* and *FANCA* mutations, but all exhibit only a partial phenotype.[124, 187, 188] The mice have decreased fertility owing to impaired germ cell formation, but lack somatic abnormalities and have normal hematopoiesis and no increase in cancer risk. Cells from *FANCC* –/– mice were sensitive to MMC *in vitro*,[189, 190] and bone marrow cells from +/+ mice had a growth advantage in –/– recipients, which was facilitated by MMC treatment of the recipients.[191] *FANCC* –/– mice also had decreased numbers of CD34+ stem and progenitor cells.[191, 192]

Gene therapy has been proposed as a method for treatment of bone marrow deficiency in patients with FA.

Patient bone marrow would be treated *in vitro* with normal FA genes and then reinfused. The selective growth advantage of normal cells in mutant mice and the ability to correct the FA phenotype of mutant cells with retroviruses containing normal FA genes provide precedents for this hypothesis. However, in a single human phase 1 gene therapy trial, the only one of four patients with FA who had a detectable *FANCC* transgene was receiving radiation therapy for a concurrent malignancy.[193] Many problems and risks are associated with gene therapy. Current methods for transduction of hematopoietic stem cells with retroviruses or lentiviruses are inefficient. Rescue of a premalignant cell might actually increase the risk of leukemic transformation. Expression of a foreign FA protein in an FA null individual might become antigenic. As for BMT, gene therapy of hematopoietic stem cells will at best cure only the bone marrow, and none of the other features of FA, including the risk of cancer (see later).

Somatic mosaicism was implied by the observation that up to 15 percent of patients with FA had clonal chromosome breakage, but a large proportion of cells did not have breaks.[72, 194] The molecular mechanisms for this phenomenon include mitotic recombination, compensatory frameshifts, gene conversion, and gene reversion.[95, 195]

Mosaicism may occur in rapidly renewing hematopoietic stem cells, and there may be false-negative diagnoses of FA by analysis of peripheral blood cells. However, chromosome breaks can be identified in skin fibroblast cultures, and FA gene mutations can be found in germline cells. Mosaicism may lead to problems with bone marrow engraftment in patients with mosaic gene-corrected T cells, which resist ablation, and ultimately lead to graft rejection.[196]

Preimplantation genetic diagnosis has now been performed successfully to treat a severely affected child in a family with the *FANCC* IVS4 + 4A→T mutation.[197] *In vitro* fertilization was performed to create a subsequent sibling. Biopsies were done on single blastomeres from day 3 embryos. Single-cell nested polymerase chain reactions were used to amplify the *FANCC* and the *HLA* genes. Four maternal ovulatory cycles were required, leading to 33 embryos, of which 30 could be analyzed. Nineteen were heterozygous carriers of FA, 6 were homozygous affected, and 5 were homozygous normal. Five of the heterozygotes were HLA matches to the patient. Implantation was accomplished with a single embryo from the last cycle, resulting in a newborn whose cord blood was recovered and used successfully for hematopoietic reconstitution of the patient. The donor was named "Adam," because his bone marrow led to life for his sister.[198] The successful use of this technique raises many ethical and moral questions that cannot be addressed here, but it does provide technical proof of the principle.

THERAPY AND OUTCOME

Prognosis. The cumulative survival for the patients with FA reported in the literature by decades is shown in Figure 8–7 and summarized in Table 8–6. The predicted median age of survival for all patients is 20 years; 25 percent are projected to live beyond age 31. The median survival age improved from 13 years for those reported before 1960 to 30 years for those reported within the past 10 years. When the only treatment option was blood transfusions, 80 percent of patients died within 2 years after the onset of aplastic anemia,[199] and almost all died within 4 years, with extended survival occurring only rarely.[200, 201] Overall, survival was much shorter for those in whom FA was diagnosed very early in life, who presumably had more severe birth defects, compared with adults in whom FA was diagnosed. The respective cumulative median ages of survival are 5 and 30 years.

Older Patients. Older females with FA have delayed menarche, irregular menses, and early menopause, resulting in the possibility of hypoestrogenemia and osteoporosis. Among the more than 100 females with FA cited in the literature or reported to the IFAR who reached at least 16 years of age, more than 20 have been pregnant.[3, 202-205] FA was diagnosed before pregnancy in less than half of the women; in the others FA was diagnosed during pregnancy or after delivery. Thirty pregnancies resulted in 21 living infants, as well as a large number of miscarriages. Nine patients required red cell transfusions, six needed platelet transfusions during the pregnancies or at delivery, six had cesarean sections for failure of labor to progress, and four had preeclampsia or eclampsia. Pregnancy in a woman with FA has complications, but these can be managed with high-risk obstetric and hematologic care. None of the mothers with FA died peripartum; although 10 died later at ages 24 to 45, 7 of the deaths were attributed to malignancies and 3 to complications of pancytopenia.

Older males with FA are small, with underdeveloped gonads and abnormal spermatogenesis.[206] Four FA males with FA were reported to be fathers.[20, 202, 207]

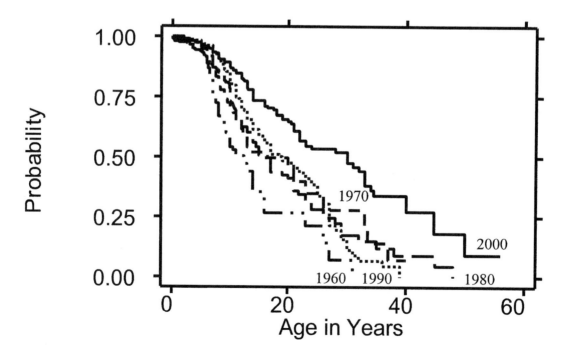

FIGURE 8–7. Kaplan-Meier plot of cumulative survival in patients with Fanconi anemia. Time is shown as age in years. −▪▪− = 118 patients reported from 1927 to 1960; - - - - = 117 patients reported from 1961 to 1970; − − − = 254 patients reported from 1971 to 1980; ▪▪▪▪▪ = 314 patients reported from 1981 to 1990; —— = 331 patients reported from 1991 to 2000. Differences are significant.

TABLE 8–6. Projected Survival Ages of Patients with Fanconi Anemia*

	Age (yrs)	
Group	50%	25%
All	20	31
Male	18	29
Female	21	33
1927–1960	13	23
1961–1970	17	33
1971–1980	16	26
1981–1990	19	27
1991–2000	30	45
Leukemia	16	22
Myelodysplastic syndrome	22	32
Solid tumor	31	36
Liver tumor	14	23
No cancer	19	33
Diagnosis ≤1 yr	5	11
Diagnosis ≥16 yrs	30	45

*Survivals are determined from Kaplan-Meier estimates: 50% means the median projected survival age; 25% means the projected survival age for 25% of patients.

Fewer than 5 percent of the males who reached age 16 were reported to be fathers, but this figure may be low because paternity is less often noted in medical histories than is maternity. Several males whose diagnosis of FA was made when they were adults did have a prior history of infertility.

Androgen Therapy. Treatment is recommended for patients with significant cytopenias, indicated by a hemoglobin level less than 8 g/dL, platelet count less than 30,000/μL, or neutrophil count less than 500/μL. Those who have an HLA-matched sibling donor for BMT have that option (see later), whereas the majority of patients with FA require medical intervention. The mechanism of action of androgens was reviewed extensively by Gardner and Besa.[208] Androgens increase erythropoietin production,[209] stimulate erythroid stem cells,[210] and increase hemoglobin levels in normal males at puberty, and in patients treated for arthritis, breast cancer, or old age. Androgen therapy for FA was initiated by Shahidi and Diamond in 1959,[211,212] who saw improvement in their first six patients. In larger series, Sanchez-Medal[213] and Najean[214] found that 75 percent of patients showed some degree of initial response. Responses usually begin with reticulocytosis, with an increase in hemoglobin level occurring within 1 to 2 months. White cell counts may increase next, whereas the platelet response is usually incomplete and may take 6 to 12 months to reach its maximum.

Almost all patients have a relapse when androgen therapy is stopped, and in fewer than 12 has treatment been discontinued successfully, often at the time of puberty.[3] Many eventually show resistance to the specific androgen they were receiving, and changing to another androgen has only occasionally provided another response. Later complications such as cancer may be seen in some because their life expectancy has been extended by androgens (see later).

Although some reports suggest that the use of androgens alone is as effective as the use of androgens combined with corticosteroids,[214] the general recommendation is that combination therapy be administered. Growth acceleration from androgens may be counterbalanced by growth retardation from corticosteroids.[215] Use of corticosteroids may also decrease bleeding at a given platelet count, perhaps by promoting vascular stability.[216] The androgen used most often is oxymetholone, an oral 17-α alkylated androgen, at 2 to 5 mg/kg/day. Prednisone is used at 5 to 10 mg every other day. If an injectable androgen is desired because of decreased risk of hepatotoxicity, the usual form is nandrolone decanoate, 1 to 2 mg/kg/wk, intramuscularly; ice packs and pressure are used to prevent hematomas.

The first sign of response to androgens may be the appearance of macrocytic red cells and an increase in the proportion of red cells containing HbF. The hemoglobin response is often seen within the first 2 to 3 months of treatment. Platelet counts may rise subsequently, and the neutrophil response, if it occurs, may be the last to appear. We recommend a trial of up to 6 months in patients who show no apparent response before a decision is made that androgens may not be effective.

Side effects of androgens include masculinization, with hirsutism as well as male-pattern baldness, deepening of the voice, enlargement of the genitalia, acne, flushing, mood swings, fluid retention, stimulation of the appetite with weight gain, and increased muscle bulk, as well as increased skeletal maturation with a growth spurt followed by growth plate fusion and thus ultimately short stature. Many of these are features of male puberty. Some of these side effects are reversed by dose reduction or discontinuation of the treatment. More serious outcomes include hepatomegaly, cholestatic jaundice, and elevated liver enzyme levels, but these are also usually reversible. The most extreme problems are peliosis hepatis, liver adenomas, and hepatocellular carcinomas (see later), but these too may resolve when androgen therapy is stopped. Patients receiving androgens should be monitored often with liver chemistry studies and ultrasound. Patients who have a response should have their androgen dose tapered very slowly but probably not discontinued. The only group of patients in whom discontinuation might be considered is the South African Afrikaners, who may have genetic distinctions.[217] In most of the experiences elsewhere, relapses occur when androgens are stopped, and subsequent remissions in patients receiving the same or a different preparation are sometimes elusive. However, there are some patients in whom androgens can be discontinued. Perhaps these are the patients who develop hematopoietic somatic mosaicism, with a "normal" stem cell, which has a selective growth advantage.

Hematopoietic Stem Cell Transplantation. Stem cell transplant offers the only possibility of cure for aplastic anemia in patients with FA and possibly a cure for or prevention of leukemia. There is a risk, however, that chemotherapy or irradiation may accelerate the appearance of secondary malignancies (see later). Several hundred transplants have now been done in patients with FA, using primarily bone marrow or cord blood as the source of stem cells. Survival is markedly better when the donor is an HLA-matched sibling than when an alternative donor, who is unrelated or is a mismatched family member, is used (e.g., 66 percent versus 29 percent in a review from the International Bone Marrow Transplant Registry) (Fig. 8–8).[218, 219]

Results of early transplants for which standard doses of cyclophosphamide were used as preparation were poor.[220, 221] Studies showing that a metabolite of cyclophosphamide is toxic to FA cells[76, 222] explained the commonly seen clinical symptoms of severe mucositis with intestinal malabsorption and hemorrhages, fluid retention, cardiac failure, and hemorrhagic cystitis.[223] Various other protocols included procarbazine, antithymocyte globulin, and fractionated total lymphoid irradiation or thoracoabdominal radiation, and T-cell depletion[3, 221, 224–226]; 66 percent survived. The cyclophosphamide dose may be reduced to 20 mg/kg divided over 4 days with the addition of 5 Gy of thoracoabdominal radiation.[223, 227] The cumulative survival with this protocol is approximately 70 percent.[218, 228] Nonmyeloablative protocols are now being introduced; these combine fludarabine with low-dose cyclophosphamide.[229, 230] However, there is a possibility of incomplete mixed chimerism with residual FA marrow cells, which might have a potential for malignancy.

Many patients do not have an HLA-compatible sibling. There is some parental sharing of haplotypes, leading to an unexpectedly high rate of HLA identity between patients and parents, who may be used as donors.[231, 232] Partially mismatched family members were donors for 10 patients[3, 226, 233] in whom the modified cyclophosphamide-thoracoabdominal radiation preparation was used. Five of these patients survived. The use of unrelated computer-matched donors was recorded in 12 patients; 5 of these survived.[3, 233, 234] All of these patients who received mismatched transplants are particularly at risk for rejection or for graft-versus-host disease. Improved matching resulting from the use of molecular tools for HLA genotyping may decrease the risks of "mismatched" transplants.[235] T-cell depletion was found to reduce the incidence of acute graft-versus-host disease, but it increased the risk of graft failure, with no net survival advantage.[219] Results were better with matched unrelated donors than with mismatched relatives.[228]

HLA-matched sibling donors need to be screened for occult FA homozygosity with thorough physical examinations, complete blood counts (including determination of red cell size and HbF level), and clastogen-induced chromosome breakage. In one unsuccessful transplant, the donor had undiagnosed FA.[236]

Umbilical cord blood contains hematopoietic progenitor cells and can be cryopreserved from a sibling identified *in utero* to not have FA for use in later transplantation.[237–240] Transplants from cord blood of unrelated donors are not as successful.[228, 241] The ultimate example of cord blood donation is the case described previously in which preimplantation genetic diagnosis was used.

Patients with FA who have an HLA-matched sibling donor might receive a transplant as soon as cytopenias warrant intervention (described earlier in the section on androgens). However, patients for whom a high-risk transplant from an alternative donor is planned might benefit from androgens, G-CSF, and supportive care. Unrelated or mismatched transplants should be considered only for patients with rapidly progressive disease caused by unmanageable aplastic anemia, severe myelodysplastic syndrome, or leukemia. In these patients the ratio of risk to benefit is on the side of the potential benefit.

Other Treatment. Supportive care must be provided as for any patient with aplastic anemia. ε-Aminocaproic acid, at 0.1 g/kg every 6 hours orally, may be used for symptomatic bleeding. No family member should be used as a blood product donor until it has been determined that a transplant will not be performed (even from an unrelated donor); this approach decreases the chance of sensitization. Leukocyte-filtered blood products should be used to reduce reactions and HLA sensitization from white cells. The possibility of BMT must be considered early. Although use of androgens and transfusions do not

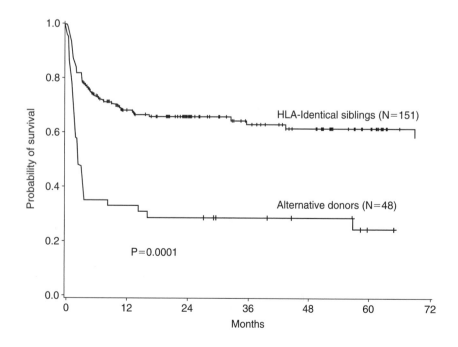

FIGURE 8–8. Kaplan-Meier plot of cumulative survival after bone marrow transplantation (BMT) for patients with Fanconi anemia. Time is shown as months from transplantation. Transplants were from HLA-identical siblings for 151 patients and from alternative donors for 48 patients. (From Gluckman E, Auerbach AD, Horowitz MM, et al. Bone marrow transplantation for Fanconi anemia. Blood 86:2856, 1995).

preclude BMT, the best results are in those with minimal medical complications. Drugs and chemicals that may be implicated as causing acquired aplastic anemia should be avoided. Medications that interfere with platelet function should not be given to thrombocytopenic patients; such medications include aspirin, antihistamines, nonsteroidal anti-inflammatory drugs, glycerol guaiacolate, vitamin E, and cod liver oil. However, if a severe allergic reaction occurs during a blood transfusion, diphenhydramine (Benadryl) can be used acutely.

Splenectomy is not indicated unless hypersplenism is clearly present. More than 40 patients were reported to have had splenectomy, resulting in no apparent long-term benefit. There was some transient improvement of pancytopenia, but at a time when the bone marrow was not yet hypocellular.[3]

The use of so-called immunotherapy has no basis. Although high-dose methylprednisolone,[242] antithymoxite globulin,[243] and cyclosporine have been used in patients with FA, there is a striking lack of success, particularly in unreported cases. Approximately 10 percent of adults in whom any of these immunomodulatory approaches failed to produce a response were shown subsequently to have previously undiagnosed FA by clastogenic stress–induced chromosome breakage studies.★

The use of lithium was reported to improve the blood counts in two of five patients with FA, presumably in those whose marrow reserve was still present.[244]

The use of hematopoietic growth factors is an area of current investigation. GM-CSF at 2.5 to 10 μg/kg/day was used in 10 patients; in 8 of these absolute neutrophil counts improved, but there was no impact on hemoglobin or platelet counts.[245–247] G-CSF given at 2.5 to 5 μg/kg/day or every other day increased the absolute neutrophil counts in 10 of 10 patients; increased hemoglobin levels were seen in 4 of these patients and increased platelet counts in 3.[248] However, use of such factors may also predispose patients to development of leukemia or hasten evolution to myelodysplastic syndrome or monosomy 7.[249, 250] Growth factors should only be used in patients with severe neutropenia, and monitoring should be done with periodic blood counts, bone marrow examinations, and marrow cytogenetic studies.

COMPLICATIONS

The *in vitro* data regarding defects in DNA repair and cellular damage suggest that FA might be a premalignant condition; this conjecture is borne out by the *in vivo* observations. More than 200 leukemias and tumors have been reported, for an overall incidence of greater than 15 percent. Because this incidence figure reflects the biased reporting of interesting cases, the true figure may be different, and thus long-term prospective analysis is needed. Among 388 patients registered by 1994, 60 (15 percent) had leukemia or myelodysplastic syndrome (MDS) (the numbers were not reported separately); solid tumors were not described.[251] At this time a detailed literature review has identified more than 100 patients with leukemia, approximately 60 with 70 solid tumors, and more than 30 with liver tumors (Table 8–7). Up to 25 percent never had aplastic anemia, and approximately half never received androgens before ascertainment of a malignant disorder.

Even a single gene for FA (heterozygosity) was thought to confer a risk of malignancy. Garriga and Crosby[252] found an increased incidence of leukemia in families with FA, and Swift[253,254] reported a predisposition to cancer in heterozygotes. These analyses were later extended from the original 8 families to 25 by Swift and colleagues,[255] and to 15 by Potter et al[256]; both groups found no increase in cancer. (Another disorder thought to occur more often in FA heterozygotes is diabetes mellitus[257, 258]). The earlier and perhaps erroneous conclusions were attributed to small numbers, incorrect assignment of heterozygotes, and biased selection. However, the question of cancer risk in FA heterozygotes should be reexamined in larger numbers in the future.

TABLE 8–7. Complications in Fanconi Anemia

	All	Leukemia	MDS	Solid Tumor	Liver Tumor
No. of patients	1206	103	74	59	34
Percentage of total	100	8.5	6.1	4.9	2.8
Male/female ratio	1.24	1.51	1.06	0.37	1.43
Age at diagnosis of FA (yrs)					
Mean	8.4	10.4	11.5	13.2	9.4
Median	7	9	9.5	9.5	7
Range	0–48	0.13–28	0.3–43	0.1–44	3–48
Age at complication (yrs)					
Mean	—	14.5	15.9	23.4	16.1
Median	—	13.8	14	26	13
Range	—	0.13–29	1.8–43	0.3–45	6–48
No. reported deceased	455	73	37	35	27
Percentage reported deceased	38	71	50	59	79
Projected median survival (yrs)	20	16	22	31	14

MDS = myelodysplastic syndrome.

★Auerbach AD, Young NS: unpublished data.

Leukemia. Leukemia was reported in more than 100 patients, representing almost 10 percent of the patients with FA in the literature. In one series of 44 patients, 9 developed leukemia (20 percent) and 5 more were preleukemic.[259] In 25 percent FA was diagnosed only when they were seen with leukemia without a preceding aplastic anemia. Approximately one third never received androgens, and thus androgens cannot be considered causative. A report cites two patients who were seen with acute myelomonocytic leukemia in whom the diagnosis of FA was not made until after BMT, when they developed toxicity from the procedure. In retrospect, these patients had increased chromosome breakage.[260]

The characteristics of the leukemic patients are summarized in Table 8–7, and the types of leukemia are shown in Table 8–8. The male-to-female ratio of occurrence is 1.5. FA was diagnosed at a median age of 9 years. This age is significantly older than the median age of 7 years in those with FA who did not develop leukemia, and leukemia itself was diagnosed at a median age of 14 years. The proportion of patients older than 16 years at diagnosis was higher in the leukemic group (16 percent compared with 9 percent of the total) and includes 10 patients in their 20s whose FA was first diagnosed when they were seen with leukemia (Fig. 8–9).

Because the most common leukemia in children is lymphocytic, it is noteworthy that until 1989 all leukemias were myeloid. Five patients with acute lymphoblastic leukemia have now been reported, but the majority of leukemias remain in the myeloid series (Table 8–8). Several patients were discussed in more than one publication, and thus the number of literature reports exceeds the actual number of cases. Five patients with leukemia had coincidental hepatic tumors discovered post mortem,[272, 281, 294, 323, 326] and one had an astrocytoma.[288]

Treatment of the leukemia was less than satisfactory, and deaths occurred on average within the first 2 months after diagnosis. Patients with FA and leukemia are exquis-itely sensitive to the toxic effects of chemotherapy, as predicted by the earlier discussion regarding agents that increase damage to DNA. The combination of leukemias that are difficult to treat (i.e., myeloid), abnormal DNA repair, and lack of marrow reserve does not provide a good prognosis. Long-term remissions are very rare.[304, 305, 317, 320,*] BMT from an unrelated donor was attempted unsuccessfully in one patient.[327] The median age of survival for those with leukemia is 16 years, not much different from the median age at diagnosis of leukemia and reflecting the high early mortality rate. More than 70 percent of those with leukemia had died by the time of the reports, and follow-up was not available for most of the rest. Will all patients develop leukemia if they do not die from aplastic anemia first? This is probably not so, because older patients have the additional risk of developing other malignancies (see later). However, only results of long-term prospective studies will answer this question properly.

Myelodysplastic Syndrome. Several patients with FA had syndromes that were called "myelodysplastic," "refractory anemia," or "preleukemia." Some of these patients developed full-blown leukemia, whereas others died or were reported on only when their disease was in the preleukemic phase. Cross-sectional studies suggest that the risk of MDS is between 10 and 35 percent.[248, 251, 259, 328] The definition of MDS within the context of FA has not been clarified and ranges from bone marrow morphologic features that meet the criteria for MDS according to the French-American-British (FAB) classification[329] to inclusion of patients with marrow cytogenetic clones and no other features of MDS. Specific types of clones have been associated with a poor prognosis within the FAB group, according to an international scoring system.[330] However, MDS in patients with FA requires clarification. In a recent systematic analysis of more than 40 patients with FA, we found a cytogenetic clone in half of these, with clonal variation

TABLE 8–8. Leukemia in Fanconi Anemia

Leukemia	Male	Female	All Patients	References
ALL	3	2	5	261–265
AML	23	14	37	36, 229, 259, 266–287*
AML M1 (acute myelocytic without maturation)	1	1	2	288, 289
AML M2 (acute myelocytic with maturation)	2	2	4	280, 290, 291
AML M3 (acute promyelocytic)	0	0	0	
AML M4 (acute myelomonocytic)	12	8	20	20, 99, 102, 292–305†
AML M5 (acute monocytic)	6	4	10	35, 285, 306–312
AML M6 (erythroleukemia)	5	2	7	266, 313–316
AML M7 (acute megakaryocytic)	1	0	1	319
AML ANLL (acute nonlymphocytic)	1	5	6	240, 312, 318–320
Other acute leukemia	8	3	11	20, 39, 259, 311, 321–325
Total	62	41	103	

*Gardner FH: Unpublished observations, 1994.
†Lux S: Unpublished observations, 1994.
ALL = acute lymphocytic; AML = acute myeloid, unspecified.

*Roozendaal KJ: personal communication, 1989.

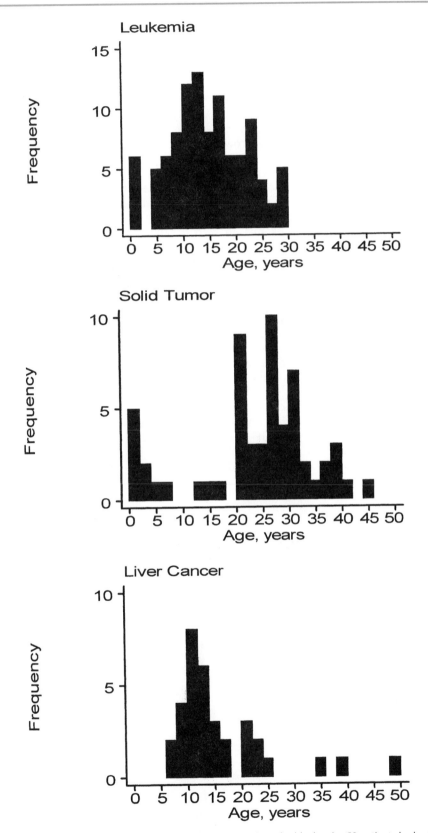

FIGURE 8–9. Age at diagnosis of cancer in patients with Fanconi anemia: 94 patients had leukemia, 60 patients had solid tumors, and 28 patients had liver cancer. Age when complications occurred was not reported for all patients with those diagnoses.

often seen over time, which included disappearance of the clone or emergence of a new and independent clone.[328] One third of the patients had morphologic

MDS, and poor outcome correlated with the presence of severe cytopenias resulting from MDS and was independent of clonality. Patients with clones have survived for more than 12 years, without development of morphologic MDS or leukemia. The clones seen most often involved chromosomes 1 and 7, but many others were involved, with partial or complete deletions, translocations, and marker chromosomes. Further cytogenetic details can be found elsewhere.[281, 284, 328, 331] Among patients with FA and leukemia, less than 10 percent had prior MDS, and in those the interval from MDS to development of leukemia was within 18 months. Marrow cytogenetic clonal assays will benefit in the future from techniques that are more sensitive than classic Giemsa banding, such as fluorescence in situ hybridization.[332] In one study, mutations were not found in N-*ras* nor *p53* oncogenes.[333]

Whether MDS inevitably evolves into leukemia in patients with FA is not known. Because patients with MDS are slightly older than those with leukemia and the median age of survival is higher in the MDS group (see Table 8–7), it is not obvious that MDS is in fact "preleukemia." Future prospective studies are required, with serial monitoring of bone marrow cytogenetics and morphologic changes, to resolve this question. It is an important issue, however, because high-risk stem cell transplants from alternative donors might not necessarily be performed for MDS per se, unless there is good evidence of its transformation into leukemia.

Three patients had Sweet syndrome (acute neutrophilic infiltration of skin, which is associated with malignancy in 20 percent of patients[334]). All had myelodysplastic bone marrows, and two had clonal chromosome abnormalities. The skin infiltrates responded to prednisone, but sustained treatment was required. This differs from responses in patients with Sweet syndrome who do not have FA, in whom permanent resolution of symptoms may occur.

Solid Tumors. In 59 patients (5 percent) a total of 70 cancers other than leukemia or liver were reported (Tables 8–7 and 8–9 and Fig. 8–9). The group with cancer differs from the entire population of FA patients in several categories. There is a large number of females, reflecting the common occurrence of gynecologic malignancies. The median age at diagnosis of FA was 9.5 years in the group with cancer, with 30 percent being 16 years or older when FA was diagnosed. Approximately 20 percent did not have a preceding aplastic anemia or diagnosis of FA. More than 80 percent of the tumors developed in patients who were at least 20 years of age, and the median age was 26 years, much younger than the age of occurrence of the same types of tumors in the general population.[335]

Most of the tumors were squamous cell, and their locations ranged from the oropharynx to the anus (see Table 8–8). One third were found in the oral cavity or oropharynx, including tumors of the tongue, gingiva, pharynx, larynx, epiglottis, and mandible. One fourth were gynecologic, including vulvar, cervical, and breast tumors. All four patients with brain tumors were younger than 5 years of age. Three patients also had acute myeloid leukemia.[270, 288, 290] Eleven patients had more than one primary cancer, including two with liver tumors.[350, 357] In several patients, more than one area was involved, and it was not always clear which was the primary tumor. A few patients were reported more than once, further

TABLE 8–9. Solid Tumors in Fanconi Anemia

Type	Male	Female	All Patients	References
NONHEPATIC				
Oropharynx	10	12	22	202, 269, 294, 307, 336–353
Esophagus	1	8	9	40, 336, 354–361
Vulva and anus	—	4	4	97, 300, 338, 362
Vulva	—	5	5	342, 363–365
Anus	—	2	2	202, 366
Cervix	—	3	3	270, 362, 363
Brain	1	3	4	12, 288, 367
Skin (nonmelanoma)	0	5	5	202, 280, 285, 366, 368
Breast	—	4	4	202, 369–371
Lung	2	0	2	20, 194
Lymphoma	1	1	2	372, 373
Gastric	2	0	2	374, 375
Renal	0	3	3	202, 367, 376, 377
Colon	0	1	1	300
Osteogenic sarcoma	0	1	1	378
Retinoblastoma	0	1	1	290
Total Cancers	17	53	70	
Total Patients	16	43	59	
HEPATIC				
Adenoma	6	5	11	203, 322, 379–385
Hepatoma	14	8	22	269, 272, 281, 294, 326, 349, 350, 357, 386–402
Not stated	0	1	1	203, 382
Total Liver Tumors	20	14	34	

complicating the identification of the actual number of patients with tumors.

The median age at onset of solid tumors of 26 years and the median projected survival age of 31 years (see Tables 8–7 and 8–9) show that cancer is a disease of "older" patients with FA, who did not die first from aplastic anemia, leukemia, or liver disease. By age 31, more than 75 percent of all of the patients with FA reported in the literature had already died. Cancer treatment is difficult in patients with FA, because of increased toxicity from chemotherapy or radiation. Surgery is performed whenever possible. Recommended surveillance for cancers·includes gynecologic examinations and Pap smears, rectal examinations, and periodic dental and oropharyngeal evaluations.

Because risk of tumors may be increased after stem cell transplantation caused by immunosuppression, graft-versus-host disease, and increased occurrence of infections from viruses, such as human papilloma virus, these tumors require separate analysis. There are at least eight reported patients (some reported more than once) between 11 and 33 years of age who had tongue cancer diagnosed at 3 to 15 years after BMT.[188, 203, 403–410] The actuarial incidence of cancers after transplant for all indications, not just FA, was 13 percent at 15 years, with a 10-fold increase in oral and esophageal cancers.[411] Thus, the combination of FA and transplant might be expected to lead to an even higher predisposition for cancer. Head and neck cancer was observed in 6 patients in a series of 50 patients with FA who had transplants; the projected incidence is 24 percent at 8 years, supporting this prediction.[412]

Liver Tumors. Liver disease was reported in almost 50 patients, with 34 patients having liver tumors (3 percent). The male-to-female ratio of occurrence was 1.4, and the median age at diagnosis of FA was 7 years, similar to that of the general population with FA (see Table 8–6). The median age at which the liver tumors were identified was 13 years, with a wide range (see Table 8–7 and Fig. 8–9). Only one patient did not have preceding androgen treatment,[389] and thus it is likely that androgen treatment increases the risk of liver disease in patients with FA. Of the tumors, 22 were called "hepatocellular carcinomas" or "hepatomas." In two patients these were called "benign." Two patients also had adenomas, and only one patient (the only one who also had an increased α-fetoprotein level) had metastases. Eleven adenomas were reported, and one tumor type was not specified. One of the adenomas had metastasized. One might speculate that the distinction between adenoma and hepatoma is not entirely clear, just as the interpretation of bone marrow as myelodysplastic is at times subjective. One patient also had tongue cancer,[350] one had esophageal cancer,[357] and five had leukemia.[272, 281, 294, 322, 326] In at least four patients the liver tumors were found only at postmortem examination.[384, 394, 396, 402] One patient had unexplained hepatic coma.[20] Several patients had peliosis hepatis (blood lakes), alone or with tumors.

Discontinuation of therapy with androgens, either alone or in combination with BMT, often led to resolution of the tumors or peliosis.[382, 393] Surgical removal of tumors was undertaken occasionally. The prognosis for these patients was very poor, and the majority had died by

the time of the reports. However, the deaths were usually not due to the liver tumors, but rather to the underlying hematologic conditions.

Summary of Malignancy in Fanconi Anemia. The absolute risk of patients with FA developing leukemia, liver tumor, or other cancer is at least 15 percent in the literature, although the true incidence may be obscured by over- or under-reporting. The risk of malignancy is particularly increased in older patients. Prolongation of survival by a combination of androgen therapy, better supportive care, BMT, and perhaps gene therapy may provide more time for malignancies to appear. In addition, FA may be diagnosed by chromosome breakage analysis in patients with malignancies but without any other stigmata of FA. Concerns about the development of malignancies in older patients should not be considered as contraindications to aggressive management, such as BMT, although cytoreductive chemotherapy and irradiation themselves may also increase the risk of malignancies. To some degree, aplastic anemia may now be considered to be the least of the problems of the patient with FA, who is also at risk for development of liver and other solid tumors, leukemia, and MDS.

Dyskeratosis Congenita

DESCRIPTION

Dyskeratosis congenita (DC; also known as *Zinsser-Cole-Engman syndrome*) is a rare form of ectodermal dysplasia. Dermatologic manifestations and nail dystrophies begin in the first decade and leukoplakia begins in the second decade; these become more extreme with increasing age. The diagnostic triad includes reticulated hyperpigmentation of the face, neck, and shoulders; dystrophic nails; and mucous membrane leukoplakia (Fig. 8–10). Aplastic anemia occurs in one half the patients with DC, usually in the second decade, and cancer develops in 10 percent in the third and fourth decades.

Inheritance and Environment. More than 275 single patients have been reported, representing all ethnic groups.[413, 414] Dokal[415] recently reviewed 148 patients from the experience at Hammersmith Hospital. Despite the general impression that DC is an X-linked recessive disorder, the male-to-female ratio of occurrence is 4.5:1. In fact, DC appears to have three patterns of inheritance (Table 8–10):

1. *Presumed X-linked recessive.* More than 200 patients, including single-case males, male sibling pairs, uncle-nephew families, and males with maternal male cousins have been reported.
2. *Autosomal recessive.* In this group are 44 patients including females with sporadic inheritance, consanguineous families, and brother-sister sets.
3. *Autosomal dominant.* Seven families had two or three generations of males and females, with passage through both sexes and consanguinity in one.

The apparently autosomal appearance in families might in fact be X-linked inheritance with X-inactivation, but this is less likely than the model of three different genes producing similar phenotypes. The X-linked recessive

A

B

C

D

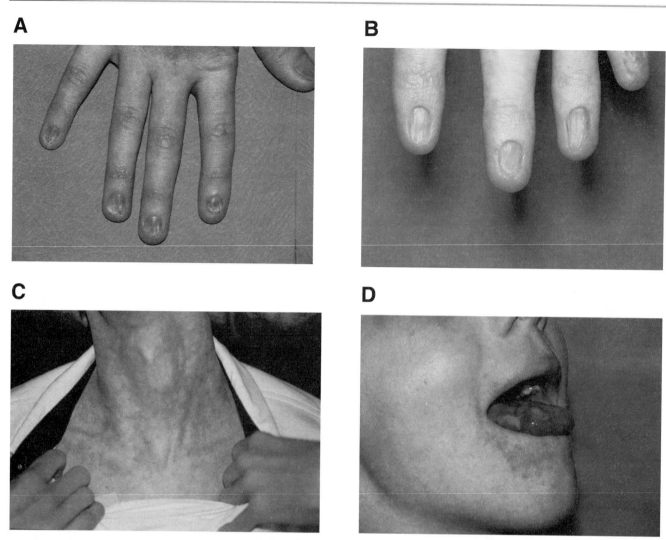

FIGURE 8–10. Physical findings in patients with dyskeratosis congenita. *A, B:* Dystrophic fingernails in two different patients. *C,* Lacy reticular pigmentation. *D,* Leukoplakia on tongue.

group might also include sporadic inheritance in males who actually have autosomal mutations. X-linked inheritance in some males may now be identified with Xq28 restriction fragment length polymorphisms and mutation analyses.[415, 416] There are white, black, and Asian patients in all groups. Those in the dominant group seem to have milder disease, with a lower incidence of findings in the diagnostic triad and fewer occurrences of cancer or aplastic anemia (Tables 8–10 through 8–14). Older age at diagnosis is also seen in the dominant group (Fig. 8–11), but this may reflect the biased retrospective ascertainment in family studies.

Physical Examination. The number of occurrences of the major physical abnormalities in the three categories of DC are compared in Table 8–11. Complete details are provided in the references cited earlier. Reticulated hyperpigmentation involves the face, neck, shoulders, and trunk. Nail dystrophy involves both hands and feet, and nail plates are small, develop longitudinal ridges, and disappear with age (see Fig. 8–10). Ocular findings include epiphora (excessive tearing caused by blocked lacrimal ducts), blepharitis, cataracts, loss of eyelashes, conjunc-

tivitis, ectropion, glaucoma, strabismus, ulcers, and Coats retinopathy. Multiple dental caries and early loss of teeth are common. Osteoporosis, fractures, aseptic necroses (most of these patients had been receiving prednisone), and scoliosis occur. Intracranial calcifications were reported. Small, delicate appearance is common. Hyperhidrosis of palms and soles is reported. Premature gray hair and early loss of hair are noted. Urinary tract disorders are predominantly mucosal and include urethral stenoses, phimosis, hypospadias, pyelonephritis, penile leukoplakia, and a horseshoe kidney. Esophageal strictures, diverticula, spasms, duodenal ulcers, anal leukoplakia, bifid uvula, and umbilical hernia have all been reported, as have hypoplastic testes in males and vaginal constriction and vulvar leukoplakia in females. Four females did have successful pregnancies. Interstitial pneumonitis was reported in four patients, and pulmonary fibrosis is a problem in several older patients with DC.

DC has sometimes been confused with FA. In a series of five patients with FA, one patient probably had DC.[201] FA can now be specifically diagnosed with chromosome breakage and mutation analyses, and DC too can be

TABLE 8–10. Dyskeratosis Congenita Literature*

Characteristic	X-Linked and Sporadic (Male)	Autosomal Recessive	Autosomal Dominant
No. of patients	200	44	30
Male/female	200	10/34	14/16
Ratio	—	0.29	0.88
Age at diagnosis (or report) (yrs)			
Mean	18.2	14.9	30
Median	15	13	25
Range	0.3–68	1.2–42	7–58
Age at nail changes (yrs)			
Mean	8.5	5.8	9.5
Median	8	5	7
Range	0–34	0–15	7–17
Age at skin pigmentation (yrs)			
Mean	9.4	7.1	13.1
Median	9	4	13
Range	0–30	0–29	7–18
Age at leukoplakia (yrs)			
Mean	12.6	9	15.3
Median	10	7	17
Range	0.7–43	2–25	12–17

*Compiled from individual case reports, not including the DCR summary.[415] Physical features were not always reported.

TABLE 8–11. Physical Abnormalities in Dyskeratosis Congenita*

Characteristic	X-Linked and Sporadic Male (%)	Autosomal Recessive (%)	Autosomal Dominant (%)
No. of patients	200	44	30
Skin pigmentation	92	86	67
Nail dystrophy	90	39	13
Leukoplakia	68	68	33
Eye abnormalities	40	43	13
Teeth abnormalities	19	30	10
Developmental delay	15	16	0
Skeletal anomalies	11	25	7
Short stature	13	23	3
Hyperhidrosis	11	9	7
Hair loss	14	30	23
Urinary tract abnormalities	8	5	3
Gastrointestinal abnormalities	13	23	7
Other conditions	10	23	10
Gonadal anomalies	4	9	3

*Physical features were not always reported.

TABLE 8–12. Projected Ages of Survival of Patients with Dyskeratosis Congenita*

Group	Age (yrs) 50 %	Age (yrs) 25 %
ALL CAUSES		
All patients	36	51
Males, XLR or sporadic	33	51
Autosomal recessive	34	—
Male	26	26
Female	34	—
Autosomal dominant	—	—
Male	—	—
Female	—	—
CANCER		
All patients	36	49
Males, XLR or sporadic	44	49
Autosomal recessive	34	—
Male	—	—
Female	34	—
Autosomal dominant	—	—
Male	—	—
Female	—	—

*Survivals are determined from Kaplan-Meier estimates.
XLR = X-linked recessive.

confirmed if mutations are found in the DC genes (see later).

Aplastic Anemia. More than one third of the patients with known X-linked and approximately 60 percent with autosomal recessive DC developed aplastic anemia at an average age of the midteens (Table 8–13). Often, the diagnosis of DC was only made after the onset of hematologic changes, although in retrospect the manifestations of DC usually occurred first but were not recognized. In the Hammersmith series bone marrow failure occurred in 86 percent of the 118 male patients, and the actuarial probability of this outcome was 94 percent by age 40 years[417]; biased referrals of patients with severe hematologic complications may have occurred in this series.

LABORATORY FINDINGS

In most patients with DC, hematologic findings begin with thrombocytopenia or anemia followed by pancytopenia. Bone marrow examinations often reveal increased cellularity at the outset, suggesting an element of hypersplenism. However, hypocellularity then ensues, consistent

TABLE 8–13. Complications in Dyskeratosis Congenita

	X-Linked and Sporadic Male	Autosomal Recessive	Autosomal Dominant
No. of patients	200	44	30
Male/female ratio	—	0.29	0.88
Age at diagnosis (or report) (yrs)			
Mean	18.2	14.9	30
Median	15	13	25
Range	0.3–68	1.2–42	7–58
Age at aplastic anemia (yrs)			
No. (%)	72 (36)	26 (59)	1 (3)
Mean	13.3	13.7	16
Median	10.5	11	16
Range	1–41	2–45	16
Age at cancer (yrs)			
No. (%)	25 (13)	6 (14)	2 (7)
Mean	30.4	27.8	30
Median	29	24.5	30
Range	13–68	21–42	17, 43
Age at death (yrs)			
No. (%)	60 (30)	12 (27)	1 (3)
Mean	21.2	21.2	39
Median	19.5	22.5	39
Range	2–70	5–34	39
Projected median survival (yrs)	33	34	—

TABLE 8–14. Cancer in Dyskeratosis Congenita

Type	X-Linked and Sporadic Male	Autosomal Recessive		Autosomal Dominant		All Patients	References*
		M	F	M	F		
Oropharyngeal	12	0	4	0	1	17	415, 417–428
Gastrointestinal	12	0	0	0	0	12	415, 417, 421, 429–440
Myelodysplastic syndrome	4	0	0	0	0	4	415, 436
Skin	3	1	0	1	0	5	415, 441–445
Hodgkin disease	2	0	0	0	0	2	446, 447
Bronchial	0	2	0	0	0	2	415, 448
Pancreatic	0	1	0	0	0	1	415, 446
Liver	1	0	0	0	0	1	449
Cervical and vaginal	0	0	1	0	0	1	450
Total cancers	37	1	5	1	1	45	
Total patients	35	1	5	1	1	43	

*Some cases were cited in more than one reference.

with the diagnosis of aplastic anemia. Macrocytosis and elevated HbF level ("stress erythropoiesis") are common.[451] Ferrokinetics are consistent with aplasia. Decreased immunoglobulin levels or cellular immunity is found inconsistently.[452]

Chromosome breakage studies were normal in more than 35 patients, including more than a dozen examined with DEB, MMC, or nitrogen mustard.[3, 9, 436, 453–457] However, increased chromosome breaks and rearrangements[3, 9, 436, 458–460] and sister chromatid exchanges[3, 9, 459, 461] were also reported. DC can be clearly distinguished from FA if clastogen-induced chromosome breakage is not seen.

PATHOPHYSIOLOGY

DC probably has at least three genotypes leading to the DC phenotype (see earlier). The Xq28 restriction fragment length polymorphism[416, 462] might be used for prenatal diagnosis,[463] but the diagnosis of the propositus may not occur until adolescence. All germ layers are affected: the ectoderm by dyskeratosis and pigmentation; the endoderm by leukoplakia; and the mesoderm by aplastic anemia. DC is also a premalignant condition.

A detailed review of DC as a chromosomal instability disorder was provided by Dokal and Luzzatto,[464] although findings are not always consistent. Evidence for a defect in DNA cross-link repair has not been confirmed, nor was an increase in sister chromatid exchange found consistently. SV40 transformation was not increased, unlike in FA. In DC, fibroblasts had decreased plating efficiency, increased MMC sensitivity, and improved growth with SOD; they also grew more rapidly than normal and had chromosomal rearrangements. Increased G_2 cell cycle phase sensitivity with decreased repair of chromatid breaks was reported in response to X-irradiation and bleomycin.[465, 466] This

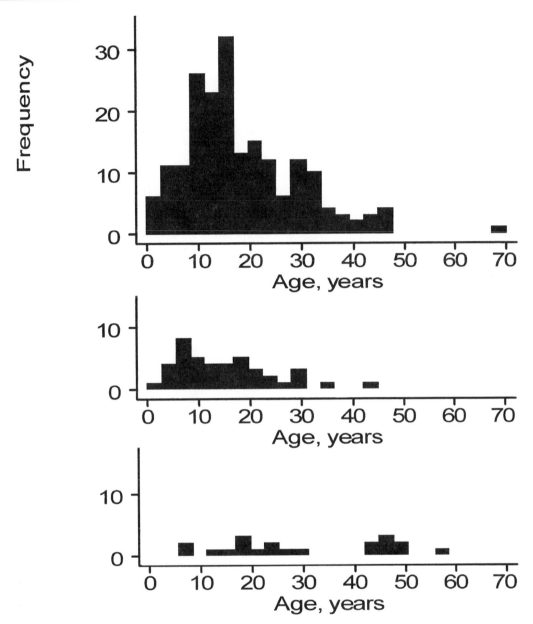

FIGURE 8–11. Age at diagnosis of dyskeratosis congenita in more than 250 published reports of patients from 1910 to 2000. *Top,* 200 males with X-linked and sporadic disease. *Middle,* 44 patients with autosomal recessive disease. *Bottom,* 30 patients with autosomal dominant disease.

sensitivity was found in both males with X-linked inherited disease and families with autosomal recessive inheritance and was also present in heterozygotes.[467]

Hematopoietic Defect. Hematopoietic cultures were usually done for patients who already had hematologic signs, and progenitors were reduced or zero in all.[3, 121, 436, 437, 455–457, 468] *In vitro,* GM-CSF or IL-3 increased the number of colonies in one study[469] but not in another,[457] and SCF did so in the culture from one patient.[121] Long-term marrow cultures suggested that the defect was in the stem cells, not in the microenvironment.[437]

One patient developed pancytopenia after chloramphenicol treatment.[470] As in other inherited syndromes, the combination of environment and genes for marrow failure may be required for aplastic anemia to appear.

Molecular Studies and Dyskeratosis Congenita Genes. The gene for the X-linked disorder was mapped to Xq28 and narrowed to 1.4 mb by restriction fragment length polymorphisms, linkage studies, and X-chromosome inactivation pattern analysis.[416, 471, 472] A deletion in one of the candidate genes in one patient and missense mutations in other patients led to the identification of the gene, now called *DKC1*.[471–474] Multiple mutations have now been detected (Fig. 8–12).[415, 477, 478]

The genomic DNA spans 15 kb, with 15 exons, and a complementary DNA of 2.6 kb (see Table 8–5), producing a protein called dyskerin, which has 514 amino acids. The function of dyskerin is not yet clear. Based on homology with rat NAP57 and yeast CBF5, dyskerin may have a role in ribosomal RNA production and in ribosome assembly.[473, 479] Dyskerin localizes to nucleoli. It may

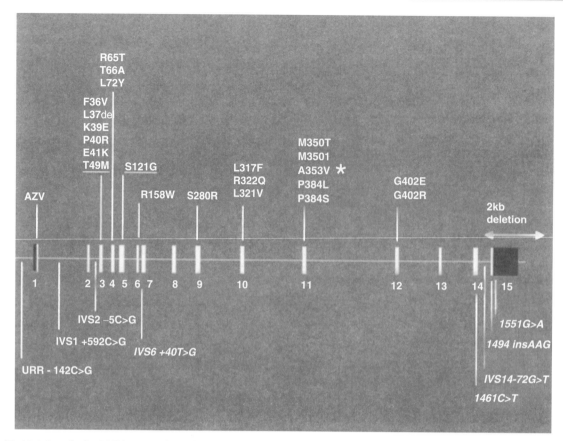

FIGURE 8–12. Mutations in the *DKC1* gene. Schematic representation of the 15 exons with patient-derived mutations shown in bold and polymorphisms in italics. * indicates the A353V mutation, which has recurred in 17 different families. Underlined mutations were found in patients with the Hoyeraal-Hreidarsson syndrome. (From Dokal I. Dyskeratosis congenita in all its forms. Br J Haematol 110:768, 2000).

have a role in survival of cells that are highly proliferative, such as skin and bone marrow, major tissues involved in the phenotype. Dyskerin binds to telomerase and may be important for maintenance of telomere length.[480] Patients with DC have blood cell telomeres that are much shorter than those in normal individuals.[481]

The gene for dominant DC, *DKC2*, was recently found to be the RNA component of telomerase (hTR).[475, 476] The authors suggest that bone marrow failure may be due to haploinsufficiency for telomerase, and that normal cells may have a selective growth advantage.

Screening for mutations is now an important addition to the evaluation of patients in whom DC is in the differential diagnosis. For example, a related syndrome, the *Hoyeraal-Hreidarsson syndrome*, results from missense mutations on *DKC1*.[482–484] These patients have microcephaly, cerebellar hypoplasia, growth retardation, immunodeficiency, and aplastic anemia. Skin and nail changes may not be prominent in these patients, particularly because they are seen when very young, and some features of the DC phenotype only appear with age.

THERAPY AND OUTCOME

Prognosis. The prognosis for patients with DC is not good, although it is possible that hematologists only know about the patients with complications. Approximately one third of males with X-linked and sporadic DC and

patients with autosomal recessive DC had died by the time of the reports (Table 8–13). The actual median age at death was 20, with a projected median survival age of 33 years for those categories of patients (Fig. 8–13). Patients with autosomal dominant DC appear to have a milder disease, with a better survival rate. Deaths were usually due to complications from aplastic anemia, BMT, or cancer. Some patients with DC have increased levels of von Willebrand factor and pulmonary complications and may show a predisposition for endothelial activation and damage.[415]

Cancer. Almost 15 percent of patients with DC reported in the literature developed cancer, mainly squamous cell carcinomas (Tables 8–13 and 8–14).[415] The most common sites were oropharyngeal (nasopharynx, larynx, lip, mouth, palate, tongue, and cheek) and gastrointestinal (esophagus, stomach, colon, and rectum). Other cancers include bronchial adenocarcinoma, Hodgkin disease, pancreatic adenocarcinoma, and skin cancers. The median age for the diagnosis of cancer was approximately 30 years, whereas the median age for emergence of aplastic anemia was 11 years (see Table 8–13). Thus, as with FA, the patients who develop cancer are older than and perhaps different from those who develop aplastic anemia in childhood. Unlike with FA, however, leukemia and MDS were reported rarely in patients with DC.

Treatment. Treatment for bone marrow failure in patients with DC is similar to that in patients with FA.

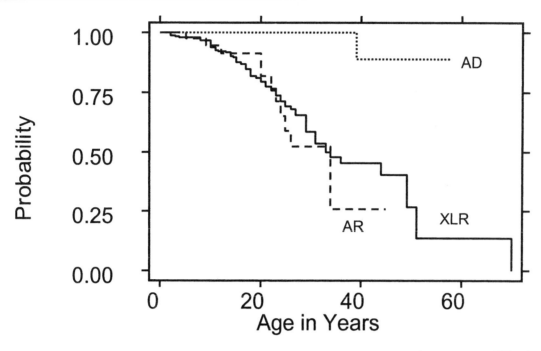

FIGURE 8–13. Kaplan-Meier plot of cumulative survival in dyskeratosis congenita. Time is shown as age in years. ——— = 195 males with X-linked recessive (XLR) and sporadic disease; - - - - = 42 patients with autosomal recessive (AR) disease; ● ● ● ● ● = 20 patients with autosomal dominant (AD) disease. Differences are significant.

Androgens, usually combined with prednisone, were given to approximately 40 patients; responses were seen in almost one half of these. Those with responses to androgen must continue treatment, and subsequent treatment failure may occur. At least eight patients had splenectomies, but only a temporary benefit was seen. Supportive care consisting of administration of blood products, antibiotics, and ε-aminocaproic acid should be provided as described earlier. Therapy with antilymphocyte globulin or cyclosporine is not expected to work (neither worked in one of our patients treated at another institution[413]).

Hematopoietic Stem Cell Transplantation. Approximately 20 BMTs were reported in males with X-linked or sporadic DC, but only six patients survived.[436, 445, 453, 455, 456, 485–493] There were four survivors among seven patients with autosomal recessive DC who were alive when reported.[445, 459, 484, 494–497] The number of reports exceeds the number of cases because of duplicate reporting. Deaths occurred from graft-versus-host disease; veno-occlusive disease, renal failure, and thrombotic microangiopathic syndrome; fungal pneumonia; graft failure (from a matched unrelated donor[456]); and pulmonary fibrosis. Because the clinical manifestations of DC appear late, it is possible that sibling donors may have undetected DC. In five patients BMT preceded the diagnosis of DC, and the skin and oral manifestations were initially thought to be graft-versus-host disease.[445, 453, 488, 490, 492, 494] Preparation for BMT in patients with DC usually involved standard doses of cyclophosphamide and irradiation, and some patients developed mucositis similar to that seen in patients with FA before the preparative regimens were modified. Transplantation in patients with DC requires caution, and irradiation may not have a role in the preparation.[487] The cumulative median survivals for patients with DC after BMT were 7 years for those with matched related donors and 1.5 years for those with alternate donors (Fig. 8–14). The median survival for males with X-linked and sporadic DC was only 1.5 years, whereas it was 8 years for patients with autosomal recessive DC. The donors reported for patients with autosomal recessive disease were all HLA-matched siblings; thus the results were biased toward a better outcome. We may speculate that BMT may also increase the risk of secondary tumors as in FA, but the number of long-term survivors is very small so far.

Hematopoietic Growth Factors. Hematopoietic growth factors may have a role in DC, which has not yet been adequately explored. Brief trials of GM-CSF led to doubling of neutrophil counts (but not above 1000/μL),[454, 498] whereas brief treatment with G-CSF at 5 μg/kg led to neutrophil counts greater than 5000,[456, 457, 499] and IL-3 produced a neutrophil response in one of three patients with DC.[500] We treated a male patient from a family with autosomal recessive disease with G-CSF combined with erythropoietin for almost 1 year; and we saw a sustained neutrophil response, and a 6-month improvement in hemoglobin and platelets.[501] Unfortunately, severe aplastic anemia recurred while the patient was receiving treatment, and BMT from an unrelated donor was not successful.* Further trials of G-CSF and erythropoietin are needed.

Disorders Related to Dyskeratosis Congenita

The possible presence of *Hoyeraal-Hreidarsson syndrome* has been reported in fewer than 12 patients. These are

---

*Unpublished observations.

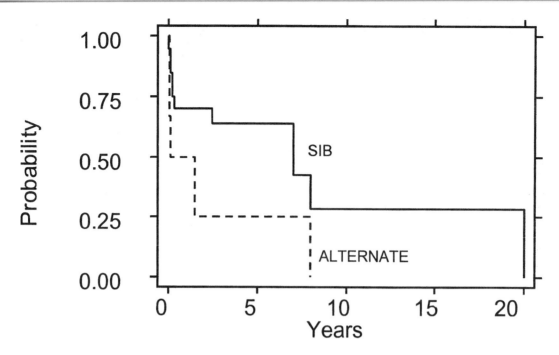

FIGURE 8–14. Kaplan-Meier plot of cumulative survival after BMT for patients with dyskeratosis congenita. Time is shown as years from transplantation. —— = 20 patients who received transplants from HLA-identical siblings; - - - - = 7 patients who received transplants from alternate donors. One patient received an unsuccessful transplant from a brother with dyskeratosis congenita (not shown). The difference between sibling and alternate donors is not significant.

small males with intrauterine growth retardation, microcephaly, cerebellar hypoplasia, developmental delay, progressive pancytopenia, and immunodeficiencies; the inheritance appears to be X-linked. Mutations in the *DKC1* gene were detected in three patients.[482, 502] Seven of the 11 reported patients died from infectious or hemorrhagic complications of aplastic anemia. The oldest survivor was alive at 5 years of age, 3 years after receiving a BMT from an unrelated donor.

Revesz syndrome has been reported in four patients, and I am aware of two more patients.[459, 503, 504]* The number of males and females was equal, and the characteristic features include intrauterine growth retardation, cerebellar hypoplasia, and microcephaly. Features of DC included dystrophic nails, oral leukoplakia, sparse hair, and reticular skin pigmentation, as well as bone marrow failure in four of the six patients. The unique feature in this syndrome is bilateral exudative retinopathy, which was called "Coats retinopathy," but which resembles Norrie disease.[505] No germline mutations were found in either the *DKC1* gene or the Norrie gene in one of our patients, however, and the genetic basis of this syndrome remains unclear. The combination of thrombocytopenia and hemorrhagic retinopathy is a potential problem, and it is recommended that platelet transfusions be provided for unresponsive thrombocytopenia to decrease further retinal hemorrhages. All patients were alive and younger than 4 when reported, although Revesz's patient subsequently died.†

The *ataxia-pancytopenia syndrome* also has some features resembling other diseases in this category. It was first described by Li et al[506, 507] in a family in which the father and all five children had ataxia. Two brothers died of aplastic anemia, two more of acute myeloblastic leukemia and acute myelomonocytic leukemia, respectively, and the only survivor was a 19-year-old girl with mild anemia. Daghistani et al[508] reported a similar family, in which the mother and her son and daughter had ataxia, and the son had pancytopenia and monosomy 7 and developed acute myeloblastic leukemia. There are a few more case reports of families or sporadic patients with ataxia in both sexes, cerebellar atrophy, microcephaly, tongue ulcers, immunodeficiencies, and aplastic anemia or leukemia[509–512]; none of these patients had monosomy 7. Eight of the 15 patients died between 3 and 10 years of age, four of leukemia and four of complications of aplastic anemia. Treatment of pancytopenia with prednisone was effective in one patient.[510] In two other patients no response was seen to antithymocyte globulin, cyclosporine, and G-CSF[509] or to prednisone plus danazol.[511]

Further cataloguing of patients with aplastic anemia and features of other syndromes will be done in the future, as more genes are identified for the known marrow failure syndromes.

Shwachman-Diamond Syndrome

DESCRIPTION

Shwachman-Diamond syndrome (SD; also known as *Bodian-Shwachman syndrome)* syndrome consists of exocrine pancreatic insufficiency combined with neutropenia.[513–515]

---

*Unpublished observations.
†Revesz T: Personal communication.

More than 300 patients have been reported (Table 8–15).[2, 3, 9] Signs of pancreatic insufficiency are apparent early in infancy and include malabsorption, steatorrhea, and failure to thrive. Neutropenia is usually detected in infancy or early childhood and is associated with skin infections or pneumonia. Approximately 40 percent of patients develop anemia or thrombocytopenia. The male-to-female ratio of occurrence is 1.6, and segregation analyses suggest that the inheritance is autosomal recessive, despite only rare reports of consanguinity.[516] Patients with SD have been reported among all racial and ethnic groups. Pregnancies and birth histories are unremarkable, except for approximately 10 percent of patients with low birth weight.

The most prominent findings on physical examination are malnourishment and short stature in more than 50 percent of patients, many of whom have metaphyseal dysostosis (Table 8–15). Mental retardation was reported in 10 percent. Other common physical findings include protuberant abdomen and an ichthyotic skin rash. Patients have also had microcephaly, hypertelorism, retinitis pigmentosa, syndactyly, cleft palate, dental dysplasia, ptosis, strabismus, short neck, coxa valga, and skin pigmentation.

The combination of pancreatic dysfunction and bone marrow failure was noted by Ozsoylu and Argun,[517] who found decreased duodenal trypsin in patients with acquired aplastic anemia or FA. However, patients with SD have decreased levels of amylase and lipase as well as of trypsin. In addition, patients with acquired aplasia or FA do not have malabsorption.

LABORATORY FINDINGS

In patients with SD, total white blood cell counts are often less than 3000/μL, and neutrophil counts are less than 1500/μL on more than one occasion. Neutropenia may be chronic, intermittent, or cyclic and is usually evident early in childhood. Anemia occurs in approximately one third of patients, but may be mild (hemoglobin level between 7 and 10 g/dL); however, transfusions are sometimes necessary. Thrombocytopenia with platelet counts less than 100,000/μL is seen in more than 20 percent of patients. The bicytopenic combination of neutropenia with anemia or thrombocytopenia also is common. Pancytopenia occurred at a median age of 3 years (range, 0 to 35 years).

TABLE 8–15. Shwachman-Diamond Syndrome Literature

	All Patients	Cytopenias	No Anemia or Thrombocytopenia
No. (%) of patients	336	134 (40)	202 (60)
Male/female	196/121	79/53	117/68
Ratio	1.6	1.5	1.7
No. (%) with metaphyseal dysostosis	124 (37)	51 (38)	73 (36)
Age at malabsorption (yrs)			
Mean	1.1	1.0	
Median	0.3	0.3	
Range	0–16	0–16	
Age at marrow failure (yrs)			
Mean		7.5	
Median		3	
Range		0–35	
No. with mental retardation	33 (10%)	20 (15%)	13 (6%)
No. with abnormal physical findings	43 (13%)	18 (13%)	25 (12%)
Age at leukemia (yrs)			
No. (%)	23 (7%)	10 (7%)	13 (6%)
Male/female	19/1	9/1	10/0
Mean	17.6	11.5	24.3
Median	14	7.8	23.5
Range	1.8–43	1.8–38	6–43
Age at MDS (yrs)			
No. (%)	30 (9%)	5 (4%)	25 (12%)
Male/female	15/11	3/2	12/9
Mean	10.3	7.6	10.8
Median	8.1	7.5	8.1
Range	2–42	3.5–12	2–42
MDS clone alone/died	5/2		
MDS morphology alone/died	6/4		
Age at death (yrs)			
No. (%)	68 (20%)	32 (24%)	36 (18%)
Male/female	37/25	20/12	17/13
Mean	7.6	8.2	7.1
Median	3.3	5.3	0.9
Range	0.3–43	0.4–35	0.3–43
Projected median survival age (yrs)			
All patients	35	25	37
Leukemia	14		
MDS	16		

Some studies have suggested a defect in neutrophil mobility that may explain the occurrence of infections even when the neutrophil count is not extremely low, but these results are inconsistent.[518–521]

Bone marrow cellularity is often decreased, and the marrow may have a myeloid maturation arrest. The erythroid series is normal or hyperplastic. HbF levels are often increased even in the absence of anemia, suggesting marrow stress.[522] Low levels of immunoglobulins were reported in a few patients. Chromosomes are normal, without increased breakage after clastogenic stress.

Hepatic dysfunction and fibrosis have been noted occasionally. Pancreatic insufficiency is documented as low levels or absence of duodenal trypsin, amylase, and lipase. The level of serum trypsinogen is low in young patients, although it may improve with age, in association with a decrease in malabsorption.[523] A fatty pancreas may be evident on ultrasound or other imaging studies. The patients do not have cystic fibrosis, and sweat chloride levels are normal.

PATHOPHYSIOLOGY

The inheritance appears to be autosomal recessive, despite the prevalence in males.[516] Although the exocrine pancreas and bone marrow hematopoiesis develop at approximately the same time *in utero*, the presence of SD in families and in only one of a pair of twins militate against an intrauterine insult as the cause.[524] A stem cell deficit was suggested by findings of decreased marrow CFU-GMs and CFU-Es in most patients, without evidence for humoral or cellular inhibitors of granulopoiesis. The reduction in the number of hematopoietic progenitor cells resembles that seen in other inherited bone marrow failure syndromes.

The SD gene has been mapped to a single locus at the chromosome 7 centromere, suggesting a monogenic disease with several mutations (see Table 8–5).[525] The gene for SD was recently identified as a novel gene in the predicted region. It is called SBDS, for Shwachman-Bodian-Diamond Syndrome. The gene has 5 exons spanning 7.9 kb, and is associated with a pseudogene which has 97% homology with the SBDS gene. Two common mutations which result from gene conversion account for ~75% of the families studied initially. Although the function of SBDS is not yet known, the authors speculated that it may be involved in aspects of RNA metabolism that are essential for the development of the exocrine pancreas, hematopoiesis, and chondrogenesis.[525a]

THERAPY AND OUTCOME

The malabsorption in patients with SD responds to treatment with oral pancreatic enzymes. Infections resulting from neutropenia are treated with the appropriate antibiotics, and anemia and thrombocytopenia are managed with transfusions of red cells or platelets as needed. Fewer than a dozen patients were treated with corticosteroids; hematologic improvement occurred in one half of these patients. Even fewer patients received androgens plus steroids (see section on FA) and showed some improvement; one patient required the addition of cyclosporine to the regimen.[526] G-CSF was used successfully in approximately 12 patients, although four developed mildly dysplastic bone marrow and clonal cytogenetics (see later).

Approximately 40 percent developed additional cytopenias (Table 8–15). The reported absolute survival was approximately 20 percent in those with neutropenia and in those with additional hematologic complications, although the projected median survival was longer in those without additional marrow involvement. Median survival was 35 years for the entire group. Those without pancytopenia, leukemia, or MDS reached a survival rate plateau of greater than 80 percent by their late teens (Fig. 8–15). Infection, bleeding, and leukemia were the causes of most deaths. As with most of the patients with inherited bone marrow failure disorders, the number of patients with mild or asymptomatic disease is underestimated from the literature, and the overall prognosis may not be as bad as implied here.

Leukemia. Leukemia was reported in 23 patients, all but one of whom was male, at a median age of 14 years (range, 2 to 43 years). Two patients had siblings with SD. Five patients had acute lymphoblastic leukemia, 17 had acute myeloblastic leukemia (types identified were M1, 4; M2, 2; M4, 3; M5, 3; and M6, 5), and 1 had juvenile chronic myelocytic leukemia.[513, 515, 527–542] Ten of these patients had prior histories of pancytopenia. The projected median survival age for those with leukemia was 14 years. Four had cytogenetic abnormalities that involved chromosomes 5, 7 (monosomy 7 in one patient), 9, and 11.[535, 538, 540] In one series of 21 patients with SD, 7 developed MDS, of whom 6 had clonal abnormalities, and 5 developed leukemia.[538]

Myelodysplastic Syndrome. Eight of 30 patients with MDS developed leukemia and are included in the analyses above.[528, 535–540, 543–552] Unlike the predominance of males seen in leukemia, the male-to-female ratio of occurrence of MDS was similar to the ratio in all patients with SD. MDS was found more often in those without prior cytopenias. The median age at diagnosis of MDS was 8 years (range, 2 to 42 years). The projected median survival age was 16 years (Table 8–15 and Fig. 8–15).

Five of the patients with MDS had marrow cytogenetic clones without morphologic evidence of MDS. Clones included monosomy 7 with t(6;13),t(4;7) and deletion 7 in patients who had received G-CSF. In those who had not received G-CSF, monosomy 7 was seen in three patients, isochromosome 7q in 11 patients, der(7) in three patients, and other clones in five patients. Chromosome 7 was involved in a total of 22 patients, an interesting observation in light of the gene localization to the centromere of chromosome 7. In a series of 88 patients, five of the six with cytogenetic clones had abnormalities of chromosome 7.[523]

Shwachman-Diamond syndrome thus resembles many of the other inherited bone marrow failure syndromes in that it predisposes patients to malignancy. Although it is not clear that MDS inevitably progresses to leukemia, leukemia does occur in patients with the syndrome. To date, no occurrences of solid tumors have been reported.

Hematopoietic Stem Cell Transplantation. One patient died from cyclophosphamide cardiotoxicity,[553] whereas another was cured after receiving the same

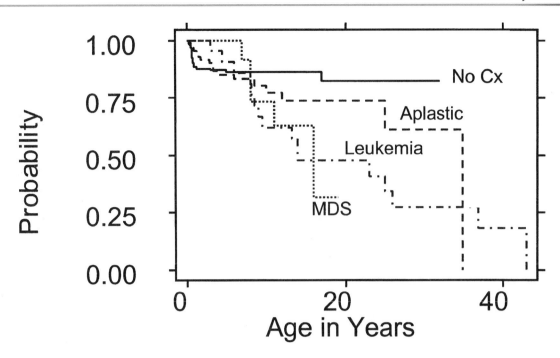

FIGURE 8–15. Kaplan-Meier plot of cumulative survival in Shwachman-Diamond syndrome. —— = 156 patients with no hematologic complications (No Cx); - - - - = 94 patients with aplastic anemia; – ● – = 18 patients with leukemia; ● ● ● ● ● = 16 patients with myelodysplastic syndrome (MDS). Differences are significant.

preparative regimen of approximately 50 mg/kg/day for 4 days.[554] Overall, more than 20 patients received a BMT, equally divided between HLA-matched sibling and alternate donors.[526, 536–541, 545–547, 549, 551, 553–557] The results are almost identical, with absolute mortalities of 50 percent, projected median survival times of 1 year, and

plateaus at 47 percent survival (Fig. 8–16). Deaths were primarily from cardiotoxicity or leukemia.

Hematopoietic Growth Factors. Most of the patients treated with G-CSF had elevated neutrophil counts.[544, 546, 557–567] In one patient no response to GM-CSF was seen.[568]

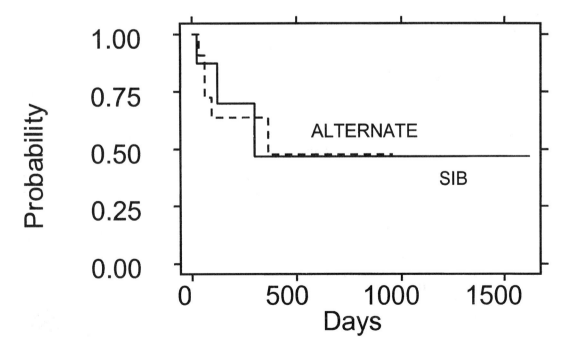

FIGURE 8–16. Kaplan-Meier plot of cumulative survival after BMT for patients with Shwachman-Diamond syndrome. Time is shown as days from transplantation. —— = 10 patients who received transplants from HLA-identical siblings; - - - - = 11 patients who received transplants from alternative donors. Differences are not significant.

Cartilage-Hair Hypoplasia

Cartilage-hair hypoplasia is an autosomal recessive chondrodysplasia characterized by metaphyseal dysostosis, short-limbed dwarfism, and fine, sparse hair that lacks the central pigment core.[569] Other skeletal findings include chest deformity, varus lower limbs, lordosis, and scoliosis. Gastrointestinal problems include aganglionic megacolon (Hirschsprung disease) and other anatomic findings. More than 300 patients have been described, primarily of Amish or Finnish background.[570, 571] Macrocytic anemia was severe in 16 percent and mild in 64 percent of patients in one Finnish series.[571] Some patients were reported initially as having Diamond-Blackfan anemia.[572–574] Lymphopenia was seen in 65 percent of patients and neutropenia in 25 percent. The presence of malignancy was increased sevenfold, including two patients with Hodgkin disease, three with non-Hodgkin lymphoma, one with testicular teratoma, and three with basal cell carcinomas.[571, 575–577] The gene was mapped to 9p21-p13,[578] and mutations have been reported in the RNA component of RNase MRP.[579] Prenatal diagnosis correctly identified one affected fetus of four examined.[580]

Similar to findings with other inherited marrow failure anemias, the numbers of CFU-Es were low and the number of BFU-Es was almost zero in eight patients.[581] The numbers of progenitors for myeloid and megakaryocytic lineages were also low. Some of the patients had normal blood counts, despite reduced numbers of progenitors. Serum erythropoietin levels were higher than predicted from the hemoglobin level, similar to those seen in patients with other marrow failure disorders.[3] An increased level of red cell adenosine deaminase, commonly seen in Diamond-Blackfan anemia (see later), was reported in a boy with cartilage-hair hypoplasia who did not have anemia.[582]

Transfusions and administration of steroids were used for anemia, and many of the patients tended to outgrow their marrow failure. Among 108 Finnish patients, 16 patients died including 3 from anemia, 4 with pneumonia, 2 with sepsis, and 2 from Hirschsprung disease.[571]

Pearson Syndrome

Pearson syndrome (refractory sideroblastic anemia with vacuolization of bone marrow precursors and exocrine pancreatic dysfunction) was astutely recognized by Dr. Howard Pearson in four patients reported in 1979.[583, 584] The pathognomonic deletion of mitochondrial DNA was identified by Rotig et al in 1990,[585] providing a molecular diagnostic test as well as an explanation for the clinical features of the syndrome, which include anemia and metabolic acidosis. More than 70 patients have been reported.[2, 3] The male-to-female ratio of occurrence is 0.7. The inheritance is maternal because mitochondria are found in ova but not in sperm. No affected siblings have been reported. One family had consanguineous disease,[586] and in another the mother had Kearns-Sayre syndrome.[587] Patients from all racial and most ethnic groups have been reported.

There was a history of low birth weight in one third of patients, and metabolic acidosis is common. Physical anomalies are rare; one patient was reported with hypoplastic mandible and large ears and another with abnormal arm skin pigmentation. One of the author's patients had metopic synostosis, inguinal hernias, and hypospadias.[588] Approximately one third of patients have exocrine pancreatic insufficiency and development of insulin-dependent diabetes is common. Metabolic problems are further complicated by liver and renal failure.

Anemia (usually macrocytic) was diagnosed at less than 1 month of age in 25 percent and by 6 months in 70 percent of affected patients. The median hemoglobin level was 5.8 g/dL (range, 2.1 to 11 g/dL). Three patients had hydrops.[585, 588] One half had absolute neutrophil counts less than 500/μL, and one half had platelet counts less than 100,000/μL. The bone marrows of essentially all patients had vacuolated myeloid or erythroid precursors, many had decreased erythroblasts, and all but one had sideroblasts; most had ringed sideroblasts (Fig. 8–17).

The majority of the patients received transfusions, and hemoglobin levels in all patients who had not died from other causes improved at a median of 2 and a maximum of 10 years. Neutropenia and thrombocytopenia were not usually of major significance. G-CSF and erythropoietin were given to two patients[588, 589]; a possible response was seen to the G-CSF. The role of growth factors is not proven, but their use on an investigative basis is probably warranted. In general, the hematologic problems are not fatal, and good supportive care should be provided.

The major problem is acidosis. The aim of specific therapy is to bypass the deleted respiratory enzymes through the use of thiamine, riboflavin, L-carnitine, and coenzyme Q. The small numbers of patients treated and the variability of the disease do not yet permit any conclusions. Deaths occurred from acidosis, renal or liver failure, sepsis, and heart block and not usually from aplastic anemia. The projected median survival time is 4 years, with a plateau of 36 percent at age 10.

A mitochondrial DNA deletion, ranging from 2.7 to 7.767 kb, was reported in all patients examined; one third had a 4.977 kb deletion (Fig. 8–18). The respiratory enzymes involved in the deletions are relevant to oxidative phosphorylation and include reduced nicotinamide adenine dinucleotide (NADH), cytochrome oxidase, adenosine triphosphatase (ATPase), as well as transfer RNAs and ribosomal RNAs.[590] Patients have organs and cells with variable numbers of deleted and normal mitochondria. Fluctuations over time (e.g., marrow improvement) might relate to selective expansion of normal or abnormal clones, explaining both inter- and intrapatient variability in phenotype. The size of the deletion does not correlate with the clinical course.[591] Excellent reviews of mitochondrial diseases are found in the literature.[584, 592]

The numbers of marrow CFU-Es and BFU-Es were decreased in several reports.[583, 588, 593, 594] CFU-GMs were normal in two patients[583] and zero in one patient.[594] Thus, the numbers of committed progenitors are usually low, at least at the time that the patients have cytopenias.

Seven patients were reported who outgrew or never had hematologic problems but did develop symptoms of Kearns-Sayre syndrome (ophthalmoplegia, pigmentary

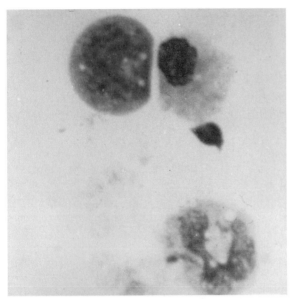

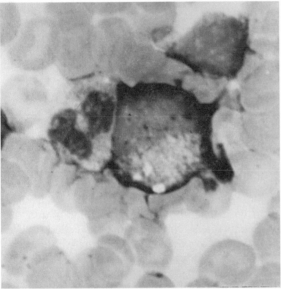

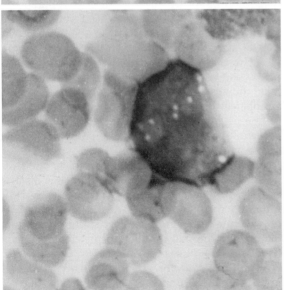

FIGURE 8–17. Bone marrow myeloid precursors in Pearson syndrome, showing cytoplasmic vacuoles.

retinopathy, ataxia, conductive heart block, and endocrinopathies) at 6 to 16 years of age.[595–602] Autopsies showed pancreatic fibrosis in a few patients. So far, no patients have developed leukemia nor has any patient undergone BMT or other organ transplantation.

Prenatal testing of fetal blood chorionic villi or amniocytes might be offered, but such testing would have a low yield (few affected mothers and no siblings were reported). The mother's DNA should be examined, however. In one family, the mother had Kearns-Sayre syndrome, with the same mitochondrial DNA deletion as her child with Pearson syndrome.[587]

Pearson syndrome should be added to the differential diagnosis of refractory anemia in children, especially for those without a clonal cytogenetic abnormality. For example, Bader-Meunier et al[603] reported two children with refractory anemia with ringed sideroblasts; both had bone marrow vacuoles, one had a mitochondrial DNA deletion, and the other did not have a deletion but did have abnormal mitochondrial enzyme activities.

Pearson syndrome can now be redefined as refractory sideroblastic anemia (or refractory anemia with ringed sideroblasts) with vacuolated marrow precursors and with deletion of mitochondrial DNA. Other findings, such as pancreatic insufficiency, acidosis, or renal tubular insufficiency, are common but not mandatory for diagnosis. DNA deletion is complicated: patients with Kearns-Sayre syndrome may have identical deletions without hematologic signs, and patients with bone marrow findings as seen in Pearson syndrome may not have DNA deletions, although they may have abnormal mitochondrial enzymes. Still other mitochondrial disorders may be due to point mutations or to deletions smaller than those that can be detected by Southern blotting.

Pearson syndrome is probably underdiagnosed and must be considered in hydropic infants and in patients with cytopenias associated with renal or liver disease, sepsis, or acidosis, as well as in children with refractory anemia or myelodysplasia and particularly in those with ringed sideroblasts.

Reticular Dysgenesis

The term *reticular dysgenesis* (thymic alymphoplasia with aleukocytosis) is used to describe infants with congenital absence of neutrophils and monocytes, lymphopenia, normal red cell counts, normal or low platelet counts, and absent cellular and humoral immunity. Since the first report in 1959,[604] approximately two dozen cases have been reported.[605] Despite a twofold preponderance among males, the identification of three sets of siblings and one of twins as well as one family with consanguinity is consistent with an autosomal recessive inheritance. These cases include one with a similar phenotype in which the mother received azathioprine for renal disease; although disease in this instance may have been acquired rather than inherited.[606, 607]

Patients usually are seen with signs of infection at birth or early infancy. Birth weights of most of these patients were less than 2500 g. On examination, no lymph nodes or tonsils were seen, and no thymic shadow was detected by radiography. At autopsy, thymus glands were extreme-

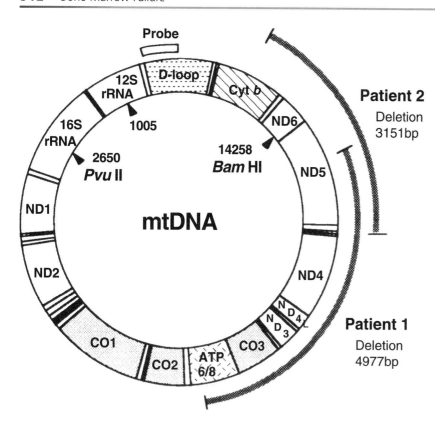

FIGURE 8–18. Schematic diagram of mitochondrial DNA, indicating an example of the type of deletion found in Pearson syndrome. (From Sano T, Ban K, Ichiki T, et al: Molecular and genetic analyses of two patients with Pearson's marrow-pancreas syndrome. Pediatr Res 1993; 34:105.)

ly small, lymph nodes were absent, and spleens did not have follicles.

Blood counts showed severe lymphopenia and granulocytopenia. Anemia was reported in most of the infants, and thrombocytopenia also occurred. Bone marrows were hypocellular, usually with no myeloid or lymphoid precursors, and occasionally a reduction in erythropoiesis was seen as well. One patient had dyserythropoietic erythroid precursors, one had a promyelocyte arrest, and one had an aplastic marrow. Bone marrow cultures from most of the studied patients had no or very low hematopoietic colonies,[2, 3] a finding that supports the stem cell model. Although the majority of the patients did not have complete aplastic anemia, they certainly exhibit neutropenia and lymphopenia.

Most patients died from infection within the first 6 months of life. One infant who survived for 17 weeks was maintained in a gnotobiotic environment.[608] BMT was often curative, when a haploidentical donor was available and T-cell depletion but not immunosuppression was part of the treatment protocol.[609–617] One patient who had a successful BMT without immunosuppression became a complete chimera, with donor erythrocytes, unlike patients with severe combined immunodeficiency, in whom only the lymphocytes become donor. This finding suggests that the defect is in the pluripotential hematopoietic stem cell. However, another patient who had BMT without immunosuppression had only lymphoid reconstitution.[612] Seven of 10 patients who received BMTs were cured.

Reticular dysgenesis is an example of a defect of an earlier stem cell than is involved in most of the other inherited aplastic anemias, because it involves the lymphoid as well as the myeloid series.

Amegakaryocytic Thrombocytopenia

DESCRIPTION

A small number of patients with inherited aplastic anemia are seen with thrombocytopenia in infancy and develop pancytopenia later. This syndrome was called *type III constitutional aplastic anemia* by O'Gorman Hughes,[297] but the term *amegakaryocytic thrombocytopenia* is more useful. The differential diagnosis of neonatal thrombocytopenia is a lengthy process; the disorder discussed here excludes thrombocytopenias in which increased numbers of bone marrow megakaryocytes are seen, as well those caused by congenital infection (particularly a viral infection, such as rubella). Immune thrombocytopenias are also excluded, despite the occasional appearance of absence of megakaryocytes presumably resulting from the reactivity of antiplatelet antibodies with megakaryocytes.[618] The syndrome of thrombocytopenia absent radii will be discussed later, in the section on single cytopenias. FA, which can begin with thrombocytopenia, was discussed earlier. Children with known associated trisomies, such as trisomies 13 and 18, are also excluded from this discussion. Table 8–16 summarizes several syndromes with associated inherited thrombocytopenias, and Table 8–17 compares patients with amegakaryocytic thrombocytopenia with congenital anomalies with patients with normal physical appearances.

The author is aware of more than 50 reports of thrombocytopenia in infants with no birth defects, in whom bone marrow megakaryocytes were absent or their numbers were decreased.[1, 2, 619, 627, 628] A smaller number of infants with amegakaryocytic thrombocytopenia did

TABLE 8–16. Inherited Thrombocytopenia Syndromes

Disorder	Genetics	Chromosome	Gene	References
Amegakaryocytic thrombocytopenia, no birth defects	AR	1p34	*mpl*	619
Amegakaryocytic thrombocytopenia, with birth defects	AR	N/A	N/A	This chapter
Thrombocytopenia absent radii	AR	N/A	N/A	
X-linked macrothrombocytopenia	X-linked	Xp11.23	*GATA–1*	620
Hoyeraal-Hreidarsson syndrome	X-linked	Xq28	*DKC1*	482
Familial platelet disorder-acute myelocytic leukemia	AD	21q22.1-.2	*CBFA2*	621
Familial dominant thrombocytopenia	AD	10p11.2–12	*THC2*	622
Amegakaryocytic thrombocytopenia, with radioulnar synostosis	AD	7p15-p14.2	*HOXA11*	623
Trisomy 13	Nondisjunction	Trisomy 13	N/A	624
Trisomy 18	Nondisjunction	Trisomy 18	N/A	625
Jacobsen syndrome	11q monosomy partial deletion	11q23	N/A	626

TABLE 8–17. Amegakaryocytic Thrombocytopenia Literature

	Without Anomalies	With Anomalies	Total
No. of patients	52	22	74
Male/female	27/24	11/10	38/34
Ratio	1.13	1.1	1.12
Age at diagnosis (days)			
Mean	301	94.3	244
Median	40	2	7
Range	0–3285	0–540	0–3285
Age at aplastic anemia (yrs)			
No. (%)	25 (48)	4 (18)	29 (39)
Mean	3.4	3.7	3.4
Median	3	3.3	3
Range	0.4–12.5	2.2–6	0.4–12.5
No. (%) with leukemia/preleukemia	2 (4)	0	2 (3)
Age at death (yrs)			
No. (%)	17 (33%)	14 (64%)	31 (42%)
Mean	5.5	2.4	4.1
Median	4	1.2	2.8
Range	0.01–21	0–10	0–21
Projected median survival age (yrs)	9	2.8	7

have physical abnormalities that fit no other specific syndrome.[2, 629, 630] The male-to-female ratio of occurrence was 1.1 for both categories. The abnormalities include microcephaly, micrognathia, intracranial structural abnormalities, congenital heart disease, failure to thrive, and developmental delays. Some of the physical findings resemble those seen in FA, which cannot always be excluded retrospectively from the reports. Reports of affected siblings and consanguinity are consistent with autosomal recessive inheritance.

Pregnancies and deliveries were essentially unremarkable, although the occurrence of spontaneous abortions was approximately 10 percent. Low birth weight was reported in 25 percent of infants without anomalies and almost one half of those with anomalies.

Bleeding in the skin, mucous membranes, or gastrointestinal tract was usually the presenting sign. Almost one half of patients, primarily those without birth defects, developed aplastic anemia.

LABORATORY FINDINGS

The first abnormality noted is thrombocytopenia. Although white blood counts and hemoglobin levels are normal, the red cells are macrocytic, and levels of HbF and i antigen are increased, findings that suggest a broader level of marrow failure. One 5-year-old boy with amegakaryocytic thrombocytopenia had increased mean cell volume and HbF level but had not yet developed aplastic anemia.[631] Platelet counts ranged from 0 to 80,000/μL at diagnosis. Bone marrow examination reveals normal cellularity with absence of or a decreased number of megakaryocytes. Megakaryocytes that are present are small and appear to be inactive. Homologous platelet survival is normal, because the defect is underproduction, not increased destruction.[632] Evolution into pancytopenia is associated with the development of hypocellular marrow with increased lymphocytes and plasma cells, as in any aplastic anemia. Peripheral blood chromosomes do not have the increased breaks characteristic of FA. In one patient who had myelodysplasia, the absence, partial deletion, or trisomy of chromosome 19 was observed in 11 of 55 marrow cells.[633]

Prenatal diagnosis may be based on platelet counts in midtrimester fetal blood. Mibashan and Millar[634] detected thrombocytopenia in one of three fetuses at risk. Cloning of the gene (see later) will permit molecular prenatal diagnoses.

PATHOPHYSIOLOGY

The thrombocytopenia is associated with absence of or a decreased number of megakaryocytes, which suggests a defect in platelet production. The number of megakaryocyte progenitors (CFU-megakaryocytes) were reduced in five patients; improvement occurred in the presence of the combination of IL-3 and GM-CSF.[627] In those with aplastic anemia, myeloid and erythroid progenitor cells are decreased in number or absent[3, 619]; these progenitor cells were also decreased in one patient who was studied during the thrombocytopenic phase.[121] Associated with megakaryocytic insufficiency are increased serum levels of thrombopoietin, IL-11, and IL-6.[635, 636] The growth of *in vitro* cultures did not improve with the addition of thrombopoietin and c-*mpl* RNA production was low.[637]

Several recent reports have demonstrated mutations in at least 15 patients in the c-*mpl* gene, which encodes the thrombopoietin receptor (Fig. 8–19 and Table 8–5). All of these were in patients without birth defects, and all had mutations in both *mpl* genes, confirming the autosomal recessive inheritance.[115, 584, 619, 628, 638]

THERAPY AND OUTCOME

Steroids are ineffective as a single modality therapy. Addition of androgens leads to transient partial improvement in platelet counts in a few patients. Splenectomy also is not helpful. The use of hematopoietic growth factors, which stimulate platelet production, theoretically has potential. In a phase I/II trial, Guinan et al[627] found a platelet response to IL-3 but not to GM-CSF in five patients. Taylor et al[630] noted slight improvements in two of six patients treated with PIXY321 (a fusion product of GM-CSF and IL-3). Neither IL-3 nor PIXY321 is currently available.

Hematopoietic stem cell transplantation was done in 15 patients without birth defects; 10 transplants came from HLA-matched sibling donors and 5 came from unrelated donors, of which two were from cord blood. Cumulative survival was 93 percent,[240, 619, 639–642] demonstrating the potential of stem cell transplants to cure thrombocytopenia and prevent aplastic anemia or leukemia.

Aplastic anemia developed in almost one half of the patients at a median age of 3 years and a maximum age of 12 years. Half of those who developed aplastic anemia died, primarily from bleeding or infection. Half of those without aplastic anemia also died from hemorrhages in the central nervous system or gastrointestinal tract. The majority of the deaths occurred before 1980, and the use of systematic platelet support was not reported. The projected median survival age in those without birth defects is 9 years, compared with 3 years in those with physical anomalies. The oldest age at death in each group was 21 and 10 years, respectively (Fig. 8–20).

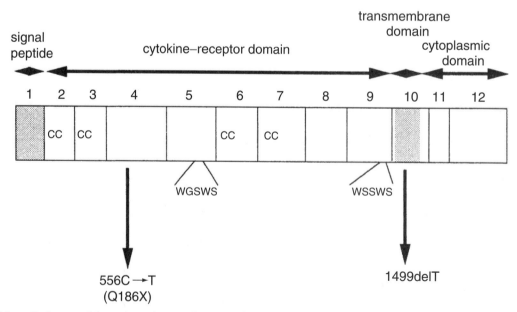

FIGURE 8–19. Schematic diagram of the *mpl* gene in amegakaryocytic thrombocytopenia. (From Ihara K, Ishii E, Eguchi M, et al: Identification of mutations in the c-*mpl* gene in congenital amegakaryocytic thrombocytopenia. Proc Natl Acad Sci USA 1999; 96:3132.)

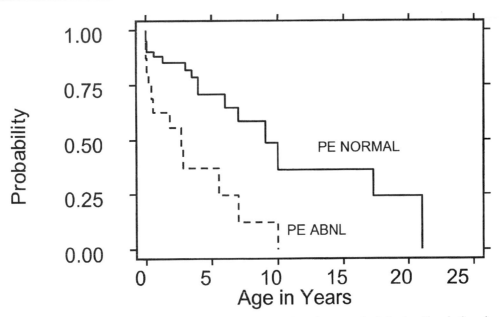

FIGURE 8–20. Kaplan-Meier plot of cumulative survival in amegakaryocytic thrombocytopenia. Patients with only thrombocytopenia and those with aplastic anemia are pooled, because the numbers are small. ——— = 42 patients without birth defects who had normal results on physical examination (PE); - - - - = 16 patients with birth defects who had abnormal results on physical examination. Differences are significant.

Development of leukemia has been rare, but the outcome for two patients who did not have birth defects suggests that a predisposition to malignancy is part of the syndrome. One male infant had amegakaryocytic thrombocytopenia from birth, developed aplastic anemia at 5 years of age, which responded poorly to androgens plus steroids and evolved further into acute myelomonocytic leukemia at age 16. He died at age 17.[297],★ A female infant had thrombocytopenia at 2 months of age, pancytopenia at 5 months, and a preleukemic condition with abnormalities involving chromosome 19.†

Familial Marrow Dysfunction

DESCRIPTION

A large group of apparently familial marrow failure syndromes do not fit any of the classifications described so far. In many, diseases in various family members include aplastic anemia, leukemia, and immunodeficiency. The ages of onset range from childhood to adult. The inheritance patterns are dominant, recessive, or X-linked; in addition, sporadic cases of aplastic anemia with physical anomalies that are not characteristic of FA or other identifiable syndromes are seen.

Autosomal Dominant with Physical Anomalies. The *IVIC syndrome,* named with the initials of the institution which first reported it (Instituto Venezolano de Investigaciones Cientificas), is characterized by radial ray hypoplasia with absent thumbs or hypoplastic radial carpal bones, hearing impairment, strabismus, imperforate anus, and thrombocytopenia. Twenty-nine members of three multigenerational families had anomalies.[643–645] Mild thrombocytopenia and leukocytosis appeared before

the age of 50 years in 13 individuals in the first family. The incidence of hematologic abnormalities is unknown because many patients are still young. Results of baseline chromosome breakage tests were normal. Despite the lack of complete aplastic anemia, the physical findings do resemble those seen in FA. It has been suggested that this syndrome be renamed "oculo-oto-radial syndrome."[646]

Three families were reported to have a disease resembling FA, but with an autosomal dominant inheritance pattern. It was called the *WT syndrome,* after the initials of the first two families in which the disorder was identified.[647, 648] The patients had radial-ulnar hypoplasia, abnormal thumbs, short fingers, clinodactyly of the fifth finger, pancytopenia or thrombocytopenia, or leukemia. These physical findings were subtly different from those of classic FA and baseline chromosome breaks were not seen. The authors suggested that several patients with "atypical FA" might have WT syndrome instead. Chromosome studies after clastogenic stress might now help to resolve this confusion.

Members of one family had dominant bone marrow failure, acute nonlymphocytic leukemia, hyperpigmented skin, warts, and immune dysfunction, and women had multiple spontaneous abortions.[649] DEB-induced chromosome breakage was not increased; thus this disorder loosely resembles FA clinically but not genetically.

Dokal et al[650] reported two families with dominant proximal fusion of the radius and ulna in which two members of each had aplastic anemia or leukemia.[650] Two additional families with radioulnar synostosis and thrombocytopenia were recently shown to have a mutation in the *HOXA11* gene, a gene involved in bone morphogenesis.[623, 651]

In another family, the son had finger-like thumbs, and he and his mother had pancytopenia; DEB-induced

---

★Potter N, Alter BP: Unpublished data.
†Harris MB, Najfeld V, Weiner MA, Shah L, Alter BP, Hirschhorn K: Unpublished data, 1984.

chromosome breakage was normal.[652] A different family was described with dominant bone marrow failure, acute nonlymphocytic leukemia, hyperpigmented skin, warts, immune dysfunction, and multiple spontaneous abortions.[649] DEB-induced chromosome breakage was not increased.

The ataxia-pancytopenia syndrome was discussed earlier in the section on dyskeratosis congenita.

Autosomal Dominant without Physical Anomalies. A five-generation family was reported with 14 members who developed mild to profound single cytopenias or pancytopenia by the third decade of life.[653] Nine members of the family had vascular occlusions. One patient had chromosome breaks in 20 percent of his cells, but his father, who also had aplastic anemia, had normal chromosomes. Kato and co-workers[654] reported a mother with aplastic anemia and her son with adult-onset neutropenia and thrombocytopenia.

A mother and child pair with idiopathic aplastic anemia was also reported.[655] Kaur et al[656] presented 5 members of a family with acute myeloid leukemia or MDS; other family members had hypoplastic anemia. In the report on 19 members of 8 families with "acquired aplastic anemia," 4 families with 9 patients had a vertical pattern—that is, a parent or aunt or uncle who also had aplasia.[657] These occurrences could be due to common environmental factors or to a genetic predisposition for bone marrow failure.

Autosomal Recessive with Physical Anomalies. Three siblings in a consanguineous family had microcephaly, short stature, immunodeficiency, skin abscesses, anemia, and increased spontaneous but not DEB-induced chromosome breaks, and increased sister chromatid exchange.[658] Another sibling pair had central nervous system malformations and hypocellular marrows, but normal results for chromosome breakage tests.[659] Two cousins (male and female) had oculocutaneous albinism, microcephaly, facial dysmorphia, immunodeficiency, neutropenia, and thrombocytopenia.[660] Three siblings with consanguineous parents had facial dysmorphia, steatorrhea, increased skin folds, congenital heart disease, vesicoureteral reflux, decreased cellular immunity, and severe neutropenia but normal chromosomes.[661] This family might belong in the SD category, despite the absence of metaphyseal dysplasia (see earlier).

Seven families with a specific pattern of inheritance have been reported: five sporadic, one consanguineous, and one with affected siblings. Diaphyseal dysplasia and anemia were observed in all and thrombocytopenia in one of the families.[662–664] The anemia responded to prednisone, suggesting that these patients might have Diamond-Blackfan anemia (see later).

Autosomal Recessive without Physical Anomalies. Abels and Reed[665] reported two brothers who were short, had macrocytosis, and developed pancytopenia at approximately 10 years of age. One had immune deficiency and multiple cutaneous squamous and basal cell carcinomas. He also had oral telangiectasias and neck and chest poikiloderma; these findings suggested but were insufficient to diagnose DC. Because both patients were male, the inheritance might also be X-linked recessive. Linsk et al[666] described a consanguineous family with associated immune disorders in which four of six

siblings had pure red cell aplasia or neutropenia, as well as unusual crystalloid structures in the neutrophils demonstrated by electron microscopy. Chitambar et al[667] described eight members (both sexes) of 14 in one generation of a large maternal kindred with aplastic anemia, acute nonlymphocytic leukemia, and monosomy 7. Two adult siblings had thrombocytopenia and a Robertsonian translocation t(13;14); however, other siblings with the translocation had normal hematologic findings.[668] In the Scandinavian report on "acquired aplastic anemia" with multiple family members (mentioned earlier),[657] 10 patients in 4 families belonged to sibships.

A clearly autosomal recessive DNA repair disorder, *xeroderma pigmentosum*, has been reported to be associated with aplastic anemia,[669] as well as with MDS[670] and acute myeloid leukemia.[671, 672] Marrow failure is not usually associated with xeroderma pigmentosum, in which skin cancer is the major problem because of sensitivity to ultraviolet light.

X-Linked Recessive without Physical Anomalies. In a family with X-linked recessive disease described by Li et al,[673] eight males in three generations had adult-onset pancytopenia, acute myelogenous leukemia, light chain disease, or acute lymphocytic leukemia (in one patient). In one of the Scandinavian families, a man and his maternal uncle had aplastic anemia.[657] The *X-linked lymphoproliferative syndrome* has been reported in more than 25 kindreds.[674] At least 17 of the boys developed fatal aplastic anemia during or after malignant infectious mononucleosis.[675] Other components of this syndrome include hypoproliferative disorders, agranulocytosis, hypogammaglobulinemia, and proliferative disorders associated with the Epstein-Barr virus (American Burkitt lymphoma, immunoblastic B cell sarcoma, plasmacytoma, and fatal mononucleosis). Restriction fragment length polymorphisms localized this gene to the region of Xq24-q27.[676]

Sporadic Cases Characterized by Aplastic Anemia and Physical Anomalies. A 16-year-old male with Friedreich ataxia, short stature, hypogonadism, and hyperreflexia had macrocytic hypoplastic anemia that responded to testosterone.[677] Peripheral blood but not marrow chromosomes showed increased breakage on baseline tests. A 3-year-old boy had cerebellar ataxia, translocation (1;20), and aplasia, without increased baseline chromosome breakage.[678] A girl had short stature, dysmorphic facies, webbed neck, and proximal thumbs, as well as pancytopenia without increased chromosome breakage.[679] A 12-year-old girl had skin pigmentation and marrow failure; results of DEB-induced chromosome breakage testing were normal.[680] Three patients with the Brachmann-de Lange syndrome had thrombocytopenia that progressed to aplastic anemia in two of them.[681, 682] Eleven children with aplastic anemia and anomalies were reported to the IFAR; in these children chromosome breakage was not increased by DEB.[69] Many patients who in fact may not have FA may have been identified as having FA in the older literature and thus are included in our own analyses (see earlier). Only modern testing for clastogen-induced chromosome breakage could properly categorize all of these.

Several cases do not fit any category.[3] In 3 of the 8 families with 19 members with aplastic anemia cited earlier,[657] the anemia might have been related to drugs. Four families had more than one patient with chloramphenicol-related aplastic anemia. Two families had siblings with aplastic anemia after hepatitis. Use of gold and methyprylon (piperidine) as well as idiopathic aplastic anemia have also each been reported in sets of siblings.

It would appear that aplastic anemia may be associated with familial (genetic) predisposition to specific adverse environments. In some cases, there may be physical abnormalities that call attention to the possibly inherited nature of the condition. The familial and inherited marrow failure syndromes are clearly heterogeneous, representing a large variety of phenotypes and inheritance patterns. Only diligent investigation will elucidate the relevant genetic and environmental factors.

LABORATORY FINDINGS

The patients in this heterogeneous group have variable degrees of pancytopenia, macrocytosis, elevated levels of HbF, and hypocellular bone marrows. Only those whose families show additional features, such as immune deficiencies, novel chromosomes, or monosomy 7, may be distinguished from those with nonfamilial aplastic anemia. Those with familial disease but without characteristic findings are more difficult to detect. Baseline chromosome breakage is usually normal in the patients with non-FA familial syndromes, but examination with clastogenic agents is required for definitive distinction. Those patients who have hypoplastic or aplastic anemia also have reduced numbers of hematopoietic stem cells, another nonspecific finding.[683]

PATHOPHYSIOLOGY

The aplastic anemia is the result of combinations of genetic and environmental factors that are unique to each family. The inheritance patterns are autosomal dominant, autosomal recessive, and X-linked recessive, as well as multifactorial. Because some of the families have features resembling some of those found in FA, we can speculate that some of the genes may be allelic. The defects may be multiple even at the hematopoietic level, because some of the patients have only single cytopenias. Thus, pluripotent or specific committed progenitor cells may be defective.

THERAPY AND OUTCOME

Many of the patients discussed in this section died of their aplastic anemia. Several were treated with transfusions, antilymphocyte globulin, androgens, or BMT, with limited success. Because each instance is practically unique, the only suggestion is that androgens might be more effective than immunosuppression. However, because immune dysfunction is part of some of the syndromes, even that statement is overly simplistic. In general, drug treatment and supportive care should be the same as those described above for FA or for acquired aplastic anemia. BMT is risky because the potential donor may have the same condition. In several families, aplastic anemia is just the first step to development of preleukemia and leukemia. The overall prognosis for patients with familial bone marrow failure is poor.

Down Syndrome

Infants with Down syndrome (trisomy 21) often have a neonatal transient myeloproliferative syndrome. Later, they also have an increased risk of developing leukemia.[684] Five patients with aplastic anemia were reported. In a 17-year-old-boy with "idiopathic" aplastic anemia and trisomy 21, an apparent response to androgens was seen.[685] A newborn with trisomy 21, cystic fibrosis, and amegakaryocytic thrombocytopenia died at 49 days; this infant had pancytopenia shortly before death.[686] A 12-year-old boy developed aplastic anemia that was unresponsive to androgen and died within 10 weeks[687]; another patient had aplastic anemia at 19 months that responded to androgens.[688] A fifth patient developed aplastic anemia at 9 months and died at 26 months of gastroenteritis.[689] Bone marrows of these patients were hypocellular. The last patient had increased numbers of CFU-GMs with both cellular and serum inhibitors of hematopoiesis. Because of the small number of patients with trisomy 21 and aplastic anemia, it is not clear whether this is a true association or merely a coincidence.

Dubowitz Syndrome

Dubowitz syndrome is a rare, apparently autosomal recessive condition in which hematologic and malignant complications were noted in approximately 10 percent of the almost 150 patients reviewed recently.[690] The major features include intrauterine and postnatal growth retardation, microcephaly, moderate mental retardation, hyperactivity, eczema, and facial anomalies such as hypertelorism, epicanthal folds, blepharophimosis, broad nose, and abnormal ears. Aplastic anemia occurred in six patients, leukopenia occurred in two patients, and single patients had acute lymphoblastic leukemia, non-Hodgkin lymphoma, malignant lymphoma, and neuroblastoma.

Autosomal recessive inheritance was supported by a summary of 17 males and 21 females,[691] with one set of twins, four sibling pairs, and one consanguineous family. This syndrome is another that is characterized by growth defects associated with hematopoietic disorders and malignancies.

Seckel Syndrome

Seckel syndrome is another rare autosomal recessive condition with aplastic anemia. The term may have been overused in the characterization of a heterogeneous group of more than 60 reported microcephalic dwarfs, and thus the true number of those affected is unclear. The stringent definition requires the presence of severe intrauterine and postnatal growth retardation, severe microcephaly, severe mental retardation, typical face with receding forehead and chin, antimongoloid slant of palpebral fissures, prominently curved nose, relatively large eyes and teeth, highly arched palate, hirsutism, and clinodactyly.[692] At least 25 percent of patients developed aplastic anemia[3, 693] or malignancies (Hodgkin disease, lymphosarcoma and neuroblastoma, acute lymphoblastic leukemia [2 patients],[694] acute myeloid leukemia,[695] and hepatoma[696]). The aplasias were noted at 4 to 16 years of age. Three patients died of sepsis (or causes not reported) at 7, 9, and 12 years of age, 2 to 5 years after diagnosis. In two patients a response to androgens was not seen, and all patients required transfusions. One patient died 2 weeks after BMT, and one was alive 1.5 years after BMT. The cancers were diagnosed at 1 to 26 years of age, and the patients did not survive. The diagnosis of FA was considered in many patients because they were small in stature, microcephalic, and retarded and had pancytopenia. Actually, patients with Seckel syndrome are much smaller and more severely microcephalic and retarded than those with FA. Results of chromosome studies were normal in five patients[693, 697, 698]; endogenous breakage was increased in one patient and increased further with MMC in a sibling.[699] However, the diagnosis of FA could not be firmly established. Two patients with Seckel syndrome without aplastic anemia had normal endogenous chromosomes and normal sister chromatid exchanges.[700] Two other patients had cells with normal sensitivity to MMC, and normal levels of FANCA and FANCC proteins.[701] Seckel syndrome is another autosomal recessive syndrome characterized by growth retardation, the occasional presence of aplastic anemia and cancer, and, probably, no increase in chromosome breakage.

Noonan Syndrome

Patients with Noonan syndrome have characteristic facies with hypertelorism, ptosis, low-set ears, and short necks, as well as short stature and congenital heart defects; they resemble patients with Turner's syndrome (45,XO). Inheritance is autosomal dominant in half of the patients, and genetic linkage has localized the gene to chromosome 12q.[702] Several patients with amegakaryocytic thrombocytopenia at birth to 30 years of age were reported[703–706]; another patient had pancytopenia and hypocellular marrow at 4 years of age.[707] Bader-Meunier et al[708] reported four patients who had a myeloproliferative disorder in the first 2 months of life that was characterized as chronic myelomonocytic leukemia. The condition gradually resolved in three patients, but developed into acute myelocytic leukemia type M1 in one patient. They also cite other reports of acute leukemia in Noonan syndrome. As in the other syndromes, the incidence of marrow failure or malignancy is unknown.

SINGLE CYTOPENIAS

Bone marrow failure disorders in which only one cell line is involved are called *single cytopenias*. Most patients with these disorders do not develop pancytopenias, unlike those described above. White cell and platelet disorders are discussed at length in other chapters of this book (see Chapters 21 and 44).

Red Blood Cells

DIAMOND-BLACKFAN ANEMIA

Description

Josephs[709] first mentioned red cell aplasia in infancy in two patients reported in 1936. Two years later four more patients were presented by Diamond and Blackfan.[710] Synonyms and eponyms have included "congenital hypoplastic anemia (CHA)," "chronic congenital aregenerative anemia," "erythrogenesis imperfecta," "chronic idiopathic erythroblastopenia with aplastic anemia (type Josephs-Diamond-Blackfan)," and "Diamond-Blackfan anemia (DBA)." Diamond and Blackfan called it "congenital hypoplastic anemia," because they thought it differed from complete aplastic anemia (pancytopenia) only in degree. The term "hypoplastic" is now used when marrow depression is only partial, and thus it is not appropriate for describing a single cytopenia. "Erythrogenesis imperfecta" is probably the most descriptive appellation, but *Diamond-Blackfan anemia (DBA)* is used here because this is the term most often encountered in the literature.

The current diagnostic criteria for DBA are as follows: (1) normochromic, usually macrocytic but occasionally normocytic anemia developing early in childhood; (2) reticulocytopenia; (3) normocellular bone marrow with selective deficiency of red cell precursors; (4) normal or slightly decreased leukocyte counts; and (5) normal or often increased platelet counts. These criteria distinguish DBA from aplastic anemia (see Chapter 7) but may not always distinguish it from transient erythroblastopenia of childhood (see later).

The data regarding the incidence of DBA are limited. A 7-year study in northern England found an annual incidence of one child per million children per year.[711] National DBA Registries are developing, with more than 350 patients registered in North America,[712] more than 200 in France and Germany,[713] and almost 100 in Italy[714] through 1999. More than 700 patients with DBA have been reported in the literature in sufficient detail for analyses (Table 8–18), and many of the references are cited elsewhere.[2, 3] An additional 500 patients are summarized in large series, some of whom may also have been the subjects of case reports.[121, 713–717]

The anemia is usually noted in infancy, but DBA has been diagnosed in patients as old as 64 years of age (Table 8–18 and Fig. 8–21). Males with DBA were slightly younger than females (medians of 2 and 3 months). Ten percent of patients were severely anemic at birth, 25 percent by 1 month of age, 50 percent by 3 months, 75 percent by 6 months, and 90 percent by 18 months. DBA was diagnosed in an additional 5 percent of patients diagnosed between 1.5 and 2.5 years of age, in 3 percent before age 6, and in another 2 percent between ages 6 and 64. The male-to-female ratio is 1.1. Patients from more than 50 countries have been reported, and the majority are whites. DBA has also been reported in blacks, Asians, and Indians.

Twelve patients with presentation at older than 6 years of age have been described. A 34-year-old male with anemia had a daughter in whom anemia was diagnosed at age 6, and subsequently classic DBA was diagnosed in his grandson in infancy.[718, 719] Anemia was diagnosed in a female at age 16, and in her son at 9 months.[720] In a family in which anemia was diagnosed in four males over three generations, the paternal grandfather's diagnosis had been made at age 20.[721] In a large consanguineous family anemia affected 7 members in one generation, including 5 male siblings and a male and a female cousin. Anemia was diagnosed in one of the males at 9 years of age.[722] Two adult females with long-standing anemia, which responded to prednisone, were short and had findings typical of DBA, including webbed

TABLE 8–18. Diamond-Blackfan Anemia Literature by Decade of First Report

	1936–1960	1961–1970	1971–1980	1981–1990	1991–2000	All Patients
No. of patients	78	113	90	115	309	705
Male/female	31/41	60/52	47/42	49/36	145/142	332/313
Ratio	0.8	1.2	1.1	1.4	1.0	1.1
Male age at diagnosis (mos)						
Mean	3.6	12.4	7.7	3.0	14.1	9.6
Median	2.3	2.0	2.0	2.0	2.5	2.0
Range	0–24	0–408	0–54	0–18	0–264	0–408
Female age at diagnosis (mos)						
Mean	6.2	6.7	8.2	37.5	15.7	14.2
Median	3.0	3.0	3.0	3	2.0	3.0
Range	0–28	0–72	0–48	0–768	0–192	0–768
No. males >1 yr	1	8	8	1	11	29
No. females >1 yr	6	5	7	6	15	39
Age at death (yrs)						
No.(%)	10 (13)	29 (26)	10 (11)	12 (10)	29 (9)	90 (13)
Mean	4.4	8.1	10.9	8.6	11.4	9.6
Median	2.3	4.8	7.5	5	8.5	6
Range	0.3–23	0.2–43	0.1–40	0–65	0–54	0–65
Projected median survival (yrs)		25	32	65	—	43

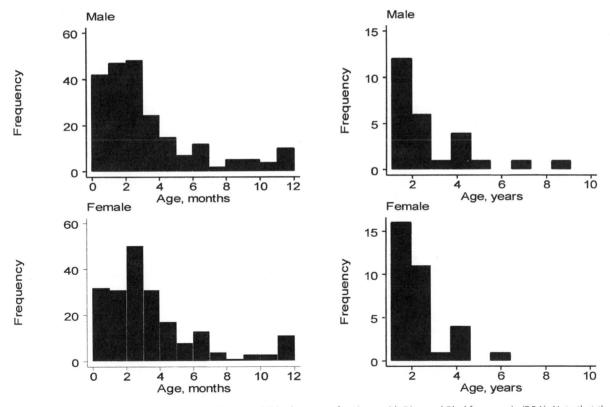

FIGURE 8–21. Age at onset of anemia in approximately 550 published reports of patients with Diamond-Blackfan anemia (DBA). Note that the scale on the abscissa is in months for the graphs on the left, for those between 0 and 12 months of age, and in years for the graphs on the right, for those between 1 and 10 years of age. Not shown are nine patients who were aged 11 to 64 years at diagnosis. *Top,* males; *bottom,* females.

necks and thenar atrophy.[723] In addition, anemia was diagnosed in two males at 7 and 22 years of age and three females at 11, 13, and 35 years of age.[716, 724–726]

Inheritance and Environment

The inheritance of DBA appears to have more than one pattern. *Dominant inheritance* is apparent in more than 30 families in whom one parent often had childhood anemia requiring transfusions, or steroid therapy, or both and one or more children have classic DBA. These dominant families involve fathers and mothers equally, and the affected parent may have only increased HbF, macrocytosis, or elevated red cell adenosine deaminase (ADA) (see later). The numbers of affected males and females in the dominant group are equal, the incidence of physical abnormalities is low, and the clinical course is generally milder than in the overall population with DBA. The large series reported by Willig et al[727, 728] had 33 families in which at least 2 generations had classic DBA. Among 154 patients with sporadic DBA, 21 had a first-degree relative with anemia, macrocytosis, or increased ADA, and these relatives had the same gene mutation as the proband in their family, suggesting that some patients with apparently sporadic inheritance may actually have autosomal dominant inheritance (see later).

Recessive inheritance might be identified in more than 30 families in which there were affected siblings with normal parents, affected cousins, or consanguinity.[2] One set of male twins was reported in a sibship with three affected males,[729] and one set of affected identical twins has also been reported.[730] Anomalies occurred more often in those with recessive inheritance than in the overall group, but the anemia was milder and more responsive to treatment. "Recessive" inheritance in these families might also be dominant with variable expression, but consanguinity makes that less likely.

The majority of the patients appear to have sporadic inheritance, suggesting new mutation dominants, acquired disease, or extremely variable penetrance.

Although data regarding pregnancies in the literature are often incomplete, approximately 1 percent of the mothers of DBA patients reported previous stillbirths or miscarriages. Problems during pregnancies include pre-eclampsia, toxemia, rashes, premature placental separation, placental infarcts, hemorrhage, spotting, positive tests for syphilis, and caesarean sections. Exposures during pregnancy involved stilbestrol, radiation, chlorothiazide, reserpine, thyroid, prednisone, phenylbutazone, chloramphenicol, and anagyrine. Seven percent of the patients with DBA weighed 2500 g or less at birth, most of whom were small for gestational age (intrauterine growth retardation). Although birth lengths were rarely recorded, several infants were less than 45 cm. The low birth weights might reflect problems during pregnancy or poor growth intrinsic to DBA itself.

Most patients were pale at birth or soon thereafter. Jaundice due to hemolytic disease of the newborn from Rh or ABO incompatibility occurred occasionally, leading to prolonged anemia that became chronic[731] or that sometimes resolved after a few months.[732] A small number of patients had nonimmune hydrops at birth, consistent with a prenatal manifestation.[733–735] Antecedent illnesses were reported, including diarrhea, respiratory infections, urinary tract infections, measles, mumps, or a reaction to smallpox vaccination. One child was treated with chloramphenicol.[736] In most children, the illness was more likely to be due to the anemia or to an unrelated cause rather than being the cause of the anemia. Signs of anemia included pallor, lethargy, irritability, and heart failure. Three infants were born after intrauterine infection with parvovirus and had B19 DNA in bone marrow cells that was detected by polymerase chain reaction,[737] but none showed a response to intravenous immunoglobulin therapy. In another series, three patients with parvovirus DNA in their bone marrow showed a response to steroid therapy and in these patients steroid-free remissions were maintained for more than 2 months, 3 years, and 9 years.[738] One patient had a parvovirus-induced relapse after spontaneous remission of his DBA.[739] The role of parvovirus in DBA is unclear, but it is probably not major.

Physical Examination

Physical appearances were abnormal in more than 25 percent of patients (Table 8–19). Abnormalities of the head and face were the most common. The typical facial appearance was described by Cathie[740] as "tow coloured hair, snub nose, wide-set eyes, thick upper lip, and an intelligent expression" and was observed in many of the children, who resemble each other more than they do their own family members. Cleft lip or palate occurred in 3 percent of patients, and three patients (two cousins and another unrelated to them) were reported who had microtia and cleft palate, features of Treacher-Collins syndrome.[741, 742] In one patient the gene mutated in Treacher-Collins syndrome was normal, as was the *RPS19* gene, which is mutated in 25 percent of patients with DBA (see later). Other facial findings in DBA include micrognathia, micro- or macrocephaly, macroglossia, wide fontanelle, and dysmorphic features.

A specific comment must be made regarding upper limb anomalies, which are found in almost 50 percent of patients with FA (see earlier), and at least 8 percent of patients with DBA. The most common feature of DBA is flattening of the thenar eminences or weakness of radial pulses, but other radial hand anomalies also are common. Triphalangeal thumbs were reported in 22 patients in whom the course of anemia was not different from that of the entire population with DBA. Although this association has been separated by some into the *Aase syndrome*,[743] it is probably an inappropriate example of splitting rather than lumping.[744] More than two dozen patients had duplicated, bifid, supernumerary, absent, or subluxed thumbs. Thumb anomalies could be unilateral or bilateral.

More than 10 percent of the patients with DBA were short, a characteristic unrelated to corticosteroid therapy. Four of eight short patients with DBA had GH deficiency and two had borderline GH deficiency; treatment with GH did improve growth.[745] There were several reports of dwarfism,[3, 9] including achondroplasia, metaphyseal

TABLE 8–19. Physical Abnormalities in Diamond-Blackfan Anemia

Abnormality	All Patients (%)	Male (%)	Female (%)
No. of patients	646	332	313
Birth weight ≤2500 g	7	5	9
Head, face, palate	7	5	8
Upper limbs	8	6	11
Short stature	12	11	14
Eyes	5	5	5
Renal	4	4	4
Neck	3	1	5
Hypogonads	2	4	0.3
Retardation	2	2	3
Cardiopulmonary	2	2	2
Nose	1	1	1
Other skeletal	4	4	5
Other	10	9	12
At least one anomaly*	25	23	25
Short stature alone	3	3	3

*Not including low birth weight or short stature. Many patients had more than one abnormality.

dysostosis, and cartilage-hair hypoplasia.[746, 747] Almost two dozen patients had short or webbed necks, including manifestations of both Klippel-Feil syndrome (fused cervical vertebrae) and Sprengel deformity (elevation of the scapula). A "Turner-like" phenotype was sometimes mentioned.

Eye anomalies in 5 percent of the patients included hypertelorism, blue sclerae, glaucoma, epicanthal folds, microphthalmos, cataracts, and strabismus. Kidney abnormalities such as horseshoe, duplicated, and absent kidneys were also noted in a few patients. Four percent of males had hypogonadism, and 2 percent of patients were retarded. Lower limb problems included dislocated hips, achondroplasia, and clubfoot. Congenital heart disease was seen occasionally. The presence of anomalies serves more to confirm the diagnosis of DBA than to provide any prognosis regarding the course of the disease.

Laboratory Findings

All patients with DBA are by definition anemic. Limited data show hemoglobin levels at birth ranging from 2.6 to 14.8 g/dL, with a median hemoglobin level of 7 g/dL. In infants in whom DBA is diagnosed within the first 2 months of life, the hemoglobin level ranged from 1.5 to 10 g/dL and the median was 4 g/dL. In infants in whom DBA was diagnosed after 2 months, the hemoglobin level was also usually approximately 4 g/dL. Macrocytosis was common (although often not reported) and reticulocyte counts were decreased or zero. The representative blood smear in Figure 8–22 shows macrocytes, anisocytosis, and teardrops. White cell counts are usually normal, although they often decrease with age. In 20 percent of patients white cell counts were 5000/μL or less at some time, and 5 percent had counts less than 3000/μL. Two older patients who had received many transfusions developed significant neutropenia.* Platelet counts, while usually normal, were less than 150,000/μL at least once in 25 percent of patients and greater than 400,000/μL in 20 percent. Buchanan et al[748] noted elevated platelet counts in one half of 38 patients and decreased platelet counts in one fourth of these on at least one occasion. Platelet function was normal.

The level of HbF is usually increased. HbF is distributed heterogeneously (Fig. 8–23), a finding indicating that the patients do not have a single clone of completely fetal cells. The HbF has a fetal composition, with the ratio of $^{G}\gamma$ to $^{A}\gamma$ exceeding 60:40. The titer of red cell membrane antigen i is also increased, as in fetuses, whereas the adult counterpart, I, remains at adult levels. These "fetal-like" erythrocyte features are seen in patients with newly diagnosed DBA, and following treatment, they persist even in those with spontaneous remissions. They are not unique to DBA, but are characteristic of the "stress erythropoiesis" seen in any type of bone marrow failure.[43]

Bone marrow aspirates and biopsies show normal cellularity, myeloid cells, and megakaryocytes. Lymphocyte counts are often increased, and lymphocytes were initially thought to be "hematogones."[749] Eosinophilia was pointed out by Gasser,[750] although it is not common. Bernard and associates[751] described three patterns of erythroid development. The most common pattern is erythroid hypoplasia or total aplasia (Fig. 8–24, *A*) which is seen in 90 percent of patients. When present, the few erythroid precursors seen are immature proerythroblasts. The next most common pattern, seen in 5 percent of patients, is one of normal numbers and maturation of erythroblasts. The remaining 5 percent have erythroid hyperplasia and also a maturation arrest, with increased numbers of immature precursors.

Despite the variable bone marrow findings, all patients have reticulocytopenia. Thus, some patients have a form of ineffective erythropoiesis and evidence of delayed precursor maturation. In addition, dyserythropoietic

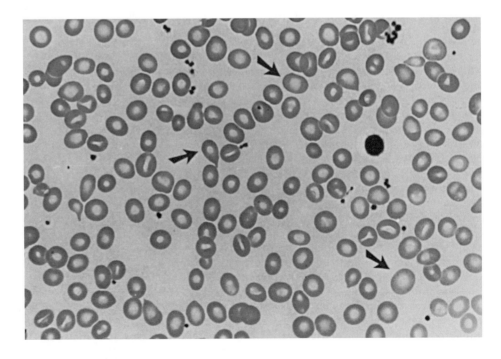

FIGURE 8–22. Peripheral blood from a patient with DBA. Note anisocytosis, with both microcytosis and macrocytosis, as well as teardrop erythrocytes *(arrows)*. (Courtesy of Dr. Gail Wolfe; with permission from Alter BP: The bone marrow failure syndromes. In Nathan DG, Oski FA (eds): Hematology of Infancy and Childhood, 3rd ed. Philadelphia, WB Saunders, 1987, p 159.)

---

*Young NS: Unpublished observations.

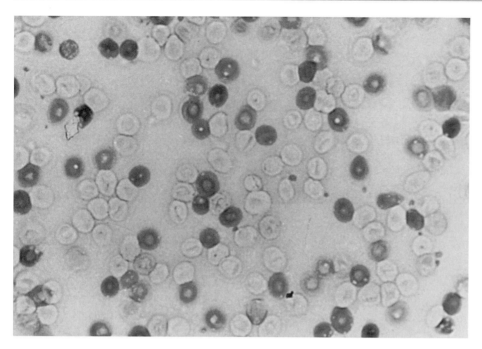

FIGURE 8–23. Kleihauer-Betke acid elution study of blood from a patient with DBA, showing the heterogeneous distribution of the fetal hemoglobin. (From Alter BP: The bone marrow failure syndromes. Nathan DG, Oski FA (eds): Hematology of Infancy and Childhood, 3rd ed. Philadelphia, WB Saunders, 1987, p 159.)

morphology has been seen occasionally (see section on congenital dyserythropoietic anemia, later in this chapter). Two patients were reported to have ringed sideroblasts that later disappeared.[752, 753] Patients who have received many transplants have accumulations of iron in their marrow (Fig. 8–24, *B*) and other organs.

Serum levels of iron, ferritin, folic acid, vitamin B_{12}, and erythropoietin[754] are all elevated. DBA is not due to a deficiency of any of the usual hematinic agents. Patients do not have antibodies to erythropoietin. Results of routine urinalyses are normal. A suggestion of an abnormality in tryptophan metabolism was not substantiated.[755] Hypocalcemia was observed once, and mild hypogammaglobulinemia was noted in several patients. These parameters are normal in many other patients, however. Low numbers of T lymphocytes and a reduction in the ratio of helper to suppressor cells were reported by Finlay and co-workers,[756] but abnormalities of T-cell function were not observed. Ferrokinetic studies showed the expected delay in plasma iron clearance and low red cell utilization. Autologous red cell survival times were slightly shortened and haptoglobin levels were low; these findings suggested a mild hemolytic component.[757–759] Patients with DBA have negative results on direct antiglobulin (Coombs') tests, and their disease is not due to red cell autoantibodies, although alloantibodies may develop after many transfusions. Results of bone marrow cultures and erythropoietic inhibitor assays are described in the section on pathophysiology.

Abnormalities involving purine or pyrimidine metabolism were observed in red cell enzymes. Giblett and colleagues[760] reported one patient with atypical DBA who also had lymphopenia and nucleoside phosphorylase deficiency, whereas other DBA patients had normal nucleoside phosphorylase levels.[761, 762] Zielke and co-workers[762] found increased erythrocyte levels of the pyrimidine enzymes orotate phosphoribosyl transferase and orotidine monophosphate decarboxylase in 5 patients. Increased orotidine monophosphate decarboxylase was observed in 5 of 10 patients in another study.[763] Because orotidine

monophosphate decarboxylase is an age-dependent enzyme, which is increased in cord blood cells, its elevation is consistent with the presence of young, fetal-like erythrocytes, as noted earlier.

Glader and his group[764] noted increased red cell ADA levels in 26 of 29 DBA patients and in 2 of 12 parents.[761] ADA is a critical enzyme in the purine salvage pathway, and it is not elevated in erythrocytes from cord blood or from patients with hemolytic or other aplastic anemias. Whitehouse et al[765] also found an increased ADA level in 9 of 19 patients and 2 of 15 relatives. The significance of the elevated ADA level is not clear, because it is also increased in some children with leukemia[764]; this increase may indicate disordered erythropoiesis that is not fetal-like. Detection of increased ADA levels may be useful in distinguishing DBA from transient erythroblastopenia of childhood (see later).[764]

Peripheral blood lymphocyte chromosomes are essentially normal in patients with DBA.[757] One patient had an achromatic area in chromosome 1,[766] and another had a pericentric inversion in chromosome 1.[767] Three of six patients in one series had an enlarged chromosome 16,[768] and one patient had breaks and endoreduplication of chromosome 16.[769] One patient had increased spontaneous and radiation-induced chromosome breakage, without increased breakage caused by MMC.[770] Others found no increased breakage in response to DEB.[652, 771] Normal chromosomes have been seen in more than 50 patients, including 20 of my own patients.[757] Sister chromatid exchange is also normal. Although some patients with DBA may have physical findings resembling those of FA, the chromosome studies are clearly distinctive.

Prenatal Diagnosis

In one fetus whose two siblings had DBA apparent high-output cardiac failure was detected with two-dimensional fetal Doppler echocardiography.[772] The specificity of this assay has been questioned, however.[773] An untested hypothesis proposes that erythrocyte ADA would be increased in a fetus with DBA. Similarly, the number of

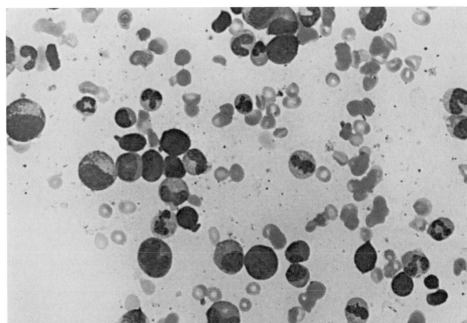

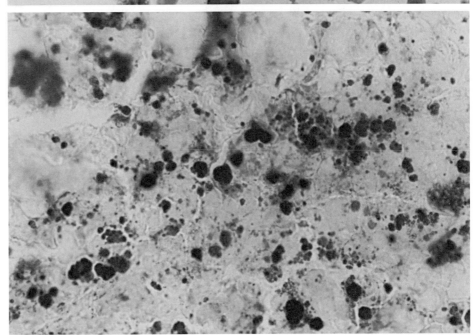

FIGURE 8–24. *A,* Bone marrow aspirate from a patient with DBA, showing normal cellularity with erythroid hypoplasia. *B,* Iron stain of bone marrow aspirate from a 2-year-old child with transfusion-dependent DBA. (Courtesy of Dr. Gail Wolfe; with permission from Alter BP: The bone marrow failure syndromes. In Nathan DG, Oski FA (eds): Hematology of Infancy and Childhood, 3rd ed. Philadelphia, WB Saunders, 1987, p 159.)

BFU-Es in blood of a fetus with DBA might be decreased (see later), but this hypothesis too has not been examined. Because DBA is familial in only approximately 10 percent of patients, the opportunities for prenatal testing are limited. In families in which the gene mutation has been identified, molecular diagnostics can be used for prenatal diagnosis (see later).

Pathophysiology

Because the genetics, time of onset of anemia, and physical appearances of patients with DBA are varied, the disease may have multiple causes. Most *in vitro* studies of erythropoiesis were limited to small numbers of patients. Differing results may be due to true variability of the disease. The consensus is that there is an intrinsic abnormality in the erythroid progenitor cell, although a few studies suggested extrinsic abnormalities in accessory cells or serum.

Erythropoietic Defect. The level of the major erythropoietic hormone erythropoietin is higher in patients with DBA than expected for the level of anemia.[3, 754] Transient improvements were seen in 6 of 10 patients given plasma infusions.[754, 774] The mechanism of response is unknown, and this observation has not been corroborated. The response was probably not due to provision of erythropoietin, because the plasmas used for the infusions were from normal individuals.

Early reports suggested that DBA might be due to red cell alloantibodies.[731, 732, 775, 776] These patients had neonatal jaundice and ABO or Rh incompatibility, and anemia persisted longer than expected; in a few of these patients true DBA was eventually diagnosed. Antibody specificity may have included erythroblasts or progenitors; blood group sensitization may have been real but unrelated. The majority of patients did not have blood group incompatibility.[777]

Ortega and co-workers[778] proposed the existence of a circulating inhibitor of erythropoiesis, but this speculation was not confirmed.[779, 780] Treatment of patient serum with an antibody to erythropoietin failed to unmask an inhibitor of erythropoiesis. In erythroid progenitor cultures in semisolid media, only one patient had a serum erythroid blocking factor that was seen only in allogeneic and not autologous cultures.[781]

Cellular inhibitors have also been proposed. Peripheral blood lymphocytes from six patients with DBA who had received multiple transfusions inhibited erythroid colony formation by normal bone marrow cells.[782] However, Nathan and co-workers[783] were unable to detect inhibitory lymphocytes from one of those patients using HLA-identical marrow as the target. Another patient with DBA had normal erythroid progenitors and no cellular inhibitors.[574] In the blood of two adults who had many transfusions as children suppressor T cells were suggested to have been overcome by a serum blocking factor.[784] Finlay et al[756] observed T-cell suppression of normal erythroid colony growth in one of five patients. Inhibitory monocytes were proposed by Zanjani and Rinehart.[785] One adult had normal bone marrow colonies, but heme synthesis was inhibited by her bone fragments; this implied a microenvironmental defect.[786]

Nathan and associates[787] found no inhibition of normal or autologous marrow CFU-Es by the lymphocytes from four transfusion-dependent patients, and no inhibition of normal or autologous blood BFU-Es by the lymphocytes of eight other patients, some of whom were transfusion-dependent and some of whom were in steroid-independent remissions.[787] Patients' T cells stimulated normal blood null cell BFU-Es, as did normal T cells.[788] The cellular suppression phenomenon may relate to transfusion sensitization, not to the pathophysiology of DBA.

Cumulative evidence indicates that the erythroid stem cell is defective in patients with DBA. Cultures of bone marrow and blood mononuclear cells in plasma clot or methyl cellulose showed a decrease in or absence of CFU-Es and BFU-Es in more than 50 patients and normal numbers of progenitors in about a dozen patients who were younger and had previously been untreated (see reference 789 and references therein). Those whose DBA subsequently responded to prednisone may have had better *in vitro* erythroid growth. Addition of steroids to cell cultures from a few patients increased colony growth and correlated with clinical response.[135, 787, 790, 791]

In some patients, unusually high concentrations of erythropoietin improved erythroid colony growth.[2] Nathan et al[787] studied two patients who had relapses and subsequently showed clinical improvement with prednisone treatment. Progenitors from these patients then responded to the usual levels of erythropoietin. Crude erythropoietin, which may have contained other erythroid growth-promoting factors, was used for these experiments. Lipton and colleagues[792] added "burst-promoting activity" and showed increased erythroid growth and increased erythropoietin sensitivity in bone marrow cultures from patients with DBA. They then enriched the cultures for erythroid progenitors by removing monocytes and lymphocytes and enhanced the burst-promoting activity effect, thus suggesting that the burst-promoting activity acts directly on progenitors and not through accessory cells.[793] The burst-promoting activity probably contains specific growth factors with erythroid activity such as GM-CSF and IL-3. Halpérin et al[794] reported that the size and number of marrow BFU-Es were enhanced with IL-3 *in vitro*. The previously reported insensitivity to erythropoietin may have reflected insensitivity to burst-promoting activity or specifically to IL-3.

Mice with mutations at the *W* or *Sl* loci have macrocytic anemia, as well as no hair pigment, mast cell deficiency, and sterility.[795] Homozygote *W* mutants have a defect in their hematopoietic stem cells, whereas the defect in *Sl* mice is in the microenvironment. The *W* mutation is in the c-*kit* proto-oncogene, a transmembrane tyrosine kinase receptor,[796] whereas the *Sl* mutation, called SCF, is in the *kit* ligand.[797] These mice provide attractive models for human DBA. In fact, the human disease resulting from a mutation in c-*kit* is piebaldism, a dominant disorder characterized by a white forelock, but the rare homozygotes are not anemic.[798, 799] The anemia of *W* but not of *Sl* mice was improved with high doses of erythropoietin,[800] but neither anemia was responsive to steroid[801] or IL-3[802] treatment (see later). The *kit* and *SCF* genes did not demonstrate structural abnormalities in 30 patients,[803–806] and *SCF* gene expression was normal,[807, 808] suggesting that the DBA defect is not present in those genes. Despite this, SCF is an effective agent *in vitro*, leading to improved or even normalized growth of marrow BFU-Es,[121, 726, 804, 809–811] and thus SCF remains a potential candidate for treatment trials.

Perdahl et al[812] described an acceleration in programmed cell death (apoptosis) in DBA marrow. They showed that progenitors were abnormally sensitive to deprivation of erythropoietin and that the typical DNA oligosomes appeared rapidly. Dianzani et al[813] found that there were no mutations in the erythropoietin receptor and that IL-9 as well as the 5q hematopoietic cluster were also normal.[814] These findings further indicate that the DBA defect is intrinsic to the erythroid progenitor cell in a manner that remains to be identified.

Molecular Studies and DBA Genes. The first clue to localization of a DBA gene was provided by a patient with a reciprocal X;19 translocation, and three patients with microdeletion syndromes involving 19q13.2.[815–819] The gene for ribosomal protein subunit 19 was involved in a translocation breakpoint.[820] Heterozygous mutations in *RPS19*, which include nonsense, frameshift, splice site, or missense mutations, have been documented in approximately 25 percent of patients with DBA (Fig. 8–25 and Table 8–5). The disease results from haploinsufficiency; presumably, biallelic mutation of *RPS19* would be lethal. The role of a dominant mutation in a ribosomal subunit in the DBA phenotype is unclear, although one might speculate that a reduced amount of one of the ribosomal

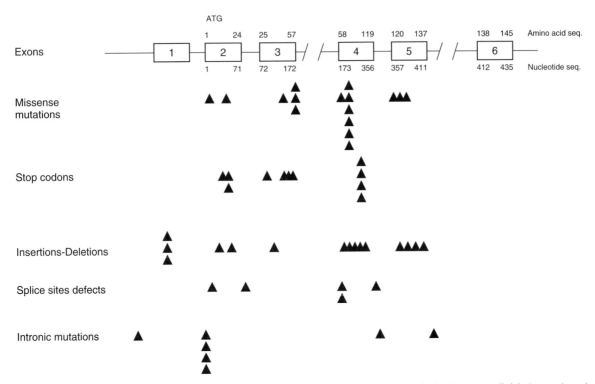

FIGURE 8–25. Point mutations in *RPS19,* one of the DBA genes. The positions of single nucleotide substitutions or small deletions or insertions in the *RPS19* gene found in patients with DBA are indicated along the six exons of the *RPS19* gene. (From Willig T-N, Draptchinskaia N, Dianzani I, et al: Mutations in ribosomal protein S19 gene and Diamond Blackfan anemia: Wide variations in phenotypic expression. Blood 1999; 94:4294.)

proteins may interfere with protein synthesis in specific target cells.

A locus for a second DBA gene was recently mapped to chromosome 8p23.2-p22, and the investigators suggested that there is at least one more gene.[821] In their study of genes in 38 families with dominantly inherited DBA, 47 percent mapped to 8p, 34 percent to 19q, and the remaining 18 percent to neither of those loci. The 8p region does not appear to encode functional ribosomal proteins, but this DBA gene may be involved in a different mechanism of cellular function.

None of the DBA gene-hunting strategies have localized the genes in families that have autosomal recessive inheritance, and some of the patients with sporadic inheritance do not have mutations in *RPS19*. Thus, there may be even more genes than the three indicated so far.

Mutation analyses in DBA genes will have important clinical applications, including clarification of diagnoses in patients, genotype/phenotype correlations, prognostic value regarding clinical outcomes, and prenatal diagnosis.

Therapy and Outcome

Transfusions. Initially, the only available treatment for DBA was blood transfusions; without this treatment affected children died of anemia.[709] Blood transfusion remains the mainstay of treatment for steroid-resistant disease. Leukocyte-depleted packed red cells should be given every 3 to 6 weeks to keep the hemoglobin level above 6 g/dL. Crossmatching for minor blood groups is only necessary if sensitization leads to the appearance of alloantibodies. The major complication from transfusions is hemosiderosis, which was the cause

of death in at least 20 percent of the more than 50 patients whose deaths were reported. The side effects of iron overload in patients with DBA are identical to those seen in patients with thalassemia major and include diabetes, cardiac failure, liver disease, growth failure, and failure to enter puberty. These complications do develop more slowly in patients with DBA than in those with thalassemia, in which a hemolytic rather than an aplastic process is involved. Chelation of iron with subcutaneous desferrioxamine should begin as soon as the patients have increased iron stores. Use of an oral chelator, which is being studied in patients with β-thalassemia, is not advised in patients with DBA because of the risk of neutropenia.[822–824]

Splenectomy was reported in approximately 40 patients, with no beneficial effect except in those who had hypersplenism related to transfusions. One half of the splenectomized patients died, often from infections. Splenectomy is no longer recommended unless there is hypersplenism.

Corticosteroids. The use of corticosteroids was first proposed by Gasser, who noted erythroblastopenia in patients with transient allergic disorders and observed increased eosinophil counts in the marrows of patients with DBA.[750, 825] The drugs used initially were cortisone or adrenocorticotropic hormone,[826] but prednisone or prednisolone is now the drug of choice. Allen and Diamond[827] were the first to treat large numbers of patients, reporting remission in 12 of 22.

The current recommended initial dose of prednisone is 2 mg/kg/day, given in three or four divided doses. Reticulocytes usually appear within 1 to 2 weeks. Some of the new erythropoiesis is apparently ineffective, because a sustained rise in hemoglobin level may not occur for several weeks, although it is often seen within a month. The high, divided dose protocol should be continued until the hemoglobin level is greater than 10 g/dL. The prednisone dose should then be tapered slowly, by sequential elimination of the divided doses, until the patient is receiving a single daily dose that still maintains the hemoglobin level. This dose is then doubled and administered on alternate days; this regimen is followed by a very slow decrease in the amount of the alternate-day dose to minimize side effects. One group managed to give their patients prednisone daily for a week, followed by 1 or 2 weeks without the drug, to permit better growth;[828] this regimen failed for the author. With the alternate-day treatment, the prednisone dose varies from as little as 1 mg to as much as 40 mg, and extreme sensitivity to small changes in dose can be seen. Steroid side effects include growth retardation (seen in more than one half of patients),[777] osteoporosis, weight gain, cushingoid appearance, hypertension, diabetes, fluid retention, and gastric ulcers. A few patients had steroid-related cataracts or glaucoma.

The patterns of response to steroid therapy are numerous and include the following:

1. Rapid response, followed by steroid-independent remission, which occurs in less than 5 percent of patients.
2. Intermittent response, also seen in less than 5 percent of patients.
3. Response followed by steroid dependence, which is seen in 60 percent of patients. In up to 20 percent of these patients hemoglobin levels may eventually be maintained without steroids.
4. Steroid response and dependence, followed by later failure to respond to the same or higher doses, seen in 5 percent of patients.
5. Requirement for very large daily doses with relapse when the dose is decreased, seen in less than 5 percent of patients. This usually means that transfusions must be resumed because of the side effects of the steroids.
6. No response, seen in 30 to 40 percent of patients.

Overall, patients who show no response to steroids, those who show a response to high doses of steroids, or patients in whom steroid treatments subsequently fail may comprise up to 50 percent. In the total group, 15 to 25 percent of patients may eventually have spontaneous remissions, regardless of their treatment response category.[829] These remissions occurred at a mean and median of 7 and 6 years of age with the range being from 1 month to 21 years of age.[3]

If prednisone therapy at 2 mg/kg/day does not induce remission, it should be followed by a trial of 4 to 6 mg/kg/day, or a trial with a different preparation such as prednisolone or dexamethasone. Use of marrow-suppressing drugs or those that might affect the metabolism of prednisone, such as phenytoin or phenobarbital, should be discontinued. Allen and Diamond[827] found that the response was better if the interval between diagnosis and treatment was short, but this result may have been seen because hemosiderosis had developed if the interval was sufficiently long for large numbers of transfusions. Actually, steroid-induced remissions have been seen after 10 years of transfusions, and a history of transfusions should not preclude an adequate trial of steroid therapy coupled with iron chelation.

Several other therapeutic approaches have also been attempted.[3, 9] Androgens (see earlier section on FA) were used in more than 50 patients, but responses were rare. Treatment with an attenuated androgen (Danazol) was effective in two patients.[830] Treatment with 6-mercaptopurine was effective in one of two patients.[779, 831] Two patients had a transient reticulocytosis after cyclophosphamide and antilymphocyte globulin treatment,* whereas others did not show a response to cyclophosphamide alone.[832] Vincristine has also been ineffective. Ozsoylu[833] reported the successful use of high doses of intravenous or oral methylprednisolone, as discussed earlier for severe acquired aplastic anemia. Bernini et al[834] also reported 50 percent efficacy with high-dose intravenous methylprednisone, but the toxicity was sufficiently high that they no longer use this approach.[834]

A few patients had a transient response to a combination of cyclosporine and prednisone. Prednisone was eliminated in only 3 patients,[835–838] but the dose was reduced in another 13 patients.[839–845] Another dozen patients did not respond to cyclosporine.[841, 843, 844, 846] Intravenous immunoglobulin was also ineffective.[737, 832, 845, 846] The rare anecdotal responses to immunosuppressive agents suggest that DBA might be an autoimmune disease, but the *in vitro* data do not support this mechanism (see earlier).

Cytokine therapy has been attempted in DBA. *In vitro* data from erythroid cultures suggested that high doses of erythropoietin might be effective, but doses of up 200 U/kg/day for up to 5 months had no therapeutic benefit.[847, 848] Because serum levels are very high, the expectation that the doses administered might be of value may have been overly enthusiastic. *In vitro* studies also suggested a role for IL-3. Only 10 percent of approximately 100 patients showed a good response to this agent, and serious side effects, which included allergic responses, fevers, chills, and deep vein thromboses, have led to removal of IL-3 from experimental use.[716, 849–852] Cytokine treatment remains experimental, and the most effective agent *in vitro*, SCF, is not in clinical trials for DBA because of toxicity *in vivo*.

Hematopoietic Stem Cell Transplantation. This is a possibility for patients who do not respond to reasonable doses of steroids. The survival rate reported in the literature was 75 percent of almost 40 patients who received transplants from HLA-matched sibling donors and 38 percent of 8 patients who had alternative donors. The results were similar in the Diamond-Blackfan Anemia Registry, with an actuarial survival of 88 percent with transplants from sibling donors and 28 percent with transplants from alternative donors.[829] Most of the transplant recipients did not show a response with steroid therapy or had a relapse while receiving steroids and had received

---

*Young NS: Unpublished observations.

transfusions. The cumulative probabilities of survival after transplant level off at 76 and 43 percent, respectively (Fig. 8–26), with the exclusion of one patient who developed metastatic osteosarcoma after transplant (see later). The actuarial survivals were similar: 59 and 63 percent for marrow donors compared with cord blood donors. Transplant-related deaths were due to infection and graft-versus-host disease. Preparation included various combinations of antilymphocyte globulin, procarbazine, total lymphoid irradiation, busulfan, and cyclophosphamide. Making the decision to perform transplantation in patients with DBA is complicated because of the possibility of spontaneous remission; in addition, BMT is generally more successful in young patients, who have received relatively few transplants (and therefore are not sensitized).

Survival Data. The cumulative survival results for more than 600 patients reported in the literature are shown in Figure 8–27 and summarized in Table 8–18. The predicted median survival ages have increased with time, reaching age 65 for the patients reported in the last decade and averaging 43 years overall. Initially, those who did not receive steroids died if transfusions were not provided or died from iron overload if transfusions were not accompanied by iron chelation. Separate analyses of males and females, those with dominant or recessive inheritance, or those with abnormal thumbs did not indicate differences in survival. Deaths were reported for almost 100 patients (13 percent), at a median age of 6 years overall and 8.5 years in the recent decade. Deaths were from complications of iron overload, as well as from pneumonia or sepsis or both. Less common causes were complications from transplant, leukemia, cancer (see later), renal disease, anesthesia, pulmonary emboli, and undefined central nervous system disorders.

The long-term prognosis remains uncertain. The group with the best prognosis is those who respond to steroids and whose condition can be maintained with relatively low doses. Those who do not respond to steroids or those in whom steroid therapy eventually fails need transfusions and chelation therapy, transplantation if there is a donor, or perhaps hematopoietic growth factors. The quality of life is usually quite good, particularly for those experiencing spontaneous remission and for those who respond to low-doses of steroids. Transfusion-dependent patients can be give chelation therapy as are patients with thalassemia major. Many patients with DBA are now adults with a good quality of life.

Pregnancy. Among 25 females with DBA who were reported to have 29 pregnancies, there were 12 normal babies, 16 babies with DBA, and 1 miscarriage.[853] In the series of 76 patients with DBA reported from the Boston experience, 5 men and 3 women had 13 children, 3 of whom had DBA.[717] Pregnancy is probably underreported and fatherhood is certainly underreported, except in clear instances of dominant inheritance. Almost one half of pregnant patients had transient worsening of anemia during pregnancy, perhaps related to marrow suppression by estrogens. We advise that the maternal hemoglobin level be maintained at greater than 8 to 9 g/dL to avoid maternal anemia, which might lead to intrauterine growth retardation, preterm delivery, or fetal distress.[853] Seven of the 28 deliveries required caesarean sections because of fetal anemia, toxemia, and failure of labor to progress; these outcomes are similar to those noted in patients with FA (see earlier).

Leukemia, MDS, and Cancer. Leukemia was described in 10 patients (Table 8–20). One girl developed acute lymphoblastic leukemia and had a history of a spontaneous remission of her DBA at the age of 5 years.[870]

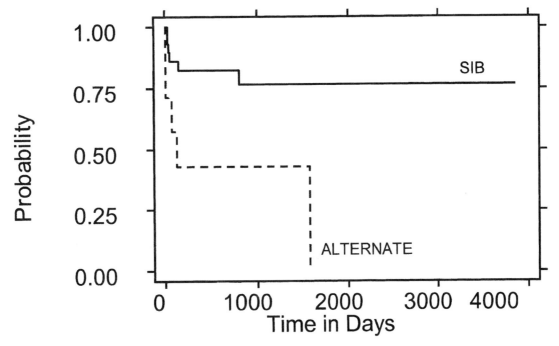

FIGURE 8–26. Kaplan-Meier plot of cumulative survival in Diamond-Blackfan anemia after BMT. Time is shown as time after BMT in days. —— = 38 patients with a sibling donor; - - - - = patients with an alternate donor (3 matched unrelated donor marrows, 3 matched unrelated donor cord blood, 1 mother, and 1 granduncle).

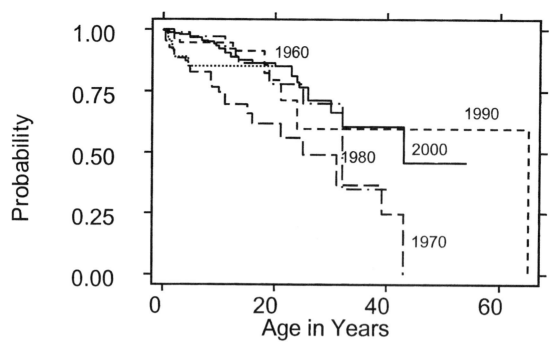

FIGURE 8–27. Kaplan-Meier plot of cumulative survival in DBA. Time is shown as age in years, because most DBA is diagnosed in infancy. ●●●●● = 78 patients reported from 1936 to 1960; – – – = 113 patients reported from 1961 to 1970; – • – = 90 patients reported from 1971 to 1980; - - - - = 115 patients reported from 1981 to 1990; —— 309 cases reported from 1991 to 2000. Differences are significant.

The acute lymphoblastic leukemia also remitted completely, and the patient had neither DBA nor leukemia at age 17 years.* The other 9 patients had acute myeloid leukemia. A female and a male from Diamond's original series[871] had intermittent remissions of DBA, but died from acute myeloblastic leukemia at ages 31 and 43.[855†] The male had received irradiation to his thymus and to his long bones to "stimulate the bone marrow." One girl who had received cyclophosphamide to treat her DBA died from acute promyelocytic leukemia at age 13.[856] A boy developed acute megakaryoblastic leukemia at age 14 months; the anemia present from 2 months of age might in fact have been a long preleukemic phase.[857] Five of the 9 patients with acute myeloid leukemia died at 2 to 43 years of age of their leukemia. In the review of 72 patients seen in Boston, 4 had acute myeloid leukemia, with a cumulative predicted risk of 23 percent by age 30 to 40 years and a relative risk of 200-fold.[872]

Among three patients with MDS, one developed AML within 1 year, whereas the other two died of complications of MDS.[712, 858]

Nonhematologic cancers developed in 17 patients (Table 8–20). There were five osteogenic sarcomas and one soft tissue sarcoma, as well as two Hodgkin and one non-Hodgkin lymphoma, two breast cancers, and one each colon cancer, fibrohistiocytoma, gastric cancer, and melanoma. Hepatomas developed in one patient who had iron overload from transfusions and one who had received androgens. Although literature series do not permit formal risk analyses, it appears that solid tumors as well as

leukemia are increased in DBA, and prospective studies are important to determine the incidence of these sequelae.

There are no well-documented instances of DBA which evolved into complete aplastic anemia, except after severe iron overload, perhaps associated with hepatitis, or during terminal sepsis. One pancytopenic patient was mentioned without details by Najean,[873] another had pancytopenia after cytomegalovirus infection,[874] and another had received multiple transfusions and perhaps the pancytopenia was viral-mediated.[875] In general, DBA remains a single cytopenia, and the prognosis is better than that of many of the other marrow failure disorders.

TRANSIENT ERYTHROBLASTOPENIA OF CHILDHOOD

Description

Acute erythroblastopenia in previously hematologically normal children was first described by Gasser in 1949,[825] who reported 12 children in whom erythroblastopenia followed toxic, allergic, or infectious episodes. Because these children recovered rapidly, they did not develop anemia. Baar then evaluated red cell life span in an 8-year-old with "complete transient aplasia of the erythropoietic tissue."[876] In 1970, Wranne[877] reported temporary red cell aplasia in four patients as "erythroblastopenia of childhood." More than 500 patients with transient erythroblastopenia of childhood (TEC) have been reported since 1970, as detailed case reports as well as series of cases without individual data.[2, 3, 789] These children have temporary peripheral blood reticulocytopenia and usually

---

*Schaison G: personal communication.
†Gardner FH: personal communication.

TABLE 8–20. Cancer in Diamond-Blackfan Anemia

Type	Male	Female	Unknown	All Patients	References
Leukemia					
Acute lymphoblastic	0	1	0	1	870
Acute myeloblastic★	5	2	2	9	278, 717, 855–860
MDS†	2	0	0	2	712, 858
Total leukemia + MDS	7	3	2	12	
Osteogenic sarcoma	2	3	0	5	712, 713, 861, 862
Sarcoma, soft tissue	1	0	0	1	712
Breast cancer	—	2	0	2	713, 863
Hodgkin's disease	2	0	0	2	713, 864, 865
Non-Hodgkin's lymphoma	0	1	0	1	866
Hepatoma	2	0	0	2	867, 868
Colon cancer	0	1	0	1	712
Fibrohistiocytoma	1	0	0	1	869
Stomach cancer	1	0	0	1	868
Melanoma	0	1	0	1	717
Total solid tumors	9	8	2	17	

★One patient had MDS that developed into AML within 1 year.
†MDS is not considered cancer in these analyses. Some patients were reported more than once. No patient had more than one cancer.

TABLE 8–21. Comparison of Diamond-Blackfan Anemia and Transient Erythroblastopenia of Childhood

	DBA	TEC
No. of reported patients	>700	>500
Male/female	1.1	1.3
Age at diagnosis, male (mos)		
Mean	10	26
Median	2	23
Range	0–408	1–120
Age at diagnosis, female (mos)		
Mean	14	26
Median	3	23
Range	0–768	1–192
Males > 1 yr	9%	82%
Females > 1 yr	12%	80%
Etiology	Genetic	Acquired
Antecedent history	None	Viral illness
Physical examination abnormal	25%	0%
Laboratory		
Hemoglobin (g/dL)	1.2–14.8	2.2–12.5
WBCs <5000/µL	15%	20%
Platelets >400,000/µL	20%	45%
Adenosine deaminase	Increased	Normal
MCV increased at diagnosis	80%	5%
During recovery	100%	90%
In remission	100%	0%
HbF increased at diagnosis	100%	20%
During recovery	100%	100%
In remission	85%	0%
i Antigen increased	100%	20%
During recovery	100%	60%
In remission	90%	0%

TEC = transient erythroblastopenia of childhood; WBCs = white blood cells; MCV = mean cell volume.

Adapted from Alter BP: The bone marrow failure syndromes. In Nathan DG, Oski FA (eds): Hematology of Infancy and Childhood, 3rd ed. Philadelphia, WB Saunders, 1987, p 159; and Link MP, Alter BP: Fetal erythropoiesis during recovery from transient erythroblastopenia of childhood (TEC). Pediatr Res 1981; 15:1036.

have anemia and bone marrow erythroblastopenia, with normal white blood cell and platelet counts. Young patients with TEC were sometimes initially diagnosed with DBA; Table 8–21 compares the features of the two conditions. An English regional study found the annual incidence of DBA was 1 and TEC was 5 per million children[711]; the comparable figure for TEC in Sweden was 4.3 per 100,000, the same as for acute lymphocytic leukemia, but five-fold higher than in England.[878]

TEC is an acquired anemia in a previously healthy child for whom prior normal blood counts are sometimes available. The male-to-female ratio of occurrence is 1.3, and the median age at diagnosis is 23 months for both sexes (Fig. 8–28). More than 80 percent of patients were 1 year of age or older; in contrast, this was true in only approximately 10 percent of those with DBA. However, only 10 percent of patients with TEC were older than 3 years of age, only 4 patients were older than 10, and the oldest was 16 years of age. There was a history of a preceding viral illness (upper respiratory or gastrointestinal) in more than one half of patients, at a median of 1 month and a range of 0 to 4 months. Because viral illnesses are common in young children, it is difficult to determine their relevance, although a viral cause for TEC has appeal (see Pathophysiology, later in this section). Neurologic manifestations of anemia—either seizures, breath-holding, or transient ischemic attacks—were reported in several patients.[880–888] Drug and toxins to which patients were exposed included piperazine, organic phosphates, penicillin, aspirin, sulfonamides, valproic acid, dilantin, phenobarbital, and insecticides.[885, 889–893]

Familial TEC has been recorded rarely. Some sets of identical twins and fraternal twins had simultaneous onset of anemia.[890, 894, 895] Four sets of siblings had TEC at similar ages, 2 to 3 years apart.[895, 896] These familial occurrences suggest that TEC may result from the combination of an environmental factor (e.g., an infection) and a genetic predisposition. All ethnic groups have been

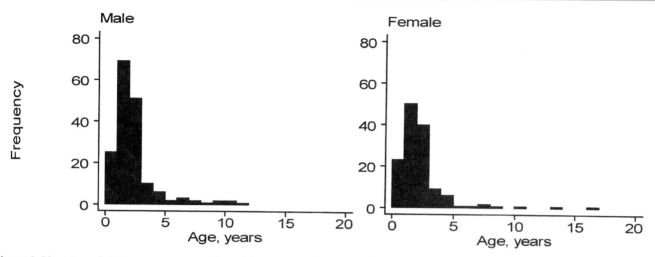

Figure 8–28. Age at diagnosis in more than 500 published reports of patients with transient erythroblastopenia of childhood. *Left*, males; *right*, females. Compare this figure with Figure 8–21 for DBA.

represented, including blacks, Hispanics, and Japanese. Most of the reports have been from temperate climates.

Seasonal TEC was suggested by the reports of apparent clusters, mostly from June to October but from November to March in one series.[3] All but one of these reports was from North America. However, the temporal clustering is not statistically significant. The number of patients is sufficiently small that the reported monthly variations may have been due to chance. There may be clusters resulting from specific local viral epidemics, but until the putative virus is identified, this possibility remains a speculation.

Physical examinations of patients with TEC are essentially normal except for pallor and signs of anemia such as tachycardia. The onset is gradual, and the pallor is often not noticed by the parents until the anemia is substantial.

Laboratory Findings

Hemoglobin levels ranged from 2.2 to 12.5 g/dL, with a median value of 5.6 g/dL. Reticulocyte counts were below 1 percent in most of the children, except those who were already recovering. White blood cell counts were often normal, but the absolute neutrophil count was less than 1000/µL in approximately 6 percent of patients. In two large series, 5 of 24 and 12 of 64 patients had neutrophil counts less than 1000/µL. Platelet counts less than 100,000/µL were reported in approximately 5 percent of patients, some of whom were also neutropenic. It is possible that whatever suppresses the erythroid marrow affects all cell lines in a few patients. Twenty percent of patients had white blood cell counts greater than 10,000/µL, perhaps because of intercurrent infections. Platelet counts were often greater than 400,000/µL as was seen in a smaller proportion of children with DBA. The mean cell volumes were usually normal when corrected for age. The mean and median were 80 fL, and the range was from 62 to 112 fL. HbF levels ranged from 0.2 to 9.2 percent, but were usually normal. One small study reported an excess of patients with blood group A,[854] but this finding was not confirmed in another small study.[879] More than 90 percent of patients had significant to profound

marrow erythroblastopenia. The erythroblasts that were seen usually had a maturation arrest. Increased marrow lymphocyte counts led to the erroneous diagnosis of acute leukemia at least once.[897] Five to 10 percent of patients were seen with reticulocytosis or with erythroid hyperplasia or with both at presentation, and they presumably were recovering without the benefit of medical attention.

Several features of the red cells distinguish TEC from DBA, if the history and age are insufficient. Wang and Mentzer[898] pointed out that the erythrocytes in TEC have normal "adult" (or at least child and not fetal) mean cell volume, and levels of HbF, i antigen, and red cell enzymes[898]; in contrast, values for these parameters are more "fetal" in DBA. These distinctions are only relevant if the patient with TEC is studied when reticulocytopenia is present. During the recovery phase, patients with TEC undergo "stress erythropoiesis," as do any patients demonstrating bone marrow recovery. They produce a transient cohort of "fetal-like" erythrocytes that can be detected as soon as reticulocytes appear, by means of a sensitive immunologic assay for F reticulocytes.[899, 900] We documented that this cohort of fetal-like erythrocytes then evolves into normal red cells.[879] Interpretation of the mean cell volume, HbF, i antigen, and red cell enzyme levels depends on the stage of the illness. The ultimate distinction between TEC and DBA is often only clear after the fact. However, macrocytosis, an elevated HbF level, and reticulocytopenia with marrow erythroblastopenia in a child younger than 1 year of age most likely indicate DBA. Red cell ADA is elevated in most patients with DBA and normal in patients with TEC.[764]

Two patients also had another transient condition, called "transient hyperphosphatasemia of infancy," characterized by temporary and unexplained elevation of alkaline phosphatase in the absence of liver or bone disease.[884]

Pathophysiology

The history of an antecedent (usually viral) illness 2 months before diagnosis of TEC suggests a viral cause. Total suppression of normal erythropoiesis would lead to symptomatic anemia in 1 to 2 months, but it is not clear why patients would then recover within another month. The prime viral suspect is parvovirus, but analyses of specific antibody in more than 50 patients yielded positive results in only 20 percent, and causality has not been demonstrated. The role of a virus that has been shown to inhibit growth of CFU-Es in patients with normal erythropoiesis[901–903] has not yet been proven in TEC, and confirmation will require sensitive assays for parvoviral antigen or DNA.

Erythropoietin levels are high, as expected for anemic patients.[904] Several laboratories examined erythroid progenitor cell cultures from blood or marrow cells from patients with TEC. One half of patients had decreased numbers of erythroid progenitor cells. Serum or IgG inhibitors of normal progenitors were found in one half of patients, and cellular inhibitors were also reported in one fourth. Only a few parameters were examined in any single patient.[789] TEC may be due to an unknown virus that infects CFU-E and that is not cleared until specific antibodies develop. An IgG directed against erythroid progenitors may develop and appear as a "serum" inhibitor. Recovery in these patients might require the development of anti-idiotype antibodies.

Therapy and Outcome

As indicated by the word "transient," all patients with TEC recover. Recurrent TEC occurred in only two patients, both within 1 year.[904, 905] Most patients are usually well within 1 to 2 months from diagnosis, and 5 to 10 percent have already begun to recover by the time they are seen for medical care. Eight months was the longest interval to recovery without recurrence, and only 10 patients took 4 months or more. No treatment was necessary for almost half of those for whom the clinical course was described. Most patients had already reached their lowest hemoglobin level by the time they received medical attention. Transfusions were given to 60 percent of patients, and a single transfusion was sufficient in 90 percent. Prednisone was administered to 20 percent, but reticulocytes often appeared within a day, and this was clearly unrelated to the steroid therapy.

The current recommendation is to observe patients with TEC, and give transfusions only if they develop cardiovascular compromise from their anemia. It is amazing how well these children cope with hemoglobin levels of 5 g/dL, and it is often the cardiovascular or mental state of the physician rather than the patient's condition that leads to transfusion. Prednisone, anabolic steroids, or other immunosuppressive therapies have no apparent role in the management of TEC. The prognosis is excellent, and the retrospective distinction of TEC from DBA is simple (Table 8–21).

CONGENITAL DYSERYTHROPOIETIC ANEMIA

Introduction

Dyserythropoiesis is the term used to describe ineffective, morphologically abnormal erythropoiesis. Conditions characterized by this dysfunction are not precisely bone marrow failure syndromes; however, they sometimes are congenital or inherited marrow disorders that may result in anemia without reticulocytosis. Ineffective erythropoiesis results from a discrepancy between erythroid output from marrow to circulation (anemia) and erythroid marrow content (erythroid hyperplasia). It implies intramedullary destruction, combining quantitative and qualitative decreases in erythropoiesis. The prefix *dys-* indicates qualitative abnormalities of the stem cell or the microenvironment. In aplastic anemia, erythropoiesis is quantitatively abnormal in the same compartments.

Approximately 1 in 1000 bone marrow erythroblasts is abnormal in normal individuals.[906] Multinucleated erythroblasts and karyorrhexis are seen occasionally in megaloblastic anemia, iron deficiency, leukemia, and hemolytic anemia and indicate bone marrow stress. The frequency of dyserythropoietic erythroblasts may be substantial in both acquired and inherited aplastic anemia. In one study of aplastic anemia, 5 to 90 percent of erythroblasts were megaloblastic or showed nuclear-to-cytoplasmic asynchrony, 1 to 3 percent were binucleate, and up to 5 percent had cytoplasmic connections or chromatin bridges.[907] During recovery from BMT, all patients had a transient wave of up to 30 percent dyserythropoietic erythroblasts.[908] These morphologic abnormalities are more extreme in *congenital dyserythropoietic anemia (CDA)* than in aplastic anemia or during recovery from BMT.

CDA was reviewed in detail in a book by Lewis and Verwilghen in 1977,[909] which remains a valuable resource. The various types are characterized by anemia with insufficient reticulocytosis and ineffective erythropoiesis. All ethnic groups are affected. The major types are as follows (Table 8–22):

Type I, macrocytosis, with bone marrow megaloblastoid changes, and internuclear chromatin bridges

Type II, normocytosis or macrocytosis, with bi- and multinucleated marrow erythroblasts, pluripolar mitoses, and karyorrhexis

Type III, macrocytosis, with erythroblastic multinuclearity of up to 12 nuclei (gigantoblasts)

The morphologic features are the major diagnostic factors for types I and III. Type II is also known by the acronym *HEMPAS* for *h*ereditary *e*rythroblastic *m*ultinuclearity with a *p*ositive *a*cidified *s*erum test, because of the positive reaction to some acidified normal sera described initially by Crookston and associates.[910] In addition, more than 50 other patients whose disease does not fit clearly into types I to III have been reported.

Type I

More than 100 patients with type I CDA have been reported (the first 20 by Heimpel[911, 912]). The age of onset of anemia or jaundice ranges from infancy to old age, with a median age of 10 years. The male-to-female ratio of occurrence is 1.1, and the inheritance is autosomal recessive. At least 15 families had consanguinity, and there were affected siblings, or cousins, or both in almost 20. Physical examination shows slight icterus and moderate splenomegaly. Almost a dozen patients had brown skin pigmentation, toe syndactyly, or abnormal fingers.

Patients with type I CDA have a mild macrocytic anemia, with a mean hemoglobin level of 9 g/dL and a range of 2 to 15 g/dL. Reticulocyte counts range from 1 to 7 percent. The median mean cell volume was 100 fL (range, 66 to 133). Peripheral blood analysis showed anisocytosis,

TABLE 8–22. Types of Congenital Dyserythropoietic Anemias

Feature	Type I	Type II	Type III
Reported patients	130	200	60
Male/female ratio	1.1	0.9	0.8
Anemia	Mild to moderate	Moderate	Mild to moderate
Red cell size	Macrocytic	Normo- or macrocytic	Macrocytic
Bone marrow erythroblasts	Megaloblastoid, binucleated (2–5%), chromatin bridges	Bi- and multinucleated (10–40%), karyorrhexis	Gigantoblasts (10–40%)
Inheritance	Recessive	Recessive	Dominant
Acid serum hemolysis	Negative	Positive	Negative
Reaction			
Anti-i	Slight	Strong	Slight
Anti-I	Slight	Strong	Slight
Effect of splenectomy	50%	96%	100%
Gene locus*	15q15.1–15.3	20q11.2	15q21–25
Gene nomenclature	*CDAI*	*CDAII*	*CDAIII*

*Gene locus for some but not all patients in each category.

poikilocytosis, punctate basophilia, and occasional Cabot's rings. White blood cells and platelets were normal. The indirect bilirubin level was elevated (1 to 4 mg/dL), as was serum lactate dehydrogenase concentration; the haptoglobin level was low, and transferrin was saturated. Further evidence for ineffective erythropoiesis was derived from the plasma iron turnover, which was as much as 10 times normal, whereas red cell utilization was reduced to less than 30 percent. Red cell survival was slightly shortened, with ^{51}Cr half-lives of 14 to 30 days (mean, 21 days). Globin synthesis studies usually showed non-α/α ratios of 1, although imbalance of 0.5 to 0.7 was observed occasionally. Normal results were seen with the acidified serum test, and the i antigen titer was usually in the adult (low) range; these results contrast with those seen in type II CDA (see later).

Bone marrow examination showed marked erythroid hyperplasia, with 25 to 80 percent erythroid precursors. The abnormalities were confined to the polychromatophilic and orthochromatic (i.e., mature) erythroblasts (Fig. 8–29). There was dissociation of nuclear and cytoplasmic maturation, with immature megaloblastoid nuclei and more mature cytoplasms. As many as 2 percent of the erythroblasts were large cells with incomplete nuclear division. Approximately 1 percent had double nuclei, with one component more mature than the other. Up to 2 percent of cells showed thin chromatin bridges connecting the nuclei of two cells. Electron microscopy confirmed that the proerythroblasts were normal. The more mature erythroblasts had widening of nuclear membrane pores, with condensation, vacuolization, and disintegration of nuclear chromatin, and cytoplasmic penetrance. There were also structural changes of the nucleolus, the appearance of microtubules, and the presence of siderotic material in the cytoplasm.[913–915]

The defect is apparently at the stem cell level. The numbers of CFU-Es and BFU-Es were normal, but electron microscopy showed that the colonies contained a mixture of normal and abnormal cells.[916] This suggests that the abnormality is expressed variably in the mature progeny of each stem cell.

A large Israeli Bedouin kinship facilitated mapping of one gene for CDA I (*CDAN1*) to chromosome

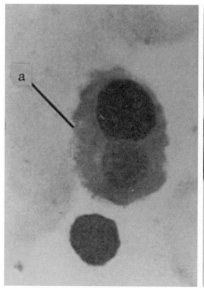
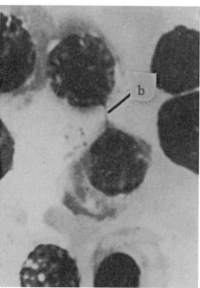

FIGURE 8–29. Bone marrow from a patient with congenital dyserythropoietic anemia type I. *A,* Small letter *a* indicates binucleate erythroblast, with nuclei of different size and maturity. *B,* Small letter *b* indicates internuclear chromatin bridges connecting two erythroblasts. (From Lewis SM, Verwilghen RL (eds): Dyserythropoiesis. London, Academic Press, 1977.)

A   B

15q15.1–15.3.[917] Genetic heterogeneity is suggested by the fact that several other unrelated patients of Lebanese and English origin did not have haplotypes that linked to this region.[918]

Treatment with the usual hematinics, such as vitamins, metals, and steroids, is without effect. Twenty percent of patients needed several or even chronic transfusions. Although splenomegaly was common, splenectomy did not improve the anemia in the 10 percent of patients in whom it was done. Some patients developed gallstones from the hemolytic anemia. Hemosiderosis was the most important long-term complication and was due to increased intestinal absorption of iron, ineffective erythropoiesis, and mild hemolysis. Phlebotomy and iron chelation warrant consideration (see Chapters 12 and 20 for details). Deaths were reported in four patients, one at age 10 from complications of splenectomy, one at age 84 from old age, and two from persistent pulmonary hypertension in infancy.[919, 920]

One patient received α-interferon during treatment of hepatitis C and became transfusion-independent.[921] This beneficial effect was subsequently confirmed in other patients.[922–924] Epstein-Barr virus–transformed B lymphoblasts from patients with type I CDA produce less interferon-α in vitro than do normal cells, which suggests a potential mechanism.[924] Addition of interferon-α to erythroid cultures improves the ultrastructural "Swiss-cheese" appearance of erythroblasts.[925]

One successful BMT was reported in which the donor was a sibling.[926]

Type II

Type II CDA (HEMPAS) has been reported in approximately 200 patients. Details for many of the early patients were summarized by Verwilghen.[927, 928] The molecular basis of type II CDA is the subject of an excellent review by Fukuda.[929] More than two dozen occurrences were in sibships and 11 were in consanguineous families. The male-to-female ratio of occurrence is 0.9, and the inheritance is autosomal recessive. The age at diagnosis ranges from infancy to adulthood, with a median age of 14 years. The anemia varies from mild to severe, such that regular transfusions are required in 15 percent of patients. Jaundice, hepatosplenomegaly, and gallstones are more common and the anemia is generally more severe in type II CDA than in type I.

The hemoglobin levels varied widely (median 9.5, range 3 to 15 g/dL), whereas reticulocyte counts were normal or inadequately elevated and averaged 4 percent. Red cells were normochromic and normocytic in half of patients and macrocytic in the rest; the median mean cell volume was 94 fL (range, 73 to 114). Smears showed anisocytosis, poikilocytosis, tear drops, and basophilic stippling—all nonspecific findings. The red cell life span was shorter in type II CDA than in type I; the ^{51}Cr half-life averaged 17 days (range, 7 to 31). Electron microscopy showed an excess of endoplasmic reticulum parallel to the cell membrane, leading to the appearance of a characteristic "double membrane," or cistern, in late erythroblasts and some erythrocytes.[914, 915] Some bone marrow reticuloendothelial cells resembled Gaucher cells, with birefringent, *p*-aminosalicylic acid-positive needle-like inclusions, which may be the products of the catabolism of erythroblasts undergoing rapid turnover. The marrow showed erythroid hyperplasia, with 45 to 90 percent erythroid precursors and with binucleated and multinucleated mature erythroblasts in 10 to 70 percent of the erythroid precursors (Fig. 8–30). The internuclear chromatin bridges of type I CDA were not present, and the multinuclearity was not as extreme as in type III CDA.

The pathognomonic findings in type II CDA are serologic.[910] In type II CDA red cells are lysed by approximately 30 percent of acidified sera from normal individuals, but not by the patient's own serum. By contrast, in PNH, the patient's cells are lysed by the patient's

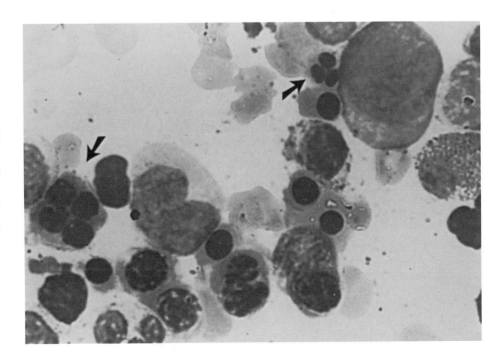

FIGURE 8–30. Bone marrow from a patient with congenital dyserythropoietic anemia type II, showing bi- and multinucleate erythroblasts. (Courtesy of Dr. Gail Wolfe; with permission from Alter BP: The bone marrow failure syndromes. In Nathan DG, Oski FA (eds): Hematology of Infancy and Childhood, 3rd ed. Philadelphia, WB Saunders, 1987, p 159.)

own acidified serum. In type II CDA, the red cells have a specific type II CDA antigen, and many normal sera contain an anti-type II CDA IgM antibody. In some instances, up to 30 normal sera must be examined before the acidified test yields positive results; some of these patients for which this was necessary were characterized as having a "type II variant" until the right serum was found.[930] Type II CDA erythrocytes are also more strongly agglutinated by anti-i antibody than are the cells of newborn infants or those of patients with stress erythropoiesis.[931] Studies with fluorescent labels demonstrated i antigen on every red cell in type II CDA. Heterozygotes also had increased expression of i antigen. Type II CDA cells are strongly agglutinated as well as lysed by anti-I antibody. Rosse and associates[932] found that type II CDA cells bind a normal amount of complement 1 (C1) but more antibody and more C4 than do those of normal subjects.[932] This causes binding of an excess of C3 with resultant hemolysis. The red cell plasma membrane abnormality in type II CDA is related to decreased N-glycan synthesis near the N-acetylglucosaminyltransferase and α-mannosidase steps in the synthetic pathway.[933] Bands 3 and 4.5 lack glycosylation with lactosaminoglycans.[934]

The numbers of erythroid progenitors in marrow and blood are probably normal. One study revealed only normal morphology of the erythroblasts produced by cultured CFU-Es,[935] but others reported multinuclearity similar to that seen *in vivo* in the bone marrow.[936, 937] As in type I CDA, the defect appears to be at the level of the erythroid stem cell, with variable expression in the mature erythroblasts.

A genome-wide search using 12 Italian families and 1 French family was successful in localizing one gene for type II CDA (*CDAN2*) to chromosome 20q11.2.[938] The genes in the majority of the Italian patients with type II CDA were linked to 20q11.2, but this linkage was not due to a founder effect[939]; however, the genes in two other Italian families were not linked to this locus.[940] Other patients had mutations in the genes for α-mannosidase II,[933] consistent with genetic heterogeneity in type II CDA.

Patients with severe anemia require blood transfusions. Unlike the situation in type I CDA, splenectomy has been effective in approximately 70 percent of patients with type II CDA in whom it was performed; an apparent increase in red cell life span and abrogation of the need for transfusions was seen. Iron accumulation does occur, both from transfusions and from increased intestinal absorption, even in patients who have not received transfusions, and death may result from cardiac compromise. Prophylactic phlebotomy, or iron chelation, or both have a definite role in the management of this disorder. Two patients died from hemochromatosis at ages 25 and 30.

It has been proposed that some of the phenotypic heterogeneity in type II CDA could be due to coinherited Gilbert's syndrome. Patients with the homozygous A(TA)7TAA box variant of the *UGT1A* gene, which leads to reduced expression of uridine diphosphate glucuronosyl transferase, had increased serum bilirubin levels and occurrence of gallstones.[941] Iron overload was increased in a patient with type II CDA who also had hereditary hemochromatosis due to a homozygous C282Y mutation in *HFE*.[942]

Type III

Approximately 70 patients in 16 families with type III CDA have been reported.[943, 944] The male-to-female ratio of occurrence is 0.8. The median age at diagnosis is 24 years, with a range from birth to old age, as for types I and II CDA. The anemia was usually macrocytic and mild to moderate. The median hemoglobin level was 9.5, and the range was from 4 to 14 g/dL. Bone marrow erythroid hyperplasia was seen, with up to 75 percent erythroblasts, multinuclearity in 10 to 40 percent of erythroblasts, and the presence of unique "gigantoblasts" with up to 12 nuclei (Fig. 8–31). The acid serum lysis test always yielded negative results, and reactions with anti-i antibody were at the level seen in stress erythropoiesis and were weaker than those seen in type II CDA. Red cell survival was slightly short, with ^{51}Cr half-lives being 21 days. As in the other types of CDA, *in vitro* culture led to formation

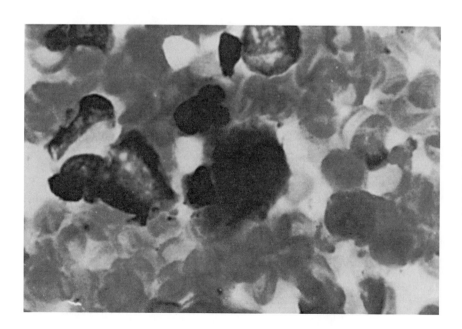

FIGURE 8–31. Bone marrow from a patient with congenital dyserythropoietic anemia type III, showing multinucleate erythroblast. (Photograph courtesy of Dr. Gail Wolfe; with permission from Alter BP: The bone marrow failure syndromes. In Nathan DG, Oski FA (eds): Hematology of Infancy and Childhood, 3rd ed. Philadelphia, WB Saunders, 1987, p 159.)

of colonies containing both normal and abnormal erythroblasts—indications of a stem cell abnormality.[945]

The gene for type III CDA, *CDAN3*, was mapped to 15q21–25 in the very large Swedish family which was reported often.[946]

Transfusions or splenectomy were rarely performed. As in the other types of CDA the major problem was hemosiderosis, which led to one death at age 42. Members of the Swedish family also have an increased occurrence of monoclonal gammopathy, myeloma, and ocular angioid streaks.[947]

Variants

There are more than 50 patients whose CDA cannot be classified as any of the types described above, and Wickramsinghe has attempted to classify these patients into discrete categories.[948] *Type IV CDA* is the classification used in reports in which the bone marrow morphology resembles that in type II CDA. Results of acidified serum tests were negative, although an insufficient number of sera may have been examined; in addition, the level of i antigen was not increased. One family had dominant inheritance; thus at least some of these cases might indeed belong to a type different from type II, in which inheritance is autosomal recessive.[949–953] Anemia appeared from infancy to adulthood and was mild in all but one patient. Ten to 40 percent of the marrow erythroblasts were binucleated, as in type II CDA. The clinical course was relatively benign, and splenectomy was required for one patient.

CDA with thalassemia is the term that has been used for another group of familial occurrences.[954–960] One family had dominant inheritance, and one had three affected siblings. The age at diagnosis of mild to moderate anemia ranged from infancy to old age. Red cell size ranged from microcytic to macrocytic, and 5 to 35 percent of the marrow erythroblasts were multinuclear. The acid serum lysis tests yielded negative results, although i antigen was found in two of the families. Globin chain synthesis was imbalanced, with β/α ratios of 0.5, similar to those seen in β-thalassemia trait. Although there may have been a coincidence of occurrence of thalassemia trait and CDA, two of the families were from ethnic groups that do not have a high incidence of thalassemia.

Almost 40 other patients had CDAs that were even harder to classify. Five families had an affected parent and child, two had consanguinity, and three had affected siblings; all of the families may have different disorders. The proportion of binucleated or multinucleated erythroblasts was usually less than 4 percent. Some erythroblasts resembled type I cells with rare internuclear bridges, and some resembled type II cells with symmetrical binuclearity, karyorrhexis, and even double membranes (as seen with electron microscopy). The ages at diagnosis of mild to severe anemia ranged from birth to adulthood, and red cell size ranged from small to large. Six infants had intrauterine hydrops; one of these infants died.[961, 962] Results of acidified serum tests were usually negative, the level of i antigen varied, and red cell ^{51}Cr survival half-lives ranged from 5 to 29 days. In one patient, CDA was associated with deficiency of erythroid CD44 and phenotype In(a–b–), Co(a–b–).[963] Eight patients had splenectomy and their condition improved.

Erythroid cultures from one patient demonstrated multinuclearity in some cells within each colony[964]; this finding suggested a stem cell disorder, as seen in the other types of CDA. The clinical variability suggests that these patients have several types of CDA; perhaps they are double heterozygotes rather than homozygotes for recessive CDA genes.

White Cells

SEVERE CONGENITAL NEUTROPENIA

Description

Infantile genetic agranulocytosis was first described by Kostmann in 1956.[965, 966] It is also called *severe congenital neutropenia (SCN)*, which does not totally distinguish all of the neutropenias of childhood (see Chapter 21 for a complete discussion of neutropenia). We previously used the eponym *Kostmann syndrome* to describe infants with extreme neutropenia (<200/mL) usually seen in the first year of life, severe pyogenic infections, and, until recently, early deaths. Because the recent identification of mutations in the neutrophil elastase 2 gene (*ELA2*)[967] has shown that inheritance is autosomal dominant in the majority of patients, it is now more appropriate to reserve use of the term Kostmann syndrome for those in whom the inheritance is in fact recessive.

There are more than 300 patients reported in the literature (Table 8–23). The male-to-female ratio of occurrence is approximately 1, and the inheritance is autosomal recessive. Most of Kostmann's original 14 and subsequent 10 patients belonged to a very large intermarried kinship in Northern Sweden.[968] Despite that founder effect, all ethnic groups are affected, including blacks, American Indians, and Asians. At least a dozen patients were found in consanguineous families, and more than 20 had affected siblings; eight families demonstrated dominant inheritance.

Half of the patients showed symptoms within the first month of life, and 90 percent had symptoms by 6 months; the few in whom the disease was diagnosed later may not have had this syndrome. Birth weights were generally normal, as were findings of physical examinations, except for signs of infection (e.g., skin abscesses). Abnormal physical findings, although rare, include short stature, mental retardation, cataracts, and microcephaly.

Laboratory Findings

Neutropenia is marked, although in several infants absolute neutrophil counts were almost normal in the first week but then declined rapidly. The average absolute neutrophil count was less than 200/μL, and neutropenia was often total. Eosinophil and monocyte counts were sometimes very high (up to 80 percent monocytes in some patients), but these cells are not as effective phagocytes as are neutrophils. Increased immunoglobulin levels were often seen. SCN is a single cytopenia, and patients with SCN usually have normal hemoglobin levels and normal or increased platelet counts. Bone marrow examinations reveal normal cellularity, with absence of or marked decreases in the number of myeloid precursors, and with a maturation arrest at the myelocyte or promyelocyte stage.

TABLE 8–23. Severe Congenital Neutropenia Literature

	Reported ≤ 1989	Reported >1989	Total
No. of patients	128	178	306
Male/female	55/68	90/81	145/149
Ratio	0.8	1.1	1
Age at leukemia (yrs)			
No. (%)	4 (3%)	23 (13%)	26 (9%)
Male/female	2/1	14/9	16/10
Mean	14	10.6	11.1
Median	14	12	12
Range	14–14	2–23	2–23
Age at MDS (yrs)			
No. (%)	0 (0%)	13 (7%)	13 (5%)
Male/female		8/5	8/5
Mean		11.3	11.8
Median		11	11
Range		1–22	1–22
Age at death (yrs)			
No. (%)	67 (52%)	15 (8%)	82 (30%)
Male/female	26/37	9/6	35/43
Mean	2.1	6.9	3
Median	0.7	3.3	0.8
Range	0.05–20	0.1–23	0.05–23
Projected median survival (yrs)			
All patients	3	—	23
Leukemia	14	23	14.8
MDS	—	23	23

*Includes four patients with bone marrow cytogenetic clones but without morphologic MDS.

Pathophysiology

SCN is a disorder that primarily affects the neutrophil series. Numbers of bone marrow CFU-C have been reported as decreased, increased, or, most often, normal. The colonies rarely contain neutrophils,[969] and more commonly comprise eosinophils, monocytes, and abnormal or arrested myeloid precursors.[970] Addition of SCF did lead to normal myeloid maturation.[971, 972] Long-term cultures from some patients also showed a block in myeloid differentiation.[969] Thus, in some patients the *in vivo* defect in myeloid differentiation was duplicated *in vitro*. The production of G-CSF and GM-CSF mRNA by patient mononuclear cells was normal,[973] and serum levels of G-CSF were usually increased,[974] findings consistent with a receptor problem or a possible intracellular signaling defect in response to G-CSF. However, the receptor for G-CSF appeared to be normal in most patients.[975, 976]

Linkage analysis by Horwitz and associates[977] in a different syndrome, familial autosomal dominant cyclic neutropenia, led to mapping of the locus to 19p13.3 and identification of mutations in the neutrophil elastase gene (*ELA2*) at that locus. The same investigators then demonstrated that 22 of 25 patients with SCN had 18 different heterozygous mutations in *ELA2* (Fig. 8–32 and Table 8–5).[967] They noted that the mutations in cyclic neutropenia cluster around the active site of the enzyme, whereas the mutations in SCN are on the opposite face. Further studies of the mutant and wild-type proteins led to the conclusion that mutant *ELA2* acts as a dominant negative inhibitor of the function of the normal enzyme.[978]

Therapy and Outcome

In the era before availability of G-CSF,[979] the prognosis for patients with SCN was very poor, with more than half of patients reported to have died at a median age of 7 months, and at ages ranging from 2 weeks to 20 years. Deaths were usually from sepsis or pneumonia. Infections were treated with antibiotics, and many patients were receiving prophylactic treatment with antibiotics. The projected median survival time was 3 years, with only 10 percent of survivors being older than 20 years (Fig. 8–33). Lithium therapy was proposed because it raises white blood cell counts in hematologically normal individuals, but it was relatively ineffective in patients with SCN.[979, 980] No patients developed pancytopenia, and thus SCN is a true single cytopenia.

The use of recombinant growth factors now offers an important prospect for patients with SCN. Subcutaneously administered G-CSF raised neutrophil counts in children with SCN in a dose-related manner. The factor must be administered chronically, has no major side effects, and markedly decreases the number and severity of infections.[981, 982] The use of GM-CSF is associated with more side effects and predominantly increases eosinophil counts rather than neutrophil counts[983]; thus, G-CSF is the treatment of choice. The dose of G-CSF is 5 to 10 µg/kg/day subcutaneously, although some patients require much higher doses. The response rate is greater than 90 percent, and the median projected survival is more than 20 years of age. Osteoporosis has been observed—either it is a side effect of G-CSF treatment or perhaps it is intrinsic to the syndrome.[984, 985]

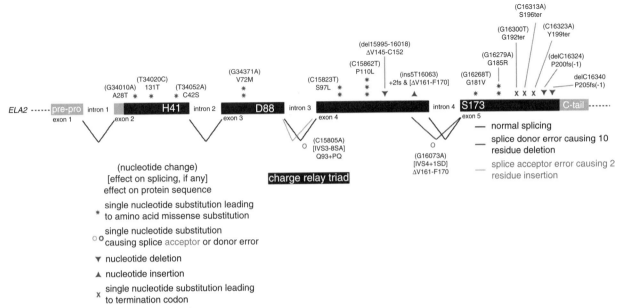

FIGURE 8–32. Mutations in *ELA2* gene associated with severe congenital neutropenia (SCN). (From Li F, Horwitz M: Characterization of mutant neutrophil elastase in severe congenital neutropenia. J Biol Chem 2001; 276:14230.)

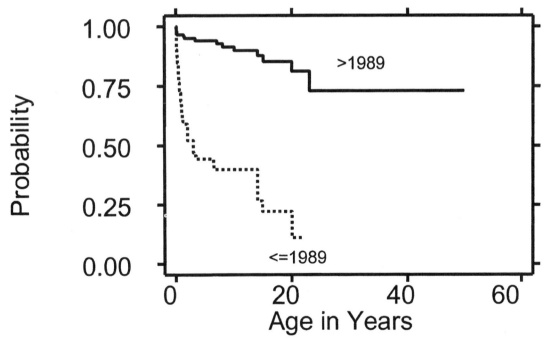

FIGURE 8–33. Kaplan-Meier plot of cumulative survival in SCN. Time is shown as age in years. - - - - = 128 patients reported in the era before availability of granulocyte colony-stimulating factor (G-CSF) (≤1989); ——— = 178 patients reported after G-CSF (>1989).

Since 1989, the death rate has been only 8 percent at a median age of 3 years (range, 1 month to 23 years), with a projected plateau of 75 percent survival at age 23. Deaths still occur from sepsis. BMT was reported in 19 patients since 1989. There were 5 deaths from complications; all of these patients received transplants from alternative donors (Fig. 8–34).[986]

Prenatal diagnosis using fetal blood obtained in the mid-trimester has been considered,[987] but the absolute neutrophil count is less than 200/µL in normal fetuses,[988] and absolute neutropenia would be required to establish the diagnosis of SCN *in utero*. Mutation analysis of *ELA2* can now be used for prenatal testing in families with autosomal dominant inheritance.

Leukemia. At least four patients developed acute myeloid leukemia (two monocytic, one myelomonocytic, and one myeloblastic without maturation) in the era before G-CSF was available. Three patients were male, one was female, and all were 13 to 14 years old and died within 18 months.[989–992] In one family, one child had

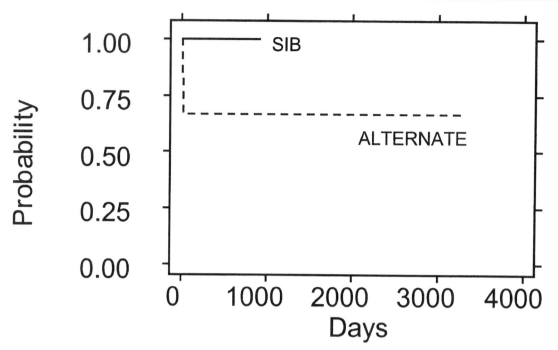

FIGURE 8–34. Kaplan-Meier plot of cumulative survival in 21 patients with SCN after BMT. Time is shown as interval from BMT in days. ——— = 13 patients with a sibling donor. - - - - = patients with alternate donors (4 matched unrelated donor marrows, 1 matched unrelated donor cord blood, and 3 alternative family members). Differences are not significant.

SCN and a sibling died of acute lymphocytic leukemia.[993] The risk of development of leukemia was 3 percent (4 of 128 patients reported). Since the initiation of the use of G-CSF, however, a cohort analysis of patients on the Severe Chronic Neutropenia International Registry indicates that the risk of development of MDS and/or leukemia is approximately 12 percent to date.[994] A summary of individual case reports identifies 13 percent of patients with leukemia and 7 percent with MDS (Table 8–23). At this time one cannot determine whether G-CSF is the cause of the malignant transformation, or whether it permits patients to live long enough to demonstrate that component of the natural history of SCN.

The most consistent cytogenetic finding in patients with SCN and acute myeloid leukemia is monosomy 7. It is also the most common finding in patients with cytogenetic marrow clones who do not have leukemia or bone marrow morphology consistent with MDS. Thus, the course of action after identification of a marrow clone in a patient with clinically stable disease is not clear. There are reports of children (who did not have SCN) who were seen with monosomy 7 and MDS, in whom spontaneous improvement was seen, with loss of the monosomy 7 clone[995]; this finding suggests that monosomy 7 itself is insufficient for leukemogenesis.

Many patients with SCN who have clonal hematopoietic complications such as MDS or acute myeloid leukemia have additional evidence for somatic cellular genetic mutations, consistent with a multistep pathogenesis. The first mutation to be reported was a heterozygous activating *ras* oncogene mutation—GGT to GAT (Gly to Asp) at codon 12.[544] It was also noted that many of the patients who developed leukemia had earlier point mutations in the G-CSF receptor, with truncation of the C-terminal cytoplasmic domain, which is critical for response to G-CSF.[996–998] The truncated receptor functions in a dominant negative manner. Prospective studies are needed to determine whether acquisition of mutations in *ras* or in the G-CSF receptor means that leukemic transformation is inevitable.

SCN is due to an abnormality in the myeloid stem cell that causes ineffective or dysmyelopoiesis; SCN predisposes patients to malignancy, as do many of the other bone marrow stem cell disorders. The potential increase in this risk associated with cytokine treatment appears real, but the magnitude is unknown. Many of the patients who received G-CSF were already "older" and thus perhaps already at increased risk. Only careful prospective studies will clarify this issue.

Platelets

THROMBOCYTOPENIA WITH ABSENT RADII

Description

More than 200 patients with *thrombocytopenia with absent radii (TAR)* have been reported and are summarized in reviews[2, 3, 999–1001] (Table 8–24). Diagnoses are usually made at birth because of the characteristic physical appearance combined with thrombocytopenia. The pathognomic physical finding is bilateral absence of the radii with thumbs present (Fig. 8–35); this feature distinguishes TAR from FA and from trisomy 18, in which thumbs are absent if radii are absent. Babies with TAR often have hemorrhagic manifestations at birth, with petechiae or bloody diarrhea being seen in 60 percent of

TABLE 8–24. Comparison of Thrombocytopenia Absent Radii and Fanconi Anemia

Feature	TAR	FA
No. of reported patients	225	1200
Median age at diagnosis (yrs)	0	8
Male/female ratio	0.8:1	1.2:1
Inheritance	Recessive	Recessive
Low birth weight	9%	11%
Stature	Short	Short
Skeletal deformities		
Absent radii, thumbs present	100%	0%
Hand anomalies	40%	43%
Lower limbs	37%	8%
Cardiac anomalies	8%	6%
Skin		
Hemangiomas	8%	0%
Pigmentation	0%	55%
Blood	Thrombocytopenia	Pancytopenia
Marrow	Absent megakaryocytes	Aplastic
Marrow colonies decreased	CFU-Mega	CFU-GM, CFU-E
HbF	Normal	Increased
Chromosome breaks	Absent	Present
Malignancies	1%	16%
Reported deaths	20%	38%
Projected median survival (yrs)	—	20
Survival plateau	~75 % at 4 yrs	None

CFU-Mega = colony-forming units-megakaryocyte; CFU-GM = colony-forming units-granulocyte-macrophage; CFU-E = colony-forming units-erythroid.

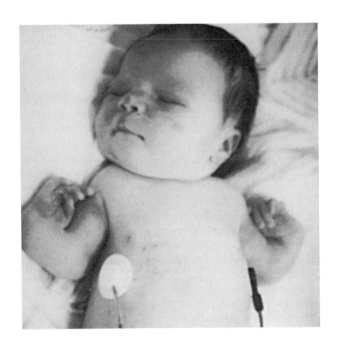

FIGURE 8–35. Newborn infant with thrombocytopenia with absent radii (TAR). Note that thumbs are present. (Courtesy of Dr. Jeffrey Lipton; with permission from Alter BP: The bone marrow failure syndromes. In Nathan DG, Oski FA (eds): Hematology of Infancy and Childhood, 3rd ed. Philadelphia, WB Saunders, 1987, p 159.)

those affected within the first week and in more than 95 percent by 4 months. Inheritance is autosomal recessive, and several families had affected siblings. Each child in two sets of identical twins had TAR,[1002, 1003] whereas only

one of a pair of fraternal twins was affected[1004]; these findings are consistent with a genetic rather than an acquired cause. However, only three patients had consanguinity,[1005–1007] which suggests that patients with TAR may be double heterozygotes for genes with similar effects, rather than true homozygotes. Parents are usually normal, and affected mothers have had normal children. In a few families more than one generation was involved (aunts or uncles and nephews or nieces, with only one example of parent-child transmission), four families had affected cousins[3, 9], one set of affected half-siblings was reported, suggesting dominant (or perhaps pseudodominant) inheritance in a few families. All ethnic groups are affected, including blacks; however, reports of Asians are rare, which may reflect a reporting rather than a genetic bias. Other inherited hematologic conditions with radial ray anomalies include FA and DBA, but no lineage other than platelets is significantly affected in TAR.

Table 8–24 compares the features of TAR with those of FA. All patients with TAR had absence of radii but presence of thumbs (Fig. 8–35). In most patients this occurred bilaterally; only five apparently bona fide patients with a typical hematologic pattern showed absence of only one radius.[1008–1012] Patients with FA were even smaller than those with TAR. The hands of patients with TAR often had shortening of the middle phalanx of the fifth finger (clinodactyly), finger syndactyly, and sometimes thumb hypoplasia. Almost half had other forearm abnormalities, such as absent ulnae and ulnar shortening or bowing, which were reported in 40 percent. Upper arms were abnormal in one third, with either short or absent humeri.

The ulnar or humeral lesions were bilateral in 90 percent of patients. Scapular hypoplasia and webbed necks in some patients contribute further to abnormal upper body appearances. Micrognathia and occasional brachycephaly or microcephaly were also seen, as were hypertelorism, epicanthal folds, strabismus, and low-set ears. Ten percent had facial hemangiomas. Lower limb abnormalities seen in 40 percent of patients included deformity, subluxation, or hypoplasia of the knees, dislocation of the hips or patellae, and varus or valgus rotation at hips, knees, or feet, as well as short legs and absent tibiae or fibulae. Ten percent of patients had congenital heart disease, such as atrial or ventricular septal defects, tetralogy of Fallot, dextrocardia, and ectopia cordis. Gonadal anomalies were also reported, including undescended testes, hypoplasia, unicornuate uterus, vaginal atresia, and absent cervix. Low birth weight was noted at term in 15 percent of patients. A detailed summary of the anomalies can be found elsewhere.[3]

In contrast, patients with FA have absence of thumbs when radii are abnormal. Also, patients with TAR have only thrombocytopenia, whereas those with FA usually develop pancytopenia. Four patients with trisomy 18 had absence or hypoplasia of radii or thrombocytopenia[3, 9]; however, trisomy 18 is characterized by other findings in addition to the cytogenetic abnormality. Robert's syndrome and SC phocomelia may have a phenotype similar to that of TAR. Other syndromes with radial anomalies are beyond the scope of this analysis.

Bloody diarrhea in infancy, which was ascribed specifically to cow's milk allergy, was reported in 20 percent of patients.[999, 1009] Removal of milk from the diet alleviated the diarrhea, and perhaps improved the thrombocytopenia.

Laboratory Findings

Platelet counts were less than 50,000/μL at the time of diagnosis in more than 75 percent of patients. Anemia was due to bleeding and was accompanied by reticulocytosis. Leukocytosis was seen, with leukocyte counts greater than 15,000/μL in more than 75 percent, greater than 20,000 in more than 60 percent, and greater than 40,000 in one-third of the infants; occasionally the leukocyte count exceeded 100,000/μL. Circulating immature myeloid precursors were reported in more than a dozen patients, but none of these had true leukoerythroblastosis (see later). This leukemoid reaction has been mistaken for congenital leukemia, but it usually subsides during infancy. Extramedullary hematopoiesis may lead to splenomegaly. Eosinophilia is not uncommon. Bone marrow cellularity is normal, and myeloid and erythroid cell lines are normal or increased in number. The majority of patients have absent megakaryocytes; and in the rest these precursors are decreased in number, hypoplastic, or immature.

Normal laboratory tests include determination of mean cell volume, HbF, and chromosome breakage, the results of which clearly distinguish TAR from FA. Karyotyping also rules out trisomy 18. Hypogammaglobulinemia was reported only in a group of Nigerian patients.[1010] Small platelets were reported only once.[1013] Platelet function is generally normal, although a few patients had abnormal platelet aggregation and storage pool defects.[1013–1015] Clinical symptoms are more likely related to quantitative rather than qualitative defects, however.

Pathophysiology

TAR is probably an autosomal recessive disorder. It is one of a group of inherited hematologic conditions, which includes FA and DBA, with radial ray anomalies. The hematopoietic defect in TAR is essentially restricted to platelets. Cultures of hematopoietic progenitor cells indicate that the other lineages are normal.[120, 1016–1019] Megakaryocytic progenitors were reported to be absent in some studies[1017–1020] and essentially normal in others.[1021] One patient had a unique megakaryocyte colony-stimulating factor in the plasma, which may have been thrombopoietin, because it is elevated in TAR.[1020, 1022] The c-mpl gene, which is mutated in amegakaryocytic thrombocytopenia, is normal in TAR.[1023, 1024] TAR is a true single cytopenia, without evolution to aplastic anemia or leukemia, and thus the hematopoietic defect presumably involves only the megakaryocytic lineage.

Therapy and Outcome

Most patients with TAR exhibit bleeding in infancy and then improvement after the first year. More than 40 deaths were reported (20 percent), 80 percent of which occurred in the first year of life and only one after age 3. The projected survival curve (Fig. 8–36) shows a plateau of 75 percent survival by age 4. These data encompass more than 50 years of TAR case reports. During this period treatment may have been of limited scope; most of the deaths were from intracranial or gastrointestinal bleeding. Patients who survived the perilous first year had an increase in platelet count to greater than 100,000/μL, adequate for the necessary orthopedic procedures. Although thrombocytopenia sometimes recurred during illnesses, usually it was not severe. Those with milk allergy benefited from dietary modification.

The most important modern therapeutic advance has been platelet transfusions. Platelet transfusion is needed during bleeding episodes or operations and should provide prophylaxis for infants with severe symptomatic thrombocytopenia. The use of single donors reduces the risk of sensitization, and HLA-matched platelets can be used, if necessary. The platelet count should be maintained at greater than 10,000 to 15,000/μL. Platelet support is usually needed for less than 1 year. Other treatments, including splenectomy, corticosteroids, and androgens, were without apparent benefit; however, a transient increase in the platelet count was seen in one adult after splenectomy.[1025] A small dose of prednisone might decrease the bleeding tendency at a given platelet count, and ε-aminocaproic acid may also be useful (see the section on FA for details).

The leukemoid reaction and eosinophilia diminish after the first year of life. There have been no reports of aplastic anemia, although the high white cell count in some infants has led to a diagnosis of so-called "congenital leukemia." Spontaneous improvement does occur, and heroic treatments such as myelotoxic drugs or BMT are usually not indicated, even though one patient with a life-threatening central nervous system hemorrhage received a successful BMT.[1026] After infancy, patients with TAR have a very good prognosis. TAR is the only bone marrow failure disorder with a plateau on the survival curve.

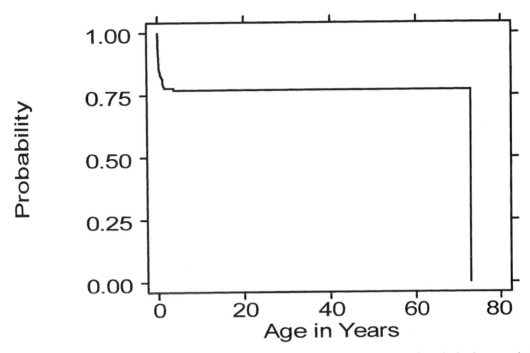

FIGURE 8–36. Kaplan-Meier plot of cumulative survival in TAR. The plateau is approximately 75 percent; the only death reported after age 4 years occurred in a 73-year-old woman with three different types of cancer.

Cancer has been rarely reported in patients with TAR. One patient had acute lymphoblastic leukemia,[1027] one had stage D(S) neuroblastoma at birth and died at 3 months of age,[1028] and one developed ileal adenocarcinoma at age 67, ovarian cancer at age 70, and bladder squamous cell carcinoma at age 73.[1029] These occurrences may all have been coincidental.

Prenatal diagnosis was performed in more than two dozen patients. Absence of radii was diagnosed with the use of radiography,[1030, 1031] ultrasound,[1032] or fetoscopy.[1033, 1034] Because unilateral radial aplasia has been reported, both forearms must be examined. In one patient, micrognathia was detected by ultrasound. Patients not known to be at risk for TAR were found to have characteristic limb abnormalities on ultrasound; in addition, fetal blood obtained by cordocentesis or fetoscopy can be used to demonstrate fetal thrombocytopenia.[634, 1034–1037] Seventy percent of the 28 fetuses at risk were found to have TAR (more than the expected 25 percent), but this result might represent reporting bias.

LEUKOERYTHROBLASTOSIS

Leukoerythroblastosis is observed in diverse disorders. The term was proposed by Vaughan in 1936 to describe "an anemia with the presence in the peripheral blood of immature red cells and a few immature white cells of the myeloid series,"[1038]—erythroblasts and leukoblasts. The blood film shows normochromic and normocytic erythrocytes, with poikilocytes, teardrops, fragments, and target cells (Fig. 8–37). Giant platelets may also be seen. Leukoerythroblastosis must be distinguished from a *leukemoid reaction*, which is a reactive leukocytosis characterized by an orderly progression of myeloid cells from immaturity through maturity. The term *leukemic hiatus*

applies when immature and mature white cells are seen without intermediate forms, producing a "gap" or "hiatus."

The disorders that may be characterized by leukoerythroblastosis are outlined in Table 8–25.[1039, 1040] Many of these involve bone marrow invasion, particularly from metastatic solid tumors, hematologic malignancies, infections, or other marrow components, with the crowding of cells out of the marrow prematurely ("myelophthisis"). Hypoxia might also stimulate premature release. In myeloproliferative disorders, the premature release of nucleated cells might be related to their intrinsic abnormality. Several other chapters in this book discuss many of the diseases associated with leukoerythroblastosis; this section will be restricted to osteopetrosis.

OSTEOPETROSIS

Description

Osteopetrosis, also known as "marble bone disease," or "Albers-Schonberg disease" was first described in 1904.[1041–1043] Variants include infantile-malignant autosomal recessive, intermediate autosomal recessive, and relatively benign autosomal dominant.[1043–1045] The milder dominant variety is diagnosed in late childhood and is characterized by dense bones that fracture easily; patients with this variant usually do not have hematologic problems. In contrast, the more severe recessive disorder is diagnosed in infancy and early childhood and is characterized by dense bones that fracture easily owing to a defect in bone resorption. These patients have large heads, sclerotic bones, and hepatosplenomegaly, and they develop blindness, deafness, and cranial nerve palsies because of bony scleroses, as well as pancytopenia. Many instances of osteopetrosis are familial, and the degree of

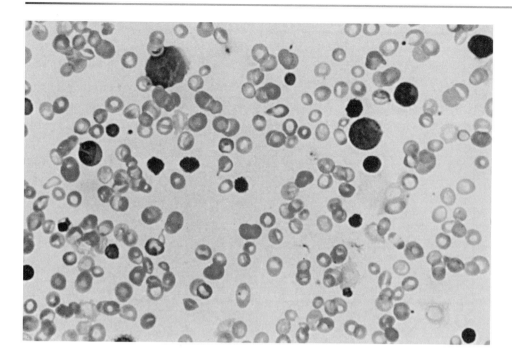

FIGURE 8–37. Peripheral blood from a patient with leukoerythroblastosis, in this case caused by osteopetrosis. (Courtesy of Dr. Gail Wolfe; with permission from Alter BP: The bone marrow failure syndromes. In Nathan DG, Oski FA (eds): Hematology of Infancy and Childhood, 3rd ed. Philadelphia, WB Saunders, 1987, p 159.)

consanguinity is high. The disease may be severe *in utero,* as there is often a history of stillbirths and spontaneous abortions. The intermediate recessive form, diagnosed in the first decade, is less severe than the infantile form. A subset of patients with this variant has a deficiency in carbonic anhydrase II.[1046]

Laboratory Findings

Patients with infantile recessive osteopetrosis have severe macrocytic anemia, reticulocytosis, teardrop red cells, circulating erythroblasts, and leukocytosis with immature myeloid elements—all of which are components of leukoerythroblastosis due to myelophthisis. High levels of HbF are a sign of stress erythropoiesis.[1047] The bone diploic spaces are small, and the marrow cavity is narrow. Bone marrow aspiration is difficult, and needles may break in attempts to penetrate the sclerotic bone. Biopsies show narrow medullary cavities, hypocellularity, fibrosis, and spindle cell stroma. Osteoblasts and osteoclasts are abundant.[1048] Hepatosplenomegaly develops because of extramedullary hematopoiesis. Hypersplenism ensues, leading to thrombocytopenia, leukopenia, and hemolytic anemia due to extracorpuscular destruction of intrinsically normal erythrocytes.[1049]

Pathophysiology

The osteoclasts are abnormal and are unable to resorb bone and perform normal remodeling. In an osteopetrotic mouse model, Walker showed that bone marrow or spleen cells from normal mice led to bone remodeling in osteopetrotic littermates, and spleen cells from affected mice led to osteopetrosis in normal mice.[1050] A cytoplasmic marker (giant lysosomes in Chédiak-Higashi mice) was used to show that marrow transplants that cured osteopetrosis in mice resulted in replacement of recipient osteoclasts with donor osteoclasts.[1050] Similar studies using donor mice with defective erythropoiesis (W^e/W^v) suggested that the osteoclast stem cell may be more primordial than the colony-forming unit spleen.[1051] The defective donor erythrocytosis was replaced by the recipient's normal erythropoiesis even though the osteopetrosis was cured and leukocytes and platelets were donor. *In vitro* studies indicate that osteoclasts are derived from hematopoietic stem cells, which are in the mononuclear light-density fraction.[1052] In humans as well, marrow transplant is curative (see later), a fact indicating that the osteoclast is contained within the transplantable stem cell population.

Hematopoiesis itself is intrinsically normal. The peripheral blood has increased numbers of CFU-GMs, BFU-Es, and even CFU-Es. The latter are normally found only in marrow and may migrate from the crowded bone marrow to sites of extramedullary hematopoiesis. Osteoclasts are numerically normal, morphologically normal or abnormal, and functionally abnormal.

Several genes that cause osteopetrosis have been identified. The gene for the autosomal dominant form mapped to chromosome 1p21, although the candidate gene *CSF-1,* which is mutant in the *op/op* mouse, was excluded in an extended Danish kindred.[1053] The milder autosomal recessive disorder, in which there is renal tubular acidosis, was shown to be associated with a deficiency of carbonic anhydrase II in 1985,[1054] and mutations in *CAII* were identified in 1992.[1055]

Severe autosomal recessive osteopetrosis appears to be multigenic. One gene maps to 11q13, syntenic with mouse chromosome 19, the site of the murine oc mutation.[1056] The murine gene is TCIRG1, which codes for the osteoclast-specific subunit of the vacuolar proton pump. Five of 9 patients were found to have mutations in *TCIRG1.*[1057] The gene is also called *OC116,* which encodes the a3 subunit of the V-ATPase from osteoclasts, and was mutant in 5 of 10 patients.[1058] Another gene in the same pathway, the CLC-7 chloride channel, was mutated in 1 of 12 patients and in mice.[1059] The

TABLE 8–25. Conditions Associated with Leukoerythroblastosis

MARROW INVASION

Tumor
Solid tumor with bone marrow metastases
Lymphoma
Hodgkin's disease
Multiple myeloma
Leukemia
Neuroblastoma
Preleukemia

Infection
Osteomyelitis
Sepsis
Tuberculosis
Congenital

Marrow Components
Osteopetrosis
Storage disease
Histiocytosis
Vasculitis, including rheumatoid arthritis

MYELOPROLIFERATIVE DISORDERS
Polycythemia vera
Myelofibrosis, myeloid metaplasia
Down syndrome transient myeloproliferative disease
Chronic myelogenous leukemia
Erythroleukemia
Thrombocythemia

HEMATOLOGIC DISEASE
Erythroblastosis fetalis
Pernicious anemia
Thalassemia major
Other hemolytic anemias

HYPOXIA
Cyanotic congenital heart disease
Congestive heart failure
Respiratory disease

disruption of the pathway of acidification of extracellular lysosomes between osteoclasts and bone leads to a defect in bone degradation and severe osteopetrosis. Thus, two or more genes are responsible for the severe form of osteopetrosis.

Therapy and Outcome

Most patients with malignant osteopetrosis die in infancy or early childhood, and none were reported to have survived beyond 20 years of age. In a longitudinal study of 33 patients, the probability of survival at age 6 was 30 percent, and the median projected survival was 4 years.[1044] Deaths occurred from the complications of bone marrow failure, infection, and hemorrhage. Host resistance may be impaired because circulating phagocytes, derived from the same lineage as osteoclasts, are defective in the generation of superoxide. Symptomatic anemia and thrombocytopenia can be treated with transfusions of red cells and platelets, but hypersplenism decreases the efficacy of such treatment. Splenectomy offers only temporary improvement because the rest of the reticuloendothelial system

remains active and the primary bone disorder is not cured. Some patients showed a response to prednisone therapy; again improvement was transient because of decreased hypersplenism and reticuloendothelial suppression.[1060, 1061] Calcitriol was not consistently effective in stimulation of bone resorption.[1062, 1063] The use of interferon-γ, which stimulates superoxide generation in chronic granulomatous disease, led to decreased trabecular bone area and significantly improved blood counts and superoxide production in 11 patients treated for 18 months.[1064] In one adult with dominant disease, erythropoietin and corticosteroids were used successfully for treating myelophthisic pancytopenia.[1065]

BMT was performed in more than 100 patients, with a median survival of 3 years.[1066] The osteoclasts and hematopoietic cells were of donor origin, whereas the osteoblasts remained host. Restoration of normal hematopoiesis, improvement of radiographic findings, and stabilization of physical changes were seen; early transplantation offers the only hope for cure. Long-term follow-up found survival of four of nine Bedouin patients, who showed hematologic improvement but persistent visual impairment.[1067] In another patient neurodegeneration progressed after BMT with a 5/6 unrelated cord.[1068] Stem cell transplant must be done early, before the bony changes have encroached on hearing and vision.

Prenatal diagnosis was first performed in 1943 using radiography,[1069] but errors were made.[1070] Currently ultrasound is used to detect increased bone density, fractures, macrocephaly, and hydrocephaly, which can then be confirmed by radiography.[1071, 1072] In Bedouin families in which the osteopetrosis was linked to 11q13, 3 of 12 fetuses were affected.[1073]

SUMMARY

The major inherited bone marrow failure disorders are summarized in Table 8–26. The diagnosis of "acquired" aplastic anemia or single cytopenia should not be made without serious consideration of these conditions. Physical anomalies may be subtle or absent, but family histories or specific laboratory investigations (e.g., chromosome breakage) may provide clues. The numbers of patients and the proportions in whom complications occur are not reflections of the true risk, because they are based on literature reports, not on epidemiologic studies. Despite underreporting and underdiagnosis, the numbers do provide some perspective about relative numbers of occurrences.

Most of these conditions are expressed in probable homozygotes (for autosomal recessive) or hemizygotes (for X-linked), although a few are inherited as dominant. Because heterozygotes cannot usually be identified (except as parents), patients with multiple bone marrow failure genes or with "acquired" diseases that may in fact be inherited cannot be defined at this time.

Treatment of marrow failure depends on the specific diagnosis. Androgen treatment may be effective in patients with pancytopenia due to FA, dyskeratosis congenita, amegakaryocytic thrombocytopenia, or Shwachman-Diamond syndrome. Patients

TABLE 8–26. Inherited Bone Marrow Failure Syndromes

Feature	Fanconi Anemia	Dyskeratosis Congenita	Shwachman-Diamond Syndrome	Amega-karyocytic Thrombocyto-penia	Diamond-Blackfan Anemia	Severe Congenital Neutropenia	Thrombocyto-penia with Absent Radii
Approximate No. of patients	1200	275	340	75	700	300	225
Male: female ratio	1.2	4.5	1.6	1.1	1.1	1	0.8
Genetics	AR	X	AR	AD, AR	AR, AD, sporadic	AR	AR
Physical abnormalities (%)	≈75	100	40	30	25	0	100
Upper limb anomalies (%)	40	1	1	0	8	0	100
Median age at diagnosis	8 yrs	16 yrs	<1 yr	≈1 mo	2 mos	≈1 mo	<1 wk
First hematologic sign	Pancytopenia	Pancytopenia	Neutropenia	Thrombocy-topenia	Anemia	Neutropenia	Thrombocy-topenia
Bone marrow	Aplastic	Aplastic	Hypocellular, myeloid arrest	Absent or small megakaryo-cytes	Erythroid hypoplasia	Promyelocyte arrest	Absent or immature megakaryo-cytes
Aplastic anemia (%)	>90	40	40	40	0	0	0
Leukemia (%)	9	0	7	3	1	9	0.4
MDS (%)	6	1	9	0	0.3	5	0
Solid tumor (%)	5	14	0	0	2	0	0
Liver tumor (%)	3	0	0	0	0.3	0	0
HbF level	Increased	Increased	Increased	Increased	Increased	Normal	Normal
Chromosomes	Breaks with clastogens	Normal	Normal	Normal	Normal	Normal	Normal
Spontaneous remissions (%)	Very rare	0	Very rare	0	15–25	0	75
Treatment	Androgens	Androgens	Androgens, G-CSF	None	Steroids	G-CSF	Platelets
Response (%)	50, transient	50, transient	50, transient	—	60, transient	Excellent	—
Prognosis	Poor	Poor	Fair	Poor	Good	Good	Good
Prenatal diagnosis	Chromosomes, mutations	Mutations	Neutropenia	Thrombocyto penia, mutations	?Anemia, ? ADA, ? BFU-E mutations	Neutropenia, mutations	Absent radii, thrombocy-topenia
Projected median survival age (yrs)	30	33	35	7	43	23	>50

AR = autosomal recessive; AD = autosomal dominant; X = X-linked recessive; FAC = Fanconi's anemia complementation group C; RFLP = restriction fragment length polymorphism.

G-CSF = granulocyte colony-stimulating factor; ADA = adenosine deaminase.

with Diamond-Blackfan anemia should receive corticosteroids. G-CSF is particularly effective in severe congenital neutropenia and may have a role in some patients with dyskeratosis congenita. Platelets provide necessary (and necessarily temporary) support for patients with TAR. BMT for FA requires modification of preparative protocols, BMT protocols for DC have not yet been developed, patients with SD may be able to undergo BMT, and patients with DBA and TAR—which might and will improve spontaneously, respectively—may not need BMT at all. The donor must be known to be unaffected by the familial disease. Immunotherapy and growth factor treatment may be provided for specific diseases. All treatments and diseases may evolve into leukemia or other malignancies, and high-risk therapies must be considered very carefully in patients whose underlying condition is premalignant. Treatment of malignant complications is difficult in these inherited disorders in which abnormalities involve more than just hematopoietic tissues.

Prenatal diagnosis is available for many of the inherited marrow failure disorders, and in many instances molecular diagnoses can be performed. Families are usually identified through a proband, and monitoring can then be offered for subsequent pregnancies. Early diagnosis of an affected fetus may eventually lead to treatment *in utero* or at birth. Diagnosis of an unaffected HLA-identical fetus may provide placental blood for treatment of the proband.

Clearly, much remains to be understood about the genetics, pathophysiology, and treatment of both inherited and acquired bone marrow failure syndromes. This understanding requires correct diagnoses as well as proper treatment and careful follow-up. The prognoses for most of these disorders have improved with recent therapeutic advances, and it is anticipated that this improvement will accelerate with the expanding knowledge of the specific molecular and cellular defects.

REFERENCES

1. O'Gorman Hughes DW: The varied pattern of aplastic anaemia in childhood. Aust Paediatr J 1966; 2:228.
2. Alter BP, Young NS: The bone marrow failure syndromes. In Nathan DG, Orkin SH (eds): Hematology of Infancy and Childhood, 5th ed. Philadelphia, WB Saunders, 1998, p 237.
3. Young NS, Alter BP: Aplastic Anemia: Acquired and Inherited. Philadelphia, WB Saunders, 1994.
4. Alter BP, Potter NU, Li FP: Classification and aetiology of the aplastic anaemias. Clin Haematol 1978; 7:431.
5. Windass B, Vowels MR, O'Gorman Hughes D, et al: Aplastic anaemia in childhood: Prognosis and approach to therapy. Med J Aust 1987; 146:15.
6. Fanconi G: Familiäre infantile perniziösaartige Anämie (perniziöses Blutbild und Konstitution). Jahrbuch Kinder 1927; 117:257.
7. Uehlinger E: Konstitutionelle infantile (perniziösaartige) Anämie. Klin Wochenschr 1929; 32:1501.
8. Fanconi G: Familial constitutional panmyelocytopathy, Fanconi's anemia (F.A.). I. Clinical aspects. Semin Hematol 1967; 4:233.
9. Alter BP, Young NS: The bone marrow failure syndromes. In Nathan DG, Oski FA (eds): Hematology of Infancy and Childhood, 4th ed. Philadelphia, WB Saunders, 1993, p 216.
10. Alter BP: Annotation: Fanconi's anaemia and its variability. Br J Haematol 1993; 85:9.
11. Liu JM, Buchwald M, Walsh CE, et al: Fanconi anemia and novel strategies for therapy. Blood 1994; 84:3995.
12. Alter BP, Tenner MS: Brain tumors in patients with Fanconi's anemia. Arch Pediatr Adolesc Med 1994; 148:661.
13. Porteous MEM, Cross I, Burn J: VACTERL with hydrocephalus: One end of the Fanconi anemia spectrum of anomalies? Am J Med Genet 1992; 43:1032.
14. Giampietro PF, Adler-Brecher B, Verlander PC, et al: The need for more accurate and timely diagnosis in Fanconi anemia: A report from the International Fanconi Anemia Registry. Pediatrics 1993; 91:1116.
15. Auerbach A, Schroeder T: First announcement of the Fanconi Anemia International Registry. Blood 1982; 60:1054.
16. Estren S, Dameshek W: Familial hypoplastic anemia of childhood. Report of eight cases in two families with beneficial effect of splenectomy in one case. Am J Dis Child 1947; 73:671.
17. Li FP, Potter NU: Classical Fanconi anemia in a family with hypoplastic anemia. J Pediatr 1978; 92:943.
18. Glanz A, Fraser FC: Spectrum of anomalies in Fanconi anaemia. J Med Genet 1982; 19:412.
19. Riley E, Caldwell R, Swift M: Comparison of clinical features in Fanconi anemia probands and their subsequently diagnosed siblings. Am J Hum Genet 1979; 31:82A.
20. Schroeder TM, Tilgen D, Kruger J, et al: Formal genetics of Fanconi's anemia. Hum Genet 1976; 32:257.
21. Rogatko A, Auerbach AD: Segregation analysis with uncertain ascertainment: Application to Fanconi anemia. Am J Hum Genet 1988; 42:889.
22. Swift M: Fanconi anaemia: Cellular abnormalities and clinical predisposition to malignant disease. In Congenital Disorders of Erythropoiesis, Ciba Foundation Symposium 37. Amsterdam, Elsevier, 1976, p 115.
23. Rosendorff J, Bernstein R, Macdougall L, et al: Fanconi anemia: Another disease of unusually high prevalence in the Afrikaans population of South Africa. Am J Med Genet 1987; 27:793.
24. Verlander PC, Kaporis A, Liu Q, et al: Carrier frequency of the IVS4 + 4 A→T mutation of the Fanconi anemia gene FAC in the Ashkenazi Jewish population. Blood 1995; 86:4034.
25. Gershanik JJ, Morgan SK, Akers R: Fanconi's anemia in a neonate. Acta Paediatr Scand 1972; 61:623.
26. Perkins J, Timson J, Emery AEH: Clinical and chromosome studies in Fanconi's aplastic anaemia. J Med Genet 1969; 6:28.
27. Reinhold JDL, Neumark E, Lightwood R, et al: Familial hypoplastic anemia with congenital abnormalities (Fanconi's syndrome). Blood 1952; 7:915.
28. O'Neill EM, Varadi S: Neonatal aplastic anaemia and Fanconi's anaemia. Arch Dis Child 1963; 38:92.
29. Welshimer K, Swift M: Congenital malformations and developmental disabilities in ataxia-telangiectasia, Fanconi anemia, and xeroderma pigmentosum families. Am J Hum Genet 1982; 34:781.
30. Dacie JV, Gilpin A: Refractory anaemia (Fanconi type). Its incidence in three members of one family, with in one case a relationship to chronic haemolytic anaemia with nocturnal haemoglobinuria (Marchiafava-Micheli disease or 'nocturnal haemoglobinuria'). Arch Dis Child 1944; 19:155.
31. Shahidi NT, Gerald PS, Diamond LK: Alkali-resistant hemoglobin in aplastic anemia of both acquired and congenital types. N Engl J Med 1962; 266:117.
32. Cassimos C, Zannos L: Congenital hypoplastic anemia associated with multiple developmental defects (Fanconi's syndrome). Am J Dis Child 1952; 84:347.
33. Beard MEJ, Young DE, Bateman CJT, et al: Fanconi's anaemia. Q J Med 1973; 42:403.
34. Jones R: Fanconi anemia: Simultaneous onset of symptoms in two siblings. J Pediatr 1976; 88:152.
35. De Vroede M, Feremans W, De Maertelaere-Laurent E, et al: Fanconi's anaemia. Simultaneous onset in 2 siblings and unusual cytological findings. Scand J Haematol 1982; 28:431.
36. Skikne BS, Lynch SR, Bezwoda WR, et al: Fanconi's anaemia, with special reference to erythrokinetic features. S Afr Med J 1978; 53:43.
37. Silver HK, Blair WC, Kempe CH: Fanconi syndrome. Multiple congenital anomalies with hypoplastic anemia. Am J Dis Child 1952; 83:14.
38. Voss R, Kohn G, Shaham M, et al: Prenatal diagnosis of Fanconi anemia. Clin Genet 1981; 20:185.
39. Gotz M, Pichler E: Zur Panmyelopathie im Kindesalter. Klin Paediatr 1972; 148:377.
40. Romero MG, Ortiz HC: Anemia de Fanconi. Respuesta a dosis bajas de anabolicos y asociacion con carcinoma de esofago. Rev Invest Clin 1984; 36:353.
41. Schroeder TM, Drings P, Beilner P, et al: Clinical and cytogenetic observations during a six-year period in an adult with Fanconi's anaemia. Blut 1976; 34:119.
42. Althoff H: Zur Panmyelopathie Fanconi als Zustandsbild multipler Abartungen. Z Kinderheilk 1953; 72:267.

43. Alter BP: Fetal erythropoiesis in stress hematopoiesis. Exp Hematol 1979; 7:200.

44. Alter BP: Fetal erythropoiesis in bone marrow failure syndromes. In Stamatoyannopoulos G, Neinhuis AW (eds): Cellular and Molecular Regulation of Hemoglobin Switching, New York, Grune and Stratton, 1979, p 87.

45. Shepard MK, Weatherall DJ, Conley CL: Semi-quantitative estimation of the distribution of fetal hemoglobin in red cell populations. Bull Johns Hopkins Hosp 1962; 110:293.

46. Cassinat B, Guardiola P, Chevret S, et al: Constitutive elevation of serum alpha-fetoprotein in Fanconi anemia. Blood 2000; 96:859.

47. Alter BP, Knobloch ME, Weinberg RS: Erythropoiesis in Fanconi's anemia. Blood 1991; 78:602.

48. Chu J-Y, Ho JE, Monteleone PL, et al: Technetium colloid bone marrow imaging in Fanconi's anemia. Pediatrics 1979; 64:635.

49. de Grouchy J, de Nava C, Marchand JC, et al: Études cytogénétique et biochimique de huit cas d'anémie de Fanconi. Ann Genet 1972; 15:29.

50. Jalbert Par P, Leger J, Bost M, et al: L'anemie de Fanconi: Aspects cytogenetiques et biochimiques. A propos d'une famille. Nouv Rev Fr Hematol 1975; 15:551.

51. Löhr GW, Waller HD, Anschütz F, et al: Hexokinasemangel in Blutzellen bei einer Sippe mit familiärer Panmyelopathie (Typ Fanconi). Klin Wochenschr 1965; 43:870.

52. Magnani M, Novelli G, Stocchi V, et al: Red blood cell hexokinase in Fanconi's anemia. Acta Haematol 1984; 71:341.

53. Schiavulli E, Gabriele S: Anemia di Fanconi. Minerva Pediatr 1978; 30:1251.

54. Cameron ES, Alleyne W, Charles W: Fanconi's aplastic anemia in two sisters in Trinidad and Tobago. West Indian Med J 1989; 38:118.

55. Schoof E, Beck JD, Joenje H, et al: Growth hormone deficiency in one of two siblings with Fanconi's anaemia complementation group FA-D. Growth Horm IGF Res 2000; 10:290.

56. Dupuis-Girod S, Gluckman E, Souberbielle J-C, et al: Growth hormone deficiency caused by pituitary stalk interruption in Fanconi's anemia. J Pediatr 2001; 138:129.

57. Wajnrajch MP, Gertner JM, Huma Z, et al: Evaluation of growth and hormonal status in patients referred to the International Fanconi Anemia Registry. Pediatrics 2001; 107:744.

58. Fisher DA, Job J-C, Preece M, et al: Leukaemia in patients treated with growth hormone. Lancet 1988; 1:1159.

59. Fradkin JE, Mills JL, Schonberger LB, et al: Risk of leukemia after treatment with pituitary growth hormone. JAMA 1993; 270:2829.

60. Blethen SL: Leukemia in children treated with growth hormone. Trends Endocrinol Metab 1998; 9:367.

61. Schroeder TM, Kurth R: Spontaneous chromosomal breakage and high incidence of leukemia in inherited disease. Blood 1971; 37:96.

62. Chaganti RSK, Schonberg S, German J: A manyfold increase in sister chromatid exchanges in Bloom's syndrome lymphocytes. Proc Natl Acad Sci USA 1974; 71:4508.

63. Kaiser TN, Lojewski A, Dougherty C, et al: Flow cytometric characterization of the response of Fanconi's anemia cells to mitomycin C treatment. Cytometry 1982; 2:291.

64. Miglierina R, le Coniat M, Gendron M, et al: Diagnosis of Fanconi's anemia by flow cytometry. Nouv Rev Fr Hematol 1991; 32:391.

65. Arkin S, Brodtman D, Naprstek B, et al: Cell cycle analysis in Fanconi anemia: A diagnostic test. Pediatr Res 1994; 35:157A.

66. Seyschab H, Friedl R, Sun Y, et al: Comparative evaluation of diepoxybutane sensitivity and cell cycle blockage in the diagnosis of Fanconi anemia. Blood 1995; 85:2233.

67. Heinrich MC, Hoatlin ME, Zigler AJ, et al: DNA Cross-linker-induced G_2/M arrest in group C Fanconi anemia lymphoblasts reflects normal checkpoint function. Blood 1998; 91:275.

68. Auerbach AD, Alter BP: Prenatal and postnatal diagnosis of aplastic anemia. In Alter BP (ed): Methods in Hematology: Perinatal Hematology. Edinburgh, Churchill Livingstone, 1989, p 225.

69. Auerbach AD, Rogatko A, Schroeder-Kurth TM: International Fanconi Anemia Registry: Relation of clinical symptoms to diepoxybutane sensitivity. Blood 1989; 73:391.

70. Arwert F, Kwee ML: Chromosomal breakage in response to cross-linking agents in the diagnosis of Fanconi anemia. In Schroeder-Kurth TM, Auerbach AD, Obe G (eds): Fanconi Anemia Clinical, Cytogenetic and Experimental Aspects. Berlin, Springer-Verlag, 1989, p 83.

71. Hasle H, Olsen JH: Cancer in relatives of children with myelodysplastic syndrome, acute and chronic myeloid leukemia. Br J Haematol 1997; 97:127.

72. Gregory JJ Jr, Wagner JE, Verlander PC, et al: Somatic mosaicism in Fanconi anemia: Evidence of genotypic reversion in lymphohematopoietic stem cells. Proc Natl Acad Sci USA 2001; 98:2532.

73. Todaro GJ, Green H, Swift MR: Susceptibility of human diploid fibroblast strains to transformation by SV40 virus. Science 1966; 153:1252.

74. Higurashi M, Conen PE: In vitro chromosomal radiosensitivity in Fanconi's anemia. Blood 1971; 38:336.

75. Sasaki MS, Tonomura A: A high susceptibility of Fanconi's anemia to chromosome breakage by DNA cross-linking agents. Cancer Res 1973; 33:1829.

76. Auerbach AD, Adler B, O'Reilly RJ, et al: Effect of procarbazine and cyclophosphamide on chromosome breakage in Fanconi anemia cells: Relevance to bone marrow transplantation. Cancer Genet Cytogenet 1983; 9:25.

77. Auerbach AD, Wolman SR: Susceptibility of Fanconi's anaemia fibroblasts to chromosome damage by carcinogens. Nature 1976; 261:494.

78. Berger R, Bernheim A, Le Coniat M, et al: Nitrogen mustard-induced chromosome breakage: A tool for Fanconi's anemia diagnosis. Cancer Genet Cytogenet 1980; 2:269.

79. Cervenka J, Arthur D, Yasis C: Mitomycin C test for diagnostic differentiation of idiopathic aplastic anemia and Fanconi anemia. Pediatrics 1981; 67:119.

80. Poll EHA, Arwert F, Joenje H, et al: Cytogenetic toxicity of antitumor platinum compound in Fanconi's anemia. Hum Genet 1982; 61:228.

81. Auerbach AD, Sagi M, Adler B: Fanconi anemia: Prenatal diagnosis in 30 fetuses at risk. Pediatrics 1985; 76:794.

82. Auerbach AD, Liu Q, Ghosh R, et al: Prenatal identification of potential donors for umbilical cord blood transplantation for Fanconi anemia. Transfusion 1990; 30:682.

83. Shipley J, Rodeck CH, Garrett C, et al: Mitomycin C induced chromosome damage in fetal blood cultures and prenatal diagnosis of Fanconi's anaemia. Prenat Diagn 1984; 4:217.

84. Trunca C, Watson M, Auerbach A, et al: Prenatal diagnosis of Fanconi anemia in a fetus not known to be at risk. Am J Hum Genet 1984; 36:198S.

85. Boue Par J, Deluchat C, Nicolas H, et al: Diagnostic prenatal des maladies geniques sur villosites choriales. J Genet Hum 1986; 34:221.

86. Auerbach AD: Fanconi anemia. Dermatol Clin 1995; 13:41.

87. Hirsch-Kauffmann M, Schweiger M: Prenatal recognition of a defect in DNA repair. Mol Gen Genet 1981; 184:17.

88. Murer-Orlando M, Llerena JC Jr, Birjandi F, et al: *FACC* gene mutations and early prenatal diagnosis of Fanconi's anaemia. Lancet 1993; 342:686.

89. Varela MA, Sternberg WH: Preanaemic state in Fanconi's anaemia. Lancet 1967; 2:566.

90. Pignatti CB, Bianchi E, Polito E: Fanconi's anaemia in infancy: Report of a case diagnosed in the pre-anaemic stage. Helv Paediatr Acta 1977; 32:413.

91. McIntosh S, Breg WR, Lubiniecki AS: Fanconi's anemia. The pre-anemic phase. Am J Pediatr Hematol Oncol 1979; 1:107.

92. Cohen MM, Simpson SJ, Honig GR, et al: The identification of Fanconi anemia genotypes by clastogenic stress. Am J Hum Genet 1982; 34:794.

93. Altay C, Sevgi Y, Pirnar T: Fanconi's anemia in offspring of patient with congenital radial and carpal hypoplasia. N Engl J Med 1975; 293:151.

94. Petridou M, Barrett AJ: Physical and laboratory characteristics of heterozygote carriers of the Fanconi aplasia gene. Acta Paediatr Scand 1990; 79:1069.

95. D'Andrea AD, Grompe M: Molecular biology of Fanconi anemia: Implications for diagnosis and therapy. Blood 1997; 90:1725.

96. Schroeder TM, Anschütz F, Knopp A: Spontane Chromosomenaberrationen bei familiärer Panmyelopathie. Humangenetik 1964; 1:194.

97. Swift MR, Hirschhorn K: Fanconi's anemia. Inherited susceptibility to chromosome breakage in various tissues. Ann Intern Med 1966; 65:496.

98. Schmid W, Schärer K, Baumann Th, et al: Chromosomenbrüchigkeit bei der familiären Panmyelopathie (Typus Fanconi). Schweiz Med Wochenschr 1965; 43:1461.

99. Bloom GE, Warner S, Gerald PS, et al: Chromosome abnormalities in constitutional aplastic anemia. N Engl J Med 1966; 274:8.

100. German J, Pugliatti Crippa L: Chromosomal breakage in diploid cell lines from Bloom's syndrome and Fanconi's anemia. Ann Genet 1966; 9:143.

101. Bloom GE: Disorders of bone marrow production. Pediatr Clin North Am 1972; 19:983.

102. Gmyrek D, Witkowski R, Syllm-Rapoport I, et al: Chromosomal aberrations and abnormalities of red-cell metabolism in a case of Fanconi's anaemia before and after development of leukaemia. Ger Med Mon 1968; 13:105.

103. Kubbies M, Schindler D, Hoehn H, et al: Endogenous blockage and delay of the chromosome cycle despite normal recruitment and growth phase explain poor proliferation and frequent endomitosis in Fanconi anemia cells. Am J Hum Genet 1985; 37:1022.

104. Schindler D, Hoehn H: Fanconi anemia mutation causes cellular susceptibility to ambient oxygen. Am J Hum Genet 1988; 43:429.

105. Korkina LG, Samochatova EV, Maschan AA, et al: Release of active oxygen radicals by leukocytes of Fanconi anemia patients. J Leuk Biol 1992; 52:357.

106. Gille JJP, Wortelboer HM, Joenje H: Antioxidant status of Fanconi anemia fibroblasts. Hum Genet 1987; 77:28.

107. Joenje H, Frants RR, Arwert F, et al: Erythrocyte superoxide dismutase deficiency in Fanconi's anaemia established by two independent methods of assay. Scand J Clin Lab Invest 1979; 39:759.

108. Mavelli I, Ciriolo MR, Rotilio G, et al: Superoxide dismutase, glutathione peroxidase and catalase in oxidative hemolysis. A study of Fanconi's anemia erythrocytes. Biochem Biophys Res Commun 1982; 106:286.

109. Bigelow SB, Rary JM, Bender MA: G2 chromosomal radiosensitivity in Fanconi's anemia. Mutat Res 1979; 63:189.

110. Rosselli F, Sanceau J, Gluckman E, et al: Abnormal lymphokine production: A novel feature of the genetic disease Fanconi anemia. II. In vitro and in vivo spontaneous overproduction of tumor necrosis factor α. Blood 1994; 5:1216.

111. Takeuchi T, Morimoto K: Increased formation of 8-hydroxy-deoxyguanosine, an oxidative DNA damage, in lymphoblasts from Fanconi's anemia patients due to possible catalase deficiency. Carcinogenesis 1993; 14:1115.

112. Fujiwara Y, Tatsumi M, Sasaki MS: Cross-link repair in human cells and its possible defect in Fanconi's anemia cells. J Mol Biol 1977; 113:635.

113. Papadopoulo D, Guillouf C, Mohrenweiser H, et al: Hypomutability in Fanconi anemia cells is associated with increased deletion frequency at the HPRT locus. Proc Natl Acad Sci USA 1990; 87:8383.

114. Willingale-Theune J, Schweiger M, Hirsch-Kauffmann M, et al: Ultrastructure of Fanconi anemia fibroblasts. J Cell Science 1989; 93:651.

115. Kupfer GM, D'Andrea AD: The effect of the Fanconi anemia polypeptide, FAC, upon p53 induction and G2 checkpoint regulation. Blood 1996; 88:1019.

116. Wang J, Otsuki T, Youssoufian H, et al: Overexpression of the Fanconi anemia group C gene (FAC) protects hematopoietic progenitors from death induced by Fas-mediated apoptosis. Cancer Res 1998; 58:3538.

117. Rosselli F, Ridet A, Soussi T, et al: P53-dependent pathway of radio-induced apoptosis is altered in Fanconi anemia. Oncogene 1995; 10:9.

118. Saunders EF, Freedman MH: Constitutional aplastic anaemia: Defective haematopoietic stem cell growth in vitro. Br J Haematol 1978; 40:277.

119. Daneshbod-Skibba G, Martin J, Shahidi NT: Myeloid and erythroid colony growth in non-anemic patients with Fanconi's anaemia. Br J Haematol 1980; 44:33.

120. Lui VK, Ragab AH, Findley HS, et al: Bone marrow cultures in children with Fanconi anemia and the TAR syndrome. J Pediatr 1977; 91:952.

121. Alter BP, Knobloch ME, He L, et al: Effect of stem cell factor on in vitro erythropoiesis in patients with bone marrow failure syndromes. Blood 1992; 80:3000.

122. Stark R, Thierry D, Richard P, et al: Long-term bone marrow culture in Fanconi's anaemia. Br J Haematol 1993; 83:554.

123. Martinez-Jaramillo G, Espinoza-Hernandez L, Benitez-Aranda H, et al. Long-term proliferation in vitro of hematopoietic progenitor cells from children with congenital bone marrow failure: Effect of rhGM-CSF and rhEPO. Eur J Haematol 2000; 64:173.

124. Whitney MA, Royle G, Low MJ, et al: Germ cell defects and hematopoietic hypersensitivity to γ-interferon in mice with a targeted disruption of the Fanconi anemia C gene. Blood 1996; 88:49.

125. Imlay JA, Linn S: DNA damage and oxygen radical toxicity. Science 1988; 240:1302.

126. Pritsos CA, Sartorelli AC: Generation of reactive oxygen radicals through bioactivation of mitomycin antibiotics. Cancer Res 1986; 46:3528.

127. Izakovic V, Strbakova E, Kaiserova E, et al: Bovine superoxide dismutase in Fanconi anaemia. Therapeutic trial in two patients. Hum Genet 1985; 70:181.

128. Liu JM, Auerbach AD, Anderson SM, et al: A trial of recombinant human superoxide dismutase in patients with Fanconi anaemia. Br J Haematol 1993; 85:406.

129. Papadopoulo D, Laquerbe A, Guillouf C, et al: Molecular spectrum of mutations induced at the HPRT locus by a cross-linking agent in human cell lines with different repair capacities. Mutat Res 1993; 294:167.

130. Digweed M, Gunthert U, Schneider R, et al: Irreversible repression of DNA synthesis in Fanconi anemia cells is alleviated by the product of a novel cyclin-related gene. Mol Cell Biol 1995; 15:305.

131. Kupfer GM, Yamashita T, Naf D, et al: The Fanconi anemia polypeptide, FAC, binds to the cyclin-dependent kinase, cdc2. Blood 1997; 90:1047.

132. Escarceller M, Buchwald M, Singleton BK, et al: Fanconi anemia C gene product plays a role in the fidelity of blunt DNA end-joining. J Mol Biol 1998; 297:375.

133. Smith J, Andrau JC, Kallenbach S, et al: Abnormal rearrangements associated with V(D)J recombination in Fanconi anemia. J Mol Biol 1998; 281:815.

134. Thyagarajan B, Campbell C: Elevated homologous recombination activity in Fanconi anemia fibroblasts. J Biol Chem 1997; 272:23328.

135. Claustres M, Margueritte G, Sultan C: In vitro CFU-E and BFU-E responses to androgen in bone marrow from children with primary hypoproliferative anaemia—A possible therapeutic assay. Eur J Pediatr 1986; 144:467.

136. Bagnara GP, Strippoli P, Bonsi L, et al: Effect of stem cell factor on colony growth from acquired and constitutional (Fanconi) aplastic anemia. Blood 1992; 80:382.

137. Butturini A, Gale RP: Long-term bone marrow culture in persons with Fanconi anemia and bone marrow failure. Blood 1994; 83:336.

138. Segal GM, Magenis E, Brown M, et al: Repression of Fanconi anemia gene (FACC) expression inhibits growth of hematopoietic progenitor cells. J Clin Invest 1994; 94:846.

139. Schultz JC, Shahidi NT: Tumor necrosis factor-α overproduction in Fanconi's anemia. Am J Hematol 1993; 42:196.

140. Rosselli F, Sanceau J, Wietzerbin J, et al: Abnormal lymphokine production: A novel feature of the genetic disease Fanconi anemia. I. Involvement of interleukin-6. Hum Genet 1992; 89:42.

141. Stark R, Andre C, Thierry D, et al: The expression of cytokine and cytokine receptor genes in long-term bone marrow culture in congenital and acquired bone marrow hypoplasias. Br J Haematol 1993; 83:560.

142. Bagnara GP, Bonsi L, Strippoli P, et al: Production of interleukin 6, leukemia inhibitory factor and granulocyte-macrophage colony stimulating factor by peripheral blood mononuclear cells in Fanconi's anemia. Stem Cells 1993; 11:137.

143. Wunder E, Mortensen BT, Schilling F, et al: Anomalous plasma concentrations and impaired secretion of growth factors in Fanconi's anemia. Stem Cells 1993; 11:144.

144. Bagby GC, Segal GM, Auerbach AD, et al: Constitutive and induced expression of hematopoietic growth factor genes by fibroblasts from children with Fanconi anemia. Exp Hematol 1993; 21:1419.

145. Jonveaux P, Le Coniat M, Grausz D, et al: Lack of mutations in the TP53 tumor suppressor gene exons 5 to 8 in Fanconi's anemia. Nouv Rev Fr Hematol 1991; 33:343.

146. Rey JP, Scott R, Muller H: Apoptosis is not involved in the hypersensitivity of Fanconi anemia cells to mitomycin C. Cancer Genet Cytogenet 1994; 75:67.

147. Rugman FP, Ashby D, Davies JM: Does *HLA-DR* predict response to specific immunosuppressive therapy in aplastic anaemia? Br J Haematol 1990; 74:545.

148. Berger R, Bernheim A, Le Coniat M, et al: Bone marrow graft of a Fanconi's anemia patient. Cytogenetic study. Cancer Genet Cytogenet 1980; 2:127.

149. Zakrzewski S, Sperling K: Genetic heterogeneity of Fanconi's anemia demonstrated by somatic cell hybrids. Hum Genet 1980; 56:81.

150. Duckworth-Rysiecki G, Cornish K, Clarke CA, et al: Identification of two complementation groups in Fanconi anemia. Somat Cell Mol Genet 1985; 11:35.

151. Digweed M, Zakrzewski-Ludcke S, Sperling K: Fanconi's anaemia: Correlation of genetic complementation group with psoralen/UVA response. Hum Genet 1988; 78:51.

152. Buchwald M: Complementation groups: One or more per gene? Nature Genet 1995; 11:228.

153. Joenje H, Oostra AB, Wijker M, et al: Evidence for at least eight Fanconi anemia genes. Am J Hum Genet 1997; 61:940.

154. Joenje H, Levitus M, Waisfisz Q, et al: Complementation analysis in Fanconi anemia: Assignment of the reference FA-H patient to group A. Am J Hum Genet 2000; 67:759.

155. Strathdee CA, Gavish H, Shannon WR, et al: Cloning of cDNAs for Fanconi's anaemia by functional complementation. Nature 1992; 356:763.

156. Strathdee CA, Duncan AMV, Buchwald M: Evidence for at least four Fanconi anaemia genes including *FACC* on chromosome 9. Nat Genet 1992; 1:196.

157. Walsh CE, Nienhuis AW, Samulski RJ, et al: Phenotypic correction of Fanconi anemia in human hematopoietic cells with a recombinant adeno-associated virus vector. J Clin Invest 1994; 94:1440.

158. Verlander PC, Lin JD, Udono MU, et al: Mutation analysis of the Fanconi anemia gene *FACC*. Am J Hum Genet 1994; 54:595.

159. Gibson RA, Ford D, Jansen S, et al: Genetic mapping of the *FACC* gene and linkage analysis in Fanconi anaemia families. J Med Genet 1994; 31:868.

160. Whitney MA, Saito H, Jakobs PM, et al: A common mutation in the *FACC* gene causes Fanconi anaemia in Ashkenazi Jews. Nat Genet 1993; 4:202.

161. Whitney MA, Jakobs P, Kaback M, et al: The Ashkenazi Jewish Fanconi anemia mutation: Incidence among patients and carrier frequency in the at-risk population. Hum Mutat 1994; 3:339.

162. Futaki M, Yamashita T, Yagasaki H, et al: The IVS4 +4 A to T mutation of the Fanconi anemia gene *FANCC* is not associated with a severe phenotype in Japanese patients. Blood 2000; 95:1493.

163. Gibson RA, Hajianpour A, Murer-Orlando M, et al: A nonsense mutation and exon skipping in the Fanconi anaemia group C gene. Hum Mol Genet 1993; 2:797.

164. Lo Ten Foe JR, Rooimans MA, Bosnoyan-Collins L, et al: Expression cloning of a cDNA for the major Fanconi anaemia gene, *FAA*. Nat Genet 1996; 14:320.

165. Timmers C, Taniguchi T, Hejna J, et al: Positional cloning of a novel Fanconi anemia gene, *FANCD2*. Mol Cell 2001; 7:241.

166. de Winter JP, Leveille F, van Berkel CGM, et al: Isolation of a cDNA representing the Fanconi anemia complementation group E gene. Am J Hum Genet 2000; 67:1306.

167. de Winter JP, Rooimans MA, van der Weel L, et al: The Fanconi anaemia gene *FANCF* encodes a novel protein with homology to ROM. Nat Genet 2000; 24:15.

168. de Winter JP, Waisfisz Q, Rooimans MA, et al: The Fanconi anaemia group G gene *FANCG* is identical with *XRCC9*. Nat Genet 1998; 20:281.

169. Elghetany MT, MacCallum JM, Nelson DA, et al: Acquired specific granule deficiency in the myelodysplastic syndromes (MDS): A study of 191 previously untreated patients entered on CALGB protocols for MDS. Blood 1995; 86:336A.

170. Liu N, Lamerdin JE, Tucker JD, et al: The human *XRCC9* gene corrects chromosomal instability and mutagen sensitivities in CHO UV40 cells. Proc Natl Acad Sci USA 1997; 94:9232.

171. Joenje H, Patel KJ: The emerging genetic and molecular basis of Fanconi anaemia. Nat Rev Genet 2001; 2:446.

172. Yamashita T, Kupfer GM, Naf D, et al: The Fanconi anemia pathway requires FAA phosphorylation and FAA/FAC nuclear accumulation. Proc Natl Acad Sci USA 1998; 95:13085.

173. Kupfer GM, Naf D, Suliman A, et al: The Fanconi anaemia proteins, FAA and FAG, interact to form a nuclear complex. Nat Genet 1997; 17:487.

174. Garcia-Higuera I, Kuang Y, Naf D, et al: Fanconi anemia proteins FANCA, FANCC, and FANCG/XRCC9 interact in a functional nuclear complex. Mol Cell Biol 1999; 19:4866.

175. Garcia-Higuera I, D'Andrea AD: Regulated binding of the Fanconi anemia proteins, FANCA and FANCC. Blood 1999; 93:1430.

176. Garcia-Higuera I, Kuang Y, Hagan R, et al: Overexpression of the Fanconi anemia protein, FANCA, functionally complements a Fanconi anemia group H cell line. Blood 1999; 94:414a.

177. Garcia-Higuera I, Kuang Y, Denham J, et al: The Fanconi anemia proteins FANCA and FANCG stabilize each other and promote the nuclear accumulation of the Fanconi anemia complex. Blood 2000; 96:3224.

178. Medhurst AL, Huber PAJ, Waisfisz Q, et al: Direct interactions of the five known Fanconi anaemia proteins suggest a common functional pathway. Hum Mol Genet 2001; 10:423.

179. Garcia-Higuera I, Taniguchi T, Ganesan S, et al: Interaction of the Fanconi anemia proteins and BRCA1 in a common pathway. Mol Cell 2001; 7:249.

180. Scully R, Chen J, Plug A, et al: Association of BRCA1 with rad51 in mitotic and meiotic cells. Cell 1997; 88:265.

181. Wu X, Petrini JHJ, Heine WF, et al: Independence of R/M/N focus formation and the presence of intact BRCA1. Science 2000; 289:11a.

182. Youssoufian H: Fanconi anemia and breast cancer: What's the connection? Nat Genet 2001; 27:352.

183. Joenje H, Arwert F: Connecting Fanconi anemia to BRCA1. Nat Med 2001; 7:406.

184. Tipping AJ, Pearson T, Organ NV, et al: Molecular and genealogical evidence for a founder effect in Fanconi anemia families of the Afrikaner population of South Africa. Proc Natl Acad Sci USA 2001; 98:5734.

185. Demuth I, Wlodarski M, Tipping AJ, et al: Spectrum of mutations in the Fanconi anaemia group G gene, FANCG/XRCC9. Eur J Hum Genet 2000; 8:861.

186. Faivre, L. Guardiola, P. Lewis, et al for the EUFAR: Association of complementation group and mutation type with clinical outcome in Fanconi anemia. Blood 2000; 96:4064.

187. Chen M, Tomkins DJ, Querbach W, et al: Inactivation of Fac in mice produces inducible chromosomal instability and reduced fertility reminiscent of Fanconi anemia. Nat Genet 1996; 12:448.

188. Cheng NC, van de Vrugt HJ, van der Valk MA, et al: Mice with a targeted disruption of the Fanconi anemia homolog Fanca. Hum Mol Genet 2000; 9:1805.

189. Haneline LS, Gobbett TA, Ramani R, et al: Loss of FancC function results in decreased hematopoietic stem cell repopulating ability. Blood 1999; 94:1.

190. Battaile KP, Bateman RL, Mortimer D, et al: In vivo selection of wild-type hematopoietic stem cells in a murine model of Fanconi anemia. Blood 1999; 94:2151.

191. Carreau M, Gan OI, Liu L, et al: Hematopoietic compartment of Fanconi anemia group C null mice contains fewer lineage-negative CD34+ primitive cells and shows reduced reconstitution ability. Exp Hematol 1999; 27:1667.

192. Walsh CE, Grompe M, Vanin E, et al: A functionally active retrovirus vector for gene therapy in Fanconi anemia group C. Blood 1994; 84:453.

193. Liu JM, Kim S, Read EJ, et al: Engraftment of hematopoietic progenitor cells transduced with the Fanconi anemia group C gene (FANCC). Hum Gene Ther 1999; 10:2337.

194. Lo Ten Foe JR, Kwee ML, Rooimans MA, et al: Somatic mosaicism in Fanconi anemia: Molecular basis and clinical significance. Eur J Hum Genet 1997; 5:137.

195. Waisfisz Q, Morgan NV, Savino M, et al: Spontaneous functional correction of homozygous Fanconi anaemia alleles reveals novel mechanistic basis for reverse mosaicism. Nat Genet 1999; 22:379.

196. MacMillan ML, Auerbach AD, DeFor TE, et al: Somatic lymphocyte mosaicism is predictive of graft failure (GF) in patients with Fanconi anemia (FA) transplanted with alternate donor hematopoietic cells. Presented at the 11th Annual International Fanconi Anemia Scientific Symposium 1999, p 41.

197. Verlinsky Y, Rechitsky S, Schoolcraft W, et al: Preimplantation diagnosis for Fanconi anemia combined with HLA matching. JAMA 2001; 285:3130.

198. Belkin L: The made-to-order savior. NY Times Mag 2001; July 1:36.
199. Bernard J, Mathé G, Najean Y: Contribution è l'étude clinique et physiopathologique de la maladie de Fanconi. Rev Fr Etudes Clin Biol 1958; 3:599.
200. Dawson JP: Congenital pancytopenia associated with multiple congenital anomalies (Fanconi type). Pediatrics 1955; 15:325.
201. McDonald R, Goldschmidt B: Pancytopenia with congenital defects (Fanconi's anaemia). Arch Dis Child 1960; 35:367.
202. Alter BP, Frissora CL, Halpérin DS, et al: Fanconi's anemia and pregnancy. Br J Haematol 1991; 77:410.
203. Flowers MED, Doney KC, Storb R, et al: Marrow transplantation for Fanconi anemia with or without leukemic transformation: An update of the Seattle experience. Bone Marrow Transplant 1992; 9:167.
204. Seaward PGR, Setzen R, Guidozzi F: Fanconi's anaemia in pregnancy: A case report. S Afr Med J 1990; 78:691.
205. Koo WH, Knight LA, Ang PT: Fanconi's anaemia and recurrent squamous cell carcinoma of the oral cavity: A case report. Ann Acad Med Singapore 1996; 25:289.
206. Bargman GJ, Shahidi NT, Gilbert EF, et al: Studies of malformation syndromes of man. XLVII: Disappearance of spermatogonia in the Fanconi anemia syndrome. Eur J Pediatr 1977; 125:163.
207. Liu JM, Auerbach AD, Young NS: Fanconi anemia presenting unexpectedly in an adult kindred with no dysmorphic features. Am J Med 1991; 91:555.
208. Gardner FH, Besa EC: Physiologic mechanisms and the hematopoietic effects of the androstanes and their derivatives. Curr Top Hematol 1983; 4:123.
209. Alexanian R: Erythropoietin and erythropoiesis in anemic man following androgens. Blood 1969; 33:564.
210. Singer JW, Adamson JW: Steroids and hematopoiesis. II. The effect of steroids on in vitro erythroid colony growth: Evidence for different target cells for different classes of steroids. J Cell Physiol 1976; 88:135.
211. Shahidi NT, Diamond LK: Testosterone-induced remission in aplastic anemia. Am J Dis Child 1959; 98:293.
212. Diamond LK, Shahidi NT: Treatment of aplastic anemia in children. Semin Hematol 1967; 4:278.
213. Sanchez-Medal L: The hemopoietic action of androstanes. Prog Hematol 1971; 7:111.
214. Najean Y: Androgen therapy in aplastic anaemia in childhood. In Congenital Disorders of Erythropoiesis, Ciba Foundation Symposium 37. Amsterdam, Elsevier, 1976, p 354.
215. Shahidi NT, Crigler JF Jr: Evaluation of growth and of endocrine systems in testosterone-corticosteroid-treated patients with aplastic anemia. J Pediatr 1967; 70:233.
216. Kitchens CS: Amelioration of endothelial abnormalities by prednisone in experimental thrombocytopenia in the rabbit. J Clin Invest 1977; 60:1129.
217. Smith S, Marx MP, Jordaan CJ, et al: Clinical aspects of a cluster of 42 patients in South Africa with Fanconi anemia. In Schroeder-Kurth TM, Auerbach AD, Obe G (eds): Fanconi Anemia Clinical, Cytogenetic and Experimental Aspects. Berlin, Springer-Verlag, 1989, p 34.
218. Gluckman E, Auerbach AD, Horowitz MM, et al: Bone marrow transplantation for Fanconi anemia. Blood 1995; 86:2856.
219. Guardiola PH, Pasquini R, Dokal I, et al: Outcome of 69 allogeneic stem cell transplantations for Fanconi anemia using HLA-matched unrelated donors: A study on behalf of the European Group for Blood and Marrow Transplantation. Blood 2000; 95:422.
220. Gluckman E, Devergie A, Schaison G, et al: Bone marrow transplantation in Fanconi Anaemia. Br J Haematol 1980; 45:557.
221. Zanis-Neto J, Ribeiro RC, Medeiros C, et al: Bone marrow transplantation for patients with Fanconi anemia: A study of 24 cases from a single institution. Bone Marrow Transplant 1995; 15:293.
222. Berger R, Bernheim A, Gluckman E, et al: In vitro effect of cyclophosphamide metabolites on chromosomes of Fanconi anaemia patients. Br J Haematol 1980; 45:565.
223. Gluckman E, Devergie A, Dutreix J: Bone marrow transplantation for Fanconi anemia. In Schroeder-Kurth TM, Auerbach AD, Obe G (eds): Fanconi Anemia: Clinical, Cytogenetic and Experimental Aspects, Berlin, Springer-Verlag, 1989, p 60.
224. Shinohara O, Kato S, Yabe H, et al: Growth after bone marrow transplantation in children. Am J Pediatr Hematol Oncol 1991; 13:263.
225. Howell RT: Evaluation of chromosomal damage following allogeneic bone marrow transplant in a patient with Fanconi's anemia. J Med Genet 1992; 29:203.
226. Yabe M, Yabe H, Matsuda M, et al: Bone marrow transplantation for Fanconi anemia. Adjustment of the dose of cyclophosphamide for preconditioning. Am J Pediatr Hematol Oncol 1993; 15:377.
227. Gluckman E, Devergie A, Dutreix J: Radiosensitivity in Fanconi anaemia: Application to the conditioning regimen for bone marrow transplantation. Br J Haematol 1983; 54:431.
228. Guardiola PH, Socie G, Pasquini R, et al: Allogeneic stem cell transplantation of Fanconi anaemia. Bone Marrow Transplant 1998; 21: s24.
229. Kapelushnik J, Or R, Slavin S, et al: A fludarabine-based protocol for bone marrow transplantation in Fanconi's anemia. Bone Marrow Transplant 1997; 20:1109.
230. Boulad F, Gillio A, Small TN, et al: Stem cell transplantation for the treatment of Fanconi anaemia using a fludarabine-based cytoreductive regimen and T-cell-depleted related HLA-mismatched peripheral blood stem cell grafts. Br J Haematol 2000; 111:1153.
231. Hansen JA, Good RA, Dupont B: HLA-D compatibility between parent and child. Transplantation 1977; 23:366.
232. O'Reilly RJ, Pollack MS, Auerbach AD, et al: HLA histocompatibility between parent and affected child in Fanconi's anemia. Pediatr Res 1982; 16:210A.
233. Socié G, Gluckman E, Raynal B, et al: Bone marrow transplantation for Fanconi anemia using low-dose cyclophosphamide/thoracoabdominal irradiation as conditioning regimen: Chimerism study by the polymerase chain reaction. Blood 1993; 82:2249.
234. Minchinton RM, Waters AH, Malpas JS, et al: Selective thrombocytopenia and neutropenia occurring after bone marrow transplantation-evidence of an auto-immune basis. Clin Lab Haematol 1984; 6:157.
235. Begovich AB, Erlich HA: HLA typing for bone marrow transplantation. New polymerase chain reaction-based methods. JAMA 1995; 273:586.
236. Deeg HJ, Storb R, Thomas ED, et al: Fanconi's anemia treated by allogeneic marrow transplantation. Blood 1983; 61:954.
237. Broxmeyer HE, Douglas GW, Hangoc G, et al: Human umbilical cord blood as a potential source of transplantable hematopoietic stem/progenitor cells. Proc Natl Acad Sci USA 1989; 86:3828.
238. Gluckman E, Broxmeyer HE, Auerbach AD, et al: Hematopoietic reconstitution in a patient with Fanconi's anemia by means of umbilical-cord blood from an HLA-identical sibling. N Engl J Med 1989; 321:1174.
239. Gluckman E, Devergie A, Bourdeau-Esperou H, et al: Transplantation of umbilical cord blood in Fanconi's anemia. Nouv Rev Fr Hematol 1991; 32:423.
240. Kurtzberg J, Laughlin M, Graham ML, et al: Placental blood as a source of hematopoietic stem cells for transplantation into unrelated recipients. N Engl J Med 1996; 335:157.
241. Johnson FL: Placental blood transplantation and autologous banking—Caveat emptor. J Pediatr Hematol Oncol 1997; 19:183.
242. Ozsoylu S: Treatment of aplastic anemia. J Pediatr 1983; 102:484.
243. Speck B, Gratwohl A, Nissen C, et al: Treatment of severe aplastic anemia with antilymphocyte globulin or bone-marrow transplantation. Br Med J 1981; 282:860.
244. Boggs DR, Joyce RA: The hematopoietic effects of lithium. Semin Hematol 1983; 20:129.
245. Ferguson L, Hoots K, Beran M, et al: Long-term bone marrow (BM) cultures with recombinant human granulocyte-macrophage colony stimulating factor (rhGM-CSF) in children with cytopenias: A correlation with clinical response. Blood 1988; 72:115a.
246. Guinan EC, Lopez ED, Huhn RD, et al: Evaluation of granulocyte-macrophage colony-stimulating factor for treatment of pancytopenia in children with Fanconi anemia. J Pediatr 1994; 124:144.
247. Kemahli S, Canatan D, Uysal Z, et al: GM-CSF in the treatment of Fanconi's anaemia. Br J Haematol 1994; 87:871.
248. Rackoff WR, Orazi A, Robinson CA, et al: Prolonged administration of granulocyte colony-stimulating factor (Filgrastim) to patients with Fanconi anemia: A pilot study. Blood 1996; 88:1588.
249. Nathan DG: Hope for hematopoietic hormones. N Engl J Med 1987; 317:626.
250. Scagni P, Saracco P, Timeus F, et al: Use of recombinant granulocyte colony-stimulating factor in Fanconi's anemia. Haematologica 1998; 83:432.

251. Butturini A, Gale RP, Verlander PC, et al: Hematologic abnormalities in Fanconi anemia: An International Fanconi Anemia Registry study. Blood 1994; 84:1650.

252. Garriga S, Crosby WH: The incidence of leukemia in families of patients with hypoplasia of the marrow. Blood 1959; 24:1008.

253. Swift M: Fanconi's anaemia in the genetics of neoplasia. Nature 1971; 230:370.

254. Swift M: Malignant disease in heterozygous carriers. Birth Defects Original Artic Ser 1976; 12(1):133.

255. Swift M, Caldwell RJ, Chase C: Reassessment of cancer predisposition of Fanconi anemia heterozygotes. J Natl Cancer Inst 1980; 65:863.

256. Potter NU, Sarmousakis C, Li FP: Cancer in relatives of patients with aplastic anemia. Cancer Genet Cytogenet 1983; 9:61.

257. Swift M, Sholman L, Gilmour D: Diabetes mellitus and the gene for Fanconi's anemia. Science 1972; 178:308.

258. Morrell D, Chase CI, Kupper LL, et al: Diabetes mellitus in ataxia-telangiectasia, Fanconi anemia, xeroderma pigmentosum, common variable immune deficiency, and severe combined immune deficiency families. Diabetes 1986; 35:143.

259. Schaison G, Leverger G, Yildiz C, et al: l'Anémie de Fanconi. Fréquence de l'évolution vers la leucémie. Presse Med 1983; 12:1269.

260. Gyger M, Perrault C, Belanger R, et al: Unsuspected Fanconi's anemia and bone marrow transplantation in cases of acute myelomonocytic leukemia. N Engl J Med 1989; 321:120.

261. Ahmed OA, Al-Rimawi HS, Al-Rashid AA, et al: Fanconi's anemia with acute lymphoblastic leukaemia in a Bedouin girl. Am Soc Hum Genet Suppl 1989; 45: A14.

262. Wada E, Murata M, Watanabe S: Acute lymphoblastic leukemia following treatment by human growth hormone in a boy with possible preanemic Fanconi's anemia. Jpn J Clin Oncol 1989; 19:36.

263. Yetgin S, Tuncer M, Guler E, et al: Acute lymphoblastic leukemia in Fanconi's anemia. Am J Hematol 1994; 45:94.

264. Tezcan I, Tuncer M, Uckan D, et al: Allogeneic bone marrow transplantation in Fanconi anemia from Turkey: A report of four cases. Pediatr Transplant 1998; 2:236.

265. Sugita K, Taki T, Hayashi Y, et al: MLL-CBP fusion transcript in a therapy-related acute myeloid leukemia with the t(11;16)(q23;p13) which developed in an acute lymphoblastic leukemia patient with Fanconi anemia. Genes Chromosomes Cancer 2000; 27:264.

266. Meisner LF, Taher A, Shahidi NT: Chromosome changes and leukemic transformation in Fanconi's anemia. In Hibino S, Takaku F, Shahidi NT (eds): Aplastic Anemia, Tokyo, University of Tokyo Press, 1976, p 253.

267. Eldar M, Shoenfeld Y, Zaizov R, et al: Pulmonary alveolar proteinosis associated with Fanconi's anemia. Respiration 1979; 38:177.

268. Perona G, Cetto GL, Bernardi F, et al: Fanconi's anaemia in adults: Study of three families. Haematologica 1977; 62:615.

269. Altay C, Alikasifoglu M, Kara A, et al: Analysis of 65 Turkish patients with congenital aplastic anemia (Fanconi anemia and non-Fanconi anemia): Hacettepe experience. Clin Genet 1997; 51:296.

270. Verbeek W, Haase D, Schoch C, et al: Induction of a hematological and cytogenetic remission in a patient with a myelodysplastic syndrome secondary to Fanconi's anemia employing the S-HAM regimen. Ann Hematol 1997; 74:275.

271. Zawartka M, Restorff-Libiszowska H, Kowalski R, et al: Bialaczka szpikowa w przebiegu anemii Fanconiego (AF). Wiad Lek 1976; 14:145.

272. Perrimond H, Juhan-Vague I, Thevenieau D, et al: Evolution médullaire et hépatique après androgenothérapie prolongée d'une anemie de Fanconi. Nouv Rev Fr Hematol 1977; 18:228.

273. van Gils JE, Mandel C, Van Weel-Sipman MH, et al: Acute leukemie bij Fanconi anemie. Tijdschr Kindergeneeskd 1987; 55:68.

274. el Mauhoub M, Sudarshan G, Banerjee G, et al: Fanconi's anemia with associated acute nonlymphocytic leukemia. Indian Pediatr 1988; 25:1124.

275. Submoke S, Kessacorn W: Fanconi's syndrome: Presentation of a case of acute myeloblastic leukemia. J Med Assoc Thailand 1985; 68:480.

276. Barton JC, Parmley RT, Carroll AJ, et al: Preleukemia in Fanconi's anemia: Hematopoietic cell multinuclearity, membrane duplication, and dysgranulopoiesis. J Submicrosc Cytol 1987; 19:355.

277. Tanzer J, Frocrain C, Desmarest MC: Anomalies du chromosome 1 dans 3 cas de leucemie compliquant une aplasie de Fanconi (FA). Nouv Rev Fr Hematol 1980; 22:XCIII.

278. Nowell P, Bergman G, Besa E, et al: Progressive preleukemia with a chromosomally abnormal clone in a kindred with the Estren-Dameshek variant of Fanconi's anemia. Blood 1984; 64:1135.

279. Woods WG, Nesbit ME, Buckley J, et al: Correlation of chromosome abnormalities with patient characteristics, histologic subtype, and induction success in children with acute nonlymphocytic leukemia. J Clin Oncol 1985; 3:3.

280. Maarek O, Jonveaux P, Le Coniat M, et al: Fanconi anemia and bone marrow clonal chromosome abnormalities. Leukemia 1996; 10:1700.

281. Obeid A, Hill FGH, Harnden D, et al: Fanconi anemia: Oxymetholone hepatic tumors, and chromosome aberrations associated with leukemic transition. Cancer 1980; 46:1401.

282. Auerbach AD, Weiner M, Warburton D, et al: Acute myeloid leukemia as the first hematologic manifestation of Fanconi anemia. Am J Hematol 1982; 12:289.

283. Berger R, Bussel A, Schenmetzler C: Somatic segregation and Fanconi anemia. Clin Genet 1977; 11:409.

284. Berger R, Le Coniat M: Cytogenetic studies in Fanconi anemia induced chromosomal breakage and cytogenetics. In Schroeder-Kurth TM, Auerbach AD, Obe G (eds): Fanconi Anemia: Clinical, Cytogenetic and Experimental Aspects, Berlin, Springer-Verlag, 1989, p 93.

285. Berger R, le Coniat M, Schaison G: Chromosome abnormalities in bone marrow of Fanconi anemia patients. Cancer Genet Cytogenet 1993; 65:47.

286. Alter BP, Scalise A, McCombs J, et al: Clonal chromosomal abnormalities in Fanconi's anemia: What do they really mean? Br J Haematol 1993; 85:627.

287. Davies SM, Khan S, Wagner JE, et al: Unrelated donor bone marrow transplantation for Fanconi anemia. Bone Marrow Transplant 1996; 17:43.

288. Griffin TC, Friedman DJ, Sanders JM, et al: Fanconi anemia complicated by acute myelogenous leukemia and malignant brain tumor. Blood 1992; 80:382a.

289. Yoshida Y, Kawabata H, Anzai N: Cell biology and programmed cell death in MDS. Leuk Res 1994; 18:5.

290. Gibbons B, Scott D, Hungerford JL, et al: Retinoblastoma in association with the chromosome breakage syndromes Fanconi's anaemia and Bloom's syndrome: Clinical and cytogenetic findings. Clin Genet 1995; 47:311.

291. Takizawa J, Kishi K, Moriyama Y, et al: Allogenic bone marrow transplantation for Fanconi's anemia with leukemic transformation from an HLA identical father. Rinsho Ketsueki 1995; 36:615.

292. Manglani M, Muralidhar HP, Bhoyar A, et al: Leukemic transformation in Fanconi's anemia. Indian Pediatr 1999; 36:1054.

293. Cowdell RH, Phizackerley PJR, Pyke DA: Constitutional anemia (Fanconi's syndrome) and leukemia in two brothers. Blood 1955; 10:788.

294. Sarna G, Tomasulo P, Lotz MJ, et al: Multiple neoplasia in two siblings with a variant form of Fanconi's anemia. Cancer 1975; 36:1029.

295. Consarino C, Magro S, Dattilo A, et al: Acute leukemia in Fanconi's anemia. In Department of Hematology of University of Rome (eds): Third International Symposium on Therapy of Acute Leukemias, Rome, University of Rome, 1982, p 492.

296. O'Gorman Hughes DW: Aplastic anaemia in childhood. III. Constitutional aplastic anaemia and related cytopenias. Med J Aust 1974; 1:519.

297. Dosik H, Hsu LY, Todaro GJ, et al: Leukemia in Fanconi's anemia: Cytogenetic and tumor virus susceptibility studies. Blood 1970; 36:341.

298. Stein AC, Blanck DM, Bennett AJ, et al: Acute myelomonocytic leukemia in a patient with Fanconi's anemia. J Oral Surg 1981; 39:624.

299. Gyger M, Bonny Y, Forest L: Childhood monosomy 7 syndrome. Am J Hematol 1982; 13:329.

300. Dosik H, Verma RS, Wilson C, et al: Fanconi's anemia and a familial stable chromosome abnormality in a family with multiple malignancies. Blood 1977; 50:190a.

301. Kunze J: Estren-Dameshek-Anämie mit myelomonocytärer Leukämie (Subtyp der Fanconi-Anämie?). In:Spranger J,

Tolksdorf M (eds): Klinische Genetik in der Pädiatrie. Stuttgart, Georg Thieme, 1980, p 213.

302. Bourgeois CA, Hill FGH: Fanconi anemia leading to acute myelomonocytic leukemia. Cytogenetic studies. Cancer 1977; 39:1163.

303. Alimena G, Avvisati G, De Cuia MR, et al: Retrospective diagnosis of a Fanconi's anemia patient by dyepoxybutane (DEB) test results in parents. Haematologica 1983; 68:97.

304. Kwee ML, Poll EHA, van de Kamp JJP, et al: Unusual response to bifunctional alkylating agents in a case of Fanconi anaemia. Hum Genet 1983; 64:384.

305. Roozendaal KJ, Nelis KOAH: Leukaemia in a case of Fanconi's anaemia. Clin Genet 1981; 25:208.

306. Ortega M, Caballin MR, Ortega JJ, et al: Follow-up by cytogenetic and fluorescence in situ hybridization analysis of allogeneic bone marrow transplantation in two children with Fanconi's anaemia in transformation. Br J Haematol 2000; 111:329.

307. Ferti A, Panani A, Dervenoulas J, et al: Cytogenetic findings in a Fanconi anemia patient with AML. Cancer Genet Cytogenet 1996; 90:182.

308. Sasaki MS: Fanconi's anemia. A condition possibly associated with a defective DNA repair. In Fox CF (ed): DNA Repair Mechanisms. New York, Academic Press, 1978, Vol 9, p 675.

309. Meddeb B, Azzouz MM, Hafsia R, et al: Transformation en leucemie aigue de l'anemia de Fanconi: A propos de 2 cas dans une serie de 21 malades. Tunis Med 1986; 64:755.

310. Ahuja HG, Advani SH, Gopal R, et al: Acute nonlymphoblastic leukemia in the first of three siblings affected with Fanconi's syndrome. Am J Pediatr Hematol Oncol 1986; 8:347.

311. Gasteama J, Giralt M, Orue MT, et al: Fanconi's anemia. Clinical study of six cases. Am J Pediatr Hematol Oncol 1986; 8:173.

312. Stivrins TJ, Davis RB, Sanger W, et al: Transformation of Fanconi's anemia to acute nonlymphocytic leukemia associated with emergence of monosomy 7. Blood 1984; 64:173.

313. Prindull G, Jentsch E, Hansmann I: Fanconi's anaemia developing erythroleukaemia. Scand J Haematol 1979; 23:59.

314. Villegas A, Aboin J, Alvarez-Sala JL, et al: Eritroleucemia en la evolucion de una anemia constitucional de Fanconi. Sangre 1983; 28:225.

315. Rotzak R, Kaplinsky N, Chaki R, et al: Giant marker chromosome in Fanconi's anemia transforming into erythroleukemia in an adult. Acta Haematol 1982; 67:214.

316. Berger R, Bernheim A, Le Coniat M, et al: Chromosomal studies of leukemic and preleukemic Fanconi's anemia patients. Examples of acquired 'chromosomal amplification.' Hum Genet 1980; 56:59.

317. Dharmasena F, Catchpole M, Erber W, et al: Megakaryoblastic leukaemia and myelofibrosis complicating Fanconi anaemia. Scand J Haematol 1986; 36:309.

318. Athale UH, Rao SR, Kadam PR, et al: Fanconi's anemia: A clinico-hematological and cytogenetic study. Indian Pediatr 1992; 28:1003.

319. Macdougall LG, Greeff MC, Rosendorff J, et al: Fanconi anemia in Black African children. Am J Med Genet 1990; 36:408.

320. Russo CL, Zwerdling T: Letter to the editor: Recognition of Fanconi's anemia eight years following treatment for acute nonlymphoblastic leukemia. Am J Hematol 1992; 40:78.

321. Shahid MJ, Khouri FP, Ballas SK: Fanconi's anaemia: Report of a patient with significant chromosomal abnormalities in bone marrow cells. J Med Genet 1972; 9:474.

322. Touraine RL, Bertrand Y, Foray P, et al: Hepatic tumours during androgen therapy in Fanconi aneaemia. Eur J Pediatr 1993; 152:691.

323. Esmer Sanchez MC, Carnevale Cantoni A, Molina Alvarez B, et al: Clinical and cytogenetic variability in 12 Mexican families with Fanconi's anemia and its relationship with complementation group assignment. Rev Invest Clin 1999; 51:273.

324. Hows JM, Chapple M, Marsh JCW, et al: Bone marrow transplantation for Fanconi's anaemia: The Hammersmith experience 1977–89. Bone Marrow Transplant 1989; 4:629.

325. Hows JM: Unrelated donor bone marrow transplantation for severe aplastic anaemia and Fanconi's anaemia. Bone Marrow Transplant 1989; 4(Suppl 4):126.

326. Bessho F, Mizutani S, Hayashi Y, et al: Chronic myelomonocytic leukemia with chromosomal changes involving 1p36 and hepatocellular carcinoma in a case of Fanconi's anemia. Eur J Haematol 1989; 42:492.

327. Gingrich RD, Ginder GD, Goeken NE, et al: Allogeneic marrow grafting with partially mismatched, unrelated marrow donors. Blood 1988; 71:1375.

328. Alter BP, Caruso JP, Drachtman RA, et al: Fanconi's anemia: Myelodysplasia as a predictor of outcome. Cancer Genet Cytogenet 2000; 117:125.

329. Bennett JM, Catovsky D, Daniel MT, et al: Proposals for the classification of the myelodysplastic syndromes. Br J Haematol 1982; 51:189.

330. Greenberg P, Cox C, LeBeau M, et al: International scoring system for evaluating prognosis in myelodysplastic syndromes. Blood 1997; 89:2079.

331. Alter BP: Fanconi's anemia and malignancies. Am J Hematol 1996; 53:99.

332. Thurston VC, Ceperich TM, Vance GH, et al: Detection of monosomy 7 in bone marrow by fluorescence in situ hybridization. A study of Fanconi anemia patients and review of the literature. Cancer Genet Cytogenet 1999; 109:154.

333. Venkatraj VS, Gaidano G, Auerbach AD: Clonality studies and N-ras and p53 mutation analysis of hematopoietic cells in Fanconi anemia. Leukemia 1994; 8:1354.

334. Baron F, Sybert VP, Andrews RG: Cutaneous and extracutaneous neutrophilic infiltrates (Sweet syndrome) in three patients with Fanconi anemia. J Pediatr 1989; 115:726.

335. Ries LAG, Kosary CL, Hankey BF, et al: SEER Cancer Statistics Review, 1973–1996. Bethesda, MD, National Cancer Institute, 1999.

336. Nara N, Miyamoto T, Kurisu A, et al: Two siblings with Fanconi's anemia developing squamous cell carcinomas. Rinshou Ketsueki 1980; 21:1944.

337. McDonough ER: Fanconi anemia syndrome. Arch Otolaryngol 1970; 92:284.

338. Swift M, Zimmerman D, McDonough ER: Squamous cell carcinomas in Fanconi's anemia. JAMA 1971; 216:325.

339. Kozarek RA, Sanowski RA: Carcinoma of the esophagus associated with Fanconi's anemia. J Clin Gastroenterol 1981; 3:171.

340. Vaitiekaitis AS, Grau WH: Squamous cell carcinoma of the mandible in Fanconi anemia: Report of case. J Oral Surg 1980; 38:372.

341. Schofield IDF, Worth AT: Malignant mucosal change in Fanconi's anemia. J Oral Surg 1980; 38:619.

342. Kennedy AW, Hart WR: Multiple squamous-cell carcinomas in Fanconi's anemia. Cancer 1982; 50:811.

343. Helmerhorst FM, Heaton DC, Crossen PE, et al: Familial thrombocytopenia associated with platelet autoantibodies and chromosome breakage. Hum Genet 1984; 65:252.

344. Kaplan MJ, Sabio H, Wanebo HJ, et al: Squamous cell carcinoma in the immunosuppressed patient: Fanconi's anemia. Laryngoscope 1985; 95:771.

345. Fukuoka K, Nishikawa K, Mizumoto Y, et al: Fanconi's anemia with squamous cell carcinoma—A case report and a review of literature. Jpn J Clin Hematol 1989; 30:1992.

346. Snow DG, Campbell JB, Smallman LA: Fanconi's anaemia and post-cricoid carcinoma. J Laryngol Otol 1991; 105:125.

347. Lustig JP, Lugassy G, Neder A, et al: Head and neck carcinoma in Fanconi's anaemia—Report of a case and review of the literature. Eur J Cancer 1995; 31B:68.

348. Halvorson DJ, McKie V, McKie K, et al: Sickle cell disease and tonsillectomy. Arch Otolaryngol Head Neck Surg 1997; 123:689.

349. Hirschman RJ, Schulman NR, Abuelo JG, et al: Chromosomal aberrations in two cases of inherited aplastic anemia with unusual clinical features. Ann Intern Med 1969; 71:107.

350. Guy JT, Auslander MO: Androgenic steroids and hepatocellular carcinoma. Lancet 1973; 1:148.

351. Reed K, Ravikumar TS, Gifford RRM, et al: The association of Fanconi's anemia and squamous cell carcinoma. Cancer 1983; 52:926.

352. Kozhevnikov BA, Khodorenko CA: Cancer of the mucous membrane of the left side of the mouth associated with congenital hypoplastic Fanconi's anemia in a 14-year-old boy. Vestn Khir 1986; 136:105.

353. Doerr TD, Shibuya TY, Marks SC: Squamous cell carcinoma of the supraglottic larynx in a patient with Fanconi's anemia. Otolaryngol Head Neck Surg 1998; 118:523.

354. Esparza A, Thompson WR: Familial hypoplastic anemia with multiple congenital anomalies (Fanconi's syndrome)—Report of three cases. RI Med J 1966; 49:103.

355. Aho S: Clinical conferences. Case of Fanconi's anemia. Kyobu Geka 1980; 33:397.

356. Rockelein G, Ulmer R, Kniewald A, et al: Osophaguskarzinom bei Fanconi-syndrom. Pathologe 1986; 7:343.

357. Linares M, Pastor E, Gomez A, et al: Hepatocellular carcinoma and squamous cell carcinoma in a patient with Fanconi's anemia. Ann Hematol 1991; 63:54.

358. Soravia C, Spilipoulos A: Carcinome épidermode de l'oesophage et anémie de Fanconi. Schweiz Med Wochenschr 1994; 124:725.

359. Goluchova M, Urban O, Chalupa J: Spinocellular carcinoma in a patient with Fanconi's anemia. Vnitr Lek 1998; 44:280.

360. Gendal ES, Mendelson DS, Janus CL, et al: Squamous cell carcinoma of the esophagus in Fanconi's anemia. Dysphagia 1988; 2:178.

361. Sicular A, Fleshner PR, Cohen LB, et al: Fanconi's anemia and esophageal carcinoma. Gullet 1993; 3:60.

362. Hersey P, Edwards A, Lewis R, et al: Deficient natural killer cell activity in a patient with Fanconi's anaemia and squamous cell carcinoma. Association with defect in interferon release. Clin Exp Immunol 1982; 48:205.

363. Arnold WJ, King CR, Magrina J, et al: Squamous cell carcinoma of the vulva and Fanconi anemia. Int J Gynaecol Obstet 1980; 18:395.

364. Ortonne JP, Jeune R, Coiffet J, et al: Squamous cell carcinomas in Fanconi's anemia. Arch Dermatol 1981; 117:443.

365. Wilkinson EJ, Morgan LS, Friedrich EG, Jr: Association of Fanconi's anemia and squamous-cell carcinoma of the lower female genital tract with condyloma acuminatum. A report of two cases. J Reprod Med 1984; 29:447.

366. Lebbé C, Pinquier L, Rybojad M, et al: Fanconi's anaemia associated with multicentric Bowen's disease and decreased NK cytotoxicity. Br J Dermatol 1993; 129:615.

367. de Chadarevian J-P, Vekemans M, Bernstein M: Fanconi's anemia, medulloblastoma, Wilms' tumor, horseshoe kidney, and gonadal dysgenesis. Arch Pathol Lab Med 1985; 109:367.

368. Puligandla B, Stass SA, Schumacher HR, et al: Terminal deoxynucleotidyl transferase in Fanconi's anaemia. Lancet 1978; 2:1263.

369. Dosik H, Steier W, Lubiniecki A: Inherited aplastic anaemia with increased endoreduplications: A new syndrome or Fanconi's anaemia variant? Br J Haematol 1979; 41:77.

370. Jacobs P, Karabus C: Fanconi's anemia. A family study with 20-year follow-up including associated breast pathology. Cancer 1984; 54:1850.

371. Zatterale A, Calzone R, Renda S, et al: Identification and treatment of late onset Fanconi's anemia. Haematologica 1995; 80:535.

372. van Niekerk CH, Jordaan C, Badenhorst PN: Pancytopenia secondary to primary malignant lymphoma of bone marrow as the first hematologic manifestation of the Estren-Dameshek variant of Fanconi's anemia. Am J Pediatr Hematol Oncol 1987; 9:344.

373. Goldsby RE, Perkins SL, Virshup DM, et al: Lymphoblastic lymphoma and excessive toxicity from chemotherapy: An unusual presentation for Fanconi anemia. J Pediatr Hematol Oncol 1999; 21:240.

374. Hill LS, Dennis PM, Fairham SA: Adenocarcinoma of the stomach and Fanconi's anaemia. Postgrad Med J 1981; 57:404.

375. Puig S, Ferrando J, Cervantes F, et al: Fanconi's anemia with cutaneous amyloidosis. Arch Dermatol 1993; 129:788.

376. Carbone P, Barbata G, Mirto S, et al: Inherited aplastic anemia with abnormal clones in bone marrow and increased endoreduplication in peripheral lymphocytes. Cancer Genet Cytogenet 1984; 13:259.

377. Ariffin H, Ariffin WA, Chan LI, et al: Wilms' tumour and Fanconi anaemia: An unusual association. J Paediatr Child Health 2000; 36:196.

378. Levinson S, Vincent KA: Multifocal osteosarcoma in a patient with Fanconi anemia. J Pediatr Hematol Oncol 1997; 19:251.

379. Mulvihill JJ, Ridolfi RL, Schultz FR, et al: Hepatic adenoma in Fanconi anemia treated with oxymetholone. J Pediatr 1975; 87:122.

380. Corberand J, Pris J, Dutau G, et al: Association d'une maladie de Fanconi et d'une tumeur hepatique. Chez une malade soumise a un traitement androgenique au long cours. Arch Fr Pediatr 1975; 32:275.

381. Resnick MB, Kozakewich HPW, Perez-Atayde AR: Hepatic adenoma in the pediatric age group. Clinicopathological observations and assessment of cell proliferative activity. Am J Surg Pathol 1995; 19:1181.

382. Schmidt E, Deeg HJ, Storb R: Regression of androgen-related hepatic tumors in patients with Fanconi's anemia following marrow transplantation. Transplantation 1984; 37:452.

383. Garel L, Kalifa G, Buriot D, et al: Multiple adenomas of the liver and Fanconi's anaemia. Ann Radiol 1980; 24:53.

384. Farrell GC: Fanconi's familial hypoplastic anaemia with some unusual features. Med J Aust 1976; 1:116.

385. Chandra RS, Kapur SP, Kelleher J, et al: Benign hepatocellular tumors in the young. A clinicopathologic spectrum. Arch Pathol Lab Med 1984; 108:168.

386. LeBrun DP, Silver MM, Freedman MH, et al: Fibrolamellar carcinoma of the liver in a patient with Fanconi anemia. Hum Pathol 1991; 22:396.

387. Ortega JJ, Olive T, Sanchez C, et al: Bone marrow transplant in Fanconi's anemia. Results in five patients. Sangre 1990; 35:433.

388. Mokrohisky ST, Ambruso DR, Hathaway WE: Fulminant hepatic neoplasia after androgen therapy. N Engl J Med 1977; 296:1411.

389. Cattan D, Kalifat R, Wautier J-L, et al: Maladie de Fanconi et cancer du foie. Arch Fr Mal App Dig 1974; 63:41.

390. Abbondanzo SL, Manz HJ, Klappenbach RS, et al: Hepatocellular carcinoma in an 11-year-old girl with Fanconi's anemia. Report of a case and review of the literature. Am J Pediatr Hematol Oncol 1986; 8:334.

391. Shapiro P, Ikeda RM, Ruebner BH, et al: Multiple hepatic tumors and peliosis hepatis in Fanconi's anemia treated with androgens. Am J Dis Child 1977; 131:1104.

392. Johnson FL, Feagler JR, Lerner KG, et al: Association of androgenic-anabolic steroid therapy with development of hepatocellular carcinoma. Lancet 1972; 2:1273.

393. Kew MC, Van Coller B, Prowse CM, et al: Occurrence of primary hepatocellular cancer and peliosis hepatis after treatment with androgenic steroids. S Afr Med J 1976; 50:1233.

394. Moldvay J, Schaff Z, Lapis K: Hepatocellular carcinoma in Fanconi's anemia treated with androgen and corticosteroid. Zentralbl Pathol 1991; 137:167.

395. Recant L, Lacy P: Fanconi's anemia and hepatic cirrhosis. Am J Med 1965; 39:464.

396. Cap J, Ondrus B, Danihel L: Focal nodular hyperplasia of the liver and hepatocellular carcinoma in children with Fanconi's anemia after long-term treatment with androgens. Bratisl Lek Listy 1983; 79:73.

397. Port RB, Petasnick JP, Ranniger K: Angiographic demonstration of hepatoma in association with Fanconi's anemia. Am J Roentgenol 1971; 113:82.

398. Bernstein MS, Hunter RL, Yachnin S: Hepatoma and peliosis hepatis developing in a patient with Fanconi's anemia. N Engl J Med 1971; 284:1135.

399. Bagheri SA, Boyer JL: Peliosis hepatis associated with androgenic-anabolic steroid therapy. A severe form of hepatic injury. Ann Intern Med 1974; 81:610.

400. Holder LE, Gnarra DJ, Lampkin BC, et al: Hepatoma associated with anabolic steroid therapy. Am J Roentgenol 1975; 124:638.

401. Sweeney EC, Evans DJ: Hepatic lesions in patients treated with synthetic anabolic steroids. J Clin Pathol 1976; 29:626.

402. Evans DIK: Aplastic anaemia in childhood. In Geary CG (ed): Aplastic Anaemia. London, Bailliere Tindall, 1979, p 161.

403. Bradford CR, Hoffman HT, Wolf GT, et al: Squamous carcinoma of the head and neck in organ transplant recipients: Possible role of oncogenic viruses. Laryngoscope 1990; 100:190.

404. Millen FJ, Rainey MG, Hows JM, et al: Oral squamous cell carcinoma after allogeneic bone marrow transplantation for Fanconi anaemia. Br J Haematol 1997; 99:410.

405. Jansisyanont P, Pazoki A, Ord RA: Squamous cell carcinoma of the tongue after bone marrow transplantation in a patient with Fanconi's anemia. J Oral Maxillofac Surg 2000; 58:1454.

406. Socie G, Henry-Amar M, Cosset JM, et al: Increased incidence of solid malignant tumors after bone marrow transplantation for severe aplastic anemia. Blood 1991; 78:277.

407. Pierga JY, Socie G, Gluckman E, et al: Secondary solid malignant tumors occurring after bone marrow transplantation for severe aplastic anemia given thoraco-abdominal irradiation. Radiother Oncol 1994; 30:55.

408. Murayama S, Manzo RP, Kirkpatrick DV, et al: Squamous cell carcinoma of the tongue associated with Fanconi's anemia: MR characteristics. Pediatr Radiol 1990; 20:347.

409. Smith CH: The anemias of early infancy. Pathogenesis and diagnosis. J Pediatr 1940; 16:375.

410. Somers GR, Tabrizi SN, Tiedemann K, et al: Squamous cell carcinoma of the tongue in a child with Fanconi anemia: A case report and review of the literature. Pediatr Pathol Lab Med 1994; 15:597.

411. Kolb H, Socie J, Duell G, et al for the Late Effects Working Party: Malignant neoplasms in long-term survivors of bone marrow transplantation. Ann Intern Med 1999; 131:738.

412. Socie G, Devergie A, Girinski T, et al: Transplantation for Fanconi's anaemia: Long-term follow-up of fifty patients transplanted from a sibling donor after low-dose cyclophosphamide and thoraco-abdominal irradiation for conditioning. Br J Haematol 1998; 103:249.

413. Drachtman RA, Alter BP: Dyskeratosis congenita: Clinical and genetic heterogeneity. Report of a new case and review of the literature. Am J Pediatr Hematol Oncol 1992; 14:297.

414. Drachtman RA, Alter BP: Dyskeratosis congenita. Dermatol Clin 1995; 13:33.

415. Dokal I: Dyskeratosis congenita in all its forms. Br J Haematol 2000; 110:768.

416. Connor JM, Gatherer D, Gray FC, et al: Assignment of the gene for dyskeratosis congenita to Xq28. Hum Genet 1986; 72:348.

417. Cole HN, Cole HN Jr, Lascheid WP: Dyskeratosis congenita. Arch Dermatol 1957; 76:712.

418. Addison M, Rice MS: The association of dyskeratosis congenita and Fanconi's anaemia. Med J Aust 1965; 1:797.

419. Krantz SB, Zaentz SD: Pure red cell aplasia. In Gordon AS, Silber R, LoBue J (eds): The Year in Hematology. New York, Plenum Press, 1977, p 153.

420. Wasylyszyn J, Kryst L, Langner A: Dyskeratosis congenita (Zinsser-Engman-Cole). Przegl Dermatol 1974; 61:687.

421. Camacho F, Moreno JC, Conejo-Mir JS, et al: Sindrome de Zinsser-Cole-Engman: Disqueratosis congenita. Med Cutan Ibero Lat Am 1982; 10:365.

422. Misawa S, Haku Y, Ifuku H, et al: Pancytopenia. Dyskeratosis congenita. A case report of dyskeratosis congenita with pancytopenia in special reference to hemopoietic stem cells. Rinsho Ketsueki 1982; 23:1222.

423. Schmidt JB, Gebhart W: Zinsser-Engman-Cole-Syndrom. Hautarzt 1983; 34:286.

424. Anil S, Beena VT, Raji MA, et al: Oral squamous cell carcinoma in a case of dyskeratosis congenita. Ann Dent 1994; 53:15.

425. Limmer RL, Zurowski SM, Swinfard RW, et al: Abnormal nails in a patient with severe anemia. Arch Derm 1997; 133:97.

426. Lespinasse J, Bourrain JL, Blanc M: Dyskeratose congenitale ou dyskeratose de Zinsser-Cole-Engman. Un cas feminin probable. Presse Med 1988; 17:1047.

427. Moretti S, Spallanzani A, Chiarugi A, et al: Oral carcinoma in a young man: A case of dyskeratosis congenita. J Eur Acad Dermatol Venereol 2000; 14:123.

428. Hyodo M, Sadamoto A, Hinohira Y, et al: Tongue cancer as a complication of dyskeratosis congenita in a woman. Am J Otolaryngol 1999; 20:405.

429. Garb J: Dyskeratosis congenita with pigmentation, dystrophia unguium, and leukoplakia oris. A follow-up report of two brothers. Arch Dermatol 1958; 77:704.

430. Cannell H: Dyskeratosis congenita. Br J Oral Surg 1971; 9:8.

431. Kubicz J: Syndroma Zinsser-Engman-Cole cum dyschromia extensiva corporis. Pezegl Dermatol 1970; 57:239.

432. Schroeder TM, Hofbauer M: Letter: Dyskeratosis congenita Zinsser-Cole-Engman form with abnormal karyotype. Dermatologica 1975; 151:316.

433. Jacobs P, Saxe N, Gordon W, et al: Dyskeratosis congenita. Haematologic, cytogenetic, and dermatologic studies. Scand J Haematol 1984; 32:461.

434. Lin TC, Lin CK, Lee JY, et al: X-linked dyskeratosis congenita with aplastic anemia: Genetic and hematologic studies. Chin Med J 1989; 43:57.

435. Kawaguchi K, Sakamaki H, Onozawa Y, et al: Dyskeratosis congenita (Zinsser-Cole-Engman syndrome). An autopsy case presenting with rectal carcinoma, non-cirrhotic hypertension, and *Pneumocystis carinii* pneumonia. Virchows Archiv A Pathol Anat 1990; 417:247.

436. Dokal I, Bungey J, Williamson P, et al: Dyskeratosis congenita fibroblasts are abnormal and have unbalanced chromosomal rearrangements. Blood 1992; 80:3090.

437. Marsh JCW, Will AJ, Hows JM, et al: "Stem cell" origin of the hematopoietic defect in dyskeratosis congenita. Blood 1992; 79:3138.

438. Chatura KR, Nadar S, Pulimood S, et al: Gastric carcinoma as a complication of dyskeratosis congenita in an adolescent boy. Digest Dis Sci 1996; 41:2340.

439. Herman TE, McAlister WH: Dyskeratosis congenita. Pediatr Radiol 1997; 27:286.

440. Baselga E, Drolet BA, van Tuinen P, et al: Dyskeratosis congenita with linear areas of severe cutaneous involvement. Am J Med Genet 1998; 75:492.

441. Auerbach AD, Lieblich LM, Ehrenbard L, et al: Dyskeratosis congenita: Cytogenetic studies in a family with an unusual pattern of inheritance. Am J Hum Genet 1979; 31:87A.

442. Costello MJ: Dyskeratosis congenita with superimposed prickle-cell epithelioma on the dorsal aspect of the left hand. Arch Dermatol 1957; 75:451.

443. Auerbach AD, Adler B, Chaganti RSK: Prenatal and postnatal diagnosis and carrier detection of Fanconi anemia by a cytogenetic method. Pediatrics 1981; 67:128.

444. Kopysc Z, Jankowska-Skrzypek A, Bielniak J, et al: Zinsser-Engman-Cole syndrome (dyskeratosis congenita) in a 13-year-old boy. Wiad Lek 1988; 41:525.

445. Langston AA, Sanders JE, Deeg HJ, et al: Allogeneic marrow transplantation for aplastic anaemia associated with dyskeratosis congenita. Br J Haematol 1996; 92:758.

446. Connor JM, Teague RH: Dyskeratosis congenita. Report of a large kindred. Br J Dermatol 1981; 105:321.

447. Baykal C, Buyukbabani N, Kavak A: Dyskeratosis congenita associated with Hodgkin's disease. Eur J Dermatol 1998; 8:385.

448. Morrison D, Rose EL, Smith AP, et al: Dyskeratosis congenita and nasopharyngeal atresia. J Laryngol Otol 1992; 106:996.

449. Vanbiervliet P, Blockmans D, Bobbaers H: Dyskeratosis congenita and associated interstitial lung disease; a case report. Acta Clin Belg 1998; 53:198.

450. Sorrow JM Jr, Hitch JM: Dyskeratosis congenita. Arch Dermatol 1963; 88:340.

451. Reichel M, Grix AC, Isseroff RR: Dyskeratosis congenita associated with elevated fetal hemoglobin, X-linked ocular albinism, and juvenile-onset diabetes mellitus. Pediatr Dermatol 1992; 9:103.

452. Ortega JA, Swanson VL, Landing BH, et al: Congenital dyskeratosis. Zinsser-Engman-Cole syndrome with thymic dysplasia and aplastic anemia. Am J Dis Child 1972; 124:701.

453. Phillips RJ, Judge M, Webb D, et al: Dyskeratosis congenita: Delay in diagnosis and successful treatment of pancytopenia by bone marrow transplantation. Br J Dermatol 1992; 127:278.

454. Putterman C, Safadi R, Zlotogora J, et al: Treatment of the hematological manifestations of dyskeratosis congenita. Ann Hematol 1993; 66:209.

455. Forni G, Melevendi C, Jappelli S, et al: Dyskeratosis congenita: Unusual presenting features within a kindred. Pediatr Hematol Oncol 1993; 10:145.

456. Pritchard SL, Junker AK: Positive response to granulocyte-colony-stimulating factor in dyskeratosis congenita before matched unrelated bone marrow transplantation. Am J Pediatr Hematol Oncol 1994; 16:186.

457. Oehler L, Reiter E, Friedl J, et al: Effective stimulation of neutropoiesis with rh G-CSF in dyskeratosis congenita: A case report. Ann Hematol 1994; 69:325.

458. Kehrer H, Krone W, Schindler D, et al: Cytogenetic studies of skin fibroblast cultures from a karyotypically normal female with dyskeratosis congenita. Clin Genet 1992; 41:129.

459. Kajtar P, Mehes K: Bilateral Coats retinopathy associated with aplastic anaemia and mild dyskeratotic signs. Am J Med Genet 1994; 49:374.

460. Kehrer H, Krone W: Letter to the editor: Chromosome abnormalities in cell cultures derived from the leukoplakia of a female patient with dyskeratosis congenita. Am J Med Genet 1992; 42:217.

461. Carter DM, Pan M, Gaynor A, et al: Psoralen-DNA cross-linking photoadducts in dyskeratosis congenita: Delay in excision and promotion of sister chromatid exchange. J Invest Dermatol 1979; 73:97.

462. Arngrimsson R, Dokal I, Luzzatto L, et al: Dyskeratosis congenita: Three additional families show linkage to a locus in Xq28. J Med Genet 1993; 30:618.

463. Mann WR, Venkatraj VS, Carter DM, et al: Use of a polymorphic DNA probe for diagnosis of dyskeratosis congenita. Clin Res 1990; 38:627A.

464. Dokal I, Luzzatto L: Dyskeratosis congenita is a chromosomal instability disorder. Leuk Lymphoma 1994; 15:1.

465. Pai GS, Yan Y, DeBauche DM, et al: Bleomycin hypersensitivity in dyskeratosis congenita fibroblasts, lymphocytes, and transformed lymphoblasts. Cytogenet Cell Genet 1989; 52:186.

466. DeBauche DM, Pai GS, Stanley WS: Enhanced G2 chromatid radiosensitivity in dyskeratosis congenita fibroblasts. Am J Hum Genet 1990; 46:350.

467. Ning Y, Yongshan Y, Pai GS, et al: Heterozygote detection through bleomycin-induced G2 chromatid breakage in dyskeratosis congenita families. Cancer Genet Cytogenet 1992; 60:31.

468. Navarro JT, Ribera JM, Milla F, et al: Hipoplasia medular asociada a disqueratosis congenita. Sangre 1994; 39:207.

469. Michalevicz R, Baron S, Nordan U, et al: Granulocytic macrophage colony stimulating factor restores in vitro growth of granulocyte-macrophage bone marrow hematopoietic progenitors in dyskeratosis congenita. Isr J Med Sci 1989; 25:193.

470. Georgouras K: Dyskeratosis congenita. Aust J Dermatol 1965; 8:36.

471. Knight SW, Vulliamy T, Forni GL, et al: Fine mapping of the dyskeratosis congenita locus in Xq28. J Med Genet 1996; 33:993.

472. Knight SW, Vulliamy TJ, Heiss NS, et al: 1.4 Mb candidate gene region for X linked dyskeratosis congenita defined by combined haplotype and X chromosome inactivation analysis. J Med Genet 1998; 35:993.

473. Heiss NS, Knight SW, Vulliamy TJ, et al: X-linked dyskeratosis congenita is caused by mutations in a highly conserved gene with putative nucleolar functions. Nat Genet 1998; 19:32.

474. Hassock S, Vetrie D, Giannelli F: Mapping and characterization of the X-linked dyskeratosis congenita (DKC) gene. Genomics 1999; 55:21.

475. Marciniak R, Guarente L: Testing telomerase. Nature 2001; 413:370.

476. Vulliamy T, Marrone A, et al. The RNA component of telomerase is mutated in autosomal dominant dyskeratosis congenita. Nature 2001; 413:432.

477. Knight SW, Heiss NS, Vulliamy TJ, et al: X-linked dyskeratosis congenita is predominantly caused by missense mutations in the DKC1 gene. Am J Hum Genet 1999; 65:50.

478. Vulliamy TJ, Knight SW, Heiss NS: Dyskeratosis congenita caused by a 3′ deletion: Germline and somatic mosaicism in a female carrier. Blood 1999; 94:1254.

479. Heiss NS, Bachner D, Salowsky R, et al: Gene structure and expression of the mouse dyskeratosis congenita gene, Dkc1. Genomics 2000; 67:153.

480. Mitchell JR, Wood E, Collins K: A telomerase component is defective in the human disease dyskeratosis congenita. Nature 1999; 402:551.

481. Vulliamy TJ, Knight SW, Mason PJ, et al: Very short telomeres in the peripheral blood of patients with X-linked and autosomal dyskeratosis congenita. Blood Cells Mol Dis 2001; 27:353.

482. Knight SW, Heiss NS, Vulliamy TJ, et al: Unexplained aplastic anaemia, immunodeficiency, and cerebellar hypoplasia (Hoyeraal-Hreidarsson syndrome) due to mutations in the dyskeratosis gene, DKC1. Br J Haematol 1999; 107:335.

483. Yaghmai R, Kimyai-Asadi A, Rostamiani K, et al: Overlap of dyskeratosis congenita with the Hoyeraal-Hreidarsson syndrome. J Pediatr 2000; 136:390.

484. Alter BP: Molecular medicine and bone marrow failure syndromes. J Pediatr 2000; 136:275.

485. Lemarchand-Venencie F, Gluckman E, Devergie A, et al: Syndrome de Zinsser-Cole-Engmann. Ann Dermatol Venereol 1982; 109:783.

486. Mahmoud HK, Schaefer UW, Schmidt CG, et al: Marrow transplantation for pancytopenia in dyskeratosis congenita. Blut 1985; 51:57.

487. Berthou C, Devergie A, D'Agay MF, et al: Late vascular complications after bone marrow transplantation for dyskeratosis congenita. Br J Haematol 1991; 79:335.

488. Chessells JM, Harper J: Bone marrow transplantation for dyskeratosis congenita. Br J Haematol 1992; 81:314.

489. Storb R, Etzioni R, Anasetti C, et al: Cyclophosphamide combined with antithymocyte globulin in preparation for allogeneic marrow transplants in patients with aplastic anemia. Blood 1994; 84:941.

490. Ivker RA, Woosley J, Resnick SD: Dyskeratosis congenita or chronic graft-versus-host disease? A diagnostic dilemma in a child eight years after bone marrow transplantation for aplastic anemia. Pediatr Dermatol 1993; 10:362.

491. Yabe M, Yabe H, Hattori K, et al: Fatal interstitial pulmonary disease in a patient with dyskeratosis congenita after allogeneic bone marrow transplantation. Bone Marrow Transplant 1997; 19:389.

492. Rocha V, Devergie A, Socie G, et al: Unusual complications after bone marrow transplantation for dyskeratosis congenita. Br J Haematol 1998; 103:243.

493. West CM, Ogden AK, Minniti C, et al: Unrelated placental/umbilical cord blood cell transplantation for dyskeratosis congenita. Pediatr Res 1999; 45:154A.

494. Ling NS, Fenske NA, Julius RL, et al: Dyskeratosis congenita in a girl simulating chronic graft-vs-host disease. Arch Dermatol 1985; 121:1424.

495. Conter V, Johnson FL, Paolucci P, et al: Bone marrow transplantation for aplastic anemia associated with dyskeratosis congenita. Am J Pediatr Hematol Oncol 1988; 10:99.

496. Lau YL, Ha SY, Chan CF, et al: Bone marrow transplant for dyskeratosis congenita. Br J Haematol 1999; 105:567.

497. Ghavamzadeh A, Alimoghadam K, Nasseri P, et al: Correction of bone marrow failure in dyskeratosis congenita by bone marrow transplantation. Bone Marrow Transplant 1999; 23:299.

498. Russo CL, Glader BE, Israel RJ, et al: Treatment of neutropenia associated with dyskeratosis congenita with granulocyte-macrophage colony-stimulating factor. Lancet 1990; 336:751.

499. Yel L, Tezcan I, Sanal O, et al: Dyskeratosis congenita: Unusual onset with isolated neutropenia at an early age. Acta Paediatr Jpn 1996; 38:288.

500. Gillio AP, Gabrilove JL: Cytokine treatment of inherited bone marrow failure syndromes. Blood 1993; 81:1669.

501. Alter BP, Gardner FH, Hall RE: Treatment of dyskeratosis congenita with granulocyte colony-stimulating factor and erythropoietin. Br J Haematol 1997; 97:309.

502. Gazda H, Lipton JM, Niemeyer CM, et al: Evidence for linkage of familial Diamond-Blackfan anemia to chromosome 8923.2-23.1 and for non-19q non-8p disease. Blood 1999; 94:673a.

503. Tolmie JL, Browne BH, McGettrick PM, et al: A familial syndrome with Coats' reaction, retinal angiomas, hair and nail defects and intracranial calcification. Eye 1988; 2:297.

504. Revesz T, Fletcher S, al-Gazali LI, et al: Bilateral retinopathy, aplastic anaemia, and central nervous system abnormalities: A new syndrome? J Med Genet 1992; 29:673.

505. Berger W: Molecular dissection of Norrie disease. Acta Anat (Basel) 1998; 162:95.

506. Li FP, Potter NU, Buchanan GR, et al: A family with acute leukemia, hypoplastic anemia and cerebellar ataxia. Association with marrow chromosome C-monosomy. Am J Med 1978; 65:933.

507. Li FP, Hecht F, Kaiser-McCaw B, et al: Ataxia-pancytopenia: Syndrome of cerebellar ataxia, hypoplastic anemia, monosomy 7, and acute myelogenous leukemia. Cancer Genet Cytogenet 1981; 4:189.

508. Daghistani D, Curless R, Toledano SR, et al: Ataxia-pancytopenia and monosomy 7 syndrome. J Pediatr 1989; 115:108.

509. Mahmood F, King MD, Smyth OP, et al: Familial cerebellar hypoplasia and pancytopenia without chromosomal breakages. Neuropediatrics 1998; 29:302.

510. Gonzalez-Del Angel A, Cervera M, Gomez L, et al: Ataxia-pancytopenia syndrome. Am J Med Genet 2000; 90:252.

511. Akaboshi S, Yoshimura M, Hara T, et al: A case of Hoyeraal-Hreidarsson syndrome: Delayed myelination and hypoplasia of corpus callosum are other important signs. Neuropediatrics 2000; 31:141.

512. Revy P, Busslinger M, Tashiro K, et al: A syndrome involving intrauterine growth retardation, microcephaly, cerebellar hypoplasia, B lymphocyte deficiency, and progressive pancytopenia. Pediatrics 2000; 105:e39.

513. Shwachman H, Diamond LK, Oski FA, et al: The syndrome of pancreatic insufficiency and bone marrow dysfunction. J Pediatr 1964; 65:645.

514. Bodian M, Sheldon W, Lightwood R: Congenital hypoplasia of the exocrine pancreas. Acta Paediatr 1964; 53:282.

515. Aggett PJ, Cavanagh NPC, Matthew DJ, et al: Shwachman's syndrome. A review of 21 cases. Arch Dis Child 1980; 55:331.

516. Ginzberg H, Shin J, Ellis L, et al: Segregation analysis in Shwachman-Diamond syndrome: Evidence for recessive inheritance. Am J Hum Genet 2000; 66:1413.

517. Ozsoylu S, Argun G: Tryptic activity of the duodenal juice in aplastic anemia. J Pediatr 1967; 70:60.

518. Thong YH: Impaired neutrophil kinesis in a patient with the Shwachman-Diamond syndrome. Aust Paediatr J 1978; 14:34.

519. Aggett PJ, Harries JT, Harvey BAM, et al: An inherited defect of neutrophil mobility in Shwachman syndrome. J Pediatr 1979; 94:391.

520. Ruutu P, Savilahati E, Repo H, et al: Constant defect in neutrophil locomotion but with age decreasing susceptibility to infection in Shwachman syndrome. Br J Haematol 1984; 70:502.

521. Repo H, Savilahti E, Leirisalo-Repo M: Aberrant phagocyte function in Shwachman syndrome. Clin Exp Immunol 1987; 69:204.

522. Shwachman H, Holsclaw D: Some clinical observations on the Shwachman syndrome (pancreatic insufficiency and bone marrow hypoplasia). Birth Defects Orig Article Ser 1972; 8(3):46.

523. Ginzberg H, Shin J, Ellis L, et al: Shwachman syndrome: Phenotypic manifestations of sibling sets and isolated cases in a large patient cohort are similar. J Pediatr 1999; 135:81.

524. Hudson E, Aldor T: Pancreatic insufficiency and neutropenia with associated immunoglobulin deficit. Arch Intern Med 1970; 125:314.

525. Goobie S, Popovic M, Morrison J, et al: Shwachman-Diamond syndrome with exocrine pancreatic dysfunction and bone marrow failure maps to the centromeric region of chromosome 7. Am J Hum Genet 2001; 68:1048.

525a. Boocock GR, Morrison JA, Popovic M, et al: Mutations in SBDS are associated with Schwachman-Diamond syndrome. Nat Genet 2003;33:97.

526. Barrios NJ, Kirkpatrick DV: Successful cyclosporin A treatment of aplastic anaemia in Shwachman-Diamond syndrome. Br J Haematol 1990; 74:540.

527. Nezeloff Ch, Watchi M: L'hypoplasie congenitale lipomateuse du pancreas exocrine chez l'enfant (deux observations et revue de la litterature). Arch Fr Pediatr 1961; 18:1135.

528. Huijgens PC, Van der Veen EA, Meijer S, et al: Syndrome of Shwachman and leukaemia. Scand J Haematol 1977; 18:20.

529. Strevens MJ, Lilleyman JS, Williams RB: Shwachman's syndrome and acute lymphoblastic leukaemia. Br Med J 1978; 2:18.

530. Caselitz J, Klöppel G, Delling G, et al: Shwachman's syndrome and leukaemia. Virchows Arch A Pathol Anat Histolol 1979; 385:109.

531. Woods WG, Roloff JS, Lukens JN, et al: The occurrence of leukemia in patients with the Shwachman syndrome. J Pediatr 1981; 99:425.

532. Woods WG, Krivit W, Lubin BH, et al: Aplastic anemia associated with the Shwachman syndrome. In vivo and in vitro observations. Am J Pediatr Hematol Oncol 1981; 3:347.

533. Gretillat F, Delepine N, Taillard F, et al: Shwachman's syndrome transformed into leukaemia. Presse Med 1985; 14:45.

534. MacMaster SA, Cummings TM: Computed tomography and ultrasonography findings for an adult with Shwachman syndrome and pancreatic lipomatosis. Can Assoc Radiol J 1993; 44:301.

535. Passmore SJ, Hann IM, Stiller CA, et al: Pediatric myelodysplasia: A study of 68 children and a new prognostic scoring system. Blood 1995; 85:1742.

536. Smith OP, Chan MY, Evans J, et al: Shwachman-Diamond syndrome and matched unrelated donor BMT. Bone Marrow Transplant 1995; 16:717.

537. Laporte J Ph, Lesage S, Portnoi MF, et al: Successful immunoadoptive therapy (IT) after allogeneic transplantation (BMT) for early relapse of myelodysplastic syndrome (MDS) in a Shwachman's Diamond syndrome (SD) patient. Blood 1995; 86:954a.

538. Smith O, Hann IM, Chessells JM, et al: Haematological abnormalities in Shwachman-Diamond syndrome. Br J Haematol 1996; 94:279.

539. Arseniev L, Diedrich H, Link H: Allogeneic bone marrow transplantation in a patient with Shwachman-Diamond syndrome. Ann Hematol 1996; 72:83.

540. Dokal I, Rule S, Chen F, et al: Adult onset of acute myeloid leukaemia (M6) in patients with Shwachman-Diamond syndrome. Br J Haematol 1997; 99:171.

541. Cipolli M, D'Orazio C, Delmarco A, et al: Shwachman's syndrome: Pathomorphosis and long-term outcome. J Pediatr Gastroenterol Nutr 1999; 29:265.

542. Spirito FR, Crescenzi B, Matteucci C, et al: Cytogenetic characterization of acute myeloid leukemia in Shwachman's syndrome. A case report. Haematologica 2000; 85:1207.

543. Maserati E, Minelli A, Olivieri C, et al: Isochromosome (7)(q10) in Shwachman syndrome without MDS/AML and role of chromosome 7 anomalies in myeloproliferative disorders. Cancer Genet Cytogenet 2000; 121:167.

544. Kalra R, Dale D, Freedman M, et al: Monosomy 7 and activating RAS mutations accompany malignant transformation in patients with congenital neutropenia. Blood 1995; 86:4579.

545. Bordigoni P: Bone marrow transplantation for inherited bone marrow failure syndromes. Int J Pediatr Hematol Oncol 1995; 2:441.

546. Davies SM, Wagner JE, Defor T, et al: Unrelated donor bone marrow transplantation for children and adolescents with aplastic anaemia or myelodysplasia. Br J Haematol 1997; 96:749.

547. Okcu F, Roberts WM, Chan KW: Bone marrow transplantation in Shwachman-Diamond syndrome: Report of two cases and review of the literature. Bone Marrow Transplant 1998; 21:849.

548. Dror Y, Squire J, Durie P, et al: Malignant myeloid transformation with isochromosome 7q in Shwachman-Diamond syndrome. Leukemia 1998; 12:1591.

549. Faber J, Lauener R, Wick F, et al: Shwachman-Diamond syndrome: Early bone marrow transplantation in a high risk patient and new clues to pathogenesis. Eur J Pediatr 1999; 158:995.

550. Sokolic RA, Ferguson W, Mark HFL: Discordant detection of monosomy 7 by GTG-banding and FISH in a patient with Shwachman-Diamond syndrome without evidence of myelodysplastic syndrome or acute myelogenous leukemia. Cancer Genet Cytogenet 1999; 115:106.

551. Pratt N, Cunningham JJP, Sales M, et al: Do chromosome 7 abnormalities mandate bone marrow transplant in Shwachman-Diamond syndrome. J Med Genet 2000; 37(Suppl 1): S27.

552. Howard J, Dunlop A, Kelly J, et al: Isochromosome 7q in two children with Shwachman-Diamond syndrome. J Med Genet 2000; 37(Suppl 1):S35.

553. Tsai PH, Sahdev I, Herry A, et al: Fatal cyclophosphamide induced congestive heart failure in a 10-year-old boy with Shwachman-Diamond syndrome and severe bone marrow failure treated with allogeneic bone marrow transplantation. Am J Pediatr Hematol Oncol 1989; 12:472.

554. Barrios N, Kirkpatrick D, Regueira O, et al: Bone marrow transplant in Shwachman Diamond syndrome. Br J Haematol 1991; 79:337.

555. Seymour JF, Escudier SM: Acute leukemia complicating bone marrow hypoplasia in an adult with Shwachman's syndrome. Leuk Lymphoma 1993; 12:131.

556. Bunin N, Leahey A, Dunn S: Related donor liver transplant for veno-occlusive disease following T-depleted unrelated donor bone marrow transplantation. Transplantation 1996; 61:664.

557. Cesaro S, Guariso G, Calore E, et al: Successful unrelated bone marrow transplantation for Shwachman-Diamond syndrome. Bone Marrow Transplant 2001; 27:97.

558. Bonilla MA, Gilmore B, Gillio AP, et al: In vivo administration of recombinant human G-CSF corrects the neutropenia associated with Shwachman-Diamond syndrome. Blood 1989; 74:324a.

559. Adachi N, Tsuchiya H, Nunoi H, et al: rhG-CSF for Shwachman's syndrome. Lancet 1990; 336:1136.

560. Adachi N, Migita M, Ohta T, et al: Depressed natural killer cell activity due to decreased natural killer cell population in a vitamin E-deficient patient with Shwachman syndrome: Reversible natural killer cell abnormality by α-tocopherol supplementation. Eur J Pediatr 1997; 156:444.

561. Paley C, Murphy S, Karayalcin G, et al: Treatment of neutropenia in Shwachman Diamond syndrome (SDS) with recombinant human granulocyte colony stimulating factor (RH-GCSF). Blood 1991; 78:3a.

562. Skapek SX, Jones WS, Hoffman KM, et al: Sinusitis and bacteremia caused by *Flavobacterium meningosepticum* in a sixteen-year-old with Shwachman Diamond syndrome. Pediatr Infect Dis J 1992; 11:411.

563. Ventura A, Dragovich D, Luxardo P, et al: Human granulocyte colony-stimulating factor (rHuG-CSF) for treatment of neutropenia in Shwachman syndrome. Haematologia 1995; 80:227.

564. Grill J, Bernaudin F, Dresch C, et al: Traitement de la neutropenie du syndrome de Shwachman par le facteur de croissance des granuleux (G-CSF). Arch Fr Pediatr 1993; 50:331.

565. Bom EP, van der Sande FM, Tjon RT, et al: Shwachman syndrome: CT and MR diagnosis. J Comput Assist Tomogr 1993; 17:474.

566. van der Sande FM, Hillen HFP: Correction of neutropenia following treatment with granulocyte colony-stimulating factor results in a decreased frequency of infections in Shwachman's syndrome. Neth J Med 1996; 48:92.

567. Dror Y, Freedman MH: Shwachman-Diamond syndrome: An inherited preleukemic bone marrow failure disorder with aberrant hematopoietic progenitors and faulty marrow microenvironment. Blood 1999; 94:3048.

568. Ferguson L, Hoots K, Beran M, et al: Long-term bone marrow (BM) cultures with recombinant human granulocyte-macrophage colony stimulating factor (rhGM-CSF) in children with cytopenias: A correlation with clinical response. Blood 1988; 72:115a.

569. Lux SE, Johnston RB, Jr, August CS, et al: Chronic neutropenia and abnormal cellular immunity in cartilage-hair hypoplasia. N Engl J Med 1970; 282:231.

570. McKusick VA, Eldridge R, Hostetler JA, et al: Dwarfism in the Amish. II. Cartilage-hair hypoplasia. Bull Johns Hopkins Hosp 1965; 116:285.

571. Makitie O, Kaitila I: Cartilage-hair hypoplasia—Clinical manifestations in 108 Finnish patients. Eur J Pediatr 1993; 152:211.

572. Sacrez R, Levy J-M, Godar G, et al: Anémie de Blackfan-Diamond associée à des malformations multiples. Med Infant (Paris) 1965; 72:493.

573. L'Hirondel J, Caen J, et al: Anémie de Blackfan-Diamond et dyostose métaphysaire récessive autosomique. Ouest Med 1967; 20:1152.

574. Harris RE, Baehner RL, Gleiser S, et al: Cartilage-hair hypoplasia, defective T-cell function, and Diamond-Blackfan anemia in an Amish child. Am J Med Genet 1981; 8:291.

575. Roberts MA, Arnold RM: Hodgkin's lymphoma in a child with cartilage-hair hypoplasia: Case report. Mil Med 1984; 149:280.

576. Gorlin RJ: Cartilage-hair-hypoplasia and Hodgkin disease. Am J Med Genet 1992; 44:539.

577. Makitie O, Pukkala E, Teppo L, et al: Increased incidence of cancer in patients with cartilage-hair hypoplasia. J Pediatr 1999; 134:315.

578. Sulisalo T, Francomano CA, Sistonen P, et al: High-resolution genetic mapping of the cartilage-hair hypoplasia (CHH) gene in Amish and Finnish families. Genomics 1994; 20:347.

579. Ridanpaa M, van Eenennaam H, Pelin K, et al: Mutations in the RNA component of RNase MRP cause a pleiotropic human disease, cartilage-hair hypoplasia. Cell 2001; 104:195.

580. Sulisalo T, Sillence D, Wilson M, et al: Early prenatal diagnosis of cartilage-hair hypooplasia (CHH) with polymorphic DNA markers. Prenat Diagn 1995; 15:135.

581. Juvonen E, Makitie O, Makipernaa A, et al: Defective in-vitro colony formation of haematopoietic progenitors in patients with cartilage-hair hypoplasia and history of anaemia. Eur J Pediatr 1995; 154:30.

582. Sanchez-Corona J, Garcia-Cruz D, Medina C, et al: Increased adenosine deaminase activity in a patient with cartilage-hair hypoplasia. Ann Genet 1990; 33:99.

583. Pearson HA, Lobel JS, Kocoshis SA, et al: A new syndrome of refractory sideroblastic anemia with vacuolization of marrow precursors and exocrine pancreatic dysfunction. J Pediatr 1979; 95:976.

584. Pearson HA: The naming of a syndrome. J Pediatr Hematol Oncol 1997; 19:271.

585. Rotig A, Cormier V, Blanche S, et al: Pearson's marrow-pancreas syndrome. A multisystem mitochondrial disorder in infancy. J Clin Invest 1990; 86:1601.

586. Gurgey A, Rotig A, Gumruk F, et al: Pearson's marrow-pancreas syndrome in 2 Turkish children. Acta Haematol 1992; 87:206.

587. Bernes SM, Bacino C, Prezant TR, et al: Identical mitochondrial DNA deletion in mother with progressive external ophthalmoplegia and son with Pearson marrow-pancreas syndrome. J Pediatr 1993; 123:598.

588. Oblender MG, Richardson CJ, Alter BP: Pearson syndrome (PS) presenting as nonimmune hydrops fetalis. Clin Res 1993; 41:803A.

589. Fleming WH, Trounce I, Krawiecki N, et al: Cytokine treatment improves the hematologic manifestations of Pearson's syndrome. Blood 1994; 84:27a.

590. Sano T, Ban K, Ichiki T, et al: Molecular and genetic analyses of two patients with Pearson's marrow-pancreas syndrome. Pediatr Res 1993; 34:105.

591. Rotig A, Bourgeron T, Chretien D, et al: Spectrum of mitochondrial DNA rearrangements in the Pearson marrow-pancreas syndrome. Hum Molec Genet 1995; 4:1327.

592. De Vivo D: The expanding clinical spectrum of mitochondrial diseases. Brain Dev 1993; 15:1.

593. Blaw ME, Mize CE: Juvenile Pearson syndrome. J Child Neurol 1993; 5:186.

594. Favareto F, Caprino D, Micalizzi C, et al: New clinical aspects of Pearson's syndrome. Report of three cases. Haematologica 1989; 74:591.

595. Larsson N-G, Holme E, Kristiansson B, et al: Progressive increase of the mutated mitochondrial DNA fraction in Kearns-Sayre syndrome. Pediatr Res 1990; 28:131.

596. McShane MA, Hammans SR, Sweeney M, et al: Pearson syndrome and mitochondrial encephalomyopathy in a patient with a deletion of mtDNA. Am J Hum Genet 1991; 48:39.

597. Baerlocher KE, Feldges A, Weissert M, et al: Mitochondrial DNA deletion in an 8-year-old boy with Pearson syndrome. J Inher Metab Dis 1992; 15:327.

598. Simonsz HJ, Bärlocher K, Rötig A: Kearns-Sayre's syndrome developing in a boy who survived Pearson's syndrome caused by mitochondrial DNA deletion. Doc Ophthalmol 1992; 82:73.

599. Nelson I, Bonne G, Degoul F, et al: Kearns-Sayre syndrome with sideroblastic anemia: Molecular investigations. Neuropediatrics 1992; 23:199.

600. Hasle H: Myelodysplastic syndromes in childhood—Classification, epidemiology, and treatment. Leuk Lymphoma 1994; 13:11.

601. Muraki K, Nishimura S, Goto Y, et al: The association between haematological manifestation and mtDNA deletions in Pearson syndrome. J Inher Metab Dis 1997; 20:697.

602. Guirado Gimenez F, Montoya Villarroya J, Olivan del Cacho MJ, et al: Paciente con sindrome de Pearson y de Kearns-Sayre y la deleción comun de 4,9 Kb del DNA mitocondrial en sangre. An Esp Pediatr 1998; 49:510.

603. Bader-Meunier B, Rotig A, Mielot F, et al: Refractory anaemia and mitochondrial cytopathy in childhood. Br J Haematol 1994; 87:381.

604. de Vaal OM, Seynhaeve V: Reticular dysgenesia. Lancet 1959; 2:1123.

605. Emile J-F, Geissmann F, de la Calle Martin O, et al: Langerhans cell deficiency in reticular dysgenesis. Blood 2000; 96:58.

606. DeWitte DB, Buick MK, Cyran SE, et al: Neonatal pancytopenia and severe combined immunodeficiency associated with antenatal administration of azathioprine and prednisone. J Pediatr 1984; 105:625.

607. Alter BP: Neonatal pancytopenia after maternal azathioprine therapy. J Pediatr 1985; 106:691.

608. Haas RJ, Niethammer D, Goldmann SF, et al: Congenital immunodeficiency and agranulocytosis (reticular dysgenesia). Acta Paediatr Scand 1977; 66:279.

609. Levinsky RJ, Tiedeman K: Successful bone-marrow transplantation for reticular dysgenesis. Lancet 1983; 1:671.

610. Roper M, Parmley RT, Crist WM, et al: Severe congenital leukopenia (reticular dysgenesis). Am J Dis Child 1985; 139:832.

611. Chin TW, Plaeger-Marshall S, Haas A, et al: Lymphokine-activated killer cells in primary immunodeficiencies and acquired immunodeficiency syndrome. Clin Immunol Immunopathol 1989; 53:449.

612. Bujan W, Ferster A, Azzi N, et al: Use of recombinant human granulocyte colony stimulating factor in reticular dysgenesis. Br J Haematol 1992; 81:128.

613. Bujan W, Ferster A, Sariban E, et al: Effect of recombinant human granulocyte colony-stimulating factor in reticular dysgenesis. Blood 1993; 82:1684.

614. Stephan JL, Vlekova V, Le Deist F, et al: Severe combined immunodeficiency: A retrospective single-center study of clinical presentation and outcome in 117 patients. J Pediatr 1993; 123:564.

615. De Stantes KB, Lai SS, Cowan MJ: Haploidentical bone marrow transplants for two patients with reticular dysgenesis. Bone Marrow Transplant 1996; 17:1171.

616. De La Calle-Martin O, Badell I, Garcia A, et al: B cells and monocytes are not developmentally affected in a case of reticular dysgenesis. Clin Exp Immunol 1997; 110:392.

617. Knutsen AP, Wall DA: Umbilical cord blood transplantation in severe T-cell immunodeficiency disorders: Two-year experience. J Clin Immunol 2000; 20:466.

618. Bizzaro N, Dianese G: Neonatal alloimmune amegakaryocytosis. Vox Sang 1988; 54:112.

619. Ballmaier M, Germeshausen M, Schulze H, et al: *c-mpl* mutations are the cause of congenital amegakaryocytic thrombocytopenia. Blood 2001; 97:139.

620. Nichols KE, Crispino JD, Poncz M et al: Familial dyserythropoietic anaemia and thrombocytopenia due to an inherited mutation in *GATA1*. Nat Genet 2000; 24:266.

621. Song W-J, Sullivan MG, Legare RD, et al: Haploinsufficiency of CBFA2 causes familial thrombocytopenia with propensity to develop acute myelogenous leukaemia. Nat Genet 1999; 23:166.

622. Savoia A, Del Vecchio M, Totaro A, et al: An autosomal dominant thrombocytopenia gene maps to chromosomal region 10p. Am J Hum Genet 1999; 65:1401.

623. Thompson AA, Nguyen LT: Amegakaryocytic thrombocytopenia and radio-ulnar synostosis are associated with *HOXA11* mutation. Nat Genet 2000; 26:397.

624. Mehes K, Bata G: Congenital thrombocytopenia in 13–15 trisomy. Lancet 1965; 1:1279.

625. Rabinowitz JG, Moseley JE, Mitty HA, et al: Trisomy 18, esophageal atresia, anomalies of the radius, and congenital hypoplastic thrombocytopenia. Radiology 1967; 89:488.

626. Jones C, Mullenbach R, Grossfeld P, et al: Co-localisation of CCG repeats and chromosome deletion breakpoints in Jacobsen syndrome: Evidence for a common mechanism of chromosome breakage. Hum Molec Genet 2000; 9:1201.

627. Guinan EC, Lee YS, Lopez KD, et al: Effects of interleukin-3 and granulocyte-macrophage colony-stimulating factor on thrombopoiesis in congenital amegakaryocytic thrombocytopenia. Blood 1993; 81:1691.

628. van den Oudenrijn S, Bruin M, Folman CC, et al: Mutations in the thrombopoietin receptor, Mpl, in children with congenital amegakaryocytic thrombocytopenia. Br J Haematol 2000; 110:441.

629. Gardner RJM, Morrison PS, Abbott GD: A syndrome of congenital thrombocytopenia with multiple malformations and neurologic dysfunction. J Pediatr 1983; 102:600.

630. Taylor DS, Lee Y, Sieff CA, et al: Phase I/II trial of PIXY321 (granulocyte-macrophage colony stimulating factor/interleukin-3 fusion protein) for treatment of inherited and acquired marrow failure syndromes. Br J Haematol 1998; 103:304.

631. Van Oostrom CG, Wilms RHH: Congenital thrombocytopenia, associated with raised concentrations of haemoglobin F. Helv Paediatr Acta 1978; 33:59.

632. Buchanan GR, Scher CS, Button LN, et al: Use of homologous platelet survival in the differential diagnosis of chronic thrombocytopenia in childhood. Pediatrics 1977; 59:49.

633. Harris MB, Najfeld V, Weiner MA, et al: Congenital amegakaryocytic thrombocytopenia: A case report with chromosomal abnormalities. Unpublished paper, 1984.

634. Mibashan RS, Millar DS: Fetal haemophilia and allied bleeding disorders. Br Med Bull 1983; 39:392.

635. Cremer M, Schulze H, Linthorst G, et al: Serum levels of thrombopoietin, IL-11, and IL-6 in pediatric thrombocytopenias. Ann Hematol 1999; 78:401.

636. Mukai HY, Kojima H, Todokoro K, et al: Serum thrombopoietin (TPO) levels in patients with amegakaryocytic thrombocytopenia are much higher than those with immune thrombocytopenic purpura. Thromb Haemost 1996; 76:675.

637. Muraoka K, Ishii E, Tsuji K, et al: Defective response to thrombopoietin and impaired expression of *c-mpl* mRNA of bone marrow cells in congenital amegakaryocytic thrombocytopenia. Br J Haematol 1997; 96:287.

638. Tonelli R, Scardovi AL, Pession A, et al: Compound heterozygosity for two different amino-acid substitution mutations in the thrombopoietin receptor (*c-mpl* gene) in congenital amegakaryocytic thrombocytopenia (CAMT). Hum Genet 2000; 107:225.

639. Alter BP: The bone marrow failure syndromes. In Nathan DG, Oski FA (eds): Hematology of Infancy and Childhood, 3rd ed. Philadelphia, WB Saunders, 1987, p 159.

640. Henter J-I, Winiarski J, Ljungman P, et al: Bone marrow transplantation in two children with congenital amegakaryocytic thrombocytopenia. Bone Marrow Transplant 1995; 15:799.

641. Margolis D, Camitta B, Pietryga D, et al: Unrelated donor bone marrow transplantation to treat severe aplastic anaemia in children and young adults. Br J Haematol 1996; 94:65.

642. MacMillan ML, Davies SM, Wagner JE, et al: Engraftment of unrelated donor stem cells in children with familial amegakaryocytic thrombocytopenia. Bone Marrow Transplant 1998; 21:735.

643. Arias S, Penchaszadeh VB, Pinto-Cisternas J, et al: The IVIC syndrome: A new autosomal dominant complex pleiotropic syndrome with radial ray hypoplasia, hearing impairment, external ophthalmoplegia, and thrombocytopenia. Am J Med Genet 1980; 6:25.

644. Sammito V, Motta D, Capodieci G, et al: IVIC syndrome: Report of a second family. Am J Med Genet 1988; 29:875.

645. Czeizel A, Goblyos P, Kodaj I: IVIC syndrome: Report of a third family. Am J Med Genet 1989; 32:282.

646. Neri G, Sammito V: Re: IVIC syndrome report by Czeizel et al. Am J Med Genet 1989; 33:284.

647. Gonzalez CH, Durkin-Stamm MV, Geimer NF, et al: The WT syndrome—A "new" autosomal dominant pleiotropic trait of radial/ulnar hypoplasia with high risk of bone marrow failure and/or leukemia. Birth Defects Orig Article Ser 1977; 13(3B):31.

648. Smith ACM, Hays T, Harvey LA, et al: WT syndrome: a third family. Am J Hum Genet 1987; 41:A84.

649. Alter CL, Levine PH, Bennett J, et al: Dominantly transmitted hematologic dysfunction clinically similar to Fanconi's anemia. Am J Hematol 1989; 32:241.

650. Dokal I, Ganly P, Riebero I, et al: Late onset bone marrow failure associated with proximal fusion of radius and ulna: a new syndrome. Br J Haematol 1989; 71:277.

651. Thompson AA, Woodruff K, Feig SA, et al: Congenital thrombocytopenia and radia-ulnar synostosis: A new familial syndrome. Br J Haematol 2001; 113:866.

652. McFarland G, Say B, Carpenter NJ, et al: A condition resembling congenital hypoplastic anemia occurring in a mother and son. Clin Pediatr 1982; 12:755.

653. Aufderheide AC: Familial cytopenia and vascular disease: A newly recognized autosomal dominant condition. Birth Defects Orig Article Ser 1972; 8(3):63.

654. Kato J, Niitsu Y, Ishigaki S, et al: Chronic hypoplastic neutropenia. A case of familial occurrence of chronic hypoplastic neutropenia and aplastic anemia. Rinsho Ketsueki 1986; 27:407.

655. Keiser G: Erworbene Panmyelopathien. Schweiz Med Wochenschr 1970; 100:1938.

656. Kaur J, Catovsky D, Valdimarsson H, et al: Familial acute myeloid leukaemia with acquired Pelger-Huet anomaly and aneuploidy of C group. Br Med J 1972; 1:1327.

657. Sleijfer D Th, Mulder NH, Niewig HO, et al: Acquired pancytopenia in relatives of patients with aplastic anaemia. Acta Med Scand 1980; 207:397.

658. Yanabe Y, Nunoi H, Tsuchiya H, et al: A disease with immune deficiency, skin abscesses, pancytopenia, abnormal bone marrow karyotype, and increased sister chromatid exchanges: An autosomal recessive chromosome instability syndrome? Jpn J Hum Genet 1990; 35:263.

659. Drachtman R, Weinblatt M, Sitarz A, et al: Marrow hypoplasia associated with congenital neurologic anomalies in two siblings. Acta Paediatr Scand 1990; 79:990.

660. Kotzot D, Richter K, Gierth-Fiebig K: Oculocutaneous albinism, immunodeficiency, hematological disorders, and minor anomalies: A new autosomal recessive syndrome? Am J Med Genet 1994; 50:224.

661. Stoll C, Alembik Y, Lutz P: A syndrome of facial dysmorphia, birth defects, myelodysplasia and immunodeficiency in three sibs of consanguineous parents. Genet Couns 1994; 5:161.

662. Ghosal SP, Mukherjee AK, Mukherjee D, et al: Diaphyseal dysplasia associated with anemia. J Pediatr 1988; 113:49.

663. Ozsoylu S: High-dose intravenous methylprednisolone therapy for anemia associated with diaphyseal dysplasia. J Pediatr 1993; 114:904.

664. Gumruk F, Besim A, Altay C: Ghosal haemato-diaphyseal dysplasia: A new disorder. Eur J Pediatr 1993; 152:218.

665. Abels D, Reed WB: Fanconi-like syndrome. Immunologic deficiency, pancytopenia, and cutaneous malignancies. Arch Dermatol 1973; 107:419.

666. Linsk JA, Khoory MS, Meyers KR: Myeloid, erythroid, and immune system defects in a family. A new stem-cell disorder? Ann Intern Med 1975; 82:659.

667. Chitambar CR, Robinson WA, Glode LM: Familial leukemia and aplastic anemia associated with monosomy 7. Am J Med 1983; 75:756.

668. Nowell P, Besa E, Emanuel B., et al: Two adult siblings with thrombocytopenia and a familial 13;14 translocation. Cancer Genet Cytogenet 1984; 11:169.

669. Salob SP, Webb DKH, Atherton DJ: A child with xeroderma pigmentosum and bone marrow failure. Br J Dermatol 1992; 126:372.

670. Berbis P, Beylot C, Noe C, et al: Xeroderma pigmentosum and refractory anaemia in two first cousins. Br J Dermatol 1989; 121:767.

671. Berlin C, Tager A: Xeroderma pigmentosum—Report of eight cases of mild to moderate type and course: A study of response to various irradiations. Dermatologica 1958; 116:27.

672. Reed WB, Landing B, Sugarman G, et al: Xeroderma pigmentosum. Clinical and laboratory investigation of its basic defect. JAMA 1969; 207:2073.

673. Li FP, Marchetto DJ, Vawter GR: Acute leukemia and preleukemia in eight males in a family: An X-linked disorder? Am J Hematol 1979; 6:61.

674. Purtilo DT, Sakamoto K, Barnabei V, et al: Epstein-Barr virus-induced diseases in boys with the X-linked lymphoproliferative syndrome (XLP). Update on studies of the registry. Am J Med 1982; 73:49.

675. Grierson H, Purtilo DT: Epstein-Barr virus infections in males with the X-linked lymphoproliferative syndrome. Ann Intern Med 1987; 106:538.

676. Skare JC, Milunsky A, Byron KS, et al: Mapping the X-linked lymphoproliferative syndrome. Proc Natl Acad Sci USA 1987; 84:2015.

677. Samad FU, Engel E, Hartmann RC: Hypoplastic anemia, Friedreich's ataxia and chromosomal breakage: Case report and review of similar disorders. South Med J 1973; 66:135.

678. Nagata M, Hara T, Sakamoto K, et al: Aplastic anemia associated with ataxia and chromosome translocation (1;20). Acta Haematol 1990; 84:198.

679. Sackey K, Sakati N, Aur RJA, et al: Multiple dysmorphic features and pancytopenia: A new syndrome? Clin Genet 1985; 27:606.

680. Muroi K, Amemiya Y, Miwa A, et al: Long-term bone marrow failure accompanied by skin pigmentation. Int J Hematol 1991; 54:281.

681. Froster UG, Gortner L: Thrombocytopenia in the Brachmann-de Lange syndrome. Am J Med Genet 1993; 46:730.

682. Fryns JP, Vinken L: Thrombocytopenia in the Brachmann-de Lange syndrome. Am J Med Genet 1994; 49:360.

683. Freedman MH: Congenital failure of hematopoiesis in the newborn infant. Clin Perinatol 1984; 11:417.

684. Weinstein HJ: Congenital leukemia and the neonatal myeloproliferative disorders associated with Down's syndrome. Clin Haematol 1978; 7:147.

685. Erdogan G, Aksoy M, Dincol K: A case of idiopathic aplastic anemia associated with trisomy-21 and partial endoreduplication. Acta Haematol 1967; 37:137.

686. Vetrella M, Barthelmai W, Matsuda H: Kongenitale amegakaryocytäre Thrombocytopenie mit finaler Pancytopenie bei Trisomie 21 mit cystischer Pankreasfibrose. Z Kinderheilk 1969; 107:210.

687. Weinblatt ME, Higgins G, Ortega JA: Aplastic anemia in Down's syndrome. Pediatrics 1981; 67:896.

688. McWilliams NB, Dunn NL: Aplastic anemia and Down's syndrome. Pediatrics 1982; 69:501.

689. Hanukoglu A, Meytes D, Fried A, et al: Fatal aplastic anemia in a child with Down's syndrome. Acta Paediatr Scand 1987; 76:539.

690. Tsukahara M, Opitz JM: Dubowitz syndrome: Review of 141 cases including 36 previously unreported patients. Am J Med Genet 1996; 63:277.

691. Kuster W, Majewski F: The Dubowitz syndrome. Eur J Pediatr 1986; 144:574.

692. Majewski F, Goecke T: Studies of microcephalic primordial dwarfism I: Approach to a delineation of the Seckel syndrome. Am J Med Genet 1982; 12:7.

693. Espérou-Bourdeau H, Leblanc T, Schaison G, et al: Aplastic anemia associated with "bird-headed" dwarfism (Seckel syndrome). Nouv Rev Fr Hematol 1993; 35:99.

694. Seemanova E, Passarge E, Beneskova D, et al: Familial microcephaly with normal intelligence, immunodeficiency, and risk for lymphoreticular malignancies: A new autosomal recessive disorder. Am J Med Genet 1985; 20:639.

695. Hayani A, Suarez CR, Molnar Z, et al: Acute myeloid leukaemia in a patient with Seckel syndrome. J Med Genet 1994; 31:148.

696. Sall MG, Badiane M, Kuakuvi N, et al: Seckel's nanism: Concerning one case. Dakar Med 1990; 35:46.

697. Lilleyman JS: Constitutional hypoplastic anemia associated with familial "bird-headed" dwarfism (Seckel syndrome). Am J Pediatr Hematol Oncol 1984; 6:207.

698. Dohlsten M, Carlsson R, Hedlund G, et al: Immunological abnormalities in a child with constitutional aplastic anemia. Pediatr Hematol Oncol 1986; 3:89.

699. Butler MG, Hall BD, Maclean RN, et al: Do some patients with Seckel syndrome have hematological problems and/or chromosome breakage? Am J Med Genet 1987; 27:645.

700. Cervenka J, Tsuchiya H, Ishiki T, et al: Seckel's dwarfism: Analysis of chromosome breakage and sister chromatid exchanges. Am J Dis Child 1979; 133:555.

701. Abou-Zahr F, Bejjani B, Kruyt FAE, et al: Normal expression of the Fanconi anemia proteins FAA and FAC and sensitivity to mitomycin C in two patients with Seckel syndrome. Am J Med Genet 1999; 83:388.

702. Jamieson CR, Van Der Burgt I, Brady AF, et al: Mapping a gene for Noonan syndrome to the long arm of chromosome 12. Nat Genet 1994; 8:357.

703. Noonan JA: Hypertelorism with Turner phenotype. A new syndrome with associated congenital heart disease. Am J Dis Child 1968; 116:373.

704. Char F, Caralis DG, Voigt GC: Noonan syndrome in 30-year-old male with cyanotic congenital heart disease. Birth Defects Orig Article Ser 1972; 8:243.

705. Evans DGR, Lonsdale RN, Patton MA: Cutaneous lymphangioma and amegakaryocytic thrombocytopenia in Noonan syndrome. Clin Genet 1991; 39:228.

706. Singer ST, Hurst D, Addiego JE, Jr: Bleeding disorders in Noonan syndrome: Three case reports and review of the literature. J Pediatr Hematol Oncol 1997; 19:130.

707. Feldman KW, Ochs HD, Price TH, et al: Congenital stem cell dysfunction associated with Turner-like phenotype. J Pediatr 1976; 88:979.

708. Bader-Meunier B, Tchernia G, Mielot F, et al: Occurrence of myeloproliferative disorder in patients with Noonan syndrome. J Pediatr 1997; 130:885.

709. Josephs HW: Anaemia of infancy and early childhood. Medicine (Baltimore) 1936; 15:307.

710. Diamond LK, Blackfan KD: Hypoplastic anemia. Am J Dis Child 1938; 56:464.

711. Kynaston JA, West NC, Ried MM: A regional experience of red cell aplasia. Eur J Pediatr 1993; 152:306.

712. Lipton JM, Federman N, Khabbaze Y, et al: Osteogenic sarcoma associated with Diamond-Blackfan anemia: A report from the Diamond-Blackfan Anemia Registry. J Pediatr Hematol Oncol 2000; 23:39.

713. Willig TN, Niemeyer CM, Leblanc T, et al: Identification of new prognosis factors from the clinical and epidemiologic analysis of a registry of 229 Diamond-Blackfan anemia patients. Pediatr Res 1999; 46:553.

714. Ramenghi U, Garelli E, Valtolina S, et al: Diamond-Blackfan anaemia in the Italian population. Br J Haematol 1999; 104:841.

715. Vlachos A, Alter BP, et al: The Diamond-Blackfan Anemia Registry (DBAR). Pediatr Res 1994; 35:171A.

716. Ball SE, Tchernia G, Wranne L, et al: Is there a role for interleukin-3 in Diamond-Blackfan anaemia? Results of a European multicentre study. Br J Haematol 1995; 91:313.

717. Janov AJ, Leong T, Nathan DG, et al: Diamond-Blackfan anemia. Natural history and sequelae of treatment. Medicine (Baltimore) 1996; 75:77.

718. Wallman IS: Hereditary red cell aplasia. Med J Aust 1956; 2:488.

719. Gray P. H.: Pure red-cell aplasia. Occurrence in three generations. Med J Aust 1982; 1:519.

720. Neilson RF, Khokhar AA: Red cell aplasia in mother and son. Clin Lab Haematol 1991; 13:224.
721. Gojic V, Van't Veer-Korthof ET, Bosch LJ, et al: Congenital hypoplastic anemia: Another example of autosomal dominant transmission. Am J Med Genet 1994; 50:87.
722. Madanat F, Arnaout M, Hasan A, et al: Red cell aplasia resembling Diamond-Blackfan anemia in seven children in a family. Am J Pediatr Hematol Oncol 1994; 16:260.
723. Balaban EP, Buchanan GR, Graham. M., et al: Diamond-Blackfan syndrome in adult patients. Am J Med 1985; 78:533.
724. Bastion Y, Campos L, Roubi N, et al: IL-3 increases marrow and peripheral erythroid precursors in chronic pure red cell aplasia presenting in childhood. Br J Haematol 1995; 89:413.
725. Cetin M, Kara A, Gurgey A, et al: Congenital hypoplastic anemia in six patients: Unusual association of short proximal phalanges with mild anemia. Pediatr Hematol Oncol 1995; 12:153.
726. Abkowitz JL, Sabo KM, Nakamoto B, et al: Diamond-Blackfan anemia: In vitro response of erythroid progenitors to the ligand for c-*kit*. Blood 1991; 78:2198.
727. Willig TN, Perignon JL, Gustavsson P, et al: High adenosine deaminase level among healthy probands of Diamond Blackfan anemia (DBA) cosegregates with the DBA gene region on chromosome 19q13. Blood 1998; 92:4422.
728. Willig T-N, Draptchinskaia N, Dianzani I, et al: Mutations in ribosomal protein S19 gene and Diamond Blackfan anemia: Wide variations in phenotypic expression. Blood 1999; 94:4294.
729. Bello A, Dorantes S, Alvarez-Amaya C: La anemia hipoplastica en la edad pediatrica. Bol Med Hosp Infant Mex 1983; 40:718.
730. Waterkotte GW, McElfresh AE: Congenital pure red cell hypoplasia in identical twins. Pediatrics 1974; 54:646.
731. Freedman MH: Diamond-Blackfan anemia. Am J Pediatr Hematol Oncol 1985; 7:327.
732. Giblett ER, Varela JE, Finch CA: Damage of the bone marrow due to Rh antibody. Pediatrics 1956; 17:37.
733. Scimeca PG, Weinblatt ME, Slepowitz G, et al: Diamond-Blackfan syndrome: An unusual cause of hydrops fetalis. Am J Pediatr Hematol Oncol 1988; 10:241.
734. van Hook JW, Gill P, Cyr D, et al: Diamond-Blackfan anemia as an unusual cause of nonimmune hydrops fetalis. A case report. J Reprod Med 1995; 40:850.
735. Rogers BB, Bloom SL, Buchanan GR: Autosomal dominantly inherited Diamond Blackfan anemia resulting in nonimmune hydrops. Obstet Gyncol 1997; 89:805.
736. Schorr JB, Cohen ES, Schwarz A, et al: Hypoplastic anemia in childhood. Jew Mem Hosp Bull 1962; 6–7:126.
737. Brown KE, Green SW, Antunez de Mayolo J, et al: Congenital anaemia after transplacental B19 parvovirus infection. Lancet 1994; 343:895.
738. Heegaard ED, Hasle H, Clausen N, et al: Parvovirus B19 infection and Diamond-Blackfan anaemia. Acta Paediatr 1996; 85:299.
739. Tchernia G, Morinet F, Congard B, et al: Diamond Blackfan anaemia: Apparent relapse due to B19 parvovirus. Eur J Pediatr 1993; 152:209.
740. Cathie IAB: Erythrogenesis imperfecta. Arch Dis Child 1950; 25:313.
741. Gripp KW, McDonald-McGinn DM, La Rossa D et al: Bilateral microtia and cleft palate in cousins with Diamond-Blackfan anemia. Am J Med Genet 2001; 101:268.
742. Hasan R, Inoue S: Diamond-Blackfan anemia associated with Treacher-Collins syndrome. Pediatr Hematol Oncol 1993; 10:261.
743. Aase JM, Smith DW: Congenital anemia and triphalangeal thumbs: A new syndrome. J Pediatr 1969; 74:471.
744. Alter BP: Thumbs and anemia. Pediatrics 1978; 62:613.
745. Becker RE, Maurer H, Bowyer FP, et al: Growth hormone deficiency (GHD) in Diamond-Blackfan anemia (DBA). Pediatr Res 1991; 29:74A.
746. Sacrez R, Levy J-M, Godar G, et al: Anémie de Blackfan-Diamond associée a des malformations multiples. Med Infant (Paris)1965; 72:493.
747. O'Gorman Hughes DW: Hypoplastic anaemia in infancy and childhood: Erythroid hypoplasia. Arch Dis Child 1961; 36:349.
748. Buchanan GR, Alter BP, Holtkamp CA, et al: Platelet number and function in Diamond-Blackfan anemia. Pediatrics 1981; 68:238.
749. Vogel P, Bassen FA: Sternal marrow of children in normal and in pathologic states. Am J Dis Child 1939; 57:245.
750. Gasser C: Aplastische Anämie (chronische Erythroblastophthise) und Cortison. Schweiz Med Wochenschr 1951; 81:1241.
751. Bernard J, Seligmann M, Chassigneux J, et al: Anémie de Blackfan-Diamond. Nouv Rev Fr Hematol 1962; 2:721.
752. Boxer LA, Hussey L, Clarke TL: Sideroblastic anemia following congenital erythroid hypoplasia. J Pediatr 1971; 79:681.
753. Girot R, Griscelli C: Erythroblastopénie a rechutes. A propos d'un cas suivi pendant 22 ans. Nouv Rev Fr Hematol 1977; 18:555.
754. Hammond D, Shore N, Movassaghi N: Production, utilization and excretion of erythropoietin. I. Chronic anemias. II. Aplastic crisis. III. Erythropoietic effects of normal plasma. Ann NY Acad Sci 1968; 149:516.
755. Price JM, Brown RR, Pfaffenbach EC, et al: Excretion of urinary tryptophan metabolites by patients with congenital hypoplastic anemia (Diamond-Blackfan syndrome). J Lab Clin Med 1970; 75:316.
756. Finlay JL, Shahidi NT, Horowitz S, et al: Lymphocyte dysfunction in congenital hypoplastic anemia. J Clin Invest 1982; 70:619.
757. Alter BP: Childhood red cell aplasia. Am J Pediatr Hematol Oncol 1980; 2:121.
758. Feldges D, Schmidt R: Erythrogenesis imperfecta (Blackfan-Diamond-Anämie). Schweiz Med Wochenschr 1971; 101:1813.
759. Fondu P, Mandelbaum IM, Stryckmans PA, et al: Un cas d'erythroblastopénie de l'enfant a début tardif. Nouv Rev Fr Hematol 1972; 12:5.
760. Giblett ER, Ammann AJ, Wara DW, et al: Nucleoside-phosphorylase deficiency in a child with severely defective T-cell immunity and normal B-cell immunity. Lancet 1975; 1:1010.
761. Glader BE, Backer K, Diamond LK: Elevated erythrocyte adenosine deaminase activity in congenital hypoplastic anemia. N Engl J Med 1983; 309:1486.
762. Zielke HR, Ozand PT, Luddy RE, et al: Elevation of pyrimidine enzyme activities in the RBC of patients with congenital hypoplastic anaemia and their parents. Br J Haematol 1979; 42:381.
763. Glader BE, Backer K: Comparative activity of erythrocyte adenosine deaminase and orotidine decarboxylase in Diamond-Blackfan anemia. Am J Hematol 1986; 23:135.
764. Glader BE, Backer K: Elevated red cell adenosine deaminase activity: A marker of disordered erythropoiesis in Diamond-Blackfan anaemia and other haematologic diseases. Br J Haematol 1988; 68:165.
765. Whitehouse DB, Hopkinson DA, Pilz AJ, et al: Adenosine deaminase activity in a series of 19 patients with the Diamond-Blackfan syndrome. Adv Exp Med Biol 1986; 195(Pt. A):85.
766. Tartaglia AP, Propp S, Amarose AP, et al: Chromosome abnormality and hypocalcemia in congenital erythroid hypoplasia (Blackfan-Diamond syndrome). Am J Med 1966; 41:990.
767. Heyn R, Kurczynski E, Schmickel R: The association of Blackfan-Diamond syndrome, physical abnormalities, and an abnormality of chromosome 1. J Pediatr 1974; 85:531.
768. Philippe N, Requin Ch., Germain D: Etudes chromosomiques dans 6 cas d'anémie de Blackfan-Diamond. Pediatrie 1971; 26:47.
769. Brizard CP, Fayard C, Fraisse J, et al: Anemie par anerythroblastose (type Blackfan-Diamond) chez une enfant porteuse d'anomalies chromosomiques constitutionnelles. Pediatrie 1971; 26:305.
770. Iskandar O, Jager MJ, Willenze R, et al: A case of pure red cell aplasia with high incidence of spontaneous chromosome breakage: A possible x-ray sensitive syndrome. Hum Genet 1980; 55:337.
771. Pfeiffer RA, Ambs E: The Aase syndrome: Autosomal-recessive hereditary, connatal erythroid hypoplasia and triphalangeal thumbs. Monatsschr Kinderheilkd 1983; 131:235.
772. Visser GHA, Desmedt MCH, Meijboom EJ: Altered fetal cardiac flow patterns in pure red cell anaemia (the Blackfan-Diamond syndrome). Prenat Diagn 1988; 8:525.
773. Van der Mooren K: Fetal anemia. Prenat Diagn 1989; 9:450.
774. Gurney CW, Pierce M. I., Schreier SE, et al: The stimulatory effect of "anemic plasma" in congenital hypoplastic anemia. J Lab Clin Med 1957; 50:821.
775. Smith CH: Chronic congenital aregenerative anemia (pure red-cell anemia) associated with isoimmunization by the blood group factor "A." Blood 1949; 4:697.
776. Moody EA: Hypoplastic anemia following exchange transfusion for erythroblastosis fetalis associated with isoimmunization to blood group factor "A." J Pediatr 1954; 44:244.

777. Diamond LK, Wang WC, Alter BP: Congenital hypoplastic anemia. Adv Pediatr 1976; 22:349.

778. Ortega JA, Shore NA, Dukes PP, et al: Congenital hypoplastic anemia inhibition of erythropoiesis by sera from patients with congenital hypoplastic anemia. Blood 1975; 45:83.

779. Geller G, Krivit W, Zalusky R, et al: Lack of erythropoietic inhibitory effect of serum from patients with congenital pure red cell aplasia. J Pediatr 1975; 86:198.

780. Freedman MH, Amato D, Saunders EF: Haem synthesis in the Diamond-Blackfan syndrome. Br J Haematol 1975; 31:515.

781. Steinberg MH, Coleman MF, Pennebaker JB: Diamond-Blackfan syndrome: Evidence for T-cell mediated suppression of erythroid development and a serum blocking factor associated with remission. Br J Haematol 1979; 41:57.

782. Hoffman R, Zanjani ED, Vila J, et al: Diamond-Blackfan syndrome: Lymphocyte-mediated suppression of erythropoiesis. Science 1976; 193:899.

783. Nathan DG, Hillman DG, Breard J: The influence of T cells on erythropoiesis. In Stamatoyannopoulos, G; Nienhuis, A W (eds): Cellular and Molecular Regulation of Hemoglobin Switching. New York, Grune and Stratton, 1979, p 291.

784. Steinberg MH, Coleman MB, Pennebaker JB: Diamond-Blackfan anemia: The role of immunoglobulin blocking factor in remission. Am J Hematol 1980; 8:213.

785. Zanjani EM, Rinehart JJ: Role of cell-cell interaction in normal and abnormal erythropoiesis. Am J Pediatr Hematol Oncol 1980; 2:233.

786. Ershler WB, Ross J, Finlay JL, et al: Bone-marrow microenvironment defect in congenital hypoplastic anemia. N Engl J Med 1980; 302:1321.

787. Nathan DG, Clarke BJ, Hillman DG, et al: Erythroid precursors in congenital hypoplastic (Diamond-Blackfan) anemia. J Clin Invest 1978; 61:489.

788. Nathan DG, Hillman DG, Chess L, et al: Normal erythropoietic helper T cells in congenital hypoplastic (Diamond-Blackfan) anemia. N Engl J Med 1978; 298:1049.

789. Alter BP: Inherited bone marrow failure syndromes. In Handin RI, Lux SE, Stossel TP (eds): Blood: Principles and Practice of Hematology. Philadelphia, JB Lippincott, 1995, p 227.

790. Chan HSL, Saunders EF, Freedman MH: Diamond-Blackfan syndrome. I Erythropoiesis in prednisone responsive and resistant disease. Pediatr Res 1982; 16:474.

791. Chan HSL, Saunders EF, Freedman MH: Diamond-Blackfan syndrome. II. In vitro corticosteroid effect on erythropoiesis. Pediatr Res 1982; 16:477.

792. Lipton JM, Kudisch M, Gross R, et al: Defective erythroid progenitor differentiation system in congenital hypoplastic (Diamond-Blackfan) anemia. Blood 1986; 67:962.

793. Tsai PH, Arkin S, Lipton JM: An intrinsic progenitor defect in Diamond-Blackfan anemia. Br J Haematol 1989; 73:112.

794. Halpérin DS, Estrov Z, Freedman MH: Diamond-Blackfan anemia: Promotion of marrow erythropoiesis in vitro by recombinant interleukin-3. Blood 1989; 73:1168.

795. Russell ES: Hereditary anemias of the mouse: A review for geneticists. Adv Gen 1979; 20:357.

796. Geissler EN, Ryan MA, Housman DE: The dominant-white spotting (W) locus of the mouse encodes the c-kit proto-oncogene. Cell 1988; 55:185.

797. Zsebo KM, Wypych J, McNiece IK, et al: Identification, purification, and biological characterization of hematopoietic stem cell factor from Buffalo rat liver-conditioned medium. Cell 1990; 63:195.

798. Spritz RA, Giebel LB, Holmes SA: Dominant negative and loss of function mutations of the c-kit (mast/stem cell growth factor receptor) proto-oncogene in human piebaldism. Am J Hum Genet 1992; 50:261.

799. Spritz RA: Lack of apparent hematologic abnormalities in human patients with c-kit (stem cell factor receptor) gene mutations. Blood 1992; 79:2497.

800. Cynshi O, Satoh K, Higuchi M, et al: Effects of recombinant human erythropoietin on anaemic W/W^v and Sl/Sl^d mice. Br J Haematol 1990; 75:319.

801. Alter BP, Gaston T, Lipton JM: Lack of effect of corticosteroids in W/W^V and Sl/Sl^D mice: These mice are not a model for steroid-responsive Diamond-Blackfan anemia. Eur J Haematol 1993; 50:275.

802. Ody C, Kindler V, Vassalli P: Interleukin 3 perfusion in W/W^V mice allows the development of macroscopic hematopoietic spleen colonies and restores cutaneous mast cell number. J Exp Med 1990; 172:403.

803. Abkowitz JL, Broudy VC, Bennett LG, et al: Absence of abnormalities of c-kit or its ligand in two patients with Diamond-Blackfan anemia. Blood 1992; 79:25.

804. Olivieri NF, Grunberger T, Ben-David Y, et al: Diamond-Blackfan anemia: Heterogenous response of hematopoietic progenitor cells in vitro to the protein product of the steel locus. Blood 1991; 78:2211.

805. Drachtman RA, Geissler EN, Alter BP: The SCF and c-kit genes in Diamond-Blackfan anemia. Blood 1992; 79:2177.

806. Spritz RA, Freedman MH: Lack of mutations of the MGF and KIT genes in Diamond-Blackfan anemia. Blood 1993; 81:3165.

807. Sieff CA, Yokoyama CT, Zsebo KM, et al: The production of steel factor mRNA in Diamond-Blackfan anaemia long-term cultures and interactions of steel factor with erythropoietin and interleukin-3. Br J Haematol 1992; 82:640.

808. McGuckin CP, Uhr MR, Liu M-M, et al: The use of recombinant SCF protein for rapid determination of c-kit expression in normal and abnormal erythropoiesis. Eur J Haematol 1996; 57:72.

809. Bagnara GP, Zauli G, Rosito P, et al: In vitro growth and regulation of bone marrow enriched CD34+ hematopoietic progenitors in Diamond-Blackfan anemia. Blood 1991; 78:2203.

810. McGuckin CP, Ball SE, Gordon-Smith EC: Diamond-Blackfan anaemia: Three patterns of in vitro response to haemopoietic growth factors. Br J Haematol 1995; 89:457.

811. Casadevall N, Croisille L, Auffray I, et al: Age-related alterations in erythroid and granulopoietic progenitors in Diamond-Blackfan anaemia. Br J Haematol 1994; 87:369.

812. Perdahl EB, Naprstek BL, Wallace WC, et al: Erythroid failure in Diamond-Blackfan anemia is characterized by apoptosis. Blood 1994; 83:645.

813. Dianzani I, Garelli E, Dompe C, et al: Mutations in the erythropoietin receptor gene are not a common cause of Diamond-Blackfan anemia. Blood 1996; 87:2568.

814. Dianzani I, Garelli E, Crescenzio N, et al: Diamond-Blackfan anemia: Expansion of erythroid progenitors in vitro by IL-9, but exclusion of a significant pathogenetic role for the IL-9 gene and the hematopoietic gene cluster on chromosome 5q. Exp Hematol 1997; 25:1270.

815. Gustavsson P, Skeppner G, Johansson B, et al: Diamond-Blackfan anaemia in a girl with a de novo balanced reciprocal X;19 translocation. J Med Genet 1997; 34:779.

816. Cario H, Bode H, Gustavsson P, et al: A microdeletion syndrome due to a 3-Mb deletion on 19q13.2—Diamond-Blackfan anemia associated with macrocephaly, hypotonia, and psychomotor retardation. Clin Genet 1999; 55:487.

817. Tentler D, Gustavsson P, Elinder G, et al: A microdeletion in 19q13.2 associated with mental retardation, skeletal malformations, and Diamond-Blackfan anaemia suggests a novel contiguous gene syndrome. J Med Genet 2000; 37:128.

818. Gustavsson P, Garelli E, Draptchinskaia N, et al: Identification of microdeletions spanning the Diamond-Blackfan anemia locus on 19q13 and evidence for genetic heterogeneity. Am J Hum Genet 1998; 63:1388.

819. Gustavsson P, Willig T-N, van Haeringen A, et al: Diamond-Blackfan anemia: Genetic homogeneity for a gene on chromosome 19q13 restricted to 1.8 Mb. J Pediatr 1997; 41:741.

820. Draptchinskaia N, Gustavsson P, Andersson B, et al: The gene encoding ribosomal protein S19 is mutated in Diamond-Blackfan anaemia. Nat Genet 1999; 21:169.

821. Gazda H, Lipton JM, Willig T-N, et al: Evidence for linkage of familial Diamond-Blackfan anemia to chromosome 8p23.3-p22 and for non-19q non-8p disease. Blood 2001; 97:2145.

822. Hoffbrand AV, Bartlett AN, Veys PA, et al: Agranulocytosis and thrombocytopenia in patient with Blackfan-Diamond anaemia during oral chelator trial. Lancet 1989; 2:457.

823. Alter BP: Agranulocytosis and thrombocytopenia, Blackfan-Diamond anaemia, and oral chelation. Lancet 1990; 335:970.

824. Berdoukas V, Bentley P, Frost H, et al: Toxicity of oral iron chelator L1. Lancet 1993; 341:1088.

825. Gasser C: Akute erythroblastopenie. Schweiz Med Wochenschr 1949; 79:838.

826. Hill JM, Hunter RB: ACTH therapy in refractory anemias. In Mote JR (Ed): Proceedings of the Second Clinical ACTH Conference, Vol. II, Therapeutics. New York, Blakiston, 1951, p 181.

827. Allen DM, Diamond LK: Congenital (erythroid) hypoplastic anemia. Am J Dis Child 1961; 102:416.

828. Sjölin S, Wranne L: Treatment of congenital hypoplastic anaemia with prednisone. Scand J Haematol 1970; 7:63.

829. Vlachos A, Federman N, Reyes-Haley C, et al: Diamond-Blackfan anaemia. Hematopoietic stem cell transplantation for Diamond Blackfan anaemia: A report from the Diamond Blackfan Anemia Registry. Bone Marrow Transplant 2001; 27:381.

830. Gomez-Almaguer D, Gonzalez-Llano O: Danazol in the treatment of Blackfan-Diamond anemia. Blood 1993; 80:382a.

831. Siegler J, Bognar I, Keleman K: Genesung einer isolierten chronischen Erythrozytenaplasie während einer Behandlung mit 6-Merkaptopurin. Kinderarztl Prax 1970; 38:145.

832. Sumimoto S-I, Kawai M, Kasajima Y, et al: Intravenous γ-globulin therapy in Diamond-Blackfan anemia. Acta Paediatr Jpn 1992; 34:179.

833. Ozsoylu S: Oral megadose methylprednisolone for the treatment of Diamond-Blackfan anemia. Pediatr Hematol Oncol 1994; 11:561.

834. Bernini JC, Carrillo JM, Buchanan GR: High-dose intravenous methylprednisolone therapy for patients with Diamond-Blackfan anemia refractory to conventional doses of prednisone. J Pediatr 1995; 127:654.

835. Williams DL, Mageed ASA, Findley H, et al: Cyclosporine in the treatment of red cell aplasia. Am J Pediatr Hematol Oncol 1987; 9:314.

836. Raghavachar A: Pure red cell aplasia: Review of treatment and proposal for a treatment strategy. Blut 1990; 61:47.

837. Gussetis ES, Peristeri J, Kitra V, et al: Clinical value of bone marrow cultures in childhood pure red cell aplasia. J Pediatr Hematol Oncol 1998; 20:120.

838. Alessandri AJ, Rogers PC, Wadsworth LD, et al: Diamond-Blackfan anemia and cyclosporine therapy revisited. J Pediatr Hematol Oncol 2000; 22:176.

839. Finlay JL, Shahidi NT: Cyclosporine A (CyA) induced remission in Diamond-Blackfan anemia (DBA). Blood 1984; 64:104A.

840. Tötterman TH, Nisell J, Killander A, et al: Successful treatment of pure red-cell aplasia with cyclosporin. Lancet 1984; 2:693.

841. Peters C, Dover GJ, Casella JE, et al: Cyclosporine A (CSA) induces transient remissions in red cell aplasias. Pediatr Res 1986; 20:285A.

842. Seip M, Zanussi GF: Cyclosporine in steroid-resistant Diamond-Blackfan anaemia. Acta Paediatr Scand 1988; 77:464.

843. Leonard EM, Raefsky E, Griffith P, et al: Cyclosporine therapy of aplastic anaemia, congenital and acquired red cell aplasia. Br J Haematol 1989; 72:278.

844. Splain J, Berman BW: Cyclosporin A treatment for Diamond-Blackfan anemia. Am J Hematol 1992; 39:208.

845. Monteserin MC, Garcia Vela JA, Ona F, et al: Cyclosporin A for Diamond-Blackfan anemia: A new case. Am J Hematol 1993; 42:406.

846. Bejaoui M, Fitouri Z, Sfar MT, et al: Failure of immunosuppressive therapy and high-dose intravenous immunoglobulins in four transfusion-dependent, steroid-unresponsive Blackfan-Diamond anemia patients. Haematologica 1993; 78:38.

847. Niemeyer CM, Baumgarten E, Holldack J, et al: Treatment trial with recombinant human erythropoietin in children with congenital hypoplastic anemia. Contrib Nephrol 1991; 88:276.

848. Fiorillo A, Poggi V, Migliorati R, et al: Letter to the editor: Unresponsiveness to erythropoietin therapy in a case of Blackfan Diamond anemia. Am J Hematol 1991; 37:65.

849. Dunbar CE, Smith DA, Kimball J, et al: Treatment of Diamond-Blackfan anaemia with haematopoietic growth factors, granulocyte-macrophage colony stimulating factor and interleukin 3: sustained remissions following IL-3. Br J Haematol 1991; 79:316.

850. Gillio AP, Faulkner LB, Alter BP, et al: Treatment of Diamond-Blackfan anemia with recombinant human interleukin-3. Blood 1993; 82:744.

851. Olivieri NF, Feig SA, Valentino L, et al: Failure of recombinant human interleukin-3 therapy to induce erythropoiesis in patients with refractory Diamond-Blackfan anemia. Blood 1994; 83:2444.

852. Bastion Y, Bordigoni P, Debre M, et al: Sustained response after recombinant interleukin-3 in Diamond Blackfan anemia. Blood 1994; 83:617.

853. Alter BP, Kumar M, Lockhart LL, et al: Pregnancy in bone marrow failure syndromes: Diamond-Blackfan anaemia and Shwachman-Diamond syndrome. Br J Haematol 1999; 107:49.

854. Wegelius R, Weber TH: Transient erythroblastopenia in childhood. A study of 15 cases. Acta Paediatr Scand 1978; 67:513.

855. Wasser JS, Yolken R, Miller DR, et al: Congenital hypoplastic anemia (Diamond-Blackfan syndrome) terminating in acute myelogenous leukemia. Blood 1978; 51:991.

856. Krishnan EU, Wegner K, Garg SK: Congenital hypoplastic anemia terminating in acute promyelocytic leukemia. Pediatrics 1978; 61:898.

857. Basso G, Cocito MG, Rebuffi L, et al: Congenital hypoplastic anaemia developed in acute megakarioblastic leukaemia. Helv Paediatr Acta 1981; 36:267.

858. Glader BE, Flam MS, Dahl GV, et al: Hematologic malignancies in Diamond Blackfan anemia. Pediatr Res 1990; 27:142A.

859. Mori PG, Haupt R, Fugazza G, et al: Pentasomy 21 in leukemia complicating Diamond-Blackfan anemia. Cancer Genet Cytogenet 1992; 63:70.

860. Haupt R, Dufour C, Dallorso S, et al: Diamond-Blackfan anemia and malignancy: A case report and a review of the literature. Cancer 1996; 77:1961.

861. Aquino VM, Buchanan GR: Osteogenic sarcoma in a child with transfusion-dependent Diamond-Blackfan anemia. J Pediatr Hematol Oncol 1996; 18:230.

862. Giri N, Kang E, Tisdale JF, et al: Clinical and laboratory evidence for a trilineage haematopoietic defect in patients with refractory Diamond-Blackfan anaemia. Br J Haematol 2000; 108:167.

863. Greinix HT, Storb R, Sanders JE, et al: Long-term survival and cure after marrow transplantation for congenital hypoplastic anaemia (Diamond-Blackfan syndrome). Br J Haematol 1993; 84:515.

864. Frappaz D, Richard O, Perrot S, et al: Maladie de Blackfan-Diamond et malignité: relations de cause à effet? Pediatrie 1992; 47:535.

865. van Dijken PJ, Verwijs W: Diamond-Blackfan anemia and malignancy. A case report and review of the literature. Cancer 1995; 76:517.

866. Hayashi AK, Kang YS, Smith BM: Non-Hodgkin's lymphoma in a patient with Diamond-Blackfan anemia. AJR Am J Roentgenol 1999; 173:117.

867. Steinherz PG, Canale VC, Miller DR: Hepatocellular carcinoma, transfusion-induced hemochromatosis and congenital hypoplastic anemia (Blackfan-Diamond syndrome). Am J Med 1976; 60:1032.

868. Seip M: Malignant tumors in two patients with Diamond-Blackfan anemia treated with corticosteroids and androgens. Pediatr Hematol Oncol 1994; 11:423.

869. Turcotte R, Bard C, Marton D, et al: Malignant fibrous histiocytoma in a patient with Blackfan-Diamond anemia. Can Assoc Radiol 1994; 45:402.

870. D'Oelsnitz M, Vincent L., De Swarte M, et al: A propos d'un cas de leucémie aigue lymphoblastique survenue après guérison d'une maladie de Blackfan-Diamond. Arch Fr Pediatr 1975; 32:582.

871. Diamond LK, Allen DM, Magill FB: Congenital (erythroid) hypoplastic anemia. Am J Dis Child 1961; 102:403.

872. Janov A, Leong T, Nathan D, et al: Natural history and sequelae of treatment in patients (Pts) with Diamond-Blackfan anemia (DBA). Blood 1993; 82:311a.

873. Hardisty RM: Diamond-Blackfan anaemia. In Congenital Disorders of Erythropoiesis, Ciba Foundation Symposium 37 (new series). Amsterdam, Elsevier, 1976, p 89.

874. Ladenstein R, Peters C, Minkov M, et al: A single centre experience with allogeneic stem cell transplantation for severe aplastic anaemia in childhood. Klin Paediatr 1997; 209:201.

875. Rossbach H-C, Grana NH, Barbosa JL: Successful management of concomitant Diamond-Blackfan anaemia and aplastic anaemia with splenectomy. Br J Haematol 1999; 106:569.

876. Baar HS: The life span of red blood corpuscles in erythronophthisis. Acta Haematol 1952; 7:17.

877. Wranne L: Transient erythroblastopenia in infancy and childhood. Scand J Haematol 1970; 7:76.

878. Skeppner G, Wranne L: Transient erythroblastopenia of childhood in Sweden: Incidence and findings at the time of diagnosis. Acta Paediatr 1993; 82:574.

879. Link MP, Alter BP: Fetal erythropoiesis during recovery from transient erythroblastopenia of childhood (TEC). Pediatr Res 1981; 15:1036.

880. Young RSK, Rannels E, Hilmo A, et al: Severe anemia in childhood presenting as transient ischemic attacks. Stroke 1983; 14:622.

881. Michelson AD, Marshall PC: Transient neurological disorder associated with transient erythroblastopenia of childhood. Am J Pediatr Hematol Oncol 1987; 9:161.

882. Beresford CH, Macfarlane SD: Temporal clustering of transient erythroblastopenia (cytopenia) of childhood. Aust Paediatr J 1987; 23:351.

883. Elian JC, Frappaz D, Pozzetto B, et al: Transient erythroblastopenia of childhood presenting with echovirus 11 infection. Acta Paediatr 1993; 62:492.

884. Hefelfinger DC: Simultaneous hyperphosphatasemia and erythroblastopenia of childhood. Clin Pediatr 1993; 32:175.

885. Chabali R: Transient erythroblastopenia of childhood presenting with shock and metabolic acidosis. Pediatr Emerg Care 1994; 10:278.

886. Colina KF, Abelson HT: Resolution of breath-holding spells with treatment of concomitant anemia. J Pediatr 1995; 126:395.

887. Chan GCF, Kanwar VS, Wilimas J: Transient erythroblastopenia of childhood associated with transient neurologic deficit: Report of a case and review of the literature. J Paediatr Child Health 1998; 34:299.

888. Tam DA, Rash FC: Breath-holding spells in a patient with transient erythroblastopenia of childhood. J Pediatr 1997; 130:651.

889. Toogood IRG, Speed IE, Cheney KC, et al: Idiopathic transient normocytic, normochromic anaemia of childhood. Aust Paediatr J 1978; 14:28.

890. Labotka RJ, Maurer HS, Honig GR: Transient erythroblastopenia of childhood. Review of 17 cases, including a pair of identical twins. Am J Dis Child 1981; 135:937.

891. Ritchey AK, Dainiak N, Hoffman R: Variable in vitro erythropoiesis in patients with transient erythroblastopenia of childhood. Yale J Biol Med 1985; 58:1.

892. Schroder H: Transient erythroblastopenia in children. Ugeskr Laeger 1983; 145:2140.

893. Douchain F, Leborgne JM, Robin M, et al: Erythroblastopenie aigue par l'intolerance au dipropyl acetate de sodium. Premiere observation. Nouv Press Med 1980; 9:1715.

894. Glader BE: Diagnosis and management of red cell aplasia in children. Hematol Oncol Clin North Am 1987; 1:431.

895. Skeppner G, Forestier E, Henter JI, et al: Transient red cell aplasia in siblings: A common environmental or a common hereditary factor? Acta Paediatr 1998; 87:43.

896. Seip M: Transient erythroblastopenia in siblings. Acta Paediatr Scand 1982; 71:689.

897. Gerrits GPJM, van Oostrom CG, de Vaan GAM: Severe anemia caused by transient erythroblastopenia in children (TEC). Tijdschr Kindergeneeskd 1982; 50:97.

898. Wang WC, Mentzer WC: Differentiation of transient erythroblastopenia of childhood from congenital hypoplastic anemia. J Pediatr 1976; 88:784.

899. Papayannopoulou Th, Vichinsky E, Stamatoyannopoulos G: Fetal Hb production during acute erythroid expansion. I. Observations in patients with transient erythroblastopenia and post-phlebotomy. Br J Haematol 1980; 44:535.

900. Dover GJ, Boyer SH, Zinkham WH: Production of erythrocytes that contain fetal hemoglobin in anemia. Transient in vivo changes. J Clin Invest 1979; 63:173.

901. Young NS, Mortimer PP, Moore JG, et al: Characterization of a virus that causes transient aplastic crisis. J Clin Invest 1984; 73:224.

902. Mortimer PP, Humphries RK, Moore JG, et al: A human parvovirus-like virus inhibits haematopoietic colony formation in vitro. Nature 1983; 302:426.

903. Mortimer PP: A virological perspective on bone marrow failure. In Young NS, Levine AS, Humphries RK (eds): Aplastic Anemia: Stem Cell Biology and Advances in Treatment. New York, Alan R. Liss, 1984, p 121.

904. Lovric VA: Anaemia and temporary erythroblastopenia in children. A syndrome. Aust Ann Med 1970; 1:34.

905. Freedman MH: 'Recurrent' erythroblastopenia of childhood. An IgM-mediated RBC aplasia. Am J Dis Child 1983; 137:458.

906. Lewis SM, Verwilghen RL: Dyserythropoiesis: Definition, diagnosis and assessment. In Lewis SM, Verwilghen RL (eds): Dyserythropoiesis, London, Academic Press, 1977, p 3.

907. Frisch B, Lewis SM: The bone marrow in aplastic anaemia: Diagnostic and prognostic features. J Clin Pathol 1974; 27:231.

908. Rozman C, Feliu E, Granena A, et al: Transient dyserythropoiesis in repopulated human bone marrow following transplantation: An ultrastructural study. Br J Haematol 1982; 50:63.

909. Lewis SM, Verwilghen RL (eds): Dyserythropoiesis. London, Academic Press, 1977, 350.

910. Crookston JH, Crookston MC, Burnie KL, et al: Hereditary erythroblastic multinuclearity associated with a positive acidified-serum test: A type of congenital dyserythropoietic anaemia. Br J Haematol 1969; 17:11.

911. Heimpel H: Congenital dyserythropoietic anaemia type I: Clinical and experimental aspects. In: Congenital Disorders of Erythropoiesis, CIBA Foundation Symposium 37. Amsterdam, Elsevier, 1976, p 135.

912. Heimpel H: Congenital dyserythropoietic anaemia, type I. In Lewis SM, Verwilghen RL (eds): Dyserythropoiesis, London, Academic Press, 1977, p 55.

913. Heimpel H, Forteza-Vila J, Queisser W, et al: Electron and light microscopic study of the erythroblasts of patients with congenital dyserythropoietic anemia. Blood 1971; 37:299.

914. Lewis SM, Frisch B: Congenital dyserythropoietic anaemias: Electron microscopy. In: Congenital Disorders of Erythropoiesis, CIBA Foundation Symposium 37. Amsterdam, Elsevier, 1976, p 171.

915. Breton-Gorius J, Daniel MT, Clauvel JP, et al: Anomalies ultrastructurales des erythroblastes et des erythrocytes dans six cas de dyserythropoiese congenitale. Nouv Rev Fr Hematol 1973; 13:23.

916. Vainchenker W, Guichard J, Bouguet J, et al: Congenital dyserythropoietic anaemia type I: Absence of clonal expression in the nuclear abnormalities of cultured erythroblasts. Br J Haematol 1980; 46:33.

917. Tamary H, Shalmon L, Shalev H, et al: Localization of the gene for congenital dyserythropoietic anemia type I to a <1-cM interval on chromosome 15q15.1–15.3. Am J Hum Genet 1998; 62:1062.

918. Hodges VM, Molloy GY, Wickramasinghe SN: Genetic heterogeneity of congenital dyserythropoietic anemia type I. Blood 1999; 94:1139.

919. Shalev H, Moser A, Kapelushnik J, et al: Congenital dyserythropoietic anemia type I presenting as persistent pulmonary hypertension of the newborn. J Pediatr 2000; 136:553.

920. Kato K, Sugitani M, Kawataki M, et al: Congenital dyserythropoietic anemia type 1 with fetal onset of severe anemia. J Pediatr Hematol Oncol 2001; 23:63.

921. Lavabre-Bertrand T, Blanc P, Navarro R, et al: Alpha-interferon therapy for congenital dyserythropoiesis type I. Br J Haematol 1995; 89:929.

922. Virjee S, Hatton C: Congenital dyserthropoiesis type I and alpha-interferon therapy. Br J Haematol 1996; 94:579.

923. Wickramasinghe SN: Response of CDA type I to alpha-interferon. Eur J Haematol 1997; 58:121.

924. Wickramasinghe SN, Hasan R, Smythe J: Reduced interferon-alpha production by Epstein-Barr virus transformed B-lymphoblastoid cell lines and lectin-stimulated lymphocytes in congenital dyserythropoietic anemia type I. Br J Haematol 1997; 98:295.

925. Menike D, Wickramasinghe SN: Effects of four species of interferon-α on cultured erythroid progenitors from congenital dyserythropoietic anemia type I. Br J Haematol 1998; 103:825.

926. Ariffin WA, Karnaneedi S, Choo K, et al: Congenital dyserythropoietic anaemia: Report of three cases. J Paediatr Child Health 1996; 32:191.

927. Verwilghen RL, Lewis SM, Dacie JV, et al: HEMPAS: Congenital dyserythropoietic anaemia (type II). Q J Med 1973; 42:257.

928. Verwilghen RL: Congenital dyserythropoietic anaemia type II (Hempas). In: Congenital Disorders of Erythropoiesis, CIBA Foundation Symposium 37. Amsterdam, Elsevier, 1976, p 151.

929. Fukuda MN: Congenital dyserythropoietic anaemia type II (HEMPAS) and its molecular basis. Bailliere's Clin Haematol 1993; 6:493.

930. Seip M, Skrede S, Bjerve K, et al: A case of variant congenital dyserythropoietic anemia revisited. Scand J Haematol 1982; 28:278.

931. Giblett ER, Crookston MC: Agglutinability of red cells by anti-i in patients with thalassaemia major and other haematological disorders. Nature 1964; 201:1138.

932. Rosse WF, Logue GL, Adams J, et al: Mechanisms of immune lysis of the red cells in hereditary erythroblastic multinuclearity with a positive acidified serum test and paroxysmal nocturnal hemoglobinuria. J Clin Invest 1974; 53:31.

933. Fukuda MN: HEMPAS. Biochim Biophys Acta 1999; 1455:231.

934. Fukuda MN, Dell A, Scartezzini P: Primary defect of congenital dyserythropoietic anemia type II. Failure in glycosylation of erythrocyte lactosaminoglycan proteins caused by lowered N-acetyl-glucosaminyltransferase II. J Biol Chem 1987; 262:7195.

935. Tebbi K, Gross S: Absence of morphological abnormalities in marrow erythrocyte colonies (CFU- E) from a patient with HEMPAS-II. J Lab Clin Med 1978; 91:797.

936. Vainchenker W, Guichard J, Breton-Gorius J: Morphological abnormalities in cultured erythroid colonies (BFU-E) from the blood of two patients with HEMPAS. Br J Haematol 1979; 42:363.

937. Roodman GD, Clare CN, Mills G: Congenital dyserythropoietic anaemia type II (CDA-II): Chromosomal banding studies and adherent cell effects on erythroid colony (CFU-E) and burst (BFU-E) formation. Br J Haematol 1982; 50:499.

938. Gasparini P, del Giudice EM, Delaunay J, et al: Localization of the congenital dyserythropoietic anemia II locus to chromosome 20q11.2 by genomewide search. Am J Hum Genet 1997; 61:1112.

939. Iolascon A, Servedio V, Carbone R, et al: Geographic distribution of CDA-II: Did a founder effect operate in Southern Italy? Haematologica 2000; 85:470.

940. Iolascon A, De Mattia D, Perrotta S, et al: Genetic heterogeneity of congenital dyserythropoietic anemia type II. Blood 1998; 92:2593.

941. Perrotta S, del Giudice M, Carbone R, et al: Gilbert's syndrome accounts for the phenotypic variability of congenital dyserythropoietic anemia type II (CDA-II). J Pediatr 2000; 136:556.

942. Fargion S, Valenti L, Fracanzani AL, et al: Hereditary hemochromatosis in a patient with congenital dyserythropoietic anemia. Blood 2000; 96:3653.

943. Wolff JA, Von Hofe FH: Familial erythroid multinuclearity. Blood 1951; 6:1274.

944. Goudsmit R: Congenital dyserythropoietic anaemia, type III. In Lewis SM, Verwilghen RL (eds): Dyserythropoiesis. London, Academic Press, 1977, p 83.

945. Vainchenker W, Breton-Gorius J, Guichard J, et al: Congenital dyserythropoietic anemia type III. Studies on erythroid differentiation of blood erythroid progenitor cells (BFU-E) in vitro. Exp Hematol 1980; 8:1057.

946. Lind L, Sandstrom H, Wahlin A, et al: Localization of the gene for congenital dyserythropoietic anemia type III, CDAN3, to chromosome 15q21-q25. Hum Mol Genet 1995; 4:109.

947. Sandstrom H, Wahlin A: Congenital dyserythropoietic anemia type III. Haematologica 2000; 85:753.

948. Wickramasinghe SN: Congenital dyserythropoietic anaemias: Clinical features, haematological morphology and new biochemical data. Blood Rev 1998; 12:178.

949. McBride JA, Wilson WEC, Baillie N: Congenital dyserythropoietic anaemia—type IV. Blood 1971; 38:837.

950. Weatherly TL, Flannery EP, Doyle WF, et al: Congenital dyserythropoietic anemia (CDA) with increased red cell lipids. Am J Med 1974; 57:912.

951. Benjamin JT, Rosse WF, Dalldorf FC, et al: Congenital dyserythropoietic anemia—type IV. J Pediatr 1975; 87:210.

952. Bird AR, Karabus CD, Hartley PS: Type IV congenital dyserythropoietic anemia with an unusual response to splenectomy. Am J Pediatr Hematol Oncol 1985; 7:196.

953. Wickramasinghe SN, Vora AJ, Will A, et al: Transfusion-dependent congenital dyserythropoietic anaemia with non-specific dysplastic changes in erythroblasts. Eur J Haematol 1998; 60:140.

954. Weatherall DH, Clegg JB, Knox-Macaulay HHM, et al: A genetically determined disorder with features both of thalassaemia and congenital dyserythropoietic anaemia. Br J Haematol 1973; 24:681.

955. Hruby MA, Mason RG, Honig GR: Unbalanced globin chain synthesis in congenital dyserythropoietic anemia. Blood 1973; 42:843.

956. Eldor A, Matzner Y, Kahane I, et al: Aberrant congenital dyserythropoietic anemia with negative acidified serum tests and features of thalassemia in a Kurdish family. Isr J Med Sci 1978; 14:1138.

957. Wickramasinghe SN, Illum N, Wimberley PD: Congenital dyserythropoietic anaemia with novel intra-erythroblastic and intra-erythrocytic inclusions. Br J Haematol 1991; 79:322.

958. Tang W, Cai S-P, Eng B, et al: Expression of embryonic ς-globin and ε-globin chains in a 10-year-old girl with congenital anemia. Blood 1993; 81:1636.

959. Dell'Orbo C, Marchi A, Quacci D: Ultrastructural findings of congenital dyserythropoietic sickle cell beta thal-associated anemia. Histol Histopathol 1992; 7:7.

960. Sansone G, Lupi L: An aberrant type of congenital dyserythropoietic anemia associated with a beta-thalassemia trait. Ann Hematol 1991; 62:184.

961. Sansone G, Masera G, Cantu-Rajnoldi, et al: An unclassified case of congenital dyserythropoietic anaemia with a severe neonatal onset. Acta Haematol 1992; 88:41.

962. Roberts DJ, Nadel A, Lage J, et al: An unusual variant of congenital dyserythropoietic anaemia with mild maternal and lethal fetal disease. Br J Haematol 1993; 84:549.

963. Parsons SF, Jones J, Anstee DJ, et al: A novel form of congenital dyserythropoietic anemia associated with deficiency of erythroid CD44 and a unique blood group phenotype [In(a-b-), Co(a-b-)]. Blood 1994; 83:860.

964. Brochstein JA, Siena S, Weinberg RS, et al: Congenital dyserythropoietic anemia (CDA) with karyorrhexis. Pediatr Res 1985; 19:258A.

965. Kostmann R: Infantile genetic agranulocytosis. A new recessive lethal disease in man. Acta Paediatr Scand 1956; 45:1.

966. Kostmann R: Infantile genetic agranulocytosis. A review with presentation of ten new cases. Acta Paediatr Scand 1975; 64:362.

967. Dale DC, Person RE, Bolyard AA, et al: Mutations in the gene encoding neutrophil elastase in congenital and cyclic neutropenia. Blood 2000; 96:2317.

968. Iselius L, Gustavson KH: Spatial distribution of the gene for infantile genetic agranulocytosis. Hum Hered 1984; 34:358.

969. Coulombel L, Morardet N, Veber F, et al: Granulopoietic differentiation in long-term bone marrow cultures from children with congenital neutropenia. Am J Hematol 1988; 27:93.

970. Zucker-Franklin D, L'Esperance P, Good RA: Congenital neutropenia: An intrinsic cell defect demonstrated by electron microscopy of soft agar colonies. Blood 1977; 49:425.

971. Hestdal K, Welte K, Lie SO, et al: Severe congenital neutropenia: Abnormal growth and differentiation of myeloid progenitors to granulocyte colony-stimulating factor (G-CSF) but normal response to G-CSF plus stem cell factor. Blood 1993; 82:2991.

972. Shitara T, Ijima H, Yugami S-I, et al: Increased cytokine levels and abnormal response of myeloid progenitor cells to granulocyte colony-stimulating factor in a case of severe congenital neutropenia. In vitro effects of stem cell factor. Am J Pediatr Hematol Oncol 1994; 16:167.

973. Bernhardt TM, Burchardt ER, Welte K: Assessment of G-CSF and GM-CSF mRNA expression in peripheral blood mononuclear cells from patients with severe congenital neutropenia and in human myeloid leukemic cell lines. Exp Hematol 1993; 21:163.

974. Mempel K, Pietsch T, Menzel T, et al: Increased serum levels of granulocyte colony-stimulating factor in patients with severe congenital neutropenia. Blood 1991; 77:1919.

975. Guba SC, Sartor CA, Hutchinson R, et al: Granulocyte colony-stimulating factor (G-CSF) production and G-CSF receptor structure in patients with congenital neutropenia. Blood 1994; 83:1486.

976. Sandoval C, Parganas E, Wang W, et al: Lack of alterations in the cytoplasmic domains of the granulocyte colony-stimulating factor receptors in eight cases of severe congenital neutropenia. Blood 1995; 85:852.

977. Horwitz M, Benson KF, Person RE, et al: Mutations in ELA2, encoding neutrophil elastase, define a 21-day biological clock in cyclic haematopoiesis. Nat Genet 1999; 23:433.

978. Li FQ, Horwitz M: Characterization of mutant neutrophil elastase in severe congenital neutropenia. J Biol Chem 2001; 276:14230.

979. Barrett AJ: Clinical experience with lithium in aplastic anemia and congenital neutropenia. Adv Exp Med Biol 1980; 127:305.

980. Chan HSL, Freedman MH, Saunders EF: Lithium therapy of children with chronic neutropenia. Am J Med 1981; 70:1073.

981. Bonilla MA, Gillio AP, Ruggeiro M, et al: Effects of recombinant human granulocyte colony-stimulating factor on neutropenia in patients with congenital agranulocytosis. N Engl J Med 1989; 320:1574.

982. Welte K, Boxer LA: Severe chronic neutropenia: Pathophysiology and therapy. Semin Hematol 1997; 34:267.

983. Welte K, Zeidler C, Reiter A, et al: Differential effects of granulo-cyte-macrophage colony-stimulating factor and granulocyte colony-stimulating factor in children with severe congenital neutropenia. Blood 1990; 75:1056.

984. Fewtrell MS, Kinsey SE, Williams DM, et al: Bone mineralization and turnover in children with congenital neutropenia, and its relationship to treatment with recombinant human granulocyte-colony stimulating factor. Br J Haematol 1997; 97:7434.

985. Yakisan E, Schirg E, Zeidler C, et al: High incidence of significant bone loss in patients with severe congenital neutropenia (Kostmann's syndrome). J Pediatr 1997; 131:592.

986. Zeidler C, Welte K, Barak Y, et al: Stem cell transplantation in patients with severe congenital neutropenia without evidence of leukemic transformation. Blood 2000; 95:1195.

987. Cividalli G, Yarkoni S, Dar H, et al: Can infantile hereditary agranulocytosis be diagnosed prenatally? Prenat Diagn 1983; 3:157.

988. Millar DS, Davis LR, Rodeck CH, et al: Normal blood cell values in the early mid-trimester fetus. Prenat Diagn 1985; 5:367.

989. Miller RW: Childhood cancer and congenital defects. A study of U.S. death certificates during the period 1960–1966. Pediat Res 1969; 3:389.

990. Gilman PA, Jackson DP, Guild HG: Congenital agranulocytosis: Prolonged survival and terminal acute leukemia. Blood 1970; 36:576.

991. Rosen RB, Kang S-J: Congenital agranulocytosis terminating in acute myelomonocytic leukemia. J Pediatr 1979; 94:406.

992. Wong W-Y, Williams D, Slovak ML, et al: Terminal acute myelogenous leukemia in a patient with congenital agranulocytosis. Am J Hematol 1993; 43:133.

993. Lui V, Ragab AH, Findley H, et al: Infantile genetic agranulocytosis and acute lymphocytic leukemia in two sibs. J Pediatr 1978; 92:1028.

994. Freedman MH, Bonilla MA, Fier C, et al: Myelodysplasia syndrome and acute myeloid leukemia in patients with congenital neutropenia receiving G-CSF therapy. Blood 2000; 96:429.

995. Mantadakis E, Shannon KM, Singer DA, et al: Transient monosomy 7. A case series in children and review of the literature. Cancer 1999; 85:2655.

996. Dong F, Brynes RK, Tidow N, et al: Mutations in the gene for the granulocyte colony-stimulating-factor receptor in patients with acute myeloid leukemia preceded by severe congenital neutropenia. N Engl J Med 1995; 333:487.

997. Tidow N, Pilz C, Kasper B, et al: Frequency of point mutations in the gene for the G-CSF receptor in patients with chronic neutropenia undergoing G-CSF therapy. Stem Cells 1997; 15:113.

998. Hermans MHA, Antonissen C, Ward AC, et al: Sustained receptor activation and hyperproliferation in response to granulocyte colony-stimulating factor (G-CSF) in mice with a severe congenital neutropenia/acute myeloid leukemia-derived mutation in the G-CSF receptor. J Exp Med 1999; 189:683.

999. Hall JG, Levin J, Kuhn JP, et al: Thrombocytopenia with absent radius (TAR). Medicine (Baltimore) 1969; 48:411.

1000. Hall JG: Thrombocytopenia and absent radius (TAR) syndrome. J Med Genet 1987; 24:79.

1001. Hedberg VA, Lipton JM: Thrombocytopenia with absent radii. A review of 100 cases. Am J Pediatr Hematol Oncol 1988; 10:51.

1002. Messen S, Vargas L, Garcia H, et al: Congenital thrombocytopenia and absent radius syndrome in identical twins. Rev Chil Pediatr 1986; 57:559.

1003. Gounder DS, Ockelford PA, Pullon HW, et al: Clinical manifestations of the thrombocytopenia and absent radii (TAR) syndrome. Aust NZ J Med 1989; 19:479.

1004. Dodesini G, Frigerio G, Cocco E: La trombocitopenia congenita ipoplastica con aplasia bilaterale del radio. Minerva Pediatr 1979; 31:1023.

1005. Teufel M, Enders H, Dopfer R: Consanguinity in a Turkish family with thrombocytopenia with absent radii (TAR) syndrome. Hum Genet 1983; 64:94.

1006. Shalev E, Weiner E, Feldman E, et al: Micrognathia—Prenatal ultrasonographic diagnosis. Int J Gynaecol Obstetr 1983; 21:343.

1007. Ceballos-Quintal JM, Pinto-Escalante D, Gongora-Biachi RA: TAR-like syndrome in a consanguineous Mayan girl. Am J Med Genet 1992; 43:805.

1008. Nilsson LR, Lundholm G: Congenital thrombocytopenia associated with aplasia of the radius. Acta Paediatr 1960; 49:291.

1009. Whitfield MF, Barr DGD: Cow's milk allergy in the syndrome of thrombocytopenia with absent radius. Arch Dis Child 1976; 51:337.

1010. Adeyokunnu AA: Radial aplasia and amegakaryocytic thrombocytopenia (TAR syndrome) among Nigerian children. Am J Dis Child 1984; 138:346.

1011. Fromm B, Niethard FU, Marquardt E: Thrombocytopenia and absent radius (TAR) syndrome. Int Orthop 1991; 15:95.

1012. Bajaj R, Jain M, Kasat L, et al: Tar syndrome with unilateral absent radius and associated esophageal atresia: A variant? Indian J Pediatr 1999; 66:460.

1013. Bessman JD, Harrison RL, Howard LC, et al: The megakaryocyte abnormality in thrombocytopenia-absent radius syndrome. Blood 1983; 62:143a.

1014. Sultan Y, Scrobohaci ML, Jeanneau C, et al: Anomalies de la lignee plaquettaire au cours du syndrome d'aplasie radiale avec thrombocytopenie. Nouv Rev Franc Hematol 1973; 13:573.

1015. Day HJ, Holmsen H: Platelet adenine nucleotide "storage pool deficiency" in thrombocytopenic absent radii syndrome. JAMA 1972; 221:1053.

1016. Linch DC, Stewart JW, West C: Blood and bone marrow cultures in a case of thrombocytopenia with absent radii. Clin Lab Haematol 1982; 4:313.

1017. Homans AC, Cohen JL, Mazur EM: Defective megakaryocytopoiesis in the syndrome of thrombocytopenia with absent radii. Br J Haematol 1988; 70:205.

1018. Michalevicz R, Baron S, Burstein Y: Osteoclast-like cells grow in cultures of multipotent hematopoietic progenitors in thrombocytopenia and absent radii (TAR) syndrome. Isr J Med Sci 1988; 24:42.

1019. Akabutu J, Vergidis D, Poololak-Doiwidziak M, et al: Studies of hematopoietic progenitor cells in thrombocytopenia with absent radii (TAR) syndrome. Blood 1988; 72:78a.

1020. Kanz L, Kostjelniak E, Welte K: Colony-stimulating activity (CSA) unique for the megakaryocytic hemopoietic cell lineage, present in the plasma of a patient with the syndrome of thrombocytopenia with absent radii (TAR). Blood 1989; 74:248a.

1021. de Alarcon PA, Graeve JLA, Levine RF, et al: Thrombocytopenia and absent radii syndrome: A defect in megakaryocyte maturation. Blood 1988; 72:321a.

1022. Ballmaier M, Schulze H, Cremer M, et al: Defective *c-Mpl* signaling in the syndrome of thrombocytopenia with absent radii. Stem Cells 1998; 16:177.

1023. Letestu R, Vitrat N, Masse A, et al: Existence of a differentiation blockage at the stage of a megakaryocyte precursor in the thrombocytopenia and absent radii (TAR) syndrome. Blood 2000; 95:1633.

1024. Strippoli P, Savoia A, Iolascon A, et al: Mutational screening of thrombopoietin receptor (*c-mpl*) in patients with congenital thrombocytopenia and absent radii (TAR). Br J Haematol 1998; 103:311.

1025. Armitage JO, Hoak JC, Elliott TE, et al: Syndrome of thrombocytopenia and absent radii: Qualitatively normal platelets with remission following splenectomy. Scand J Haematol 1978; 20:25.

1026. Brochstein JA, Shank B, Kernan NA, et al: Marrow transplantation for thrombocytopenia-absent radii syndrome. J Pediatr 1992; 121:587.

1027. Camitta BM, Rock A: Acute lymphoidic leukemia in a patient with thrombocytopenia/absent radii (TAR) syndrome. Am J Pediatr Hematol Oncol 1993; 15:335.

1028. Katzenstein HM, Bowman LC, Brodeur GM, et al: Prognostic significance of age, *MYCN* oncogene amplification, tumor cell ploidy, and histology in 110 infants with stage D(S) neuroblastoma: The Pediatric Oncology Group Experience—A Pediatric Oncology Group Study. J Clin Oncol 1998; 16:2007.

1029. Symonds RP, Clark BJ, George WD, et al: Thrombocytopenia with absent radii (TAR) syndrome: A new increased cellular radiosensitivity syndrome. Clin Oncol 1995; 7:56.

1030. Omenn GS, Figley MM, Graham CB, et al: Prospects for radiographic intrauterine diagnosis—The syndrome of thrombocytopenia with absent radii. N Engl J Med 1973; 288:777.

1031. Luthy DA, Hall JG, Graham CB: Prenatal diagnosis of thrombocytopenia with absent radii. Clin Genet 1979; 15:495.

1032. Hobbins JC, Bracken MB, Mahoney MJ: Diagnosis of fetal skeletal dysplasias with ultrasound. Am J Obstet Gynecol 1982; 142:306.

1033. Filkins K, Russo J, Bilinki I, et al: Prenatal diagnosis of thrombocytopenia absent radius syndrome using ultrasound and fetoscopy. Prenat Diagn 1984; 4:139.

1034. Labrune PH, Pons JC, Khalil M, et al: Antenatal thrombocytopenia in three patients with TAR (thrombocytopenia with absent radii) syndrome. Prenat Diagn 1993; 13:463.

1035. Donnenfeld AE, Wiseman B, Lavi E, et al: Prenatal diagnosis of thrombocytopenia absent radius syndrome by ultrasound and cordocentesis. Prenat Diagn 1990; 10:29.

1036. Weinblatt M, Petrikovsky B, Bialer M, et al: Prenatal evaluation and in utero platelet transfusion for thrombocytopenia absent radii syndrome. Prenat Diagn 1994; 14:892.

1037. Daffos F, Forestier F, Kaplan C, et al: Prenatal diagnosis and management of bleeding disorders with fetal blood sampling. Am J Obstet Gynecol 1988; 158:939.

1038. Vaughan JM: Leuco-erythroblastic anaemia. J Pathol Bacteriol 1936; 42:541.

1039. Weick JK, Hagedorn AB, Linman JW: Leukoerythroblastosis. Diagnostic and prognostic significance. Mayo Clin Proc 1974; 49:110.

1040. Sills RH, Hadley RAR: The significance of nucleated red blood cells in the peripheral blood of children. Am J Pediatr Hematol Oncol 1983; 5:173.

1041. Albers-Schonberg H: Roentgenbilder einer seltenen Knochenerkrankung. Munch Med Wochenschr 1904; 51:365.

1042. Johnston CC, Jr, Lavy N, Lord T, et al: Osteopetrosis. A clinical, genetic, metabolic, and morphologic study of the dominantly inherited, benign form. Medicine (Baltimore) 1968; 47:149.

1043. Shapiro F: Osteopetrosis. Current clinical considerations. Clin Orthop Rel Res 1993; 294:34.

1044. Gerritsen EJA, Vossen JM, van Loo IHG, et al: Autosomal recessive osteopetrosis: Variability of findings at diagnosis and during the natural course. Pediatrics 1994; 93:247.

1045. Bollerslev J, Mosekilde L: Autosomal dominant osteopetrosis. Clin Orthop Rel Res 1993; 294:45.

1046. Sly WS, Hewett-Emmett D, Whyte MP, et al: Carbonic anhydrase II deficiency identified as the primary defect in the autosomal recessive syndrome of osteopetrosis with renal tubular acidosis and cerebral calcification. Proc Natl Acad Sci USA 1983; 80:2752.

1047. Schiliro G, Musumeci S, Pizzarelli G, et al: Fetal haemoglobin in early malignant osteopetrosis. Br J Haematol 1978; 38:339.

1048. Farber S, Vawter GF: Clinical pathological conference. J Pediatr 1965; 67:133.

1049. Sjölin S: Studies on osteopetrosis. II. Investigations concerning the nature of the anaemia. Acta Paediatr 1959; 48:529.

1050. Ash P, Loutit JF, Townsend KMS: Osteoclasts derived from haematopoietic stem cells. Nature 1980; 283:669.

1051. Marshall MJ, Nisbet NW, Menage J, et al: Tissue repopulation during cure of osteopetrotic (*mi/mi*) mice using normal and defective (*Wᵉ/Wᵛ*) bone marrow. Exp Hematol 1982; 10:600.

1052. Scheven BAA, Visser JWM, Nijweide PJ: In vitro osteoclast generation from different bone marrow fractions, including a highly enriched haematopoietic stem cell population. Nature 1986; 321:79.

1053. van Hul W, Bollerslev J, Gram J, et al: Localization of a gene for autosomal dominant osteopetrosis (Albers-Schonberg disease) to chromosome 1p21. Am J Hum Genet 1996; 61:363.

1054. Sly WS, Whyte MP, Sundaram V, et al: Carbonic anhydrase II deficiency in 12 families with the autosomal recessive syndrome of osteopetrosis with renal tubular acidosis and cerebral calcification. N Engl J Med 1985; 313:139.

1055. Hu PY, Roth DE, Skaggs LA, et al: A splice junction mutation in intron 2 of the carbonic anhydrase II gene of osteopetrosis patients from Arabic countries. Hum Mutat 1992; 1:288.

1056. Heaney C, Shalev H, Elbedour K, et al: Human autosomal recessive osteopetrosis maps to 11q13, a position predicted by comparative mapping of the murine osteosclerosis (oc) mutation. Hum Mol Genet 1998; 7:1407.

1057. Frattini A, Orchard PJ, Sobacchi C, et al: Defects in TCIRG1 subunit of the vacuolar proton pump are responsible for a subset of human autosomal recessive osteopetrosis. Nat Genet 2000; 25:343.

1058. Kornak U, Schulz A, Friedrich W, et al: Mutations in the a3 subunit of the vacuolar H⁺-ATPase cause infantile malignant osteopetrosis. Hum Mol Genet 2000; 9:2059.

1059. Kornak U, Kasper D, Bosl MR, et al: Loss of the ClC-7 chloride channel leads to osteopetrosis in mice and man. Cell 2001; 104:205.

1060. Moe PJ, Skjaeveland A: Therapeutic studies in osteopetrosis. Report of 4 cases. Acta Paediatr Scand 1969; 58:593.

1061. Reeves J, Huffer W, August CS, et al: The hematopoietic effects of prednisone therapy in four infants with osteopetrosis. J Pediatr 1979; 94:210.

1062. Key L, Carnes D, Cole S, et al: Treatment of congenital osteopetrosis with high-dose calcitriol. N Engl J Med 1984; 310:409.

1063. van Lie Peters EM, Aronson DC, Everts V, et al: Failure of calcitriol treatment in a patient with malignant osteopetrosis. Eur J Pediatr 1993; 152:818.

1064. Key LL, Rodriguiz RM, Willi SM, et al: Long-term treatment of osteopetrosis with recombinant human interferon gamma. N Engl J Med 1995; 332:1594.

1065. Meletis J, Samarkos M, Michali E, et al: Correction of anaemia and thrombocytopenia in a case of adult type I osteopetrosis with recombinant human erythropoietin (rHuEPO). Br J Haematol 1995; 89:911.

1066. Fasth A, Porras O: Human malignant osteopetrosis: Pathophysiology, management and the role of bone marrow transplantation. Pediatr Transplant 1999; 3:102.

1067. Kapelushnik J, Shalev C, Yaniv I, et al: Osteopetrosis: a single centre experience of stem cell transplantation and prenatal diagnosis. Bone Marrow Transplant 2001; 27:129.

1068. Locatelli F, Beluffi G, Giorgiani G, et al: Transplantation of cord blood progenitor cells can promote bone resorption in autosomal recessive osteopetrosis. Bone Marrow Transplant 1997; 20:701.

1069. Jenkinson EL, Pfisterer WH, Latteier KK, et al: A prenatal diagnosis of osteopetrosis. Am J Roentgenol 1943; 49:455.

1070. Golbus MS, Koerper MA, Hall BD: Failure to diagnose osteopetrosis in utero. Lancet 1976; 2:1246.

1071. Khazen NE, Faverly D, Vamos E, et al: Lethal osteopetrosis with multiple factures in utero. Am J Med Genet 1986; 23:811.

1072. Dini G, Floris R, Garaventa A, et al: Long-term follow-up of two children with a variant of mild autosomal recessive osteopetrosis undergoing bone marrow transplantation. Bone Marrow Transplant 2000; 26:219.

1073. Shalev H, Mishori-Dery A, Kapelushnik J, et al: Prenatal diagnosis of malignant osteopetrosis in Bedouin families by linkage analysis. Prenat Diagn 2001; 21:183.

9 | Principles of Bone Marrow and Stem Cell Transplantation

Leslie Lehmann • W. Nicholas Haining • Eva C. Guinan

Stem cell transplantation (SCT) has become an accepted therapeutic modality for a wide variety of diseases, including hematologic malignancies, aplastic anemia, immunodeficiency disorders, congenital hematologic defects, and some solid tumors. Preparation for SCT has traditionally involved delivery of chemotherapy and radiation therapy to ablate normal (and abnormal) hematopoiesis and provide sufficient immunosuppression to allow donor cell engraftment. Subsequent protracted immune compromise and risk for opportunistic infections as well as the sequelae of other complications such as graft rejection, graft-verus-host disease (GVHD), and the recurrence of the primary disease have limited the success of SCT. However, advances in understanding the biology of SCT coupled with advances in the supportive care and clinical management of stem cell transplant recipients have made this approach an increasingly effective therapy.

Infusion of bone marrow in an effort to restore hematopoiesis was first reported in 1939: a patient with aplastic anemia was treated by regular transfusions as well as the infusion of a small aliquot of bone marrow from his brother.[1] Subsequently, Jacobson and his colleagues[2, 3] demonstrated that normal hematopoiesis could be restored in lethally irradiated mice by shielding their spleens from radiation. Later, it became clear that the protective effect came from elements in the bone marrow or spleen that could reconstitute hematopoiesis in irradiated animals.[4] These hematopoietic stem cells (HSCs) could function after cryopreservation and thawing.[5] Investigators subsequently demonstrated that animals did well if histocompatible HSCs were infused, but they suffered from GVHD, then termed *secondary disease*, if given cells from a histoincompatible donor.[6] Better understanding of the biology of the immune response coupled with the observation that administration of methotrexate was effective in both the prophylaxis and treatment of GVHD[7] provided both the theoretical and practical tools to enable human SCT studies.

HISTORY AND OVERVIEW

The first attempt to transplant human bone marrow was carried out in 1957 by E. Donnall Thomas, whose body of work in this area was later recognized by a Nobel Prize. In 1959, lethal doses of total-body irradiation (TBI) and bone marrow from an identical twin were used to perform transplants in two patients with advanced acute lymphoblastic leukemia.[8] Hematopoiesis was established within weeks, although again the patients had relapses and died later. These first experiments demonstrated that chemotherapy followed by intravenous marrow infusion could result in a transient graft, although all patients subsequently died of progressive disease.[9] Longer survival after allogeneic SCT was first achieved in 1968 and 1969 with the survival of three patients given transplants for different congenital immunodeficiencies although clinical responses were not yet optimal.[10–13]

SCT is currently used in a number of malignant and nonmalignant disorders in which replacement of HSC-derived populations of cells is necessary or may be beneficial. Although bone marrow was initially considered the only source of pluripotent HSCs, more recently it has become clear that other sources exist. For example, self-renewing HSCs can be collected from umbilical cord blood (UCB). The low absolute number of HSCs in peripheral blood can be increased after chemotherapy or administration of hematopoietic growth factors and collected as mobilized peripheral blood stem cells (PBSCs). Exploration of the potential for cell populations derived from tissues such as liver, nervous system, and muscle to provide HSC has been initiated.[14–18]

Reinfusion of a patient's own HSCs after administration of high-dose chemotherapy, radiation therapy, or both is referred to as autologous SCT. Both tumor contamination and preexisting damage to HSCs from prior therapy limit its application in patients with malignant disease in whom lack of autologous immunologic response against any residual or recurrent tumor may further limit success. For most patients with benign diseases, the intrinsic abnormalities of the HSCs prevent autologous SCT from being a meaningful option. Allogeneic SCT involves the infusion of HSCs from a related or unrelated donor (UD). Complications of allogeneic SCT, such as graft rejection and GVHD, are generally more common or severe with increasing histoincompatibility between donor and host, and a histocompatible sibling, if available, remains the preferred donor. However, it is estimated that only 15 to 40 percent of patients will have a matched related donor,[19, 20] a number likely to decrease with the current socioeconomic pressures that lead to limited nuclear family size. Alternatives available include a transplant that is mismatched (haploidentical) from a related donor[21, 22] and transplants from donors in the UD pool,[23–25] including UD UCB collections.[26–28] Finally, the patient may undergo autologous SCT if the disease is appropriate or the HSCs are not involved with the disease process.

The specific conditioning regimens used to prepare patients are reviewed in the next section. In brief, the preparative regimen must reduce or eliminate tumor burden and recipient hematopoietic cells and provide sufficient immunosuppression to permit engraftment. These directives must be modified for patients with congenital immunodeficiencies and benign hematopoietic disorders. After conditioning, HSCs are infused into the host; the day of HSC infusion is generally referred to as day 0. Neutrophil engraftment occurs approximately 10 to 24 days after infusion, with red cell and platelet recovery being somewhat more delayed. A number of peritransplant and post-transplant complications influence not only survival but also quality of life after transplantation (Table 9–1). There is a risk of early graft rejection and of late graft failure. Early complications of SCT are due to profound pancytopenia, regimen-related toxicity, immunologic reaction of the graft against host tissues (acute GVHD) if the transplant is allogeneic, and protracted immune incompetence. Late complications of SCT are due to chronic end organ damage from drug and immune insults, ongoing or *de novo* manifestations of immune dysregulation such as poor immune function or chronic GVHD, and the consequences of disease recurrence. Each of these factors and complications is considered in detail below.

Given these obstacles, the evolution of SCT into a practical and curative therapy has depended on a number of important advances. These include improved knowledge of the human histocompatibility system and

---

TABLE 9–1. Complications of Bone Marrow Transplantation

SHORT TERM

Graft rejection
Infection
Bleeding
Acute graft-versus-host disease
Veno-occlusive disease of the liver
Idiopathic pneumonitis
Side effects of radiation therapy, chemotherapy, and immunosuppressive therapy (e.g., radiation nephritis, azotemia)

LONG TERM

Late graft failure
Chronic graft-versus-host disease and its sequelae (e.g., bronchiolitis obliterans)
Pulmonary disorders
Infection
Altered intellectual and growth development in children
Reduced stamina
Endocrine dysfunction
   Hypothyroidism
   Growth retardation (children)
   Pubertal delay; gonadal failure
   Sexual dysfunction (both sexes)
Complications secondary to radiation therapy (e.g., cataracts, radiation nephritis)
Complications caused by immunosuppressive therapy (e.g., aseptic necrosis of bone (hips, ankles, shoulders), hemolytic uremic syndrome)
Dental problems
Psychosocial problems
Increased risk of second malignancies

development of more exact methods to establish the degree of histocompatibility between the donor and recipient. Ability to deliver the preparative regimen with greater accuracy, as illustrated both by improvements in TBI dosimetry and strategy and by the ability to monitor busulfan pharmacokinetics, has significantly decreased regimen-related toxicity. Early and aggressive use of antibiotics, antifungal agents, and antiviral agents has improved survival during the early neutropenic period and during the period of profound and persistent immunosuppression after engraftment. Advances in transfusion support, including viral screening tests and irradiation of blood products and the availability of leukopheresed platelet products, have had an enormous impact. Nutritional and other supportive therapies including the ability to establish long-term vascular access with indwelling lines has significantly changed the experience and comfort of stem cell transplant recipients. Whereas SCT was originally offered only to the rare patient with end-stage disease, improved outcomes because of these and other advances have markedly increased the indications for which the procedure is recommended.

Although improvement in supportive care issues, broadly speaking, has been the major focus in the past, current efforts have turned increasingly to graft engineering initiatives. For example, despite the difficulties of translating successful gene transfer into murine HSCs to larger animal models, substantial clinical experience has accumulated regarding gene transfer into human cells, and clinical trials of gene therapy have begun to generate important observations. Brenner and colleagues[29-32] marked bone marrow cells with a retrovirus carrying the *Neo-resistance* gene in pediatric patients with acute myeloblastic leukemia or neuroblastoma to identify the origin of hematopoiesis and relapse after autologous SCT. The first steps in gene therapy have been taken for patients with congenital diseases of the HSC. The cells of immunodeficient patients with adenosine deaminase deficiency have been transduced with retroviral vectors containing a normal adenosine deaminase gene and reinfused into patients.[33-35] Many issues have confounded interpretation of the results and limited detection of virus has been reported. Greater success has been achieved with transduction of autologous HSCs from patients with X-linked severe combined immunodeficiency.[36] Introduction of the defective common cytokine receptor γ-chain contained in a retroviral vector has resulted in appearance of a normal number of T cells with diverse repertoire and, most importantly, sustained resolution of clinical disease. Given the limitations of current approaches, the value of gene therapy as an adjunct or competitor to SCT remains unsettled. Additional graft engineering strategies involving cell separation, *ex vivo* cell expansion, collection of "mega" HSC doses, and infusion of donor lymphocytes as well as other initiatives are in various stages of clinical exploration and are noted below.

CONDITIONING REGIMENS

The first human bone marrow transplantation (BMT) for leukemia carried out by Thomas and colleagues in 1957[8] and a subsequent experience using UD marrow to treat victims of a radiation accident in Belgrade in 1959[37] established the basic principle of TBI-based conditioning. In the 1960s work initiated by Santos, Owens, and Sensenbrenner first delineated the potential utility of cyclophosphamide.[38] However, preparation of patients who had advanced leukemia with cyclophosphamide alone resulted in relapse in all survivors. Relapse was also commonly seen in patients prepared with TBI alone.[38-40] Spurred by inadequate access to costly radiation facilities, busulfan was developed in the early to mid-1970s as an alternative ablative agent.[41]

Over the next decade, the desired effects of conditioning for SCT were generally defined to be threefold: (1) hematopoietic ablation of recipient bone marrow to create space or competitive advantage for donor HSCs, (2) host immunosuppression to prevent graft rejection, and (3) eradication of diseased cells. It became clear that the relative importance of these ends differed among patient populations. For example, persistent significant relapse rates after SCT stimulated attempts to increase antileukemic efficacy by the use of additional high-dose chemotherapy in place of or in combination with cyclophosphamide. In contrast, the emergence of graft failure/rejection as a prominent limitation to T-cell depletion and alternative donor SCT spurred development of new regimens intended to increase recipient immunosuppression. Preparative approaches for patients with aplastic anemia and children with severe combined immunodeficiency disease capitalized on, respectively, their preexisting aplasia and immunosuppression whereas different regimens were developed for benign hematologic diseases.[42] In addition, as autologous HSC support for high-dose chemotherapy became more common, many new conditioning regimens were developed emphasizing potential antitumor effects. Although individual studies demonstrated acceptable or even favorable outcomes related to some of these changes, no consensus on the optimal preparation of the recipient for either autologous or allogeneic SCT has emerged. More recently, alternative concepts regarding the relative roles of conditioning regimens and the donor immune system in achieving recipient hematopoietic ablation have been applied in preclinical and clinical studies of nonmyeloablative or "minitransplantation." Some key issues are highlighted below.

Total-Body Irradiation. Total dose, dose rate, fraction size, interfraction interval, and shielding are among the TBI parameters most manipulated in preparation for SCT. An ideal schedule would maximize killing of malignant cells, hematopoietic ablation, and, in the case of allogeneic SCT, immunosuppression while limiting acute and chronic toxicity. In principle, higher total dose, higher dose rate, and larger fraction size are associated with greater hematopoietic ablative effect (and therefore potentially greater antileukemic efficacy) and with better immunosuppression. Toxicity of TBI in general increases with total dose but depends on fractionation and dose rate.[43, 44] Fractionation theoretically yields improved tissue tolerance, leading to decreased acute toxicity and reduced late effects, but carries the risk of decreased antileukemic efficacy. In 1982[45] and 1986,[46] results of the first randomized trial of single-fraction (1000 cGy) versus fractionated (200 cGy daily for 6 days) radiation therapy were reported. A short- and long-term survival advantage was seen with the fractionated schedule. Studies from Seattle have demonstrated increased antileukemic efficacy with increased total dose, but lung, liver, and kidney tolerances were limiting factors.[47, 48] Just as the relative requirements for immunosuppression and ablation differ between types of SCT, (e.g., immunosuppression is inconsequential in autologous SCT), toxicity considerations vary considerably depending on recipient condition and age. It may be that alternative TBI strategies would be advantageous for children, but in fact little has been accomplished to date in resolving the issues of total dose, fractionation, dose rate, and schedule as they apply to children or adults.[49, 50]

Busulfan. Developed in the mid-1970s, busulfan-/cyclophosphamide (BU/CY) rapidly became an established preparative regimen for either allogeneic[38] or autologous SCT in patients with acute myeloblastic leukemia (AML).[51–53] The original regimen, called BU/CY4 (big BU/CY, BU 4 mg/kg/day for 4 days followed by CY 50 mg/kg/day for 4 days), was joined by BU/CY2 (little BU/CY, in which the CY was delivered as 60 mg/kg/day for 2 days).[51–55] Use of this regimen has expanded to include patients with acute lymphoblastic leukemia (ALL) and chronic myelogenous leukemia (CML).[56, 57] The BU/CY regimen has been used extensively in pediatric patients, particularly those with nonmalignant diseases[58–63] in an attempt to avoid radiation-mediated toxicity.

Total-Body Irradiation Versus Busulfan. Several randomized studies and meta-analyses have compared BU/CY and TBI-based regimens.[64–72] Overall, results are similar although they suggest that both relapse rates and hepatic veno-occlusive disease (VOD) may be decreased with the TBI-containing regimens. Although recent data support these observations, variability of the chemotherapy component of TBI-based regimens and potential differences in the antileukemic efficacy of BU/CY4 and BU/CY2 regimens[73] render definitive generalizations difficult. Reports of decreased bioavailability, increased volume of distribution, and increased clearance rate of busulfan in children raise the question of how to interpret studies in which such data are unavailable.[74–77] Alternative busulfan dosing, based on plasma levels, has been suggested,[78, 79] and comparison of "optimal" BU/CY with CY/TBI has not been reported. BU-containing regimens have often been reported to result in greater toxicity compared with TBI-based regimens; thus, increases in the busulfan dose may further increase regimen-related morbidity.[64, 65, 67, 70, 80, 81] Monitoring of busulfan pharmacokinetics has generally, but not always, demonstrated an association of increased area under the curve with increased VOD.[78, 82] Individualizing BU dosing may possibly increase the risk/benefit ratio. Recent approval of an intravenous form of busulfan and growing amounts of clinical data on its use will permit more predictable dosing and subsequent evaluation of relative toxicity and efficacy.[83] The relative differences in late toxicity, reviewed in the section on late complications in pediatric patients receiving either TBI or busulfan, have not been completely studied.

Alternative Myeloablative Regimens. The addition or substitution of a variety of chemotherapeutic agents to the backbone of CY/TBI, and less commonly BU/CY, has produced mixed success. Etoposide, cytarabine, and busulfan have been added to or substituted for cyclophosphamide in TBI-based regimens.[68, 84–91] Etoposide (VP-16) and melphalan have also replaced cyclophosphamide in some busulfan-based protocols.[92–95] Fluorouracil, high-dose methotrexate, doxorubicin, cisplatin, carboplatin, thiotepa, melphalan, and many other agents have been used in a variety of high-dose chemotherapeutic regimens supported by autologous SCT. Common conditioning regimens referred to by acronyms are: CBV (cyclophosphamide, carmustine, VP-16); BACT (carmustine [BCNU], cytarabine [Ara-C], cyclophosphamide, 6-thioguanine); BEAM (carmustine [BCNU], etoposide, cytarabine [Ara-C], melphalan); and CBP (cyclophosphamide, BCNU, cisplatin). In the setting of allogeneic transplantation, alternative regimens have often shown benefits in terms of disease control equivalent to those with "conventional" regimens. Some cause increased toxicity, but no regimen has shown unequivocal superiority in terms of disease-free or overall survival. Given the more limited follow-up and the extraordinary diversity of diseases and regimens in use, establishment of relative efficacy in the realm of autologous SCT is likely to be a prolonged process.[96–100]

Nonmyeloablative Regimens. Based on improved understanding of graft-versus-host HSC activity gained from observing aplasia after donor lymphocyte infusion or transfusional GVHD, numerous studies examining the ability of donor T cells to participate in ablation of host hematopoiesis or malignancy or both have been initiated.[101–107] The object is to use donor-derived lymphoid cells to eradicate recipient HSCs and in some instances tumor, thus allowing decreased dosing of conventional myeloablative therapy and sparing the patient from related toxicity. However, aggressive immunosuppression of the host is still required to eliminate potential host rejection of donor cells. This approach, generally referred to as *nonmyeloablative SCT* (also called minitransplant), has been applied to both malignant and benign diseases. Adequate host immunosuppression has been achieved by either purine analog chemotherapy or low-dose TBI (or both), and a variety of agents, including lower-dose busulfan, melphalan, and cytarabine have been used for additional effect and partial HSC depletion.[101–107] Thus far, the utility of nonmyeloablative regimens appears greatest for patients with CML, low-grade lymphomas, and perhaps myeloma, and considerable attention has been turned to this approach for second transplant.[101–108] The utility of this approach for other diseases, especially acute leukemias such as those of childhood, is very unclear. The experience to date in patients with benign hematologic disease is highly variable.[103, 109, 110]

SOURCES OF STEM CELLS

Selection of an appropriate source of stem cells for the patient undergoing SCT has become a more complex undertaking in recent years. For each disease entity, the clinician must consider what sources of stem cells are available and what are the relative risks and benefits associated with each potential stem cell source.

Autologous Stem Cell Transplantation

Over the past decade, increasing numbers of patients with cancer who have either hematologic malignancies or solid tumors have elected to undergo autologous SCT. In fact, this number is now in the tens of thousands worldwide. The fundamental hypothesis supporting this therapeutic approach is the belief that tumor cells are responsive to very high doses of cytotoxic agents (dose intensification) and that a high-dose treatment regimen can be devised in which the major dose-limiting toxicity is marrow aplasia. This toxicity can be ameliorated by autologous stem cells obtained either by bone marrow harvest or by apheresis of peripheral blood to collect PBSCs. Use of autologous cells to support and reconstitute the host after aggressive ablative or near-ablative therapy has been most thoroughly explored in both Hodgkin and non-Hodgkin lymphomas. It is less well developed in acute and chronic leukemias, and is still considered experimental, albeit relatively widely applied, for a growing number of solid tumors in children and adults. However, the relative merits and drawbacks of each autologous cell source are still not firmly established.

Method of Collection. Bone marrow is harvested with the patient under general or regional anesthesia in an operating room. Most often, the entire volume can be aspirated from the posterior iliac crests, but aspiration of the anterior iliac crests and even sternum may be required to obtain an adequate cell concentration. Prior radiation to the pelvis or severe myelofibrosis may significantly limit the yield of marrow cells. Multiple aspirations are performed, usually through a limited number of skin holes (two to three per side), to a total volume of 10 to 15 mL/kg of recipient body weight. The marrow is filtered through a fine wire mesh to rid the product of aggregates and bony spicules. Bone marrow harvest is a very safe and well-tolerated procedure with an extremely low probability of complications.[111] However, the heavily pretreated donor of autologous stem cells may have an increased potential for operative morbidity because of end-organ compromise. Stem cells may also be more difficult to harvest owing to either underlying disease or prior therapy. PBSCs are collected by leukapheresis. In the pediatric patient leukapheresis requires special attention to volume and access issues[112] and often requires the placement of a specialized pheresis catheter. Thus, the patient still requires an operative procedure, which in pediatric patients is almost always performed with the use of general anesthesia. Although PBSCs can be collected from patients without prior intervention, the yield is low and many hours of collection over several days are usually necessary to obtain an adequate yield. Optimization of yield is achieved by collection after chemotherapy; agents used most often are high-dose cyclophosphamide plus hematopoietic growth factors granulocyte colony-stimulating factor (G-CSF) or granulocyte-macrophage colony-stimulating factor or growth factors alone.[113–116] The best schedules of both priming and collection have not yet been established for children or adults although experience in pediatric patients is growing.[117] However, successful engraftment using a single apheresis product has been reported.[118] In the future, UCB cells collected and cryopreserved at the time of delivery may provide a source of autologous stem cells for both hematopoietic reconstitution and, potentially, gene therapy.

Contamination by Tumor Cells. A major limitation of autologous SCT is contamination of the stem cell product with residual malignant cells. Although the relative contributions of either residual tumor within the host or tumor reinfused with stem cells to subsequent relapse remain unknown, increasing evidence from gene-marking studies suggests that reinfused cells contribute to relapse.[119] In addition, *in vitro* assays of tumor cell colony formation and minimal residual disease detection by polymerase chain reaction suggest that contamination of the stem cell source by tumor cells is associated with an increased relapse rate after SCT.[120] No large randomized clinical trial to compare disease-free survival (DFS) after use of PBSCs versus bone marrow has been reported. However, paired samples of PBSCs and bone marrow have been examined in a variety of settings (e.g., breast cancer and non-Hodgkin lymphoma) in which lower levels of tumor cell contamination have been seen in PBSCs in the steady-state setting.[121] More recent data suggest that the advantage of PBSCs may be abrogated after mobilization,[122–126] although the impact on DFS remains unclear.

A variety of methodologies have been developed to eliminate, or purge, tumor cells from stem cell collections. These are based on either positive or negative selection. The major positive selection strategy in clinical use is stem cell enrichment, most often selection of CD34+ cells. Negative selection is based on technologies that deplete tumor cells to a greater degree than normal stem cells. Strategies include the use of pharmacologic agents (e.g., mafosfamide), immunologic reagents targeting tissue-specific antigens (e.g., neural crest antigens in neuroblastoma), and manipulation of physical or culture properties of cells. Combinations of both negative and positive selection strategies may improve both the yield and purity of stem cell collections.[127, 128] Increasing evidence in multiple clinical settings demonstrates an association between minimal residual tumor contamination and relapse[120] and, conversely, suggests that the more effective purging strategies may be associated with improved DFS. However, results of randomized studies comparing purged and unpurged stem cells have not yet been reported, and elimination of tumor from the stem cells before reinfusion does not address the more complex problem of eradicating residual tumor resident within the recipient.

Engraftment. Trilineage hematologic reconstitution has been achieved after the infusion of autologous bone marrow, bone marrow and PBSCs, and PBSCs alone. The most mature studies are of patients in whom hematopoiesis was reconstituted with autologous marrow. In these patients engraftment after bone marrow infusion is both reliable and durable whereas the durability of PBSC-reconstituted hematopoiesis, undertaken more recently, has not been fully evaluated. The best predictor of engraftment and rate of hematologic recovery has not been established. Although numbers of colony-forming units and burst-forming units-erythroid, nucleated cell count, and other measures have correlated with time to engraftment in some studies, correlations have not been universal and may additionally depend on the patient population, method of cell procurement, and subsequent cell manipulation. Although the pluripotent HSCs may be CD34– or CD34dim, **CD34**+ counts have emerged empirically as the most reliable and practical method to date for predicting engraftment after PBSC infusion.[129, 130]

Reconstitution of hematopoiesis after autologous bone marrow infusion has shown some tendency to be delayed compared with that after allogeneic bone marrow infusion. This delay is presumed to be due to the extent, nature, and duration of prior therapy. In addition, cell manipulation *ex vivo* (purging) may also contribute to delayed engraftment. Reconstitution after SCT with autologous bone marrow can be hastened somewhat by the addition of hematopoietic growth factors to the supportive care regimen after SCT, although the extent and nature of prior therapy may limit response to growth factors. Preliminary information in both the preclinical and clinical arenas suggests that prior aggressive chemotherapy may limit the potential for hematologic recovery.[131–133] Prior intensive chemotherapy supported by use of growth factors may also contribute to poor engraftment after autologous transplantation. In fact, despite recovery of peripheral blood cell counts, hematologic marrow reserves as assessed by *in vitro* measures of hematopoiesis may be blunted for many years after autologous SCT.[134]

Addition of mobilized PBSC to bone marrow has resulted in a dramatic decrease in days of neutropenia and thrombocytopenia in patients in most series with or without subsequent growth factor support. Further, use of mobilized PBSCs as the sole stem cell source has been almost universally associated with more rapid hematologic recovery, particularly of the peripheral platelet count. Whether the use of hematopoietic growth factors in this setting further enhances the rate of engraftment is still being debated, but available data suggest that it may do so. Whether the process of PBSC transplantation will result in durable hematopoiesis over decades cannot yet be evaluated, but graft failure has not been reported as a commonly seen complication. Most studies suggest that the increased rate of engraftment observed with PBSCs results in decreases in time in the hospital, use of antibiotics, and use of associated supportive services. The overall impact of the use of PBSCs versus bone marrow as a stem cell source on the efficacy, toxicity, and cost of transplantation has yet to be determined.

Myelodysplasia as a Late Complication. Intensive chemotherapy, particularly with alkylating agents, may result in an increased risk of subsequent myelodysplasia (MDS). Many patients who undergo autologous transplantation have received treatment with such agents. Over the past several years, increases in the numbers of patients developing MDS after autologous transplantation have been reported. The MDS usually occurs from 4 to 7 years after SCT.[135] The actuarial incidence ranges from 5 to 10 percent in most series,[136–138] although the incidence has been reported to be as high as 18 percent at 5 to 6 years after SCT in single-center experiences.[139, 140] Risk factors identified have included etoposide use for stem cell mobilization,[138] conditioning regimens using TBI,[136, 141, 142] the amount of chemotherapy received before SCT, and the interval between diagnosis and SCT.[142, 143] Whether

the MDS results from previously damaged reinfused hematopoietic cells or from residual hematopoietic cells sustaining further injury during conditioning is unresolved. Cytogenetic analysis of bone marrow before autologous SCT can reveal preexisting abnormalities and should be a standard component of patient evaluation before SCT.[144] However, results of cytogenetic analysis in most patients developing MDS have been reported to be normal at the time of transplant.[137] With the current availability of more sensitive techniques, such as fluorescence *in situ* hybridization, the majority of patients who develop MDS after SCT have been shown to harbor the same cytogenetic abnormality in specimens taken before SCT.[145] Similarly, using a clonality assay based on an X-inactivation, clonal hematopoiesis was demonstrated in a small percentage of female patients before SCT; those patients had a significant risk of developing MDS after SCT.[135] This finding suggests that MDS after SCT in many patients evolves from an abnormal clone already present before SCT. The appropriate evaluation of hematopoietic status before autologous stem cell collection and transplantation are performed has not been fully determined.

Allogeneic Stem Cell Transplantation

To date, most allogeneic SCT procedures have used HSCs from a matched sibling donor. However, with improvements in immunosuppression and the ability to prevent or treat GVHD, alternative and increasing disparate allogeneic sources of HSCs have been used. These include mismatched family members, in so-called "haploidentical SCT," as well as UD SCT. There are now approximately 7 million UDs listed in more than 72 registries worldwide, including registries of banked UD UCB collections.

The selection of an allogeneic HSC source depends on many variables, including the aggressiveness of the underlying disorder, the accessibility of a donor, and, particularly, the degree of histocompatibility between host and potential donor. Historically, increases in histoincompatibility have contributed to both an increased rate of graft rejection and severe acute and chronic GVHD. The best results are reported when fully histocompatible sibling donors are used, but only approximately 25 percent of patients will have such a donor available.[146] Even in this matched setting, selection can be further refined according to sex, history of donor parity, donor infectious disease status, donor age, and other variables. For the majority of patients who do not have a matched sibling donor, potential sources include a phenotypically matched but genotypically distinct family member, a more disparate family member, or a volunteer unrelated donor. The likelihood of the first is low, although more mismatched family members are available to the vast majority of the population. The likelihood of locating an appropriate UD depends both on the patient's ethnicity (inasmuch as it determines histocompatibility antigen and haplotype occurrence) and on the composition of the donor pool. For example, for whites of mid and northern European descent the likelihood of finding a six-antigen matched UD approaches 50 to 70 percent.[147] In contrast, the extreme genetic heterogeneity of the African-American population coupled with under-representation of this population in volunteer registries makes the likelihood of finding a similar donor approximately 10 to 15 percent. Molecular typing techniques demonstrate that the allelic disparities in both whites and nonwhites are much higher than previously expected, thus making the ascertainment of a truly "matched" UD less likely even as the donor pool expands.[148] Although the implications of specific human leukocyte antigen (HLA) mismatches are not completely understood, most studies suggest that high-resolution HLA matching is associated with improved outcome in UD SCT.[149, 150] Thus, additional strategies to broaden the donor base by using alternative sources of HSCs, such as PBSCs and UCB, which may have different biologic properties, are being explored.

Typing. The initial identification of antigens involved in allograft rejection or acceptance resulted from experimentation in inbred mouse strains. The genes encoding for the antigens most associated with allograft rejection became known as the major histocompatibility complex (MHC). In humans, the MHC maps to a region of the short arm of chromosome 6, which is known as the HLA system. The MHC codes for many genes, and the identification and exploration of the functional importance of some of these gene products are ongoing. Among the best characterized gene products are proteins comprising the class I and class II antigens. Classically, MHC class I molecules were identified serologically whereas MHC class II antigens were defined both serologically and cellularly (see later). In the human, MHC class I molecules include HLA-A, B, and C whereas MHC class II molecules are called HLA-D. The MHC class I antigens are present on nearly all human cells (with rare exceptions such as the erythrocyte and corneal endothelium). MHC class II proteins have much more restricted expression. They are constitutively expressed on "professional" antigen-presenting cells, which include dendritic cells, B cells, and monocytic cells (including monocytes, macrophages, and Langerhans cells), and may be induced on a variety of human cells, most notably activated T cells and endothelium. These genes are highly polymorphic, and both MHC class I and II molecules play a central role in the presentation of antigen to T lymphocytes. It is generally accepted that antigen-presenting cells present peptide antigens in the groove of the MHC class II molecules to the T-cell receptor complex on CD4+ helper T cells. In contrast, all nucleated cells are capable of presenting peptide antigens in the groove of the MHC class I molecule to the T-cell receptor complex on CD8+ cytotoxic/suppressor T cells. In addition to MHC class I and class II antigens, ever-increasing evidence demonstrates the existence of minor histocompatibility antigens in humans.[151] Although these antigens may not be directly responsible for organ and bone marrow rejection, human typing studies suggest that these minor antigens may be critical in the generation of GVHD.[152, 153]

Historically, HLA typing was performed by using antibodies derived from postpartum sera, from persons who have undergone transplants or transfusions, or even from persons immunized for the purpose of generating specific serologic reagents. These antibodies were used in a standardized complement-dependent, microcytotoxicity assay with purified T or B lymphocytes as their target cell.[154] The extensive cross-reactivity among products coded by the alleles of the HLA-A and HLA-B loci, known as cross-reactive groups, makes precise delineation of the MHC class I antigens by this technique difficult. In contrast, HLA-D specificities were originally defined by their ability to stimulate T-lymphocyte proliferation in a mixed leukocyte culture.[155] It has become increasingly clear that the HLA-D region is a complex region composed of many loci that in aggregate induce the mixed leukocyte culture reaction.[156] There are at least five subregions, including DR, DQ, and DP, but the number of genes transcribed differs between different HLA class II haplotypes. Considering the importance of major and minor HLAs in transplant biology, the development of increasingly sophisticated methods to identify distinct alleles encoding both class I, class II, and, in the future, minor antigens, is not surprising. Of these, molecular analyses have rapidly become the new standard. The first attempts to use molecular genetic techniques were based on application of restriction fragment length polymorphism analysis of genomic DNA by Southern blotting using HLA region probes. This soon gave way to current technology in which sequence-specific oligonucleotide probes and, in some cases, direct sequence analysis are performed. Generation of appropriate probes and sequence data has resulted in more accurate and detailed description of MHC class I and II alleles. This has already led to a great multiplication in the known HLA specificities. This fine analysis is increasingly being used to determine the haplotypes of individuals. The implications of more exact typing within families, in which the haplotypes are "conserved," are probably confined to the potential identification of minor histocompatibility antigen differences, allowing for better selection among possible donors.[152, 153] In the UD setting, high-resolution HLA matching appears to improve outcome,[149, 150] but which antigens and what degree of matching are most acceptable where mismatch is inevitable have not yet been established.

Methods of Collection. The physical methodology of bone marrow collection is identical to that described earlier for autologous SCT. If there is ABO incompatibility, the red cells may be removed before infusion.[157] The marrow may be manipulated *ex vivo* to remove donor T lymphocytes (see later) or tumor cells. It is estimated that only 1 percent of the donor's pluripotent HSC population is removed in a typical bone marrow harvest. Risks to the donor are minimized by the fact that the donor is generally a healthy individual undergoing an elective procedure. Potential short- and long-term complications include risks of anesthesia, blood loss, and the potential for transfusion, pain, neurologic deficits, and psychosocial complications. In the most truly altruistic setting, UD marrow harvest, only 5 to 8 percent of donors later expressed any ambivalence about their participation. This situation was most marked if the transplant was subsequently unsuccessful.[158]

Although bone marrow has been used as the HSC source in the overwhelming majority of allogeneic SCTs, interest in the use of allogeneic PBSC transplants is increasing.[159–163] Mobilization and collection of stem cells from normal donors have generally been accomplished by administration of high doses of G-CSF for 4 to 5 days followed by pheresis using peripheral venous access. Complications have included bone pain, as a side effect of administration of G-CSF, and inability to establish adequate peripheral access, resulting in central line placement.[164, 165] Access issues are likely to be more significant with pediatric donors than with adult donors. The implications of mobilizing and harvesting PBSCs from pediatric donors have not been fully explored[116, 166]; however, cytopenias and hemostatic changes of unknown short- and long-term significance have been observed in healthy adult donors.[167, 168]

Since the first description of its use in a child with Fanconi anemia in 1988,[169] UCB has become an increasingly investigated source of HSCs. Placental blood is recovered from the umbilical vein by drainage or catheterization, and techniques to optimize collection of HSCs from UCB are being investigated.[27, 170] If indicated, the HLA type of the fetus can be determined before delivery. Otherwise, typing and analysis are performed on intrapartum or postpartum samples.

Selection of a UD, whether for bone marrow or UCB, is facilitated by the availability of a database of epidemiologic information (e.g., age and sex) as well as HLA typing that is accessible through electronic mail. Complementary databases exist on CD-ROMs that are updated often. By comparing a patient's HLA type with that of donors listed and categorized in the registries, one can estimate the likelihood of a successful search, devise search strategies for patients with uncommon HLA types, and sort among potential HSC sources. Although stored UCB can be readily supplied after confirmatory typing, obtaining bone marrow from an UD is more involved. A potential donor must be contacted and give consent to proceed. Then the donor center must arrange for appropriate confirmatory studies and medical and other evaluations and schedule the harvest. The time from formal search to actual BMT averages 4 months, although in some instances the time is much shorter.

Engraftment. After allogeneic SCT, donor stem cells must expand to repopulate hematopoietic tissue and differentiate to form mature blood cells. Stem cell transplant recipients show accelerated telomere shortening in peripheral blood cells, which is presumably caused by the increased replicative demand of donor stem cells.[171] Donor hematopoietic engraftment after allogeneic SCT can be documented both by analysis of chimerism as well as by the recovery of peripheral blood cell counts. However, sensitive DNA amplification technologies have demonstrated residual host hematopoiesis for variable periods of time, certainly up to 1 year.[172–174] Mixed lymphoid chimerism is also well documented.[172–175] The implications of mixed chimerism for subsequent relapse remain a subject of controversy, probably because current extremely sensitive assays generate data that are difficult to interpret uniformly and because outcome may differ by disease type.[176] For example, chimerism after BMT for CML is quite reliably related to subsequent relapse, but this relationship may not be true for other diseases.[175–177]

The rate of engraftment after allogeneic BMT varies somewhat with the prophylactic regimen used for GVHD. In general, neutrophil recovery is achieved within 2 to 3 weeks and platelet recovery occurs 1 to 2 weeks thereafter. The use of methotrexate in the prophylactic regimen is associated with a delay in cell count recovery; conversely, recovery after T-cell–depleted BMT is more rapid. Use of colony-stimulating factors after BMT is associated with more rapid neutrophil recovery after related donor BMT, a finding confirmed in a small pediatric series.[175–183] No change in platelet recovery has been noted. Interestingly, preliminary data do not show any colony-stimulating factor–mediated acceleration of engraftment in patients undergoing UD BMT.[183]

With the use of allogeneic PBSCs, a far higher CD34+ cell dose can be collected and administered than with bone marrow.[184] Neutrophil engraftment occurs between 1 and 6 days earlier with PBSC transplantation than with BMT, and platelet engraftment occurs between 4 and 7 days earlier.[185] Whether the increased rate of engraftment will translate into a survival advantage in all patients remains to be seen.[163, 186] Neutrophil and platelet engraftment after UCB transplantation is significantly delayed compared with that expected with other SCT.[187–191] The use of hematopoietic growth factors after UCB transplantation has not been associated with accelerated hematopoietic reconstitution.[26]

Immune Reconstitution

The presence of mature, functional T cells capable of antigen-specific responses is critical to the maintenance of normal cellular and humoral immunity. Initial hematopoiesis is usually identified within 2 to 4 weeks of SCT; however, the development of a broad repertoire of functional T cells can take considerably longer. For this reason, the period after SCT is characterized by a variable degree of immunoincompetence.

Several studies have shown that recovery of normal numbers of CD4+ and CD8 T+ cells can take between 6 and 12 months after SCT.[192] T-cell reconstitution probably occurs initially as a result of expansion of mature donor T cells transferred with the graft. After this, naïve T cells that have differentiated from HSCs migrate to and colonize lymphoid organs, including the thymus gland. Parkman and Weinberg[193] have demonstrated that the ability of T cells to respond to a mitogen challenge after T-cell depleted SCT (in which few mature donor T cells are transferred) may take as long as 4 to 6 months. During this period of recovery, T cells with a naïve phenotype predominate in the peripheral blood, suggesting repopulation of the T-cell compartment with recent thymic emigrants.[192, 194, 195] New techniques have been developed to measure the relative numbers of recent thymic emigrants in the peripheral blood T-cell pool by the quantitative detection of genomic DNA that is present only in thymocytes (T-cell receptor excision circle DNA). Using these methods, researchers have shown that increased thymic output contributes to the expanding peripheral T-cell pool for 12 to 24 months after SCT.[196] This thymic output occurs even in adult patients whose thymus glands have presumably involuted. The rate of increase in T cells is usually much more rapid in pediatric patients after SCT, consistent with the presence of more robust thymic function.[192] In fact, one study demonstrated a marked decrease in the fraction of naïve peripheral blood T cells after SCT in a 15-year-old patient who had previously had a thymectomy compared with other patients who still had intact thymus glands.[197] Using quantitative molecular measures of T-cell repertoire, several researchers have shown that it can take as long as 12 to 24 months after SCT for a full range of T-cell receptor diversity to be present in the T-cell compartment.[194, 195, 198] This finding underscores the critical role of naïve thymic emigrants in restoring the full complement of T-cell receptor specificities.

Several factors influence the length of time for immunologic recovery. The age of bone marrow transplant recipients profoundly affects the rate of immune reconstitution, and there is an inverse correlation between recipient age and the absolute number of T cells 1 year after SCT.[199] Use of mobilized PBSCs as the source of stem cells appears to be associated with a faster rate of recovery than use of HSCs from bone marrow, possibly as a result of a large cell dose.[160, 200] However, increasingly intensive conditioning regimens are delaying immune recovery in autologous SCT to a degree comparable with that in allogeneic SCT.[199] Although hematopoietic engraftment appears to be delayed in recipients of UCB SCT, immune reconstitution in children after UCB SCT is comparable to that in children receiving UD BMT.[201] The presence of GVHD can significantly delay immune reconstitution as a result of both disruption of normal T-cell development and the added immunosuppression that is required for management of disease.[193] The consequences of factors that delay immunologic recovery is significant: slow recovery of immune function is associated with an increase in the cumulative incidence of infections.[160, 202] Reagents now available, such as HLA tetramers, can measure the number of T cells specific for known antigens and will allow analysis of the recovery of host immunity to opportunistic pathogens.[203]

PERITRANSPLANT SUPPORTIVE CARE

Transfusion Support

The intensive myeloablative preparative regimens used for tumor eradication and successful engraftment result in an extended period of aplasia that lasts until robust engraftment occurs. Virtually all patients require red cell and platelet transfusions during transplant. All blood products should be irradiated to prevent transfusion-induced GVHD from lymphocyte contamination of the blood product.[204–206] In addition, it is recommended that blood products be administered through an in-line filter to remove lymphocytes and leukocytes that may harbor latent viruses such as cytomegalovirus (CMV).[207] The use of such leukocyte-poor blood products has been shown to be equivalent to the use of CMV-seronegative blood products in preventing transmission of CMV by transfusion.[208] It is generally recommended that all stem cell transplant recipients continue to receive irradiated, leukocyte-poor blood products regardless of the interval after transplant.

Whether platelet and red cell transfusions should be given prophylactically during the period of cytopenia remains an area of controversy. No recommendations can supplant the need for clinical judgment in individual situations. Historically, platelet counts less than $20,000/\mu L$ were associated with an increased risk of spontaneous hemorrhage in patients with leukemia although the effect on patient outcome was not clear.[209] As supportive care measures have improved and the risks of transfusions have been identified, the threshold for transfusion in a patient with a stable condition has been lowered.[210] A recent summary of the data has led to new recommendations,[211] and now platelet counts of $10,000/\mu L$ are often accepted in an patient without complications of transplantation because the desire to prevent untoward bleeding is balanced by the risk of platelet alloimmunization, the finite risk of transfusion-associated infection, and the cost of blood products. However, this practice has not been investigated in stem cell transplant recipients whose many comorbid conditions, including fever, mucositis, hypertension, liver dysfunction, and uremia, may affect hemostasis and dictate more conservative management.

Infection Prophylaxis and Treatment

After engraftment, patients continue to have depressed T-cell function and decreased antibody production and remain at risk for a variety of infections. This risk is particularly prolonged in recipients of allogeneic transplants Although these patients have phenotypically normal circulating lymphocytes, they often continue to have depressed cellular immunity for at least 1 year after SCT. During this time viral infections continue to present a major risk to patients. Both CMV-seropositive and -seronegative patients who have received grafts from seropositive donors are at risk for CMV disease, although the risk is greater when the recipient is seropositive.[212, 213] Common manifestations of CMV disease after SCT include interstitial pneumonitis, diarrhea, hepatitis, and CMV-related cytopenias. With the availability of antiviral therapies, almost all patients at risk for CMV disease received ganciclovir prophylaxis during the first 3 months after SCT because randomized studies had demonstrated both a decrease in CMV disease and a survival advantage with this approach.[214, 215] However, associated toxicities (cytopenias and renal toxicity)[214] and costs were problems. Although no consensus on optimal management exists,[216] many centers have begun to use prophylactic ganciclovir only in high-risk patients. The remainder undergo weekly screening tests using methods based on either a polymerase chain reaction[217] or a CMV antigen.[218] CMV-seropositive patients undergoing autologous SCT have not generally received either screening tests or prophylaxis. Newer modalities of peripheral stem cell collection using CD34 selection markedly decreases the numbers of infused lymphocytes and has been reported to be associated with an increase in viral infections after SCT.[219]

Up to 50 percent of patients receiving either autologous and allogeneic transplants experience varicella-zoster virus reactivation, usually within the first year after SCT.[220] In children the onset of reactivation may be earlier, but children rarely experience visceral dissemination or associated mortality.[221] Fungal infection remains a problem, especially in patients receiving steroids. A randomized trial demonstrated that administration of prophylactic fluconazole for 75 days after allogeneic SCT resulted in ongoing protection against disseminated candidal infections and improved survival.[222] However, prophylactic fluconazole has been associated with the emergence of resistant species such as *Candida krusei*.[223] Although less studied, low doses of amphotericin B have also been used prophylactically and appear to be effective and nontoxic.[224] All patients are also at risk for the development of infection from *Pneumocystis carinii* after SCT. Standard practice is to administer prophylaxis for some period, which ranges from 3 to 12 months, to recipients of allogeneic SCT until they are no longer receiving immunosuppressive therapy. In contrast, recipients of autologous stem cell transplants generally receive prophylaxis for a shorter interval.

Nutrition Support

Provision of nutritional support during SCT requires an appreciation of the metabolic needs of the individual patient that are, in turn, influenced by comorbid complications of transplant. Cytoreductive therapy induces gastrointestinal damage that may progress further with the onset of GVHD. Several studies have demonstrated the efficacy of total parenteral nutrition when enteral nutrition is no longer possible.[225, 226] In addition, a prospective randomized trial demonstrated a survival advantage for patients given total parenteral nutrition during SCT compared with control subjects.[227] However, in addition to expense, total parenteral nutrition has potential attendant complications, including vascular access difficulties, abnormal liver function, and episodes of hyperglycemia and hyperlipidemia. Some patients may be able to maintain their nutritional needs orally throughout transplant, and both enteral and total parenteral nutrition routes may be used on occasion.[228] Resumption of enteral feeding should be encouraged, and continued monitoring of nutritional intake and weight is necessary not only through engraftment but also after discharge from the hospital. Malnutrition appears to occur relatively often after SCT, and even patients with no or limited GVHD may have significant nutritional problems.[229]

EARLY COMPLICATIONS OF STEM CELL TRANSPLANTATION

Graft Rejection

Failure of hematopoietic recovery is a rare event after matched sibling SCT for hematologic malignancy.[22] Although graft failure and graft rejection are not always easy to separate, failure to recover hematopoiesis ("graft failure") occurs more often as the genetic disparity between donor and recipient increases, in the presence of a positive crossmatch for antidonor lymphocytotoxic antibody, and with the use of T-cell depletion for GVHD prophylaxis.[22, 230–232] In addition, patients with aplastic anemia, particularly if they previously were given transfusions, have a high rate of apparent graft rejection.[233, 234] Patients with storage disorders and osteopetrosis (see later

discussions) may also have an increased failure rate, presumably due in part to disordered microenvironment and also perhaps to their immunocompetent status before SCT. Adjustments to both chemotherapy and radiotherapy components of conditioning regimens,[235] the use of monoclonal antibodies targeting selected effector cell populations in the recipient,[236] and increases in cell dose (including the use of PBSCs in addition to bone marrow)[237] are among the manipulations that have shown some promise in reducing graft failure. The increased risk of graft failure after T-cell depletion of the marrow suggests that mature donor T cells facilitate alloengraftment although the immunologic mechanism by which this occurs has not been elucidated. Mature donor T cells may themselves secrete or induce the secretion by bone marrow stromal cells of essential cytokines that promote engraftment. A number of approaches have been explored to overcome graft failure associated with T-cell depletion.[238] First, an increase in the number of cells in the graft decreases the risk of graft failure.[239, 240] Second, intensification of the conditioning regimen has been successful, implying that residual host hematopoietic elements are involved in mediating graft rejection. However, such intensification is associated with increased transplant-related morbidity and mortality.[241] Third, because the risk of graft failure appears to increase with more exhaustive T-cell depletion, less extensive T-cell removal such as removal of selective T-cell subsets from the graft has been attempted.[242–244]

Veno-Occlusive Disease of the Liver

VOD is a clinical syndrome characterized by hepatomegaly and/ right upper quadrant pain, jaundice, and fluid retention,[245–247] and it remains one of the most common toxic reactions related to the preparative regimen for both autologous and allogeneic SCT.[246, 248, 249] Injury to sinusoidal endothelial cells and hepatocytes in zone 3 of the liver acinus appears to be the initial event, and it is characterized by subendothelial edema and endothelial cell damage with microthromboses, fibrin deposition, and the expression of factor VIII/von Willebrand factor within venular walls.[250] Later features include collagen deposition in the sinusoids, sclerosis of the venular walls, and the development of collagen deposits within venular lumens and abluminally with eventual venular obliteration and further hepatocyte necrosis.[251] Higher plasma levels of some of the cytotoxic drugs used in SCT have been associated with an increased risk of VOD.[75, 82, 83, 252–254] In this regard, it is intriguing that hepatocytes in zone 3 contain both a high concentration of cytochrome P450 enzymes, which metabolize many chemotherapeutic agents used in SCT, and glutathione *S*-transferase enzymes, which catalyze the reaction of glutathione with electrophilic compounds.[255, 256] There is some experimental evidence to support the role of glutathione depletion in the pathogenesis of VOD.[257–259]

Hepatomegaly and right upper quadrant pain and fluid retention are the first clinical signs of VOD, typically occurring relatively soon after completion of conditioning therapy. Jaundice, ascites, and encephalopathy occur somewhat later.[248] Additional clinical markers of VOD include marked renal sodium retention, another early event; peripheral edema, mild and then worsening ascites, appearance of pulmonary infiltrates, and the need for supplemental oxygen follow later if the VOD is severe.[246] Frank hepatorenal syndrome occurs in nearly half of patients with severe disease.[248] Exclusion of other causes for these findings is essential in establishing the diagnosis of VOD. Transvenous liver biopsy may have considerable morbidity but remains the gold standard for diagnosis. Concurrent measurement of the wedged hepatic venous pressure gradient is useful. Values greater than 10 mm Hg have been reported to have good specificity and positive predictive value but only moderate sensitivity.[260] Other modalities with significantly less potential morbidity include ultrasound and computer tomographic imaging to exclude other etiologies and to confirm hepatomegaly or the presence of ascites and, together with Doppler studies, to determine whether or not there is attenuation or reversal of venous flow.[261] Doppler measurement of hepatic arterial resistance has been studied prospectively in a limited number of patients.[262] Once the diagnosis is established, the most useful prognostic data are the rate of rise in bilirubin and weight and the presence of multiorgan failure.[248] The latter is typically associated with a very high rate of death.[263, 264] Other measures helpful in predicting the severity of VOD include the degree of sodium avidity and the presence of renal impairment.[248, 265, 266] A risk model, based on total serum bilirubin level and percentage of weight gain at specific times after particular SCT regimens, has been used to generate risk curves to predict severe VOD. These in turn are associated with more than 98 percent fatality by day +100 after SCT.[267] Similar models have not yet been proposed for other temporal or therapeutic settings.

Treatment options for patients with severe VOD remain limited,[246, 247] and meticulous fluid and blood product management remains the cornerstone of supportive care. Based upon the histologic observation of microthromboses and fibrin deposition, the goal of most therapeutic strategies has been to promote fibrinolysis with or without concomitant anticoagulant therapy.[268–270] The use of thrombolytic therapy with or without anticoagulation (generally heparin and tissue plasminogen activator) has been reported in many small series. Although 20 to 30 percent of patients respond in some manner, no patient with renal insufficiency or hypoxemia or both at the time of treatment responded and a substantial number of patients developed significant and sometimes fatal hemorrhage.[270] The administration of antithrombin III and activated protein C has shown no clear effect.[271–273] Liver transplantation has resulted in clinical improvement in about 30 percent of the small numbers of patients whose conditions are stable enough to undergo this procedure, although the immediate and long-term issues are formidable.[274] Transjugular intrahepatic portosystemic shunting has also been tested, although it probably has no merit unless fluid retention and ascites are relatively isolated issues.[275, 276] These studies prompted a search for agents that could modulate endothelial cell injury without enhancing systemic bleeding, particularly because elevations in markers of endothelial injury have been observed in patients with VOD.[277–281]

Defibrotide, a single-stranded polydeoxyribonucleotide with a molecular mass of 15 to 30 kD emerged as a candidate based on significant inhibition of fibrin deposition without significant systemic anticoagulant effects.[282] In a pilot clinical trial a response was seen in approximately 40 percent of patients with excellent day +100 survival in those who responded and no attributable toxicity.[283] Additional trials have produced similar results in patients with severe VOD and multiorgan failure.[247, 284] Prospective, multi-institutional trials of defibrotide in the treatment of severe VOD are underway.

Many prophylactic strategies have been examined.[245–247, 284] Of these, the simplest may be the recognition of patients at highest risk by using epidemiologic and other criteria to identify patients in whom alternative regimens should be used or SCT delayed or declined.[245–247] Preliminary studies of genetic polymorphisms have suggested a possible association between a mutation of glutathione *S*-transferase synthesis and increased risk of VOD.[285] In contrast, in a large, prospective study of allelic variants for tumor necrosis factor (TNF)-α in patients receiving SCT, a high incidence of multiorgan failure was seen in association with a specific allelic variant (TNF d3), which causes increased TNF-α production in response to injury.[286] A number of alternative prophylactic strategies have been investigated in pilot studies, although few have been studied extensively. The use of pharmacokinetics to monitor drug levels with the intent of minimizing hepatic injury may be helpful.[78, 82] The prophylactic administration of ursodeoxycholic acid, a hydrophilic water-soluble bile acid, has been studied in randomized placebo-controlled prospective trials with divergent results.[287–289] The significant decline in use of glutathione and other antioxidants after SCT suggests that further evaluation of supportive nutrition and antioxidants is needed[290] as is exploration of the recent report of successful treatment of VOD with *N*-acetylcysteine supplementation.[291]

Acute Graft-Versus-Host Disease

First reported by Barnes and Loutit in 1954,[6] the syndrome of acute GVHD (then termed *secondary disease* because it followed radiation sickness, which occurred first) was observed in lethally irradiated animals given allogeneic spleen cells. The animals developed skin abnormalities and diarrhea and eventually succumbed to a wasting illness. Criteria for the development of GVHD were presented by Billingham,[292] who asserted that (1) "the graft must contain immunologically competent cells," (2) "the host must possess important transplantation alloantigens that are lacking in the donor graft, so that the host appears foreign to the graft and is, therefore, capable of stimulating it antigenically," and (3) "the host itself must be incapable of mounting an effective immunologic reaction against the graft, at least for sufficient time for the latter to manifest its immunologic capabilities; that is, it must have the security of tenure." GVHD is caused by donor alloreactivity in an immunoincompetent host and results from T lymphocytes contained in the marrow graft that proliferate and differentiate in the host. These T cells then recognize host alloantigens as foreign and, through both direct effector mechanisms and by inflammatory mediators released by T cells and host tissues, mediate tissue damage.[293-295] Animal studies and later human clinical trials demonstrated that T-cell depletion from the marrow inocula can abrogate the development of GVHD, albeit at an increased risk of graft rejection and relapse of initial disease.[296] Donor cells contain T (or other) cells capable of recognizing malignant cells and mediating a graft-versus-leukemia and, perhaps, a graft-versus-tumor effect.[297-299] Indeed, patients with hematologic malignancies who develop mild to moderate GVHD have a decreased risk of disease relapse.[300-303] Efforts to distinguish both the populations of T cells and the different cytotoxic pathways that mediate GVHD from those that mount a graft-versus-leukemia response are topics of current research.[304]

The clinical syndrome of acute GVHD develops within 100 (and usually within 60) days of allogeneic SCT. Chronic GVHD is a distinctive clinical syndrome that occurs after day 100 and is discussed later. Acute GVHD classically involves the skin, liver, and lower gastrointestinal tract, although the degree of involvement of each organ varies. For that reason, a grade is assigned to indicate the overall severity of acute GVHD by determining the involve-

ment of individual organs and the clinical performance of the patient. Table 9–2 presents the modified Glucksberg criteria, introduced in 1974[305] and, with several revisions and additions,[39, 306, 307] this is the system historically used for assessing acute GVHD. As newer methods of both preventing and treating acute GVHD were developed, there was concern about the ability of the Glucksberg staging system to accurately reflect transplant outcome. The International Bone Marrow Transplant Registry (IBMTR) constructed a severity index based on organ involvement alone with no need for subjective performance assessment. This index has been shown to correlate well with outcome and is the staging system used in most current studies[308] (Table 9–3).

The first manifestation of GVHD is often a skin rash, presenting as a maculopapular eruption, commonly involving the palms and soles, the back of the neck and ears at first, and later the trunk and extremities. Biopsy specimens from involved areas often demonstrate epidermal basal cell vacuolization, followed by epidermal basal cell apoptotic death with lymphoid infiltration.[309] Characteristic eosinophilic bodies may be seen. Unfortunately, the sensitivity of skin biopsy is not high, and often it is not possible to differentiate GVHD from a drug allergy or reaction to the conditioning regimen with skin biopsy results.[310] As

TABLE 9–2. Glucksberg Criteria for Staging and Grading of Acute Graft-Versus-Host Disease

Organ System	Stage	Extent of Organ Involvement
Skin	1	<25%
	2	25%–50%
	3	Generalized erythema
	4	Desquamation, bullous
Liver	1	2–3 mg/dL*
	2	3.1–6 mg/dL
	3	6.1–15 mg/dL
	4	>15 mg/dL
Gastrointestinal tract (children)	1	10–15 mL stool/kg/day
	2	16–20 mL stool/kg/day
	3	21–25 mL stool/kg/day
	4	>25 mL stool/kg/day; severe pain with or without ileus
Gastrointestinal tract (adult)	1	500–1000 mL stool/day; nausea, anorexia
	2	1000–1500 mL stool/day; histologic diagnosist of upper gastrointestinal tract GVHD
	3	1500–2000 mL stool/day
	4	>2000 mL stool/day; ileus, severe pain

Overall Clinical Grade	Organ System	Clinical Stage
I (mild)	Skin	1–2
	Liver	1
	Gastrointestinal tract	0
II (moderate)	Skin	1–3
	Liver	1–2
	Gastrointestinal tract	1
III (severe)	Skin	2–4
	Liver	2–4
	Gastrointestinal tract	2–4
IV (life threatening)‡	Skin	2–4
	Liver	2–4
	Gastrointestinal tract	2–4

*Modified Glucksberg scale[305] to prevent overlap in categories.

†Data from Weisdorf DJ, Snover DC, et al: Acute upper gastrointestinal graft-versus-host disease: Clinical significance and response to immunosuppressive therapy. Blood 1990; 76:624.

‡With severe constitutional symptoms.

GVHD = Graft-versus-host disease

TABLE 9–3. International Bone Marrow Transplant Registry (IBMTR) Severity Index for Acute Graft-Versus-Host Disease

Severity Index	Maximum Organ Stage	RR Treatment-Related Mortality (95% CI)	RR Treatment Failure (95% CI)	Glucksberg
0	No GVHD	1.00	1.00	0
A	Skin 1 only	0.84 (0.6, 1.18)	0.85 (0.68, 1.05)	I
B	Any organ stage 2*	1.90 (1.5, 2.42)	1.21 (1.02–1.43)	I, II, III, IV
C	Any organ stage 3	4.34 (3.33, 5.67)	2.19 (1.78, 2.71)	II, III, IV
D	Any organ stage 4	11.9 (9.12, 15.5)	5.68 (4.57, 7.08)	IV

*Any organ stage 1 other than skin alone (e.g., skin 1, gut 1 = Severity Index B).
CI = confidence interval; RR = relative risk.

GVHD increases in severity, formation of bullae with epidermal separation and necrosis is observed.[311] Hepatic involvement in GVHD often presents as cholestatic jaundice, which must be differentiated from VOD, infection, and drug toxicity.[312, 313] Although not without attendant risks of bleeding and pain, liver biopsy may be helpful because characteristic pathologic changes are often observed that aid in differential diagnosis.[314, 315] The classic manifestation of gastrointestinal involvement is watery diarrhea with a "seedy" component that may progress to include crampy abdominal pain, bleeding, and even ileus.[312, 313] By convention, stool volume is used to quantitate the severity of gut involvement. Rectal or colonic biopsy may reveal crypt cell necrosis with lymphocytic infiltration, and, with increasing severity, crypt abscess or loss and mucosal denudation.[316] Skin, liver, and the gastrointestinal tract are assessed individually and graded for severity of involvement, after which an overall grade of GVHD is assigned according to criteria developed by Glucksberg and coworkers (Table 9–2) or the IBMTR (Table 9–3). However, other symptoms and findings may be indicative of acute GVHD. Involvement of the upper gastrointestinal tract is manifested by symptoms of anorexia, inanition, and vomiting.[306] The differential diagnosis of these symptoms also includes viral or fungal infection, dyspepsia, and gastritis, all common conditions in the immunosuppressed stem cell transplant recipient. Endoscopy with biopsy is a minimally invasive diagnostic procedure; the presence of crypt cell apoptosis with dropout indicates GVHD. Fever, thrombocytopenia, anemia, pulmonary involvement, and vascular leak may accompany acute GVHD.

Several risk factors for the development of acute GVHD have been identified. As the genetic disparity between the donor and host increase, so do the incidence and severity of GVHD.[317–320] Thus, genetic disparity is the single most important predictor of acute GVHD. Increasing age of the recipient has a negative impact on the development of acute GVHD.[318, 321, 322] Other factors reported to affect the incidence of GVHD are use of a female donor for a male recipient, a history of parity in female donors, and a history of prior herpes virus infections in the recipient.[318, 319, 321, 323] The source of allogeneic stem cells may also influence the risk for subsequent GVHD. For example, the number of T cells collected during pheresis is significantly greater than the number collected during bone marrow harvest. Despite this, it appears that the rate of severe acute GVHD in patients receiving T cell–rich PBSCs with standard GVHD prophylaxis may not be greater than that seen after BMT.[163, 166, 186] Insufficient data are available to comment definitively on the alloreactivity and GVHD potential of UCB, whether matched or mismatched. Results from large series of UCB SCT procedures indicate that there may be a decrease in the severity of acute GVHD, although whether this is due to the T-cell dose, T-cell repertoire, or some other variable is unknown.[26, 188–190]

Therapeutic strategies aimed to prevent (prophylaxis) of acute GVHD begin with selection of the best available donor. When a matched sibling donor is not available, HLA matching using molecular techniques is the single most important factor in preventing severe GVHD.[320, 324] Considerations of donor sex and parity are advisable if there is a choice of donors. If the patient is seronegative for CMV, use of a CMV-negative donor appears to reduce the risk of GVHD as well as the risk of CMV infection after transplant.[323] Whether the source of hematopoietic stem cells (i.e., bone marrow, PBSCs, or UCB) modifies the risk of acute GVHD is an area of controversy. Supportive care measures such as the use of protective isolation and gut decontamination also protect against the development of GVHD.[325–327]

Conventional prophylactic approaches have been used in an attempt to inhibit T-cell responses by relying on *in vivo* immunosuppression. Essentially all current pharmacologic regimens use combinations of immunosuppressive agents that target different molecular intermediates of T-cell signaling. Cyclosporine (Sandimmune) and tacrolimus (Prograf) both inhibit activity of calcineurin, a serine-threonine phosphatase whose activity is essential for T-cell cytokine transcription.[328] Methotrexate prevents T-cell proliferation,[329] whereas high doses of corticosteroids are lympholytic. Current combinations are cyclosporine or tacrolimus plus methotrexate and/or prednisone.[330–332] A common prophylactic regimen includes cyclosporine given intravenously at a dose of 1.5 mg/kg every 12 hours until oral administration at a dose of 6.25 mg/kg every 12 hours is tolerated. Doses are adjusted to achieve desired blood levels. Cyclosporine is continued on a tapering schedule through day 180 after SCT. Methotrexate is given at 15 mg/m² on day 1 and at 10 mg/m² on days 3, 6, and 11 after HSC infusion. This regimen has been shown to reduce the incidence and severity of acute GVHD and improve long-term survival compared with single-agent therapy in comparable patient cohorts.[333, 334]

As discussed earlier, selective depletion of T lymphocytes from the donor HSC inoculum effectively prevents GVHD. T cells can be removed by a variety of techniques; some of these are lectin depletion or anti–T-cell monoclonal antibodies plus complement, coupling to immunotoxin derivatives, or purging with magnetic beads. Each of these techniques may effect up to a 3 log or more depletion of T cells. Unfortunately, T-cell depletion is associated with an increased risk of graft failure, lymphoproliferative disease after SCT, and, for patients with hematologic malignancies undergoing SCT with identical regimens, of leukemic relapse. Thus, the long-term survival rates of patients who have received T cell–depleted grafts are similar to those of patients who have received conventional *in vivo* immunosuppression after transplantation.[335-337] Strategies using "add-back" of donor T-cells at various time points after SCT are being explored.[338-341] The ultimate role of T-cell depletion in SCT has not been completely delineated.

The outcome and long-term survival of patients with acute GVHD vary directly with the grade of GVHD and response to treatment. The mainstay of treatment of established, acute GVHD remains the administration of glucocorticoids. Glucocorticoids (generally methylprednisolone) have been used in a variety of schedules and doses.[330, 342] The lympholytic effects of very high doses of corticosteroids must be balanced against the increased risk of infections,[343] and doses greater than 2 mg/kg/day may not have increased efficacy.[344] A number of agents have been tried for patients in whom corticosteroid therapy fails or who have disease progression, but secondary treatment of GVHD is often unsuccessful.[345] Generally, cyclosporine is continued at therapeutic levels in patients who develop acute GVHD, and cyclosporine treatment may be initiated in patients who have never received the drug. Antithymocyte globulin, extracorporeal photochemotherapy,[346] newer immunosuppressive agents such as mycophenolate mofetil,[347] and methods targeting CD5, CD3, the interleukin-2 receptor,[307] and TNF-α and its receptor have all been used with varying, incomplete, or unpredictable responses. Novel and reproducible methods of approaching the treatment of patients with corticosteroid-resistant acute GVHD that do not compromise the ability to mount an immune response against infection are needed because the outcome for these patients remains poor.

LATE COMPLICATIONS OF TREATMENT

The number of long-term survivors of SCT continues to grow as transplantation is offered to an increasing number of patients as a therapeutic modality. In addition, advances in supportive care and improved patient selection have contributed to the growth of this population. Thus, delayed complications caused by both the chemoradiotherapy used to prepare patients for SCT and the transplant process itself (e.g., GVHD and a propensity for infection) are being better defined with regard to incidence, severity, and outcome.

Chronic Graft-Versus-Host Disease

GVHD was initially characterized as occurring in two phases; acute GVHD generally presented within the first 100 days after transplant, whereas chronic GVHD occurred after day 100 (Table 9–4). It has become evident that in certain patients chronic GVHD is seen as early as day 50 to 60 after marrow infusion, defined by both clinical and histopathologic criteria.[348] The morbidity and mortality of chronic GVHD are most severe in patients who have chronic GVHD that has progressed directly from acute GVHD.[349] Alternatively, patients may develop chronic GVHD after a period without active GVHD (quiescent) or without any antecedent acute GVHD *(de novo)*. The pathogenesis of chronic GVHD is not completely understood, and it appears to be related to both alloreactivity from donor T cells and dysregulation of peripheral T-cell tolerance caused by thymic dysfunction, which leads to symptoms resembling those of autoimmune disorders.

Risk factors for development of chronic GVHD include HLA disparity between donor and host, prior acute GVHD, increasing patient age, and possibly latent herpes virus in donor or recipient.[349] Additionally, the use of female donors for male recipients and the use of sensitized donors (by prior pregnancy or transfusions) may increase the risk of chronic GVHD.[350] An increased number of T cells in the stem cell inoculum, as occurs with the use of PBSCs as a stem cell source[351] or with T-cell infusions after SCT,[352, 353] appear to result in a higher incidence of chronic GVHD as well.

The diagnosis of chronic GVHD is made by a combination of clinical and pathologic features. The syndrome resembles autoimmune systemic collagen vascular

TABLE 9–4. Comparison of Acute and Chronic Graft-Versus-Host Disease

	Acute GVHD	Chronic GVHD
Incidence	40%–60%	20%–40%
Onset	Day 7–60 (up to 100)	Day >100 (often >60)
Manifestations:		
Skin	Erythematous rash	Sclerodermatous changes
Gut	Secretory diarrhea	Dry mouth; sicca syndrome
Liver	Hepatitis	Esophagitis, malabsorption, cholestasis
Other	Fever	Pulmonary dysfunction
	?Diffuse alveolar hemorrhage	Contractures
		Alopecia
		Thrombocytopenia

diseases with protean manifestations involving essentially every organ (Table 9–5). The majority of patients with chronic GVHD have some cutaneous involvement. Skin involvement may present as lichen planus, patchy erythema, and areas of hyperpigmentation or hypopigmentation. The skin may be dry, freckled, or ulcerated, and the findings are often aggravated by exposure to sunlight. Pathologic changes in the skin involve epithelial cell damage characterized by basal cell degeneration and necrosis, and, later, epidermal atrophy and dermal fibrosis.[354, 355] Sclerodermatous changes may evolve to flexion contractures. Hair follicles may be involved, resulting in areas of alopecia. Eye involvement is common; decreased tearing is quantitated by a Schirmer test. Xerostomia can be problematic and contribute to poor oral intake and the risk of dental caries. There is often scalloping of the lateral margins of the tongue and areas of depapillation. The tongue, buccal mucosa, and gums may have lichen planus–like lesions, which should not be confused with, but may co-occur with, oral candidiasis. A biopsy specimen typically shows lichenoid changes with epithelial cell necrosis and salivary gland inflammation, lymphocytic infiltrate, and fibrosis. Involvement of the liver in chronic GVHD usually manifests as obstructive jaundice, which may progress,

if untreated, to bridging necrosis and cirrhosis. Gastrointestinal signs include inanition with progressive weight loss, chronic malabsorption, diarrhea, anorexia, nausea, and vomiting. Biopsy of the gastrointestinal tract demonstrates single cell apoptosis with crypt destruction and may show fibrosis of the lamina propria. Esophageal webs can contribute to malnutrition by causing dysphagia. Early chronic GVHD may present as diffuse myositis and tendonitis. Progressive joint involvement, which may result from the myositis and tendonitis or simply from overlying skin fibrosis, results in decreased range of motion and flexion contractures. Chronic GVHD may involve the lungs with signs and symptoms of obstructive lung disease progressing to bronchiolitis obliterans (see later). Persistent immunodeficiency with profoundly depressed B- and T-cell responses predisposes patients to recurrent and severe infections. Patients may have reduced immunoglobulin (Ig) G_2 and IgG_4, decreased mucosal IgA, diminished delayed-type hypersensitivity, and hyposplenism. They are susceptible to opportunistic infections with encapsulated organisms (primarily *Pneumococcus*),[356] *P. carinii*, varicella-zoster, and herpes simplex and may have a variety of chronic infections, including sinusitis, bronchitis, and conjunctivitis.

TABLE 9–5. Clinicopathologic Features of Chronic Graft-Versus-Host Disease

System	Features
Systemic	Recurrent infections with immunodeficiency
	Weight loss
	Sicca syndrome
	Debility
Skin	Lichen planus, scleroderma, hyperpigmentation or hypopigmentation
	Dry scale, ulcerated, erythema, freckling
	Flexion contractures
	Biopsy: Epithelial cell damage
	Basal cell degeneration and necrosis
	Epidermal atrophy and dermal fibrosis
Hair	Alopecia
Mouth	Sicca syndrome, depapillation of tongue with variegations
	Scalloping of lateral margins
	Lichen planus and ulcer, angular tightness
	Biopsy: Lichenoid changes with mononuclear infiltrates
	Epithelial cell necrosis
	Salivary gland inflammation, lymphocytic infiltrate, fibrosis
Joints	Decreased range of motion, diffuse myositis/tendonitis
Eyes	Decreased tearing, injected sclerae, conjunctivae
Liver	↑ Alkaline phosphatase > transaminases and bilirubin
	Cholestasis, cirrhosis
	Biopsy: Focal portal inflammation with bile ductule obliteration
	Chronic aggressive hepatitis
	Bridging necrosis
	Cirrhosis
Gastrointestinal	Failure to thrive (children), weight loss (adults)
	Esophageal strictures, malabsorption, chronic diarrhea
	Biopsy: Crypt destruction, single cell dropout
	Fibrosis of lamina propria
Lung	Bronchiolitis obliterans, chronic rales
	Cough, dyspnea, wheezing
	Pneumothorax
	Pulmonary function tests: Decreased forced expiratory volume
Heme	Refractory thrombocytopenia
	Eosinophilia
Spleen	Howell-Jolly bodies

Staging of chronic GVHD is based on the degree of organ involvement (Table 9–6). Limited chronic GVHD consists of localized skin involvement with or without hepatic dysfunction. All other manifestations of chronic GVHD are classified as extensive chronic GVHD. Limited chronic GVHD may resolve spontaneously without specific therapy, and patients with limited chronic GVHD have a favorable outcome.[357] Patients with extensive chronic GVHD have an increased risk of mortality. Specific risk factors for poor outcome include progressive chronic GVHD, lichenoid skin changes, elevated bilirubin levels,[358] and thrombocytopenia.[359]

The most effective prophylactic measure for chronic GVHD is effective prevention of acute GVHD. Once extensive chronic GVHD occurs, it is difficult to resolve. First-line therapy is corticosteroids (usually oral prednisone) that may be given simultaneously or on an alternate-day schedule with cyclosporine.[360] The addition of azathioprine may be help for patients unable to taper the primary corticosteroid therapy without recurrence of disease. A number of other approaches are being tested, including psoralen plus ultraviolet radiation,[346] thalidomide,[361] and clofazimine.[362, 363] Despite new strategies, treatment of extensive chronic GVHD remains a difficult problem with much attendant medical and psychologic morbidity.[364]

Supportive care and symptomatic management are critical in management of chronic GVHD. For example, patients with sicca syndrome are advised to use artificial tears with careful ophthalmologic follow-up and artificial saliva with periodic dental examinations. Oral pilocarpine hydrochloride may relieve the symptoms of xerostomia.[365] Regular and aggressive physical therapy with range of motion exercises is essential to prevent flexion contractures. Finally infection prophylaxis against *P. carinii* and against encapsulated bacteria should be continued well after cessation of treatment with immunosuppressive agents.

Ophthalmologic Problems

A number of ophthalmologic complications may accompany SCT. Decreased lacrimation in chronic GVHD may contribute to ophthalmologic problems, including punctate keratopathy, scar formation, and corneal perforation.[366] Patients may develop infectious complications (particularly from herpes simplex viruses) at any time after SCT. Cyclosporine usage is associated with a number of eye complaints, including an increasingly well-described syndrome of headache, hypertension, seizures, or visual impairment (see section on neurologic complications for a detailed description).[367, 368] In addition, there are numerous reports of symptoms that can be grouped loosely as transplant-related retinopathy. Optic disc edema, either asymptomatic or presenting with visual blurring, has been described in patients who received cyclosporine for GVHD prophylaxis after either busulfan or TBI-based conditioning.[369, 370] Ischemic fundal lesions, detected as "cotton-wool spots" or optic disc edema, have been reported in 13 percent of patients receiving both TBI and cyclosporine.[370] Lesions appeared 3 to 6 months after SCT, and the majority of patients had complaints of decreased visual acuity or other visual disturbance. Most discontinued cyclosporine treatment and half were treated with systemic corticosteroids. In the majority of patients visual acuity recovered and ischemic lesions resolved over time, but little further information is available about the course of or prognosis for patients with this complication. Occlusive microvascular retinopathy has also been described after autologous SCT with high doses of cytarabine and TBI,[371] suggesting that certain high-dose chemotherapy regimens may predispose patients to vascular injury at radiation doses not otherwise associated with toxicity, an argument analogous to that for the development of hemolytic-uremic syndrome after SCT.[372, 373]

A substantial risk of cataract development has been described as a consequence of SCT. Cataracts occur in up to 80 percent of patients given TBI as a single dose, whereas fractionated TBI or chemotherapy-only regimens still result in a 10 to 50 percent incidence of cataracts at 5 to 6 years after SCT.[374–376] A higher chemotherapy dose rate is also associated with an increased incidence.[377] The relative risk of cataracts and the need for subsequent cataract surgery may also be related to prior therapy or to glucocorticoid use for prophylaxis or management of GVHD.[375, 378]

Dental Problems

Disturbances in dental development have been described in children conditioned for SCT with TBI, particularly if SCT occurred before age 6.[379] Characteristic findings include short dental roots, absence of root development, and microdontia. Subsequent decreased alveolar bone growth may lead to additional compromise of dental development. Oral sicca syndrome (occurring as a complication of either TBI, chronic GVHD, or both) may result in chronic oral mucosal injury, poor oral hygiene, and subsequent dental decay. The effects of prophylactic interventions are not well reported.

Pulmonary Complications

Pulmonary dysfunction of both restrictive and obstructive nature can occur after autologous and allogeneic

TABLE 9–6. Staging of Chronic Graft-Versus-Host Disease

LIMITED CHRONIC GVHD

Localized skin involvement and/or
Hepatic dysfunction caused by chronic GVHD

EXTENSIVE CHRONIC GVHD

Generalized skin involvement, or
Localized skin involvement and/or hepatic dysfunction caused by chronic GVHD, plus:
    Liver histology showing chronic aggressive hepatitis, bridging necrosis, or cirrhosis, or
    Eye involvement: Schirmer test (<5 mm wetting), or
    Involvement of minor salivary glands or oral mucosa demonstrated by buccal biopsy, or
    Involvement of any other target organ

SCT in children. Obstructive lung disease, characterized by either interstitial fibrosis or bronchiolitis obliterans pathologically,[380] has been reported in up to 20 percent of children after allogeneic SCT,[381] which is similar to the rate of occurrence in adult patients.[382] Rarely described after autologous SCT, obstructive lung disease has been associated most firmly with chronic GVHD[382, 383] although associations with concurrent viral infections[383] and gastroesophageal reflux[384] have also been reported. There is no clear relationship between TBI-based conditioning and obstructive lung disease.[383] Obstructive lung disease may not be permanent or progressive because in some patients pulmonary function recovers to the pretransplant level in the first months after SCT.[383, 385] Poor survival of chronically affected patients has been suggested,[386] although symptomatic and radiographic improvement with immunosuppression has been described, particularly in those without other concurrent symptoms or signs of active GVHD.[382, 385] The cause of restrictive abnormalities described after SCT is unclear. Modest decreases in total lung capacity, vital capacity, and forced expiratory volume in 1 second at 6 months after SCT have been described in cohorts of both adults and children.[387–389] These values reverted to normal or near normal over time. Because restrictive changes can be asymptomatic,[390] assessment of the occurrence of this complication depends on the intensity of follow-up after SCT. Excluding patients with GVHD, no difference among patients receiving autologous and allogeneic transplants has been described. There may be a relationship to TBI-based conditioning, and fractionation may decrease the adverse effects. The specific effects of prior drug exposure, particularly to nitrosoureas and bleomycin, or underlying pulmonary disease (e.g., asthma) on long-term pulmonary functioning in patients who underwent SCT as children are unknown.

Hematologic Complications

Patients who undergo ABO-incompatible allogeneic SCT are at risk for immune hemolytic anemias caused by donor lymphocyte–produced antibodies. This type of hemolysis is seen most commonly in patients who have received minor ABO-mismatched sibling or UD bone marrow.[391–393] In this latter setting, hemolysis of transfused group O erythrocytes was also observed. This type of hemolysis usually occurs within weeks of SCT, but occasionally its onset may be delayed and it may be prolonged. A relationship to use of cyclosporine without methotrexate for posttransplant immunosuppression has been suggested.[391] In the setting of partially mismatched donors, immune-mediated hemolytic anemia may be the principal manifestation of chronic GVHD.[394] Prolonged red cell aplasia lasting up to 8 months after SCT with ABO major-mismatched bone marrow, also presumably on an immune basis, has been reported.[395, 396] Cytopenias with demonstrable antiplatelet and antineutrophil antibodies have been identified after both autologous and allogeneic SCT.[397–400] These autoimmune cytopenias may be seen early after transplant or up to several years later and may respond to corticosteroids, intravenous γ-globulin, or

other therapy including the use of an anti-CD20 monoclonal antibody (Rituximab).[401] Pancytopenia, unrelated to graft rejection or graft failure, has been noted to occur more often in patients with histories of either acute or chronic GVHD.[358, 402] In addition, even when peripheral blood cell counts are normal, function may be aberrant. For example, neutrophil chemotaxis, superoxide production, and phagocytic capacity have been demonstrated to be abnormal for up to 12 months after SCT,[403] and ultrastructural and immunophenotypic changes in granulocytes have been reported after both autologous and allogeneic SCT.[404] These defects may contribute to the increased susceptibility to infections that exists after SCT.

Coagulation factor deficiencies, specifically deficiencies of factors VII and XII, protein C, and antithrombin III, have been reported after autologous SCT.[405–407] A variety of microangiopathic syndromes have also been described after SCT; some of these have delayed onset. The use of cyclosporine for GVHD prophylaxis or treatment has been associated with both thrombotic thrombocytopenic purpura and hemolytic-uremic syndromes, which can occur either acutely or after periods of exposure to cyclosporine.[408, 409] Specific therapeutic maneuvers have not been shown to be efficacious in either circumstance nor do the syndromes necessarily resolve with discontinuation of cyclosporine. A hemolytic-uremic syndrome, apparently related to the use of TBI in the conditioning regimen, may also occur with onset generally between 4 and 9 months after SCT (see the section on renal and urinary tract complications).

Renal and Urinary Tract Complications

Patients may develop a hemolytic-uremic syndrome, which may occur from 4 to 9 months after SCT.[372, 373, 410] This disorder generally presents as moderate hemolysis and renal dysfunction, although some patients have a more aggressive presentation with hypertension and seizures. In the majority of patients reported, the condition resolves spontaneously over time, although modest persistent anemia as well as decrements in renal function have been reported. Occasionally patients have protracted, severe hematologic and renal manifestations.[411] This syndrome probably reflects toxicity to the endothelium, and the long-term sequelae with respect to renal or other end-organ function in pediatric patients remain unknown.

Chronic nephropathy is occasionally observed. This is most often related to nephrotoxic drugs delivered in the peritransplant period. Patients may develop acute, reversible renal insufficiency related to cyclosporine (often in the setting of elevated blood levels).[408, 412] Less often, patients receiving cyclosporine may develop chronic, irreversible renal insufficiency.[413, 414] Hematoma is another complication seen after SCT. Patients who have received cyclophosphamide as part of their conditioning regimen and also potentially those having received ifosfamide may have continuous or recurrent episodes of hemorrhagic cystitis for up to 10 years after treatment. Such patients may experience chronic dysuria and may have a risk for bladder fibrosis or the development of bladder cancer.[415, 416] Hematuria can also have an infectious cause. Predominant organisms are adenovirus, papovaviruses, and CMV.[417] In most patients, hematuria resolves with time and appropriate supportive care.

Neurologic Complications

Patients undergoing SCT may experience a variety of neurologic complications either directly or more indirectly related to their treatment. Drug toxicity is a major contributor to these problems. Acyclovir is often used after SCT for either prophylaxis or treatment of herpes simplex virus infection. Confusion, tremors, delusion, and frank psychosis have been associated with the use of this drug.[418] Similarly, mental status changes, paresthesias, and, rarely, seizures have been reported with the antiviral agents ganciclovir and foscarnet.[419, 420] Impaired renal function may potentiate the occurrence of these symptoms. Both prednisone and cyclosporine may have neurologic side effects. Psychosis or mood swings accompanying high-dose corticosteroid therapy are well described in the general medical literature. Calcineurin inhibitor administration may be associated with depression, tremors, seizures, and visual impairment.[421–424] Less commonly, hallucinations and ataxia have been observed.[425, 426] It has been postulated that both seizures and acute visual loss arise from hydrostatic changes accompanying drug-associated hypertension. These changes affect white matter in the brain, most commonly in the occipital area, and are accompanied by characteristic radiologic findings on magnetic resonance imaging.[367] In general, symptoms abate rapidly with control of hypertension. It has been suggested that hypomagnesemia potentiates or predisposes patients to cyclosporine-mediated neurotoxicity.[426] Thalidomide, under investigation for treatment of chronic GVHD, may produce sedation and, less commonly, severe peripheral neuropathy.[362] Cerebrovascular accidents, most often caused by thrombocytopenia, may also be observed after SCT.[427] Decreased production of the clotting factor protein C (referred to in the section on hematologic complications) may be another risk factor, and one such instance has been reported.[407]

Central nervous system (CNS) infectious complications related to either immunosuppression, chronic GVHD, or both occur after SCT. Several autopsy series in the 1970s to 1980s demonstrated an incidence of CNS infection ranging from 5 to 7 percent.[427–429] A significant proportion (30 to 50 percent) of these infections were due to *Aspergillus* species; mortality from *Aspergillus* infections involving the CNS is greater than 90 percent.[430] The increased immunosuppression accompanying many current SCT regimens, especially those using T-cell–depleted or alternative donors, may well exacerbate this problem. Infection with *Toxoplasma gondii* also occurs after SCT and has been the second most common CNS pathogen found after *Aspergillus* in recent series.[431, 432] Patients may experience additional neurologic infections, including bacterial meningitis. The presentation of meningitis or of any CNS infection may differ from that in an immunocompetent patient because localizing signs and symptoms may be less dramatic. Patients may also develop encephalitis or meningoencephalitis from a variety of

viruses, including CMV, herpes simplex types 1 and 6, adenovirus, and varicella-zoster.

Leukoencephalopathy can be seen 4 to 5 months after SCT, presenting as lethargy, slurred speech, ataxia, seizures, confusion, decreased sensorium, dysphagia, spasticity, or decerebrate posturing. Consistent objective correlates are found on magnetic resonance imaging or biopsy. In a series of 415 patients from Seattle, a 7 percent incidence was found, and leukoencephalopathy was observed only in patients who had received CNS radiation or intrathecal therapy or both before SCT and methotrexate intrathecal therapy after SCT.[433]

The effects of SCT during childhood on subsequent neuropsychologic functioning have been incompletely investigated. In particular, results from analysis of very young patients are limited. Nonetheless, it is clear in small series that very young children, including those younger than 2 years of age, can undergo SCT with high doses of preparatory chemotherapy or radiotherapy and subsequently perform well in areas such as sensorimotor and cognitive functioning,[434–436] social development,[437] and school performance.[438] Preliminary identification of risk factors that may predict negative neuropsychologic sequelae has been initiated. One large prospective series found that only age younger than 3 years at SCT correlated with subsequent impaired cognitive test performance.[439] Other factors that may influence neuropsychologic outcome include prior cranial radiation,[440] radiation dose rate and cumulative dose, cumulative methotrexate dosing before and after SCT, and exposure to other chemotherapeutic agents.

Endocrine Disorders

Endocrine dysfunction after SCT is often, although not exclusively, associated with radiation therapy, and its incidence and severity are attenuated when fractionated radiation therapy is used. Endocrine evaluation of children having received BU/CY-containing regimens is less well reported. Thyroid dysfunction is well documented in radiation-containing regimens, with compensated hypothyroidism in up to 40 percent of patients and overt hypothyroidism in from 3 to 20 percent.[441, 442] Both are reduced when children received fractionated rather than single-fraction TBI.[442] Conditioning with BU/CY resulted in normal thyroid function 1 year after SCT in a small cohort of patients,[442] although in a larger series a 10 percent incidence of hypothyroidism was found.[443] The incidence of thyroid dysfunction increases over time after SCT and screening should occur on a regular basis.

Children undergoing SCT for an underlying malignancy have a risk for both growth failure and growth hormone deficiency.[444–447] Concomitant factors such as prior treatment, corticosteroid use, chronic GVHD, and renal disease may complicate both the assessment of linear growth and the determination of the cause of poor growth. In some studies, the relationship of low growth hormone levels to observed poor growth is unclear, and it is possible that direct radiation effects on bone and cartilage affect subsequent growth.[448] Fractionated TBI may have a lesser effect, whereas prior cranial radiation seems to be a particularly strong predictor of poor growth.[446, 449, 450] Reports of linear growth of children after BU/CY treatment have been conflicting with some studies demonstrating less growth impairment compared with use of fractionated TBI[449, 451] and some showing equivalent decreases in growth rate.[450] As greater systemic exposure to busulfan occurs through the use of surface-area dosing and monitoring of levels, changes in the toxicity profile of this regimen may become evident.[446]

Gonadal failure is a common sequela of SCT. In both prepubertal male and female patients, delayed puberty associated with hypergonadotropic hypogonadism often occurs.[442] Primary gonadal failure has been described in approximately three fourths of postpubertal females after TBI-containing regimens and is also documented in the same population after BU/CY and other chemotherapy-only regimens.[442, 452, 453] Reduced uterine size and ovarian volume have been observed.[452–454] Other abnormalities noted in a majority of females who are postpubertal at the time of SCT include reduced vaginal elasticity, decreased vaginal and cervical size, atrophic vulvovaginitis, introital stenosis, and loss of pubic hair.[454] These findings appear to be more common in but not confined to patients who had received radiation therapy. No comparable data are published for patients who are prepubertal at the time of SCT. Thus, female patients should be followed closely for gynecologic complications. Hormone replacement should be considered for alleviation of discomfort as well as for chemical indications.[454, 455] In postpubertal males, SCT with or without radiation-based conditioning often results in azoospermia. Significant Leydig cell damage with decreased testosterone levels, decreased testicular volume, and decreased libido appears less often.[442, 451–453, 456, 457] In both sexes, spontaneous recovery of gonadal function has occurred years after SCT, particularly in those who are very young at the time of SCT.[457–459] Fertility resulting in liveborn infants has been reported for both male and female patients receiving SCT. Although it is more common in patients receiving chemotherapy-only conditioning regimens, it has been reported in patients who received radiation therapy as well. Pregnancies in female patients after SCT appear to be accompanied by an increased risk of preterm labor and low-birth-weight infants, although no increase in congenital anomalies in offspring was observed.[460]

Bone Problems

The most prominent bone-related complication of SCT, aseptic (avascular) necrosis, is a known effect of corticosteroid therapy. Therefore it should most likely be seen as a complication of allogeneic SCT when corticosteroids are used for prevention or treatment of GVHD.[461–463] Up to 5 percent of patients may develop aseptic necrosis, with half ultimately requiring joint replacement. Risk factors include acute or chronic GVHD, steroid exposure, and age older than 16 years at the time of SCT.[464] Patients receiving chronic corticosteroid therapy may also be prone to osteoporosis. In addition, gonadal failure and hypoestrogenism related to conditioning therapy may increase the risk for early onset and severe osteoporosis in female patients.[465, 466] The incidence and severity of this potential complication and the long-term consequences

for children are unclear. Growth of craniofacial bones in children undergoing SCT may be impaired, particularly those treated with TBI.[379] Patients developing chronic obstructive airway disease (bronchiolitis obliterans) may develop a pronounced pectus carinatum.

TRANSPLANTATION IN ACQUIRED DISEASES

Aplastic Anemia

Severe aplastic anemia (SAA) is a syndrome characterized by peripheral pancytopenia and marrow hypoplasia (see Chapter 7). Mortality associated with this disorder in children can be as high as 50 percent in the first 6 months.[467] Although a number of immunosuppressive and marrow stimulatory therapies have shown reasonable activity, the only curative treatment is SCT. The potential efficacy of allogeneic SCT for patients with SAA was established with the initial publication in 1972 of results achieved in four patients.[468] Randomized studies have since established the superiority of matched allogeneic SCT over supportive care (androgens in the 1970s, immunosuppressive therapy with antithymocyte globulin in the 1980s and 1990s) in both children[469, 470] and, more recently, adults.[471] In addition, large retrospective series have demonstrated a significant survival advantage for patients older than 40 years of age who received SCT compared with those who received immunosuppressive therapies.[472, 473] The survival of patients with SAA receiving SCT from a matched sibling donor has steadily improved over the past three decades.[474] Most series report long-term DFS of more than 60 percent, and survival approaches 90 percent for select low-risk patients such as young patients,[474, 475] patients receiving transplants during the last decade,[476] and those without chronic GVHD.[477]

Notwithstanding its demonstrated efficacy, application of SCT in the treatment of SAA has been fraught with problems. Most prominent of these has been the high rate of graft rejection. In fact, the patterns observed in syngeneic twins undergoing SCT for SAA suggest three general pathophysiologic bases for graft failure: (1) stem cell abnormality (twin engrafts without conditioning), (2) other hematopoietic cell or immune-mediated defect (twin rejects simple infusion but accepts graft if conditioned with cytoreductive or immunosuppressive therapy), and (3) microenvironmental defect (complete failure of engraftment despite aggressiveness of preparative approach).[478] Graft rejection rates as high as 40 percent are seen when patients are given cyclophosphamide alone[479] and hover around 10 percent with current approaches to conditioning. Risk factors identified for graft failure after SCT include low donor cell dose, positive crossmatch of recipient against donor in a lymphocytotoxicity assay, previous transfusion, a non–radiation-containing regimen, a non-cyclosporine GVHD prophylaxis regimen, or the use of T-cell depletion.[480] The addition of buffy coat cells[481] and the inclusion of additional immunosuppressive medications such as antithymocyte globulin in chemotherapy-only conditioning regimens, use of alternative radiotherapy schedules such as total lymphoid irradiation or low-dose TBI or thoracoabdominal irradiation, more widespread use of cyclosporine, and more conservative transfusion practices before SCT have led to increasingly successful outcomes.[234, 334, 480, 482, 483] The potential impact of decreased transfusion-associated allosensitization associated with depletion of leukocytes through filters has not yet been assessed. No randomized trials of different conditioning regimens have been reported. Results from approximately 600 patients who underwent transplantation in the 1980s have been analyzed in aggregate through the IBMTR[334] as well as results from more than 2000 patients from the European group.[474] Although the incidence of graft failure differed among the different approaches used, overall survival did not.

Many studies have shown that causes of treatment failure after allogeneic SCT for SAA vary significantly and depend on patient- and disease-related variables as well as on the regimen chosen.[480] Multivariate analyses support the impression that children with SAA do particularly well after SCT.[474] The administration of donor buffy coat cells at the time of SCT decreases graft rejection but is associated with increased occurrence of chronic GVHD.[481] Use of a conditioning regimen containing radiation also appears to be associated with less graft rejection but with increased occurrence of interstitial pneumonitis and GVHD.[334] In addition, TBI-based regimens may be associated with a substantially increased risk of secondary solid malignancy compared with chemotherapy-only regimens.[484-485] The impact of GVHD prophylaxis on outcome is pronounced. In several large analyses, use of cyclosporine was associated with a significant improvement in overall survival, which may be attributable to either effects on rejection or GVHD or both.[334, 474, 486-488]

The overall good outcome, coupled with the paucity of other therapeutic options, the incidence of relapse, and growing concern over the evolution of MDS and AML in long-term survivors of treatment with immunosuppressive agents has encouraged use of SCT in patients without a matched family donor.[489-491] Results have been mixed. Survival had historically been less than 30 percent with mismatched family and matched and mismatched unrelated donors. Recent results are more encouraging and reflect advances in HLA typing, better supportive care, more aggressive conditioning regimens that decrease the incidence of graft rejection,[492] and a shorter interval between diagnosis and SCT.[493] The majority of patients without a matched sibling donor receive at least one trial of immunosuppressive therapy before a decision is made to proceed with SCT.

Myelodysplasia

Myelodysplasia has been estimated to account for about 6 percent of childhood hematologic malignancies, although this figure is probably an underestimate because a subset of children with AML presumably had antecedent MDS.[494] Allogeneic SCT remains the only curative modality for MDS.[495-498] Both busulfan- and TBI-based regimens have been used, with no discernible difference in outcome.[499] In combined adult and pediatric series, prognostic variables associated with favorable outcome are younger age, shorter duration of disease,

and SCT before the appearance of excess numbers of blasts.[497, 500, 501] SCT in patients with secondary AML is uniformly associated with poor DFS, primarily because of the high incidence of relapse but also because of high rates of regimen-related toxicity.[501] Although prior reports implicated marrow fibrosis as a particular risk factor for impaired hematologic recovery and poor outcome, more recent analyses do not substantiate this concern, and fibrosis should not preclude consideration of SCT.[502, 503] The decision to offer SCT to patients with MDS is controversial. This is especially true for older individuals because in adult patients the course of MDS is often indolent, and 5-year survival is appreciable with conservative management. These issues may be less pertinent for children who more often are seen with increased numbers of blasts and generally develop acute leukemia if untreated.

Acute Lymphoblastic Leukemia

The treatment of children with newly diagnosed ALL has become more effective over the last four decades. However, despite this improvement, 25 to 30 percent of pediatric patients with ALL have a relapse of their disease. In recent years the efficacy of SCT has been studied in this group of patients. The DFS of children in second or subsequent remissions treated with matched sibling allogeneic SCT has been reported to range from 40 to 75 percent.[64, 504-508] Although the role of SCT in the treatment of relapses of ALL is still not completely decided, there are some clinical situations in which SCT appears to be more effective than treatment with chemotherapy alone.

Children who have a relapse less than 18 to 30 months after their first complete remission have an especially poor prognosis. The best outcome after use of chemotherapy for a second remission has been reported by Henze et al.[509] In a cohort of intensively treated patients, the event-free survival (EFS) was 18 percent in patients who had a bone marrow relapse less than 6 months after completing treatment compared with 30 percent in who have relapses thereafter. An analysis of 36 published studies found a DFS rate of less than 5 percent in patients who had relapses within 18 months of the first remission when treated with chemotherapy.[510] In a large cohort of British children with ALL the survival of patients with an early bone marrow relapse was only 3 percent regardless of method of treatment.[508] Several studies have addressed the efficacy of use of SCT in this group of patients. One study of a group of 44 children with ALL in second remission after an early relapse showed a DFS of 36 percent in those who received a BMT from HLA-identical siblings compared with 7 percent in those who were treated with chemotherapy.[511] Other studies of matched sibling donor BMT in the setting of early relapse have shown EFS rates as high as 47 percent.[506] In the majority of studies, the superiority of SCT is largely due to a reduction in the risk of relapse, a gain that is partly offset by the increase in treatment-related mortality associated with SCT.

In patients who have a late relapse (i.e., more than 24 to 36 months after first remission), the benefit of treatment with SCT is less clear. The DFS of patients treated with chemotherapy alone has been reported to be between 30 and 50 percent.[509, 512, 513] Several studies suggest that treatment with SCT from an HLA-identical sibling may not substantially increase this number,[506, 511, 514], although others have reported that the outcome with SCT is still superior even in patients with a long first remission.[515]

For patients whose ALL is refractory to primary induction or reinduction therapy but who subsequently have a remission, the most likely potentially curative modality is allogeneic SCT. Children with ALL in first remission with certain high-risk disease characteristics may also benefit from allogeneic SCT. For example, the prognosis for children with Philadelphia chromosome (Ph[1])–positive ALL appears to be particularly poor. Analysis of a large cohort of children with Ph[1]-positive ALL in first remission has shown a substantial benefit with SCT; children treated with SCT had a DFS of 65 percent at 7 years compared with 25 percent for those treated with chemotherapy.[516] Moreover in this series, the advantage of SCT became more apparent with each succeeding year from treatment, suggesting a greater protection from late relapse than that seen with chemotherapy alone.[516] The IBMTR has reported the results for 67 patients with Ph[1]-positive ALL who had HLA-matched sibling allografts. The probability of 2-year DFS was approximately 38 percent if SCT was performed in the first clinical remission and 41 percent if performed thereafter.[517, 518] Another sizable series reported DFS of 46 percent if SCT was performed in the first clinical remission and 28 percent if performed after the first relapse.[84] This suggests that allogeneic SCT is an effective treatment that may be advantageous to pursue in the first clinical remission, although it is still likely to be effective after relapse. Insufficient data exist to perform similar analyses of outcome for patients with other high-risk features such as the presence of t(4;11) or t(8;14) translocations or hypodiploidy. Some centers pursue aggressive chemotherapy for such patients, whereas others uniformly attempt SCT in the first clinical remission.

A major obstacle to SCT remains the availability of matched family donors. For those children without related donors, autologous SCT, UD SCT, and mismatched family donor SCT remain therapeutic options. Concerns about autologous SCT include the damage inflicted on autologous stem cells and stroma by prior chemotherapy and the potential contamination of HSCs by leukemic cells. Techniques to purge leukemic cells using either pharmacologic or immunologic methodologies were established a long time ago and are relatively safe.[519] Billett and colleagues[520, 521] reported an EFS of 53 percent at 3 years for 51 children who had this procedure. No studies have directly addressed the role of purging in autologous SCT, but one retrospective analysis of children with relapsed ALL found no difference in relapse rates or outcome among those who received purged as opposed to unpurged autologous marrow.[522] The relative efficacy of autologous SCT, allogeneic SCT, and chemotherapy as treatments for children in second remission has not been examined in a randomized fashion. A retrospective analysis of data from the United Kingdom showed that the outcome with autologous SCT and chemotherapy was equivalent (EFS of 34 percent versus 26 percent),[508] although there was a significantly higher rate of relapse in the autologous SCT and chemotherapy groups than in those patients who received a matched family donor SCT.

Published experience with SCT from UDs in patients with relapsed ALL is still limited. However, its role has been examined in several studies, in which DFS rates of 42 to 67 percent have been achieved.[232, 508, 523] Future studies will be needed to show that these results can be generalized to larger patient populations. A retrospective comparison of patients with acute leukemia treated with an UCB transplant showed that the outcome was comparable with that for those treated with BMT.[524] Studies of mismatched family (haploidentical) donor SCT do not contain sufficient numbers of patients with ALL to permit generalizations about efficacy.

Acute Myeloblastic Leukemia

Successive clinical trials over the last 20 years have firmly established the role of intensive postremission therapy in the treatment of AML. However, during that time there has been much debate as to whether allogeneic SCT or intensive chemotherapy without stem cell support is the optimal postremission therapy. Allogeneic SCT offers dose intensity and the possibility of a graft-versus-leukemia effect. Alternatively, intensive chemotherapy without stem cell support is feasible in the majority of patients and may be less toxic. The issue of using allogeneic SCT in the first clinical remission was first addressed in a series of prospective trials in the mid-1980s. In 111 consecutive patients, the Seattle group performed matched sibling allogeneic SCT for patients who had a donor, whereas the remaining patients received conventional chemotherapy dose intensification. The probability of 5-year DFS was 49 percent for patients receiving SCT compared with 20 percent for patients receiving chemotherapy alone.[525] However, since that time, more intensive postremission chemotherapy regimens have been associated with improved disease control in some pediatric and adult clinical trials.[526] This result has raised the question of whether allogeneic SCT remains more effective than intensive chemotherapy in the postremission setting. To address this issue the Children's Cancer Group conducted a large, randomized trial of allogeneic SCT versus chemotherapy or autologous SCT in 652 children and adolescents whose AML was in remission. At the end of induction chemotherapy, patients with five or six HLA-antigen matched relatives were assigned to receive allogeneic BMT. All others were randomly assigned to receive either autologous SCT with 4-hydroperoxycyclophosphamide purging or four courses of chemotherapy. The results of this trial showed that the outcome with allogeneic SCT was superior to that achieved with either chemotherapy or autologous SCT. For the subgroup of patients treated with a more intensive induction regimen overall survival improved for all groups; the DFS with allogeneic SCT was 66 percent compared with 53 percent with chemotherapy and 48 percent with autologous SCT.[528] These data underscore the benefit of both intensive induction chemotherapy and first-remission matched family donor SCT in the management of newly diagnosed AML.

For patients who have no allogeneic donor, autologous SCT remains a treatment option. In many trials, autologous marrow was purged of residual leukemic cells with 4-hydroperoxycyclophosphamide, although no direct benefit of this technique has been proven. Early reports of trials in adults and adolescents with AML suggested that autologous SCT might offer additional therapeutic efficacy over chemotherapy.[529, 530] However, pediatric trials have not demonstrated any advantage to this modality in patients with AML in first remission, and there is insufficient data to assess the influence of AML subclass on outcome.[526, 528, 531]

In most studies of patients with relapsed AML, the duration of the first remission strongly predicts outcome; the DFS of patients having a relapse less than 1 year after diagnosis is 10 to 20 percent regardless of treatment modality used.[532, 533] Patients with relapsed AML are often treated with allogeneic SCT from an HLA-matched sibling. Early studies reported the DFS of patients receiving transplants in the untreated first ("early") relapse to be as high as 25 to 30 percent.[85, 534] In contrast, a more recent report of 379 adults with relapsed or refractory AML found the DFS of patients receiving transplants in the untreated first relapse to be no better than 13 percent.[535] Patients with treatment-refractory disease had an equivalently poor prognosis. However, the DFS for patients who had a second remission was significantly better at 32 percent. The outcome of children with relapsed AML was studied by the Medical Research Council Childhood Leukemia Working Party.[532] Of the 81 patients in whom reinduction chemotherapy therapy was attempted, 69 percent had a second remission. Approximately two thirds of these patients were treated with allogeneic SCT and the overall survival of the group was 44 percent at 3 years. In addition, patients treated with SCT had a longer second remission than those treated with chemotherapy alone.[532] These data suggest a role for allogeneic SCT in the treatment of relapsed AML, especially for those patients who have a second remission. Results of UD SCT in children with relapsed AML have not been extensively reported. One report of 18 pediatric patients with AML in first or second remission found an EFS of 70 percent at 2 years, suggesting that in selected groups of patients in second remission UD SCT may also be an effective treatment option.[536]

Chronic Myelogenous Leukemia and Juvenile Myelomonocytic Leukemia

CML is a relatively uncommon disorder in children, but its clinical course and outcome with the use of allogeneic SCT seem indistinguishable from results in adults. The DFS and overall outcome of patients receiving SCT in the first chronic phase of the disease are excellent.[537] BMT in either the accelerated phase of the disease or blast crisis is less effective.[538] Transplant within a year of diagnosis is associated with better outcome.[539, 540] Use of T-cell depletion has been associated with a marked rate of relapse, suggesting a very significant role for allogeneic T cells in control of this disorder,[301] and relapse after BMT has been successfully treated with infusion of donor lymphocytes.[541]

There is no curative chemotherapy for juvenile chronic myelomonocytic leukemia (see Chapter 27). Allogeneic SCT from both conventional and alternative donors has been used successfully.[542–547] Longer follow-up of larger patient cohorts shows that as many as half of patients have a relapse after the transplant and that relapse often occurs soon after SCT.[542, 547] However, very limited data suggest that the rapid withdrawal of immunosuppression or administration of donor leukocytes may result in a second remission.[542, 548] Alternative approaches to preparative regimens and patient management are being evaluated in an attempt to improve the success of SCT as a treatment for this disorder.

Hodgkin and Non-Hodgkin Lymphoma

SCT has been used in children with Hodgkin disease (HD) or aggressive non-Hodgkin lymphoma (NHL) who either have a relapse or demonstrate refractory disease after initial treatment with conventional chemotherapy. The most efficacious conditioning regimen remains uncertain, as DFS appears to be equivalent among series using either TBI-based or chemotherapy-only approaches.[549] With regard to stem cell source, there has been increasing consensus about the use of autologous PBSCs rather than bone marrow, based on the favorable engraftment characteristics reviewed earlier. The potential for survival of pediatric patients with lymphoma was established in 1986, when results from a 5-year French study demonstrated approximately 50 percent DFS in children with Burkittt lymphoma treated with high-dose chemotherapy followed by autologous BMT.[550] Similar results in children with aggressive NHL and HD have been reported more recently from other centers and in larger combined pediatric and adult series.[551–554] Paralleling the findings in adult patients, DFS in children with NHL is most consistently predicted by disease responsiveness to chemotherapy before SCT; virtually no long-term survivors are seen among patients with refractory disease before conditioning.[555] In contrast, long-term survival is seen for some patients with refractory progressive HD after SCT.[556, 557] The role of allogeneic SCT in the treatment of NHL and HD has not been completely elucidated.[558] Retrospective case-control studies in adult/pediatric series suggest comparable results.[559, 560] A prospective trial revealed a lower relapse rate in those undergoing allogeneic BMT but no overall survival advantage.[561] Whether this decrease in relapse rate reflects a graft-versus-lymphoma effect or merely the infusion of uncontaminated HSCs is not clear. Characterization of patients with a particularly high risk for treatment failure after autologous SCT may serve to identify those for whom alternative treatment approaches should be developed.

Neuroblastoma and Other Solid Tumors

The most extensive experience using SCT to treat solid tumors in pediatric patients has been with advanced-stage neuroblastoma. DFS in this group of children has repetitively been shown to be less than 20 percent when they are treated with conventional chemotherapy. Thus, several studies suggested that more intensive induction therapy followed by dose intensification with autologous HSC support could favorably affect DFS.[562, 563] A randomized trial of conventional chemotherapy versus myeloablative therapy and purged autologous BMT in high-risk patients with newly diagnosed neuroblastoma confirmed these findings with a DFS of 34 percent in the transplant cohort.[564] Because regimen-related toxicity was acceptable and dose intensification appeared to improve DFS, current strategies are focused on further chemotherapy dose intensification. Sequential ("tandem") SCT over a short period of time (4 to 6 weeks) using non–cross-resistant agents and CD34+ selected PBSCs has been studied. The reported DFS is 58 percent with median follow-up of less than 2 years.[565] Small numbers of patients have undergone allogeneic SCT with no clear improvement in outcome over that achieved with autologous SCT.[566]

Little has been published on the use of either allogeneic or autologous SCT for other pediatric nonhematologic malignancies. Some promise in terms of initial response has been observed for patients with sarcomas who have minimal disease at SCT that is also chemosensitive.[567, 568] The generalizability and durability of these responses will need to be established before widespread application of SCT can be supported.

TRANSPLANTATION IN GENETIC DISEASES

Allogeneic SCT is the best treatment option for some inherited diseases, whereas for other diseases, it has been proven to have no role. The most common inherited diseases that have been treated with SCT are reviewed, and the experience with less common diseases is summarized in Table 9–7.

Immunodeficiency Disorders

SEVERE COMBINED IMMUNODEFICIENCY SYNDROMES

Since the late 1960s, allogeneic BMT has been used successfully to cure children with a number of lethal immunodeficiency diseases (see Table 9–7), including severe combined immunodeficiency disease (SCID) and

TABLE 9–7. Immunodeficiency Disorders Treated with Stem Cell Transplantation

Classic severe combined immunodeficiency disease (B⁻)
Common severe combined immunodeficiency disease (B⁺)
Adenosine deaminase deficiency
Reticular dysgenesis
Omenn syndrome
Severe combined immunodeficiency disease associated with short-limbed dwarfism and ectodermal dysplasia
Familial erythrophagocytic lymphohistiocytosis
HLA class II deficiency (bare lymphocyte syndrome)
Purine nucleoside phosphorylase deficiency
X-linked lymphoproliferative disease
Leukocyte adhesion deficiency (CD11/18 deficiency)
Wiskott-Aldrich syndrome

Wiskott-Aldrich syndrome. SCID is a clinical syndrome resulting from one or more defects in the molecules responsible for T-cell function. Without question, conventional, matched sibling allogeneic SCT for SCID is one of the major success stories of the use of SCT. Unlike most other forms of SCT, transplantation in patients with SCID does not necessarily require conditioning because recipients may be incapable of rejecting donor cells. However, some patients such as those with purine nucleoside phosphorylase deficiency, Omenn syndrome,[569] and reticular dysgenesis[570] may require both myeloablative and immunosuppressive conditioning regimens to ensure engraftment.

After conventional matched SCT without cytoreduction, phenotypic and functional T-cell immune reconstitution may take up to 4 months.[571] B-cell engraftment is variable and a proportion of these children will require chronic intravenous immune γ-globulin therapy.[572, 573] Grade II or greater acute GVHD is rarely observed and contributes little to treatment-related mortality.[574] Similarly, chronic GVHD is uncommon. Dramatically improved long-term survival of patients ranging from approximately 50 percent in the 1970s to nearly 90 percent by the end of the 1980s[574] appears to be attributable to more rapid and precise diagnosis, followed by SCT of younger patients with better medical conditions as well as improved supportive care for infectious complications.[574, 575]

In the context of the remarkable successes observed in patients with SCID and other severe immunodeficiency disorders who were treated with matched sibling SCT, studies using HSCs from mismatched family and unrelated donors were initiated. The early experience using conventional grafts from haploidentical donors was characterized by graft failure, severe GVHD, and opportunistic infection and resulted in poor long-term survival.[572, 576] The development of T-cell depletion protocols combined either with no conditioning[573, 577] or with modified conditioning regimens[578] significantly reduced the rate of graft rejection and significantly improved both hematopoietic and immunologic engraftment in the majority of patients.[572, 579] Most patients develop functional donor T lymphocytes, although reconstitution of B-cell immunity is seen less often and, when present, it is delayed. This situation seems particularly true if cytoreduction is not used and has led, particularly in Europe, to more frequent adoption of complete cytoreduction to encourage the evolution of a fully functional donor immune and hematopoietic system.[580] Overall, survival of patients who received SCT from HLA-disparate donors after T-cell depletion has risen substantially, to the range of 60 to 80 percent.[573] Nonetheless, treatment failure because of infection, graft failure, poor immune reconstitution, and B-cell lymphoproliferative disease after SCT persists. Experience with the use of matched UD SCT has been limited.[581] The advantage of such donors over haploidentical family donors is not clear: standard ablative regimens are necessary and the time required to identify an appropriate UD is a concern in this vulnerable population. More recent approaches have involved greater use of cytoreductive but not nonmyeloablative preparative regimens.[582] Although these regimens are potentially less toxic and thus are suited for patients with severe organ dysfunction that precludes the use of standard conditioning regimens, the likelihood and extent of durable immunologic reconstitution are unknown. Alternative sources of stem cells including UD human fetal liver or thymus have also been evaluated in the treatment of patients with SCID.[583] Less than one third of patients demonstrated durable engraftment, and even fewer had meaningful immunologic reconstitution.[584] Although intriguing, these studies have not significantly contributed to the treatment of patients with SCID, and alternative treatments have been superseded by T cell– and B cell–depleted haploidentical SCT.

WISKOTT-ALDRICH SYNDROME

Wiskott-Aldrich syndrome is an X-linked recessive disorder in which progressive T-cell immunodeficiency is associated with eczema, small platelets, and thrombocytopenia. The pathogenesis of this disorder is associated with aberrant expression of the CD43 molecule.[585, 586] This disorder is reviewed in detail in Chapters 23 and 44. As for SCID, matched sibling allogeneic SCT was first undertaken in children with Wiskott-Aldrich syndrome in the late 1960s, and full correction of the disorder was reported in 1978.[587] Both TBI- and busulfan-based regimens have been used successfully. The overall outcome (almost 90 percent DFS) of this group of patients is among the best of any patient cohort undergoing allogeneic SCT.[60, 574, 588] This success led to extension of this approach to the use of mismatched family and unrelated donors, but historically the outcomes have been less successful. Significant problems related to graft rejection and the development of posttransplant B-cell lymphoproliferative disease have been difficult to surmount.[581, 589, 590] More recent registry data suggest that the outcome for UD SCT approaches that for sibling SCT if patients are young (younger than 5 years of age) at the time of SCT, whereas the outcome remains suboptimal using family members other than matched siblings as donors.[591]

Inherited Hematopoietic Disorders

THALASSEMIA

Until 20 years ago, thalassemia was managed solely by red cell transfusion (see Chapter 21) Only 50 percent of patients survived to age 15, and few, if any, survived beyond age 25.[592] Although hypertransfusion regimens initiated in the 1960s virtually abolished both mortality directly related to severe anemia and bony deformity caused by marrow expansion, death due to iron overload persisted. Acquisition of blood-borne infection became an additional risk. The advent of subcutaneously administered iron chelation therapy with deferoxamine in the 1970s substantially altered the fatal course of transfusional hemosiderosis. Hypertransfusion and chelation have been demonstrated to prolong cardiac DFS.[593–596] Although results to date strongly suggest that patients with thalassemia who comply with routine self-administration of desferrioxamine will remain free of cardiac and other iron-related toxicity for at least one to two decades,

follow-up is insufficient to assess either long-term efficacy or toxicity.

The successful application of SCT as an alternative treatment for thalassemia major was first reported in 1982.[597, 598] Subsequently, experience with a very large group reported by Lucarelli and coworkers[59] has unquestionably established the feasibility of SCT for thalassemia in children younger than age 16, with EFS hovering around 75 percent.[59] Although the generalizability of these findings is unclear because of the highly selected patient groups analyzed, portal fibrosis, hepatomegaly, and history of inadequate chelation have been used to define a class of patients with poor outcome.[59] Nonetheless, older patients, those with more extensive hepatic damage, and those who have had transfusions more often appear to fare worse.[599, 600] Both CY/TBI and BU/CY conditioning regimens have been used successfully. The use of reduced doses of CY has recently been investigated in an attempt to make conditioning less toxic for adults and other high-risk patients.[601] In addition to common causes of SCT-related morbidity and mortality, rejection followed by persistence or recurrence of host (thalassemic) hematopoiesis remains a major cause of treatment failure. Thus, although matched donor SCT can be curative, the decision to pursue conservative chelation programs or allogeneic BMT in individual patients with suitable matched sibling donors remain difficult. The experience using donors other than matched siblings is limited; complications of graft rejection, infection, and GVHD have resulted in unacceptable toxicity and EFS of only 20 percent.[602] The deliberate use of a nonmyeloablative approach to reduced mixed chimerism is being explored.

SICKLE CELL DISEASE

Because the clinical course of sickle cell disease is highly variable, acceptance of SCT as a treatment modality has been relatively slow and is still not widespread. Debate about the factors necessary to identify appropriate candidates for SCT is vigorous and centers on defining markers of severity, delineating prognostic factors, evaluating potential synergistic damage to end organs already damaged by sickle cell disease, and defining the relative merits of alternative treatments such as hydroxyurea.[603–605] Additional constraints have inhibited more widespread use of SCT for this disorder. In addition, the number of times that parental consent for allogeneic SCT would have been granted has been assessed, and it is clear that there is significant resistance to such an approach given its potential acute morbidity and long-term sequelae.[606] Models based on sibling number and exclusion of affected siblings suggest that less than 15 percent of patients have an appropriate sibling donor.[607]

Nonetheless, several substantial series as well as case reports of the use of BMT to treat sickle cell disease are found in the literature,[608–611] and some patients have been followed for many years.[612] Survival is very good, and resolution of vascular crises and hemolysis and evidence of correction of prior splenic reticuloendothelial dysfunction are seen.[609, 613] However, graft rejection remains a problem with an incidence of autologous recovery and recurrent sickle cell disease reported in 10 percent of patients.[612] Expected rates of both acute and chronic GVHD have been observed. Neurologic complications, both hemorrhage and seizure, have been reported, and the incidence may be increased, particularly in patients with a previous history of CNS complications.[611, 614, 615] The best therapeutic intervention for a given child with sickle cell disease remains a difficult decision.

FANCONI ANEMIA

Fanconi anemia is an autosomal recessive disorder characterized clinically by a highly variable physical phenotype, progressive marrow failure, and a marked propensity for development of AML and certain solid tumors (see Chapter 8). Although patients with Fanconi anemia may exhibit excessive toxicity after exposure to alkylating agents, such as cyclophosphamide, and irradiation, the development of specialized conditioning regimens has spurred the use of SCT as a treatment option.[616] In addition to successful BMT, the first reported UCB transplant was successfully undertaken for a child with Fanconi anemia using UCB cells of an HLA-identical sibling.[169] Earlier intervention results in excellent outcomes, supported by single center data for 18 children with Fanconi anemia who received transplants from HLA-matched siblings relatively early in their disease course, with a DFS at 2 years of 95 percent.[617]

In contrast, the outcome using alternative donors is significantly worse.[616] A large retrospective study of 199 patients reported to the IBMTR demonstrated a 2-year probability of survival of 66 percent after HLA-identical sibling BMT and 29 percent after alternative donor BMT.[618] The rate of graft rejection appears to be very high in the UD setting, with several studies reporting graft failure in 17 to 33 percent of patients.[619, 620] Graft failure has contributed to the low overall survival rate of approximately 30 percent.[618–620] However, newer regimens that emphasize more robust immunosuppression may be more promising.[621, 622] Although improvement in conditioning regimens and GVHD prophylaxis may reduce the acute toxicities of SCT in patients with Fanconi anemia, long-term follow-up shows that they have a significant risk for second tumors, particularly squamous cell carcinomas.[623] Patients with Fanconi anemia already have a high risk for development of neoplasia, which may be increased by exposure to radiation and chemotherapy. However, the paucity of other effective therapies makes SCT the most successful modality in current use.

DIAMOND-BLACKFAN ANEMIA

Diamond-Blackfan anemia is a rare, heritable marrow failure syndrome. The condition is generally diagnosed in the first months of life. Patients often exhibit macrocytosis and reticulocytopenia and also have a bone marrow that shows a selective decrease in erythroid precursors (see Chapter 8). Although approximately two thirds of patients show an initial response to corticosteroid therapy, failure to respond to therapy or a loss of response over time is seen in significant numbers of patients.[624] The toxicity of treatment, whether sequelae of chronic transfusion

or corticosteroid use, is significant. In addition, there is a potential for development of leukemia in early to mid adulthood.[624] For these reasons, allogeneic SCT has been explored as a therapeutic option. The majority of patients, reported either individually or to registries, have had successful engraftment and are long-term survivors.[625–630] Reports of matched sibling SCT significantly outnumber those of alternative donor SCT. Both TBI- and busulfan-based regimens have been used.

GRANULOCYTE AND PLATELET DISORDERS

Limited numbers of patients with various disorders of myeloid function and number have had successful reconstitution of hematopoietic function by allogeneic SCT (Table 9–8 and specific diseases in Chapter 21). In general, the conditioning regimen used was BU/CY, although TBI-based regimens have also been used. Individualized determination of the relative toxicity and benefit of available treatment options influences the decision to transplant. The advent of cytokine therapy has also changed the outlook for patients with many of the neutropenic disorders; this is seen most dramatically for patients with severe congenital neutropenia and chronic granulomatous disease.[631] Nonetheless, SCT, from both matched and mismatched donors, remains an option for patients with high-risk diseases such as CD11/18 deficiency (leukocyte adhesion deficiency) and Chédiak-Higashi syndrome as well as for those with other granulocyte disorders that respond poorly to more conservative treatment.[24, 574, 583, 632, 633]

Similarly, but in even smaller numbers, allogeneic SCT has successfully corrected platelet number and function in patients with congenital platelet disorders (see specific diseases in Chapter 44). Because other therapeutic options are limited, consideration of both matched and alternative donor SCT for disorders such as amegakaryocytic thrombocytopenia and Glanzmann thrombasthenia is warranted.[634–638]

OSTEOPETROSIS

This rare disorder results from dysfunction of osteoclasts with resulting formation of excessive mineralized osteoid and cartilage. In addition to encroachment on optic and other cranial nerve foramina, eradication of the marrow space ensues. Thus, progressive neurologic and hematologic dysfunction develops early in childhood. Studies in osteopetrotic mice revealed that the phenotype could be reversed by BMT from unaffected animals.[639] These and other studies confirmed that osteoclasts were macrophages with specialized functions, thus providing a

TABLE 9–8. White Blood Cell Disorders Treated with Stem Cell Transplantation

Chédiak-Higashi syndrome[632]
Severe congenital neutropenia
Chronic granulomatous disease[110]
CD11/18 deficiency (leukocyte adhesion deficiency)
Neutrophil actin defects
Shwachman-Diamond syndrome

rationale for the potential efficacy of SCT. Successful human SCT for this disorder was begun in the late 1970s.[575, 640, 641] Both busulfan- and TBI-based regimens have been used. Significant problems in engraftment have been described, attributed in part to disruption of the underlying marrow microenvironment.[642] However, most graft failures have been associated with the use of T cell–depleted, histoincompatible grafts, which are themselves risk factors for graft failure.[575, 642, 643] Several cases of hypercalcemia occurring in the first months after SCT have been described, especially in children beyond infancy at the time of SCT, and appropriate monitoring for this complication is essential.[642, 644] Because neurologic damage occurs early and is rarely reversible, the decision to perform SCT should be made rapidly. Depending on the future success of ongoing efforts to explore the efficacy of cytokines, such a decision may include a prior trial of alternative therapy.

STORAGE DISORDERS

Disruption of cellular function and subsequent organ impairment caused by substrate accumulation from an underlying enzymatic deficiency characterize the storage disorders (see Chapter 33). Historically, few treatment options other than palliative and supportive modalities have been available. More recently, the availability of alglucerase (Ceredase) enzyme infusion has dramatically altered the course of Gaucher disease.[645] Although similar inroads have not yet been made in other diseases, the concepts of gene transfer and somatic cell therapy as well as infusion of enzymes produced by recombinant techniques are being investigated in various animal models of such diseases.

Several excellent reviews of the results of SCT for specific storage disorders have been published.[61, 646–651] The rationale for SCT as a therapeutic maneuver is based on the belief that the most affected cell population is hematopoietic in origin or that sufficient transfer of enzyme via enzyme-replete cells will reverse existing damage and prevent subsequent damage (Table 9–9). However, the capacity for repair or arrest of damage to affected organ systems, especially the CNS, remains

unproven for many storage disorders. Age and neurodevelopmental status before SCT consistently predict outcome. Children severely affected at the time of SCT are unlikely to experience meaningful gains in neurocognitive function. Patients with Hurler disease, globoid cell leukodystrophy, and adrenoleukodystrophy appear to benefit from SCT if they have more indolent forms of disease or if SCT is performed before symptoms of dementia occur.[652–654] In addition, availability of donors is a significant issue in all genetic disorders, because siblings may be homozygotes or heterozygotes for the defective gene. Although transplantation from a heterozygotic donor for hematopoietic disorders such as thalassemia is therapeutic, transplantation from a donor with limited enzyme levels may be less effective in patients with storage disorders; acceptable levels of heterozygosity have not been well defined.[651, 655] Furthermore, the relative risks of allogeneic SCT are very difficult to measure against the uncertain therapeutic gain with SCT for many of these disorders. Because use of alternative donors is associated with an increase in morbidity and mortality of SCT, the decision is particularly problematic when a matched sibling donor is not available.[656] Thus, although a subset of patients with storage disorders can clearly benefit from SCT, notably those who are young or have no symptoms or who have indolent forms of disease, patients with aggressive infantile forms or those with significant neurologic impairment will need alternative therapeutic modalities to affect outcome.

REFERENCES

1. Osgood EE, Riddle MC, Mathews TJ: Aplastic anemia treated with daily transfusions and intravenous marrow: case report. Ann Intern Med 1939; 13:357–367.
2. Jacobson LO, Marks EK, Gaston EO, et al: Effect of spleen protection on mortality following x-irradiation. J Lab Clin Med 1949; 34:1538–1543.
3. Jacobson LO, Simmons EL, Marks EK, et al: Recovery from radiation injury. Science 1951; 113:510–511.
4. Ford CE, Hamerton JL, Barnes DWH, et al: Cytological identification of radiation-chimaeras. Nature 1956; 177:452–454.
5. Barnes DWH, Loutit JF: The radiation recovery factor: Preservation by the Polge-Smith-Parkes techniques. J Natl Cancer Inst 1955; 15:901–905.
6. Barnes DWH, Loutit JF: Spleen protection: The cellular hypothesis. In Bacq ZM, Alexander P (eds): Radiobiology Symposium 1954. New York, Academic Press, 1954, pp 134–135.
7. Uphoff DE: Alteration of homograft reaction by A-methopterin in lethally irradiated mice treated with homologous marrow. Proc Soc Exp Biol Med 1958; 99:651–653.
8. Thomas ED, Lochte HL Jr, Cannon JH, et al: Supralethal whole body irradiation and isologous marrow transplantation in man. J Clin Invest 1959; 38:1709–1716.
9. Thomas ED, Lochte HL, Jr, Lu WC, et al: Intravenous infusion of bone marrow in patients receiving radiation and chemotherapy. N Engl J Med 1957; 257:491–496.
10. Bach FH, Albertini RJ, Anderson JL, et al: Bone marrow transplantation in a patient with the Wiskott-Aldrich syndrome. Lancet 1968; 2:1364.
11. de Koning J, van Bekkum DW, Dicke KA, et al: Transplantation of bone marrow cells and fetal thymus in an infant with lymphopenic immunological deficiency. Lancet 1969; 1:1223.
12. Good RA, Meuwissen HJ, Hong R, et al: Bone marrow transplantation: Correction of immune deficit in lymphopenic immunologic deficiency and correction of an immunologically induced pancytopenia. Trans Assoc Am Physicians 1969; 82:278–285.
13. Good RA, Gatti A, Hong R, et al: Successful marrow transplantation for correction of immunological deficit in lymphopenic

TABLE 9–9. Storage Disorders Treated with Stem Cell Transplantation

Hurler syndrome[650, 656]
Hunter syndrome[649]
Sanfilippo syndrome
Adrenoleukodystrophy[650]
Metachromatic leukodystrophy[646]
Globoid cell leukodystrophy (Krabbe disease)[650]
Maroteaux-Lamy syndrome
Gaucher disease[647]
Niemann-Pick disease
Glycogen storage disease (type II, Pompe disease)
Farber disease
Fucosidosis
I-cell disease
Morquio disease
Batten disease

agammaglobulinemia and treatment of immunologically induced pancytopenia. Exp Hematol 1969; 19:4.

14. Bjornson CR, Rietze RL, Reynolds BA, et al: Turning brain into blood: A hematopoietic fate adopted by adult neural stem cells in vivo. Science 1999; 283:534–537.

15. Pang W: Role of muscle-derived cells in hematopoietic reconstitution of irradiated mice. Blood 2000; 95:1106–1108.

16. Jackson KA, Mi T, Goodell MA: Hematopoietic potential of stem cells isolated from murine skeletal muscle. Proc Natl Acad Sci USA 1999; 96:14482–14486.

17. Seale P, Rudnicki MA: A new look at the origin, function, and "stem-cell" status of muscle satellite cells. Dev Biol 2000; 218:115–124.

18. Weissman IL: Translating stem and progenitor cell biology to the clinic: Barriers and opportunities. Science 2000; 287:1442–1446.

19. Armitage JO: Bone marrow transplantation. N Engl J Med 1994; 330:827–838.

20. Mentzer WC, Heller S, Pearle PR, et al: Availability of related donors for bone marrow transplantation in sickle cell anemia. Am J Hematol Oncol 1994; 16:27–29.

21. Beatty PG, Clift RA, Mickelson EM, et al: Marrow transplantation from related donors other than HLA-identical siblings. N Engl J Med 1985; 313:765–771.

22. Anasetti C, Amos D, Beatty PG, et al: Effect of HLA compatibility on engraftment of bone marrow transplants in patients with leukemia or lymphoma. N Engl J Med 1989; 320:197–204.

23. Champlin R, Coppo P, Howe C: National marrow donor program: Progress and challenges. Bone Marrow Transplant 1993; 33:567.

24. Kernan NA, Bartsch G, Ash RC, et al: Analysis of 462 transplantation from unrelated donors facilitated by the national marrow donor program. N Engl J Med 1993; 328:593–601.

25. Anasetti C, Etzioni R, Petersdorf EW, et al: Marrow transplantation from unrelated volunteer donors. Annu Rev Med 1995; 46:169.

26. Wagner JE, Kernan NA, Steinbuch M, et al: Allogeneic sibling umbilical-cord-blood transplantation in children with malignant and non-malignant disease. Lancet 1995; 346:214–219.

27. Rubinstein P, Rosenfield RE, Adamson JW, et al: Stored placental blood for unrelated bone marrow reconstitution. Blood 1993; 81:1679–1690.

28. Kurtzberg J, Laughlin M, Graham ML, et al: Placental blood as a source of hematopoietic stem cells for transplantation into unrelated recipients. N Engl J Med 1996; 335:157–166.

29. Brenner MK, Rill DR, Moen RC, et al: Gene-marking to trace origin of relapse after autologous bone-marrow transplantation. Lancet 1993; 341:85–86.

30. Brenner MK, Rill DR, Holladay MS, et al: Gene marking to determine whether autologous marrow infusion restores long-term haemopoiesis in cancer patients. Lancet 1993; 342:1134–1137.

31. Rill DR, Buschle M, Foreman NK, et al: Retrovirus-mediated gene transfer as an approach to analyze neuroblastoma relapse after autologous bone marrow transplantation. Hum Gene Ther 1992; 3:129–136.

32. Rill DR, Moen RC, Buschle M, et al: An approach for the analysis of relapse and marrow reconstitution after autologous marrow transplantation using retrovirus-mediated gene transfer. Blood 1992; 79:2694–2700.

33. Blaese RM, Culver KW: Gene therapy for primary immunodeficiency. Immunodefic Rev 1992; 3:329–349.

34. Kohn DB, Weinberg KI, Parkman R, et al: Gene therapy for neonates with ADA-deficient SCID by retroviral-mediated transfer of the human ADA cDNA into umbilical cord CD34+ cells. Blood 1993; 82:315a.

35. Hoogerbrugge PM, Beusecchem VV, Valerio D, et al: Gene therapy in 3 children with adenosine deaminase deficiency. Blood 1993; 82:315a.

36. Cavazzana-Calvo M, Hacein-Bey S, de Saint Basile G, et al: Gene therapy of human severe combined immunodeficiency (SCID)-X1 disease. Science 2000; 288:669–672.

37. Mathe G, Jammet H, Pendic B, et al: Transfusions et greffes de moelle osseuse homologue chez des humains irradies a haute dause accidentellement. Rev Fr Etud Clin Biol 1959; 4:226–238.

38. Santos GW: History of bone marrow transplantation. Clin Haematol 1983; 12:611–639.

39. Thomas ED, Storb R, Clift RA, et al: Bone marrow transplantation. N Engl J Med 1975; 16:832–843,895–902.

40. Graw RG Jr, Yankee RA, Rogentine GN, et al: Bone marrow transplantation from HL-A matched donors to patient with acute leukemia: Toxicity and antileukemic effect. Transplantation 1972; 14:79–90.

41. Tutschka PJ, Santos GW, Elfenbein GJ: Marrow transplantation in acute leukemia following busulfan and cyclophosphamide. Blut 1980; 25:375.

42. Storb R, Yu C, Deeg HJ, et al: Current and future preparative regimens for bone marrow transplantation in thalassemia. Ann NY Acad Sci 1998; 850:276–287.

43. Rosen EM, Fan S, Goldberg ID, et al: Biological basis of radiation sensitivity. Part 2: Cellular and molecular determinants of radiosensitivity. Oncology (Huntingt) 2000; 14:741–757; discussion 757–758, 761–766.

44. Rosen EM, Fan S, Goldberg ID, et al: Biological basis of radiation sensitivity. Part 1: Factors governing radiation tolerance. Oncology (Huntingt) 2000; 14:543–550.

45. Thomas E, Clift R, Hersman J, et al: Marrow transplantation for acute nonlymphoblastic leukemia in first remission using fractionated or single dose irradiation. Int J Radiat Oncol Biol Phys 1982; 8:817.

46. Deeg H, Sullivan K, Buckner C, et al: Marrow transplantation for ANLL in first remission: Toxicity and long-term follow-up of patients conditioned with single dose or fractionated total body irradiation. Bone Marrow Transplant 1986; 1:151.

47. Buckner C, Clift R, Appelbaum F, et al: A randomized trial of 12 or 15.75 Gy of total body irradiation (TBI) in patients with ANLL and CML followed by marrow transplantation. Exp Hematol 1989; 17:522.

48. Clift R, Buckner C, Appelbaum F, et al: Allogeneic marrow transplantation in patients with chronic myeloid leukemia in the chronic phase: A randomized trial of two irradiation regimens. Blood 1991; 77:1660.

49. Lawton C: Total-body irradiation for bone marrow transplantation. Oncology (Huntingt) 1999; 13:972, 975–978, 981–982.

50. Chou RH, Wong GB, Kramer JH, et al: Toxicities of total-body irradiation for pediatric bone marrow transplantation. Int J Radiat Oncol Biol Phys 1996; 34:843–851.

51. Santos GW: Antonio Raichs lecture. Autologous bone marrow transplantation. Sangre 1992; 37:471–474.

52. Yeager AM, Kaizer H, Santos GW, et al: Autologous bone marrow transplantation in patients with acute nonlymphocytic leukemia using ex vivo marrow treatment with 4 hydroperoxycyclophosphamide. N Engl J Med 1986; 315:141–147.

53. Beelen DW, Quabeck K, Graeven U, et al: Acute toxicity and first clinical results of intensive postinduction therapy using a modified busulfan and cyclophosphamide regimen with autologous bone marrow rescue in first remission of acute myeloid leukemia. Blood 1989; 74:1507–1516.

54. Copelan EA, Biggs JC, Thompson JM, et al: Treatment for acute myelocytic leukemia with allogeneic bone marrow transplantation following preparation with BuCy2. Blood 1991; 78:838.

55. Tutschka PJ, Copelan EA, Klein JP: Bone marrow transplantation for leukemia following a new busulfan and cyclophosphamide regimen. Blood 1987; 70:1382.

56. Copelan EA, Deeg HJ: Conditioning for allogeneic marrow transplantation inpatients with lymphohematopoietic malignancies without the use of total body irradiation. Blood 1992; 80:1648–1658.

57. Copelan EA, Biggs JC, Avalos BR, et al: Radiation-free preparation for allogeneic bone marrow transplantation in adults with acute lymphoblastic leukemia. J Clin Oncol 1992; 10:237–242.

58. Lucarelli G, Clift RA: Bone marrow transplantation in thalassemia. In Forman SJ, Blume KG, Thomas ED (eds): Bone Marrow Transplantation. Boston, Blackwell Scientific, 1994, pp 829–838.

59. Lucarelli G, Galimberti M, Polchi P, et al: Bone marrow transplantation in patients with thalassemia. N Engl J Med 1990; 322:417–421.

60. Rimm IJ, Rappeport JM: Bone marrow transplantation for the Wiskott-Aldrich syndrome. Transplantation 1990; 50:617–620.

61. Hoogerbrugge PM, Brouwer OF, Bordigoni P, et al: Allogeneic bone marrow transplantation for lysosomal storage diseases. Lancet 1995; 345:1398–1402.

62. Blanche S, Caniglia M, Girault D, Landman J, et al: Treatment of hemophagocytic lymphohistiocytosis with chemotherapy and bone marrow transplantation: A single-center study of 22 cases. Blood 1991; 78:51–54.

63. Hasle H, Arico M, Basso G, et al: Myelodysplastic syndrome, juvenile myelomonocytic leukemia, and acute myeloid leukemia associated with complete or partial monosomy 7. European Working Group on MDS in Childhood (EWOG-MDS). Leukemia 1999; 13:376–385.

64. Davies SM, Ramsay NK, Klein JP, et al: Comparison of preparative regimens in transplants for children with acute lymphoblastic leukemia. J Clin Oncol 2000; 18:340–347.

65. Shank B: Can total body irradiation be supplanted by busulfan in cytoreductive regimens for bone marrow transplantation? Int J Radiat Oncol Biol Phys 1995; 31:195–196.

66. Hartman AR, Williams SF, Dillon JJ: Survival, disease-free survival and adverse effects of conditioning for allogeneic bone marrow transplantation with busulfan/cyclophosphamide vs total body irradiation: A meta-analysis. Bone Marrow Transplant 1998; 22:439–443.

67. Ringden O, Remberger M, Ruutu T, et al: Increased risk of chronic graft-versus-host disease, obstructive bronchiolitis, and alopecia with busulfan versus total body irradiation: Long-term results of a randomized trial in allogeneic marrow recipients with leukemia. Nordic Bone Marrow Transplantation Group. Blood 1999; 93:2196–2201.

68. Blume KG, Kopecky KJ, Henslee-Downey JP, et al: A prospective randomized comparison of total body irradiation-etoposide versus busulfan-cyclophosphamide as preparatory regimens for bone marrow transplantation in patients with leukemia who were not in first remission: A Southwest Oncology Group study. Blood 1993; 81:2187–2193.

69. Clift RA, Buckner CD, Thomas ED, et al: Marrow transplantation for chronic myeloid leukemia: A randomized study comparing cyclophosphamide and total body irradiation with busulfan and cyclophosphamide. Blood 1994; 84:2036–2043.

70. Ringden O, Ruutu T, Remberger M, et al: A randomized trial comparing busulfan with total body irradiation as conditioning in allogeneic marrow transplant recipients with leukemia: A report from the Nordic Bone Marrow Transplantation Group. Blood 1994; 83:2723–2730.

71. Devergie A, Blaise D, Attal M, et al: Allogeneic bone marrow transplantation for chronic myeloid leukemia in first chronic phase: A randomized trial of busulfan-Cytoxan versus Cytoxan-total body irradiation as preparative regimen: A report from the French Society of Bone Marrow Graft (SFGM). Blood 1995; 85:2263–2268.

72. Blaise D, Maraninchi D, Archimbaud E, et al: Allogeneic bone marrow transplantation for acute myeloid leukemia in first remission: A randomized trial of a busulfan-Cytoxan versus Cytoxan-total body irradiation as preparative regimen: A report from the Groupe d'Etudes de la Greffe de Moelle Osseuse. Blood 1992; 79:2578–2582.

73. Michel G, Gluckman E, Esperou-Bourdeau H, et al: Allogeneic bone marrow transplantation for children with acute myeloblastic leukemia in first complete remission: Impact of conditioning regimen without total-body irradiation—A report from the Societe Francaise de Greffe de Moelle. J Clin Oncol 1994; 12:1217–1222.

74. Hassan M, Ljungman P, Bolme P, et al: Busulfan bioavailability. Blood 1994; 84:2144–2150.

75. Grochow LB, Krivit W, Whitley CB, et al: Busulfan disposition in children. Blood 1990; 75:1723–1727.

76. Yeager AM, Wagner JE Jr, Graham ML, et al: Optimization of busulfan dosage in children undergoing bone marrow transplantation: A pharmacokinetic study of dose escalation. Blood 1992; 80: 2425–2428.

77. Vassal G, Deroussent A, Challine D, et al: Is 600 mg/m^2 the appropriate dosage of busulfan in children undergoing bone marrow transplantation? Blood 1992; 79:2475–2479.

78. Schuler U, Schroer S, Kuhnle A, et al: Busulfan pharmacokinetics in bone marrow transplant patients: Is drug monitoring warranted? Bone Marrow Transplant 1994; 14:759–765.

79. Shaw PJ, Scharping CE, Brian RJ, et al: Busulfan pharmacokinetics using a single daily high-dose regimen in children with acute leukemia. Blood 1994; 84:2357–2362.

80. Spitzer TR, Peters C, Ortlieb M, et al: Etoposide in combination with cyclophosphamide and total body irradiation or busulfan as conditioning for marrow transplantation in adults and children. Int J Radiat Oncol Biol Phys 1994; 29:39–44.

81. Teinturier C, Hartmann O, Valteau-Couanet D, et al: Ovarian function after autologous bone marrow transplantation in childhood: High-dose busulfan is a major cause of ovarian failure. Bone Marrow Transplant 1998; 22:989–994.

82. Grochow LB, Jones RJ, Brundrett RB, et al: Pharmacokinetics of busulfan: Correlation with veno-occlusive disease in patients undergoing bone marrow transplantation. Cancer Chemother Pharmacol 1989; 25:55–61.

83. Olavarria E, Hassan M, Eades A, et al: A phase I/II study of multiple-dose intravenous busulfan as myeloablation prior to stem cell transplantation. Leukemia 2000; 14:1954–1959.

84. Chao NJ, Forman SJ, Schmidt GM, et al: Allogeneic bone marrow transplantation for high-risk acute lymphoblastic leukemia during first complete remission. Blood 1991; 78:1923–1927.

85. Brown RA, Wolff SN, Fay JW, et al: High-dose etoposide, cyclophosphamide, and total body irradiation with allogeneic bone marrow transplantation for patients with acute myeloid leukemia in untreated first relapse: A study by the North American Marrow Transplant Group. Blood 1995; 85:1391–1395.

86. Petersen FB, Lynch MHE, Clift RA, et al: Autologous marrow transplantation for patients with acute myeloid leukemia in untreated first relapse or in second complete remission. J Clin Oncol 1993; 11:1353–1360.

87. Petersen FB, Buckner CD, Appelbaum FR, et al: Etoposide, cyclophosphamide and fractionated total body irradiation as a preparative regimen for marrow transplantation in patients with advanced hematological malignancies: A phase I study. Bone Marrow Transplant 1992; 10:83–88.

88. Krance RA, Forman SJ, Blume KG: Total-body irradiation and high-dose teniposide: A pilot study in bone marrow transplantation for patients with relapsed acute lymphoblastic leukemia. Cancer Treat Rep 1987; 71:645–647.

89. Coccia PF, Strandjord SE, Warkentin PI, et al: High-dose cytosine arabinoside and fractionated total-body irradiation: An improved preparative regimen for bone marrow transplantation of children with acute lymphoblastic leukemia. Blood 1988; 71:888–893.

90. Blume KG, Forman SJ, O'Donnell MR, et al: Total body irradiation and high dose etoposide: A new preparatory regimen for bone marrow transplantation in patients with advanced hematologic malignancies. Blood 1987; 69:1015–1020.

91. Bostrom B, Brunning RD, McGlave P, et al: Bone marrow transplantation for acute nonlymphocytic leukemia in first remission: Analysis of prognostic factors. Blood 1985; 65:1191–1196.

92. Chao NJ, Stein AS, Long GD, et al: Busulfan/etoposide—Initial experience with a new preparatory regimen for autologous bone marrow transplantation in patients with acute nonlymphoblastic leukemia. Blood 1993; 81:319–323.

93. Linker CA, Ries CA, Damon LE, Rugo HS, Wolf JL: Autologous bone marrow transplantation for acute myeloid leukemia using busulfan plus etoposide as a preparative regimen. Blood 1993; 81:311–318.

94. Matsuyama T, Kojima S, Kato K: Allogeneic bone marrow transplantation for childhood leukemia following a busulfan and melphalan preparative regimen. Bone Marrow Transplant 1998; 22:21–26.

95. Vey N, De Prijck B, Faucher C, et al: A pilot study of busulfan and melphalan as preparatory regimen prior to allogeneic bone marrow transplantation in refractory or relapsed hematological malignancies. Bone Marrow Transplant 1996; 18:495–499.

96. Ayash LJ, Antman K, Cheson BD: A perspective on dose-intensive therapy with autologous bone marrow transplantation for solid tumors. Oncology (Huntingt) 1991; 5:25–33.

97. Dicke KA, Spitzer G: Evaluation of the use of high-dose cytoreduction with autologous marrow rescue in various malignancies. Transplantation 1986; 41:4–20.

98. Cheson BD, Lacerna L, Leyland-Jones B, et al: Autologous bone marrow transplantation. Ann Intern Med 1989; 110:51–65.

99. Dallorso S, Manzitti C, Morreale G, et al: High dose therapy and autologous hematopoietic stem cell transplantation in poor risk solid tumors of childhood. Haematologica 2000; 85:66–70.

100. Burnett AK, Kell J, Rowntree C: Role of allogeneic and autologous hematopoietic stem cell transplantation in acute myeloid leukemia. Int J Hematol 2000; 72:280–284.

101. Giralt S, Estey E, Albitar M, et al: Engraftment of allogeneic hematopoietic progenitor cells with purine analog-containing

chemotherapy: Harnessing graft-versus-leukemia without myeloablative therapy. Blood 1997; 89:4531–4536.

102. Giralt S, Khouri I, Champlin R: Non myeloablative "mini transplant." Cancer Treat Res 1999; 101:97–108.

103. Slavin S, Nagler A, Naparstek E, et al: Nonmyeloablative stem cell transplantation and cell therapy as an alternative to conventional bone marrow transplantation with lethal cytoreduction for the treatment of malignant and nonmalignant hematologic diseases. Blood 1998; 91:756–763.

104. Storb R, Yu C, Sandmaier BM, et al: Mixed hematopoietic chimerism after marrow allografts. Transplantation in the ambulatory care setting. Ann NY Acad Sci 1999; 872:372–375; discussion 375–376.

105. Storb R, Yu C, Wagner JL, et al: Stable mixed hematopoietic chimerism in DLA-identical littermate dogs given sublethal total body irradiation before and pharmacological immunosuppression after marrow transplantation. Blood 1997; 89:3048–3054.

106. Sandmaier BM, McSweeney P, Yu C, et al: Nonmyeloablative transplants: Preclinical and clinical results. Semin Oncol 2000; 27:78–81.

107. Champlin R, Khouri I, Kornblau S, et al: Reinventing bone marrow transplantation: Reducing toxicity using nonmyeloablative, preparative regimens and induction of graft-versus-malignancy. Curr Opin Oncol 1999; 11:87–95.

108. Nagler A, Aker M, Or R, et al: Low-intensity conditioning is sufficient to ensure engraftment in matched unrelated bone marrow transplantation. Exp Hematol 2001; 29:362–370.

109. Kapelushnik J, Or R, Slavin S, et al: A fludarabine-based protocol for bone marrow transplantation in Fanconi's anemia. Bone Marrow Transplant 1997; 20:1109–1110.

110. Horwitz ME, Barrett AJ, Brown MR, et al: Treatment of chronic granulomatous disease with nonmyeloablative conditioning and a T-cell-depleted hematopoietic allograft. N Engl J Med 2001; 344:881–888.

111. Jin NR, Hill RS, Peterson FB, et al: Marrow harvesting for autologous marrow transplantation. Exp Hematol 1985; 13:879–884.

112. Lasky LC, Bostrom B, Smith J, et al: Clinical collection and use of peripheral blood stem cells in pediatric patients. Transplantation 1989; 47:613–616.

113. Makino S, Haylock DN, Dowse T, et al: Ex vivo culture of peripheral blood CD34+ cells: Effects of hematopoietic growth factors on production of neutrophilic precursors. J Hematother 1997; 6:475–489.

114. Haylock DN, Horsfall MJ, Dowse TL, et al: Increased recruitment of hematopoietic progenitor cells underlies the ex vivo expansion potential of FLT3 ligand. Blood 1997; 90:2260–2272.

115. To LB, Haylock DN, Simmons PJ, et al: The biology and clinical uses of blood stem cells. Blood 1997; 89:2233–2258.

116. Kanold J, Rapatel C, Berger M, et al: Use of G-CSF alone to mobilize peripheral blood stem cells for collection from children. Br J Haematol 1994; 88:633–635.

117. Kletzel M, Longino R, Rademaker AW, et al: Peripheral blood stem cell transplantation in young children: Experience with harvesting, mobilization and engraftment. Pediatr Transplant 1998; 2:191–196.

118. Negrin RS, Kusnierz-Glaz CR, Still BJ, et al: Transplantation of enriched and purged peripheral blood progenitor cells from a single apheresis product in patients with non-Hodgkin's lymphoma. Blood 1995; 85:3334–3341.

119. Rill DR, Santana VM, Roberts WM, et al: Direct demonstration that autologous bone marrow transplantation for solid tumors can return a multiplicity of tumorigenic cells. Blood 1994; 84:380–383.

120. Freedman AS, Neuberg D, Mauch P, et al: Long-term follow-up of autologous bone marrow transplantation in patients with relapsed follicular lymphoma. Blood 1999; 94:3325–3333.

121. Ross AA, Cooper BW, Lazarus HM, et al: Detection and viability of tumor cells in peripheral blood stem cell collections from breast cancer patients using immunocytochemical and clonogenic assay techniques. Blood 1993; 82:2605.

122. Brugger W, Bross KJ, Glatt M, et al: Mobilization of tumor cells and hematopoietic progenitor cells into peripheral blood of patients with solid tumors. Blood 1994; 83:636–640.

123. Lopez M, Lemoine FM, Firat H, et al: Bone marrow versus peripheral blood progenitor cells CD34 selection in patients with non-Hodgkin's lymphomas: Different levels of tumor cell reduction. Implications for autografting. Blood 1997; 90:2830–2838.

124. Kanteti R, Miller K, McCann J, et al: Randomized trial of peripheral blood progenitor cell vs bone marrow as hematopoietic support for high-dose chemotherapy in patients with non-Hodgkin's lymphoma and Hodgkin's disease: A clinical and molecular analysis. Bone Marrow Transplant 1999; 24:473–481.

125. Leung W, Chen AR, Klann RC, et al: Frequent detection of tumor cells in hematopoietic grafts in neuroblastoma and Ewing's sarcoma. Bone Marrow Transplant 1998; 22:971–979.

126. Jacquy C, Soree A, Lambert F, et al: A quantitative study of peripheral blood stem cell contamination in diffuse large-cell non-Hodgkin's lymphoma: One-half of patients significantly mobilize malignant cells. Br J Haematol 2000; 110:631–637.

127. Humpe A, Riggert J, Wolf C, et al: Successful transplantation and engraftment of peripheral blood stem cells after cryopreservation, positive and negative purging procedures, and a second cryopreservation cycle. Ann Hematol 2001; 80:109–112.

128. Tchirkov A, Kanold J, Giollant M, et al: Molecular monitoring of tumor cell contamination in leukapheresis products from stage IV neuroblastoma patients before and after positive CD34 selection. Med Pediatr Oncol 1998; 30:228–232.

129. Weaver CH, Hazelton B, Birch R, et al: An analysis of engraftment kinetics as a function of the CD34 content of peripheral blood progenitor cell collections in 692 patients after the administration of myeloablative chemotherapy. Blood 1995; 86:3961–3969.

130. Shpall EJ, Champlin R, Glaspy JA: Effect of CD34+ peripheral blood progenitor cell dose on hematopoietic recovery. Biol Blood Marrow Transplant 1998; 4:84–92.

131. Haas R, Mohle R, Fruhauf S, et al: Patient characteristics associated with successful mobilizing and autografting of peripheral blood progenitor cells in malignant lymphoma. Blood 1994; 83:3787–3794.

132. Tricot G, Jagannath S, Vesole D, et al: Peripheral blood stem cell transplants for multiple myeloma: Identification of favorable variables for rapid engraftment in 255 patients. Blood 1995; 85:588–596.

133. O'Day SJ, Rabinowe SN, Neuberg D, et al: A phase II study of continuous infusion recombinant human granulocyte-macrophage colony-stimulating factor as an adjunct to autologous bone marrow transplantation for patients with non-Hodgkin's lymphoma in first remission. Blood 1994; 83:2707–2714.

134. Domenech J, Linassier C, Gihana E, et al: Prolonged impairment of hematopoiesis after high-dose therapy followed by autologous bone marrow transplantation. Blood 1995; 85:3320–3327.

135. Mach-Pascual S, Legare RD, Lu D, et al: Predictive value of clonality assays in patients with non-Hodgkin's lymphoma undergoing autologous bone marrow transplant: A single institution study. Blood 1998; 91:4496–4503.

136. Darrington DL, Vose JM, Anderson JR, et al: Incidence and characterization of secondary myelodysplastic syndrome and acute myelogenous leukemia following high-dose chemoradiotherapy and autologous stem cell transplantation for lymphoid malignancies. J Clin Oncol 1994; 12:2527–2534.

137. Traweek ST, Slovak ML, Nademanee AP, et al: Clonal karyotypic hematopoietic cell abnormalities occurring after autologous bone marrow transplantation for Hodgkin's disease and non-Hodgkin's lymphoma. Blood 1994; 84:957–963.

138. Krishnan A, Bhatia S, Slovak ML, et al: Predictors of therapy-related leukemia and myelodysplasia following autologous transplantation for lymphoma: An assessment of risk factors. Blood 2000; 95:1588–1593.

139. Miller JS, Arthur DC, Litz CE, et al: Myelodysplastic syndrome after autologous bone marrow transplantation: An additional late complication of curative cancer therapy. Blood 1994; 83:3780–3786.

140. Stone RM: Myelodysplastic syndrome after autologous transplantation for lymphoma: The price of progress? Blood 1994; 83:3437–3440.

141. Travis LB, Weeks J, Curtis RE, et al: Leukemia following low-dose total body irradiation and chemotherapy for non-Hodgkin's lymphoma. J Clin Oncol 1996; 14:565–571.

142. Milligan DW, Ruiz De Elvira MC, Kolb HJ, et al: Secondary leukaemia and myelodysplasia after autografting for lymphoma: Results from the EBMT. EBMT Lymphoma and Late Effects Working Parties. European Group for Blood and Marrow Transplantation. Br J Haematol 1999; 106:1020–1026.

143. Micallef IN, Lillington DM, Apostolidis J, et al: Therapy-related myelodysplasia and secondary acute myelogenous leukemia after high-dose therapy with autologous hematopoietic progenitor-cell support for lymphoid malignancies. J Clin Oncol 2000; 18:947–955.

144. Chao NJ, Nademanee AP, Long GD, et al: Importance of bone marrow cytogenetic evaluation before autologous bone marrow transplantation for Hodgkin's disease. J Clin Oncol 1991; 9:1575–1579.

145. Abruzzese E, Radford JE, Miller JS, et al: Detection of abnormal pretransplant clones in progenitor cells of patients who developed myelodysplasia after autologous transplantation. Blood 1999; 94:1814–1819.

146. Schipper RF, D'Amaro J, Oudshoorn M: The probability of finding a suitable related donor for bone marrow transplantation in extended families. Blood 1996; 87:800–804.

147. Beatty PG, Dahlberg S, Mickelson EM, et al: Probability of finding HLA-matched unrelated marrow donors. Transplantation 1988; 45:714–718.

148. Prasad VK, Heller G, Kernan NA, et al: The probability of HLA-C matching between patient and unrelated donor at the molecular level: Estimations based on the linkage disequilibrium between DNA typed HLA-B and HLA-C alleles. Transplantation 1999; 68:1044–1050.

149. Speiser DE, Tiercy JM, Rufer N, et al: High resolution HLA matching associated with decreased mortality after unrelated bone marrow transplantation. Blood 1996; 87:4455–4462.

150. Petersdorf EW, Gooley TA, Anasetti C, et al: Optimizing outcome after unrelated marrow transplantation by comprehensive matching of HLA class I and II alleles in the donor and recipient. Blood 1998; 92:3515–3520.

151. Goulmy E: Minor histocompatibility antigens: From T cell recognition to peptide identification. Hum Immunol 1997; 54:8–14.

152. Goulmy E, Schipper R, Pool J, et al: Mismatches of minor histocompatibility antigens between HLA-identical donors and recipients and the development of graft-verus-host disease after bone marrow transplantation. N Engl J Med 1996; 334:281–285.

153. den Haan JM, Sherman NE, Blokland E, et al: Identification of a graft versus host disease-associated human minor histocompatibility antigen. Science 1995; 268:1476–1480.

154. Terasaki PI, McClelland JD: Microdroplet assay of human serum cytotoxins. Nature 1964; 204:998.

155. Yunis EJ, Amos DB: Three closely linked genetic systems relevant to transplantation. Proc Natl Acad Sci USA 1971; 68:3031–3035.

156. Dupont B, Jersild C, Hansen GS, et al: Typing for MLC determinants by means of LD-homozygous and LD-heterozygous test cells. Transplant Proc 1973; 5:1543–1549.

157. Clift RA: Cellular support of the marrow transplant recipient. Prog Clin Biol Res 1990; 337:87–92.

158. Butterworth VA, Simmons RG, Bartsch G, et al: Psychosocial effects of unrelated bone marrow donation: Experiences of the national marrow donor program. Blood 1993; 81:1947–1959.

159. Goldman J: Peripheral blood stem cells for allografting. Blood 1995; 85:1413–1415.

160. Storek J, Gooley T, Siadak M, et al: Allogeneic peripheral blood stem cell transplantation may be associated with a high risk of chronic graft-versus-host disease. Blood 1997; 90:4705–4709.

161. Przepiorka D, Anderlini P, Ippoliti C, et al: Allogeneic blood stem cell transplantation in advanced hematologic cancers. Bone Marrow Transplant 1997; 19:455–460.

162. Bensinger WI, Weaver CH, Appelbaum FR, et al: Transplantation of allogeneic peripheral blood stem cells mobilized by recombinant human granulocyte colony-stimulating factor. Blood 1995; 85:1655–1658.

163. Bensinger WI, Martin PJ, Storer B, et al: Transplantation of bone marrow as compared with peripheral-blood cells from HLA-identical relatives in patients with hematologic cancers. N Engl J Med 2001; 344:175–181.

164. Korbling M, Przepiorka D, Huh YO, et al: Allogeneic blood stem cell transplantation for refractory leukemia and lymphoma: Potential advantage of blood over marrow allografts. Blood 1995; 85:1659–1665.

165. Schmitz N, Dreger P, Suttorp M, et al: Primary transplantation of allogeneic peripheral blood progenitor cells mobilized by filgrastim (granulocyte colony-stimulating factor). Blood 1995; 85:1666–1672.

166. Korbling M, Chan KW, Anderlini P, et al: Allogeneic peripheral blood stem cell transplantation using normal patient-related pediatric donors. Bone Marrow Transplant 1996; 18:885–890.

167. Falanga A, Marchetti M, Evangelista V, et al: Neutrophil activation and hemostatic changes in healthy donors receiving granulocyte colony-stimulating factor. Blood 1999; 93:2506–2514.

168. Anderlini P, Korbling M, Dale D, et al: Allogeneic blood stem cell transplantation: Considerations for donors. Blood 1997; 90:903–908.

169. Gluckman E, Broxmeyer HE, Auerbach AD, et al: Hematopoietic reconstitution in a patient with Fanconi's anemia by means of umbilical cord blood from an HLA-identical sibling. N Engl J Med 1989; 321:1174–1178.

170. Bertolini F, Lazzari L, Lauri E, et al: Comparative study of different procedures for the collection and banking of umbilical cord blood. J Hematother 1995; 4:29–36.

171. Wynn RF, Cross MA, Hatton C, et al: Accelerated telomere shortening in young recipients of allogeneic bone-marrow transplants. Lancet 1998; 351:178–181.

172. van Leeuwen JEM, van Tol MJD, Joosten AM, et al: Persistence of host-type hematopoiesis after allogeneic bone marrow transplantation for leukemia is significantly related to the recipient's age and/or the conditioning regimen, but it is not associated with an increased risk of relapse. Blood 1994; 83:3059–3067.

173. Hill RS, Petersen FB, Storb R, et al: Mixed hematologic chimerism after allogeneic marrow transplantation for severe aplastic anemia is associated with a higher risk of graft rejection and a lessened incidence of acute graft-versus-host disease. Blood 1986; 67:811–816.

174. Petit T, Raynal B, Socie G, et al: Highly sensitive polymerase chain reaction methods show the frequent survival of residual recipient multipotent progenitors after non-T-cell-depleted bone marrow transplantation. Blood 1994; 84:3575–3583.

175. Mackinnon S, Barnett L, Heller G, et al: Minimal residual disease is more common in patients who have mixed T-cell chimerism after bone marrow transplantation for chronic myelogenous leukemia. Blood 1994; 83:3409–3416.

176. Bertheas MF, Lafage M, Levy P, et al: Influence of mixed chimerism on the results of allogeneic bone marrow transplantation for leukemia. Blood 1991; 78:3103–3106.

177. Roux E, Helg C, Chapuis B, et al: Evolution of mixed chimerism after allogeneic bone marrow transplantation as determined on granulocytes and mononuclear cells by the polymerase chain reaction. Blood 1992; 79:2775–2783.

178. Locatelli F, Zecca M, Ponchio L, et al: Pilot trial of combined administration of erythropoietin and granulocyte colony-stimulating factor to children undergoing allogeneic bone marrow transplantation. Bone Marrow Transplant 1994; 14:929–935.

179. Tsuchiya S, Minegishi M, Fujie H, et al: Allogeneic bone marrow transplantation for malignant hematologic disorders in children. Tohoku J Exp Med 1992; 168:345–350.

180. Masaoka T, Takaku F, Kato S, et al: Recombinant human granulocyte colony-stimulating factor in allogeneic bone marrow transplantation. Exp Hematol 1989; 17:1047–1050.

181. Powles R, Smith C, Milan S, et al: Human recombinant GM-CSF in allogeneic bone marrow transplant for leukemia: Double blind placebo controlled trial. Lancet 1990; 336:1417.

182. Schriber JR, Chao NJ, Long GD, et al: Granulocyte colony-stimulating factor after allogeneic bone marrow transplantation. Blood 1994; 84:1680–1684.

183. Nemunaitis J, Buckner CD, Appelbaum FR, et al: Phase I/II trial of recombinant granulocyte-macrophage colony stimulating factor following allogeneic bone marrow transplantation. Blood 1991; 77:2065.

184. Singhal S, Powles R, Kulkarni S, et al: Comparison of marrow and blood cell yields from the same donors in a double-blind, randomized study of allogeneic marrow vs blood stem cell transplantation. Bone Marrow Transplant 2000; 25:501–505.

185. Cutler C, Antin JH: Peripheral blood stem cells for allogeneic transplantation: A review. Stem Cells 2001; 19:108–117.

186. Ringden O, Remberger M, Runde V, et al: Peripheral blood stem cell transplantation from unrelated donors: A comparison with marrow transplantation. Blood 1999; 94:455–464.

187. Gluckman E, Rocha V, Boyer-Chammard A, et al: Outcome of cord-blood transplantation from related and unrelated donors.

Eurocord Transplant Group and the European Blood and Marrow Transplantation Group. N Engl J Med 1997; 337:373–381.

188. Thomson BG, Robertson KA, Gowan D, et al: Analysis of engraftment, graft-versus-host disease, and immune recovery following unrelated donor cord blood transplantation. Blood 2000; 96:2703–2711.

189. Rocha V, Wagner JE Jr, Sobocinski KA, et al: Graft-versus-host disease in children who have received a cord-blood or bone marrow transplant from an HLA-identical sibling. Eurocord and International Bone Marrow Transplant Registry Working Committee on Alternative Donor and Stem Cell Sources. N Engl J Med 2000; 342:1846–1854.

190. Rubinstein P, Carrier C, Scaradavou A, et al: Outcomes among 562 recipients of placental-blood transplants from unrelated donors. N Engl J Med 1998; 339:1565–1577.

191. Barker JN, Davies SM, DeFor T, et al: Survival after transplantation of unrelated donor umbilical cord blood is comparable to that of human leukocyte antigen-matched unrelated donor bone marrow: Results of a matched-pair analysis. Blood 2001; 97:2957–2961.

192. Small TN, Papadopoulos EB, Boulad F, et al: Comparison of immune reconstitution after unrelated and related T-cell-depleted bone marrow transplantation: Effect of patient age and donor leukocyte infusions. Blood 1999; 93:467–480.

193. Parkman R, Weinberg KI: Immunological reconstitution following bone marrow transplantation. Immunol Rev 1997; 157:73–78.

194. Roux E, Dumont-Girard F, Starobinski M, et al: Recovery of immune reactivity after T-cell-depleted bone marrow transplantation depends on thymic activity. Blood 2000; 96:2299–3303.

195. Dumont-Girard F, Roux E, van Lier RA, et al: Reconstitution of the T-cell compartment after bone marrow transplantation: Restoration of the repertoire by thymic emigrants. Blood 1998; 92:4464–4471.

196. Douek DC, Vescio RA, Betts MR, et al: Assessment of thymic output in adults after haematopoietic stem-cell transplantation and prediction of T-cell reconstitution. Lancet 2000; 355:1875–1881.

197. Heitger A, Neu N, Kern H, et al: Essential role of the thymus to reconstitute naive (CD45RA+) T-helper cells after human allogeneic bone marrow transplantation. Blood 1997; 90:850–857.

198. Verfuerth S, Peggs K, Vyas P, et al: Longitudinal monitoring of immune reconstitution by CDR3 size spectratyping after T-cell-depleted allogeneic bone marrow transplant and the effect of donor lymphocyte infusions on T-cell repertoire. Blood 2000; 95:3990–3995.

199. Mackall CL, Stein D, Fleisher TA, et al: Prolonged CD4 depletion after sequential autologous peripheral blood progenitor cell infusions in children and young adults. Blood 2000; 96:754–762.

200. Talmadge JE, Reed E, Ino K, et al: Rapid immunologic reconstitution following transplantation with mobilized peripheral blood stem cells as compared to bone marrow. Bone Marrow Transplant 1997; 19:161–172.

201. Moretta A, Maccario R, Fagioli F, et al: Analysis of immune reconstitution in children undergoing cord blood transplantation. Exp Hematol 2001; 29:371–379.

202. Small TN, Avigan D, Dupont B, et al: Immune reconstitution following T-cell depleted bone marrow transplantation: Effect of age and posttransplant graft rejection prophylaxis. Biol Blood Marrow Transplant 1997; 3:65–75.

203. Marshall NA, Howe JG, Formica R, et al: Rapid reconstitution of Epstein-Barr virus-specific T lymphocytes following allogeneic stem cell transplantation. Blood 2000; 96:2814–2821.

204. Anderson KC, Goodnough LT, Sayer M: Variation in blood component irradiation practice: Implications for prevention of transfusion-associated graft-versus-host disease. Blood 1991; 77:2096–2102.

205. Leitman SF, Holland PV: Irradiation of blood products. Indications and guidelines. Transfusion 1985; 25:293–300.

206. Greenbaum BH: Transfusion-associated graft-versus-host disease: Historical perspectives, incidence, and current use of irradiated blood products. J Clin Oncol 1991; 9:1889–1902.

207. Adler SP: Cytomegalovirus and transfusions. Transfus Med Rev 1988; 2:235–244.

208. Bowden RA, Slichter SJ, Sayers MH, et al: Use of leukocyte-depleted platelets and cytomegalovirus-seronegative red blood cells for prevention of primary cytomegalovirus infection after marrow transplant. Blood 1991; 78:246–250.

209. Slichter SJ: Controversies in platelet transfusion therapy. Annu Rev Med 1980; 31:509–540.

210. Consensus conference. Platelet transfusion therapy. JAMA 1987; 257:1777–1780.

211. Beutler E: Platelet transfusions: The 20,000/microL trigger. Blood 1993; 81:1411–1413.

212. Winston DJ, Huang ES, Miller MJ, et al: Molecular epidemiology of cytomegalovirus infections associated with bone marrow transplantation. Ann Intern Med 1985; 102:16–20.

213. Meyers JD, Flournoy N, Thomas ED: Risk factors for cytomegalovirus infection after human marrow transplantation. J Infect Dis 1986; 153:478–488.

214. Goodrich JM, Bowden RA, Fisher L, et al: Ganciclovir prophylaxis to prevent cytomegalovirus disease after allogeneic marrow transplant. Ann Intern Med 1993; 118:173–178.

215. Winston DJ, Ho WG, Bartoni K, et al: Ganciclovir prophylaxis of cytomegalovirus infection and disease in allogeneic bone marrow transplant recipients. Results of a placebo-controlled, double-blind trial. Ann Intern Med 1993; 118:179–184.

216. Avery RK, Adal KA, Longworth DL, et al: A survey of allogeneic bone marrow transplant programs in the United States regarding cytomegalovirus prophylaxis and pre-emptive therapy. Bone Marrow Transplant 2000; 26:763–767.

217. Boeckh M, Gallez-Hawkins GM, Myerson D, et al: Plasma polymerase chain reaction for cytomegalovirus DNA after allogeneic marrow transplantation: Comparison with polymerase chain reaction using peripheral blood leukocytes, pp65 antigenemia, and viral culture. Transplantation 1997; 64:108–113.

218. Boeckh M, Bowden RA, Gooley T, et al: Successful modification of a pp65 antigenemia-based early treatment strategy for prevention of cytomegalovirus disease in allogeneic marrow transplant recipients. Blood 1999; 93:1781–1782.

219. Sica S, Sora F, Chiusolo P, et al: Early viral complications after autologous CD34-selected peripheral blood stem cell transplantation. Bone Marrow Transplant 2000; 26:587–588.

220. Koc Y, Miller KB, Schenkein DP, et al: Varicella zoster virus infections following allogeneic bone marrow transplantation: Frequency, risk factors, and clinical outcome. Biol Blood Marrow Transplant 2000; 6:44–49.

221. Kawasaki H, Takayama J, Ohira M: Herpes zoster infection after bone marrow transplantation in children. J Pediatr 1996; 128:353–356.

222. Marr KA, Seidel K, Slavin MA, et al: Prolonged fluconazole prophylaxis is associated with persistent protection against candidiasis-related death in allogeneic marrow transplant recipients: Long-term follow-up of a randomized, placebo-controlled trial. Blood 2000; 96:2055–2061.

223. Wingard JR, Merz WG, Rinaldi MG, et al: Increase in *Candida krusei* infection among patients with bone marrow transplantation and neutropenia treated prophylactically with fluconazole. N Engl J Med 1991; 325:1274–1277.

224. Riley DK, Pavia AT, Beatty PG, et al: The prophylactic use of low-dose amphotericin B in bone marrow transplant patients. Am J Med 1994; 97:509–514.

225. Szeluga DJ, Stuart RK, Brookmeyer R, et al: Nutritional support of bone marrow transplant recipients: A prospective, randomized clinical trial comparing total parenteral nutrition to an enteral feeding program. Cancer Res 1987; 47:3309–3316.

226. Uderzo C, Rovelli A, Bonomi M, et al: Total parenteral nutrition and nutritional assessment and leukaemic children undergoing bone marrow transplantation. Eur J Cancer 1991; 27:758–762.

227. Weisdorf SA, Lysne J, Wind D: Positive effect of prophylactic total parenteral nutrition on long-term outcome of bone marrow transplantation. Transplantation 1987; 43:833–838.

228. Herrmann VM, Petruska PJ: Nutrition support in bone marrow transplant recipients. Nutr Clin Pract 1993; 8:19–27.

229. Lenssen P, Sherry ME, Cheney CL, et al: Prevalence of nutrition-related problems among long-term survivors of allogeneic marrow transplantation. J Am Diet Assoc 1990; 90:835–842.

230. Martin PJ, Hansen JA, Buckner CD, et al: Effects of in vitro depletion of T cells in HLA-identical allogeneic marrow grafts. Blood 1985; 66:664–672.

231. Kernan NA, Bordignon C, Heller G, et al: Graft failure after T-cell-depleted human leukocyte antigen identical marrow transplants for leukemia: I. analysis of risk factors and results of secondary transplants. Blood 1989; 74:2227–2236.

232. Green A, Clarke E, Hunt L, et al: Children with acute lymphoblastic leukemia who receive T-cell-depleted HLA mismatched marrow allografts from unrelated donors have an increased incidence of primary graft failure but a similar overall transplant outcome. Blood 1999; 94:2236–2246.

233. Champlin RE, Horowitz MM, van Bekkum DW, et al: Graft failure following bone marrow transplantation for severe aplastic anemia: Risk factors and treatment results. Blood 1989; 73:606–613.

234. Smith BR, Guinan EC, Parkman RP, et al: Efficacy of a cyclophosphamide procarbazine antithymocyte serum regimen for prevention of graft rejection following marrow transplantation of transfused patients with aplastic anemia. Transplantation 1985; 39:671–673.

235. Aversa F, Terenzi A, Carotti A, et al: Improved outcome with T-cell-depleted bone marrow transplantation for acute leukemia. J Clin Oncol 1999; 17:1545–1550.

236. Hale G, Waldmann H: Control of graft-versus-host disease and graft rejection by T cell depletion of donor and recipient with Campath-1 antibodies. Results of matched sibling transplants for malignant diseases. Bone Marrow Transplant 1994; 13:597–611.

237. Aversa F, Tabilio A, Terenzi A, et al: Successful engraftment of T-cell-depleted haploidentical "three-loci" incompatible transplants in leukemia patients by addition of recombinant human granulocyte colony-stimulating factor-mobilized peripheral blood progenitor cells to bone marrow inoculum. Blood 1994; 84:3948–3955.

238. Drobyski WR, Baxter-Lowe LA, Truitt RL: Detection of residual leukemia by the polymerase chain reaction and sequence-specific oligonucleotide probe hybridization after allogeneic bone marrow transplantation for AKR leukemia: A murine model for minimal residual disease. Blood 1993; 81:551–559.

239. Shizuru JA, Jerabek L, Edwards CT, Weissman IL: Transplantation of purified hematopoietic stem cells: Requirements for overcoming the barriers of allogeneic engraftment. Biol Blood Marrow Transplant 1996; 2:3–14.

240. Davies SM, Kollman C, Anasetti C, et al: Engraftment and survival after unrelated-donor bone marrow transplantation: A report from the national marrow donor program. Blood 2000; 96:4096–4102.

241. Bozdech MJ, Sondel PM, Trigg ME, et al: Transplantation of HLA-haploidentical T-cell-depleted marrow for leukemia: Addition of cytosine arabinoside to the pretransplant conditioning prevents rejection. Exp Hematol 1985; 13:1201–1210.

242. Antin J, Bierer N, Smith B, et al: Selective depletion of bone marrow T lymphocytes with anti-CD5 monoclonal antibodies: Effective prophylaxis for graft-versus-host disease in patients with hematologic malignancies. Blood 1991; 76:1464–1472.

243. Soiffer RJ, Ritz J: Selective T cell depletion of donor allogeneic marrow with anti-CD6 monoclonal antibody: Rationale and results. Bone Marrow Transplant 1993; 12:S7–S10.

244. Verdonck LF, Dekker AW, de Gast GC, et al: Allogeneic bone marrow transplantation with a fixed low number of T cells in the marrow graft. Blood 1994; 83:3090–3096.

245. McDonald GB, Sharma P, Matthews DE, et al: Venoclusive disease of the liver after bone marrow transplantation: Diagnosis, incidence, and predisposing factors. Hepatology 1984; 4:16.

246. Bearman SI: The syndrome of hepatic veno-occlusive disease after marrow transplantation. Blood 1995; 85:3005–3020.

247. Richardson P, Guinan E: The pathology, diagnosis, and treatment of hepatic veno-occlusive disease: Current status and novel approaches [published erratum appears in Br J Haematol 2000 109:254]. Br J Haematol 1999; 107:485–493.

248. McDonald GB, Hinds MS, Fisher LD, et al: Veno-occlusive disease of the liver and multiorgan failure after bone marrow transplantation: A cohort study of 355 patients. Ann Intern Med 1993; 118:255.

249. Ayash LJ, Hunt M, Antman K, et al: Hepatic venoocclusive disease in autologous bone marrow transplantation of solid tumors and lymphomas. J Clin Oncol 1990; 8:1699–1706.

250. Shulman HM, Gown AM, Nugent DJ: Hepatic veno-occlusive disease after bone marrow transplantation. Immunohistochemical identification of the material within occluded central venules. Am J Pathol 1987; 127:549–558.

251. Shulman HM, Fisher LB, Schoch JG, et al: Venoocclusive disease of the liver after marrow transplantation: Histological correlates of clinical signs and symptoms. Hepatology 1994; 19:1171.

252. Hassan M, Ljungman P, Ringden O, et al: The effect of busulphan on the pharmacokinetics of cyclophosphamide and its 4-hydroxy metabolite: Time interval influence on therapeutic efficacy and therapy-related toxicity. Bone Marrow Transplant 2000; 25:915–924.

253. Hassan M, Oberg G, Bekassy AN, et al: Pharmacokinetics of high-dose busulphan in relation to age and chronopharmacology. Cancer Chemother Pharmacol 1991; 28:130–134.

254. Slattery JT, Kalhorn TF, McDonald GB, et al: Conditioning regimen-dependent disposition of cyclophosphamide and hydroxycyclophosphamide in human marrow transplantation patients. J Clin Oncol 1996; 14:1484–1494.

255. Traber PG, Chianale J, Gumucio JJ: Physiologic significance and regulation of hepatocellular heterogeneity. Gastroenterology 1988; 95:1130–1143.

256. Mouelhi M, Kauffman FC: Sublobular distribution of transferases and hydrolases associated with glucuronide, sulfate and glutathione conjugation in human liver. Hepatology 1986; 6:450–456.

257. Teicher BA, Crawford JM, Holden SA, et al: Glutathione monoethyl ester can selectively protect liver from high dose BCNU or cyclophosphamide. Cancer 1988; 62:1275–1281.

258. Wang X, Kanel GC, DeLeve LD: Support of sinusoidal endothelial cell glutathione prevents hepatic veno-occlusive disease in the rat. Hepatology 2000; 31:428–434.

259. Deleve LD: Dacarbazine toxicity in murine liver cells: A model of hepatic endothelial injury and glutathione defense. J Pharmacol Exp Ther 1994; 268:1261–1270.

260. Shulman HM, Gooley T, Dudley MD, et al: Utility of transvenous liver biopsies and wedged hepatic venous pressure measurements in sixty marrow transplant recipients. Transplantation 1995; 59:1015–1022.

261. Brown BP, Abu-Yousef M, Farner R, et al: Doppler sonography: A noninvasive method for evaluation of hepatic venocclusive disease. Am J Roentgenol 1990; 154:721–724.

262. Sonneveld P, Lameris JS, Cornelissen J, et al: Color-flow imaging sonography of portal and hepatic vein flow to monitor fibrinolytic therapy with r-TPA for veno-occlusive disease following myeloablative treatment. Bone Marrow Transplant 1998; 21:731–734.

263. Haire WD, Ruby EI, Gordon BG, et al: Multiple organ dysfunction syndrome in bone marrow transplantation. JAMA 1995; 274:1289–1295.

264. Rubenfeld GD, Crawford SW: Withdrawing life support from mechanically ventilated recipients of bone marrow transplants: A case for evidence-based guidelines. Ann Intern Med 1996; 125:625–633.

265. Fink J, Cooper M, Burkhart K, et al: Marked enzymuria following bone marrow transplantation: A correlate of veno-occlusive disease-induced "hepato-renal syndrome." J Am Soc Nephrol 1995; 6:1655–1660.

266. Zager RA, O'Quigley J, Zager BK, et al: Acute renal failure following bone marrow transplantation: A retrospective study of 272 patients. Am J Kid Dis 1989; 13:210–216.

267. Bearman SI, Anderson GL, Mori M, et al: Venoocclusive disease of the liver: Development of a model for predicting fatal outcome after marrow transplantation. J Clin Oncol 1993; 11:1729–1736.

268. Leahey AM, Bunin NJ: Recombinant human tissue plasminogen activator for the treatment of severe hepatic veno-occlusive disease in pediatric bone marrow transplant patients. Bone Marrow Transplant 1996; 17:1101–1104.

269. Bearman SI, Shuhart MC, Hinds MS, et al: Recombinant human tissue plasminogen activator for the treatment of established severe venocclusive disease of the liver after bone marrow transplantation. Blood 1992; 80:2458.

270. Bearman SI, Lee JL, Baron AE, et al: Treatment of hepatic venocclusive disease with recombinant human tissue plasminogen activator and heparin in 42 marrow transplant patients. Blood 1997; 89:1501–1506.

271. Haire WD, Stephens LC, Ruby EI: Antithrombin III (AT3) treatment of organ dysfunction during bone marrow transplantation (BMT)—Results of a pilot study [abstract]. Blood 1996; 88:458a.

272. Morris JD, Harris RE, Hashmi R, et al: Antithrombin-III for the treatment of chemotherapy-induced organ dysfunction following bone marrow transplantation. Bone Marrow Transplant 1997; 20:871–878.

273. Strasser SI, McDonald GB: Gastrointestinal and hepatic complications. In Forman SJ, Blume KG, Thomas ED (eds): Hematopoietic Cell Transplantation, 2nd ed. Boston, Blackwell Scientific, 1998.

274. Schlitt HJ, Tischler HJ, Ringe B, et al: Allogeneic liver transplantation for hepatic veno-occlusive disease after bone marrow transplantation—Clinical and immunological considerations. Bone Marrow Transplant 1995; 16:473–478.

275. Smith FO, Johnson MS, Scherer LR, et al: Transjugular intrahepatic portosystemic shunting (TIPS) for the treatment of severe hepatic veno-occlusive disease. Bone Marrow Transplant 1996; 18:643–646.

276. Fried MW, Connaghan DG, Sharma S, et al: Trans jugular intrahepatic portosystemic shunt for the management of severe venocclusive disease following bone marrow transplantation. Hepatology 1996; 24:588–591.

277. Catani L, Gugliotta L, Vianelli N, et al: Endothelium and bone marrow transplantation. Bone Marrow Transplant 1996; 17:277–280.

278. Salat C, Holler E, Reinhardt B, et al: Parameters of the fibrinolytic system in patients undergoing BMT: Elevation of PAI-1 in veno-occlusive disease. Bone Marrow Transplant 1994; 14:747–750.

279. Salat C, Holler E, Hans-Jochem K, et al: Plasminogen activator inhibitor-1 confirms the diagnosis of hepatic veno-occlusive disease in patients with hyperbilirubinemia after bone marrow transplant. Blood 1997; 89:2184–2188.

280. Richardson PG, Hoppensteadt D, Elias AD, et al: Elevation of endothelial stress products and trends seen in patients with severe veno-occlusive disease treated with defibrotide. Thromb Hemost 1999; 628:1982.

281. Nurnberger W, Michelmann I, Burdach S, et al: Endothelial dysfunction after bone marrow transplantation: Increase of soluble thrombomodulin and PAI-1 in patients with multiple transplant-related complications. Ann Hematol 1998; 76:61–65.

282. Palmer KJ, Goa KL: Defibrotide: A review of its pharmacodynamic and pharmacokinetic properties, and therapeutic use in vascular disorders. Drugs 1993; 45:259–294.

283. Richardson PG, Elias AD, Krishnan A, et al: Treatment of severe veno-occlusive disease with defibrotide: Compassionate use results in response without significant toxicity in a high-risk population. Blood 1998; 92:737–744.

284. Chopra R, Eaton JD, Grassi A, et al: Defibrotide for the treatment of hepatic veno-occlusive disease: Results of the European compassionate-use Study. Br J Haematol 2000; 111:1122–1129.

285. Tse WT, Beyer W, Pendleton JD, et al: Genetic polymorphisms in glutathione s-transferase and plasminogen activator inhibitor and risk of veno-occlusive disease (VOD). Blood 2000; 96(Suppl):390a.

286. Haire WD, Cavet J, Pavletic SZ, et al: Tumor necrosis factor d3 allele predicts for organ dysfunction after allogeneic blood stem cell transplantation (ABSCT). Blood 2000; 96(Suppl):584a.

287. Essell JH, Thompson JM, Harman GS, et al: Pilot trial of prophylactic ursodiol to decrease the incidence of veno-occlusive disease of the liver in allogeneic bone marrow transplant patients. Bone Marrow Transplant 1994; 10:367.

288. Ruutu T, Eriksson B, Remes K, et al: Ursodiol for the prevention of hepatic complications in allogeneic stem cell transplantation [abstract]. Bone Marrow Transplant 1999; 23:756.

289. Ohashi K, Tanabe J, Watanabe R, et al: The Japanese multicenter open randomized trial of ursodeoxycholic acid prophylaxis for hepatic veno-occlusive disease after stem cell transplantation. Am J Hematol 2000; 64:32–38.

290. Jonas CR, Puckett AB, Jones DP, et al: Plasma antioxidant status after high-dose chemotherapy: A randomized trial of parenteral nutrition in bone marrow transplantation patients. Am J Clin Nutr 2000; 72:181–189.

291. Ringden O, Remberger M, Lehmann S, et al: N-acetylcysteine for hepatic veno-occlusive disease after allogeneic stem cell transplantation. Bone Marrow Transplant 2000; 25:993–996.

292. Billingham RE: The biology of graft-versus-host disease. Harvey Lect 1966; 62:21–78.

293. Ferrara JLM, Deeg HJ: Graft-versus-host disease. N Engl J Med 1991; 324:667–674.

294. Antin JH, Ferrara JLM: Cytokine dysregulation and acute graft-versus-host disease. Blood 1992; 80:2964–2968.

295. Ferrara JL, Levy R, Chao NJ: Pathophysiologic mechanisms of acute graft-vs.-host disease. Biol Blood Marrow Transplant 1999; 5:347–356.

296. Martin PJ, Kernan NA: T-cell depletion for GVHD prevention in humans. In Ferrara JLM, Deeg HJ, Burakoff SJ (eds): Graft-vs.-Host Disease. New York, Marcel Dekker, 1997, pp 615–637.

297. Antin JH: Graft-versus-leukemia: No longer an epiphenomenon. Blood 1993; 82:2273–2277.

298. Barrett AJ, Malkovska V: Graft-versus-leukaemia: Understanding and using the alloimmune response to treat haematological malignancies. Br J Haematol 1996; 93:754–761.

299. Truitt RL, Johnson BD, McCabe CM, et al: Graft versus leukemia. In Ferrara JLM, Deeg HJ, Burakoff SJ (eds): Graft-vs.-host disease. New York, Marcel Dekker, 1997, pp 385–423.

300. Sullivan KM, Weiden PL, Storb R, et al: Influence of acute and chronic graft-versus-host disease on relapse and survival after bone marrow transplantation from HLA-identical siblings as treatment of acute and chronic leukemia. Blood 1989; 73:1720–1728.

301. Horowitz MM, Gale RP, Sondel PM, et al: Graft-versus-leukemia reactions after bone marrow transplantation. Blood 1990; 75:555–562.

302. Ringden O, Hermans J, Labopin M, et al: The highest leukaemia-free survival after allogeneic bone marrow transplantation is seen in patients with grade I acute graft-versus-host disease. Acute and Chronic Leukaemia Working Parties of the European Group for Blood and Marrow Transplantation (EBMT). Leuk Lymphoma 1996; 24:71–79.

303. Locatelli F, Zecca M, Rondelli R, et al: Graft versus host disease prophylaxis with low-dose cyclosporine-A reduces the risk of relapse in children with acute leukemia given HLA-identical sibling bone marrow transplantation: Results of a randomized trial. Blood 2000; 95:1572–1579.

304. Schmaltz C, Alpdogan O, Horndasch KJ, et al: Differential use of Fas ligand and perforin cytotoxic pathways by donor T cells in graft-versus-host disease and graft-versus-leukemia effect. Blood 2001; 97:2886–2895.

305. Glucksberg H, Storb R, Fefer A, et al: Clinical manifestations of graft-versus-host disease in human recipients of marrow from HLA-matched sibling donors. Transplantation 1974; 18:295–304.

306. Weisdorf DJ, Snover DC, Haake R, et al: Acute upper gastrointestinal graft-versus-host disease: Clinical significance and response to immunosuppressive therapy. Blood 1990; 76:624–629.

307. Przepiorka D, Weisdorf D, Martin P, et al: Consensus conference on acute GVHD grading. Bone Marrow Transplant 1995; 15:825–828.

308. Rowlings PA, Przepiorka D, Klein JP, et al: IBMTR Severity Index for grading acute graft-versus-host disease: Retrospective comparison with Glucksberg grade. Br J Haematol 1997; 97:855–864.

309. Sale GE, Lerner KG, Barker EA, et al: The skin biopsy in the diagnosis of acute graft-versus-host disease in man. Am J Pathol 1977; 89:621–635.

310. Kohler S, Hendrickson MR, Chao NJ, et al: Value of skin biopsies in assessing prognosis and progression of acute graft-versus-host disease. Am J Surg Pathol 1997; 21:988–996.

311. Peck GL, Elias PM, Graw RG: Graft-versus-host reaction and toxic epidermal necrolysis. Lancet 1972; 2:1151.

312. McDonald GB, Shulman HM, Sullivan KM, et al: Intestinal and hepatic complications of human bone marrow transplantation. Part II. Gastroenterology 1986; 90:770–784.

313. McDonald GB, Shulman HM, Sullivan KM, et al: Intestinal and hepatic complications of human bone marrow transplantation. Part I. Gastroenterology 1986; 90:460–477.

314. Snover DC, Weisdorf SA, Ramsay NK, et al: Hepatic graft-versus-host disease: A study of the predictive value of liver biopsy in diagnosis. Hepatology 1984; 4:123–130.

315. Shulman HM, Sharma P, Amos D, et al: A coded histologic study of hepatic graft-versus-host disease after human bone marrow transplantation. Hepatology 1988; 8:463–470.

316. Sale GE, McDonald GB, Shulman HM, et al: Gastrointestinal graft-versus-host disease in man: A clinicopathologic study of the rectal biopsy. Am J Surg Pathol 1979; 3:291–299.

317. Beatty PG, Hansen JA, Longton GM, et al: Marrow transplantation from HLA-matched unrelated donors for treatment of hematologic malignancies. Transplantation 1991; 51:443–447.

318. Weisdorf D, Hakke R, Blazar B: Risk factors for acute graft versus host disease in histocompatible donor bone marrow transplantation. Transplantation 1991; 51:1197–1203.

319. Nash RA, Pepe MS, Storb R, et al: Acute graft-versus-host disease: Analysis of risk factors after allogeneic marrow transplantation and prophylaxis with cyclosporine and methotrexate. Blood 1992; 80:1838–1845.

320. Petersdorf EW, Longton GM, Anasetti C, et al: The significance of HLA-DRB1 matching on clinical outcome after HLA-A, B, DR identical unrelated donor marrow transplantation. Blood 1995; 86:1606–1613.

321. Gale RP, Bortin MM, Van Bekkum DW, et al: Risk factors for acute graft-versus-host disease. Br J Haematol 1987; 67:397–406.

322. Hansen JA, Gooley TA, Martin PJ, et al: Bone marrow transplants from unrelated donors for patients with chronic myeloid leukemia. N Engl J Med 1998; 338:962–968.

323. Hagglund H, Bostrom L, Remberger M, et al: Risk factors for acute graft-versus-host disease in 291 consecutive HLA-identical bone marrow transplant recipients. Bone Marrow Transplant 1995; 16:747–753.

324. Nademanee A, Schmidt GM, Parker P, et al: The outcome of matched unrelated donor bone marrow transplantation in patients with hematologic malignancies using molecular typing for donor selection and graft-versus-host disease prophylaxis regimen of cyclosporine, methotrexate, and prednisone. Blood 1995; 86:1228–1234.

325. Storb R, Prentice RL, Buckner CD, et al: Graft-versus-host disease and survival in patients with aplastic anemia treated by marrow grafts from HLA-identical siblings: Beneficial effect of a protective environment. N Engl J Med 1983; 308:302–306.

326. Petersen FB, Buckner CD, Clift RA, et al: Laminar air flow isolation and decontamination: A prospective randomized study of the effects of prophylactic systemic antibiotics in bone marrow transplant patients. Infection 1986; 14:115–121.

327. Beelen DW, Elmaagacli A, Muller KD, et al: Influence of intestinal bacterial decontamination using metronidazole and ciprofloxacin or ciprofloxacin alone on the development of acute graft-versus-host disease after marrow transplantation in patients with hematologic malignancies: Final results and long-term follow-up of an open-label prospective randomized trial. Blood 1999; 93:3267–3275.

328. Crum Vander Woude A, Bierer BE: Immunosuppression and immunophilin ligands: Cyclosporin A, FK506, and rapamycin. In Ferrara JLM, Deeg HJ, Burakoff SJ (eds): Graft-vs.-Host Disease. New York, Marcel Dekker, 1997, pp 111–149.

329. Jolivet J, Cowan KH, Curt GA, et al: The pharmacology and clinical use of methotrexate. N Engl J Med 1983; 309:1094–1104.

330. Chao NJ, Deeg HJ: In vivo prevention and treatment of GVHD: In Ferrara JLM, Deeg HJ, Burakoff SJ (eds): Graft-vs.-Host Disease. New York, Marcel Dekker, 1997, pp 639–666.

331. Ruutu T, Niederwieser D, Gratwohl A, et al: A survey of the prophylaxis and treatment of acute GVHD in Europe: A report of the European Group for Blood and Marrow Transplantation (EBMT). Chronic Leukaemia Working Party of the EBMT: Bone Marrow Transplant 1997; 19:759–764.

332. Peters C, Minkov M, Gadner H, et al: Statement of current majority practices in graft-versus-host disease prophylaxis and treatment in children. Bone Marrow Transplant 2000; 26:405–411.

333. Storb R, Deeg HJ, Pepe M, et al: Methotrexate and cyclosporine versus cyclosporine alone for prophylaxis of graft-versus-host disease in patients given HLA-identical marrow grafts for leukemia: Long-term follow-up of a controlled trial. Blood 1989; 73:1729–1734.

334. Gluckman E, Horowitz MM, Champlin RE, et al: Bone marrow transplantation for severe aplastic anemia: Influence of conditioning and graft-versus-host disease prophylaxis regimens on outcome. Blood 1992; 79:269–275.

335. Blaise D, Gravis G, Marinichi D: Long-term follow-up of T-cell depletion for bone marrow transplantation. Lancet 1993; 341:51–52.

336. Marmont AM, Horowitz MM, Gale RP, et al: T-cell depletion of HLA-identical transplants in leukemia. Blood 1991; 78:2120–2130.

337. Champlin RE, Passweg JR, Zhang MJ, et al: T-cell depletion of bone marrow transplants for leukemia from donors other than HLA-identical siblings: Advantage of T-cell antibodies with narrow specificities. Blood 2000; 95:3996–4003.

338. Hale G, Zhang MJ, Bunjes D, et al: Improving the outcome of bone marrow transplantation by using CD52 monoclonal antibodies to prevent graft-versus-host disease and graft rejection. Blood 1998; 92:4581–4590.

339. Clark RE, Pender N: Transplantation of T-lymphocyte depleted marrow with an addback of T cells. Hematol Oncol 1995; 13:219–224.

340. Sehn LH, Alyea EP, Weller E, et al: Comparative outcomes of T-cell-depleted and non-T-cell-depleted allogeneic bone marrow transplantation for chronic myelogenous leukemia: Impact of donor lymphocyte infusion. J Clin Oncol 1999; 17:561–568.

341. Drobyski WR: Evolving strategies to address adverse transplant outcomes associated with T cell depletion. J Hematother Stem Cell Res 2000; 9:327–337.

342. Aschan J: Treatment of moderate to severe acute graft-versus-host disease: A retrospective analysis. Bone Marrow Transplant 1994; 14:601–607.

343. Sayer HG, Longton G, Bowden R, et al: Increased risk of infection in marrow transplant patients receiving methylprednisolone for graft-versus-host disease prevention. Blood 1994; 84:1328–1332.

344. Van Lint MT, Uderzo C, Locasciulli A, et al: Early treatment of acute graft-versus-host disease with high- or low-dose 6-methylprednisolone: A multicenter randomized trial from the Italian Group for Bone Marrow Transplantation. Blood 1998; 92:2288–2293.

345. Martin PJ, Schoch G, Fisher L, et al: A retrospective analysis of therapy for acute graft-versus-host disease: Secondary treatment. Blood 1991; 77:1821–1828.

346. Greinix HT, Volc-Platzer B, Kalhs P, et al: Extracorporeal photochemotherapy in the treatment of severe steroid-refractory acute graft-versus-host disease: A pilot study. Blood 2000; 96:2426–2431.

347. Basara N, Blau WI, Romer E, et al: Mycophenolate mofetil for the treatment of acute and chronic GVHD in bone marrow transplant patients. Bone Marrow Transplant 1998; 22:61–65.

348. Atkinson K, Horowitz MM, Gale RP, et al: Consensus among bone marrow transplanters for diagnosis, grading and treatment of chronic graft-versus-host disease. Bone Marrow Transplant 1989; 4:247–254.

349. Siadak M, Sullivan KM: The management of chronic graft-versus-host disease. Blood Rev 1994; 8:154–160.

350. Ochs LA, Miller WJ, Filipovich AH, et al: Predictive factors for chronic graft-versus-host disease after histocompatible sibling donor bone marrow transplantation. Bone Marrow Transplant 1994; 13:455–460.

351. Brown RA, Adkins D, Khoury H, et al: Long-term follow-up of high-risk allogeneic peripheral-blood stem-cell transplant recipients: Graft-versus-host disease and transplant-related mortality. J Clin Oncol 1999; 17:806–812.

352. Porter DL, Collins RH Jr, Hardy C, et al: Treatment of relapsed leukemia after unrelated donor marrow transplantation with unrelated donor leukocyte infusions. Blood 2000; 95:1214–1521.

353. Dazzi F, Szydlo RM, Craddock C, et al: Comparison of single-dose and escalating-dose regimens of donor lymphocyte infusion for relapse after allografting for chronic myeloid leukemia. Blood 2000; 95:67–71.

354. Shulman HM, Sale GE, Lerner KG, et al: Chronic cutaneous graft-versus-host disease in man. Am J Pathol 1978; 91:545–570.

355. Shulman HM, Sullivan KM, Weiden P, et al: Chronic graft-versus-host syndrome in man: A long-term clinicopathologic study of 20 Seattle patients. Am J Med 1980; 69:204–217.

356. Kulkarni S, Powles R, Treleaven J, et al: Chronic graft versus host disease is associated with long-term risk for pneumococcal infections in recipients of bone marrow transplants. Blood 2000; 95:3683–3686.

357. Sullivan KM, Shulman HM, Storb R, et al: Chronic graft-versus-host disease in 52 patients: Adverse natural course and successful treatment with combination immunosuppression. Blood 1981; 57:267–277.

358. Wingard JR, Piantadosi S, Vogelsang GB, et al: Predictors of death from chronic graft-versus-host disease after bone marrow transplantation. Blood 1989; 74:1428–1435.

359. First LR, Smith BR, Lipton J, et al: Isolated thrombocytopenia after allogeneic bone marrow transplantation: Existence of transient and chronic thrombocytopenic syndromes. Blood 1985; 65:368–374.

360. Sullivan KM, Witherspoon RP, Storb R, et al: Alternating-day cyclosporine and prednisone for treatment of high-risk chronic graft-v-host disease. Blood 1988; 72:555–561.

361. Parker PM, Chao N, Nademanee A, et al: Thalidomide as salvage therapy for chronic graft-versus-host disease. Blood 1995; 86:3604–3609.

362. Lee SJ, Wegner SA, McGarigle CJ, et al: Treatment of chronic GVUD with clofazimine. Blood 1997; 89:2298–2302.

363. Busca A, Saroglia EM, Lanino E, et al: Mycophenolate mofetil (MMF) as therapy for refractory chronic GVHD (cGVHD) in children receiving bone marrow transplantation. Bone Marrow Transplant 2000; 25:1067–1071.

364. Schiller G, Gale RP: Is there an effective therapy for chronic graft-versus-host disease? Bone Marrow Transplant 1993; 11:189–192.

365. Singhal S, Mehta J, Rattenbury H, et al: Oral pilocarpine hydrochloride for the treatment of refractory xerostomia associated with chronic graft-versus-host disease. Blood 1995; 85:1147–1148.

366. Livesey SJ, Holmes JA, Whittaker JA: Ocular complications of bone marrow transplantation. Eye 1989; 3:271–276.

367. Truwit CL, Denaro CP, Lake JR, et al: MR imaging of reversible cyclosporin A-induced neurotoxicity. Am J Neuroradiol 1991; 12:651–659.

368. Schwartz RB, Jones KM, Kalina P, et al: Hypertensive encephalopathy: Findings on CT, MR imaging, and SPECT imaging in 14 cases. Am J Roentgenol 1992; 159:379–383.

369. Avery R, Jabs DA, Wingard JR, et al: Optic disc edema after bone marrow transplantation. Ophthalmology 1991; 98:1294–1301.

370. Bernauer W, Gratwohl A, Keller A, et al: Microvasculopathy in the ocular fundus after bone marrow transplantation. Ann Intern Med 1991; 115:925–930.

371. Lopez PF, Sternberg P, Dabbs CK, et al: Bone marrow transplant retinopathy. Am J Ophthalmol 1991; 112:635–646.

372. Guinan EC, Tarbell NJ, Niemeyer CM, et al: Intravascular hemolysis and renal insufficiency after bone marrow transplantation. Blood 1988; 72:451–455.

373. Rabinowe SN, Soiffer RJ, Tarbell NJ, et al: Hemolytic-uremic syndrome following bone marrow tranplantation in adults for hematologic malignancies. Blood 1991; 77:1837–1844.

374. Deeg HJ, Flournoy N, Sullivan KM, et al: Cataracts after total body irradiation and marrow transplantation: A sparing effect of dose fractionation. Int J Oncol Biol Phys 1984; 10:957–964.

375. Benyunes MC, Sullivan KM, Deeg HJ, et al: Cataracts after bone marrow transplantation: Long-term follow-up of adults treated with fractionated total body irradiation. Int J Radiat Oncol Biol Physiol 1995; 32:661–670.

376. Zierhut D, Lohr F, Schraube P, et al: Cataract incidence after total-body irradiation. Int J Radiat Oncol Biol Phys 2000; 46:131–135.

377. Ozsahin M, Belkacemi Y, Pene F, et al: Total-body irradiation and cataract incidence: A randomized comparison of two instantaneous dose rates. Int J Radiat Oncol Biol Physiol 1993; 28:343–347.

378. Fife K, Milan S, Westbrook K, et al: Risk factors for requiring cataract surgery following total body irradiation. Radiother Oncol 1994; 33:93–98.

379. Dahllof G, Forsberg CM, Ringden O, et al: Facial growth and morphology in long-term survivors after bone marrow transplantation. Eur J Orthod 1989; 11:332–340.

380. Johnson FL, Stokes DC, Ruggiero M, et al: Chronic obstructive airways disease after bone marrow transplantation. J Pediatr 1984; 105:370–375.

381. Schultz KR, Green GJ, Wensley D, et al: Obstructive lung disease in children after allogeneic bone marrow transplantation. Blood 1994; 84:3212–3220.

382. Palmas A, Tefferi A, Myers JL, et al: Late-onset noninfectious pulmonary complications after allogeneic bone marrow transplantation. Br J Haematol 1998; 100:680–687.

383. Gore EM, Lawton CA, Ash RC, et al: Pulmonary function changes in long-term survivors of bone marrow transplantation. Int J Radiat Oncol Biol Phys 1996; 36:67–75.

384. Schultz KR, Fernandez CV, Israel DM, et al: Association of gastroesophageal reflux with obstructive lung diseases in children after allogeneic bone marrow transplantation [letter]. Blood 1995;3763–3766.

385. Sanchez J, Torres A, Serrano J, et al: Long-term follow-up of immunosuppressive treatment for obstructive airways disease after allogeneic bone marrow transplantation. Bone Marrow Transplant 1997; 20:403–408.

386. Crawford SW, Pepe M, Lin D, et al: Abnormalities of pulmonary function tests after marrow transplantation predict nonrelapse mortality. Am J Respir Crit Care Med 1995; 152:690–695.

387. Tait RC, Burnett AK, Robertson AG, et al: Subclinical pulmonary function defects following autologous and allogeneic bone marrow transplant: Relationship to total body irradiation and graft-versus-host disease. Int J Radiat Oncol Biol Physiol 1991; 20:1219–1227.

388. Arvidson J, Bratteby L-E, Carson K, et al: Pulmonary function after autologous bone marrow transplantation in children. Bone Marrow Transplant 1994; 14:117–123.

389. Kaplan EB, Wodell RA, Wilmott RW, et al: Late effects of bone marrow transplantation on pulmonary function in children. Bone Marrow Transplant 1994; 14:613–621.

390. Nysom K, Holm K, Hesse B, et al: Lung function after allogeneic bone marrow transplantation for leukaemia or lymphoma. Arch Dis Child 1996; 74:432–436.

391. Gajewski JL, Petz LD, Calhoun L, et al: Hemolysis of transfused group O red blood cells in minor ABO-incompatible unrelated-donor bone marrow transplants in patients receiving cyclosporine without posttransplant methotrexate. Blood 1992; 79:3076–3085.

392. Hows J, Beddow K, Gordon-Smith E, et al: Donor-derived red blood cell antibodies and immune hemolysis after allogeneic bone marrow transplantation. Blood 1986; 67:177–181.

393. Petz LD: Hemolysis associated with transplantation. Transfusion 1998; 38:224–228.

394. Godder K, Pati AR, Abhyankar SH, et al: De novo chronic graft-versus-host disease presenting as hemolytic anemia following partially mismatched related donor bone marrow transplant. Bone Marrow Transplant 1997; 19:813–817.

395. Gmur JP, Burger J, Schaffner A, et al: Pure red cell aplasia of long duration complicating major ABO-incompatible bone marrow transplantation. Blood 1990; 75:290–295.

396. Benjamin RJ, Connors JM, McGurk S, et al: Prolonged erythroid aplasia after major ABO-mismatched transplantation for chronic myelogenous leukemia. Biol Blood Marrow Transplant 1998; 4:151–156.

397. Klumpp TR, Block CC, Caligiuri MA, et al: Immune-mediated cytopenia following bone marrow transplantation: Case reports and review of the literature. Medicine (Baltimore) 1992; 71:73.

398. Klumpp TR, Herman JH, Macdonald JS, et al: Autoimmune neutropenia following peripheral blood stem cell transplantation. Am J Hematol 1992; 41:214.

399. Bashey A, Owen I, Lucas GF, et al: Late onset immune pancytopenia following bone marrow transplantation. Br J Haematol 1991; 78:268.

400. Lambertenghi-Deliliers GL, Annaloro C, Della Volpe A, et al: Multiple autoimmune events after autologous bone marrow transplantation. Bone Marrow Transplant 1997; 19:745–747.

401. Ratanatharathorn V, Carson E, Reynolds C, et al: Anti-CD20 chimeric monoclonal antibody treatment of refractory immune-mediated thrombocytopenia in a patient with chronic graft-versus-host disease. Ann Intern Med 2000; 133:275–279.

402. Peralvo J, Bacigalupo A, Pittaluga PA, et al: Poor graft function associated with graft-versus-host disease after allogeneic marrow transplantation. Bone Marrow Transplant 1987; 2:279–285.

403. Zimmerli W, Zarth A, Gratwohl A, et al: Neutrophil function and pyogenic infections in bone marrow transplant recipients. Blood 1991; 77:393–399.

404. Masat T, Feliu E, Villamor N, et al: Immunophenotypic and ultrastructural study in peripheral blood neutrophil granulocytes following bone marrow transplantation. Br J Haematol 1997; 98:299–307.

405. Kaufman PA, Jones RB, Greenberg CS, et al: Autologous bone marrow transplantation and factor XII, factor VII, and protein C deficiencies. Cancer 1990; 66:515–521.

406. Gordon B, Haire W, Kessinger A, et al: High frequency of antithrombin 3 and protein C deficiency following autologous bone marrow transplantation and lymphoma. Bone Marrow Transplant 1991; 8:497–502.

407. Gordon BG, Saving KL, McCallister JAM, et al: Cerebral infarction associated with protein C deficiency following allogeneic bone marrow transplantation. Bone Marrow Transplant 1991; 8:323–325.

408. Shulman H, Striker G, Deeg HJ, et al: Nephrotoxicity of cyclosporin A after allogeneic marrow transplantation. N Engl J Med 1981; 305:1392–1395.

409. Holler E, Kolb HJ, Hiller E, et al: Microangiopathy in patients on cyclosporine prophylaxis who developed acute graft-versus-host

disease after HLA-identical bone marrow transplantation. Blood 1989; 73:2018–2024.

410. Bergstein J, Andreoli SP, Provisor AJ, et al: Radiation nephritis following total-body irradiation and cyclophosphamide in preparation for bone marrow transplantation. Transplantation 1986; 41:63–66.

411. Butcher JA, Hariharan S, Adams MB, et al: Renal transplantation for end-stage renal disease following bone marrow transplantation: A report of six cases, with and without immunosuppression. Clin Transplant 1999; 13:330–335.

412. Hows JM, Palmer S, Gordon SE: Use of cyclosporin A in allogeneic bone marrow transplantation for severe aplastic anemia. Transplantation 1982; 33:382–386.

413. Hows JM, Chipping PM, Fairhead S, et al: Nephrotoxicity in bone marrow transplant recipients treated with cyclosporin A. Br J Haematol 1983; 54:69–78.

414. Feutren G, Mihatsch J: Risk factors for cyclosporine-induced nephropathy inpatients with autoimmune diseases. N Engl J Med 1992; 326:1654–1660.

415. Fairchild W, Spence C, Solomon H, et al: The incidence of bladder cancer after cyclophophamide therapy. J Urol 1979; 122:163–164.

416. Stillwell TJ, Benson RCJ: Cyclophosphamide-induced hemorrhagic cystitis. A review of 100 patients. Cancer 1988; 61:451–457.

417. Russell SJ, Vowels MR, Vale T: Haemorrhagic cystitis in paediatric bone marrow transplant patients: An association with infective agents, GVHD and prior cyclophosphamide. Bone Marrow Transplant 1994; 13:533–539.

418. Wade JC, Meyers JD: Neurologic symptoms associated with parenteral acyclovir treatment after marrow transplantation. Ann Intern Med 1983; 98:921–925.

419. Davis CL, Springmeyer S, Gmerek BJ: Central nervous system side effects of ganciclovir. N Engl J Med 1990; 322:933–934.

420. Chrisp P, Clissold SP: Foscarnet: A review of its antiviral activity, pharmacokinetic properties and therapeutic use in immunocompromised patients with cytomegalovirus retinitis. Drugs 1991; 41:104–129.

421. Kahan BD: Cyclosporine. N Engl J Med 1989; 321:1725–1738.

422. Schwartz RB, Bravo SM, Klufas R, et al: Cyclosporine neurotoxicity and its relationship to hypertensive encephalopathy. AJR Am J Roentgenol 1995; 165:627–631.

423. Woo M, Przepiorka D, Ippoliti C, et al: Toxicities of tacrolimus and cyclosporin A after allogeneic blood stem cell transplantation. Bone Marrow Transplant 1997; 20:1095–1098.

424. Tezcan H, Zimmer W, Fenstermaker R, et al: Severe cerebellar swelling and thrombotic thrombocytopenic purpura associated with FK506. Bone Marrow Transplant 1998; 21:105–109.

425. Noll RB, Kulkarni R: Complex visual hallucinations and cyclosporine. Arch Neurol 1984; 41:329–330.

426. Thompson CB, June CH, Sullivan KM, et al: Association between cyclosporine neurotoxicity and hypomagnesaemia. Lancet 1984:1116–1120.

427. Mohrmann R, Mah V, Vinters HV: Neuropathologic findings after bone marrow transplantation: An autopsy study. Hum Pathol 1990; 21:630–639.

428. Patchell RA, White CL, Clark AW, Beschorner WE, Santos GW: Neurologic complications of bone marrow transplantation. Neurology 1985; 35:300–306.

429. Winston DJ, Gale RP, Meyer DV, et al: Infectious complications of human bone marrow transplantation. Medicine (Baltimore) 1979; 58:1–31.

430. Denning DW, Stevens DA: Antifungal and surgical treatment of invasive aspergillosis: Review of 2,121 published cases. Rev Infect Dis 1990; 12:1147–1201.

431. Maschke M, Dietrich U, Prumbaum M, et al: Opportunistic CNS infection after bone marrow transplantation. Bone Marrow Transplant 1999; 23:1167–1176.

432. de Medeiros BC, de Medeiros CR, Werner B, et al: Central nervous system infections following bone marrow transplantation: An autopsy report of 27 cases. J Hematother Stem Cell Res 2000; 9:535–540.

433. Thompson CB, Sanders JE, Flournoy N, et al: The risks of central nervous system relapse and leukoencephalopathy in patients receiving marrow transplants for acute leukemia. Blood 1986; 67:195–199.

434. Smedler A-C, Ringden K, Bergman H, et al: Sensory-motor and cognitive functioning in children who have undergone bone marrow transplantation. Acta Paediatr Scand 1990; 79:613–621.

435. Kaleita TA, Shields WD, Tesler A, et al: Normal neurodevelopment in four young children treated with bone marrow transplantation for acute leukemia or aplastic anemia. Pediatrics 1989; 83:753–757.

436. van den Berg H, Gerritsen EJA, Noordijk EM, et al: Major complications of the central nervous system after bone marrow transplantation in children with acute lymphoblastic leukemia. Radiother Oncol 1990; 18(Suppl 1):94–97.

437. Van Weel-Sipman MH, Van't Veer-Korthof ET, Van Den Berg H, et al: Late effects of total body irradiation and cytostatic preparative regimen for bone marrow transplantation in children with hematological malignancies. Radiother Oncol 1990; 1:155–157.

438. Johnson FL, Rubin CM: Allogeneic marrow transplantation in the treatment of infants with cancer. Br J Cancer Suppl 1992; 18.

439. Phipps S, Dunavant M, Srivastava DK, et al: Cognitive and academic functioning in survivors of pediatric bone marrow transplantation. J Clin Oncol 2000; 18:1004–1011.

440. Gordon BG, Warkentin PI, Strandjord SE, et al: Allogeneic bone marrow transplantation for children with acute leukemia: Long-term follow-up of patients prepared with high-dose cytosine arabinoside and fractionated total body irradiation. Bone Marrow Transplant 1997; 20:5–10.

441. Borgstrom B, Bolme P: Thyroid function in children after allogeneic bone marrow transplantation. Bone Marrow Transplant 1994; 13:59–64.

442. Sanders JE: Endocrine problems in children after bone marrow transplant for hematologic malignancies. The long-term follow-up team. Bone Marrow Transplant 1991; 8(Suppl 1):2–4.

443. Toubert ME, Socie G, Gluckman E, et al: Short- and long-term follow-up of thyroid dysfunction after allogeneic bone marrow transplantation without the use of preparative total body irradiation. Br J Haematol 1997; 98:453–457.

444. Huma Z, Boulad F, Black P, et al: Growth in children after bone marrow transplantation for acute leukemia. Blood 1995; 86:819–824.

445. Sklar CA: Growth following therapy for childhood cancer. Cancer Invest 1995; 13:511–516.

446. Giorgiani G, Bozzola M, Locatelli F, et al: Role of busulfan and total body irradiation on growth of prepubertal children receiving bone marrow transplantation and results of treatment with recombinant human growth hormone. Blood 1995; 86:825–831.

447. Holm K, Nysom K, Rasmussen MH, et al: Growth, growth hormone and final height after BMT: Possible recovery of irradiation-induced growth hormone insufficiency. Bone Marrow Transplant 1996; 18:163–170.

448. Brauner R, Fontoura M, Zucker JM, et al: Growth and growth hormone secretion after bone marrow transplantation. Arch Dis Child 1993; 68:458–463.

449. Cohen A, Rovelli A, Bakker B, et al: Final height of patients who underwent bone marrow transplantation for hematological disorders during childhood: A study by the Working Party for Late Effects—EBMT. Blood 1999; 93:4109–1415.

450. Wingard JR, Plotnick LP, Freemer CS, et al: Growth in children after bone marrow transplantation: Busulfan plus cyclophosphamide versus cyclophosphamide plus total body irradiation. Blood 1992; 79:1068–1073.

451. Michel G, Socie G, Gebhard F, et al: Late effects of allogeneic bone marrow transplantation for children with acute myeloblastic leukemia in first complete remission: The impact of conditioning regimen without total-body irradiation—A report from the Societe Francaise de Greffe de Moelle. J Clin Oncol 1997; 15:2238–2246.

452. Liesner RJ, Leiper AD, Hann IM, et al: Late effects of intensive treatment for acute myeloid leukemia and myelodysplasia in childhood. J Clin Oncol 1994; 12:916–924.

453. Chatterjee R, Mills W, Katz M, et al: Prospective study of pituitary-gonadal function to evaluate short-term effects of ablative chemotherapy or total body irradiation with autologous or allogeneic marrow transplantation in post-menarcheal female patients. Bone Marrow Transplant 1994; 13:511–517.

454. Schubert MA, Sullivan KM, Schubert MM, et al: Gynecological abnormalities following allogeneic bone marrow transplantation. Bone Marrow Transplant 1990; 5:425–430.

455. Chiodi S, Spinelli S, Cohen A, et al: Cyclic sex hormone replacement therapy in women undergoing allogeneic bone marrow transplantation: Aims and results. Bone Marrow Transplant 1991; 8:47–49.

456. Sanders JE, Buckner CD, Leonard JM, et al: Late effects on gonadal function of cyclophosphamide total-body irradiation and marrow transplantation. Transplantation 1983; 36:252–255.

457. Sarafoglou K, Boulad F, Gillio A, et al: Gonadal function after bone marrow transplantation for acute leukemia during childhood. J Pediatr 1997; 130:210–216.

458. Schimmer AD, Quatermain M, Imrie K, et al: Ovarian function after autologous bone marrow transplantation. J Clin Oncol 1998; 16:2359–2363.

459. Thibaud E, Rodriguez-Macias K, Trivin C, et al: Ovarian function after bone marrow transplantation during childhood. Bone Marrow Transplant 1998; 21:287–290.

460. Sanders JE, Hawley J, Levy W, et al: Pregnancies following high-dose cyclophosphamide with or without high-dose busulfan or total-body irradiation and bone marrow transplantation. Blood 1996; 87:3045–3052.

461. Mascarin M, Giavitto M, Zanazzo GA, et al: Avascular necrosis of bone in children undergoing allogeneic bone marrow transplantation. Cancer 1991; 68:655–659.

462. Atkinson K, Cohen M, Biggs J: Avascular necrosis of femoral head secondary to corticosteroid therapy for graft-versus-host disease after marrow transplantation: Effective therapy with hip arthroplasty. Bone Marrow Transplant 1987; 2:421–426.

463. Russel JA, Blaley WB, Stuart TA, et al: Avascular necrosis of bone in bone marrow transplant patients. Med Pediatric Oncol 1989; 17:140–143.

464. Socie G, Cahn JY, Carmelo J, et al: Avascular necrosis of bone after allogeneic bone marrow transplantation: Analysis of risk factors for 4388 patients by the Societe Francaise de Greffe de Moelle (SFGM). Br J Haematol 1997; 97:865–870.

465. Schimmer AD, Minden MD, Keating A: Osteoporosis after blood and marrow transplantation: Clinical aspects. Biol Blood Marrow Transplant 2000; 6:175–181.

466. Kashyap A, Kandeel F, Yamauchi D, et al: Effects of allogeneic bone marrow transplantation on recipient bone mineral density: A prospective study. Biol Blood Marrow Transplant 2000; 6:344–351.

467. Li FP, Alter BP, Nathan DG: The mortality of acquired aplastic anemia in children. Blood 1972; 40:153–161.

468. Thomas ED, Buckner CD, Storb R, et al: Aplastic anaemia treated by marrow transplantation. Lancet 1972; 1:284.

469. Camitta BM, Thomas ED, Nathan DG, et al: A prospective study of androgens and bone marrow transplantation for treatment of severe aplastic anemia. Blood 1979; 53:504.

470. Werner EJ, Stout RD, Valdez LP, Harris RE: Immunosuppressive therapy versus bone marrow transplantation for children with aplastic anemia. Pediatrics 1989; 83:61–65.

471. Paquette RL, Tebyani N, Frane M, et al: Long-term outcome of aplastic anemia in adults treated with antithymocyte globulin: Comparison with bone marrow transplantation. Blood 1995; 85:283–290.

472. Doney K, Leisenring W, Storb R, Appelbaum FR: Primary treatment of acquired aplastic anemia: Outcomes with bone marrow transplantation and immunosuppressive therapy. Seattle Bone Marrow Transplant Team. Ann Intern Med 1997; 126:107–115.

473. Fouladi M, Herman R, Rolland-Grinton M, et al: Improved survival in severe acquired aplastic anemia of childhood. Bone Marrow Transplant 2000; 26:1149–1156.

474. Bacigalupo A, Oneto R, Bruno B, et al: Current results of bone marrow transplantation in patients with acquired severe aplastic anemia. Report of the European Group for Blood and Marrow Transplantation. On behalf of the Working Party on Severe Aplastic Anemia of the European Group for Blood and Marrow Transplantation. Acta Haematol 2000; 103:19–25.

475. Bunin N, Leahey A, Kamani N, et al: Bone marrow transplantation in pediatric patients with severe aplastic anemia: Cyclophosphamide and anti-thymocyte globulin conditioning followed by recombinant human granulocyte-macrophage colony stimulating factor. J Pediatr Hematol Oncol 1996; 18:68–71.

476. Storb R, Leisenring W, Anasetti C, et al: Long-term follow-up of allogeneic marrow transplants in patients with aplastic anemia conditioned by cyclophosphamide combined with antithymocyte globulin. Blood 1997; 89:3890–3891.

477. Deeg HJ, Leisenring W, Storb R, et al: Long-term outcome after marrow transplantation for severe aplastic anemia. Blood 1998; 91:3637–3645.

478. Champlin RE, Feig SA, Sparkes RS, et al: Bone marrow transplantation from identical twins in the treatment of aplastic anemia: Implication for the pathogenesis of the disease. Br J Haematol 1984; 56:455–463.

479. Storb R, Longton G, Anasetti C, et al: Changing trends in marrow transplantation for aplastic anemia. Bone Marrow Transplant 1992; 10:45–52.

480. Horowitz MM: Current status of allogeneic bone marrow transplantation in acquired aplastic anemia. Semin Hematol 2000; 37:30–42.

481. Storb R, Doney KC, Thomas ED, et al: Marrow transplantation with or without donor buffy coat cells for 65 transfused aplastic anemia patients. Blood 1982; 59:236–246.

482. Shank B, Brochstein JA, Castro-Malaspina H, et al: Immunosuppression prior to marrow transplantation for sensitized aplastic anemia patients: Comparison of TLI with TBI: Int J Radiat Oncol Biol Phys 1988; 14:1133–1141.

483. Storb R, Etzioni R, Anasetti C, et al: Cyclophosphamide combined with antithymocyte globulin in preparation for allogeneic marrow transplants in patients with aplastic anemia. Blood 1994; 84:941–949.

484. Socie G, Gluckman E, Devergie A, et al: Bone marrow transplantation (BMT) for acquired severe aplastic anaemia (SAA): Long term follow-up of 107 consecutive patients. Bone Marrow Transplant 1991; 7:102.

485. Witherspoon RP, Storb R, Pepe M, et al: Cumulative incidence of secondary solid malignant tumors in aplastic anemia patients given marrow grafts after conditioning with chemotherapy alone. Blood 1992; 79:289–292.

486. Pierga J-Y, Socie G, Gluckman E, et al: Secondary solid malignant tumors occurring after bone marrow transplantation for severe aplastic anemia given thoraco-abdominal irradiation. Radiother Oncol 1994; 30:55–58.

487. Storb R, Deeg HJ, Farewell V, et al: Marrow transplantation for severe aplastic anemia: Methotrexate alone compared with a combination of methotrexate and cyclosporine for prevention of acute graft-versus-host disease. Blood 1986; 68:119–125.

488. Storb R, Champlin RE: Bone marrow transplantation for severe aplastic anemia. Bone Marrow Transplant 1991; 8:69–72.

489. Young NS: The problem of clonality in aplastic anemia. Dr. Damshek's riddle, restated. Blood 1992; 79:1385.

490. Tichelli A, Gratwohl A, Wursch A, et al: Late haematological complications in severe aplastic anaemia. Br. J:Haematol 1988; 69:413.

491. Socie G, Henry-Amar M, Bacigalupo A, et al: Malignant tumors occurring after treatment of aplastic anemia. N Engl J Med 1993; 329:1152–1157.

492. Wagner JL, Deeg HJ, Seidel K, et al: Bone marrow transplantation for severe aplastic anemia from genotypically HLA-nonidentical relatives. An update of the Seattle experience. Transplantation 1996; 61:54–61.

493. Margolis DA, Casper JT: Alternative-donor hematopoietic stem-cell transplantation for severe aplastic anemia. Semin Hematol 2000; 37:43–55.

494. Hasle H, Wadsworth LD, Massing BG, et al: A population-based study of childhood myelodysplastic syndrome in British Columbia, Canada. Br J Haematol 1999; 106:1027–1032.

495. Guinan EC, Tarbell NJ, Tantravahi R, et al: Bone marrow transplantation for children with myelodysplastic syndromes. Blood 1989; 73:619–622.

496. Nichols K, Parsons SK, Guinan EC: Long-term follow-up of twelve pediatric patients with primary myelodysplastic syndrome treated with HLA-identical sibling donor bone marrow transplantation. Blood 1996; 87:4020–4022.

497. Runde V, de Witte T, Arnold R, et al: Bone marrow transplantation from HLA-identical siblings as first-line treatment in patients with myelodysplastic syndromes: Early transplantation is associated with improved outcome. Chronic Leukemia Working Party of the European Group for Blood and Marrow Transplantation. Bone Marrow Transplant 1998; 21:255–261.

498. Locatelli F, Zecca M, Niemeyer C, et al: Role of allogeneic bone marrow transplantation for the treatment of myelodysplastic syndromes in childhood. The European Working Group on Childhood Myelodysplastic Syndrome (EWOG-MDS) and the Austria-Germany-Italy (AGI) Bone Marrow Transplantation Registry. Bone Marrow Transplant 1996; 18(Suppl 2):63–68.

499. Anderson JE, Appelbaum FR, Schoch G, et al: Allogeneic marrow transplantation for refractory anemia: A comparison of two preparative regimens and analysis of prognostic factors. Blood 1996; 87:51–58.

500. Sutton L, Chastang C, Ribaud P, et al: Factors influencing outcome in de novo myelodysplastic syndromes treated by allogeneic bone marrow transplantation: A long-term study of 71 patients Societe Francaise de Greffe de Moelle. Blood 1996; 88:358–365.

501. Anderson JE, Gooley TA, Schoch G, et al: Stem cell transplantation for secondary acute myeloid leukemia: Evaluation of transplantation as initial therapy or following induction chemotherapy. Blood 1997; 89:2578–2585.

502. Rajantie J, Sale GE, Deeg HJ, et al: Adverse effect of severe marrow fibrosis on hematologic recovery after chemoradiotherapy and allogeneic bone marrow transplantation. Blood 1986; 67:1693–1697.

503. Soll E, Massumoto C, Clift RA, et al: Relevance of marrow fibrosis in bone marrow transplantation: A retrospective analysis of engraftment. Blood 1995; 86:4667–4673.

504. Barrett AJ, Horowitz MM, Pollock BH, et al: Bone marrow transplants from HLA-identical siblings as compared with chemotherapy for children with acute lymphoblastic leukemia in a second remission. N Engl J Med 1994; 331:1253–1258.

505. Weisdorf DJ, Woods WG, Nesbit ME Jr, et al: Allogeneic bone marrow transplantation for acute lymphoblastic leukaemia: Risk factors and clinical outcome. Br J Haematol 1994; 86:62–69.

506. Dopfer R, Henze G, Bender-Gotze C, et al: Allogeneic bone marrow transplantation for childhood acute lymphoblastic leukemia in second remission after intensive primary and relapse therapy according to the BFM- and CoALL-protocols: Results of the German Cooperative Study. Blood 1991; 78:2780–2784.

507. Bacigalupo A, Van Lint M, Frassoni F, et al: Allogeneic bone marrow transplantation versus chemotherapy for childhood acute lymphoblastic leukemia in second remission: An update. Bone Marrow Transplant 1990; 6:353–354.

508. Wheeler K, Richards S, Bailey C, Chessells J: Comparison of bone marrow transplant and chemotherapy for relapsed childhood acute lymphoblastic leukaemia: The MRC UKALL X experience. Medical Research Council Working Party on Childhood Leukaemia. Br J Haematol 1998; 101:94–103.

509. Henze G, Fengler R, Hartmann R, et al: Six-year experience with a comprehensive approach to the treatment of recurrent childhood acute lymphoblastic leukemia (ALL-REZ BFM 85). A relapse study of the BFM group. Blood 1991; 78:1166–1172.

510. Butturini A, Rivera GK, Bortin MM, Gale RP: Which treatment for childhood acute lymphoblastic leukemia in second remission? Lancet 1987; 1:429–432.

511. Torres A, Alvarez MA, Sanchez J, et al: Allogeneic bone marrow transplantation vs chemotherapy for the treatment of childhood acute lymphoblastic leukaemia in second complete remission (revisited 10 years on). Bone Marrow Transplant 1999; 23:1257–1260.

512. Rivera GK, Buchanan G, Boyett JM, et al: Intensive retreatment of childhood acute lymphoblastic leukemia in first bone marrow relapse. A Pediatric Oncology Group Study. N Engl J Med 1986; 315:273–278.

513. Sadowitz PD, Smith SD, Shuster J, et al: Treatment of late bone marrow relapse in children with acute lymphoblastic leukemia: A Pediatric Oncology Group study. Blood 1993; 81:602–609.

514. Uderzo C, Valsecchi MG, Bacigalupo A, et al: Treatment of childhood acute lymphoblastic leukemia in second remission with allogeneic bone marrow transplantation and chemotherapy: Ten-year experience of the Italian Bone Marrow Transplantation Group and the Italian Pediatric Hematology Oncology Association. J Clin Oncol 1995; 13:352–358.

515. Boulad F, Steinherz P, Reyes B, et al: Allogeneic bone marrow transplantation versus chemotherapy for the treatment of childhood acute lymphoblastic leukemia in second remission: A single-institution study. J Clin Oncol 1999; 17:197–207.

516. Arico M, Valsecchi MG, Camitta B, et al: Outcome of treatment in children with Philadelphia chromosome-positive acute lymphoblastic leukemia. N Engl J Med 2000; 342:998–1006.

517. Barrett AJ, Horowitz MM, Ash RC, et al: Bone marrow transplantation for Philadelphia chromosome-positive acute lymphoblastic leukemia. Blood 1992; 79:3067–3070.

518. Barrett AJ, Pollock B, Horowitz MM, et al: Chemotherapy versus bone marrow transplantation for children with acute lymphoblastic leukemia in second remission. Blood 1993; 82:194a.

519. Ramsay N, LeBien T, Nesbit M, et al: Autologous bone marrow transplantation for patients with acute lymphoblastic leukemia in second or subsequent remission: Results of bone marrow treated with monoclonal antibodies BA-1, BA-2, and BA-3 plus complement. Blood 1985; 66:508–513.

520. Billett AL, Sallan SE: Autologous bone marrow transplantation in childhood acute lymphoid leukemia with use of purging. Am J Pediatr Hematol Oncol 1993; 15:162–168.

521. Billett A, Tarbell N, Donnelly M, et al: Autologous bone marrow transplantation for relapsed childhood acute lymphoblastic leukemia after a short remission. Blood 1992; 80:24a.

522. Granena A, Castellsague X, Badell I, et al: Autologous bone marrow transplantation for high risk acute lymphoblastic leukemia: Clinical relevance of ex vivo bone marrow purging with monoclonal antibodies and complement. Bone Marrow Transplant 1999; 24:621–627.

523. Lausen BF, Heilmann C, Vindelov L, et al: Outcome of acute lymphoblastic leukaemia in Danish children after allogeneic bone marrow transplantation. Superior survival following transplantation with matched unrelated donor grafts. Bone Marrow Transplant 1998; 22:325–330.

524. Rocha V, Cornish J, Sievers EL, et al: Comparison of outcomes of unrelated bone marrow and umbilical cord blood transplants in children with acute leukemia. Blood 2001; 97:2962–2971.

525. Appelbaum FR, Dahlberg S, Thomas ED, et al: Bone marrow transplantation or chemotherapy after remission induction for adults with acute nonlymphoblastic leukemia. Ann Intern Med 1984; 101:591–588.

526. Stevens RF, Hann IM, Wheatley K, et al: Marked improvements in outcome with chemotherapy alone in paediatric acute myeloid leukemia: Results of the United Kingdom Medical Research Council's 10th AML trial. MRC Childhood Leukaemia Working Party. Br J Haematol 1998; 101:130–140.

527. Reference deleted in proofs.

528. Woods WG, Neudorf S, Gold S, et al: A comparison of allogeneic bone marrow transplantation, autologous bone marrow transplantation, and aggressive chemotherapy in children with acute myeloid leukemia in remission. Blood 2001; 97:56–62.

529. Burnett AK, Goldstone AH, Stevens RM, et al: Randomised comparison of addition of autologous bone-marrow transplantation to intensive chemotherapy for acute myeloid leukaemia in first remission: Results of MRC AML 10 trial. UK Medical Research Council Adult and Children's Leukaemia Working Parties. Lancet 1998; 351:700–708.

530. Zittoun RA, Mandelli F, Willemze R, et al: Autologous or allogeneic bone marrow transplantation compared with intensive chemotherapy in acute myelogenous leukemia. N Engl J Med 1995; 332:217–223.

531. Ravindranath Y, Yeager AM, Chang MN, et al: Autologous bone marrow transplantation versus intensive consolidation chemotherapy for acute myeloid leukemia in childhood. N Engl J Med 1996; 334:1428–1434.

532. Webb DK, Wheatley K, Harrison G, et al: Outcome for children with relapsed acute myeloid leukaemia following initial therapy in the Medical Research Council (MRC) AML 10 trial. MRC Childhood Leukaemia Working Party. Leukemia 1999; 13:25–31.

533. Estey EH: Treatment of relapsed and refractory acute myelogenous leukemia. Leukemia 2000; 14:476–479.

534. Clift RA, Buckner CD, Appelbaum FR, et al: Allogeneic marrow transplantation during untreated first relapse of acute myeloid leukemia. J Clin Oncol 1992; 10:1723–1729.

535. Michallet M, Thomas X, Vernant JP, et al: Long-term outcome after allogeneic hematopoietic stem cell transplantation for advanced stage acute myeloblastic leukemia: A retrospective study of 379 patients reported to the Societe Francaise de Greffe de Moelle (SFGM). Bone Marrow Transplant 2000; 26:1157–1163.

536. Chown SR, Marks DI, Cornish JM, et al: Unrelated donor bone marrow transplantation in children and young adults with acute myeloid leukaemia in remission. Br J Haematol 1997; 99:36–40.

537. Mauro MJ, Druker BJ: Chronic myelogenous leukemia. Curr Opin Oncol 2001; 13:3–7.

538. Gratwohl A, Hermans J, Niederwieser D, et al: Bone marrow transplantation for chronic myeloid leukemia: Long-term results.

Chronic Leukemia Working Party of the European Group for Bone Marrow Transplantation. Bone Marrow Transplant 1993; 12:509–516.

539. Lee SJ, Anasetti C, Horowitz MM, Antin JH: Initial therapy for chronic myelogenous leukemia: Playing the odds. J Clin Oncol 1998; 16:2897–2903.

540. Goldman JM, Szydlo R, Horowitz MM, et al: Choice of pretransplant treatment and timing of transplants for chronic myelogenous leukemia in chronic phase. Blood 1993; 82:2235–2238.

541. Collins RH, Shpilberg O, Drobyski WR, et al: Donor leukocyte infusions in 140 patients with relapsed malignancy after allogeneic bone marrow transplantation. J Clin Oncol 1997; 15:433–444.

542. Matthes-Martin S, Mann G, Peters C, et al: Allogeneic bone marrow transplantation for juvenile myelomonocytic leukaemia: A single centre experience and review of the literature. Bone Marrow Transplant 2000; 26:377–382.

543. Sanders JE, Buckner CD, Thomas ED, et al: Allogeneic marrow transplantation for children with juvenile chronic myelogenous leukemia. Blood 1988; 71:1144–1146.

544. Locatelli F, Niemeyer C, Angeluccu E, et al: Allogeneic bone marrow transplantation (BMT) for chromic myelomonocytic leukemia (CMML) in childhood: A report of the European working group on childhood myelodysplastic syndrome (EWOG-MDS) [abstract]. Blood 1995; 86:93a.

545. MacMillan ML, Davies SM, Orchard PJ, et al: Haemopoietic cell transplantation in children with juvenile myelomonocytic leukaemia. Br J Haematol 1998; 103:552–558.

546. Smith FO, Sanders JE, Robertson KA, et al: Allogeneic marrow transplantation (BMT) for children with juvenile chronic myelogenous leukemia (JCML) [abstract]. Blood 1994; 84:201a.

547. Niemeyer CM, Arico M, Basso G, et al: Chronic myelomonocytic leukemia in childhood: A retrospective analysis of 110 cases. European Working Group on Myelodysplastic Syndromes in Childhood (EWOG-MDS). Blood 1997; 89:3534–3543.

548. Orchard PJ, Miller JS, McGlennen R, et al: Graft-versus-leukemia is sufficient to induce remission in juvenile myelomonocytic leukemia. Bone Marrow Transplant 1998; 22:201–203.

549. Stockerl-Goldstein KE, Horning SJ, Negrin RS, et al: Influence of preparatory regimen and source of hematopoietic cells on outcome of autotransplantation for non-Hodgkin's lymphoma. Biol Blood Marrow Transplant 1996; 2:76–85.

550. Philip T, Biron P, Philip I, et al: Massive therapy and autologous bone marrow transplantation in pediatric and young adults: Burkitt's lymphoma (30 courses in 28 patients: A 5-year experience). Eur J Cancer Clin Oncol 1986; 22:1015–1027.

551. Ladenstein R, Pearce R, Hartmann O, et al: High-dose chemotherapy with autologous bone marrow rescue in children with poor-risk Burkitt's lymphoma: A report from the European Lymphoma Bone Marrow Transplantation Registry. Blood 1997; 90:2921–2930.

552. Loiseau HA, Hartmann O, Valteau D, et al: High-dose chemotherapy containing busulfan followed by bone marrow transplantation in 24 children with refractory or relapsed non-Hodgkin's lymphoma. Bone Marrow Transplant 1991; 8:465–472.

553. Baker KS, Gordon BG, Gross TG, et al: Autologous hematopoietic stem-cell transplantation for relapsed or refractory Hodgkin's disease in children and adolescents. J Clin Oncol 1999; 17:825–831.

554. Sureda A, Arranz R, Iriondo A, et al: Autologous stem-cell transplantation for Hodgkin's disease: Results and prognostic factors in 494 patients from the Grupo Espanol de Linfomas/Transplante Autologo de Medula Osea Spanish Cooperative Group. J Clin Oncol 2001; 19:1395–1404.

555. Kewalramani T, Zelenetz AD, Hedrick EE, et al: High-dose chemoradiotherapy and autologous stem cell transplantation for patients with primary refractory aggressive non-Hodgkin's lymphoma: An intention-to-treat analysis. Blood 2000; 96:2399–2404.

556. Josting A, Reiser M, Rueffer U, et al: Treatment of primary progressive Hodgkin's and aggressive non-Hodgkin's lymphoma: Is there a chance for cure? J Clin Oncol 2000; 18:332–339.

557. Lazarus HM, Rowlings PA, Zhang MJ, et al: Autotransplants for Hodgkin's disease in patients never achieving remission: A report from the Autologous Blood and Marrow Transplant Registry. J Clin Oncol 1999; 17:534–545.

558. Bierman PJ: Allogeneic bone marrow transplantation for lymphoma. Blood Rev 2000; 14:1–13.

559. Milpied N, Fielding AK, Pearce RM, et al: Allogeneic bone marrow transplant is not better than autologous transplant for patients with relapsed Hodgkin's disease. J Clin Oncol 1996; 14:1291–1296.

560. Dhedin N, Giraudier S, Gaulard P, et al: Allogeneic bone marrow transplantation in aggressive non-Hodgkin's lymphoma (excluding Burkitt and lymphoblastic lymphoma): A series of 73 patients from the SFGM database. Societ Francaise de Greffe de Moelle. Br J Haematol 1999; 107:154–161.

561. Ratanatharathorn V, Uberti J, Karanes C, et al: Prospective comparative trial of autologous versus allogeneic bone marrow transplantation in patients with non-Hodgkin's lymphoma. Blood 1994; 84:1050–1055.

562. Garaventa A, Rondelli R, Lanino E, et al: Myeloablative therapy and bone marrow rescue in advanced neuroblastoma. Report from the Italian Bone Marrow Transplant Registry. Italian Association of Pediatric Hematology-Oncology, BMT Group. Bone Marrow Transplant 1996; 18:125–130.

563. Stram DO, Matthay KK, O'Leary M, et al: Consolidation chemoradiotherapy and autologous bone marrow transplantation versus continued chemotherapy for metastatic neuroblastoma: A report of two concurrent Children's Cancer Group studies. J Clin Oncol 1996; 14:2417–2426.

564. Matthay KK, Villablanca JG, Seeger RC, et al: Treatment of high-risk neuroblastoma with intensive chemotherapy, radiotherapy, autologous bone marrow transplantation, and 13-cis-retinoic acid. Children's Cancer Group. N Engl J Med 1999; 341:1165–1173.

565. Grupp SA, Stern JW, Bunin N, et al: Tandem high-dose therapy in rapid sequence for children with high-risk neuroblastoma. J Clin Oncol 2000; 18:2567–2575.

566. Matthay KK, Seeger RC, Reynolds CP, et al: Allogeneic versus autologous purged bone marrow transplantation for neuroblastoma: A report from the Childrens Cancer Group. J Clin Oncol 1994; 12:2382–2389.

567. Kushner BH, Meyers PA: How effective is dose-intensive/myeloablative therapy against Ewing's sarcoma/primitive neuroectodermal tumor metastatic to bone or bone marrow? The Memorial Sloan-Kettering experience and a literature review. J Clin Oncol 2001; 19:870–880.

568. Carli M, Colombatti R, Oberlin O, et al: High-dose melphalan with autologous stem-cell rescue in metastatic rhabdomyosarcoma. J Clin Oncol 1999; 17:2796–2803.

569. Gomez L, Le Deist F, Blanche S, et al: Treatment of Omenn syndrome by bone marrow transplantation. J Pediatr 1995; 127:76–81.

570. De Santes KB, Lai SS, Cowan MJ: Haploidentical bone marrow transplants for two patients with reticular dysgenesis. Bone Marrow Transplant 1996; 17:1171–1173.

571. Wijnaendts L, Le Deist F, Griscelli C, et al: Development of immunologic functions after bone marrow transplantation in 33 patients with severe combined immunodeficiency. Blood 1989; 74:2212–2219.

572. Fischer A, Landais P, Friedrich W, et al: European experience of bone-marrow transplantation for severe combined immunodeficiency. Lancet 1990; 336:850–854.

573. Buckley RH, Schiff SE, Schiff RI, et al: Hematopoietic stem-cell transplantation for the treatment of severe combined immunodeficiency [see comments]. N Engl J Med 1999; 340:508–516.

574. Fischer A, Landais P, Friedrich W, et al: Bone marrow transplantation (BMT) in Europe for primary immunodeficiencies other than severe combined immunodeficiency: A report from the European Group for BMT and the European Group for Immunodeficiency. Blood 1994; 83:1149–1154.

575. Fischer A, Friedrick W, Levinsky R: Bone marrow transplantation for immunodeficiencies and osteopetrosis: European survey, 1968–1985. Lancet 1986; 2:1080–1084.

576. Kenny AB, Hitzig WH: Bone marrow transplantation for severe combined immunodeficiency disease. Reported from 1968 to 1977. Eur J Pediatr 1979; 131:155–177.

577. Reisner Y, Kapoor N, Kirkpatrick D, et al: Transplantation for severe combined immunodeficiency with HLA-A,B,D,DR incompatible parental marrow cells fractionated by soybean agglutinin and sheep red blood cells. Blood 1983; 61:341–347.

578. Dror Y, Gallagher R, Wara DW, et al: Immune reconstitution in severe combined immunodeficiency disease after lectin-treated, T-cell-depleted haplocompatible bone marrow transplantation. Blood 1993; 81:2021–2030.

579. O'Reilly RJ, Keever CA, Small TN, et al: The use of HLA-non-identical T-cell-depleted marrow transplants for correction of severe combined immunodeficiency disease. Immunodefic Rev 1989; 1:279–309.

580. Fischer A, Friedrich W, Fasth A, et al: Reduction of graft failure by a monoclonal antibody (anti-LFA-1-CD11a) after HLA noniden-tical bone marrow transplantation in children with immunodefi-ciencies, osteopetrosis, and Fanconi's anemia: A European Group for Immunodeficiency/European Group for Bone Marrow Transplantation report. Blood 1991; 77:249–256.

581. Filipovich AH, Shapiro RS, Ramsay NKC, et al: Unrelated donor bone marrow transplantation for correction of lethal congenital immunodeficiencies. Blood 1992; 80:270–276.

582. Amrolia P, Gaspar HB, Hassan A, et al: Nonmyeloablative stem cell transplantation for congenital immunodeficiencies. Blood 2000; 96:1239–1246.

583. Buckley RH, Whisnant KJ, Schiff RI, et al: Correction of severe combined immunodeficiency by fetal liver cells. N Engl J Med 1976; 294:1076–1081.

584. Touraine JL, Laplace S, Rezzoug F, et al: The place of fetal liver transplantation in the treatment of inborn errors of metabolism. J Inherit Metab Dis 1991; 14:619–626.

585. Remold-O'Donnell E, Rosen FS: Sialophorin (CD34) and the Wiskott-Aldrich syndrome. Immunodefic Rev 1990; 2:151–174.

586. Remold-O'Donnell E, Rosen FS, Kenney DM: Defects in Wiskott-Aldrich syndrome blood cells. Blood 1996; 87:2621–2631.

587. Parkman R, Rappeport J, Geha R, et al: Complete correction of the Wiskott-Aldrich syndrome by allogeneic bone-marrow transplant-ation. 1978; 298:921–927.

588. Mullen CA, Anderson KD, Blaese RM: Splenectomy and/or bone marrow transplantation in the management of the Wiskott-Aldrich syndrome: Long-term follow-up of 62 cases. Blood 1993; 82:2961–2966.

589. Brochstein JA, Gillio AP, Ruggiero M, et al: Marrow transplant-ation from human leukocyte antigen-identical or haploidentical donors for correction of Wiskott-Aldrich syndrome. J Pediatr 1991; 119:907–912.

590. Ozsahin H, Le Deist F, Benkerrou M, et al: Bone marrow trans-plantation in 26 patients with Wiskott-Aldrich syndrome from a single center. J Pediatr 1996; 129:238–244.

591. Filipovich AH, Stone JV, Tomany SC, et al: Impact of donor type on outcome of bone marrow transplantation for Wiskott-Aldrich syndrome: Collaborative study of the International Bone Marrow Transplant Registry and the National Marrow Donor Program. Blood 2001; 97:1598–1603.

592. Modell B, Berdoukas VA: The Clinical Approach to Thalassemia. New York, Grune & Stratton, 1984.

593. Wolfe LC, Olivieri NF, Sallan D, et al: Prevention of cardiac dis-ease with subcutaneous deferoxamine in patients with thalassemia major. N Engl J Med 1985; 312:1600–1603.

594. Ehlers KH, Giardina PJ, Lesser ML, et al: Prolonged survival in patients with beta-thalassemia major treated with deferoxamine. J Pediatr 1991; 118:540–545.

595. Brittenham GM, Griffith PM, Nienhuis AW, et al: Efficacy of deferoxamine in preventing complications of iron overload in patients with thalassemia major. N Engl J Med 1994; 331:567–573.

596. Olivieri NF, McGee A, Liu P, et al: Cardiac disease-free survival in patients with thalassemia major treated with subcutaneous defer-oxamine. Ann NY Acad Sci 1990; 612:585–586.

597. Thomas ED, Buckner CD, Sanders JE, et al: Marrow transplant-ation for thalassaemia. Lancet 1982; 2:227–229.

598. Thomas ED: Allogeneic bone marrow transplantation for blood cell disorders. Birth Defects 1982; 18:361–369.

599. Lucarelli G, Galimberti M, Polchi P, et al: Bone marrow transplant-ation in adult thalassemia. Blood 1992; 80:1603–1607.

600. Lucarelli G, Galimberti M, Polchi P, et al: Marrow transplantation in patients with thalassemia responsive to iron chelation therapy. N Engl J Med 1993; 329:840–844.

601. Lucarelli G, Clift RA, Galimberti M, et al: Bone marrow transplantation in adult thalassemic patients. Blood 1999; 93:1164–1167.

602. Gaziev D, Galimberti M, Lucarelli G, et al: Bone marrow trans-plantation from alternative donors for thalassemia: HLA-pheno-typically identical relative and HLA-nonidentical sibling or parent transplants. Bone Marrow Transplant 2000; 25:815–821.

603. Davies SC: Bone marrow transplant for sickle cell disease—The dilemma. Blood Rev 1993; 7:4–9.

604. Roberts IAG, Davies SC: Sickle cell: The transplant issue. Bone Marrow Transplant 1993; 11:253–254.

605. Platt OS, Guinan EC: Bone marrow transplantation in sickle cell anemia—The dilemma of choice. N Engl J Med 1996; 335:426–428.

606. Kodish E, Lantos J, Stocking C, et al: Bone marrow transplantation for sickle cell anemia. N Engl J Med 1991; 325:1349–1353.

607. Walters MC, Patience M, Leisenring W, et al: Barriers to bone mar-row transplantation for sickle cell anemia. Biol Blood Marrow Transplant 1996; 2:100–104.

608. Ferster A, De Valck C, Azzi N, et al: Bone marrow transplantation for severe sickle cell anaemia. Br J Haematol 1992; 80:102–105.

609. Vermylen C, Cornu G: Bone marrow transplantation in sickle cell anaemia. Blood Rev 1993; 7:1–3.

610. Bernaudin F, Souillet G, Vannier JP, et al: Bone marrow transplant-ation (BMT) in 14 children with severe sickle cell disease (SCD): The French experience. Bone Marrow Transplant 1993; 12:118–121.

611. Walters MC, Patience M, Leisenring W, et al: Bone marrow trans-plantation for sickle cell disease. N Engl J Med 1996; 335:369–376.

612. Walters MC, Storb R, Patience M, et al: Impact of bone marrow transplantation for symptomatic sickle cell disease: An interim report. Blood 2000; 95:1918–1924.

613. Ferster A, Bujan W, Corazza F, et al: Bone marrow transplantation corrects the splenic reticuloendothelial dysfunction in sickle cell anemia. Blood 1993; 81:1102–1105.

614. Walters MC, Sullivan KM, Bernaudin F, et al: Neurologic compli-cations after allogeneic marrow transplantation for sickle cell ane-mia. Blood 1995; 85:879–884.

615. Giardini C, Galimberti M, Lucarelli G, et al: Bone marrow trans-plantation in sickle-cell anemia in pesaro. Bone Marrow Transplant 1993; 12:122–123.

616. Guardiola P, Socie G, Pasquini R, et al: Allogeneic stem cell trans-plantation for Fanconi anaemia. Severe Aplastic Anaemia Working Party of the EBMT and EUFAR: European Group for Blood and Marrow Transplantation. Bone Marrow Transplant 1998; 21(Suppl 2):S24–S27.

617. Kohli-Kumar M, Morris C, DeLaat C, et al: Bone marrow trans-plantation in Fanconi anemia using matched sibling donors. Blood 1994; 84:2050–2054.

618. Gluckman E, Auerbach AD, Horowitz MM, et al: Bone marrow transplantation for Fanconi anemia. Blood 1995; 86:2856–2862.

619. MacMillan ML, Auerbach AD, Davies SM, et al: Haematopoietic cell transplantation in patients with Fanconi anaemia using alter-nate donors: Results of a total body irradiation dose escalation trial. Br J Haematol 2000; 109:121–129.

620. Guardiola P, Pasquini R, Dokal I, et al: Outcome of 69 allogeneic stem cell transplantations for Fanconi anemia using HLA-matched unrelated donors: A study on behalf of the European Group for Blood and Marrow Transplantation. Blood 2000; 95:422–429.

621. Boulad F, Gillio A, Small TN, et al: Stem cell transplantation for the treatment of Fanconi anaemia using a fludarabine-based cytoreduc-tive regimen and T-cell-depleted related HLA-mismatched peripher-al blood stem cell grafts. Br J Haematol 2000; 111:1153–1157.

622. McCloy M, Almeida A, Daly P, et al: Fludarabine-based stem cell transplantation protocol for Fanconi's anaemia in myelodysplastic transformation. Br J Haematol 2001; 112:427–429.

623. Socie G, Devergie A, Girinski T, et al: Transplantation for Fanconi's anaemia: Long-term follow-up of fifty patients trans-planted from a sibling donor after low-dose cyclophosphamide and thoraco-abdominal irradiation for conditioning. Br J Haematol 1998; 103:249–255.

624. Janov A, Leong T, Nathan DG, Guinan EC: Diamond-Blackfan anemia. Natural history and sequelae of treatment. Medicine (Baltimore) 1996; 76:1–11.

625. Iriondo A, Garijo J, Baro J, et al: Complete recovery of hemopoiesis following bone marrow transplant in a patient with unresponsive congenital hypoplastic anemia (Blackfan-Diamond syndrome). Blood 1984; 64:348–351.

626. Lenarsky C, Weinber K, Guinan E, et al: Bone marrow transplant-ation for constitutional pure red cell aplasia. Blood 1988; 71:226–229.

627. Greinix HT, Storb R, Sanders JE, et al: Long-term survival and cure after marrow transplantation for congenital hypoplastic anaemia (Diamond-Blackfan syndrome). Br J Haematol 1993; 84:515–520.

628. Mugishima H, Gale RP, Rowlings PA, et al: Bone marrow transplantation for Diamond-Blackfan anemia. Bone Marrow Transplant 1995; 15:55–58.

629. Wiktor-Jedrzejczak W, Szcczlik C, Pojda C, et al: Success of bone marrow transplantation in congenital Diamond-Blackfan anaemia: A case report. Eur J Haematol 1987; 38:204–206.

630. Willig TN, Niemeyer CM, Leblanc T, et al: Identification of new prognosis factors from the clinical and epidemiologic analysis of a registry of 229 Diamond-Blackfan anemia patients. DBA Group of Societe d'Hematologie et d'Immunologie Pediatrique (SHIP), Gesellschaft fur Padiatrische Onkologie und Hamatologie (GPOH), and the European Society for Pediatric Hematology and Immunology (ESPHI). Pediatr Res 1999; 46:553–561.

631. Bonilla MA: Cytokine treatment of severe chronic neutropenia. Int J Pediatr Hematol Oncol 1994; 2:117–124.

632. Haddad E, Le Deist F, Blanche S, et al: Treatment of Chédiak-Higashi syndrome by allogenic bone marrow transplantation: Report of 10 cases. Blood 1995; 85:3328–3333.

633. Thomas C, Le Deist F, Cavazzano-Calvo M, et al: Results of allogeneic bone marrow transplantation in patients with leukocyte adhesion deficiency. Blood 1995; 86:1629–1635.

634. Bellucci S, Damaj G, Boval B, et al: Bone marrow transplantation in severe Glanzmann's thrombasthenia with antiplatelet alloimmunization. Bone Marrow Transplant 2000; 25:327–230.

635. Bellucci S, Devergie A, et al: Complete correction of Glanzmann's thrombasthenia by allogeneic bone-marrow transplantation. Br J Haematol. 1985; 59:635.

636. Lackner A, Basu O, Bierings M, et al: Haematopoietic stem cell transplantation for amegakaryocytic thrombocytopenia. Br J Haematol 2000; 109:773–775.

637. Lonial S, Bilodeau PA, Langston AA, et al: Acquired amegakaryocytic thrombocytopenia treated with allogeneic BMT: A case report and review of the literature. Bone Marrow Transplant 1999; 24:1337–1341.

638. Gillio AP, Guinan EC: Cytokine treatment of inherited bone marrow failure syndromes. Int J Pediatr Hematol Oncol 1995; 2:125–133.

639. Walker DG: Bone resorption restored in osteopetrotic mice by transplants of normal bone marrow and spleen cells. Science 1975; 190:784–786.

640. Ballet JJ, Griscelli C, Coutris C, et al: Bone-marrow transplantation in osteopetrosis. Lancet 1977; 2:1137.

641. Coccia PF, Krivit W, Cervenka J, et al: Successful bone-marrow transplantation for infantile malignant osteopetrosis. N Engl J Med 1980; 302:701–708.

642. Gerritsen EJ, Vossen JM, Fasth A, et al: Bone marrow transplantation for autosomal recessive osteopetrosis. A report from the Working Party on Inborn Errors of the European Bone Marrow Transplantation Group. J Pediatr 1994; 125:896–902.

643. Jabado N, Le Deist F, Cant A, et al: Bone marrow transplantation from genetically HLA-nonidentical donors in children with fatal inherited disorders excluding severe combined immunodeficiencies: Use of two monoclonal antibodies to prevent graft rejection. Pediatrics 1996; 98:420–428.

644. O'Reilly RJ, Brochstein J, Dinsmore R, et al: Marrow transplantation for congenital disorders. Semin Hematol 1984; 21:188–221.

645. Barton NW, Brady RO, Dambrosia JM, et al: Replacement therapy for inherited enzyme deficiency: Macrophage-targeted glucocerebrosidase for Gaucher's disease. N Engl J Med 1991; 324:1464–1470.

646. Krivit W, Shapiro E, Kennedy W, et al: Treatment of late infantile metachromatic leukodystrophy by bone marrow transplantation. N Engl J Med 1990; 322:28–32.

647. Tsai P, Lipton JM, Sahdev I, et al: Allogeneic bone marrow transplantation in severe Gaucher disease. Pediatr Res 1992; 31:503–507.

648. Krivit W: Maroteaux-Lamy syndrome (mucopolysaccharidosis type VI) treatment by allogeneic BMT in 6 patients and potential for autotransplantation bone marrow gene insertion. Int Pediatr 1992; 7:47–52.

649. Bergstrom SK, Quinn JJ, Greenstein R, Ascensao J: Long-term follow-up of a patient transplanted for Hunter's disease type IIB: A case report and literature review. Bone Marrow Transplant 1994; 14:653–658.

650. Krivit W, Lockman LA, Watkins PA, et al: The future for treatment by bone marrow transplantation for adrenoleukodystrophy, metachromatic leukodystrophy, globoid cell leukodystrophy and Hurler syndrome. J Inherit Metab Dis 1995; 18:398–412.

651. Peters C, Shapiro EG, Anderson J, et al: Hurler syndrome: II: Outcome of HLA-genotypically identical sibling and HLA-haploidentical related donor bone marrow transplantation in fifty-four children. The Storage Disease Collaborative Study Group. Blood 1998; 91:2601–2608.

652. Shapiro EG, Lockman LA, Balthazor M, et al: Neuropsychological outcomes of several storage diseases with and without bone marrow transplantation. J Inherit Metab Dis 1995; 18:413–429.

653. Krivit W, Shapiro EG, Peters C, et al: Hematopoietic stem-cell transplantation in globoid-cell leukodystrophy. N Engl J Med 1998; 338:1119–1126.

654. Shapiro E, Krivit W, Lockman L, et al: Long-term effect of bone-marrow transplantation for childhood-onset cerebral X-linked adrenoleukodystrophy. Lancet 2000; 356:713–718.

655. Guffon N, Souillet G, Maire I, et al: Follow-up of nine patients with Hurler syndrome after bone marrow transplantation. J Pediatr 1998; 133:119–125.

656. Peters C, Balthazor M, Shapiro EG, et al: Outcome of unrelated donor bone marrow transplantation in 40 children with Hurler syndrome. Blood 1996; 87:4894–4902.

IV | Disorders of Erythrocyte Production

10 | A Diagnostic Approach to the Anemic Patient

Frank A. Oski[†] • Carlo Brugnara • David G. Nathan

Most of the chapters thus far have been devoted to descriptions of specific disorders that result in anemia. The purpose of this chapter is to provide both a more general classification of the anemias and an initial diagnostic approach to the patient with this laboratory finding. Details of the diagnostic procedures used in the ultimate diagnosis of the various anemias are omitted because they are presented in their respective chapters.

DEFINITION OF ANEMIA

Anemia is generally defined as a reduction in red cell mass or blood hemoglobin concentration. The limit for differentiating anemic from normal states is generally set at two standard deviations below the mean for the normal population. This definition will result in 2.5 percent of the normal population being classified as anemic. Conversely, the values for hemoglobin-deficient individuals are distributed in such a fashion that some are placed within the normal range. These individuals, who have the potential for a hemoglobin concentration in the upper part of the normal range, may be recognized only after a response to treatment.

Because the primary function of the red cell is to deliver and release adequate quantities of oxygen to the tissues to meet their metabolic demands, it is apparent that some measures of both body oxygen metabolism and accompanying cardiovascular compensations are required to complement the current laboratory definition of anemia. The fact that hemoglobin concentration alone is insufficient to judge whether a patient is "functionally anemic" is best illustrated in a patient with cyanotic congenital heart disease or chronic respiratory insufficiency or in a patient with mutant hemoglobins that alter hemoglobin's affinity for oxygen (see Chapter 18).

With these caveats in mind, a useful statistical definition of anemia that recognizes the effect of age and sex on the designation of anemia is provided in Table 10–1.[1]

CLASSIFICATION OF ANEMIAS

Anemias may be classified on a physiologic or a morphologic basis. A combination of both approaches is often used in the initial differential diagnosis.

The best approach for providing an understanding of the multiple disorders capable of producing anemia is to

TABLE 10–1. Values (Normal Mean and Lower Limits of Normal) for Hemoglobin, Hematocrit, and Mean Corpuscular Volume (MCV) Determinations

Age (yrs)	Hemoglobin (g/dL)		Hematocrit (%)		MCV (μ^3)	
	Mean	Lower Limit	Mean	Lower Limit	Mean	Lower Limit
0.5–1.9	12.5	11.0	37	33	77	70
2–4	12.5	11.0	38	34	79	73
5–7	13.0	11.5	39	35	81	75
8–11	13.5	12.0	40	36	83	76
12–14:						
Female	13.5	12.0	41	36	85	78
Male	14.0	12.5	43	37	84	77
15–17:						
Female	14.0	12.0	41	36	87	79
Male	15.0	13.0	46	38	86	78
18–49:						
Female	14.0	12.0	42	37	90	80
Male	16.0	14.0	47	40	90	80

[†]Deceased.

separate the causes of anemia into two categories of functional disturbances[2]:

1. Disorders of effective red cell production, in which the net rate of red cell production is depressed. This can be due to disorders of erythrocyte maturation, in which erythropoiesis is largely ineffectual, or to an absolute failure of erythropoiesis. In the former, the marrow contains many erythroblasts that die *in situ* before reaching the reticulocyte stage. In the latter, there is absolute erythroblastopenia.
2. Disorders in which rapid erythrocyte destruction or red cell loss is primarily responsible for the anemia.

These two categories are not mutually exclusive. More than one mechanism may be present in some anemias, but one functional disorder is generally the major reason for the patient's anemia. Table 10–2 lists the anemias most commonly encountered in infancy and childhood and classifies them into three categories of functional disturbance.

Anemias may also be classified on the basis of red cell size and then further subdivided, according to red cell morphology. In this type of classification, anemias are subdivided into microcytic anemias, normocytic anemias, and macrocytic anemias. This classification is also arbitrary, and categories are not mutually exclusive. For example, macrocytic reticulocytes abound in the hemolytic anemias. Therefore, although the mature erythrocytes in the various hemolytic anemias may be normocytic, the mean corpuscular volume (MCV) of all the cells may be larger than normal, owing to the contribution of reticulocytes to the volume measurement.[6] Volume distribution curves may reveal the contribution of a subset of large cells to the MCV. Furthermore, during the course of a disease, classification of the patient's anemia may change from one category to another as a result of other clinical or pathologic variables. In Table 10–3 the more common anemias of infancy and childhood are classified on the basis of their characteristic cell size.

EVALUATION OF THE ANEMIC PATIENT

The initial diagnostic approach to the anemic patient includes a detailed history and physical examination and a minimum of essential laboratory tests. Tables 10–4 and 10–5 list those features of the history and physical examination that are most helpful in providing clues to the etiology of anemia. The initial laboratory tests should include determination of hemoglobin and hematocrit concentration, and measurement of red cell indices, platelet count, white blood cell count and differential, reticulocyte count, and examination of a peripheral blood smear. After this initial assessment, other useful and simple laboratory procedures may be employed. These include, when indicated, measurement of erythrocyte porphyrin concentration and serum ferritin concentration, supravital stains of

TABLE 10–2. Physiologic Classification of Anemia

A. DISORDERS OF RED CELL PRODUCTION IN WHICH THE RATE OF RED CELL PRODUCTION IS LESS THAN EXPECTED FOR THE DEGREE OF ANEMIA 　1. Marrow failure 　　a. Aplastic anemia 　　　Congenital 　　　Acquired 　　b. Pure red cell aplasia 　　　Congenital 　　　　Diamond-Blackfan syndrome 　　　Aase syndrome 　　　Acquired 　　　　Transient erythroblastopenia of childhood 　　　Other 　　c. Marrow replacement 　　　Malignancies 　　　Osteopetrosis 　　　Myelofibrosis[3] 　　　Chronic renal disease[4] 　　　Vitamin D deficiency[5] 　　d. Pancreatic insufficiency-marrow hypoplasia syndrome 　2. Impaired erythropoietin production 　　a. Chronic renal disease 　　b. Hypothyroidism, hypopituitarism 　　c. Chronic inflammation 　　d. Protein malnutrition 　　e. Hemoglobin mutants with decreased affinity for oxygen	B. DISORDERS OF ERYTHROID MATURATION AND INEFFECTIVE ERYTHROPOIESIS 　1. Abnormalities of cytoplasmic maturation 　　a. Iron deficiency 　　b. Thalassemia syndromes 　　c. Sideroblastic anemias 　　d. Lead poisoning 　2. Abnormalities of nuclear maturation 　　a. Vitamin B_{12} deficiency 　　b. Folic acid deficiency 　　c. Thiamine-responsive megaloblastic anemia 　　d. Hereditary abnormalities in folate metabolism 　　e. Orotic aciduria 　3. Primary dyserythropoietic anemias (types I, II, III, IV) 　4. Erythropoietic protoporphyria 　5. Refractory sideroblastic anemia with vacuolization of marrow precursors and pancreatic dysfunction deficiency C. HEMOLYTIC ANEMIAS 　1. Defects of hemoglobin 　　a. Structural mutants 　　b. Synthetic mutants (thalassemia syndromes) 　2. Defects of the red cell membrane 　3. Defects of red cell metabolism 　4. Antibody-mediated 　5. Mechanical injury to the erythrocyte 　6. Thermal injury to the erythrocyte 　7. Oxidant-induced red cell injury 　8. Infectious agent-induced red cell injury 　9. Paroxysmal nocturnal hemoglobinuria 　10. Plasma-lipid-induced abnormalities of the red cell membrane

TABLE 10–3. Classification of Anemias Based on Red Cell Size

A. MICROCYTIC ANEMIAS
  1. Iron deficiency (nutritional, chronic blood loss)
  2. Chronic lead poisoning
  3. Thalassemia syndromes
  4. Sideroblastic anemias
  5. Chronic inflammation
  6. Some congenital hemolytic anemias with unstable hemoglobin

B. MACROCYTIC ANEMIAS
  1. With megaloblastic bone marrow
    a. Vitamin B_{12} deficiency
    b. Folic acid deficiency
    c. Hereditary orotic aciduria
    d. Thiamine-responsive anemia[5]
  2. Without megaloblastic bone marrow
    a. Aplastic anemia
    b. Diamond-Blackfan syndrome
    c. Hypothyroidism
    d. Liver disease
    e. Bone marrow infiltration
    f. Dyserythropoietic anemias

C. NORMOCYTIC ANEMIAS
  1. Congenital hemolytic anemias
    a. Hemoglobin mutants
    b. Red cell enzyme defects
    c. Disorders of the red cell membrane
  2. Acquired hemolytic anemias
    a. Antibody-mediated
    b. Microangiopathic hemolytic anemias
    c. Secondary to acute infections
  3. Acute blood loss
  4. Splenic pooling
  5. Chronic renal disease (usually)

TABLE 10–4. Historical Factors of Importance in Evaluating the Patient with Anemia

Age	Nutritional iron deficiency is never responsible for anemia in term infants before 6 months of age; rarely seen in premature infants prior to the time they have doubled their birth weight. Anemia manifesting itself in the neonatal period generally is the result of recent blood loss, isoimmunization, or initial manifestation of a congenital hemolytic anemia or congenital infection. Anemia first detected at ages 3 to 6 months suggests a congenital disorder of hemoglobin synthesis or hemoglobin structure.
Gender	Consider x-linked disorders in males (glucose-6-phosphate dehydrogenase (G6PD) deficiency, pyruvate kinase deficiency).
Race	Hemoglobins S and C more common in blacks; β-thalassemia more common in whites; α-thalassemia trait most common among black and yellow races.
Ethnicity	Thalassemia syndromes most common among patients of Mediterranean origin. G6PD deficiency is observed more often among Sephardic Jews, Filipinos, Greeks, Sardinians, and Kurds.
Neonatal	History of hyperbillirubinemia in the newborn period suggests the presence of congenital hemolytic anemia, such as hereditary spherocytosis of G6PD deficiency. Prematurity predisposes to early development of iron deficiency.
Diet	Document sources of iron, vitamin B_{12}, folic acid, or vitamin E in the diet. History of pica, geophagia, or pagophagia suggests presence of iron deficiency.
Drugs	Oxidant-induced hemolytic anemia, phenytoin (Dilantin)-induced megaloblastic anemia, drug-induced aplastic anemia.
Infection	Hepatitis-induced aplastic anemia, infection-induced red cell aplasia, or hemolytic anemia.
Inheritance	Family history of anemia, jaundice, gallstones, or splenomegaly.
Diarrhea	Suspect small bowel disease with malabsorption of folate or vitamin B_{12}. Suspect inflammatory bowel disease with blood loss. Suspect exudative enteropathy with blood loss.

the erythrocytes, hemoglobin electrophoresis, a screening test for the presence of unstable hemoglobins, a direct and an indirect Coombs' test, a screening test for glucose-6-phosphate dehydrogenase deficiency, and an examination of the bone marrow.

Electronic Cell Counting

The most widely used methods for determination of hemoglobin, hematocrit, and red cell indices are electronic. Compared with manual techniques, electronic methods have the advantages of greater precision and reproducibility and the capacity for completing a large number of measurements quickly.

One of two general principles is used in most of the more popular electronic counting systems. These may be simply classified as the *electrical impedance principle* and the *light scatter principle*.

The electrical impedance principle is used in the Coulter Counter (Coulter Electronics, Hialeah, FL). With this technique, cells passing through an aperture cause changes in electrical resistance that are counted as voltage pulses, which are proportional to cell volume. The electrical pulses are amplified and are counted during the time an accurately metered volume of the suspension is drawn through the aperture. These devices can directly measure the MCV and compute the hematocrit from the MCV and red blood cell count.

The light scatter principle is used in the Technicon H★1, H★2, and H★3 Autoanalyzers (Bayer Diagnostics, Tarrytown, NY).[10-13] With this flow cytometric technique, red cells first undergo isovolumetric sphering and then MCV and mean corpuscular hemoglobin concentration (MCHC) are measured from the low-angle forward light scattering and the high-angle (refractive index) light scattering, respectively.

Readers are encouraged to consult other references[14-16] for details of operation of electronic counters and to familiarize themselves with potential sources of error. Some of these potential errors are listed in Table 10–6. Cold agglutinins in high titer tend to cause spurious macrocytosis with low red cell counts and very high

TABLE 10–5. Physical Findings as Clues to the Etiology of Anemia

Skin	Hyperpigmentation	Fanconi aplastic anemia
	Petechiae, purpura	Autoimmune hemolytic anemia with thrombocytopenia, hemolytic-uremic syndrome, bone marrow aplasia, bone marrow infiltration
	Carotenemia	Suspect iron deficiency in infants
	Jaundice	Hemolytic anemia, hepatitis, and aplastic anemia
	Cavernous hemangioma	Microangiopathic hemolytic anemia
	Ulcers on lower extremities	S and C hemoglobinopathies, thalassemia
Facies	Frontal bossing, prominence of the malar and maxillary bones	Congenital hemolytic anemias, thalassemia major, severe iron deficiency
Eyes	Microcornea	Fanconi's aplastic anemia
	Tortuosity of the conjunctival and retinal vessels	S and C hemoglobinopathies
	Microaneurysms of retinal vessels	S and C hemoglobinopathies
	Cataracts	Glucose-6-phosphate dehydrogenase deficiency, galactosemia with hemolytic anemia in newborn period
	Vitreous hemorrhages	S hemoglobinopathy
	Retinal hemorrhages	Chronic, severe anemia
	Edema of the eyelids	Infectious mononucleosis, exudative enteropathy with iron deficiency, renal failure
	Blindness	Osteopetrosis
Mouth	Glossitis	Vitamin B_{12} deficiency, iron deficiency
	Angular stomatitis	Iron deficiency
Chest	Unilateral absence of the pectoral muscles	Poland syndrome (increased incidence of leukemia)[7–9]
	Shield chest	Diamond-Blackfan syndrome
Hands	Triphalangeal thumbs	Red cell aplasia
	Hypoplasia of the thenar eminence	Fanconi aplastic anemia
	Spoon nails	Iron deficiency
Spleen	Enlargement	Congenital hemolytic anemia, leukemia, lymphoma, acute infection, portal hypertension

TABLE 10–6. Sources of Error in Blood Cell Counts Specific for Electronic Counters

1. *Incorrect diluent or lysis agent* for particular instrument
2. *Extraneous particles in diluting fluid* (or containers, at any step)
3. *Presence of cell type that was not to be counted*
4. *Destruction of cell type that was to be counted*
5. *Error in metered delivery of cells after dilution*: pump, valves, tubing, connections, cut-off switch
6. *Partial obstruction of aperture* (impedance type instrument)
7. *Coincidence loss*
8. *Threshold setting*, sensitivity or potentiometer setting not determined by proper calibration
9. *Carry-over* from one specimen to the next
10. *Spurious pulses from sensing region* of equipment, owing to air bubbles
11. *Spurious signals* from electrical or radiofrequency interference
12. *Instability*, or intermittent failure of electronic components

MCHCs. Warming either the blood or the diluent eliminates this problem.[17]

Electronic cell counting provides a useful means of categorizing anemias based on the MCV and MCHC. The red cell volume distribution width (RDW) is derived from the red blood cell histogram that accompanies each analysis. The RDW is an index of the variation in red cell size and thus can be used to detect anisocytosis. In the normal patient, the histogram is virtually symmetric. The RDW is calculated as a standard statistical value, the coefficient of variation of the red cell volume distribution. The formula can be expressed as:

$$RDW = SD/MCV \times 100$$

Because RDW reflects the ratio of standard deviation (SD) and MCV, a wide red cell distribution curve in a patient with a markedly increased MCV may still generate a normal RDW number. The RDW in normal individuals ranges from 11.5 to 14.5 percent, but it may vary as a function of the model of the electronic cell counter used. Normal values for infants and children appear to range from 1.5 to 15.0 percent.[18] The hemoglobin distribution width (HDW) is calculated in a similar manner from the histogram for MCHC. Coulter instruments do not directly measure cell hemoglobin concentration. MCHC and HDW provided by these instruments are sensitive to variations in MCV and should be used with caution in the differential diagnosis of anemias.

Bessman and associates[19] have provided a classification of anemias based on MCV and RDW. An updated version that includes MCHC and HDW appears in Table 10–7.

Visual analysis of the red cell histograms generated by automated cell counters provides essential clues for the diagnosis of anemias. The presence of either microcytes or macrocytes and of increased RDW can be readily appreciated. Histograms for MCHC are particularly useful because they allow prompt identification of dehydrated hyperchromic cells in sickle cell disease, hereditary spherocytosis, hereditary xerocytosis, and immune

TABLE 10–7. The Relationship of Mean Corpuscular Volume and Red Cell Volume Distribution Width in a Variety of Disease States

RDW	MCV		
	Low	**Normal**	**High**
Normal	Heterozygous α- and β-thalassemia	Normal Lead poisoning	Aplastic anemia
High	Iron deficiency Hemoglobin H disease S β-thalassemia	Early iron deficiency Liver disease Mixed nutritional deficiencies	Newborns, prematurity Vitamin B_{12} or folate deficiency
		HIGH MCHC/HDW: Immune hemolytic anemia SS and SC disease Hereditary spherocytosis/xerocytosis	**HIGH MCHC/HDW:** Immune hemolytic anemia

hemolytic anemias. Moreover, a careful study of volume and hemoglobin concentration histograms allows rapid differentiation of iron deficiency and β-thalassemia trait and of hemoglobin H and hemoglobin H/CS disease. Figure 10–1 provides the histograms for MCV and MCHC in a normal control and in patients with β-thalassemia trait, iron deficiency, and sickle cell disease.

Automated reticulocyte counting is also available in several hematology analyzers. Automated counting is more precise and accurate compared with manual counting.[20–22] Absolute reticulocyte counts are easily obtained with these instruments, obviating the limitations of counting reticulocytes only as a percentage or correcting for the changes in hematocrit (corrected reticulocyte count). An additional useful feature of automated reticulocyte counters is that the presence of stress reticulocytes can easily be identified based on their increased volume and RNA content. Cellular indices for reticulocytes such as volume, hemoglobin concentration, and hemoglobin content are also available in the Technicon H★3 instrument.[23]

The Blood Film

Films made on coverslips are preferable to those made on glass slides because a greater proportion of the blood on the film is technically suitable for microscopic examination. The proper processing of blood films on coverslips is fast becoming a lost art. The details of preparation and examination can be found in manuals of laboratory hematology,[24] but the lucid and succinct instructions of Wintrobe[25] deserve reproduction here:

1. Use a small drop of blood, only 2 to 3 mm in diameter, taken either from a stylet wound, as described earlier, or from a syringe or needle tip used in venipuncture immediately after the venipuncture has been performed (anticoagulants are not to be used because they will alter the morphologic appearance).
2. Hold the coverslips only by their edges, placing one crosswise over the other, and allow the blood to spread between them for about 2 seconds.
3. Quickly but gently separate the coverslips by pulling them laterally, in opposite directions to one another

but in the plane of the spreading film, just before the film reaches the edges (do not squeeze or lift the coverslips from one another).
4. Quickly air-dry the films, either by placing them face up on a clean surface if the humidity is low or by moving them through the air while holding them by their edges with your fingertips.

If the procedure has been carried out successfully, the blood will be spread evenly, and there will be no holes or thick areas in the preparation. A multicolored sheen will be seen on the surface of the dried, unstained film if light glances off from it at the proper angle, because the thin layer of closely fitting cells acts like a diffraction grating. Later, under the microscope, after staining, the red cells will be seen next to each other, but neither overlapping, nor in rouleau formation, and central pallor will be visible; lymphocytes will have a readily distinguished cytoplasm, rather than a minimal zone bearing closely on the nucleus as occurs in thick films or those that dry too slowly.

The examination of the peripheral blood film is the single most useful procedure in the initial evaluation of the patient with anemia. The blood film should first be examined under low power to determine the adequacy of cell distribution and staining. Signs of poor blood film preparation include loss of central pallor in red blood cells, polygonal shapes, and artifactual spherocytes. Artifactual spherocytes, in contrast to true spherocytes, show no variation in central pallor and are larger than normal red cells. One should never attempt to interpret a poorly prepared blood film.

After the adequacy of the blood film is determined by low-power examination, the blood film should be examined under 1000 × magnification. Cells should be graded as to size, staining intensity, variation in color, and abnormalities of shape. A classification of red cell hemolytic disorders based on their predominant morphology can be accomplished. An approach to such a classification is presented in Table 10–8 and is discussed in detail in Chapter 15.

The blood film should also be examined for the presence of basophilic stippling and red cell inclusions. The significance of some of these findings is described in Table 10–9.

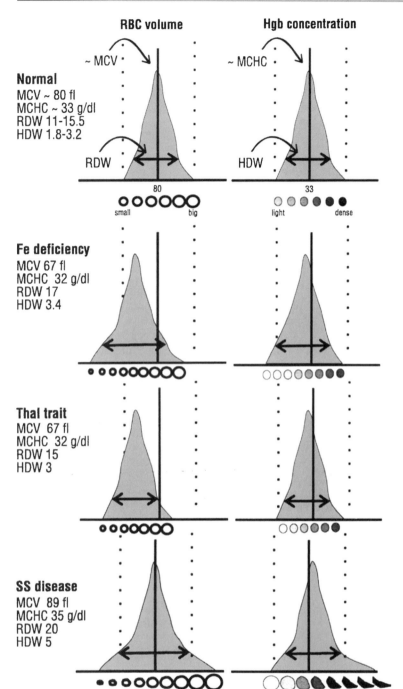

FIGURE 10–1. Histograms for mean value of red cell volume (MCV, *left column*) and of red cell hemoglobin concentration (MCHC, *right column*) in a normal control subject *(first row)*, a patient with iron deficiency *(second row)*, a subject with heterozygous β-thalassemia *(third row)*, and a patient with homozygous hemoglobin S disease *(bottom row)*. Goal posts are placed at 60 and 120 fL for MCV and at 28 and 41 g/dL for MCHC. RDW = red cell volume distribution width; HDW = hemoglobin distribution width.

A DIAGNOSTIC APPROACH TO THE ANEMIC PATIENT

After the laboratory tests have been obtained, results may be used in an initial attempt to diagnostically characterize the patient's anemia, as illustrated by the simple algorithm in Figure 10–2. This algorithm provides for two additional diagnostic steps after the initial characterization of anemia based on the complete blood cell count, reticulocyte count, and cellular indices.

If the diagnosis of hemolytic anemia is considered, it is useful to consider the potential pathophysiology before ordering useless and expensive screening tests. The authors have used a simple and reliable approach to pathophysiologic analysis that involves consideration of the potential assaults on the red cell from the farthest point to the inner core of the erythrocyte (Fig. 9–3).

The most common cause of rapid red cell loss with reticulocytosis is hemorrhage. In infants and children, unusual causes of hemorrhage include hemorrhage beneath the scalp and intra-abdominal, urinary tract, and pulmonary hemorrhage. In the latter two causes, hyperbilirubinemia is not present. Indeed, if the hemorrhage is chronic, leading to iron deficiency, the plasma will be pale.

Sequestration in an abnormal spleen will usually cause spherocytosis, but if the hypersplenism is associated with

TABLE 10–8. Classification of Red Cell Hemolytic Disorders by Predominant Morphology (Nonhemolytic Disorders of Similar Morphology Are Enclosed in Parentheses for Reference)

SPHEROCYTES

Hereditary spherocytosis
ABO incompatibility in neonates
Immunohemolytic anemias with IgG- or C3-coated red cells*
Acute oxidant injury (hexose monophosphate shunt defects during hemolytic crisis, oxidant drugs and chemicals)
Hemolytic transfusion reactions*
Clostridium welchii septicemia
Severe burns, other red cell thermal injury
Spider, bee, and snake venoms
Severe hypophosphatemia
Hypersplenism[†]

BIZARRE POIKILOCYTES

Red cell fragmentation syndromes (micro- and macroangiopathic hemolytic anemias)
Acute oxidant injury[†]
Hereditary elliptocytosis in neonates
Hereditary pyropoikilocytosis

ELLIPTOCYTES

Hereditary elliptocytosis
Thalassemias
(Other hypochromic-microcytic anemias)
(Megaloblastic anemias)

STOMATOCYTES

Hereditary stomatocytosis
Rh$_{null}$ blood group
Stomatocytosis with cold hemolysis
(Liver disease, especially acute alcoholism)
(Mediterranean stomatocytosis)

IRREVERSIBLY SICKLED CELLS

Sickle cell anemia
Symptomatic sickle syndromes

INFRAERYTHROCYTIC PARASITES

Malaria
Babesiasis
Bartonellosis

SPICULATED OR CRENATED RED CELLS

Acute hepatic necrosis (spur cell anemia)
Uremia
Red cell fragmentation syndromes[†]
Infantile pyknocytosis
Embden-Meyerhof pathway defects[†]
Vitamin E deficiency[†]
Abetalipoproteinemia
Heat stroke[†]
McLeod blood group
(Postsplenectomy)
(Transiently after massive transfusion of stored blood)
(Anorexia nervosa)[†]

TARGET CELLS

Hemoglobins S, C, D, and E
Hereditary xerocytosis
Thalassemias
(Other hypochromic-microcytic anemias)
(Obstructive liver disease)
(Postsplenectomy)
(Lecithin: cholesterol acyltransferase deficiency)

PROMINENT BASOPHILIC STIPPLING

Thalassemias
Unstable hemoglobins
Lead poisoning[†]
Pyrimidine 5′-nucleotidase deficiency

NONSPECIFIC OR NORMAL MORPHOLOGY

Embden-Meyerhof pathway defects
Hexose monophosphate shunt defects
Unstable hemoglobins
Paroxysmal nocturnal hemoglobinuria
Dyserythropoietic anemias
Copper toxicity (Wilson's disease)
Cation permeability defects
Erythropoietic porphyria
Vitamin E deficiency
Hemolysis with infections[†]
Rh hemolytic disease in neonates*
Paroxysmal cold hemoglobinuria*[†]
Cold hemagglutinin disease*
Hypersplenism
Immunohemolytic anemia*[†]

*Usually associated with positive Coombs' test.
[†]Disease sometimes associated with this morphology.

liver disease, target cells are also present. In this condition, the osmotic fragility test will reveal a sensitive and a resistant population of erythrocytes.

Vascular damage to erythrocytes may be associated with thrombocytopenia and be caused by hemangiomas (the Kasabach-Merritt syndrome); intravascular coagulation, usually due to sepsis; damaged artificial heart valves; and renal vascular disease and severe hypertension. Schistocytes that resemble military helmets of various nationalities are usually present, and siderinuria and hemoglobinuria are often detected.

Abnormalities of plasma are frequent causes of hemolysis. Antibodies usually induce spherocytosis by causing splenic sequestration but sometimes merely fix complement and cause hemoglobinuria without morphologic change. Many drugs and toxins can damage red cells either by oxidant injury with resultant schistocytosis or by direct lysis, as illustrated by bacterial lipases in septic shock. Acute hemolysis also may be caused by excessive release of hepatic copper in Wilson disease. No morphologic change is noted.

Primary membrane abnormalities that cause hemolysis are usually congenital and are associated with specific morphologic changes. An exception is paroxysmal nocturnal hemoglobinuria, which is an acquired membrane defect associated with no morphologic change. The

TABLE 10–9. Diagnostic Significance of Red Cell Inclusions

Inclusion	Staining Agent	Diagnostic Significance
Basophilic stippling	Wright's stain	Represent aggregated ribosomes. May be observed in thalassemia syndromes, iron deficiency, syndromes accompanied by ineffective erythropoiesis and pyrimidine 5′-nucleotidase deficiency, particularly prominent in unstable hemoglobinopathies and lead poisoning.
Howell-Jolly bodies	Wright's stain	Represent nuclear remnants. Observed in asplenic and hyposplenic states, pernicious anemia, dyserythropoietic anemias, and severe iron deficiency anemia.
Cabot rings	Wright's stain	Appear as basophilic rings, circular, or twisted figures-of-eight. Considered to be nuclear remnants or artifacts. Observed in lead poisoning, pernicious anemia and hemolytic anemias.
Heinz bodies	Brilliant cresyl blue, methyl violet	Represent denatured or aggregated hemoglobin. Observed in patients with thalassemia syndromes or unstable hemoglobins, after oxidant stress in patients with enzyme deficiencies of the pentose phosphate pathway, and in patients with asplenia or chronic liver disease.
Siderocytes	Prussian blue counterstained with safranin O	Represent nonhemoglobin iron within erythrocytes. Seen in increased numbers in peripheral circulation after splenectomy. Observed in increased numbers in patients with chronic infection, aplastic anemias, or hemolytic anemias.

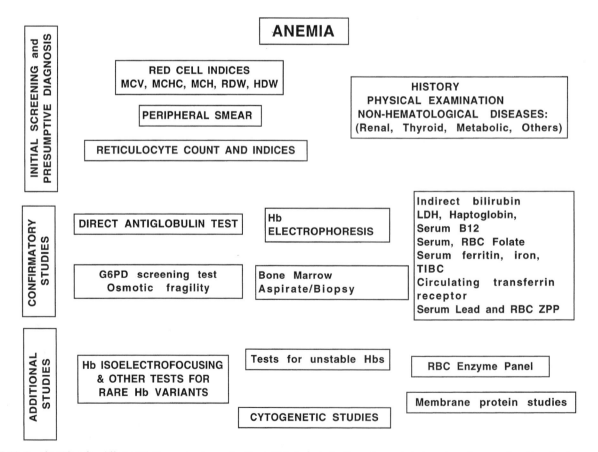

FIGURE 10–2. Algorithm for differential diagnosis of anemia. The initial characterization of anemia is based on the complete blood cell count, reticulocyte count, cellular indices, erythrocyte morphology, and history. This first step is followed by two additional diagnostic steps: to confirm a relatively common kind of anemia or to diagnose one of the uncommon types of anemia. Hb = hemoglobin; LDH = lactate dehydrogenase; RBC = red blood cell; G6PD = glucose-6-phosphate dehydrogenase; TIBC = total iron-binding capacity; ZPP = zinc protoporphyrin.

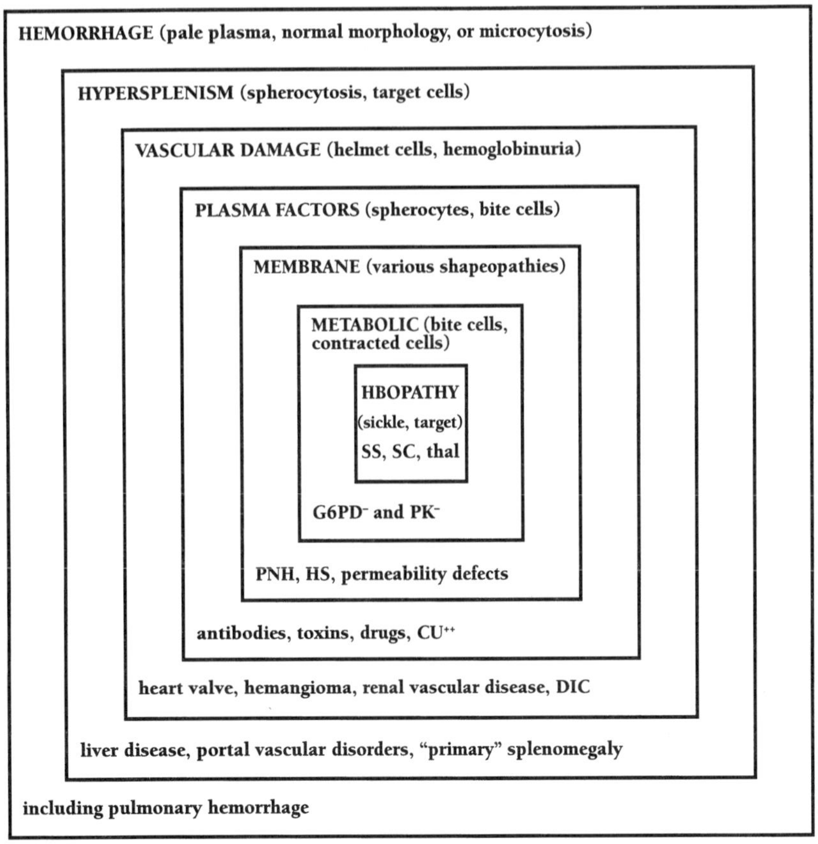

FIGURE 10–3. The assaults on the red cell from the vasculature to the "center" of the cell. The site of damage is in capital letters, the laboratory findings in parentheses, and the common causes in the lower part of the square. HBOPATHY = hemoglobinopathy; SS = hemoglobin SS; SC = hemoglobin SC; thal = thalassemia; PK = pyruvate kinase; PNH = paroxysmal nocturnal hemoglobinuria; HS = hereditary spherocytosis; CU^{++} = copper; DIC = disseminated intravascular coagulation.

congenital membrane defects are usually due to abnormalities of structural membrane proteins, such as in hereditary spherocytosis, but may involve cation channels (hydrocytosis and xerocytosis) and, rarely, membrane lipids (abetalipoproteinemia).

The red cell itself may contribute to its own quietus, as exemplified by glucose-6-phosphate dehydrogenase deficiency, pyruvate kinase deficiency, and deficiencies of the other enzymes involved in erythrocyte metabolic pathways. Morphologic alterations are not predictable.

Finally, the red cell may be sabotaged by its own hemoglobin, such as in sickle cell anemia, the thalassemias, and the unstable hemoglobinopathies.

If the clinician considers these options in an inclusive but systematic fashion, direct screening tests can be ordered and expert consultation avoided.

REFERENCES

1. Dallman PR, Siimes MA: Percentile curves for hemoglobin and red cell volume in infancy and childhood. J Pediatr 1979; 94:26.
2. Finch CA: Red Cell Manual. Seattle, University of Washington, 1970.
3. Beguin Y, Fillet G, et al: Ferrokinetic study of splenic erythropoiesis: Relationships among clinical diagnosis, myelofibrosis, splenomegaly, and extramedullary erythropoiesis. Am J Hematol 1989; 32:123.
4. Geary DG, Fennel RS, et al: Hyperparathyroidism and anemia in chronic renal failure. Eur J Pediatr 1982; 139:296.
5. Abboud MR, Alexander D, et al: Diabetes mellitus, thiamine-dependent megaloblastic anemia, and sensorineural deafness associated with deficient β-ketoglutarate dehydrogenase activity. J Pediatr 1985; 107:537.
6. d'Onofrio G, Chirillo R, et al: Simultaneous measurement of reticulocyte and red blood cell indices in healthy subjects and patients with microcytic and macrocytic anemia. Blood 1995; 85:818.
7. Parikh PM, Karandikar SM, et al: Poland's syndrome with acute lymphoblastic leukemia in an adult. Med Pediatr Oncol 1988; 16:290.
8. Sackey K, Odone V, et al: Poland's syndrome associated with childhood non-Hodgkin's lymphoma. Am J Dis Child 1984; 138:600.
9. Parikh T, Karandikar SM, et al: Poland's syndrome with acute lymphoblastic leukemia in an adult. Med Pediatr Oncol 1988; 16:290.
10. Tycko DH, Metz MH, et al: A flow-cytometric light scattering measurement of red blood cell volume and hemoglobin concentration. J Appl Opt 1985; 24:1355.
11. Fossat G, David M, et al: New parameters in erythrocyte counting. Arch Pathol Lab Med 1987; 111:1150.
12. Mohandas N, Kim YR, et al: Accurate and independent measurement of volume and hemoglobin concentration of individual red cells by laser light scattering. Blood 1986; 68:506.
13. Mohandas N, Johnson A, et al: Automated quantitation of cell density distribution and hyperdense cell fraction in RBC disorders. Blood 1989; 74:442.
14. Brittin GM, Brecher G: Instrumentation and automation in clinical hematology. In Brown E, Moore CV (eds): Progress in Hematology, Vol. VII. New York, Grune & Stratton, 1971, p 299.
15. Nelson DA, Morris MW: Basic examination of blood. In Henry JB (ed): Clinical Diagnosis and Management by Laboratory Methods, 18th ed. Philadelphia, WB Saunders, 1991, p 553.
16. Simson E: Hematology beyond the Microscope. Tarrytown, NY, Technicon Instruments Corporation, 1984.
17. Hattersley PG, Gerard PW, et al: Erroneous values on the Model S Coulter due to high titer cold agglutinins. Am J Clin Pathol 1971; 55:442.
18. Novak RW: Red blood cell distribution width in pediatric microcytic anemias. Pediatrics 1987; 80:251.
19. Bessman JD, Gilmer PR Jr, et al: Improved classification of anemias by MCV and RDW. Am J Clin Pathol 1983; 80:322.

20. Savage RA, Skoog DP, Rabinovitch A: Analytic inaccuracy and imprecision in reticulocyte counting: A preliminary report from the College of American Pathologists reticulocyte project. Blood Cells 1985; 11:97.
21. National Committee for Clinical Laboratory Standards: Methods for Reticulocyte Counting, Proposed Standards. NCCLS document H16-P, Villanova, PA, 1985.
22. Schimenti KJ, Lacerna K, et al: Reticulocyte quantification by flow cytometry, image analysis and manual counting. Cytometry 1992; 13:853.
23. Brugnara C, Hipp MJ, et al: Automated reticulocyte counting and measurement of reticulocyte cellular indices: Evaluation of the Miles H*3 blood analyzer. Am J Clin Pathol 1994; 102:623.
24. Cartwright GE: Diagnostic Laboratory Hematology, 4th ed. New York, Grune & Stratton, 1968.
25. Wintrobe MM: Clinical Hematology, 7th ed. Philadelphia, Lea & Febiger, 1974, p 24.

11 | Megaloblastic Anemia

V. Michael Whitehead • David S. Rosenblatt • Bernard A. Cooper

Before the mid-1920s, *pernicious anemia* was a disease dreaded as much as drug-resistant leukemia is today. With its characteristic megaloblastic bone marrow, pernicious anemia was a fatal illness until it was successfully treated with dietary liver in 1926.[1] It is now known that megaloblastic anemia is caused most frequently by a nutritional deficiency of folates or by a specific malabsorption of cobalamin known as pernicious anemia (Table 11–1). Precise means for diagnosing and treating these deficiencies are now available. Over the past 70 years, hematologists have gained detailed knowledge of the synthesis, biology, biochemistry, and molecular biology of both vitamin B$_{12}$ and folate. It is extraordinary that this knowledge base is continuing to grow as new discoveries are made.

TABLE 11–1. Causes of Megaloblastic Anemia

VITAMIN B₁₂ (COBALAMIN)

Defects in Absorption

Inadequate Gastric Intrinsic Factor Due to
Pernicious anemia
Gastritis
Total gastrectomy
Intrinsic factor gene mutations

Achlorhydria and Pepsin Deficiency (?)
Disease of the Small Intestine
Surgical resection or bypass of the terminal ileum
Regional enteritis (Crohn's disease)
Tropical and nontropical sprue
Infiltrative diseases (Whipple's syndrome, lymphoma)
Competition by parasites (fish tapeworm, blind loop
  syndrome)
Imerslund-Gräsbeck syndrome
Drugs (colchicine, PAS, neomycin)
Transcobalamin II deficiency
Secondary to megaloblastic anemia

Inadequate Nutrition
Strict vegetarians (vegans)
Maternal deficiency affecting the fetus or infant

Defects in Transport
Transcobalamin II deficiency

Defects in Metabolism
Nitrous oxide intoxication
Inherited (cbIC, cbID, cbIE, cbIF, and cbIG diseases)

FOLATES

Defects in Absorption
Inherited (hereditary folate malabsorption)
Tropical and nontropical sprue
Infiltrative diseases of the small bowel (Whipple's sydrome,
  lymphoma)

Inadequate Nutrition
Insufficient or poorly selected diet
Maternal deficiency affecting the fetus or infant

Increased Requirement
Alcoholism
Pregnancy
Lactation
Hemolytic anemia
Hyperthyroidism
Anticonvulsant therapy
Lesch-Nyhan syndrome
Prematurity
Homocystinuria
First trimester during neural tube development

Folate Inhibitors
Antifolates (methotrexate, pyrimethamine, trimethoprim)
Sulfones

Inherited Defects
Methylenetetrahydrofolate reductase deficiency
Methionine synthase deficiency (cbIE and cbIG disease)
Others

OTHER CAUSES

Defects in Purine and Pyrimidine Synthesis

Inherited
Orotic aciduria

Acquired
Myelodysplasia and leukemia
Drug-induced
HIV infection

Other
Thiamine-responsive anemia
Scurvy
Pyridoxine-responsive anemia

This chapter reviews aspects of this knowledge as it pertains in particular to pediatric patients. Emphasis is placed on the clinical and laboratory diagnosis of overt deficiencies of vitamin B₁₂ and folates as well as on their treatment. Also, attention is focused on subclinical deficiency states as they relate to populations at increased risk, including premature newborns, the elderly, those with HIV infection, and those with elevated plasma total homocysteine levels. Consideration is given to the role of these vitamins in the prevention of neural tube defects and of cardiovascular disease and in the pathogenesis of cancer. Finally, current knowledge of inborn errors of cobalamin and folate metabolism is presented.

cobalamin are used interchangeably to refer to corrins that have coenzyme activity or that can be converted to coenzymes in cells (see later). The term *folates* refers to synthetic folic acid and to the various natural folate coenzymes, which are reduced dihydro-folates (DHFs) and tetrahydrofolates (THFs) and their single-carbon substituted forms. *Natural folate coenzymes* are substrates for the enzyme folate polyglutamate synthetase and are converted by it to folate polyglutamates containing predominantly 6 or 7 γ-linked glutamate residues. Most folates in nature are present as reduced and substituted folate polyglutamates. These, too, are included under the general term *folates*.

DEFINITIONS

Megaloblastic anemia is a macrocytic anemia that is usually accompanied by leukopenia and thrombocytopenia. It is characterized by a specific megaloblastic bone marrow morphology, affecting erythroid, myeloid, and platelet precursors. In this chapter, the terms *vitamin B₁₂* and

HISTORY

Anemia associated with morphologically abnormal erythrocytes had been observed in pernicious anemia from 1876 to 1877.[2–4] By 1883, macrocytosis had been described in patients with pernicious anemia. In 1891, Ehrlich stained and described megaloblastic erythroid precursors.[5] The presence of increased numbers of nuclear segments in circulating neutrophils ("hypersegmentation") was described in 1923, and giant myeloid band forms were observed in megaloblastic bone marrow in 1920. Megaloblastic changes in the bone marrow during relapse, with the return of normal morphology during remission, were reported in 1921, 5 to 6 years before therapy for the disease was developed. In 1926, Minot and Murphy[1] described conversion of megaloblastic bone marrow to normoblastic bone marrow along with reticulocytosis and correction of the anemia following treatment with dietary liver. The sequence of these events has been summarized in several reviews.[3,6]

Among many subsequent observations, the following are among the most important:

1. Similar clinical syndromes (pernicious anemia of pregnancy and tropical anemia) were described in 1931 and subsequently were shown to be due to deficiency in folates.[7]

2. In pernicious anemia, because of atrophy (destruction) of the gastric mucosa,[8] the stomach does not contain enough of the gastric intrinsic factor needed for absorption of vitamin B_{12} from the gut.[9] The disease is caused by failure to absorb adequate quantities of vitamin B_{12}.[2,10]

3. Cobalamin injections were found to correct pernicious anemia,[11] and folate administration to resolve the anemia described by Wills. Each vitamin, when given in large doses, could produce some effect on the hematologic abnormalities caused by deficiency of the other.[12,13]

4. The cobalamin-binding protein transcobalamin II functions as an "intrinsic factor" within the body, permitting endocytosis-mediated utilization of cobalamin by cells.[14,15]

5. Assays for cobalamin and folates in serum and tissues of patients with megaloblastic anemia permitted chemical definition of the deficiency.[16–18]

6. Subacute combined degeneration of the spinal cord, a neurologic syndrome, often accompanied classic pernicious anemia but not the megaloblastic anemia caused by folate deficiency.[2,19]

7. Pernicious anemia is probably an autoimmune disease[20] caused by lymphocyte-mediated destruction of gastric parietal cells, with the possible immunologic target being the Na^+, K^+ ATPase on the parietal cell membrane.[21–23]

8. Inherited defects of the metabolism of cobalamin and folates may cause abnormal development in addition to megaloblastic anemia.[24–27]

9. The purification and subsequent cloning of intrinsic factor and the transcobalamins, the accumulation of information about their structure, and the study of their receptors define the function of these proteins.[28–33]

10. The complete pathway of cobalamin biosynthesis by bacteria has been elucidated.[34]

11. Elevated plasma methylmalonic acid and total homocysteine reflect tissue functional deficiency of cobalamin and of either folates or cobalamin, respectively, even in patients with vitamin levels within the normal range.[35]

12. Neural tube defects including spina bifida can be prevented by maternal folate supplementation during the periconceptual interval.[36,37]

13. Folate supplementation can reduce the elevated plasma total homocysteine level, recognized to be a risk factor for arteriosclerotic vascular disease,[38] and it may decrease the incidence of bowel and other cancers.[39]

HEMATOLOGIC DESCRIPTION

Bone Marrow and Blood

The causes of megaloblastic anemia are classified in Table 11–1.

The megaloblastic bone marrow is hyperplastic, with erythropoiesis being stimulated by increased levels of erythropoietin acting on erythroid progenitor cells. Megaloblastic erythroid cells are more prone to undergo programmed cell death or apoptosis during maturation than when they are mature[40,41]; this results in a predominance of young erythroid cells in the bone marrow. This "ineffective erythropoiesis" is the cause of elevated serum levels of lactate dehydrogenase, bile pigments, and iron (derived from dying erythroid precursors). Mature erythrocytes have abnormal shapes and are of various sizes, and their mean cell volume (MCV) is much greater than normal. Macrocytic and misshapen erythrocytes survive for a shorter time in the blood than do normal erythrocytes.

In megaloblastic anemia, erythroid precursors have a normal DNA content together with an elevated RNA content. For this reason, they have more cellular RNA per unit of DNA and, thus, are larger than normal cells of the same level of maturation.[42] Their nuclear chromatin appears looser than normal on stained smears (Fig. 11–1), giving the characteristic appearance of the megaloblast. There is asynchrony of maturation of nucleus and cytoplasm, with the nucleus appearing less mature than the cytoplasm. For example, polychromatophilic erythroblasts with considerable accumulation of hemoglobin in the cytoplasm may have vesicular, open, or immature nuclei, and more mature orthochromic erythroblasts may contain nuclei that are not the dense, small, purple-staining nuclei of normal orthochromes. Experienced observers usually recognize megaloblastic erythropoiesis by noting the vesicular and open nuclear pattern in the earliest erythroblasts (proerythroblasts and basophilic erythroblasts) (see Fig. 11–1).

Myeloid precursors are larger than normal; the most striking are the giant metamyelocytes and band neutrophils in the megaloblastic bone marrow. These cells may persist in bone marrow for 10 to 14 days after the start of treatment.[43] Giant metamyelocytes and band neutrophils are not seen in the megaloblastoid bone marrow of patients with leukemia or myelodysplasia. Similar abnormalities probably affect megakaryocyte precursors, but these changes have not been well described. Neutropenia and thrombocytopenia are more common in patients with severe than with mild anemia associated with megaloblastic bone marrow, but they may both occur in cobalamin-deficient patients who are not anemic.

Multilobar neutrophils are seen in the peripheral blood (Fig. 11–2). *Neutrophil hypersegmentation* is defined as the

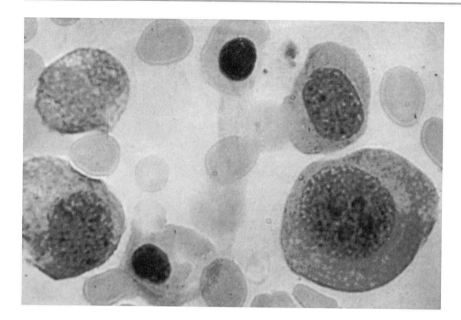

FIGURE 11–1. Megaloblasts in the bone marrow. (See the text for details.)

presence of one or more six-lobed neutrophils or of five or more neutrophils with five or more well-separated lobes among 100 segmented neutrophils. Hypersegmentation is a characteristic feature of cobalamin and folate deficiencies.

Other Tissues

Macrocytosis of buccal cells has been reported in patients with megaloblastic anemia. Similar abnormalities have been described in cells of the tongue, vaginal epithelium, urinary tract, nasal epithelium, and other lining tissues. Decreased height of gastric cells and enterocytes also has been described. These changes reverse after treatment of the megaloblastic anemia and are not found in all patients.[44,45]

VITAMIN B$_{12}$ (COBALAMIN)

Nutritional Sources and Requirements

Cobalamin is synthesized by bacteria and algae. The entire bacterial biosynthetic pathway for cobalamin synthesis has been elucidated and involves 20 different enzy-

matic steps.[34] Cobalamin is required as a vitamin by animals but is not required by higher plants. Plants neither synthesize nor accumulate cobalamin and, thus, do not contribute it to the diet. The presence of cobalamin in ground water is used as an index of fecal contamination.

Because all of the cobalamin needed by humans is provided through the diet, inadequate intake causes deficiency. Neither the dietary cobalamin needs nor the frequency of dietary cobalamin deficiency in different populations are well defined, but some published data do exist.[46,47] In India, the concentration of vitamin B$_{12}$ in serum and tissues is low[48–52]—both in vegetarians, who eat no meat but do eat dairy products, and in strict vegetarians (vegans) who consume no animal products whatever and in whom megaloblastic anemia due to inadequate cobalamin intake does occur. Neuro-logic disease, subacute combined degeneration of the spinal cord (SCDSC), due to cobalamin deficiency, has been described in vegans, but its frequency appears to be very low.[53,54] It is not known why the frequency of neurologic disease in vegans with very low plasma cobalamin levels is low. Insight might be gained from studies of the frequency of neurologic disease and of biologic cobalamin deficiency as reflected by elevated plasma levels of total homocysteine and of methylmalonic acid in such vegan communities.

The World Health Organization has recommended a daily intake of cobalamin of 1 µg for normal adults; 1.3 and 1.4 µg daily for lactating and pregnant women, respectively; and 0.1 µg per day for infants, on the basis of the known physiology and turnover of cobalamin, the quantity required to treat deficiency, and a variety of other factors. The World Health Organization has calculated that mean adult cobalamin intake per day was less than 1 µg in many countries.[55]

Chemistry of Cobalamins

Cobalamins have the chemical structure shown in Figure 11–3. They belong to a class of compounds known as *cor-*

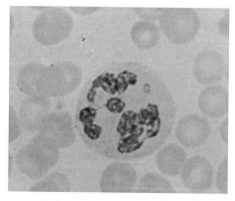

FIGURE 11–2. Multilobar neutrophil.

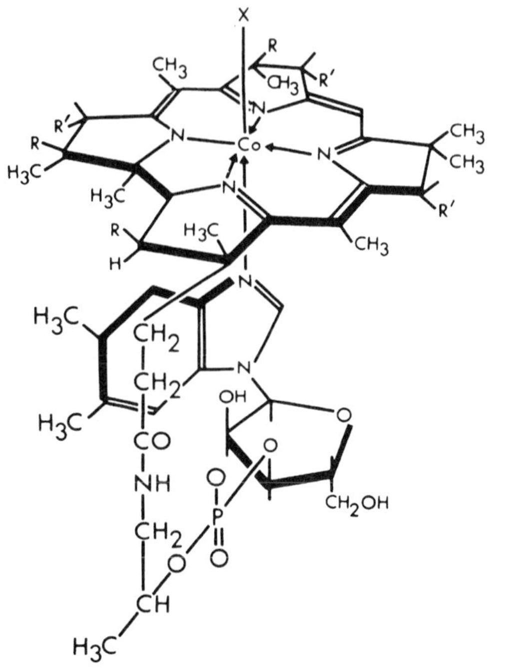

FIGURE 11–3. Cobalamin (vitamin B_{12}, Cbl). When X is methyl, the compound is methylcobalamin (MeCbl); when it is adenosyl, the compound is 5'-deoxyadenosylcobalamin (AdoCbl); when it is CN, the compound is cyanocobalamin (CNCbl), and so forth.

rins, which contain a ringlike structure resembling but distinct from that of porphyrins (including hemoglobin) and a nucleotide, 5,6-dimethylbenzimidazole, that is set almost at right angles to the corrin ring. Corrins that have coenzyme activity or can be converted to coenzymes in cells include cobalamins with CN, OH, H_2O, SH, SO_3, glutathione, methyl, or 5'-deoxyadenosyl bound to the cobalt, as well as cobalamins with the cobalt atom reduced to divalent cob(II)alamin (vitamin B_{12R}) or to monovalent cob(I)alamin (vitamin B_{12S}). When the cobalt atom is in its oxidized, trivalent state, the compounds are known as *cob(III)alamins* or are named for the group binding to the cobalt (e.g., cyanocobalamin [CNCb1], hydroxocobalamin [OHCb1], aquocobalamin [H_2OCb1]).[56–58]

Biochemistry of Vitamin B_{12}

Vitamin B_{12} functions as a coenzyme in two reactions:

1. As methylcobalamin (MeCbl) in the synthesis of methionine from homocysteine and 5-methyltetrahydrofolate (5-methyl-THF),[59] which is mediated by the cobalamin-requiring enzyme methionine synthase (5-methyl-THF-homocysteine S-methyltransferase, EC 2.1.1.13)[60]:
   Reaction 1

   Homocysteine + 5-methyl-THF → methionine + THF

2. As 5'-deoxyadenosylcobalamin (AdoCbl, Ado-B_{12}) in the conversion of methylmalonyl coenzyme A (CoA) to succinyl CoA,[2,61] which is mediated by the cobalamin-requiring enzyme methylmalonyl-CoA mutase (MMA mutase, EC 5.4.99.2)[62–69]:

Reaction 2.

   Methylmalonyl CoA → succinyl CoA

In prokaryotes, a variety of other enzymes utilize cobalamin for reactions that appear not to occur in mammalian cells.

Reaction 1 is the major pathway for resynthesis of methionine in humans, and low plasma levels of methionine develop when it is impaired. Interruption of this reaction, which requires both folate and cobalamin cofactors, is considered to be the common lesion that results in megaloblastic anemia with both cobalamin and folate deficiencies (known as the "methylfolate trap" hypothesis). In addition, both cobalamin-dependent reactions reduce plasma levels of two potentially toxic materials: (1) homocysteine, which has been associated with vascular endothelial damage; and (2) methylmalonate, which can cause metabolic acidosis (limited to inborn errors of cobalamin metabolism).

Cobalamin that enters the cytoplasm does not appear to be retained in the cell unless it binds to a high-affinity binder. Methionine synthase[60] is the major such binder in the cytoplasm. Cobalamin also enters the mitochondria, in which it reacts with adenosine triphosphate (ATP)-cob(II)alamin transferase to form Ado-Cbl, which binds to MMA mutase (Fig. 11–4).[70–75] In mitochondria from rat liver, most of the cobalamin appears to be AdoCbl.[74] Cytoplasmic cobalamin is probably reduced to cob(II)alamin before binding to methionine synthase.[60] It is possible that entry into mitochondria also requires reduction or chemical modification of cobalamins because intact (unswollen) mitochondria from rat liver appear to be impermeable to cob(III)alamins.[76]

METHIONINE SYNTHESIS

Methionine is consumed in the diet and is absorbed. Plasma methionine enters cells and the cerebrospinal fluid by similar membrane transport systems. Cellular methionine may be incorporated into protein or may be adenosylated to *S*-adenosylmethionine (SAMe) by the enzyme ATP-L-methionine *S*-adenosyltransferase (EC 2.5.1.6):
Reaction 3

   Methionine + adenosine → SAMe

SAMe donates methyl groups in many reactions, leaving *S*-adenosylhomocysteine (AHCy):
Reaction 4

   SAMe + R → AHCy + CH_3-R

AHCy is hydrolyzed to homocysteine and adenosine by the enzyme *S*-adenosylhomocysteine hydrolase (EC 3.3.1.1):
Reaction 5

   AHCy → homocysteine + adenosine

The homocysteine may then be remethylated to methionine by methionine synthase (see Reaction 1, presented earlier) or in hepatocytes by betaine-L-homocysteine methyltransferase (EC 2.1.1.5), or it may react with cystathionine. β-synthase (EC 4.2.1.22) and serine to form

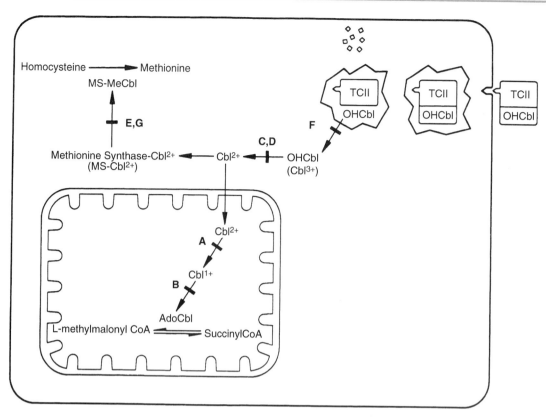

FIGURE 11–4. Scheme of cobalamin (vitamin B_{12}, Cbl) metabolism. The letters A through G represent the sites of known inherited defects (cblA through cblG). Cbl = cobalamin; $Cbl^{1+,2+,3+}$ = cobalamin with 1+, 2+, or 3+ oxidation states of the central cobalt; OHCbl = hydroxycobalamin; MS = methionine synthase; TC II = transcobalamin II; CoA = coenzyme A.

cystathionine. Pyridoxal phosphate is a cofactor in this last reaction.[77–81]

The crystalline structure of a 27-kd MeCbl-containing fragment of methionine synthase from *Escherichia coli* was determined at a resolution of 0.3 nm[81a] (Fig. 11–5). This structure depicts cobalamin-protein interactions and reveals that the corrin macrocycle lies between a helical NH_2-terminal domain and an $\alpha\beta$ carboxyl-terminal domain that is a variant of the Rossmann fold. MeCbl undergoes a conformational change on binding the protein; the dimethylbenzimidazole group, which is coordinated to the cobalt in the free cofactor, moves away from the corrin and is replaced by a histidine contributed by the protein.

Methionine synthase requires cobalamin bound to the enzyme as a prosthetic group or coenzyme. If cob(I)alamin is bound to the enzyme, it is readily methylated by 5-methyl-THF to form MeCbl. The methionine synthase then mediates transfer of this methyl from MeCbl to homocysteine to form methionine. Cob(I) alamin is readily oxidized and appears to spontaneously undergo oxidation to cob(II)alamin. Methylation of cob(II)alamin requires SAMe as a methyl donor. In *E. coli*, two flavoproteins have been described that maintain cob(I)alamin in its reduced state or provide other necessary reduction in the reaction.[82] In mammalian cells, this function may be provided by an iron atom that is a part of the methionine synthase enzyme,[60] whereas a

copper atom appears to serve this function in the *E. coli* enzyme.[83] Evidence for the importance of some type of reduction reaction associated with methionine synthesis is provided by patients with cblE disease (described later), in whom this activity appears to be abnormal.[84]

METHYLMALONYL-COA MUTASE

For this intramitochondrial reaction to occur (see Reaction 2, presented earlier), cobalamin must undergo reduction to cob(I)alamin (either before entry or in the mitochondria), enter the mitochondria (by an unknown mechanism), and receive a 5'-deoxyadenosyl group from ATP:

Reaction 6

$$ATP + Cob(I)alamin \rightarrow AdoCbl + Triphosphate$$

The resulting AdoCbl then binds to MMA mutase to produce the active enzyme.

The biochemical effects associated with impairment of this pathway due to cobalamin deficiency include (1) elevated plasma and urine methylmalonic acid levels to an extent determined by the flow of odd-chain fatty acids, valine, and threonine through the pathway; and (2) the secondary effects of MMA accumulation, which include acidosis, hyperglycinemia, the possible inhibition of other enzymes, and perhaps inhibition of proliferation of bone marrow stem cells.[85–89]

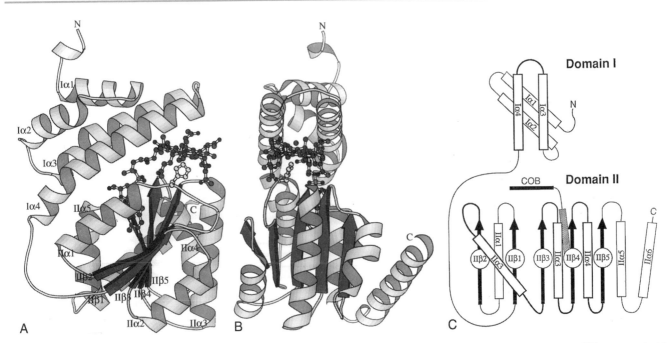

FIGURE 11–5. The cobalamin-binding domains of methionine synthase. *A,* A ribbon drawing with atoms of the cobalamin and His[759] in ball-and-stick mode. The drawing was generated with the use of MOLSCRIPT (see Kraulis PJ: MOLSCRIPT. A program to produce both detailed and schematic plots of protein structures. J Appl Crystallogr 1991; 24:946). The NH$_2$-terminal helical bundle domain is shown "above" the corrin. Kinks in helices in 1α3 and 1α4, evident in the drawing, occur at Pro[696] and Pro[734]. *B,* A ribbon drawing in an orientation 90 degrees from that shown in *A.* This orientation corresponds approximately to the topology diagram of *C.* In this view, a striking feature is the narrow first domain, which is similar in width to the corrin macrocycle. In the intact enzyme, substrate-binding segments are expected to adjoin this domain. *C,* Topology diagram. The helices of the first domain form a bundle according to defined criteria (see Harris NL, Presnell SR, Cohen FE: Four helix bundle diversity in globular proteins. J Mol Biol 1994; 236:1356), with the front and back pair of helices inclined at angles of 50 and 55 degrees, respectively. In domain II, a doubly wound α/β fold, helices IIα1 and IIα5 are behind the sheet and IIα2, IIα3, and IIα4 are in front. Helix IIα6 makes substantial contacts with helix IIα5 but may also pack against other domains in intact methionine synthase. The corrin (COB) is indicated above the cleft between β-sheet strands 1 and 3; the dimethylbenzimidazole tail (*shaded*) adjoins strands IIβ3 and IIβ4. (Adapted from Drennan CL, Huang S, et al: How a protein binds B$_{12}$: A 3.0 Å X-ray structure of B$_{12}$-binding domains of methionine synthase. Science 1994; 266:1669–1674.)

Physiology of Cobalamins

TRANSPORT

Effective transmembrane transport of cobalamins into mammalian cells at the low cobalamin levels found in nature requires mediation of a cobalamin-binding protein reacting with a receptor on the cell surface that recognizes the cobalamin-protein complex. These transporters are *intrinsic factor (IF)*, which binds to the IF-Cbl receptor on the small intestinal mucosa, and *transcobalamin II (TC II)*, which binds to the TC II–Cbl receptor, located on the surface of many cells.

COBALAMIN-BINDING PROTEINS

Intrinsic Factor. IF, a glycoprotein, is synthesized in gastric parietal cells in humans and guinea pigs and in chief (pepsinogen) cells in the rat stomach. It may also be secreted by pancreatic cells in dogs.[90] It is readily digested by pepsin but not by trypsin.[91] The Cbl-IF in the gut lumen is available for absorption, whereas unbound IF is not absorbed. IF binds cobalamins less tightly ($K_d = 0.1$ to 1.0 nmol/L)[92] than do the transcobalamins. However, its binding affinity for cobalamins is far greater than that for nonfunctional corrin analogues, such that the latter are

not absorbed from the intestine. The gene for IF is located on chromosome 11.[93]

Transcobalamin II. TC II mediates the entry of cobalamin into cells. It is found in plasma, cerebrospinal fluid, seminal fluid, and transudates. It is synthesized in a variety of cells, including fibroblasts, macrophages, enterocytes, renal cells, hepatocytes, spleen, heart, gastric mucosa, and endothelium.[94] It is a nonglycosylated protein with a molecular weight of 43,000.[95] It polymerizes with itself or with another protein when it binds cobalamin. Plasma turnover of TC II is rapid.[96] It binds cobalamin tightly ($K_d = 5$ to 18 pmol/L) but has low affinity for corrins without vitamin B$_{12}$ activity. A complementary DNA (cDNA) for TC II has been characterized.[28]

Haptocorrins. Haptocorrins (also variously called *TC 0, TC I, TC III, R binder,* and *cobalophilin*) are a family of proteins with similar structure but different degrees of glycosylation. They are synthesized by myeloid cells and probably by many other cells. Haptocorrins are present in many secretions, including plasma, bile, saliva, tears, breast milk, amniotic fluid, and seminal fluid, and in extracts of granulocytes, salivary gland, platelets, hepatoma cells, and breast tumors.[94, 97, 98] The fully glycosylated haptocorrin found in plasma has a low isoelectric point and a half-life of 9 days; those haptocorrins with higher pIs are cleared more rapidly from the plasma into the bile. Seventy to 90% of the cobalamin in plasma is bound to haptocorrin, with the remainder associated with TC II. Haptocorrins have the greatest affinity for cobalamins of all of the cobalamin-binding proteins (K_d = 3 to 7 pmol/L). In addition, they have considerable binding affinity for other corrins that lack vitamin B_{12} activity. It has been suggested that an important function of haptocorrins *in vivo* is the binding and excretion of such cobalamin analogues into the bile.[99] Gastric juice contains both haptocorrins, which are probably derived from saliva and perhaps gastric parietal cells,[98] and IF.

ABSORPTION OF COBALAMINS

Cobalamin in meat and fish is released from intracellular enzymes and binds to haptocorrin present in saliva or the food. Haptocorrin is digested by trypsin in the stomach and duodenum, permitting binding of cobalamin to IF. The IF-Cbl complex binds to receptors on the brush border of the ileal enterocyte; after binding, the cobalamin slowly enters the portal vein bound to TC II. Whereas cobalamin fed in large quantities without IF appears in the portal vein 1 hour after feeding, cobalamin bound to IF appears about 12 hours after feeding and 8 to 12 hours after reaching the ileal lumen (Fig. 11–6).[100] Synthesis of TC II by ileal cells may be required for transport.[101, 102] The distribution of the ileal IF-Cbl receptor varies in different subjects. In some, removal of a small segment of ileum removes the majority of the absorptive surface and causes malabsorption of vitamin B_{12}; in other subjects, the absorptive mechanism extends through a considerable portion of the ileum.

The maximum quantity of IF-Cbl that can be bound to receptor in the human intestine is about 1.5 μg.[2] The IF-Cbl receptor appears to disappear from the surface of the enterocyte during IF-Cbl absorption; this limits the

absorption of large doses of cobalamin bound to IF. However, receptor activity reappears rapidly, so that a second bolus can be absorbed soon after the first. When massive quantities of cobalamin (100 to 1000 μg) are fed to patients lacking IF in the gut, a small proportion (0.1% to 1%) is absorbed from the jejunum, presumably by means of a nonspecific mechanism such as diffusion. The receptor for IF-Cbl has been purified.[103, 104]

Malabsorption of cobalamin caused by competition for the cobalamin in the intestinal lumen has generated some quite exotic studies. Following the demonstration that megaloblastic anemia could be corrected by removal of massive quantities of fish tapeworm *(Diphyllobothrium latum)* from some patients in Finland, the worm was studied and shown to be capable of accumulating cobalamin after releasing it from IF.[105, 106] Although this competition by 100 m of worm length was well documented, it is likely that the cobalamin deficiency caused by the worm occurred only in patients with marginal secretion of IF, and not in subjects with normal gastric secretion. The recent increase in ingestion of raw fish among some social groups may provide us with new cases for additional studies.

Cobalamin malabsorption has been observed in some patients with intestinal blind loops or with stenotic areas of the small bowel.[107] This malabsorption decreased after treatment with antibiotics (e.g., tetracyclines); this finding suggests that bacteria proliferating in stagnant intestinal areas competed with the host for cobalamin in the intestinal lumen, but the exact nature of the process remains unclear. An increased serum folate level is observed in many of these patients and is attributed to the synthesis of large amounts of folates by the intestinal bacteria.

How cobalamin is transported across the ileal cell is unknown. Indirect evidence suggests that the transport occurs by means of endocytosis,[108–112] with release of the cobalamin from IF in lysosomes. The subsequent trans-

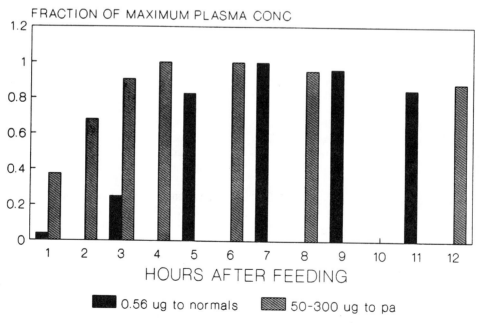

FIGURE 11–6. Absorption of labeled cyanocobalamin (vitamin B_{12}) with the intrinsic factor mechanism (*black bars*) or without intrinsic factor (*shaded bars*). (Adapted from Doscherholmen A, Hagen PS: Delay of absorption of radiolabeled cyanocobalamin in the intestinal wall in the presence of intrinsic factor. J Lab Clin Med 1959; 54:434.)

port of the vitamin appears to require the correct chemical configuration of the cobalamin[113] and, thus, probably involves specific binding to a transporter, possibly TC II. Chemical modification of absorbed cobalamin is not required for passage through the intestinal cell, although cobalamin may be reduced and metabolized to coenzyme forms in ileal cells, as described earlier.

Cobalamin is excreted in the bile, binds to IF in the small intestine, and is reabsorbed. Reabsorption does not occur in pernicious anemia; as a result, depletion of cobalamin stores occurs more rapidly than when absorption is unimpaired. Normal body losses have been estimated to be in the range of 2 to 4 μg cobalamin per day.

ENTRY OF COBALAMIN INTO CELLS

Cobalamin bound to TC II enters cells by endocytosis after the complex associates with receptors on the cell surface.[14, 15, 92, 114] The TC II–Cbl receptor has been purified.[115] No chemical modification of cobalamin is required for transport. Entry into the cytoplasm is probably from lysosomes[14] and requires lysosome-mediated digestion of the TC II before the free cobalamin can enter the cell. Treatment of cells with lysosomotropic agents (e.g., chloroquine or ammonium chloride), which prevent generation of low pH in endosomes, prevents entry of cobalamin into the cytoplasm[14, 116]; as a result, TC II–Cbl accumulates in endosomes. Penetration of free cobalamin from the lysosome into the cytoplasm appears to require a specific transport system, which is defective in children with cobalamin F disease (cblF disease; see later in this chapter).[117, 118] Excretion or loss of cobalamin from cells has not been studied.

Pernicious Anemia

Pernicious anemia is a disease that results from the destruction of IF-producing gastric parietal cells by lymphocyte-mediated immune activity. The consequent lack of IF results in vitamin B$_{12}$ malabsorption. Patients who lack IF following gastric resection and those few in whom a presumed genetic mutation yields defective or undetectable IF are not considered to have pernicious anemia.

AGE, GENDER, AND RACE*

The frequency of pernicious anemia increases with age, with most new cases detected in the fifth to seventh decades of life. Men and women have been shown to be equally affected in most surveys. Studies in Sweden, Denmark, and the United Kingdom conducted between 1942 and 1968 found the incidence to be between 100 and 130 cases per 100,000. As American and European populations age, the frequency of pernicious anemia will probably exceed this reported incidence. In the seventh decade and later, the incidence of pernicious anemia may be as great as 250 to 500 cases per 100,000.

Pernicious anemia occurs predominantly in whites. It is less common in blacks, in whom it may appear at a younger age than in whites, and in East Indians. It is very rare in Asians. Pernicious anemia is more common among those of northern European origin than among those originating in the Mediterranean area. Such a north-south gradient of case incidence has even been reported within the United Kingdom and Holland.[2]

GENETICS

The hereditary nature of pernicious anemia is unknown. Attempts to link pernicious anemia with HLA phenotypes have been inconclusive. There is an increased risk of pernicious anemia in identical twins.†

CLINICAL PRESENTATIONS

Cobalamin deficiency is manifested clinically through its effects on rapidly proliferating tissues, principally the bone marrow and the lining of the intestinal tract, as well as on the nervous system. This can give rise to three clinical pictures in which megaloblastic anemia, gastrointestinal symptoms, or neurologic degeneration predominate.

Megaloblastic Anemia. Pernicious anemia often presents as severe macrocytic anemia accompanied by neutropenia and thrombocytopenia. The gradual onset of the anemia, to which the patient adjusts by gradually curtailing activity, means that the patient may be largely asymptomatic, except for some weakness. Impending or actual congestive heart failure may be present, as may postural or activity-induced shortness of breath. Usually, some neurologic or mental symptoms and signs also are present, as are glossitis and other intestinal symptoms.

Gastrointestinal Features. In some patients, the anemia and neurologic deficits are relatively mild, and the predominant symptoms are gastrointestinal. These symptoms include loss of appetite with minor weight loss (5% to 10% of body weight), nausea, constipation, occasional diarrhea, and soreness of the tongue (glossitis) or "cankers" of the tongue that are aggravated by the eating of spicy or "acid" foods. Failure to notice an accompanying mild macrocytic anemia or to elicit neurologic abnormalities may result in unwarranted intestinal visualization and imaging. Although gastrointestinal symptoms may be secondary to "megaloblastic" changes in gut cells, the relationship of such morphologic changes in buccal, esophageal, and enteric cells to glossitis, anorexia, constipation, and diarrhea is uncertain.[45]

Neurologic Disease. The neurologic syndrome of cobalamin deficiency is known as *subacute combined degeneration of the spinal cord* (SCDSC). The syndrome consists of degeneration of posterior and lateral columns of the cord and a peripheral nerve lesion,[119, 120] which is more severe in the lower than in the upper extremities. Demyelination may be secondary to axonal degeneration. Decreased vibration and position sense are usually the first objective manifestations of SCDSC, with pyramidal tract signs being observed later. The latter may be masked by a decrease in tendon reflexes secondary to the peripheral nerve lesion.[121–123] Cerebral symptoms and optic

---

*See reference 2, pp 316–321.

†See reference 2, p 483.

nerve degeneration also occur. SCDSC can occur with little evidence of anemia and includes some or all of the following features*:

- Degeneration of the posterior spinal columns, which results in decreased vibration sense below the iliac crests in 48%, loss of position sense in the feet in 42%, and ataxia in 64% of patients
- Degeneration of pyramidal tracts, which causes spasticity and dorsiflexion of the toes (Babinski's reflex) in 56% of patients
- Peripheral neuropathy with distal paresthesia, anesthesia, and muscular weakness in 90% of patients
- Dementia mimicking Alzheimer's disease
- Depression, with or without dementia, in 90% of patients and affecting virtually all symptomatic patients
- Optic atrophy, which is very rare in pernicious anemia

Decreased vibration sense and paresthesias in the legs probably affect most patients with symptomatic pernicious anemia, but SCDSC affects no more than 30%. In one series,† paresthesias were noted in 30% of patients, whereas SCDSC was present in only 6% to 9%.

In many of these patients with SCDSC, the MCV is elevated, and the serum cobalamin level is in the deficient range. However, patients without anemia and mainly neurologic disease may have serum cobalamin levels above the range of deficiency. The diagnosis of cobalamin deficiency in patients with neurologic problems should not be excluded only on the basis of a normal serum cobalamin level. The same applies to patients with a syndrome of senile dementia or Alzheimer's disease. In such patients, elevated levels of plasma methylmalonic acid and total homocysteine should be sought.

The pathogenesis of the neurologic lesions is not clear. A neurologic lesion similar to that in SCDSC can be produced in primates (including humans) and pigs by chronic exposure to nitrous oxide.[124] Nitrous oxide also produces megaloblastic anemia in humans. Nitrous oxide penetrates cells readily and oxidizes MeCbl bound to methionine synthase when it transfers its methyl. The cob(I)alamin remaining after the methyl group has been transferred to homocysteine is oxidized irreversibly by nitrous oxide to cobalamin catabolites, which remain bound to and inactivate methionine synthase.[125, 126] The neurologic lesion can be prevented in monkeys and pigs with methionine supplements. How this inactivation of methionine synthase causes neurologic disease and how it is prevented by methionine is unknown, but SCDSC probably is caused by the same mechanism. It should be noted that the concentration of methylmalonic acid in spinal fluid exceeds that in plasma.[127, 128]

Subclinical or Preclinical Pernicious Anemia. Many patients with pernicious anemia now come to medical attention because of erythrocyte macrocytosis detected on routine electronic blood cell analysis. Other patients are identified through screening programs in at-risk populations, such as the institutionalized and the elderly. The diagnosis is based on the detection of a low serum vitamin B_{12} level, an increased plasma holotranscobalamin II level, an elevated plasma level of methylmalonic acid, or an elevated plasma total homocysteine level.[129–134] Whether or not clinical manifestations of cobalamin deficiency are detectable, many patients who show biochemical evidence of deficiency volunteer that they "feel better" following treatment with vitamin B_{12}.

The frequency of the neurologic syndrome of SCDSC as the presenting symptoms and signs of pernicious anemia in adult patients appears to have increased over the past 30 years. In a study published in 1961,‡ 10% to 15% reported neurologic symptoms. Hall reported finding neurologic signs in 35% of patients with this disease.[135] In a study in California reported in 1986, neurologic or mental disorders were present in 50% of patients with cobalamin deficiency.[136] Because no data on change of incidence of pernicious anemia have been published during this interval, it is unclear whether the spectrum of the disease has changed or whether patients without anemia are now being recognized because of the universal availability of the red cell volume determination (MCV), as well as the availability of assays for serum cobalamin.

Maternal and Pediatric Vitamin B_{12} Deficiency

In well-nourished subjects, cobalamin deficiency takes many months to develop because of the long half-life of cobalamin within the body (about 0.05% to 0.2% is lost per day)[137] and of the large hepatic stores of the vitamin. The earliest manifestations of impending deficiency are related to loss of gastric IF in pernicious anemia, with reduced capacity to absorb vitamin B_{12} from the diet. At this stage, the proportion of cobalamin in plasma that is associated with TC II is decreased to below normal.[138]

During development of the deficiency, the quantities of cobalamin in the liver and in the plasma decrease progressively. In most subjects, the plasma cobalamin level falls below the normal range before other manifestations of deficiency are detected. In some, however, other manifestations of deficiency may appear before the concentration of cobalamin in the plasma reaches the levels that are usually associated with deficiency.[139, 140]

The appearance of hypersegmented neutrophils in the peripheral blood smear and the presence of increased methylmalonic acid and total homocysteine levels in the plasma may precede the development of classic megaloblastic anemia. However, bone marrow morphology, if it is examined, probably is abnormal, and oval macrocytes may be observed on blood smears. Neurologic and mental disease may develop at this stage and may not be recognized as resulting from cobalamin deficiency in the absence of anemia, elevated MCV, or decreased concentration of cobalamin in the plasma.[139, 140]

More prolonged deficiency results in anemia with a megaloblastic bone marrow accompanied by neutropenia and thrombocytopenia. These are most commonly (but not exclusively) seen in patients with the most severe anemia.[141]§

---

*See reference 2, pp 472–473.
†See reference 2, pp 468–469.

‡See reference 2, pp 320–322.
§See reference 2, pp 202–204.

From the previous discussion, it is apparent that patients with deficiency of cobalamin without symptoms may be identified by laboratory testing, may present with unexplained neurologic signs or dementia, or may develop the full picture of megaloblastic anemia. The progression is more rapid in patients with low cobalamin stores and in those with an additional metabolic insult (exposure to nitrous oxide, simultaneous deficiency of folate, or exposure to antifols).

MATERNAL VITAMIN B$_{12}$ DEFICIENCY

Pernicious anemia, the most common cause of vitamin B$_{12}$ deficiency, has its greatest incidence after the childbearing years. However, it has been described in young women. When it is recognized, diagnosed, and treated, the infant suffers no ill effects. However, apparently asymptomatic, nonanemic cases of maternal pernicious anemia have been described.[52, 142] Such mothers have low serum and milk vitamin B$_{12}$ levels, and the infants are born with low cobalamin stores. These stores are not repleted during breast-feeding. If the mother has circulating anti-IF antibodies, these antibodies can cross the placenta and enter the fetus and impair intestinal cobalamin absorption during the first few weeks of life, particularly if the antibody titer is high.[143]

Nutritional deficiency of vitamin B$_{12}$ is seen in strict vegan mothers, whose diets contain no animal-derived components and, therefore, no source of vitamin B$_{12}$.[144] This is particularly so in immigrants to the West, where improved hygienic standards in food handling and preparation minimize the bacterial and fungal content of food, which is believed to be the source of vitamin B$_{12}$ in Asian countries.[145] Food faddists also can consume a diet deficient in vitamin B$_{12}$.

Other less common causes of maternal vitamin B$_{12}$ deficiency are secondary to gastric resection, which results in loss of IF-producing mucosa; the presence of fish tapeworms or small intestinal bacterial overgrowth; and bowel disease resulting in malabsorption of vitamin B$_{12}$ from the terminal ileum (see Table 11–1). Crohn's disease, ulcerative colitis, and surgical resection of the terminal ileum all can result in vitamin B$_{12}$ malabsorption, leading to deficiency. Because of the enterohepatic circulation of vitamin B$_{12}$, such deficiency may develop more rapidly in those with malabsorption than in those whose diet is deficient because vitamin B$_{12}$ entering the gut from the bile will not be reabsorbed.

Inhalation of the anesthetic gas nitrous oxide inactivates MeCbl, the vitamin B$_{12}$ coenzyme involved in methionine synthesis. Repeated exposure to nitrous oxide produces a full-blown clinical picture of vitamin B$_{12}$ deficiency with megaloblastic anemia and SCDSC.[124] The effect of nitrous oxide exposure on the fetus during maternal nitrous oxide inhalation is unknown.

VITAMIN B$_{12}$ DEFICIENCY IN NEWBORNS AND INFANTS

Newborn infants born to mothers who are deficient in cobalamin may develop severe deficiency in the early weeks of life. Severely deficient mothers probably are sterile,[146] but those with marginal cobalamin stores due to diet or early pernicious anemia may produce cobalamin-deficient infants. This deficiency, if unrecognized, may cause permanent neurologic damage in the infant. The clinical manifestations in young children are predominantly those of "failure to thrive" and slow mental development.

Deficiency of vitamin B$_{12}$ is rarely recognized in newborns, presenting most often as failure to thrive, including developmental delay and mental retardation, after several months of life. The most common cause is maternal vitamin B$_{12}$ deficiency (see earlier), which may go unrecognized. There may be no anemia or macrocytosis in the infant, and variable degrees of pancytopenia may be present. The bone marrow may not show florid megaloblastic changes. The extent to which dietary folates or folate supplements may mask the clinical picture is unknown. The diagnosis is based on a high index of suspicion leading to demonstration of a low serum vitamin B$_{12}$ level, other confirmatory tests, response to treatment, and investigation of the mother's diet and vitamin B$_{12}$ status.

The other major causes of inadequate vitamin B$_{12}$ availability in newborns, detected within the first year of life or sometimes some years later, are inborn errors of vitamin B$_{12}$ metabolism. These are described in a later section.

VITAMIN B$_{12}$ DEFICIENCY IN OLDER CHILDREN AND ADOLESCENTS

Deficiency in older children and adolescents has the same causes as that in adults. Pernicious anemia has been reported in children younger than 10 years of age but is very rare. Cases are also encountered in teenagers, but again, uncommonly. Diets lacking vitamin B$_{12}$ prepared by parents or selected by teenagers[147] may be the cause. Gastric and intestinal diseases may result in vitamin B$_{12}$ malabsorption. Vitamin B$_{12}$ deficiency has been reported following surgery for necrotizing enterocolitis, particularly when resection has included part of the terminal ileum.[148] Low serum vitamin B$_{12}$ levels and decreased vitamin B$_{12}$ absorption as determined with the Schilling test have been reported in patients with HIV infection with and without AIDS.[149]

Diagnosis of Vitamin B$_{12}$ Deficiency

Commonly, macrocytic anemia occurs and is accompanied by neutropenia and thrombocytopenia. The MCV is 120 fL or greater, unless the increase in MCV is balanced by a decrease due to a coexisting iron deficiency or a chronic inflammatory process.[150–153] The blood smear contains oval macrocytes and multilobar neutrophils. For a variety of reasons, including the use of newer automated cell counters and the varying competence of technicians analyzing blood smears, oval macrocytes and multilobar neutrophils may not be reported even if present. The bone marrow usually is megaloblastic.

Abnormal biochemical findings in the serum include increased levels of lactate dehydrogenase, bilirubin, and iron, as well as increased transferrin saturation, which reflects "ineffective erythropoiesis." Serum cholesterol, lipid, and immunoglobulin levels may be decreased. These changes are not specific to cobalamin deficiency but are corrected after cobalamin therapy.[154, 155] Equally nonspecific is the finding of increased serum gastrin levels and antibody to gastric parietal cells, which signal the presence of atrophic gastritis but do not distinguish those who lack IF from those who do not. The presence of antibody to IF in serum means that the patient has or will develop cobalamin deficiency.[20, 156]

SERUM LEVELS OF VITAMIN B$_{12}$

The most direct evidence of cobalamin deficiency is an abnormally low serum cobalamin level. Although early studies using microbiologic assays showed that serum cobalamin level was almost always less than 100 pg/mL[141] (78 pmol/L) in patients with megaloblastic anemia due to cobalamin deficiency, megaloblastic bone marrow is found in only 20% to 30% of patients with serum cobalamin levels less than 100 pg/mL. Therefore, significant cobalamin deficiency can occur without hematologic manifestations. In some patients with deficiency of cobalamin, megaloblastic anemia and a decrease in serum cobalamin level into the deficient range occur with longer periods of deficiency. Neurologic manifestations of cobalamin deficiency may appear before macrocytic erythrocytes and classic megaloblastic anemia develop.[140]

Serum cobalamin level has been shown to reflect hepatic cobalamin in reports that describe studies of a small number of subjects,[157] but the clinical significance of isolated low levels of cobalamin in serum without other evidence of cobalamin deficiency, such as abnormal metabolism of methylmalonate or homocysteine, or a definitely abnormal deoxyuridine suppression test result, has not been determined. In many cases, these patients are treated with vitamin B$_{12}$, but without obvious clinical benefit.

In contrast, significant cobalamin deficiency may occur in the absence of low serum cobalamin levels in patients who do not have megaloblastic anemia. In one study, serum cobalamin level was greater than 100 pg/mL in 30% to 40% of patients demonstrated to have significant cobalamin deficiency; in 3% to 5%, the serum cobalamin level was in the normal range.[139, 140] This failure of the assay to provide a near-perfect clinical correlation[158] is due in part to technical defects in the specificity of the cobalamin binder used in some commercial ligand-binding assays. It also reflects the limits of sensitivity and specificity of the assay when used as the sole measure of cobalamin deficiency, particularly when the assay is applied to populations in which florid clinical features of cobalamin deficiency are not present. In patients with megaloblastic anemia, the finding of a normal to increased level of serum folate, together with a reduced ratio of erythrocyte to serum folate level, provides strong but indirect evidence of cobalamin deficiency.[159]

These studies suggest that evidence of functional cobalamin deficiency other than serum cobalamin levels (e.g., macrocytosis, multilobar neutrophils, and elevated levels of plasma methylmalonic acid and total homocysteine) must be sought when cobalamin sufficiency is evaluated in such populations, as well as in individuals in whom deficiency is strongly suspected.

The diagnosis of cobalamin deficiency is confirmed by the finding of increased serum levels of methylmalonic acid and total homocysteine, which is evidence of functional cobalamin deficiency, and by the demonstration of cobalamin malabsorption, which can be corrected by the administration of cobalamin with a source of IF (urinary excretion test, or Schilling test; Fig. 11–7). Indeed, correction of the cobalamin malabsorption with the feeding of IF together with radiolabeled cobalamin confirms that a lack of IF is the cause, proving that the patient has pernicious anemia. The diagnosis can also be established on the basis of a positive therapeutic test result (described in the next section).

In patients who cannot absorb vitamin B$_{12}$, there is some evidence that the amount of cobalamin bound to TC II decreases before the decrease in total serum cobalamin (mostly bound to haptocorrin) occurs.[138] In such patients, the neutrophil lobe count (number of lobes per 100 cells) may increase within 6 to 8 weeks after discontinuation of cobalamin injections and will decrease again after injection of CNCbl. Plasma homocysteine and methylmalonic acid levels sometimes increase into the abnormal range in less than 6 months. Decreased TC II–Cbl might then signal a failure of vitamin B$_{12}$ absorption, whereas increased neutrophil lobe count and homocysteine and methylmalonic acid levels would indicate tissue cobalamin functional deficiency.

A Positive Therapeutic Test Result

A positive therapeutic test result is the correction of hematologic, biochemical, and neurologic abnormalities following vitamin treatment. If cobalamin deficiency is apparent and the megaloblastic anemia is not severe, then treatment consists of the administration of one or more injections of 100 to 1000 μg of CNCbl or OHCbl (to confirm the diagnosis if megaloblastic changes in the erythroid series in the bone marrow disappear within 48 hours) and at least two of the following:

1. A decrease in serum iron by 50% over 24 hours
2. An increase in the reticulocyte count 5 to 10 days after treatment
3. The correction of thrombocytopenia over 2 weeks
4. The correction of neutropenia over 2 weeks
5. A decrease in the MCV by 5 fL or more over 2 weeks (after the reticulocytosis has subsided)
6. The correction of anemia over 2 to 4 weeks
7. A decrease in the neutrophil lobe count from the elevated to the normal range over 4 weeks
8. A decrease in elevated plasma methylmalonic acid and total homocysteine levels over 2 weeks

To establish the diagnosis of cobalamin deficiency and avoid severe metabolic disturbances, the patient should receive 10 μg CNCbl subcutaneously daily for 2 days. This therapy is sufficient for normalizing metabolic derangements such as elevated levels of serum lactate dehydrogenase and serum iron and for inducing an increase in the reticulocyte count, with a maximum level being attained at 5 to 7 days. For children, the dose of CNCbl is 0.2 μg/kg per day subcutaneously for 2 days.

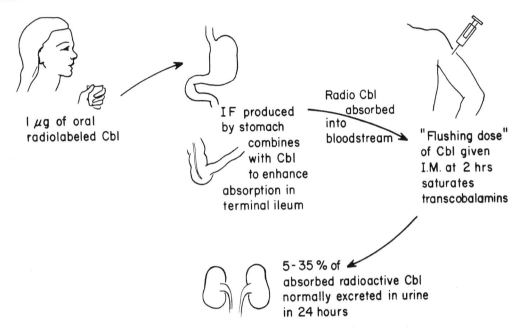

FIGURE 11–7. The urinary excretion (Schilling) test. Labeled cyanocobalamin is fed, and a proportion of absorbed label is flushed into the urine by subsequent injection of a large quantity (1000 μg) of unlabeled vitamin B_{12}. The oral dose must be standardized, other radioactivity must be absent from the urine, and renal function and urine collection must be adequate. If excretion is low, then the test may be repeated with the use of a source of intrinsic factor.

The clinician can establish a diagnosis of folate deficiency by treating the patient with a low dose of folic acid (in the range of 0.5 mg/d by mouth for 2 to 3 days) and then by monitoring for metablic normalization and reticulocytosis in the succeeding 2 weeks (see earlier). It should be noted that the administration of 2 to 5 mg of folic acid will induce reticulocytosis in almost all patients with cobalamin deficiency, whereas giving 100 to 1000 μg of cobalamin will induce reticulocytosis in some patients with folate deficiency.

SERUM COBALAMIN IN FOLATE DEFICIENCY

The serum cobalamin level is decreased in a proportion of patients with folate deficiency and megaloblastic anemia and may be in the range of deficiency. This cobalamin level increases over 7 days when folate is administered; the level does not increase in patients deficient in cobalamin.[160] The mechanism involved is unknown but may represent redistribution of cobalamin between cells and plasma.

URINARY EXCRETION TEST (THE SCHILLING TEST)

In performing this standard test for the measurement of cobalamin absorption, the clinician feeds the fasting patient 0.5 μg of ^{57}Co-labeled CNCbl in water, waits 2 hours, gives a subcutaneous injection of 1000 μg of CNCbl to block tissue uptake of ^{57}Co-CNCbl, and measures the amount of ^{57}Co-CNCbl excreted in the urine in 24 hours. If malabsorption is found, the test is repeated 1 week later, with the addition of a source of IF to the 0.5 μg of oral ^{57}Co-CNCbl to demonstrate correction of the malabsorption by IF; such correction establishes the diagnosis of pernicious anemia (see Fig. 11–7).

FOOD SCHILLING TEST

In patients with atrophic gastritis and inadequate gastric peptic activity, vitamin B_{12} may be absorbed when it is fed in water; however, cobalamin in food may not be adequately absorbed. Cobalamin in a variety of cooked foods has been demonstrated to be poorly absorbed by such patients, and this may produce decreased body stores of cobalamin and sometimes even true deficiency. In such patients, the results of the Schilling test are normal.

In the *food Schilling test*, ^{57}Co-CNCbl is incorporated into or added to eggs, meat, or liver and fed to the patient. Tests for this abnormality are not well standardized. Those utilizing cobalamin naturally incorporated into eggs, meat, or liver may require performance of the fecal excretion test (see the next section) because the OHCbl produced by breakdown of the natural coenzymes of cobalamin (mostly 5′-deoxyadenosyl cobalamin) binds to plasma and other proteins and may not be as well excreted into the urine as during the routine Schilling test. Absorption of 1 μg of labeled CNCbl added to eggs and fed, either cooked or uncooked, or mixed with 3 mL of chicken serum[161–163] can be tested with the standard protocol for the Schilling test; however, clinical studies remain inadequate for defining normal ranges, reliability (reproducibility, and the ability to detect abnormality, such as malabsorption), and precise procedures (with respect to types of food, food amount, and interaction of ^{57}Co-CNCbl with food [added or incorporated], details of feeding, B_{12} flushing, urine collection). At this time, such tests must be standardized within the institution that uses them, with development of normal ranges for each batch of cobalamin-containing food produced. If possible, the total amount of cobalamin fed in the test should not exceed 2 μg.

SINGLE-SAMPLE FECAL EXCRETION TEST

The single-sample fecal excretion test of cobalamin absorption is convenient and simple, and it probably avoids the pitfalls of tests that rely on urinary excretion. The basis of this test of vitamin B_{12} absorption is the simultaneous feeding of labeled cobalamin (free or bound to food) with 2 g of a nonabsorbable dye (carmine) and 10 µCi (1 mg) of ^{51}Cr–chromic chloride. The ^{51}Cr is not absorbed. A 2- to 3-g sample of the first or second carmine (red)–stained stool is added to a counting vial, shaken with 1 to 3 mL of water, and counted for ^{51}Cr and ^{57}Co. The ratio of counts is compared with the ratio in the sample fed. In normal subjects, 36% to 88% of a 1- to 2-µg dose of ^{57}Co-labeled cobalamin is absorbed.[164]

DEOXYURIDINE SUPPRESSION TEST

The deoxyuridine suppression test[165, 166] was developed (Fig. 11–8) on the basis of the hypothesis that the activity of thymidylate synthase is decreased in cells deficient in cobalamin or folates because of lack of the required folate coenzyme, 5,10-methylene-THF polyglutamate. Such deficient cells may have an expanded intracellular pool of

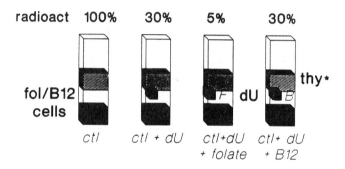

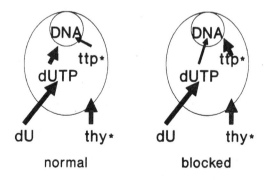

FIGURE 11–8. Deoxyuridine suppression test. This test, effective only with bone marrow cells, evaluates the capacity of the cells to convert deoxyuridine into thymidylate. Four test tubes containing bone marrow from a patient deficient in folate are illustrated. Labeled thymidine (*hatched area*, radioactivity) is incorporated into DNA in the presence of excess deoxyuridine (*dotted cubes*) because thymidylate synthesis from deoxyuridine is limited by the folate deficiency. Thymidylate synthesis is corrected by the addition of folate to tube 3 but not by the addition of cobalamin to tube 4. The presumed phenomenon occurring in the cells is illustrated below, with reaction rates shown as thick or thin arrows. fol = folate; dU = deoxyuridine; thy = thymidine; ctl = control; dUTP = deoxyuridine triphosphate; ttp = thymidine triphosphate.

deoxyuridylate, which reflects the decreased activity of thymidylate synthase. Incubation of deficient cells with deoxyuridine would be expected to further expand this pool. The test involves incubation of fresh washed bone marrow cells with deoxyuridine for 1 hour, followed by incubation with ^{3}H-labeled thymidine for 1 hour. The quantity of ^{3}H-thymidine incorporated into cell DNA is then determined.

In normal cells, thymidylate synthase converts the deoxyuridine to thymidylate during the initial incubation. This reduces the amount of ^{3}H-thymidine subsequently incorporated into DNA to less than 10% of that observed when the preincubation with deoxyuridine is not carried out. In bone marrow cells from a patient who is deficient in cobalamin or folates, preincubation with deoxyuridine reduces incorporation of ^{3}H-thymidine into DNA to only 30% to 40% of that observed in the absence of preincubation with deoxyuridine.

The defect in suppression of the incorporation of ^{3}H-thymidine into DNA by preincubation with deoxyuridine in cobalamin-deficient cells is corrected by the addition of either MeCbl or 5-formyl-THF (folinic acid) during the preincubation with deoxyuridine. Addition of N-5-methyl-THF to deoxyuridine during the preincubation corrects the defect in folate-deficient cells but not in cells deficient in cobalamin. There is uncertainty regarding the details of the actual biochemical processes being modulated during this test, but the deoxyuridine suppression test as described has proved reliable in discriminating between cobalamin and folate deficiency. The exception to this is in patients who have concomitant iron deficiency.

METHYLMALONIC ACID AND TOTAL HOMOCYSTEINE LEVELS IN COBALAMIN DEFICIENCY

Tissues deficient in cobalamin may not adequately metabolize substrates of cobalamin-dependent enzymes, such as methylmalonic acid. The presence of methylmalonic acid in the urine of some patients with pernicious anemia and its slow disappearance following treatment with doses of cobalamin that corrected the anemia was described in 1962.[167] It is now known that almost all subjects who are cobalamin deficient, both children and adults,[168] accumulate methylmalonic acid in the plasma.[35, 169–172] Indeed, elevated plasma levels of methylmalonic acid may be found before the appearance of macrocytosis or anemia, or of other clinical features of cobalamin deficiency. These levels return to the normal range after several days or weeks of cobalamin treatment.

Homocysteine accumulates in the plasma of patients deficient in cobalamin, as well as in that of patients who are deficient in folates.[35, 132, 139, 140, 168, 173, 174] Plasma homocysteine binds to free SH groups on proteins. Thus, it may not be detected when it is present in low concentrations unless it is released from the proteins by reducing agents to yield a measure of total plasma homocysteine. Elevated plasma total homocysteine levels are found in more than 80% of patients who are deficient in cobalamin or folates. As with elevated plasma methylmalonic acid levels, the total plasma homocysteine concentration returns to normal after several days or weeks of therapy with the appropriate vitamin. Raised plasma total homocysteine may not decrease if the vitamin in which the patient is not deficient is given. Methylmalonic acid and total homocysteine may also accumulate in the plasma of patients with renal insufficiency. The implications of elevated levels of total homocysteine in plasma in relation to neural tube defects, cerebral and cardiovascular disease, and the incidence of cancer are discussed later in this chapter.

Treatment of Cobalamin Deficiency

GENERAL

Patients admitted to a hospital with severe anemia may have heart failure due to a combination of factors, including tachycardia, increased cardiac output, sodium retention, and inadequate oxygenation of the myocardium. The aim of emergency treatment is stabilization of the patient with the use of oxygen, diuretics, and limited slow red cell transfusion. Rapid or generous transfusion may exacerbate the cardiac failure. Immediate administration of vitamin B$_{12}$ or folate in large doses is not required because several days must elapse before hematologic improvement can be detected. Clinical disasters sometimes occur during therapy. Treatment of severely anemic adults with pernicious anemia has been associated with immediate death in 14%[175]; however, more recent studies do not appear to confirm this.[176] Disasters include life-threatening hypokalemia and cerebral and cardiovascular accidents (usually strokes due to thrombosis or embolism).

Severe hypokalemia is most likely to occur following the administration of a large dose of cobalamin in a patient who is severely anemic. This results from a rapid recovery and retention of intracellular potassium that is accompanied by a delay in renal potassium conservation, which in turn shifts potassium from the extracellular to the intracellular compartment. Although hypokalemia may not have been the primary cause of the reported deaths, the clinician should anticipate and avoid it, if possible, by providing potassium supplements (sometimes in large doses), as needed; by initiating treatment with a low dose of cobalamin (e.g., 10 µg of CNCbl given daily subcutaneously for 2 to 3 days); and by transfusion to achieve partial correction of the anemia.

The risk of occurrence of an acute thrombotic episode may be reduced by these maneuvers, but this has not been documented. The role of potentially thrombogenic homocystinemia in causing these thrombotic episodes is not known. Also, these complications of initial therapy may affect children with severe cobalamin deficiency.

INITIAL THERAPY

Bone marrow aspiration should be performed early to establish the presence of megaloblastic anemia because erythroid hyperplasia will decrease and cell morphology will change within a few hours following transfusion. Serum cobalamin and folate values are not significantly altered by transfusion but should be obtained before the procedure is performed. However, a whole blood sample for red cell folate determination must be collected (in citrate or ethylenediaminetetra-acetic acid [EDTA]) before transfusion. Otherwise, the red cell folate level will be that of the mixture of the patient's and donor's red cells.

A dose of 10 µg CNCbl given subcutaneously daily for 2 days is sufficient to correct metabolic abnormalities, such as the elevated serum lactate dehydrogenase and iron levels, and to induce an increase in the reticulocyte count, with a maximum count attained 5 to 7 days after the start of treatment. For children, the dose of CNCbl is 0.2 µg/kg subcutaneously daily for 2 days. Such doses given over 5 to 7 days usually do not restore elevated plasma MMA and total homocysteine levels to normal.

Complete correction of megaloblastic erythropoiesis and associated metabolic changes can occur with as little as 15 µg of CNCbl in some adults, whereas as much as 150 µg may be required in others. Dementia and depression may improve rapidly with therapy, whereas other neurologic abnormalities usually show slow improvement over 6 months and may not return to normal. However, one of the authors of this chapter (BAC) has observed complete recovery from SCDSC in a patient who was bedridden and had positive Babinski's reflexes within as short a time as 1 to 2 weeks after institution of cobalamin treatment.

Subsequently, injections of CNCbl of 1000 µg should be given daily for 1 week, followed by 100 µg of CNCbl weekly for 1 month. This therapy is required to replete body cobalamin stores.

Patients proven to be deficient in cobalamin and who cannot absorb the vitamin (i.e., those with pernicious anemia) require monthly injections of CNCbl. A prudent monthly dose is 100 µg injected subcutaneously. Failure of this regimen to maintain normal body stores is extremely rare. Similar maintenance of stores and repletion appears to follow injections of 1000 µg (1 mg) of OHCbl every 3 months[177] or of 1 mg of OHCbl daily for 1 to 2 weeks every 6 to 12 months. The binding of OHCbl to tissues permits such infrequent injection, but a small proportion of patients do develop antibodies against the TC II-Cbl complex.[178] These antibodies have not been found to affect health but do cause the accumulation of very large concentrations of TC II in plasma. It is unclear whether this rare allergy to cobalamin is more common after injections of OHCbl or of CNCbl.

In some patients with pernicious anemia, cobalamin levels in serum or plasma can be maintained in the normal range with daily ingestion of 50 to 200 µg of CNCbl, taken remote from meals. Efficacy of therapy should be monitored biochemically.

In patients with apparent deficiency of cobalamin secondary to defective peptic digestion (normal results obtained on Schilling test but abnormal absorption of cobalamin bound to food), normal cobalamin levels and stores can be maintained through feeding 10 to 25 µg/d of CNCbl; however, the efficacy of such treatment should be verified periodically by the demonstration of normal levels of serum cobalamin, methylmalonic acid, and total homocysteine. In children with inherited defects of cobalamin metabolism, injections of 1000 µg OHCbl 2 to 3 times per week should be used. The effectiveness of therapy in such cases can be monitored with the measurement of serum levels of total homocysteine, methylmalonic acid, and methionine, and perhaps of additional metabolites.

ASSOCIATED DISEASES

Patients with pernicious anemia are at increased risk of developing carcinoma of the stomach.[179, 180] Cancer may be diagnosed before, at the same time as, or many years after the diagnosis of pernicious anemia. Currently, patients undergo follow-up that includes annual gastroscopy, with biopsy of suspicious areas. Evidence of mucosal dysplasia or the presence of chromosomal changes suggesting a premalignant state would warrant more frequent assessment. Pernicious anemia is also associated with other autoimmune diseases, particularly those involving the thyroid. Hypothyroidism is common and should be evaluated clinically and with measurement of hormone levels, as needed.[181] Pernicious anemia is associated with type I diabetes as well.[182]

Inborn Errors of Vitamin B$_{12}$ Transport and Metabolism

TRANSPORT DISORDERS

Intrinsic Factor Deficiency

A small number of children have been recognized to have megaloblastic anemia and developmental delay as a result of an absence of effective IF. Evidence of vitamin B$_{12}$ deficiency usually appears after the first year but before the fifth year of life, although clinical deficiency has appeared as late as age 12 years in patients with partially defective IF.[183] These patients have normal gastric acid secretion and normal findings on gastric cytologic examination. In some cases, immunologically active but nonfunctional IF is produced, whereas in others none is found at all. An IF labile to destruction by acid and pepsin and having a low affinity for vitamin B$_{12}$ has been reported.[184] In children with IF deficiency, absorption of cobalamin is abnormal but is normalized when the vitamin is mixed with a source of normal IF, such as human gastric juice from an unaffected individual. The gene for human IF is on chromosome 11. Southern blot analysis of DNA from patients with inherited IF deficiency has not revealed any large deletions,[93] suggesting that most mutations are the result of point mutations. As with the other disorders of cobalamin transport, inheritance appears to be autosomal recessive.

Defective Transport of Vitamin B$_{12}$ by Enterocytes

Defective transport of vitamin B$_{12}$ by enterocytes, also known as the *Imerslund-Gräsbeck syndrome*, usually presents with clinical manifestations of vitamin B$_{12}$ deficiency in children between the ages of 1 and 15 years.[2, 185, 186] At least 150 cases have been described; they most commonly occur among Finns and Sephardic Jews. All patients who were investigated had normal IF, no evidence of antibodies to IF, and normal intestinal morphology. They had a selective defect in vitamin B$_{12}$ absorption that was not corrected by treatment with IF. In some patients, proteinuria of the tubular type was found.

In one sibship,[187] normal quantities of IF–vitamin B$_{12}$ receptor were found in ileal biopsy specimens. Ileal homogenates bound IF–vitamin B$_{12}$ normally; this finding suggests that the basic defect is not an absence of receptors. In other patients,[188] an apparent absence of the ileal receptor has been observed. A canine model exists for this disorder.[189, 190]

The inheritance is autosomal recessive. Therapy with systemic vitamin B$_{12}$ corrects the anemia but not the proteinuria.

R Binder (Haptocorrin, TC I) Deficiency

The deficiency or complete absence of R binder in the plasma, saliva, and leukocytes of six individuals has been described.[191–196] It is unclear whether R binder deficiency is the cause of disease in any of these patients. Although serum cobalamin levels are low, TC II–vitamin B$_{12}$ levels are normal, and the patients are not clinically deficient in vitamin B$_{12}$.

The original report described two brothers, only one of whom had optic atrophy, ataxia, long tract signs, and dementia.[196] A more recently described patient had findings resembling those seen in SCDSC.[196] A role for R binders has been postulated in the scavenging of cobalamin analogues that may be toxic to the brain.[99]

Transcobalamin II Deficiency (see Fig. 11–4)

Clinical Findings. At least 30 patients with TC II deficiency are known.[191, 197] Although all of the TC II in fetal and cord blood is of fetal origin, infants with no detectable TC II in their plasma do not develop manifestations of cobalamin deficiency until several days after birth. TC II–deficient patients develop severe anemia much earlier than do patients with other causes of cobalamin malabsorption, usually in the first few months of life. Other symptoms include failure to thrive, weakness, and diarrhea in addition to pallor. The anemia usually is clearly megaloblastic, but some patients present with pancytopenia or even isolated erythroid hypoplasia.[198] The presence of immature white cell precursors in a marrow that is otherwise hypocellular can lead to the misdiagnosis of leukemia. Neurologic disease has appeared from 6 months to 30 months following the onset of symptoms.[199–202] Severe immunologic deficiency with defective cellular and humoral immunity has been seen, as has defective granulocyte function. Homocystinuria has been sought in at least two patients prior to their receiving vitamin B$_{12}$ therapy. In three of five patients[191] who were tested before the initiation of therapy, methylmalonic aciduria was found. Following discontinuation of therapy, methylmalonic aciduria may return.

In all patients except one, no TC II competent to bind cobalamin was detected. However, immunologically reactive TC II was found in three patients. In one patient, TC II was able to bind cobalamin, but the complex did not mediate vitamin uptake into cells. An abnormal Schilling test result was usually found in TC II deficiency (five of seven patients); in two patients in whom the absorption of cobalamin was normal, immunoreactive TC II was present. This suggests that the TC II molecule may have a role in the IF–vitamin B$_{12}$–mediated transport across the ileal cell even if it is not functional in transporting the vitamin in the circulation or in delivering it to cells.

Inheritance. On the basis of electrophoretic polymorphisms,[203, 204] the TC II gene (*TCN2*) was originally linked to the P blood group on chromosome 22.[205] The cDNA for *TCN2* has now been cloned[206] and the molecular basis of some of the variants defined.[207] The first mutant alleles in TC II deficiency have included deletions[197] and nonsense mutations.[208] Autosomal recessive inheritance for TC II deficiency has been confirmed. TC II is synthesized by cultured cells, and prenatal diagnosis is possible even when the specific mutation in a family is not yet known.

Treatment. Serum vitamin B_{12} levels must be kept very high if TC II–deficient patients are to be treated successfully. Levels ranging from 1000 to 10,000 pg/mL have been required and are achieved with doses of oral OHCbl or CNCbl twice weekly (500 to 1000 μg) or with systemic administration of CNCbl or OHCbl (1000 μg) weekly or more often. Folate in the form of folic acid or folinic acid in milligram doses has been successful in reversing the hematologic findings in most patients. Folate should not be given as the only therapy because of the danger of hematologic relapse and of neurologic damage, which has been induced in one such patient by folate supplementation without cobalamin.[191]

DISORDERS OF UTILIZATION

The Methylmalonic Acidurias

Those disorders causing methylmalonic aciduria[209] are characterized by severe metabolic acidosis and the accumulation of large amounts of MMA in the blood, urine, and cerebrospinal fluid. Levels are much higher than those seen in adults with cobalamin deficiency. Patients with methylmalonic acidurias have a defect in the mitochondrial matrix enzyme methylmalonyl CoA mutase, which requires AdoCbl as a cofactor and catalyses the conversion of L-methylmalonyl CoA to succinyl CoA. Classification of the methylmalonic acidurias has been made largely on the basis of studies in cultured fibroblasts. Complementation groups have been defined on the basis of whether two lines partially correct a defect in propionate incorporation following cell fusion.

Mutase Deficiency (Deficiency of Methylmalonyl CoA Mutase)

Background. Disorders of the mutase apoenzyme result in methylmalonic aciduria, which is not responsive to vitamin B_{12} therapy. Mature mutase purified from human liver is a 77,000-dalton homodimer that is coded by a nuclear gene, is found in the cytoplasm as a precursor with a leader sequence, and is processed to a mature protein in the mitochondria.[67] There are at least two separate types of mutase deficiency. The mut° cell lines have no residual mutase activity, whereas the mut⁻ cell lines show some residual mutase activity when AdoCbl is added, and the mutase in mut⁻ cell lines show decreased affinity for AdoCbl. Several of the mut° cell lines synthesize no detectable protein, whereas some synthesize unstable proteins, and at least one has a mutation that interferes with transfer of the mutase to the mitochondria.[210] Similarly, variable levels of mRNA have been demonstrated in different mut° lines. Usually, there is no complementation between mut° and mut⁻ cell lines, but intragenic (interallelic) complementation has been seen among some mut lines.[211,212]

Clinical Syndromes. Clinically well at birth, patients with mutase deficiency rapidly become symptomatic with protein feeding. They usually come to medical attention because of lethargy, vomiting, failure to thrive, muscular hypotonia, respiratory distress, and recurrent vomiting and dehydration. In normal children, MMA level usually is less than 15 to 20 μg per gram of creatinine; in contrast, in methylmalonic aciduria, excretion is usually more than 100 mg and as much as several grams per day. In addition to methylmalonic aciduria, these patients may have ketones and glycine in both blood and urine and metabolic acidosis with elevated levels of ammonia. Many also have hypoglycemia, leukopenia, and thrombocytopenia. One study[213] has demonstrated that MMA inhibits bone marrow stem cells in a concentration-dependent manner. It is interesting that follow-up of children identified by newborn screening[214] has revealed a number of individuals who excrete MMA and have mutase deficiency as demonstrated by complementation analysis, and yet who are clinically well and have never developed acidosis. It is unclear whether these children are at risk for catastrophic acidosis later in life. The incidence of all forms of methylmalonic aciduria in Massachusetts is about 1 in 29,000.

Inheritance. The gene for the mutase is located on the short arm of chromosome 6, 6p12-21.2, spans 40 kb, and consists of 13 exons.[63,66,215,216] At least 15 point mutations have been found, including a large number near the carboxyl terminus that appear to alter AdoCbl binding to the enzyme.[217,218] A premature stop codon has been found in the mitochondrial leader sequence,[219] and a common mutation has been detected in three African-American patients who had a similar phenotype.[220] In Japan, 6 of 16 patients studied shared 1 mutation.[221] Mutase deficiency is an autosomal recessive disease, and prenatal diagnosis is possible.

Treatment. Therapy consists of protein restriction, with the goal of limiting the amino acids that use the propionate pathway. Formula deficient in valine, isoleucine, methionine, and threonine is used. Mutase-deficient patients are not responsive to vitamin B_{12}. Therapy with carnitine has been advocated in patients who are deficient.[222,223] Lincomycin and metronidazole have been used to reduce enteric propionate production by anaerobic bacteria.[224–226] Even with therapy, prognosis is guarded, and brain infarcts and renal dysfunction have been reported as late complications.[209]

Adenosylcobalamin Deficiency (cblA and cblB Diseases)

Background. Two disorders result in vitamin B_{12}–responsive methylmalonic aciduria and an intracellular deficiency in AdoCbl. They are distinguished by complementation analysis and by the fact that cblA is capable of AdoCbl synthesis in cell extracts but not in intact cells, whereas cblB is deficient in both systems. The defect in cblA disease is in a reducing system, presumably in mitochondria, and results in the conversion of cob(III)alamin to cob(I)alamin. The defect in cblB disease lies in the adenosyltransferase, which is the final step in the synthesis of AdoCbl (see Fig. 11–4, Points A and B).

Clinical Syndromes. Most children with cblA disease become ill either in the first week of life or before the end of the first year. Similarly, most patients with cblB disease present in the first year of life. Symptoms are similar to those seen in mutase deficiency but usually are less severe and depend on the clinical response to vitamin B_{12} therapy.[227] Most cblA disease patients (90%) respond to vitamin B_{12}, with almost 70% being well by the age of 14 years. Fewer than half of cblB disease patients (40%) respond to therapy, and only 30% have long-term survival. Therapy has been with either OHCbl or CNCbl systemically. It is not clear whether AdoCbl offers any therapeutic advantage.

Inheritance. The inheritance of both cblA and cblB diseases is presumed to be autosomal recessive. Roughly equal numbers of patients of both sexes have been reported, and obligate heterozygotes of patients with cblB disease show decreased adenosyltransferase activity.[203] The mutations behave as recessive in complementation analyses.

Management. One report of prenatal therapy with vitamin B_{12} with a good therapeutic result has been published.[228] However, it is not certain whether therapy at birth would not have been equally effective.

Combined Deficiencies of Adenosylcobalamin and Methylcobalamin (cblC, cblD, and cblF Diseases)

Background. The precise defect in the cblC, cblD, and cblF disorders is not known, but all three result in failure of the cell to synthesize both cobalamin cofactors, MeCbl and adenosylcobalamin (AdoCbl).[203] Patients have a functional deficiency in both methionine synthase and MMA-CoA mutase, leading to homocystinuria and hypomethioninemia along with methylmalonic aciduria. The three defects occur subsequent to the endocytosis of TC II–vitamin B_{12} and to hydrolysis of the TC II–vitamin B_{12} complex (see Fig. 11–4, Points C, D, and F). In cblF disease, the defect appears to block the transfer of free vitamin B_{12} from the lysosome to the cytoplasm, whereas in cblC and cblD diseases, the defect is presumed to be in a cytosolic cob(III)alamin reductase or reductases, which are needed to reduce the trivalent cobalt of vitamin B_{12} before further vitamin B_{12} metabolism can occur.[229] Partial deficiencies of CNCbl β-ligand transferase and microsomal cob(III)alamin reductase in cblC and cblD fibroblasts have been described.[230,231] When incubated with labeled CNCbl, fibroblasts from cblC and cblD accumulate very little intracellular vitamin B_{12} and virtually no AboCbl or MeCbl. In contrast, cblF fibroblasts accumulate excess vitamin B_{12}, but all of it is unmetabolized, non-protein bound, and localized to lysosomes.[117,118]

Clinical Syndromes. There are more than 90 known cases of cblC disease[232]; 2 patients in 1 sibship with cblD disease; and 5 unrelated patients with cblF disease.

Most of the patients with cblC disease present in the first month or before the end of the first year of life with poor feeding, failure to thrive, and lethargy.[233] Most but not all have megaloblastic macrocytic anemia, and some have hypersegmented neutrophils and thrombocytopenia. Others have onset later in childhood or adolescence with spasticity, delirium, and psychosis.[234] For example, a boy presented at the age of 4 years with fatigue, delirium, and spasticity,[235] and a girl presented at the age of 14 years

with mental deterioration and myelopathy.[234] In four patients, pigmentary retinopathy with perimacular degeneration was described.[191,233,236,237] Other reported findings in cblC disease include hydrocephalus, cor pulmonale, and hepatic failure.[232,238,239] Neonatal screening for MMA was the method by which the diagnosis was made in some cases. In these patients, the MMA levels are lower than those seen in mutase deficiency but higher than those reported for the defects in vitamin B_{12} transport. Elevated serum cobalamin and folate levels have been reported in several patients.

The patients with cblD disease were more mildly affected, having come to attention because of mild mental retardation and behavioral problems.[240] Cerebrovascular disease due to thromboembolism was found at the age of 18 years in one of the brothers.[203]

The findings common to the first two patients with cblF disease include their being small for gestational age, poor feeding, growth retardation, and persistent stomatitis.[241,242] The first patient had glossitis and an abnormal Schilling test result,[243] and the second had a persistent skin rash. Both patients had minor facial abnormalities, and the first had dextrocardia. Only the second patient had macrocytosis and homocystinemia as reflected by elevated total blood homocysteine level.[241] Both patients are female. The second patient died suddenly despite apparent clinical response to therapy with vitamin B_{12}. The third patient with cblF, a boy, had recurrent stomatitis in infancy, arthritis at the age of 4 years, and confusion, disorientation, and a pigmentary skin abnormality at the age of 10 years. He was subequently found to have pancytopenia, an increased MCV, low serum cobalamin levels, and abnormal cobalamin absorption.[244] The fourth patient, also a boy, had aspiration pneumonia at birth and then hypotonia, lethargy, hepatomegaly, hypoglycemia, neutropenia, and thrombocytopenia.[244] Both patients had a good response to cobalamin treatment. The fifth patient with cblF, a Native Canadian girl, was diagnosed at the age of 6 months with anemia, failure to thrive, developmental delay, and recurrent infections. Serum cobalamin levels and cobalamin absorption were both low.[245]

Inheritance. The numbers of males and females affected with cblC disease are roughly equal, and both sexes are affected with equal severity. Thus, cblC disease is probably inherited as an autosomal recessive disorder. Both of the two siblings with cblD disease are males, so the possibility of sex linkage cannot be excluded. Inheritance of cblF disease also is thought to be autosomal recessive.

Laboratory Findings. The Cbl disorders can be differentiated by the results of studies of cultured fibroblasts (Table 11–2). Uptake of labeled CNCbl can distinguish the cblC and cblD diseases from all other cobalamin mutations because its level in these two disorders is reduced. The incorporation of the substrates propionate and methyl-THF is reduced in all three disorders, as is the synthesis of the two vitamin B_{12} cofactors, AdoCbl and MeCbl. Direct measurements of total mutase and methionine synthase activity in cell extracts should be low (they are not measured in cblF disease). Complementation analysis with an unknown cell line and previously defined groups provides the specific diagnosis.[117] Prenatal diag-

TABLE 11–2. Diagnostic Studies in cbl Diseases: Correlation of Genetic Complementation Group with Biochemical Phenotype and Major Clinical Manifestations

Complementation Group	cb1A	cb1B	cb1C	cb1D	cb1E	cb1G	cb1F
MAJOR CLINICAL FINDINGS							
Megaloblastic anemia	N	N	D	D	D	D	N†
Methylmalonic aciduria	D	D	D	D	N*	N	D
Homocystinuria	N	N	D	D	D	D	N†
LABORATORY FINDINGS							
Studies in Intact Fibroblasts							
(^{57}Co)-cyano-B$_{12}$ uptake:	N	N	D	D	N	N	I
AdoCbl (%)	D	D	D	D	N	N	D
MeCbl (%)	N	N	D	D	D	D	D
Propionate incorporation	D	D	D	D	N	N	D
Methyltetrahydrofolate incorporation	N	N	D	D	D	D	D
STUDIES IN CELL EXTRACTS							
Methylmalony-CoA mutase holoenzyme	D	D	D	D	N	N	–
Methionine synthase holonenzyme	N	N	D	D	N‡	D	D

*Transient methylmalonic aciduria reported in one patient.
†Seen in one of two cases reported.
‡Under standard reducing conditions.
N = Normal for laboratory findings, not seen for clinical findings; D = decreased for laboratory findings, detected for clinical findings; I = increased; AdoCbl = 5′ deoxyadenosyl cobalamin; MeCbl = methylcobalamin.

nosis of cblC disease has been successfully accomplished with the use of amniocytes, and the diagnosis ruled out with the use of chorionic villus biopsy material and cells.[246,247]

Management. Therapy in cblC disease can be difficult, particularly in the patient with early onset. Many patients with onset in the first month of life die.[203] Many patients have improved with OHCbl therapy, 1 mg per day by injection, by reducing MMA and homocystine excretion. Results from studies of cultured cells[248] and from clinical studies suggest that OHCbl rather than CNCbl should be used.[249] Therapy with MeCbl and AdoCbl has been employed, but it is unclear whether these agents offer a therapeutic advantage. In a detailed study of therapy,[249] the effectiveness of oral OHCbl and systemic OHCbl was compared along with the effect of carnitine, folinic acid, and betaine (250 mg/kg per day). Systemic OHCbl treatment was much more effective than oral therapy, and betaine appeared to be helpful when used in combination with OHCbl. Neither folinic acid nor carnitine had any effect. The result of therapy with daily oral betaine and biweekly injections of OHCbl was a reduction in MMA, normalization of serum methionine and homocysteine concentrations, and resolution of lethargy, irritability, and failure to thrive. However, complete reversal of the neurologic and retinal findings did not occur; this emphasizes the need for early diagnosis and treatment. Even with good metabolic control, surviving patients usually have moderate to severe developmental delay.[191, 203] The prognosis appears to be better in patients with a later age of onset.

The patients with cblF disease appeared to respond to systemic therapy with OHCbl, though the first patient responded to oral Cbl.[242, 244, 245, 250] A theoretic concern in cblF disease is that patients may have accumulation of vitamin B$_{12}$ in lysosomes to an extent that it in itself causes symptoms. The disease has been excluded in twins and in a single pregnancy by the results of studies on amniocytes.

Methylcobalamin Deficiency (cblE and cblG Diseases)

Background. Functional methionine synthase deficiency is characterized by homocystinuria and hypomethioninemia without methylmalonic aciduria. On the basis of complementation analysis, two distinct groups of patients have been identified: those with cblE disease, and those with cblG disease (see Fig. 11–4, Points E and G).

Clinical Syndromes. The patients usually come to medical attention in the first 2 years of life; in one case, however, the patient presented at age 21 years with symptoms that caused her to be diagnosed as having multiple sclerosis. Both males and females have been described as having cblE and cblG diseases, although there is predominance in males in cblE disease.[232] The most common findings in both cblE and cblG diseases included megaloblastic anemia and various neurologic problems, of which developmental delay and cerebral atrophy were the most common.[251] Other findings included electroencephalographic abnormalities, nystagmus, hypotonia, hypertonia, seizures, blindness, and ataxia.

Laboratory Findings. Fibroblasts from both cblE and cblG patients show decreased intracellular levels of MeCbl and normal levels of adenosylmethionine.[252] Total CNCbl uptake and binding to the intracellular enzymes are normal in cblE fibroblasts and in fibroblasts from most cblG patients. In fibroblasts from a minority of cblG patients, binding of labeled Cbl to methionine synthase does not occur.[253] In both cblE and cblG diseases, there is decreased incorporation of methyl-THF, reflecting the functional methionine synthase deficiency. The standard assay for methionine synthase in cell extracts gives activities within the range of controls in cblE patients, but most cblG patients have low methionine synthase activity in cell extracts. In cblE cells, a relative deficiency in methionine synthase activity can be seen when the assay is performed under suboptimal reducing conditions, suggesting that the defect lies in a reducing system associated with methionine synthase.[254, 255] It has been suggested that the defect in cblG disease lies in the interaction of the enzyme with S-adenosylmethionine.[256]

One patient with cblE disease has had transient methylmalonic aciduria.[84] The clinical heterogeneity is evidenced by several patients who did not present for therapy until adulthood. Their disease was mainly neurologic, and the anemia was recognized only later.

Inheritance. The cblE and cblG diseases are thought to be inherited in an autosomal recessive pattern. Decreased MeCbl levels have been seen in obligate heterozygotes for cblE.[257]

Management. Generally, systemic therapy with OHCbl, at first daily and then once or twice weekly, has been used. Usually, therapy with cobalamin results in correction of the anemia and metabolic abnormalities. The neurologic findings have been difficult to reverse, particularly in cblG disease; this stresses the importance of early diagnosis and therapy.

Prenatal diagnosis of cblE disease has been successfully performed in amniocytes, and the mother carrying the affected fetus was treated from the second trimester with systemic vitamin B_{12}.[257] The baby was treated from birth and, throughout the first decade of life, has done very well. It is uncertain, however, whether prenatal therapy is needed.

FOLATE

Nutritional Sources and Requirements

SOURCES

Folate is widespread in food.[2, 258–260] Foods with very high folate content include liver, kidney, orange juice, and spinach.[261–264] In studies of replete adult populations, about one third of the daily folate intake is provided by cereals and bread, another one third by fruits and vegetables, and the remaining one third by meats and fish.[265] Human milk provides enough folate for the infant, but heat-sterilized bovine milk may be inadequate. Goat's milk contains little folate, and children maintained on it alone develop severe folate deficiency.[266]

REQUIREMENTS

Inadequate folate intake is the commonest cause of folate deficiency causing megaloblastic anemia. The reduced folates in food are labile to light and oxidation and are partly destroyed during cooking. The dietary folate requirement is a matter of dispute, but the daily intake recommended by the World Health Organization is listed in Table 11–3. It should be noted, however, that the assay of folate in diets is not standardized and that different results are obtained through the use of different techniques. Within these limits, in populations in which clinical folate deficiency is unusual, mean dietary folate intake has been about 3 μg of total folates per kg of body weight.

TABLE 11–3. Recommended Intake of Folate and Cobalamin*

Age	Folate (μg/kg/day)	Cobalamin (μg/day)
Infants	3.6	0.1
Age 1–16	3.3	
Adults	3.1†	1.0†

*World Health Organization, Food and Agriculture Organization of the United States, 1989.
†For pregnant or lactating women: folate, supplementation with 300–1000 μg/day; cobalamin, 0.3–0.4 μg/day.

This is about 150 μg/d for women and 200 μg/d for men. In such a population, folate levels were measured in 500 liver specimens, most of which were obtained from victims of trauma. The concentrations of hepatic folates appeared to be adequate.[267] In volunteers ingesting diets of known folate content,[268, 269] plasma and erythrocyte folate levels remained within the normal range when intakes were from 150 to 200 μg/d. Intakes of this magnitude were calculated for normal subjects by measurement of a catabolite of folate (p-acetamidobenzoyl glutamate) that is excreted in urine.[270,271]

SUBJECTS WITH INCREASED FOLATE REQUIREMENTS

Although folate deficiency can be recognized through its hematologic effects and the lack of these combined with normal plasma methylmalonic acid and total homocysteine levels interpreted as folate sufficiency, studies linking folate status with neural tube defects and with arteriosclerotic vascular disease (see later) suggest the need to re-examine what is meant by "folate sufficiency." Intakes of folate in excess of those recommended to maintain normal red cell and serum folate levels may be necessary for maximum birth-weight gain, for prevention of neural tube defects, and for reduction of the risk of cardiovascular and cerebrovascular disease. Whether this represents a greater need for folate in the population in general or is restricted to one or more specific subpopulations with altered folate metabolism remains to be determined.

Folate requirements appear greatest per kilogram in the newborn infant and the young child,[55] in pregnant women in whom folate is shunted to the developing fetus and urinary folate loss is increased, and in lactating women who secrete 50 μg or more into each liter of milk. The folate content of milk does not correlate with the level of plasma folate,[272] folate being concentrated in milk above the level of plasma folate. Some milk folate is bound to the folate-binding protein, as described later.

Other groups with greater than normal folate requirements include patients with sprue and other diseases of the small intestine; patients chronically taking antiepileptic medication[273]; women taking the birth control pill[274]; and patients with hemolytic anemia, including those with sickle cell anemia and thalassemia.

Chemistry of Folates

Folates or pteroylglutamates are conjugates of pterin, p-aminobenzoate, and glutamate, and they have a molecular weight of about 450. *Folic acid* is an oxidized folate that is synthesized chemically as a stable yellow powder and sold commercially. It requires reduction to a DHF or THF to function as a coenzyme in cells. Folic acid has a low solubility in aqueous solutions and at acid pH. Reduced folates are photolabile and susceptible to destruction by oxidation. THF is very labile and readily breaks at the carbon 9–nitrogen 10 bond, producing inactive catabolites.[275]

Biochemistry of Folates

Folates bind to and act as coenzymes for enzymes that mediate single-carbon metabolism. They accept and donate single-carbon atoms at different states of oxidation (e.g., formaldehyde, formate, and methyl).[2,275] Folate-dependent enzymes are inactive without their folate cofactors.[276] A scheme of folate metabolism is illustrated in Figure 11–9. The concentrations of folates found within cells are far lower than the affinity constants of most of the folate-dependent enzymes for them.[277-279] Intracellular metabolism would not occur if these affinities were not increased. This appears to depend on the enzyme *folate polyglutamate synthetase*, which converts folates to folate polyglutamates. Almost all intracellular folates in animals and humans are in the form of polyglutamates, which usually contain a total of six or seven glutamates.[279] The affinity of folate polyglutamates for most of these enzymes is much greater than that of folate monoglutamates, and this greater affinity permits intracellular folate-dependent enzyme reactions to occur.

FOLATE-DEPENDENT REACTIONS

Folate (PteGlu) enters cells as folic acid, as 5-methyl-THF, or as 5-formyl-THF. Folic acid is successively reduced to DHF and THF by the enzyme DHF reductase (EC 1.2.1.3.):
Reaction 1

$$PteGlu + H_2 \rightarrow H_2PteGlu + H_2 \rightarrow H_4PteGlu$$

5-Methyl-THF is the predominant folate in plasma and extracellular fluids. It enters cells and gives its CH_3 to homocysteine to form methionine, through the action of the cobalamin-dependent enzyme methionine synthase (see earlier). A decrease in this reaction that is related to cobalamin deficiency or a lack of folate results in increased homocysteine and decreased methionine levels:
Reaction 2

$$5\text{-}CH_3\text{—}H_4PteGlu + homocysteine \rightarrow H_4PteGlu + methionine$$

5-Formyl-THF (folinic acid, leucovorin) is a stable, reduced folate that is available commercially. It also is a natural folate and is converted to 5,10-methenyl-THF by the enzyme 5,10-methenyl-THF synthetase:
Reaction 3

$$5\text{-}CHO\text{—}H_4PteGlu \rightarrow 5,10\text{-}CH{=}H_4PteGlu$$

THF has a central role in folate metabolism, arising from 5-methyl-THF (see above) and from 10-formyl-THF during purine synthesis. It is a principal substrate for the enzyme folate polyglutamate synthetase (EC 6.3.2.17):

Reaction 4

$$H_4PteGlu + Glu \rightarrow H_4PteGlu_n$$

THF polyglutamate accepts a single carbon from serine to become 5,10-methylene-THF polyglutamate through the action of cytosolic and mitochondrial serine hydroxymethyltransferase enzymes (EC 2.1.2.1):
Reaction 5

$$H_4PteGlu_n + serine \rightarrow 5,10\text{-}CH_2\text{—}H_4PteGlu_n + glycine$$

5,10-Methylene-THF polyglutamate has a central regulatory role in folate metabolism through its reaction with thymidylate synthase (dTMP synthase) to form thymidylate and DHF polyglutamate and through the following two reactions[7,8]:
Reaction 6

$$5,10\text{-}CH_2\text{—}H_4PteGlu_n + dUMP \rightarrow H_2PteGlu_n + dTMP$$

5,10-Methylene-THF polyglutamate is converted to 5,10-methenyl-THF polyglutamate and then to 10-for-myl-THF polyglutamate, which is required for purine synthesis by a trifunctional enzyme referred to as C_1 *synthase* (methylene-THF dehydrogenase [EC 1.5.1.5], 5,10-methenyl-THF cyclohydrolase [EC 3.5.4.9], formyl-THF synthetase [EC 6.3.4.4]):
Reaction 7

$$5,10\text{-}CH_2\text{—}H_4PteGlu_n \text{ - } H_2 \rightarrow 5,10\text{-}CH^+\text{—}H_4PteGlu_n \rightarrow 10\text{-}CHO\text{—}H_4PteGlu_n \leftrightarrows H_4PteGlu_n + CHO$$

5,10-Methylene-THF polyglutamate is reduced to 5-methyl-THF polyglutamate by the enzyme methylene-THF reductase. Polymorphism in this gene has been linked to elevated plasma total homocysteine levels and to both arteriosclerotic vascular disease and neural tube birth defects[280,281]:
Reaction 8

$$5,10\text{-}CH_2\text{—}H_4PteGlu_n + H_2 \rightarrow 5\text{-}CH_3\text{—}H_4PteGlu_n$$

10-Formyl-THF polyglutamate is the coenzyme for the bifunctional enzyme phosphoribosylglycinamide (GAR) transformylase (EC 2.1.2.2) and phosphoribosyl-aminoimidazolecarboxamide (AICAR) transformylase (EC 2.1.2.3) involved in purine synthesis:
Reaction 9

$$10\text{-}CHO\text{—}H_4PteGlu_n + GAR \text{ or } AICAR \rightarrow H_4PteGlu_n + CHO\text{-}GAR \text{ or } CHO\text{-}AICAR$$

Histidine catabolism involves a bifunctional enzyme (formimino transferase–cyclodeaminase) that transfers a formimino (FI) group from glutamate to $H_4PteGlu_n$, with its subsequent deamination. Increased urinary excretion of formiminoglutamic acid (FIGlu) is a biochemical feature of folate deficiency. It is not measured frequently because of technical difficulties and lack of specificity.
Reaction 10

$$FIGlu + H_4PteGlu_n \rightarrow FIH_4PteGlu_n + Glu \rightarrow 5,10\text{-}CH^+\text{—}H_4PteGlu_n + NH_3$$

Folate polyglutamates are converted to monoglutamates by the enzyme γ-glutamylhydrolase (EC 3.4.22.12), which is located in lysosomes and in the intestinal brush border.[282, 283] Folate monoglutamates cross cell membranes

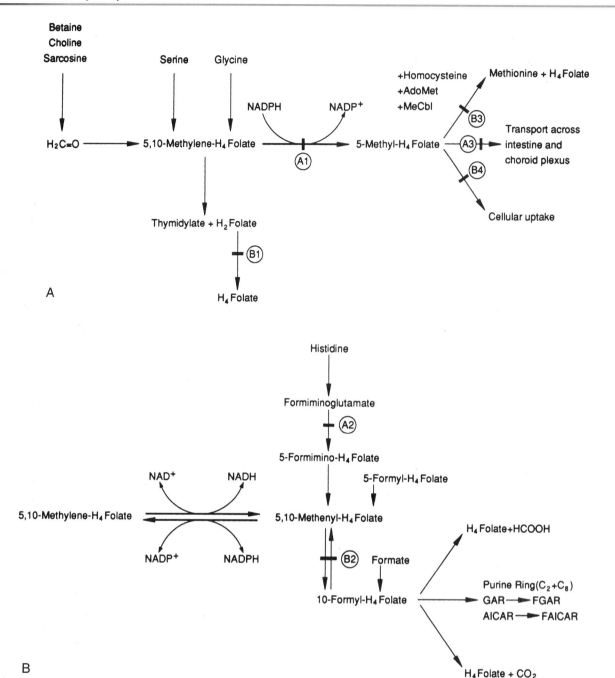

FIGURE 11–9. Folate metabolism. *A,* The generation of methyltetrahydrofolate and its disposition. *B,* The remainder of the folate pathway. The sites of the confirmed (A series) and suspected (B series) inborn errors of folate metabolism and transport are indicated (see text for details). NAD = nicotinamide adenine dinucleotide; NADH = reduced nicotinamide adenine dinucleotide; NADP = nicotinamide adenine dinucleotide phosphate; NADPH = reduced nicotinamide adenine dinucleotide phosphate; GAR = phosphoribosylglycinamide; FGAR = phosphoriboformylglycinamide; AICAR = phosphoribosylaminoimidazolecarboxamide; FAICAR = AICAR + 10-formyltetrahydrofolate.

much better than do polyglutamates, and adequate cellular nutrition is impossible without this hydrolysis.
Reaction 11

$$R\text{-}H_4PteGlu_n \rightarrow R\text{—}H_4PteGlu$$

Physiology of Folates

ABSORPTION OF FOLATES FROM THE GUT

Dietary folates are principally folate polyglutamates. They are hydrolyzed within the gut lumen or brush border or in the lysosomes of enterocytes to folate monoglutamates. The monoglutamates are transported by a carrier-mediated transport system from the proximal small intestine into the portal venous plasma. In addition to this transport system, folate can diffuse across the intestine *in vitro* by unidentified pathways. The saturable system utilizes a folate binder on the enterocyte surface that binds most folate monoglutamates with equal affinity. Transport is affected by pH and sodium transport[284–288] and does not require metabolism of the folate.[289] Folate appears in the portal venous blood within 15 minutes of entering the stomach and reaches a maximum level in portal venous plasma about 1 hour later. Reduced folates, such as 5-formyl-THF, are rapidly converted to 5-methyl-THF during absorption.[290]

Some folates that are presented to the liver, and some hepatic folates, are excreted into the bile and reabsorbed.[2,291,292] This enterohepatic circulation of folates provides a slow and more even absorption than would occur in its absence. There is evidence that the enterohepatic circulation of folates is disturbed by alcohol ingestion (i.e., it occurs more rapidly),[292,293] and this contributes to folate deficiency.[294–296] The efficiency of utilization of folic acid, of folate polyglutamates, and of food folate is variable in different subjects. In general, folate polyglutamates are absorbed about 80% as effectively as are monoglutamates,[297] but food folate availability varies, depending on the diet. Folate absorption from a mixed diet is, on average, about 50% as efficient as absorption of synthetic folic acid—that is, about twice as much folate in food is required as is folic acid.[55, 261]

TRANSPORT OF FOLATES IN PLASMA

Plasma folate consists almost entirely of 5-methyl-THF.[298] It is mostly unbound, although some of it may be bound to albumen. When absorption of food folate ceases, plasma folate decreases rapidly over days, becoming very low within 1 to 2 weeks.[299]

A small amount of plasma folate is bound to a folate-binding protein[300–303] that is homologous or identical to a folate receptor protein present on the surfaces of many cells.[303–305] Plasma folate-binding protein levels are increased in pregnancy, during folate deficiency, in renal failure, in the presence of breast and ovarian cancers, and during some types of inflammation. Its function in plasma is unclear.[306–309] In milk, it may function to improve the utilization of milk folate by the newborn animal.[307, 310, 311]

ENTRY OF FOLATES INTO CELLS

Folates enter cells principally by an anion-coupled, energy-independent, reduced folate carrier that also transports methotrexate, a widely used folate antagonist, but not folic acid. The gene for the human reduced folate carrier (*RFC1*) has been cloned.[311a, 311b] It is located on the long arm of chromosome 21. The reduced folate carrier also is involved in the countertransport of folates from cells.[312–315]

The folate receptor is a 38- to 39-kd glycoprotein attached to the cell membrane via a glycosylphosphatidylinositol anchor. There are three isoforms, two of which have been mapped to the human chromosomal locus 11q13. It binds 5-methyl-THF and folic acid and mediates their entry into cells by a process known as *potocytosis*.[316] The folate receptor increases greatly on the surface of cells grown in very low folate concentrations.[317] The extent of its contribution to total folate uptake by cells is not known. It is not expressed on hematopoietic cells.

Folate Deficiency

Folate deficiency worldwide is extremely prevalent, coexisting with poverty, malnutrition, and chronic parasitic, bacterial, and viral infections. Inadequate diet, overcooking of vegetables with loss of folates, and malabsorption secondary to tropical sprue are important contributors. Additional populations at increased risk in society are the elderly, the very young, and pregnant and lactating mothers. In Europe and North America, significant groups of the population fail to consume 200 µg of folates daily and are at increased risk of being folate deficient. Megaloblastic anemia due to folate deficiency is common worldwide, as is anemia with megaloblastosis in patients with multifactorial malnutrition and ill health. The recent findings of (1) elevated plasma total homocysteine levels in association with cerebral and cardiovascular disease, as well as their reduction with folate supplements; and (2) that a folate supplement in the periconceptual period prevents many cases of neural tube defects (even when given to mothers whose serum and red cell folate levels fall within the normal range) have raised questions about how much folate constitutes dietary sufficiency (see later).

Maternal and Pediatric Folate Deficiency

MATERNAL FOLATE DEFICIENCY

Folate deficiency is common in mothers, particularly where poverty or malnutrition are common and dietary supplements are not provided.[318] It is usually accompanied by iron deficiency. The growing fetus imposes an increased demand for folate, which is often not met by the diet. Increased demand for folates in mothers with thalassemia minor and sickle cell disease increases further the risk of folate deficiency with fullblown megaloblastic anemia. Folate deficiency may also result from malabsorption due to disease of the small intestine. An increased need for folates in the first trimester of pregnancy has been implicated in the occurrence of neural tube defects (anencephaly, sphingomyelocele, and spina bifida) in infants (see later).

DEFICIENCY IN NEWBORNS AND INFANTS

The level of serum folates is higher in cord blood than maternal blood. This means that the fetus is privileged in extracting adequate folate from the mother even in the face of developing maternal folate deficiency. Therefore, clinical folate deficiency is not present at birth. The newborn has increased demands for folate for growth, which must be met by the diet. Maternal milk folate levels remain elevated during development of maternal folate deficiency, but they decrease when deficiency is present. Folate deficiency is common in premature infants unless folate supplements are given.[319] Folate must be added to hyperalimentation solutions given to newborns receiving care in intensive care units. Other factors contributing to increased folate needs are infections or other illnesses. Hemolysis due to vitamin E deficiency or due to enzyme defects, such as glucose-6-phosphate dehydrogenase deficiency, or to rarer red cell enzyme deficiencies, results in an increased demand for folates. Folate absorption is reduced in chronic diarrhea. As mentioned earlier, infants fed goat's milk develop folate deficiency because goat's milk contains almost no folate.[266]

Folate deficiency in infants may not present as classic megaloblastic anemia. Rather, the baby likely will have been transfused, and neutropenia and thrombocytopenia may be the only hematologic features. Where general malnutrition exists, features of folate deficiency may be overshadowed by the clinical picture of marasmus or protein-calorie malnutrition. The increased requirement for growth and the lack of long-term folate stores makes folate deficiency a regular component of starvation. Because folate is stored principally in the liver, hepatitis and other diseases of the liver may disturb stores and precipitate folate deficiency. Inborn errors of folate metabolism are rare but of considerable interest (discussed later).

DEFICIENCY IN OLDER CHILDREN AND ADOLESCENTS

The most common cause of folate deficiency in older children is malnutrition. Some subgroups are particularly at risk because of increased demands, including those with sickle cell disease, thalassemia major, hepatitis, HIV infection, and malabsorption.

Certain drugs and medications predispose to folate deficiency. Alcohol abuse is associated with folate deficiency and affects a proportion of children and adolescents. Antifolate drugs such as triamterene and sulfisoxazole-trimethoprim can inhibit human DHF reductase to some degree and, in the presence of marginal folate stores, induce folate deficiency. Similarly, folate deficiency has been reported in patients taking chronic antiepileptic medication and oral contraceptives.[273,274]

Diagnosis of Folate Deficiency

The diagnosis of folate deficiency is similar to that for cobalamin deficiency. The bone marrow is indistinguishable from that in deficiency of cobalamin, and the same abnormalities may be noted in clinical chemistry data. In most patients who are deficient in folate, serum folate and erythrocyte folate levels are low. The level of serum folate (normal range, 4 to 20 ng/mL [8.8 to 44.0 nmol/L]) decreases rapidly during folate deprivation and falls into the range of deficiency (less than 3 ng/mL [less than 6.6 nmol/L]) within 2 weeks of cessation of folate intake.[299] The erythrocyte folate level decreases slowly (normal, 200 to 800 ng/mL [440 to 1800 nmol/L]) as deficient erythrocytes replace sufficient ones (most deficient subjects have erythrocyte folate values that are less than 150 ng/mL [less than 330 nmol/L]) during the 3 to 4 months' turnover of red cells. In patients who are folate deficient because of poor intake or absorption, both values will usually be in the deficient range. In patients who develop deficiency while taking alcohol, intravenous amino acids, or possibly some antibiotics, serum folate levels are deficient but erythrocyte folate levels may not have decreased out of the range of normal. The level of FIGlu in a 24-hour sample of urine collected in acid following a histidine load is elevated in folate deficiency. This test is infrequently performed today.

Total plasma homocysteine is increased above normal in 80% to 90% of patients with proven deficiency of folate; however, large groups of patients have not yet been studied. The level of methylmalonic acid is normal.[127,320]

The result of the deoxyuridine suppression test with bone marrow cells is abnormal and is corrected by the addition of 5-formyl-THF, 5-methyl-THF, or other folates during the preincubation with deoxyuridine (see earlier; see also Fig. 11–8).

ERYTHROCYTE FOLATE LEVELS IN COBALAMIN DEFICIENCY

Erythroid precursors in the bone marrow accumulate 5-methyl-THF from plasma and convert it to THF by means of the cobalamin-dependent enzyme methionine synthase. THF is converted to THF polyglutamates and retained in mature red cells as 5-methyl-THF polyglutamates. This reaction is impaired in cobalamin-deficient cells, with the result that patients deficient in cobalamin have lower erythrocyte folate levels together with normal or raised serum folate levels.[159] This interpretation of the cause of erythrocyte folate changes in cobalamin deficiency is known as the "methylfolate trap hypothesis."[321]

Treatment of Folate Deficiency

In patients deficient in folate, the diet should be corrected. In those with intestinal disease, 5 mg of folic acid taken daily by mouth (or 100 µg/kg of body weight for children) is sufficient.

Folate deficiency megaloblastic anemia responds to very small doses of folic acid (200 to 500 µg/d). The response provides verification of the diagnosis, because cobalamin deficiency does not respond to such low doses of folate. Daily treatment with 1 mg is more than adequate. However, larger doses are frequently given because folic acid is manufactured in 5-mg tablets. Such treatment is without risk if cobalamin deficiency can be excluded. There is concern that large doses of folate can exacerbate neurologic damage in patients with cobalamin deficiency. Certainly, the diagnosis of megaloblastic anemia can be delayed, with the result that the duration of neurologic damage is extended and the risk of incomplete neurologic recovery increased after the correct diagnosis has been made. In some patients with inborn errors of cobalamin metabolism, neurologic degeneration has appeared during prolonged treatment with folate.[322]

The primary treatment modality for patients with nutritional folate deficiency is correction of the dietary abnormality. For patients with sprue, 5 to 15 mg/d of folate suffice and can be verified by the detection of normal or high serum and erythrocyte folate levels after therapy.

Clinical responses have been reported in a small number of patients with dementia, restless leg syndrome, and other neurologic defects following the administration of large doses of folic acid or folinic acid.[323–325] How common these responses are is unknown.

Folates and Neural Tube Defects

In North America and Europe, the population incidence of neural tube defects (anencephaly, sphingomyelocele, and spina bifida) ranges from 0.6 to 3.7 cases per 1000 live births.[326] Folate deficiency (or insufficiency) in the first trimester of pregnancy has been implicated in the occurrence of neural tube defects in infants.[327] The United Kingdom and the Hungarian studies of recurrent and occurrent neural tube defects, respectively, confirmed the findings of earlier and later studies and proved that a folate supplement taken in the periconceptual period (to include the time from initiation of pregnancy to that of closure of the neural tube at about 1 month of gestation) reduced the incidence of neural tube defects by 50% to 70%.[36,37] Both folate and cobalamin status have been implicated in the causation of neural tube defects.[328] The incidence of neural tube defects was inversely correlated with the red cell folate level.[329] Until it is determined who is at particular risk in the population, perhaps by maternal total plasma homocysteine level or methylene-THF reductase polymorphism status,[281,330,331] the problem of how to provide adequate folate to mothers planning a pregnancy remains. Folate supplements are the most effective way to deliver folate, but half of all pregnancies are unplanned. Fortifying the diet (e.g., by adding folate to wheat) to increase the mean folate intake of the population has been recommended.[332] The Food and Drug Administration has recommended that folate be added to prepared foods in sufficient amounts to provide an additional intake of 150 to 200 µg/d of folate. This supplementation is likely to be more effective in improving folate nutriture in the population than would the consumption of a diet higher in natural folates.[333]

Folates and Arteriosclerotic Vascular Disease

In addition to known major risk factors for the development of atherosclerotic vascular disease involving peripheral, coronary, and cerebral arteries, such as increased serum cholesterol and low-density lipoprotein levels, the premature occurrence of arteriosclerosis in patients with severe homocystinuria has suggested that an elevated plasma homocysteine might be an atherogenic factor.[334] Subsequently, a thermolabile (at 46°C) variant of methylene-THF reductase was described and found to be associated with higher plasma homocysteine concentration and with the development of atherosclerotic vascular disease.[335] A polymorphism involving an alanine-to-valine substitution in methylene-THF reductase correlates with reduced enzyme activity and increased thermolability; individuals homozygous for the polymorphism have significantly elevated plasma homocysteine levels[280] (Fig. 11–10). Being a heterozygosity for cystathionine β-synthase may account for a small number of cases of elevated plasma homocysteine as well.[38] Treatment of subjects with elevated total plasma homocysteine levels with either vitamin B_6 or folic acid or, occasionally, betaine normalizes the homocysteine level.[336] It appears likely that such therapy can prevent recurrent or occurrent arteriosclerotic disease.[337] In fact, a recent review of the Framingham Heart Study population shows a strong correlation between plasma homocysteinemia levels, carotid stenosis, and low folate levels.[337a]

Folates and Cancer

A number of epidemiologic studies suggest an association between folate deficiency and premalignant changes in sev-

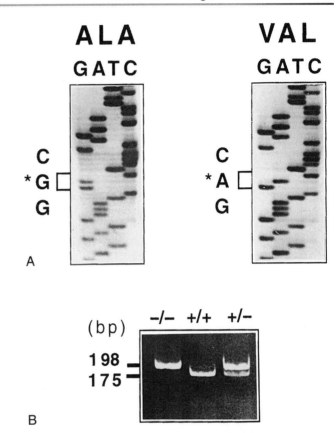

FIGURE 11–10. Sequence change and restriction enzyme analysis for the alanine (ALA)-to-valine (VAL) substitution in methylenetetrahydrofolate reductase. *A,* Sequence of two individuals, a homozygote for the alanine residue and a homozygote for the valine residue. The antisense strands are depicted. The primers for analysis of the A→V change are: 5'-TGAAGGAGAA GGTGTCTGCGGGA-3' (exonic) and 5'-AGGACG-GTGC GGTGAGAGTG-3' (intronic); these primers generate a fragment of 198 bp. *B,* The substitution creates a *Hin*F1 recognition sequence, which digests the 198-bp fragment into 175- and 23-bp fragments; the latter fragment has been run off the gel. All three possible genotypes are shown. (From Frosst P, Blom HJ, et al: A candidate genetic risk factor for vascular disease: A common methylenetetrahydrofolate reductase mutation causes thermoinstability. Nat Genet 1995; 10:111.)

eral epithelial tissues, including the cervix,[338] bronchus,[339] and colon.[39] Some of these studies have demonstrated an apparent reversal of the pathologic lesions with folate supplementation. However, difficulty in differentiating between megaloblastic and dysplastic changes tends to confound these results. A causal relationship between folate deficiency and the development of colon cancer has been established by comparison of folate-deficient and folate-replete rats fed the carcinogen dimethylhydrazine.[340]

Ribofolate Peptide

A thymic factor that stimulates DNA synthesis of immature thymocytes has been found to recruit G1-phase cells synchronously into the S phase, thereby functioning as a progression growth factor.[341] This thymic growth peptide consists of a formyl pteroyl group bound to the N-terminal glutamyl of a nonapeptide. The pterin part of the thymic growth peptide molecule has a ribitol substituent, in analogy with riboflavin.[342] This represents a novel folate structure with unexpected properties.

Folate Antimetabolites

Antifolates are analogues of folic acid that block folate metabolism, interrupting DNA synthesis and causing cell death. They inhibit the enzyme DHF reductase as the primary target.

Methotrexate is an effective anticancer agent widely used in combination chemotherapy of carcinomas of the breast, lung, bone, ovary, and head and neck, as well as of other cancers. It contributes to cure of chorio-carcinoma and childhood acute lymphoblastic leukemia. Methotrexate is also used for its immunosuppressive and antiproliferative properties in the treatment of psoriasis, rheumatoid arthritis, and graft-versus-host disease following bone marrow transplanation.

Pyrimethamine is an antimalarial drug having greater affinity for parasitic than human DHF reductase. Trimethoprim is another antifolate with antibacterial activity and a higher affinity for bacterial than human DHF reductase. It is combined with sulfisoxazole, a sulfa drug that interferes with bacterial synthesis of folic acid, to deliver a double-dose synergistic antifolate attack on bacteria. Bactrim and Septra are such combinations widely used to treat urinary tract and other infections. They are also used to prevent *Pneumocystis carinii* pneumonia in immunocompromised patients receiving chemotherapy or in persons infected with HIV.

Newer antifolates have been synthesized and tested for the past 40 years. Currently, trimetrexate and piritrexim are two lipid-soluble antifolates that enter cells by transport routes different from those used by methotrexate. Trimetrexate appears to be useful against *P. carinii*; this is because host toxicity can be prevented with leucovorin, whereas *P. carinii* is unable to take up this folate. A series of novel antifolates that specifically inhibit thymidylate synthesis are being developed in Great Britain. The prototype, CB3717, has been proved toxic to the liver and kidneys. Newer analogues, including D-1694,[343] do not seem to be so toxic. Dideaza-THF is a new antifolate that specifically inhibits GAR transformylase, a folate-requiring enzyme involved in purine synthesis.[344]

RESISTANCE TO METHOTREXATE

Cancer and leukemia cells develop resistance to methotrexate in a variety of ways, including the following[345]:

1. Diminished transport of methotrexate (and of reduced folates) into the cell
2. Amplification of the DHF reductase gene, with overproduction of DHF reductase
3. Mutations of the DHF reductase gene resulting in a DHF reductase, with decreased binding affinity for methotrexate
4. Decreased folate polyglutamate synthetase activity, with diminished polyglutamylation of methotrexate
5. Increased γ-glutamyl hydrolase activity, with decreased retention of methotrexate polyglutamates

Inborn Errors of Folate Metabolism and Transport

METHYLENETETRAHYDROFOLATE REDUCTASE DEFICIENCY

Description. Methylene-THF reductase deficiency is the most common inborn error of folate metabolism, with more than 40 cases being recognized[26, 346] (Table 11–4). It is not associated with megaloblastic anemia because the block is in the conversion of methylene-THF to methyl-THF. There is no "trapping" of folates as methyl-THF, and reduced folates are available for purine and pyrimidine metabolism. Since methyl-THF serves as a methyl donor for the conversion of homocysteine to methionine, methylene-THF reductase deficiency results in elevated homocysteine levels and decreased levels of methionine (see Fig. 11–9, Point A1).

Clinical Syndromes. This disorder may be diagnosed at any time from infancy to adulthood, and clinically asymptomatic but biochemically affected individuals have been reported.[27, 347] In general, clinical severity is related to the proportion of methyl-THF in cells. Most of the patients are brought to medical attention in infancy, with the most common clinical manifestation being developmental delay. Most of the patients have been diagnosed during the first year of life. Breathing disorders, seizures, and microcephaly are often present, and motor and gait abnormalities and psychiatric manifestations have been reported. The report of two patients with schizophrenia and methylene-THF reductase deficiency leads to speculation on the role of methylene-THF reductase deficiency in psychiatric disease.[348, 349]

Laboratory Investigation. Homocystinuria is seen in all patients, with homocystine level ranging from 15 to 667 μmol per 24 hours[350] and having a mean of 130 μmol per 24 hours. These values are much lower than those found in homocystinuria due to cystathionine synthase deficiency. If methylene-THF reductase deficiency is suspected, more than one determination of homocystine excretion should be performed to eliminate the possibility of a false-negative value. Recently, there has been interest in measurements of both protein-bound and total homocysteine. These measurements are performed by treating plasma or serum with reducing agents to free the homocysteine from proteins to which it is bound. These measurements have defined several patients[351] with elevated levels of homocysteine and an increased risk for cardiovascular disease.[335, 352] Measurement of methylene-THF reductase in cell extracts has revealed unusual thermolability, and the term "intermediate homocystinuria"[351] has been coined. These patients were adults without the usual manifestations of methylene-THF reductase deficiency—in particular, the absence of neurologic manifestations. An alanine-to-valine substitution in a conserved residue of the methylene-THF reductase gene on chromosome 1 has been identified as the polymorphism associated with both thermolability and susceptibility to cardiovascular disease.[280]

Plasma methionine levels have been found to be low in this deficiency. Values ranged from 0 to 18 μmol/L (mean, 12 μmol/L)[350]; normal fasting plasma methionine levels

TABLE 11–4. Inherited Defects of Folate Metabolism

	Hereditary Folate Malabsorption	Methylenetetrahydrofolate Reductase Deficiency	Glutamate Formimino transferase Deficiency
CLINICAL FINDINGS			
Prevalence	*15 cases*	*>25 cases*	*13 cases*
Megaloblastic anemia	A	N	N*
Developmental delay	A	A	N*
Seizures	A	A	N*
Speech abnormalities	N	N	A*
Gait abnormalities*	N	A	N*
Peripheral neuropathy	N	A	N*
Apnea	N	A	N*
BIOCHEMICAL FINDINGS			
Homocystinuria(emia)	N	A	N
Hypomethioninemia	N	A	N
Formiminoglutamic aciduria	A*	N	A
Folate absorption	A	N	N
Serum folate	A	A	N*
Red cell folate	A	A*	N*
DEFECTS DETECTABLE IN CULTURED FIBROBLASTS			
Whole cells			
CH$_3$-H$_4$PteGlu uptake	N	N	N
CH$_3$-H$_4$PteGlu content	N	A	N
Extracts			
Glutamate formiminotranferase	*Activity undetectable in cultured fibroblasts*		
?Abnormal in liver and erythrocytes			
Methylene-H$_4$PteGlu reductase	N	A	N

*Exceptions described in some cases.

N = normal; A = abnormal (i.e., clinical findings or laboratory findings present); PteGlu = folate.

are usually in the range of 23 to 35 μmol/L. Neurotransmitter levels have been measured in the cerebrospinal fluid of only a few patients, and they usually have been low.[350] The diagnosis of methylene-THF reductase deficiency has been confirmed by direct measurement of enzyme activity in the liver, leukocytes, and cultured fibroblasts and lymphocytes. The specific activity of methylene-THF reductase in cultured fibroblasts is dependent on the stage of the culture cycle, being several-fold greater at confluence than during logarithmic growth. It is important to compare activities of unknown samples and control cell lines at confluence. A rough correlation exists between residual enzyme activity and the clinical severity.[353] In cultured fibroblasts, the proportion of total folate that is methyl-THF and the extent of labeled formate incorporated into methionine provide better correlations with clinical severity.[353, 354] Cultured fibroblasts from patients with methylene-THF reductase deficiency do not grow on tissue culture medium in which homocysteine replaces methionine.[355, 356] This methionine auxotrophy is shared by the inborn errors of vitamin B$_{12}$ metabolism that affect methionine synthase activity (cblC, cblD, cblE, cblF, and cblG diseases). The clinical heterogeneity in methylene-THF reductase deficiency is reflected at the biochemical level. Enzyme from fibroblasts of the first reported case of methylene-THF reductase deficiency had increased thermolability compared with control enzyme, especially when the assay was performed in the presence of the cofactor flavin-adenine din-

ucleotide.[356] As already discussed, studies have demonstrated increased thermolability in enzyme from adults who have been detected on the basis of increased total plasma homocysteine levels or of plasma protein-bound homocysteine levels. The patients were detected during screening of either patients with coronary heart disease or those with low folate and cobalamin levels. These patients had none of the other manifestations of methylene-THF reductase deficiency.

Autopsy Findings. The findings at autopsy in methylene-THF reductase deficiency[357–364] include dilation of cerebral vessels, internal hydrocephalus, and microgyria. Perivascular changes, demyelination, macrophage infiltration, gliosis, and astrocytosis have been reported. The major factor in the death of some patients was thrombosis, both of arteries and of cerebral veins.[357] The neurovascular findings in methylene-THF reductase deficiency are not dissimilar to those seen in classic homocystinuria due to cystathionine synthase deficiency. Two reports of patients with classic findings of subacute combined degeneration of the spinal cord similar to that described for vitamin B$_{12}$ deficiency have been published.[363,364] Methionine deficiency may cause demyelination by interfering with methylation. Because methylene-THF reductase is present in the mammalian brain, and since only methyl-THF can cross the blood-brain barrier, methylene-THF reductase deficiency may result in functionally low levels of folate in the brain. Because neurologic findings in methylene-THF reductase deficiency may be present in the absence of low methionine levels, it is possible that they are due to impaired purine and pyrimidine synthesis, as opposed to methionine depletion. Also, because methylene-THF reductase has dihydropteridine reductase activity,[365] it may have a direct role in neurotransmitter synthesis. Whether most of the neuropathologic disorder arises from decreased methionine levels, elevated homocysteine levels, or the effects of low folate level other than the methylation of homocysteine to methionine has not been resolved.

Inheritance and Prenatal Diagnosis. More than one case have been reported in several families. Both affected males and females have been born to unaffected parents, and consanguinity has been reported. Methylene-THF reductase deficiency shows autosomal recessive inheritance. Phenotypic heterogeneity is associated with genotypic heterogeneity, and at least nine different mutations are known.[366, 367] Prenatal diagnosis has been reported using amniocytes,[368] and the enzyme is present in chorionic villi.

Treatment. This disease has been very difficult to treat, and the prognosis is poor once evidence of neurologic involvement has been detected. Therefore, it is important to diagnose methylene-THF reductase deficiency as early as possible. The following agents have been used for therapy:

1. Folates, to maximize any residual enzyme activity
2. Methyl-THF, to replace specifically the missing product of methylene-THF reductase
3. Methionine, to correct the deficiency of this amino acid, which requires methyl-THF for synthesis
4. Pyridoxine, because it is a cofactor for cystathionine synthase and thus may lower homocysteine levels
5. Vitamin B_{12}, because MeCbl is a cofactor for methionine synthase
6. Carnitine, because of its requirement for adenosylmethionine
7. Betaine, because it—along with homocysteine—is a substrate for betaine methyltransferase, an enzyme that also converts homocysteine to methionine but which is primarily active in the liver.

Betaine has the advantage of both raising methionine levels and decreasing homocysteine levels. It is to be noted, however, that because betaine methyltransferase is a liver enzyme, the effects of betaine on the brain are thought to be mediated through changes in circulating levels of metabolites. A summary of the treatment protocols for the individual patients with methylene-THF reductase deficiency has been published.[350] These protocols have been highly variable and, for the most part, unsuccessful until the introduction of betaine. Therapy either with methionine alone or with methyl-THF has not been effective. The authors[369] have suggested a regimen consisting of oral betaine, folinic acid, vitamin B_{12}, and vitamin B_6. Therapy with betaine following prenatal diagnosis has resulted in the best outcome reported to date.[370]

GLUTAMATE FORMIMINOTRANSFERASE DEFICIENCY

Clinical Syndromes. It is still uncertain whether glutamate formiminotransferase deficiency (GFD) is associated with any consistent clinical findings. Only 13 patients have been described. Formiminoglutamate (FIGlu) excretion is the one constant feature of GFD. Patients with GFD range in age from 3 months to 42 years at diagnosis. Several patients had macrocytosis and hypersegmentation of neutrophils. Three patients had delayed speech, two had seizures, and two had mental retardation as their presenting signs. Two patients were studied because they were siblings of known patients. Mental retardation was described in the majority of the original patients from Japan,[371] but only three of the remaining eight patients showed mental retardation.

A mild phenotype and a severe phenotype have been described. The severe form of GFD is characterized by mental and physical retardation, abnormal electroencephalographic activity, and dilatation of the cerebral ventricles with cortical atrophy. No mental retardation occurs in the mild form, but excretion of FIGlu is greater. It has been proposed,[372] without direct enzyme measurements, that the mild form is due to a defect in the formiminotransferase enzyme, whereas the severe form results from a block in the cyclodeaminase enzyme.

Laboratory Investigation. The catabolism of histidine is associated with the transfer of a formimino group to THF, followed by the release of ammonia and the formation of 5,10-methenyl-THF (see Fig. 11–9, Point A2). Glutamate formiminotransferase and formimino-THF cyclodeaminase, two activities that share a single octameric enzyme, are involved in these reactions. These activities are found only in the liver and kidneys, and defects in these activities result in the excretion of FIGlu.

In most cases in which enzyme activity in the liver has been examined, it was higher than would be expected for an enzymatic block causing disease. This activity, measured in five patients, ranged from 14% to 54% of control values. Because the enzyme activity is expressed in the liver only, it has not been possible to confirm the diagnosis of GFD through the use of cultured cells. There has also been considerable debate as to whether the enzyme is expressed in erythrocytes.[350, 373]

Elevated FIGlu excretion as well as increased FIGlu levels in the blood following histidine load, as well as high to normal serum folate levels, have been reported in GFD. Amino acid levels, including those of histidine, were usually normal in the plasma; however, hyperhistidinemia and hyperhistidinuria have been found on occasion, as have low plasma methionine levels. The excretion of two other metabolites—hydantoin-5-propionate, the stable oxidation product of the FIGlu precursor 4-imidazolone-5-propionate; and 4-amino-5-imidazolecarboxamide, an intermediate in purine synthesis—has also been reported.

Inheritance. Offspring of both sexes with unaffected parents have been reported; however, neither enzyme levels in the livers of the parents nor reports of consanguinity have been published. Autosomal recessive inheritance is the probable means of transmission. Because GFD is not expressed in cultured cells, definitive understanding of the genetics of this disorder awaits the cloning of the gene and the localization of the molecular defect.

Treatment. Two patients in one family[374] responded with decreased FIGlu excretion to therapy with folates, whereas six other patients did not.[350] One of two patients responded to methionine supplementation.[375, 376] As the relationship between clinical expression and FIGlu excretion has not been easy to define, it is uncertain whether reducing FIGlu excretion is of any value.

HEREDITARY FOLATE MALABSORPTION

Clinical and Laboratory Studies. Megaloblastic anemia, diarrhea, mouth ulcers, failure to thrive, and usually progressive neurologic deterioration characterize hereditary folate malabsorption (HFM). Fifteen patients with HFM have been reported, 12 of whom were females.[322,377] Megaloblastic anemia in the first few months of life associated with low serum folate levels is the most important diagnostic feature.

FIGlu and orotic acid excretion may be found in patients with HFM. All patients have a severe abnormality in the absorption of oral folic acid or of reduced folates. The patients with HFM provide the best evidence for a specific transport system of folates across both the intestine and the choroid plexus (see Fig 11–9, Point A3). Even when blood folate levels are raised sufficiently to correct the anemia, levels in the cerebrospinal fluid may remain low.[378] This provides evidence that the carrier system in both the intestine and the brain is coded by a single gene product. The uptake of folate into other cells is probably not defective in HFM, and uptake of folate into cultured cells is not abnormal. The hematologic findings are reversed by relatively low levels of folate.

Management. The clinical response to therapy with folates has varied among patients. Oral administration of folate in pharmacologic doses did elicit a therapeutic response in some patients through correction of the hematologic abnormality. Parenterally administered folates have been effective in reversing the anemia but have been less effective in correcting the low level of folate in the cerebrospinal fluid. Folinic acid or methyltetrahydrofolic acid may be more effective in entering the cerebrospinal fluid in HFM. In some cases, seizures were reduced in number, and in others, seizures worsened with folate therapy.[322, 379]

In treating these patients, it is essential to maintain levels of folate in the blood and in the cerebrospinal fluid in the range that is associated with folate sufficiency. Oral doses of folates may be increased to 100 mg or more daily if necessary; if oral therapy is not effective, systemic therapy must be instituted. It may be necessary to give intrathecal folate if cerebrospinal fluid levels cannot be normalized. As mentioned previously, it is thought that the reduced folates, such as folinic acid and methyl-THF, may be more effective than folic acid in treating HFM.

Inheritance. All but three of the 15 HFM patients have been female. One male had atypical clinical findings, including a lack of mental retardation and correction of cerebrospinal fluid folate levels in conjunction with correction of serum folate levels.[380] Cases of HFM may have gone unrecognized, as several of the patients had siblings who died. Consanguinity has been reported in four families, and the father of one patient has intermediate levels of folate absorption. This makes autosomal recessive inheritance probable. The need to explain the preponderance of this disorder among females remains.

CELLULAR UPTAKE DEFECTS

A series of patients with well-characterized abnormalities of folate uptake into cells have been described (see Fig. 10–9, Point B4). It remains unclear whether any of these abnormalities represent primary defects.

In one large family,[381, 382] the prevalence of severe hematologic disease was very high, with the disorders including anemia, pancytopenia, and leukemia in 34 individuals that resulted in the death of 18. The proband had severe aplastic anemia that responded to folate therapy. The uptake of methyl-THF was markedly reduced, despite the normal uptake of folic acid in stimulated lymphocytes from the proband and from four family members. The proband and his son also had a lesser reduction of methyl-THF uptake in bone marrow cells. One son only developed the transport defect after becoming neutropenic, suggesting that the abnormality may not be the primary defect. In another family, the proband and three daughters had dyserythropoiesis without anemia.[383] An abnormality of methyl-THF uptake was detected in red cells and bone marrow cells but not in lymphocytes. There was no clear correlation in the family between the clinical findings and the disorder of cellular uptake.

OTHER POSSIBLE INBORN ERRORS OF FOLATE METABOLISM

Individual cases suggesting defects in the function of DHF reductase (see Fig. 11–9, Point B1), the synthesis of 10-formyl-THF (see Fig. 11–9, Point B2), and methionine synthase (see Fig. 11–9, Point B3) are insufficiently documented for comment at the present time.

Thiamine-Responsive Megaloblastic Anemia

Thiamine-responsive megaloblastic anemia with deafness and diabetes (TRMA) is a rare autosomal recessive disorder of thiamine transport now known to be due to mutations in a gene on chromosome 1q23 encoding a high-affinity thiamine transporter.[384–388]

REFERENCES

1. Minot GR, Murphy WP: Treatment of pernicious anemia by special diet. JAMA 1926; 87:470.
2. Chanarin I: The Megaloblastic Anaemias. London, Blackwell Scientific Publications, 1979.
3. Wintrobe MM: Hematology, the Blossoming of a Science: A Story of Inspiration and Effort. Philadelphia, Lea & Febiger, 1985.
4. Castle WB: The conquest of pernicious anemia. In Wintrobe MM (ed): Blood, Pure and Eloquent. New York, McGraw-Hill Book Co., 1979, pp 283–318.
5. Ehrlich P: Untersuchungen zur Histologie und Klinik des Blutes. Berlin, Hirschwald, 1891.
6. Chanarin I: The Megaloblastic Anaemias. London, Blackwell Scientific Publications, 1979, pp 329–340.
7. Wills L: Treatment of "pernicious anaemia of pregnancy" and "tropical anaemia" with special reference to yeast extract as curative agent. BMJ 1931; 1:1059.
8. Fenwick S: On atrophy of the stomach. Lancet 1870; 2:78.
9. Castle WB: Observations on the etiologic relationship of achylia gastrica to pernicious anemia. I. The effect of administration to patients with pernicious anemia of the contents of the normal human stomach recovered after ingestion of beef muscle. Am J Med Sci 1929; 178:748.

10. Cooper BA, Castle WB: Sequential mechanisms in the enhanced absorption of vitamin B_{12} by intrinsic factor in the rat. J Clin Invest 1960; 39:199.

11. Ungley CC: Vitamin B_{12} in pernicious anaemia. Parenteral administration. BMJ 1949; 2:1370.

12. Zalusky R, Herbert V, Castle WB: Cyanocobalamin therapy effect in folic acid deficiency. Arch Intern Med 1962; 109:545.

13. Hall BE, Watkins CH: Experience with pteroylglutamate synthetic folic acid in treatment of pernicious anemia. J Lab Clin Med 1947; 32:622.

14. Youngdahl-Turner P, Rosenberg LE: Binding and uptake of transcobalamin II by human fibroblasts. J Clin Invest 1978; 61:133.

15. Cooper BA, Paranchych W: Selective uptake of specifically-bound cobalt-58 vitamin B_{12} by human and mouse tumour cells. Nature 1961; 191:393.

16. Mollin DL, Ross GIM: The vitamin B_{12} concentrations of serum and urine of normals and of patients with megaloblastic anaemias and other diseases. J Clin Pathol 1952; 5:129.

17. Gottlieb CW, Lau K-S, et al: Rapid charcoal assay for intrinsic factor (IF), gastric juice unsaturated binding capacity, antibody to IF, and serum unsaturated binding capacity. Blood 1965; 25:875.

18. Adams JF, Tankel HI, Macewan F: Estimation of the total body vitamin B_{12} in the live subject. Clin Sci 1970; 39:107.

19. Russell JSR, Batten FE, Collier J: Subacute combined degeneration of the spinal cord. Brain 1900; 23:39.

20. Jeffries GH, Hoskins DW, Sleisinger MH: Antibody to intrinsic factor in serum of patients with pernicious anemia. J Clin Invest 1962; 41:1106.

21. Dow CA, Aizpura HJ, et al: 65–70kd protein identified by immunoblotting as the presumptive gastric microsomal autoantigen in pernicious anaemia. Clin Exp Immunol 1985; 62:732.

22. Aizpura HJ, Ungar B, Toh B-H: Autoantibody to the gastric receptor in pernicious anaemia. N Engl J Med 1985; 313:479.

23. Burman P, Måardh S, et al: Parietal cell antibodies in pernicious anemia inhibit H^+, K^+-adenosine triphosphatase, the proton pump of the stomach. Gastroenterology 1989; 96:1434.

24. Hakami N, Nieman PE, et al: Neonatal megaloblastic anemia due to inherited transcobalamin II deficiency in two siblings. N Engl J Med 1971; 285:1163.

25. Levy HL, Mudd SH, et al: A derangement in B_{12} metabolism associated with homocystinemia, cystathioninemia, hypomethioninemia and methylmalonic aciduria. Am J Med 1970; 48:390.

26. Erbe RW: Inborn errors of folate metabolism. In: Blakley RL, Whitehead VM (eds): Folates and Pterins: Nutritional, Pharmacological and Physiological Aspects. Vol 3. New York, John Wiley & Sons, 1986, pp 413–466.

27. Marquet J, Chadefaux B, et al: Methylenetetrahydrofolate reductase deficiency: prenatal diagnosis and family studies. Prenatal Diagn 1994; 14:29.

28. Platica O, Geneczko R, et al: Isolation of the complementary DNA for human transcobalamin II. Proc Soc Exp Biol Med 1989; 192:95.

29. Johnston J, Bollekens J, et al: Structure of the cDNA encoding transcobalamin I, a neutrophil granule protein. J Biol Chem 1989; 264:15754.

30. Hansen MR, Nexo E, et al: Human intrinsic factor. Its primary structure compared to the primary structure of rat intrinsic factor. Scand J Clin Lab Invest 1989; 49(Suppl 194):19.

31. Gueant JL, Jokinen O, et al: Purification of intrinsic factor receptor from pig ileum using as affinity medium human intrinsic factor covalently bound to Sepharose. Biochim Biophys Acta 1989; 992:281.

32. Dieckgraefe BK, Seetharam B, et al: Isolation and structural characterization of a cDNA clone encoding rat gastric intrinsic factor. Proc Natl Acad Sci U S A 1988; 85:46.

33. Gräsbeck R, Simons K, Sinkkonen I: Isolation of intrinsic factor and its probable degradation product, as their vitamin B_{12} complexes, from human gastric juice. Biochim Biophys Acta 1968; 158:292.

34. Chen P, Ailion M, et al: The end of the *cob* operon: evidence that the last gene (*cob T*) catalyses synthesis of the lower ligand of vitamin B_{12}, dimethylbenzimidazole. J Bacteriol 1995; 177:1461.

35. Savage DG, Lindenbaum J, et al: Sensitivity of serum methylmalonic acid and total homocysteine determinations for diagnosing cobalamin and folate deficiencies. Am J Med 1994; 96:239.

36. MRC Vitamin Study Research Group: Prevention of neural tube defects: results of the Medical Research Council Vitamin Study. Lancet 1991; 338:131.

37. Czeizel AE, Dudas I: Prevention of the first occurrence of neural-tube defects by periconceptional vitamin supplementation. N Engl J Med 1992; 327:1832.

38. Dudman NP, Wilcken DE, et al: Disordered methionine/homocysteine metabolism in premature vascular disease. Its occurrence, cofactor therapy, and enzymology. Arterioscler Thromb 1993; 13:1253.

39. Lashner BA, Heidenreich PA, et al: The effect of folate supplementation on the incidence of dysplasia and cancer in chronic ulcerative colitis: a case control study. Gastroenterology 1989; 97:255.

40. Finch CA, Coleman DH, et al: Erythrokinetics in pernicious anemia. Blood 1956; 11:807.

41. London IM, West R: The formation of bile pigments in pernicious anemia. J Biol Chem 1950; 184:359.

42. Glazer HS, Mueller JF, et al: Effect of vitamin B_{12} and folic acid on nucleic acid composition of bone marrow of patients with megaloblastic anemia. J Lab Clin Med 1954; 43:905.

43. Nath BJ, Lindenbaum J: Persistence of neutrophil hypersegmentation during recovery from megaloblastic granulopoiesis. Ann Intern Med 1979; 90:757.

44. Chanarin I: The Megaloblastic Anaemias. London, Blackwell Scientific Publications, 1979, pp 225–226.

45. Mitchell K, Ferguson MM, et al: Epithelial dysplasia in the oral mucosa associated with pernicious anaemia. Br Dent J 1986; 161:259.

46. Levine AS, Doscherholmen A: Vitamin B_{12} bioavailability from egg yolk and egg white: relationship to binding proteins. Am J Clin Nutr 1983; 38:436.

47. Doscherholmen A, McMahon J, Economon P: Vitamin B_{12} absorption from fish. Proc Soc Exp Biol Med 1981; 167:480.

48. Bakker HD, van Gennip AH, et al: Methylmalonate excretion in a pregnancy at risk for methylmalonic acidaemia. Clin Chim Acta 1978; 86:349.

49. Baker SJ, Mathan VI: Evidence regarding the minimal daily requirement of dietary vitamin B_{12}. Am J Clin Nutr 1981; 34:2423.

50. Roberts RD, Webb JKG, et al: Vitamin B_{12} deficiency in Indian infants. BMJ 1973; 3:67.

51. Banerjee DK, Chatterjea JB: Vitamin B_{12} content of some articles of Indian diets and effect of cooking on it. Br J Nutr 1963; 17:385.

52. Chanarin I, Stephenson E: Vegetarian diet and cobalamin deficiency: their association with tuberculosis. J Clin Pathol 1988; 41:759.

53. Armstrong BK, Davis RE, et al: Hematological vitamin B_{12} and folate studies on seventh day-adventist vegetarians. Am J Clin Nutr 1974; 27:712.

54. Abdulla M, Anderson I, et al: Nutrient uptake and health status of vegans. Chemical analyses of diets using the duplicate portion sampling technique. Am J Clin Nutr 1981; 34:2464.

55. Beaton G: Requirements of Vitamin A, Iron, Folate and Vitamin B_{12}: Report of a Joint FAO/WHO Expert Consultation. Rome, Food and Agriculture Organization of the United Nations, 1988.

56. Dolphin D: B_{12}: Chemistry. Vol. 1. New York, John Wiley & Sons, 1982.

57. Pratt JM: Inorganic Chemistry of Vitamin B_{12}. New York, Academic Press, 1972.

58. Hogenkamp HPC: The chemistry of cobalamins and related compounds. In Babior BM (ed): Cobalamin: Biochemistry and Pathophysiology. New York, Wiley-Interscience, 1975, pp 21–74.

59. Taylor RT: B_{12}-dependent methionine biosynthesis. In Dolphin D (ed): B_{12}: Biochemistry and Medicine. Vol 2. New York, John Wiley & Sons, 1982, pp 307–355.

60. Utley CS, Marcell PD, et al: Isolation and characterization of methionine synthetase from human placenta. J Biol Chem 1985; 260:13656.

61. Retey J: Methylmalonyl-CoA mutase. In Dolphin D (ed): B_{12}: Biochemistry and Medicine. Vol 2. New York, John Wiley & Sons, 1982, pp 357–380.

62. Kolhouse JF, Utley C, et al: Immunochemical studies on cultured fibroblasts from patients with inherited methylmalonic acidemia. Proc Natl Acad Sci U S A 1981; 78:7737.

63. Ledley FD, Lumetta M, et al: Molecular cloning of L-methylmalonyl-CoA mutase: gene transfer and analysis of mut cell lines. Proc Natl Acad Sci U S A 1988; 85:3518.

64. Marsh EN, McKie N, et al: Cloning and structural characterization of the genes coding for adenosylcobalamin-dependent methylmalonyl-CoA mutase from *Propionibacterium shermanii*. Biochem J 1989; 260:345.

65. Cameron B, Briggs K, et al: Cloning and analysis of genes involved in coenzyme-B_{12} biosynthesis in *Pseudomonas denitrificans*. J Bacteriol 1989; 171:547.

66. Ledley FD, Lumetta MR, et al: Mapping of human methylmalonyl CoA mutase (MUT) locus on chromosome 6. Am J Hum Genet 1988; 42:839.

67. Fenton WA, Hack AM, et al: Biogenesis of the mitochondrial enzyme methylmalonyl-CoA mutase: synthesis and processing of a precursor in a cell-free system and in cultured cells. J Biol Chem 1984; 259:6616.

68. Barness LA, Morrow G 3d: Methylmalonic aciduria. A newly discovered inborn error. Ann Intern Med 1968; 69:633.

69. Morrow G 3d, Revsin B, et al: A new variant of methylmalonic acidemia: defective coenzyme-apoenzyme binding in cultured fibroblasts. Clin Chim Acta 1978; 85:67.

70. Fenton WA, Ambani LM, Rosenberg LE: Uptake of hydroxocobalamin by rat liver mitochondria. Binding to a mitochondrial protein. J Biol Chem 1976; 251:6616.

71. Fenton WA, Rosenberg LE: Genetic and biochemical analysis of human cobalamin mutants in cell culture. Ann Rev Genet 1978; 12:223.

72. Fenton WA, Rosenberg LE: The defect in the cbl B class of human methylmalonic acidemia: deficiency of cob(I)alamin adenosyltransferase activity in extracts of cultured fibroblasts. Biochem Biophys Res Commun 1981; 98:283.

73. Abe T, Gibbs B, Cooper BA: Forms of vitamin B_{12} in blood and bone marrow in patients with pernicious anaemia. Br J Haematol 1975; 31:493.

74. Beck WS, Cohen R, Jorgensen J: Mitochondrial cobalamins: evidence of their noninvolvement in mitochondrial DNA synthesis. In Zagalak B, Friedrich W (eds): Vitamin B_{12}. Berlin, Walter de Gruyter, 1979, pp 975–977.

75. Quadros EV, Jackson B, Linnell JC: Interconversion of cobalamins in human lymphocytes *in vitro* and the influence of nitrous oxide on synthesis of cobalamin coenzymes. In Zagalak B, Friedrich W (eds): Vitamin B_{12}. Berlin, Walter de Gruyter, 1979, pp 1045–1054.

76. Fenton WA, Rosenberg LE: Mitochondrial metabolism of hydroxocobalamin: synthesis of adenosylcobalamin by intact rat liver mitochondria. Arch Biochem Biophys 1978; 189:441.

77. Finkelstein JD: Regulation of methionine metabolism in mammals. In Usdin E, Borchardt RT, Creveling CR (eds): Transmethylation. New York, Elsevier North-Holland, 1978, pp 49–68.

78. Storch KJ, Wagner DA, et al: Quantitative study *in vivo* of methionine cycle in humans using [*methyl*-$^2H_3$]- and [1^{13}C]methionine. Am J Physiol 1988; 255:E322.

79. Gahl WA, Finkelstein JD, et al: Hepatic methionine adenosyl-transferase deficiency in a 31-year-old man. Am J Hum Genet 1987; 40:39.

80. Gahl WA, Bernardini I, et al: Transsulfuration in an adult with hepatic methionine adenosyltransferase deficiency. J Clin Invest 1988; 81:390.

81. Blom HJ, Boers GHJ, et al: Cystathionine-synthase-deficient patients do not use the transamination pathway of methionine to reduce hypermethioninemia and homocystinemia. Metabolism 1989; 38:577.

81a. Drennan CL, Huang S, et al: How a protein binds B_{12}: a 3.0 Å X-ray structure of B_{12}-binding domains of methionine synthase. Science 1994; 266:1669.

82. Fujii K, Galivan JH, Huennekens FM: Activation of methionine synthase: further characterization of the flavoprotein system. Arch Biochem Biophys 1979; 178:662.

83. Frasca V, Dunham WR, et al: Studies of cobalamin-dependent methionine synthase from *Escherichia coli*. In Cooper BA, Whitehead VM (eds): Chemistry and Biology of Pteridines: Pteridines and Folic Acid Derivatives. Berlin, Walter de Gruyter, 1986, pp 917–920.

84. Tuchman M, Kelly P, et al: Vitamin B_{12}-responsive megaloblastic anemia, homocystinuria, and transient methylmalonic aciduria in cblE disease. J Pediatr 1988; 113:1052.

85. Rosenberg LE: The inherited methylmalonic acidemias. Prog Clin Biol Res 1982; 103:187.

86. Kinnally KW, Tedeschi H: Adenosine triphosphate synthesis coupled to K$^+$ influx in mitochondria. Science 1982; 216:742.

87. Coulombe JT, Shih VE, Levy HL: Massachusetts Metabolic Disorders Screening Program. II. Methylmalonic aciduria. Pediatrics 1981; 67:26.

88. Halperin ML, Schiller CM, Fritz IB: The inhibition by methylmalonic acid of malate transport by the dicarboxylate carrier in rat liver mitochondria. A possible explanation for hypoglycemia in methylmalonic aciduria. J Clin Invest 1971; 50:2276.

89. Montgomery JA, Mamer OA, Scriver CR: Metabolism of methylmalonic acid in rats. J Clin Invest 1983; 72:1937.

90. Batt RM, Horadagoda NU: Gastric and pancreatic intrinsic factor–mediated absorption of cobalamin in the dog. Am J Physiol 1989; 257:G344.

91. Allen RH, Seetharam B, et al: Effect of proteolytic enzymes on the binding of cobalamin to R protein and intrinsic factor. J Clin Invest 1978; 61:47.

92. Sennett C, Rosenberg LE, Mellman IS: Transmembrane transport of cobalamin in prokaryotic and eukaryotic cells. Ann Rev Biochem 1981; 50:1053.

93. Hewitt JE, Gordon MM, et al: Human gastric intrinsic factor: characterization of cDNA and genomic clones and localization to human chromosome 11. Genomics 1991; 10:432.

94. Fernandez-Costa F, Metz J: Vitamin B_{12} binders (transcobalamins) in serum. CRC Crit Rev Clin Lab Sci 1982; 18:1.

95. Quadros EV, Rothenberg SP, et al: Purification and molecular characterization of human transcobalamin II. J Biol Chem 1986; 261:15455.

96. Pletsch QA, Coffey JW: Intracellular distribution of radioactive vitamin B_{12} in rat liver. J Biol Chem 1971; 246:4619.

97. Ogawa K, Kudo H, et al: Expression of vitamin B_{12} R-binder in breast tumors: an immunohistochemical study. Arch Pathol 1988; 112:1117.

98. Lee EY, Seetharam B, et al: Immunohistochemical survey of cobalamin-binding proteins. Gastroenterology 1989; 97:1171.

99. Kolhouse JF, Kondo H, et al: Cobalamin analogues are present in human plasma and can mask cobalamin deficiency because current radioisotope dilution assays are not specific for true cobalamin. N Engl J Med 1978; 299:785.

100. Doscherholmen A, Hagen PS: Delay of absorption of radiolabeled cyanocobalamin in the intestinal wall in the presence of intrinsic factor. J Lab Clin Med 1959; 54:434.

101. Rothenberg SP, Weiss JP, Cotter R: Formation of transcobalamin II–vitamin B_{12} complex by guinea-pig ileal mucosa in organ culture after *in vivo* incubation with intrinsic factor–vitamin B_{12}. Br J Haematol 1978; 40:401.

102. Chanarin I, Muir M, et al: Evidence for an intestinal origin of transcobalamin II during vitamin B_{12} absorption. BMJ 1978; 1:1453.

103. Katz M, Cooper BA: Solubilization of the receptor for intrinsic factor–B_{12} complex from guinea pig intestinal mucosa. Methods Enzymol 1980; 67:67.

104. Seetharam B, Levine JS, et al: Purification, properties, and immunochemical localization of a receptor for intrinsic factor-cobalamin complex in the rat kidney. J Biol Chem 1988; 263:4443.

105. Von Bonsdorf B: On the remission after removal of the worm in pernicious anemia in presence and absence of extrinsic factor in the food. Acta Med Scand 1943; 116:77.

106. Nyberg W, Gräsbeck R, et al: Serum vitamin B_{12} levels and incidence of tape worm anemia in a population heavily infected with *Diphyllobothrium latum*. Am J Clin Nutr 1961; 9:606.

107. Seetharam B: Gastrointestinal absorption and transport of cobalamin (vitamin B_{12}). In Johnson LR (ed): Physiology of the Gastrointestinal Tract. New York, Raven Press, 1994, pp 1997–2026.

108. Robertson JA, Gallagher ND: Intrinsic factor–cobalamin accumulates in the ilea of mice treated with chloroquine. Gastroenterology 1985; 89:1353.

109. Robertson JA, Gallagher ND: *In vivo* evidence that cobalamin is absorbed by receptor-mediated endocytosis in the mouse. Gastroenterology 1985; 88:908.

110. Kapadia CR, Serfilippi D, et al: Intrinsic factor–mediated absorption of cobalamin by guinea pig ileal cells. J Clin Invest 1983; 71:440.

111. Gueant JL, Monin GB, et al: Radioautographic localisation of iodinated human intrinsic factor in the guinea pig ileum using electron microscopy. Gut 1988; 29:1370.

112. Cooper BA: Complex of intrinsic factor and B_{12} in human ileum during vitamin B_{12} absorption. Am J Physiol 1968; 214:832.

113. Kolhouse JF, Allen RH: Absorption, plasma transport and cellular retention of cobalamin analogues. J Clin Invest 1977; 60:1381.

114. Kishimoto T, Tavassoli M, et al: Receptors for transferrin and transcobalamin II display segregated distribution on microvilli of leukemia L1210 cells. Biochem Biophys Res Commun 1987; 146:1102.

115. Seligman PA, Allen RH: Characterization of the receptor for transcobalamin II isolated from human placenta. J Biol Chem 1978; 253:1766.

116. Rosenblatt DS, Hosack A, Matiaszuk N: Expression of transcobalamin II by amniocytes. Prenat Diagn 1987; 7:35.

117. Rosenblatt DS, Cooper BA: Inherited disorders of vitamin B_{12} metabolism. Blood Rev 1987; 1:177.

118. Vassiliadis A, Rosenblatt DS, et al: Lysosomal cobalamin accumulation in fibroblasts from a patient with an inborn error of cobalamin metabolism (cbIF complementation group): visualization by electron microscope radioautography. Exp Cell Res 1991; 195:295.

119. Botez MI: Neuropsychiatric illness and deficiency of vitamin B_{12} and folate. In Zittoun JA, Cooper BA (eds): Folates and Cobalamins. Berlin, Springer-Verlag, 1989, pp 145–159.

120. Ditrapani G, Barone C, et al: Dementia–peripheral neuropathy during combined deficiency of vitamin B_{12} and folate. Light microscopy and ultrastructural study of sural nerve. Ital J Neurol Sci 1986; 7:545.

121. Steiner I, Kidron D, et al: Sensory peripheral neuropathy of vitamin B_{12} deficiency: a primary demyclinating disease? J Neurol 1988; 235:163.

122. Zegers de Beyl D, Delecluse F, et al: Somatosensory conduction in vitamin B_{12} deficiency. Electrophysiol Clin Neurophysiol 1988; 69:313.

123. Perkin GD, Roche SW, et al: Delayed somatosensory evoked potentials in pernicious anaemia with intact peripheral nerves. J Neurol Neurosurg Psychiatry 1989; 52:1017.

124. Weir DG, Keating S, et al: Methylation deficiency causes vitamin B_{12}–associated neuropathy in the pig. J Neurochem 1988; 51:1949.

125. Drummond JT, Matthews RG: Nitrous oxide inactivation of cobalamin-dependent methionine synthase from Escherichia coli: characterization of the damage to the enzyme and prosthetic group. Biochemistry 1994; 33:3742.

126. Drummond JT, Matthews RG: Nitrous oxide degradation by cobalamin-dependent methionine synthase: characterization of the reactants and products in the inactivation reaction. Biochemistry 1994; 33:3732.

127. Stabler SP, Allen RH, et al: Marked elevation of methylmalonic acid in cerebrospinal fluid (CSF) of patients with cobalamin (CbI) deficiency. Clin Res 1989; 37:550a.

128. Stabler SP, Allen RH, et al: Cerebrospinal fluid methylmalonic acid levels in normal subjects and patients with cobalamin deficiency. Neurology 1991; 41:1627.

129. Nilsson K, Gustafson L, et al: Plasma homocysteine in relation to serum cobalamin and blood folate in a psychogeriatric population. Eur J Clin Invest 1994; 24:600.

130. Lindenbaum J, Rosenberg IH, et al: Prevalence of cobalamin deficiency in the Framingham elderly population. Am J Clin Nutr 1994; 60:2.

131. Herbert V: Staging vitamin B_{12} (cobalamin) status in vegetarians. Am J Clin Nutr 1994; 59(5 Suppl):1213S.

132. Joosten E, Pelemans W, et al: Cobalamin absorption and serum homocysteine and methylmalonic acid in elderly subjects with low serum cobalamin. Eur J Haematol 1993; 51:25.

133. Norman EJ, Morrison JA: Screening elderly populations for cobalamin (vitamin B_{12}) deficiency using the urinary methylmalonic acid assay by gas chromatography mass spectrometry. Am J Med 1993; 94:589.

134. Pennypacker LC, Allen RH, et al: High prevalence of cobalamin deficiency in elderly outpatients. J Am Geriatr Soc 1992; 40:1197.

135. Hall CA: The nondiagnosis of pernicious anemia. Ann Intern Med 1965; 63:951.

136. Carmel R, Karnaze DS, Weiner JM: Neurologic abnormalities in cobalamin deficiency are associated with higher cobalamin "analogue" values than are hematologic abnormalities. J Lab Clin Med 1988; 111:57.

137. Reizenstein PG, Ek G, Matthews CME: Vitamin B_{12} kinetics in man: implications on total-body-B_{12}-determinations, human requirements, and normal and pathological cellular B_{12} uptake. Physics Med Biol 1966; 11:295.

138. Herzlich B, Herbert V, Drivas G: Depletion of serum homotranscobalamin-II. An early sign of negative vitamin-B_{12} balance. Lab Invest 1988; 58:332.

139. Lindenbaum J, Healton EB, et al: Neuropsychiatric disorders caused by cobalamin deficiency in the absence of anemia or macrocytosis. N Engl J Med 1988; 318:1720.

140. Lindenbaum J, Savage DG, et al: Diagnosis of cobalamin deficiency II. Relative sensitivities of serum cobalamin, methylmalonic acid and total homocysteine concentrations. Am J Hematol 1990; 34:99.

141. Mollin DL, Anderson BB, Burman JF: The serum vitamin B_{12} level: its assay and significance. Clin Haematol 1976; 5:521.

142. Danielsson L, Enocksson E, et al: Failure to thrive due to sub-clinical maternal pernicious anemia. Acta Paediatr Scand 1988; 77:310.

143. Bar-Shany S, Herbert V: Transplacentally acquired antibody to intrinsic factor with vitamin B_{12} deficiency. Blood 1967; 30:777.

144. Specker BL, Miller D, et al: Increased urinary methylmalonic acid excretion in breast-fed infants of vegetarian mothers and identification of an acceptable dietary source of vitamin B_{12}. Am J Clin Nutr 1988; 47:89.

145. Herbert V: Vitamin B_{12}: plant sources, requirements, and assay. Am J Clin Nutr 1988; 48(Suppl 3):852.

146. Sanfilipo JS, Liu YK: Vitamin B_{12} deficiency and infertility: report of a case. Int J Fertility 1991; 36:36.

147. Ashkenazi S, Weitz R, et al: Vitamin B_{12} deficiency due to a strictly vegetarian diet in adolescence. Clin Pediatr 1987; 26:662.

148. Skidmore MD, Shenker N, et al: Biochemical evidence of asymptomatic vitamin B_{12} deficiency in children after ileal resection for necrotizing enterocolitis. J Pediatr 1989; 115:102.

149. Harriman GR, Smith PD, et al: Vitamin B_{12} malabsorption in patients with acquired immunodeficiency syndrome. Arch Intern Med 1989; 149:2039.

150. Saxena S, Weiner JM, Carmel R: Red blood cell distribution width in untreated pernicious anemia. Am J Clin Pathol 1988; 89:660.

151. Thong KL, Hanley SA, McBride JA: Clinical significance of a high mean corpuscular volume in nonanemic patients. Can Med Assoc J 1977; 117:908.

152. Pierce HI, Hillman RS: The value of serum vitamin B_{12} level in diagnosing B_{12} deficiency. Blood 1974; 43:915.

153. Carmel R, Karnaze DS: Physician response to low serum cobalamin levels. Arch Intern Med 1986; 146:1161.

154. Kafetz K: Immunoglobulin deficiency responding to vitamin B_{12} in two elderly patients with megaloblastic anaemia. Postgrad Med J 1985; 61:1065.

155. Wright PE, Sears DA: Hypogammaglobulinemia and pernicious anemia. South Med J 1987; 80:243.

156. Nimo R, Carmel R: Increased sensitivity of detection of the blocking (type I) anti-intrinsic factor antibody. Am J Clin Pathol 1987; 88:729.

157. Chanarin I: The Megaloblastic Anaemias. London, Blackwell Scientific Publications, 1979, pp 144–146.

158. Cooper BA, Whitehead VM: Evidence that some patients with pernicious anemia are not recognized by radiodilution assay for cobalamin in serum. N Engl J Med 1978; 299:816.

159. Cooper BA, Lowenstein L: Relative folate deficiency of erythrocytes in pernicious anemia. Blood 1964; 24:502.

160. Cooper BA, Lowenstein L: Vitamin B_{12}-folate interrelationships in megaloblastic anaemia. Br J Haematol 1966; 12:283.

161. Carmel R, Sinow RM, et al: Food cobalamin malabsorption occurs frequently in patients with unexplained low serum cobalamin levels. Arch Intern Med 1988; 148:1715.

162. Gozzard DI, Dawson DW, Lewis MJ: Experiences with dual protein-bound aqueous vitamin B_{12} absorption test in subjects with low serum vitamin B_{12} concentrations. J Clin Pathol 1987; 40:633.

163. Jones BP, Broomhead AF, et al: Incidence and clinical significance of protein-bound vitamin B_{12} malabsorption. Eur J Haematol 1987; 38:131.

164. Hippe E, Gimsing P, Hollander NH: A simplified method for quantitative determination of vitamin B_{12} absorption. In Zagalak B, Friedrich W (eds): Vitamin B_{12}. Berlin, Walter de Gruyter, 1979, pp 939–944.

165. Waxman S, Metz J, Herbert V: Defective DNA synthesis in human megaloblastic marrow: effects of homocysteine and methionine. J Clin Invest 1969; 48:284.

166. Wickramasinghe SN: The deoxyuridine suppression test. In Hall CA (ed): The Cobalamins. Edinburgh, Churchill Livingstone, 1983, pp 196–208.

167. Cox EV, White AM: Methylmalonic acid excretion: an index of vitamin-B_{12} deficiency. Lancet 1962; 2:853.

168. Schneede J, Dagnelie PC, et al: Methylmalonic acid and homocysteine in infants on macrobiotic diets. Pediatr Res 1994; 36:194.

169. Norman EJ: New urinary methylmalonic acid test is a sensitive indicator of cobalamin (vitamin B_{12}) deficiency: a solution for a major unrecognized medical problem. J Lab Clin Med 1987; 110:369.

170. Stabler SP, Marcell PD, et al: Assay of methylmalonic acid in the serum of patients with cobalamin deficiency using capillary gas chromatography mass spectrometry. J Clin Invest 1986; 77:1606.

171. Ho CH, Chang HC, Yeh SF: Quantitation of urinary methylmalonic acid by gas chromatography mass spectrometry and its clinical applications. Eur J Haematol 1987; 38:80.

172. Matchar DB, Feussner JR, et al: Isotope-dilution assay for urinary methylmalonic acid in the diagnosis of vitamin B_{12} deficiency. A prospective clinical evaluation. Ann Intern Med 1987; 106:707.

173. Kang S-S, Wong PWK, Norusis M: Homocystinemia due to folate deficiency. Metabolism 1987; 36:458.

174. Refsum H, Ueland PM, Svardal AM: Fully automated fluorescence assay for determining total homocysteine in plasma. Clin Chem 1989; 35:1921.

175. Lawson DH, Parker JWL: Deaths from severe megaloblastic anaemia in hospitalised patients. Scand J Haematol 1976; 17:347.

176. Carmel R: Treatment of severe pernicious anemia: no association with sudden death. Am J Clin Nutr 1988; 48:1443.

177. Skouby AP: Hydroxocobalamin for initial and long-term therapy for vitamin B_{12} deficiency. Acta Med Scand 1987; 221:399.

178. Olesen H, Hom B, Schwartz M: Antibody to transcobalamin II in patients treated with long-acting vitamin B_{12} preparations. Scand J Haematol 1968; 5:5.

179. Berendt RC, Jewell LD, et al: Multicentric gastric carcinoids complicating pernicious anemia: origin from the metaplastic endocrine cell population. Arch Pathol Lab Med 1989; 113:399.

180. Hsing AW, Hansson L-E, et al: Pernicious anemia and subsequent cancer: a population-based cohort study. Cancer 1993; 71:745.

181. Ottesen M, Feldt-Rasmussen U, et al: Thyroid function and autoimmunity in pernicious anemia before and during cyanocobalamin treatment. J Endocrinol Invest 1995; 18:91.

182. Davis RE, McCann VJ, Stanton KG: Type I diabetes and latent pernicious anemia. Med J Aust 1992; 156:160.

183. Katz M, Lee SK, Cooper BA: Vitamin B_{12} malabsorption due to a biologically inert intrinsic factor. N Engl J Med 1972; 287:425.

184. Yang Y-M, Ducos R, et al: Cobalamin malabsorption in three siblings due to abnormal intrinsic factor that is markedly susceptible to acid and proteolysis. J Clin Invest 1985; 76:2057.

185. Gräsbeck R: Familial selective vitamin B_{12} malabsorption. N Engl J Med 1972; 287:358.

186. Wulffraat NM, De Schryver J, et al: Failure to thrive is an early symptom to the Imerslund-Gräsbeck syndrome. Am J Hematol Oncol 1994; 16:177.

187. Mackenzie IL, Donaldson RM Jr, et al: Ileal Mucosa in familial selective vitamin B_{12} malabsorption. N Engl J Med 1972; 286:1021.

188. Burman JF, Walker WJ, et al: Absent ileal uptake of IF-bound-vitamin B_{12} in the Imerslund-Gräsbeck syndrome (familial vitamin B_{12} malabsorption with proteinuria). Gut 1985; 26:311.

189. Fyfe JC, Ramanujam KS, et al: Defective brush-border expression of intrinsic factor–cobalamin receptor in canine inherited intestinal cobalamin malabsorption. J Biol Chem 1991; 266:4489.

190. Fyfe JC, Giger U, et al: Inherited selective intestinal cobalamin malabsorption and cobalamin deficiency in dogs. Pediatr Res 1991; 29:24.

191. Cooper BA, Rosenblatt DS: Inherited defects of vitamin B_{12} metabolism. Ann Rev Nutr 1987; 7:291.

192. Carmel R: A new case of deficiency of the R binder for cobalamin, with observations on minor cobalamin binding proteins in serum and saliva. Blood 1982; 59:152.

193. Carmel R: R-binder deficiency. A clinically benign cause of cobalamin pseudodeficiency. J Am Med Assoc 1983; 250:1886.

194. Carmel R, Herbert V: Deficiency of vitamin B_{12} α-globulin in two brothers. Blood 1969; 33:1.

195. Jenks J, Begley J, Howard L: Cobalamin–R binder deficiency in a woman with thalassemia. Nutr Rev 1983; 41:277.

196. Sigal SH, Hall CA, Antel JP: Plasma R binder deficiency and neurologic disease. N Engl J Med 1988; 317:1330.

197. Li N, Rosenblatt DS, et al: Identification of two mutant alleles of transcobalamin II in an affected family. Hum Molec Genet 1994; 3:1835.

198. Nierbrugge DJ, Benjamin DR, et al: Hereditary transcobalamin II deficiency presenting as red cell hypoplasia. J Pediatr 1982; 101:732.

199. Burman JF, Mollin DL, et al: Inherited lack of transcobalamin II in serum and megaloblastic anemia: a further patient. Br J Haematol 1979; 43:27.

200. Meyers PA, Carmel R: Hereditary transcobalamin II deficiency with subnormal serum cobalamin levels. Pediatrics 1984; 74:866.

201. Thomas PK, Hoffbrand AV, Smith IS: Neurological involvement in hereditary transcobalamin II deficiency. J Neurol Neurosurg Psychiatry 1982; 45:74.

202. Zeitlin HC, Sheppard K, et al: Homozygous transcobalamin II deficiency maintained on oral hydroxocobalamin. Blood 1985; 66:1022.

203. Fenton W, Rosenberg LE: Inherited disorders of cobalamin transport and metabolism. In Scriver CR, Beaudet AL, et al (eds): The Metabolic and Molecular Basis of Inherited Disease. New York, McGraw-Hill Book Co., 1995, pp 3129–3149.

204. Daiger SP, Labowe ML, et al: Detection of genetic variation with radioactive ligands. III. Genetic polymorphism of transcobalamin II in human plasma. Am J Hum Genet 1978; 30:202.

205. Eiberg H, Moller N, et al: Linkage of transcobalamin II (TC2) to the P blood group system and assignment to chromosome 22. Clin Genet 1986; 29:354.

206. Platica O, Janeczko R, et al: The cDNA sequence and the deduced amino acid sequence of human transcobalamin II show homology with rat intrinsic factor and human transcobalamin I. J Biol Chem 1991; 266:7860.

207. Li N, Seetharam S, et al: Isolation and sequence analysis of variant forms of human transcobalamin II. Biochim Biophys Acta 1993; 1172:21.

208. Li N, Rosenblatt DS, Seetharam B: Nonsense mutations in human transcobalamin II deficiency. Biochem Biophys Res Commun 1994; 204:1111.

209. Mahoney MJ, Bick D: Recent advances in the inherited methylmalonic acidemias. Acta Paediatr Scand 1987; 76:689.

210. Fenton WA, Hack AM, et al: Immunochemical studies of fibroblasts from patients with methylmalonyl-CoA mutase apoenzyme deficiency: detection of a mutation interfering with mitochondrial import. Proc Natl Acad Sci U S A 1987;84:1421.

211. Raff ML, Crane AM, et al: Genetic characterization of a *mut* locus mutation discriminating heterogeneity in mut° and mutmethylmalonic aciduria by interallelic complementation. J Clin Invest 1991; 87:203.

212. Qureshi AA, Crane AM, et al: Cloning and expression of mutations demonstrating intragenic complementation in mut°methylmalonic aciduria. J Clin Invest 1994; 93:1812.

213. Inoue S, Krieger I, et al: Inhibition of bone marrow stem cell growth *in vitro* by methylmalonic acid: a mechanism for pancytopenia in a patient with methylmalonic acidemia. Pediatr Res 1981; 15:95.

214. Ledley FD, Levy HL, et al: Benign methylmalonic aciduria. N Engl J Med 1984; 311:1015.

215. Zoghbi HY, O'Brien WE, Ledley FD: Linkage relationships of the human methylmalonyl-CoA mutase to the *HLA* and *D6S4* loci on chromosome 6. Genomics 1988; 3:396.

216. Jansen R, Kalousek F, et al: Cloning of full-length methylmalonyl-CoA mutase from a cDNA library using the polymerase chain reaction. Genomics 1989; 4:198.

217. Crane AM, Ledley FD: Cluster of mutations in methylmalonyl CoA mutase associated with mut⁻ methylmalonic acidemia. Am J Hum Genet 1994; 55:42.

218. Crane AM, Jansen R, et al: Cloning and expression of a mutant methylmalonyl coenzyme A mutase with altered cobalamin affinity that causes mut⁻ methylmalonic aciduria. J Clin Invest 1992; 89:385.

219. Ledley FD, Jansen R, et al: Mutation eliminating mitochondrial leader sequence of methylmalonyl CoA mutase causes mut° methylmalonic aciduria. Proc Natl Acad Sci 1991; 87:3147.

220. Crane AM, Martin LS, et al: Phenotype of disease in three patients with identical mutations in methylmalonyl CoA mutase. Human Genet 1992; 89:259.

221. Ogasawara M, Matsubara Y, et al: Identification of two novel mutations in the methylmalonyl-CoA mutase gene with decreased levels of mutant mRNA in methylmalonic acidemia. Hum Mol Genet 1994; 3:867.

222. Chalmers RA, Stacey TE, et al: L-Carnitine insufficiency in disorders of organic acid metabolism: response to L-carnitine by patients with methylmalonic aciduria and 3-hydroxy-3-methylglutaric aciduria. J Inherit Metab Dis 1984; 7:109.

223. Wolff JA, Carroll JE, et al: Carnitine reduces fasting ketogenesis in patients with disorders of propionate metabolism. Lancet 1986; 1:289.

224. Bain MD, Jones M, et al: Contribution of gut bacterial metabolism to human metabolic disease. Lancet 1988; 1:1078.

225. Snyderman SE, Sansaricq C, et al: The use of neomycin in the treatment of methylmalonic aciduria. Pediatrics 1972; 50:925.

226. Koletzko B, Bachmann C, Wendel U: Antibiotic treatment for improvement of metabolic control in methylmalonic aciduria. J Pediatr 1990; 117:99.

227. Matsui SM, Mahoney MJ, Rosenberg LE: The natural history of the inherited methylmalonic acidemias. N Engl J Med 1983; 308:857.

228. Ampola MG, Mahoney MJ, et al: Prenatal therapy of a patient with vitamin B$_{12}$ responsive methylmalonic acidemia. N Engl J Med 1975; 293:313.

229. Mellman I, Willard HF, et al: Cobalamin coenzyme synthesis in normal and mutant fibroblasts: evidence for a processing enzyme activity deficient in cblC cells. J Biol Chem 1979; 254:11847.

230. Pezacka EH: Identification and characterization of two enzymes involved in the intracellular metabolism of cobalamin. Cyanocobalamin β-ligand transferase and microsomal cob(III)alamin reductase. Biochim Biophys Acta 1993; 1157:167.

231. Pezacka EH, Rosenblatt DS: Intracellular metabolism of cobalamin. Altered activities of β-axial-ligand transferase and microsomal cob(III)alamin reductase in cblC and cblD fibroblasts. In Bhatt HR, James VHT, et al (eds): Advances in Thomas Addison's Diseases. Vol. 1. Bristol, England: Journal of Endocrinology Ltd., 1994, pp 315–323.

232. Rosenblatt DS: Inherited errors of cobalamin metabolism: an overview. In Bhatt HR, James VHT, et al (eds): Advances in Thomas Addison's Diseases. Vol. 1. Bristol, England: Journal of Endocrinology Ltd., 1994, pp 303–313.

233. Mitchell GA, Watkins D, et al: Clinical heterogeneity in cobalamin C variant of combined homocystinuria and methylmalonic aciduria. J Pediatr 1986; 108:410.

234. Shinnar S, Singer HS: Cobalamin C mutation (methylmalonic aciduria and homocystinuria) in adolescence. A treatable cause of dementia and myelopathy. N Engl J Med 1984; 311:451.

235. Mitchell GA, Watkins D, et al: Clinical heterogeneity in cobalamin C variant of combined homocystinuria and methylmalonic aciduria. J Pediatr 1986;108:410.

236. Robb RM, Dowton SB, et al: Retinal degeneration in vitamin B$_{12}$ disorder associated with methylmalonic aciduria and sulfur amino acid abnormalities. Am J Ophthalmol 1984; 97:691.

237. Traboulski EI, Silva JC, et al: Ocular histopathologic characteristics of cobalamin C type vitamin B$_{12}$ defect with methylmalonic aciduria and homocystinuria. Am J Ophthalmol 1992; 113:269.

238. Weintraub L, Tardo C, et al: Hydrocephalus as a possible complication of the cblC type of methylmalonic aciduria. Am J Hum Genet 1991; 49:108. Abstract.

239. Caouette G, Rosenblatt D, Laframboise R: Hepatic dysfunction in a neonate with combined methylmalonic aciduria and homocystinuria. Clin Invest Med 1992; 15:A112. Abstract.

240. Goodman SI, Moe PG, et al: Homocystinuria with methylmalonic aciduria: two cases in a sibship. Biochem Med 1970; 4:500.

241. Shih VE, Axel SM, et al: Defective lysosomal release of vitamin B$_{12}$ (cb1F): a hereditary cobalamin metabolic disorder associated with sudden death. Am J Med Genet 1989; 33:555.

242. Rosenblatt DS, Laframboise R, et al: New disorder of vitamin B$_{12}$ metabolism (cobalamin F) presenting as methylmalonic aciduria. Pediatrics 1986; 78:51.

243. Laframboise R, Cooper BA, Rosenblatt DS: Malabsorption of vitamin B$_{12}$ from the intestine in a child with cblF disease: evidence for lysosomal-mediated absorption. Blood 1992; 80:291. Letter.

244. MacDonald MR, Wiltse HE, et al: Clinical heterogeneity in two patients with cblF disease. Am J Hum Genet 1992; 15:A353. Abstract.

245. Wong LTK, Rosenblatt DS, et al: Diagnosis and treatment of a child with cblF disease. Clin Invest Med 1992; 15:A111. Abstract.

246. Zammarchi E, Lippi A, et al: cblC disease: case report and monitoring of a pregnancy at risk by chorionic villus sampling. Clin Invest Med 1990; 13:139.

247. Chadefaux-Vekemans B, Rolland MO, et al: Prenatal diagnosis of combined methylmalonic aciduria and homocystinuria (CblC or CblD mutant). Prenat Diagn 1994; 14:417. Letter.

248. Wallis J, Clark DM, Bain BJ: The use of hydroxocobalamin in the Schilling test. Scand J Haematol 1986; 37:337.

249. Bartholomew DW, Batshaw ML, et al: Therapeutic approaches to cobalamin-C methylmalonic acidemia and homocystinuria. J Pediatr 1988; 112:32.

250. Shih VE, Axel SM, et al: Defective lysosomal release of vitamin B$_{12}$ (cblF) a hereditary metabolic disorder associated with sudden death. Am J Hum Genet 1989; 33:555.

251. Watkins D, Rosenblatt DS: Functional methionine synthase deficiency (cblE and cblG): clinical and biochemical heterogeneity. Am J Med Genet 1989; 34:427.

252. Watkins D, Rosenblatt DS: Genetic heterogeneity among patients with methylcobalamin deficiency. J Clin Invest 1988; 81:1690.

253. Sillaots SL, Hall CA, et al: Heterogeneity in cblG: differential retention of cobalamin on methionine synthase. Biochem Med Metab Biol 1992; 47:242.

254. Rosenblatt DS, Cooper BA, et al: Altered vitamin B$_{12}$ metabolism in fibroblasts from a patient with megaloblastic anemia and homocystinuria due to a new defect in methionine biosynthesis. J Clin Invest 1984; 74:2149.

255. Rosenblatt DS, Cooper BA: Selective deficiencies of methyl B$_{12}$ (cblE and cblG). Clin Invest Med 1989; 12:270.

256. Hall CA, Lindenbaum RH, et al: The nature of the defect in cobalamin G mutation. Clin Invest Med 1989; 12:262.

257. Rosenblatt DS, Cooper BA, et al: Prenatal vitamin B$_{12}$ therapy of a fetus with methylcobalamin deficiency (cobalamin E disease). Lancet 1985; 1:1127.

258. Chung ASM, Pearson WN, et al: Folic acid, vitamin B$_6$, pantothenic acid and vitamin B$_{12}$ in human dietaries. Am J Clin Nutr 1961; 9:573.

259. Collins RA, Harper AE, et al: The folic acid and vitamin B$_{12}$ content of the milk of various species. J Nutr 1951; 43:313.

260. Moscovitch LF, Cooper BA: Folate content of diets in pregnancy: comparison of diets collected at home and diets prepared from dietary records. Am J Clin Nutr 1973; 26:707.

261. Cooper BA: Reassessment of folic acid requirements. In White PL, Selvey N (eds): Nutrition in Transition: Proceedings, Western Hemisphere Nutrition Congress V. Monroe, WI, American Medical Association, 1978, pp 281–288.

262. Zittoun J: Folate and nutrition. Chemioterapia 1985; 4:388.

263. Senti FR, Pilch SM: Analysis of folate data from the second National Health and Nutrition Examination Survey (NHANES II). J Nutr 1985; 115:1398.

264. Herbert V: Making sense of laboratory tests of folate status: folate requirements to sustain normality. In Zittoun J, Cooper BA (eds): Folates and Cobalamins. Berlin, Springer-Verlag, 1989, pp 119–127.

265. Canada Department of National Health and Welfare: Food Consumption Patterns Report. A Report from Nutrition Canada by the Bureau of Nutritional Sciences, Health Protection Branch, Department of Health and Welfare. Ottawa, Ontario, Canada, Health and Welfare Canada, 1976.

266. Taitz LS, Armitage BL: Goats' milk for infants and children. BMJ [Clin Res] 1984; 288:428. Editorial.

267. Hoppner K, Lampi B: Folate levels in human liver from autopsies in Canada. Am J Clin Nutr 1980; 33:862.

268. Milne DB, Johnson L, et al: Folate status of adult males living in a metabolic unit: possible relationships with iron nutriture. Am J Clin Nutr 1983; 37:768.
269. Banerjee DK, Maitra A, et al: Minimal daily requirement of folic acid in normal Indian subjects. Ind J Med Sci 1975; 63:45.
270. McNulty H, McPartlin JM, et al: Folate catabolism in normal subjects. Hum Nutr Appl Nutr 1987; 41:338.
271. Scott JM: Catabolism of folates. In Blakley RL, Benkovic SJ (eds): Folates and Pterins: Chemistry and Biochemistry of Folates. Vol. 1. New York, John Wiley & Sons, 1984, pp 307–344.
272. Ek J: Plasma, red cell, and breast milk folacin concentration in lactating women. Am J Clin Nutr 1983; 38:929.
273. Dansky LV, Rosenblatt DS, Andermann E: Mechanisms of teratogenesis: folic acid and antiepileptic therapy. Neurology 1992; 42:32.
274. Shojania AM: Oral contraceptives: effect of folate and vitamin B_{12} metabolism. Can Med Assoc J 1982; 126:244.
275. Blakley RL, Benkovic SJ (eds): Folates and Pterins: Chemistry and Biochemistry of Folates. Vol. 1. New York, John Wiley & Sons, 1984.
276. Mackenzie RE: Biogenesis and interconversion of substituted tetrahydrofolates. In Blakley RL, Benkovic SJ (eds): Folates and Pterins: Chemistry and Biochemistry of Folates. New York, John Wiley & Sons, 1984, pp 255–306.
277. Matthews RG, Lu Y-Z, et al: The polyglutamate specificities of four folate-dependent enzymes from pig liver. In Goldman ID (ed): Proceedings of the Second Workshop on Folyl and Antifolyl Polyglutamates. New York, Praeger Publishers, 1985, pp 65–75.
278. Hilton JG, Cooper BA, Rosenblatt DS: Folate polyglutamate synthesis and turnover in cultured human fibroblasts. J Biol Chem 1979; 254:8398.
279. Foo SK, Shane B: Regulation of folypoly-γ-glutamate synthesis in mammalian cells *in vivo* and *in vitro* synthesis of pteroylpoly-γ-glutamates by Chinese hamster ovary cells. J Biol Chem 1982; 257:13587.
280. Frosst P, Blom HJ, et al: A candidate genetic risk factor for vascular disease: a common methylenetetrahydrofolate reductase mutation causes thermoinstability. Nat Genet 1995; 10:111.
281. van der Put NMJ, Steegers-Theunissen RPM, et al: Mutated methylenetetrahydrofolate reductase as a risk factor for spina bifida. Lancet 1995; 346:1070.
282. Chandler CJ, Wang TT, Halsted CH: Pteroylpolyglutamate hydrolase from human jejunal brush borders. Purification and characterization. J Biol Chem 1986; 261:928.
283. McGuire JJ, Coward JK: Pteroylpolyglutamates: biosynthesis, degradation, and function. In Blakley RL, Benkovic SJ (eds): Folates and Pterins: Chemistry and Biochemistry of Folates. Vol. 1. New York, John Wiley & Sons, 1984, pp 135–190.
284. Rosenberg IH, Zimmerman J, Selhub J: Folate transport. Chemioterapia 1985; 4:354.
285. Selhub J, Rosenberg IH: Folate transport in isolated brush border membrane vesicles from rat intestine. J Biol Chem 1981; 256:4489.
286. Schron CM, Washington C Jr, Blitzer BL: Anion specificity of the jejunal folate carrier: effects of reduced folate analogues on folate uptake and efflux. J Membr Biol 1988; 102:175.
287. Blakeborough P, Salter DN: Folate transport in enterocytes and brush-border-membrane vesicles isolated from the small intestine of the neonatal goat. Br J Nutr 1988; 59:485.
288. Browman BB, McCormick DB, Rosenberg IH: Epithelial transport of water-soluble vitamins. Ann Rev Nutr 1989; 9:187.
289. Whitehead VM, Cooper BA: Absorption of unaltered folic acid from the gastro-intestinal tract in man. Br J Haematol 1967; 13:679.
290. Whitehead VM, Pratt R, et al: Intestinal conversion of folinic acid to 5-methyltetrahydrofolate in man. Br J Haematol 1972; 22:63.
291. Herbert V: Excretion of folic acid in the bile. Lancet 1965; 1:913.
292. Hillman RS, McGuffin R, Campbell C: Alcohol interference with the folate enterohepatic cycle. Trans Assoc Am Physicians 1977; 90:145.
293. Eisenga BH, Collins TD, McMartin KE: Differential effects of acute ethanol on urinary excretion of folate derivatives in the rat. J Pharmacol Exp Ther 1989; 248:916.
294. Blocker EB, Thenen SW: Intestinal absorption, liver uptake, and excretion of ^{3}H-folic acid in folic acid–deficient, alcohol consuming nonhuman primates. Am J Clin Nutr 1987; 46:503.
295. Eichner ER, Pierce HI, Hillman RS: Folate balance in dietary induced megaloblastic anemia. N Engl J Med 1971; 284:933.
296. Lane F, Goff P, et al: Folic acid metabolism in normal, folate deficient and alcoholic man. Br J Haematol 1976; 34:489.
297. Halsted CH: The intestinal absorption of folates. Am J Clin Nutr 1979; 32:846.
298. Herbert V, Larrabee AR, Buchanan JM: Studies on the identification of a folate compound of human serum. J Clin Invest 1962; 41:1134.
299. Herbert V: Experimental nutritional folate deficiency in man. Trans Assoc Am Physicians 1962; 75:307.
300. Waxman S, Schreiber C: Characteristics of folic acid-binding protein in folate deficient serum. Blood 1973; 42:291.
301. Wagner C: Folate-binding proteins. Nutr Rev 1985; 43:293.
302. Eichner ER, McDonald CR, Dickson VL: Elevated serum levels of unsaturated folate-binding protein: clinical correlates in a general hospital population. Am J Clin Nutr 1978; 31:1988.
303. Sadasivan E, Rothenberg SP: The complete amino acid sequence of a human folate-binding protein from KB cells determined from the cDNA. J Biol Chem 1989; 264:5806.
304. Sadasivan E, Rothenberg SP: Molecular cloning of the complementary DNA for a human folate-binding protein. Proc Soc Exp Biol Med 1988; 189:240.
305. Lacey SW, Sanders JM, et al: Complementary DNA for the folate-binding protein correctly predicts anchoring to the membrane by glycosyl-phosphatidylinositol. J Clin Invest 1989; 84:715.
306. Deutsch JC, Elwood PC, et al: Role of the membrane-associated folate-binding protein (folate receptor) in methotrexate transport by human KB cells. Arch Biochem Biophys 1989; 274:327.
307. Anonymous: Transport properties of folate bound to human milk folate-binding protein. Nutr Rev 1988; 46:230. Editorial.
308. Ratnam M, Marquardt H, et al: Homologous membrane folate-binding proteins in human placenta: cloning and sequence of a cDNA. Biochemistry 1989; 28:8249.
309. Hansen SI, Holm J, Hoier-Madsen M: A high-affinity folate-binding protein in human urine. Radioligand binding characteristics, immunological properties and molecular size. Biosci Rep 1989; 9:93.
310. Lonnerdal B: Biochemistry and physiological function of human milk proteins. Am J Clin Nutr 1985; 42:1299.
311. Said HM, Horne DW, Wagner C: Effect of human milk folate-binding protein on folate intestinal transport. Arch Biochem Biophys 1986; 251:114.
311a. Moscow JA, Gong M, et al: Isolation of a gene encoding a human reduced folate carrier (RFC1) and analysis of its expression in transport-deficient, methotrexate-resistant human breast cancer cells. Cancer Res 1995; 55:3790.
311b. Wong SC, Proefke SA, et al: Isolation of human cDNAs that restore methotrexate sensitivity and reduced folate carrier activity in methotrexate transport-defective Chinese hamster ovary cells. J Biol Chem 1995; 270:17468.
312. Henderson GB, Tsuji JM, Kumar HP: Mediated uptake of folate by a high-affinity binding protein in sublines of L1210 cells adapted to nanomolar concentrations of folate. J Membr Biol 1988; 101:247.
313. Henderson GB: Transport of folate compounds by hematopoietic cells. In Zittoun J, Cooper BA (eds): Folates and Cobalamins. Berlin, Springer-Verlag, 1989, pp 231–245.
314. Freisheim JH, Ratnam M, et al: Photoaffinity analogues of methotrexate as folate antagonist binding probes. Adv Enzyme Regul 1988; 27:15.
315. Price EM, Freisheim JH: Photoaffinity analogues of methotrexate as folate antagonist binding probes. 2. Transport studies, photoaffinity labeling, and identification of the membrane carrier protein for methotrexate from murine L1210 cells. Biochemistry 1987; 26:4757.
316. Anderson RG, Kamen BA, et al: Potocytosis: sequestration and transport of small molecules by caveolae. Science 1992; 255:410.
317. Matsue H, Rothberg KG, et al: Folate receptor allows cells to grow in low concentrations of 5-methyltetrahydrofolate. Proc Natl Acad Sci U S A 1992; 89:6006.
318. Subar AF, Block G, James LD: Folate intake and food sources in the US population. Am J Clin Nutr 1989; 50:508.
319. Worthington-White DA, Behnke M, Gross S: Premature infants require additional folate and vitamin-B_{12} to reduce the severity of the anemia of prematurity. Am J Clin Nutr 1994; 60:930.

320. Stabler SP, Marcell PD, et al: Elevation of total homocysteine in the serum of patients with cobalamin and folate deficiency detected by capillary gas chromatography-mass spectrometry. J Clin Invest 1988; 810:4660.

321. Scott JM, Weir DG: Hypothesis: the methyl folate trap. Lancet 1981; 2:337.

322. Rosenblatt DS: Inherited disorders of folate transport and metabolism. In Scriver CR, Beaudet AL, et al (eds): The Metabolic and Molecular Basis of Inherited Disease. New York, McGraw-Hill Book Co., 1995, pp 3111–3128.

323. Reynolds EH: Neurological aspects of folate and vitamin B_{12} metabolism. Clin Haematol 1976; 5:661.

324. Lever EG, Elwes RDC, et al: Subacute combined degeneration of the cord due to folate deficiency: response to methyl folate treatment. J Neurol Neurosurg Psychiatry 1986; 49:1203.

325. Brockner P, Lods JC: Folate deficiency in geriatric patients. In Zittoun J, Cooper BA (eds): Folates and Cobalamins. Berlin, Springer-Verlag, 1989, pp 179–189.

326. Christensen B, Rosenblatt DS: Effects of folate deficiency on embryonic development. In Wickramasinghe SN (ed): Baillière's Clinical Haematology: Megaloblastic Anemia. London, Baillière Tindall, 1995, pp 617–637.

327. Schorah CJ, Smithells RW, Scott J: Vitamin B_{12} and anencephaly. Lancet 1980; 1: 880.

328. Kirke PN, Molloy AM, et al: Maternal plasma folate and vitamin B_{12} are independent risk factors for neural tube defects. Q J Med 1993; 86:703.

329. Daly LE, Kirke PN, et al: Folate levels and neural tube defects. JAMA 1995; 274:1698.

330. Steegers-Theunissen RPM, Boers GHJ, et al: Maternal hyperhomocysteinemia: a risk factor for neural tube defects. Metabolism 1994; 43:1475.

331. Mills JL, McPartlin JM, et al: Homocysteine metabolism in pregnancies complicated by neural-tube defects. Lancet 1995; 345:149.

332. Oakley GP, Erickson JD, Adams MJ: Urgent need to increase folic acid supplementation. JAMA 1995; 274:1717.

333. Cuskelly GJ, McNulty H, Scott JM: Effect of increasing dietary folate on red-cell folate: implications for prevention of neural tube defects. Lancet 1996; 347:657.

334. McCully KS: Vascular pathology of homocysteinemia: implications for the pathogenesis of arteriosclerosis. Am J Pathol 1969; 56:111.

335. Kang S-S, Wong PWK, et al: Thermolabile methylenetetrahydrofolate reductase: an inherited risk factor for coronary artery disease. Am J Hum Genet 1991; 48:536.

336. Franken DG, Boers GH, et al: Treatment of mild hyperhomocysteinemia in vascular disease patients. Arterioscler Thromb 1994; 14:465.

337. Boushey CJ, Beresford SAA, et al: A quantitative assessment of plasma homocysteine as a risk factor for vascular disease: probable benefits of increasing folic acid intakes. JAMA 1995; 274:1049.

337a. Selhub J, Jacques PF, et al: Relationship between plasma homocysteine and vitamin status in the Framingham study population. Impact of folic acid fortification. Public Health Rev 2000; 28:117–145.

338. Butterworth CE Jr, Hatch KD, et al: Improvement in cervical dysplasia associated with folic acid therapy in users of oral contraceptives. Am J Clin Nutr 1982; 35:73.

339. Heimberger DC, Alexander CB, et al: Improvement in bronchial squamous metaplasia in smokers treated with folate and vitamin B_{12}. JAMA 1988; 259:1525.

340. Cravo ML, Mason JB, et al: Folate deficiency enhances the development of colonic neoplasia in dimethylhydrazine-treated rats. Cancer Res 1992; 52:5002.

341. Soder O, Ernstrom U: Recruitment of thymocytes from G1 into S phase by a thymic factor. Int Arch Allergy Appl Immunol 1984; 74:186.

342. Ernstrom U: Identification of a mammalian growth factor as a ribofolate peptide. Biosci Rep 1991; 11:119.

343. Jackman AL, Taylor GA, et al: ICI D1694, a quinazoline antifolate thymidylate synthase inhibitor that is a potent inhibitor of L1210 tumor cell growth in vitro and in vivo: a new agent for clinical study. Cancer Res 1991; 51:5579.

344. Beardsley GP, Moroson BA, et al: A new folate antimetabolite, 5,10-dideaza-5,6,7,8-tetrahydrofolate is a potent inhibitor of de novo purine synthesis. J Biol Chem 1989; 264:328.

345. Jolivet J: Methotrexate and 5-fluorouracil: cellular interactions with folates. In Zittoun J, Cooper BA (eds): Folates and Cobalamins. Berlin, Springer-Verlag, 1989, pp 247–254.

346. Marquet J, Chadefaux B, et al: Methylenetetrahydrofolate reductase deficiency: prenatal diagnosis and family studies. Prenat Diagn 1994; 14:29.

347. Haworth JC, Dilling LA, et al: Symptomatic and asymptomatic methylenetetrahydrofolate reductase deficiency in two adult brothers. Am J Med Genet 1993; 45:572.

348. Freeman JM, Finkelstein JD, et al: Homocystinuria presenting as reversible "schizophrenia": a new defect in methionine metabolism with reduced 5,10-methylenetetrahydrofolate reductase activity. Pediatr Res 1972; 6:423.

349. Pasquier F, Lebert F, et al: Methylenetetrahydrofolate reductase deficiency revealed by a neuropathy in a psychotic adult. J Neurol Neurosurg Psychiatry 1994; 57:765. Letter.

350. Erbe RW: Inborn errors of folate metabolism. In Blakley RL, Whitehead VM (eds): Folates and Pterins: Nutritional, Pharmacological and Clinical Aspects. Vol. 3. New York, John Wiley & Sons, 1986, pp 413–466.

351. Kang SS, Zhou J, et al: Intermediate homocysteinemia: a thermolabile variant of methylenetetrahydrofolate reductase. Am J Hum Genet 1988; 43:414.

352. Engbersen AMT, Franken DG, et al: Thermolabile 5,10-methylenetetrahydrofolate reductase as a cause of mild hyperhomocysteinemia. Am J Hum Genet 1995; 56:142.

353. Rosenblatt DS, Cooper BA, et al: Folate distribution in cultured human cells: studies on 5,10-CH_2-H_4PteGlu reductase deficiency. J Clin Invest 1979; 63:1019.

354. Boss GR, Erbe RW: Decreased rates of methionine synthesis by methylenetetrahydrofolate reductase–deficient fibroblasts and lymphoblasts. J Clin Invest 1981; 67:1659.

355. Mudd SH, Uhlendorf BW, et al: Homocystinuria associated with decreased methylenetetrahydrofolate reductase activity. Biochem Biophys Res Commun 1972; 46:905.

356. Rosenblatt DS, Erbe RW: Methylenetetrahydrofolate reductase in cultured human cells. II. Studies of methylenetetrahydrofolate reductase deficiency. Pediatr Res 1977; 11:1141.

357. Kanwar YS, Manaligod JR, Wong PWK: Morphologic studies in a patient with homocystinuria due to 5,10-methylenetetrahydrofolate reductase deficiency. Pediatr Res 1976; 10:598.

358. Wong PWK, Justice P, et al: Folic acid nonresponsive homocystinuria due to methylenetetrahydrofolate reductase deficiency. Pediatrics 1977; 59:749.

359. Baumgartner ER, Schweizer K, Wick H: Different congenital forms of defective remethylation in homocystinuria. Clinical, biochemical, and morphological studies. Pediatr Res 1977; 11:1015.

360. Haan EA, Rogers JG, et al: 5,10-Methylenetetrahydrofolate reductase deficiency: clinical and biochemical features of a further case. J Inherit Metab Dis 1985; 8:53.

361. Hyland K, Smith I, et al: The determination of pterins, biogenic amino metabolites, and aromatic amino acids in cerebrospinal fluid using isocratic reverse phase liquid chromatography within series dual cell coulometric electrochemical and fluorescence determinations—use in the study of inborn errors of dihydropteridine reductase and 5,10-methylenetetrahydrofolate reductase. In Wachter H, Curtius H, Pfleiderer W (eds): Biochemical and Clinical Aspects of Pteridines. Vol. 4. Berlin, Walter de Gruyter, 1985, p 85.

362. Baumgartner ER, Stokstad ELR, et al: Comparison of folic acid coenzyme distribution patterns in patients with methylenetetrahydrofolate reductase and methionine synthetase deficiencies. Pediatr Res 1985; 19:1288.

363. Clayton, PT, Smith, et al: Subacute combined degeneration of the cord, dementia, and Parkinsonism due to an inborn error of folate metabolism. J Neurol Neurosurg Psychiatry 1986; 49:920.

364. Beckman DR, Hoganson G, et al: Pathological findings in 5,10-methylenetetrahydrofolate reductase deficiency. Birth Defects 1987; 23:47.

365. Matthews RG, Kaufman S: Characterization of dihydropteridine reductase activity of pig liver methylenetetrahydrofolate reductase. J Biol Chem 1980; 255:6014.

366. Goyette P, Frosst P, et al: Seven novel mutations in the methylenetetrahydrofolate reductase gene and genotype/phenotype corre-

lations in severe methylenetetrahydrofolate reductase deficiency. Am J Hum Genet 1995; 56:1052.

367. Goyette P, Milos R, et al: Human methylenetetrahydrofolate reductase: isolation of cDNA, mapping and mutation identification. Nat Genet 1994; 7:195.

368. Christensen E, Brandt NJ: Prenatal diagnosis of 5,10-methylenetetrahydrofolate reductase deficiency. N Engl J Med 1985; 313:50.

369. Cooper BA: Anomalies congénitales du métabolisme des folates. In Zittoun J, Cooper BA (eds): Folates et Cobalamines. Paris, Doin, 1987, pp 193–208.

370. Brandt NJ, Christensen E, et al: Treatment of methylenetetrahydrofolate reductase deficiency from the neonatal period. The Society for the Study of Inborn Errors of Metabolism. The Netherlands, Amersfoort, 1986, p 23. Abstract.

371. Arakawa T: Congenital defects in folate utilization. Am J Med 1970; 48:594.

372. Rowe PB: Inherited disorders of folate metabolism. In Stanbury JB, Wyngaarden JB, et al (eds): The Metabolic Basis of Inherited Diseases. 5th ed. New York, McGraw-Hill Book Co., 1983, p 498.

373. Shin YS, Reiter S, et al: Orotic aciduria, homocystinuria, formiminoglutamic aciduria and megaloblastosis associated with the formiminotransferase / cyclodeaminase deficiency. In Nyhan WL, Thompson LF, Watts RWE (eds): Purine and Pyrimidine Metabolism in Man. New York, Plenum Publishing Corp., 1986, p 71.

374. Perry TL, Applegarth DA, et al: Metabolic studies of a family with massive formiminoglutamic aciduria. Pediatr Res 1975; 9:117.

375. Russel A, Statter M, Abzug S: Methionine-dependent formiminoglutamic acid transferase deficiency: human and experimental studies in its therapy. Hum Hered 1977; 27:205.

376. Duran M, Ketting D, et al: A case of formiminoglutamic aciduria. Eur J Pediatr 1981; 136:319.

377. Lankowsky P: Congenital malabsorption of folate. Am J Med 1970; 48:580.

378. Steinschneider M, Sherbany A, et al: Congenital folate malabsorption: reversible clinical and neurophysiologic abnormalities. Neurology 1990; 40:1315.

379. Buchanan JA: Fibroblast Plasma Membrane Vesicles to Study Inborn Errors of Transport. Montréal, Québec, Canada, McGill University, 1984. Doctoral thesis.

380. Urbach J, Abrahamov A, Grossowicz N: Congenital isolated folate acid malabsorption. Arch Dis Child 1987; 62:78.

381. Branda RF, Moldow CF, et al: Folate-induced remission in aplastic anemia with familial defect of cellular folate uptake. N Engl J Med 1978; 298:469.

382. Arthur DC, Danzyl TJ, Branda FR: Cytogenetic studies of a family with a hereditary defect of cellular folate uptake and high incidence of hematologic disease. In Butterworth CE, Hutchinson M (eds): Nutritional Factors in the Induction and Maintenance of Malignancy: Symposium. New York, Academic Press, 1983, pp 101–111.

383. Howe RB, Branda RF, et al: Hereditary dyserythropoiesis with abnormal membrane folate transport. Blood 1979; 54:1080.

384. Fleming JC, Steinkamp MP, et al: Characterization of a murine high-affinity thiamine transporter Slc19a2. Mol Genet Metab 2001; 74:273–280.

385. Gritli S, Omar S, et al: A novel mutation in the Slc19a2 gene in a Tunisian family with thiamine-responsive megaloblastic anaemia, diabetes and deafness syndrome. Br J Haematol 2001; 113:508–513.

386. Neufeld EJ, Fleming JC, et al: Thiamine-responsive megaloblastic anemia syndrome: a disorder of high-affinity thiamine transport. Blood Cells Mol Dis 2001; 27:135–138.

387. Fleming JC, Tartaglini E, et al: The gene mutated in thiamine-responsive anaemia with diabetes and deafness (TRMA) encodes a functional thiamine transporter. Nat Genet 1999; 22:305–308.

388. Stagg AR, Fleming JC, et al: Defective high-affinity thiamine transporter leads to cell death in thiamine-responsive megaloblastic anemia syndrome fibroblasts. J Clin Invest 1999; 103:723–729.

12 | Disorders of Iron Metabolism and Sideroblastic Anemia

Nancy C. Andrews

Iron lacks the glitter of gold and the sparkle of silver but outshines both in biologic importance. This plebeian metal is vital to the function of a number of critical enzymes, including catalases, aconitases, ribonucleotide reductase, peroxidases, and cytochrome oxidases, that exploit the flexible redox chemistry of iron to execute a variety of chemical reactions essential for our survival (Table 12–1). In addition, we depend on hemoglobin, another iron-containing protein, to transport inhaled oxygen from the lungs to peripheral tissues. Human existence is inextricably linked to iron, and disturbances in its metabolism may have dire consequences.

PHYSIOLOGIC CHEMISTRY OF IRON

Iron and Oxidation

The key to the biologic utility of iron is its ability to exist in either of two stable oxidation states: Fe^{2+} (ferrous) or Fe^{3+} (ferric). This property permits iron to act as a redox catalyst by reversibly donating or accepting electrons. An excellent example is the electron transport chain of oxidative phosphorylation, in which adenosine triphos-

phate (ATP) is generated from glucose by the orderly transfer of high-energy electrons through a network of iron-containing mitochondrial cytochromes.

When dissolved in aqueous solution, ferrous iron rapidly oxidizes to its ferric form, which is insoluble at physiologic pH. The resulting ferric hydroxide salts (rust) are of no metabolic utility. To achieve solubility under physiologic conditions, iron must be complexed to iron-binding agents termed *chelators*. Chelators are synthesized by all organisms ranging from microbes (e.g., desferrioxamine produced by *Streptomyces pilosis*) to humans (e.g., transferrin in human plasma). These molecules are crucial to the acquisition of iron from the environment and to its transport and storage within the body.

Iron-Protein Complexes

Iron-protein complexes capitalize on the properties of the metal to perform metabolic functions. Stable coordination complexes form between iron and electron-donating amino acids in proteins. Iron acts as the chemical workhorse, and protein structure dictates biologic specificity.

TABLE 12–1. Iron-Containing Proteins

HEME-CONTAINING PROTEINS

Hemoglobin
Myoglobin
Cytochromes *a*, *b*, and *c*
Cytochrome P-450
Tryptophan-1,2-dioxygenase
Catalase
Myeloperoxidase

IRON-DEPENDENT ENZYMES

Aldehyde oxidase
NADH dehydrogenase
Tyrosine hydroxylase
Succinate dehydrogenase
Prolyl hydroxylase
Tryptophan hydrolase
Xanthine oxidase
Ribonucleotide reductase
Aconitase
Phosphoenolpyruvate carboxykinase

NADH = reduced nicotinamide adenine nucleotide.
Adapted from Griffin IJ, Abrams SA: Iron and breastfeeding. Pediatr Clin North Am 2001; 48:401.

Individual iron atoms can interact directly with amino acid side groups in proteins, as in ribonucleotide reductase. Alternatively, iron may form coordination complexes with other small molecules. Protoporphyrin IX donates four of the six electrons needed to form a stable coordination complex with iron. Heme, the iron-protoporphyrin IX complex, is so stable that removal of the iron moiety requires the enzyme heme oxygenase. The functional properties of heme are determined by the nature of the associated protein or small molecule ligands supplying the remaining two electrons. The best-characterized heme protein is hemoglobin, in which a globin histidine residue donates the fifth electron and the sixth comes from molecular oxygen.[1] This configuration enables hemoglobin to transport oxygen safely throughout the body.

Iron and sulfur atoms can form stable complexes ("clusters") that catalyze enzymatic reactions. The Krebs cycle enzyme aconitase, for example, contains an iron-sulfur cluster. As discussed later in this chapter, the iron content of the iron-sulfur cluster of a related aconitase-like molecule allows it to "sense" iron concentrations within the cell and to act as an iron regulatory protein to modulate the translation of genes of iron metabolism.

Iron Toxicity

The ability of iron to catalyze redox reactions also explains its toxicity. As an enzymatic cofactor, the metal is involved in the restructuring of cellular components, including proteins, carbohydrates, and nucleic acids. Unbound iron has unbridled redox activity, however, and may wreak havoc. We live in an oxygen-rich atmosphere and our bodies require oxygen for many metabolic processes. However, oxygen is extraordinarily reactive and thus is toxic. Reactive oxygen intermediates superoxide (O_2^-) and hydrogen peroxide (H_2O_2) are generated by normal cellular reactions. Oxidative stress develops when production of reactive oxygen species exceeds the body's processing capacity. Under these circumstances, reactive oxygen intermediates may be converted to injurious free radicals by the iron-catalyzed Fenton reaction[2]:

$$O_2^- + Fe^{3+} \rightarrow O_2 + Fe^{2+}$$

$$Fe^{2+} + H_2O_2 \rightarrow Fe^{3+} + HO\bullet + OH^-$$

$$O_2^- + H_2O_2 \rightarrow O_2 + HO\bullet + OH^-$$

Hydroxyl radicals (HO•) attack many biologic macromolecules, including proteins and DNA. They also promote peroxidation of membrane lipids, a problem exacerbated by iron overload and pathologic membrane binding of iron. Intracellular structures are particularly susceptible to iron-dependent peroxidation. In iron-overloaded cells, injured lysosomes become fragile and leaky.[3] Release of lysosomal proteases causes further cell injury and may ultimately lead to cell death. This process contributes to the severe tissue damage seen in the liver, heart, joints, and pancreas of patients with iron overload disorders (see later).

Iron is not normally present in cell membranes. However, both sickle cell disease and thalassemia promote adherence of iron, heme, ferritin, and denatured hemoglobin to the inner surface of the red cell plasma membrane.[4, 5] The membrane complex containing denatured hemoglobin has been termed *hemichrome*.[6] The red cell anion transport protein band 3 appears to nucleate the formation of these iron aggregates.[7, 8] Injured cells decorated with membrane iron deposits are removed by a functioning spleen in patients with thalassemia and hemoglobin SC disease, but they circulate in functionally asplenic patients with homozygous hemoglobin SS disease. Membrane-associated iron promotes free radical formation and further membrane damage, marked by generation of the lipid peroxidation product malonyldialdehyde and by cross-linking of membrane proteins.[4, 5] Membranes become rigid, contributing to the formation of irreversibly sickled cells that occlude the microcirculation.

Sometimes reactive oxygen intermediates can be beneficial. Neutrophils contain a membrane-associated reduced nicotinamide adenine dinucleotide phosphate (NADPH) oxidase that produces superoxide to kill ingested microorganisms (reviewed in reference 9). Superoxide and secondary reactive oxygen intermediates are potent antimicrobial agents. Congenital defects in this NADPH oxidase, collectively termed *chronic granulomatous disease* (see Chapter 21), are characterized by a serious defect in defense against bacterial pathogens.

Neutrophils and iron also injure tissues in inflammatory diseases such as rheumatoid arthritis.[10] Synovial macrophages ingest red cell hemoglobin introduced by intermittent joint hemorrhage. Iron is deposited in the synovial membrane, proximate to superoxide and hydrogen peroxide generated by neutrophils and macrophages participating in the inflammatory reaction. Iron catalyzes the conversion of these compounds into free radical species, which promote lipid peroxidation. Iron therapy exacerbates this process. In contrast, antioxidants and iron chelators retard free radical generation, thereby affording some theoretical protection against injury in rheumatoid arthritis.[11, 12]

These deleterious properties of iron are threatening only when the element is in a "free" state or in an abnormal compartment within the cell. Protection of cell structures from iron-dependent free radical damage is crucial to survival. When iron is bound to protein either directly or in the form of heme, the generation of free radicals is largely abrogated. Thus, tight chelation of iron is a means of controlling its reactivity. As discussed later, cytoplasmic ferritin allows iron to be stored safely within cells by sequestering it in an innocuous form. Ferritin expression is induced by oxidative stress.[13] Both prokaryotic and eukaryotic cells contain ferritins, and mice lacking one of the two ferritin genes do not develop past early embryonic stages.[14] Thus, ferritin appears to be necessary for most, if not all, living cells.

ACQUISITION AND DISTRIBUTION OF IRON

Although the average adult has 4 to 5 g of iron, a meticulous balance exists between dietary uptake and loss. About 1 mg of iron is lost each day through sloughing of cells from skin and mucosal surfaces (Fig. 12–1).[15] Menstruating females lose an average of an additional 1 mg of iron daily, increasing their dietary iron requirement.[16] Neither the liver nor the kidney has a significant capability to excrete iron in humans. Consequently, absorption appears to be the sole means of regulating body iron stores.[17] During neonatal and childhood growth spurts, iron requirements increase in response to augmentation of body mass.

Iron Absorption

Iron absorption occurs predominantly in the duodenum (Fig. 12–2).[18, 19] The physical state of iron entering the duodenum greatly influences its absorption. At physiologic pH, ferrous iron is rapidly converted to the insoluble ferric form. Acid production by the stomach serves to lower the pH in the duodenum, enhancing the solubility and uptake of iron (see later). Heme is absorbed separately from and more efficiently than inorganic iron,[18] independent of duodenal pH. Consequently, meat is an excellent nutritive source of iron. Heme iron absorption is poorly understood, but a heme oxygenase inhibitor has been shown to block heme catabolism in the intestine, resulting in an iron-deficient state.[20]

A number of dietary factors influence iron absorption.[21] Ascorbate and citrate increase iron uptake in part

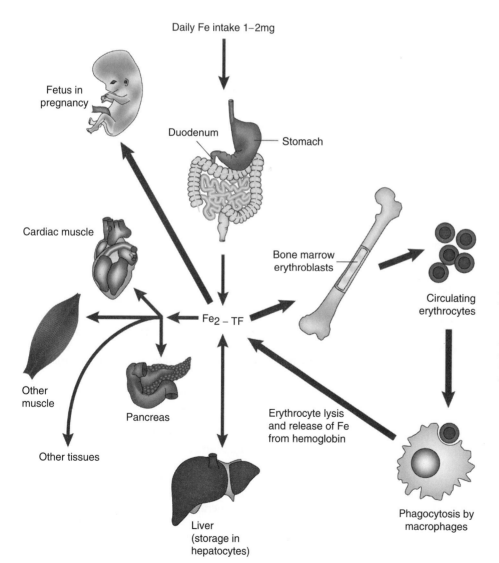

FIGURE 12–1. The body's iron economy. Although the average adult has 3 to 5 g of body iron, only 1 mg of dietary iron enters and leaves the iron economy on an average day. Dietary iron enters through the duodenum and becomes bound to plasma transferrin for delivery to the tissues. The erythron is the largest site of iron utilization, but all cells require the metal. Storage iron is primarily found in the liver. Reticuloendothelial macrophages carry out iron recycling. Iron is lost from the body with bleeding and with exfoliation of skin and mucosal cells. (Adapted from Andrews NC: Iron homeostasis: Insights from genetics and animal models. Nat Rev Genet 2000; 1:208.)

Daily Fe intake 1–2mg

Fetus in pregnancy

Duodenum

Stomach

Cardiac muscle

Bone marrow erythroblasts

Circulating erythrocytes

$Fe_2 - TF$

Other muscle

Pancreas

Erythrocyte lysis and release of Fe from hemoglobin

Other tissues

Liver (storage in hepatocytes)

Phagocytosis by macrophages

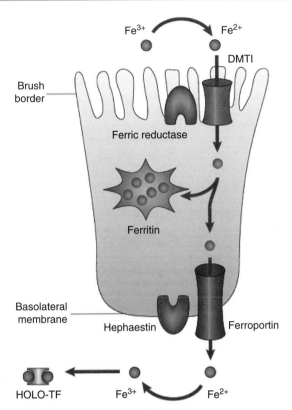

Fe³⁺ Fe²⁺

DMTI

Brush border

Ferric reductase

Ferritin

Basolateral membrane

Hephaestin   Ferroportin

HOLO-TF   Fe³⁺   Fe²⁺

FIGURE 12–2. Duodenal iron transfer. The microstructure of the iron absorption apparatus is depicted in this cartoon. Iron is taken up by enterocytes lining the duodenal villi. These absorptive cells start out as undifferentiated precursors in the intestinal crypts. Crypt cells appear to be programmed for an iron absorption "set-point" that is determined in response to iron needs. As the cells differentiate they migrate up the villi and begin to express iron transporter proteins. According to current models, nonheme iron uptake occurs in mature enterocytes, through the enzymatic reduction of iron by duodenal cytochrome b, transmembrane import into the cell by DMT1, transmembrane export from the cell by ferroportin and enzymatic oxidation by hephaestin before loading on to apotransferrin to produce diferric transferrin (HOLO-TF). (Adapted from Andrews NC: Iron homeostasis: Insights from genetics and animal models. Nat Rev Genet 2000; 1:208.)

by acting as weak chelators to help to solubilize the metal in the duodenum. Iron is readily transferred from these compounds into the mucosal lining cells. Conversely, plant phytates, bran, and tannins inhibit iron absorption.[21–23] These compounds also chelate iron but prevent its uptake by the absorption machinery (see later).

Much has been learned about the absorption of nonheme iron over the past decade, through a combination of genetic and biochemical approaches. Nonheme iron arrives at the apical surface of the absorptive duodenal enterocyte in its ferric (Fe³⁺) form. It is reduced through the action of a brush border ferric reductase. This enzyme is probably duodenal cytochrome b, a heme protein that is homologous to b561 cytochromes.[24] Expression of duodenal cytochrome b is significantly greater in the proximal duodenum than elsewhere, and it increases in iron deficiency.

Ferrous (Fe²⁺) iron is then taken up by the enterocyte, through the action of divalent metal transporter 1 (DMT1, formerly known as Nramp2, DCT1). This transporter was identified and characterized by two groups simultaneously, using complementary cloning strategies. Gunshin and

colleagues[25] injected expressible complementary DNA (cDNA) molecules derived from iron-deficient rats into *Xenopus* oocytes and isolated a unique clone that stimulated iron uptake. The cDNA corresponded to the rat *Nramp2* gene transcript. Nramp2 had previously been identified, but its function was unknown.[26] Gunshin et al. designated their rat protein product DCT1, for divalent cation transporter 1, because it also mediated uptake of other divalent metal ions including Cd²⁺, Co²⁺, Cu²⁺, Mn²⁺, Pb²⁺, and Zn²⁺. Transport requires movement of protons along with metal ions in the same direction (symport), generating an electrical gradient. DMT1 only functions at low pH; it has little or no activity at neutral pH. It is widely expressed, but duodenal levels increase dramatically in iron-deficient animals.[25]

Although this biochemical evidence indicated that DMT1 was a good candidate for the apical iron transporter involved in iron absorption by duodenal cells, proof of its importance *in vivo* came from concurrent genetic experiments. Fleming and colleagues[27] hypothesized that a strain of mice with inherited microcytic anemia (gene *mk*) carried a mutation in the major intestinal iron transporter. Earlier characterization of homozygous *mk* mice had shown that they were severely iron deficient, with defects in iron transport both at the apical surface of intestinal epithelial cells and in erythroid precursor cells.[28–34] Fleming and colleagues bred *mk* homozygotes to wild-type mice of a distinct strain and then backcrossed the first generation of hybrid offspring to *mk* homozygotes to generate progeny that would be informative for genetic mapping. Data derived from analysis of 1000 backcross pups were used to localize the *mk* mutation to a small genetic interval near the end of mouse chromosome 15. The *Nramp2* gene lies within this interval. Although its function was not known and the oocyte expression experiment had not yet been reported, a yeast homolog, SMF1, had been shown to function as a manganese transporter.[35] The observations that the Nramp2 protein encoded a transporter-like protein with 12 predicted transmembrane domains and that SMF1 transported a related divalent metal made Nramp2 an attractive candidate for the site of the *mk* mutation. In fact, *mk* mice were shown to carry a missense mutation that resulted in substitution of an arginine residue for glycine at position 185 of the Nramp2 protein.[27] Functional studies confirmed that the wild-type protein could mediate iron uptake when expressed in transfected cells, but the mutant form had very little activity.[36] Taken together, data from both biochemical and genetic experiments provided compelling evidence that DMT1 (Nramp2, DCT1) is the major intestinal nonheme iron uptake protein in the rodent intestine. It is highly likely that this is also true in humans, although formal proof may require the identification of human mutations affecting DMT1 function. To date, none have been described.

Most investigators use the name DMT1 because it is more descriptive than earlier designations. The first name, Nramp2, was given because the gene encodes a protein homologous to natural resistance associate macrophage protein 1 (Nramp1), a macrophage-specific protein important for attenuating infections by intracellular pathogens in mice.[37] Although Nramp1 is now also presumed to be a metal transporter, the pattern of expression and functional properties of the two homologous proteins are different. Although the name DCT1 is more descriptive than Nramp2, it does not indicate the unique importance of this molecule in the transmembrane transport of transition metals. Therefore, by consensus, the molecule is now termed DMT1. Unfortunately, its gene symbol in both humans and mice was determined independently; it is designated *SLC11A2* in humans and *Slc11a2* in mice, adding to the confusion.

Competition studies suggest that several other heavy metals may share the intestinal absorption pathway used by iron. These include lead, manganese, cobalt, and zinc. Increased iron absorption induced by iron deficiency also enhances the uptake of these elements. Because iron deficiency often coexists with lead intoxication, this interaction has vast public health significance and can produce particularly serious medical complications in children.[38] Interestingly, copper absorption and metabolism appear to be handled by different mechanisms, as discussed later.

After iron enters the absorptive enterocyte through the action of DMT1, it has at least two possible fates. It can be retained by the cell and subsequently lost when the enterocyte dies and is sloughed into the intestinal lumen, or it can be transported across the basolateral membrane to enter the body. Iron retained by the enterocyte is used for cellular metabolism or incorporated into ferritin. Exported iron leaves the cell through the action of a distinct, basolateral transmembrane iron transporter.

Once again, a strong candidate for the basolateral transporter was identified simultaneously by different laboratories. This molecule, designated ferroportin (also IREG1, MTP1, gene *SLC11A3* in humans and *Slc11a3* in mice), has 10 predicted transmembrane domains and is not homologous to any previously identified protein. Donovan and colleagues[39] showed that it is mutated in *weissherbst* (*weh*) mutant zebrafish, which have severe iron deficiency due to a defect in transport of iron from the yolk sac to the developing embryo. They noted that the mammalian homolog is expressed in placental syncytiotrophoblasts, liver Kupffer cells, and duodenal enterocytes, in a pattern consistent with a role in cellular iron egress. McKie and colleagues[40] isolated a cDNA encoding the same protein using a subtraction strategy to identify molecules expressed at high levels in the duodenum of mice with increased intestinal iron absorption. They showed that ferroportin (designated IREG1 in their report) localized to the basolateral surface of polarized epithelial cells and contained a consensus iron regulatory element (discussed later in this chapter) in the 5′ untranslated region of its messenger RNA (mRNA). Abboud and Haile[41] isolated ferroportin (designated MTP1 in their report) because of this iron regulatory element, using a cloning strategy designed to isolate mRNAs containing such elements. All three groups presented functional data in support of the conclusion that ferroportin serves as an iron exporter. Two of them developed *Xenopus* oocyte transport assays[39, 40] and the third showed that intracellular ferritin levels decreased when ferroportin was overexpressed in mammalian cells.[41] Unfortunately, however, all of the assays are cumbersome, and none is ideal for quantitative analysis.*

Based on the observations described earlier, ferroportin is a compelling candidate for a basolateral iron transporter. However, it is not yet clear whether it is the only (or even the major) basolateral transporter functioning in mammalian enterocytes because no animals or human patients have been identified in which loss-of-function mutations in ferroportin interrupt intestinal iron absorption. In fact, human patients heterozygous for missense mutations in ferroportin have been shown to develop iron overload.[42, 43] Further insight may await the study of mice carrying deliberate mutations in the ferroportin gene.

Regardless of the exact mechanism of basolateral iron transfer, there is evidence that it also requires a change in the oxidation state of the metal. This comes from studies of mice carrying the sex-linked anemia (*sla*) mutation. These mice have iron deficiency anemia due to inefficient transfer of iron across the placenta and inefficient absorption of iron through the intestine.[44–48] The mutation was found to be a deletion within the gene encoding hephaestin, a multicopper protein with homology to the ferroxidase, ceruloplasmin.[49] The size of the deletion suggests that it results in a total loss of protein function, although this has not yet been validated experimentally. Although mice homozygous (females) or hemizygous (males) for the X-linked *sla* mutation are iron deficient, their phenotype is far less severe than that of *mk* mutants. This suggests that hephaestin function is not absolutely required. Either another ferroxidase (e.g., ceruloplasmin) may substitute, nonenzymatic oxidation may occur, or oxidation need not be coupled to basolateral iron transfer.

A comprehensive model of intestinal iron absorption, including most available information, is shown in Figure 12–2. It should be noted that the membrane localization of hephaestin is based on what is known about its function rather than on direct experimental data. Furthermore, this model only pertains to nonheme iron transport; details of heme iron uptake have not yet been worked out. Although this is probably a good representation of what takes place in mice, it is possible that human iron absorption is significantly different.

Normally only about 10 percent of dietary nonheme iron entering the duodenum is absorbed. However, this value increases significantly with iron deficiency.[50] In contrast, iron overload reduces but does not eliminate absorption, reaffirming the fact that body iron stores regulate absorption. Finch[50] and later investigators have designated this modulation the "stores regulator." In addition, both iron deficiency anemia and anemia associated with ineffective erythropoiesis induce a marked increase in iron absorption. This effect is greater than that seen with variations in iron stores, and it has been designated the "erythroid regulator."[50] In addition, hypoxia increases iron absorption. The molecular mechanisms involved in each of these regulators are currently unknown.

Most of the total body iron is ultimately incorporated into hemoglobin in erythroid precursors. An average adult produces 200 billion red cells daily, for a red cell renewal rate of 0.8 percent/day. Each red cell contains more than 1 billion atoms of iron, and each milliliter of packed red blood cells contains 1 mg of iron. To meet this daily need for 2×10^{20} atoms (or 20 mg) of elemental iron, iron is recycled from senescent red cells and returned to the

---

*Donovan A, Andrews N, unpublished data.

circulation. Plasma iron turnover (PIT) represents the mass turnover of transferrin-bound iron in the circulation (expressed as milligrams per kilogram per day).[51] Accelerated erythropoiesis increases the PIT and enhances iron uptake from the gastrointestinal tract.[52] The pathophysiologic mechanism is unknown. A circulating factor that modulates iron absorption (the erythroid regulator, see earlier) has been hypothesized but not identified.[50, 53] Several candidate factors have been excluded, including transferrin[54] and erythropoietin.[55] The humoral communication between the marrow and the intestine is particularly apparent in patients with thalassemia intermedia who develop marked iron overload even without transfusions. The accelerated (but ineffective) erythropoiesis taking place in thalassemia substantially boosts iron absorption. Increased PIT also leads to increased gastrointestinal iron absorption in pregnancy, in which PIT is accelerated by placental removal of iron. This increases the availability of the element to meet the needs of the growing and developing fetus.

Intercellular Iron Transport

As illustrated in Figure 12–1, only a small proportion of total body iron enters and leaves the body each day. Consequently, intercellular iron transport is quantitatively more important than intestinal absorption. The greatest mass of iron is found in erythroid cells, making up about 60 to 80 percent of the total body endowment in normal individuals. The reticuloendothelial system recycles a substantial amount of iron from effete red cells, approximating the amount used by the erythron for new hemoglobin production.

Approximately 0.1 percent (4 mg) of the total body iron circulates in the plasma as an exchangeable pool. In normal individuals, nearly all circulating plasma iron is bound to transferrin. Transferrin serves three purposes: (1) it renders iron soluble under physiologic conditions, (2) it prevents iron-mediated free radical toxicity, and (3) it facilitates transport into cells. Transferrin is by far the most important physiologic supplier of iron to red cells.[56] In fact, plasma transferrin serves to deliver iron to most tissues of the body. It is an 80-kD glycoprotein that has homologous N-terminal and C-terminal iron-binding domains.[57] The molecule is related to several other proteins, including ovotransferrin in bird and reptile eggs,[58] lactoferrin in extracellular secretions and neutrophil granules,[59, 60] and melanotransferrin (p97), a protein produced by melanoma cells.[61] The functions of these related proteins are poorly understood.

The liver is the major site of transferrin synthesis and secretion.[62] Other tissues can produce the protein, however; these include Sertoli cells of the testes, oligodendrocytes of the central nervous system (CNS), lymphocytes, muscle cells, and mammary cells.[63–68] Local synthesis within brain and testis apparently provides transferrin for those tissues, because serum transferrin does not penetrate their unique capillary barriers. The blood-testis barrier prevents the free flow of proteins from the circulation into the lumen of the seminiferous tubules. The Sertoli cells of the testis synthesize a significant quantity of transferrin that bathes developing germ cells.[64, 66] These rapidly dividing cells require substantial amounts of iron for normal growth and differentiation. Transferrin supplied by the Sertoli cells is believed to be vital to spermatocyte development.

Transferrin mRNA and protein have also been detected in oligodendrocytes.[67] Like the testis, the CNS has limited access to serum molecules because of the blood-brain barrier. Unlike the testis, however, the CNS has no cohort of rapidly proliferating cells. Iron may be needed instead to support a vast array of redox reactions that produce specialized neurotransmitter compounds such as γ-aminobutyric acid. The question of whether transferrin synthesis by oligodendrocytes is absolutely required for iron distribution to neural tissues remains unanswered. Interestingly, however, mice with an inactivating mutation in the transferrin gene[69] have been reported to have subtle abnormalities of CNS architecture.[70]

Activated T lymphocytes also synthesize and secrete transferrin.[68] At rest, mature T cells do not generate transferrin and do not express surface transferrin receptors. After mitogenic stimulation, however, both proteins are produced.[68, 71] The synthesis of transferrin is restricted to the CD4+ helper lymphocytes. Transferrin mRNA production and transferrin receptor synthesis by these cells precede cell division and have been postulated to be part of an autocrine regulatory loop.[68] Additional data are required to confirm this hypothesis.

Transferrin genes have been cloned from several different species. A basic similarity exists both in the protein structure of the transferrin molecule and in its genomic organization. Human transferrin mRNA is 2.3 kb in length and encodes 679 amino acids including a 19-amino acid leader sequence.[72] It is located on chromosome 3q, near genes for the transferrin receptor and melanotransferrin (p97).

Transferrin production is regulated at multiple levels. Several *cis*-acting control regions exist upstream of the gene. The transferrin promoter contains binding sites for tissue-specific nuclear factors, which activate transcription differentially in liver and other tissues (e.g., Sertoli cells).[73–78] Transferrin gene expression is also modulated by iron, hormones, and inflammatory stimuli.[79–82] In the setting of iron deficiency, serum transferrin levels rise substantially, owing to enhanced transferrin mRNA synthesis by the liver.[83] In contrast, inflammation depresses levels of both serum transferrin and serum iron.

Control of transferrin gene expression contrasts with that of the transferrin receptor in which iron deficiency is thought to increase message levels largely by message stabilization. Transferrin is an abundant, secreted protein involved in iron homeostasis of the whole organism. Consequently, its expression does not have to be altered acutely to respond to external events. Primary control of transferrin expression at the level of message transcription allows modulation of systemic iron metabolism in response to a variety of factors such as inflammation or the hormonal changes of pregnancy. Liver-derived serum transferrin levels fall in patients with genetic or acquired iron overload, although mRNA levels have been reported to be unchanged.[84] This suggests that hepatic transferrin is also controlled at the level of translation or secretion.

Interestingly, the quantity of transferrin mRNA in non-hepatic tissues (including the testis, kidney, and spleen) is not affected by iron deficiency. The liver-derived transferrin, therefore, appears to have the unique responsibility of responding to iron status.

X-ray crystal structures have been determined for a portion of human transferrin, human lactoferrin, and rabbit transferrin.[85, 86] All members of the transferrin protein superfamily have similar polypeptide folding. N-terminal and C-terminal domains are globular moieties of about 330 amino acids; each of these is divided into two sub-domains, with the iron- and anion-binding sites in the intersubdomain cleft on either side of a central plane of symmetry, suggesting an origin by gene duplication from a primordial protein containing a single iron-binding site. The binding cleft opens with iron release and closes with iron binding. N-terminal and C-terminal binding sites are very similar. No cooperativity exists in iron binding by the two sites, and the protein can be proteolytically cleaved into two halves, each of which retains iron-binding capability.[87, 88] Transferrin binds ferric iron much more avidly than ferrous iron.[89]

The precise mechanism by which iron is loaded onto transferrin as it leaves intestinal epithelial cells or reticuloendothelial cells is unknown. Ferroportin has been postulated to mediate iron export from those cells. The copper-dependent ferroxidase ceruloplasmin probably also plays a role. Compelling evidence indicates that ceruloplasmin is involved in mobilizing tissue iron stores to produce diferric transferrin.[90–95] Transferrin binds iron avidly with a dissociation constant of approximately 10^{22} mol/L^{-1}.[89] Ferric iron binds only in the company of an anion (usually carbonate) that serves as a bridging ligand between the metal and the protein, excluding water from two coordination sites.[89, 96, 97] Without the anion cofactor, iron binding is negligible; with it, ferric transferrin is resistant to all but the most potent chelators. The remaining four coordination sites provided by the transferrin protein are a histidine nitrogen, an aspartic acid carboxylate oxygen, and two tyrosine phenolate oxygens.[85, 98, 99] Available evidence suggests that anion binding takes place before iron binding. Iron release from transferrin involves protonation of the carbonate anion, loosening the metal-protein bond.

The sum of all iron-binding sites on transferrin constitutes the total iron-binding capacity of plasma. Thus, on a molar basis, the total iron-binding capacity is approximately twice the concentration of transferrin protein, because each transferrin molecule can bind two iron atoms. Under normal circumstances, about one third of transferrin iron-binding pockets are filled. Consequently, except for the situation of iron overload in which all transferrin-binding sites are occupied, non–transferrin-bound iron in the circulation is present at very low concentrations.[100] Distribution of plasma and tissue iron can be traced using ^{59}Fe as a radioactive tag by reinfusing a subject with autologous transferrin loaded with radiolabeled iron. Blood samples can be analyzed at timed intervals to determine the rate of loss of the radioactive label. Such ferrokinetic studies indicate that the normal half-life of iron in the circulation is about 75 minutes.[51] The absolute amount of iron released from transferrin per unit time is the PIT (see earlier).

Such radioactive tracer studies indicate that at least 80 percent of the iron bound to circulating transferrin is delivered to the bone marrow and incorporated into newly formed reticulocytes (see Fig. 12–1).[101, 102] Other major sites of iron delivery include the liver, which is a primary depot for stored iron, and the spleen. Hepatic iron is found in both reticuloendothelial cells and hepatocytes. Reticuloendothelial cells acquire iron primarily by phagocytosis and breakdown of aging red cells, extracting it from heme and returning it to the circulation bound to transferrin. Hepatocytes take up iron by at least two different pathways. The relative amounts of iron in each of these cell types depend on clinical circumstances, as discussed in detail later.

Given the preeminent role of the bone marrow in the clearance of labeled iron from the circulation, ferrokinetic studies provide a window on erythropoietic activity. Conditions that augment erythrocyte production increase the PIT. For example, hemolytic anemias such as hereditary spherocytosis and sickle cell disease induce rapid delivery of transferrin-bound iron to the marrow. In contrast, disorders that reduce red cell production prolong the PIT. Such a picture is seen, for example, in Diamond-Blackfan anemia and aplastic anemia.

When erythrocytes are produced and released into the circulation in a normal fashion, the process of erythropoiesis is termed *effective*. In patients with certain hemolytic anemias, however, the abnormal, nascent red cells are destroyed before they leave the marrow cavity. In this circumstance, the erythropoiesis is *ineffective*, meaning simply that the erythropoietic precursors have failed to accomplish their primary task: the delivery of intact erythrocytes to the circulation. The ferrokinetic profile in this case shows rapid removal of iron from transferrin with a delayed entry of label into the pool of circulating red cell hemoglobin. β$^+$-Thalassemia is an important example of this pattern. In β$^+$-thalassemia, ineffective erythropoiesis is coupled with a markedly enhanced PIT.

Intracellular Iron Metabolism

Although transferrin was first characterized more than 50 years ago,[103] its receptor eluded investigators until the early 1980s when monoclonal antibodies prepared against tumor cells were found to recognize the transferrin receptor glycoprotein.[104] Subsequently, receptor-mediated endocytosis of iron bound to transferrin has been characterized in detail. A diagram showing key features of the transferrin receptor is shown in Figure 12–3. Each subunit of the disulfide-linked homodimer contains 760 amino acids.[105–107] Oligosaccharides account for about 5 percent of the 90-kD subunit molecular mass.[108] Four glycosylation sites (three N-linked and one O-linked) are found in the protein.[109, 110] Glycosylation-defective mutants have fewer disulfide bridges, less transferrin binding, and less cell surface expression. The transmembrane domain, between amino acids 62 and 89, functions as an internal signal peptide, because there is none at the N-terminal end.[111] A molecule of fatty acid (usually palmitate) is also covalently linked to each subunit at the internal edge of the transmembrane domain and may play a role in membrane localization. Interestingly, nonacylated mutants

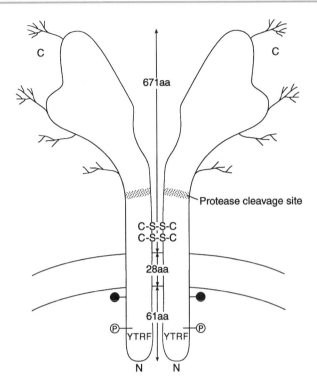

FIGURE 12–3. Structure of the dimeric transferrin receptor. The N termini of both subunits are inside the cell, and the C termini are outside. The 61-amino acid intracellular domain has three structural features that appear to play a role in endocytosis: a tyrosine-threonine-arginine-phenylalanine *(YTRF)* amino acid motif, a phosphorylated serine residue *(encircled "P")*, and a covalently linked molecule of palmitic acid *(solid circle)*. The transmembrane domain is 28 amino acids long. The extracellular domain has 671 amino acids, including disulfide linkages (C-S-S-C) as well as four glycosylation sites *(branched lines)*. A potential protease cleavage site is located between amino acids 100 and 101.

mediate faster iron uptake.[112, 113] The transferrin binding regions of the protein have not been definitively identified. However, the crystal structure of the ectodomain of the transferrin receptor was recently reported[114] Although no one has yet succeeded in cocrystallizing the receptor with transferrin, binding studies of mutant transferrin receptor proteins have yielded important insights.[115]

Iron is taken into cells by receptor-mediated endocytosis of monoferric and diferric transferrin (Fig. 12–4).[116–118] Receptors on the outer face of the plasma membrane bind iron-loaded transferrin with a very high affinity. The C-terminal domain of transferrin appears to mediate receptor binding.[119] Diferric transferrin binds with higher affinity than that of monoferric transferrin or apotransferrin.[120–122] The dissociation constant (K_d) for bound diferric transferrin ranges from 10^{-7} to 10^{-9} mol/L at physiologic pH, depending on the species and tissue. The K_d of monoferric transferrin is approximately 10^{-6} mol/L. The concentration of circulating transferrin is about 25 μmol/L. Therefore, cellular transferrin receptors are ordinarily fully saturated.

After binding to its receptor on the cell surface, transferrin is rapidly internalized by invagination of clathrin-coated pits and formation of endocytic vesicles. This process requires the short, 61-amino acid intracellular tail of the transferrin receptor molecule.[123–126] Receptors with truncated N-terminal cytoplasmic domains do not recycle properly. This portion of the molecule contains a

conserved tyrosine-threonine-arginine-phenylalanine (YTRF) sequence that functions as a signal for endocytosis. Genetically engineered addition of a second YTRF sequence enhances receptor endocytosis.[127] A number of stimuli reversibly phosphorylate the serine residue adjacent to the YTRF sequence at position 24 by the action of protein kinase C.[128] The role of receptor phosphorylation is unclear. Despite removal of the phosphorylation site by site-directed mutagenesis, the transferrin receptor recycles normally.[123]

An ATP-dependent proton pump lowers the pH of the internalized endosome to about 5.5.[129–131] The acidification of the endosome weakens the association between iron and transferrin[132] and promotes a conformational change in the transferrin receptor to enhance binding of apotransferrin and facilitate iron release.[133, 134] It is likely that an endosomal oxidoreductase reduces transferrin-bound iron from the Fe^{3+} state to Fe^{2+}, directly or indirectly facilitating the removal of iron from the protein.[135–137]

Iron released from transferrin must leave the endosome to enter the cytoplasm, where it is used for heme biosynthesis and other purposes. Available data suggest that this transmembrane transport step is also mediated by DMT1. The Belgrade *(b)* rat was shown to take up transferrin-bound iron into endosomes, but the iron was not appropriately transferred to the cytoplasm, suggesting a defect in a transmembrane endosomal transporter.[138–141] Genetic

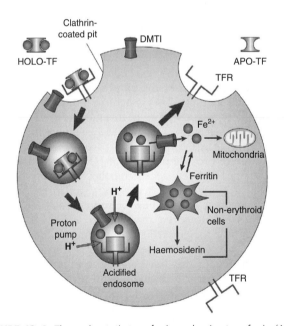

FIGURE 12–4. The endocytotic transferrin cycle. Apotransferrin (APO-TF) binds two atoms of iron per molecule to form diferric transferrin (HOLO-TF). Diferric transferrin binds to the transferrin receptor (TFR) on the cell surface. The complex is internalized by invagination of clathrin-coated pits to form specific endosomes. The endosomes import protons, thus lowering the pH within the organelle and decreasing the affinity of transferrin for iron. Liberated iron is translocated through the endosome membrane to the cytoplasm by DMT1. Released iron is shuttled to mitochondria for heme synthesis and to ferritin for storage. The apotransferrin-transferrin receptor complex recycles to the cell surface, where neutral pH promotes release of apotransferrin into the serum for reuse. Details are given in the text. (Adapted from Andrews NC: Iron homeostasis: Insights from genetics and animal models. Nat Rev Genet 2000; 1:208.)

mapping and analysis of the rat gene encoding DMT1 revealed that *b* rats, like *mk* mice, carry a glycine to arginine missense mutation at codon 185 in the protein.[142] This was a remarkable finding because the same mutation was shown to have occurred in two different species. In retrospect, it is clear that *mk* mice and *b* rats have very similar phenotypes, including defects in both intestinal iron absorption and erythroid iron assimilation. The similarity was not initially appreciated because the two animal models were studied using different approaches. DMT1 is unusual in that it is expressed on two very different types of membranes—the apical membrane of intestinal enterocytes[143] and the endosomal membrane of transferrin-uptake vesicles in nonpolarized cells.[36, 144]

The fates of the transferrin and transferrin receptor are distinct from that of the iron. Rather than entering lysosomes for degradation, as do ligands in other receptor-mediated endocytosis pathways, intact receptor-bound apotransferrin recycles to the cell surface, where neutral pH promotes detachment into the circulation. Thus, the preservation and reuse of transferrin are accomplished by pH-dependent changes in the affinity of transferrin for its receptor.[118, 129, 130] Exported apotransferrin binds additional iron atoms and undergoes further rounds of iron delivery to cells. The average transferrin molecule, with a half-life of 8 days, may be used hundreds of times for iron delivery.[145]

Topologically, the cell exterior and the endosome interior are equivalent compartments. The primary role of the transferrin-transferrin receptor interaction is to sequester iron into the vicinity of the cell membrane, thereby increasing the likelihood of iron uptake. DMT1 may reside on the plasma membrane of the cell before endocytosis. If so, it should be oriented to transport iron directly into the cell, without the assistance of transferrin (as diagrammed in Fig. 12–4). Such non–transferrin-bound iron uptake activities have been characterized in tissue culture cells (see later). This uptake system could function constitutively but inefficiently in tissues in which pH is low enough to provide protons for DMT1 function.

It was once a widely accepted belief that the transferrin cycle was important, if not necessary, for iron uptake by all mammalian cells with the exception of mature intestinal enterocytes. However, two lines of evidence indicate that this is not the case. First, mice and human patients who have severe deficiencies of plasma transferrin have iron deficiency anemia but excess iron in nonhematopoietic tissues.[69, 146–152] This finding indicates that the uptake of iron bound to transferrin is important for red blood cell hemoglobinization and maturation, but transferrin is not needed for iron delivery to most other tissues. Second, mouse embryos lacking transferrin receptor die midway through gestation from severe anemia, but non-hematopoietic tissues are generally intact.[153] Aside from the erythron, only the developing CNS shows an apparent requirement for transferrin receptor. In its absence, primitive neuroepithelial cells undergo apoptosis at a greatly increased rate. Taken together, these observations indicate that the transferrin cycle is of primary importance in erythropoiesis and neurogenesis but of lesser importance in other mammalian tissues, at least early in embryonic development.

Non–Transferrin-Bound Iron Uptake

Both hypotransferrinemia and iron overload lead to complete saturation of available plasma transferrin, and non–transferrin-bound iron circulates in a chelatable, low-molecular-weight form (reviewed in reference 100). This iron is weakly complexed to albumin, citrate, amino acids, and sugars and other small molecules, and it behaves differently from iron associated with transferrin. Nonhematopoietic tissues (particularly the liver, endocrine organs, kidneys, and heart) preferentially take up non–transferrin-bound iron.

Radiolabeled iron administered to mice with and without available transferrin-binding capacity is distributed in markedly different patterns.[147, 151] In normal animals with excess plasma iron-binding capacity, hematopoietic tissues are the primary sites of uptake. When free transferrin iron-binding sites are absent, however, most iron is deposited in the liver and pancreas, indicating that these organs serve as initial iron reservoirs in the situation of iron overload. Notably, this pattern of distribution is similar to that seen in idiopathic hemochromatosis.

Kaplan and co-workers[154, 155] have studied cellular assimilation of iron from $FeNH_4$ citrate in HeLa cells. Intriguingly, they find that its transferrin-independent uptake increases in direct proportion to the concentration of this compound, similar to hepatic uptake of non–transferrin-bound iron in patients with saturated transferrin. They speculated that this is a protective alternative pathway that removes the toxic metal from the circulation. Other investigators have described similar uptake in HepG2 cells and have shown that it is interrupted by addition of chelating compounds.[156]

A non-transferrin iron uptake mechanism with different properties has been described in K562 erythroleukemia cells.[157, 158] In the absence of ferric transferrin, iron uptake into K562 cells is sensitive to treatment with trypsin, suggesting that it requires a protein carrier. Higher ambient iron concentrations do not increase cellular iron uptake. As discussed earlier, this transport may be accomplished by the same machinery responsible for passage of iron out of transferrin cycle endosomes into the cytoplasm. These two processes accomplish essentially the same task. However, the fact that DMT1 only functions at acidic pH suggests that it cannot, by itself, account for all non–transferrin-bound iron transport.

Non–transferrin-bound iron is highly toxic to cells.[159] Plasma non–transferrin-bound iron can potentiate formation of free radicals through the Fenton reaction (see earlier) and thus induce damage of cell membranes. Cardiac cells are particularly susceptible to this damage. Hence, therapeutic removal of iron, through chelation, must effectively remove plasma non–transferrin-bound iron.

Role of Iron in Cell Proliferation and Differentiation

Iron is indispensable for DNA synthesis and a host of metabolic processes. Iron starvation arrests proliferation, presumably because ribonucleotide reductase and other enzymes require the metal.[160] Although transferrin receptors are expressed on all dividing cells in numbers that roughly reflect growth rate,[161] the erythron is the tissue that relies most heavily on iron delivery by transferrin, as discussed in detail earlier. However, the transferrin cycle also appears to play a significant, if sometimes expendable, role in other cell types.

Studies of mature T lymphocytes exemplify the general relationship between transferrin receptor expression and cell proliferation. Transferrin receptors, absent from resting T cells, have long been recognized as a marker of T-cell activation. The initiation of cell division by a mitogen such as phytohemagglutinin dramatically increases both transferrin receptor surface expression and iron uptake.[162] Along the same lines, tumor cells up-regulate transferrin receptor expression to optimize iron acquisition for proliferation.

Blockade of transferrin receptor function can halt cell division. For instance, certain monoclonal antibodies against the transferrin receptor curb proliferation of tumor cells *in vitro* and *in vivo*.[163–165] Some of these antibodies actually prevent binding of transferrin to its receptor, whereas others suppress receptor recycling but do not abrogate ligand binding.[166] Interestingly, some reports have suggested that the transferrin receptor may have an additional role in activated T cells, apart from its iron uptake function. Anti–transferrin receptor monoclonal antibodies have been described that can trigger T-cell activation and interleukin-2 secretion.[167–169] These antibodies presumably activate a signal transduction pathway beginning with the transferrin receptor but independent of iron trafficking. The transferrin receptor also appears to have a role in early lymphocyte development. Embryonic stem cells in which both transferrin receptor genes have been inactivated fail to differentiate into circulating lymphocytes *in vivo* in chimeric mice.* It is not yet clear whether this is due to defective iron delivery or perturbation of some other, as yet unknown, function of the transferrin receptor.

Chelators that can deplete intracellular iron and limit its bioavailability in extracellular fluids further demonstrate the central role of iron in cell proliferation. Agents such as desferrioxamine, desferrithiocin, and pyridoxal isonicotinoyl hydrazone inhibit the growth of a variety of tumor cells in culture[170, 171] and greatly reduce T-cell proliferation.[172–175] A likely inhibitory mechanism is iron deprivation, with reduced ribonucleotide reductase activity and lower levels of deoxyribonucleotides. This, in turn, leads to mitotic arrest in the S phase of the cell cycle.[176] The addition of iron to the medium reverses the growth inhibition. Chelators may also induce apoptosis or programmed cell death through other mechanisms that are not yet understood.

Erythroid precursors need an extraordinary amount of iron to support hemoglobin synthesis and differentiation into mature red cells. The density of transferrin receptors on the cell surface is modulated during erythroid development. Transferrin receptors first appear in measurable numbers on the colony-forming unit-erythroid (CFU-E), increasing to 300,000 per cell on proerythroblasts and as many as 800,000 per cell on basophilic erythroblasts at the time of maximal iron uptake. Numbers then fall to 100,000 per cell on circulating reticulocytes and to negligible levels on mature red cells.[177] A precise correlation

exists between iron requirement and transferrin receptor number, indicating that the abundance of transferrin receptors on the cell surface is a major determinant of erythroid iron uptake. In culture, a monoclonal antibody to the transferrin receptor that permits ligand binding but subsequently slows receptor recycling partially blocks erythroid burst cell iron uptake. The level of iron uptake is sufficient for cell division but not hemoglobin synthesis.[178]

Beug and co-workers[179] demonstrated that an anti–transferrin receptor monoclonal antibody blocked differentiation of chick erythroid cells at the erythroblast or early reticulocyte stage and promoted premature, pyknotic cell death. The antibody apparently prevented normal cycling of transferrin receptors and inhibited efficient iron uptake. Its effects were specific for erythroid differentiation because it did not inhibit proliferation of a variety of other cell lines. Ferric salicylaldehyde-isonicotinyl-hydrazone (Fe-SIH) was added to antibody-treated cells to determine whether direct delivery of iron by this compound could rescue the normal erythroid program. Interestingly, the Fe-SIH only partially restored maturation of antibody-treated avian cells. The investigators postulated that insufficient levels of heme or hemoglobin might shut off production of proteins required for differentiation. These data are in accord with those of Ponka and Schulman,[56] who have shown that the rate of heme synthesis is influenced by the efficiency of an unknown step in iron uptake. They localized the critical step distal to the interaction of ferric transferrin with the transferrin receptor but proximal to insertion of iron into heme by ferrochelatase. A wealth of literature demonstrates that oxidized heme (hemin) promotes differentiation of erythroleukemia cell lines in tissue culture.[180–183] Conversely, deficient heme biosynthesis abrogates chemical induction of differentiation in an erythroleukemia cell line subclone.[184]

Other reports indicate that heme biosynthesis indirectly regulates the transcription of globin, transferrin receptor, and ferritin genes.[185–187] Heme also regulates globin mRNA translation. Whereas the onset of globin protein synthesis precedes that of heme in developing erythroblasts *in vivo*,[188] the intracellular concentration of heme directly modulates globin synthesis *in vitro*.[189] Although the precise mechanisms remain to be elucidated, it is clear that iron uptake, heme biosynthesis, and globin protein production are coordinately regulated. Interrelated regulatory networks apparently allow red cell precursors to maximize hemoglobin formation without accumulating excess globin proteins, unbound iron, or toxic protoporphyrin intermediates.

REGULATION OF PROTEINS OF IRON METABOLISM

Ferritin

Once inside the cell cytoplasm, iron is probably bound by unidentified carrier molecules, which may assist in delivery to various intracellular locations including mitochondria (for heme biosynthesis) and ferritin (for storage; reviewed in reference 190). The identities of the intracellular iron carrier molecules remain unknown. The amount of iron in transit within the cell at any given time is small

---

*Ned R, Andrews N, unpublished data.

and difficult to measure. This minute pool of transit iron, which is believed to be in the Fe^{2+} oxidation state, is the biologically active and potentially toxic form of the element. Metabolically inactive iron, stored in ferritin and hemosiderin, is nontoxic and is in equilibrium with this exchangeable transit iron.

Both prokaryotes and eukaryotes produce ferritin molecules for iron storage. Mammalian ferritins are complex 24-subunit heteropolymers of H (for heavy or heart) and L (for light or liver) protein subunits. L subunits are 19.7 kD in mass, with isoelectric points of 4.5 to 5.0; H subunits are 21 kD in mass with isoelectric points of 5.0 to 5.7. The subunits of the ferritin molecule probably arose by gene duplication, although the degree of nucleotide sequence homology between the two is only about 50 percent. They assemble to form a sphere with a central cavity in which up to several thousand atoms of crystalline iron can be stored in the form of poly-iron-phosphate oxide.[191] Eight channels through the sphere are lined by hydrophilic amino acid residues (along the threefold axes of symmetry), and six more are lined by hydrophobic residues (along the fourfold axes).[192] Strong interspecies amino acid conservation is seen in the residues that line the hydrophilic channels, whereas marked variation is seen in those along the hydrophobic passages. Hydrophilic channels terminate with aspartic acid and glutamic acid residues and are lined by serine, histidine, and cysteine residues (all of which potentially bind metal ligands).

Although the two ferritin chains are homologous, only H ferritin has ferroxidase activity. A mechanism involving dioxygen converts ferrous to ferric iron, promoting incorporation into ferritin.[193, 194] The composition of ferritin shells varies from H-subunit homopolymers to L-subunit homopolymers and includes all possible combinations between the two. Isoelectric focusing of ferritin from a particular tissue reveals multiple bands representing shells with different subunit compositions. These isoferritins, as they are called, show tissue-specific variation. Ferritin from liver, for instance, is rich in L subunits, as is that from the spleen. In contrast, the heart has ferritin rich in H subunits. Increased H-subunit content correlates with increased iron utilization, whereas increased L-subunit content correlates with increased iron storage.[195] The H-to-L ratio increases with increased cell proliferation.[196] Thus, ferritin provides a flexible reserve of iron.

Ferritin molecules aggregate over time to form clusters, which are engulfed by lysosomes and degraded. The end product of this process, hemosiderin, is an amorphous agglomerate of denatured protein and lipid interspersed with iron oxide molecules.[197] In cells overloaded with iron, lysosomes accumulate large amounts of hemosiderin, which can be visualized by Prussian blue staining. Although the iron enmeshed in this insoluble compound constitutes an end-stage product of cellular iron storage, it remains in equilibrium with soluble ferritin. Ferritin iron, in turn, is in equilibrium with iron complexed to low-molecular-weight carrier molecules. Therefore, the introduction into the cell of an effective chelator captures iron from the low-molecular-weight "toxic" iron pool, draws iron out of ferritin, and eventually depletes iron from hemosiderin as well, although only very slowly. As might

be expected, the bioavailability of hemosiderin iron is much lower than that of iron stored in ferritin.

The large number of processed pseudogenes that exist for each subunit initially confounded pinpointing the chromosomal location of ferritin genes.[198–200] Functional ferritin genes have now been located on human chromosomes 11 and 19 for the H and L subunits, respectively.[201] In addition, there is an intron-less gene encoding a mitochondrion-specific ferritin molecule located in human chromosome 5q.[202] The function of mitochondrial ferritin remains uncertain, although the fact that its expression is increased in erythroid precursors from patients with sideroblastic anemia suggests that it is involved in mitochondrial iron storage.

Ferritin formation is controlled at multiple levels—transcription, message stabilization, translation, and subunit assembly.[203, 204] In the liver and in HeLa cells, iron rapidly induces L-subunit mRNA synthesis, with no effect on H-subunit transcription.[204, 205] In contrast, induced differentiation of HL-60 promyelocytic leukemia cells and mouse erythroleukemia cells increases H-subunit mRNA production.[206, 207] Tumor necrosis factor induces H-chain transcription in human myoblasts.[208] Iron, heme, reactive oxygen species, and oxidative stress all enhance transcription and translation of the ferritin heavy chain.[13, 187, 203]

Cytoplasmic ferritin mRNA forms a stable complex with several proteins. Both iron and interleukin-1β enhance translation of ferritin messenger ribonucleoprotein (mRNP).[209, 210] The influx of iron into cells shifts the message onto the ribosomes, thereby enhancing the synthesis of ferritin subunits. This translational control mechanism involves an RNA-protein interaction that links the expression of genes encoding ferritin, the transferrin receptor, enzymes of heme biosynthesis, DMT1, and ferroportin. Munro and colleagues[210] initially showed that ferritin synthesis was regulated at the level of message translation. Comparison of the 5′-untranslated regions of ferritin mRNAs encoding both heavy and light chains showed striking conservation of a 28-bp sequence motif that was predicted to form a stable RNA stem-loop structure and was necessary for ferritin translational control (Fig. 12–5, *inset*).[211, 212]

Subsequently designated the iron response element (IRE), this RNA stem-loop is recognized by at least two specific RNA-binding proteins. These are called IRP-1 and IRP-2 for iron regulatory proteins-1 and -2. IRP-1 is a 98-kD soluble polypeptide with striking homology to the mitochondrial tricarboxylic acid cycle enzyme, aconitase.[213] IRP-1 and mitochondrial aconitase have identical amino acid residues in the region corresponding to the aconitase active site, and IRP-1 probably serves as the major cytosolic aconitase. The enzymatic active site of IRP-1 contains a [4Fe/4S] cluster. When the iron concentration in the cytosol is high, the cluster is complete, and this form of IRP-1 has aconitase activity but cannot bind mRNA. Under those circumstances, the ferritin message is translated efficiently. Conversely, when the iron concentration is low, aconitase activity is absent, RNA binding is avid, and ferritin message translation is blocked because translation initiation complexes cannot form properly[214–219] Thus, IRP-1 is a dual-function protein, with ambient iron controlling the switch by its participa-

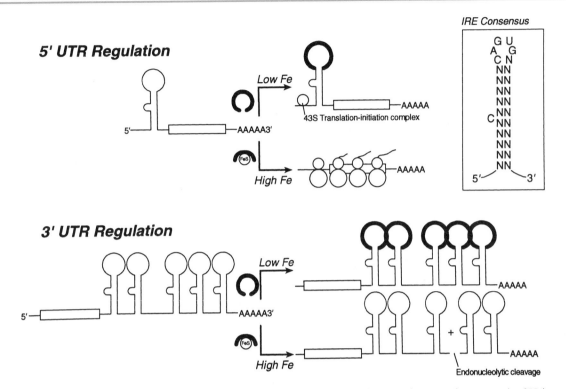

FIGURE 12–5. Iron response element/iron regulatory protein regulation. Two mechanisms of action of iron regulatory proteins (IRPs) are shown. An IRP molecule binds to an iron response element (IRE) stem-loop structure located in noncoding mRNA sequences. A consensus IRE structure is shown in the *inset*. Under low iron conditions, IRP binds avidly to RNA. With abundant iron, no binding occurs. IRP binding to IRE elements in the 5'-untranslated region (UTR) (e.g., in ferritin mRNAs) blocks translation. In contrast, IRP binding to 3'-UTR IRE elements (e.g., in transferrin receptor mRNA) prevents site-specific nucleolytic cleavage, thereby stabilizing the message. In this way, a single regulatory element plays two different roles in the translational regulation of proteins involved in cellular iron metabolism.

tion in the [Fe/4S] cluster. Other molecules that modulate the switch include ascorbic acid, nitric oxide, and heme.[220–222] This mechanism allows ferritin protein expression to be rapidly down-regulated without mRNA degradation. The importance of this mechanism of translational control is underscored by the fact that human patients with mutations in the L-ferritin IRE develop hyperferritinemia and ferritin-containing cataracts (without abnormalities in iron homeostasis).[223, 224] Also, it appears that patients with mutations in the H-ferritin IRE develop an iron overload disorder resembling hereditary hemochromatosis, presumably because increased H-ferritin expression leads to increased cellular iron assimilation.[225]

A second IRE-binding protein, IRP-2, also modulates post-transcriptional expression of mRNAs by binding to IREs in much the same way. Initially isolated in liver, IRP-2 has been found in all tissues examined and is more abundant than IRP-1 in some.[226–228] Although the two proteins differ in molecular mass (90 kD for IRP-1 and 118 kD for IRP-2), the key difference is that IRP-2 lacks aconitase activity[228] and does not contain an Fe/•S cluster to function as a "ferrostat." Rather, IRP-2 protein levels are modulated directly by iron, and the molecule is actively degraded when iron is abundant.[229]

The Transferrin Receptor

IRPs also modulate expression of the transferrin receptor gene. The gene encoding the transferrin receptor is located on human chromosome 3q26.2-qter, near the gene encoding transferrin at 3q21.[230, 231] It consists of 19 exons spread over 31 kb.[232] The transferrin receptor mRNA is approximately twice the length needed to encode the receptor protein. Its lengthy 3'-untranslated region contains five potential RNA stem-loop structures that are structurally similar to those of the ferritin IREs.[233–235] These conserved regions of the transferrin receptor mRNA bind the same proteins as the IREs of the ferritin mRNAs.[235] The attached protein increases the stability of the transferrin receptor message by obscuring a potential site of endonucleolytic cleavage.[236] The result is a larger amount of transferrin receptor mRNA in the cell. A deficit of cellular iron, then, raises transferrin receptor mRNA levels at least in part through enhanced message stability. However, IRE regulation is probably not responsible for the primary increases in transferrin receptor numbers in erythroid cells, because this occurs at the transcriptional level and is unaffected by iron status. Relatively little is understood about the tissue-specific transcriptional regulation of the transferrin receptor, although there has been some recent progress in this area.[237]

The versatile regulatory functions of IREs may also confer iron-dependent regulation on other proteins. IREs have been detected in the 5'-untranslated regions of the mRNAs encoding the erythroid form of the heme biosynthetic enzyme δ-aminolevulinic acid synthase, mitochondrial aconitase, and ferroportin.[39–41, 238–240] A single 3' IRE is found in one splicing isoform of DMT1 mRNA.[25] As the rate-limiting enzyme in heme biosynthesis, the IRE in the erythroid form of δ-aminolevulinic acid synthase produces a conceptually satisfying link between iron and heme production. However, the functions of the IREs in the other mRNAs are not yet understood. It is postulated that all IREs serve the common purpose of coupling changes in the iron status of the cell with its ability to utilize and store the element (Fig. 12–5). When the intracellular iron concentration is low, the IRE of ferritin mRNA binds IRP, reducing ferritin synthesis, because additional iron storage capacity is not needed in this circumstance. Simultaneously, the level of transferrin receptor mRNA increases as the IRP stabilizes the message, thereby increasing transferrin receptor expression. Together these events increase the flow of iron into cells while protecting against iron toxicity. When iron levels in the cell are high, the opposite scenario is operative. Although the IRPs accomplish these regulatory feats under extremes of iron status, the importance of IREs and IRPs in modulating gene expression in normal humans and animals has not yet been established.

In an attempt to sort out the unique functions of IRP-1 and IRP-2 and to evaluate their roles *in vivo*, targeted mutagenesis was used to generate mutant mice lacking each of the proteins.[241] Surprisingly, IRP-1 knockout mice had no identifiable defects, but IRP-2 knockout mice had abnormalities in several tissues. The most striking aspect of the IRP-2 knockout phenotype was a late-onset neurologic disorder associated with abnormal deposition of iron in white matter tracts and nuclei throughout the brain. The mice demonstrated ataxia, bradykinesia, and tremors. These findings could not readily be explained by known activities of IRP-2 and will require further investigation. The IRP-2 knockout mice also showed accumulation of iron in their duodenal enterocytes. Again, the significance of this finding is presently unclear.

Plasma Ferritin and Transferrin Receptors

Ferritin. Although most ferritin is located within cells, a measurable amount of the protein exists in serum. The source of extracellular ferritin is unclear. Some apparently leaks from necrotic cells. Intracellular concentrations are several orders of magnitude higher than plasma concentrations. Therefore, a small amount of cellular lysis could liberate a relatively large amount of ferritin. However, the vast majority of plasma ferritin appears to be secreted. Circulating ferritin is iron-poor and consists almost exclusively of L-chain subunits.[242] In contrast, intracellular ferritin contains a mixture of H and L subunits. Also, circulating ferritin is glycosylated, unlike intracellular ferritin, suggesting that it passes through the endoplasmic reticulum and Golgi apparatus as do other secreted proteins.[243, 244]

Serum ferritin levels decline with iron deficiency and rise with iron loading.[245] They reasonably reflect total body iron stores in the absence of liver disease, infection, or chronic inflammation. The correlation between serum ferritin levels and body iron stores is useful in the evaluation of patients with possible iron deficiency or iron overload. A low serum ferritin level (less than 12 mg/L) invariably represents iron deficiency, and high serum ferritin levels are found in patients with iron overload.

Extreme plasma ferritin levels should be interpreted cautiously, however, because the correlation between plasma ferritin levels and body iron stores is approximately linear only for storage reserves of iron ranging between 1 and 3 g.[244] In addition, normal plasma ferritin values vary with sex and age. These considerations must be factored into any evaluation of iron stores based on plasma ferritin values, particularly in children.

Various conditions modify plasma ferritin levels. Inflammation increases the plasma ferritin concentration several fold.[246] Infections, particularly chronic conditions such as tuberculosis or osteomyelitis, may increase plasma ferritin levels substantially, presumably because of the associated inflammatory response. Chronic renal disease and chronic liver disease are also associated with elevated levels. A number of tumors variably raise the level of circulating ferritin.[247, 248] For example, ferritin is an important prognostic factor in childhood neuroblastoma, in which serum ferritin levels correlate with disease severity.[249]

The mechanisms by which inflammation and tumors increase the quantity of plasma ferritin are unknown. Treatment with interleukin-1β, a prime mediator of the inflammatory response, increases ferritin synthesis in human hepatoma cells,[209] whereas tumor necrosis factor has been shown to increase ferritin mRNA levels in murine cells in culture.[208] These cytokines may also increase ferritin synthesis in cells secreting the protein.

Soluble Transferrin Receptor. Soluble transferrin receptors are also found in the plasma. Small vesicles containing transferrin receptors are shed from reticulocytes during their maturation to erythrocytes.[250–252] In addition to these vesicle-associated receptors, the extracellular portion of the transferrin receptor lacking its transmembrane anchor can be found in the circulation.[253, 254] One mechanism by which soluble transferrin receptors are generated is a membrane-associated protease activity that clips the molecule between amino acids 100 and 101, at the base of its extracellular stem.[255–257] This cleavage is potentiated by mutation of an O-linked glycosylation site at amino acid 104, suggesting that differential glycosylation may play a regulatory role.[258] The transferrin-binding domain is intact in these soluble receptors, and they are likely to be complexed with transferrin in the plasma.

Because maturing red cells shed their transferrin receptors, the amount of soluble transferrin receptor in plasma reasonably reflects erythropoiesis. Measurement of plasma levels of soluble transferrin receptor provides a means of estimating erythropoietic activity, which is simpler than the relatively cumbersome PIT determination.[259] The protein exists in substantially lower amounts in patients with aplastic anemia relative to normal individuals. In contrast, the values in patients with anemias caused by ineffective erythropoiesis are markedly increased. Patients with iron deficiency also have increased levels of circulating soluble transferrin receptors. This may result in part from the increase in cellular transferrin receptor expression produced by iron starvation and in part from the increased erythroid turnover associated with the ineffective erythropoiesis of iron deficiency. Serum transferrin receptor and serum ferritin values can be considered together as the ratio of sTfR to the log of ferritin (sTfR-F index). Values greater than 1.5 suggest iron deficiency alone or in combination with an inflammatory condition; values less than 1.5 are characteristic of the anemia of chronic disease.[260] The sTfR-F index also appears to be sensitive enough to detect iron deficiency before iron-restricted erythropoiesis is clinically apparent.[261] Serum transferrin receptor and the sTfR-F index are both decreased in patients with iron overload.[262, 263]

COPPER METABOLISM

Nutritional Copper Deficiency

Like iron, copper is essential for normal cell growth and metabolism but toxic in excess. Copper deficiency commonly causes hypochromic anemia among farm animals in areas of the world where the soil is copper-poor.[264–267] Nutritional copper deficiency in humans usually results from extraordinary dietary circumstances,[268, 269] such as inadvertent omission of copper from intravenous alimentation formulations for an extended time, treatment of severely malnourished patients with a copper-deficient milk diet,[270] or impaired copper absorption resulting from immense amounts of dietary zinc.[268] Despite their potential susceptibility to copper deficiency, preterm infants have been found to have the condition only when they were given a milk diet.[271] Hypocupremia has also been reported with iron deficiency and hypoproteinemia[272] and in active celiac disease,[273] but it is extremely uncommon.

Copper balance, in contrast to iron balance, is regulated by excretion as well as by absorption.[268, 269] The gastrointestinal tract absorbs daily about 30 percent of the copper present in an average diet. The liver promptly disposes of much of that copper in the bile, whereas a lesser amount is lost through the intestinal mucosa. Experimental animals fed copper-deficient diets conserve the element by a decrease in biliary copper excretion.

The normal net copper intake is 2 to 5 mg in an adult and 0.04 to 0.15 mg/kg in the growing child. Because of milk's low copper content (about 0.12 mg/L), a risk of consumption of a diet consisting of milk to the exclusion of other foods during late infancy is marginal copper nutrition or deficiency. Premature infants with low copper stores are at particular risk. Iron deficiency or severe malnutrition can obscure the manifestations of copper deficiency. Depressed plasma copper levels are seen early in copper deficiency. After about 6 months of age, normal plasma copper levels range between 70 and 140 mg/dL. The values are lower in early infancy.[274] Copper deficiency is sometimes associated with a mild, hypochromic anemia. Leukopenia with very marked neutropenia is particularly prevalent with copper deficiency. Osteoporosis may occur with severe copper deficiency.

Oral treatment with 0.1 to 0.3 mg/kg of copper per day (two or three times the estimated daily requirement) as 0.5 percent copper sulfate (containing about 2 mg of copper per mL) produces prompt reticulocytosis and correction of the anemia and neutropenia. Generally, the dietary imbalance that produced the deficiency can be corrected when the problem is recognized.

A total of 100 to 150 mg of copper is present in the adult human. As with iron, the fetus accumulates large amounts of copper near the end of gestation, particularly in the liver, where concentrations are 5 to 10 times greater at birth than in adulthood. Normally these stores do not decrease to adult levels until 5 to 15 years of age. The liver has the highest copper content, which, together with muscle and bone, accounts for 50 percent to 75 percent of total body copper. Plasma copper, which is held much more constant than plasma iron, exists in two forms. Albumin and amino acids loosely bind 10 to 15 percent of circulating copper. Ceruloplasmin, a multicopper ferroxidase, tightly binds the remaining copper in the plasma. Although ceruloplasmin was once thought to be a copper transport protein, it is now clear that it primarily functions to change the oxidation state of iron, aiding in the release of iron from storage cells, including hepatocytes and macrophages (as discussed earlier). Human patients[92, 93, 275, 276] and mice[94] lacking ceruloplasmin develop a distinct clinical syndrome, characterized by gradual neurodegeneration, hepatic iron overload, diabetes, and mild iron deficiency anemia.

Copper is an essential component of cytochrome oxidase, the terminal oxidase of the electron transport chain required for the combination of hydrogen with oxygen to form water. As such, the element is essential for the oxidative production of ATP. The enzyme tyrosinase is a copper-containing protein required for melanin synthesis. Thus, copper-deficient animals have depressed levels of cytochrome oxidase in most tissues, along with a loss of hair pigment. Another copper metalloenzyme, lysyl oxidase, plays a role in the cross-linking of collagen and elastin. Lysyl oxidase deficiency may cause the vascular defects, including aortic aneurysm, seen in copper-deficient animals.[268]

Copper Transport

Copper trafficking is relatively well understood. A multi-transmembrane domain protein, CTR1, appears to be the major transporter that brings copper into mammalian cells.[277–279] Knockout mice lacking CTR1 die early in gestation with findings that may be attributable to severe copper deficiency. Once copper is inside cells, it moves to its sites of utilization escorted by specific chaperone proteins. (reviewed in references 280 and 281). These appear to be conserved from yeast to mammals. One of them, Atox1, was disrupted by gene targeting to make knockout mice.[282] Atox1 knockout mice have a copper-deficient phenotype, but some animals live, indicating that the chaperone function is important but not essential.

Two inherited defects of human copper metabolism have given insight into copper export from cells. Menkes disease, or kinky hair syndrome, is a congenital disorder characterized by a low serum copper concentration, reduced activity of copper metalloenzymes, slow growth, gray kinky hair, cerebral degeneration, and an X-linked pattern of inheritance.[283] Interestingly, anemia is not a prominent feature of the syndrome. Death before 3 years of age is usual. Despite a low serum copper level, the disease is characterized by copper sequestration in several tissues, particularly the kidney. Parenteral copper administration, like all other attempts to treat the disease, is ineffective.

Wilson disease, in contrast, produces copper toxicity. Patients are unable to excrete copper. Systemic copper overload results, with pathologic changes caused by deposition of the metal in the liver, kidneys, and CNS.[284]

Positional cloning led to the identification of the genes mutated in Menkes and Wilson diseases.[285–290] Both encode transmembrane proteins that are highly homologous to P-type ATPases involved in the transport of calcium ions, sodium ions, and protons. Their N termini have repeats of the amino acid motif Gly-Met-Thr-Cys-X-X-Cys, forming copper-binding domains. Both Menkes and Wilson proteins function as transmembrane copper transporters. Menkes protein is involved in basolateral transport of copper in intestinal enterocytes, whereas Wilson protein participates in ceruloplasmin production and hepatobiliary copper excretion. Remarkably, these human proteins share extensive homology with bacterial proteins and yeast that transport copper ions into and out of single-celled organisms.

EXTREMES OF IRON BALANCE

Iron disorders are invariably abnormalities of iron balance and/or distribution. Iron deficiency is primarily due to acquired causes. In contrast, primary iron overload usually results from genetic abnormalities that perturb the regulation of intestinal iron absorption. Disorders affecting other steps in transport may be manifested by inappropriate iron accumulation in some tissues and iron deficiency in other tissues.

Iron Deficiency

ETIOLOGY

Abnormal Iron Uptake from the Alimentary Tract

Poor Bioavailability. Although iron is the second most abundant metal in the earth's crust, it is nearly insoluble in aqueous solution, making acquisition of the element a major challenge. Most environmental iron exists as insoluble salts. Gastric acidity assists in conversion to absorbable forms, but the efficiency of this process is limited.[291] Many plant products contain iron, but absorption often is limited both by low solubility and powerful natural chelators that bind ambient iron. The phytates (organic polyphosphates) found in wheat products, for example, bind iron with tremendous avidity. The challenge of acquiring sufficient iron from the environment may have been an important factor in the spread of genes for hemochromatosis disorders (see later).

High gastric pH reduces the solubility of inorganic iron, impeding absorption. Surgical interventions, such as vagotomy or hemigastrectomy for peptic ulcer disease, formerly were the major causes of impaired gastric acidification with secondary iron deficiency. Today, the histamine-2 blockers and the more recently introduced acid pump blockers, used to treat peptic ulcer disease and acid reflux, are among the most common causes of defective iron absorption. Use of these medications is widespread, but peptic ulcer disease is rare in children. Therefore, treatment with these drugs (and their attendant complications) is relatively uncommon in children.

The impaired function of gastric parietal cells associated with pernicious anemia not only reduces the production of intrinsic factor but also lessens gastric acidity, compromising iron absorption. In addition, megaloblastic enterocytes absorb iron poorly. Frank iron deficiency can accompany the anemia produced by cobalamin deficiency. However, the rarity of pernicious anemia in children makes this complication uncommon in pediatric populations.

Heme, derived from animal tissues, is the most readily absorbed form of iron. Uptake occurs independently of gastric pH and, like the uptake of nonheme iron, is increased in patients with high marrow erythroid activity. Much of the world's population eats little or no meat, deriving their nutrition from cultivated grasses, such as rice. These plants are relatively poor sources of iron,[23] contributing to the fact that iron deficiency anemia is the most common nutritional anemia worldwide.

Inhibition of Iron Absorption. A number of environmental factors can produce dietary iron deficiency by interfering with iron absorption. These include metals, such as cobalt, that share the iron absorption machinery. Lead may fall into this category, though it remains to be established whether DMT1 is the primary intestinal transporter for lead in vivo.[25] Regardless of the mechanism, it is clear that iron deficiency increases the rate of uptake both of iron and lead from the gastrointestinal tract. Iron deficiency and lead intoxication often coexist.

Disruption of the Enteric Mucosa. Some disorders disrupt the integrity of the enteric mucosa, thereby hampering iron absorption (Table 12–2). Inflammatory bowel disease, particularly Crohn disease, may injure extensive segments of the small intestine, including the jejunum and duodenum. Invasion of the submucosa by inflammatory cells and disruption of the tissue architecture impair iron absorption and uptake of dietary nutrients.[292] Occult gastrointestinal bleeding exacerbates the problem. The result is iron deficiency anemia complicated by the anemia of chronic inflammation. Furthermore, Crohn disease often involves the terminal ileum, producing concurrent cobalamin deficiency. These disorders are not diagnostic enigmas. Patients with extensive bowel involvement are very ill. Diminishing the underlying inflammatory process best treats the iron deficiency.

Tropical sprue and celiac disease can also interfere with iron absorption.[293] Degeneration of the intestinal lining cells along with chronic inflammation causes profound malabsorption, although some patients with deranged iron absorption lack gross or even histologic changes in the structure of the bowel mucosa. The anemia in these patients is often complicated by a superimposed, generalized nutritional deficiency.[294] Celiac disease often improves when the patient is fed a gluten-free diet, with secondary correction of the anemia.

Loss of Functional Bowel. Iron absorption may be disrupted when substantial segments of bowel are removed surgically. Intractable inflammatory bowel disease, traumatic abdominal injury, and structural complications such as intestinal volvulus or intussusception, all may necessitate intestinal resection. Iron deficiency develops slowly afterward and may not become evident for several years after the surgical procedure.

Malabsorption of iron is rare in the absence of structural defects of the intestine, but it has been described in

TABLE 12–2. Causes of Iron Deficiency Anemia

INADEQUATE ABSORPTION

Poor bioavailability (absorption of heme Fe > Fe^{2+} > Fe^{3+})
Antacid therapy/high gastric pH
Bran, tannins, phytates, starch
Other metals (Co, Pb)
Loss/dysfunction of absorptive enterocytes

INSUFFICIENT/INACCESSIBLE IRON STORES

Bleeding

Gastrointestinal
Epistaxis
Gastritis
Ulcer
Meckel diverticulum
Milk-induced enteropathy
Parasitosis
Varices
Tumor or polyps
Inflammatory bowel disease
Arteriovenous malformation
Colonic diverticuli
Hemorrhoids

Vaginal
Increased menstrual flow
Tumor

Urinary
Chronic infection
Tumor

Pulmonary
Pulmonary hemosiderosis
Tuberculosis
Bronchiectasis
Inflammation/infection

INADEQUATE PRESENTATION TO ERYTHROID PRECURSORS

Atransferrinemia
Anti–transferrin receptor antibodies

ABNORMAL INTRACELLULAR TRANSPORT/UTILIZATION

Erythroid iron trafficking defects
Defects of heme biosynthesis

several families with autosomal recessive inheritance of marked iron deficiency.[295–297] To date, the gene(s) that are mutated in these patients has not been discovered. Obvious candidates such as DMT1 and ferroportin have been excluded in some of these families.*

Blood Loss

Gastrointestinal Blood Loss. Blood loss is the world's leading cause of iron deficiency. The gastrointestinal tract is both the site of iron uptake and the most common site of blood loss, particularly when bleeding is not readily apparent. However, bleeding from other sites should also be considered if iron deficiency has not otherwise been explained.

Anatomic defects of the gastrointestinal tract commonly cause blood loss and consequent iron deficiency. The most common congenital defect is Meckel diverticulum, resulting from a persistent omphalomesenteric duct. This abnormality can produce abdominal pain and, occasionally,

intestinal obstruction in young children. Adolescents with Meckel diverticulum may be seen with occult blood loss and secondary iron deficiency. Peptic ulcer disease is extremely uncommon in children, but it should be considered as a cause for gastrointestinal blood loss when the clinical setting suggests it. The stomach and duodenum are affected most often. Inflammation and erosion are prominent at affected sites.

Other structural defects of the gastrointestinal tract are much less likely to cause bleeding. Arteriovenous malformations involving the superficial blood vessels occur in patients with hereditary hemorrhagic telangiectasia (the Osler-Weber-Rendu syndrome). These defective vessels often bleed to a degree that engenders iron deficiency. Although the disorder is transmitted as an autosomal dominant trait, the pathognomonic lesions rarely attain clinical significance before young adulthood. The condition is easily recognized because the mucosal linings of the oropharynx and nasal cavity exhibit characteristic telangiectasias.

Although cow's milk and human milk both have low iron contents, the bioavailability of iron in human milk is greater.[298] Furthermore, whole cow's milk contains proteins that may irritate the lining of the gastrointestinal tract in infants. Low-grade, chronic hemorrhage may produce significant iron deficiency.[299] The prodigious neonatal growth spurt requires a tremendous quantity of iron, compounding the disadvantages of cow's milk. For these reasons, current recommendations exclude cow's milk from the infant diet in the first year of life, suggest that non–breast-fed infants should receive iron-fortified formulas and recommend some additional source of iron for infants that are breast-fed after 4 to 6 months of age, when the excess iron that was present in newborn stores and erythrocytes is depleted.[300, 301]

The world's leading cause of gastrointestinal blood loss is parasitic infestation. Hookworm infection, caused primarily by *Necator americanus* or *Ancylostoma duodenale*, is endemic to much of the world and is often asymptomatic. Microscopic blood loss leads to significant iron deficiency, particularly in children.[302] Over 1 billion people, mostly living in tropical or subtropical areas, are infested with parasites. Their total daily blood losses exceed 11 million liters. The larvae spawn in moist soil and penetrate the skin of unprotected feet. The incidence of hookworm infection, once prevalent in the southeastern United States, declined precipitously with better sanitation and the routine use of footwear when outside.

Trichuris trichiura, the culprit in trichuriasis or whipworm infection, is believed to infest the colon of 600 to 700 million people. Only 10 to 15 percent of these have worm burdens great enough to produce clinical disease. However, most are children between the ages of 2 and 10 years. Growth retardation, in addition to iron deficiency, occurs with heavy infestation. Trichuriasis is the most common helminthic infection encountered in Americans returning from visits to tropical or subtropical regions of the world.

Urinary Blood Loss. Occasionally, blood loss into the urinary tract outstrips iron absorption. However, urinary blood loss is usually apparent and sufficiently alarming that patients seek medical attention before substantial iron

---

*Andrews N, unpublished data.

deficiency develops. Iron deficiency resulting from hematuria caused by renal disease is relatively uncommon.

The best characterized cause of significant renal blood loss is Berger disease, which produces relapsing episodes of gross or microscopic hematuria. The disorder occurs most commonly in older children and young adults. It is characterized by diffuse mesangial proliferation or focal and segmental glomerulonephritis. Diffuse mesangial deposits of IgA are the hallmark of the disorder. Although the disease spontaneously remits in some children, progression to end-stage renal disease may occur. Occasionally, Goodpasture syndrome produces substantial urinary blood loss. Immunofluorescent staining of biopsy specimens reveals the characteristic antibodies to basement membrane lining the glomeruli. Blood loss into the urinary bladder can occur in association with infectious cystitis. Hematuria to the point of iron deficiency is extremely uncommon, however.

Pulmonary Blood Loss. Although pulmonary blood loss may be severe enough to produce iron deficiency, it is distinctly rare. Chronic pulmonary hemosiderosis primarily affects children and young adolescents (reviewed in reference 303). This potentially deadly disorder is characterized by slow but intractable hemorrhage into the bronchioles and alveoli. Iron deficiency anemia is a major part of the clinical picture of pulmonary hemosiderosis. Because the pulmonary macrophages are distinct from the normal iron recycling circuit, iron trapped within these cells is effectively lost to body metabolism. A paradoxical situation occurs in which patients develop iron deficiency anemia in the presence of a surfeit of total body iron. Bronchoalveolar lavage reveals hemosiderin-laden macrophages that are pathognomonic of the disorder. Chronic pulmonary infection with bronchiectasis, once considered to be a common cause of this problem, is now rare. Formation of toxic products is induced by the iron that accumulates in these cells, leading to the activation of the macrophages. These cells begin to damage the delicate lining of the bronchoalveolar tree, producing severe fibrosis. Oxygen exchanges poorly across the damaged alveolar surfaces, lowering the efficiency of oxygen/carbon dioxide exchange. Late in the course of pulmonary hemosiderosis the radiographic picture of the lungs is striking and commonly shows marked retraction and scarring.[304] The restrictive lung disease and substantial pulmonary arterial shunting across the lung may eventually be fatal.

Most often the cause of pulmonary hemosiderosis evades elucidation. In a number of patients, it occurs in conjunction with disorders of immune dysfunction, including celiac disease[305] and Goodpasture syndrome.[306, 307] Treatment of the associated disorder can lead to remission of the pulmonary process, consistent with an immunologic mechanism for the lung injury.[308] Chloroquine treatment has been used with modest success in some patients.[309] Cyclophosphamide treatment has produced responses in a number of patients.[310] A combination of prednisone and azathioprine has also been used.[311] Other immunosuppressive agents may prove to be even more effective as immunologic suppressers in the treatment of this condition, but the rarity of the disorder means that a large, multicenter trial is needed to collect

definitive treatment information. Although the prognosis was once believed to be very poor for all patients with idiopathic pulmonary hemosiderosis, a recent study suggests that this may not be the case.[307]

CONSEQUENCES

Although anemia is the most prominent manifestation of iron deficiency, there may be other clinically significant sequelae. Some of these abnormalities, such as cognitive dysfunction in young children, are important but not well understood.

Anemia

Because most of the body's iron is directed to hemoglobin synthesis, erythrocyte production is among the first casualties of iron deficiency to become clinically apparent. However, it actually represents a late stage of iron depletion. Iron deficiency progresses through three discernible phases:

1. Prelatent iron deficiency occurs when tissue stores are depleted without a change in hematocrit or serum iron levels. This stage of iron deficiency may be detected by low serum ferritin measurements.

2. Latent iron deficiency occurs when reticuloendothelial macrophage iron stores are depleted. The serum iron level drops and the total iron-binding capacity increases without a change in the hematocrit. This stage may be detected by a routine check of the fasting, early morning transferrin saturation. Erythropoiesis begins to be limited by a lack of available iron, and serum transferrin receptor levels increase. The reticulocyte hemoglobin content decreases because newly produced erythrocytes are iron deficient.[312] However, the bulk erythrocyte population appears normal.

3. Frank iron deficiency anemia is associated with erythrocyte microcytosis and hypochromia. It is detected when iron deficiency has persisted long enough that a large proportion of circulating erythrocytes were produced after iron became limiting.

The microcytic, hypochromic anemia of iron deficiency impairs tissue oxygenation, producing weakness, fatigue, palpitations, and lightheadedness. Thalassemia trait (see Chapter 20) also produces microcytic cells and is sometimes confused with iron deficiency. Iron deficiency alters red cell size unevenly. Electronic blood analyzers determine the mean red cell volume as well as the range of variation in red cell size (expressed as the red cell distribution width). The red cell distribution width and the cell hemoglobin distribution width (both determined as part of electronically processed complete blood cell counts) are normal in patients with thalassemia trait but high in those with iron deficiency.[313] Other common features of thalassemia trait are basophilic stippling and target cells. These characteristics are not sufficiently distinctive to be diagnostically useful, however. A simple, reliable approach is to examine the color of plasma. It is watery in iron deficiency and straw colored in thalassemia trait.

The plasma membranes of iron-deficient red cells are abnormally stiff, and the cells are more prone to hemolysis.[314] This rigidity could contribute to poikilocytic changes, seen particularly with severe iron deficiency. Small, stiff, misshapen cells are cleared by the reticuloendothelial system, further contributing to low-grade hemolysis. The cause of this alteration in membrane fluidity is unknown.

Unexplained thrombocytosis with platelet counts in the range of 500,000 to 700,000 cells/fL occurs often in iron-deficient patients. Megakaryocytes and normoblasts are derived from a common committed progenitor cell, the colony-forming unit granulocyte-erythroid-monocyte-macrophage (CFU-GEMM). Thrombopoietin, the molecule that stimulates the growth of megakaryocytes and the production of platelets, is structurally homologous to erythropoietin (see Chapter 6). The high levels of erythropoietin produced in iron deficiency anemia conceivably could cross-react with megakaryocyte thrombopoietin receptors, modestly raising the platelet count. However, this hypothesis has not been proven experimentally.

Growth and Developmental Retardation

Iron deficiency, with or without concomitant anemia, can impair growth and intellectual development in children.[315, 316] However, studies of cognitive development in the setting of iron deficiency have produced disparate results. In some investigations, dietary iron supplementation for infants reversed cognitive dysfunction,[317] whereas others failed to show improvement.[318] Some of the disparities may have resulted from differences in the instruments used for the analyses and differences in the populations examined (reviewed in reference 319).

When tested using the Bayley Scale of Infant Development, abnormalities were uncovered in children as young as 9 to 12 months of age. Developmental abnormalities occur with or without anemia. In one study, iron replacement increased the Mental Development Index scores substantially in only 7 days.[320] Iron deficiency does not impair motor development even in infants with low scores on the tests of cognitive development.[321] Concomitant lead exposure can further hamper the psychological development of these children.[322] Information on the long-term effects of iron deficiency during infancy highlights the importance of early intervention. Health care providers, therefore, must actively work to prevent iron deficiency during infancy.

The mechanism by which iron deficiency impairs neurologic function is unknown. Iron deficiency has been shown to decrease expression of dopamine receptors in the rat brain.[323] Several enzymes in neural tissue require iron for normal function.[324] The cytochromes involved in energy production, for example, are predominantly heme proteins. The effect of iron deficiency on childhood growth is often difficult to separate from overall nutritional deficiency. However, when the two factors have been separated, correction of iron deficiency improves growth independently of nutritional status.[325, 326]

Epithelial Changes

Iron deficiency produces significant gastrointestinal tract abnormalities, reflecting the enormous proliferative capacity of this tissue. Patients may develop angular stomatitis and glossitis with painful swelling of the tongue. The flattened, atrophic, lingual papillae make the tongue smooth and shiny. A rare complication of iron deficiency is Plummer-Vinson syndrome with the formation of a postcricoid esophageal web. Longstanding, severe iron deficiency affects the cells that generate the fingernails, producing koilonychia, or spooning. The nail substance is soft, so that ordinary pressure on the fingertips, such as with writing, for instance, produces a concave deformity. Most of these abnormalities are now uncommon in industrialized nations.

Pica

Pica, the compulsive consumption of non-nutritive substances, occurs variably in patients with iron deficiency, but the precise pathophysiology of this symptom is unknown. Patients often consume laundry starch, ice, soil, or clay. Both clay and starch can bind iron in the gastrointestinal tract, exacerbating the deficiency.[327, 328] A dramatic example of the problems produced with clay consumption occurred in the 1950s in iron-deficient children along the border between Iran and Turkey.[329, 330] These youngsters had other, peculiar abnormalities, including massive hepatosplenomegaly, poor wound healing, and a bleeding diathesis. Presumably, the children initially had simple iron deficiency associated with pica, including geophagia. The soil contained compounds that bound both iron and zinc.[331] Secondary zinc deficiency was thought to cause the hepatomegaly and other unusual features.[330]

TREATMENT

The most important steps in the evaluation and treatment of iron deficiency are determining the cause and correcting the abnormality. Malignancy of the gastrointestinal tract, the most worrisome etiology in adults with iron deficiency, is rarely seen in children. Growth spurts, poor dietary patterns, and benign gastrointestinal bleeding are much more common. After initial diagnostic investigations, oral iron supplementation usually replaces stores most efficiently.

Oral Supplementation

Iron salts are an inexpensive, effective therapy for iron deficiency. Although ferrous sulfate is most often recommended, patients often complain of gastrointestinal discomfort, bloating, and other distress, making its use unacceptable to many. Administration of low doses of ferrous sulfate, such as a single 325-mg tablet (containing 65 mg of elemental iron) on an empty stomach at night, will lessen the gastrointestinal difficulties. The decreased gastrointestinal motility of sleep will also enhance absorption. The absorptive capacity for iron in the normal duodenum is essentially saturated with about 25 mg of elemental iron in ionic form. Ferrous gluconate, which costs approximately the same, contains about 50 mg of elemental iron per tablet. This form of replacement may produce fewer problems than those seen with ferrous sulfate and is excellent as the initial treatment of iron deficiency. Ascorbic acid supplementation enhances iron absorption, although it has a relatively minor effect in individuals ingesting normal, balanced diets.[332] Combination tablets containing iron salts and ascorbic acid are significantly more expensive than separate tablets for each. Even with faithful use of oral iron, adequate replacement of body stores in patients with moderate iron deficiency anemia requires several months. With ongoing blood loss, replacement of stores with oral iron becomes very difficult.

Polysaccharide/iron complex differs from the iron salts. Polar oxygen groups in the sugars form coordination complexes with iron atoms. The well-hydrated microspheres of polysaccharide iron remain in solution over a wide pH range. Most patients tolerate this form of iron better than the iron salts, even though the 150 mg of elemental iron per tablet is substantially greater than that provided by iron salts.

Table 12–3 lists potential causes of a poor response to oral iron supplementation.

Parenteral Iron Replacement

Parenteral iron is now available in the United States in three intravenous forms: iron dextran, iron gluconate, and iron sucrose.[333-336] This medication is indicated when (1) oral iron is poorly tolerated, (2) rapid replacement of iron stores is needed, (3) gastrointestinal iron absorption is compromised, or (4) erythropoietin therapy is necessary, particularly in patients undergoing renal dialysis. Iron dextran can also be administered by intramuscular injection, but this is discouraged because the injection can be painful, and leakage into the subcutaneous tissue produces longstanding skin discoloration. A "Z-track" injection into the muscle minimizes the chance of subcutaneous leak. Suboptimal muscle mass usually associated with nutritional deficiency further complicates this mode of replacement. Intravenous infusion circumvents these problems altogether. With either route of administration, a small test dose should be given, and the patient should be observed by a physician for 30 minutes to rule out an anaphylactic reaction to the medication. Such reactions do occur but are seen rarely. The newer iron sucrose and iron gluconate preparations are believed to be less likely to cause complications, but there is less accumulated experience with those preparations, and many practitioners still use iron dextran routinely.

Ten to 15 percent of patients experience transient mild to moderate arthralgias the day after intramuscular or intravenous administration of iron dextran.

TABLE 12–3. Poor Response to Oral Iron

Noncompliance
Ongoing blood loss
Insufficient duration of therapy
High gastric pH
    Antacids
    Histamine-2 blockers
    Gastric acid pump inhibitors
Inhibitors of iron absorption/utilization
    Lead
    Aluminum intoxication (hemodialysis patients)
    Chronic inflammation
    Neoplasia
Incorrect diagnosis
    Thalassemia
    Sideroblastic anemia

Acetaminophen usually relieves the discomfort effectively. Iron dextran is generally avoided in patients with rheumatoid arthritis, because it may provoke painful flares of their disease.[12] The symptoms may result from release of inflammatory cytokines such as interleukin-1 and tumor necrosis factor. Iron dextran is cleared from the circulation by fixed tissue macrophages, which are probably activated to release proinflammatory peptides.

In patients with uncomplicated iron deficiency, intravenous replacement produces subjective improvement within a few days. Peak reticulocytosis occurs after about 10 days, and complete correction of the anemia takes 4 to 6 weeks, although the hematocrit rises sufficiently in 1 or 2 weeks to provide symptomatic relief for most patients.[337] Reticulocyte hemoglobin content is a very sensitive measure of response.[338]

Refractory bleeding that cannot be prevented, such as that with hereditary hemorrhagic telangiectasias, presents a management problem. Oral iron supplementation often fails to keep pace with losses. Blood transfusions replace red cells in the short term and iron in the long term, but infection and alloimmunization make the use of transfusions unacceptable for many patients. Intermittent iron replacement with infusions of intravenous iron is the most reasonable alternative. Replacements should occur over short intervals two or three times a year, with the aim of repleting the body stores. A simple formula can be used to determine the replacement dose of iron dextran:

$$\text{Dose (mL)} = 0.0442 \times (\text{desired Hb} - \text{observed Hb}) \times \text{LBW (kg)} + (0.26 \times \text{LBW}) \text{ (kg)}$$

where LBW = lean body weight.

Alternatively, there is a calculator provided on the Internet at http://www.globalrph.com/irondextran.htm. The maximum adult dose of iron dextran is 14 mL.

Over many years, this treatment can produce massive deposition of hemosiderin (from iron dextran) in macrophages, liver, and pancreas, despite the fact that plasma transferrin is iron deficient because of increased iron delivery to erythroid precursors. This supports the concept that tissue iron content is unimportant for erythropoiesis and that erythropoiesis relies exclusively on iron from transferrin.[101, 153]

Iron Replacement in Infants

Infants and children from disadvantaged families are the most conspicuous victims of iron deficiency in the United States, despite a decline in the incidence of the condition over the past three decades. Without consumption of iron-fortified formula, 20 percent of infants from inner city families develop iron deficiency; frank iron deficiency anemia is seen in nearly 10 percent of these children.[299] Routine use of iron-fortified infant formulas reduces the incidence of iron deficiency to about 1 percent. Because the fetus accumulates iron at the mother's expense in the third trimester of pregnancy, full-term infants are born with iron stores that are adequate to last for approximately 6 months. Preterm infants have a greater risk for development of iron deficiency, depleting their stores by 3 to 4 months of age.

Human breast milk initially contains relatively high amounts of iron, but the level decreases, independent of maternal iron status, to approximately 0.3 mg/L after 5 months of lactation (reviewed in reference 339). The iron is present in several forms: in casein, in whey, in fat, and, to a small extent, in the abundant protein lactoferrin. Absorption of iron from human milk has been estimated to be 20 to 50 percent, which is adequate early in life when iron stores are still high, but is inadequate to meet an older infant's needs. Based on all available information, the Committee on Nutrition of the American Academy of Pediatrics has recommended the following[300]:

1. Breast milk should be provided for at least 5 to 6 months when feasible. During that period young infants can mobilize iron from their large stores. Iron supplementation of 1 mg/kg/day should be provided to infants who are exclusively fed breast milk beyond 6 months of age.
2. Infants who are not breast-fed should be nourished with an iron-supplemented formula (at least 12 mg/L) until the end of the first year of life.
3. Iron-enriched cereals should be among the first foods introduced with a solid diet.
4. Cow's milk should be avoided during the first year because it contains substances that chelate iron, and it sometimes induces occult gastrointestinal hemorrhage in young infants.

Iron Overload

ETIOLOGY

Hereditary Hemochromatosis

Hereditary hemochromatosis is a condition that originates from a genetic predisposition to iron overload, resulting from mutations in one of several genes involved in iron metabolism (see later). It results from an alteration in the iron absorption mechanism that fractionally increases the uptake of dietary iron.[340–342] Although the rate and extent of iron loading vary widely among patients, many develop dangerous levels of tissue iron by middle age. Iron deposits in cells of the liver, heart, endocrine tissues, and skin. It promotes oxidative cell damage, leading to fibrosis, and, when unrecognized, to the classical presentation of "bronze diabetes" with liver dysfunction, increased melanization of the epidermis, and pancreatic insufficiency.[343] Erythropoiesis is normal, allowing removal of iron through phlebotomies performed regularly. If untreated, hemochromatosis may be a lethal disease, resulting in death from cirrhotic liver failure or, less often, from cardiomyopathy.

Pediatricians are often asked to evaluate children who have close relatives with hemochromatosis. This is a complicated task, because iron loading occurs gradually over many years and may not be apparent before adulthood. Although the genes responsible for several forms of hemochromatosis have been identified recently, at this time commercial laboratories only test for one form of the disease. However, this situation is likely to change over the next few years, simplifying presymptomatic diagnosis. Until then, assessment should take into account family history, serum transferrin saturation, serum ferritin levels, and, if indicated, quantitative liver iron determined by analysis of a biopsy sample.

In the United States, Canada, Australia, and the northwestern part of Europe, most patients with hemochromatosis are homozygous for a unique missense mutation, designated C282Y (for cysteine 282 to tyrosine), in the gene encoding HFE, a protein that resembles class I major histocompatibility molecules.[344] Like its relatives, the *HFE* gene lies on chromosome 6p, near to the HLA-A locus. It was discovered through a positional cloning approach[344] that took advantage of the fact that most or all patients with the C282Y mutation are descended from a common ancestor, who probably lived in a Celtic population in the British isles 60 to 70 generations ago.[345]

Like other class I proteins, HFE forms a heterodimer with β_2-microglobulin and is expressed on the cell surface. However, unlike other family members, HFE cannot bind a small peptide. It structure, as determined by X-ray crystallography, does not allow enough space within the groove that is involved in peptide binding by other class I molecules.[346] Some insight into the function of HFE was gained from observations that it forms a high-affinity complex with the transferrin receptor.[115, 346–353] HFE binds to a site that overlaps the binding site for ferric transferrin, resulting in a competition between HFE and transferrin for transferrin receptor occupancy. Studies in transfected cells overexpressing HFE indicate that the HFE-transferrin receptor association decreases cellular iron uptake. Despite all this information, however, no model for the function of HFE that takes into account all known information has been presented thus far.

Although the normal function of HFE has not yet been elucidated, it is presumed to be involved in restricting absorption of iron through the intestine. Serum transferrin becomes saturated with iron before clinical signs appear. The increased serum iron is deposited in parenchymal cells of the liver, heart, pancreas, and other tissues. Knockout mice, lacking murine Hfe, develop an iron overload disorder that closely resembles human hemochromatosis.[354–356]

The prevalence of the mutant allele for HLA-linked hemochromatosis in the United States was originally estimated by analysis of samples from healthy, primarily white, blood donors before identification of the *HFE* gene.[357] The estimated carrier occurrence was approximately 10 to 12 percent. This number was confirmed in a later investigation, carried out by direct screening for C282Y mutations. Studying a cross-section of the American population, Steinberg and colleagues[358] found that 9.5 percent of non-Hispanic whites, 2 percent of non-Hispanic blacks, and approximately 5 percent of the population overall were C282Y carriers.[358]

Testing for the *HFE* C282Y mutation offers a new, genetic approach to identifying patients who may develop clinical hemochromatosis. Heterozygotes rarely have clinically significant iron overload, but homozygotes are at risk. Published data give conflicting estimates of what proportion of patients homozygous for C282Y will develop complications of the disease,[359–362] but it is clear that some individuals have severe iron loading as young adults, whereas others may never manifest signs or symptoms of hemochromatosis. There must be both environmental and genetic modifiers that affect the extent of iron loading. Current efforts are aimed at defining these modifiers, to aid in prognosis.

Other polymorphisms and potential mutations have been described in the *HFE* coding sequence. One of these polymorphisms, H63D (histidine 63 to aspartic acid) is prevalent throughout the world, and found in one quarter to one third of asymptomatic patients. Although clinical laboratories currently test for and report the H63D polymorphism, whether this change causes hemochromatosis by itself or whether it is simply associated with another, yet to be defined, mutation is still an area of controversy. Clinicians should be cautious in their interpretation and assume that most patients with one or two copies of the H63D allele are probably not at risk for iron loading. Other polymorphisms associated with altered amino acids or altered mRNA splicing have also been reported (reviewed in reference 363). Some of these do appear to be associated with iron overload, but most clinical laboratories do not look exhaustively for them. If doubt exists, liver biopsy is still a useful test to diagnose hemochromatosis.

Since the identification of *HFE*, it has become clear that there are at least three other types of hemochromatosis. One of these, referred to as type 3 hemochromatosis, may be clinically indistinguishable from HFE-associated hemochromatosis. To date, it has only been described in Italy. This disorder results from homozygosity for mutations in the gene encoding transferrin receptor-2 (*TFR2*).[364, 365] TFR2 is highly homologous to the transferrin receptor, particularly in its extracellular domain. However, in contrast to transferrin receptor, TFR2 is not regulated in response to iron levels,[366] and it binds transferrin with much lower affinity.[367, 368] It is primarily expressed in the liver and in erythroid cells, where it is made at very high levels. Its function remains unclear, as does the reason why loss of the protein results in iron overload. In contrast to the transferrin receptor, TFR2 does not appear to form a complex with HFE.[368] Further understanding of this disease awaits better understanding of the protein and the generation of a mouse model.

Two other types of hemochromatosis are easier to distinguish from HFE-associated hemochromatosis. Juvenile hemochromatosis, also called type 2 hemochromatosis, is a more severe disorder, with accelerated iron loading that typically leads to death by the third decade.[369–374] Patients have iron deposition in the same pattern as that seen in patients with HFE-associated hemochromatosis, but the rapid accumulation of metal leads to a different clinical picture, dominated by cardiac disease and endocrine dysfunction. Patients are often identified when they fail to enter puberty. If these patients are recognized before end-stage organ disease develops, they can be treated by aggressive phlebotomy. Juvenile hemochromatosis is inherited in an autosomal recessive pattern, but the causative gene has been mapped to chromosome 1q, away from all known genes involved in iron metabolism.[375] The juvenile hemochromatosis gene is likely to be identified within the next few years.

Finally, there is an autosomal dominant form of hemochromatosis (type 4 hemochromatosis) that is characterized by increased iron loading of macrophages, an early rise in serum ferritin levels, and comparatively less saturation of transferrin with iron.[376] This disorder was first described in Italy, but it has subsequently been found elsewhere. Patients carry mutations in the ferroportin gene

that are presumed to alter the function of the protein.[42, 43] Although a simple model, taking into account the dominant inheritance pattern, might be that the mutations result in an increase in ferroportin function, several observations suggest that this is probably not the case. First, macrophage iron loading is not readily explained by a simple increase in intestinal ferroportin function. Second, preliminary functional assays suggest that one of the mutations, A77D, results in decreased transport activity.* Third, gain-of-function mutations are rare.

How might autosomal dominant hemochromatosis be caused by a deleterious mutation altering one ferroportin allele? The current hypothesis is based on the idea that an abnormality in iron distribution leads to indirect induction of intestinal iron absorption. As discussed earlier, most of the body's iron is normally found in the erythron. There is an unknown signal between the bone marrow and the intestine that increases iron absorption in response to increased erythroid iron needs. Most available iron is supplied to the erythron through macrophage recycling and recovery from senescent erythrocytes. If loss of one ferroportin allele resulted in decreased macrophage ferroportin activity, recycling might be impaired, resulting in iron-restricted erythropoiesis and a compensatory increase in iron absorption. If intestinal iron absorption is not limited by haploinsufficiency for ferroportin, but macrophage iron release is, increased flux of dietary iron into the body might occur. Some iron would be used to derive erythropoiesis, but the remaining excess iron would be deposited in the tissues. Under these circumstances, patients might not be clinically anemic if compensation is sufficient. Iron loading need not be greatly increased; in fact, a small but chronic increment in absorption of dietary iron would be most consistent with the gradual onset of this form of iron overload.

Our understanding of hemochromatosis is advancing rapidly, but much remains to be learned. Until there are laboratory tests that can predict development of this disorder, evaluation of children from families with hemochromatosis will continue to be complicated. An algorithm for investigating these children is presented in Figure 12–6.

African Iron Overload Syndrome

During the 1960s, several groups of investigators reported that iron overload occurred at a very high rate among sub-Saharan Africans.[377–380] Many patients had massive iron stores, approaching or exceeding those seen in individuals with hereditary hemochromatosis. Some indigenous inhabitants of the region prepared alcoholic beverages in nongalvanized steel drums, raising the possibility that iron overload resulted from the high iron content of these beverages. Iron loading was thought to be exacerbated by an increase in gastrointestinal iron absorption induced by alcohol. The term *Bantu siderosis* was coined to describe the condition.[379]

Later reports suggested that African iron overload was not simply the result of increased intake.[381–383] Only a fraction of the group who drank the beverage developed iron overload. In fact, a more extensive study showed that

---

*Donovan A, Andrews N, unpublished data.

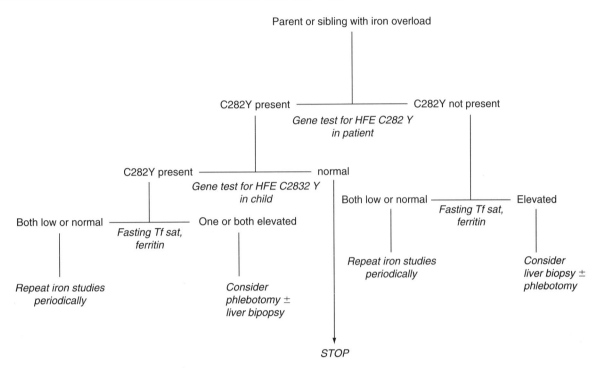

FIGURE 12–6. Algorithm for workup of children at risk for iron overload. Tf sat = transferrin saturation. (Adapted from Andrews NC: Inherited iron overload disorders. Curr Opin Pediatr 2000; 12:596.)

similar degrees of iron overload occurred in people who consumed little, if any, of this brew. Although the pattern of inheritance has not been definitively worked out, the disorder appears to be autosomal codominant, with obligate heterozygotes expressing an intermediate level of iron loading. African iron overload does not appear to be associated with *HFE* mutations, but the location of the responsible gene has not yet been reported.[384]

Intriguingly, African iron overload syndrome most closely resembles type 4 hemochromatosis in the cellular distribution of iron. In contrast with other forms of hereditary hemochromatosis, in which the iron is almost entirely confined to parenchymal cells, reticuloendothelial macrophages display massive iron deposition in the African variety of iron overload.[377] To date, it has not been established whether ferroportin mutations may similarly be responsible for this disorder. However, the ultimate clinical consequences of iron overload are similar to those seen in all other forms of hemochromatosis, irrespective of the cause of the accumulation. The African iron overload syndrome is not confined to any ethnic group, although it appears to be restricted to the inhabitants of sub-Saharan Africa. In some areas, the incidence of heterozygosity may be as high as 10 percent, making it one of the most common, clinically significant, inherited defects in any population.

An important unanswered question is whether the mutated gene or genes that cause this syndrome are found in people of African descent elsewhere in the world. No comprehensive study exists of iron overload in African Americans, but preliminary data suggest that a substantial portion of that population may be at risk.[385, 386] Because the gene pool of black Americans includes genes of European origin as well as those derived from Africa, any study of iron overload must account for possible mutations in other genes associated with hereditary hemochromatosis.

The Evolutionary Advantage of Iron Overload

The fact that multiple mutations in diverse populations all lead to iron overload raises the possibility that these conditions once conferred a selective advantage. As previously noted, iron deficiency is the most common nutritional cause of anemia in the world. Anemia was probably a selective disadvantage earlier in human history. A genetic change that increased the efficiency of iron absorption, therefore, may have been an advantage. A person who survived into the third decade would have reproduced and passed his or her genes on to the next generation, including those that increase iron absorption. Survival into the fifth decade, when iron overload begins to produce problems, was uncommon until recently.

A problem develops with this tidy theory when the inhabitants of Asia are considered. The incidence of iron overload is reportedly quite low in this region of the world, the home to most of the Earth's population. However, Asian medical information is underrepresented in the English literature, and concepts may be revised as more is learned about iron overload in that part of the world.

Neonatal Iron Overload Syndrome

The role of the placenta in regulating transfer of iron to the fetus is dramatically demonstrated in infants with the neonatal iron overload syndrome (also called neonatal hemochromatosis). Affected newborns have massive iron deposits in many body tissues (reviewed in reference 387). Although some survive for a few months, many die within days of birth of multisystem organ failure, primarily of the liver, pancreas, and heart. At necropsy, histologic examination shows abnormal hepatocyte morphology with extensive iron deposition both in parenchymal and reticuloendothelial cells.[388–390] The heavy and widespread iron deposition is accompanied by organ necrosis and fibrosis. Regenerating hepatic nodules (cirrhosis) frequently develop in newborns who survive for more than a few weeks.

The neonatal iron overload syndrome superficially resembles hereditary hemochromatosis. However, the disorders are clearly distinguishable. The pathologic appearance of the liver is distinct.[390] The most important difference is that iron is deposited *in utero* with neonatal iron overload syndrome, indicating that the defect involves iron transport across the placenta. Hereditary hemochromatosis, in contrast, arises from an alteration in gastrointestinal iron absorption. Placental iron transport is poorly understood and difficult to study, particularly because there are significant differences between the structures of human placentas compared with those of other mammals.

The cause of neonatal iron overload is not known. It is likely that more than one defect may result in similar clinical presentations. Neonatal iron overload syndrome often occurs sporadically, but families with several affected children have been described. Interestingly, women have produced affected children by two or more different fathers, suggesting that the defect may be inherited only from the mother, perhaps because of a mitochondrial mutation.[391–393] Alternatively, the disorder may result from acquired maternal conditions, such as an aberrant immune reaction. Unfortunately, there is currently no genetic means for determining early in pregnancy whether the fetus is at risk.

Acute Iron Poisoning

Acute iron poisoning due to accidental ingestion of large doses of medicinal iron is a medical emergency. Significant gastrointestinal symptoms occur with doses as low as 20 mg/kg of elemental iron and systemic toxicity becomes evident with ingestions of 60 mg/kg (reviewed in reference 394). Treatment consists of removing as much residual iron as possible from the gastrointestinal tract and administering intravenous desferrioxamine, which chelates the toxic non–transferrin-bound iron.[394, 395] It is appropriate to consult a toxicologist or poison center for assistance.

Erythroid Hyperplasia

The connection between hematopoiesis and iron absorption is most strikingly apparent in patients with ineffective erythropoiesis. With disorders such as β^+-thalassemia (thalassemia intermedia) and X-linked sideroblastic anemia the fractional absorption of ingested iron is increased. Patients with these disorders can develop iron overload without transfusion.[396]

The mechanism by which bone marrow activity modulates gastrointestinal iron absorption is unknown. A soluble factor appears to be released that stimulates iron uptake. In one study, reticulocytosis was induced in rats either by feeding iron-rich food to animals with severe dietary iron deficiency or by injecting phenylhydrazine, a compound that lyses circulating erythrocytes.[102] Internal iron exchange doubled, and iron absorption increased dramatically. Infusion of reticulocyte-rich blood from these animals into normal rats increased internal iron exchange and gastrointestinal iron absorption. In contrast, blood from normal animals did not have this effect.

In humans, robust absorption of iron from the gastrointestinal tract is associated most often with ineffective erythropoiesis. Some patients with pyruvate kinase deficiency, a condition frequently associated with reticulocyte counts as high as 70 percent, develop iron overload without transfusion. Hemolytic anemias with effective erythropoiesis rarely lead to iron loading. Without some compounding variable, such as hereditary hemochromatosis trait, iron loading without transfusion is not generally seen with conditions such as sickle cell anemia or hereditary spherocytosis, in which the erythroid cells mature and leave the bone marrow before they are destroyed.

CONSEQUENCES

The effects of iron overload on some organs, such as the skin, are trivial, whereas hemosiderotic harm to others, such as the liver, can be fatal. Few notable symptoms precede advanced injury. Abdominal discomfort, lethargy, depression, arthralgias, erectile dysfunction, and fatigue are common but nonspecific complaints. Dyspnea with exertion and peripheral edema indicate significant cardiac compromise and reflect advanced iron loading.

Liver

As the major site of iron storage, the liver is a conspicuous target for excess iron deposition. Mild to moderate hepatomegaly develops early, followed by shrinkage produced by fibrosis and micronodular cirrhosis. Hepatic tenderness may be present, but hemosiderotic liver damage produces little inflammation. Consequently, significant hepatic iron deposition and even fibrosis can occur with very little increase in the serum transaminase levels. Disturbances in liver synthetic function indicate advanced disease. Liver biopsy is still the "gold standard" for determining the extent of hepatic iron deposition. Hematoxylin and eosin staining reveals a brownish pigment in the hepatocytes that staining with Perls' Prussian blue unmasks as iron. Large amounts of iron are also deposited in Kupffer cells in patients with type 4 hemochromatosis, African iron overload syndrome, or transfusional iron overload. Electron microscopy reveals substantial hemosiderin aggregates in addition to large quantities of ferritin.

Heart

Congestive cardiomyopathy is the most common heart problem that occurs with iron overload, but other abnormalities have been described, including pericarditis, restrictive cardiomyopathy, and angina without coronary artery disease.[397–400] There is a strong correlation between the cumulative number of blood transfusions and functional cardiac derangements in children with thalassemia.[401] Findings on physical examination are surprisingly benign even in patients with heavy cardiac iron deposition. Once evidence of cardiac failure appears, however, heart function deteriorates rapidly, and medical intervention is frequently ineffective. Biventricular failure produces pulmonary congestion, peripheral edema, and hepatic engorgement. These potentially lethal cardiac complications have occasionally been reversed by vigorous iron extrication.[402]

Iron deposition in the bundle of His and the Purkinje system can lead to conduction defects.[403, 404] Sudden death is common in these patients, presumably owing to arrhythmias. At one time, patients treated with the chelator desferrioxamine for transfusional iron overload received supplements of ascorbic acid in the range of 15 to 30 mg/kg/day to promote iron mobilization. Reports of sudden death prompted cessation of this practice.[405] At lower doses (2 to 4 mg/kg), ascorbic acid is a safe adjunct to chelation therapy in patients with transfusional iron overload.

Cardiac dysfunction can occur with very little tissue iron deposition. The total quantity of iron is less important than the unbound, or "toxic," iron fraction in the circulation. The concentration of unbound iron in tissues is extremely small and virtually impossible to measure. This toxic iron is precisely the component that is bound and neutralized by iron chelators. Therefore, cardiac damage is best prevented in patients with transfusional iron overload by maintaining a constant, low level of chelator in the circulation (and consequently in the tissues, where the protection is rendered).

Endocrine Organs

Dysfunction of the endocrine pancreas is common in patients with iron overload.[406, 407] Some patients develop overt diabetes mellitus requiring insulin therapy. The disturbances in carbohydrate metabolism may be more subtle, however. An oral glucose tolerance test often unmasks abnormal insulin production. Vigorous removal of excess iron occasionally reverses islet cell dysfunction.[408] Exocrine pancreatic function, in contrast, is usually well preserved.

Pituitary dysfunction may produce several endocrine disturbances.[409] Reduced gonadotropin levels are common. When coupled with primary reductions in gonadal synthesis of sex steroids, sexual maturation is delayed in children with transfusional iron overload.[410] Secondary infertility is common. Although Addison syndrome is uncommon with iron overload, production of adrenocorticotropic hormone is occasionally deficient. A metapyrone stimulation test shows delayed or diminished pituitary secretion of this hormone.[411]

Thyroid function is usually well preserved in patients with iron overload. In contrast, parathyroid activity is frequently compromised. Functional hypoparathyroidism can be demonstrated in many patients by inducing hypocalcemia with an intravenous bolus of ethylenediaminetetraacetic acid (EDTA) while monitoring the production of parathyroid hormone.[412]

Miscellaneous Abnormalities Associated with Iron Overload

Hyperpigmentation is a nonspecific skin response to a variety of insults, including excessive exposure to ultraviolet light (tanning), thermal injury, and drug eruptions. Cutaneous iron deposition damages the skin and enhances melanin production by melanocytes. Ultraviolet light exposure and iron are often synergistic in the induction of skin pigmentation, so that many patients with siderosis tan very readily. Fair-skinned people who tan poorly may never develop hyperpigmentation despite very large body iron burdens, highlighting the genetic contribution to skin pigmentation. In contrast, patients with moderate baseline pigmentation frequently develop a striking, almond-colored hue. With particularly heavy iron overload, visible iron deposits sometimes appear in the skin as a grayish discoloration.

Arthropathy is a common problem in patients with hereditary hemochromatosis, but rare in patients with secondary iron overload.[413,414] Patients with hemochromatosis typically have involvement of small joints, particularly in the hands, but may also have involvement of large joints, such as the hips. Chondrocalcinosis is a late but characteristic feature of the arthropathy seen in hereditary hemochromatosis. Other troubling musculoskeletal problems include severe, recurrent cramps and disabling myalgias. Muscle biopsy shows iron deposits in the myocytes, but the pathophysiologic connection to the pain and cramps is unclear.

Iron Overload and Opportunistic Infections

Withholding iron from potential pathogens is believed to be one strategy used in host defense.[415] Because transferrin binds iron with extremely high affinity, and two thirds of the iron-binding sites of the protein are normally unoccupied, there is very little free iron available in plasma and extracellular fluids. Not surprisingly, both transferrin and its homolog lactoferrin are bacteriostatic *in vitro* for many bacteria.[416–418] However, the very high transferrin saturations attained in patients with iron overload compromise the bacteriostatic properties of the proteins, and transferrin can serve as a source of iron for some microorganisms.[419] Various infections with unusual organisms have been reported in patients with iron overload (Table 12–4).[420–423] Host defense is compromised even further in patients with sideroblastic anemia and secondary iron overload because of abnormal neutrophil function. Although aggressive antimicrobial therapy is often successful, some infections, such as the mucormycosis produced by *Rhizopus oryzae*, are usually fatal.

The iron chelator desferrioxamine may promote opportunistic infections with unusual organisms (e.g., *R. oryzae)* in patients with iron overload.[424–427] Desferrioxamine is a natural compound that is synthesized as a siderophore by *Streptomyces pilosis* when it is grown in an iron-deficient

---

TABLE 12–4. Infectious Agents Associated with Iron Overload

BACTERIAL

Listeria monocytogenes
Yersinia enterocolitica
Salmonella typhimurium
Klebsiella pneumoniae
Vibrio vulnificus
Escherichia coli

FUNGAL

Cunninghamella bertholeatiae
Rhizopus oryzae
Mucor sp.

environment. Siderophores are low-molecular-weight molecules that are released locally by microbes to bind iron, facilitate its uptake, and make the metal available for growth and replication. Siderophores tend to be promiscuous in their activity, and some pathogenic bacteria and fungi can utilize desferrioxamine-bound iron to promote their own growth. Thus, pharmacologic administration of desferrioxamine can, on occasion, enhance the risk of severe infection. However, serious infections are still uncommon in patients treated with desferrioxamine, and the benefits of therapy to prevent iron-induced organ damage generally outweigh the risk of infectious complications. There is no simple answer to the question of when to begin chelation therapy in a patient with transfusional siderosis.[428] The decision must be carefully made for each individual.

TREATMENT

Phlebotomy

Phlebotomy is the most effective means of removing excess iron from patients with all forms of hereditary hemochromatosis. A single unit of blood contains about 200 mg of iron. Otherwise healthy individuals can often tolerate initial phlebotomy sessions as often as twice a week. Most commonly, a weekly schedule of phlebotomy is used to deplete excess iron load. The process can be continued at this rate for months if necessary. Rapid compensatory synthesis of new red blood cells empties iron stores. Phlebotomy is safe for adolescents and young adults. However, because most forms of hereditary hemochromatosis do not cause iron overload earlier in life, phlebotomy of small children is rarely indicated.

The endpoint of phlebotomy is the removal of all excess iron. Iron-deficient erythropoiesis, characterized by hypochromic, microcytic red cells, marks the achievement of this objective. When phlebotomy therapy is initiated, the hematocrit changes very little from week to week. Meanwhile, the plasma ferritin level and the transferrin saturation fall. Phlebotomy therapy should not be stopped in response to normalization of those parameters, however, because the rapid changes in iron stores greatly compromise their diagnostic value.

When the mean corpuscular volume and mean corpuscular hemoglobin concentration of the erythrocytes begin to fall, the iron stores have been exhausted. At the very least, the rate of iron egress from stores along with iron intake from food does not match the rate of utilization. At this point, the rate of phlebotomy should be reduced to two to four times per year. Because erythropoiesis is the physiologic process that is most heavily dependent on iron availability, iron-deficient erythropoiesis is the best biologic indicator of depleted iron stores.

Patients with ineffective erythropoiesis (e.g., thalassemia intermedia or pyruvate kinase deficiency) sometimes develop substantial iron overload without transfusion.[396, 429, 430] Phlebotomy can be attempted if the patient's steady-state hematocrit is in the range of 28 to 30 percent and no concomitant cardiovascular disease exists. An initial regimen of 1 unit removed every 2 weeks is reasonable. This rate of phlebotomy would remove about 450 mg of iron per month or 15 mg/day. Often this is enough to cause negative iron balance in the patient, without the trouble

associated with chelation therapy. The caveat to this approach is that phlebotomy can exacerbate marrow hyperplasia. Bone deformities can occur in young children. Another concern is cord compression caused by compromise of the spinal canal by hyperplastic marrow. This approach to iron overload demands constant vigilance.

Iron Chelation

Desferrioxamine (Desferal) is the only chelator available in the United States to treat chronic iron overload. Several characteristics of the drug place severe constraints on its use. First, absorption from the gastrointestinal tract is limited, mandating parenteral administration. Second, the compound is excreted from the circulation with a half-life of only 10 to 15 minutes.[431] Therefore, slow continuous parenteral administration is required to draw iron out of tissues. Third, desferrioxamine is irritating to subcutaneous tissue; consequently, only a small amount can be administered at a given site.

For these reasons, desferrioxamine is usually administered by continuous subcutaneous infusion using a rate-controlled pump.[432, 433] Skin irritation, manifested as raised, painful, erythematous welts, is less severe in children than in adults. Nonetheless, the sites of infusion are rotated each day to minimize the problem. The infusion is given over 12 to 16 hours, allowing freedom from the pump for part of the day. Iron mobilization often falls to unacceptable levels when the infusion time is less than 12 hours. Desferrioxamine therapy is most effective when the pump is used daily, but few patients can conform to such a rigid schedule. As a compromise, the infusion should be administered at least 5 days each week.

Subcutaneous infusion of desferrioxamine is unacceptable to some patients, most often because of intolerable skin irritation. The drug mobilizes iron more efficiently when administered as a continuous intravenous infusion, usually by way of a permanent, indwelling central venous catheter, but this method is rarely practical. Other complications include otovestibular toxicity and bone abnormalities when the drug is given in large doses.[434, 435] Immunologic reactions to the drug are rare and include urticaria and anaphylaxis. Desensitization procedures, similar to those used for patients with penicillin hypersensitivity, have allowed chelation treatment of some individuals with immunologic intolerance.[436] In these situations, desferrioxamine must be continued without a break to prevent recovery of immune sensitivity.

The urine of chelated patients acquires an orange color, reflecting the excretion of the iron-desferrioxamine complex (ferrioxamine) by the kidneys. Desferrioxamine has been used in peritoneal dialysis fluids in some patients receiving chronic ambulatory peritoneal dialysis, with effective removal of excess iron.[437] However, aggressive opportunistic infections may be problematic in these patients, as discussed earlier.

An effective oral iron chelator is the "Holy Grail" of chelation.[438] Many agents have been suggested, but none has yet met the exacting requirements. In the last decade, several clinical trials were performed with 1,2-dimethyl-3-hydroxypyrid-4-one, also called L1 or deferiprone. Early results led to concerns that the drug induced reversible granulocytopenia. More recent trials have questioned the efficacy of this compound.[439] Although there is still some controversy,[440] deferiprone should not currently be considered as an alternative to desferrioxamine. Additional chelators are under development but, to date, none can be considered a replacement for desferrioxamine.

MATERNAL-FETAL IRON BALANCE

Iron Delivery to the Fetus

Approximately 1 g of iron is required for full-term fetal development, with about 300 mg incorporated into fetal tissues. Iron transport to the fetus is entirely dependent upon the placenta. This organ removes from the maternal circulation all the iron necessary for fetal development, even at the cost of maternal iron deficiency.[441, 442] PIT is a major determinant of gastrointestinal iron absorption. Ordinarily, the erythroid cells in the bone marrow have the predominant effect on the PIT. During pregnancy, however, placental iron uptake increases the PIT, thereby boosting gastrointestinal iron absorption. This physiologic increase in iron absorption by the maternal gut increases the availability of the element to the developing fetus. Transferrin receptor, DMT1, and ferroportin are all expressed at substantial levels in the placenta, but the detailed mechanics of iron transport across the placenta remain unknown. The expression of transferrin receptors by the placenta increases in response to fetal iron demand, suggesting the existence of a regulatory mechanism in the placental-fetal unit. Equally mysterious is the mechanism by which iron is placed onto transferrin in the fetal circulation. Unlike the situation with hemoglobin, no fetal-specific transferrin exists. Therefore the driving force for iron delivery to the fetal circulation is not an electrochemical gradient from low-affinity to high-affinity transferrin molecules.

Although iron transport across the placenta superficially resembles the uptake of the element from the gastrointestinal tract, significant differences exist between the two processes. An important fact is that the placenta takes up iron that is coupled to transferrin, whereas iron in the alimentary tract is bound to inorganic molecules. It is remarkably efficient at acquiring iron from the maternal circulation. The placenta is programmed to take up iron without signals or cues from the fetus. In one study, the placentas of pregnant rats continued to remove iron efficiently from the maternal circulation for several days after excision of the fetuses.[443] Because the iron could no longer be transferred to the fetus, it accumulated abnormally in the placenta.

Effects on the Fetus of Maternal Iron Deficiency

Even when maternal iron deficiency exists, the placenta is concerned only with the welfare of the fetus. It will continue to remove iron from the mother to support fetal development even at the cost of negative maternal iron balance. For years, investigators debated the effect of maternal iron deficiency on the fetus. The controversy was fueled by the indirect and imprecise assays of neonatal iron status, such as the cord blood ferritin level or transferrin saturation. These parameters in cord blood are subject to all the vicissitudes that affect their values in later life. Accurate determination of neonatal iron status was difficult, if not impossible. The one point on which nearly universal agreement existed was that neonatal anemia resulting from maternal iron deficiency is rare.

The most compelling data came from a study of women who had elective abortions.[444, 445] The iron status of the mothers was determined from transferrin saturation, plasma ferritin levels, and hemoglobin values. This information was correlated with the iron status of the fetuses, which was determined by atomic absorption spectroscopy of the complete abortus. This procedure determined the absolute fetal iron content. Fetal iron stores varied linearly with maternal hemoglobin, which ranged between 6 g/dL (severe iron deficiency) and 13 g/dL (adequate, although possibly low, iron stores). Although neonatal iron deficiency anemia is quite uncommon, maternal iron status over a wide range of values does affect the iron stores of the neonate.

DISORDERS OF IRON DISTRIBUTION

Transferrin Abnormalities

Congenital atransferrinemia is a rare disorder in which transferrin is virtually absent.[149, 150, 152, 446] Causative mutations have been described within the transferrin gene.[446] With insufficient transferrin, most plasma iron is loosely bound to other plasma constituents, such as albumin.[100] The normal pattern of iron distribution is dramatically altered. Cells that depend upon transferrin-mediated iron uptake, such as erythroid normoblasts, are severely affected, resulting in hypochromic, microcytic anemia, whereas other cells such as hepatocytes (with transferrin-independent iron uptake) have a surfeit. The non–transferrin-mediated iron uptake system deposits much of the plasma iron in the liver and other organs. The heavy hepatic iron deposition eventually leads to cellular necrosis and fibrosis. Affected patients typically die from liver failure if not treated with transferrin or red blood cell transfusions. A similar disorder has been reported in hypotransferrinemic (*hpx*) mice, which carry a spontaneous mutation that disrupts a critical splice donor site in the transferrin gene.[69, 146]

Defective transferrin molecules are extremely rare. These proteins disrupt the delivery of iron to the bone marrow and other tissues. In some instances, iron is weakly bound and tends to dissociate. In other instances, the transferrin protein fails to bind properly to the transferrin receptor. Affected patients have a hypochromic, microcytic anemia. Infusion of normal transferrin has not been reported but presumably would correct the defect.

An antibody against the transferrin receptor was identified in a patient with a lymphoproliferative disorder who acquired a refractory hypochromic, microcytic anemia.[447] The antibody blocked transferrin-mediated iron uptake. It had a disproportionate effect on normoblast development, but other cell types were relatively unaffected.

Siblings in another report were seen with congenital hypochromic, microcytic anemia associated with a high transferrin saturation.[448, 449] Liver biopsy revealed elevated hepatic iron stores. Their transferrin was shown to deliver iron normally to cultured cells *in vitro*, ruling out a problem with the protein. Impaired transferrin receptor activity of some type may have led to relative iron starvation of the normoblasts despite hepatic iron overload. The number of receptors on the cells was normal, raising the possibility of physiologically dysfunctional receptors or a defect at some later step in the transferrin cycle. A second, similar kindred has been reported.[450, 451] These case reports emphasize the importance of transferrin-mediated iron uptake for erythropoiesis.

SIDEROBLASTIC ANEMIAS

The sideroblastic anemias are a heterogeneous group of disorders characterized by anemia, a low reticulocyte count, and ineffective erythropoiesis with distinctive morphology (Table 12–5).[452–456] They may be due to genetic or acquired causes. Although the anemia is most commonly normochromic and normocytic, some patients have microcytosis and hypochromia. Ineffective erythropoiesis frequently produces elevated body iron stores. All patients are anemic, and thrombocytopenia and neutropenia develop in some. About 30 percent of patients with sideroblastic anemia have elevated levels of erythrocyte protoporphyrins, reflecting disturbances in heme biosynthesis.

Bone marrow examination frequently reveals erythroid hyperplasia despite profound anemia. This is the *sine qua non* of ineffective erythropoiesis, a condition in which the normoblasts fail to supply mature erythrocytes to the circulation. The key to the recognition of sideroblastic anemia is staining of iron in bone marrow erythroid cells with Perls' Prussian blue. This procedure highlights the characteristic ring sideroblast, a normoblast with a perinuclear halo of Prussian blue-stained material (Fig. 12–7; see color section at the front of this volume). Electron microscopic examination reveals the rings to be juxtanuclear

TABLE 12–5. Classification of Sideroblastic Anemias

CONGENITAL

X-linked
Erythroid delta-aminolevulinic acid synthase defects
ATP7 defects

Autosomal
SLC19A2 defects
Mutations in other, as yet unidentified, genes

ACQUIRED

Idiopathic
Alkylating agents (e.g., nitrogen mustard)
Other drugs
Ethanol
Isoniazid
Chloramphenicol

mitochondria containing large deposits of inorganic iron.[457] In congenital sideroblastic anemia the rings predominate in late normoblasts, whereas rings occur in early cells in the acquired form. A recent report suggests that the iron deposits may contain a mitochondrial ferritin molecule, encoded by a nuclear gene that is distinct from those encoding H- and L-ferritin polypeptides.[202] The nucleus and the cytoplasm of the affected normoblasts commonly mature asynchronously. However, these megaloblastic changes (often termed *megaloblastoid*) are less pronounced than those seen with deficiencies of cobalamin or folic acid.

Mild to moderate hemolysis exacerbates the anemia produced by ineffective erythropoiesis. The cause of the peripheral red cell destruction is unknown. Some patients with sideroblastic anemia develop an acquired form of hemoglobin H disease, which contributes to the hemolysis. Hemoglobin H (tetramers of hemoglobin β chains) forms in a subpopulation of the developing normoblasts owing to

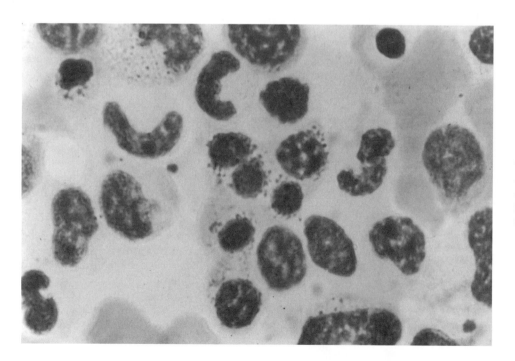

FIGURE 12–7. Prussian blue stain of a bone marrow aspirate from a patient with sideroblastic anemia. The greenish blue flecks that circle the nucleus of the normoblasts are iron-laden mitochondria (see color section at the front of this volume).

a shutdown of α-globin production. Consequently, its distribution in the circulating erythrocytes is heterogeneous (see Chapter 11).

Congenital Sideroblastic Anemias

Congenital sideroblastic anemia disproportionately affects males. This is not surprising, because both well-characterized forms are X-linked recessive disorders. However, female patients with Turner syndrome (XO karyotype), X-chromosome aberrations, or severely skewed X chromosome inactivation[458] make up a significant, and often undiagnosed, portion of the total group. Mutations have been described in two proteins that are important in mitochondrial iron homeostasis—erythroid δ-aminolevulinic acid synthase (eALAS, also known as ALAS2) and ATP7.

Missense mutations in the *eALAS* gene have been identified in many patients with X-linked sideroblastic anemia.[459–462] *eALAS* mutations result in impaired heme biosynthesis because ALAS is the first and rate-limiting enzyme in that process, and the erythroid form of the enzyme is critically important for normal red blood cell development. Mutations may affect enzyme activity, cofactor binding, protein production, or interactions with succinyl coenzyme A synthetase, a protein necessary for normal enzyme function and localization.[461, 462] The impaired production of heme presumably leads to mitochondrial iron accumulation and the formation of ring sideroblasts. Disturbed heme biosynthesis reduces hemoglobin production, leading to the microcytic, hypochromic anemia. Interestingly, the kindred described by Cooley in the initial report of familial sideroblastic anemia was analyzed using molecular techniques and found to have a defect in *eALAS*.[460]

The age at clinical onset of X-linked sideroblastic anemia varies greatly in the patients. Some children develop anemia within a few months of birth, whereas manifestations of the full-blown disorder do not appear in others before the age of 7 or 8 years.[463] Generally, the anemia is progressive, often requiring transfusions to maintain an adequate hematocrit. Frequent transfusions can hasten the development of iron overload. Oral pyridoxine therapy is useful in many patients with congenital sideroblastic anemia resulting from *eALAS* mutations, because it is a cofactor for eALAS and pharmacologic doses help to compensate for the defect in δ-aminolevulinic acid synthase activity.[462] Often, however, the correction of the anemia is incomplete. Some patients show more response to pyridoxine after their excess body iron stores are depleted.[459] A few children in whom pyridoxine therapy failed have shown a response to the parenteral administration of pyridoxal 5-phosphate.[464] Unfortunately, many children with congenital sideroblastic anemia improve little, if at all, with either of these interventions. Because pyridoxine is inexpensive and lacks deleterious side effects, all children with sideroblastic anemia should receive a trial of vitamin therapy. Pyridoxal 5-phosphate is not commercially available. There is one case report of successful allogeneic peripheral stem cell transplantation for refractory sideroblastic anemia.[465]

A distinct form of X-linked sideroblastic anemia is milder and is associated with ataxia.[466] Patients rarely need transfusion therapy and do not develop systemic iron overload. This disorder is due to mutations in ABC7, an ATP-binding cassette transporter protein that localizes to mitochondria.[455, 456] To date, all mutations have been relatively conservative substitutions, but their functional significance has been confirmed by taking advantage of the fact that yeast have a homologous protein, Atm1p, that is necessary for normal cellular function.[455] The normal human ABC7 protein can substitute for yeast Atm1p, but the mutant protein is less active. The function of the human protein is incompletely understood, but, like its yeast homolog, it appears to be involved in the formation and transfer of iron-sulfur clusters produced within mitochondria.[456, 467–471]

Occasionally, sideroblastic anemia appears as a component of syndromes with disturbances in cellular metabolism. A rare cohort of children with sideroblastic anemia has an inherited defect in thiamine transport. These patients with thiamine-responsive megaloblastic anemia (also known as Rogers syndrome) are seen with a characteristic triad of megaloblastic anemia with ringed sideroblasts, diabetes mellitus, and deafness (see Chapter 11).[472, 473] The manifestations of this rare syndrome are progressive, and may include optic atrophy and non-thrombotic, non-embolic strokes. Hematopoiesis is markedly disturbed, with prominent sideroblastic changes in the normoblasts. Therapy with pharmacological doses of thiamine ameliorates the disorder. The gene responsible for thiamine-responsive megaloblastic anemia has been identified and shown to encode a transmembrane thiamine transporter designated SLC19A2.[474] The pathogenesis of the unusual anemia has not yet been reported.

Another metabolic defect produces Pearson syndrome, a fatal disorder of infancy with marked disturbances in bone marrow and pancreatic function.[475] The initial manifestation is often a severe, transfusion-dependent, macrocytic anemia plus a variable degree of neutropenia and thrombocytopenia. Striking vacuolization occurs in the erythroid and myeloid precursors, along with hemosiderosis and ringed sideroblasts.[476] Exocrine pancreatic dysfunction occurs frequently. Necropsy reveals prominent pancreatic fibrosis. Some patients develop hepatic, renal, and neurologic dysfunction as well. Pearson marrow-pancreas syndrome is a mitochondrial cytopathy.[477, 478] Defective energy production appears to be the central disturbance. The variable expression in the reported patients may result from the inconstant inheritance of defective mitochondria, which are derived stochastically from the mother. No treatment exists.

Acquired Sideroblastic Anemias

A number of drugs and toxins that impair heme biosynthesis or perturb mitochondrial iron metabolism can produce sideroblastic anemia (Table 12–5). The most important of these is lead. This element inhibits enzymes in the heme biosynthetic pathway. Screening for lead, therefore, is mandatory in any child suspected of having sideroblastic anemia, because lead poisoning can be treated. Isoniazid also produces sideroblastic anemia by causing functional depletion of pyridoxine, inhibiting heme biosynthesis. Prophylactic treatment with pyridoxine is now part of the standard therapeutic regimen with this drug.

Chromosomal aberrations occur frequently in acquired sideroblastic anemias, which are rare in children unless they have previously received chemotherapy for cancer. Some changes, such as the loss of the long arm of chromosomes 5 or 7 (5q- and 7q-, respectively), may have pathophysiologic importance, as discussed elsewhere (Chapter 27). It is not known how these karyotypic changes are related to the development of sideroblastic anemia. In adult patients, karyotype analysis frequently reveals random chromosomal losses and breaks. Hypodiploid karyotypic changes indicate a poor prognosis.[479] Intriguingly, some patients have been shown to have mutations within the mitochondrial genome, altering the coding sequence for cytochrome *c* oxidase.[454]

Although anemia is usually the initial manifestation of acquired sideroblastic anemia, stem cell dysfunction may produce significant thrombocytopenia and neutropenia. Polymorphonuclear leukocytes and platelets may function poorly even when their counts are normal.[480, 481] The platelet defect produces abnormal aggregation patterns *in vitro*, including impaired responses to epinephrine, arachidonic acid, and collagen. Clinically, these changes may be manifested as a prolonged bleeding time and a tendency to frank hemorrhage. Neutrophil dysfunction, along with neutropenia, often means that patients have an increased risk of serious infection.

Development of acute myelogenous leukemia occurs in 15 to 20 percent of adult patients with acquired sideroblastic anemia.[482–484] The rate of leukemic conversion in children is unknown. Patients who have received chemotherapy containing alkylating agents have an increased risk for later development of myelodysplastic disorders, including sideroblastic anemia.[485] Often the secondary leukemias are very aggressive and resistant to chemotherapy.

DISORDERS OF IRON UTILIZATION

Anemia of Chronic Inflammation

The anemia of chronic inflammation, also called the anemia of chronic disease, is a well-recognized condition associated with a broad spectrum of maladies (reviewed in references[486–489]). The mild to moderate anemia (hemoglobin level of 10 to 11 g/dL) is typically normochromic and normocytic with a slightly elevated red cell distribution width, reflecting a mild anisocytosis. Serum iron and serum transferrin levels are usually low, although the transferrin saturation need not be. Serum ferritin levels are usually, but not always, increased. The levels of serum transferrin receptor are normal unless iron deficiency accompanies the disorder. Not surprisingly, the diagnosis of anemia of chronic inflammation may be quite challenging to make. Inflammation is the key to the condition. Chronic disorders that lack an inflammatory component, such as congestive heart failure due to essential hypertension, for instance, do not produce the anemia of chronic inflammation.

Bone marrow examination with Perls' Prussian blue stain reveals large deposits of iron in the reticuloendothelial cells.

This characteristic feature of the anemia of chronic inflammation reflects ineffective iron recycling. Normoblasts that fail to mature properly and effete erythrocytes are engulfed by reticuloendothelial macrophages in the marrow, liver, and spleen. The phagocytes degrade the protein and lipid and recycle the iron from hemoglobin onto transferrin for reuse. The anemia of chronic inflammation disturbs this cycle, leaving iron trapped in the reticuloendothelial cells.

The cause of these disturbances is unknown, although recent *in vitro* experiments have provided clues. Proinflammatory cytokines, such as interleukin-1 and interleukin-6, activate ferritin synthesis in cultured cells in the absence of iron. This synthesis has been proposed to be causally related to the pathogenesis of anemia of chronic disease. Empty ferritin shells may provide excess iron storage capacity, leading to iron sequestration through simple trapping.[490, 491] Eventually, the ferritin would be converted into hemosiderin. Alternatively, the anemia of chronic disease may result from inflammation-induced or cytokine-induced alterations in the expression of iron transporters.

Patients with the anemia of chronic inflammation have unusually low plasma erythropoietin levels for their degree of anemia.[489] This finding is consistent with *in vitro* data in which proinflammatory cytokines suppress erythropoietin production by cells in culture (see Chapter 6).[492] The involvement of erythropoietin in the anemia of chronic inflammation reflects the multifactorial nature of the condition. Control of the inflammation (e.g., by colectomy in patients with ulcerative colitis) usually eliminates the anemia and corrects the disturbances in iron metabolism. The anemia is recalcitrant when inflammation is uncontrolled.

Erythropoietin and Functional Iron Deficiency

Human erythropoietin was one of the first biologic agents of widespread clinical use produced by recombinant DNA technology. Used to correct the anemia of end-stage renal disease, prematurity, cancer, chronic disease, and other disorders, this hormone has provided new insight into the kinetic relationship between iron and erythropoietin in red cell production (reviewed in reference 493). Erythropoietin treatment of anemia in patients with end-stage renal disease has also underscored the variable nature of storage iron. The shifting states of storage iron contribute to the inconsistency with which erythropoietin corrects the anemia of renal failure.

With steady-state erythropoiesis, iron and erythropoietin flow to the bone marrow at constant, low rates. In patients with end-stage renal disease, recombinant human erythropoietin is administered in intermittent surges.[494] The resulting kinetics of erythropoiesis are markedly unphysiologic and strain the production process. Erythropoietin, the accelerator of erythroid proliferation, is not coordinated with the supply of iron, the fuel for erythroid proliferation. This imbalance almost never occurs naturally. The intense erythropoietin signal jars previously quiescent cells to proliferate and produce hemoglobin. The requirement for iron rises dramatically and outstrips its rate of delivery by transferrin.[495]

Erythropoietin stimulates proliferation and differentiation of erythroid precursors, with an upsurge in heme synthesis (see Chapter 6). Primitive erythroid cells have relatively few transferrin receptors. The number increases with differentiation, peaking at more than 10^6/cell in the late pronormoblasts. The number subsequently declines to the point that mature erythroid cells lack transferrin receptors altogether. This variable expression of transferrin receptors means that iron delivery must be synchronized both with proliferation and stage of erythroid development.[496] Late normoblasts, for instance, cannot compensate for iron that was not delivered during the basophilic normoblast stage. These cells have fewer transferrin receptors, and those receptors are busy supplying iron for *currently* produced heme molecules.

As discussed earlier, transferrin-bound iron is the only important source of the element for erythroid precursors. Even with normal body iron stores and transferrin saturation, robust proliferation of erythroid precursors can create a demand that outstrips the capacity of the iron-delivery system.[497] Transferrin iron saturation falls as the available iron on plasma transferrin is stripped off by voracious erythroid precursors. PIT rises, as does erythron iron turnover and erythron transferrin uptake.[494] The late arrival of newly mobilized storage iron fails to prevent production of hypochromic cells. This is "functional iron deficiency" or "iron-erythropoietin kinetic imbalance." Therefore, even when initial iron stores are substantial, patients with end-stage renal disease benefit from the administration of iron along with erythropoietin (or newer erythropoietin analogs), particularly when the iron is given intravenously.[498] In this setting, the rate-limiting factor in erythrocyte synthesis is the proliferative capacity of the erythroid precursors. Current studies are investigating the role of iron administration in other groups of patients treated with erythropoietin and an erythropoietin analog.

LEAD POISONING

Sources of Lead

Lead (Pb) is a toxic metal without any function in the human body. Because of its useful properties, lead has been mined for several centuries. As a result, progressively larger amounts have been removed from the depths of the earth and introduced into the biosphere. Enough lead has found its way into humans that, at least in the industrialized parts of the world, all people have some lead in the body and hence in the blood. Thus, it has become customary to refer to the blood lead values found in apparently healthy populations as "normal" blood lead levels. This term is an obvious misnomer, because it implies some kind of minimum physiologic requirement for lead.

Airborne lead enters the human body through inhalation; about 35 percent is absorbed and 15 to 18 percent is retained.[499] The intake of airborne lead is greater in children, because they breathe at a lower height, where the lead concentration is greater, and have a greater respiratory rate per unit of body weight.[500] Sources of inhaled lead include combustion engines that burn leaded fuel and primary and secondary (recycling) lead smelters. Lead can also be ingested through the intake of contaminated food,

water, and beverages. Lead absorption is increased by deficiencies of essential minerals, such as iron and calcium.[501] High maternal lead levels can result in fetal lead toxicity.[502]

Children living in older houses are exposed to the additional risk of lead in paint. Although lead in air, food, and beverages can be considered "low-dose" sources, lead in paint is by far the most concentrated source. As much as 40 percent lead by weight is present in dried paint that was manufactured before World War II. Since then, lead levels in paint have been progressively reduced. For many years, it was believed that lead poisoning in children occurred primarily as a result of pica (the urge to ingest nonfood material), with consequent ingestion of paint chips.[503] Although this is not an uncommon occurrence, it is neither the only nor even the prevailing mechanism of ingestion of lead from paint. Small children, through their ordinary hand-to-mouth activities (such as thumb sucking) directly ingest dust and thus take in large amounts of lead. Despite legislative efforts and scientific advances in the United States, millions of dwellings still contain lead-based paint. These dwellings present an obvious risk, particularly to the children of the poor, who tend to live in the oldest houses. The state of repair of the dwelling is almost as important as the lead content of the paint; peeling or flaking paint is obviously more accessible to small children. Because iron deficiency often induces pica, lead poisoning is more common in iron-deficient children.

Less common sources of lead include fumes from old battery casings; illegally distilled whiskey; printed paper, particularly colored magazines; and toys painted with lead-based paint. An uncommon source of lead that may result in severe poisoning is improperly glazed earthenware vessels used to store acidic beverages (such as fruit juices or cider).

Biochemical and Hematologic Effects of Lead

Lead has a strong affinity for the sulfhydryl groups of cysteine, the amino group of lysine, the carboxyl groups of glutamic and aspartic acids, and the hydroxyl group of tyrosine. Lead binds to proteins, modifies their tertiary structure, and inactivates enzymatic properties. Enzymes that are rich in sulfhydryl groups appear to be the most sensitive. Mitochondria are particularly sensitive to lead. Many prominent effects of lead on heme synthesis are mediated through the alterations of the mitochondrial membrane. Heme synthesis starts and ends inside the mitochondria; intermediate steps take place in the cytoplasm. In all cells, heme is an essential component of molecules of the cytochrome system, also located inside the mitochondria. Additionally, in erythropoietic precursors, very large amounts of heme are formed to make hemoglobin. Lead interferes at several points in the heme synthetic pathway in all cells. The two most important steps affected are those catalyzed by δ-aminolevulinic acid dehydratase (a cytoplasmic enzyme) and ferrochelatase (an intramitochondrial enzyme). Both of these enzymes depend on critical sulfhydryl groups for their activities. The inhibition by lead of ferrochelatase, which catalyzes the ultimate insertion of iron into protoporphyrin, results in the accumulation of protoporphyrins in maturing erythrocytes. Furthermore, iron transport through the mitochondrial membrane requires energy-dependent mechanisms, inhibited by lead.[504] Ultimately, despite the presence of a normal or an increased intracellular content of iron, the mitochondria are starved for iron. Metalloporphyrins inhibit several mitochondrial enzymes and the increased concentration of zinc protoporphyrin resulting from lead toxicity further impairs mitochondrial function.[505] There is a relationship between the concentration of lead that inhibits ferrochelatase in mitochondria and the ambient concentration of iron in the medium. At any concentration of lead, ferrochelatase inhibition is most marked when the iron concentration is the lowest.[38] This biochemical mechanism explains the greater elevation of erythrocyte protoporphyrin observed, at equal lead exposure, in children with concomitant iron deficiency.[506] A progressive, exponential increase in erythrocyte protoporphyrin concentration is observed at blood lead levels from 5 to 90 μg/dL.[507] The erythrocyte protoporphyrin level is an indicator of adverse metabolic effects. It is very effective as a screening test for severe lead poisoning, but it cannot be used to screen for blood lead levels less than 40 to 50 μg/dL.

The bulk of lead in blood (greater than 90 percent) is in the erythrocytes, but blood lead content is independent of the hematocrit. Basophilic stippling results from deposition of ribosomal DNA and mitochondrial fragments.[508] Moderate basophilic stippling may be seen in iron deficiency and thalassemia trait, but the stippling is particularly prominent in the polychromatophilic erythrocytes in lead poisoning and unstable hemoglobinopathies including severe β-thalassemia and pyrimidine 5′-nucleotidase deficiency. Anemia is observed primarily in children with severe lead poisoning or with presence of concomitant iron deficiency.[38] This is not an unexpected finding, because the defect in heme synthesis affects only a very small fraction of the total protoporphyrin production, and clinically significant anemia usually develops in the late stages. It is not uncommon to observe severe neurologic toxicity in the absence of anemia in children. On the other hand, lead intoxication and iron deficiency anemia tend to occur in the same lower socioeconomic population and are aggravated by each other. Iron-deficient children are more severely affected because iron deficiency increases lead ingestion through pica, increases lead absorption, enhances the defect in heme synthesis, and increases the toxicity of lead.

Other enzymes of heme biosynthesis are also affected by lead but less severely. Uroporphyrinogen synthetase activity is inhibited only by rather high (10^{-4} mol/L) lead concentrations.[505] Coproporphyrinogen decarboxylase, another mitochondrial enzyme, also is inhibited by lead.[505] There is a marked increase in the urinary coproporphyrin level in lead intoxication. Measurement of urinary coproporphyrin has been widely used for the diagnosis of childhood lead poisoning, particularly in emergency departments. Although this test has been superseded by the easier measurement of erythrocyte protoporphyrin, it is important to recognize its usefulness in discriminating between recent and past exposure to lead. Because of the long persistence of protoporphyrin within erythrocytes, significant elevations may be observed as long as 2 to 3 months after expo-

sure to lead.[509] On the other hand, increased coproporphyrin production, because of its high solubility, is immediately reflected in excess urinary excretion. Hence, when exposure to lead is current, both the erythrocyte protoporphyrin level and urinary coproporphyrin excretion are increased; when exposure to lead is no longer present, there is a discrepancy between the elevated erythrocyte protoporphyrin level and the normal urinary coproporphyrin excretion.

The process of heme synthesis is not exclusive to the erythron. All cells contain essential heme proteins, particularly in the respiratory cytochrome system, also located in the mitochondria. The most visible effects of lead on heme synthesis are those detectable in the peripheral blood, because this is the easiest tissue to sample. However, the ubiquitous presence of active heme synthesis in the mitochondria of all body cells and the affinity of lead for mitochondria result in widespread impairment of cellular function. Lead intoxication inhibits the synthesis of cytochrome P-450, the key enzyme in the mixed oxidase system. It appears likely that toxic effects of lead, particularly in the nervous system, reflect the derangement of heme synthesis.[510]

In adults, peripheral neuropathy, abdominal colic, and anemia are the most common initial signs of lead poisoning. In children, the clinical effects of excessive exposure to lead are apparent primarily in the CNS; alterations of renal function and anemia occur only with the most severe poisoning. Acute encephalopathy can be the first presentation of severe childhood lead poisoning. The onset is usually marked by seizures, that are often intractable, followed by coma and cardiorespiratory arrest. The syndrome may be fatal within 24 to 48 hours. Survivors often suffer permanent neurologic damage.[511] Acute encephalopathy may be accompanied by Fanconi syndrome with aminoaciduria, glycosuria, and hyperphosphaturia.[512]

The chronic symptoms of lead toxicity are vague, including abdominal pain, vomiting, general malaise, and behavioral changes. These symptoms are nonspecific and of little diagnostic help, particularly in the youngest children, aged 1 to 3 years, who are the most frequently affected. The threshold blood lead level at which encephalopathy occurs in children is difficult to define. *Acute lead poisoning* with clinical signs other than encephalopathy has been observed at blood lead levels ranging between 60 and 450 μg/dL. On the other hand, it is possible to observe children with blood lead levels as high as 200 μg/dL who do not have overt neurologic symptoms. The probability of overt neurologic problems increases with the blood lead level and becomes significant when the blood lead level rises to greater than 70 μg/dL. For these reasons and because of the impending risk of unpredictable clinical deterioration, blood lead levels of 70 μg/dL or more in children should be treated as medical emergencies, even in the absence of symptoms.[513]

As a result of the greater awareness of childhood lead poisoning by physicians, extensive screening programs in large cities, and the reduction of lead in the air subsequent to the wider use of lead-free gasoline, severe lead poisoning is extremely rare. On the other hand, there is a greater awareness of the subclinical effects of lead and the fact that there is no threshold below which body lead levels can be considered safe. In view of the evidence of adverse effects of exposure to lead, even at low levels, there has been a progressive lowering of the "acceptable" blood lead level. Therefore, it is important not to confuse "intervention levels" (decided on pragmatic considerations) with "safe" levels.

The insidious nature of lead toxicity mandates the detection of excessive exposure in apparently asymptomatic children before irreparable damage occurs. Screening for lead poisoning is made particularly difficult by the fact that the most commonly affected children are those of preschool age who are also the least accessible, as a group, to mass testing. Screening in this age group is most often performed by pediatricians during routine office visits. It would be desirable, instead, for screening programs to reach out to the community, focusing on the most economically deprived children, who have the least access to medical care as well as the highest risk.

Nationwide programs for screening children must be primarily focused on identifying those in need of medical attention. The definition of *lead poisoning* now includes the category of children with blood lead levels of 10 to 19 μg/dL. Yet it has been shown that, at this level, the potential loss of IQ is so low that most people would agree it is trivial.[514, 515] Although medical intervention is not necessary for this group, educational and dietary advice are recommended. Children in need of medical attention are those with blood lead levels of 20 μg/dL or greater. Above this level, cognitive issues become significant.[514, 515] Severe lead poisoning is defined as levels greater than 45 μg/dL.

Treatment of Lead Poisoning

The first and most essential step in treating lead poisoning in children is the identification and removal of the source of lead. Without elimination of the exposure, any treatment is futile. Environmental analysis, including home visits, is recommended to ascertain and remove the source of lead. Although complete removal of lead from the environment remains a formidable task for modern society, it offers the only viable solution to prevent lead toxicity in children. Many studies have shown that neurotoxicity is unlikely to be reversible, regardless of the treatment used, once lead intoxication is discovered. Because lead exposures are additive, the removal of automobile-generated lead from the air has already had a profound impact on the problem of urban lead poisoning. However, residual lead-based paint continues to be a major problem.

Children who are symptomatic require urgent treatment. However, because the symptoms of lead poisoning may be elusive, treatment is indicated even in their absence when there is clear evidence of an excessive body burden of lead. The goal of treatment is prevention of subclinical damage without producing complications of the therapy itself; it is necessary to achieve judicious compromise. Two parenteral treatments are used for severe lead poisoning: dimercaprol (formerly called BAL for British anti-lewisite) and calcium-sodium EDTA (CaNaEDTA). Both of these agents chelate lead and induce its excretion. Dimercaprol is an oily, malodorous compound that is unpleasant to patients. It forms an emetic compound with iron; thus, iron therapy should not be given to a patient receiving dimercaprol.[516] It is dissolved in peanut oil and thus is contraindicated in children allergic to peanuts. Approximately half of patients treated with dimercaprol have side effects, many of which can be ameliorated by concurrent use of antihistamines.[513]

CaNaEDTA is water soluble. It is best administered by continuous intravenous infusion. When administered intramuscularly (a less preferable and much more painful option), 2 percent procaine should be added to avoid severe local pain. CaNaEDTA may itself be toxic, particularly to the kidneys. Overdosage may induce tubular necrosis directly or renal toxicity because of hypercalcemia. CaNaEDTA is also able to chelate zinc, presenting another risk. Because δ-aminolevulinic acid dehydratase, a zinc-dependent enzyme, is already damaged by lead, the additional removal of zinc leads to its complete paralysis. This leads to a burst of neurotoxic δ-aminolevulinic acid into the plasma, which may aggravate (and even induce) convulsions. For these reasons, CaNaEDTA should never be given alone to symptomatic children or to asymptomatic children with blood lead levels of 70 μg/dL or more; instead, it should be given after administration of dimercaprol to prevent these acute effects.[516] An additional note of caution is necessary with regard to the use of EDTA. Besides CaNaEDTA, a commercial preparation of disodium EDTA is also available and is occasionally used for treatment of hyperparathyroidism. Disodium EDTA should never be used for treatment of lead poisoning, because it may induce acute hypocalcemia, which may be fatal. Only CaNaEDTA should be used for the treatment of lead poisoning. Hospital pharmacies should exercise maximum caution in dispensing disodium EDTA, which could be fatal if erroneously given to a child with lead poisoning but without hypercalcemia.

Because of their different pharmacologic properties, dimercaprol and CaNaEDTA are advantageously used in combination to treat children with symptomatic lead poisoning, with or without concomitant encephalopathy, and asymptomatic children with blood lead levels greater than 70 μg/dL.[513] The combined use of dimercaprol and CaNaEDTA is both safer and more effective than the use of CaNaEDTA alone. Treatment should always start first with dimercaprol, to avoid precipitation of encephalopathy.[516] The involvement of an experienced toxicologist is strongly advised for safe, effective management of these patients.

Succimer is a derivative of dimercaprol in which the methyl groups are replaced by carboxylic groups. This results in excellent water solubility, allowing it to be used orally. Whereas the advantages of an oral chelator are obvious, caution in its use is crucial, because, owing to its great water solubility and affinity for lead, it may result in increased absorption if used in a lead-laden environment. For this reason, succimer should only be used when it is absolutely certain that the child has been removed from the lead-containing environment and is in a safe home. In a recent trial, succimer was shown to be effective in reducing blood lead levels in patients who had levels of 20 to 45 μg/dL.[517] Importantly, however, it did not reverse neurologic and cognitive deficits. For that reason, the authors concluded that its use was not indicated in children with moderate lead levels (20 to 45 µg/dL). Experience with this drug in treating children with blood lead levels of 70 µg/dL or more is very limited. It may still be prudent to treat these children, as well as symptomatic children, with a combination of dimercaprol and CaNaEDTA.

Regardless of the treatment, it is important to remember that a decrease in the blood lead level does not mean that all lead has been removed. Blood levels are likely to rebound 1 to 2 weeks after therapy as tissue lead (particularly from bone) enters the circulation. Children with a large body burden of lead, such as those with clinical symptomatology or blood lead levels greater than 70 µg/dL, invariably require several cycles of chelation therapy before substantial reduction of the body burden of lead is obtained.[516] The need for additional cycles of therapy can be established by the measurement of urinary lead excretion during the first days of treatment. The lead excreted should be related to the amount of CaNaEDTA given. Children who excrete lead in larger proportions are in greater need of additional cycles of therapy. It is not uncommon for a child to require several months of chelation therapy, initially with both dimercaprol and CaNaEDTA, and later with CaNaEDTA alone, before the urinary lead excretion declines and the blood lead level stabilizes at a value less than 30 µg/dL. Only at that point can chelation therapy be stopped.[516]

ACKNOWLEDGMENT

I am grateful to Ms. Karyn Giarla for her help in preparing this chapter and to Dr. Sergio Piomelli, who contributed a chapter on lead poisoning to the previous edition; portions of his chapter are now incorporated into this one.

REFERENCES

1. Karlin KD: Metalloenzymes, structural motifs, and inorganic models. Science 1993; 261:701.
2. Gutteridge JMC, Rowley DA, Halliwell B: Superoxide-dependent formation of hydroxyl radicals in the presence of iron salts. Biochem J 1981; 199:263.
3. Frigerio R, Mela Q, et al: Iron overload and lysosomal stability in β_0-thalassemia intermedia and trait: Correlation between serum ferritin and serum N-acetyl-β-D-glucosaminidase levels. Scand J Haematol 1984; 33:252.
4. Hebbel RP: The sickle erythrocyte in double jeopardy: Autoxidation and iron decompartmentalization. Semin Hematol 1990; 27:51.
5. Repka T, Shalev O, Reddy R, et al: Nonrandom association of free iron with membranes of sickle and β-thalassemic erythrocytes. Blood 1993; 82:3204.
6. Kuross SA, Rank BH, Hebbel RP: Iron compartments associated with sickle cell RBC membranes: A mechanism for targeting of oxidative damage. Prog Clin Biol Res 1989; 319:601.
7. Schluter K, Drenckhan D: Co-clustering of denatured hemoglobin with band 3: Its role in binding of autoantibodies against band 3 to abnormal and aged erythrocytes. Proc Natl Acad Sci USA 1986; 83:6137.
8. Waugh SM, Willardson BM, Kannan R, et al: Heinz bodies induce clustering of band 3, glycophorin and ankyrin in sickle cell erythrocytes. J Clin Invest 1988; 78:1155.
9. Clark RA: Activation of the neutrophil respiratory burst oxidase. J Infect Dis 1999; 179(Suppl 2):S309.
10. Dabbagh AJ, Trenam CW, Morris CJ, et al: Iron in joint inflammation. Ann Rheum Dis 1993; 52:67.
11. Blake DR, Hall ND, et al: Protection against superoxide and hydrogen peroxide in synovial fluid from rheumatoid patients. Clin Sci 1981; 68:483.
12. Winyard PG, Blake DR, Chirico S, et al: Mechanism of exacerbation of rheumatoid synovitis by total dose iron dextran infusion. In vivo demonstration of iron promoted oxidant stress. Lancet 1987; 1:69.
13. Cairo G, Tacchini L, Pogliaghi G, et al: Induction of ferritin synthesis by oxidative stress. J Biol Chem 1995; 270:700.
14. Ferreira C, Bucchini D, Martin ME, et al: Early embryonic lethality of H ferritin gene deletion in mice. J Biol Chem 2000; 275:3021.
15. Cook JD, Skikne BS, et al: Estimates of iron sufficiency in the US population. Blood 1986; 68:726.
16. Bothwell TH, Charlton RW: A general approach of the problems of iron deficiency and iron overload in the population at large. Semin Hematol 1982; 19:54.
17. McCance RA, Widdowson EM: The absorption and excretion of iron following oral and intravenous administration. J Phys 1938; 94:148.
18. Gitlin D, Cruchaud A: On the kinetics of iron absorption in mice. J Clin Invest 1962; 41:344.
19. Muir A, Hopfer U: Regional specificity of iron uptake by small intestinal brush-border membranes from normal and iron-deficient mice. Gastrointest Liver Pathol 1985; 11:6376.
20. Kappas A, Drummond GS, Galbraith RA: Prolonged clinical use of a heme oxygenase inhibitor: Hematological evidence for an inducible but reversible iron-deficiency state. Pediatrics 1993; 91:537.
21. Zijp IM, Korver O, Tijburg LB: Effect of tea and other dietary factors on iron absorption. Crit Rev Food Sci Nutr 2000; 40:371.
22. Gillooly M, Bothwell TH, Torrance JD, et al: The effects of organic acids, phytates and polyphenols on the absorption of iron from vegetables. Br J Nutr 1983; 49:331.
23. Gillooly M, Bothwell TH, Charlton RW, et al: Factors affecting the absorption of iron from cereals. Br J Nutr 1984; 51:37.
24. McKie AT, Barrow D, Latunde-Dada GO, et al: An iron-regulated ferric reductase associated with the absorption of dietary iron. Science 2001; 291:1755.
25. Gunshin H, Mackenzie B, Berger UV, et al: Cloning and characterization of a mammalian proton-coupled metal-ion transporter. Nature 1997; 388:482.
26. Gruenheid S, Cellier M, Vidal S, et al: Identification and characterization of a second mouse *Nramp* gene. Genomics 1995; 25:514.
27. Fleming MD, Trenor CCI, Su MA, et al: Microcytic anemia mice have a mutation in *Nramp2*, a candidate iron transporter gene. Nat Genet 1997; 16:383.
28. Nash DJ, Kent E, Dickie MM, et al: The inheritance of "mick," a new anemia in the house mouse [abstract]. Am Zoologist 1964; 4:404.
29. Russell ES, McFarland EC, Kent EL: Low viability, skin lesions, and reduced fertility associated with microcytic anemia in the mouse. Transplant Proc 1970; 2:144.
30. Russell ES, Nash DJ, Bernstein SE, et al: Characterization and genetic studies of microcytic anemia in house mouse. Blood 1970; 35:838.
31. Bannerman RM, Edwards JA, Kreimer-Birnbaum M, et al: Hereditary microcytic anaemia in the mouse; studies in iron distribution and metabolism. Br J Haematology 1972; 23:235.
32. Edwards JA, Hoke JE: Defect of intestinal mucosal iron uptake in mice with hereditary microcytic anemia. Proc Soc Exp Biol Med 1972; 141:81.
33. Edwards JA, Hoke JE: Red cell iron uptake in hereditary microcytic anemia. Blood 1975; 46:381.
34. Harrison DE: Marrow transplantation and iron therapy in mouse hereditary microcytic anemia. Blood 1972; 40:893.
35. Supek F, Supekova L, Nelson H, et al: A yeast manganese transporter related to the macrophage protein involved in conferring resistance to mycobacteria. Proc Natl Acad Sci USA 1996; 93:5105.
36. Su MA, Trenor CC, Fleming JC, et al: The G185R mutation disrupts function of iron transporter Nramp2. Blood 1998; 92:2157.
37. Vidal SM, Malo D, Vogan K, et al: Natural resistance to infection with intracellular parasites: Isolation of a candidate for Bcg. Cell 1993; 73:469.
38. Piomelli S, Seaman C, Kapoor S: Lead-induced abnormalities of porphyrin metabolism. The relationship with iron deficiency. Ann NY Acad Sci 1987; 514:278.
39. Donovan A, Brownlie A, Zhou Y, et al: Positional cloning of zebrafish ferroportin1 identifies a conserved vertebrate iron exporter. Nature 2000; 403:776.

40. McKie AT, Marciani P, Rolfs A, et al: A novel duodenal iron-regulated transporter, IREG1, implicated in the basolateral transfer of iron to the circulation. Mol Cell 2000; 5:299.
41. Abboud S, Haile DJ: A novel mammalian iron-regulated protein involved in intracellular iron metabolism. J Biol Chem 2000; 275:19906.
42. Montosi G, Donovan A, Totaro A, et al: Autosomal-dominant hemochromatosis is associated with a mutation in the ferroportin (SLC11A3) gene. J Clin Invest 2001; 108:619.
43. Njajou OT, Vaessen N, Joosse M, et al: A mutation in SLC11A3 is associated with autosomal dominant hemochromatosis. Nat Genet 2001; 28:213.
44. Bannerman RM, Cooper RG: Sex-linked anemia: A hypochromic anemia of mice. Science 1966; 151:581.
45. Edwards JA, Bannerman RM: Hereditary defect of intestinal iron transport in mice with sex-linked anemia. J Clin Invest 1970; 49:1869.
46. Manis J: Intestinal iron-transport defect in the mouse with sex-linked anemia. Am J Physiol 1971; 220:135.
47. Bedard YC, Pinkerton PH, Simon GT: Ultrastructure of the duodenal mucosa of mice with a hereditary defect in iron absorption. J Pathol 1971; 104:45.
48. Kingston PJ, Bannerman CE, Bannerman RM: Iron deficiency anaemia in newborn *sla* mice: A genetic defect of placental iron transport. Br J Haematol 1978; 40:265.
49. Vulpe CD, Kuo YM, Murphy TL, et al: Hephaestin, a ceruloplasmin homologue implicated in intestinal iron transport, is defective in the *sla* mouse. Nat Genet 1999; 21:195.
50. Finch C: Regulators of iron balance in humans. Blood 1994; 84:1697.
51. Huff RL, Hennessey TG, Austin RE, et al: Plasma and red cell iron turnover in normal subjects and in patients having various hematopoietic disorders. J Clin Invest 1950; 29:1041.
52. Weintraub LR, Conrad ME, Crosby WH: Regulation of the intestinal absorption of iron by the rate of erythropoiesis. Br J Hematol 1965; 2:432.
53. Beutler E, Buttenweiser E: The regulation of iron absorption. I. A search for humoral factors. J Lab Clin Med 1960; 55:274.
54. Aron J, Baynes R, Bothwell TH, et al: Does plasma transferrin regulate iron absorption? Scand J Haematol 1985; 35:451.
55. Raja KN, Pippard MJ, Simpson RJ, et al: Relationship between erythropoiesis and the enhanced intestinal uptake of ferric iron in hypoxia in the mouse. Br J Haematol 1986; 64:587.
56. Ponka P, Schulman HM: Regulation of heme biosynthesis: Distinct features in erythroid cells. Stem Cells 1993; 11(Suppl 1):24.
57. Huebers HA, Finch CA: The physiology of transferrin and transferrin receptors. Physiol Rev 1987; 67:520.
58. Williams J, Ellerman TC, et al: The primary structure of hen ovotransferrin. Eur J Biochem 1982; 122:297.
59. Mazurier J, Metz-Boutigue M, et al: Human lactotransferrin: Molecular, functional and evolutionary comparisons with human serum transferrin and hen ovotransferrin. Experientia 1983; 39:135.
60. Metz-Boutigue MH, Jolies J, et al: Human lactotransferrin: Amino acid sequence and structural comparison with other transferrins. Eur J Biochem 1984; 145:659.
61. Brown JP, Henwick RM, et al: Human melanoma-associated antigen p97 is structurally and functionally related to transferrin. Nature 1982; 296:171.
62. Aisen P, Leibman A, Zweier J: Stoichiometric and site characteristics of the binding of iron to human transferrin. J Biol Chem 1978; 253:1930.
63. Levin MJ, Tuil D, et al: Expression of transferrin gene during development of non-hepatic tissues: High level of transferrin mRNA in fetal muscle and adult brain. Biochem Biophys Res Commun 1984; 122:212.
64. Skinner MK, Cosand WL, Griswold MD: Purification and characterization of testicular transferrin secreted by rat Sertoli cells. Biochem J 1984; 218:313.
65. Chen L-H, Bissel MJ: Transferrin mRNA level in the mouse mammary gland is regulated by pregnancy and extracellular matrix. J Biol Chem 1987; 262:17247.
66. Sylvester SR, Griswold MD: Localization of transferrin and transferrin receptors in rat testes. Biol Reprod 1984; 31:195.
67. Gerber MR, Connor JR: Do oligodendrocytes mediate iron regulation in the human brain? Ann Neurol 1989; 26:95.
68. Lum JB, Infante AJ, et al: Transferrin synthesis by inducer T-lymphocytes. J Clin Invest 1986; 77:841.
69. Trenor CCI, Campagna DR, Sellers VM, et al: The molecular defect in hypotransferrinemic mice. Blood 2000; 96:1113.
70. Dickinson T, Connor JR: Histological analysis of selected brain regions of hypotransferrinemic mice. Brain Res 1994; 635:169.
71. Pattanapanyasat K, Hoy TG: Expression of cell surface transferrin receptor and intracellular ferritin after in vitro stimulation of peripheral blood T lymphocytes. Eur J Haematol 1991; 47:140.
72. Schaeffer E, Lucero MA, Jeltsch JM, et al: Complete structure of the human transferrin gene. Comparison with analogous chicken gene and human pseudogene. Gene 1987; 56:109.
73. Brunel F, Ochoa A, et al: Interactions of DNA-binding proteins with the 5′ region of the human transferrin gene. J Biol Chem 1988; 263:10180.
74. Griswold MD, Hugly S, Morales C, et al: Evidence for in vitro transferrin synthesis and the relationship between transferrin mRNA levels and germ cells for the testes. Ann NY Acad Sci 1988; 513:302.
75. Guillou F, Zakin MM, Part D, et al: Sertoli cell-specific expression of the human transferrin gene. Comparison with liver-specific expression. J Biol Chem 1991; 266:9876.
76. Ochoa A, Brunel F, Mendelzon D, et al: Different liver nuclear proteins bind to similar DNA sequences in the 5′ flanking regions of three hepatic genes. Nucleic Acids Res 1989; 17:119.
77. Schaeffer E, Boissier F, et al: Cell type-specific expression of the human transferrin gene. J Biol Chem 1989; 264:7153.
78. Mendelzon D, Boissier F, Zakin MM: The binding site for the liver-specific transcription factor Tf-LF1 and the TATA box of the human transferrin gene promoter are the only elements necessary to direct liver-specific transcription in vitro. Nucleic Acids Res 1991; 18:5717.
79. Adrian GS, Korinek BW, Bowman BH, et al: The human transferrin gene: 5′ region contains conserved sequences which match the control elements regulated by heavy metals, glucocorticoids and acute phase reaction. Gene 1986; 490:167.
80. Lucerno MA, Schaeffer E, et al: The 5′ region of the human transferrin gene: Structure and potential regulatory sites. Nucleic Acids Res 1986; 14:8692.
81. Huggenvik JI, Idzerda RL, et al: Transferrin messenger ribonucleic acid: Molecular cloning and hormonal regulation in rat Sertoli cells. Endocrinology 1987; 120:332.
82. Tsutsumi M, Skinner MK, Sanders-Bush E: Transferrin gene expression and synthesis by cultured choroid plexus epithelial cells. Regulation by serotonin and cyclic adenosine 3′,5′-monophosphate. J Biol Chem 1989; 264:9226.
83. Idzerda RL, Huebers H, et al: Rat transferrin gene expression: Tissue-specific regulation by iron deficiency. Proc Natl Acad Sciences USA 1986; 83:3723.
84. Pietrangelo A, Rocchi E, Ferrari A, et al: Regulation of hepatic transferrin, transferrin receptor and ferritin genes in human siderosis. Hepatology 1991; 14:1083.
85. Baker EN, Lindley PF: New perspectives on the structure and function of transferrins. J Inorg Biochem 1992; 47:147.
86. MacGillivray RT, Moore SA, Chen J, et al: Two high-resolution crystal structures of the recombinant N-lobe of human transferrin reveal a structural change implicated in iron release. Biochemistry 1998; 37:7919.
87. Williams J: The formation of iron-binding fragments of hen ovotransferrin by limited proteolysis. Biochem J 1974; 141:745.
88. Zak O, Aisen P: Preparation and properties of a single-sited fragment from the C-terminal domain of human transferrin. Biochim Biophys Acta 1985; 829:348.
89. Aisen P, Listowsky I: Iron transport and storage proteins. Annu Rev Biochem 1980; 49:357.
90. Osaki S, Johnson DA: Mobilization of liver iron by ferroxidase (ceruloplasmin). J Biol Chem 1969; 244:5757.
91. Osaki S, Johnson DA, Frieden E: The mobilization of iron from the perfused mammalian liver by a serum copper enzyme, ferroxidase I. J Biol Chem 1971; 246:3018.
92. Yoshida K, Furihata K, Takeda S, et al: A mutation in the ceruloplasmin gene is associated with systemic hemosiderosis in humans. Nat Genet 1995; 9:267.
93. Harris ZL, Takahashi Y, Miyajima H, et al: Aceruloplasminemia: Molecular characterization of this disorder of iron metabolism. Proc Natl Acad Sci USA 1995; 92:2539.

94. Harris ZL, Durley AP, Man TK, et al: Targeted gene disruption reveals an essential role for ceruloplasmin in cellular iron efflux. Proc Natl Acad Sci USA 1999; 96:10812.

95. Harris ZL, Klomp LW, Gitlin JD: Aceruloplasminemia: An inherited neurodegenerative disease with impairment of iron homeostasis. Am J Clin Nutr 1998; 67:972S.

96. Harris DC, Aisen P: Physical biochemistry of the transferrins. In Loehr TM, Gray HB, Lever ABP (eds): Iron Carriers and Iron Proteins. Weinheim, VCH, 1989, pp 239–349.

97. Shongwe MS, Smith CA, Ainscough EW, et al: Anion binding by human lactoferrin: Results from crystallographic and physico-chemical studies. Biochemistry 1992; 31:4451.

98. Bailey S, Evans RW, Garatt RC, et al: Molecular structure of serum transferrin at 3.3-A resolution. Biochem 1988; 27:5804.

99. Anderson BF, Baker HM, Norris GE, et al: Structure of human lactoferrin: Crystallographic structure analysis and refinement at 2.8 A resolution. J Mol Biol 1989; 209:711.

100. Breuer W, Hershko C, Cabantchik ZI: The importance of non-transferrin bound iron in disorders of iron metabolism. Transfus Sci 2000; 23:185.

101. Jandl JH, Katz JH: The plasma-to-cell cycle of transferrin. J Clin Invest 1963; 42:314.

102. Finch CA, Huebers H, Eng M, et al: Effect of transfused reticulocytes on iron exchange. Blood 1982; 59:364.

103. Laurell C, Ingelman B: The iron-binding protein of swine serum. Acta Chem Scand 1947; 1:770.

104. Sutherland R, Delia D, Schneider C, et al: Ubiquitous cell-surface glycoprotein on tumor cells is proliferation-associated receptor for transferrin. Proc Natl Acad Sci USA 1980; 78:4515.

105. Kuhn LC, McClelland A, Ruddle FH: Gene transfer, expression and molecular cloning of the human transferrin receptor gene. Cell 1984; 37:95.

106. Schneider C, Kurkinen M, Greaves M: Isolation of cDNA clones for the human transferrin receptor. EMBO J 1983; 2:2259.

107. Jing SQ, Trowbridge IS: Identification of the intermolecular disulfide bonds of the human transferrin receptor and its lipid-attachment site. EMBO J 1987; 6:327.

108. Reckhow CL, Enns CA: Characterization of the transferrin receptor in tunicamycin-treated A431 cells. J Biol Chem 1988; 263:7297.

109. Hayes GR, Enns CA, Lucas JJ: Identification of the O-linked glycosylation site of the human transferrin receptor. Glycobiology 1992; 2:355.

110. Williams AM, Enns CA: A region of the C-terminal portion of the human transferrin receptor contains an asparagine-linked glycosylation site critical for receptor structure and function. J Biol Chem 1993; 268:12780.

111. Zerial M, Melancon P, Schneider C, et al: The transmembrane segment of the human transferrin receptor functions as a signal peptide. EMBO J 1986; 5:1543.

112. Alvarez E, Girones N, Davis RJ: Inhibition of receptor-mediated endocytosis of diferrin transferrin is associated with covalent modification of the transferrin receptor with palmitic acid. J Biol Chem 1990; 265:16644.

113. Jing SQ, Trowbridge IS: Nonacylated human transferrin receptors are rapidly internalized and mediate iron uptake. J Biol Chem 1990; 265:11555.

114. Lawrence CM, Ray S, Babyonyshev M, et al: Crystal structure of the ectodomain of human transferrin receptor. Science 1999; 286:779.

115. Ramalingam TS, West AP Jr, Lebron JA, et al: Binding to the transferrin receptor is required for endocytosis of HFE and regulation of iron homeostasis. Nat Cell Biol 2000; 2:953.

116. Iacopetta BJ, Morgan EH: The kinetics of transferrin endocytosis and iron uptake from transferrin in rabbit reticulocytes. J Biol Chem 1983; 258:9108.

117. Karin M, Mintz B: Receptor-mediated endocytosis of transferrin in developmentally totipotent mouse teratocarcinoma stem cells. J Biol Chem 1981; 256:3245.

118. Klausner RD, van Renswoude J, Ashwell G, et al: Receptor-mediated endocytosis of transferrin in K562 cells. J Biol Chem 1983; 258:4715.

119. Zak O, Trinder D, Aisen P: Primary receptor-recognition site of human transferrin is in the C-terminal lobe. J Biol Chem 1994; 269:7110.

120. Huebers HA, Huebers E, Csiba E, et al: Heterogeneity of the plasma iron pool: Explanation of the Fletcher-Huehns phenomenon. Am J Physiol 1984; 247:R280.

121. Huebers H, Csiba E, Huebers E, et al: Molecular advantage of diferric transferrin in delivering iron to reticulocytes: A comparative study. Proc Soc Exp Biol Med 1985; 179:222.

122. Young SP, Bomford A, Williams R: The effect of the iron saturation of transferrin on its binding and uptake by rabbit reticulocytes. Biochem J 1984; 219:505.

123. Rothenberger S, Iacopetta BJ, Kuhn LC: Endocytosis of the transferrin receptor requires the cytoplasmic domain but not its phosphorylation site. Cell 1987; 49:423.

124. McGraw TE, Maxfield FR: Human transferrin receptor internalization is partly dependent upon an aromatic amino acid in the cytoplasmic domain. Cell Regul 1990; 1:369.

125. Girones N, Alvarez E, Seth A, et al: Mutational analysis of the cytoplasmic tail of the human transferrin receptor. Identification of a sub-domain that is required for rapid endocytosis. J Biol Chem 1991; 266:19006.

126. Miller K, Shipman M, Trowbridge IS, et al: Transferrin receptors promote the formation of clathrin lattices. Cell 1991; 65:621.

127. Collawn JF, Lai A, Domingo D, et al: YTRF is the conserved internalization signal of the transferrin receptor, and a second YTRF signal at position 30–34 enhances endocytosis. J Biol Chem 1993; 268:21686.

128. Davis RJ, Johnson GL, Kelleher DJ, et al: Identification of serine 24 as the unique site on the transferrin receptor phosphorylated by protein kinase C. J Biol Chem 1986; 261:9034.

129. Van Renswoude J, Bridges KR, Harford JB, et al: Receptor-mediated endocytosis and the uptake of iron in K562 cells: Identification of a non-lysosomal acidic compartment. Proc Natl Acad Sci USA 1982; 79:6186.

130. Dautry-Varsat A, Ciechanover A, Lodish HF: pH and the recycling of transferrin during receptor-mediated endocytosis. Proc Natl Acad Sci USA 1983; 80:2258.

131. Paterson S, Armstrong NJ, Iacopetta BJ, et al: Intravesicular pH and iron uptake by immature erythroid cells. J Cell Physiol 1984; 120:225.

132. Yamashiro DJ, Tycko B, Fluss SR, et al: Segregation of transferrin to a mildly acidic (pH 6.5) para-Golgi compartment in the recycling pathway. Cell 1984; 37:789.

133. Bali PK, Zak O, Aisen P: A new role for the transferrin receptor in the release of iron from transferrin. Biochemistry 1991; 30:324.

134. Sipe DM, Murphy RF: Binding to cellular receptors results in increased iron release from transferrin at mildly acidic pH. J Biol Chem 1991; 266:8002.

135. Low H, Grebing C, Lindgren A, et al: Involvement of transferrin in the reduction of iron by the transplasma membrane electron transport system. J Bioenerg Biomembr 1987; 19:535.

136. Thorstensen K, Romslo I: Uptake of iron from transferrin by isolated rat hepatocytes. A redox-mediated plasma membrane process? J Biol Chem 1988; 263:8844.

137. Nunez M-T, Gaete V, Watkins JA, et al: Mobilization of iron from endocytic vesicles. The effects of acidification and reduction. J Biol Chem 1990; 265:6688.

138. Edwards JA, Garrick LM, Hoke JE: Defective iron uptake and globin synthesis by erythroid cells in the anemia of the Belgrade laboratory rat. Blood 1978; 51:347.

139. Edwards JA, Sullivan AL, Hoke JE: Defective delivery of iron to the developing red cell of the Belgrade laboratory rat. Blood 1980; 55:645.

140. Farcich EA, Morgan EH: Uptake of transferrin-bound and non-transferrin-bound iron by reticulocytes from the Belgrade laboratory rat: Comparison with Wistar rat transferrin and reticulocytes. Am J Hematol 1992; 39:9.

141. Garrick MD, Gniecko K, Liu L, et al: Transferrin and the transferrin cycle in Belgrade rat reticulocytes. J Biol Chem 1993; 268:14867.

142. Fleming MD, Romano MA, Su MA, et al: Nramp2 is mutated in the anemic Belgrade (b) rat: Evidence of a role for Nramp2 in endosomal iron transport. Proc Natl Acad Sci USA 1998; 95:1148.

143. Canonne-Hergaux F, Gruenheid S, Ponka P, et al: Cellular and subcellular localization of the Nramp2 iron transporter in the intestinal brush border and regulation by dietary iron. Blood 1999; 93:4406.

144. Gruenheid S, Canonne-Hergaux F, Gauthier S, et al: The iron transport protein NRAMP2 is an integral membrane glycoprotein that colocalizes with transferrin in recycling endosomes. J Exp Med 1999; 189:831.

145. Harford JB, Rouault TA, Huebers HA, et al: Molecular mechanisms of iron metabolism. In Stamatoyannopoulos G, Nienhuis AW, Majerus PW, et al (eds): The Molecular Basis of Blood Diseases. Philadelphia, WB Saunders, 1994, p 351.

146. Bernstein SE: Hereditary hypotransferrinemia with hemosiderosis, a murine disorder resembling human atransferrinemia. J Lab Clin Med 1987; 110:690.

147. Kaplan J, Craven C, Alexander J, et al: Regulation of the distribution of tissue iron. Lessons learned from the hypotransferrinemic mouse. Ann NY Acad Sci 1988; 526:124.

148. Simpson RJ, Konijn AM, Lombard M, et al: Tissue iron loading and histopathological changes in hypotransferrinaemic mice. J Pathol 1993; 171:237.

149. Heilmeyer L, Keller W, Vivell O, et al: Congenital transferrin deficiency in a seven-year old girl. Ger Med Mon 1961; 86:1745.

150. Goya N, Miyazaki S, Kodate S, et al: A family of congenital atransferrinemia. Blood 1972; 40:239.

151. Craven CM, Alexander J, Eldridge M, et al: Tissue distribution and clearance kinetics of non-transferrin-bound iron in the hypotransferrinemic mouse: A rodent model for hemochromatosis. Proc Natl Acad Sci USA 1987; 84:3457.

152. Hamill RL, Woods JC, Cook BA: Congenital atransferrinemia: A case report and review of the literature. Am J Clin Pathol 1991; 96:215.

153. Levy JE, Jin O, Fujiwara Y, et al: Transferrin receptor is necessary for development of erythrocytes and the nervous system. Nat Genet 1999; 21:396.

154. Kaplan J, Jordan I, Sturrock A: Regulation of the transferrin-independent iron transport system in cultured cells. J Biol Chem 1991; 266:2997.

155. Sturrock A, Alexander J, Lamb J, et al: Characterization of a transferrin-independent uptake system for iron in HeLa cells. J Biol Chem 1990; 265:3139.

156. Randell EW, Parkes JG, Olivieri NF, et al: Uptake of non-transferrin bound iron by both reductive and non-reductive processes is modulated by intracellular iron. J Biol Chem 1994; 269:16046.

157. Inman RS, Coughlan MM, Wessling-Resnick M: Extracellular ferrireductase activity of K562 cells is coupled to transferrin-independent iron transport. Biochemistry 1994; 33:11850.

158. Inman RS, Wessling-Resnick M: Characterization of transferrin-independent iron transport in K562 cells. Unique properties provide evidence for multiple pathways of iron uptake. J Biol Chem 1993; 268:8521.

159. Hershko C, Graham G, Bates GW, et al: Non-specific serum iron in thalassemia: An abnormal serum iron fraction of potential toxicity. Br. J. Haematol 1978; 40:255.

160. Hoffbrand AV, Ganeshaguru K, Hooton JW, et al: Effect of iron deficiency and desferrioxamine on DNA synthesis in human cells. Br J Haematol 1976; 33:517.

161. Frazier JL, Caskey JH, Yoffe M, et al: Studies of the transferrin receptor on both human reticulocytes and nucleated human cells in culture. J Clin Invest 1982; 69:853.

162. Larrick JW, Cresswell P: Modulation of cell surface iron transferrin receptors by cellular density and state of activation. J Supramol Struct 1979; 11:579.

163. Trowbridge IS, Lopez F: Monoclonal antibody to transferrin receptor blocks transferrin binding and inhibits tumour cell growth in vitro. Proc Natl Acad Sci USA 1982; 79:1175.

164. Lesley JF, Schulte RJ: Inhibition of cell growth by monoclonal antitransferrin receptor antibodies. Mol Cell Biol 1985; 5:1814.

165. White S, Taetle R, Seligman PA, et al: Combinations of anti-transferrin receptor monoclonal antibodies inhibit human tumor cell growth in vitro and in vivo: Evidence for synergistic anti-proliferative effects. Cancer Res 1990; 50:6295.

166. Trowbridge IS, Lesley JF, Domingo D, et al: Monoclonal antibodies to transferrin receptor and assay of their biological effects. Methods Enzymol 1987; 147:265.

167. Cano E, Pizarro A, Redondo JM, et al: Induction of T cell activation by monoclonal antibodies specific for the transferrin receptor. Eur J Immunol 1990; 20:765.

168. Keyna U, Platzer E, Woith W, et al: Differential effects of transferrin receptor antibodies on growth and receptor expression of human lymphocytic and myelocytic cell lines. Eur J Haematol 1994; 52:169.

169. Manger B, Weiss A, Hardy KJ, et al: A transferrin receptor antibody represents one signal for the induction of IL-2 production by a human T cell line. J Immunol 1987; 136:532.

170. Reddel RR, Hedley DW, Sutherland RL: Cell cycle effects of iron depletion on T-47D human breast cancer cells. Exp Cell Res 1985; 161:277.

171. Gao J, Richardson DR: The potential of iron chelators of the pyridoxal isonicotinoyl hydrazone class as effective antiproliferative agents. IV. The mechanisms involved in inhibiting cell-cycle progression. Blood 2001; 98:842.

172. Bierer BE, Nathan DG: The effect of desferrithiocin, an oral iron chelator, on T cell function. Blood 1990; 76:2052.

173. Chaudri G, Clark IA, et al: Effect of antioxidants on primarily alloantigen-induced T-cell activation and proliferation. J Immunol 1986; 137:2646.

174. Pattanapanyasat K, Webster HK, Tongtawe P, et al: Effect of orally active hydroxypyridinone iron chelators on human lymphocyte function. Br J Haematol 1992; 82:13.

175. Polson RJ, Jenkins R, Lombard M, et al: Mechanisms of inhibition of mononuclear cell activation by the iron-chelating agent desferrioxamine. Immunology 1990; 71:176.

176. Lederman HM, Cohen A, Lee JW, et al: Deferoxamine: A reversible S-phase inhibitor of human lymphocyte proliferation. Blood 1984; 64:748.

177. Brittenham GM: The red cell cycle. In Brock JH, Halliday JW, Pippard MJ, et al (eds): Iron Metabolism in Health and Disease. London, WB Saunders, 1994, p 31.

178. Shannon KM, Larrick JW, et al: Selective inhibition of the growth of human erythroid bursts by monoclonal antibodies against transferrin or transferrin receptor. Blood 1986; 67:1631.

179. Schmidt JA, Marshall J, Hayman MJ, et al: Control of erythroid differentiation. Cell 1986; 46:41.

180. Bonanou-Tzedaki SA, Sohi M, Arnstein HR: Regulation of erythroid cell differentiation by haemin. Cell Differ 1981; 10:267.

181. Mager D, Bernstein A: The role of heme in the regulation of the late program of Friend cell erythroid differentiation. J Cell Physiol 1979; 100:467.

182. Ross J, Sautner D: Induction of globin mRNA accumulation by hemin in cultured erythroleukemic cells. Cell 1976; 8:513.

183. Rutherford TR, Clegg JB, Weatherall DJ: K562 human leukaemic cells synthesise embryonic haemoglobin in response to haemin. Nature 1979; 280:164.

184. Rutherford TR, Weatherall DJ: Deficient heme synthesis as the cause of noninducibility of hemoglobin synthesis in a Friend erythroleukemia cell line. Cell 1979; 16:415.

185. Battistini A, Coccia EM, Marziali G, et al: Intracellular heme coordinately modulates globin chain synthesis, transferrin receptor number, and ferritin content in differentiating Friend erythroleukemia cells. Blood 1991; 78:2098.

186. Battistini A, Marziali G, Albertini R, et al: Positive modulation of hemoglobin, heme and transferrin receptor synthesis by murine interferon-α and -β in differentiating Friend cells. Pivotal role of heme synthesis. J Biol Chem 1991; 266:528.

187. Coccia E, Profita V, Fiorucci G, et al: Modulation of ferritin H-chain expression in Friend erythroleukemia cells: Transcriptional and translational regulation by hemin. Mol Cell Biol 1992; 12:3015.

188. Nathan DG, Piomelli S, Gardner FH, et al: The synthesis of heme and globin in the maturing human erythroid cell. J Clin Invest 1961; 40:940.

189. London IM, Levin DH, Matts RL, et al: Regulation of protein synthesis. In Boyer PD (ed): The Enzymes. New York, Academic Press, 1987, p 359.

190. Richardson DR, Ponka P: The molecular mechanisms of the metabolism and transport of iron in normal and neoplastic cells. Biochim Biophys Acta 1997; 1331:1.

191. Harrison PM, Fischbach FA, Hoy TG, et al: Ferric oxyhydroxide core of ferritin. Nature 1967; 216:1188.

192. Harrison PM, Arosio P: The ferritins: Molecular properties, iron storage function and cellular regulation. Biochim Biophys Acta 1996; 1275:161.

193. Levi S, Luzzago A, Cesareni G, et al: Mechanism of ferritin iron uptake: Activity of the H-chain and deletion mapping of the ferro-oxidase site. A study of iron uptake and ferro-oxidase activity of

human liver, recombinant H-chain ferritins, and two H-chain deletion mutants. J Biol Chem 1988; 263:18086.

194. Theil EC, Takagi H, Small GW, et al: The ferritin iron entry and exit problem. Inorg Clin Acta 1999; 297:242.

195. Drysdale J, Jain SK, Boyd D: Human ferritins: Genes and proteins. In Spik G, Montreuil J, Crichton RR, et al (eds): Proteins of Iron Storage and Transport. New York, Elsevier, 1985, p 343.

196. McClarty G, Chan AK, Choy BK, et al: Increased ferritin gene expression is associated with increased ribonucleotide reductase gene expression and the establishment of hydroxyurea resistance in mammalian cells. J Biol Chem 1990; 265:7539.

197. Wixom RL, Prutkin L, Munro HN: Hemosiderin: Nature, formation and significance. Int Rev Exp Pathol 1980; 22:193.

198. Costanzo F, Colombo M, et al: Structure of gene and pseudogenes of human apoferritin H. Nucleic Acids Res 1986; 14:721.

199. Cragg SJ, Drysdale J, Worwood M: Genes for the `H' subunit of human ferritin are present on a number of human chromosomes. Hum Gene 1985; 71:108.

200. McGill JR, Naylor SL, Sakaguchi AY, et al: Human ferritin H and L sequences lie on ten different chromosomes. Hum Genet 1987; 76:66.

201. Worwood M, Brook JD, et al: Assignment of human ferritin genes to chromosomes 11 and 19q13.3-19 qter. Hum Genet 1985; 69:371.

202. Levi S, Corsi B, Bosisio M, et al: A human mitochondrial ferritin encoded by an intronless gene. J Biol Chem 2001; 276:24437.

203. Coulson RM, Cleveland DW: Ferritin synthesis is controlled by iron-dependent translational derepression and by changes in synthesis/transport of nuclear ferritin RNAs. Proc Natl Acad Sci USA 1993; 90:7613.

204. White K, Munro HN: Induction of ferritin synthesis by iron is regulated at both transcriptional and translational levels. J Biol Chem 1988; 263:8938.

205. Cairo G, Bardella L, Schiaffonata L, et al: Multiple mechanisms of iron-induced ferritin synthesis in HeLa cells. Biochem Biophys Res Commun 1985; 133:314.

206. Beaumont C, Jain SK, Bogard M, et al: Ferritin synthesis in differentiating Friend erythroleukemia cells. J Biol Chem 1987; 262:10619.

207. Chou CC, Gatti RA, Fuller ML, et al: Structure and expression of ferritin genes in a human promyelocytic cell line that differentiates in vitro. Mol Cell Biol 1986; 6:566.

208. Torti SV, Kwak EL, et al: The molecular cloning and characterization of murine ferritin heavy chain, a tumor necrosis factor-inducible gene. J Biol Chem 1988; 263:12638.

209. Rogers J, Bridges KR, et al: Translational control during the acute phase response: Ferritin synthesis in response to interleukin-1. J Biol Chem 1990; 265:14572.

210. Zahringer J, Baliga BS, Munro HN: Novel mechanism for translation control in regulation of ferritin synthesis by iron. Proc Natl Acad Sci USA 1976; 73:857.

211. Aziz N, Munro HN: Iron regulates ferritin mRNA translation through a segment of its 5'-untranslated region. Proc Natl Acad Sci USA 1987; 84:8478.

212. Hentze MW, Rouault TA, et al: A cis-acting element is necessary and sufficient for translational regulation of human ferritin expression in response to iron. Proc Natl Acad Sci USA 1987; 84:6730.

213. Rouault TA, Tang CK, Kaptain S, et al: Cloning of the cDNA encoding an RNA regulatory protein—The human iron-responsive element-binding protein. Proc Natl Acad Sci USA 1990; 87:7958.

214. Constable A, Quick S, Gray NK, et al: Modulation of the RNA-binding activity of a regulatory protein by iron in vitro: Switching between enzymatic and genetic function? Proc Natl Acad Sci USA 1992; 89:4554.

215. Emory-Goodman A, Hirling H, Scarpellino L, et al: Iron regulatory factor expressed from recombinant baculovirus: Conversion between the RNA-binding apoprotein and Fe-S cluster containing aconitase. Nucleic Acids Res 1993; 21:1457.

216. Haile DJ, Rouault TA, Tang CK, et al: Reciprocal control of RNA-binding and aconitase activity in the regulation of the iron-responsive element binding protein: Role of the iron-sulfur cluster. Proc Natl Acad Sci USA 1992; 89:7536.

217. Kaptain S, Downey WE, Tang C, et al: A regulated RNA binding protein also possesses aconitase activity. Proc Natl Acad Sci USA 1991; 88:10109.

218. Gray NK, Hentze MW: Iron regulatory protein prevents binding of the 43S translation initiation complex to ferritin and eALAS mRNAs. EMBO J 1994; 13:3882.

219. Muckenthaler M, Gray NK, Hentze MW: IRP-1 binding to ferritin mRNA prevents the recruitment of the small ribosomal subunit by the cap-binding complex eIF4F. Mol Cell 1998; 2:383.

220. Hentze MW, Kuhn LC: Molecular control of vertebrate iron metabolism: mRNA-based regulatory circuits operated by iron, nitric oxide, and oxidative stress. Proc Natl Acad Sci USA 1996; 93:8175.

221. Lin J-J, Daniels-McQueen S, Patino MM, et al: Derepression of ferritin messenger RNA translation by hemin in vitro. Science 1990; 247:74.

222. Toth I, Bridges KR: Ascorbic acid enhances ferritin mRNA translation by an IRP/aconitase switch. J Biol Chem 1995; 270:19540.

223. Beaumont C, Leneuve P, Devaux I, et al: Mutation in the iron responsive element of the L ferritin mRNA in a family with dominant hyperferritinemia and cataract. Nat Genet 1995; 11:444.

224. Girelli D, Corrocher R, Bisceglia L, et al: Molecular basis for the recently described hereditary hyperferritinemia-cataract syndrome: A mutation in the iron-responsive element of ferritin L-subunit gene (the "Verona mutation"). Blood 1995; 86:4050.

225. Kato J, Fujikawa K, Kanda M, et al: A mutation in the iron-responsive element of H ferritin mRNA, causing autosomal dominant iron overload. Am J Hum Genet 2001; 69:191.

226. Samaniego F, Chin J, Iwai K, et al: Molecular characterization of a second iron-responsive element binding protein, iron regulatory protein 2. Structure, function, and post-translational regulation. J Biol Chem 1994; 269:30904.

227. Guo B, Brown FM, Phillips JD, et al: Characterization and expression of iron regulatory protein 2 (IRP2). J Biol Chem 1995; 270:16529.

228. Guo B, Yu Y, Leibold EA: Iron regulates cytoplasmic levels of a novel iron-responsive element-binding protein without aconitase activity. J Biol Chem 1994; 269:24252.

229. Guo B, Phillips JD, Yu Y, et al: Iron regulates the intracellular degradation of iron regulatory protein 2 by the proteasome. J Biol Chem 1995; 270:21645.

230. Huerre C, Uzan G, et al: The structural gene for transferrin (Tf) maps to 3q21 m3qter. Ann Genet (Paris) 1984; 27:5.

231. Rabin M, McClelland A, et al: Regional localization of the human transferrin receptor gene to 3q26mqter. Am J Hum Genet 1985; 37:1112.

232. McClelland A, Kuhn LC, Ruddle FH: The human transferrin receptor gene: Genomic organization, and the complete primary structure of the receptor deduced for a cDNA sequence. Cell 1984; 39:267.

233. Koeller DM, Casey JL, et al: A cytosolic protein binds to structural elements within the iron-responsive regulatory region of the transferrin receptor mRNA. Proc Natl Acad Sci USA 1989; 86:3574.

234. Mullner EW, Kuhn LC: A stem-loop in the 3'-untranslated region mediates iron-dependent regulation of transferrin receptor mRNA stability in the cytoplasm. Cell 1988; 53:815.

235. Mullner EW, Neupert B, Kuhn LC: A specific mRNA binding factor regulates the iron-dependent stability of cytoplasmic transferrin receptor mRNA. Cell 1989; 58:373.

236. Binder R, Horowitz JA, Basilion JP, et al: Evidence that the pathway of transferrin receptor mRNA degradation involves an endonucleolytic cleavage within the 3' UTR and does not involve poly(A) tail shortening. EMBO J 1994; 13:1969.

237. Lok CN, Ponka P: Identification of an erythroid active element in the transferrin receptor gene. J Biol Chem 2000; 275:24185.

238. Cox TC, Bawden MJ, Martin A, et al: Human erythroid 5'-aminolevulinate synthase: Promoter analysis and identification of an iron-responsive element in the mRNA. EMBO J 1991; 10:1891.

239. Dandekar T, Stripecke R, Gray NK, et al: Identification of a novel iron-responsive element in murine and human erythroid δ-aminolevulinic acid synthase mRNA. EMBO J 1991; 10:1903.

240. Zheng L, Kennedy MC, Blondin GA, et al: Binding of cytosolic aconitase to the iron responsive element of porcine mitochondrial aconitase mRNA. Archiv Biochem Biophys 1992; 299:356.

241. LaVaute T, Smith S, Cooperman S, et al: Targeted deletion of the gene encoding iron regulatory protein-2 causes misregulation of iron metabolism and neurodegenerative disease in mice. Nat Genet 2001; 27:209.

242. Worwood M: Serum ferritin. Clin Sci 1986; 70:215.

243. Cragg SJ, Wagstaff M, Worwood M: Detection of a glycosylated subunit in human serum ferritin. Biochem J 1981; 199:565.

244. Worwood M: Laboratory determination of iron status. In Brock JH, Halliday JW, Pippard MJ, et al (eds): Iron Metabolism in Health and Disease. London, WB Saunders, 1994, p 449.

245. Lipschitz DA, Cook JD, Finch CA: A clinical evaluation of serum ferritin as an index of iron stores. N Engl J Med 1974; 290:1213.

246. Elin RJ, Wolff SM, Finch CA: Effect of induced fever on serum iron and ferritin concentrations in man. Blood 1977; 49:147.

247. Pojaznik D, de Sousa M, et al: Ferritin in neuroblastoma. Impact of tumor load and blood transfusions. Cancer Invest 1985; 3:327.

248. Zhou XD, Stahlhut MW, et al: Serum ferritin in hepatocellular carcinoma. Hepatogastroenterology 1988; 35:1.

249. Brodeur GM, Pritchard J, Berthold F, et al: Revisions of the international criteria for neuroblastoma diagnosis, staging and response to treatment. J Clin Oncol 1993; 11:1466.

250. Johnstone RM, Biachini, A. and Teng, K.: Reticulocyte maturation and exosome release: Transferrin receptor containing exosomes show multiple plasma membrane functions. Blood 1989; 74:1844.

251. Pan BT, Johnstone RM: Fate of the transferrin receptor during maturation of sheep reticulocytes in vitro: Selective externalization of the receptor. Cell 1983; 33:967.

252. Pan BT, Teng K, et al: Electron microscopic evidence for externalization of the transferrin receptor in vesicular form in sheep erythrocytes. J Cell Biol 1985; 101:942.

253. Beguin Y, Huebers HA, Josephson B, et al: Transferrin receptors in rat plasma. Proc Natl Acad Sci USA 1988; 85:637.

254. Kohgo Y, Nishisato T, et al: Circulating transferrin receptors in human serum. Br J Haematol 1986; 64:277.

255. Baynes RD, Shih YJ, Cook JD: Production of soluble transferrin receptor by K562 erythroleukemia cells. Br J Haematol 1991; 78:450.

256. Baynes RD, Shih YJ, Hudson BG, et al: Production of the serum form of the transferrin receptor by a cell membrane-associated serine protease. Proc Soc Exp Biol Med 1993; 204:65.

257. Shih YJ, Baynes RD, Hudson BG, et al: Serum transferrin receptor is a truncated form of tissue receptor. J Biol Chem 1990; 265:19077.

258. Rutledge EH, Root BJ, Lucas JJ, et al: Elimination of the O-linked glycosylation site at Thr 104 results in the generation of a soluble human transferrin receptor. Blood 1994; 83:580.

259. Cook JD: The measurement of serum transferrin receptor. Am J Med Sci 1999; 318:269.

260. Punnonen K, Irjala K, Rajamaki A: Serum transferrin receptor and its ratio to ferritin in the diagnosis of iron deficiency. Blood 1997; 89:1052.

261. Suominen P, Punnonen K, Rajamaki A, et al: Serum transferrin receptor and transferrin receptor-ferritin index identify healthy subjects with subclinical iron deficits. Blood 1998; 92:2934.

262. Looker AC, Loyevsky M, Gordeuk VR: Increased serum transferrin saturation is associated with lower serum transferrin receptor concentration. Clin Chem 1999; 45:2191.

263. Baynes RD, Cook JD, Bothwell TH, et al: Serum transferrin receptor in hereditary hemochromatosis and African siderosis. Am J Hematol 1994; 45:288.

264. Gubler CJ, Lahey ME, Chase MS, et al: Studies on copper metabolism. III. The metabolism of iron in copper deficient swine. Blood 1952; 7:1075.

265. Lahey ME, Gubler CJ, Chase MS, et al: Studies on copper metabolism. II. Hematologic manifestations of copper deficiency in swine. Blood 1952; 7:1053.

266. Cartwright GE, Gubler CJ, Bush JA, et al: Studies on copper metabolism. XVII. Further observations on the anemia of copper deficiency in swine. Blood 1956; 11:143.

267. Lee GR, Nacht S, Lukens JN, et al: Iron metabolism in copper-deficient swine. J Clin Invest 1968; 47:2058.

268. Danks DM: Copper deficiency in humans. Annu Rev Nutr 1988; 8:235.

269. Williams DM: Copper deficiency in humans. Semin Hematol 1983; 20:118.

270. Castillo-Duran C, Uauy R: Copper deficiency impairs growth of infants recovering from malnutrition. Am J Clin Nutr 1988; 47:710.

271. Levy Y, Zeharia A, et al: Copper deficiency in infants fed cow milk. J Pediatr 1985; 106:786.

272. Celsing F, Blomstrand E, et al: Effects of iron deficiency on endurance and muscle enzyme activity in man. Med Sci Sports Exerc 1986; 18:156.

273. Goyens P, Brasseur D, et al: Copper deficiency in infants with active celiac disease. J Pediatr Gastroenterol Nutr 1985; 4:677.

274. Salmenpera L, Perheentupa J, et al: Cu nutrition in infants during prolonged exclusive breast-feeding: Low intake by rising serum concentrations of Cu and ceruloplasmin. Am J Clin Nutr 1986; 43:251.

275. Okamoto N, Wada S, Oga T, et al: Hereditary ceruloplasmin deficiency with hemosiderosis. Hum Genet 1996; 97:755.

276. Takahashi Y, Miyajima H, Shirabe S, et al: Characterization of a nonsense mutation in the ceruloplasmin gene resulting in diabetes and neurodegenerative disease. Hum Mol Genet 1996; 5:81.

277. Kuo Y-M, Zhou B, Cosco D, et al: The copper transporter CTR1 provides an essential function in mammalian embryonic development. Proc Natl Acad Sci USA 2001; 98:6836.

278. Lee J, Prohaska JR, Thiele DJ: Essential role for mammalian copper transporter Ctr1 in copper homeostasis and embryonic development. Proc Natl Acad Sci USA 2001; 98:6842.

279. Andrews NC: Mining copper transport genes. Proc Natl Acad Sci USA 2001; 98:6543.

280. Culotta VC, Lin SJ, Schmidt P, et al: Intracellular pathways of copper trafficking in yeast and humans. Adv Exp Med Biol 1999; 448:247.

281. Rosenzweig AC, O'Halloran TV: Structure and chemistry of the copper chaperone proteins. Curr Opin Chem Biol 2000; 4:140.

282. Hamza I, Faisst A, Prohaska J, et al: The metallochaperone Atox1 plays a critical role in perinatal copper homeostasis. Proc Natl Acad Sci USA 2001; 98:6848.

283. Menkes JH, Alter M, Steigleder GK, et al: A sex-linked recessive disorder with retardation of growth, peculiar hair and focal cerebral and cerebellar degeneration. Pediatrics 1962; 29:764.

284. Wilson SAK: Progressive lenticular degeneration: A familial nervous disease associated with cirrhosis of the liver. Brain 1912; 34:295.

285. Bull PC, Thomas GR, Rommens JM, et al: The Wilson's disease gene is a putative copper transporting P-type ATPase similar to the Menkes gene. Nat Genet 1993; 5:327.

286. Chelly J, Tumer S, Tonnesen T, et al: Isolation of a candidate gene for Menkes disease that encodes a potential heavy metal binding protein. Nat Genet 1993; 3:14.

287. Mercer JF, Livingston J, Hall B, et al: Isolation of a partial candidate gene for Menkes disease by positional cloning. Nat Genet 1993; 3:20.

288. Vulpe C, Levinson B, Whitney S, et al: Isolation of a candidate gene for Menkes disease and evidence that it encodes a copper-transporting ATPase. Nat Genet 1993; 3:7.

289. Yamaguchi Y, Heiny ME, Gitlin JD: Isolation and characterization of a human liver cDNA as a candidate gene for Wilson's disease. Biochem Biophys Res Commun 1993; 197:271.

290. Tanzi RE, Petrukhin K, Chernov I, et al: The Wilson's disease gene is a copper transporting ATPase with homology to the Menkes disease gene. Nat Genet 1993; 5:344.

291. Conrad ME, Barton JC: Factors affecting iron balance. Am J Hematol 1981; 10:199.

292. Beeken WL: Absorptive defects in young people with regional enteritis. Pediatrics 1973; 52:69.

293. Anand BS, Callender ST, Warner GT: Absorption of inorganic and haemoglobin iron in coeliac disease. Br J Haematol 1977; 37:409.

294. Sutton DR, Stewart JS, Baird IM, et al: "Free" iron loss in atrophic gastritis, post-gastrectomy states, and adult coeliac disease. Lancet 1970; 2:387.

295. Buchanan GR, Sheehan RG: Malabsorption and defective utilization of iron in three siblings. J Pediatr 1981; 98:723.

296. Hartman KR, Barker JA: Microcytic anemia with iron malabsorption: An inherited disorder of iron metabolism. Am J Hematol 1996; 51:269.

297. Pearson HA, Lukens JN: Ferrokinetics in the syndrome of familial hypoferremic microcytic anemia with iron malabsorption. J Pediatr Hematol Oncol 1999; 21:412.

298. Picciano MF, Deering RH: The influence of feeding regimens on iron status during infancy. Am J Clin Nutr 1980; 33:746.

299. Tunnessen WW, Jr., Oski FA: Consequences of starting whole cow milk at 6 months of age. J Pediatr 1987; 111:813.

300. American Academy of Pediatrics Committee on Nutrition: The use of whole cow's milk in infancy. Pediatrics 1992; 89:1105.

301. American Academy of Pediatrics. Committee on Nutrition: Iron fortification of infant formulas. Pediatrics 1999; 104:119.

302. Crompton DW: The public health importance of hookworm disease. Parasitology 2000; 121:S39.

303. Specks U: Diffuse alveolar hemorrhage syndromes. Curr Opin Rheumatol 2001; 13:12.

304. Buschman DL, Ballard R: Progressive massive fibrosis associated with idiopathic pulmonary hemosiderosis. Chest 1993; 104:293.

305. Bouros D, Panagou P, Rokkas T, et al: Bronchoalveolar lavage findings in a young adult with idiopathic pulmonary haemosiderosis and coeliac disease. Eur Respir J 1994; 7:1009.

306. van der Ent CK, Walenkamp MJ, Donckerwolcke RA, et al: Pulmonary hemosiderosis and immune complex glomerulonephritis. Clin Nephrol 1995; 43:339.

307. Le Clainche L, Le Bourgeois M, Fauroux B, et al: Long-term outcome of idiopathic pulmonary hemosiderosis in children. Medicine (Baltimore) 2000; 79:318.

308. Saeed MM, Woo MS, MacLaughlin EF, et al: Prognosis in pediatric idiopathic pulmonary hemosiderosis. Chest 1999; 116:721.

309. Bush A, Sheppard MN, Warner JO: Chloroquine in idiopathic pulmonary haemosiderosis. Arch Dis Child 1992; 67:625.

310. Colombo JL, Stolz SM: Treatment of life-threatening primary pulmonary hemosiderosis with cyclophosphamide. Chest 1992; 102:959.

311. Rossi GA, Balzano E, Battistini E, et al: Long-term prednisone and azathioprine treatment of a patient with idiopathic pulmonary hemosiderosis. Pediatr Pulmonol 1992; 13:176.

312. Brugnara C, Zurakowski D, DiCanzio J, et al: Reticulocyte hemoglobin content to diagnose iron deficiency in children. JAMA 1999; 281:2225.

313. Liu TC, Seong PS, Lin TK: The erythrocyte cell hemoglobin distribution width segregates thalassemia traits from other nonthalassemic conditions with microcytosis. Am J Clin Pathol 1997; 107:601.

314. Anderson C, Aronson I, Jacobs P: Erythropoiesis: Erythrocyte deformability is reduced and fragility increased by iron deficiency. Hematology 2000; 4:457.

315. Kretchmer N, Beard JL, Carlson S: The role of nutrition in the development of normal cognition. Am J Clin Nutr 1996; 63:997S.

316. Halterman JS, Kaczorowski JM, Aligne CA, et al: Iron deficiency and cognitive achievement among school-aged children and adolescents in the United States. Pediatrics 2001; 107:1381.

317. Oski FA, Honig AS: The effects of therapy on the developmental scores of iron-deficient infants. J Pediatr 1978; 92:21.

318. Deinard AS, List A, Lindgren B, et al: Cognitive deficits in iron-deficient and iron-deficient anemic children. J Pediatr 1986; 108:681.

319. Grantham-McGregor S, Ani C: A review of studies on the effect of iron deficiency on cognitive development in children. J Nutr 2001; 131:649S.

320. Oski FA, Honig AS, Helu B, et al: Effect of iron therapy on behavior performance in nonanemic, iron-deficient infants. Pediatrics 1983; 71:877.

321. Pollitt E, Saco-Pollitt C, Leibel RL, et al: Iron deficiency and behavioral development in infants and preschool children. Am J Clin Nutr 1986; 43:555.

322. Wasserman G, Graziano JH, Factor-Litvak P, et al: Independent effects of lead exposure and iron deficiency anemia on developmental outcome at age 2 years. J Pediatr 1992; 121:695.

323. Erikson KM, Jones BC, Hess EJ, et al: Iron deficiency decreases dopamine D_1 and D_2 receptors in rat brain. Pharmacol Biochem Behav 2001; 69:409.

324. Beard JL: Iron biology in immune function, muscle metabolism and neuronal functioning. J Nutr 2001; 131:568S.

325. Aukett MA, Parks YA, Scott PH, et al: Treatment with iron increases weight gain and psychomotor development. Arch Dis Child 1986; 61:849.

326. Angeles IT, Schultink WJ, Matulessi P, et al: Decreased rate of stunting among anemic Indonesian preschool children through iron supplementation. Am J Clin Nutr 1993; 58:339.

327. Thomas FB, Falko JM, Zuckerman K: Inhibition of intestinal iron absorption by laundry starch. Gastroenterology 1976; 71:1028.

328. Crosby WH: Clay ingestion and iron deficiency anemia. Ann Intern Med 1982; 97:456.

329. Cavdar AO, Arcasoy A: Hematologic and biochemical studies of Turkish children with pica. A presumptive explanation for the syndrome of geophagia, iron deficiency anemia, hepatosplenomegaly and hypogonadism. Clin Pediatr (Phila) 1972; 11:215.

330. Prasad AS: Recognition of zinc-deficiency syndrome. Nutrition 2001; 17:67.

331. Cavdar AO, Arcasoy A, Cin S, et al: Geophagia in Turkey: Iron and zinc deficiency, iron and zinc absorption studies and response to treatment with zinc in geophagia cases. Prog Clin Biol Res 1983; 129:71.

332. Cook JD, Reddy MB: Effect of ascorbic acid intake on nonheme-iron absorption from a complete diet. Am J Clin Nutr 2001; 73:93.

333. Charytan C, Levin N, Al-Saloum M, et al: Efficacy and safety of iron sucrose for iron deficiency in patients with dialysis-associated anemia: North American clinical trial. Am J Kidney Dis 2001; 37:300.

334. Fishbane S, Kowalski EA: The comparative safety of intravenous iron dextran, iron saccharate, and sodium ferric gluconate. Semin Dial 2000; 13:381.

335. Kosch M, Bahner U, Bettger H, et al: A randomized, controlled parallel-group trial on efficacy and safety of iron sucrose (Venofer) vs iron gluconate (Ferrlecit) in haemodialysis patients treated with rHuEpo. Nephrol Dial Transplant 2001; 16:1239.

336. Yorgin PD, Belson A, Sarwal M, et al: Sodium ferric gluconate therapy in renal transplant and renal failure patients. Pediatr Nephrol 2000; 15:171.

337. Stein ML, Gunston KD, May RM: Iron dextran in the treatment of iron-deficiency anaemia of pregnancy. Haematological response and incidence of side-effects. S Afr Med J 1991; 79:195.

338. Brugnara C, Laufer MR, Friedman AJ, et al: Reticulocyte hemoglobin content (CHr): Early indicator of iron deficiency and response to therapy. Blood 1994; 83:3100.

339. Griffin IJ, Abrams SA: Iron and breastfeeding. Pediatr Clin North Am 2001; 48:401.

340. Cox TM, Peters TJ: Uptake of iron by duodenal biopsy specimens from patients with iron-deficiency anaemia and primary haemochromatosis. Lancet 1978; 1:123.

341. Cox TM, Peters TJ: Cellular mechanisms in the regulation of iron absorption by the human intestine: Studies in patients with iron deficiency before and after treatment. Br J Haematol 1980; 44:75.

342. Lynch SR, Skikne BS, Cook JD: Food iron absorption in idiopathic hemochromatosis. Blood 1989; 74:2187.

343. von Recklinghausen FD: Uber haemochromatose. Tageblatt Versammlung Deut Naturforsch Artze Herdelbert 1889; 62:324.

344. Feder JN, Gnirke A, Thomas W, et al: A novel MHC class I-like gene is mutated in patients with hereditary haemochromatosis. Nat Genet 1996; 13:399.

345. Jazwinska EC, Pyper WR, Burt MJ, et al: Haplotype analysis in Australian hemochromatosis patients: Evidence for a predominant ancestral haplotype exclusively associated with hemochromatosis. Am J Hum Genet 1995; 56:428.

346. Lebron JA, Bennett MJ, Vaughn DE, et al: Crystal structure of the hemochromatosis protein HFE and characterization of its interaction with transferrin receptor. Cell 1998; 93:111.

347. Parkkila S, Waheed A, Britton RS, et al: Association of the transferrin receptor in human placenta with HFE, the protein defective in hereditary hemochromatosis. Proc Natl Acad Sci USA 1997; 94:13198.

348. Feder JN, Penny DM, Irrinki A, et al: The hemochromatosis gene product complexes with the transferrin receptor and lowers its affinity for ligand binding. Proc Natl Acad Sci USA 1998; 95:1472.

349. Lebron JA, Bjorkman PJ: The transferrin receptor binding site on HFE, the class I MHC-related protein mutated in hereditary hemochromatosis. J Mol Biol 1999; 289:1109.

350. Lebron JA, West AP, Jr., Bjorkman PJ: The hemochromatosis protein HFE competes with transferrin for binding to the transferrin receptor. J Mol Biol 1999; 294:239.

351. Roy CN, Penny DM, Feder JN, et al: The hereditary hemochromatosis protein, HFE, specifically regulates transferrin-mediated iron uptake in HeLa cells. J Biol Chem 1999; 274:9022.

352. Bennett MJ, Lebron JA, Bjorkman PJ: Crystal structure of the hereditary haemochromatosis protein HFE complexed with transferrin receptor. Nature 2000; 403:46.

353. Roy CN, Carlson EJ, Anderson EL, et al: Interactions of the ectodomain of HFE with the transferrin receptor are critical for iron homeostasis in cells. FEBS Lett 2000; 484:271.

354. Zhou XY, Tomatsu S, Fleming RE, et al: *HFE* gene knockout produces mouse model of hereditary hemochromatosis. Proc Natl Acad Sci USA 1998; 95:2492.

355. Levy JE, Montross LK, Cohen DE, et al: The C282Y mutation causing hereditary hemochromatosis does not produce a null allele. Blood 1999; 94:9.

356. Bahram S, Gilfillan S, Kuhn LC, et al: Experimental hemochromatosis due to MHC class I HFE deficiency: Immune status and iron metabolism. Proc Natl Acad Sci USA 1999; 96:13312.

357. Edwards CQ, Griffen LM, Goldgar D, et al: Prevalence of hemochromatosis among 11,065 presumably healthy blood donors. N Engl J Med 1988; 318:1355.

358. Steinberg KK, Cogswell ME, Chang JC, et al: Prevalence of C282Y and H63D mutations in the hemochromatosis (*HFE*) gene in the United States. JAMA 2001; 285:2216.

359. Olynyk JK, Cullen DJ, Aquilia S, et al: A population-based study of the clinical expression of the hemochromatosis gene. N Engl J Med 1999; 341:718.

360. Bulaj ZJ, Ajioka RS, Phillips JD, et al: Disease-related conditions in relatives of patients with hemochromatosis. N Engl J Med 2000; 343:1529.

361. Beutler E, Felitti V, Gelbart T, et al: The effect of HFE genotypes on measurements of iron overload in patients attending a health appraisal clinic. Ann Intern Med 2000; 133:329.

362. Sham RL, Raubertas RF, Braggins C, et al: Asymptomatic hemochromatosis subjects: Genotypic and phenotypic profiles. Blood 2000; 96:3707.

363. Camaschella C, De Gobbi M, Roetto A: Hereditary hemochromatosis: Progress and perspectives. Rev Clin Exp Hematol 2001; 4:302.

364. Camaschella C, Roetto A, Cali A, et al: The gene TFR2 is mutated in a new type of haemochromatosis mapping to 7q22. Nat Genet 2000; 25:14.

365. Roetto A, Totaro A, Piperno A, et al: New mutations inactivating transferrin receptor 2 in hemochromatosis type 3. Blood 2001; 97:2555.

366. Fleming RE, Migas MC, Holden CC, et al: Transferrin receptor 2: Continued expression in mouse liver in the face of iron overload and in hereditary hemochromatosis. Proc Natl Acad Sci USA 2000; 97:2214.

367. Kawabata H, Germain RS, Vuong PT, et al: Transferrin receptor 2-α supports cell growth both in iron-chelated cultured cells and in vivo. J Biol Chem 2000; 275:16618.

368. West AP, Jr., Bennett MJ, Sellers VM, et al: Comparison of the interactions of transferrin receptor and transferrin receptor 2 with transferrin and the hereditary hemochromatosis protein HFE. J Biol Chem 2000; 275:38135.

369. Cazzola M, Ascari E, Barosi G, et al: Juvenile idiopathic haemochromatosis: A life-threatening disorder presenting as hypogonadotropic hypogonadism. Hum Genet 1983; 65:149.

370. Camaschella C, Roetto A, Cicilano M, et al: Juvenile and adult hemochromatosis are distinct genetic disorders. Eur J Hum Genet 1997; 5:371.

371. Camaschella C: Juvenile haemochromatosis. Baillieres Clin Gastroenterol 1998; 12:227.

372. Kaltwasser JP, Gottschalk R, Seidl CH: Severe juvenile haemochromatosis (JH) missing HFE gene variants: Implications for a second gene locus leading to iron overload. Br J Haematol 1998; 102:1111.

373. Kelly AL, Rhodes DA, Roland JM, et al: Hereditary juvenile haemochromatosis: A genetically heterogeneous life-threatening iron-storage disease. Q J Med 1998; 91:607.

374. Rivard SR, Mura C, Simard H, et al: Clinical and molecular aspects of juvenile hemochromatosis in Saguenay-Lac-Saint-Jean (Quebec, Canada). Blood Cells Mol Dis 2000; 26:10.

375. Roetto A, Totaro A, Cazzola M, et al: Juvenile hemochromatosis locus maps to chromosome 1q. Am J Hum Genet 1999; 64:1388.

376. Pietrangelo A, Montosi G, Totaro A, et al: Hereditary hemochromatosis in adults without pathogenic mutations in the hemochromatosis gene. N Engl J Med 1999; 341:725.

377. Bothwell TH, Bradlow BA: Siderosis in the Bantu: A combined histopathological and chemical study. Arch Pathol 1960; 70:279.

378. Bothwell TH, Charlton RW, Seftel HC: Oral iron overload. S Afr Med J 1965; 39:892.

379. Seftel HC, Malkin C, Schmaman A, et al: Osteoporosis, scurvy, and siderosis in Johannesburg Bantu. Br Med J 1966; 5488:642.

380. Gordeuk VR, Boyd RD, Brittenham GM: Dietary iron overload persists in rural sub-Saharan Africa. Lancet 1986; 1:1310.

381. Gordeuk V, Mukiibi J, Hasstedt SJ, et al: Iron overload in Africa. Interaction between a gene and dietary iron content. N Engl J Med 1992; 326:95.

382. Moyo VM, Gangaidzo IT, Gomo ZA, et al: Traditional beer consumption and the iron status of spouse pairs from a rural community in Zimbabwe. Blood 1997; 89:2159.

383. Moyo VM, Mandishona E, Hasstedt SJ, et al: Evidence of genetic transmission in African iron overload. Blood 1998; 91:1076.

384. McNamara L, MacPhail AP, Gordeuk VR, et al: Is there a link between African iron overload and the described mutations of the hereditary haemochromatosis gene? Br J Haematol 1998; 102:1176.

385. Barton JC, Edwards CQ, Bertoli LF, et al: Iron overload in African Americans. Am J Med 1995; 99:616.

386. Wurapa RK, Gordeuk VR, Brittenham GM, et al: Primary iron overload in African Americans. Am J Med 1996; 101:9.

387. Shneider BL: Neonatal liver failure. Curr Opin Pediatr 1996; 8:495.

388. Witzleben CL, Uri A: Perinatal hemochromatosis: Entity or end result? Hum Pathol 1989; 20:335.

389. Silver MM, Beverley DW, Valberg LS, et al: Perinatal hemochromatosis. Clinical, morphologic, and quantitative iron studies. Am J Pathol 1987; 128:538.

390. Moerman P, Pauwels P, Vandenberghe K, et al: Neonatal haemochromatosis. Histopathology 1990; 17:345.

391. Verloes A, Temple IK, Hubert AF, et al: Recurrence of neonatal haemochromatosis in half sibs born of unaffected mothers. J Med Genet 1996; 33:444.

392. Krahenbuhl S, Kleinle S, Henz S, et al: Microvesicular steatosis, hemosiderosis and rapid development of liver cirrhosis in a patient with Pearson's syndrome. J Hepatol 1999; 31:550.

393. Brown MD, Chitayat D, Allen J, et al: Mitochondrial DNA mutations associated with neonatal hemochromatosis [abstract]. Am J Hum Genet 1999; 45:A45.

394. McGuigan MA: Acute iron poisoning. Pediatr Ann 1996; 25:33.

395. Mills KC, Curry SC: Acute iron poisoning. Emerg Med Clin North Am 1994; 12:397.

396. Pippard MJ, Callender ST, Warner GT, et al: Iron absorption and loading in β-thalassaemia intermedia. Lancet 1979; 2:819.

397. Fitchett DH, Coltart DJ, Littler WA, et al: Cardiac involvement in secondary haemochromatosis: A catheter biopsy study and analysis of myocardium. Cardiovasc Res 1980; 14:719.

398. Sanyal SK, Johnson W, Jayalakshmamma B, et al: Fatal "iron heart" in an adolescent: Biochemical and ultrastructural aspects of the heart. Pediatrics 1975; 55:336.

399. Schellhammer PF, Engle MA, Hagstrom JW: Histochemical studies of the myocardium and conduction system in acquired iron-storage disease. Circulation 1967; 35:631.

400. Liu P, Olivieri N: Iron overload cardiomyopathies: New insights into an old disease. Cardiovasc Drugs Ther 1994; 8:101.

401. Wolfe L, Olivieri N, Sallan D, et al: Prevention of cardiac disease by subcutaneous deferoxamine in patients with thalassemia major. N Engl J Med 1985; 312:1600.

402. Rahko PS, Salerni R, Uretsky BF: Successful reversal by chelation therapy of congestive cardiomyopathy due to iron overload. J Am Coll Cardiol 1986; 8:436.

403. Buja LM, Roberts WC: Iron in the heart. Etiology and clinical significance. Am J Med 1971; 51:209.

404. Olson LJ, Edwards WD, McCall JT, et al: Cardiac iron deposition in idiopathic hemochromatosis: Histologic and analytic assessment of 14 hearts from autopsy. J Am Coll Cardiol 1987; 10:1239.

405. Nienhuis AW: Vitamin C and iron. N Engl J Med 1981; 304:170.

406. Oerter KE, Kamp GA, Munson PJ, et al: Multiple hormone deficiencies in children with hemochromatosis. J Clin Endocrinol Metab 1993; 76:357.

407. Flynn DM, Fairney A, Jackson D, et al: Hormonal changes in thalassaemia major. Arch Dis Child 1976; 51:828.

408. Bomford A, Williams R: Long term results of venesection therapy in idiopathic haemochromatosis. Q J Med 1976; 45:611.

409. Costin G, Kogut MD, Hyman CB, et al: Endocrine abnormalities in thalassemia major. Am J Dis Child 1979; 133:497.

410. Schafer AI, Cheron RG, Dluhy R, et al: Clinical consequences of acquired transfusional iron overload in adults. N Engl J Med 1981; 304:319.

411. Schafer AI, Rabinowe S, Le Boff MS, et al: Long-term efficacy of deferoxamine iron chelation therapy in adults with acquired transfusional iron overload. Arch Intern Med 1985; 145:1217.

412. Gertner JM, Broadus AE, Anast CS, et al: Impaired parathyroid response to induced hypocalcemia in thalassemia major. J Pediatr 1979; 95:210.

413. Ines LS, da Silva JA, Malcata AB, et al: Arthropathy of genetic hemochromatosis: A major and distinctive manifestation of the disease. Clin Exp Rheumatol 2001; 19:98.

414. von Kempis J: Arthropathy in hereditary hemochromatosis. Curr Opin Rheumatol 2001; 13:80.

415. Weinberg ED: The iron-withholding defense system. ASM News 1993; 59:559.

416. Bullen JJ, Rogers HJ, Lewin JE: The bacteriostatic effect of serum on *Pasteurella septica* and its abolition by iron compounds. Immunology 1971; 20:391.

417. Reiter B, Brock JH, Steel ED: Inhibition of *Escherichia coli* by bovine colostrum and post-colostral milk. II. The bacteriostatic effect of lactoferrin on a serum susceptible and serum resistant strain of *E. coli.* Immunology 1975; 28:83.

418. Lawrence TH 3rd, Biggers CJ, Simonton PR: Bacteriostatic inhibition of *Klebsiella pneumoniae* by three human transferrins. Ann Hum Biol 1977; 4:281.

419. Otto BR, Verweij-van Vught AM, MacLaren DM: Transferrins and heme-compounds as iron sources for pathogenic bacteria. Crit Rev Microbiol 1992; 18:217.

420. Abbott M, Galloway A, Cunningham JL: Haemochromatosis presenting with a double *Yersinia* infection. J Infect 1986; 13:143.

421. Brennan RO, Crain BJ, Proctor AM, et al: *Cunninghamella:* A newly recognized cause of rhinocerebral mucormycosis. Am J Clin Pathol 1983; 80:98.

422. Bullen JJ, Spalding PB, Ward CG, et al: Hemochromatosis, iron and septicemia caused by *Vibrio vulnificus.* Arch Intern Med 1991; 151:1606.

423. Capron JP, Capron-Chivrac D, Tossou H, et al: Spontaneous *Yersinia enterocolitica* peritonitis in idiopathic hemochromatosis. Gastroenterology 1984; 87:1372.

424. Boelaert JR, van Roost GF, Vergauwe PL, et al: The role of desferrioxamine in dialysis-associated mucormycosis: Report of three cases and review of the literature. Clin Nephrol 1988; 29:261.

425. Daly AL, Velazquez LA, Bradley SF, et al: Mucormycosis: Association with deferoxamine therapy. Am J Med 1989; 87:468.

426. Rex JH, Ginsberg AM, Fries LF, et al: *Cunninghamella bertholletiae* infection associated with deferoxamine therapy. Rev Infect Dis 1988; 10:1187.

427. Robins-Browne RM, Prpic JK: Effects of iron and desferrioxamine on infections with *Yersinia enterocolitica.* Infect Immun 1985; 47:774.

428. Fargion S, Taddei MT, Gabutti V, et al: Early iron overload in β-thalassaemia major: When to start chelation therapy? Arch Dis Child 1982; 57:929.

429. Pippard MJ, Weatherall DJ: Iron absorption in non-transfused iron loading anaemias: Prediction of risk for iron loading, and response to iron chelation treatment, in beta thalassaemia intermedia and congenital sideroblastic anaemias. Haematologia 1984; 17:17.

430. Zanella A, Berzuini A, Colombo MB, et al: Iron status in red cell pyruvate kinase deficiency: Study of Italian cases. Br J Haematol 1993; 83:485.

431. Keberle H: The biochemistry of desferrioxamine and its relation to iron metabolism. Ann NY Acad Sci 1964; 119:758.

432. Propper RD, Cooper B, Rufo RR, et al: Continuous subcutaneous administration of deferoxamine in patients with iron overload. N Engl J Med 1977; 297:418.

433. Cooper B, Bunn HF, Propper RD, et al: Treatment of iron overload in adults with continuous parenteral desferrioxamine. Am J Med 1977; 63:958.

434. Orzincolo C, Scutellari PN, Castaldi G: Growth plate injury of the long bones in treated β-thalassemia. Skeletal Radiol 1992; 21:39.

435. Olivieri NF, Buncic JR, Chew E, et al: Visual and auditory neurotoxicity in patients receiving subcutaneous deferoxamine infusions. N Engl J Med 1986; 314:869.

436. Bousquet J, Navarro M, Robert G, et al: Rapid desensitisation for desferrioxamine anaphylactoid reaction. Lancet 1983; 2: 859.

437. Falk RJ, Mattern WD, Lamanna RW, et al: Iron removal during continuous ambulatory peritoneal dialysis using deferoxamine. Kidney Int 1983; 24:110.

438. Nathan DG, Piomelli S: Oral iron chelators. Semin Hematol 1990; 27:83.

439. Olivieri NF, Brittenham GM, McLaren CE, et al: Long-term safety and effectiveness of iron-chelation therapy with deferiprone for thalassemia major. N Engl J Med 1998; 339:417.

440. Pippard MJ, Weatherall DJ: Oral iron chelation therapy for thalassaemia: An uncertain scene. Br J Haematol 2000; 111:2.

441. MacPhail AP, Charlton RW, Bothwell TH, et al: The relationship between maternal and infant iron status. Scand J Haematol 1980; 25:141.

442. Murray MJ, Murray AB, Murray NJ, et al: The effect of iron status of Nigerian mothers on that of their infants at birth and 6 months, and on the concentration of Fe in breast milk. Br J Nutr 1978; 39:627.

443. McArdle HJ, Morgan EH: Transferrin and iron movements in the rat conceptus during gestation. J Reprod Fertil 1982; 66:529.

444. Ahmad SH, Amir M, Ansari Z, et al: Influence of maternal iron deficiency anemia on the fetal total body iron. Indian Pediatr 1983; 20:643.

445. Ahmad SH, Ansari Z, Matto GM, et al: Serum iron in babies of anemic mothers—II. Indian Pediatr 1984; 21:759.

446. Beutler E, Gelbart T, Lee P, et al: Molecular characterization of a case of atransferrinemia. Blood 2000; 96:4071.

447. Larrick J, Hyman E: Acquired iron-deficiency anemia caused by an antibody against the transferrin receptor. N Engl J Med 1984; 311:214.

448. Shahidi NT, Nathan DG, Diamond LK: Iron deficiency anemia associated with an error of iron metabolism in two siblings. J Clin Invest 1964; 43:510.

449. Parsons SK, Fleming MD, Nathan DG, et al: Iron deficiency anemia associated with an error of iron metabolism in two siblings: A thirty year follow up. Hematology 1996; 1:65.

450. Stavem P, Romslo T, Hovig K, et al: Ferrochelatase deficiency of the bone marrow in a syndrome of congenital microcytic anemia with iron overload of the liver and hyperferraemia. Scand J Hematol 1985; 34:204.

451. Stavem P, Saltveldt E, Elgjo K, et al: Congenital hypochromic microcytic anemia with iron overload of liver and hyperferraemia. Scand J Hematol 1973; 10:153.

452. Cox TC, Bottomley SS, Wiley JS, et al: X-linked pyridoxine-responsive sideroblastic anemia due to a Thr388-to-Ser substitution in erythroid 5-aminolevulinate synthase. N Engl J Med 1994; 330:675.

453. Fitzsimons EJ, May A: The molecular basis of the sideroblastic anemias. Curr Opin Hematol 1996; 3:167.

454. Gatterman N, Retzlaff S, Wang Y-L, et al: Heteroplasmic point mutations of mitochondrial DNA affecting subunit I of cytochrome *c* oxidase in two patients with acquired idiopathic sideroblastic anemia. Blood 1997; 90:4961.

455. Allikmets R, Raskind WH, Hutchinson A, et al: Mutation of a putative mitochondrial iron transporter gene (ABC7) in X-linked sideroblastic anemia and ataxia (XLSA/A). Hum Mol Genet 1999; 8:743.

456. Bekri S, Kispal G, Lange H, et al: Human ABC7 transporter: Gene structure and mutation causing X-linked sideroblastic anemia with ataxia with disruption of cytosolic iron-sulfur protein maturation. Blood 2000; 96:3256.

457. Bessis MC, Jensen WN: Sideroblastic anemia, mitochondria and erythroblast iron. Br J Haematol 1965; 11:49.

458. Cazzola M, May A, Bergamaschi G, et al: Familial-skewed X-chromosome inactivation as a predisposing factor for late-onset X linked sideroblastic anemia in carrier females. Blood 2000; 96:4363.

459. Cotter PD, May A, Li L, et al: Four new mutations in the erythroid-specific 5-aminolevulinate synthase (ALAS2) gene causing X-linked sideroblastic anemia: increased pyridoxine responsiveness after removal of iron overload by phlebotomy and coinheritance of hereditary hemochromatosis. Blood 1999; 93:1757.

460. Cotter PD, Rucknagel DL, Bishop DF: X-linked sideroblastic anemia: Identification of the mutation in the erythroid-specific delta-aminolevulinate synthase gene (ALAS2) in the original family described by Cooley. Blood 1994; 84:3915.

461. Furuyama K, Sassa S: Interaction between succinyl CoA synthetase and the heme-biosynthetic enzyme ALAS-E is disrupted in sideroblastic anemia. J Clin Invest 2000; 105:757.

462. May A, Bishop DF: The molecular biology and pyridoxine responsiveness of X-linked sideroblastic anaemia. Haematologica 1998; 83:56.

463. Hamel BC, Schretlen ED: Sideroblastic anaemia. A review of seven paediatric cases. Eur J Pediatr 1982; 138:130.

464. Mason DY, Emerson PM: Primary acquired sideroblastic anaemia: Response to treatment with pyridoxal-5-phosphate. Br Med J 1973; 1:389.

465. Gonzalez MI, Caballero D, Vazquez L, et al: Allogeneic peripheral stem cell transplantation in a case of hereditary sideroblastic anaemia. Br J Haematol 2000; 109:658.

466. Pagon RA, Bird TD, Detter JC, et al: Hereditary sideroblastic anaemia and ataxia: An X linked recessive disorder. J Med Genet 1985; 22:267.

467. Leighton J, Schatz G: An ABC transporter in the mitochondrial inner membrane is required for normal growth of yeast. EMBO J 1995; 14:188.

468. Leighton J: ATP-binding cassette transporter in *Saccharomyces cerevisiae* mitochondria. Methods Enzymol 1995; 260:389.

469. Kispal G, Csere P, Guiard B, et al: The ABC transporter Atm1p is required for mitochondrial iron homeostasis. FEBS Lett 1997; 418:346.

470. Csere P, Lill R, Kispal G: Identification of a human mitochondrial ABC transporter, the functional orthologue of yeast Atm1p. FEBS Lett 1998; 441:266.

471. Kispal G, Csere P, Prohl C, et al: The mitochondrial proteins Atm1p and Nfs1p are essential for biogenesis of cytosolic Fe/S proteins. EMBO J 1999; 18:3981.

472. Porter FS, Rogers LE, Sidbury JB, Jr.: Thiamine-responsive megaloblastic anemia. J Pediatr 1969; 74:494.

473. Neufeld EJ, Fleming JC, Tartaglini E, et al: Thiamine-responsive megaloblastic anemia syndrome: A disorder of high-affinity thiamine transport. Blood Cells Mol Dis 2001; 27:135.

474. Fleming JC, Tartaglini E, Steinkamp MP, et al: The gene mutated in thiamine-responsive anaemia with diabetes and deafness (TRMA) encodes a functional thiamine transporter. Nat Genet 1999; 22:305.

475. Pearson HA, Lobel JS, Kocoshis SA, et al: A new syndrome of refractory sideroblastic anemia with vacuolization of marrow precursors and exocrine pancreatic dysfunction. J Pediatr 1979; 95:976.

476. Stoddard RA, McCurnin DC, Shultenover SJ, et al: Syndrome of refractory sideroblastic anemia with vacuolization of marrow precursors and exocrine pancreatic dysfunction presenting in the neonate. J Pediatr 1981; 99:259.

477. McShane MA, Hammans SR, Sweeney M, et al: Pearson syndrome and mitochondrial encephalomyopathy in a patient with a deletion of mtDNA. Am J Hum Genet 1991; 48:39.

478. Rotig A, Cormier V, Blanche S, et al: Pearson's marrow-pancreas syndrome. A multisystem mitochondrial disorder in infancy. J Clin Invest 1990; 86:1601.

479. Clark R, Peters S, Hoy T, et al: Prognostic importance of hypodiploid hemopoietic precursors in myelodysplastic syndromes. N Engl J Med 1986; 314:1472.

480. Ruutu P, Ruutu T, Vuopio P, et al: Function of neutrophils in preleukaemia. Scand J Haematol 1977; 18:317.

481. Sultan Y, Caen JP: Platelet dysfunction in preleukemic states and in various types of leukemia. Ann NY Acad Sci 1972; 201:300.

482. Lewy RI, Kansu E, Gabuzda T: Leukemia in patients with acquired idiopathic sideroblastic anemia: An evaluation of prognostic indicators. Am J Hematol 1979; 6:323.

483. Bolwell BJ, Cassileth PA, Gale RP: Low dose cytosine arabinoside in myelodysplasia and acute myelogenous leukemia: A review. Leukemia 1987; 1:575.

484. Estey EH, Keating MJ, Dixon DO, et al: Karyotype is prognostically more important than the FAB system's distinction between myelodysplastic syndrome and acute myelogenous leukemia. Hematol Pathol 1987; 1:203.

485. Kitahara M, Cosgriff TM, Eyre HJ: Sideroblastic anemia as a preleukemic event in patients treated for Hodgkin's disease. Ann Intern Med 1980; 92:625.

486. Freireich EJ, Miller A, Emerson CP, et al: The effect of inflammation on the utilization of erythrocyte and transferrin bound radio-iron for red cell production. Blood 1957; 12:972.

487. Cartwright GE: The anemia of chronic disorders. Semin Hematol 1966; 3:351.

488. Sears DA: Anemia of chronic disease. Med Clin North Am 1992; 76:567.

489. Means RT: Pathogenesis of the anemia of chronic disease: A cytokine-mediated anemia. Stem Cells 1995; 13:32.

490. Konijn AM, Hershko C: Ferritin synthesis in inflammation. I. Pathogenesis of impaired iron release. Br J Haematol 1977; 37:7.

491. Konijn AM, Carmel N, Levy R, et al: Ferritin synthesis in inflammation. II. Mechanism of increased ferritin synthesis. Br J Haematol 1981; 49:361.

492. Faquin WC, Schneider TJ, Goldberg MA: Effect of inflammatory cytokines on hypoxia-induced erythropoietin production. Blood 1992; 79:1987.

493. Goodnough LT, Skikne B, Brugnara C: Erythropoietin, iron, and erythropoiesis. Blood 2000; 96:823.

494. Means RT Jr.: Erythropoietin in the treatment of anemia in chronic infectious, inflammatory, and malignant diseases. Curr Opin Hematol 1995; 2:210.

495. Adamson JW: The relationship of erythropoietin and iron metabolism to red blood cell production in humans. Semin Oncol 1994; 21:9.

496. Chan RY, Seiser C, Schulman HM, et al: Regulation of transferrin receptor mRNA expression. Distinct features in erythroid cells. Eur J Biochem 1994; 220:683.

497. Brugnara C, Colella GM, Cremins J, et al: Effects of subcutaneous recombinant human erythropoietin in normal subjects: Development of decreased reticulocyte hemoglobin content and iron-deficient erythropoiesis. J Lab Clin Med 1994; 123:660.

498. Macdougall IC: Strategies for iron supplementation: Oral versus intravenous. Kidney Int 1999; 69(Suppl):S61.

499. Lin-Fu JS: Vulnerability of children to lead exposure and toxicity (first of two parts). N Engl J Med 1973; 289:1229.

500. Knelson JH: Problem of estimating respiratory lead dose in children. Environ Health Perspect 1974; 7:53.

501. Mahaffey KR: Exposure to lead in childhood. The importance of prevention. N Engl J Med 1992; 327:1308.

502. Hamilton S, Rothenberg SJ, Khan FA, et al: Neonatal lead poisoning from maternal pica behavior during pregnancy. J Natl Med Assoc 2001; 93:317.

503. Chisolm JJ, Harrison HE: The exposure of children to lead. Pediatrics 1956; 18:943.

504. Flatmark T, Romslo I: Energy-dependent accumulation of iron by isolated rat liver mitochondria. Requirement of reducing equivalents and evidence for a unidirectional flux of Fe(II) across the inner membrane. J Biol Chem 1975; 250:6433.

505. Sassa S: Toxic effects of lead, with particular reference to porphyrin and heme metabolism. In DeMatteis F, Aldridge W (eds): Handbook of Experimental Pharmacology, New Series. Berlin, Springer-Verlag, 1973, vol 44, p 333.

506. Piomelli S: The diagnostic utility of measurements of erythrocyte porphyrins. Hematol Oncol Clin North Am 1987; 1:419.

507. Piomelli S: A micromethod for free erythrocyte porphyrins: The FEP test. J Lab Clin Med 1973; 81:932.

508. Bessis MC, Breton-Gorius J: Ferritin and ferruginous micelles in normal erythroblsts and hypochromic hypersideremic anemias. Blood 1959; 14:423.

509. Piomelli S, Lamola AA, Poh-Fitzpatrick MF, et al: Erythropoietic protoporphyria and lead intoxication: The molecular basis for difference in cutaneous photosensitivity. I. Different rates of disappearance of protoporphyrin from the erythrocytes, both in vivo and in vitro. J Clin Invest 1975; 56:1519.

510. Silbergeld EK: Mechanisms of lead neurotoxicity, or looking beyond the lamppost. FASEB J 1992; 6:3201.

511. Byers RK, Lord EE: Late effects of lead poisoning on mental development. Am J Dis Child 1943; 6:471.

512. Chisolm JJ: Aminoaciduria as a manifestation of renal tubular injury in lead intoxication and a comparison with patterns of aminoaciduria seen in other disease. J Pediatr 1962; 60:1.

513. American Academy of Pediatrics Committee on Drugs: Treatment guidelines for lead exposure in children. Pediatrics 1995; 96: 155.

514. Pocock SJ, Smith M, Baghurst P: Environmental lead and children's intelligence: A systematic review of the epidemiological evidence. BMJ 1994; 309:1189.

515. Schwartz J: Low-level lead exposure and children's IQ: A meta-analysis and search for a threshold. Environ Res 1994; 65:42.

516. Piomelli S, Rosen JF, et al: Management of childhood lead poisoning. J Pediatr 1984; 105:523.

517. Rogan WJ, Dietrich KN, Ware JH, et al: The effect of chelation therapy with succimer on neuropsychological development in children exposed to lead. N Engl J Med 2001; 344:1421.

13 | The Porphyrias

Shigeru Sassa ● Attallah Kappas

The porphyrias are a group of disorders caused by deficiencies in the activities of the enzymes of the heme biosynthetic pathway. The enzyme deficiencies can be either partial or nearly complete. As a result, porphyrins or their precursors, such as δ-aminolevulinic acid (ALA) and porphobilinogen (PBG), are abnormally produced in excess, accumulate in tissues, and are excreted in urine and stool. Two cardinal symptoms of the porphyrias are cutaneous photosensitivity and neurologic disturbances.

ENZYMES AND INTERMEDIATES IN THE HEME BIOSYNTHETIC PATHWAY

Outline of the Pathway

The enzymatic and intermediate steps in the heme biosynthetic pathway are illustrated in Figure 13–1. In animal cells, the first step and the last three steps occur in mitochondria; the intermediate steps take place in the cytosol. The two major organs that are active in heme synthesis are the liver and the erythroid bone marrow, and inherited enzymatic defects in the porphyrias are mainly expressed in these tissues.

DELTA-AMINOLEVULINATE SYNTHASE

δ-Aminolevulinate synthase (ALAS) is the first enzyme of the heme biosynthetic pathway and catalyzes the condensation of glycine and succinyl coenzyme A to form ALA (Fig. 13–1). The enzyme is localized in the inner membrane of mitochondria and requires pyridoxal 5′-phosphate as a cofactor.[1] ALAS activity is very low and is rate-limiting for heme formation.[2] Hepatic (or nonspecific) and erythroid ALASs are isozymes that are encoded by two distinct nuclear genes,[3, 4] *ALAS1* and *ALAS2*, respectively. The two human *ALAS* genes appear to have evolved by duplication of a common ancestral gene that encoded a primitive catalytic site, with subsequent addition of DNA sequences encoding variable functions.[5] The locus for human gene *ALAS1* is at chromosome 3p21.1 and that for *ALAS2* is at Xp11.21.[4] Inherited deficiency of *ALAS2* is associated with X-linked sideroblastic anemia.[6]

DELTA-AMINOLEVULINATE DEHYDRATASE

Two molecules of ALA are converted by a cytosolic enzyme, δ-aminolevulinate dehydratase (ALAD), to a monopyrrole, PBG, with the removal of two molecules of water (Fig. 13–1). ALAD deficiency porphyria (ADP) is due to an almost complete lack of enzyme activity. The human *ALAD* gene is localized at chromosome 9q34.[7] The enzyme is a homo-octamer with a subunit size of 36,274 D[8] and requires an intact sulfhydryl group and a zinc atom per subunit for full activity.[9] Zinc is the essential metal for enzyme activity. The human *ALAD* genomic structure is 16 kb in length with two promoter regions and two alternative noncoding exons, 1A and 1B, that generate housekeeping and erythroid-keeping transcripts.[10] Both transcripts encode the same amino acid sequence because translation begins in exon 2. The novel expression of nonspecific and erythroid-specific transcripts apparently evolved to ensure sufficient heme synthesis for the high-level tissue-specific production of hemeproteins in the liver and in erythroid cells.[10] Lead displaces zinc from the enzyme; the result is neurologic disturbances, some of which resemble those of ADP.[11] The most potent inhibitor of the enzyme is succinylacetone,[12] a structural analog of ALA, which is found in urine and blood of patients with hereditary tyrosinemia who often develop symptoms similar to those of ADP.[13]

PORPHOBILINOGEN DEAMINASE

Porphobilinogen deaminase (PBGD) catalyzes the condensation of four molecules of PBG to yield a linear tetrapyrrole, hydroxymethylbilane. In the absence of the subsequent enzyme, uroporphyrinogen III cosynthase, hydroxymethylbilane is spontaneously converted into a ring-form tetrapyrrole, uroporphyrinogen I. In contrast, in the presence of the cosynthase, uroporphyrinogen III, which has an inverted D-ring pyrrole, is formed (Fig. 13–1).

The gene locus for human *PBGD* is at chromosome 11q23→ 11qter.[14] The human *PBGD* gene is split into 15 exons, spread over 10 kb of DNA.[15] There are two isozymes of PBGD: erythroid specific and nonspecific.[16] The two isoforms of PBGD are produced by distinct messenger RNAs (mRNAs), which are transcribed from a single gene by alternate transcription and splicing of its mRNA. The human erythroid-specific *PBGD* consists of 344 amino acid residues; nonspecific *PBGD* contains 17 additional amino acid residues at its N terminus, and the remainder is identical to the erythroid enzyme. A partial (or heterozygous) deficiency of PBGD is associated with acute intermittent porphyria (AIP).

UROPORPHYRINOGEN III COSYNTHASE

Uroporphyrinogen III cosynthase (UCS) catalyzes the formation of uroporphyrinogen III from hydroxymethylbilane. This involves an intramolecular rearrangement that affects only the D-ring of the uroporphyrinogen (Fig. 13–1). Human UCS predicted from its complementary DNA (cDNA) consists of 265 amino acid residues.[17] Using the cDNA as a probe, a single *UCS* gene has been assigned to 10q25.3→q26.3.[18] The genomic structure of the human *UCS* gene indicates that the gene is approximately 34 kb in length and contains 10 exons, and all exon/intron boundaries conform to the GT-AG rule.[19] Similar to *ALAD* and *PBGD*, the *UCS* gene has alternative promoters that generate housekeeping and erythroid transcripts, which are apparently under separate tissue-specific control.[19] Homozygous deficiency of *UCS* is associated with congenital erythropoietic porphyria (CEP).

UROPORPHYRINOGEN DECARBOXYLASE

Uroporphyrinogen decarboxylase (UROD) is a cytosolic enzyme that catalyzes the sequential removal of the four carboxylic groups of the carboxymethyl side chains in uroporphyrinogen to yield coproporphyrinogen (Fig. 13–1). Human *UROD* cDNA encodes a polypeptide of 367 amino acid residues.[20] The *UROD* gene has been mapped to chromosome 1p34.[21, 22] Porphyria cutanea tarda (PCT) is due to a partial (or heterozygous) deficiency of UROD, whereas hepatoerythropoietic porphyria (HEP) is due to a homozygous deficiency of the enzyme.

COPROPORPHYRINOGEN OXIDASE

Coproporphyrinogen oxidase (CPO) is a mitochondrial enzyme that catalyzes the removal of the carboxyl group and two hydrogens from the propionic groups of pyrrole

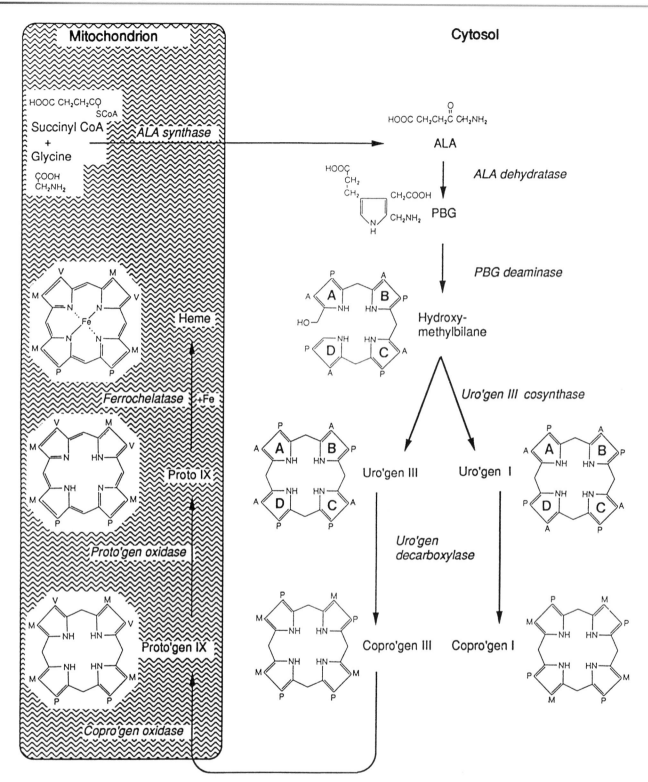

FIGURE 13–1. Enzymes *(italics)* and intermediates *(plain letters)* in the heme biosynthetic pathway. Pyrrole ring designation is shown in the structures of hydroxymethylbilane and uroporphyrinogen (uro'gen) I and III. In uroporphyrinogen III, substituent groups in the D ring have undergone "flipping"; that is, the pyrrole ring is reversed. A = –CH$_2$COOH; ALA = δ-aminolevulinic acid; copro'gen = coproporphyrinogen; M = –CH$_3$; P = –CH$_2$CH$_2$COOH; PBG = porphobilinogen; proto = protoporphyrin; proto'gen = protoporphyrinogen; uro'gen = uroporphyrinogen; V = –CHCH$_2$.

rings A and B of coproporphyrinogen to form vinyl groups at these positions (Fig. 13–1). The gene for human CPO is localized to chromosome 3q12.[23] Although a unique erythroid-specific promoter is not present, *CPO* transcripts increase during erythroid cell differentiation.

Functional analysis of the mouse *CPO* promoter demonstrated that the synergistic action of an Sp-1–like element, a GATA-1 site, and a novel regulatory element, *CPO* promoter regulatory element, were prerequisite for the promoter activity in erythroid cells.[24] In contrast, in nonerythroid cells, the GATA-1 site was not required, whereas the *CPO* promoter regulatory element was necessary. These findings indicate that a single promoter contains elements for both the housekeeping and erythroid-specific expression of the *CPO* gene.[24] Human CPO predicted from its cDNA is a protein of 354 amino acid residues.[25] Hereditary coproporphyria (HCP) is due to a partial (or heterozygous) deficiency of CPO.

PROTOPORPHYRINOGEN OXIDASE

The oxidation of protoporphyrinogen to protoporphyrin is mediated by a mitochondrial enzyme, protoporphyrinogen oxidase (PPO), which catalyzes the removal of six hydrogen atoms from the porphyrinogen nucleus (see Fig. 13–1). The human *PPO* gene is 5.5 kb in length and contains 1 noncoding and 12 coding exons, and the exon/intron boundaries all conform to the consensus acceptor (GTN) and donor (NAG) sequences.[26, 27] The human *PPO* coding sequence encodes a 477-amino acid polypeptide. The gene for human *PPO* has been mapped to chromosomal region 1q22→q23.[27, 28] Variegate porphyria (VP) is due to a partial (or heterozygous) deficiency of PPO. This is the only enzyme in the heme pathway for which no cDNA cloning has been reported.

FERROCHELATASE

The final step of heme biosynthesis is the insertion of iron into protoporphyrin (see Fig. 13–1). This reaction is cat-alyzed by a mitochondrial enzyme, ferrochelatase. Unlike other steps in the heme biosynthetic pathway, this enzyme utilizes protoporphyrin IX as substrate, rather than its reduced form. However, the enzyme specifically requires ferrous, not ferric, iron. The gene for human ferrochelatase has been assigned to chromosome 18q21.3.[29] The human *ferrochelatase* gene contains 11 exons and has a minimum size of about 45 kb.[29] The human *ferrochelatase* cDNA encodes a polypeptide of 423 amino acid residues, including a leader sequence of 54 residues (molecular mass 47.9 kD) and a mature enzyme of 369 amino acid residues.[30] Erythropoietic protoporphyria (EPP) is due to a partial (or heterozygous) ferrochelatase deficiency.

CONTROL OF HEME SYNTHESIS IN THE LIVER AND ERYTHROID CELLS

Biosynthesis of heme in the liver is controlled largely by the rate of formation of ALAS,[2] that is, ALAS1 (Fig. 13–2). The level of enzyme activity in normal liver cells is very low, whereas its level increases dramatically when the liver needs to make more heme in response to various chemical treatments.[31] The synthesis of the enzyme is also regulated in a feedback fashion by heme, which is the end product of the biosynthetic pathway.[32] At higher heme concentrations than those that repress the synthesis of ALAS1, heme induces microsomal heme oxygenase, resulting in an enhancement of its own catabolism.[33, 34] Therefore, the hepatic heme concentration is maintained

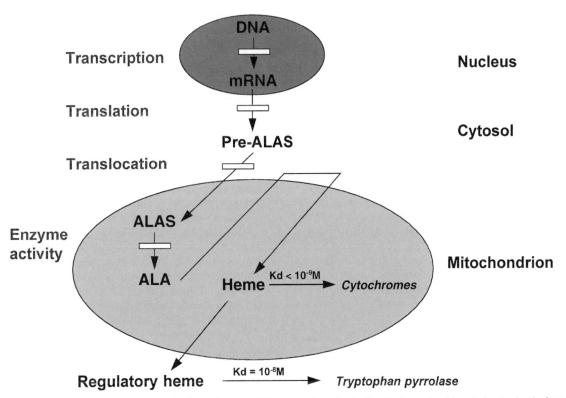

FIGURE 13–2. Regulation of heme synthesis in the liver. The rate of heme synthesis in the liver is determined largely by the level of ALA synthase (ALAS). The regulatory function of heme can be exerted by the regulatory heme concentration, which is in equilibrium with the heme moiety of tryptophan pyrrolase. Excess heme may be degraded by microsomal heme oxygenase; heme also may induce heme oxygenase *(not shown)*. All of these changes ultimately result in the normalization of the concentration of regulatory heme when all pools that require heme (e.g., cytochromes) have been filled. mRNA = messenger RNA.

by a balance between the synthesis of ALAS1 and heme oxygenase, both of which are under the regulatory influence of heme.(Fig. 13–2)

In contrast to the liver, the high rate of heme formation in erythroid cells requires ALAS2, and the enzyme is either refractory to or stimulated by heme treatment or is developmentally increased when heme content increases in the cell. Thus, regulation of heme synthesis in erythroid cells is different from that in the liver.[35] The human *ALAS2* promoter/enhancer region contains numerous erythroid-specific elements, and deletion analysis has shown that maximal erythroid-specific expression is supported by the first 300 nucleotides (nt) upstream of the transcription start site.[36] In addition, the 5′-untranslated region of *ALAS2* mRNA contains an iron-responsive element (IRE) that coordinates ALAS2 synthesis with iron availability.[37, 38] A 28-nt region (spanning most of *ALAS2* intron 1) forms a stem-loop structure that acts as a binding site for the IRE-binding protein 1 (IRP1).[39] This protein-mRNA complex blocks translation in iron-deficient erythroid cells[38] whereas in iron-replete cells, the iron-IRP1 complex is released from the *ALAS2* IRE, allowing translation to proceed. Not much is known about regulation of heme biosynthesis in other tissues and cell types, but it might be different from that in the liver and erythroid cells.[40]

PATHOPHYSIOLOGY OF PORPHYRINS AND THEIR PRECURSORS

Photosensitivity

Photosensitivity in cutaneous forms of porphyria is due to the accumulation of free porphyrins in the skin. Free porphyrins occur only in small amounts in normal tissues, but their levels may become markedly elevated in the porphyrias. On illumination at wavelengths of about 400 nm (Soret band) and in the presence of oxygen, porphyrins cause photodynamic damage to tissues, cells, subcellular elements, and biomolecules through the formation of singlet oxygen.[41]

Neurologic Disturbances

Acute hepatic porphyrias (ADP, AIP, HCP, and VP) are characterized by neurologic disturbances. The most common symptoms are abdominal pain, disturbances in intestinal motility (e.g., diarrhea and constipation), dysesthesias, muscular paralysis, and respiratory failure, which can be fatal. Despite the fact that a few theories have been put forth, the exact nature of the neurologic disturbances in the porphyrias remains obscure.[42]

CLASSIFICATION OF PORPHYRIAS

Porphyrias were traditionally classified as either hepatic or erythropoietic, depending on the principal site of expression of the specific enzymatic defect. They can also be classified as acute hepatic or cutaneous porphyrias. *Acute hepatic porphyrias* are characterized clinically by neurologic disturbances and biochemically by an overproduction of porphyrin precursors (e.g.,

ALA or PBG), whereas *cutaneous porphyrias* are characterized clinically by cutaneous photosensitivity and biochemically by an excessive production of porphyrins. These classifications are not necessarily absolute, because some porphyrias (e.g., HEP) show a major biochemical expression in both the liver and the bone marrow or are associated with both cutaneous and neurologic disturbances, as are HCP and VP. Eight enzymes are involved in the synthesis of heme and, with the exception of the first enzyme (i.e., ALAS), an enzymatic defect at each step of heme synthesis is associated with each form of porphyria (Fig. 13–3 and Table 13–1). In this chapter, each porphyria is described according to the order of the enzymes in the heme biosynthetic sequence (Fig. 13–3). Cardinal symptoms and laboratory findings of each porphyria are summarized in Table 13–2.

Delta-Aminolevulinate Dehydratase Deficiency Porphyria

ADP is an autosomal recessive disorder resulting from a homozygous ALAD deficiency (see Fig. 13–3 and Table 13–1). This is the rarest form of the porphyrias; ADP as confirmed by molecular diagnosis has been reported in only four patients. The symptomatology is similar to that seen in AIP, but ADP can be differentiated from AIP by the lack of PBG overproduction.

CLINICAL FINDINGS

Signs and symptoms of ADP include vomiting, pain in the arms and legs, and neuropathy, which are exacerbated after stress, alcohol use, or decreased food intake[43] (Table 13–2). One infant with ADP has been described whose condition had an unusual clinical course from birth onward that included general muscle hypotonia and respiratory insufficiency.[44]

BIOCHEMICAL FINDINGS

Urinary ALA excretion is highly elevated, whereas urinary PBG excretion is within the normal range (see Table 13–2). Urinary and erythrocyte porphyrin levels are also markedly elevated (≈100-fold), but PBG excretion is normal; no satisfactory explanation has been advanced to account for these observations. A primary block in a distal enzyme is unlikely. Fecal porphyrin excretion is normal or marginally elevated. Furthermore, patients with ADP display markedly decreased activity of ALAD in erythrocytes as well as in nonerythroid cells (≤2 percent of normal), and their parents show approximately 50 percent decreases in enzyme activity.

MOLECULAR BIOLOGY

ALAD point mutations in the four reported patients have been defined (Fig. 13–4). In the two original German patients with ADP,[45] patient H had *ALAD* missense mutation V153M and a two-base deletion, 818delTC, that resulted in a frameshift and premature truncation after residue 294.[46] Patient B had *ALAD* missense mutations

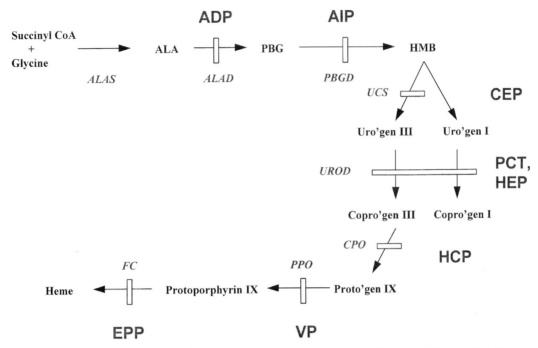

FIGURE 13–3. Porphyrias and their enzymatic defects *(open bars)* are shown. ALA = δ-aminolevulinic acid; ADP = ALAD deficiency porphyria; AIP = acute intermittent porphyria; ALAD = ALA dehydratase; CEP = congenital erythropoietic porphyria; copro'gen = coproporphyrinogen; CPO = copro'gen oxidase; EPP = erythropoietic protoporphyria; FC = ferrochelatase; HCP = hereditary coproporphyria; HEP = hepatoerythropoietic porphyria; HMB = hydroxymethylbilane; PBG = porphobilinogen; PBGD = PBG deaminase; proto'gen = protoporphyrinogen; PCT = porphyria cutanea tarda; PPO = proto'gen oxidase; uro'gen = uroporphyrinogen; UCS = uro'gen III cosynthase; UROD = uro'gen decarboxylase; VP = variegate porphyria.

TABLE 13–1. The Porphyrias and Their Enzymatic Defects

Enzyme Deficiency	Porphyria	Principal Site of Expression	Mode of Transmission	Remarks
ALAD	ADP	Liver	Recessive	
PBGD	AIP	Liver	Dominant	
	Type I			CRIM (−)
	Type II			Normal erythrocyte PBGD
	Type III			CRIM (+)
UCS	CEP	Bone marrow	Recessive	
UROD	PCT	Liver		
	Type I		None	Acquired
	Type II		Dominant	UROD decreased in all tissues
	Type III		Dominant	UROD decreased in the liver, but not in erythrocytes
	HEP	Liver and bone marrow	Recessive	
CPO	HCP	Liver	Dominant	
PPOX	VP	Liver	Dominant	
FECH	EPP	Bone marrow	Dominant	

ALAD = δ-aminolevulinate dehydratase; ADP = δ-aminolevulinate dehydratase deficiency porphyria; PBGD = porphobilinogen deaminase; AIP = acute intermittent porphyria; UCS = uroporphyrinogen III cosynthase; CEP = congenital erythropoietic porphyria; UROD = uroporphyrinogen decarboxylase; PCT = porphyria cutanea tarda; HEP = hepatoerythropoietic porphyria; CPO = coproporphyrinogen oxidase; HCP = hereditary coproporphyria; PPOX = protoporphyrinogen oxidase; VP = variegate porphyria; FECH = ferrochelatase; EPP = erythropoietic protoporphyria; CRIM = cross-reactive immunologic material.

R240W and A274T,[47] yielding a mutant enzyme with little catalytic activity and a mutant protein with thermal instability.[47] Molecular analysis of the *ALAD* gene in a Swedish child with severe ADP also revealed two missense mutations, G133R and V275M.[48] Molecular analysis of a 63-year-old Belgian male patient identified the lesion in one allele, G133R, which was the same mutation identified in the Swedish child.[49] Although the Belgian patient was heterozygous for ALAD deficiency, he developed clinical ADP at the age of 63 when he suffered from polycythemia vera. It was concluded that his porphyria was presumably due to clonal expansion of bone marrow cells that carried the ADP mutation.[50] Another point mutation, F12L, was identified in an asymptomatic Swedish girl who had only 12 percent of ALAD activity in erythrocytes.[51] Bacterial expression studies revealed the highly

TABLE 13–2. Clinical and Laboratory Features of the Porphyrias

Porphyria	Clinical Features	Laboratory Features			
		Erythrocytes	Plasma	Urine	Stool
ADP	Neurologic (as in AIP)	ZnPP	—	ALA	—
AIP	Neurologic: nausea, vomiting, abdominal pain, diarrhea, constipation, ileus, dysuria, muscle hypotonia, respiratory failure, sensory neuropathy, seizures	—	—	ALA, PBG	—
CEP	Photosensitivity: bullae, crusts, scar formation, sclerodermoid change,hyperpigmentation and hypopigmentation, hypertrichosis, erythrodontia, hemolytic anemia, splenomegaly	Uro I, copro I	Uro I, copro I	Uro, 7-carboxyl	—
PCT	Photosensitivity: skin fragility, bullae, crusts, scar formation, sclerodermoid change, hyperpigmentation and hypopigmentation, hypertrichosis	—	Uro, 7-carboxyl	Uro, 7-carboxyl	Uro, 7-carboxyl, isocopro
HEP	Photosensitivity (as in CEP)	ZnPP	Uro, 7-carboxyl	Uro, 7-carboxyl	Uro, 7-carboxyl, isocopro
HCP	Neurologic (as in ADP, AIP, and VP) and photosensitivity (as in VP)	—	Copro	Copro, ALA, PBG	Copro
VP	Neurologic (as in ADP, AIP, and HCP) and photosensitive (as in HCP)	—	Proto	ALA, PBG	Proto
EPP	Photosensitivity: burning sensation, edema, erythema, itching, scarring, vesicles	Proto	Proto	—	Proto

PBG = porphobilinogen; 7-carboxyl = 7-carboxylporphyrin; copro = coproporphyrin; isocopro = isocoproporphyrin; uro = uroporphyrin; ZnPP = zinc protoporphyrin.

heterogeneous nature of enzyme phenotypes of these mutant proteins[52](see Fig. 13–4).

DIAGNOSIS

Definitive diagnosis depends on the demonstration of markedly decreased ALAD activity and deficiency of enzyme protein in erythrocytes. Supporting evidence for the diagnosis includes massive elevations of urinary ALA (but not PBG) and substantial elevations of porphyrins in urine and erythrocytes. Clinical symptoms of ADP occur typically only in homozygotes, whereas heterozygotes (i.e., parents and certain siblings of the proband) remain clinically unaffected.

TREATMENT

The clinical management of ADP is the same as that described later for AIP.

Acute Intermittent Porphyria

AIP, which is also known as *Swedish porphyria, pyrroloporphyria,* or *intermittent acute porphyria,* is an autosomal dominant disorder resulting from a partial PBGD deficiency (see Fig. 13–3 and Table 13–1). The deficient enzyme activity (≈50 percent of normal) is found in all tissues, including erythrocytes, in the great majority of patients (≥95 percent). However, a subset of patients (≤5 percent) shows deficient enzyme activity only in nonerythroid cells. The majority (≈90 percent) of individuals with this genetic enzyme deficiency remain clinically normal throughout life. Clinical expression of the disease is usually linked to environmental or acquired factors (e.g., nutritional status, drugs, corticosteroids, and other chemicals of endogenous or exogenous origin). The cardinal pathobiologic defect of the disease is a neurologic dysfunction that may affect the peripheral, autonomic, and central nervous systems (see Table 13–2).

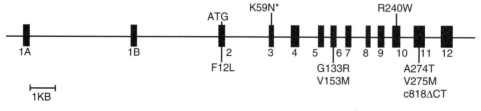

FIGURE 13–4. The human *ALAD* gene and locations of mutations causing ADP. (Courtesy Dr. K. H. Astrin.)

PREVALENCE

AIP is the severest form of the acute hepatic porphyrias and probably the most common of the genetic porphyrias. The highest incidence of AIP occurs in Lapland, Scandinavia, and the United Kingdom, although it has been reported in many population groups. The prevalence of AIP was estimated to be 1 to 2 per 100,000 in Europe[53] and 2.4 per 100,000 in Finland.[54] The prevalence of low PBGD activity, which includes both patients with clinically manifest AIP and latent gene carriers, is, however, as high as 1 per 500 in the general population of Finland.[55] The disorder is seen clinically almost invariably after puberty and more often in women than in men.

CLINICAL FINDINGS

AIP is a severely debilitating form of acute hepatic porphyria. Abdominal pain, which may be generalized or localized, is the most common symptom and is often the initial sign of an acute attack. Other gastroenterologic features may include nausea, vomiting, constipation or diarrhea, abdominal distention, and ileus. Urinary retention, incontinence, and dysuria may commonly be observed. Tachycardia and hypertension and less often fever, sweating, restlessness, and tremor also are observed. In up to 40 percent of patients, hypertension may become sustained between acute attacks.

Peripheral neuropathy is a common feature of AIP. Muscle weakness often begins proximally in the legs but may involve the arms or the distal extremities. Motor neuropathy also may involve the cranial nerves or lead to bulbar paralysis, respiratory impairment, and death. Sensory, patchy neuropathy also may occur. Acute attacks of AIP may be accompanied by seizures, especially in patients with hyponatremia due to vomiting, inappropriate fluid therapy, or the syndrome of inappropriate antidiuretic hormone release. The course of an acute attack of AIP is highly variable both in individuals and among patients, with attacks lasting from a few days to several months. No cutaneous manifestations are associated with this enzyme deficiency.

PRECIPITATING FACTORS

Asymptomatic heterozygotes (≈90 percent of subjects with documented PBGD deficiency) may display neither abnormalities in concentrations of porphyrin precursors nor clinical symptoms. Endogenous or exogenous environmental factors may precipitate an acute attack in individuals with both latent or previously clinically expressed AIP. There are at least five different classes of precipitating factors in this disease.[42]

ALAS1 Inducers

Most precipitating factors can be related to an associated increase in the activity of ALAS1 in the liver.[42] Overproduction of ALA then makes the partially deficient PBGD activity rate-limiting.

Endocrine Factors

The clinical disease is more common in women, especially at the time of menses. A subset of female patients experiences cyclical premenstrual exacerbations of the disease.[56] It has been shown that C_{19} and C_{21} steroids, particularly of the 5β-configuration, potently induce ALAS1 activity in the liver.[57, 58]

Calorie Intake

Loss of appetite or reduced calorie intake often leads to exacerbations of AIP.[59] Caloric supplementation may reduce PBG excretion and suppress clinical symptoms.[60]

Drugs and Foreign Chemicals

Many chemicals (e.g., barbiturates, certain steroids, and other foreign substances) that exacerbate porphyria have the potential to induce cytochrome P-450.[42] The result is enhanced demand for heme synthesis that may lead to induction of hepatic ALAS1.

Stress

Various forms of stress, including intercurrent illnesses, infections, alcoholic excess, and surgery, are known to upregulate the heme oxygenase gene, leading to excessive heme catabolism and derepression of ALAS1, with clinical expression of AIP.

BIOCHEMICAL FINDINGS

In patients with clinically expressed AIP and a few individuals with latent AIP, variably increased amounts of ALA and PBG are excreted in the urine between attacks. In the majority of patients, the onset of an acute attack is accompanied by further marked increases in excretion of these precursors. In severe attacks, the urine develops a port-wine color from a high content of porphobilin, an auto-oxidation product of PBG. Acute attacks may also be associated with elevations in the serum concentrations of ALA, PBG, and porphyrins, which are normally undetectable. Stool porphyrin levels are usually normal or only slightly elevated. The Watson-Schwartz test is widely used as a screening test for urinary PBG. The column method of Mauzerall and Granick[61] is the most specific and quantitative test. Hemoglobin levels and bilirubin production are normal in patients with AIP.

MOLECULAR BIOLOGY

Patients with AIP can be classified into three subsets (Table 13–3):

1. Patients with type I mutations are characterized by cross-reactive immunologic material (CRIM)-negative *PBGD* mutations; they exhibit both reduced

TABLE 13–3. Subsets of Acute Intermittent Porphyria

Type	Erythrocyte PBGD			CRIM
	Activity (% of Control)	Mass (% of Control)	Mass / Activity	
I	50	50	1	(−)
II	100	100	1	(−)
III	50	>50	>1	(+)

enzyme activity and reduced PBGD protein content (≈ 50 percent of normal).

2. Type II mutations are observed in fewer than 5 percent of all patients with AIP and are characterized by decreased PBGD activity in nonerythroid cells, such as liver (≈ 50 percent of normal), but with normal erythroid PBGD activity.

3. Patients with type III mutations are characterized by CRIM-positive mutations, that is, decreased enzyme activity (≈ 50 percent of normal) with the presence of structurally abnormal enzyme protein.[62]

More than 170 different mutations of the human *PBGD* gene have been described in patients with AIP (Fig. 13–5). Mutations found in type I AIP are single-base substitutions or deletions that lead to a single amino acid change or to truncated proteins, which result in the loss of expression of the enzyme protein. The mutations found in type II AIP are single-base substitutions that occur in the exon/intron boundary of exon 1, resulting in a splicing defect that affects only the nonspecific form of *PBGD*, but not the erythroid-specific *PBGD*, because the transcription of the gene in erythroid cells starts downstream of the site of mutation. Mutations characterizing type III AIP, mostly occurring in exons 10 and 12, are observed in the region that is thought to be essential for catalytic activity (Fig. 13–5). In addition to these mutations or deletions, a few intragenic restriction fragment length polymorphisms that are unique to certain families with AIP have been reported, but their mutations have not yet been identified.[63–70] (see Fig. 13–5)

DIAGNOSIS

The diagnosis of types I and III AIP can be made by the demonstration of decreased PBGD activity in erythrocytes (seen in ≥95 percent of patients), whereas the distinction between carrier or latent status and clinically expressed AIP requires demonstration of elevated urinary excretion of PBG and ALA. Elevated urinary levels of both ALA and PBG also may be seen in HCP and VP; measurement of urinary and stool porphyrins usually differentiates these conditions from AIP. The diagnosis of type II AIP requires either the demonstration of PBGD deficiency in nonerythroid cells (e.g., lymphocytes or fibroblasts) or DNA hybridization with allele-specific oligonucleotides specific for the mutation.

TREATMENT

The treatment for AIP is essentially identical to that for ADP, HCP, and VP. Between attacks, treatment comprises adequate nutritional intake, avoidance of drugs and chemicals known to exacerbate porphyria, and prompt treatment of other intercurrent diseases or infections. Patients with unresponsive severe disease should be treated with intravenous administration of carbohydrate initiated with dextrose to provide a minimum of 300 g of carbohydrate per day. Intravenous hematin (4 mg/kg every 12 hours) is probably most effective in reducing ALA and PBG excretion as well as in curtailing acute attacks.[71] Nasal or subcutaneous administration of long-acting agonistic analogs of luteinizing hormone–releasing hormone has been shown to inhibit ovulation and greatly reduce the incidence of perimenstrual attacks of AIP in some women with cyclic exacerbations of the disease.[72] Administration of synthetic heme analogs (e.g., tin mesoporphyrin, which inhibits heme catabolism) has also been shown to diminish the output of ALA, PBG, or porphyrins in patients with AIP and VP.[73]

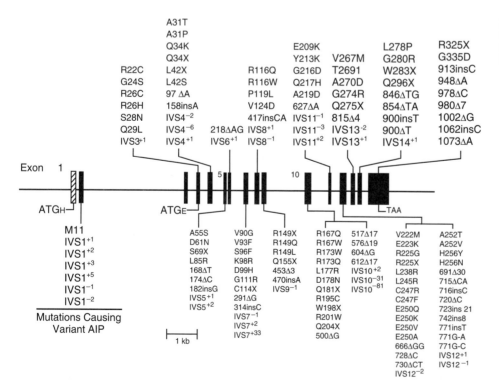

FIGURE 13–5. The human *PBGD* gene and locations of some of the many mutations causing AIP. (Courtesy of Dr. K. H. Astrin.)

Congenital Erythropoietic Porphyria

CEP, which is also referred to as Günther disease, is an autosomal recessive disorder (see Fig. 13–3 and Table 13–1). The primary abnormality is decreased activity of UCS that results in accumulation and hyperexcretion of predominantly type I porphyrins (see Table 13–2). A fetus with this enzymatic defect shows brownish amniotic fluid from excessive amounts of porphyrins, and after birth, homozygous gene carriers manifest cutaneous photosensitivity, hemolysis, and a decreased life expectancy.

PREVALENCE

Fewer than 200 patients have been reported, and some of these patients may actually have had PCT or HEP. No clear racial or sexual predilection is apparent.

CLINICAL FINDINGS

The first clue suggesting the diagnosis of CEP at birth is pink to dark-brown staining of diapers, which is caused by large amounts of porphyrins in the urine. Early onset of cutaneous photosensitivity is characteristic and is exacerbated by exposure to sunlight. Subepidermal bullous lesions progress to crusted erosions that heal with scarring and either hyperpigmentation or, less commonly, hypopigmentation. Hypertrichosis and alopecia are common, and erythrodontia (with red fluorescence under ultraviolet light) is virtually pathognomonic of CEP (Fig. 13–6; see color section at front of this volume). Patients may display symptoms and signs of hemolytic anemia with splenomegaly and porphyrin-rich gallstones. Occasionally, anemia may be severe and require transfusion. Bone marrow shows erythroid hyperplasia, which may result in pathologic fractures or vertebral compression-collapse and shortness of stature. Although the onset of symptoms of CEP is most often observed in early infancy, a few patients may first be seen with the syndrome as adults.

PATHOGENESIS

The primary site of expression of the enzymatic defect is the bone marrow, wherein fluorescence secondary to porphyrin accumulation is variably distributed but invariably present. Many marrow normoblasts (30 to 70 percent) display fluorescence, principally localized in the nuclei of the cells.[74] Massive accumulations of porphyrins systemically in CEP are derived from porphyrin-laden erythrocytes, which account for the multiple lesions of the integument.

BIOCHEMICAL FINDINGS

Urinary levels of uroporphyrins and coproporphyrins are always elevated (20- to 60-fold), with predominant elevations of type I isomers. Erythrocyte concentrations of uroporphyrins and coproporphyrins also are elevated.

MOLECULAR BIOLOGY

A heterogeneity of mutations in the *UCS* gene exists in patients with CEP (Fig. 13–7). The first molecular analysis in a patient with CEP revealed compound heterozygosity: a T→C transition resulting in an amino acid

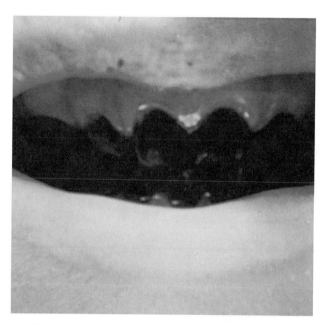

FIGURE 13–6. Erythrodontia of a patient with CEP. Dark reddish-brown discoloration of the teeth is noted. When the teeth are exposed to ultraviolet light they emit the intense red fluorescence of porphyrins. Discoloration is usually more pronounced in decidual teeth than in permanent teeth (see color section at front of this volume). (Courtesy of H. M. Nitowsky, MD.)

FIGURE 13–7. The human *UCS* gene and locations of mutations causing CEP. (Courtesy of Dr. K. H. Astrin.)

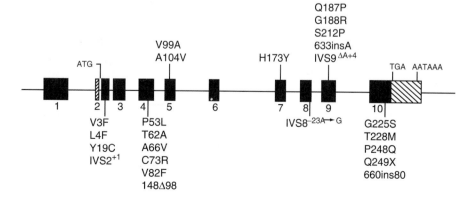

change of Cys[73]→Arg and a Cr→T transition resulting in Pro[53]→Leu[75]. The second patient was, however, homozygous for the mutation Cys[73]→Arg[52]. This point mutation appears to occur often because it has been found in 8 of 21 unrelated patients with CEP (about 21 percent of CEP alleles).[76] Subsequently, however, other mutations have been found in CEP, indicating that the nature of the enzymatic defect in CEP is heterogeneous, as is the case in other porphyrias.

DIAGNOSIS

Pink urine or the onset of severe cutaneous photosensitivity in infancy (or rarely in adults) suggests the diagnosis of CEP. Demonstration of elevated levels of urinary, fecal, and erythrocyte porphyrins with elevated type I isomers of uroporphyrin and coproporphyrin establishes the diagnosis of CEP. Demonstration of a deficiency of UCS activity constitutes the definitive diagnosis.

TREATMENT

The avoidance of precipitating factors such as sunlight, trauma to the skin, and infections is the most important preventive measure. Topical sunscreens may be of some help, as may oral treatment with β-carotene.[77] Transfusions with packed erythrocytes transiently decrease hemolysis and its attendant drive to increased erythropoiesis and also decrease porphyrin excretion.[78] Splenectomy has been used fairly often and has produced short-term reductions in hemolysis, porphyrin excretion, and skin manifestations, but not all patients respond.[79] Treatment with charcoal in a man with CEP was reported to have lowered porphyrin excretion levels and induced complete clinical remission during therapy.[80]

Porphyria Cutanea Tarda

PCT refers to a heterogeneous group of cutaneous porphyric diseases caused by UROD deficiency, which may be either inherited or, more commonly, acquired.[81] Reductions in hepatic UROD activity are seen in both forms of the disease, but erythrocyte UROD activity may or may not be decreased, depending on the clinical subtype of the disease as discussed below (Table 13–4).

Type I PCT is an acquired disease that typically presents in adults as decreased hepatic, but not erythrocyte, UROD activity. The disease may occur spontaneously but more commonly occurs in conjunction with precipitating environmental factors, such as alcohol, estrogen, or drug use, or in association with other disorders.[81]

Type II PCT is, in contrast, inherited in an autosomal dominant fashion and is associated with decreased UROD activity in all tissues.

Type III PCT is also inherited, but the defect is confined to the liver[82–84]; erythrocyte UROD activity and its protein concentrations are normal.[84]

PREVALENCE

PCT is probably the most common of all forms of the porphyrias, but its exact incidence is not clear. The disease is recognized worldwide, and there is no racial predilection except among the Bantus in South Africa, in whom it is secondary to their high incidence of hemosiderosis. Type I PCT is generally more common than type II PCT in Europe, South Africa, and South America, although the trend may be less obvious in North America. Previously, PCT was thought to be more common in men, perhaps because their alcohol intake is greater than that of women; the incidence in females has recently increased to the level seen in males, perhaps from increased use of steroids for contraception, estrogens for postmenopausal symptoms, and alcohol.

CLINICAL FINDINGS

The pathognomonic clinical feature of PCT is the formation of vesicles on sun-exposed areas of the skin, particularly the dorsum of the hands (Fig. 13–8; see color section at front of this volume). The vesicles are superseded by crusting, superficial scarring, or milia formation and by residual pigmentation. Facial hypertrichosis may be

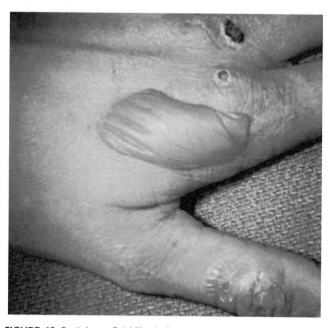

FIGURE 13–8. A large fluid-like bulla, crusted erosions, and unsightly scarring are typical findings in patients with PCT. These changes may also be seen in patients with other forms of the cutaneous porphyrias, but adult onset of lesions suggests either PCT, HEP, HCP, or VP (see color section at front of this volume). (From Poh-Fitzpatrick MB: Porphyrin-sensitized cutaneous photosensitivity. Pathogenesis and treatment. Clin Dermatol 1985; 3:41.)

TABLE 13–4. Subsets of Porphyria Cutanea Tarda

| Type | Familial Occurrence | UROD Activity | |
		Liver	Erythrocytes
I	(−)	Decreased	Normal
II	(+)	Decreased	Decreased
III	(+)	Decreased	Normal

present (Fig. 13–9; see color section at front of this volume) and is conspicuous in women. Hypopigmented indurated plaques of skin may develop and resemble those seen in scleroderma. Photo-onycholysis is occasionally present. In contrast to the acute hepatic porphyrias, neurologic dysfunction does not occur in PCT.

PATHOGENESIS

Porphyrins in the skin may be largely derived from the liver and, to some extent, are formed locally in the skin. Porphyrin-mediated activation of the complement system after light irradiation has been demonstrated in patients with PCT both *in vivo*[85, 86] and *in vitro* in sera[87, 88] and is presumed to result from the generation of reactive oxygen species, most likely singlet oxygen. Bullous fluid is known to contain prostaglandin E_2 and photoactivation of uroporphyrin damages lysosomes.[89] Livers from patients with PCT almost invariably display siderosis with fatty changes, necrosis, chronic inflammatory changes, and granuloma formation.[89] Iron, estrogens, alcohol, and

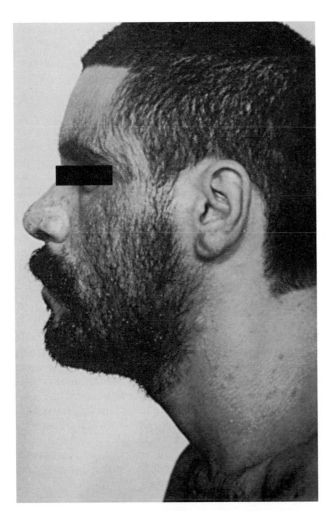

FIGURE 13–9. Hypertrichosis of the face of a patient with PCT. Note the erosions and pigmentations over the nose and cheeks (see color section at front of this volume). (From Poh-Fitzpatrick MB: Porphyrin-sensitized cutaneous photosensitivity. Pathogenesis and treatment. Clin Dermatol 1985; 3:41.)

chlorinated hydrocarbons, which are all potential hepatotoxins, may also aggravate PCT. The incidence of hepatitis B and C infection may also be higher than normal in patients with PCT.[90] The incidence of hepatocellular carcinoma in patients with PCT is known to be greater than that in the general population.[91] Several patients with PCT who were infected with the human immunodeficiency virus have been reported.[92–94]

BIOCHEMICAL FINDINGS

Increased concentrations of uroporphyrin (mainly isomer I) and 7-carboxylic porphyrins (isomer III) are found in the urine in PCT, with lesser increases of coproporphyrin and 5-carboxylic and 6-carboxylic porphyrins. Small quantities of isocoproporphyrin may be detected in serum or in urine, but in feces this is often the dominant porphyrin and represents the most important diagnostic criterion for PCT (Fig. 13–10).[95] Total daily fecal porphyrin excretion exceeds total urinary porphyrin excretion. Skin porphyrin levels are increased, especially in areas that are protected from photoactivation. Serum iron and ferritin concentrations are commonly elevated.

DIAGNOSIS

The clinical manifestations of PCT are fairly specific but can be confused with those of other porphyric (e.g., VP) and nonporphyric (e.g., systemic lupus erythematosus or scleroderma) diseases. Urinary fluorescence under ultraviolet light illumination and quantification and separation and identification of porphyrins by thin-layer chromatography and high-performance liquid chromatography assist the diagnosis. Plasma porphyrin levels are elevated in PCT and in other porphyrias that cause photosensitivity. Serum ferritin levels are also typically elevated in patients with PCT compared with levels in normal subjects and in patients with other porphyrias. Fecal porphyrin levels are often elevated; isocoproporphyrin (or an isocoproporphyrin-to-coproporphyrin ratio ≥0.1) is diagnostic for PCT.

TREATMENT

In type I PCT, the identification and avoidance of precipitating factors represent the first line of treatment.[96] The clinical response to cessation of alcohol ingestion is highly variable; nonetheless, abstinence should be recommended. Phlebotomy is usually effective in reducing urinary porphyrin concentrations and in induction of clinical remissions.[97] Strong evidence exists that the beneficial effects of phlebotomy result from a diminution in the stores of body iron.[98] If phlebotomy is ineffective or contraindicated owing to the presence of other diseases such as anemia, low-dose chloroquine therapy may be effective.[99] The efficacies of chloroquine therapy and phlebotomy are probably similar and a combined approach may diminish the incidence of side effects. The mechanism of action of chloroquine therapy is thought to be related to its ability to chelate porphyrins in a water-soluble, and hence more easily excretable, form.

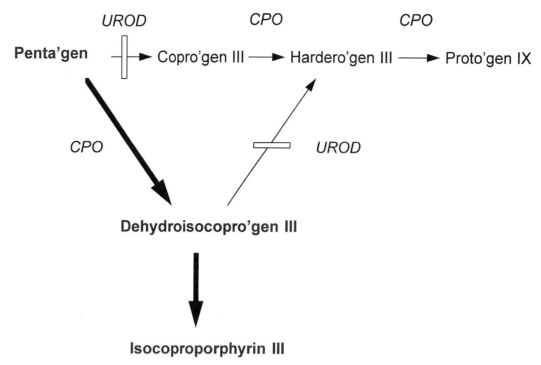

FIGURE 13–10. The formation of isocoproporphyrin in PCT and HEP. The normal route in heme biosynthesis is shown in the top line. In patients with PCT and HEP, the conversion of 5-carboxylate porphyrinogen (penta'gen) III to coproporphyrinogen (copro'gen) III is impaired because of a deficiency of UROD. Increased 5-carboxylate porphyrinogen III is metabolized by CPO, yielding dehydroisocoproporphyrinogen (dehydroisocopro'gen). The latter accumulates and autoxidizes to isocoproporphyrin, because its further metabolism to harderoporphyrinogen (hardero'gen) is impaired owing to the decarboxylase defect. The enzymatic block is shown by an *open bar*, and abnormally elevated intermediates are shown in *bold*.

Hepatoerythropoietic Porphyria

HEP is a rare form of porphyria probably resulting from a homozygous defect of *UROD*.[100] Clinically, HEP is characterized by the childhood onset of severe photosensitivity and skin fragility and is indistinguishable from CEP. Some 20 patients have been reported worldwide.[101]

CLINICAL FINDINGS

The clinical findings in HEP are very similar to those seen in CEP. Pink urine, severe photosensitivity leading to scarring and mutilation of sun-exposed areas of skin, sclerodermoid changes, hypertrichosis, erythrodontia, anemia (often hemolytic), and hepatosplenomegaly are characteristic findings. Onset is usually in early infancy or childhood, but adult onset has also been described. In contrast to PCT, serum iron concentrations are usually normal and phlebotomy has no beneficial effects in patients with HEP.

BIOCHEMICAL FINDINGS

Elevations in the levels of urinary porphyrins—predominantly uroporphyrin of isomer type I with lesser quantities of 7-carboxylic porphyrins, mainly type III—are commonly found. Isocoproporphyrin concentrations equal to or greater than those of coproporphyrin are also found in urine and feces. An elevated erythrocyte zinc protoporphyrin concentration is commonly observed (see Table 13–2). Anemia and biochemical evidence of impaired hepatic function are highly variable findings.

MOLECULAR BIOLOGY

The full-length human *UROD* cDNA contained a coding region of 1104 bp and 5'- and 3'-untranslated regions of 18 and 72 bp, respectively, encoding a polypeptide of 367 amino acid residues. The human *UROD* gene has been mapped to chromosome 1p34.[21, 22] The human *UROD* genome is approximately 3 kb in length and contains 10 exons, and all intron/exon boundaries are consistent with the boundary consensus sequences.[102] In contrast to the unique erythroid expression mechanism for the first four enzymes of the heme biosynthetic pathway, the *UROD* gene has only a single promoter and the gene is transcribed as a single mRNA.[20]

A variety of *UROD* mutations causing type II familial PCT have been identified, including missense, nonsense, and splice site mutations, several small and large deletions, and a small insertion (Fig. 13–11).[103–108] With the exception of the G281E, IVS6[+1], and g10insA mutations, each of which has been identified in several families, the other *UROD* mutations were individual, each having been found in only one family.[103, 106, 108] *UROD* mutations have not been found in type I PCT.[109, 110] Mutations in type III PCT have not been identified, and it is unclear whether type III represents a distinct subtype due to a familial predisposing gene encoding a protein that inactivates hepatic UROD activity.

A variety of *UROD* mutations have been identified in HEP patients, indicating the molecular heterogeneity of the disease.[103, 104, 111, 112] Of note, with a few exceptions, the *UROD* mutations causing HEP were unique and were not found in type II PCT.[103, 109, 113]

FIGURE 13–11. The human *UROD* gene and locations of mutations causing familial (type II) PCT and HEP. (Courtesy of Dr. K. H. Astrin.)

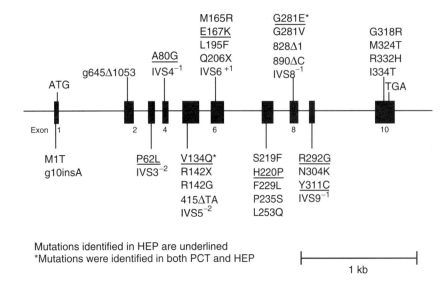

Mutations identified in HEP are underlined
*Mutations were identified in both PCT and HEP

1 kb

DIAGNOSIS

The diagnosis must be suspected in patients with severe photosensitivity and especially considered in the differential diagnosis of CEP. Diagnostic criteria include elevated levels of fecal or urinary isocoproporphyrin and erythrocyte zinc protoporphyrin. Differential diagnosis of HEP includes EPP, in which the erythrocyte protoporphyrin concentration also is elevated but, in contrast to HEP, urinary porphyrin levels are normal. EPP is a clinically milder disease than HEP. Measurement of erythrocyte or fibroblast UROD activity typically shows reductions to 2 to 10 percent of normal control values with intermediate reductions of UROD activities in family members.[114]

TREATMENT

Avoidance of the sun and the use of topical sunscreens are essentially the only recommendations that can be made to these patients. Unlike in patients with PCT, phlebotomy provides no beneficial response.

Hereditary Coproporphyria

HCP is a disease caused by a heterozygous deficiency of CPO activity that is inherited in an autosomal dominant manner (see Fig. 13–3 and Table 13–1). Clinically, the disease is similar to ADP or AIP, although it is often milder; additionally, HCP may be associated with photosensitivity. Expression of the disease is variable and influenced by the same precipitating factors responsible for the exacerbation of AIP. Very rarely, homozygous deficiency of this enzyme may occur, and this is associated with a more severe form of the disease.[115]

PREVALENCE

Clinically expressed HCP is much less common than is clinically expressed AIP, but as in the latter disease, latent HCP or HCP gene carriers are being recognized more

often since the advent of improved molecular laboratory techniques for their detection.

CLINICAL FINDINGS

Neurovisceral symptoms are predominant and are essentially indistinguishable from those of ADP, AIP, or VP. Abdominal pain, vomiting, constipation, neuropathies, and psychiatric manifestations are common. Cutaneous photosensitivity is a feature in about 30 percent of patients. Attacks can be precipitated by pregnancy, the menstrual cycle, and use of steroids for contraception, but the most common precipitating factor is drug administration, most notably of barbiturates.

BIOCHEMICAL FINDINGS

The biochemical hallmark of HCP is hyperexcretion of coproporphyrin (predominantly type III) in urine and feces. Fecal coproporphyrin may be chelated with copper and the fecal protoporphyrin level may be modestly elevated. Hyperexcretion of ALA, PBG, and uroporphyrin into the urine may accompany exacerbations of the disease, but in contrast to AIP these high excretion levels generally return to normal between attacks. CPO activity is typically reduced by about 50 percent in heterozygotes and by 90 to 98 percent in rare homozygotes.[115]

MOLECULAR BIOLOGY

Molecular analysis of several families with HCP has revealed a variety of mutations in the CPO gene (Fig. 13–12). These include missense, nonsense, and splicing mutations, as well as insertions and deletions.[113, 116] A K404E mutation was found in two unrelated families with the harderoporphyria variant. All other CPO mutations found to date are private, each occurring in only one affected family.[113, 116] Mutations G197W, Q306X, Q385X, and W427R occur in highly conserved amino

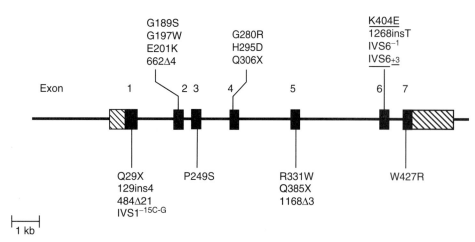

FIGURE 13–12. The human *CPO* gene and localizations of mutations causing HCP. (Courtesy of Dr. K. H. Astrin.)

Underlined Mutations Found in Patients with Harderoporphyria

acids.[117] A homozygous R331W mutation was found in a consanguineous patient with homozygous HCP.[118]

DIAGNOSIS

A diagnosis of HCP should be suspected in patients with the signs, symptoms, and clinical course characteristic of the acute hepatic porphyrias but in whom PBGD activity is normal. Urinary excretion of heme precursors is similar in HCP and VP, but the predominant or exclusive presence of fecal coproporphyrin is highly suggestive of HCP. Fecal or urinary predominance of harderoporphyrin, with greatly reduced CPO activity, was reported in a patient with harderoporphyria,[119] a variant form of HCP.

TREATMENT

The identification and avoidance of precipitating factors are essential. Treatment of acute attacks is similar to the treatment of AIP.

Variegate Porphyria

VP, which is also known as *porphyria variegata, protocoproporphyria, South African genetic porphyria,* or *royal malady* (referring to George III and the House of Hanover), is caused by a heterozygous deficiency in PPO activity and is inherited in an autosomal dominant manner (see Fig. 13–3 and Table 13–1). Patients with this disorder may show neurovisceral symptoms or photosensitivity or both (see Table 13–2). Very rare forms of VP are seen with homozygous deficiencies in PPO activity.[120–122]

PREVALENCE

The incidence of VP of 3 per 1000 in South Africa is substantially higher than that seen elsewhere.[123] In 1980, it was estimated that there were 10,000 affected individuals in South Africa and there is good evidence to suggest that they are all descendants of a single union between two Dutch settlers in 1688.[124] However, the disease is recognized worldwide, and, with the exception of South Africa, there is probably no racial or geographic predilection. The incidence in Finland is reported to be 1.3 per 100,000. Other than in South Africa, VP is probably less common than AIP.

CLINICAL FINDINGS

The neurovisceral symptoms of VP are identical to those observed in ADP, AIP, and HCP, which have been described previously. Photosensitivity is more common, and the resulting lesions tend to be more chronic in VP than in HCP. Cutaneous manifestations include vesicles, bullae, hyperpigmentation, milia, hypertrichosis, and increased skin fragility. Lesions are clinically and histologically indistinguishable from those of PCT. Skin manifestations are less often observed in cold climates than in hot climates. The same spectrum of factors that leads to activation of ADP, AIP, and HCP may also exacerbate VP. Thus, barbiturates, dapsone, lead from "moonshine" whiskey, steroids for contraception, pregnancy, and decreased carbohydrate intake have all been reported to induce or exacerbate VP.

PATHOGENESIS

PPO activity in most patients with VP is decreased by about 50 percent. In rare patients with homozygous VP, however, a virtual absence of PPO activity has been documented[120]; symptoms in these patients were severe photosensitivity, growth and mental retardation, and marked neurologic abnormalities. Onset of the homozygous disease was in childhood in all patients.

BIOCHEMICAL FINDINGS

The biochemical hallmark of VP is an elevated fecal porphyrin level, with the level of protoporphyrin usually exceeding that of coproporphyrin (mostly isomer III). Fecal X-porphyrins (ether-acetic acid–insoluble, extracted with urea-Triton), a heterogeneous group of porphyrin-peptide conjugates, are elevated in VP more than in any other type of porphyria. Urinary coproporphyrin (type III), ALA, and PBG values are often normal between attacks but may become markedly elevated during acute exacerbations of the disease. Plasma invariably shows a fluorescence emission when excited by long ultraviolet light (maximum ≈ 400 nm) that probably represents a protoporphyrin-peptide conjugate.[125]

MOLECULAR BIOLOGY

Mutations causing VP are summarized in Fig. 13–13. These include missense, nonsense, and splice-site mutations, as well as insertions and deletions. Of note, a missense mutation, R59W, is prevalent in South Africa (≈20,000 individuals), which suggests a common founder, as most patients with VP can be traced back to a Dutch immigrant couple who married in Cape Town in 1688.[124, 126] Rare patients with homozygous dominant VP have been identified; these patients had *PPO* mutations that were not found in heterozygous VP, suggesting that they were hypomorphs encoding enzyme proteins with residual activity.[126–128]

DIAGNOSIS

VP should be considered in the differential diagnosis of acute porphyria, especially if PBGD activity is normal. Characteristic plasma porphyrin fluorescence, having a different emission maximum from PCT, is seen in VP.[129] The differentiation of VP from HCP is also possible by fecal porphyrin analysis, because VP is characterized by increased protoporphyrin levels, whereas in HCP predominantly coproporphyrin is seen. The demonstration of urinary 8-uro- and 7-carboxylic porphyrins as well as isocoproporphyrin in PCT is usually sufficient for differentiation from VP. PPO deficiency can be demonstrated in fibroblasts or lymphocytes.

TREATMENT

Identification and avoidance of precipitating factors are essential. Photosensitivity can be minimized by the wearing of protective clothing, and the use of canthaxanthrin (a β-carotene analog) may be of some help. The treatment of neurovisceral symptoms is identical to that described for AIP.

Erythropoietic Protoporphyria

EPP, which is also referred to as *protoporphyria* or *erythrohepatic protoporphyria,* is associated with a partial deficiency of ferrochelatase and is inherited in an autosomal dominant fashion (see Fig. 13–3 and Table 13–1). Biochemically, this defect results in massive accumulations of protoporphyrin in erythrocytes, plasma, and feces. Clinically, the disease is characterized by the childhood onset of cutaneous photosensitivity in light-exposed areas, but skin lesions are milder and less disfiguring than those seen in CEP.

PREVALENCE

EPP is the most common form of erythropoietic porphyria. Three hundred case reports were found in the literature as of 1976. There is no racial or sexual predilection and onset is typically in childhood.

CLINICAL FINDINGS

Cutaneous photosensitivity of EPP is quite different from that seen in CEP or PCT. Stinging or painful burning sensations in the skin occur within 1 hour of exposure to the sun and are followed several hours later by erythema and edema. Some patients experience only burning sensations in the absence of such objective signs of cutaneous phototoxicity, resulting in the erroneous diagnosis of a psychiatric illness. Petechiae, or, more rarely, purpura, vesicles, and crusting may develop and persist for several days after sun exposure. Artificial lights also may cause photosensitivity, especially operating theater lights. Symptoms are usually worse during spring and summer

FIGURE 13–13. The human *PPO* gene and localizations of mutations causing VP. (Courtesy of Dr. K. H. Astrin.)

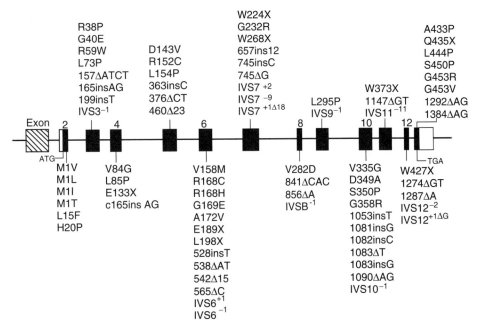

and occur in light-exposed areas, especially on the face and hands. Intense and repeated exposure to the sun may result in onycholysis, leathery hyperkeratotic skin over the dorsum of the hands, and mild scarring. Gallstones, sometimes appearing at an unusually early age, are fairly common, and hepatic disease, although unusual, may be severe and associated with significant morbidity. Anemia is uncommon. There are no known precipitating factors and no neurovisceral manifestations.

PATHOGENESIS

The peak light absorption range for porphyrins corresponds well to the wavelength of light (≈400 nm) known to trigger photosensitivity reactions in the skin of patients with EPP. Light-excited porphyrins generate free radicals and singlet oxygen.[130] Such radicals, notably singlet oxygen, may lead to peroxidation of lipids and cross-linking of membrane proteins, which, in erythrocytes, may result in reduced deformability and thus hemolysis. Protoporphyrin, but not zinc protoporphyrin, can be released from erythrocytes after irradiation.[131] This finding may explain why patients with EPP with elevated levels of free protoporphyrin manifest photosensitivity, whereas patients with lead intoxication and iron deficiency, which are predominantly associated with elevated zinc protoporphyrin levels, do not.[131] Forearm irradiation in patients with EPP leads to complement activation and polymorphonuclear chemotaxis. Similar results have been obtained *in vitro* and these events may also contribute to the pathogenesis of skin lesions in EPP.[85]

BIOCHEMICAL FINDINGS

The biochemical hallmark of EPP is excessive concentrations of protoporphyrin in erythrocytes, plasma, bile, and feces but, because of its poor solubility in water, not in urine. The bone marrow and the newly released erythrocytes appear to be the major source of elevated protoporphyrin concentrations,[132] although the liver may contribute in certain instances.

MOLECULAR BIOLOGY

Molecular analysis of *ferrochelatase* mutations causing EPP has revealed a variety of alterations including missense, nonsense, and splice-site mutations, as well as insertions and deletions (Fig. 13–14).[113] Among these alterations, splice-site mutations were seen most often.[113] Patients with EPP were found to have only 10 to 25 percent of normal ferrochelatase activity, whereas their asymptomatic family members typically have 50 percent ferrochelatase activity. In several EPP families, it was found also that a normal coding *ferrochelatase* sequence allele was expressed at a lower than normal level.[133, 134] The low expression normal allele, which had a particular 5′-haplotype (−251A/G, IVS1–23C/T, IVS2μsat:An, 798G/C, and 1520C/T) was present in about 10 percent of the white population. Inheritance of a *ferrochelatase* mutation in *cis* and the low expression allele in *trans* may thus account for the low ferrochelatase activity and clinical expression of the disease.

DIAGNOSIS

Photosensitivity should suggest the diagnosis, which can be confirmed by the demonstration of elevated concentrations of free protoporphyrin in erythrocytes, plasma, and stools with normal urinary porphyrins. The presence of protoporphyrin in both plasma and erythrocytes is a finding specific for EPP. The presence of fluorescent reticulocytes in a peripheral blood smear may also suggest the diagnosis.

TREATMENT

Avoidance of the sun and use of topical sunscreen agents may be helpful. Oral administration of β-carotene may afford systemic protection against photosensitivity, resulting in improved, although highly variable, tolerance to the sun. The recommended serum β-carotene level of 600 to 800 μg/dL is usually achieved with oral doses of 120 to 180 mg daily, and beneficial effects are typically seen 1 to 3 months after the onset of therapy.[135, 136] The mechanism of this beneficial effect of β-carotene probably involves quenching of activated oxygen radicals.[137]

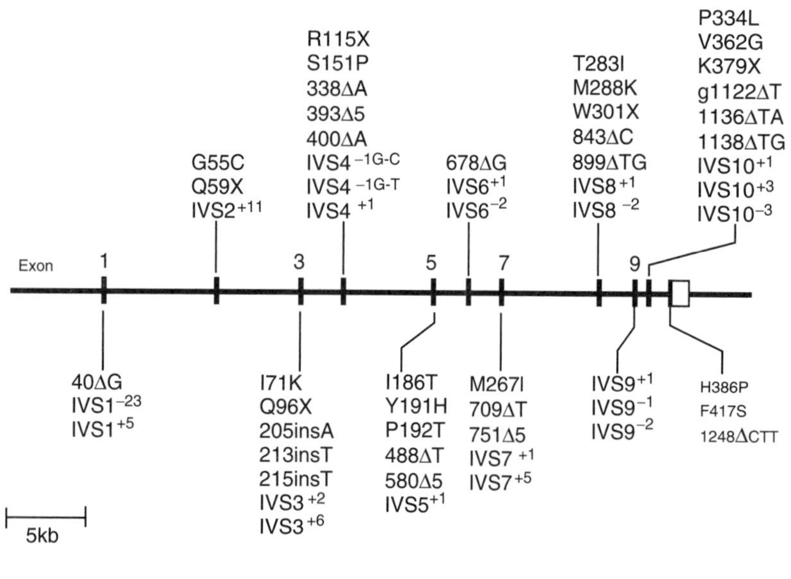

FIGURE 13–14. The human *ferrochelatase* gene and locations of mutations causing EPP. (Courtesy of Dr. K. H. Astrin.)

REFERENCES

1. McKay R, Druyan R, Getz GS, et al: Intramitochondrial localization of δ-aminolevulinate synthase and ferrochelatase in rat liver. Biochem J 1969; 114:455.
2. Granick S, Urata G: Increase in activity of δ-aminolevulinic acid synthetase in liver mitochondria induced by feeding of 3,5-dicarbethoxy–1,4-dihydrocollidine. J Biol Chem 1963; 238:821.
3. Riddle RD, Yamamoto M, Engel JD: Expression of δ-aminolevulinate synthase in avian cells: Separate genes encode erythroid-specific and nonspecific isozymes. Proc Natl Acad Sci USA 1989; 86:792.
4. Bishop DF, Astrin KH, Ioannou YA: Human δ-aminolevulinate synthase: Isolation, characterization, and mapping of house-keeping and erythroid-specific genes. Am J Hum Genet 45:A176, 1989.
5. Cox TC, Bawden MJ, Martin A, et al: Human erythroid 5-aminolevulinate synthase: Promoter analysis and identification of an iron-responsive element in the mRNA. EMBO J 1991; 10:1891.
6. Cotter PD, Baumann M, Bishop DF: Enzymatic defect in "X-linked" sideroblastic anemia: Molecular evidence for erythroid delta-aminolevulinate synthase deficiency. Proc Natl Acad Sci USA 1992; 89:4028.
7. Potluri VR, Astrin KH, Wetmur JG, et al: Human 5-aminolevulinate dehydratase: Chromosomal localization to 9q34 by in situ hybridization. Hum Genet 1987; 76:236.
8. Wetmur JG, Bishop DF, Ostasiewicz L, et al: Molecular cloning of a cDNA for human δ-aminolevulinate dehydratase. Gene 1986; 43:123.
9. Sassa S: δ-Aminolevulinic acid dehydratase assay. Enzyme 1982; 28:133.
10. Kaya AH, Plewinska M, Wong DM, et al: Human δ-aminolevulinate dehydratase (ALAD) gene: Structure and alternative splicing of the erythroid and housekeeping mRNAs. Genomics 1994; 19: 242–248.
11. Granick JL, Sassa S, Kappas A: Some biochemical and clinical aspects of lead intoxication. In Bodansky O, Latner AL (eds): Advances in Clinical Chemistry. New York, Academic Press, 1978, p 287.
12. Sassa S, Kappas A: Hereditary tyrosinemia and the heme biosynthetic pathway. Profound inhibition of δ-aminolevulinic acid dehydratase activity by succinylacetone. J Clin Invest 1983; 71:625.
13. Lindblad B, Lindstedt S, Steen G: On the genetic defects in hereditary tyrosinemia. Proc Natl Acad Sci USA 1977; 74:4641.
14. Meisler M, Wanner L, Eddy RE, et al: The UPS locus encoding uroporphyrinogen I synthase is located on human chromosome 11. Biochem Biophys Res Commun 1980; 95:170.
15. Chretien S, Dubart A, Beaupain D, et al: Alternative transcription and splicing of the human porphobilinogen deaminase gene result either in tissue-specific or in housekeeping expression. Proc Natl Acad Sci USA 1988; 85:6.
16. Grandchamp B, Beaumont C, de Verneuil H, et al: Genetic expression of porphobilinogen deaminase and uroporphyrinogen decarboxylase during the erythroid differentiation of mouse erythroleukemic cells. In Nordmann Y (ed): Porphyrins and Porphyrias. London, John Libbey, 1986, p 35.
17. Tsai SF, Bishop DF, Desnick RJ: Human uroporphyrinogen III synthase: Molecular cloning, nucleotide sequence, and expression of a full-length cDNA. Proc Natl Acad Sci USA 1988; 85:7049.
18. Astrin KH, Warner CA, Yoo HW, et al: Regional assignment of the human uroporphyrinogen III synthase (UROS) gene to chromosome 10q25.2—q26.3. Hum Genet 1991; 87:18.
19. Aizencang G, Solis C, Bishop DF, et al: Human uroporphyrinogen-III synthase: Genomic organization, alternative promoters, and erythroid-specific expression. Genomics 2000; 70:223.
20. Romeo P-H, Raich N, Dubart A, et al: Molecular cloning and nucleotide sequence of a complete human uroporphyrinogen decarboxylase cDNA. J Biol Chem 1986; 261:9825.
21. de Verneuil H, Grandchamp B, Foubert C, et al: Assignment of the gene for uroporphyrinogen decarboxylase to human chromosome 1 by somatic cell hybridization and specific enzyme immunoassay. Hum Genet 1984; 66:202.
22. Dubart A, Mattei MG, Raich N, et al: Assignment of human uroporphyrinogen decarboxylase (URO-D) to the p34 band of chromosome 1. Hum Genet 1986; 73:277.
23. Cacheux V, Martasek P, Fougerousse F, et al: Localization of the human coproporphyrinogen oxidase gene to chromosome band 3q12. Hum Genet 1994; 94:557.
24. Takahashi S, Taketani S, Akasaka J, et al: Differential regulation of mouse coproporphyrinogen oxidase gene expression in erythroid and non-erythroid cells. Blood 1998; 92:3436–3444.
25. Taketani S, Kohno H, Furukawa T, et al: Molecular cloning, sequencing and expression of cDNA encoding human coproporphyrinogen oxidase. Biochim Biophys Acta 1994; 1183:547.
26. Puy H, Robreau AM, Rosipal R, et al: Protoporphyrinogen oxidase: Complete genomic sequence and polymorphisms in the human gene. Biochem Biophys Res Commun 1996; 226:226.
27. Taketani S, Inazawa J, Abe T, et al: The human protoporphyrinogen oxidase gene (PPOX): Organization and location to chromosome 1. Genomics 1995; 29:698.
28. Roberts AG, Whatley SD, Daniels J, et al: Partial characterization and assignment of the gene for protoporphyrinogen oxidase and variegate porphyrias to human chromosome 1q23. Human Mol Genet 1995; 4:2387–2390.
29. Taketani S, Inazawa J, Nakahashi Y, et al: Structure of the human ferrochelatase gene: Exon/intron gene organization and location of the gene to chromosome 18. Eur J Biochem 1992; 205:217.
30. Nakahashi Y, Taketani S, Okuda M, et al: Molecular cloning and sequence analysis of cDNA encoding human ferrochelatase. Biochem Biophys Res Commun 1990; 173:748.
31. Sassa S, Granick S: Induction of δ-aminolevulinic acid synthetase in chick embryo liver cells in culture. Proc Natl Acad Sci USA 1970; 67:517.
32. Granick S, Sinclair P, Sassa S, et al: Effects by heme, insulin, and serum albumin on heme and protein synthesis in chick embryo liver cells cultured in a chemically defined medium, and a spectrofluorometric assay for porphyrin composition. J Biol Chem 1975; 250:9215.
33. Tenhunen R, Marver HS, Schmid R: The enzymatic catabolism of hemoglobin: Stimulation of microsomal heme oxygenase by hemin. J Lab Clin Med 1970; 75:410.
34. Shibahara S: Regulation of and physiological implication in heme catabolism. In Regulation of Heme Protein Synthesis. Miamisburg, OH, AlphaMed Press, 1994, p 103.
35. Sassa S: Heme biosynthesis in erythroid cells: The distinctive aspects of the regulatory mechanism. In Goldwasser E (ed): Regulation of Hemoglobin Biosynthesis. Harvard, MA, Elsevier/North Holland, 1983, p 359.
36. Sadlon TJ, Dell'Oso T, Surinya KH, et al: Regulation of erythroid 5-aminolevulinate synthase expression during erythropoiesis [review]. Int J Biochem Cell Biol 1999; 31:1153.
37. Dierks P: Molecular biology of eukaryotic 5-aminolevulinate synthase. In Dailey HA (ed): Biosynthesis of Heme and Chlorophylls, New York, McGraw-Hill, 1990, p 201.
38. Bhasker CR, Burgiel G, Neupert B, et al: The putative iron-responsive element in the human erythroid 5-aminolevulinate synthase mRNA mediates translational control. J Biol Chem 1993; 268:12699.
39. Ke Y, Wu J, Leibold EA, et al: Loops and bulge/loops in iron-responsive element isoforms influence iron regulatory protein binding. Fine-tuning of mRNA regulation? J Biol Chem 1998; 273:23637.
40. Nagai M, Nagai T, Yamamoto M, et al: Novel regulation of delta-aminolevulinate synthase in the rat harderian gland. Biochem Pharmacol 1997; 53:643.
41. Lim HW, Sassa S: The porphyrias. In Lim HW, Soter NA (eds): Photomedicine for Clinical Dermatologists. New York, Marcel Dekker, 1993, p 241.
42. Kappas A, Sassa S, Galbraith RA, et al: The porphyrias. In Scriver CR, Beaudet AL, Sly WS, et al (eds): The Metabolic and Molecular Basis of Inherited Disease. New York, McGraw-Hill, 1995, p 2103.
43. Doss M, von Tiepermann R, Schneider J, et al: New type of hepatic porphyria with porphobilinogen synthase defect and intermittent acute clinical manifestation. Klin Wochenschr 1979; 57:1123.
44. Thunell S, Holmberg L, Lundgren J: Aminolevulinate dehydratase porphyria in infancy. A clinical and biochemical study. J Clin Chem Clin Biochem 1987; 25:5.
45. Doss M, Schneider J, von Tiepermann R, et al: New type of acute porphyria with porphobilinogen synthase (δ-aminolevulinic acid dehydratase) defect in the homozygous state. Clin Biochem 1982; 15:52.
46. Akagi R, Shimizu R, Furuyama K, et al: Novel molecular defects of the δ-aminolevulinate dehydratase gene in a patient with inherited acute hepatic porphyria. Hepatology 2000; 31:704–708.

47. Ishida N, Fujita H, Fukuda Y, et al: Cloning and expression of the defective genes from a patient with δ-aminolevulinate dehydratase porphyria. J Clin Invest 1992; 89:1431.

48. Plewinska M, Thunell S, Holmberg L, et al: δ-Aminolevulinate dehydratase deficient porphyria: Identification of the molecular lesions in a severely affected homozygote. Am J Hum Genet 1991; 49:167.

49. Imagawa M, Tsuchiya T, Nishihara T: Identification of inducible genes at the early stage of adipocyte differentiation of 3T3-L1 cells. Biochem Biophys Res Commun 1999; 254:299.

50. Akagi R, Nishitani C, Harigae H, et al: Molecular analysis of δ-aminolevulinate dehydratase deficiency in a patient with an unusual late-onset porphyria. Blood 2000; 96:3618–3623.

51. Akagi R, Yasui Y, Harper P, et al: A novel mutation of δ-aminolaevulinate dehydratase in a healthy child with 12 percent erythrocyte enzyme activity. Br J Haematol 1999; 106:931.

52. Maruno M, Furuyama K, Akagi R, et al: Highly heterogenous nature of δ-aminolevulinate dehydratase (ALAD) deficiencies in ALAD porphyria. Blood 2001; 97:2972–2978.

53. Goldberg A, Moore MR, McColl KEL, et al: Porphyrin metabolism and the porphyrias. In Ledingham JGG, Warrell DA, Weatherall DJ (eds): Oxford Textbook of Medicine. Oxford, UK, Oxford University Press, 1987, p 9136.

54. Mustajoki P, Koskelo P: Hereditary hepatic porphyrias in Finland. Acta Med Scand 1976; 200:171.

55. Mustajoki P, Kauppinen R, Lannfelt L, et al: Frequency of low porphobilinogen deaminase activity in Finland. J Intern Med 1992; 231:389.

56. McColl KEL, Wallace AM, et al: Alterations in haem biosynthesis during the human menstrual cycle: Studies in normal subjects and patients with latent and active acute intermittent porphyria. Clin Sci 1982; 62:183.

57. Kappas A, Song CS, Levere RD, et al: The induction of δ-aminolevulinic acid synthetase in vivo in chick embryo liver by natural steroids. Proc Natl Acad Sci USA 1968; 61:509.

58. Sassa S, Bradlow HL, Kappas A: Steroid induction of δ-aminolevulinic acid synthase and porphyrins in liver. Structure-activity studies and the permissive effects of hormones on the induction process. J Biol Chem 1979; 254:10011.

59. Felsher BF, Redeker AG: Acute intermittent porphyria: Effect of diet and griseofulvin. Medicine (Baltimore) 1967; 46:217.

60. Welland FH, Hellman ES, Gaddis EM, et al: Factors affecting the excretion of porphyrin precursors by patients with acute intermittent porphyria. I. The effects of diet. Metabolism 1964; 13:232.

61. Mauzerall D, Granick S: The occurrence and determination of δ-aminolevulinic acid and porphobilinogen in urine. J Biol Chem 1956; 219:435.

62. Grandchamp B, Picat C, de Rooij F, et al: A point mutation G→A in exon 12 of the porphobilinogen deaminase gene results in exon skipping and is responsible for acute intermittent porphyria. Nucleic Acids Res 1989; 17:6637.

63. Llewellyn DH, Kalsheker NA, Elder GH, et al: A *MspI* polymorphism for the human porphobilinogen deaminase gene. Nucleic Acids Res 1987; 15:1349.

64. Lee JS, Anvret M: A *PstI* polymorphism for the human porphobilinogen deaminase gene (PBG). Nucleic Acids Res 1987; 15:6307.

65. Picat C, Bourgeois F, Grandchamp B: PCR detection of a C/T polymorphism in exon 1 of the porphobilinogen deaminase gene (PBGD). Nucleic Acids Res 1988; 19:5099.

66. Gu X-F, Lee JS, Delfau MH, et al: PCR detection of a G/T polymorphism at exon 10 of the porphobilinogen deaminase gene (PBG-D). Nucleic Acids Res 1991; 19:1966.

67. Lee JS, Anvret M, Lindsten J, et al: DNA polymorphisms within the porphobilinogen deaminase gene in two Swedish families with acute intermittent porphyria. Hum Genet 1988; 79:379.

68. Daimon M, Morita Y, Yamatani K, et al: Two new polymorphisms in introns 2 and 3 of the human porphobilinogen deaminase gene. Hum Genet 1993; 92:115.

69. Schreiber WE, Jamani A, Ritchie B: Detection of a T/C polymorphism in the porphobilinogen deaminase gene by polymerase chain reaction amplification of specific alleles [letter]. Clin Chem 1992; 38:2153.

70. Sagen E, Laegreid A, Anvret M, et al: Genetic carrier detection in Norwegian families with acute intermittent porphyria. Scand J Clin Lab Invest 1993; 53:687.

71. Mustajoki P, Tenhunen R, Pierach C, et al: Heme in the treatment of porphyrias and hematological disorders. Semin Hematol 1989; 26:1.

72. Anderson KE, Spitz IM, Sassa S, et al: Prevention of cyclical attacks of acute intermittent porphyria with a long-acting agonist of luteinizing hormone-releasing hormone. N Engl J Med 1984; 311:643.

73. Galbraith RA, Kappas A: Pharmacokinetics of tin-mesoporphyrin in man and the effects of tin-chelated porphyrins on hyperexcretion of heme pathway precursors in patients with acute inducible porphyria. Hepatology 1989; 9:882.

74. Schmid R, Schwartz S, Sundberg RD: Erythropoietic (congenital) porphyria: A rare abnormality of normoblasts. Blood 1955; 10:416.

75. Deybach J-C, de Verneuil H, Boulechfar S, et at: Point mutations in the uroporphyrinogen III synthase gene in congenital erythropoietic porphyria (Gunther's disease). Blood 1990; 75:1763.

76. Warner CA, Yoo HW, Roberts AG, et al: Congenital erythropoietic porphyria: Identification of exonic mutations in the uroporphyrinogen III synthase gene. J Clin Invest 1992; 89:693.

77. Seip M, Thune PO, Eriksen L: Treatment of photosensitivity in congenital erythropoietic porphyria (CEP) with beta-carotene. Acta Derm Venereol 1974; 54:239.

78. Haining RG, Cowger ML, Labbe RF, et al: Congenital erythropoietic porphyria. II. The effects of induced polycythemia. Blood 1970; 36:297.

79. Varadi S: Haemotological aspects in a case of erythropoietic porphyria. Br J Haematol 1958; 4:270.

80. Pimstone NR, Gandhi SN, Mukerji SK: Therapeutic efficacy of oral charcoal in congenital erythropoietic porphyria. N Engl J Med 1987; 316:390.

81. de Verneuil H, Nordmann Y, Phung N, et al: Familial and sporadic porphyria cutanea: Two different diseases. Int J Biochem 1978; 9:927.

82. Elder GH, Lee GB, Tovey JA: Decreased activity of hepatic uroporphyrinogen decarboxylase in sporadic porphyria cutanea tarda. N Engl J Med 1978; 299:274.

83. Elder GH: Human uroporphyrinogen decarboxylase defects. In Orfanos CS, Stadler R, Gollnick H (eds): Dermatology in Five Continents. Berlin, Springer-Verlag, 1988, p 857.

84. Held JL, Sassa S, Kappas A, et al: Erythrocyte uroporphyrinogen decarboxylase activity in porphyria cutanea tarda: A study of 40 consecutive patients. J Invest Dermatol 1989; 93:332.

85. Lim HW, Poh-Fitzpatrick MB, Gigli I: Activation of the complement system in patients with porphyrias after irradiation in vivo. J Clin Invest 1984; 74:1961.

86. Meurer M, Schulte C, Weiler A, et al: Photodynamic action of uroporphyrin on the complement system in porphyria cutanea tarda. Arch Dermatol Res 1985; 277:293.

87. Torinuki W, Miura T, Tagami H: Activation of complement by 405-nm light in serum from porphyria cutanea tarda. Arch Dermatol Res 1985; 277:174.

88. Pigatto PD, Polenghi MM, Altomare GF, et al: Complement cleavage products in the phototoxic reaction of porphyria cutanea tarda. Br J Dermatol 1986; 114:567.

89. Sandberg S, Romslo I, Hovding G, et al: Porphyrin-induced photodamage as related to the subcellular localization of the porphyrins. Acta Derm Venereol Suppl 1982; 100:75.

90. Herrero C, Vicente A, Bruguera M, et al: Is hepatitis C virus infection a trigger of porphyria cutanea tarda? Lancet 1993; 341:788–789.

91. Pierach CA: Porphyria and hepatocellular carcinoma. Br J Cancer 1987; 55:111.

92. Wissel PS, Sordillo P, Anderson KE, et al: Porphyria cutanea tarda associated with the acquired immune deficiency syndrome. Am J Hematol 1987; 25:107.

93. Lobato MN, Berger TG: Porphyria cutanea tarda associated with the acquired immunodeficiency syndrome. Arch Dermatol 1988; 124:1009.

94. Blauvelt A, Harris HR, Hogan DJ, et al: Porphyria cutanea tarda and human immunodeficiency virus infection. Int J Dermatol 1992; 31:474.

95. Lockwood WH, Poulos V, Rossi E, et al: Rapid procedure for fecal porphyrin assay. Clin Chem 1985; 31:1163.

96. Topi GC, Amantea A, Griso D: Recovery from porphyria cutanea tarda with no specific therapy other than avoidance of hepatic toxins. Br J Dermatol 1984; 111:75.

97. Ippen H: Allgemeine Symptome. Der späten Hautporphyrie (porphyria cutanea tarda) als Hinweise für deren Behandlung. Dtsch Med Wochenschr 1961; 86:127.

98. Ippen H: Treatment of porphyria cutanea tarda by phlebotomy. Semin Hematol 1977; 14:253.

99. Felsher BF, Redeker AG: Effect of chloroquine on hepatic uroporphyrin metabolism in patients with porphyria cutanea tarda. Medicine (Baltimore) 1966; 45:575.

100. Elder GH, Smith SG, Herrero C, et al: Hepatoerythropoietic porphyria: A new uroporphyrinogen decarboxylase defect or homozygous porphyria cutanea tarda? Lancet 1981;1:916.

101. Toback AC, Sassa S, Poh Fitzpatrick MB, et al: Hepatoerythropoietic porphyria: Clinical, biochemical, and enzymatic studies in a three-generation family lineage. N Engl J Med 1987; 316:645.

102. Romeo P-H, Raich N, Dubart A, et al: Molecular cloning and tissue-specific expression analysis of human porphobilinogen deaminase and uroporphyrinogen decarboxylase. In Nordmann Y (ed): Porphyrins and Porphyrias London, John Libbey, 1986, p 25.

103. Roberts AG, Elder GH, De Salamanca RE, et al: A mutation (G281E) of the human uroporphyrinogen decarboxylase gene causes both hepatoerythropoietic porphyria and overt familial porphyria cutanea tarda: Biochemical and genetic studies on Spanish patients. J Invest Dermatol 1995; 104:500.

104. Moran-Jimenez MJ, Ged C, Romana M, et al: Uroporphyrinogen decarboxylase: Complete human gene sequence and molecular study of three families with hepatoerythropoietic porphyria. Am J Hum Genet 1996; 58:712.

105. Garey JR, Hansen JL, Harrison LM, et al: A point mutation in the coding region of uroporphyrinogen decarboxylase associated with familial porphyria cutanea tarda. Blood 1989; 73:892.

106. Garey JR, Harrison LM, Franklin KF, et al: Uroporphyrinogen decarboxylase: A splice site mutation causes the deletion of exon 6 in multiple families with porphyria cutanea tarda. J Clin Invest 1990; 86:1416.

107. McManus JF, Begley CG, Sassa S, et al: Five new mutations in the uroporphyrinogen decarboxylase gene identified in families with cutaneous porphyria. Blood 1996; 88:3589.

108. Mendez M, Sorkin L, Rossetti MV, et al: Familial porphyria cutanea tarda: Characterization of seven novel uroporphyrinogen decarboxylase mutations and frequency of common hemochromatosis alleles. Am J Hum Genet 1998; 63:1363.

109. Elder GH: Porphyria cutanea tarda [review]. Semin Liver Dis 1998; 18:67.

110. Garey JR, Franklin KF, Brown DA, et al: Analysis of uroporphyrinogen decarboxylase complementary DNAs in sporadic porphyria cutanea tarda. Gastroenterology 1993; 105:165.

111. de Verneuil H, Grandchamp B, Beaumont C, et al: Uroporphyrinogen decarboxylase structural mutant (Gly281 Glu) in a case of porphyria. Science 1986; 234:732.

112. de Verneuil H, Grandchamp B, Romeo P-H, et al: Molecular analysis of uroporphyrinogen decarboxylase deficiency in a family with two cases of hepatoerythropoietic porphyria. J Clin Invest 1986; 77:431.

113. Human Gene Mutation Database: Available at www.uwcm.ac.uk/uwcm/mg/hgmd0.html.

114. Meguro K, Fujita H, Ishida N, et al: Molecular defects of uroporphyrinogen decarboxylase in a patient with mild hepatoerythropoietic porphyria. J Invest Dermatol 1994; 102:681.

115. Grandchamp B, Phung N, Nordmann Y: Homozygous case of hereditary coproporphyria [letter]. Lancet 1977; 2:1348.

116. Martasek P: Hereditary coproporphyria [review]. Semin Liver Dis 1998; 18:25.

117. Rosipal R, Lamoril J, Puy H, et al: Systematic analysis of coproporphyrinogen oxidase gene defects in hereditary coproporphyria and mutation update. Hum Mutat 1999; 13:44.

118. Martasek P, Nordmann Y, Grandchamp B: Homozygous hereditary coproporphyria caused by an arginine to tryptophane substitution in coproporphyrinogen oxidase and common intragenic polymorphisms. Hum Mol Genet 1994; 3:477.

119. Nordmann Y, Grandchamp B, de Verneuil H, et al: Harderoporphyria: A variant hereditary coproporphyria. J Clin Invest 1983; 72:1139.

120. Kordac V, Martasek P, Zeman J, et al: Increased erythrocyte protoporphyrin in homozygous variegate porphyria. Photo-Dermatology 1985; 2:257.

121. Murphy GM, Hawk JL, Magnus IA, et al: Homozygous variegate porphyria: Two similar cases in unrelated families. J R Soc Med 1986; 79:361.

122. Mustajoki P, Tenhunen R, Niemi KM, et al: Homozygous variegate porphyria. A severe skin disease of infancy. Clin Genet 1987; 32:300.

123. Eales L, Day RS, Blekkenhorst GH: The clinical and biochemical features of variegate porphyria: An analysis of 300 cases studied at Groote Schuur Hospital, Cape Town. Int J Biochem 1980; 12:837.

124. Dean G: The Porphyrias. A Study of Inheritance and Environment. London, Pitman Medical, 1971.

125. Rimington C, Lockwood WH, Belcher RV: The excretion of porphyrin-peptide conjugates in porphyria variegata. Clin Sci 1968; 35:211.

126. Meissner PN, Dailey TA, Hift RJ, et al: A R59W mutation in human protoporphyrinogen oxidase results in decreased enzyme activity and is prevalent in South Africans with variegate porphyria. Nat Genet 1996; 13, 95–97.

127. Roberts AG, Puy H, Dailey TA, et al: Molecular characterization of homozygous variegate porphyria. Hum Mol Genet 1998; 7:1921–1925.

128. Frank J, McGrath J, Lam H, et al: Homozygous variegate porphyria: Identification of mutations on both alleles of the protoporphyrinogen oxidase gene in a severely affected proband [review]. J Invest Dermatol 1998; 110:452.

129. Romana M, Grandchamp B, Dubart A, et al: Identification of a new mutation responsible for hepatoerythropoietic porphyria. Eur J Clin Invest 1991; 21:225.

130. Spikes JD: Porphyrins and related compounds as photodynamic sensitizers. Ann NY Acad Sci 1975; 244:496.

131. Sandberg S, Talstad I, Hovding G, et al: Light-induced release of protoporphyrin, but not of zinc protoporphyrin, from erythrocytes in a patient with greatly elevated erythropoietic protoporphyria. Blood 1983; 62:846.

132. Bottomley SS, Tanaka M, Everett MA: Diminished erythroid ferrochelatase activity in protoporphyria. J Lab Clin Med 1975; 86:126.

133. Gouya L, Deybach JC, Lamoril J, et al: Modulation of the phenotype in dominant erythropoietic protoporphyria by a low expression of the normal ferrochelatase allele. Am J Hum Genet 1996; 58:292.

134. Gouya L, Puy H, Lamoril J, et al: Inheritance in erythropoietic protoporphyria: A common wild-type ferrochelatase allelic variant with low expression accounts for clinical manifestation. Blood 1999; 93:2105.

135. Lamoril J, Boulechfar S, de Verneuil H, et al: Human erythropoietic protoporphyria: Two point mutations in the ferrochelatase gene. Biochem Biophys Res Commun 1991; 181:594.

136. Mathews-Roth MM: Systemic photoprotection. Dermatol Clin 1986; 4:335.

137. Mathews-Roth MM, Pathak MA, Fitzpatrick TB, et al: Beta carotene therapy for erythropoietic protoporphyria and other photosensitivity diseases. Arch Dermatol 1977; 113:1229.

V | Hemolytic Anemias

Autoimmune Hemolytic Anemia

Disorders of the Erythrocyte Membrane

Pyruvate Kinase Deficiency and Disorders of Glycolysis

Glucose-6-Phosphate Dehydrogenase Deficiency and Hemolytic Anemia

14 | Autoimmune Hemolytic Anemia

Russell E. Ware

The vast majority of erythrocyte disorders that occur in the pediatric age-group result from abnormalities within the red blood cell; that is, they are intracorpuscular defects. These intrinsic red cell defects include a wide variety of inherited genetic mutations as well as acquired nutritional deficiencies and lead to defects in globin chain and heme synthesis, abnormal membrane structural proteins, or defective intracellular enzymes. Particularly in the congenital conditions, intracorpuscular defects often lead to a shortened erythrocyte life span, premature destruction of the erythrocytes (hemolysis), and anemia.

A less common category of erythrocyte disorders includes conditions characterized by abnormalities external to the red cells, known as extracorpuscular defects. Examples include environmental stress (oxidation, heat, or mechanical injury), microangiopathic erythrocyte damage (hemolytic-uremic syndrome or thrombotic thrombocytopenic purpura), or immune-mediated red blood cell destruction. Like many of the intrinsic condi-

tions, extrinsic erythrocyte disorders are typically associated with hemolysis and anemia.

Conditions that result from abnormal interactions between erythrocytes and the immune system are collectively referred to as immune-mediated hemolytic anemia. The most common type is *autoimmune hemolytic anemia (AIHA)*, characterized by the presence of autoantibodies that bind to the erythrocyte surface membrane and lead to premature red cell destruction. Specific characteristics of the autoantibodies, particularly the isotype, thermal reactivity, and ability to fix complement, help shape the resulting clinical picture. In all patients with AIHA, however, the autoantibody leads to a shortened red blood cell survival, hemolysis, and anemia. The reticuloendothelial system, primarily the spleen, plays a critical role in the premature destruction of erythrocytes in immune-mediated hemolytic anemia.

This chapter begins with a description of the spleen, whose anatomy and physiology provide a unique environment for the clearance of normal and abnormal erythrocytes.

Three important clinical forms of AIHA are then described: (1) *warm-reactive AIHA,* characterized by an autoantibody (usually immunoglobulin [Ig] G) that binds preferentially to erythrocyte antigens at 37°C, fixes complement in some cases, and leads to extravascular hemolysis; (2) *paroxysmal cold hemoglobinuria (PCH),* in which an IgG erythrocyte autoantibody binds optimally at 4°C, fixes complement efficiently, and causes intravascular hemolysis; and (3) *cold agglutinin disease,* characterized by an autoantibody (typically IgM) that binds optimally to erythrocytes below 37°C, fixes complement efficiently, and also leads primarily to intravascular hemolysis. These three disorders are discussed together because of their many similarities, although differences in pathophysiology and therapy are emphasized. The next section describes *paroxysmal nocturnal hemoglobinuria (PNH),* a rare and fascinating acquired hematologic disorder that features hemolysis due to abnormal interactions between erythrocytes and the complement system. Unlike true AIHA, the defect in PNH is intracorpuscular, but the presentation and clinical manifestations may be similar. Advances in the understanding of PNH are described, including its recognition as an acquired clonal stem cell disorder and the identification of specific acquired mutations in the phosphatidylinositol glycan Class A *(PIGA)* gene in affected patients. Finally, miscellaneous extracorpuscular disorders that lead to *schistocytic hemolytic anemia* are described, including microangiopathy, preeclampsia, and environmental stress such as heat or mechanical injury.

THE SPLEEN

Historical Perspective

Since ancient times, the spleen has occupied a mysterious niche among organs of the human body. Its proposed functions and necessity for good health were a subject of debate and discussion for centuries, as recently reviewed.[1] Only in the last few decades has this enigmatic organ begun to yield its secrets, revealing its prominent and vital role in providing important hematologic and immunologic functions.

Hippocrates believed that the spleen helped balance the body's "humors," a process necessary to promote harmony and stability. Plato and Aristotle agreed with this notion of the spleen absorbing unhealthy body fluids, but further suggested it assisted or balanced the liver, based on its location. Galen noted the anatomical connections among the spleen, liver, and stomach and concluded that the spleen had true digestive functions that included the filtering of humoral impurities. Subsequently, the spleen gained a reputation for controlling feelings and emotions including laughter, ill temper, melancholy, and others. Shakespeare often referred to the spleen as an organ of anger, merriment, or other strong emotion.

During the Renaissance, when the study of anatomy and physiology became popularized, the spleen's microscopic patterns supported a role for filtration; however, only circulatory connections between the spleen and the stomach, liver, and other digestive organs could be identified. Moreover, the survival of both animals and humans after surgical splenectomy demonstrated that the spleen

was not absolutely required for life. Only in the modern era, with the discovery of individual blood cells, have investigators begun to elucidate the true functions of the spleen. We now recognize that the spleen has vital roles for blood filtration and immunologic competence.

Anatomy and Physiology

The spleen can be identified in human embryogenesis during week 5 of gestation, although the development of characteristic splenic architecture with influx of red and white blood cells occurs much later in gestation. At birth the spleen weighs about 10 g and then it grows steadily to 30 g at 1 year of age, to 60 g by age 5 years, and finally to the adult size of approximately 200 g.[2] The spleen is located under the confines of the left anterior ribcage, and can have a triangular, crescent, or rhomboidal shape. Although not accurate as a measure of total splenic volume, spleen size is usually estimated based on length alone, specifically how far below the left costal margin the tip of the spleen can be palpated.

The spleen receives about 6 percent of the total cardiac output, making it a highly perfused organ.[3] Blood enters and leaves the spleen primarily through the splenic artery and vein, respectively, both located at the hilum on the concave (medial) side of the organ. Within the splenic parenchyma, the splenic arterial branches have little overlap, allowing classification of the spleen into lobes and segments that are separated by relatively avascular planes.

Histologically, the spleen can be separated into two distinct regions, the red pulp and the white pulp, so named because of the blood cells most commonly found in each area. The red pulp represents a large open circulation within the spleen, through which the erythrocytes pass slowly for filtration and culling functions. In contrast, the white pulp consists primarily of collections of lymphocytes and macrophages, which form small white nodules (1 to 2 mm in diameter) distributed throughout the splenic parenchyma. These two regions provide the vital functions of blood filtration and immunologic response, respectively, which are made possible through a unique circulation pattern found within the spleen. In Figure 14–1 the arterial and venous circulations of the spleen are diagrammed, illustrating the close proximity of the red and white pulp.

As the largest arteries within the spleen branch progressively into the smallest arterioles, the white pulp can be recognized as a circumferential ring of leukocytes that surround the vessel, also known as the periarterial (or periarteriolar) lymphoid sheath (PALS). The PALS consists primarily of T lymphocytes, and this cylindrical cuff of cells becomes thinner as the artery becomes smaller. Spheroidal lymphoid follicles arise at intervals from the PALS, usually where arterial branch points occur, and these follicles contain primarily B lymphocytes (Fig. 14–2). When immunologically stimulated, these primary lymphoid follicles develop into secondary follicles with germinal centers, similar to the processes and architecture observed within lymph nodes. Lymphocytes within the white pulp are the beneficiaries of plasma "skimmed" from the central arterial blood supply. Whereas the blood cells tend to continue within the vessel, plasma elements

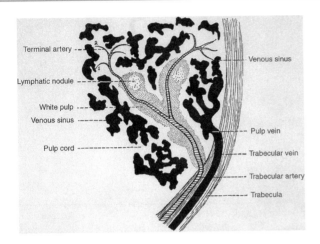

FIGURE 14–1. Blood circulation in the spleen. As blood enters the spleen, the arterial vessels are surrounded by lymphatic sheaths and nodules that comprise the white pulp. The majority of the arterial blood terminates into venous sinuses (red pulp) that allow filtration and quality control of erythrocytes. Erythrocytes return to the venous circulation via the venous sinuses. (From Fawcett D: A Textbook of Histology, 11th ed. Philadelphia, WB Saunders, 1985, p 474.)

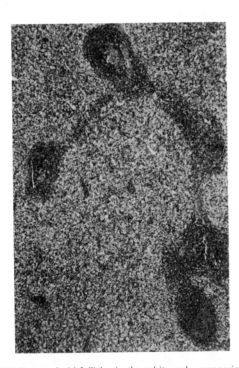

FIGURE 14–2. Lymphoid follicles in the white pulp, appearing as bud-like outgrowths from the periarteriolar lymphoid sheath. (From Neiman RS, Orazi A (eds): Disorders of the Spleen, 2nd ed. Philadelphia, WB Saunders 1999, p 10.)

enter the PALS via tiny vessels that arise perpendicular to the blood flow. Soluble antigens are thus herded into the white pulp, where they encounter dendritic cells and macrophages that function as professional antigen-presenting cells, allowing proper immune stimulation of the T and B lymphocytes.

After plasma is redirected toward the white pulp, the blood cells that continue through the splenic circulation are mostly erythrocytes, and they form the red pulp as

they exit the arteries. Occasionally, erythrocytes pass directly from the arterial to the venous circulation via traditional endothelialized capillaries, a process known as the closed (rapid) splenic circulation that is primarily nutritive. Much more commonly, however, erythrocytes leave the arterial circulation and empty into large pools called the splenic cords, in which they encounter macrophages and other immune effector cells. The erythrocytes must survive these intimate encounters in this hypoxic and acidic environment and then pass from the cords through an endothelialized barrier into the splenic sinuses and finally back to the venous circulation. This open (slow) circulation allows careful filtration of individual erythrocytes, with repair or phagocytosis of cells that cannot successfully negotiate this return trip.

Important Functions of the Spleen

All red blood cells pass through the spleen many times each day.[4, 5] The spleen serves as an efficient filter for erythrocytes and is able to perform grooming (removal of antibodies or other surface molecules), culling (destruction of cells), and pitting functions (removal of intracellular material). While moving slowly through the hostile environment of the splenic cords, erythrocytes are carefully examined for abnormalities, a process constituting a biologic form of quality control. Macrophages in the red pulp identify abnormal erythrocytes, such as those that have IgG or complement on their surface, and either remove a portion of their membrane or fully engulf them. Newly made reticulocytes spend their first day or two in the spleen,[6] during which the cells appear to be groomed with removal of cytoplasmic organelles and surface adhesion molecules. Normal mature erythrocytes, in contrast, typically endure macrophage scrutiny without difficulties. To leave the red pulp, erythrocytes must then pass from the splenic cords through potential spaces in the endothelial lining of the splenic sinuses. To negotiate these tiny apertures, known as the cords of Billroth, the erythrocytes must deform themselves substantially (Fig. 14–3). Cordal macrophages phagocytose erythrocytes that cannot deform themselves sufficiently, such as senescent cells; as erythrocytes age, they lose volume and gain density and eventually lose deformability that allows reentry into the splenic sinus. In certain pathologic conditions such as immune-mediated hemolytic anemia, as well as a variety of erythrocyte membrane, hemoglobin, or enzyme disorders, younger erythrocytes also can be trapped in the splenic cords. Erythrocytes with intracellular inclusions such as nuclear remnants (Howell-Jolly bodies), denatured hemoglobin (Heinz bodies), siderotic granules (Pappenheimer bodies), or malarial parasites have their inclusions "pitted" out because they cannot pass through the endothelial slits.

The spleen also provides several important immunologic functions. Skimming of plasma into the PALS allows particulate antigens to interact with dendritic cells and other antigen-presenting cells, which initiates the immune response for T and B lymphocyte proliferation. Polysaccharide antigens in particular require this unique immunologic environment for optimal antibody responses.[7, 8] Intravenous antigens, such as those found

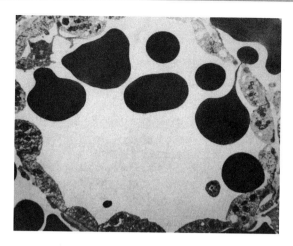

FIGURE 14–3. Deformation of erythrocytes returning from the splenic cords (red pulp) back into the venous sinus. The erythrocytes must pass through very small potential spaces in the sinus wall known as the cords of Billroth. (From Neiman RS, Orazi A (eds): Disorders of the Spleen, 2nd ed. Philadelphia, WB Saunders 1999, p 18.)

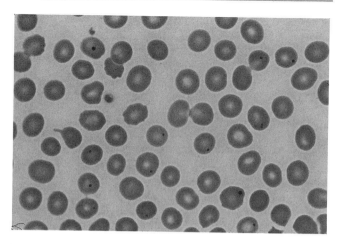

FIGURE 14–4. Howell-Jolly bodies in peripheral blood erythrocytes. These nuclear remnants are identified as small inclusions within circulating erythrocytes and have several characteristic and required features by light microscopy: (1) they are spherical inclusions that are 0.5 to 2.0 μ in diameter, about the size of a small platelet; (2) they have a smooth contour and no surrounding halo, thereby distinguishing them from platelets juxtaposed to an erythrocyte; (3) they are always in the same focal plane as the erythrocyte, because they are intracellular; (4) they are never refractile, unlike talc or dust particles; and (5) they are homogeneous in appearance, unlike other intracellular inclusions such as Pappenheimer bodies or malarial parasites. Howell-Jolly bodies are normally removed when the erythrocytes pass through the cords of Billroth into the venous sinus. Their presence in the peripheral blood indicates a lack of splenic function (see color section at front of this volume).

during an infection or after an immunization, are primarily processed by the spleen.[9] Not surprisingly, normal splenic function is required for an optimal early (IgM) response, as well as the secondary (IgG) response, to most intravenous antigens.[10] In contrast, antigens administered by intramuscular or subcutaneous routes do not require normal splenic function for robust immune response.[11, 12] Finally, blood-borne bacteria, particularly encapsulated organisms, are removed by splenic macrophages located in the PALS and in the cords. Without a functioning spleen, patients are susceptible to overwhelming bacterial sepsis and to exaggerated parasitemia from *Plasmodium*, *Babesia*, or other organisms.[13, 14]

To a much lesser extent, the human spleen also can serve as a reservoir for circulating blood cells. About 50 mL of blood are normally contained in the normal spleen, as well as 30 percent of the platelet mass. In the abnormal state (see later), the spleen can enlarge and trap a larger portion of the circulating blood cells. The spleen also may serve a small role in iron metabolism and homeostasis. Unlike the spleen in other species, however, the spleen has no appreciable role in human hematopoiesis.

Abnormalities of the Spleen

Congenital asplenia is found in children with the rare Ivemark syndrome, in which the body has bilateral "right-sidedness" with trilobed lungs and a centralized liver.[15] Cardiac defects are common, as well as a risk of infection.[16] The uptake of radionuclide by functioning splenic tissue can be difficult to document, because anatomic features are distorted, and liver tissue can obscure any splenic uptake. Circulating erythrocytes with Howell-Jolly bodies or intracellular vesicles that appear as "pits" or "pocks" allow the diagnosis of asplenia to be made noninvasively.[17] Figure 14–4 illustrates the Howell-Jolly bodies that are found in the peripheral blood smear of an asplenic person. The converse arrangement of bilateral "left-sidedness" leads to congenital polysplenia, with several spleens of varying sizes. In most patients the splenic

tissue in polysplenia has normal function. Cardiac defects are common, however, as well as hepatobiliary abnormalities.[18, 19]

Accessory spleens can be identified in 15 percent of normal persons.[20] In most of these, a single accessory spleen, measuring only 1 to 2 cm in diameter, is present either in the splenic hilum or in the tail of the pancreas. Multiple accessory spleens can exist, however, as well as ectopic spleens in locations ranging from the abdomen to the pelvis to the scrotum. The function of accessory spleens depends upon the quality and quantity of blood flow; in most instances the filtration capabilities are minimal but antibody responses may be present.

Splenoptosis, or wandering spleen, occurs when the spleen is not fixed within the retroperitoneum.[21] The resulting mass can be palpated anywhere in the abdomen and may require reattachment (splenopexy) or even splenectomy if symptoms of sequestration or torsion develop.[22] Splenosis refers to the autotransplantation of splenic tissue into the omentum or peritoneal surfaces of the abdominal cavity. Splenosis typically occurs after fracture or rupture of the spleen, from spillage and subsequent implantation of splenocytes. Although some protection against infection may be afforded by splenosis,[23] filtering functions and immunologic responses are limited by the relatively small total amount of splenic tissue and reduced blood supply.

Sequestration refers to enlargement of the spleen that occurs when blood enters the organ but is unable to exit properly. This condition is most often observed in children with sickle cell anemia, when venous return of blood is hindered by intrasplenic sickling of erythrocytes in the red pulp. Splenic sequestration can also occur in other settings with abnormal erythrocytes, however, including congenital spherocytosis. Splenic sequestration can develop acutely with sudden pooling of blood within the spleen, causing rapid and painful expansion of the splenic parenchyma and capsule. Children are seen with pallor, fatigue, severe anemia, and occasionally hypovolemic shock.[24] Occasionally, splenic sequestration develops over a period of days or weeks and is then termed subacute or chronic because it presents with relatively asymptomatic splenomegaly.

Hypersplenism refers to the condition of splenomegaly with nonimmune-mediated trapping of peripheral blood cells, resulting in mild to moderate cytopenia.[25] Hypersplenism can develop in patients with abnormal erythrocytes, metabolic storage disorders, or other causes of chronic congestive splenomegaly. In these clinical settings, the spleen first enlarges because of progressive trapping of erythrocytes or storage material, then subsequently becomes a reservoir for all circulating blood cells. Typically, both the peripheral platelet and leukocyte counts are less than normal, but the former especially is seen. If surgery is required, peripheral blood counts normalize after splenectomy.

Surgery Involving the Spleen

Although the spleen has important hematologic and immunologic functions, there are occasions when its surgical removal is beneficial. A variety of congenital anomalies of the spleen, as well as numerous pathophysiologic processes, are indications for splenectomy.

Benign tumors of the spleen are relatively rare in childhood, but primarily include congenital cysts (epidermoid or lymphangiomatous) or pseudocysts that reflect liquefaction of splenic parenchyma after infarction or hemorrhage. These tumors may require splenectomy, depending upon their size. Malignant splenic tumors are almost always lymphomatous or leukemic in origin, with cancerous cells found diffusely or in a nodular pattern throughout the splenic parenchyma. Somewhat surprisingly, very few solid tumors metastasize to the spleen. Overall, splenectomy is usually not indicated in the setting of malignancy.

Splenomegaly requiring splenectomy may develop in a variety of clinical settings, including metabolic storage disorders such as Gaucher disease, transfusion-acquired iron overload from chronic erythrocyte transfusions, or splenic congestion resulting from portal hypertension. Commonly, splenectomy is the recommended therapeutic option for splenic enlargement in patients with erythrocyte abnormalities. Congenital hemoglobin, enzyme, and membrane disorders lead to trapping of the abnormal erythrocytes within the splenic cords and expansion of the red pulp. In these settings, splenectomy can relieve the signs and symptoms of splenomegaly including abdominal discomfort, anemia, hypersplenism, and dependence on transfusions.

Total surgical splenectomy is usually performed via an open laparotomy using a left subcostal incision. Laparoscopic splenectomy is becoming a popular alternative, but requires careful attention to technical details[26]

and may not be appropriate for large spleens.[27] With the laparoscopic approach occasionally small amounts of residual splenic tissue may be left or accessory spleens may be missed,[28] which can be a problem for patients with immune-mediated hematologic disorders. When splenectomy is necessary for AIHA or immune thrombocytopenia purpura, all splenic tissue must be removed to prevent recurrent autoantibody production. Over the past decade, subtotal (partial) splenectomy has become a viable therapeutic alternative to total splenectomy. The partial splenectomy approach is possible because the spleen can be divided into distinct lobes and segments.[29] Removal of 80 to 90 percent of the enlarged spleen usually provides relief from splenomegaly while retaining sufficient splenic tissue for immune competence. Partial splenectomy has been used successfully in children with spherocytosis,[30] homozygous β-thalassemia,[31] and sickle cell disease,[32] although splenic regrowth may limit its long-term efficacy.[33] Based on animal studies, one third of the normal spleen mass is required for normal plasma filtration and antibody formation.[34] Compared with reimplanted splenic tissue, either by surgical autotransplantation or splenosis, partial splenectomy provides superior retained immune function.[35–37]

The primary danger after total splenectomy is the risk of fatal bacterial sepsis, sometimes referred to as overwhelming postsplenectomy infection (OPSI). First recognized 50 years ago,[38] the patient without splenic function can abruptly develop bacteremia that evolves rapidly into fatal sepsis with or without meningitis. Pathogens associated with OPSI are primarily encapsulated bacterial organisms including *Streptococcus pneumoniae*, *Haemophilus influenzae* type b, and *Neisseria meningitidis*. The presumed pathophysiologic origin of OPSI is the loss of plasma filtration by the spleen, which allows bacteria to multiply within the bloodstream from a low-grade bacteremia to fulminant sepsis. Risk factors for OPSI include a younger age at clinical presentation, a younger age at splenectomy, and failure to comply with prophylactic antibiotics or vaccinations. The true risk of development of OPSI has been estimated in two large studies, although many of the patients are from the prevaccination era. First, in a literature review covering 35 years from 1952 to 1987 (5902 patients), the incidence of infection after splenectomy in children younger than 16 years old was 4.4 percent with a mortality rate of 2.2 percent; for adults the corresponding values were 0.9 percent and 0.8 percent, respectively. Children younger than age 5 years, and especially infants, had a much higher risk of sepsis.[39] In a survey of 226 splenectomized patients with hereditary spherocytosis with 5461 years of postoperative follow-up, the estimated mortality rate was 0.73/1000 years for the entire group, but somewhat higher for children.[40] Since these earlier times, the introduction of polysaccharide pneumococcal vaccination has helped greatly to decrease the incidence of bacteremia and sepsis. The advent of protein-conjugated vaccines against *S. pneumoniae* and *H. influenzae* type b will help offset the lack of splenic filtration function for children undergoing splenectomy. However, even with the use of presplenectomy immunizations, prophylactic antibiotics, and prompt medical attention for fever, the splenectomized child still has a finite risk of developing OPSI with substantial morbidity and mortality.

IMMUNE-MEDIATED HEMOLYTIC ANEMIA

Historical Perspective

Erythrocyte hemolysis characterized by anemia, shortened red blood cell survival, jaundice, and occasionally hemoglobinuria, has been recognized as a clinical entity for more than a century.[41, 42] In the early 1900s, it was noted that the serum from some patients with hemolytic anemia had the ability to agglutinate or hemolyze erythrocytes *in vitro*; such sera contained "agglutinins" or "hemolysins," respectively, which suggested an immunologic basis for the hemolysis.[43] The majority of patients with hemolytic anemia did not have these laboratory findings, however, and the mechanism by which their erythrocytes were destroyed was unknown. In fact, it was quite difficult to distinguish acquired immune hemolytic anemia (an extracorpuscular defect) from the intracorpuscular defect known as congenital hemolytic jaundice (now called hereditary spherocytosis).

A major advance occurred in 1945, when Coombs and co-workers reported the use of a rabbit antihuman globulin serum to detect Rh agglutinins.[44] This substance called Coombs reagent amplified weak agglutinins present on sensitized red cells and allowed serologic identification of previously undetectable autoantibodies on the erythrocyte surface. The authors presciently noted that their reagent "promises to be of practical use" but probably did not foresee that it would completely revolutionize the field of immunohematology. Their subsequent demonstration that the sensitizing agent on the erythrocytes was γ-globulin strengthened the idea of an autoimmune process,[45] and it was later documented that IgG warm-reactive antibodies were the most common form of AIHA.[46] By the late 1950s, it was finally possible to distinguish accurately between intrinsic erythrocyte defects and immune-mediated extrinsic erythrocyte destruction.[47]

Over the next two decades, several additional important advances were reported. Complement components as well as γ-globulins were found on the red cell surface of patients with immune-mediated hemolytic anemia, and by the late 1960s, the role of complement in immune-mediated destruction of erythrocytes was established.[48–52] Interactions between IgG-sensitized red cells and monocytes were investigated,[53–55] including differences related to IgG subtypes[56, 57] or erythrocyte antigens.[58] These studies started to elucidate the immune mechanisms of erythrocyte clearance by the reticuloendothelial system.

The development of an animal model, using guinea pigs deficient in complement components C3 or C4, represented an experimental breakthrough that led to a greater understanding of both the pathophysiology[59–61] and therapy[62, 63] of immune-mediated hemolytic anemia. With this model, the important contributions of antibody, complement, and the reticuloendothelial system to the pathophysiology of erythrocyte hemolysis could be studied. Taken together, these laboratory investigations led to models of the immune-mediated clearance of erythrocytes by the reticuloendothelial system that are still accepted today.

Over the next 15 years, there were relatively fewer advances in the field, chiefly ones involving increased precision of serologic diagnosis,[64, 65] occasional new therapeutic options,[66–68] or large clinical reviews of patient outcome.[69–71] Within the past 10 years, however, there has been a rapid increase in our knowledge of the immunologic abnormalities that may be important in the generation and expansion of erythrocyte autoantibodies in AIHA. In addition, novel therapies directed at specific targets in the immune system have emerged. The stage is now set for focused research on the T and B lymphocytes in patients with AIHA, with the goal of understanding the pathogenesis of AIHA at the molecular level. Specific questions remain unanswered regarding the formation of autoreactive antibodies, the loss of self-tolerance, and the lack of regulation and suppression of these autoantibodies by the immune system. In addition, novel targeted therapies that are being developed will expand the treatment armamentarium for AIHA.

Classification of AIHA

AIHA can be classified in a variety of ways, such as by the thermal sensitivity or isotype of the autoantibodies, but a simple and convenient classification scheme separates the disorders into a primary versus a secondary process (Table 14–1). In primary AIHA, hemolytic anemia is the only clinical finding, and there is no identifiable ongoing systemic illness to explain the presence of erythrocyte autoantibodies. Some children with this form of AIHA will, however, have had a recent viral-like illness. Warm-reactive AIHA is the most common form of primary AIHA in children and usually involves IgG autoantibodies that sensitize erythrocytes and lead to extravascular immune clearance and hemolysis. A second category of primary AIHA is PCH, which is particularly common in children after a viral-like illness. PCH is a particularly interesting form of AIHA characterized by an IgG autoantibody that binds at cold temperatures, fixes complement efficiently, and causes intravascular hemolysis. The third major form of primary AIHA, cold agglutinin

---

TABLE 14–1. Classification of Autoimmune Hemolytic Anemia (AIHA) in Children

PRIMARY AIHA*

Warm-reactive autoantibodies, usually IgG
Paroxysmal cold hemoglobinuria, usually IgG
Cold-agglutinin disease, usually IgM

SECONDARY AIHA†

Systemic autoimmune disease (e.g., lupus)
Malignancy (Hodgkin's and non-Hodgkin's lymphoma)
Immunodeficiency
Infection (*Mycoplasma*, viruses)
Drug-induced

*Occurs in majority of affected children and often follows a nonspecific viral-like syndrome but in the absence of another systemic illness.
†Occurs in association with another systemic process.

disease, is more commonly observed in adults, but in children it commonly follows *Mycoplasma* infections. In this disorder, an IgM autoantibody binds to erythrocytes optimally below 37°C and fixes complement; erythrocytes either undergo intravascular hemolysis or immune-mediated clearance from surface-bound complement components.

Secondary AIHA occurs in the context of another clinical diagnosis, with hemolytic anemia being only one manifestation of a systemic illness. Secondary AIHA can occur in patients with generalized autoimmune disease, such as systemic lupus erythematosus or other autoimmune inflammatory disorders. AIHA also occurs in patients with malignancy, immunodeficiency states, exposure to drugs, or specific infections. Because the AIHA may be the initial presenting manifestation, however, it is imperative to evaluate each patient with AIHA for the presence of an underlying illness. As discussed later, Evans syndrome is a unique entity that features autoimmune pancytopenia, although the erythrocytes and platelets are most often involved. Evans syndrome often has a severe clinical course, and patients require aggressive systemic therapy.

PRIMARY AUTOIMMUNE HEMOLYTIC ANEMIA

Incidence

Primary AIHA is not a rare disorder. The annual incidence of the disease has been estimated to be 1 in 80,000 persons in the general population,[72] making it more common than acquired aplastic anemia[73, 74] but less common than immune thrombocytopenic purpura.[75] In the pediatric age-group, AIHA may even occur in infants and toddlers, especially after an infection[69, 71, 76]; teenagers with AIHA are more likely to have an associated underlying systemic illness and therefore have secondary disease.[77–79] Cold agglutinin disease can occur in the pediatric age-group but is particularly common in older persons.[80–83] In summary, it can be said that AIHA can affect persons of any age, race, or nationality. The issue of gender preference is somewhat more controversial; in children, males may be affected more often, whereas affected teenagers are more commonly female.[69, 76, 84]

Natural History

The prognosis for the majority of children with primary AIHA is good.[70, 78, 85–87] Overall, young patients with cold-reactive erythrocyte autoantibodies appear to have a better clinical outcome than those with warm-reactive antibodies. The former patients tend to have an acute self-limited illness but may require aggressive short-term supportive care. In contrast, the clinical course in children with warm-reactive AIHA often is chronic, characterized by intermittent remissions and relapses, and these patients usually require long-term therapy.

Older series reported a high mortality rate for patients with AIHA, but these studies included many adults with AIHA secondary to malignancy.[46, 88] More recent series, including several that focused exclusively on children,

have demonstrated a much better prognosis. Buchanan and colleagues[85] reported that 77 percent of children with AIHA had an acute self-limited disease and that the majority of children responded well to short-term therapy; these results were later confirmed in a review of 42 children.[71] In the modern era, mortality of children with primary AIHA appears to be no more than 10 percent, with death occurring primarily in older children with chronic refractory disease.[69, 71, 76]

Heisel and Ortega[77] attempted to define prognostic factors for AIHA in childhood. They concluded that children between 2 and 12 years of age had the best prognosis; these patients tended to have an abrupt onset of symptoms with low numbers of reticulocytes but otherwise normal blood counts. The children who fared worse were either infants younger than 2 years of age or teenagers; these patients had a more prolonged onset of symptoms, had higher reticulocyte counts with nucleated erythrocyte precursors in the peripheral blood, and often had decreased platelet counts.[77] Other studies have confirmed the observation that younger children with an abrupt onset of symptoms have a better prognosis than older patients.[69, 76, 84]

Clinical Presentation

The proper evaluation of a pediatric patient with AIHA begins with a careful history and physical examination. Many children with AIHA are seen with signs and symptoms referable to anemia, such as pallor and weakness and less commonly dizziness or exercise intolerance. The anemia is usually well compensated from a cardiovascular standpoint, so that symptoms of congestive heart failure or circulatory collapse are rare. Occasionally, a patient is seen with jaundice, typically noted in the sclerae, owing to accelerated erythrocyte destruction and increased bilirubin turnover. The symptom of dark urine usually reflects intravascular hemolysis rather than bilirubin, and has been described by patients using a variety of colorful and flavorful terms including cola, iced tea, mahogany, or even motor oil. Less commonly, the patient will describe abdominal pain or fever.

Children with AIHA often have a benign previous medical history, although questions should be asked regarding prior similar episodes. The review of systems should include a query about recent or concurrent medications and careful questioning regarding the possibility of an underlying illness such as a systemic autoimmune disease, inflammatory disorder, or malignancy. The family history is usually negative in AIHA; rare instances of apparent familial AIHA[69, 89, 90] probably reflect a tendency toward a generalized autoimmune disorder such as systemic lupus erythematosus.

On physical examination, the child with AIHA is often pale and jaundiced, with pallor and icterus especially apparent in the conjunctivae and palms. The patient should have no physical stigmata of congenital disorders such as Blackfan-Diamond anemia, Fanconi anemia, or constitutional aplastic anemia. Jaundice may be apparent, especially if hemolysis is brisk, reflecting the breakdown and recycling of unconjugated bilirubin from the destroyed erythrocytes. Depending upon the skill of the examiner, scleral icterus can be detected at a bilirubin concentration of 2 to 4 mg/dL. Examination of the heart typically reveals tachycardia and an early systolic flow murmur that results from the high-output anemic state. The liver and spleen may be palpable, owing in the latter case to an increase in red pulp.[91] However, the presence of massive splenomegaly, hepatomegaly, or enlarged lymph nodes should suggest an underlying infection or malignant process.

Routine Laboratory Evaluation

Similar to that seen with other forms of anemia in young patients, such as aplastic anemia or transient erythroblastopenia of childhood, the degree of anemia in AIHA may be surprisingly marked at presentation. A child with AIHA often has a hemoglobin concentration of 4 to 7 g/dL with no apparent cardiovascular compromise. Red blood cell indices are not generally helpful in establishing the diagnosis, because a normal mean corpuscular volume may reflect the weighted average of small microspherocytes and large reticulocytes. Erythrocyte agglutination within the sample tube may give an artificially large mean corpuscular volume on an automated counter.[92] An elevated mean corpuscular hemoglobin concentration (>36 g/dL) is more suggestive of hereditary spherocytosis, because the spherocyte has a smaller volume than the normal erythrocyte but contains the normal amount of hemoglobin (see Chapter 15). The leukocyte count and platelet count should be within the normal range. Concurrent thrombocytopenia may indicate a bone marrow failure syndrome (e.g., aplastic anemia) or microangiopathic hemolytic anemia (e.g., hemolytic uremic syndrome or thrombotic thrombocytopenic purpura). The combination of AIHA and thrombocytopenia is referred to as Evans syndrome and is characterized by a broader immune dysregulation.[93] Granulocytopenia also may be present in Evans syndrome, reflecting immune pancytopenia.

Evaluation of the peripheral blood smear is very useful in establishing the diagnosis of AIHA. Numerous small spherocytes are usually present in warm-reactive AIHA; splenic ingestion of a portion of the erythrocyte allows the cell to "sphere," that is, to re-form into the entropically favored spherical shape.[53] Surface complement also may induce erythrocyte sphering.[94] Occasionally, teardrop shapes or even schistocytes may be observed[95]; the presence of target cells is more consistent with a hemoglobinopathy or primary hepatic disease. Polychromasia is a common finding in AIHA, because the bone marrow releases large numbers of reticulocytes and even nucleated red blood cells to compensate for the accelerated erythrocyte destruction. Figure 14–5A shows the peripheral blood smear from a patient with warm-reactive AIHA that has numerous small microspherocytes and large reticulocytes (see color section at the front of this volume). Numerous Howell-Jolly bodies are present, because this patient had previously undergone splenectomy. In contrast, Fig. 5B shows the blood smear of a patient with hereditary spherocytosis and illustrates the morphologic similarities between these two conditions. Spherocytes are seen less commonly in cold-reactive AIHA, but erythro-

cyte agglutination can be observed on the blood film if the binding affinity of the antibody reaches room temperature. Figure 5C illustrates agglutinated red cells in a patient with cold-reactive (IgM-mediated) AIHA; at higher power (Fig. 5D) the nucleated cells are seen to be immature erythroid cells prematurely released from the bone marrow.

Reticulocytosis is usually present in AIHA, owing to the bone marrow's compensation for the shortened red cell survival in the peripheral blood.[96] Absolute reticulocyte counts are typically 200 to 600×10^9/L, representing 10 to 30 percent of circulating erythrocytes. However, reticulocytopenia is well described in AIHA and probably occurs in 10 percent of pediatric patients.[97–99] Several explanations have been offered for a low reticulocyte count in the presence of accelerated erythrocyte clearance. The autoantibody may react with antigens on erythroid precursors, which leads to immune-mediated clearance within the marrow by resident macrophages. Alternatively, erythrocyte autoantibodies may induce apoptosis of bone marrow erythroblasts.[100] Finally, AIHA may be well compensated for and subclinical, until infection with parvovirus B19 temporarily shuts off erythropoiesis and leads to worse and symptomatic anemia.[101, 102] Regardless of its mechanism, however, the presence of reticulocytopenia should not influence therapy or prognosis.

Aspiration of the bone marrow is not generally necessary for children with AIHA but may be helpful to exclude a malignant process, myelodysplasia, or a bone marrow failure syndrome. In AIHA, the marrow aspirate usually reveals erythroid hyperplasia, with a myeloid/erythroid ratio below unity. Dyserythropoiesis is not a common finding but has been reported in an adult with AIHA and reticulocytopenia.[103]

Results of urine examination may be unremarkable. In patients with AIHA with intravascular hemolysis, however, free plasma hemoglobin is cleared through the renal filtration system, which leads to darkened urine. When hemoglobinuria is present, urine dipstick analysis will indicate the presence of blood, but microscopic examination will reveal few if any red blood cells. Chronic hemoglobinuria will lead to hemosiderin accumulation in uroepithelial cells, which can be detected in the urinary sediment.

The results of a variety of serum chemistry analyses may be abnormal owing to erythrocyte hemolysis, but their routine measurement should not be essential to establish the diagnosis of AIHA. Elevations in levels of lactate dehydrogenase and aspartate aminotransferase reflect the release of intraerythrocyte enzymes; in contrast, the level of serum alanine aminotransferase or other hepatic enzymes should not be elevated in AIHA. The serum haptoglobin level is almost always low, because this protein acts as a scavenger for free plasma hemoglobin. However, haptoglobin is not synthesized well in young infants and is an acute phase reactant[104]; for these reasons, quantitation of serum haptoglobin may not be helpful in the evaluation of a patient with AIHA (or for that matter, in any patient). The serum total bilirubin concentration is elevated in most patients with AIHA, although levels greater than 5 mg/dL are unusual and suggest hepatic impairment or the

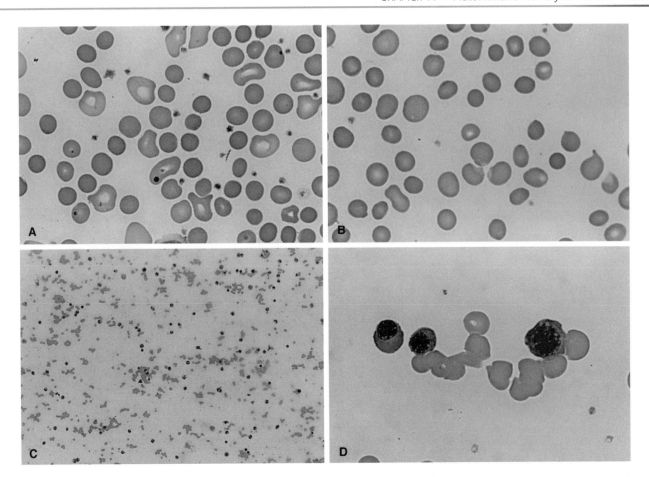

FIGURE 14–5. Examination of the peripheral blood in autoimmune hemolytic anemia (AIHA). *A,* Blood from a patient with IgG (warm-reactive) AIHA illustrates many small microspherocytes and larger reticulocytes (× 1000). *B,* Blood from a patient with hereditary spherocytosis illustrates the morphologic similarities between these two conditions. *C,* Agglutinated erythrocytes from a patient with IgM (cold-reactive) AIHA are clearly visible at low power (× 400). *D,* At higher power (× 1000) the nucleated cells in the peripheral blood from this patient are identified as erythroid progenitor cells prematurely released from the bone marrow (see color section at the front of this volume).

presence of Gilbert syndrome. Because the elevated bilirubin concentration in AIHA reflects accelerated erythrocyte destruction rather than intrinsic hepatic disease, virtually all of the bilirubin is unconjugated. The direct (conjugated) fraction should not exceed 10 to 20 percent of the total bilirubin concentration.

Specialized Laboratory Evaluation

The most important and useful laboratory test to establish the diagnosis of AIHA is the direct antiglobulin test (DAT or Coombs test), which identifies antibodies and complement components on the surface of circulating erythrocytes. Therefore, a thorough understanding of the individual laboratory steps that constitute the DAT is essential for the accurate interpretation of the test results.

Anticoagulated erythrocytes from the patient are first washed several times to remove all plasma proteins and then are incubated at 37°C with polyclonal rabbit antiserum that binds to human γ-globulin and human complement (usually C3). First described more than 50 years ago,[44] this Coombs reagent is clearly the most important diagnostic laboratory tool for the patient with AIHA. IgM autoantibodies are pentameric and can act as a bridge

between adjacent erythrocytes (Fig. 6*A*). In contrast, IgG autoantibodies are smaller and are unable to bridge the surface repulsion between adjacent erythrocytes known as the zeta potential (Fig. 6*B*), unless the distance imposed by the zeta potential is reduced (Fig. 6*C*). The broad-spectrum Coombs reagent binds to erythrocyte autoantibodies, bridges the zeta potential, and causes agglutination (Fig. 6*D*).

A positive DAT result with the Coombs reagent leads to testing with more specific antisera to discriminate between IgG and complement on the red blood cell surface. The presence of IgG on the erythrocyte is sufficient evidence for an IgG autoantibody; simultaneous detection of complement indicates that the antibody can fix complement as well. In contrast, the presence of complement alone (with no IgG detected) suggests a cold-reactive autoantibody that fixes complement at lower temperatures but binds poorly to the erythrocyte at 37°C; in this setting, the serum should be analyzed either for the presence of an IgM autoantibody or the unique IgG Donath-Landsteiner autoantibody described in a later section.

The DAT report for a patient with AIHA should describe the agglutination results of the polyspecific Coombs reagent and, if positive, the results of testing with

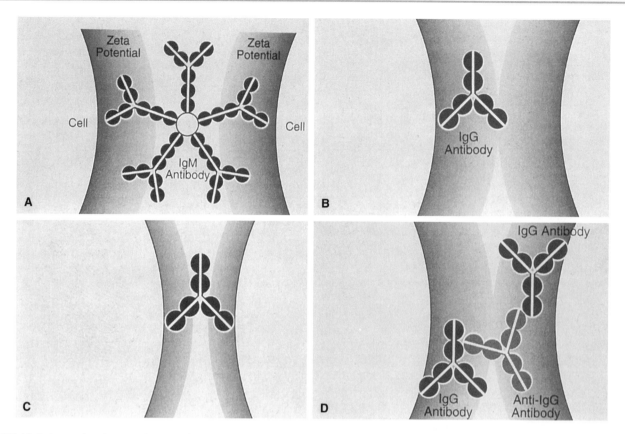

FIGURE 14–6. Interactions between immunoglobulin molecules and the erythrocyte during agglutination tests and the direct antiglobulin test (DAT). *A,* An IgM autoantibody can simultaneously bind two erythrocytes owing to its multiple antigen-binding sites. The large size of the IgM molecule allows it to bridge the zeta potential between erythrocytes and cause agglutination. *B,* An IgG autoantibody is too small to bridge the zeta potential. *C,* Hence, there is no agglutination of erythrocytes unless the zeta potential is reduced. *D,* On the addition of the Coombs reagent, which is a rabbit antiglobulin that recognizes human IgG, the zeta potential is successfully bridged and red cells agglutinate.

the specific IgG and C3 reagents. The DAT can be performed at temperatures lower than 37°C such as 4°C, 10°C, or room temperature (23°C), to assist with the detection of cold-reactive autoantibodies and characterization of their thermal reactivity and amplitude. The DAT results are scored on the basis of the amount of agglutination, usually on a scale of 1 to 4.

On occasion, results for the DAT are negative despite good clinical evidence for autoimmune hemolysis. One explanation for this apparent paradox is that the amount of IgG present on the erythrocyte may be below the threshold for detection by standard Coombs reagent testing. In this setting, a more sensitive assay for surface-bound IgG such as a radioimmunoassay,[105] enzyme-linked immunosorbent assay,[106, 107] or rosette formation[108] may be helpful in identifying IgG on the cell surface. Alternatively, the lack of surface IgG may indicate the presence of a surface antibody other than an IgG molecule, such as an IgA autoantibody[65, 109–111] or even a warm-reactive IgM autoantibody.[112–114]

Also of interest is the observation that results of the DAT may be positive in an otherwise normal person. This is apparently a biologically false-positive result, because these individuals develop no evidence of AIHA even with extended follow-up.[115, 116] Analysis of the immune system of such persons revealed normal T-cell subsets, although the number of B cells was significantly increased.[117]

Differential Diagnosis

The typical patient with AIHA is seen with clear evidence of hemolytic anemia, including jaundice and splenomegaly on physical examination and spherocytes with reticulocytosis on the peripheral blood smear. In this setting, the differential diagnosis includes certain forms of nonimmune hemolytic anemia, including intrinsic red blood cell membrane or enzyme defects, as well as other rare extrinsic causes of hemolysis. Hereditary spherocytosis, described more fully in Chapter 15, can be confused with AIHA. A positive result for the osmotic fragility test, often erroneously considered to be pathognomonic for the diagnosis of hereditary spherocytosis, is also observed in patients with AIHA or congestive splenomegaly. Patients with other rare disorders such as clostridial sepsis, early stages of Wilson disease,[118] or hyperlipoproteinemic liver disease[119] also can have numerous spherocytes and hemolytic anemia. Patients with microangiopathic hemolytic anemia, such as hemolytic uremic syndrome or thrombotic thrombocytopenic purpura, typically have schistocytes rather than spherocytes and usually have severe thrombocytopenia as well. In all clinical settings, the diagnosis of AIHA is most easily and accurately made on the basis of the positive DAT results.

If the patient is seen with anemia and reticulocytopenia, the differential diagnosis should include other acquired forms of hypoplastic anemia, such as transient erythroblastopenia of childhood or acquired aplastic anemia. In addition, patients with nonimmune hemolytic anemia who develop transient hypoplastic anemia from parvovirus B19 infection may be seen with this clinical picture.[120] In these patients, the underlying hemolytic anemia may not be clinically recognizable until the parvovirus infection worsens the anemia and leads to clinical symptoms.

Characteristics of Erythrocyte Autoantibodies

The *sine qua non* of both primary and secondary AIHA is the presence of antibodies that bind to erythrocytes. As a direct consequence of the binding of these erythrocyte autoantibodies, circulating erythrocytes have a shortened life span with hemolysis or accelerated clearance by the reticuloendothelial system. However, the clinical complexity and variability of AIHA depends in large part upon immunologic characteristics of the autoantibody including its isotype, thermal reactivity, ability to fix complement, binding affinity, and antigenic specificity. Elucidation of each of these characteristics is important to an understanding of the pathophysiology and clinical course of AIHA in a given patient.[83, 121–126] Table 14–2 summarizes the important characteristics of erythrocyte autoantibodies in AIHA, emphasizing the differences among the three major clinical conditions: warm-reactive AIHA, PCH, and cold agglutinin disease.

ANTIBODY ISOTYPE

One of the most important tasks for the immunohematology laboratory in the evaluation of a new patient with AIHA is to determine the isotype of the erythrocyte autoantibody. In most cases, the pathogenic antibody is identified as an IgG molecule.[71, 86, 127, 128] In general, IgG autoantibodies bind to red blood cell antigens optimally at 37°C, hence the descriptive term *warm-reactive* autoantibodies. All IgG molecules are heterodimers, with two heavy chains linked noncovalently to two light chains. The heavy and light chains together form two variable antigen-binding sites known as the Fab portions, and the heavy chains also contain a constant structural domain (the Fc portion) that includes the binding site for complement and the binding site for the Fc receptor.

There are four subtypes of IgG antibodies, which are designated IgG1, IgG2, IgG3, and IgG4. These different subtypes have important implications for the fixation of complement, hemolysis, and clearance by the reticuloendothelial system. IgG1 and IgG3 antibodies fix complement better than IgG2 and IgG4 antibodies.[129, 130] A patient who had only IgG4 autoantibody on his erythrocytes was reported to have little hemolysis, presumably due to weak interactions with the FcR on macrophages.[131] Adapted from the review of several thousand patients with AIHA by Engelfriet and colleagues,[128] Table 14–3 lists the relative occurrence of each IgG subclass identified in patients with warm IgG autoantibody AIHA. IgG1 autoantibodies were by far the predominant subclass identified, followed by multiple subclasses that typically included IgG1.

Less commonly, IgG antibodies are cold reactive; these autoantibodies are characteristic of childhood PCH but also have been reported rarely in cold hemagglutinin disease.[132] In the unusual setting of a pregnant woman with AIHA, certain IgG autoantibodies can cross the placenta and cause acquired neonatal AIHA.[133–135]

In other patients with AIHA, IgM autoantibodies are identified, particularly after an infection with an organism such as *Mycoplasma pneumoniae*.[136] In one series, IgM autoantibodies characterized a significant proportion of instances of AIHA in early childhood.[137] The IgM molecule is a pentameric structure that contains five covalently linked domains, each of which is structurally similar to a single IgG molecule. Because of their large size, IgM autoantibodies can span the zeta potential between adjacent erythrocytes. Erythrocytes that are connected by a bridging IgM molecule become too dense to remain in suspension and thus agglutinate.

IgG and IgM autoantibodies characterize the vast majority of instances of AIHA, but rarely an IgA autoantibody is identified.[65, 110, 111, 138] IgA antibodies do not react with the standard Coombs reagent, and special research reagents must be used, therefore, for their identification. Testing for IgA autoantibodies should be considered and

TABLE 14–2. Common Characteristics of Erythrocyte Autoantibodies in Autoimmune Hemolytic Anemia

Characteristic*	Warm-Reactive	Paroxysmal Cold Hemoglobinuria	Cold Agglutinin
Immunoglobulin isotype	IgG	IgG	IgM
Thermal reactivity	37°C	4°C	4°C
Fixes complement	Variable	Yes	Yes
Direct antiglobulin test			
4°C	Not performed	IgG, C3	C3
37°C	IgG, ± C3	C3	C3
Plasma titer	Low/absent	Moderate	High
Hemolysin	No	Yes	Variable
Antigenic specificity	Rh and others	P	I/i
Site of red blood cell destruction	Spleen	Intravascular	Liver, intravascular
Common therapy	Corticosteroids	Avoidance of cold	Avoidance of cold
	Splenectomy	Corticosteroids	Plasmapheresis

*Many characteristics of the autoantibodies differ between warm-reactive AIHA, paroxysmal cold hemoglobinuria, and cold agglutinin disease. See text for additional descriptions and details.

TABLE 14–3. Frequency of IgG Subclasses Identified in Warm-Reactive (IgG Autoantibody) Autoimmune Hemolytic Anemia

IgG Subclass	Percentage of Total Cases
IgG1	74.0
IgG2	0.7
IgG3	2.1
IgG4	0.9
Multiple, including IgG1	20.1
Multiple, not including IgG1	0.3
None detectable	1.9

Adapted from Engelfriet CP, Overbeeke MAM, von dem Borne AE: Autoimmune hemolytic anemia. Semin Hematol 1992; 29:3.

specifically requested whenever the DAT fails to detect surface-bound IgG or C3 in a patient who otherwise appears to have AIHA. Finally, a combination of different isotypes, especially simultaneous IgG and IgM autoantibodies, has been reported on several occasions.[139–145]

THERMAL REACTIVITY

The thermal reactivity (sometimes called the thermal amplitude) of an erythrocyte autoantibody is another important parameter to determine. Although the core temperature of humans is 37°C, temperatures in superficial vessels (particularly in the face and digits) may fall below 30°C. Binding of antibody to erythrocytes can be considered a process of dynamic equilibrium, depending upon the location of a given erythrocyte within the circulation. The thermal reactivity of most IgG autoantibodies is 37°C, meaning that binding to erythrocytes occurs best at normal body temperature. These antibodies are therefore referred to as warm-reactive autoantibodies. Occasionally, warm-reactive IgM autoantibodies are identified, although these are rare.[112–114, 137]

Cold-reactive (Donath-Landsteiner) IgG autoantibodies bind optimally at 4°C and are clinically important as the cause of PCH. Because of their unusual characteristics, results of the DAT are often negative or demonstrate only the presence of complement, because the cold-reacting antibodies are removed during the washing of the erythrocytes. A special procedure must therefore be followed to detect the Donath-Landsteiner antibody characteristic of PCH. Specific testing for this antibody should be performed early in the clinical course, ideally before therapy is initiated.

The Donath-Landsteiner autoantibody is a biphasic hemolysin, meaning it binds to erythrocytes and fixes complement at 4°C, but upon warming to 37°C the complement cascade is amplified and leads to hemolysis. Two samples of blood should be drawn simultaneously from the patient and kept at 37°C to prevent *in vitro* autoantibody binding and hemolysis. The serum samples are separated from the erythrocytes by centrifugation (preferably at a warm temperature) and then incubated with normal erythrocytes and a source of complement, either in a melting ice bath or at 37°C. Both reactions are then warmed to 37°C and analyzed for the presence of hemolysis. In the first sample, the cold incubation allows the IgG autoanti-

body to bind and fix complement, after which the subsequent warming step allows complement amplification to occur with resultant red blood cell lysis. In contrast, the sample maintained at 37°C shows no lysis, because no significant IgG autoantibody binding occurred at the warmer temperature to allow complement fixation.

In contrast to many IgG autoantibodies, IgM autoantibodies typically bind optimally to erythrocytes at 0 to 4°C and hence are called *cold-reactive* antibodies. The thermal range over which the autoantibody is active is crucial and determines the amount of hemolysis observed (Fig. 14–7). An IgM autoantibody binds optimally in the cold, but complement activation proceeds optimally at warmer temperatures. The overlap between the range of antibody activity and complement activation is the so-called "zone of hemolysis."[146]

COMPLEMENT FIXATION

The ability of an erythrocyte autoantibody to fix complement plays a critical role in the pathophysiology of immune clearance and the clinical manifestations of hemolysis, because complement augments the destructive effects of the autoantibody. The process of complement deposition, amplification, and pore formation involves a complex series of intravascular enzymatic events.

In the classical complement activation pathway, the Fc portion of the bound immunoglobulin molecule interacts with C1q, the first component of the complement cascade. Two IgG molecules in close proximity are required to bind C1q to the erythrocyte (Fig. 8A), whereas a single IgM molecule is sufficient to bind C1q (Fig. 8B). Components C1r and C1s then bind to C1q to form a multiunit protein complex on the red cell surface. This active complex binds and enzymatically cleaves C4, followed by additional enzymatic events that lead to the deposition of component C3b on the surface of the

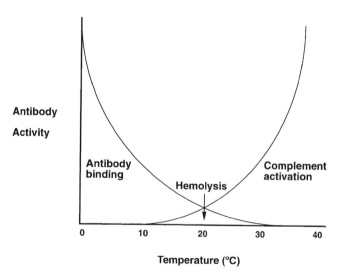

FIGURE 14–7. Thermal reactivity curve of a cold-reactive IgM autoantibody. The antibody is optimally reactive at 0 to 4°C, whereas complement is fixed most efficiently at 37°C. The overlap area is the so-called "zone of hemolysis" and determines the amount of hemolysis observed. (Adapted from Issitt PD, Anstee DJ: Applied Blood Group Serology, 3rd ed. Miami, Montgomery Scientific Publications, 1985, p 545.)

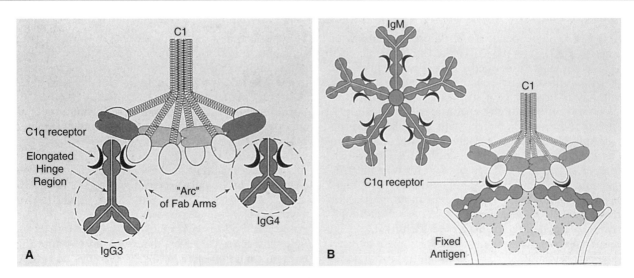

FIGURE 14–8. The binding of C1, the first component of complement, to antibodies. *A,* Binding of C1 to IgG molecules occurs through the Fc portion of the immunoglobulin molecule. Binding is inhibited by interference from the Fab arms, which is minimized when the hinge region is elongated, as in an IgG3 molecule; hence, IgG3 fixes complement more efficiently than IgG4. *B,* Complement binding sites of IgM molecules are not available when the antibody is in its fluid-phase planar form. When two of the monomers are affixed, however, the IgM molecule assumes an arched form and the C1 binding sites become available for reaction.

erythrocyte. At this point, the erythrocyte may be cleared by the spleen, liver, or other parts of the reticuloendothelial system that recognize C3b via specific surface receptors. Alternatively, amplification of the complement cascade may continue, leading to the formation of the C5b–7 membrane attack complex followed by fixation of C8 and C9, and finally by the polymerization of C9 to form pores within the cell membrane (Fig. 14–9). These pores breach the erythrocyte membrane integrity and cause hemolysis of the cell.

IgM autoantibodies fix complement very efficiently, because distinct binding sites within the IgM pentamer are close enough to bind C1q (see Fig. 8B). In fact, the "hemolysins" that were identified at the turn of the century were actually IgM autoantibodies that fixed complement efficiently and completely, resulting in membrane pore formation and erythrocyte lysis. Rarely, IgM antibodies that do not fix complement have been reported.[137, 147] In contrast, IgG autoantibodies do not fix complement as efficiently as their IgM counterparts, owing in part to the necessity of two distinct IgG molecules being in close proximity to allow the initial binding of C1q.[51] If the target autoantigens on the erythrocyte membrane are not mobile or are spaced too far apart, complement cannot be fixed. Moreover, all IgG molecules do not have equivalent complement-fixing abilities; the IgG1 and IgG3 subclasses are able to fix complement far better than the IgG2 and IgG4 subtypes.[129, 130] The Donath-Landsteiner antibodies, even though they are IgG autoantibodies, fix complement very efficiently, which leads to brisk intravascular lysis.

ANTIBODY BINDING AFFINITY

The binding affinity of an erythrocyte autoantibody for its antigen has implications both for the likelihood of *in vitro* detection and for the pathophysiologic process of ery-

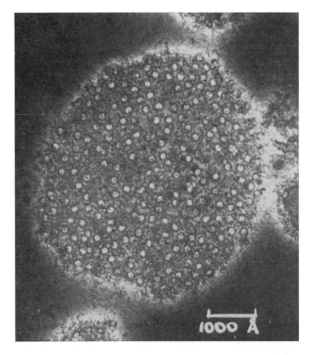

FIGURE 14–9. Electron micrograph of the lesions that appear in the cell membrane after completion of the membrane attack complex. The dark lesions are hydrophilic complexes of protein about 10 nm in diameter.

throcyte clearance.[122, 126] An IgG autoantibody typically has a high affinity for its antigen on the erythrocyte surface and therefore can be identified readily by the DAT. For this same reason, the indirect antiglobulin test may fail to detect an IgG autoantibody, because there is very little unbound antibody circulating in the plasma. In contrast, most IgM autoantibodies have little binding affinity at 37°C and therefore are more easily detected as high-titer unbound antibody within the plasma.

ANTIGENIC SPECIFICITY

When the serologic specificity in most patients with warm-reactive AIHA is tested, reactivity with all cells tested is commonly identified. This "panreactive" or "nonspecific" pattern of reactivity suggests that the autoantibody is binding to a surface antigenic structure that is common to all human erythrocytes. Interestingly, the autoantibody may not react with cells that lack the entire Rh protein complex; experiments with these rare Rh$_{null}$ erythrocytes provide evidence that the Rh protein cluster is the main antigenic determinant for many warm-reactive autoantibodies.[50, 146] Other studies have confirmed that autoantibodies bind to Rh in about 50 percent of patients with warm-reactive AIHA,[124, 125, 148] although other candidate autoantigens have been identified.[149]

Occasionally, reactivity against a particular Rh antigen such as c or e is identified,[82, 150] although this is not common. Warm autoantibodies with defined specificity against unusual protein antigens, including protein 4.1,[151] Ge,[152] Wr^b,[64] Sc1,[153] Kpb[154], and many others, have been described. Reactivity with the ABO blood group antigens[155, 156] or with other major systems such as Lewis or Kell is extremely rare in warm-reactive AIHA.[128, 146, 157] In contrast, IgM autoantibodies often have reactivity against polysaccharides on the red cell rather than surface proteins. The I/i surface structure is a prototypic polysaccharide autoantigen on the red cell surface and is the target of many IgM antibodies that develop in response to infections.[136] In addition to the important I/i surface antigens, other autoantigens have also been reported in cold-reactive AIHA,[82, 83, 158–160] including the polysaccharide P autoantigen in PCH.[161]

Elucidation of the antigenic specificity of autoreactive erythrocyte antibodies provides information that is useful for several reasons. One is the likelihood of finding compatible blood for transfusion. If an autoantibody is a panreactive antibody that binds to all cells with no apparent specificity, then fully compatible blood will probably not be found. Identification of the antigenic specificity may also help predict intravascular lysis resulting from complement activation. If the antigen is within the Rh complex, then the antigenic density on the erythrocytes makes complement activation remote and complement-mediated intravascular hemolysis less likely. The P antigen system, in contrast, is densely populated on the erythrocyte surface and capable of binding sufficient Donath-Landsteiner IgG antibodies to fix complement efficiently and lead to substantial intravascular lysis.[51]

Immune Clearance of Sensitized Erythrocytes

Much of our understanding about the pathophysiology of immune-mediated erythrocyte clearance derives from experiments performed more than 25 years ago. An elegant series of *in vitro* and *in vivo* studies by Jandl and associates[47, 53, 54, 56] and by Rosse[51, 52, 58] clarified the roles of antibody, complement, and the reticuloendothelial system in the pathophysiology of autoimmune erythrocyte clearance. In the early 1970s, Frank and colleagues developed a guinea pig model for AIHA that permitted dissection of the steps involved in the clearance of erythrocytes coated with antibody or complement. Using ^{51}Cr-labeled red blood cells that were sensitized *in vitro* using rabbit IgG or IgM anti-guinea pig erythrocyte antibodies, these investigators analyzed the rates and patterns of clearance, as well as the sites of sequestration. IgG-coated erythrocytes were removed predominantly by the spleen, regardless of concurrent complement activation, and the amount of surface IgG was correlated with the rate of splenic clearance. The liver was the predominant clearance site when very large amounts of IgG were present. Fc receptors on macrophages were responsible for the binding and phagocytosis of IgG-coated erythrocytes.[59, 60] In contrast to these findings for IgG-mediated hemolysis, IgM-coated erythrocytes were cleared rapidly within the liver and the amount of bound IgM correlated with the rate of erythrocyte clearance. However, there was an absolute dependence upon complement for the clearance of IgM-coated cells, and macrophage receptors for the C3b molecule were responsible for binding and phagocytosis of erythrocytes.[59, 61] Several investigators have attempted to mimic erythrocyte-monocyte interactions and correlate *in vitro* results with *in vivo* hemolysis,[162–165] but with limited success.

These and other laboratory experiments, coupled with careful clinical observations, have led to the development of a general understanding about immune-mediated clearance of erythrocytes in AIHA (Fig. 14–10). In warm-reactive AIHA, the IgG autoantibodies coat autologous erythrocytes and may fix complement. The sensitized cells pass through the spleen and other parts of the reticuloendothelial system, where they interact with complement and Fc receptors on the macrophages. The human macrophage has three distinct classes of receptor for the Fc portion of the IgG molecule, designated FcγRI, FcγRII, and FcγRIII. Although each form of FcR binds IgG with similar specificity, the binding affinity varies for

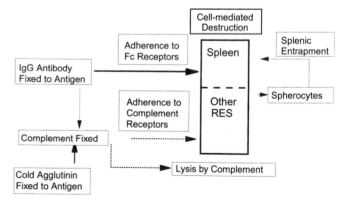

FIGURE 14–10. Immune-mediated clearance of erythrocytes in AIHA. In warm-reactive disease, the IgG autoantibodies are bound to erythrocytes but typically do not fix complement efficiently. The coated cells enter the spleen and other parts of the reticuloendothelial system (RES), where they interact with Fc receptors on macrophages. Erythrocytes may be completely engulfed and destroyed by this interaction or may have only a portion of their membrane removed. In this case, the red cells will reshape into spherocytes, which are then doomed upon their next passage through the spleen. In cold-reactive disease, complement is typically fixed very efficiently, and intravascular lysis by the complement cascade can occur. Alternatively, the presence of surface-bound complement (C3) can lead to extravascular red cell destruction by the spleen and RES.

individual subclasses of IgG autoantibodies.[166] The sensitized erythrocytes may be fully ingested by macrophages; however, if only a portion of the surface membrane is removed, the erythrocyte re-forms into a spherocyte that is identifiable on the peripheral blood smear. For IgG-coated erythrocytes, the majority of immune clearance occurs within the cords of the spleen[167]; hence the hemolysis is extravascular. If the IgG antibody fixes complement, the erythrocyte can also be cleared by macrophages bearing receptors for complement receptors.[59, 63, 168]

In cold agglutinin disease or PCH, the autoreactive antibody binds preferentially at 4°C and fixes complement efficiently. At normal body temperature, there is virtually no antibody identifiable on the cell surface, but complement components, particularly C3b, can be identified using the Coombs reagent. If complement is activated to completion on the cell surface *in vivo*, the erythrocytes will hemolyze intravascularly and cause hemoglobinemia followed by hemoglobinuria. When C3b is present on the red cell surface without further activation of complement, however, then macrophages within the reticuloendothelial system can bind the erythrocytes via specific complement receptors and engulf them in a manner similar to that in warm-reactive AIHA.[169, 170] Complement-coated erythrocytes are cleared by macrophages located primarily within the liver rather than the spleen.

Therapy

The need to treat a patient with AIHA depends upon the severity and rapidity with which the anemia develops. A child with relatively mild anemia (hemoglobin concentration 9 to 12 g/dL), especially one who has had a recent viral infection, will benefit from observation alone. If the patient has a more severe degree of anemia (hemoglobin concentration 6 to 9 g/dL) or if the hemoglobin concentration is observed to fall precipitously, then therapy should be instituted. Optimal therapy depends upon the clinical picture as well as on the form of AIHA. If the autoantibodies are cold reactive, for example, then the patient should be kept warm with avoidance of all cold stimuli. Strict adherence to this recommendation is difficult, but it is often the best therapy for a patient with cold-reactive autoantibodies. If severe intravascular hemolysis is present, it is imperative that good renal blood flow and urine output be maintained.[87]

Therapy for acute warm-reactive AIHA in children should begin with close observation, the judicious use of erythrocyte transfusions, and use of corticosteroids. Second-line therapy includes administration of intravenous immunoglobulin (IVIG) and plasma (exchange) transfusion. Other therapeutic modalities such as cyclosporine, vinblastine, danazol, azathioprine, cyclophosphamide, and other agents are not yet widely accepted for the pediatric age group and therefore have no therapeutic role for acute AIHA in children. Table 14–4 lists these various treatment modalities; clinical responses and mechanisms of action are described in later sections.

When the anemia is severe enough to cause cardiovascular compromise, usually at a hemoglobin level less than 5 g/dL, the use of erythrocyte transfusions to provide additional oxygen-carrying capacity should be strongly considered. Although the transfusion process is complicated and can be somewhat intimidating, an erythrocyte transfusion may be life-saving for a patient with AIHA who may die as a result of complications related to anemia.[171] If clinically warranted, erythrocyte transfusions should never be withheld because of a fear of a hemolytic transfusion reaction. The fate of transfused cells probably will not be worse than that of the patient's own erythrocytes, and they may provide temporary support until additional therapy slows the rate of hemolysis.

The first problem related to the transfusion of a patient with AIHA is the identification of compatible erythrocytes. It is important to provide a relatively large amount

TABLE 14–4. Treatment Modalities for Autoimmune Hemolytic Anemia

Treatment*	Dose	Comments
Red blood cell transfusions	Sufficient to reach 6–8 g/dL	Incompatibility may cause hemolysis
		Alloantibodies may be present
Corticosteroids	1–2 mg/kg IV q6h acutely	Useful for IgG more than IgM
	5–30 mg PO qod chronically	High doses for short-term use only
Intravenous immunoglobulin	1.0 g/kg per day for 1–5 days	Expensive, inconvenient to administer
		Effective in one third of patients
Exchange transfusion or plasmapheresis	Daily until stable	Useful for IgM more than IgG
		Requires large-caliber intravenous access
Splenectomy	—	Curative in 60–80% of patients
		Risk of postsplenectomy sepsis
Danazol	50–800 mg/day PO	Hepatic dysfunction
		Androgenic side effects
Vincristine	1 mg/m² IV every week	Neurotoxicity
Cyclophosphamide	50–100 mg/day PO	Carcinogenesis
Azathioprine	25–200 mg/day PO	Immunosuppression
Cyclosporin A	2–10 mg/kg per day PO	Nephrotoxicity, hypertension
		Immunosuppression
Rituximab	375 mg/m² IV every week	Anecdotal, experimental

IV = Intravenously; PO = perorally.
*See text for further description and discussion of each therapeutic agent.

of serum and cells for testing, well in advance of an anticipated erythrocyte transfusion. Particularly if the antigenic specificity is panreactive, the crossmatch will probably identify no units of blood that are compatible. In this instance, certain units that are "least incompatible" with the patient's serum will be identified. For patients who have previously received transfusions, it is critical to identify alloantibodies that may be masked by the stronger autoantibody.[172–174] Adsorption techniques are designed to remove autoantibodies and allow the identification of clinically important alloantibodies.[175, 176]

The second difficulty associated with transfusion of a patient with AIHA is the actual transfusion itself. Fortunately, acute symptomatic transfusion reactions are not seen often, even with transfusion of units of blood that may have a strong *in vitro* reactivity with the patient's serum.[172, 177] The transfused cells have an *in vivo* survival that is approximately equivalent to that of endogenous erythrocytes and so often have a beneficial effect even if they circulate only for a short time. On occasion, however, the transfusion results in severe hemolysis with hemoglobinemia, hemoglobinuria, and renal failure. For this reason, it is prudent to begin the transfusion at a slow rate, checking both plasma and urine samples periodically for free hemoglobin. For patients with cold-reactive antibodies, it is useful to warm the patient and the entire room; a blood warmer should be used to raise the temperature of the transfused blood.

A recent report described the successful use of polymerized bovine hemoglobin to provide life-saving oxygen-carrying capacity in a woman dying of AIHA.[178] Although intriguing as an alternative to erythrocyte transfusions, the use of erythrocyte substitutes such as perfluorochemicals or cell-free hemoglobin-based oxygen carriers must be considered highly experimental at this time.[179] Additional research in this area is likely to identify safe alternatives to transfusions that may eventually benefit children with AIHA.

The use of corticosteroids is widely accepted therapy for AIHA, particularly for patients with IgG antibodies. From the initial report more than 50 years ago,[180] glucocorticoids have been used to interfere with the basic pathophysiologic process and immune destruction observed in AIHA. The guinea pig model of AIHA demonstrated that steroids increased the survival of both IgG- and IgM-sensitized erythrocytes by decreasing sequestration within the spleen and liver, respectively.[60, 61] Corticosteroids are believed to inhibit the FcR-mediated clearance of sensitized erythrocytes,[63, 181] which probably accounts for their effect within 24 to 48 hours of administration. Corticosteroids may also inhibit autoantibody synthesis, although this effect requires several weeks to occur.

For the patient with warm-reactive AIHA or PCH, a typical dosing regimen of corticosteroids is 1 to 2 mg/kg of methylprednisolone given intravenously every 6 hours for the first 24 to 72 hours, usually while the patient is the sickest. Oral prednisone at 2 mg/kg/day may then be used when the patient's clinical condition is more stable. Typically, these high doses of therapy are required only for 2 to 4 weeks, followed by a slow tapering of dose that may take 3 months or more. Tapering of the corticosteroid

dose should be aimed toward the use of a single morning dose, preferably every other day, but must be based upon the patient's hemoglobin concentration, reticulocyte count, and DAT result. In general, tapering should be slower when active disease is evident. An overall response rate of approximately 80 percent has been reported.[182] On occasion, corticosteroid therapy may be beneficial in cold-agglutinin disease.[183]

IVIG became a popular therapy for immune thrombocytopenic purpura in the 1980s.[184] Able to induce a potent blockade of the reticuloendothelial system,[185] IVIG was therefore an attractive option for the therapy of AIHA as well. Unfortunately, AIHA in many patients in early trials appeared to be refractory to IVIG therapy.[186, 187] Bussel and colleagues[68] then reported that very high doses of IVIG (5 g/kg over 5 days) were necessary to produce a therapeutic benefit, perhaps because the reticuloendothelial system was enlarged in AIHA patients.[68] Even at this high dose, however, only approximately one third of patients with warm-reactive AIHA had a response to IVIG therapy.[68, 188] Prognostic factors that predicted IVIG response included a lower pretreatment hemoglobin concentration and the presence of hepatomegaly.[189] Based on these results, as well as on a variety of safety and cost issues,[190] IVIG should not be considered standard treatment of AIHA in children. However, continued investigation of its potential role in modulation of the immune response may shed light on important mechanisms of autoantibody production and immune-mediated erythrocyte clearance.[191]

Exchange transfusion is a reasonable therapeutic option for AIHA in the acute setting, because circulating erythrocyte autoantibodies, soluble activated complement components, and sensitized erythrocytes can all be removed from the patient simultaneously.[192] More commonly, however, plasmapheresis or plasma exchange has been used,[193–196] even for very small infants.[197–199] It is generally accepted that patients with IgM autoantibodies respond better to plasmapheresis than those with IgG autoantibodies,[195, 200] presumably because of differences in the size and binding characteristics of the two molecules. The larger size of IgM molecules keeps them within the intravascular space and amenable to removal by plasmapheresis. In contrast, IgG autoantibodies can diffuse into the extravascular space; thus plasmapheresis removes only a fraction of the total IgG autoantibodies. In addition, IgM autoantibodies are less tightly affixed to erythrocytes than are IgG autoantibodies at warm temperatures and are more likely to be removed by plasmapheresis. For this reason, the extracorporeal circuit should be warmed during exchange transfusion of a patient with cold-reactive autoantibodies.[201]

For the child with chronic or refractory AIHA, more aggressive therapy is often required to alleviate the symptoms of anemia and to help the child achieve a more normal lifestyle. Long-term use of corticosteroids or immunoglobulin is generally unacceptable, because of side effects, costs, and inconvenience. A variety of additional therapeutic agents are available, however, as well as surgical intervention. No simple treatment algorithm can be proposed that is correct for all children with AIHA. The clinician should individualize therapy for each patient, based on the hematologic response and side effects.

Splenectomy is the time-honored therapy for the patient with chronic AIHA.[182, 202] The rationale for splenectomy is based in part upon the animal model of AIHA, which demonstrated that IgG-sensitized erythrocytes were cleared almost exclusively within the spleen, regardless of whether or not complement was activated.[62] In keeping with this model, patients with IgG autoantibodies respond better to splenectomy than do patients with IgM autoantibodies.[203] However, preoperative prediction of the clinical response to splenectomy, based on splenic uptake of radiolabeled red cells,[204] is variable at best.[69, 88] In 12 patients with AIHA, Parker and colleagues[205] found a poor correlation between ^{51}Cr-labeled red cell survival and eventual response to splenectomy. Only 3 of 5 patients with a highly elevated spleen-to-liver uptake ratio had a clinical remission after splenectomy, whereas 3 of 5 with a very low ratio also had a remission after splenectomy. The authors concluded that radiolabeled red cell survival studies were not reliable indicators of the clinical response to splenectomy in AIHA.[205] Splenectomy also may benefit the patient with AIHA by removing a major site of autoantibody production, similar to the pathophysiologic effect of anti-platelet autoantibody production in immune thrombocytopenic purpura.[75]

Coon[206] reported on 52 patients with AIHA who underwent splenectomy. There was no surgical mortality and low morbidity, and an excellent response was seen in 64 percent and an improved status in another 21 percent of patients. However, splenectomy should be avoided in young children if possible, because of the risk of postsplenectomy sepsis due to encapsulated bacterial organisms. Before splenectomy, children should receive immunization with polyvalent polysaccharide vaccines against *S. pneumoniae*, *H. influenzae* type b, and *N. meningitidis* to enhance the humoral immune response against these potentially lethal pathogens. The addition of protein-conjugated vaccines against *S. pneumoniae* and *H. influenzae* type b into the routine infant immunization series will help provide effective immunity against these organisms. Children who undergo splenectomy should be given penicillin twice daily for at least 2 years after surgery; some clinicians prefer life-long penicillin prophylaxis because fatal sepsis occurring years after splenectomy has been described.[207, 208] Erythromycin should be used if the patient is allergic to penicillin. After splenectomy, prompt medical attention should be sought for children with fever (temperature greater than 38.5°C [101.5°F]) because of the possibility of bacterial sepsis.

Additional therapeutic agents have been used less often in children with AIHA. High-dose pulse dexamethasone, which caused initial but fleeting excitement for patients with chronic immune thrombocytopenic purpura, has been reported to have beneficial effect for some adults with warm-reactive AIHA.[209] Danazol, a semisynthetic androgen, also has efficacy in some patients with AIHA[67, 210, 211] although no young children were included in these reports. One report suggested that danazol was more effective when used as first-line therapy in conjunction with corticosteroids,[211] whereas another demonstrated

excellent responses even in patients with refractory AIHA who had received previous therapy including splenectomy.[67] The mechanisms of action of danazol are not known, but decreased titers of cell-bound IgG and complement were noted in most patients who had a response.[67] Danazol has been shown to decrease IgG production,[212] suggesting that this therapy may have multiple mechanisms of action that could be beneficial for the patient with AIHA. The primary side effects of danazol are elevations in the hepatic transaminases and mild masculinizing effects, however, that essentially preclude its routine use in young or female patients.

Cytotoxic agents have been used in the treatment of AIHA, with the presumed intent of reducing autoantibody formation. Vincristine and vinblastine have limited use in the pediatric age-group but should be considered for the patient with refractory AIHA.[66, 213, 214] *In vitro* incubation of platelets with *Vinca* alkaloids followed by transfusion of these "loaded" platelets has been used to poison the reticuloendothelial macrophages directly.[213] The success of other cytotoxic agents, including cyclophosphamide, 6-mercaptopurine, and 6-thioguanine, has been limited in adults, but no trials in children with AIHA have been reported. A typical daily dose of cyclophosphamide for an adult with AIHA is 50 to 100 mg orally. Because these agents are generally myelosuppressive and potentially mutagenic,[215] they should be used with great caution in children. The use of high-dose cyclophosphamide, designed to provide immunoablation without complete myeloablation, has been reported anecdotally for severe refractory AIHA.[216, 217] One of the side effects of this immunoablative therapy is profound myelosuppression, and its long-term efficacy remains unproved at the current time. Similarly, combination chemotherapy for autoimmune disease has significant side effects related to severe granulocytopenia and thrombocytopenia.

Azathioprine is an immunosuppressive agent that affects both the humoral and cellular arms of the immune response, but its greatest effects are on the T lymphocytes.[182] By affecting T-cell helper function, azathioprine can interfere with autoantibody synthesis. Azathioprine is unlikely to induce a clinical remission as a single agent but could be used as a corticosteroid-sparing agent. A treatment dose of azathioprine ranges from 25 to 200 mg/day orally, and side effects include leukopenia, thrombocytopenia, and hepatic injury. Because the goal of azathioprine therapy is a reduction in autoantibody synthesis, responses may not be noted until after 3 months of therapy.[182]

Cyclosporine, another immunosuppresive agent that focuses primarily on T lymphocytes, has been reported to have been successful in a few patients with steroid-resistant AIHA.[218] Because of the significant side effects associated with long-term use of cyclosporine, however, including nephrotoxicity, hypertension, and even the risk of malignancy, it should not be used routinely in children with AIHA.

Several additional miscellaneous agents have been reported anecdotally to have had beneficial effects in the treatment of AIHA. The response of a patient with cold agglutinin disease to α-interferon therapy merits additional investigation.[219] The effects of soluble growth factors on erythrocyte phagocytosis by macrophages in AIHA suggests a potential role for cytokine therapy.[220] As with many other autoimmune diseases, therapy with specific action on autoreactive T or B lymphocytes is clearly needed and potentially would allow clinical benefit without hazardous side effects.

Targeted therapy against the source of autoantibody production (plasma cells) may soon be possible. Rituximab (Rituxan) is a humanized murine monoclonal antibody directed against the human CD20 antigen, which is present only on B lymphocytes. Rituximab induces B-cell apoptosis[221] and is highly effective for B-cell lymphoma.[222] Although rituximab is not currently licensed as a therapeutic agent for autoimmune diseases, its restricted action against B lymphocytes makes it an attractive drug for autoantibody-mediated disorders such as AIHA. Anecdotal accounts of success with rituximab have been reported for adults with immune thrombocytopenia[223, 224] and cold agglutinin disease[225–227] and for children with refractory warm-reactive AIHA.[228] Trials with this exciting new agent will no doubt be forthcoming.

Finally, complete lymphoid ablation and myeloablation, followed by reconstitution with compatible healthy hematopoietic stem cells, could theoretically cure systemic autoimmune diseases. The use of stem cell transplantation for autoimmune disorders such as AIHA has been proposed, and suggested guidelines have been published.[229] For children with refractory AIHA, transplantation using autologous stem cells has been attempted but with limited success.[230, 231] Human leukocyte antigen (HLA)-matched allogeneic stem cells may provide an additional graft-versus-autoimmunity effect,[230] although the current morbidity and mortality of allogeneic bone marrow transplantation must be carefully weighed against the adverse effects of conventional therapy. Moreover, AIHA can actually develop after bone marrow transplantation for other indications,[232, 233] presumably in the setting of a weakened immune system with lymphocyte dysregulation. At this time, stem cell transplantation should not be considered a reasonable therapeutic option for children with AIHA unless they have refractory and life-threatening disease.

Pathogenesis of Autoantibody Formation

The autoantibodies produced in AIHA are clearly pathogenic, and the amount of antibody bound to the cell surface is proportional to the rate of erythrocyte removal by the reticuloendothelial system. Much less is known about the origin of autoantibody formation and why certain individuals have *in vivo* expansion of autoreactive lymphocytes that should normally be suppressed or eliminated by the immune system.

Case reports have suggested an association between AIHA and certain immune response genes, especially the HLA-B locus.[234] Patients with HLA-B8 may have an increased risk for AIHA[235] and a linkage with HLA-B27 also has been reported.[236] HLA-DQ6 may confer protection against AIHA.[237,238] One large investigation of familial autoimmune cytopenias concluded that genetic factors were present, but they were not linked to the HLA complex.[239] In cold agglutinin disease, trisomy 3 has been

identified as a commonly seen chromosomal abnormality, and the autoantibodies are produced by defined abnormal clones of B lymphocytes.[240, 241]

The erythrocyte autoantibodies that develop in most patients with AIHA represent a polyclonal B-lymphocyte response. The mechanisms by which these autoreactive B cells proliferate without proper immune surveillance are still poorly understood at this time, although new data are beginning to shed light on these processes. Expansion of autoreactive B cells could result from *in vivo* stimulation of normal B lymphocytes[242]; two reports support this idea.[243, 244] Furthermore, altered control of normal self IgG in AIHA has been postulated.[245] However, a considerable amount of data suggests that autoreactive antibodies develop after a specific immune stimulation, rather than as a consequence of nonspecific polyclonal antibody formation.[246, 247] Sequence analysis of the immunoglobulin gene rearrangements used by autoreactive autoantibodies has demonstrated a restricted repertoire of variable gene usage and evidence of somatic mutations.[248–251] These results suggest that autoreactive B lymphocytes in AIHA undergo *in vivo* antigen-driven selection and mutation. The ability to clone individual autoreactive B cells, either by Epstein-Barr virus transformation[251, 252] or by hybridoma formation,[253] should facilitate additional molecular analysis of the immunoglobulin response.

Although the pathogenic autoantibodies are produced by B lymphocytes, it is quite possible that the underlying immune defect in many patients with AIHA lies within the cellular immune compartment.[254] T lymphocytes orchestrate the immune response by interacting with antigen-presenting mononuclear cells and helping B cells produce specific antibody. Experimental results from a murine model of AIHA have implicated T lymphocytes in the pathogenesis of the disorder.[255, 256] In humans, previous reports documented a variety of T-lymphocyte abnormalities in patients with AIHA, including an increase in activated T lymphocytes,[257] an imbalance in T-cell subsets,[258] a deficiency in the autologous mixed lymphocyte reaction,[259] and a deficiency of T-suppressor function.[260, 261] T-lymphocyte reactivity with Rh cryptic epitopes has been recently described.[262] AIHA has been reported in several patients with T-lymphocyte immunosuppression from cyclosporine treatment[263, 264]; in these patients AIHA may result from dysregulation of transplanted donor lymphocytes.[265, 266] AIHA also is a well-recognized clinical manifestation of infection with the human immunodeficiency virus.[267, 268]

The role of monocytes and macrophages in AIHA has only recently begun to be elucidated. Increased levels of regulatory cytokines including interleukin (IL)-4, IL-6, IL-10, and IL-13 have been reported in AIHA.[269, 270] Altered expression of FcγRIII on macrophages appears to influence the clearance of antibody-sensitized erythrocytes, further illustrating the importance of macrophages in the pathophysiologic origin of AIHA and the potential for targeted therapy. Taken together, these data support the hypothesis that autoreactive B lymphocytes are present in the immune repertoire of normal individuals but expand and proliferate only in certain clinical settings, such as genetically susceptible individuals or those with T-lymphocyte dysregulation or monocyte/macrophage abnormalities.

SECONDARY AUTOIMMUNE HEMOLYTIC ANEMIA

The classification scheme described in Table 14–1 indicates that AIHA can be a primary disorder or can occur in association with another systemic illness. The latter cases are known as secondary AIHA, because they occur in the setting of a much broader immune dysregulation. In one large series composed mostly of adults, patients with secondary AIHA represented more than one half of the total patients with warm-reactive AIHA.[128] All patients with AIHA should be evaluated for the presence of another underlying illness.

A common form of secondary AIHA occurs in the presence of another recognized autoimmune disease such as systemic lupus erythematosus.[271] Other generalized autoimmune and inflammatory disorders, including Sjögren syndrome,[272, 273] scleroderma,[274] dermatomyositis,[275] ulcerative colitis,[276, 277] rheumatoid arthritis, autoimmune thyroiditis, and others,[128] also have been associated with AIHA. The belief is that patients with these disorders have a genetic susceptibility for immune dysregulation, which leads to the expansion and proliferation of autoreactive B lymphocytes.

A special association exists between AIHA and other autoimmune cytopenias, especially thrombocytopenia.[278, 279] First noted by Evans and colleagues,[93] the combination of autoimmune anemia and thrombocytopenia (and occasionally granulocytopenia) is known as Evans syndrome. In a large review of childhood Evans syndrome, the typical clinical course was noted to be chronic and relapsing, and the therapy was generally unsatisfactory.[280] A variety of immunoregulatory abnormalities have been suggested in this disorder,[279, 281] although no single underlying specific immune defect has been identified. The autoantibodies are apparently directed against specific antigens on each of the various blood cell types; that is, the antibodies against erythrocytes, platelets, and occasionally granulocytes are not cross-reactive.[282] Because many children with Evans syndrome have refractory life-threatening disease, aggressive therapy is often warranted. High-dose or combination chemotherapy has been used, but success has been limited.[283–285] Similarly, bone marrow transplantation for children with Evans syndrome has been associated with a poor clinical outcome.[286–288]

AIHA can occur in the setting of malignancy, sometimes presenting clinically before the diagnosis of cancer. In adults, the erythrocyte autoantibodies may reflect an abnormal B-lymphocyte clone found in chronic lymphocytic leukemia,[289, 290] lymphoma,[289, 291] or multiple myeloma.[292] AIHA may also occur in young patients with Hodgkin disease,[293–296] leukemia,[297] or myelodysplasia.[298] Survival for patients with lymphoma who develop AIHA is poor.[291] Although the cause of AIHA in patients with cancer is not known, an underlying immune deficiency may be the origin of both the autoimmune phenomenon and the malignancy.

Children with congenital immunodeficiency can develop AIHA, probably due to the lack of proper immune regulation.[299–301] Similarly, patients with acquired immunosuppression can develop AIHA.[264, 302] Patients infected with the human immunodeficiency virus are particularly susceptible to the development of erythrocyte autoantibodies,[267, 268] probably due to both the polyclonal B-lymphocyte activation and lack of immune regulation by T lymphocytes.

The majority of young children who are seen with PCH have had a recent viral-like illness,[76, 84, 87] although an infectious pathogen is rarely identified. Historically, PCH developed in patients with syphilis, although this is rarely observed today. On occasion, however, a well-defined infection triggers an episode of AIHA. Numerous infectious agents have been reported, including *M. pneumoniae*,[303] Epstein-Barr virus,[304, 305] measles, varicella, mumps, rubella,[306] and parvovirus.[307] Most of these autoantibodies are IgM with a specificity for the I/i polysaccharide antigen system on the red cells,[136] although occasionally specificity against the P polysaccharide antigen has been reported.[308] Reactivity of anti-I antibodies with mycoplasmal antigens suggests that autoantibodies may result from immunologic cross-reactivity.[309]

Acute bacterial infections can cause hemolytic anemia from a different mechanism. The T antigen on the erythrocyte surface is known as a "cryptic" antigen, because it is not normally available for binding. In the presence of bacteria with neuraminidase activity, such as clostridial or pneumococcal species, however, sialic acid removal leads to exposure of the T antigen. Because many people have naturally occurring cold-reactive IgM antibodies with anti-T specificity, hemolysis can result.[310] Although the practice is somewhat controversial, transfusions of erythrocytes should be washed in this clinical setting to avoid transfusing additional anti-T antibodies.[311]

Although they are not common in childhood, drug-induced autoantibodies should be mentioned as an cause of secondary AIHA. Classically described after therapy with methyldopa,[312] red cell antibodies have been reported in association with dozens of different pharmaceutical agents.[313] Medications of particular importance in the pediatric age range that can cause AIHA include a variety of antibiotics: penicillins,[314, 315] cephalosporins,[316, 317] tetracycline,[318] erythromycin,[319] and probenecid.[320] Common agents such as acetaminophen[321] and ibuprofen[322] also have been implicated in hemolysis. Drug-induced hemolytic anemia typically results from generation of antidrug antibodies that cross-react with erythrocytes, although the drug may be required to form a hapten or even a ternary complex with the erythrocyte.[313, 323]

Therapy for patients with secondary AIHA must be twofold: the hemolytic anemia must be treated, and for best results the underlying systemic illness must be addressed as well. For example, treatment for a generalized autoimmune or inflammatory disorder or administration of antibiotics for a specific infection also can have a beneficial effect on the AIHA. Discontinuation of the offending drug will help ameliorate hemolysis from drug-induced autoantibodies. For most cases of warm-reactive secondary AIHA, administration of corticosteroids is effective in reducing hemolysis. Short bursts or tapering courses of steroids can be used safely in patients with secondary AIHA, even if they are immunodeficient. In contrast, splenectomy is less likely to be successful for adults with secondary AIHA in association with malignancy, compared with those with primary AIHA.[324]

PAROXYSMAL NOCTURNAL HEMOGLOBINURIA

A rare condition, PNH has fascinated hematologists for more than a century. In its classical presentation, patients with PNH have ongoing hemolysis with intermittent episodes of dark urine (hemoglobinuria), most commonly on awakening in the morning. The hemolysis of PNH is due to abnormal interactions between the erythrocytes and the complement system. However, unlike AIHA, PNH is an intracorpuscular defect, because the hemolysis results from an increased sensitivity of the patient's erythrocytes to physiologic complement-mediated lysis. In addition, PNH is a complex disease with protean clinical manifestations, only one of which is hemolytic anemia. The secrets of this enigmatic disorder have only recently yielded to the efforts of modern molecular biology, culminating with the identification of the *PIGA* gene that is mutated in patients with PNH.

Historical Perspective

Clinicians first described PNH in the latter part of the 19th century,[325, 326] although it took many years to recognize several important facts: (1) the dark pigment in the urine was actually hemoglobin; (2) the serum of patients with PNH did not induce hemolysis of normal erythrocytes, thus distinguishing PNH from PCH; (3) the hemolysis was due to an intrinsic defect in the patient's own erythrocytes; and (4) the hemolysis was due to the lytic action of serum complement. Many of the initial insights into the pathophysiology of the hemolysis were due to the efforts of Dr. Thomas Ham, who first clearly demonstrated that acidified serum enhanced the hemolysis of PNH erythrocytes[327–329]; the test that bears his name was for many years the definitive laboratory method to establish the diagnosis of PNH. It was later recognized that the complement lysis sensitivity was not all or none; patients often had a population of erythrocytes with a 15- to 25-fold increased complement sensitivity (type III cells), another population with a 3- to 5-fold increased sensitivity (type II cells), and a population of normal type I erythrocytes.[330–332] Flow cytometry has now replaced the time-honored Ham test, as well as the sucrose lysis and complement lysis sensitivity tests, as the preferred diagnostic laboratory method for the diagnosis of PNH.[333]

Clinical Manifestations

The passing of dark urine is the classical symptom for which the disorder is named. Patients with PNH have hemoglobinuria rather than hematuria, resulting from chronic intravascular hemolysis from complement. Although the original descriptions accurately indicated that dark urine occurs more often on awakening, the cause for this temporal variation is not clear. Moreover, many patients have dark urine throughout the day whereas some never develop this symptom. The typical patient with PNH reports an episode every few weeks, although some have chronic unrelenting hemolysis. Patients may describe hemoglobinuria using colorful language, ranging from iced tea to cola to mahogany to motor oil, or may describe the urine as various combinations of red, orange, brown, and black (Fig. 14–11*A*). Stress or infections tend to trigger hemolysis, although often there is no identifiable reason. Therapy with oral corticosteroids (1 to 2 mg/kg/day of prednisone) can ameliorate the hemolysis and is often recommended for 24 to 72 hours around the time of a hemolytic episode.

The clinical manifestations of PNH include much more than simply hemolytic anemia.[334] Table 14–5 lists the more common signs and symptoms observed in patients with PNH. In addition to hemolysis, patients with PNH tend to have an increased number of infections, particularly those that are sinopulmonary and blood-borne. A more severe clinical complication is venous thrombosis, which often occurs in unusual locations such as the hepatic veins, leading to the Budd-Chiari syndrome (Fig. 11*B*); mesenteric veins; or sagittal veins (Figure 14–11*C*). The complications of venous thrombosis are often fatal, because the hypercoagulability observed in PNH is very difficult to treat even with thrombolytic agents. The development of venous thrombosis is a risk factor for poor long-term survival, at least for caucasian patients.[335] Patients of Asian ancestry with PNH rarely develop venous thrombosis, however, suggesting a genetic predisposition for the hypercoagulable state in PNH.

Defective hematopoiesis is present in the majority of patients with PNH, either at presentation or during the course of the disease. Most patients have peripheral macrocytic anemia with erythroid hyperplasia in the bone marrow, but some evolve into severe aplastic anemia and suffer the clinical consequences of pancytopenia. Treatment with antithymocyte globulin seems to help in a portion of patients. Finally, PNH can evolve into myelodysplasia or acute nonlymphoblastic leukemia, which typically occurs within the first 5 years of disease.[336] The incidence of leukemic transformation is only 1 to 3 percent, but this rate far exceeds that of the general population.

Although primarily a disease of adults, PNH definitely occurs in children and adolescents, and the diagnosis should be considered for any child with unexplained cytopenia or thrombosis. In a cohort of 26 young patients with PNH, several important differences were noted compared with the clinical descriptions of adults.[337] In many children PNH was initially misdiagnosed, with an average of almost 2 years from initial symptoms to the correct diagnosis. Very few children had dark urine as a presenting symptom, and only 65 percent of children ever developed clinically evident hemoglobinuria. Thrombosis occurred in approximately one third of patients, and some died of this dreaded complication. All patients had laboratory evidence of defective or ineffective hematopoiesis, either at diagnosis or over the course of their disease. The survival curve for these patients indicated that the 10-year survival was only 60 percent, although several deaths were

TABLE 14–5. Signs and Symptoms Commonly Observed in Paroxysmal Nocturnal Hemoglobinuria

Intravascular hemolysis
 Dark urine
 Iron deficiency
 Acute renal failure
Infections
 Sinopulmonary
 Bloodborne
Venous thrombosis
 Occurs in one third of patients
 Unusual locations
Defective hematopoiesis
 Macrocytosis, pancytopenia
 Association with aplastic anemia
Transition to malignancy
 Nonlymphoblastic leukemia

CD55 (decay accelerating factor, DAF)[340] and CD59 (membrane inhibitor of reactive lysis),[341] in the 1980s. The abnormal peripheral blood cells in patients with PNH were noted to be lacking both CD55 and CD59. As a result of these deficiencies, randomly deposited complement factors and C3 convertase complexes cannot be cleared from the erythrocyte membrane, which leads to the formation of the membrane attack complex, pores, and cell lysis.[330]

The commonality of these two complement regulatory proteins goes beyond function, because both use a novel motif for anchoring into the plasma membrane (Fig. 14–12). Unlike the majority of surface proteins that contain a highly hydrophobic domain that serves as a transmembrane region between the intracellular domain and the extracellular domain of the polypeptide, certain proteins use a glycosylphosphatidylinositol (GPI) anchor for

due to complications of pancytopenia in an era before modern antibiotic and transfusion therapy. Because bone marrow transplantation can be curative therapy for PNH,[338, 339] it should be considered for selected patients with this disorder if an HLA-matched sibling donor is available. Transplants from unrelated stem cell donors are associated with substantial morbidity and mortality, however, and currently cannot be recommended routinely for patients with PNH.

Biochemical Basis

Important clues to the etiology of PNH emerged with the identification of two complement regulatory proteins,

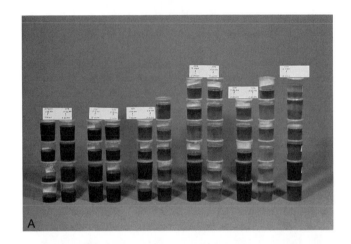

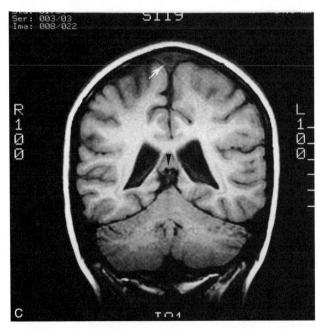

FIGURE 14–11. Clinical manifestations of paroxysmal nocturnal hemoglobinuria (PNH). *A,* Hemoglobinuria produced over several days, with urine samples ranging from normal yellow to black. (Photograph courtesy of Dr. Wendell Rosse). *B,* Massive hepatosplenomegaly that developed in a 14-year-old child with PNH and Budd-Chiari syndrome. *C,* A fatal superior sagittal sinus thrombosis that developed in a 16-year-old female with PNH. In this T$_1$-weighted coronal image at the level of the posterior internal cerebral veins, the normally expected black flow signal void in the superior sagittal sinus *(white arrow)* is replaced with an intermediate signal owing to the thrombus. This appearance contrasts with the normal black venous flow void that is preserved in the internal cerebral veins *(black arrowhead).* (Photograph courtesy of Drs. Frank Keller and Jeffrey Hogg.)

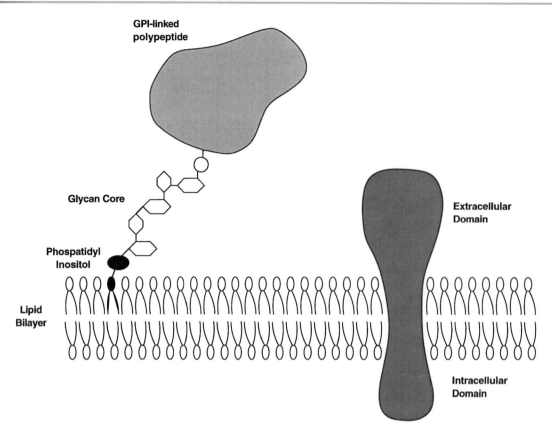

FIGURE 14–12. The glycosylphosphatidylinositol (GPI) anchor for attachment of surface proteins to the cell membrane. The structure of a GPI-linked protein is shown on the *left*. The GPI anchor consists of a phosphatidylinositol molecule in the outer leaflet of the lipid bilayer, which is connected to a glycan core consisting of multiple sugars and side chains. The polypeptide is then linked to the anchor at its C terminus via an amide bond. The result is a surface protein with a fluid and mobile attachment to the cell surface. The entire polypeptide is present in the extracellular milieu. In contrast, a transmembrane protein is shown on the *right,* with an extracellular domain, a short transmembrane domain, and an intracellular domain.

TABLE 14–6. Surface Proteins Absent from Affected Hematopoietic Cells in Paroxysmal Nocturnal Hemoglobinuria

Complement regulatory proteins
  Decay accelerating factor (CD55)
  Membrane inhibitor of reactive lysis (CD59)
Immunologically important proteins
  Lymphocyte function antigen-3 (LFA-3, CD58)
  Fc receptor gamma III (FcγRIII, CD16)
  Endotoxin binding protein receptor (CD14)
Receptors
  Urokinase receptor (UPAR)
  Folate receptor
Enzymes
  Alkaline phosphatase
  Acetylcholinesterase
  5′-*ecto*nucleotidase
Proteins with unknown functions
  CD24
  CD48
  CD52 (Campath-1)
  CD66c
  CD67
  JMH-bearing protein

Adapted from Rosse WF, Ware RE: The molecular basis of paroxysmal nocturnal hemoglobinuria. Blood 1995; 86:3277.

membrane attachment.[342, 343] GPI-linked proteins are covalently attached at their C terminus to a variable glycan moiety, which is itself attached to a phosphatidylinositol molecule in the outer leaflet of the cell membrane lipid bilayer. This glycolipid structure is assembled within the endoplasmic reticulum and is coupled to the protein precursor as a preformed unit.[343, 344] Initially described for the alkaline phosphatase enzyme,[345] GPI linkage is now known to be used by a diverse set of surface proteins (Table 14–6), including acetylcholinesterase,[346] Thy–1,[347] lymphocyte function-associated antigen 3,[348] Fcγ receptor type III,[349] the complement regulatory proteins CD55 and CD59,[340, 341] and others.[350, 351] The functional advantages of GPI-linkage for surface proteins are speculative but include increased lateral diffusional mobility,[352, 353] second messenger generation,[354] signal transduction,[355, 356] and the ability to be cleaved from the cell surface into the extracellular milieu.[357]

The primary defect in PNH resides in the incomplete bioassembly of GPI anchors, because all GPI-linked surface proteins have absent or diminished expression on the surface of the abnormal PNH cells.[358–364] Biochemical analysis of GPI-deficient cells localized the defect in PNH to an early step in GPI anchor biosynthesis.[365–368] Mammalian mutant cell lines deficient in GPI-linked surface proteins have been established and can be classified into different complementation classes.[369, 370] Class A, C, and H mutants cannot transfer the initial *N*-acetylglu-

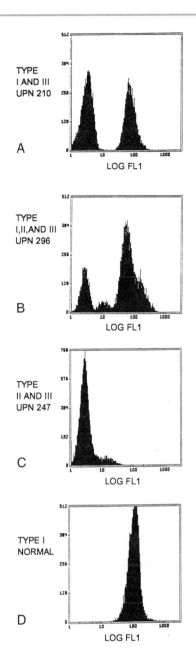

FIGURE 14–13. Immunophenotype analysis of erythrocytes in PNH by flow cytometry. Examples of surface CD59 expression are shown for three patients and a control subject. *A*, Data for unique patient number (UPN) 210, who had both type I and Type III erythrocytes. *B*, Data for UPN 296 with type I, II, and III cells. *C*, Data for UPN 247, who had predominantly type III erythrocytes and a few type II cells. *D*, Normal expression from a control subject. (Data from Ware RE, Rosse WF, Hall SE: Immunophenotypic analysis of reticulocytes in paroxysmal nocturnal hemoglobinuria. Blood 1995; 86:1586.)

cosamine to the phosphatidylinositol acceptor, suggesting that at least three genes control this step. Fusion experiments of PNH cells with murine GPI-deficient cell lines further identified the defect as a class A mutation in all patients tested.[367, 371, 372] Thus, despite the possibility of various enzymatic defects along the GPI anchor biosynthetic pathway, all patients with PNH reported to date have a class A defect.[373]

Altered expression of GPI-linked surface proteins on the abnormal cells in PNH has led to a simpler and more accurate diagnostic test than older methods of complement-mediated lysis. Peripheral blood erythrocytes and granulocytes can be analyzed by flow cytometry for surface expression of GPI-linked proteins such as CD16, CD48, CD55, or CD59.[333, 374] Erythrocytes that are completely deficient in GPI-linked surface proteins are present in almost all patients and correspond to the PNH type III cells. Partially deficient cells can be detected in approximately 50 percent of patients and correspond to type II cells.[333, 375] Cells with normal GPI-linked surface expression (type I cells) are typically present as well. Identification of these cell populations by flow cytometric analysis is illustrated in Figure 14–13. The surface CD59 expression on circulating erythrocytes from a patient with type I and type III cells is shown in Figure 14–13*A*, that for a patient with type I, II, and III cells in Figure 14–13*B*, and that for a patient with predominantly type III cells but a few type II cells in Figure 14–13*C*. Flow cytometry for a normal control is shown in Figure 13*D*.

Molecular Basis

Analyses of glucose-6-phosphate dehydrogenase allozymes[376] and a monoclonal pattern of X chromosome inactivation[377, 378] have documented that PNH is a clonal hematologic disorder. The abnormal clone is believed to originate at the level of a primitive multipotent bone marrow progenitor cell, in that all cells of the myeloerythroid lineage, including erythrocytes, granulocytes, platelets, and monocytes are affected.[364] Lymphocytes[371, 379] and natural killer cells[380] also are GPI-deficient to varying degrees, however, suggesting that PNH is actually a clonal stem cell disorder. The abnormal PNH clone may be relatively small, affecting 10 to 25 percent of circulating erythrocytes and granulocytes or may become dominant with more than 95 percent GPI-deficient circulating cells.

The recognition that all patients with PNH have a class A complementation defect suggested that a single gene was responsible for this disorder. By using the strategy of a human cDNA expression library, a gene was identified that repaired the defect in a class A GPI-deficient cell line.[381] Designated *PIGA* because it repaired the *phos-phatidylinositolglycan* defect in a class *A* mutant, this cDNA encoded a novel polypeptide with homology to other known glycosyltransferases. The cloned cDNA was 3589 nucleotides in length and encoded a predicted protein of 484 amino acids. No N-terminal leader or signal peptide sequence was apparent, but a highly hydrophobic region near the C terminus might form a transmembrane domain for insertion through the endoplasmic reticulum membrane. Northern blot analysis indicated a single transcript of approximately 4.2 kb.[381]

PIGA was subsequently considered to be a candidate gene for PNH, so several groups analyzed their patients for genetic mutations. *PIGA* abnormalities in PNH have now been reported from laboratories around the world, confirming that *PIGA* is the gene defective in PNH.[382–389] Interestingly, the majority of mutations are short (one to two nucleotide) insertions or deletions that

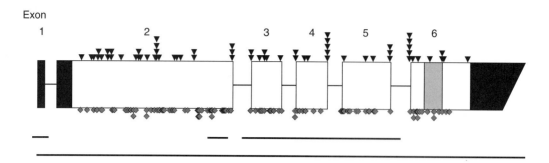

▼ : Base substitution

◆ : Deletion/insertion

— : Large deletion/insertion

FIGURE 14–14. Summary of *PIGA* mutations identified in patients with PNH. The *PIGA* exons are illustrated, along with the location and type of mutations previously reported. The majority of the *PIGA* mutations are small frameshift mutations, either from insertion or deletion of one or two nucleotides. (From Nishimura J, Murakami Y, Kinoshita T: Paroxysmal nocturnal hemoglobinuria: An acquired genetic disease. Am J Hematol 1999; 62:175.)

occur throughout the coding region of the *PIGA* gene.[390] These nucleotide changes cause frameshift mutations, as the triplet nucleotide coding sequence is altered; usually a premature termination codon follows the frameshift mutation. Missense mutations that substitute a single amino acid residue account for the minority of *PIGA* abnormalities reported, but may be clustered toward the 5' end of the coding region.[391] Figure 14–14 illustrates the known *PIGA* mutations that have been identified and reported to date in patients with PNH.

The chromosomal assignment of *PIGA* to the X chromosome[382, 392] and the assignment of other genes involved in GPI anchor biosynthesis (*PIGF* and *PIGH*) to autosomes[392] help to explain the predominant class A defect in PNH. Whereas a single *PIGA* mutation could result in abnormal GPI anchor biosynthesis, mutations in both alleles of other genes involved in GPI anchor biosynthesis would be required to produce clinically overt disease. It is possible that a patient with PNH will be identified with a complementation other than class A and a gene mutation other than *PIGA*.

Do *PIGA* Mutations Cause Paroxysmal Nocturnal Hemoglobinuria?

The pathophysiology of the various clinical manifestations of PNH presumably reflects the absence or diminished expression of specific GPI-linked surface proteins. Hemoglobinuria is readily explained by the absence of surface CD55 and CD59, which allows chronic complement-mediated intravascular hemolysis. In contrast, the cause of the hypercoagulable state in PNH is not well understood. PNH platelets lack the GPI-linked complement regulatory proteins CD55 and CD59 and respond to the deposition of terminal complement components by vesiculation of portions of their plasma membrane. The resultant platelet microparticles have increased procoagulant properties.[393] PNH cells also lack the receptor for the GPI-linked uroki-

nase plasminogen activator, which may result in impaired fibrinolysis.[394] However, patients with PNH have normal plasma levels of natural anticoagulants including proteins C and S, thrombomodulin, and antithrombin III.[395]

The defective hematopoiesis that affects so many patients with PNH is also not well understood. Although GPI-linked surface proteins are likely to be important for normal hematopoiesis, no specific molecule has been identified whose absence leads to marrow hypoplasia. An unusual association exists between PNH and aplastic anemia, however, in that one usually evolves clinically into the other.[396, 397] For example, some patients will have severe aplastic anemia and eventually develop PNH, often after immunosuppressive therapy such as antithymocyte globulin or cyclosporine.[398] In contrast, others with near-normal blood counts and a hypercellular bone marrow will slowly develop hypoplasia, usually as a terminal event.

Several models have been proposed for the pathogenesis and development of PNH. A one-step model was originally proposed more than 30 years ago, stating that a single genetic defect leads directly to PNH.[399] Although this model was attractive because of its simplicity, laboratory evidence using embryonic stem cells[400, 401] and murine models[402, 403] indicated that an acquired *PIGA* mutation did not lead to aplastic anemia or clonal dominance by the abnormal cells. A subsequent two-step model[404, 405] suggested that aplastic anemia occurs first, then a *PIGA* mutation develops within a remaining stem cell. The resulting PNH progeny are then able to either grow preferentially compared with their normal hematopoietic counterparts. However, the identification of multiple clones with distinct *PIGA* mutations in a single patient with PNH,[388, 389, 406, 407] coupled with the recent observation that normal healthy persons have rare hematopoietic cells that harbor *PIGA* mutations,[408, 409] indicate that the two-step model also is too simplistic. As illustrated in Figure 14–15, a newer multistep model has been recently proposed in which *PIGA* mutations initially

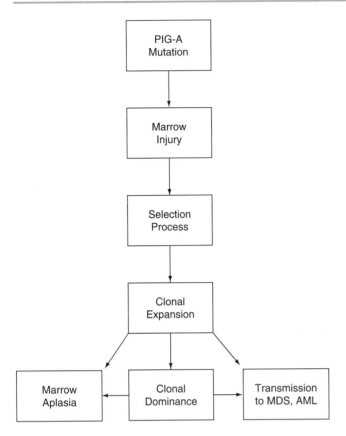

FIGURE 14–15. Multistep model for the pathogenesis and evolution of PNH. In contrast to previous models that hypothesized either a one-step or two-step model; a multistep process is proposed. *PIGA* mutations are acquired randomly and are present in most normal healthy persons. In the setting of an aplastogenic event with marrow injury, such as an autoimmune attack on hematopoiesis, surviving cells undergo a selection process. Genetic mechanisms, including those conferring resistance to apoptosis, allow continued clonal expansion and sometimes clonal dominance of the abnormal PNH clone. Additional genetic events occasionally lead to myelodysplasia or aplasia. (From Ware RE, Heeney MM, Pickens CV, et al: A multistep model for the pathogenesis and evolution of PNH. In Paroxysmal Nocturnal Hemoglobinuria and Related Disorders: Molecular Aspects of Pathogenesis, Omine M, Kinoshita T (eds.). Heidelberg, Springer-Verlag, 2003.

develop as randomly acquired events in normal persons.[410] The *PIGA* mutant cells do not proliferate, however, unless marrow damage then occurs, perhaps in the form of an autoimmune attack against hematopoietic progenitor cells or a further mutation in normal stem cells that arrests their development. Additional genetic events, perhaps including those that confer a resistance to apoptosis,[411–413] then lead to a growth advantage with clonal expansion and eventual clonal dominance. Later genetic events can lead to evolution to myelodysplasia or even malignant transformation into leukemia.

SCHISTOCYTIC HEMOLYTIC ANEMIA

Overview

The term *schistocyte* derives from the Greek word σχιζω (*schizo*), which translates "to tear" and describes erythrocytes that are broken, torn, or sheared. These bizarre poikilocytes are sometimes referred to as schizocytes, but

because this term might be confused with the schizont phase of malarial erythrocyte infection, the term schistocyte is generally preferred. Schistocytic hemolytic anemia is characterized by red cell fragments that develop after erythrocytes are exposed to excessive environmental stresses or shearing forces. This unusual form of hemolytic anemia arises in various pathophysiologic settings, but each clinical condition features increased external forces on the erythrocytes.

Red blood cells encounter tremendous forces as they travel normally through the circulation, including collisions, turbulence, pressure fluctuations, shearing stresses, and interactions with a variety of solid surfaces. Erythrocytes are exposed to some of the highest forces in the left ventricle, as they pass through the aortic valve and flow into the aorta. Among these various forces, experiments have shown that shearing forces are the most difficult for erythrocytes to withstand, and hemolysis occurs after a threshold is reached. Erythrocytes can withstand shear forces up to 15,000 dynes/cm^2 without hemolysis if these forces arise at a fluid-fluid interface,[414] but hemolysis occurs at much lower shear forces at a fluid-solid interface. *In vitro*, hemolysis occurs between 1500 and 3000 dynes/cm^2, especially if the solid surface has any irregularities.[415, 416] Moreover, the mechanical fragility of erythrocytes is affected by temperature, lipids, viscosity, and plasma proteins.[414]

The clinical presentation of schistocytic hemolytic anemia reflects primarily intravascular hemolysis, because the erythrocytes are damaged within the blood vessels. Anemia with pallor and fatigue is more common than jaundice, and dark urine is often present as the primary manifestation of intravascular hemolysis. Erythrocyte fragmentation leads to hemoglobinemia and hemoglobinuria, as well as to elevation of serum lactate dehydrogenase. The serum bilirubin level is usually modestly elevated, reflecting extravascular clearance of the damaged erythrocytes. Examination of the peripheral blood smear (Fig. 14–16) reveals schistocytes with characteristic triangular or crescent shapes, representing

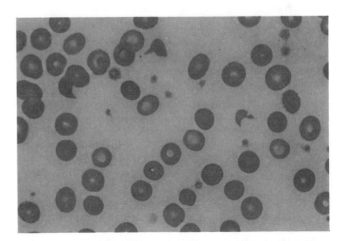

FIGURE 14–16. Schistocytic hemolytic anemia. The peripheral blood smear (× 1000) contains several erythrocytes with characteristic triangular or crescent shapes reflecting cells that have recently undergone fragmentation. Spherocytes are also identified, representing broken cells that have resealed their membranes and adopted a spherical shape (see color section at front of this volume).

erythrocytes that have recently undergone fragmentation. Spherocytes (sometimes called spheroschistocytes) also can be present, which represent broken cells that have resealed their membranes and formed into a sphere, analogous to the process that occurs in immune-mediated hemolytic anemia. Teardrop shapes may be seen, along with polychromasia (reticulocytosis), as a response to the anemia. Depending upon the pathophysiologic changes, there may also be laboratory evidence of intravascular coagulation and thrombocytopenia from platelet trapping or consumption. Schistocytic hemolytic anemia with renal failure and thrombocytopenia is called hemolytic-uremic syndrome (HUS); the additional presence of fever and neurologic dysfunction is called thrombotic thrombocytopenic purpura (TTP).

Microangiopathic Hemolytic Anemia

The term *microangiopathic hemolytic anemia* was used 40 years ago by Brain and co-workers[417] to describe schistocytic hemolysis in conjunction with "disease of small blood vessels." Studying a large cohort of patients with schistocytic hemolytic anemia and acute or chronic renal failure, these authors demonstrated that the amount of erythrocyte fragmentation correlated with the degree of microangiopathic disease, and they postulated that schistocytes developed as a direct consequence of vascular injury. Histologically, microangiopathy was most prominent in the kidney, where arteriolar damage and intraluminal thrombi were noted.[417] An instructive case report of a patient with fatal microangiopathic hemolytic anemia appeared some years later, in which large numbers of microclots composed of fine fibrin strands were identified within the renal and pulmonary arterioles.[418] With scanning electron microscopy, individual erythrocytes were found to be tangled in the fibrin strands, which caused cellular deformation, breakage, and sphering. Figure 14–17 illustrates a "hanged" red blood cell in this destructive intraluminal milieu.[418] Identification of these fine fib-

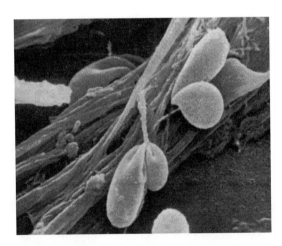

FIGURE 14–17. Hanged red blood cell. A dense fibrin band is seen with several finer strands, over which erythrocytes can be found hanging. With the shearing forces available within the arterial circulation, such erythrocytes will be broken across these thin fibrin strands, resulting in schistocytes. (From Bull BS, Kuhn IN: The production of schistocytes by fibrin strands (a scanning electron microscope study). Blood 1970; 35:104.)

rin strands within the small arteriolar circulation provides a pathophysiologic mechanism for schistocyte formation: the small clots do not fully occlude the vessel; hence, blood flow continues with arterial speed and pressure, thereby shearing erythrocytes at this irregular fluid-solid interface. Microangiopathic schistocytic hemolytic anemia can occur, therefore, in any disorder of the small blood vessels.

Genetic Basis

In the vast majority of patients, microangiopathic schistocytic hemolytic anemia appears sporadically, although sometimes a trigger or associated medical condition can be identified. However, the rare occurrence of congenital or familial microangiopathic hemolytic anemia in conjunction with thrombocytopenia and renal dysfunction (HUS/TTP), with a clinical course that tends to be chronic and relapsing,[419–423] suggests a genetic basis. Mutations in two unrelated genes have recently been identified in patients with familial disease, which provide insight into the pathophysiologic mechanism of microangiopathic schistocytic hemolysis.

Abnormally large circulating multimers of von Willebrand factor (VWF) have been recognized for many years in patients with HUS/TTP.[419, 424, 425] Endothelial cells normally release VWF as very large multimers (sometimes reaching 5 to 20 million D) and a VWF-cleaving protease that is responsible for the continuous limited proteolytic degradation of plasma VWF was recently identified.[426, 427] The gene encoding this protease is located on chromosome 9q34 and is named *ADAMTS13*, a new member of the *ADAMTS* (a *d*isintegrin-like *a*nd *m*etalloproteinase with *t*hrombo*s*pondin motifs) family of zinc metalloproteinase genes. Mutations in *ADAMTS13* that lead to a deficiency of VWF-cleaving protease activity were recently identified in families with relapsing TTP,[428] demonstrating that physiologic degradation of VWF is essential for normal *in vivo* hemostasis. In cases of familial relapsing HUS/TTP, very large undegraded VWF multimers presumably initiate or participate in intravascular coagulation that leads to arteriolar fibrin deposition, platelet trapping, and microangiopathic schistocytic hemolytic anemia. Whether or not this pathophysiologic process occurs in all patients with microangiopathic hemolytic anemia and thrombocytopenia is not known at this time, although an instance of TTP mediated by an autoantibody against the VWF-cleaving protease suggests a common pathway.[429] Recently, however, very large VWF multimers have also been identified in other thrombocytopenic disorders, including immune thrombocytopenic purpura, disseminated intravascular coagulation, and systemic lupus erythematosus, which suggests that this abnormality is not specific to microangiopathic disorders.[430] Currently, the importance of *ADAMTS13* gene mutations in microangiopathic hemolytic anemia is not known; inactivating mutations may be present in familial or relapsing HUS/TTP, whereas less severe gene mutations or polymorphisms could be present in some patients with sporadic disease.

A potentially different pathophysiologic process for the development of schistocytic hemolytic anemia derives from patients with familial disease in whom abnormalities of complement factor H have been identified. Factor H is a 150-kD plasma protein that normally regulates the alternative pathway of complement activation. Without proper binding and inhibition of factor H, C3b produced by C3 convertase is allowed to activate the alternative pathway unchecked. In a porcine model, factor H deficiency is associated with dysregulated complement activation and the development of fatal glomerulonephritis.[431] In humans, missense mutations in the factor H gene *(HF1)* have been identified in both dominant and recessive familial cases of microangiopathic hemolytic anemia.[432, 433] The *HF1* mutations reported to date are clustered in the C-terminal region of factor H, which is the moiety that binds to C3b.[434] Whether *HF1* mutations lead directly to complement deposition within the kidney, which then leads to microangiopathy, is not proven, but damage to the endothelium appears to be important.[435] Perhaps complement activation and deposition onto the renal endothelium leads to exaggerated local release of VWF, which then promotes microangiopathy in an mechanism analogous to that observed in patients with deficiency of VWF-cleaving protease activity. Damage to the renal endothelium also creates an irregular fluid-solid interface against which the erythrocytes must pass, making schistocyte formation more likely.

Clinical Settings

As noted above, when microangiopathic schistocytic hemolytic anemia occurs with acute renal failure and severe thrombocytopenia, this triad is referred to as HUS; the concomitant presence of fever and neurologic deterioration is known as TTP. Both of these related clinical syndromes typically occur sporadically and are associated with substantial morbidity and mortality. These disorders are discussed more fully in Chapter 44.

Schistocytic microangiopathy has also been reported in the setting of immune vasculitis. Patients with a variety of connective tissue disorders including systemic lupus erythematosus,[436] systemic sclerosis,[437] diabetes mellitus,[438] Kawasaki disease,[439] Wegener granulomatosis,[440] and antiphospholipid antibody syndrome[441] can develop schistocytic hemolytic anemia. The pathophysiologic process is believed to reflect renal involvement by the systemic process, especially small vessel (renal arteriolar) damage. Correlation of autoantibody titers with the degree of microangiopathy,[441] coupled with a case report of neonatal lupus erythematosus with severe microangiopathic hemolytic anemia,[442] suggests that autoantibodies can mediate this process.

On some occasions, microangiopathic schistocytic hemolytic anemia occurs in clinical settings that are associated with widespread microangiopathy. Disseminated malignancy, especially adenocarcinoma of the breast or stomach, can lead to schistocytic hemolysis and thrombocytopenia.[443–446] In patients with cancer, laboratory evidence of ongoing intravascular coagulation consistent with a widespread microangiopathic process is typically seen. Similarly, patients with systemic infections can occasionally develop schistocytic microangiopathic hemolysis.[447, 448] Disseminated intravascular coagulation can lead to schistocytic hemolysis as erythrocytes encounter systemic intravascular fibrin deposition. Schistocytic hemolytic anemia has also been described after allogeneic or autologous stem cell transplantation, usually in conjunction with thrombocytopenia and renal dysfunction.[449, 450] Microangiopathic hemolytic anemia that occurs as a late complication after transplantation is associated with a high mortality rate.[449] The etiology is unclear but could reflect systemic endothelial damage that occurs during pretransplant conditioning with total body irradiation.[450]

Microangiopathic disorders associated with pregnancy include pre-eclampsia, characterized by hypertension and proteinuria, and the more dangerous eclampsia that can lead to severe hypertension, seizures, and even death. In pregnant women, the development of schistocytic *h*emolytic anemia, *e*levated *l*iver enzymes, and *l*ow *p*latelet count is known as the HELLP syndrome.[451, 452] This triad of abnormalities is considered to be a severe form of pre-eclampsia that necessitates aggressive management. Transfusions are often required for anemia and thrombocytopenia. Plasmapheresis may be beneficial in reducing hemolysis, even if symptoms continue postpartum.[453] Perhaps the best "therapy" is elective delivery of the infant, which usually leads to complete resolution of the syndrome. The etiology and pathophysiology of microangiopathic hemolytic anemia during pregnancy are unknown; the presence of proteinuria indicates intrinsic renal disease, and laboratory tests do not suggest disseminated intravascular coagulation. Quantitative analysis of carboxyhemoglobin levels has documented that even in mild pre-eclampsia, there is increased destruction of maternal erythrocytes.[454] Immune mechanisms or severe vasospasm with subsequent endothelial damage may also be present in some patients, leading to platelet consumption.[455] The improvement after delivery suggests that the process relates directly to the pregnancy, perhaps from circulating placentally derived factors. Taken together, clinical and laboratory observations indicate that schistocytic hemolytic anemia during pregnancy is an ominous development that warrants aggressive intervention during gestation but usually resolves completely after delivery.

Microangiopathic hemolytic anemia can occur after exposure to a variety of drugs. Cocaine abuse[456] and the therapeutic use of quinine,[457] immunosuppressants cyclosporine[458] and FK506 (tacrolimus),[459, 460] and various antineoplastic agents,[461–464] have all been associated with the development of microangiopathic schistocytic hemolytic anemia. The pathophysiologic process of drug-induced microangiopathy is not known, but it probably follows nephrotoxicity with drug-induced renal endothelial and microvascular damage.

Finally, schistocytic hemolysis can occur with hypertension. In patients with pulmonary hypertension, either as a primary disorder[465] or secondary to congenital heart disease,[466] microangiopathic hemolytic anemia can develop from changes within the pulmonary vasculature. Fibrin deposition in the pulmonary arterial and arteriolar circulation can shear erythrocytes efficiently and lead to schistocyte formation. Severe systemic hypertension, sometimes referred to as "malignant" hypertension, also can lead to schistocytic hemolysis.[467–469] The proposed pathophysiologic process in this setting involves not only intrinsic renal arteriolar changes, but also elevated arterial pressure that increases the shearing forces.[469] Pharmacologic treatment of malignant hypertension can reverse the schistocytic hemolytic process,[468, 469] although in rare patients bilateral nephrectomy is required to control the hypertension and ameliorate the hemolytic anemia.[467, 469]

Therapy

Treatment for patients with microangiopathic schistocytic hemolytic anemia should be individualized, based on the degree of anemia and on the presence of an associated medical condition. Whenever possible, specific therapy for the underlying process leading to the microangiopathic anemia should be instituted. Transfusion support is warranted if the schistocytic hemolysis is massive, or if the anemia is severe enough to be symptomatic. The fate of transfused erythrocytes will probably be the same as that of endogenous red blood cells; thus, transfusions should be administered carefully and judiciously. However, erythrocyte transfusions can be life-saving for patients with schistocytic hemolytic anemia and cardiovascular compromise.

Although a low platelet count can accompany microangiopathic hemolytic anemia, hemorrhagic bleeding is not the norm, even with severe thrombocytopenia. Platelet transfusions are usually unnecessary and can actually lead to worsening of the patient's condition due to *in vivo* aggregation and consumption.

For patients with congenital schistocytic hemolytic anemia, regular infusions of fresh frozen plasma can help ameliorate laboratory abnormalities and prevent clinical complications.[419, 470, 471] Particularly in patients with documented deficiency of VWF-cleaving protease, prophylactic treatment with fresh frozen plasma can be effective even with long-term use.[472]

Exchange plasmapheresis has emerged as the most effective acute intervention for patients with severe microangiopathic schistocytic hemolytic anemia. The beneficial effects of plasmapheresis derive from both the infusion of fresh frozen plasma and the removal of free hemoglobin, fragments of broken erythrocyte membranes, and any plasma substances promoting intravascular coagulation and platelet aggregation. For patients who develop life-threatening disease, plasmapheresis is the therapy of choice[473, 474] and is more effective than corticosteroids, aspirin, dipyridamole, or splenectomy.[475] Exchange plasmapheresis is now recommended early in the clinical course, soon after the diagnosis of microangiopathic hemolytic anemia.[476] However, the patient should be weaned from this therapeutic intervention slowly over several weeks, because relapses and periodic exacerbations are often observed when daily plasmapheresis is discontinued.

Large Vessel Schistocytic Hemolytic Anemia

In addition to the microangiopathic processes that can lead to schistocyte formation, there are several large vessel or "macrovascular" disorders that cause mechanical shearing of erythrocytes. The most common of these large vessel schistocytic disorders occurs in association with hemangiomas, which can lead to hemolytic anemia with intravascular coagulation and severe thrombocytopenia (Kasabach-Merritt syndrome). Most of the cutaneous lesions that lead to the Kasabach-Merritt syndrome are not actually hemangiomas at all; they have a kaposiform (spindle cell) hemangioendothelioma pattern on histologic examination, consistent with their aggressive vascular proliferation.[477, 478] True capillary hemangiomas, although common in infancy, do not cause erythrocyte fragmentation. In contrast, large cavernous hemangiomas can develop in the liver, spleen, or other organs and cause schistocytic hemolytic anemia at any age.[479–481] However, no single effective therapy has been identified for hemangiomas causing schistocytic hemolysis. Improvement has been reported anecdotally and in small series with use of steroids and antifibrinolytic agents,[482] embolization,[481] laser therapy,[483] local radiation,[484] and chemotherapy.[485, 486] The initial success of α-interferon therapy has been dampened by reports of spastic diplegia in association with its use.[487] Newer approaches directed against the angiogenesis itself, such as the use of angiostatin,[488] may eventually prove to be a successful targeted therapy for hemangiomas.

Schistocytic hemolytic anemia is also a well-described complication of valvular heart disease, resulting from excessive shearing forces on the erythrocytes at the interface with the abnormal heart valve. Although mild hemolysis can occur with both congenital and acquired abnormalities of the heart valves,[489, 490] "cardiac" schistocytic hemolysis is most severe after the insertion or failure of a prosthetic heart valve.[491, 492] In the immediate postoperative period, erythrocytes are sheared on the valvular surfaces that lack smooth endothelium, leading to schistocyte formation, hemoglobinuria, and anemia. Occasionally, intravascular hemolysis is severe enough to cause massive hemolysis with profound anemia. Transfusions may be required in the short-term, while the patient awaits endothelialization of the prosthetic valve. When schistocytic hemolytic anemia develops after heart surgery, the clinician should suspect heart valve abnormalities. Echocardiography is relatively insensitive for this clinical diagnosis compared with cardiac catheterization.[492] Surgical correction is generally required for patients with chronic or life-threatening transfusion-dependent intravascular hemolysis. The successful use of pentoxifylline for this condition warrants further investigation.[493]

Finally, an infant with fetal schistocytic hemolytic anemia in association with an umbilical vein varix was reported.[494] Turbulent flow through this large vessel was noted by ultrasonographic examination, and severe schistocytic hemolytic anemia was identified at birth. The infant received aggressive support care including erythrocyte transfusions and survived.

Miscellaneous Forms of Schistocytic Hemolytic Anemia

The term "march hemoglobinuria" refers to transient intravascular hemolysis that can occur after strenuous exercise.[495] This relatively rare form of schistocytic hemolytic anemia was originally noted in soldiers after prolonged marching drills and has been attributed to physical trauma of the erythrocytes within the soles of the feet. The phenomenon seems to occur only in selected individuals, but it can be associated with severe hemoglobinuria and even renal failure.[496] A better name for this form of hemolysis might be "exertional hemoglobinuria," because it can occur after a variety of exercises including running, swimming, karate, and even playing of conga drums.[497–499] One study reported that transfused erythrocytes also had a shortened survival after exercise, documenting the extracorpuscular nature of the defect.[500] Avoidance of the offending physical trauma is usually sufficient to resolve the hemolysis. For persons who develop hemoglobinuria after running, the insertion of protective insoles also may protect against the physical pounding of the erythrocytes.[501]

Thermal burns are the most common form of burn injury that causes anemia, although chemical burns also can induce hemolysis.[502] Erythrocytes that are directly exposed to the burn become injured, and this damage leads either to their immediate lysis or results in shape changes that shorten their survival *in vivo*. If the damage is severe, the erythrocytes circulating through the skin at the time of the injury undergo intravascular hemolysis within hours and cause hemoglobinemia, hemoglobinuria, and anemia. Less damaged erythrocytes continue to circulate but undergo shape changes and are prematurely removed by the spleen.[503] This extravascular hemolysis may occur several days or weeks after the burn injury and may lead to marked late-onset hemolytic anemia. Despite earlier reports suggesting a high incidence of a positive DAT results after burn injury, there is little evidence for immune-mediated hemolytic anemia in this setting.[504]

Although an initial burn injury may be sufficient to cause anemia, concomitant therapies also can contribute to hemolytic anemia.[505] For example, the liberal use of silver sulfadiazine provides an oxidative stress that can induce hemolysis, especially in patients with glucose-6-phosphate dehydrogenase deficiency.[506] Many burn patients require transfusions of fresh frozen plasma, which can induce hemolysis via passively acquired isohemagglutinins. Finally, infections and the antibiotics used to treat these infections can induce hemolysis. Thus, hemolytic anemia associated with burns is often multifactorial. Immediate and delayed hemolytic anemia occurs as a direct consequence of the burn injury, whereas additional therapies can lead to further hemolysis.

REFERENCES

1. McClusky DA III, Skandalakis LJ, Colborn G, et al: Tribute to a triad: History of splenic anatomy, physiology, and surgery—Part 1. World J Surg 1999; 23:311.
2. Neiman RS, Orazi A: Embryology and anatomy. In Disorders of the Spleen, 2nd ed. Philadelphia, WB Saunders, 1999, p 3.
3. Lavender JP, Maseri A, et al: The distribution of cardiac output in man recorded by intravenous injection of microspheres [abstract]. J Nucl Med 1981; 22:P30.
4. Hirasawa Y, Tokuhiro H: Electron microscopic studies on the normal spleen: Especially on the red pulp and the reticuloendothelial cells. Blood 1970; 35:201.
5. Weiss L, Tavassoli M: Anatomical hazards to the passage of erythrocytes through the spleen. Semin Hematol 1970; 7:372.
6. Berendes M: The proportion of reticulocytes in the erythrocytes of the spleen as compared with those of circulating blood, with special reference to hemolytic states. Blood 1959; 14:558.
7. Hosea SW, Burch CG, et al: Impaired immune response of splenectomized patients to polyvalent pneumococcal vaccine. Lancet 1981; 1:804.
8. Ruben FL, Hankins WA, et al: Antibody responses to meningococcal polysaccharide vaccine in adults without a spleen. Am J Med 1984; 76:115.
9. Rowley DA: The formation of circulating antibody in the splenectomized human being following intravenous injection of heterologous erythrocytes. J Immunol 1950; 65:515.
10. Sullivan JL, Ochs HD, et al: Immune response after splenectomy. Lancet 1978; 1:178.
11. Saslaw S, Bouroncle BA, et al: Studies on the antibody response in splenectomized persons. N Engl J Med 1959; 261:120.
12. Motohashi SJ: The effect of splenectomy on the production of antibodies. J Med Res 1972; 43:473.
13. Schnitzer B, Sodeman TM, et al: An ultrastructural study of the red pulp of the spleen in malaria. Blood 1973; 41:207.
14. Rosner F, Zarrabi MH, et al: Babesiosis in splenectomized adults. Review of 22 reported cases. Am J Med 1984; 76:696.
15. Ivemark BI: Implications of agenesis of the spleen on the pathogenesis of cono-truncus anomalies in childhood: Analysis of the heart malformations of the splenic agenesis syndrome, with fourteen new cases. Acta Paediatr 1955; 44(Suppl 104):1.
16. Phoon CK, Neill CA: Asplenia syndrome: Insight into embryology through an analysis of cardiac and extra cardiac anomalies. Am J Cardiol 1994; 73:581.
17. Holroyde CP, Oski FA, Gardner FH: The "pocked" erythrocyte: Red cell alterations in the reticuloendothelial immaturity of the neonate. N Engl J Med 1960; 281:516.
18. Moller JH, Nakib A, et al: Congenital cardiac disease associated with polysplenia: A developmental complex of bilateral "left-sidedness." Circulation 1967; 36:789.
19. Karrer FM, Hall RJ, Lilly JR: Biliary atresia and the polysplenia syndrome. J Pediatr Surg 1991; 26:524.
20. Eraklis AJ, Filler RM: Splenectomy in childhood: A review of 1413 cases. J Pediatr Surg 1972; 7:382.
21. Balik E, Yazici M, Taneli C, et al: Splenoptosis (wandering spleen). Eur J Pediatr Surg 1993; 3:174.
22. Balm R, Willekens FG: Torsion of a wandering spleen. Eur J Surg 1993; 159:249.
23. Schwartz AD, Dadash-Zadeh M, et al: Antibody response to intravenous immunization following splenic tissue autotransplantation in Sprague-Dawley rats. Blood 1977; 49:779.
24. Emond AM, Collis R, Darvill D, et al: Acute splenic sequestration crisis in homozygous sickle cell disease: Natural history and management. J Pediatr 1985; 107:201.
25. Jandl JH, Aster RH: Increased splenic pooling and the pathogenesis of hypersplenism. Am J Med 1967; 253:383.
26. Trias M, Targarona EM, Espert JJ, et al: Laparoscopic surgery for splenic disorders. Lessons learned from a series of 64 cases. Surg Endosc 1998; 12:66.
27. Poulin EC, Mamazza J: Laparoscopic splenectomy: Lessons from the learning curve. Can J Surg 1998; 41:28.
28. Targarona EM, Espert JJ, Balague C, et al: Residual splenic function after laparoscopic splenectomy: A clinical concern. Arch Surg 1998; 133:56.
29. Liu DL, Xia S, Xu W, et al: Anatomy of vasculature of 850 spleen specimens and its application in partial splenectomy. Surgery 1996; 119:27.
30. Bader-Meunier B, Gauthier F, Archambaud F, et al: Long-term evaluation of the beneficial effect of subtotal splenectomy for management of hereditary spherocytosis. Blood 2001; 97:399.
31. de Montalembert M, Girot R, Revillon Y, et al: Partial splenectomy in homozygous β thalassemia. Arch Dis Child 1990; 65:304.
32. Svarch E, Vilorio P, Nordet I, et al: Partial splenectomy in children with sickle cell disease and repeated episodes of splenic sequestration. Hemoglobin 1996; 20:393.
33. Rice HE, Oldham KT, Hillery CA, et al: Clinical and hematological benefits of partial splenectomy for congenital hemolytic anemias in children. Ann Surg.

34. Zer M, Freud E: Subtotal splenectomy in Gaucher's disease: Towards a definition of critical splenic mass. Br J Surg 1992; 79:742.

35. Malangoni MA, Dawes LG, Droege KA, et al: Splenic phagocytic function after partial splenectomy and splenic autotransplantation. Arch Surg 1985; 120:275.

36. Traub A, Giebink GS, Smith C, et al: Splenic reticuloendothelial function after splenectomy, spleen repair, and spleen autotransplantation. N Engl J Med 1987; 317:1559.

37. Ludtke FE, Schuff-Werner P, Lion KA, et al: Immunorestorative effects of reimplanted splenic tissue and splenosis. J Surg Res 1990; 49:413.

38. King H, Shumacker HB Jr: Susceptibility to infection after splenectomy performed in infancy. Ann Surg 1951; 136:239.

39. Holdsworth RJ, Irving AD, Cuschieri A: Postsplenectomy sepsis and its mortality rate: Actual versus perceived risks. Br J Surg 1991; 78:1031.

40. Schilling RF: Estimating the risk for sepsis after splenectomy in hereditary spherocytosis. Ann Intern Med 1995; 122:187.

41. Hayem G: Sur une variete particuliere d'ictere chronique. Ictere infectieux chronique splenomegalique. Presse Med 1898; 6:121.

42. Donath J, Landsteiner K: Ueber paroxysmale Hamoglobinurie. Munch Med Wochenschr 1904; 51:1590.

43. Landsteiner K: Uber Beziehungen zwischen dem Blutserum und den Korperzellen. Munch Med Wochenschr 1903; 50:1812.

44. Coombs RRA, Mourant AE, Race RR: A new test for the detection of weak and "incomplete" Rh agglutinins. Br J Exp Pathol 1945; 26:255.

45. Coombs RRA, Mourant AE: On certain properties of antisera prepared against human serum and its various protein fractions: Their use in the detection of sensitization of human red cells with "incomplete" Rh antibody, and on the nature of this antibody. J Pathol Bacteriol 1947; 59:105.

46. Dausset J, Colombani J: The serology and the prognosis of 128 cases of autoimmune hemolytic anemia. Blood 1959; 14:1280.

47. Jandl JH, Jones AR, Castle WB: The destruction of red cells by antibodies in man. I. Observations on the sequestration and lysis of red cells altered by immune mechanisms. J Clin Invest 1957; 30:1428.

48. Borsos T, Rapp HJ: Complement fixation on cell surfaces by 19S and 7S antibodies. Science 1965; 150:505.

49. Eyster ME, Jenkins DE Jr: Erythrocyte coating substances in patients with positive antiglobulin reactions. Correlation of γG globulin and complement coating with underlying diseases, overt hemolysis and response to therapy. Am J Med 1969; 46:360.

50. Eyster ME, Jenkins DE Jr: γG erythrocyte autoantibodies: Comparison of in vivo complement coating and in vitro "Rh" specificity. J Immunol 1970; 105:221.

51. Rosse WF: Fixation of the first component of complement (C'1a) by human antibodies. J Clin Invest 1968; 47:2430.

52. Rosse WF: Quantitative immunology of immune hemolytic anemia. I. The fixation of C1 by autoimmune antibody and heterologous anti-IgG antibody. J Clin Invest 1971; 50:727.

53. LoBuglio AF, Cotran RS, Jandl JH: Red cells coated with immunoglobulin G: Binding and sphering by mononuclear cells in man. Science 1967; 158:1582.

54. Abramson N, LoBuglio AF, Jandl JH, et al: The interaction between human monocytes and red cells. Binding characteristics. J Exp Med 1970; 132:1191.

55. Kay NE, Douglas SD: Monocyte-erythrocyte interaction in vitro in immune hemolytic anemias. Blood 1977; 50:889.

56. Abramson N, Gelfand EW, Jandl JH, et al: The interaction between human monocytes and red cells. Specificity for IgG subclasses and IgG fragments. J Exp Med 1970; 132:1207.

57. Huber H, Douglas SD, Nusbacher J, et al: IgG subclass specificity of human monocyte receptor sites. Nature 1971; 229:419.

58. Kurlander RJ, Rosse WF, Logue GL: Quantitative influence of antibody and complement coating of red cells on monocyte-mediated cell lysis. J Clin Invest 1978; 61:1309.

59. Schreiber AD, Frank MM: Role of antibody and complement in the immune clearance and destruction of erythrocytes. I. In vivo effects of IgG and IgM complement-fixing sites. J Clin Invest 1972; 51:575.

60. Atkinson JP, Frank MM: Complement-independent clearance of IgG-sensitized erythrocytes: Inhibition by cortisone. Blood 1974; 44:629.

61. Atkinson JP, Frank MM: Studies on in vivo effects of antibody: Interaction of IgM antibody and complement in the immune clearance and destruction of erythrocytes in man. J Clin Invest 1974; 54:339.

62. Atkinson JP, Schreiber AD, Frank MM: Effects of corticosteroids and splenectomy on the immune clearance and destruction of erythrocytes. J Clin Invest 1973; 52:1509.

63. Schreiber AD, Parsons J, McDermott P, et al: Effect of corticosteroids on the human monocyte IgG and complement receptors. J Clin Invest 1975; 56:1189.

64. Issitt PD, Pavone BG, Goldfinger D, et al: Anti-Wr^b, and other autoantibodies responsible for positive direct antiglobulin tests in 150 individuals. Br J Haematol 1976; 34:5.

65. Reusser P, Osterwalder B, Burri H, et al: Autoimmune hemolytic anemia associated with IgA—Diagnostic and therapeutic aspects in a case with long-term follow-up. Acta Haematol 1987; 77:53.

66. Ahn YS, Harrington WJ, Byrnes JJ, et al: Treatment of autoimmune hemolytic anemia with Vinca-loaded platelets. JAMA 1983; 249:2189.

67. Ahn YS, Harrington WJ, Mylvaganam R, et al: Danazol therapy for autoimmune hemolytic anemia. Ann Intern Med 1985; 102:298.

68. Bussel JB, Cunningham-Rundles C, Abraham C: Intravenous treatment of autoimmune hemolytic anemia with very high dose gammaglobulin. Vox Sang 1986; 51:264.

69. Habibi B, Homberg J-C, Schaison G, et al: Autoimmune hemolytic anemia in children. A review of 80 cases. Am J Med 1974; 56:61.

70. Carapella de Luca E, Casadei AM, di Piero G, et al: Auto-immune haemolytic anaemia in childhood. Follow-up in 29 cases. Vox Sang 1979; 36:13.

71. Sokol RJ, Hewitt S, Stamps BK, et al: Autoimmune haemolysis in childhood and adolesence. Acta Haematol 1984; 72:245.

72. Schreiber AD: Autoimmune hemolytic anemia. In Austen KF, Frank MM, Atkinson JP, Cantor H (eds): Samter's Immunologic Diseases, 6th ed, vol II. Philadelphia, Lippincott Williams & Wilkins, 2001, pp 738–749.

73. Clausen N: A population study of severe aplastic anemia in children. Acta Paediatr Scand 1986; 75:58.

74. Szklo M, Sensenbrenner L, et al: Incidence of aplastic anemia in metropolitan Baltimore: A population-based study. Blood 1985; 66:115.

75. Ware R, Kinney TR: Immunopathology of childhood idiopathic thrombocytopenia. CRC Crit Rev Oncol Hematol 1987; 7:169.

76. Sokol RJ, Hewitt S, Stamps BK: Autoimmune haemolysis associated with Donath-Landsteiner antibodies. Acta Haematol 1982; 68:268.

77. Heisel MA, Ortega JA: Factors influencing prognosis in childhood autoimmune hemolytic anemia. Am J Pediatr Hematol Oncol 1983; 5:147.

78. Zupanska B, Lawkowicz W, Gorska B, et al: Autoimmune haemolytic anaemia in children. Br J Hematol 1976; 34:511.

79. Wolach B, Heddle N, Barr RD, et al: Transient Donath-Landsteiner hemolytic anemia. Br J Haematol 1981; 48:425.

80. Schubothe H: The cold hemagglutinin disease. Semin Hematol 1966; 3:27.

81. Schreiber AD, Herskovitz BS, Goldwein M: Low-titer cold-hemagglutinin disease. N Engl J Med 1977; 296:1490.

82. Sokol RJ, Hewitt S, Stamps BK: Autoimmune haemolysis: An 18-year study of 865 cases referred to a regional transfusion centre. Br Med J 1981; 282:2023.

83. Nydegger UE, Kazatchkine MD, Miescher PA: Immunopathologic and clinical features of hemolytic anemia due to cold agglutinins. Semin Hematol 1991; 28:66.

84. Gottsche B, Salama A, Mueller-Eckhardt C: Donath-Landsteiner autoimmune hemolytic anemia in children. A study of 22 cases. Vox Sang 1990; 58:281.

85. Buchanan GR, Boxer LA, Nathan DG: The acute and transient nature of idiopathic immune hemolytic anemia in childhood. J Pediatr 1976; 88:780.

86. Nordhagen R, Stensvold K, Winsnes A, et al: Paroxysmal cold hemoglobinuria. The most frequent autoimmune hemolytic anemia in children? Acta Paediatr Scand 1984; 73:258.

87. Warren RW, Collins ML: Immune hemolytic anemia in children. CRC Crit Rev Oncol Hematol 1988; 8:65.

88. Allgood JW, Chaplin H Jr: Idiopathic acquired autoimmune hemolytic anemia. A review of forty-seven cases treated from 1955 through 1965. Am J Med 1967; 43:254.

89. Dobbs CE: Familial auto-immune hemolytic anemia. Arch Intern Med 1965; 116:273.

90. Toolis F, Parker AC, White A, et al: Familial autoimmune haemolytic anaemia. Br Med J 1977; 1:1392.

91. Jensen OM, Kristensen J: Red pulp of the spleen in autoimmune haemolytic anaemia and hereditary spherocytosis: Morphometric light and electron microscopy studies. Scand J Haematol 1986; 36:263.

92. Weiss GB, Bessman JD: Spurious automated red cell values in warm autoimmune hemolytic anemia. Am J Hematol 1984; 17:433.

93. Evans RS, Takahashi K, Duane RT, et al: Primary thrombocytopenic purpura and acquired hemolytic anemia. Evidence for a common etiology. Arch Intern Med 1951; 87:48.

94. Brown DL, Nelson DA: Surface microfragmentation of red cells as a mechanism for complement-mediated immune spherocytosis. Br J Haematol 1973; 24:301.

95. Farolino DL, Rustagi PK, Currie MS, et al: Teardrop-shaped red cells in autoimmune hemolytic anemia. Am J Hematol 1986; 21:415.

96. Stefanelli M, Barosi G, Cazzola M, et al: Quantitative assessment of erythropoiesis in haemolytic disease. Br J Haematol 1980; 45:297.

97. Greenberg J, Curtis-Cohen M, Gill FM, et al: Prolonged reticulocytopenia in autoimmune hemolytic anemia of childhood. J Pediatr 1980; 97:784.

98. Hauke G, Fauser A A, Weber S, et al: Reticulocytopenia in severe autoimmune hemolytic anemia (AIHA) of the warm antibody type. Blut 1983; 46:321.

99. Liesveld JL, Rowe JM, Lichtman MA: Variability of the erythropoietic response in autoimmune hemolytic anemia: Analysis of 109 cases. Blood 1987; 69:820.

100. Van De Loosdrecht AA, Hendriks DW, Blom NR, et al: Excessive apoptosis of bone marrow erythroblasts in a patient with autoimmune haemolytic anaemia with reticulocytopenia. Br J Haematol 2000; 108:313.

101. Bertrand Y, Lefrere J J, Leverger G, et al: Autoimmune haemolytic anaemia revealed by human parvovirus linked erythroblastopenia [letter]. Lancet 1985; 2:382.

102. Smith MA, Shah NS, Lobel JS: Parvovirus B19 infection associated with reticulocytopenia and chronic autoimmune hemolytic anemia. Am J Pediatr Hematol Oncol 1989; 11:167.

103. Roush GR, Rosenthal NS, Gerson SL, et al: An unusual case of autoimmune hemolytic anemia with reticulocytopenia, erythroid dysplasia, and an IgG2 autoanti-U. Transfusion 1996; 36:575.

104. Javid J: Human serum haptoglobins. Semin Hematol 1967; 4:35.

105. Yam P, Petz LD, Spath P: Detection of IgG sensitization of red cells with ^{125}I staphylococcal protein A. Am J Hematol 1982; 12:337.

106. Bodensteiner D, Brown P, Skikne B, et al: The enzyme-linked immunosorbent assay: Accurate detection of red blood cell antibodies in autoimmune hemolytic anemia. Am J Clin Pathol 1983; 79:182.

107. Sokol RJ, Hewitt S, Booker DJ, et al: Small quantities of erythrocyte bound immunoglobulins and autoimmune haemolysis. J Clin Pathol 1987; 40:254.

108. Galili U, Manny N, Izak G: EA rosette formation: A simple means to increase sensitivity of the antiglobulin test in patients with anti red cell antibodies. Br J Haematol 1981; 47:227.

109. Angevine CD, Anderson BR, Barnett EV: A cold agglutinin of the IgA class. J Immunol 1966; 96:578.

110. Suzuki S, Amano T, Mitsunaga M, et al: Autoimmune hemolytic anemia associated with IgA autoantibody. Clin Immunol Immunopathol 1981; 21:247.

111. Kowal-Vern A, Jacobson P, Okuno T, et al: Negative direct antiglobulin test in autoimmune hemolytic anemia. Am J Pediatr Hematol Oncol 1986; 8:349.

112. Freedman J, Wright J, Lim FC, et al: Hemolytic warm IgM autoagglutinins in autoimmune hemolytic anemia. Transfusion 1987; 27:464.

113. Shirey RS, Kickler TS, Bell W, et al: Fatal immune hemolytic anemia and hepatic failure associated with a warm-reacting IgM autoantibody. Vox Sang 1987; 52:219.

114. Friedmann AM, King KE, Shirey RS, et al: Fatal autoimmune hemolytic anemia in a child due to warm-reactive immunoglobulin M antibody. J Pediatr Hematol Oncol 1998; 20:502.

115. Worlledge SM: The interpretation of a positive direct antiglobulin test. Br J Haematol 1978; 39:157.

116. Gorst DW, Rawlinson VI, Merry AH, et al: Positive direct antiglobulin test in normal individuals. Vox Sang 1980; 38:99.

117. Bareford D, Longster G, Gilks L, et al: Follow-up of normal individuals with a positive antiglobulin test. Scand J Haematol 1985; 35:348.

118. Forman SJ, Kumar KS, et al: Hemolytic anemia in Wilson disease: Clinical findings and biochemical mechanisms. Am J Hematol 1980; 9:269.

119. Zieve L: Jaundice, hyperlipemia and hemolytic anemia: A heretofore unrecognized syndrome associated with alcoholic fatty liver and cirrhosis. Ann Intern Med 1958; 48:471.

120. Ware R: Human parvovirus infection. J Pediatr 1989; 114:343.

121. Rubin H: Autoimmune hemolytic anemias. Warm and cold antibody types. Am J Clin Pathol 1977; 68:638.

122. Joshi SR, Iyer YS, Bhatia HM: Serological and immunoglobulin studies in autoimmune haemolytic anaemia with emphasis on the nature of biphasic antibodies. Acta Haematol 1980; 64:31.

123. Garratty G: Mechanisms of immune red cell destruction, and red cell compatibility testing. Hum Pathol 1983; 14:204.

124. Wolf MW, Roelcke D: Incomplete warm hemolysins. I. Case reports, serology, and immunoglobulin classes. Clin Immunol Immunopathol 1989; 51:55.

125. Wolf MW, Roelcke D: Incomplete warm hemolysins. II. Corresponding antigens and pathogenetic mechanisms in autoimmune hemolytic anemias induced by incomplete warm hemolysins. Clin Immunol Immunopathol 1989; 51:68.

126. Andrzejewski C Jr, Young PJ, Cines DB, et al: Heterogeneity of human red cell autoantibodies assessed by isoelectric focusing. Transfusion 1991; 31:236.

127. Bell CA, Zwicker H, Sacks HJ: Autoimmune hemolytic anemia: Routine serologic evaluation in a general hospital population. Am J Clin Pathol 1973; 60:903.

128. Engelfriet CP, Overbeeke MAM, von dem Borne AEGKr: Autoimmune hemolytic anemia. Semin Hematol 1992; 29:3.

129. Ishizaka T, Ishizaka K, Salmon S, et al: Biologic activities of aggregated γ-globulin. VIII. Aggregated immunoglobulins of different classes. J Immunol 1967; 99:82.

130. Augener W, Grey HM, Cooper N, et al: The reaction of monomeric and aggregated immunoglobulins with C1. Immunochemistry 1971; 8:1011.

131. von dem Borne AEGKr, Beckers D, van der Meulen FW, et al: IgG$_4$ autoantibodies against erythrocytes, without increased haemolysis: A case report. Br J Haematol 1977; 37:137.

132. Silberstein LE, Berkman EM, Schreiber AD: Cold hemagglutinin disease associated with IgG cold-reactive antibody. Ann Intern Med 1987; 106:238.

133. Chaplin H Jr, Cohen R, Bloomberg G, et al: Pregnancy and idiopathic autoimmune haemolytic anaemia: A prospective study during 6 months gestation and 3 months post-partum. Br J Haematol 1973; 24:219.

134. Sacks DA, Platt LD, Johnson CS: Autoimmune hemolytic disease during pregnancy. Am J Obstet Gynecol 1981; 140:942.

135. Sokol RJ, Hewitt S, Stamps BK: Erythrocyte autoantibodies, autoimmune haemolysis and pregnancy. Vox Sang 1982; 43:169.

136. Bell CA, Zwicker H, Rosenbaum DL: Paroxysmal cold hemoglobinuria (P.C.H.) following mycoplasma infection: Anti-I specificity of the biphasic hemolysin. Transfusion 1973; 13:138.

137. Salama A, Mueller-Eckhardt C: Autoimmune haemolytic anaemia in childhood associated with non-complement binding IgM autoantibodies. Br J Haematol 1987; 65:67.

138. Gottsche B, Salama A, Mueller-Eckhardt C: Autoimmune hemolytic anemia associated with an IgA autoanti-Gerbich. Vox Sang 1990; 58:211.

139. Sokol RJ, Hewitt S, Stamps BK: Autoimmune hemolysis: Mixed warm and cold antibody type. Acta Haematol 1983; 69:266.

140. Silberstein LE, Shoenfeld Y, Schwartz RS, et al: Combination of IgG and IgM autoantibodies in chronic cold agglutinin disease: Immunologic studies and response to splenectomy. Vox Sang 1985; 48:105.

141. Shulman IA, Branch DR, Nelson JM, et al: Autoimmune hemolytic anemia with both cold and warm autoantibodies. JAMA 1985; 253:1746.

142. Nusbaum NJ, Khosla S: Autoimmune hemolytic anemia with both cold and warm autoantibodies. JAMA 1985; 254:1175.

143. Freedman J, Lim FC, Musclow E, et al: Autoimmune hemolytic anemia with concurrence of warm and cold red cell autoantibodies and a warm hemolysin. Transfusion 1985; 25:368.

144. Szymanski IO, Teno R, Rybak ME: Hemolytic anemia due to a mixture of low-titer IgG lambda and IgM lambda agglutinins reacting optimally at 22°C. Vox Sang 1986; 51:112.

145. McCann EL, Shirey RS, Kickler TS, et al: IgM autoagglutinins in warm autoimmune hemolytic anemia: A poor prognostic feature. Acta Haematol 1992; 88:120.

146. Issitt PD, Anstee DJ: Applied Blood Group Serology, 4th ed. Durham NC, Montgomery Scientific Publications, 1998, p 1004.

147. Szymanski IO, Huff SR, Selbovitz LG, et al: Erythrocyte sensitization with monomeric IgM in a patient with hemolytic anemia. Am J Hematol 1984; 17:71.

148. Barker RN, Casswell KM, Reid ME, et al: Identification of autoantigens in autoimmune haemolytic anaemia by a non-radioisotope immunoprecipitation method. Br J Haematol 1992; 82:126.

149. Leddy JP, Falany JL, Kissel GE, et al: Erythrocyte membrane proteins reactive with human (warm-reacting) anti-red cell autoantibodies. J Clin Invest 1993; 91:1672.

150. van't Veer MB, van Wieringen PMV, van Leeuwen I, et al: A negative direct antiglobulin test with strong IgG red cell autoantibodies present in the serum of a patient with autoimmune haemolytic anaemia. Br J Haematol 1981; 49:383.

151. Wakui H, Imai H, Kobayashi R, et al: Autoantibody against erythrocyte protein 4.1 in a patient with autoimmune hemolytic anemia. Blood 1988; 72:408.

152. Shulman IA, Vengelen-Tyler V, Thompson JC, et al: Autoanti-Ge associated with severe autoimmune hemolytic anemia. Vox Sang 1990; 59:232.

153. Owen I, Chowdhury V, Reid ME, et al: Autoimmune hemolytic anemia associated with anti-Sc1. Transfusion 1992; 32:173

154. Win N, Kaye T, Mir N, et al: Autoimmune haemolytic anaemia in infancy with anti-Kpb specificity. Vox Sang 1996; 71:187.

155. Szymanski IO, Roberts PL, Rosenfield RE: Anti-A autoantibody with severe intravascular hemolysis. N Engl J Med 1976; 294:995.

156. Sokol RJ, Booker DJ, Stamps R, et al: Autoimmune haemolysis and red cell autoantibodies with ABO blood group specificity. Haematologia 1995; 26:121.

157. Marsh WL, Oyen R, Alicea E, et al: Autoimmune hemolytic anemia and the Kell blood groups. Am J Hematol 1979; 7:155.

158. von dem Borne AEGKr, Mol JJ, Joustra-Maas N, et al: Autoimmune haemolytic anemia with monoclonal IgM (K) anti-P cold autohaemolysins. Br J Haematol 1982; 50:345.

159. Longster GH, Johnson E: IgM anti-D as autoantibody in a case of "cold" autoimmune haemolytic anaemia. Vox Sang 1988; 54:174.

160. Rousey SR, Smith RE: A fatal case of low titer anti-Pr cold agglutinin disease. Am J Hematol 1990; 35:286.

161. Levine P, Celano MJ, Falkowski F: The specificity of the antibody in paroxysmal cold hemoglobinuria (P.C.H.). Transfusion 1963; 3:278.

162. Gallagher MT, Branch DR, Mison A, et al: Evaluation of reticuloendothelial function in autoimmune hemolytic anemia using an in vitro assay of monocyte-macrophage interaction with erythrocytes. Exp Hematol 1983; 11:82.

163. Zupanska B, Brojer E, Thomson EE, et al: Monocyte-erythrocyte interaction in autoimmune haemolytic anaemia in relation to the number of erythrocyte-bound IgG molecules and subclass specificity of autoantibodies. Vox Sang 1987; 52:212.

164. Garratty G, Nance SJ: Correlation between in vivo hemolysis and the amount of red cell-bound IgG measured by flow cytometry. Transfusion 1990; 30:617.

165. Zupanska B, Sokol RJ, Booker DJ, et al: Erythrocyte autoantibodies, the monocyte monolayer assay and in vivo haemolysis. Br J Haematol 1993; 84:144.

166. Anderson CL, Looney RJ: Human leukocyte IgG Fc receptors. Immunol Today 1986; 7:264.

167. Ferreira JA, Feliu E, Rozman C, et al: Morphologic and morphometric light and electron microscopic studies of the spleen in patients with hereditary spherocytosis and autoimmune haemolytic anaemia. Br J Haematol 1989; 72:246.

168. Fischer JT, Petz LD, Garratty G, et al: Correlations between quantitative assay of red cell-bound C3, serologic reactions, and hemolytic anemia. Blood 1974; 44:359.

169. Logue GL, Rosse WF, Gockerman JP: Measurement of the third component of complement bound to red blood cells in patients with the cold agglutinin syndrome. J Clin Invest 1973; 52:493.

170. Jaffe CH, Atkinson JP, Frank MM: The role of complement in the clearance of cold agglutinin-sensitized erythrocytes in man. J Clin Invest 1976; 58:942.

171. Garratty G, Petz LD: Transfusing patients with autoimmune haemolytic anaemia. Lancet 1993; 341:1220.

172. Sokol RJ, Hewitt S, Booker DJ, et al: Patients with red cell autoantibodies: Selection of blood for transfusion. Clin Lab Haematol 1988; 10:257.

173. James P, Rowe GP, Tozzo GG: Elucidation of alloantibodies in autoimmune haemolytic anaemia. Vox Sang 1988; 54:167.

174. Engelfriet CP, Reesink HW, Garratty G, et al: The detection of alloantibodies against red cells in patients with warm-type autoimmune haemolytic anaemia. Vox Sang 2000; 78:200.

175. Petz LD: Transfusing the patient with autoimmune haemolytic anemia. Clin Lab Med 1982; 2:193.

176. Wallhermfechtel MA, Pohl BA, Chaplin H: Alloimmunization in patients with warm autoantibodies. A retrospective study employing three donor alloabsorptions to aid in antibody detection. Transfusion 1984; 24:482.

177. Salama A, Berghofer H, Mueller-Eckhardt C: Red blood cell transfusion in warm-type autoimmune haemolytic anaemia. Lancet 1992; 340:1515.

178. Mullon J, Giacoppe G, Clagett C, et al: Transfusions of polymerized bovine hemoglobin in a patient with severe autoimmune hemolytic anemia. N Engl J Med 2000; 342:1638.

179. Klein HG: The prospects for red-cell substitutes. N Engl J Med 2000; 342:1666.

180. Dameshek W, Rosenthal MC, Schwartz LI: The treatment of acquired hemolytic anemia with adrenocorticotrophic hormone (ACTH). N Engl J Med 1951; 244:117.

181. Fries LF, Brickman CM, Frank MM: Monocyte receptors for the Fc portion of IgG increase in number in autoimmune hemolytic anemia and other hemolytic states and are decreased by glucocorticoid therapy. J Immunol 1983; 131:1240.

182. Collins PW, Newland AC: Treatment modalities of autoimmune blood disorders. Semon Hematol 1992; 29:64.

183. Meytes D, Adler M, Virag I, et al: High dose methylprednisolone in acute immune cold hemolysis. N Engl J Med 1985; 312:318.

184. Ware R, Kinney TR: Therapeutic considerations in childhood idiopathic thrombocytopenic purpura. Crit Rev Oncol Hematol 1987; 7:169.

185. Fehr J, Hofmann V, Kappeler U: Transient reversal of thrombocytopenia in idiopathic thrombocytopenic purpura by high-dose intravenous gamma globulin. N Engl J Med 1982; 306:1254.

186. Salama A, Mueller-Eckhardt C, Kiefel V: Effect of intravenous immunoglobulin in immune thrombocytopenia: Competitive inhibition of reticuloendothelial system function by sequestration of autologous red blood cells? Lancet 1983; 2:193.

187. Mueller-Eckhardt C, Salama A, Mahn I, et al: Lack of efficacy of high-dose intravenous immunoglobulin in autoimmune hemolytic anemia: A clue to its mechanism. Scand J Hematol 1985; 34:394.

188. Hilgartner MW, Bussel J: Use of intravenous gamma globulin for the treatment of autoimmune neutropenia of childhood and autoimmune hemolytic anemia. Am J Med 1987; 83:25.

189. Flores G, Cunningham-Rundles C, Newland AC, et al: Efficacy of intravenous immunoglobulin in the treatment of autoimmune hemolytic anemia: Results in 73 patients. Am J Hematol 1993; 44:237.

190. Ware RE: The use of intravenous immunoglobulin in hematologic disorders. Semin Pediatr Infect Dis 1992; 3:179.

191. Klaesson S, Ringden O, Markling L, et al: Immune modulatory effects of immunoglobulins on cell-mediated immune responses in vitro. Scand J Immunol 1993; 38:477.

192. Heidemann SM, Sarnaik SA, Sarnaik AP: Exchange transfusion for severe autoimmune hemolytic anemia. Am J Pediatr Hematol Oncol 1987; 9:302.

193. Bernstein ML, Schneider BK, Naiman JL: Plasma exchange in refractory acute autoimmune hemolytic anemia. J Pediatr 1981; 98:774.

194. Brooks BD, Steane EA, Sheehan RG, et al: Therapeutic plasma exchange in the immune hemolytic anemias and immunologic thrombocytopenic purpura. Prog Clin Biol Res 1982; 106:317.

195. Silberstein LE, Berkman EM: Plasma exchange in autoimmune hemolytic anemia (AIHA). J Clin Apheresis 1983; 1:238.
196. McConnell ME, Atchison JA, Kohaut E, et al: Successful use of plasma exchange in a child with refractory immune hemolytic anemia. Am J Pediatr Hematol Oncol 1987; 9:158.
197. Fosburg M, Dolan M, Propper R, et al: Intensive plasma exchange in small and critically ill pediatric patients: Techniques and clinical outcome. J Clin Apheresis 1983; 1:215.
198. Greuth M, Wagner HP, Pipczynski-Suter K, et al: Plasma exchange: An important part of the therapeutic procedure of a small child with autoimmune hemolytic anemia. Acta Pediatr Scand 1986; 75:1037.
199. McCarthy LJ, Danielson CF, Fernandez C, et al: Intensive plasma exchange for severe autoimmune hemolytic anemia in a four-month-old infant. J Clin Apheresis 1999; 14:190.
200. Council on Scientific Affairs: Current status of therapeutic plasmapheresis and related techniques. Report of the AMA panel on therapeutic plasmapheresis. JAMA 1985; 253:819.
201. Andrzejewski, C Jr, Gault E, Briggs M, et al: Benefit of a 37°C extracorporeal circuit in plasma exchange therapy for selected cases with cold agglutinin disease. J Clin Apheresis 1988; 4:13.
202. Chertkow G, Davie JV: Results of splenectomy in auto-immune haemolytic anaemia. Br J Haematol 1956; 2:237.
203. Dacie JV: Autoimmune hemolytic anaemia. Arch Intern Med 1975; 135:1293.
204. Mollison PL: Survival curves of incompatible red cells. An analytical review. Transfusion 1986; 26:43.
205. Parker AC, Macpherson AIS, Richmond J: Value of radiochromium investigation in autoimmune haemolytic anaemia. Br Med J 1977; 1:208.
206. Coon WW: Splenectomy in the treatment of hemolytic anemia. Arch Surg 1985; 120:625.
207. Grinblat J, Billoa Y: Overwhelming pneumococcal sepsis 25 years after splenectomy. Am J Med Sci 1975; 270:523.
208. McMullen M, Johnston G: Long term management of patients after splenectomy. Br Med J 1993; 307:1372.
209. Meyer O, Stahl D, Beckhove P, et al: Pulsed high-dose dexamethasone in chronic autoimmune haemolytic anaemia of warm type. Br J Haematol 1997; 98:860.
210. Chan AC, Sack K: Danazol therapy in autoimmune hemolytic anemia associated with systemic lupus erythematosus. J Rheumatol 1991; 18:280.
211. Pignon J-M, Poirson E, Rochant H: Danazol in autoimmune haemolytic anaemia. Br J Haematol 1993; 83:343.
212. Agnello V, Pariser K, Gell J, et al: Preliminary observations on danazol therapy of systemic lupus erythematosus: Effects on DNA antibodies, thrombocytopenia and complement. J Rheumatol 1983; 10:682.
213. Gertz MA, Petitt RM, Pineda AA, et al: Vinblastine-loaded platelets for autoimmune hemolytic anemia. Ann Intern Med 1981; 95:325.
214. Medellin PL, Patten E, Weiss GB: Vinblastine for autoimmune hemolytic anemia. Ann Intern Med 1982; 96:123.
215. Seiber SM, Adamson RH: Toxicity of antineoplastic agents in man: Chromosomal aberrations, antifertility effects, congenital malformations, and carcinogenic potential. Adv Cancer Res 1975; 22:57.
216. Brodsky TA, Petri M, Smith BD, et al: Immunoablative high-dose cyclophosphamide without stem-cell rescue for refractory, severe autoimmune disease. Ann Intern Med 1998; 129:1031.
217. Panceri R, Fraschini D, Tornotti G, et al: Successful use of high-dose cyclophosphamide in a child with severe autoimmune hemolytic anemia. Haematologica 1992; 77:76.
218. Dundar S, Ozdemir O, Ozcebe O: Cyclosporin in steroid-resistant autoimmune haemolytic anaemia. Acta Haematol 1991; 86:200.
219. O'Connor BM, Clifford JS, Lawrence WD, et al: Alpha-interferon for severe cold agglutinin disease. Ann Intern Med 1989; 111:255.
220. Berney T, Shibata T, Merino R, et al: Murine autoimmune hemolytic anemia resulting from Fcg receptor-mediated erythrophagocytosis: Protection by erythropoietin but not by interleukin–3, and aggravation by granulocyte-macrophage colony-stimulating factor. Blood 1992; 79:2960.
221. Shan D, Ledbetter JA, Press OW: Signaling events involved in anti-CD20-induced apoptosis of malignant human B cells. Can Immunol Immunother 2000; 48:673.
222. Davis TA, Grillo-Lopez AJ, White CA, et al: Rituximab anti-CD20 monoclonal antibody therapy in non-Hodgkin's lymphoma: Safety and efficacy of re-treatment. J Clin Oncol 2000; 18:3135.
223. Faurschou M, Hasselbalch HC, Nielsen OJ: Sustained remission of platelet counts following monoclonal anti-CD20 antibody therapy in two cases of idiopathic autoimmune thrombocytopenia and neutropenia. Eur J Haematol 2001; 66:408.
224. Stasi R, Pagano A, Stipa E, et al: Rituximab chimeric anti-CD20 monoclonal antibody treatment for adults with chronic idiopathic thrombocytopenic purpura. Blood 2001; 98:952.
225. Lee EJ, Kueck B: Rituxan in the treatment of cold agglutinin disease. Blood 1998; 92:3490.
226. Treon SP, Anderson KC: The use of rituximab in the treatment of malignant and nonmalignant plasma cell disorders. Semin Oncol 2000; 27:79.
227. Layios N, Van Den Neste E, Jost E, et al: Remission of severe cold agglutinin disease after rituximab therapy. Leukemia 2001; 15:187.
228. Quartier P, Brethon B, Philippet P, et al: Treatment of childhood autoimmune haemolytic anaemia with rituximab. Lancet, 2001; 358:1511.
229. Tyndall A, Gratwohl A: Blood and marrow stem cell transplants in auto-immune disease: A consensus report written on behalf of the European League against Rheumatism (EULAR) and the European Group for Blood and Marrow Transplantation (EBMT). Bone Marrow Transplant 1997; 19:643.
230. De Stefano P, Zecca M, Giorgiani G, et al: Resolution of immune haemolytic anaemia with allogeneic bone marrow transplantation after an unsuccessful autograft. Br J Haematol 1999; 106:1063.
231. Paillard C, Kanold J, Halle P, et al: Two-step immunoablative treatment with autologous peripheral blood CD34+ cell transplantation in an 8 year old boy with autoimmune haemolytic anaemia. Br J Haematol 2000; 110:900.
232. Horn B, Viele M, Mentzer W, et al: Autoimmune hemolytic anemia in patients with SCID after T cell-depleted BM and PBSC transplantation. Bone Marrow Transplant 1999; 24:1009.
233. Azuma E, Nishihara H, Hanada M, et al: Recurrent cold hemagglutinin disease following allogeneic bone marrow transplantation successfully treated with plasmapheresis, corticosteroid and cyclophosphamide. Bone Marrow Transplant 1996; 18:243.
234. Abdel-Khalik A, Paton L, White AG, et al: Human leucocyte antigens A, B, C, and DRW in idiopathic "warm" autoimmune haemolytic anaemia. Br Med J 1980; 280:760.
235. Kleiner-Baumgarten A, Schlaeffer F, Keynan A: Multiple autoimmune manifestations in a splenectomized subject with HLA-B8. Arch Intern Med 1983; 143:1987.
236. Lortholary O, Valeyre D, Gayraud M, et al: Autoimmune haemolytic anaemia and idiopathic pulmonary fibrosis associated with HLA-B27 antigen. Eur J Haematol 1990; 45:112.
237. Wang-Rodriguez J, Rearden A: Reduced frequency of HLA-DQ6 in individuals with a positive direct antiglobulin test. Transfusion 1996; 36:979.
238. Nomura S, Okamae F, Matsuzaki T, et al: Autoimmune hemolytic anemia and HLA-DQ6. Autoimmunity 1998; 28:57.
239. Lippman SM, Arnett FC, Conley CL, et al: Genetic factors predisposing to autoimmune diseases. Autoimmune hemolytic anemia, chronic thrombocytopenic purpura, and systemic lupus erythematosus. Am J Med 1982; 73:827.
240. Silberstein LE, Robertson GA, Hannam Harris AC, et al: Etiologic aspects of cold agglutinin disease: Evidence for cytogenetically defined clones of lymphoid cells and the demonstration that an anti-Pr cold autoantibody is derived from a chromosomally aberrant B cell clone. Blood 1986; 67:1705.
241. Gordon J, Silberstein L, Moreau L, et al: Trisomy 3 in cold agglutinin disease. Cancer Genet Cytogenet 1990; 46:89.
242. Haneberg B, Matre R, Winsnes R, et al: Acute hemolytic anemia related to diphtheria-pertussis-tetanus vaccination. Acta Paediatr Scand 1978; 67:345.
243. Stevenson FK, Smith GJ, North J, et al: Identification of normal B-cell counterparts of neoplastic cells which secrete cold agglutinins of anti-I and anti-i specificity. Br J Haematol 1989; 72:9.
244. Stellrecht KA, Vella AT: Evidence for polyclonal B cell activation as the mechanism for LCMB-induced autoimmune hemolytic anemia. Immunol Lett 1992; 31:273.

245. Stahl D, Lacroix-Desmazes S, Heudes D, et al: Altered control of self-reactive IgG by autologous IgM in patients with warm autoimmune hemolytic anemia. Blood 2000; 95:328.

246. Reininger L, Shibata T, Schurmans S, et al: Spontaneous production of anti-mouse red blood cell autoantibodies is independent of the polyclonal activation in NZB mice. Eur J Immunol 1990; 20:2405.

247. Scott BB, Sadigh S, Stow M, et al: Molecular mechanisms resulting in pathogenic anti-mouse erythrocyte antibodies in New Zealand black mice. Clin Exp Immunol 1993; 93:26.

248. Sanz I, Casali P, Thomas JW, et al: Nucleotide sequences of eight human natural autoantibody V_H regions reveals apparent restricted use of V_H families. J Immunol 1989; 142:4054.

249. Silverman GJ, Carson DA: Structural characterization of human monoclonal cold agglutinins: Evidence for a distinct primary sequence-defined V_H4 idiotype. Eur J Immunol 1990; 20:351.

250. Friedman DF, Cho EA, Goldman J, et al: The role of clonal selection in the pathogenesis of an autoreactive human B cell lymphoma. J Exp Med 1991; 174:525.

251. Silberstein LE, Jefferies LC, Goldman J, et al: Variable region gene analysis of pathologic human autoantibodies to the related i and I red blood cell antigens. Blood 1991; 78:2372.

252. Andrzejewski C, Young PJ, Goldman J, et al: Production of human warm-reacting red cell monoclonal autoantibodies by Epstein-Barr virus transformation. Transfusion 1989; 29:196.

253. Shoenfeld Y, Hsu-Lin SC, Gabriels JE, et al: Production of autoantibodies by human-human hybridomas. J Clin Invest 1982; 70:205.

254. Parkman R: Cellular basis of autoimmune hemolytic anemia. Am J Pediatr Hematol Oncol 1981; 3:105.

255. Calkins CE, Cochran SA, Miller RD, et al: Evidence for regulation of the autoimmune antierythrocyte response by idiotype-specific suppressor T cells in NZB mice. Int Immunol 1990; 2:127.

256. Young JL, Hooper DC: Characterization of autoreactive helper T cells in a murine model of autoimmune haemolytic disease. Immunology 1993; 80:13.

257. Parker AC, Stuart AE, Dewar AE: Activated T-cells in autoimmune haemolytic anaemia. Br J Haematol 1977; 36:337.

258. Phan-Dinh-Tuy F, Habibi R, Bach MA, et al: T cell subpopulations defined by monoclonal antibodies in autoimmune hemolytic anemia. Biomed Pharmacother 1983; 37:75.

259. Conte R, Tazzari PL, Finelli C: Deficiency of autologous mixed lymphocyte reaction in patients with idiopathic autoimmune hemolytic anemia. Vox Sang 1985; 49:285.

260. Soyano A, Romano E, Linares J: Abnormal generation of concanavalin A-induced suppressor cell function in human autoimmune hemolytic anemia. Clin Immunol Immunopathol 1982; 23:70.

261. Horowitz SD, Borcherding W, Hong R: Autoimmune hemolytic anemia as a manifestation of T-suppressor-cell deficiency. Clin Immunol Immunopathol 1984; 33:313.

262. Barker RN, Hall AM, Standen GR, et al: Identification of T-cell epitopes on the rhesus polypeptides in autoimmune hemolytic anemia. Blood 1997; 90:2701.

263. Albrechtsen D, Solheim BG, Flatmark A, et al: Autoimmune hemolytic anemia in cyclosporine-treated organ allograft recipients. Transplant Proc 1988; 20:959.

264. Sniecinski IJ, Oien L, Petz LD, et al: Immunohematologic consequences of major ABO-mismatched bone marrow transplantation. Transplantation 1988; 45:530.

265. Solheim BG, Albrechtsen D, Egeland T, et al: Auto-antibodies against erythrocytes in transplant patients produced by donor lymphocytes. Transplant Proc 1987; 19:4520.

266. Tamura T, Kanamori H, Yamazaki E, et al: Cold agglutinin disease following allogeneic bone marrow transplantation. Bone Marrow Transplant 1994; 13:321.

267. Puppo F, Torresin A, et al: Autoimmune hemolytic anemia and human immunodeficiency virus (HIV) infection. Ann Intern Med 1988; 1:249.

268. Scadden DT, Zon LI, Groopman JE: Pathophysiology and management of HIV-associated hematologic disorders. Blood 1988; 74:1455.

269. Fagiolo E, Terenzi CT: Enhanced IL–10 production in vitro by monocytes in autoimmune haemolytic anaemia. Immunol Invest 1999; 28:347.

270. Barcellini W, Clerici G, Montesano R, et al: In vitro quantification of anti-red blood cell antibody production in idiopathic autoimmune haemolytic anaemia: Effect of mitogen and cytokine stimulation. Br J Haematol 2000; 111:452.

271. Fong KY, Loisou S, Boey ML, et al: Anticardiolipin antibodies, haemolytic anaemia and thrombocytopenia in systemic lupus erythematosus. Br J Rheumatol 1992; 31:453.

272. Boling EP, Wen J, Reveille JD, et al: Primary Sjogren's syndrome and autoimmune hemolytic anemia in sisters. Am J Med 1983; 74:1066.

273. Kondo H, Sakai S, Sakai Y: Autoimmune haemolytic anaemia, Sjogren's syndrome and idiopathic thrombocytopenic purpura in a patient with sarcoidosis. Acta Haematol 1993; 89:209.

274. Jones E, Jones JV, Woodbury JFL, et al: Scleroderma and hemolytic anemia in a patient with deficiency of IgA and C4: A hitherto undescribed association. J Rheumatol 1987; 14:609.

275. Kay EM, Makris M, Winfield J, et al: Evans' syndrome associated with dermatomyositis. Ann Rheum Dis 1990; 49:793.

276. Veloso T, Fraga J, Carvalho J, et al: Autoimmune hemolytic anemia in ulcerative colitis. A case report with review of the literature. J Clin Gastroenterol 1991; 13:445.

277. Yates P, Macht LM, Williams NA, et al: Red cell autoantibody production by colonic mononuclear cells from a patient with ulcerative colitis and autoimmune haemolytic anaemia. Br J Haematol 1992; 82:753.

278. Fagiolo E: Platelet and leukocyte antibodies in autoimmune hemolytic anemia. Acta Haematol 1976; 56:97.

279. Miller BA, Beardsley DS: Autoimmune pancytopenia of childhood associated with multisystem disease manifestations. J Pediatr 1983; 103:877.

280. Pui C-H, Wilimas J, Wang W: Evans syndrome in childhood. J Pediatr 1980; 97:754.

281. Wang W, Herrod H, Pui C-H, et al: Immunoregulatory abnormalities in Evans syndrome. Am J Hematol 1983; 15:381.

282. Pegels JG, Helmerhorst FM, van Leeuwen EF, et al: The Evans syndrome: Characterization of the responsible autoantibodies. Br J Haematol 1982; 51:445.

283. Gombakis N, Trahana M, Athanassiou M, et al: Evans syndrome: Successful management with multi-agent treatment including intermediate-dose intravenous cyclophosphamide. J Pediatr Hematol Oncol 1997; 19:433.

284. Ucar B, Akgun N, Aydogdu SD, et al: Treatment of refractory Evan's syndrome with cyclosporine and prednisone. Pediatr Int 1999; 41:104.

285. Scaradavou A, Bussel J: Evans syndrome. Results of a pilot study utilizing a multiagent treatment protocol. J Pediatr Hematol Oncol 1995; 17:290.

286. Raetz E, Beatty PG, Adams RH: Treatment of severe Evans syndrome with an allogeneic cord blood transplant. Bone Marrow Transplant 1997; 20:427.

287. Martino R, Sureda A, Brunet S: Peripheral blood stem cell mobilization in refractory autoimmune Evans syndrome: A cautionary case report. Bone Marrow Transplant 1997; 20:521.

288. Marmont AM: Immune ablation and stem cell transplantation for severe Evans syndrome and refractory thrombocytopenic purpura. Bone Marrow Transplant 1999; 23:1215.

289. Sthoeger ZM, Sthoeger D, Shtalrid M, et al: Mechanism of autoimmune hemolytic anemia in chronic lymphocytic leukemia. Am J Hematol 1993; 43:259.

290. Mauro FR, Foa R, Cerretti R, Giannarelli D, et al: Autoimmune hemolytic anemia in chronic lymphocytic leukemia: Clinical, therapeutic, and prognostic features. Blood 2000; 95:2786.

291. Sallah S, Sigounas G, Vos P, et al: Autoimmune hemolytic anemia in patients with non-Hodgkin's lymphoma: Characteristics and significance. Ann Oncol 2000; 11:1571.

292. Pereira A, Mazzara R, Escoda L, et al: Anti-Sa cold agglutinin of IgA class requiring plasma-exchange therapy as early manifestation of multiple myeloma. Ann Hematol 1993; 66:315.

293. Kedar A, Khan AB, Mattern JQA, et al: Autoimmune disorders complicating adolescent Hodgkin's disease. Cancer 1979; 44:112.

294. Chu J-Y: Autoimmune hemolytic anemia in childhood Hodgkin's disease. Am J Pediatr Hematol Oncol 1982; 4:125.

295. Xiros N, Binder T, Anger B, et al: Idiopathic thrombocytopenic purpura and autoimmune hemolytic anemia in Hodgkin's disease. Eur J Haematol 1988; 40:437.

296. Strickland DK, Ware RE: Urticarial vasculitis: An autoimmune disorder following therapy for Hodgkin's disease. Med Pediatr Oncol 1995, 25:208.

297. Arbaje YM, Beltran G: Chronic myelogenous leukemia complicated by autoimmune hemolytic anemia. Am J Med 1990; 88:197.

298. Sokol RJ, Hewitt S, Booker DJ: Erythrocyte autoantibodies, autoimmune haemolysis, and myelodysplastic syndromes. J Clin Pathol 1989; 42:1088.

299. Blanchette VS, Hallett JJ, Hemphill JM, et al: Abnormalities of the peripheral blood as a presenting feature of immunodeficiency. Am J Hematol 1978; 4:87.

300. Rich KC, Arnold WJ, Palella T, et al: Cellular immune deficiency with autoimmune hemolytic anemia in purine nucleoside phosphorylase deficiency. Am J Med 1979; 67:172.

301. Leickly FE, Buckley RH: Successful treatment of autoimmune hemolytic anemia in common variable immunodeficiency with high-dose intravenous gamma globulin. Am J Med 1987; 82:159.

302. Bapat AR, Schuster SJ, Dahlke M, et al: Thrombocytopenia and autoimmune hemolytic anemia following renal transplantation. Transplantation 1987; 44:157.

303. Murray HW, Masur H, Senterfit LB, et al: The protean manifestations of *Mycoplasma pneumoniae* infection in adults. Am J Med 1975; 58:229.

304. Rollof J, Eklund PO: Infectious mononucleosis complicated by severe immune hemolysis. Eur J Haematol 1989; 43:81.

305. Terada K, Tanaka H, Mori R, et al: Hemolytic anemia associated with cold agglutinin during chickenpox and a review of the literature. J Pediatr Hematol Oncol 1998; 20:149.

306. Miyazaki S, Ohtsuka M, Ueda K, et al: Coombs positive hemolytic anemia in congenital rubella. J Pediatr 1979; 94:759.

307. De la Rubia J, Moscardo F, Arriaga F, et al: Acute parvovirus B19 infection as a cause of autoimmune hemolytic anemia. Haematologica 2000; 85:995.

308. Boccardi V, D'Annibali S, Di Natale G, et al: *Mycoplasma pneumoniae* infection complicated by paroxysmal cold hemoglobinuria with anti-P specificity of biphasic hemolysin. Blut 1977; 34:211.

309. Costea N, Yakulis VJ, Heller P: Inhibition of cold agglutinins (anti-I) by *M. pneumoniae* antigens. Proc Soc Exp Biol Med 1972; 139:476.

310. Richard KA, Robinson RJ, et al: Acute acquired haemolytic anaemia associated with polyagglutination. Arch Dis Child 1969; 44:102.

311. Williams RA, Brown EF, et al: Transfusion of infants with activation of T antigen. J Pediatr 1989; 115:949.

312. Murphy WG, Kelton JG: Methyldopa-induced autoantibodies against red blood cells. Blood Rev 1988; 2:36.

313. Petz LD: Drug-induced immune haemolytic anaemia. Clin Haematol 1980; 9:455.

314. Petz LD, Fudenberg HH: Coombs-positive hemolytic anemia caused by penicillin administration. N Engl J Med 1966; 274:171.

315. Seldon MR, Bain B, Johnson CA, et al: Ticarcillin-induced immune haemolytic anaemia. Scand J Haematol 1982; 28:459.

316. Branch DR, Berkowitz LR, Becker RL, et al: Extravascular hemolysis following the administration of cefamandole. Am J Hematol 1985; 18:213.

317. Arndt PA, Leger RM, Garratty G: Serology of antibodies to second- and third-generation cephalosporins associated with immune hemolytic anemia and/or positive direct antiglobulin tests. Transfusion 1999; 39:1239.

318. Simpson MB, Pryzbylik J, Innis B, et al: Hemolytic anemia after tetracycline therapy. N Engl J Med 1985; 312:840.

319. Wong KY, Boose GM, Issitt CH: Erythromycin-induced hemolytic anemia. J Pediatr 1981; 98:647.

320. Sosler SD, Behzad O, Garratty G, et al: Immune hemolytic anemia associated with Probenecid. Am J Clin Pathol 1985; 84:391.

321. Manor E, Marmor A, Kaufman S, et al: Massive hemolysis caused by acetaminophen. JAMA 1976; 236:2777.

322. Korsager S, Sorensen H, Jensen OH, et al: Antiglobulin-tests for detection of auto-immunohaemolytic anaemia during long-term treatment with ibuprofen. Scand J Rheumatol 1981; 10:174.

323. Salama A, Mueller-Eckhardt C: On the mechanisms of sensitization and attachment of antibodies to RBC in drug-induced immune hemolytic anemia. Blood 1987; 69:1006.

324. Akpek G, McAneny D, Weintraub L: Comparative response to splenectomy in Coombs-positive autoimmune hemolytic anemia with or without associated disease. Am J Hematol 1999; 61:98.

325. Gull WW: A case of intermittent haematinuria, with remarks. Guy's Hosp Rep 1866; 12:381.

326. Strubing P: Paroxysmale haemoglobinurie. Dtsch Med Wochenschr 1882; 8:1.

327. Ham TH: Chronic hemolytic anemia with paroxysmal nocturnal hemoglobinuria. A study of the mechanism of hemolysis in relation to acid-base equilibrium. N Engl J Med 1937; 217:915.

328. Ham TH: Studies on the destruction of red blood cells. I. Chronic hemolytic anemia with paroxysmal nocturnal hemoglobinuria: An investigation of the mechanism of hemolysis with observations on five cases. Arch Intern Med 1939; 64:127

329. Ham TH and Dingle JH: Studies on destruction of red blood cells. II. Chronic hemolytic anemia with paroxysmal nocturnal hemoglobinuria: Certain immunological aspects of the hemolytic mechanism with special reference to serum complement. J Clin Invest 1939; 18:657.

330. Rosse WF, Dacie JV: Immune lysis of normal human and paroxysmal nocturnal hemoglobinuria red blood cells. I. The sensitivity of PNH red cells to lysis by complement and specific antibody. J Clin Invest 1966; 45:736.

331. Rosse WF: Variations in the red cells in paroxysmal nocturnal hemoglobinuria. Br J Hematol 1973; 24:327.

332. Rosse WF, Adams JP, Thorpe AM: The population of cells in paroxysmal nocturnal hemoglobinuria of intermediate sensitivity to complement lysis—Significance and mechanism of increased immune lysis. Br J Haematol 1974; 28:181.

333. Hall SE, Rosse WF: The use of monoclonal antibodies and flow cytometry in the diagnosis of paroxysmal nocturnal hemoglobinuria. Blood 1996; 87:5332.

334. Rosse WF: Evolution of clinical understanding: Paroxysmal nocturnal hemoglobinuria as a paradigm. Am J Hematol 1993; 42:122.

335. Socie G, Mary J-Y, de Gramont A, et al: Paroxysmal nocturnal haemoglobinuria: long-term follow-up and prognostic factors. Lancet 1996; 348:573.

336. Devine DV, Gluck WL, Rosse WF, et al: Acute myeloblastic leukemia in paroxysmal nocturnal hemoglobinuria: Evidence of evolution from the abnormal paroxysmal nocturnal hemoglobinuria clone. J Clin Invest 1987; 79:314.

337. Ware RE, Hall SG and Rosse WF: Paroxysmal nocturnal hemoglobinuria with onset in childhood and adolescence. N Engl J Med 1991; 325:991.

338. Saso R, Marsh J, Cevreska L, et al: Bone marrow transplants for paroxysmal nocturnal haemoglobinuria. Br J Haematol 1999; 104:392.

339. Raiola AM, Van Lint MT, Lamparelli T, et al: Bone marrow transplantation for paroxysmal nocturnal hemoglobinuria. Haematologica 2000; 85:59.

340. Medof ME, Walter EI, Roberts WL, et al: Decay accelerating factor of complement is anchored to cells by a C-terminal glycolipid. Biochemistry 1986; 25:6740.

341. Stefanova I, Hilgert I, Kristofova H, et al: Characterization of a broadly expressed human leucocyte surface antigen MEM43 anchored in membrane through phosphatidylinositol. Mol Immunol 1989; 26:153.

342. Low MG: Biochemistry of the glycosylphosphatidyl-inositol membrane protein anchors. Biochem J 1987; 244:1.

343. Low MG, Saltiel AR: Structural and functional roles of glycosylphosphatidylinositol in membranes. Science 1988; 239:268.

344. Bangs JD, Hereld D, Krakow JL, et al: Rapid processing of the carboxyl terminus of a trypanosome variant surface glycoprotein. Biochemistry 1985; 82:3207.

345. Low MG, Zilversmit DB: Role of phosphatidylinositol in attachment of alkaline phosphatase to membranes. Biochemistry 1980; 19:3913.

346. Haas R, Brandt PT, Knight J et al: Identification of amine components in a glycolipid membrane-binding domain at the C-terminus of human erythrocyte acetylcholinesterase. Biochemistry 1986; 25:3098.

347. Fatemi SH, Haas R, Jentoft N, et al: The glyco-phospholipid anchor of Thy–1. J Biol Chem 1987; 262:4728.

348. Dustin ML, Selvaraj P, Mattaliano RJ, et al: Anchoring mechanisms for LFA–3 cell adhesion glycoprotein at membrane surface. Nature 1987; 329:846.

349. Selvaraj P, Rosse WF, Silber R, et al: The major Fc receptor in blood has a phosphatidylinositol anchor and is deficient in paroxysmal nocturnal haemoglobinuria. Nature 1988; 333:565.

350. Reiser H, Oettgen H, Yeh ETH, et al: Structural characterization of the TAP molecule: A phosphatidylinositol-linked glycoprotein

distinct from the T cell receptor T3 complex and Thy–1. Cell 1986; 47:365.

351. Stiernberg J, Low MG, Flaherty L, et al: Removal of lymphocyte surface molecules with phosphatidylinositol-specific phospholipase C: Effects on mitogen responses and evidence that ThB and certain Qa antigens are membrane-anchored via phosphatidylinositol. J Immunol 1987; 38:3877.

352. Ishihara A, Hou Y and Jacobson K: The Thy–1 antigen exhibits rapid lateral diffusion in the plasma membrane of rodent lymphoid cells and fibroblasts. Proc Natl Acad Sci USA 1987; 84:1290.

353. Noda M, Yoon K, Rodan GA, et al: High lateral mobility of endogenous and transfected alkaline phosphatase: A phosphatidylinositol-anchored membrane protein. J Cell Biol 1987; 105:1671.

354. Romero G, Luttrell L, Rogol A, et al: Phosphatidyl-inositol-glycan anchors of membrane proteins: Potential precursors of insulin mediators. Science 1988; 240:509.

355. Yeh ETH, Reiser H, Bamezai A, et al: TAP transcription and phosphatidylinositol linkage mutants are defective in activation through the T cell receptor. Cell 1988; 52:665.

356. Presky DH, Low MG and Shevach EM: The role of phosphatidylinositol (PI)-anchored proteins in T cell activation. FASEB J 1989; A1654.

357. Roy-Choudhury S, Mishra VS, Low MG, et al: A phospholipid is the membrane-anchoring domain of a protein growth factor of molecular mass 34 kDa in placental trophoblasts. Proc Natl Acad Sci USA 1988; 85:2014.

358. Auditore JV, Hartmann RC, Flexner JM, et al: The erythrocyte acetylcholinesterase enzyme in paroxysmal nocturnal hemoglobinuria. Arch Pathol 1960; 69:534.

359. Tanaka KR, Valentine WN and Fredricks RE: Diseases or clinical conditions associated with low leukocyte alkaline phosphatase. N Engl J Med 1960; 262:912.

360. Nicholson-Weller A, March JP, Rosenfeld SI, et al: Affected erythrocytes of patients with paroxysmal nocturnal hemoglobinuria are deficient in the complement regulatory protein, decay accelerating factor. Proc Natl Acad Sci USA 1983; 80:5066.

361. Selvaraj P, Dustin ML, Silber R, et al: Deficiency of lymphocyte function-associated antigen 3 (LFA-3) in paroxysmal nocturnal hemoglobinuria. J Exp Med 1987; 166:1011.

362. Holguin MH, Fredrick LR, Bernshaw NJ, et al: Isolation and characterization of a membrane protein from normal human erythrocytes that inhibits reactive lysis of the erythrocytes of paroxysmal nocturnal hemoglobinuria. J Clin Invest 1989; 84:7.

363. Simmons DL, Tan S, Tenen DG, et al: Monocyte antigen CD14 is a phospholipid anchored membrane protein. Blood 1989; 73:284.

364. Rosse, WF: Phosphatidylinositol-linked proteins and paroxysmal nocturnal hemoglobinuria. Blood 1990; 75:1595.

365. Hirose S, Ravi L, Prince GM, et al: Synthesis of mannosylglucosaminylinositol phospholipids in normal but not paroxysmal nocturnal hemoglobinuria cells. Proc Natl Acad Sci USA 1992; 89:6025.

366. Mahoney JF, Urakaze M, Hall S, et al: Defective glycosylphosphatidylinositol anchor synthesis in paroxysmal nocturnal hemoglobinuria granulocytes. Blood 1992; 79:1400.

367. Takahashi M, Takeda J, Hirose S, et al: Deficient biosynthesis of N-acetylglucosaminyl-phosphatidylinositol, the first intermediate of glycosyl phosphatidylinositol anchor biosynthesis, in cell lines established from patients with paroxysmal nocturnal hemoglobinuria. J Exp Med 1993; 177:517.

368. Hillmen P, Bessler M, Mason PJ, et al: Specific defect in N-acetylglucosamine incorporation in the biosynthesis of the glycosylphosphatidylinositol anchor in cloned cell lines from patients with paroxysmal nocturnal hemoglobinuria. Proc Natl Acad Sci USA 1993; 90:5272.

369. Hyman R: Somatic genetic analysis of the expression of cell surface molecules. Trends Genet 1988; 4:5.

370. Sugiyama E, DeGasperi R, Urakaze M, et al: Identification of defects in glycosylphosphatidylinositol anchor biosynthesis in the Thy-1 expression mutants. J Biol Chem 1991; 266:12119.

371. Armstrong C, Schubert J, Ueda E, et al: Affected paroxysmal nocturnal hemoglobinuria T lymphocytes harbor a common defect in assembly of N-Acetyl-D-glucosamine inositol phospholipid corresponding to that in class A Thy-1⁻ murine lymphoma mutants. J Biol Chem 1992; 267:25347.

372. Norris J, Hoffman S, Ware RE, et al: Glycosyl-phosphatidylinositol anchor synthesis in paroxysmal nocturnal hemoglobinuria: Partial or complete defect in an early step. Blood 1994; 83:816.

373. Yeh ETH, Rosse WF: Paroxysmal nocturnal hemoglobinuria and the glycosylphosphatidylinositol anchor. J Clin Invest 1994; 93:2305.

374. Schubert J, Alvarado M, Uciechowski P, et al: Diagnosis of paroxysmal nocturnal hemoglobinuria using immunophenotyping of peripheral blood cells. Br J Haematol 1991; 79:487.

375. Ware RE, Rosse WF, Hall SE: Immunophenotypic analysis of reticulocytes in paroxysmal nocturnal hemoglobinuria. Blood 1995; 86:1586.

376. Oni SB, Osunkoya BO, Luzzato L: Paroxysmal nocturnal hemoglobinuria: Evidence for monoclonal origin of abnormal red cells. Blood 1970; 36:145.

377. Josten KM, Tooze JA, Borthwick-Clarke C, et al: Acquired aplastic anemia and paroxysmal nocturnal hemoglobinuria: Studies on clonality. Blood 1991; 78:3162.

378. Ohashi H, Hotta T, Ichikawa A, et al: Peripheral blood cells are predominantly chimeric of affected and normal cells in patients with paroxysmal nocturnal hemoglobinuria: Simultaneous investigation on clonality and expression of glycophosphatidylinositol-anchored proteins. Blood 1994; 83:853.

379. Tseng JE, Hall SE, Howard TA, et al: Phenotypic and functional analysis of lymphocytes in paroxysmal nocturnal hemoglobinuria. Am J Hematol 1995; 50:244.

380. Nicholson-Weller A, Russian DA, Austen KF: Natural killer cells are deficient in the surface expression of the complement regulatory protein, decay accelerating factor (DAF). J Immunol 1986; 137:1275.

381. Miyata T, Takeda J, Iida Y, et al: The cloning of *PIG-A*, a component in the early step of GPI-anchor biosynthesis. Science 1993; 259:1318.

382. Takeda J, Miyata T, Kawagoe K: Deficiency of the GPI anchor caused by a somatic mutation of the *PIG-A* gene in paroxysmal nocturnal hemoglobinuria. Cell 1993; 73:703.

383. Bessler M, Mason PJ, Hillmen P, et al: Paroxysmal nocturnal haemoglobinuria (PNH) is caused by somatic mutations in the *PIG-A* gene. EMBO J 1994; 13:110.

384. Miyata T, Yamada N, Iida Y, et al: Abnormalities of *PIG-A* transcripts in granulocytes from patients with paroxysmal nocturnal hemoglobinuria. N Engl J Med 1994; 330:249.

385. Schwartz RS: *PIG-A*—The target gene in paroxysmal nocturnal hemoglobinuria. N Engl J Med 1994; 330:283.

386. Ware RE, Rosse WF, Howard TA: Mutations within the *Piga* gene in patients with paroxysmal nocturnal hemoglobinuria. Blood 1994; 83:2418.

387. Bessler M, Mason PJ, Hillmen P, et al: Mutations in the *PIG-A* gene causing partial deficiency of GPI-linked surface proteins (PNH II) in patients with paroxysmal nocturnal hemoglobinuria. Br J Haematol 1994; 87:863.

388. Yamada N, Miyata T, Maeda K, et al: Somatic mutations of the *PIG-A* gene found in Japanese patients with paroxysmal nocturnal hemoglobinuria. Blood 1995; 85:885.

389. Ostendorf T, Nischan C, Schubert, et al: Heterogeneous *PIG-A* mutations in different cell lineages in paroxysmal nocturnal hemoglobinuria. Blood 1995; 85:1640.

390. Rosse WF, Ware RE: The molecular basis of paroxysmal nocturnal hemoglobinuria. Blood 1995; 86:3277.

391. Nishimura J, Murakami Y, Kinoshita T: Paroxysmal nocturnal hemoglobinuria: An acquired genetic disease. Am J Hematol 1999; 62:175.

392. Ware RE, Howard TA, Kamitani T, et al: Chromosomal assignment of genes involved in glycosylphosphatidylinositol anchor biosynthesis: Implications for the pathogenesis of paroxysmal nocturnal hemoglobinuria. Blood 1994; 83:3753.

393. Wiedmer T, Hall SE, Ortel TL, et al: Complement-induced vesiculation and exposure of membrane prothrombinase sites in platelets of paroxysmal nocturnal hemoglobinuria. Blood 1993; 82:1192.

394. Ploug M, Plesner T, Ronne E, et al: The receptor for urokinase-type plasminogen activator is deficient on peripheral blood leukocytes in patients with paroxysmal nocturnal hemoglobinuria. Blood 1992; 79:1447.

395. Griscelli-Bennaceur A, Gluckman E, Scrobohaci ML, et al: Aplastic anemia and paroxysmal nocturnal hemoglobinuria: Search for a pathogenetic link. Blood 1995; 85:1354.

396. Rosse WF: Paroxysmal nocturnal hemoglobinuria in aplastic anemia. Clin Haematol 1985; 14:105.
397. Lewis SM, Dacie JV: The aplastic anaemia-paroxysmal nocturnal haemoglobinuria syndrome. Br J Haematol 1967; 13:236.
398. Schubert J, Vogt HG, Zielinska-Skowronek M, et al: Development of the glycosylphosphatidylinositol-anchoring defect characteristic for paroxysmal nocturnal hemoglobinuria in patients with aplastic anemia. Blood 1994; 83:2323.
399. Lewis SM, Dacie JV: The aplastic anemia—Paroxysmal nocturnal hemoglobinuria syndrome. Br J Haematol 1967; 13:236.
400. Kawagoe K, Kitamura D, Okabe M, et al: Glycosylphosphatidylinositol-anchor-deficient mice: Implications for clonal dominance of mutant cells in paroxysmal nocturnal hemoglobinuria. Blood 1996; 87:3600.
401. Rosti V, Tremml G, Soares V, et al: Murine embryonic stem cells without pig-a gene activity are competent for hematopoiesis with the PNH phenotype but not for clonal expansion. J Clin Invest 1997; 100:1028.
402. Tremml G, Dominguez C, Rosti V, et al: Increased sensitivity to complement and a decreased red blood cell life span in mice mosaic for a nonfunctional Piga gene. Blood 1999; 94:2945.
403. Murakami Y, Kinoshita T, Maeda Y, et al: Different roles of glycosylphosphatidylinositol in various hematopoietic cells as revealed by a mouse model of paroxysmal nocturnal hemoglobinuria. Blood 1999; 94:2963.
404. Rotoli B, Luzzatto L: Paroxysmal nocturnal haemoglobinuria. Bailliere's Clin Haematol 1989; 2:113.
405. Young NS: Hematopoietic cell destruction by immune mechanisms in acquired aplastic anemia. Semin Hematol 2000; 37:3.
406. Bessler M, Mason P, Hillmen P, et al: Somatic mutations and cellular selection in paroxysmal nocturnal haemoglobinuria. Lancet 1994; 343:951.
407. Nishimura J, Inoue N, Wada H, et al: A patient with paroxysmal nocturnal hemoglobinuria bearing four independent PIG-A mutant clones. Blood 1997; 89:3470.
408. Araten DJ, Nafa K, Pakdeesuwan K, et al: Clonal populations of hematopoietic cells with paroxysmal nocturnal hemoglobinuria genotype and phenotype are present in normal individuals. Proc Natl Acad Sci USA 1999; 96:5209.
409. Ware RE, Pickens CV, DeCastro DM, et al: Circulating PIG-A mutant T lymphocytes in healthy adults and patients with bone marrow failure syndromes. Exp Hematol 2001; 29:1403.
410. Ware RE, Heeney MM, Pickens CV, et al: A multistep model for the pathogenesis and evolution of PNH. In Paroxysmal Nocturnal Hemoglobinuria and Related Disorders: Molecular Aspects of Pathogenesis, Omine M, Kinoshita T (eds.). Heidelberg, Springer-Verlag, 2003.
411. Brodsky RA, Vala MS, Barber JP, et al: Resistance to apoptosis caused by PIG-A gene mutations in paroxysmal nocturnal hemoglobinuria. Proc Natl Acad Sci USA 1997; 94:8756.
412. Horikawa K, Nakakuma H, Kawaguchi T, et al: Apoptosis resistance of blood cells from patients with paroxysmal nocturnal hemoglobinuria, aplastic anemia, and myelodysplastic syndrome. Blood 1997; 90:2716.
413. Ware RE, Nishimura J, Moody MA, et al: The PIG-A mutation and absence of glycosylphosphatidylinositol-linked proteins do not confer resistance to apoptosis in paroxysmal nocturnal hemoglobinuria. Blood 1998; 92:2541.
414. Blackshear PL Jr, Dorman FD, et al: Shear wall interaction and hemolysis. Trans Am Soc Artif Intern Organs 1966; 12:113.
415. Nevaril CG, Lynch EC, et al: Erythrocyte destruction and damage induced by shearing stress. J Lab Clin Med 1968; 71:784.
416. Monroe JM, True DE, et al: Surface roughness and edge geometrics in hemolysis with rotating disc flow. J Biomed Mater Res 1981; 15:923.
417. Brain MC, Dacie JV, Hourihane: Microangiopathic haemolytic anaemia: The possible role of vascular lesions in pathogenesis. Br J Haematol 1962; 8:358.
418. Bull BS, Kuhn IN: The production of schistocytes by fibrin strands (a scanning electron microscope study). Blood 1970; 35:104.
419. Saitoh H, Murakami H, Mori C: Upshaw-Schulman syndrome in two siblings. Acta Paediatr Jpn 1990; 32:373.
420. Chintagumpala MM, Hurwitz RL, Moake JL, et al: Chronic relapsing thrombotic thrombocytopenic purpura in infants with large von Willebrand factor multimers during remission. J Pediatr 1992; 120:49.
421. Azuno Y, Kaku K, Shino K, et al: A congenital variant of thrombotic thrombocytopenic purpura in two siblings. Intern Med 1994; 33:752.
422. Daghistani D, Jimenez JJ, Moake JL, et al: Familial infantile thrombotic thrombocytopenic purpura. J Pediatr Hematol Oncol 1996; 18:171.
423. Savasan S, Taub JW, Buck S, et al: Congenital microangiopathic hemolytic anemia and thrombocytopenia with unusually large von Willebrand factor multimers and von Willebrand factor-cleaving protease. J Pediatr Hematol Oncol 2001; 23:364.
424. Moake JL, McPherson PD: Abnormalities of von Willebrand factor multimers in thrombotic thrombocytopenic purpura and the hemolytic-uremic syndrome. Am J Med 1989; 87:9N.
425. Furlan M, Robles R, Galbusera M, et al: von Willebrand factor-cleaving protease in thrombotic thrombocytopenic purpura and the hemolytic-uraemic syndrome. N Engl J Med 1998; 339:1578.
426. Gerritsen HE, Robles R, Lammle B, et al: Partial amino acid sequence of purified von Willebrand factor-cleaving protease. Blood 2001; 98:1654.
427. Fujikawa K, Suzuki H, McMullen B, et al: Purification of human von Willebrand factor-cleaving protease and its identification as a new member of the metalloproteinase family. Blood 2001; 98:1662.
428. Levy GG, Nichols WC, Lian EC, et al: Mutations in a member of the ADAMTS gene family cause thrombotic thrombocytopenic purpura. Nature 2001; 413:488.
429. Tsai H-M, Lian EC-Y: Antibodies to von Willebrand factor-cleaving protease in acute thrombotic thrombocytopenic purpura. N Engl J Med 1998; 339:1585.
430. Moore JC, Haymward CP, Warkentin TE, et al: Decreased von Willebrand factor protease activity associated with thrombocytopenic disorders. Blood 2001; 98:1842.
431. Hogasen K, Jansen JH, Mollnes TE, et al: Hereditary porcine membranoproliferative glomerulonephritis type II is caused by factor H deficiency. J Clin Invest 1995; 95:1054.
432. Warwicker P, Goodship THJ, Donne RL, et al: Genetic studies into inherited and sporadic hemolytic uremic syndrome. Kidney Int 1998; 53:836.
433. Ying L, Katz Y, Schlesinger M, et al: Complement factor H gene mutation associated with autosomal recessive atypical hemolytic uremic syndrome. Am J Hum Genet 2000; 66:1721.
434. Perez-Caballero D, Gonzales-Rubio C, Gallardo ME, et al: Clustering of missense mutations in the C-terminal region of factor H in atypical hemolytic uremic syndrome. Am J Hum Genet 2001; 68:478.
435. Zipfel PF: Hemolytic uremic syndrome: How do factor H mutants mediate endothelial damage? Trends Immunol 2001; 22:345.
436. Jain R, Chartash E, Susin M, et al: Systemic lupus erythematosus complicated by thrombotic microangiopathy. Semin Arthritis Rheum 1994; 24:173.
437. Steen VD: Renal involvement in systemic sclerosis. Clin Dermatol 1994; 12:253.
438. James SH, Meyers AM: Microangiopathic hemolytic anemia as a complication of diabetes mellitus. Am J Med Sci 1998; 315:211.
439. Tucker LB: Vasculitis, Kawasaki disease, and hemolytic uremic syndrome. Curr Opin Rheum 1994; 6:530.
440. Boudes P, Andre C, Belghiti D, et al: Microscopic Wegener's disease: A particular form of Wegener's granulomatosis. J Rheumatol 1990; 17:1412.
441. Durand JM, Lefevre P, Kaplanski G, et al: Thrombotic microangiopathy and the antiphospholipid antibody syndrome. J Rheumatol 1991; 18:1916.
442. Hariharan D, Manno CS, Seri I: Neonatal lupus erythematosus with microvascular hemolysis. J Pediatr Hematol Oncol 2000; 22:351.
443. Bancroft-Lesesne J, Rothschild N, et al: Cancer-associated hemolytic-uremic syndrome: Analysis of 85 cases from a national registry. J Clin Oncol 1989; 7:781.
444. Nordstrom B, Strang P: Microangiopathic hemolytic anemias (MAHA) in cancer. A case report and review. Anticancer Res 1993; 13:1845.
445. Schiller D: Malignancy-associated microangiopathic hemolytic anemia. J Clin Oncol 1997; 15:2474.

446. Ataga KI, Graham ML: Microangiopathic hemolytic anemia associated with metastatic breast carcinoma. Am J Hematol 1999; 61:254.

447. Rarick MU, Espina B, Mocharnuk R: Thrombotic thrombocytopenic purpura in patients with human immunodeficiency virus infection: A report of three cases and review of the literature. Am J Hematol 1992; 40:103.

448. Myers KA, Marrie TJ: Thrombotic microangiopathy associated with *Streptococcus pneumoniae* bacteremia: case report and review. Clin Infect Dis 1995; 20:720.

449. Juckett M, Perry EH, Daniels BS, et al: Hemolytic uremic syndrome following bone marrow transplantation. Bone Marrow Transplant 1991; 7:405.

450. Kondo M, Kojima S, Horibe K, et al: Hemolytic uremic syndrome after allogeneic or autologous hematopoietic stem cell transplantation for childhood malignancies. Bone Marrow Transplant 1998; 21:281.

451. Weinstein L. Syndrome of hemolysis, elevated liver enzymes, and low platelet count: a severe consequence of hypertension in pregnancy. Am J Obstet Gynol 1982; 142:159.

452. Erkkola R, Ekblad U, Kero P, et al: HELLP syndrome. Ann Chir Gynaecol Suppl 1987; 202:26.

453. Schwartz ML, Brenner W. Severe preeclampsia with persistent postpartum hemolysis and thrombocytopenia treated by plasmapheresis. Obstet Gynecol 1985; 65:53S.

454. Entman SS, Kambam JR, Bradley CA, et al: Increased levels of carboxyhemoglobin and serum iron as an indicator of increased red cell turnover in preeclampsia. Am J Obstet Gynecol 1987; 156:1169.

455. Gibson B, Hunter D, Neame PB, et al: Thrombocytopenia in preeclampsia and eclampsia. Semin Thromb Hemost 1982; 8:234.

456. Volcy J, Nzerue Cm, Oderinde A, et al: Cocaine-induced acute renal failure, hemolysis, and thrombocytopenia mimicking thrombotic thrombocytopenic purpura. Am J Kidney Dis 2000; 35:E3.

457. Crum NF, Gable P: Quinine-induced hemolytic-uremic syndrome. South Med J 2000; 93:726.

458. Oteo JF, Alonso-Pulpon L, Diez JL: Microangiopathic hemolytic anemia secondary to cyclosporine therapy in a heart and liver transplant recipient. J Heart Lung Transplant 1996; 15:322.

459. Mach-Pascual S, Samii K, Beris P: Microangiopathic hemolytic anemia complicating FK506 (tacrolimus) therapy. Am J Hematol 1996; 52:310.

460. Trimarchi HM, Truong LD, Brennan S, et al: FK506-associated thrombotic microangiopathy: Report of two cases and review of the literature. Transplantation 1999; 67:539.

461. Canpolat C, Pearson P, Jaffe N: Cisplatin-associated hemolytic uremic syndrome. Cancer 1994; 74:3059.

462. Sakai C, Takagi T, Wakatsuki S, et al: Hemolytic-uremic syndrome due to deoxycoformycin: A report of the second case. Intern Med 1995; 34:593.

463. Cantrell JE, Phillips TM, Schein PS: Carcinoma-associated hemolytic-uremic syndrome: A complication of mitomycin C chemotherapy. J Clin Oncol 1985; 3:723.

464. Fung MC, Storniolo AM, Nguyen B, et al: A review of hemolytic uremic syndrome in patients treated with gemcitabine therapy. Cancer 1999; 85:2023.

465. Jubelirer SJ: Primary pulmonary hypertension. Its association with microangiopathic hemolytic anemia and thrombocytopenia. Arch Intern Med 1991; 151:1221.

466. Suzuki H, Nakasato M, Sato S, et al: Microangiopathic hemolytic anemia and thrombocytopenia in a child with atrial septal defect and pulmonary hypertension. Tohoku J Exp Med 1997; 181:379.

467. Otsuka Y, Abe K, Sato Y, et al: Malignant hypertension and microangiopathic hemolytic anemia. Jpn Heart J 1976; 17:258.

468. Becker CE, Benowitz NL: Hypertensive emergencies. Med Clin North Am 1979; 63:127.

469. Ruggenenti P, Remuzzi G: Malignant vascular disease of the kidney: Nature of the lesions, mediators of disease progression, and the case for bilateral nephrectomy. Am J Kidney Dis 1996; 27:459.

470. Chintagumpala MM, Hurwitz RL, Moake JL, et al: Chronic relapsing thrombotic thrombocytopenic purpura in infants with large von Willebrand factor multimers during remission. J Pediatr 1992; 120:49.

471. Savasan S, Taub JW, Buck S, et al: Congenital microangiopathic hemolytic anemia and thrombocytopenia with unusually large von Willebrand factor multimers and von Willebrand factor-cleaving protease. J Pediatr Hematol Oncol 2001; 23:364.

472. Barbot J, Costa E, Guerra M, et al: Ten years of prophylactic treatment with fresh-frozen plasma in a child with chronic relapsing thrombotic thrombocytopenic purpura as a result of a congenital deficiency of von Willebrand factor-cleaving protease. Br J Haematol 2001; 113:649.

473. Maes P, Brichard B, Vermylen C, et al: Chronic relapsing thrombotic thrombocytopenic purpura: Three case reports and update of the pathogenesis and therapeutic modalities. Eur J Pediatr 1998; 157:468.

474. Haberle J, Kehrel B, Ritter J, et al: New strategies in diagnosis and treatment of thrombotic thrombocytopenic purpura: Case report and review. Eur J Pediatr 1999; 158:883.

475. Bell WR, Braine JG, Ness PM, et al: Improved survival in thrombotic thrombocytopenic purpura-hemolytic uremic syndrome. Clinical experience in 108 patients. N Engl J Med 1991; 325:398.

476. George JN, Gilcher RO, Smith JW, et al: Thrombotic thrombocytopenic purpura-hemolytic uremic syndrome: Diagnosis and management. J Clin Apheresis 1998; 13:120.

477. Enjolras O, Wassef M, Mazoyer E, et al: Infants with Kasabach-Merritt syndrome do not have "true" hemangiomas. J Pediatr 1997; 130:631.

478. Vin-Christian K, McCalmont TH, Frieden IJ: Kaposiform hemangioendothelioma. An aggressive, locally invasive vascular tumor that can mimic hemangioma of infancy. Arch Dermatol 1997; 133:1573.

479. Shimizu M, Miura J, Itoh H, et al: Hepatic giant cavernous hemangioma with microangiopathic hemolytic anemia and consumption coagulopathy. Am J Gastroenterol 1990; 85:1411.

480. Pampin C, Devillers A, Treguier C, et al: Intratumoral consumptions of indium-111-labeled platelets in a child with splenic hemangioma and thrombocytopenia. J Pediatr Hematol Oncol 2000; 22:256.

481. Billio A, Pescosta N, Rosanelli C, et al: Treatment of Kasabach-Merritt syndrome by embolisation of a giant liver hemangioma. Am J Hematol 2001; 66:140.

482. Morad AB, McClain KL, Ogden AK: The role of tranexamic acid in the treatment of giant hemangiomas in newborns. J Pediatr Hematol Oncol 1995; 15:383.

483. Waldschmidt J, Schier F, Bein U, et al: The use of the laser in the treatment of aerterio-venous malformations and vascular tumours of the liver. Eur J Pediatr Surg 1993; 3:217.

484. Hall GW: Kasabach-Merritt syndrome: pathogenesis and management. Br J Haematol 2001; 112:851.

485. Hu B, Lachman R, Phillips J, et al: Kasabach-Merritt syndrome-associated kaposiform hemangioendothelioma successfully treated with cyclophosphamide, vincristine, and actinomycin D. J Pediatr Hematol Oncol 1998; 20:567.

486. Moore J, Lee M, Garzon M, et al: Effective therapy of a vascular tumor of infancy with vincristine. J Pediatr Surg 2001; 36:1273.

487. Powell J: Update on hemangiomas and vascular malformations. Curr Opin Pediatr 1999; 11:457.

488. Lannutti BJ, Gately St, Quevedo ME, et al: Human angiostatin inhibits murine hemangioendothelioma tumor growth in vivo. Cancer Res 1997; 57:5277.

489. Westphal RG, Azem EA: Macroangiopathic hemolytic anemia due to congenital cardiac anomalies. JAMA 1971; 216:1477.

490. Westring DW: Aortic valve disease and hemolytic anemia. Ann Intern Med 1966; 65:203.

491. Marsh GW, Lewis SM: Cardiac haemolytic anaemia. Semin Hematol 1969; 6:133.

492. Enzenauer RJ, Berenberg JL, Cassell PF: Microangiopathic hemolytic anemia as the initial manifestation of porcine valve failure. South Med J 1990; 83:912.

493. Geller S, Gelber R: Pentoxifylline treatment for microangiopathic hemolytic anemia caused by mechanical heart valves. Maryland Med J 1999; 48:173.

494. Batton DG, Amanullah A, Comstock C: Fetal schistocytic hemolytic anemia and umbilical vein varix. J Pediatr Hematol Oncol 2000; 22:259.

495. Davidson RJL: March or exertional haemoglobinuria. Semin Hematol 1969; 6:150.

496. Pollard TD, Weiss IW: Acute tubular necrosis in a patient with march hemoglobinuria. N Engl J Med 1970; 283:803.

497. Streeton JA: Traumatic haemoglobinuria caused by karate exercises. Lancet 1967; 2:191.

498. Schwartz KA, Flessa HC: March hemoglobinuria. Report of a case after basketball and congo drum playing. Ohio State Med J 1973; 69:448.

499. Abarbanel J, Benet AE, Lask D, et al: Sports hematuria. J Urol 1990; 143:887.

500. Joshua H, DeVries A: Effect of exercise of red blood cell in march hemoglobinuria. Am J Clin Pathol 1966; 46:341.

501. Sagov SE: March hemoglobinuria treated with rubber insoles: two case reports. J Am Coll Health Assoc 1970; 19:146.

502. Sigurdsson J, Bjornsson A, Gudmundsson ST: Formic acid burn— Local and systemic effects. Report of a case. Burns 1983; 9:358.

503. Bhargava M, Agarwal KN, Kumar S: Site of red cell destruction in the anaemia of experimental burns. Br J Haematol 1969; 17:179.

504. Vertel RM, Summerlin WT, Pruitt BA Jr, et al: Coombs' tests after thermal burns. J Trauma 1967; 7:871.

505. Sevitt S, Stone P, Jackson D, et al: Acute Heinz-body anaemia in burned patients. Lancet 1973; 2:471.

506. Eldad A, Neuman A, Weinberg A, et al: Silver sulphadiazine-induced haemolytic anaemia in a glucose-6-phosphate dehydrogenase-deficient burn patient. Burns 1991; 17:430.

15 | Disorders of the Erythrocyte Membrane

Patrick G. Gallagher • Samuel E. Lux

The erythrocyte membrane is the most thoroughly studied biologic membrane. Its easy accessibility has enabled researchers to characterize both its primary structure and a number of its important functions. Although it constitutes only about 1 percent of the total weight of the red cell, the membrane plays a pivotal role in the maintenance of erythrocyte integrity in a number of ways. It responds to erythropoietin during erythropoiesis and imports the iron required by the cell for hemoglobin synthesis. It retains vital compounds such as organic phosphates and removes metabolic waste. The erythrocyte membrane sequesters the reductants required to prevent corrosion by oxygen. It helps regulate erythrocyte metabolism by selectively and reversibly binding and inactivating glycolytic enzymes. It exchanges chloride and bicarbonate ions and helps the body maintain an adequate pH. The membrane maintains a slippery exterior so that erythrocytes do not adhere to endothelial cells or aggregate and occlude the microcirculation, and it provides strength and flexibility to the red cell to allow it to maintain its integrity while enduring circulatory stresses during its 4-month life span.

The red cell membrane was originally characterized as an example of the fluid mosaic model, proposed by Singer and Nicolson, more than 30 years ago.[1] In this model, the erythrocyte membrane is composed of mobile, asymmetrically distributed proteins and lipids that interact in a variety of ways. This model has been revised, because many membrane proteins are not freely mobile, but instead diffuse in complicated patterns, sometimes confined to discrete domains.[2-4] In this chapter, the normal erythrocyte membrane is discussed, with particular emphasis placed on aspects that are critical in the genesis of membrane abnormalities. The focus then shifts to the defects that lead to abnormalities of red cell shape, particularly hereditary spherocytosis and elliptocytosis. These are two of the most common and best-understood disorders of the erythrocyte membrane.

COMPOSITION OF THE ERYTHROCYTE MEMBRANE

Membrane Lipids

LIPID COMPOSITION

Lipids compose about 50 percent by weight of the red cell membrane (Table 15–1). Phospholipids and unesterified (free) cholesterol predominate and are present in nearly equal proportions (cholesterol-to-phospholipid molar ratio is 0.80).[5-7] Small amounts of glycolipids, principally globoside, are also present (Fig. 15–1).[5] The average red cell contains approximately 250 million phospholipid molecules, 195 million cholesterol molecules, 10 million glycolipid molecules, and 4 million protein molecules in a membrane whose total surface area is approximately 140 mm^2.[8,9] Phosphatidylcholine (PC), phosphatidylethanolamine (PE), sphingomyelin (SM), and phosphatidylserine (PS) are the predominant phospholipids. Their structures are shown in Figure 15–1. Small amounts of phosphatidic acid (PA), phosphatidylinositol (PI), and lysophosphatidylcholine (lyso-PC) are also present. At physiologic pH, PS, PA, and PI have a net negative charge, whereas the other phospholipids are electrically neutral. With the exception of SM and lyso-PC, these lipids have two fatty acids attached to a glycerol backbone. These are usually in ester linkage, although sometimes, particularly in PE, one of the fatty acids is a vinyl ether (plasmalogen).[10] The lysophospholipids have only one fatty acid and are named for the hemolysis induced because of their detergent-like properties.

LIPID ORGANIZATION

The majority of the phospholipids in the red cell membrane are in a planar bilayer with their polar head groups exposed at each surface and their hydrophobic fatty acyl side chains buried in the bilayer core. The phospholipid head groups tend to adopt regular, superlattice-like lateral distributions.[11] Glycolipids and cholesterol are intercalated between the phospholipids in the bilayer with their long axes perpendicular to the bilayer plane. Red cell glycolipids are located entirely in the external half of the bilayer with their carbohydrate moieties extending into the aqueous phase. They carry many important red cell antigens, including A, B, H, Le^a, Le^b, and P and serve other important functions such as enhancing membrane stability. Cholesterol is present in about equal proportions on both sides of the bilayer,[12] although some data suggest that it is somewhat more prevalent in the outer half.[13, 14] However, because all of the membrane cholesterol is available for exchange within 24 hours,[15] inner and outer membrane cholesterol must also be exchangeable. Measurements indicate that this transfer occurs rapidly, with a half-time of only seconds.[16] Cholesterol molecules are relatively buried, because the 3-OH group, the part of the molecule that is closest to the aqueous interface, lies approximately at the level of the carbonyl group of the phospholipid fatty acids.[17]

Phospholipid Asymmetry

Red cell membrane lipids, like membrane proteins (to be discussed), are asymmetrically distributed across the bilayer plane (*trans* asymmetry).[18-20] The asymmetric distribution of phospholipids reflects a steady state involving a constant exchange (flip/flop) of phospholipids between the two bilayer hemileaflets. Maintenance of asymmetry appears to depend on the fact that "flipping" occurs at a much higher rate than "flopping" and on membrane potential.[21] In pure phospholipid bilayers, this transmembrane diffusion is slow, lasting several hours to days. In contrast, the transmembrane shuttle of phospholipids in biologic membranes is very fast. In addition to enzymatic phospholipid translocation, described in the next paragraph, phospholipid flip/flop is accelerated by transmembrane proteins, which produce localized discontinuities in the bilayer, or, in the case of neutral phospholipids, by transmembrane pH gradients.[22]

Trans Asymmetry. *Trans* asymmetry of phospholipids is produced and maintained by an adenosine triphosphate (ATP)-dependent transport system, called the aminophospholipid translocase or "flippase."[23-26] This enzyme translocates PS, and to a lesser extent PE, from the outer to the inner bilayer. The half-times for PS and PE are about 5 and 60 minutes, respectively, at 37°C.[27] A similar activity exists in all mammalian red cells and in at least some nonerythroid cells and cell organelles. A 130-kD integral membrane protein that is a member of the magnesium (Mg^{2+})-dependent P-glycoprotein adenosine triphosphatase (ATPase) family mediates flippase activity.[28] Closely related enzymes exist in yeast, the malaria parasite *Plasmodium falciparum*, and the worm *Caenorhabditis elegans*. A yeast strain that lacks the homologous enzyme cannot transport PS from the outer to the inner membrane surface,[28] which confirms the function of this family of proteins. This protein may also play a role in toxin clearance.[29]

PC and SM are not transported inward by the flippase enzyme[28, 30]; however, red cells are able to transport PC,

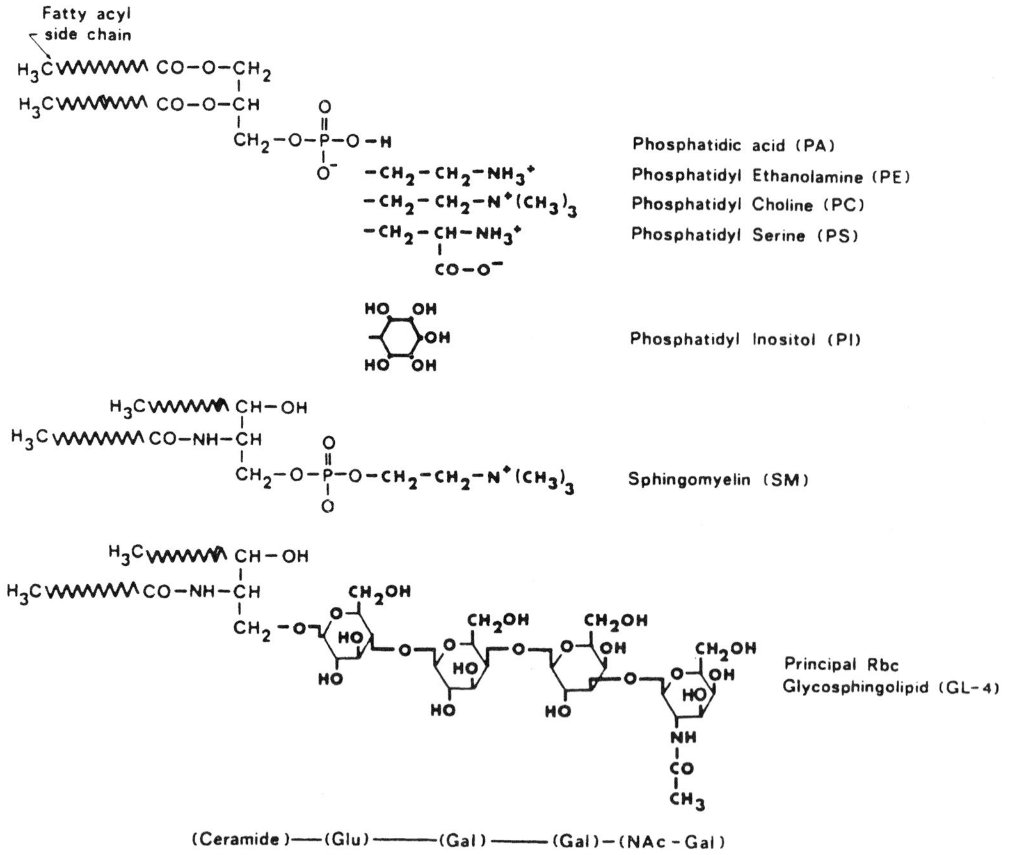

FIGURE 15–1. Chemical structures of the major phospholipids and the principal glycosphingolipid (GL-4) of the red cell (RBC) membrane. Note that phosphatidylcholine (PC) and sphingomyelin (SM) share the same polar moiety (choline) and that SM and GL-4 share the same nonpolar moiety (ceramide).

TABLE 15–1. Composition of Normal Human Red Cell Membranes

Component	Weight (%)	Grams per Membrane ($\times 10^{-13}$)	Approximate Number of Molecules per Membrane ($\times 10^6$)	Percentage in Outer Half of Bilayer	Percentage in Inner Half of Bilayer
Proteins and glycoproteins	55	5.7	6		
Lipids	45	4.7	475		
Phospholipids	28	3.0	250		
Sphingomyelin	6.8	0.73	60	80	20
Phosphatidylcholine	7.0	0.75	65	75	25
Phosphatidylethanolamine	7.4	0.79	65	20	80
Phosphatidylserine	4.3	0.46	40	0	100
Phosphatidylinositol (PI)	1.0	0.10	8	0	100
PI	0.34	0.036	3		
PI-4-P	0.22	0.024	2		
PI-4,5-PP	0.39	0.042	3		
Phosphatidic acid	1.0	0.10	8	Unknown	Unknown
Lysophosphatidylcholine	0.3	0.03	3	Unknown	Unknown
Lysophosphatidylethanolamine	0.3	0.03	3	Unknown	Unknown
Cholesterol	13	1.3	195	50	50
Glycolipids	3	0.3	10	100	0
Free fatty acids	1	0.1	20	Unknown	Unknown
	100	10.4	481		

From Lux SE, Palek J: Disorders of the red cell membrane. In Handin RI, Lux SE, Stossel TP (eds): Blood: Principles and Practice of Hematology. Philadelphia, JB Lippincott, 1995, pp 1701–1818.

along with PS and PE, from the inner to the outer bilayer. This floppase activity in red cell membranes appears to be mediated by the multidrug resistance protein, MRP1, a distantly related member of the P-glycoprotein ATPase family.[31–33] A series of experiments with targeted disruption of the multidrug resistance proteins—Mdr1a/1b,

Mdr2, and MRP1—revealed that MRP1 is responsible for the flop of labeled lipid analogs in the membrane.[34]

Membrane skeletal proteins such as spectrin help stabilize phospholipid asymmetry through interactions with inner membrane lipids. Spectrin interacts weakly with anionic phospholipids *in vitro*,[35–37] and phospholipid asymmetry is lost when spectrin is oxidized and cross-linked.[38–41] However, it is now known that the translocase is also sensitive to oxidation and would have been damaged by the treatments used to oxidize spectrin.[38–42] In addition, heat-treated ghosts, heat-induced vesicles that are spectrin depleted, and spectrin-deficient hereditary spherocytes are capable of translocating aminophospholipids with the same efficiency as normal ghosts.[43, 44] It appears that the aminophospholipid flippase can maintain phospholipid asymmetry without help from the membrane skeleton, at least under normal conditions.

An increase in intracellular calcium (Ca^{2+}) leads to activation of a "scramblase" that promotes randomization and loss of asymmetry in which both PS and PE flip to the outer bilayer leaflet while PC flops inside.[45–47] This scramblase, which has been cloned and characterized,[48, 49] mediates redistribution of membrane phospholipids in activated, injured, or apoptotic cells and is activated by calcium via an EF-hand motif.[50–53] Derangements within the red cell often raise intracellular calcium by direct or indirect damage to ion channels and pumps. Scott syndrome is a congenital bleeding disorder in which red cells and platelets expose subnormal amounts of PS on the outer surface in response to calcium, but it does not appear to be due to scramblase deficiency.[54, 55]

Phospholipid asymmetry results from the balance of the active translocation of PS and PE and the passive, slow bidirectional flip/flop of phospholipids. Changes in the equilibrium distribution of phospholipids could occur by inhibition of the translocase, acceleration of basal flip/flop rates to a degree that overwhelms the translocase, or both. Phospholipid asymmetry is lost in sickle cells[56, 57] with PS exposure correlating with the loss of translocase activity.[58] Phospholipid asymmetry is also altered in diabetic red cells,[59, 59a] which, like sickle cells, tend to adhere to endothelial cells.[56, 59a, 60] In one study, normal membrane phospholipid distribution was demonstrated in the erythrocytes of patients with hereditary spherocytosis and elliptocytosis.[61] Abnormal PS exposure has been found on Rh-deficient erythrocytes[62] and hydrocytosis erythrocytes.[63]

Maintenance of phospholipid asymmetry is important in maintaining membrane mechanical properties[64] in the regulation of a number of important cellular events such as membrane budding and endocytosis, and in the sequestration of aminophospholipids on the cytoplasmic side of the membrane. The disruption of asymmetry can have effects including creation of a procoagulant state and activation of the alternate complement pathway.[57, 65] In addition, macrophages bind and ingest red cells or even liposomes that have PS exposed on their outer surfaces.[66, 67] Several adhesive surface receptors on macrophages, including CD14, CD36, CD68, and the class B scavenger proteins SR-BI,[57] mediate the recognition and removal of PS-exposing cells during apoptosis. These receptors do not discriminate between PS and other anionic phospholipids. A PS-specific receptor has been identified.[68]

Studies have shown that phagocytosis of apoptotic cells requires tethering of the cells to the receptor, followed by PS-stimulated, PS receptor–mediated macropinocytosis.[69–71] Whether mature erythrocytes undergo caspase-mediated apoptosis is controversial.[72, 73]

***Cis* Asymmetry.** Red cell lipids exist in different domains within each of the bilayer planes (*cis* asymmetry).

Macroscopic Domains. Fluorescent phospholipids partition into doughnut-shaped lipid domains up to several microns in diameter within the membrane of red cells or ghosts.[74, 75] These lipid-rich domains are intrinsic structural features of the membrane, not just "gel-phase" or "fluid-phase" domains.[74] They increase in size when membrane proteins aggregate, and they are lacking in large liposomes made solely of membrane lipids, which suggests that proteins play a role in their formation. How and why this occurs is a mystery.

Microscopic Domains: Protein-Bound Lipids. Lipids may also partition on a more microscopic scale within the membrane. Early experiments[76] detected a layer of tightly associated "boundary lipids" attached to membrane proteins that intruded into the bilayer core, but subsequent work[77] suggested that such lipids were bound only transiently ($<10^{-7}$ second) and probably were not distinguishable from other lipids in the bilayer on the time scale of enzyme reactions and other cellular events. However, there are probably exceptions to this generalization, because specific lipids are required for the enzymatic functions of some transport proteins, such as the sodium (Na^+) and Ca^{2+} pumps, and because some membrane proteins, such as glycophorin A (to be discussed later), bind anionic (PS and PI) but not choline (PC and SM) phospholipids. Positively charged amino acids are concentrated on the cytoplasmic side of the bilayer-spanning domains of glycophorins and other membrane proteins, in part because their position determines the orientation of the protein.[78, 79] Although it is not well documented, anionic phospholipids probably cluster near these regions of positive charge. Surface-bound membrane proteins such as spectrin and protein 4.1, which bind preferentially to anionic phospholipids,[35–37] may also contribute to the nonrandom topography of inner membrane phospholipids.

Bilayer Couple Hypothesis and the Protein Scaffold Theory. The shape of the lipid bilayer is responsive to very slight variations (<0.4 percent) in the surface area of its inner and outer halves.[80, 81] This is termed the *bilayer couple effect*.[82] It reflects the tight packing of membrane lipids, the independent motion of lipids in each half of the bilayer, and the extreme thinness of the membrane (<0.1 percent of the diameter of the cell). Processes that expand the outer bilayer (or contract the inner) will produce uniform membrane spiculation, called *echinocytosis*. Conversely, relative expansion of the inner bilayer will lead to membrane invagination and cup-shaped red cells, *stomatocytosis*. Strongly charged amphipathic compounds, such as phospholipids, cause echinocytosis.[81, 83] They are trapped in the outer bilayer by their fixed charge. Permeable amphipaths (e.g., weak acids and bases that can cross the membrane in their uncharged form) will cause the membrane to extend toward the side of greater accumulation.[84, 85] In general, cationic compounds accumulate in the negatively charged inner bilayer and anionic compounds partition to the neutral outer bilayer. Even subtle effects, such as differences in the cross-sectional area of lipid head groups or fatty acyl tails, can lead to changes in membrane curvature.[83]

The bilayer couple hypothesis predicts that shape changes resulting from expansion of one lipid leaflet can be reversed by a commensurate alteration in the other. For example, the intensely spiculated red cells of patients with abetalipoproteinemia can be almost completely converted to biconcave disks by the addition of small amounts (0.1 mmol/L) of chlorpromazine, a cationic amphipath.[86] Unfortunately, this simple test has not been widely applied to red cells showing pathologic changes, so it is difficult to estimate how often bilayer couple effects dictate cell shape *in vivo*.

Evidence has accumulated against the lipid bilayer coupled hypothesis[87]; this includes the behavior of red cell ghosts and triton shells, various erythrocyte protein manipulations, and fixation of erythrocyte shape by the addition of large reagents outside the cell.[88-90] In addition, erythrocytes from patients with hereditary spherocytosis demonstrate normal, asymmetrically distributed phospholipids[61] and despite changes in the shapes of red cells during storage in citrate phosphate glucose at 4°C, phospholipid asymmetry was maintained.[91] These findings have led some researchers to support a protein scaffold theory, in which complex interactions of the spectrin-actin network, the lipid bilayer, and intracellular water interact to shape the erythrocyte.[87]

Glycolipids and Cholesterol. Glycolipids and cholesterol are intercalated between the phospholipids in the bilayer with their long axes perpendicular to the bilayer plane. Red cell glycolipids are located entirely in the external half of the bilayer with their carbohydrate moieties extending into the aqueous phase. They carry several important red cell antigens, including A, B, H, Le[a], Le[b], and P, and may serve other important functions. The P glycolipid, for example, serves as the receptor for parvovirus B19,[92] the agent responsible for most aplastic crises (see later).

Cholesterol is present in about equal proportions on both sides of the bilayer[12] (Table 15–1) and equilibrates between them in seconds or less. This facilitates membrane bending, because the movement of cholesterol can offset the difference in surface pressure caused by bending and compressing one of the bilayers relative to the other. Cholesterol depletion promotes inward curvature of the membrane, whereas cholesterol enrichment favors outward deflection.[93] Cholesterol molecules are relatively buried, because the 3-OH group (the part of the molecule that is closest to the aqueous interface) lies approximately at the level of the carbonyl group of the phospholipid fatty acids.[94]

Membrane Phosphoinositides. The polar head group of this interesting class of phospholipids contains PI, or its phosphorylated forms, PI-4-monophosphate and PI-4,5-bisphosphate. In nucleated cells, phosphoinositides are precursors of important intracellular second messengers such as inositol-1,4,5-trisphosphate (IP$_3$) and diacylglycerol.[95] In mature erythrocytes, phosphoinositides represent 2 to 5 percent of the total phospholipids. They reside largely at the inner membrane surface and undergo rapid phosphoryla-

tion and dephosphorylation. They help regulate Ca^{2+} transport, interact with membrane proteins such as glycophorin C and protein 4.1 (see later), and may influence discocyte-echinocyte shape transformation.

Lipid Mobility

Purified phospholipids exhibit discrete, liquid crystalline to gel phase transitions that depend on the length and degree of unsaturation of their acyl side chains. At temperatures greater than the temperature of this transition, the acyl side chains waggle very rapidly (10^8 to 10^9 times/sec) from side to side, with progressively greater excursions as one proceeds from the glycerol ester linkage to the terminal methyl group.[96, 97] The presence of a double bond in the acyl chain increases the disorder and flexibility all along the hydrocarbon chain,[98, 99] especially toward the terminal methyl end.[99] At temperatures less than the temperature of the liquid crystalline to gel phase transition, acyl chains of purified lipids are extended in stiff, parallel, hexagonally packed arrays that are more nearly solid than liquid.

Cholesterol as an Intermediate. Cholesterol buffers the extremes of the gel and liquid crystalline states. At temperatures greater than that of the gel to liquid phase transition, cholesterol partially immobilizes the acyl chains of phospholipids, particularly the proximal 8 to 10 carbons that are adjacent to the bulky steroid nucleus.[97] At temperatures less than that of this transition, cholesterol disrupts the ordering of the acyl chains, in effect preserving membrane fluidity.[100] The net result is that cholesterol tends to abolish the gel to liquid crystalline transition and create a condition of intermediate fluidity in which the proximal ends of the hydrocarbon chains are extended and relatively rigid and the distal ends are disordered and fluid. The red cell membrane contains relatively large amounts of cholesterol (cholesterol-to-phospholipid ratio is 0.8 mol/mol) and is relatively less fluid than other plasma membranes.[101] The inner bilayer is somewhat more fluid than the outer layer, probably because it contains more unsaturated fatty acids.[10] The significance of this difference is unknown.

Spectroscopic techniques are available for assessing the motion of various lipid-soluble probes and are widely used to measure lipid "fluidity." Decreased red cell lipid fluidity due to membrane cholesterol accumulation has been implicated in the pathogenesis of acanthocytosis associated with abetalipoproteinemia[102] or liver disease (spur cell anemia)[103, 104] and with a number of other conditions; however, whether these changes are due to true alterations in lipid fluidity or to changes in lipid organization that alter the location and spectroscopic properties of the probe has not yet been determined.

Lateral Diffusion. Phospholipids move about rapidly within each plane of model lipid bilayers.[101, 105, 106] From the measured lateral diffusion constants (2 to 5 × 10^{-8} cm^2/sec), one can calculate that phospholipids exchange places with each other about 10^7 times/sec. This rate is somewhat damped in the red cell membrane (estimated diffusion constant of 1.4 × 10^{-8} cm^2/s),[107] but this difference is not unexpected. Differences between diffusion rates *in vivo* and *in vitro* have been attributed to compartmentalization of the membrane formed by proteins of the actin-based membrane skeleton.[107a]

Lipid Renewal Pathways

Mature erythrocytes are unable to synthesize fatty acids, phospholipids, or cholesterol *de novo* and depend on lipid exchange and fatty acid acylation as mechanisms for phospholipid repair and renewal (Fig. 15–2). Outer bilayer phospholipids (PC and SM) exchange slowly (approximate turnover time of 5 days)[108] with the phospholipids of plasma lipoproteins.[109, 110] Inner bilayer phospholipids (PS and PE) are unable to participate in this process and are virtually unexchangeable.[108]

Fatty acids and lysophosphatides exchange more rapidly. Red cell membrane cholesterol (unesterified) also exchanges readily with the unesterified cholesterol in plasma lipoproteins (half-life is 7 hours), where it is partially converted to esterified cholesterol by the action of lecithin:cholesterol acyltransferase (LCAT). Because the newly formed cholesteryl ester cannot return to the red cell membrane (there is virtually no esterified cholesterol in the membrane), LCAT catalyzes a unidirectional pathway that depletes the membrane of cholesterol and decreases its surface area. Conversely, if LCAT is absent or inhibited, excess membrane cholesterol accumulates, expanding the membrane surface area.[111]

The fatty acid acylation pathway is an active metabolic pathway and requires ATP energy. This system combines fatty acids with lysophosphatides (principally lyso-PC) to remake the native phospholipid.[112–114] The acylase enzyme and its phospholipid products are located in the inner bilayer.[115] In theory, this enzyme should facilitate the renewal of lost or damaged fatty acid side chains and should prevent the accumulation of deleterious lysophosphatides within the membrane; however, it is not certain that the phospholipases necessary to remove damaged fatty acids operate in the red cell.

These renewal pathways, although limited, permit a slow replacement of membrane lipid components. Approximately 30 days are required before erythrocyte lipids reach equilibrium after a change in dietary fatty acids. Theoretically, this could be pathologically significant in persons consuming unusual diets (e.g., infants receiving a high intake of medium-chain triglycerides); however, no pathologic consequences have been reported.

Membrane Proteins

The red cell membrane contains at least a dozen major proteins[116] and hundreds of minor ones.[117] The major proteins of the red cell membrane (Fig. 15–3) and their disorders have been intensively studied,[118–120] and, in most cases, their genes have been cloned. It is important to realize that the enumeration and characterization of all the proteins of the red cell membrane may never be achieved because the membrane is not a separate, discontinuous structure but one that extends into both the cytoplasm and the extracellular space. Isolation of many of these minor proteins may be technically challenging because some of these proteins may be sensitive to even minor variations in isolation conditions, as are some of the proteins already characterized.

Traditionally, components of the erythrocyte membrane have been analyzed after hypotonic hemolysis[116, 121] and separation by sodium dodecyl sulfate (SDS) polyacrylamide gel electrophoresis (PAGE) (Fig. 15–4).[116, 122, 123] Various classifications for proteins of the erythrocyte membrane exist based on electrophoretic mobility, protein function, location, and so on (Table 15–2). For example, the network of proteins on the inner surface of the red cell that is responsible for maintaining the shape and deformability of the erythrocyte is called the erythrocyte membrane skeleton. The principal proteins of the membrane skeleton include spectrin, actin, and protein 4.1. In another classification that uses location for classification, membrane proteins of the red cell may be classified as either integral or peripheral. Integral membrane proteins penetrate or traverse the lipid bilayer and interact with the hydrophobic lipid core. They include glycophorins

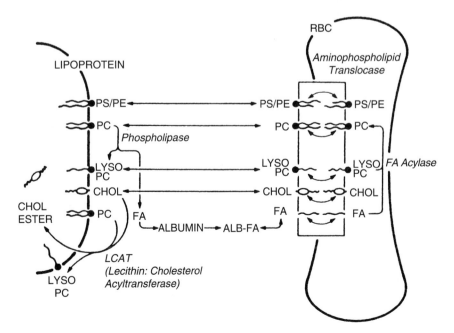

FIGURE 15–2. Fatty acid (FA) renewal and lipid exchange pathways in the human erythrocyte. PS, phosphatidylserine; PE, phosphatidylethanolamine; CHOL, cholesterol; LYSO, lysophosphatides.

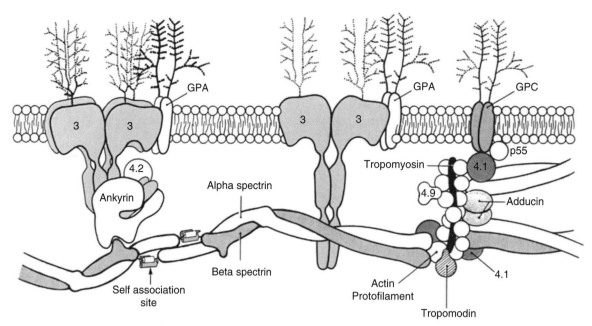

FIGURE 15–3. Schematic model of the red cell membrane. The relative position of the various proteins is correct, but the proteins and lipids are not drawn to scale. (Adapted with permission from Lux SE, Palek J.: Disorders of the red cell membrane. In Handin RJ, Lux SE, Stossel, TP (eds.): Blood: Principles and Practice of Hematology. Philadelphia, Lippincott-Raven, 1995, pp 1701–1818.)

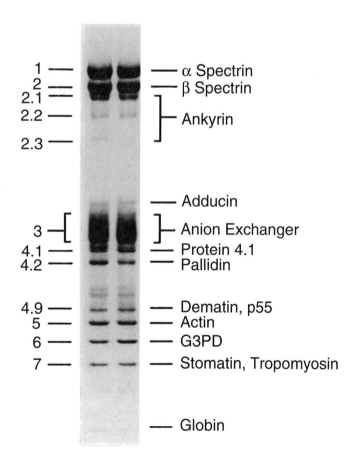

FIGURE 15–4. Protein composition of the red blood cell membrane skeleton. The major components of the erythrocyte membrane as separated by sodium dodecyl sulfate polyacrylamide gel electrophoresis (SDS-PAGE) and revealed by Coomassie blue staining. (Adapted from Gallagher PG, Tse WT, Forget BG: Clinical and molecular aspects of disorders of the erythrocyte membrane skeleton. Semin Perinatol 14:352, 1990.)

A, B, C, and D, which possess membrane receptors and antigens, and transport proteins such as band 3, the erythrocyte anion exchanger. Peripheral proteins interact with integral proteins or lipids at the membrane surface but do not penetrate into the bilayer core. In the red cell, the major peripheral membrane proteins are located on the cytoplasmic membrane face and include enzymes such as glyceraldehyde-3-phosphate dehydrogenase and structural proteins such as spectrin. With this classification as a guide, significant features of the major erythrocyte membrane proteins are delineated.

INTEGRAL MEMBRANE PROTEINS

Glycophorins

Study of red cell antigens has led to our knowledge of the glycophorin proteins. Glycophorins A, B, and E[124, 125] are associated with the MNSs antigens, and glycophorins C and D are associated with the Gerbich (Ge) blood groups.[126–129]

Glycophorin A. Glycophorin A (GpA), the major sialoglycoprotein of the red cell, is present in approximately 1 million copies per cell. Three GpA complementary DNA (cDNA) transcripts are expressed from the gene (transcripts of 2.8, 1.7, and 1.0 kb) that vary only by usage of alternate polyadenylation sites. GpA is synthesized with a cleavable leader sequence that produces a mature protein of 181 amino acids (Fig. 15–5). The 36-kD protein has an extracellular NH_2 terminus, a single transmembrane region, and a cytoplasmic COOH terminus.[130–132] The extracellular domain (residues 1 to 61) contains 15 tetrasaccharides that are O-glycosidically linked to serine or threonine residues and one complex oligosaccharide attached to asparagine 26.[133] Overall, the carbohydrate accounts for about 60 percent of the mass of

TABLE 15–2. Major Human Erythrocyte Membrane Proteins

SDS Gel Band[‡]	Protein	Peripheral or Integral	Molecular Wt. × 10³ (Gel/Calculated)	Approx Proportion (Wt%)	Monomer Copies per Cell (× 10⁻³)[†]	Oligomeric State	Chromosome Location
1	α spectrin	P	240/281	14	242 ± 20	Heterodimer/tetramer	1q22 q23
2	β spectrin	P	220/246	13	242 ± 20		14q23 p24.2
2.1[¶]	Ankyrin	P	210/206	6[¶]	124 ± 11[¶]	Monomer	8p 11.2
2.9	α adducin	P	103/81	<1	≈30	Heterodimer/tetramer	4p16.3
	β adducin	P	97/80	<1	≈30		2p 13 p14
3[#]	AE1[$]	1	90–100**/102[††]	29	≈1200	Dimer or tetramer	17q12 p21
4.1	Protein 4.1	P	80 + 78[‡‡]/66[§§]	5	≈200	Monomer	1p33 p34.2
4.2	Protein 4.2	P	72/77	5	≈250	Dimer or trimer	15q15 q21
4.9[#]	Dematin	P	48 + 52/43 + 46	1	≈140	Trimer[¶¶]	8p21.1
	p55	P	55/53		≈80	Dimer	Xq28
5[#]	β actin	P	43/42	6	≈500	Oligomer (≈14)	7pter q22
	Tropomodulin	P	43/41		≈30	Monomer	9q22
6	G3PD[$]	P	35/36	5[##]	≈500	Tetramer	12p 13
7[#]	Stomatin	I	31/32	4	—	—	9q33 q34
	Tropomyosin	P	27 + 29/28***		≈70	Heterodimer***	1q31
8	Protein 8	P	23/—	1–2	≈200	—	—
PAS-1	Glycophorin A[†††]	I	36[‡‡‡]/14[††]	1.6	≈1000	Dimer	4q31
PAS-2	Glycophorin C[†††]	I	32[‡‡‡]/14[††]	0.1	≈200(C + D)[§§§]	—	2q14 q21
PAS-3	Glycophorin B[†††]	I	20[‡‡‡]/8[††]	0.2	≈200	Dimer	4q31
	Glycophorin D[†††]	I	23[‡‡‡]/11[††]	0.02	≈200(C + D)[§§§]	—	2q14 q21
	Glycophorin E[†††]	I	—[§§§]21/6[††]	—[§§§]	—[§§§]	—[§§§]	—4q31

*Calculated from amino acid sequences.

[†]Based on an estimate of 5.7 × 10⁻¹³ g protein/ghost[117] and on the approximate proportions of each protein, estimated from densitometry of SDS gels. The data for spectrin and ankyrin were measured directly by radioimmunoassay.

[‡]Proteins 1 to 8 were estimated from the data in Fairbanks et al,[116] Palek and Jarolim,[593] and from unpublished data.

[§]Numbering system of Fairbanks et al[116] and Steck.[123] Bands 1 to 8 refer to Coomassie blue–stained gels. PAS-1 to PAS-3 refer to periodic acid-Schiff–stained gels.

[$]HE, hereditary elliptocytosis; HS, hereditary spherocytosis; HPP, hereditary pyropoikilocytosis; HAc, hereditary acanthocytosis; HSt, hereditary stomatocytosis; SAO, Southeast Asian ovalocytosis; AE1, anion exchange protein 1 (erythroid anion exchange protein); G3PD, glyceraldehyde-3-phosphate dehydrogenase.

[¶]Protein 2.1 is full-length ankyrin. Other isoforms are evident on SDS gels including band 2.2, 195 kd; band 2.3, 175 kd; and band 2.6, 145 kd. Band 2.2 is produced by alternate splicing. The origin of the other bands is unknown. The data shown are for ankyrin 2.1 except for the number of copies/cell and approximate proportion (wt%), which include all isoforms.

[#]The α and β adducins lie in the upper part of SDS gel band 3. Band 4.9 contains both dematin and p55; band 5 contains β actin and tropomodulin; band 7 contains stomatin and tropomyosin.

**The protein runs as a broad band on SDS gels due to heterogeneous glycosylation.

[††]The calculated molecular weight does not include the contribution of the carbohydrate chains.

the molecule. This includes much of the sialic acid on the red cell membrane as well as the M and N blood group antigens. The M and N antigens on GpA are determined by polymorphic amino acids at residues 1 and 5 of the mature protein.[130] The M antigen is defined by a serine at residue 1 and a glycine at residue 5, whereas the N antigen is defined by a leucine at position 1 and a glutamine at position 5 (Table 15–3). M and N antibodies usually recognize these peptide determinants exclusively, but some may exhibit carbohydrate-dependent recognition characteristics.

Little is known about the membrane domain (amino acids 62 to 95), except that it binds negatively charged phospholipids,[134–137] such as PS and PI, and is probably the site of GpA dimerization.[124, 134–137] The dimeric interaction is strong due to a series of complex interactions that are difficult to dissociate, even in detergents.[138–140] Conventional SDS gels contain monomers, dimers, and heterodimers of GpA and similar oligomers of some of the other glycophorins. All of these species run anomalously on SDS gels because the large amount of carbohydrate interferes with SDS binding.[141] The carbohydrate also interferes with Coomassie blue staining to the extent that the glycophorins are invisible unless special stains (e.g., periodic acid–Schiff) are used. The function of the cytoplasmic domain (residues 96 to 131) is also largely unknown. The protein is first detectable in proerythroblasts and is a specific marker for erythroid cells.[142]

Glycophorin B. Glycophorin B (GpB) is structurally similar to GpA but is present at a much lower level than GpA, with only about 150,000 copies per cell. A single 0.6-kb cDNA transcript gives rise to a protein with a cleavable leader sequence yielding a mature protein 72 amino acids in length (Fig. 15–5). The protein is almost identical to the N blood group form of GpA for the first 26-amino acid residues except that it lacks the complex oligosaccharide at position 21.[130, 143] Subsequently, it lacks a piece of the extracellular domain of GpA corresponding

Gene Size (kb)	Number of Exons	Amino Acids	Gene Symbol	Associated Diseases[§]
80	52	2429	*SPTA1*	HE, HPP, HS
>100	≈32	2137	*SPTB*	HE, HPP, HS, HAc
>120	42	1880	ANK1	HS
—	—	737	*ADDA*	—
—	—	726	*ADDB*	—
17	20	911	EPB3	HS, SAO, HAc
>250	23	588	*EL1*	HE
20	13	691	*ELB42*	HS[§§]
—	—	383[¶]	—	—
—	—	466	*MPP1*	—
>4	6	375	*ACTB*	—
—	—	359	*TMOD*	—
5	9	335	*GAPD*	—
12	7	288	*STOM*	HSt
—	—	239[***]	*TPM3*	—
—	—	—	—	—
>40	7	131	*GYPA*	—
14	4	128	*GYPC*	HE
>30	5	72	*GYPB*	None
14	4	107	*GYPD*	HE
>30	4	59	*GYPE*	—

[‡‡11]Protein 4.1 is a doublet (4.1a and 4.1b) on SDS gels. Protein 4.1a is derived from 4.1b by slow deamidation. Its proportion is a measure of RBC age.

[§§]Protein 4.1 exists in a very large number of isoforms. The major erythroid isoform is listed here. It is not known why its calculated molecular weight deviates so much from the apparent molecular weight on SDS gels.

[$$]Deficiency of protein 4.2 is associated with a variety of morphologies (see text), but spherocytes predominate.

[¶]Although dematin is present as a trimer in solution, the 48- and 52-kD subunits have an apparent stoichiometry of 3:1 on SDS gels.

[##]The amount of G3PD (band 6) associated with the membrane varies from person to person (≈3 to 6 wt%).

[***]Tropomyosin is a heterodimer of the 27-kD and 29-kD subunits. There are about 70,000 copies of each chain per RBC. Data for the calculated molecular weight and the number of amino acids are for fibroblast tropomyosin.

[†††]The glycophorins (GPA to GPD) are visible only on PAS-stained gels.

[‡‡]Molecular weights, including carbohydrate, estimated from mobilities on SDS gels.

[§§§]Glycophorins C and D are probably synthesized from the same mRNA using different translational start sites. The total number of GPC and GPD molecules is about 200,000.

[$$$]Glycophorin E mRNA has been identified but it is not certain that the mRNA is translated.

From Lux SE, Palek J: Disorders of the red cell membrane. In Handin RI, Lux SE, Stossel TP (eds): Blood: Principles and Practice of Hematology. Philadelphia. J.B. Lippincott Co., 1995, pp 1701–1818.

to exon 3 and almost all of the cytoplasmic domain. Thus, there are no asparagine-linked carbohydrate chains on GpB, but there are about 11 serine/threonine-linked oligosaccharide chains. Besides the peptide sequence that carries the N antigen reactivity, which is also found on GpA, GpB carries the S, s, and U antigens. The S and s antigens differ by an amino acid polymorphism at residue 29; S is a methionine, and s is a threonine.[144–146] There is evidence that GpB forms a macromolecular complex with the Rh glycoproteins, which form the Rh antigens, the Rh50 glycoprotein, CD47, and proteins bearing the Duffy and LW antigens.[147–150]

Glycophorin E. Glycophorin E (GpE) is a glycophorin identified by molecular cloning.[151, 152] It resides on chromosome 4 just beyond GpB, which it resembles in structure, except that it lacks amino acid residues 27 to 39 of GpB, and it contains an in-frame insertion of 8 amino acids in the region corresponding to the transmembrane domain of GpA. The function of GpE is unknown. In fact it is not even known if the GpE messenger RNA (mRNA) is translated. The GpA, GpB, and GpE genes are oriented in tandem on chromosome 4. They apparently arose by gene duplication during primate evolution.

Glycophorins C and D. Glycophorins C (GpC) and D (GpD) have a general domain structure similar to GpA, GpB, and GpE, but they are located on a different chromosome and their amino acid sequences are unique.[153] GpC contains one N-linked and about 12 O-linked oligosaccharides as well as the Gerbich (Ge:3) blood group antigens (amino acids 41 to 50). The GpC cDNA predicts a protein of about 14 kD (Fig. 15–6), a size substantially smaller than the observed size of 32 kD on SDS polyacrylamide gels. This discrepancy is thought to be due to extensive glycosylation at sites within a 57-amino acid stretch at the NH_2 terminus predicted to be at the surface of the erythrocyte membrane. Unlike GpA, GpC is not erythroid specific. Monoclonal antibodies to GpC stain neural tissue in a distinctive fibrillar pattern.[154]

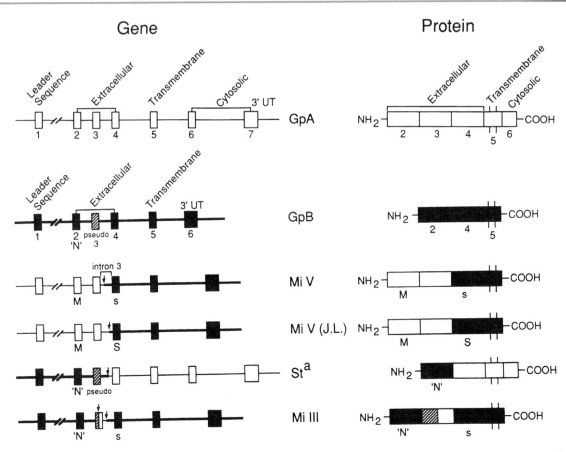

FIGURE 15–5. Genomic structures and polypeptides of glycophorins A and B and representative variants. GpA, glycophorin A; GpB, glycophorin B; Mi, Miltenberger; St^a. (From Lowe JB: In Stamatoyannopoulos G, Majerus PW, Perlmutter RM, Varmus H (eds.): The Molecular Basis of Blood Diseases, 3rd ed. Philadelphia, WB Saunders, 2000, pp 315–361.)

In red cells a desialylated form of GpC is exposed on the surface of very early progenitors (erythrocyte burst-forming unit) and can be a useful marker of early normal or leukemic erythroid differentiation.[155] Normally glycosylated GpC first appears in the erythrocyte colony-forming unit.[124] GpD is a shortened form of GpC, lacking its NH$_2$-terminal 21 amino acids. It arises from the same mRNA as GpC by use of an alternate initiation codon.[156, 157] There are 143,000 copies of GpC and 82,000 copies of GpD per red cell.[158]

TABLE 15-3. Variants of Glycophorins A, B, and E

Variant	Defect	References
Amino terminal	Amino terminal sequence	
M	Ser-Ser*-Thr*-Thr*-Gly-Val...	130, 144
N	Leu-Ser*-Thr*-Thr*-Glu-Val...	130, 144
M^c	Ser-Ser*-Thr*-Thr*-Glu-Val...	127–129
M^g	Leu-Ser-Thr-Asn-Glu-Val...	127–129
H^e (Henshaw)	Trp-Ser*-Thr*-Ser*-Gly-Val...	145
Other	Structural defects	
En(a–)	Absence of glycophorin A†	125, 130, 181–184
S-s-U–	Absence of glycophorin B†	125, 178–181
M^k	Absence of glycophorin A and B†	125, 182
MiII (Miltenberger I). MiII, MiVII, MiVIII	Variants of glycophorin A that differ by one or two amino acids.	127, 188
MiII, MiJ.L., MiV, MiVI, MiIX, MiX, Ph, Pj, Dantu, St^a (types A, B, and C)	Variants due to formation of Lepore-like and anti-Lepore-like hybrids of glycophorins A, B, and E	125, 127, 188–195
Cad	Carbohydrate variant with an abnormal O-linked oligosaccharide containing an extra β(1 → 4)-linked galactosamine on the penultimate galactose residue of both glycophorins A and B	127

*O-glycosylation site.
†Due to homologous recombination and unequal crossover → partial gene deletions.

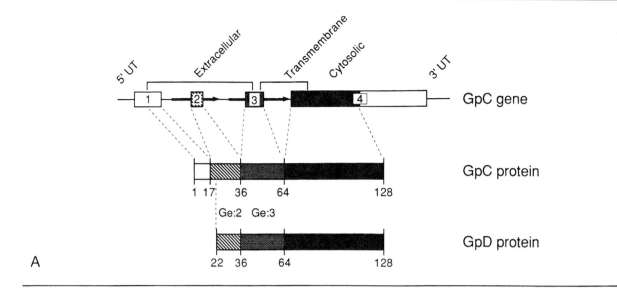

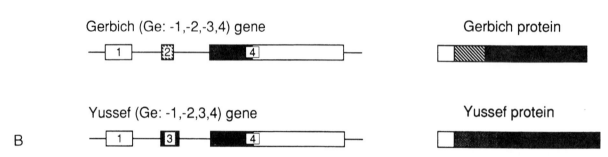

FIGURE 15–6. Genomic structures and polypeptides of glycophorins C and D and representative variants. *A,* Wild-type glycophorin C (GpC) gene and derived protein products. The GpC gene comprises four exons. The extracellular domain of GpC is encoded by exons 1 and 2. Its transmembrane segment is encoded by exons 3 and 4, and the cytosolic portion by exon 4. *Arrows* encompassing exons 2 and 3 represent repeat sequences believed to be involved in recombination events that have deleted exon 2 or 3 in some glycophorin C variants (see *B*). Glycophorin D (GpD) is believed to be derived from the same transcript that yields GpC, via translation initiation at an internal methionine residue corresponding to residue 22 of GpC. Positions of amino acid residues corresponding to exon boundaries are indicated below the GpC and GpD proteins. The Ge:2 and Ge:3 determinants have been localized to positions corresponding to exons 2 and 3, respectively. *B,* Variant GpC proteins. The Gerbich-type variant GpC gene lacks sequences corresponding to exon 3, via a postulated recombination event occurring between repeated sequences depicted in *A*. This variant gene encodes a shortened GpC molecule deficient in amino acid residues corresponding to exon 3. The Yussef-type variant GpC gene lacks sequences corresponding to exon 2, via a similar mechanism, and is predicted to express a shortened protein deficient in amino acid residues corresponding to exon 2. (Reprinted with permission from Lowe JB: In Stamatoyannopoulos G, Majerus PW, Perlmutter RM, Varmus H (eds.): The Molecular Basis of Blood Diseases, 3rd ed. Philadelphia, WB Saunders, 2000, pp 315–361.)

Association of Glycophorin A with Band 3. GpA and band 3 are associated in the membrane.[159] The Wright b (Wr[b]) antigen is caused by interaction of a site on band 3 (Glu[658]) with a site or sites located near the end of the extracellular domain of GpA or in the adjacent transmembrane domain.[160, 161] A monoclonal antibody to the Wr[b] blood group antigen immunoprecipitates both GpA and band 3.[162, 163] Antibodies to glycophorin, including monovalent Fab fragments, decrease the lateral[164] and rotational[165] mobility of band 3. The coexpression of GpA in *Xenopus* oocytes enhances expression of band 3 by facilitating transport of band 3 from the endoplasmic reticulum to the cell surface.[166]

Glycophorin Functions. The functions of the glycophorins are uncertain, except for the observation that they provide most of the negative surface charge red cells require to avoid sticking to each other and to the vascular wall. GpC binds to protein 4.1 and p55 and

may help anchor the membrane skeleton to the lipid bilayer.[167]

The glycophorins have been considered as conduits for transmembrane signaling and carry receptors for *P. falciparum* and for a number of viruses and bacteria.[168, 169] When wheat germ agglutinin or specific antibodies are attached to the external domain of GpA, the protein binds to the underlying membrane skeleton,[157, 170] probably through its interactions with band 3.[164, 171] The effect seems to involve transmembrane communication rather than antibody or lectin cross-linking, because it is also observed with monovalent Fab fragments but is not observed in red cells bearing variant glycophorins that lack a cytoplasmic domain (e.g., Miltenberger V). The increased cross-links dramatically rigidify the membrane and cause it to acquire irreversible, plastic-like properties on deformation. The reason why red cells have this interesting property is a mystery. Chasis and Mohandas[124] note that a number of pathogens adhere to red cells and suggest that the consequently stiffened erythrocytes may hasten reticuloendothelial removal of the invaders.

GpA bears receptors for *P. falciparum* as demonstrated by either direct competition experiments, using the purified sialoglycoproteins, or by the inability of *P. falciparum* to infect red cells with various glycophorin abnormalities.[172–175] The principal ligand appears to be sialic acid attached through an $\alpha2$–3 linkage to galactose,[176] but recognition also requires the peptide backbone of GpA.[177] GpA binds to EBA-175, a 175-kD erythrocyte-binding antigen located on the surface of *P. falciparum* merozoites.[177]

Glycophorin Variants. The realization that the MNSs blood group antigens are carried by the glycophorins led to the discovery of a large number of glycophorin defects in persons with variants of this blood group system, some of which are listed in Table 15–3.

Glycophorin A-B-E Variants. Variants of the *GpA-GpB-GpE* locus have been classified according to the mechanism that brought about the alteration, including deletions of the GpA or GpB gene or both, recombination due to genetic crossover or gene replacement (either double crossover events or gene conversion), and variants with altered antigenic properties due to alterations in the glycans attached to otherwise normal GpA or GpB proteins. Variants derived from complete or partial deletion of the GpA or GpB genes lead to the most dramatic phenotypes. Red cells with little or no detectable MN antigens, En(a–) cells, have been described with the underlying genetic defect being homozygous GpA gene deletion or the creation of a chimeric molecule with the 5′ end of the GpA gene linked to the 3′ end of the GpB gene. En(a–) red cells have very weak MN blood group antigens and, as expected from the gene defect, lack GpA.[178–181] Surprisingly, the red cell compensates for this loss of surface charge by increasing the glycosylation of band 3.[178, 180, 182] As a result the surface charge is only about 20 percent less than expected.

Erythrocytes lacking the Ss and U determinants are found in individuals from some regions of Africa[183] but are rarely seen in North Americans. These cells are deficient in GpB or express a defective, nonglycosylated form of GpB.[184, 185] In most instances, Southern blot analysis of DNA from S-s-U– individuals with GpB deficiency has identified large GpB gene deletions.[186, 187] Rarely, S-s-U– individuals have been identified without detectable GpB gene deletions on Southern blotting. In these individuals, point mutations or microdeletions have been hypothesized to be the cause.

Recombination events leading to hybrid glycophorin molecules are relatively common among the glycophorin A-B-E variants, as would be expected for a cluster of recently duplicated genes.[125–127, 188, 189] They are believed to result from chromosomal misalignment during meiosis and subsequent nonhomologous crossing over of the chromosomes in the region of GpA and GpB. A similar process is known to be responsible for the Lepore hemoglobins. Both Lepore-like and anti-Lepore-like unequal crossover of the glycophorins occur. In the former, illustrated by the Miltenberger (Mi) V (MiV) variants,[190–192] the normal GpA gene is replaced by a fusion gene containing the NH$_2$-terminal end of GpA (first three exons)

and the COOH-terminal end of GpB (last three exons). These two phenotypes vary in the particular *Ss* allele derived from the GpB gene. In the St^a variant,[192–195] the hybrid protein is reversed and is derived from the NH$_2$-terminal end of GpB (first two exons) and the COOH-terminal of GpA (last three exons). Variants produced by sequence replacements include the MiIII, MiX, and MiVI types.

Individuals with homozygous deletions of both GpA and GpB genes have been described. Red cells from these individuals lack GpA and GpB proteins, as well as the MN, Ss, and En^a antigens and the Wr^b determinants. It is important to note that none of the GpA or GpB variants produce any detectable change in erythropoiesis or in the shape, function, or life span of the affected red cells. This is true even in the rare individuals with complete absence of both GpA and GpB. This observation indicates either that GpA, GpB, and GpE have no essential function or that such functions are redundant or can be performed by another protein such as band 3 or GpC.

Glycophorin C-D Variants. Antigens of the Gerbich blood group correspond to determinants on GpC and GpD. The four most common variants are

1. The Melanesian type. This variant lacks the Ge:1 determinant (Ge: –1, 2, 3, 4). Its molecular basis is not known.
2. The Yussef type (Ge: –1, –2, 3, 4) lacks exon 2 due to a 3.4-kb DNA deletion.
3. The Gerbich type (–1, –2, –3, 4) which lacks exon 3 also due to a 3.4-kb DNA deletion.
4. The Leach variant (see later).

Other less common variants include the Webb type, a trypsin-sensitive antigen created by a single nucleotide substitution that changes an asparagine to a serine, removing the single asparagine-linked glycosylation site on GpC.[196] This, in turn, is responsible for the smaller size of W$_b$ GpC. Red cells of the Yussef, Gerbich, and Webb phenotypes have mutations in the extracellular domain of GpC, and in all three cases the mutant GpC protein is present, although its antigenicity is altered. In the rare Ls^a phenotype, erythrocytes display elongated GpC and GpD, owing to a duplication of exon 3.

In the Leach phenotype, GpC protein is absent, owing either to deletion of both exons 3 and 4[197–199] or to a frameshift mutation.[199] The Leach phenotype does not result in significant anemia, but it does cause elliptocytosis, as well as a decrease in membrane deformability and mechanical stability.[200–203] In contrast, red cells with the extracellular Ge-mutants and red cells that lack GpA or GpB have normal mechanical properties.[124, 204] Studies suggest that the deficiency of GpC is not directly responsible for the altered mechanical properties observed in Leach erythrocytes. Instead, the mechanical instability appears to be due to a concomitant partial deficiency of protein 4.1.[205] The instability is fully corrected by introducing protein 4.1 or its spectrin-binding domain (which facilitates spectrin-actin interactions) into GpC-deficient red cells. Why protein 4.1 and another recently described protein, p55, are deficient is not completely clear. However, the cytoplasmic domain of GpC interacts with both proteins[206] and presumably helps bind them to the membrane.

Band 3 (Anion Exchanger-1)

Band 3 (or AE1), the erythroid anion-exchange protein, is the major integral protein of the red cell, comprising 25 to 30 percent of the membrane protein (see Fig. 15–3).[207] It is expressed in great abundance, about 1.2 million copies per cell. The human band 3 cDNA is about 4.7 kb in length and encodes a 911-amino acid polypeptide (Fig. 15–7).[208, 209] Band 3 migrates as a diffuse band on SDS gels due to heterogeneous glycosylation (see Fig. 15–4). In addition to its critical role as the conduit for chloride-bicarbonate exchange,[207, 210–213] there is some evidence that band 3 may be a flippase[214, 215] and considerable evidence that it influences red cell deformability, intermediary metabolism, senescence, and possibly even shape.[216, 217] Band 3 is also a major binding site for a variety of enzymes and cytoplasmic membrane components. Two of these functions, transport and binding, are relegated to structurally separate protein domains.[207, 218–220]

Structure and Functions of Band 3.

The NH₂-Terminal Domain (Cytoplasmic Domain) of Band 3. The NH₂-terminal domain of band 3, consisting of the first 403 amino acids, binds glycolytic enzymes, hemoglobin, and skeletal proteins. The majority of this domain can be released from the membrane by treatment with chymotrypsin or trypsin as a 43-kD fragment. Crystallographic studies demonstrate that the band 3 dimer is stabilized by interlocking dimerization arms contributed by both monomers.[221] Each subunit also includes a large, peripheral protein binding domain with a β-fold. The binding sites of several peripheral proteins are in the structure.[221] These include sites for the glycolytic enzymes glyceraldehyde-3-phosphate dehydrogenase (G3PD),[222, 223] phosphoglycerate kinase (PGK),[224] and aldolase.[225, 226] About 65 percent of G3PD, 50 percent of PGK, and 40 percent of aldolase are bound in the intact red cell.[222, 225] Membrane attachment inhibits enzyme

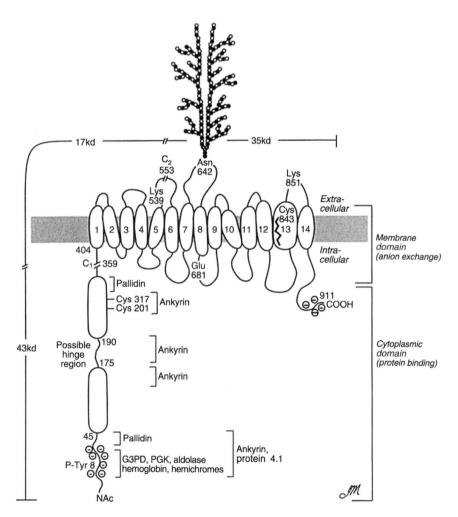

FIGURE 15–7. Organizational model of the human erythrocyte anion-exchange protein, band 3. The protein is divided into two structurally and functionally distinct domains: an approximately 43-kD cytoplasmic domain (amino acids 1 to 359), which contains binding sites for several cellular proteins, and an approximately 52-kD (17 kD + 35 kD) transmembrane domain (amino acids 360 to 911), which forms the anion-exchange channel. The two regions can be separated by chymotrypsin cleavage at the inner membrane (C1). A second chymotryptic site (C2) is accessible at the external surface. *Cytoplasmic Domain.* The highly acidic NH₂-terminal region (amino acids 1 to 45) binds hemoglobin, hemichromes, protein 4.1, and the glycolytic enzymes phosphoglycerate kinase (PGK), aldolase, and glyceraldehyde-3-phosphate dehydrogenase (G3PD). Enzyme attachment is blocked by phosphorylation of tyrosine 8. Ankyrin and probably protein 4.2 binding involves several noncontiguous regions scattered throughout the cytoplasmic domain, which suggests that these binding sites are formed by protein folding. A functional hinge exists in the middle of the domain. *Transmembrane Domain.* Band 3 may contain as many as 14 transmembrane segments. Their orientation with respect to the inside and outside of the membrane has been extensively studied; almost nothing is known about how they are positioned, relative to each other, to form the anion channel. Lys^{539} and Lys^{851} are probably the sites where H₂-4,4'-diisothiocyanostilbene-2,2'-disulfonate, a covalent inhibitor of anion transport, attaches to band 3. Lys^{851} and Glu^{681} (in its protonated form) are candidates for the specific sites involved in monovalent and divalent anion transport, respectively. A fatty acid, indicated by the *zig-zag* symbol, is esterified to Cys^{843}, and a complex carbohydrate structure is attached to Asn^{642}. Solid circles, *N*-acetylglucosamine; hatched circles, mannose; open circles, galactose. (From Lux SE, Palek J: Disorders of the red cell membrane. In Handin RJ, Lux SE, Stossel, TP (eds.): Blood: Principles and Practice of Hematology. Philadelphia, Lippincott-Raven, 1995, pp 1701–1818.)

activity[223, 226] and is regulated by substrates, cofactors, and inhibitors of the three enzymes and by phosphorylation of tyrosine 8 and tyrosine21.[227–229] The phosphorus is added by the kinase p72syk and SHP-2 tyrosine phosphatase[228, 228a] and is removed by a phosphotyrosine phosphatase that is bound to band 3.[229, 229a] These observations suggest that band 3 may be an important regulator of red cell glycolysis. In fact, mild oxidants, which stimulate tyrosine phosphorylation in intact red cells, elevate glycolytic rates.[230] A casein kinase I phosphorylation site has been identified as threonine 42.[231] This site may influence band 3–protein interactions.

The NH_2 terminus also weakly ($K_d = 10^{-4}$ mol/L) binds hemoglobin,[232, 233] deoxyhemoglobin binds better than the oxyhemoglobin, but 2,3-diphosphoglycerate (2,3-DPG) inhibits deoxyhemoglobin binding.[232] This is understandable from x-ray diffraction studies, which show that the first five to seven amino acids of band 3 insert deeply into the 2,3-DPG–binding cleft of hemoglobin.[233] However, owing to high hemoglobin concentrations, approximately one half of the band 3 molecules have hemoglobin attached under physiologic conditions. Hemichromes, a partially denatured form of hemoglobin, bind much better and copolymerize with band 3, forming an aggregate.[234–236] These aggregates play a role in red cell senescence.

Band 3 Cytoplasmic Domain–Peripheral Membrane Protein Interactions. Three peripheral membrane proteins—ankyrin,[220, 237–240] protein 4.1,[241, 242] and protein 4.2[243, 244]—also bind to the cytoplasmic domain of band 3. The ankyrin-binding site has been partially characterized and includes sequences from the proximal, middle, and distal portions of the cytoplasmic domain.[238, 239, 245] This and other evidence suggest that the cytoplasmic domain has a complex folded structure and that this conformation is reversible.[246] Ankyrin binds to the flexed conformations of band 3, preferably to band 3 tetramers.[240, 247] Proteins 4.1 and 4.2 may also have more than one site of attachment. Protein 4.1 binds to the tetrameric form of band 3.[248] Protein 4.1 competes with antibodies specific for the NH_2 terminus, protects NH_2-terminal sites from proteolysis, and inhibits ankyrin binding, which occurs partly at the NH_2 terminus.[242] However, it also binds to peptides containing clustered basic residues (LRRRY and IRRRY) that are located at the COOH-terminal end of the domain.[249] Protein 4.2 binding to band 3 has been localized to the NH_2 terminus in a region containing amino acids 187 to 211.[250]

The COOH-Terminal Domain of Band 3. The 52-kD COOH-terminal domain of band 3 (amino acids 404 to 911) contains the anion-exchange channel. The 1.2 million channels in each red cell can exchange 10^{10} to 10^{11} bicarbonate and chloride anions per second. This allows most of the bicarbonate produced in red cells by carbonic anhydrase to be carried in the plasma and increases carbon dioxide transport from the tissues to the lungs by about 60 percent.[251] The hydrogen (H^+) byproduct of the carbonic anhydrase reaction binds to hemoglobin and facilitates oxygen (O_2) release to the tissues (Bohr effect). All of these reactions are reversed in the lungs.

The relationship of band 3 structure and the ion transport mechanism is under investigation.[252–254] The COOH-terminal membrane domain is composed of 12 or 14 transmembrane helices connected by hydrophilic segments.[207–209] The location and orientation of these structures (i.e., which are cytoplasmic and which are extracellular) has been studied in great detail.[207, 255–257] The helices form the transport channel, but how they do so is unknown. Low-resolution structure image analysis of negatively stained two-dimensional crystals of the membrane domain revealed that two different conformations exist, represented by two crystal structures.[258] Perhaps these are the inward- and outward-facing transporters. The basic structural unit in both is an oblong band 3 dimer (~40 × 11 Å). At the center of the dimer, the two monomers abut and appear to form a channel, presumably the transport channel.[258] There is also a flexible subdomain on the far side of each monomer, which might be formed by one or more of the large cytoplasmic loops between the transmembrane helices.[256] Nuclear magnetic resonance (NMR) solution studies of a cytoplasmic surface loop predicted that the related transmembrane helices are in close proximity.[259] The cytoplasmic loop exhibited local order but was mobile with respect to the rest of the peptide.

It is unknown whether the apparent morphologic channel is actually one or two functional channels. A variety of studies suggest that each monomer contains a functional anion channel.[260, 261] If two channels exist, their location at the interface of band 3 monomers raises the possibility that two anions may be translocated simultaneously in opposite directions or that allosteric interactions between the subunits may regulate transport.[262, 263]

Anion exchange probably occurs by a ping-pong mechanism in which an intracellular anion enters the transport channel and is translocated outward and released, with the channel remaining in the outward conformation until an extracellular anion enters and triggers the reverse cycle.[264, 265] Whatever the mechanism, it probably involves a fairly large conformational change, because anion transport has a high energy and volume of activation.[266, 267] The specific residues involved in transport have not been identified, although there is evidence that a glutamic acid, four histidines, and one or more arginines are involved.[268–270] Anion exchange is extremely rapid (half-life is 50 msec) for chloride and bicarbonate, the physiologic anions. The specificity of the channel is quite broad, and larger anions such as sulfate, phosphate, pyruvate, and superoxide are also transported, although at much slower rates.

A large number of potent and useful anion transport inhibitors are known, especially various stilbene disulfonates such as 4,4′-diisothiocyanostilbene-2,2′-disulfonate. These bind to two lysine residues, probably Lys^{539} and Lys^{851}, on externally exposed portions of the protein in or near the entrance of the channel.[211, 271, 272] These inhibitors have been of great benefit in the study of normal and mutant band 3 states.

Band 3-Related Antigens and Polymorphisms. Four to 20 percent of individuals are heterozygous for a polymorphic, but functionally normal, band 3 called band 3 Memphis (Lys^{56} to Glu).[273, 274] Band 3 also carries the Diego (Dia) blood group (Pro^{854} to Leu plus Lys^{56} to Glu)[273] and several low-incidence blood group antigens, as well as the Wright a (Wr^a)/Wright b (Wr^b) blood groups (Lys^{658}/Glu^{658}, respectively).[161, 275, 276]

Self-Association of Band 3. Band 3 is extracted from the membrane by the nonionic detergent octaethylene glycol *n*-dodecyl monoether as stable dimers, tetramers, and higher-order oligomers. Quantitation of these species after separation on sizing columns shows that 70 percent of band 3 is in the dimer form and 30 percent is tetramers and oligomers. Almost all of the latter is associated with the membrane skeleton. This correlates with studies that show ankyrin binds preferentially to band 3 tetramers.[240, 247, 277] Isolated membrane domains only form dimers[278]; thus, tetramers are probably assembled by cross-linking of neighboring dimers through the cytoplasmic domain, either with ankyrin (the physiologic cross-linker) or by oxidation (disulfide cross-linking),[245] hemichromes,[234–236] or other means.

Association of Band 3 with Glycophorin A. As noted earlier, GpA and band 3 are associated in the membrane. GpA facilitates migration of band 3 from its site of synthesis in the endoplasmic reticulum to the plasma membrane under experimental conditions[166, 279] but probably is not critical *in vivo* because M^{k}M^k red cells, which lack GpA and GpB, contain normal amounts of band 3.[280] Band 3, on the other hand, does seem to be critical for GpA synthesis or stability because red cells that lack band 3 (described later in the section on band 3 defects in hereditary spherocytosis) also lack GpA.

Intramembranous Particles. Freeze-cleave electron microscopy of erythrocyte membranes reveals randomly distributed intramembranous particles (IMPs) of 80 to 100 Å on both the inner (P, protoplasmic) and outer (E, external) bilayer faces. Some studies suggest the more numerous IMP$_P$ are primarily band 3 dimers and tetramers and that IMP$_E$ are mostly glycophorins or the glucose transport protein.[281, 282]

Defects of Band 3 and Human Disease. Defects of band 3 have been identified in several disorders: (1) hereditary spherocytosis, owing to decreased synthesis, membrane insertion, or stability of band 3, or to mutations in the protein-binding sites; (2) Southeast Asian ovalocytosis, owing to deletion of amino acids 400 to 408; (3) rare forms of inherited acanthocytosis in which band 3 variants exhibit increased anion transport[283, 284]; (4) renal tubular acidosis; and (5) congenital dyserythropoietic anemias, in which the lactosaminoglycan side chain is improperly constructed, owing to a lack of the relevant glycosyl transferases.[285–287]

Anion Exchangers in Nonerythroid Tissues. Erythroid band 3 (AE1 or SLC4a1) is a member of the *SLC4* multigene family of bicarbonate transporters. Two other genes encoding band 3-related anion-exchange proteins have been identified: *AE2* and *AE3*.[288–294] AE2 is widely distributed and is probably the general tissue anion antiporter. AE3 expression is restricted to the heart and the brain. Both proteins are larger than AE1, owing to addition of about 300 amino acids at the NH$_2$ terminus. There is distinct homology between the three transporters, particularly in the membrane domain.[293–295] AE1 itself is expressed outside the red cell, in the acid-secreting, type A-intercalated cells in the collecting ducts of the kidney,[296, 297] and in cardiac myocytes.[298, 299] The kidney

transcript lacks the first 66 amino acids and is unable to bind glycolytic enzymes, protein 4.1, or ankyrin.[300, 301] In the heart, AE1 is expressed as a novel splice variant.[298]

Other Integral Membrane Proteins

The red cell membrane contains more than 100 other integral proteins. These include the Rh protein(s); the Kell antigen; the Duffy antigen; transporters for glucose, urea, and amino acids; ATPases including Na$^+$,K$^+$-ATPase, Ca^{2+}-ATPase, and Mg^{2+}-ATPase; various kinases and phosphatases; acetylcholinesterase; decay-accelerating factor; complement proteins (C3b and C4b); receptors for transferrin, insulin, insulin-like growth factors, thyroid hormone, parathyroid hormone, β-adrenergic agonists, cholinergic agents, diphtheria toxin, ceruloplasmin, and opiates; and many more.

PERIPHERAL MEMBRANE PROTEINS

The erythrocyte membrane skeleton (see Fig. 15–3) comprises 55 to 60 percent of the membrane protein mass and includes spectrin, actin, tropomyosin, tropomodulin, adducin, ankyrin, protein 4.1, dematin (protein 4.9), a portion of band 3, protein 4.2, and the proteins in the band 7 region of the SDS gel. Spectrin, actin, protein 4.1, and dematin (and perhaps tropomodulin and adducin) form the core of the structure because the skeleton retains its shape when other components are eluted with hypertonic KCl but disintegrates if spectrin or actin is removed. Operationally, the red cell membrane skeleton is the insoluble proteinaceous residue that remains after extraction of red cells[302] or their ghosts[303] with the nonionic detergent Triton X-100.

Spectrin

Structure and Function of Erythrocyte Spectrin. Spectrin is composed of two subunits, α and β, that, despite some similarities, are structurally distinct (Fig. 15–8) and are encoded by separate genes.[304, 305] On SDS polyacrylamide gels,[116] α-spectrin (~280 kD) and β-spectrin (~246 kD) (see Fig. 15–4) are the most abundant proteins of the red cell membrane skeleton, comprising 25 to 30 percent of total membrane protein and are present in approximately 200,000 copies per cell. The α- and β-spectrin chains intertwine in an antiparallel manner to form 100-nm long heterodimers, which in turn self-associate head to head to form tetramers and some larger oligomers.[306–309] Spectrin is highly flexible[308, 309] and is able to assume a variety of configurations, a property that may be critical for normal membrane function.[310]

Spectrin tetramers, which have a contour length of 200 nm,[308, 309] are tightly coiled *in vivo*, with an end-to-end distance of only about 76 nm.[311] Spectrin molecules condense by twisting their α and β subunits around a common axis and regulate the degree of condensation by varying the pitch and diameter of the twisted double strand.[312] The native molecule has about 10 turns with a pitch of 7 nm and a diameter of 5.9 nm. The coiled spectrin tetramers can extend reversibly when the membrane is stretched but cannot exceed their contour length without rupturing.

α-Spectrin migrates on SDS polyacrylamide gels as a 240-kD polypeptide. It begins with an isolated, unpaired

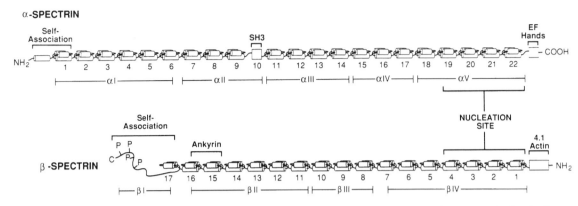

FIGURE 15–8. Spectrin structure. The α and β chains are aligned antiparallel with respect to their NH₂- and COOH-terminal ends. The approximately 106 amino acid "spectrin repeats" are numbered from the NH₂ terminus of each chain. In this model, each repeat is composed of three α helices (A, B, and C). The spectrin self-association site is formed by joining parts of a repeat that are left over at the "head" ends of the two chains. The α chain contributes helix C; the β chain contributes helices A and B. Some repeats are specialized, such as β15 and part of β16, which form the ankyrin-binding site, and the first four repeats at the "tail" of each chain, which nucleate interchain interactions. Rectangles denote peptide segments that differ from the repeats. They include the actin/protein 4.1 binding sites, a potential Ca²⁺ binding region (EF hands), and an SH3 domain. Each chain can be further divided into large structural domains by gentle proteolysis with trypsin. These domains are marked below each chain. In patients with hereditary elliptocytosis or pyropoikilocytosis due to defects in spectrin, the defects lie in the αI, αII, or βI domains. (From Lux SE, Palek J: Disorders of the red cell membrane. In Handin RJ, Lux SE, Stossel, TP (eds.): Blood: Principles and Practice of Hematology. Philadelphia, Lippincott-Raven, 1995, pp 1701–1818.)

helix (helix C) followed by nine typical 106-amino acid repeats (conformational segments 1 to 9), a short central segment that lacks homology to the repeats, but is related to SH3 domains (segment 10), followed by 12 more repeats (segments 11 to 22) and ends in a longer COOH-terminal segment that potentially encodes Ca²⁺-binding EF-hand structures.[304, 313] The function of the spectrin SH3 domain is unknown, but it appears to bind a member of the tyrosine kinase–binding family of proteins.[314] The COOH terminus of α-spectrin contains two EF hands, structures that participate in Ca²⁺ binding and regulate Ca²⁺ action in other proteins, including α-actinin[315, 316] and probably fodrin.[317, 318] Whereas one of the EF hands can bind Ca²⁺ at high concentrations (millimoles),[319–321] there is no evidence that spectrin binds Ca²⁺ *in vivo* or that its interactions with actin and protein 4.1 are regulated by Ca²⁺.

β-Spectrin migrates on SDS polyacrylamide gels as a 220-kD polypeptide. It consists of 17 homologous 106-amino acid repeat segments,[305, 322] a nonhomologous NH₂-terminal segment that contains an actin-binding domain,[323–326] the putative protein 4.1–binding site,[324, 327] and a short nonhomologous COOH-terminal segment that contains a consensus sequence for at least four casein kinase I phosphorylation sites.[328, 329] Evidence shows that membrane mechanical stability is sensitive to the state of phosphorylation.[330] Increased phosphorylation decreases and decreased phosphorylation increases membrane stability. Repeat 15 and part of repeat 16 are arranged in a β-sheet structure and form the binding site for ankyrin.[322]

Seminal studies using limited tryptic digestion of spectrin showed that the α- and β-spectrin chains are divided into five and four domains, respectively, designated α-I to α-V and β-I to β-IV (Fig. 15–9).[312, 331] This technique allowed the isolation and characterization of functional domains of normal spectrin and the identification of mutant spectrins from patients with hereditary elliptocytosis and pyropoikilocytosis (see later).

Spectrin Is Composed of Homologous Triple-Helical Repeats. The homologous 106-amino acid repeats in α- and β-spectrin fold into α-helical segments containing three antiparallel helices connected by short nonhelical segments (Fig. 15–10).[303, 304, 310, 313, 332–336] Each repeat forms a triple-helical structure that is about 5 nm long, is 2 nm wide, and is rotated 60° (right-handed) relative to the neighboring repeats.[313] Evidence for this model comes from circular dichroism measurements of spectrin length, biochemical analyses, comparison of spectrin flexibility in solution with other coiled-coil α-helical proteins, expression studies, and x-ray crystallography.

Each repeat begins with a straight, 28-amino acid α helix (helix A) (Fig. 15–10). The polypeptide chain then reverses itself and forms a second, 34-amino acid long α helix (helix B). This is followed by another reverse turn and the 31-amino acid C helix, which bends in the middle. The helices are in a triangular array and are held together by both hydrophobic and electrostatic interactions.[313] One face of each helix is lined with mostly hydrophobic amino acids. Because an α helix makes one turn every 3.6 residues, the hydrophobic amino acids are spaced every third or fourth residue, at the positions designated "a" and "d" in Figure 15–10. Additional salt bonds occur between the mostly polar amino acids at positions "e" and "g" of the helices, particularly between helices A and C and B and C.[313] The three helices are tilted away from each other by 10° to 20° so that the COOH-terminal end of each repeat is wider than the NH₂-terminal end. This allows for the attachment of the following repeat without any adjustment of the structure. The repeats connect to each other through the A and C helices, forming one long α helix. Because of the tight connection, the B helix of the proximal repeat overlaps the A helix of the distal repeat. Varying degrees of bending at the linker region were observed in chicken α-spectrin,[310]

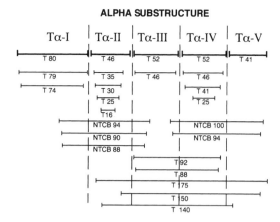

ALPHA SUBSTRUCTURE

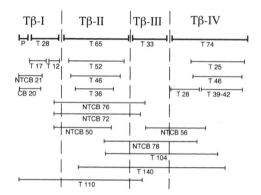

BETA SUBSTRUCTURE

A

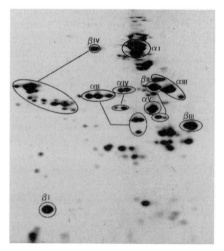

B

FIGURE 15–9. Domain maps of erythrocyte spectrin generated by limited tryptic digestion. Spectrin was subjected to mild tryptic digestion at 0°C, cleaving the protein into a reproducible number of well-characterized fragments. *A,* The alignment of the various tryptic fragments, as determined by high-resolution peptide mapping, is shown. Also shown is the alignment of some of the fragments generated by 2-nitroa-5-thiocyanobenzoic acid (NTCB) digestion of spectrin. *B,* The pattern after tryptic digestion. Peptide fragments are resolved by two-dimensional isoelectric focusing–SDS-PAGE analysis and visualized by Coomassie blue staining. The pattern that results is of limited complexity, facilitating the identification of the sites of functional domains, post-translational modifications, and inherited mutations in this very large protein. (From Morrow JS, Rimm DL, Kennedy SP, et al: In Hoffman J, Jamieson J (eds): Handbook of Physiology. London, Oxford University Press, 1997, pp 485–540.)

different from *Drosophila* tissue spectrin (also called fodrin), in which interactions between the two helices appeared to restrict the mobility of the repeats.

Speicher and Marchesi[333] note that several residues appeared to be highly conserved in the repeat segments, particularly at position 45, where there is an invariant tryptophan, and position 26, where there is almost always a leucine. Other conserved residues include positions 1, 12, 15, 26, 35, 46, 68 (hydrophobic amino acids), 22 (arginine), 38 (aspartate), 41 (aspartate or glutamate), 71 (lysine), 72, and 101 (histidine). Studies of spectrin mutations in hereditary elliptocytosis and pyropoikilocytosis highlight the importance of these conserved residues.

The presence of homologous 106-amino acid repeats suggests that spectrin evolved from duplication of a single ancestral minigene.[337–340] However, the genomic organization of both human α- and β-spectrin genes reveals that, with only a few exceptions, the size and position of exons do not correspond with the structural or conformational unit of spectrin repeats.[341, 342] This lack of correlation suggests that if an ancestral minigene did exist very early in evolution, the original distribution of introns within the minigene has been lost owing to the subsequent loss or acquisition of various introns.

Spectrin Functions. The functions of erythrocyte spectrin are to maintain cellular shape, regulate the lateral mobility of integral membrane proteins, and provide structural support for the lipid bilayer. In nonerythroid cells, spectrin has many roles which include establishing or maintaining local concentrations of proteins of the plasma membrane, participating in the early stages of cell junction formation, regulating access of secretory vesicles to the plasma membrane, serving as a membrane adaptor for cytoplasmic proteins, interacting with various ion channels, and participating in the secretory pathway.[343–345] Many of these important functions are mediated through the interactions of spectrin repeats and other proteins forming complex, multiproteins structures involved in cytoskeletal scaffolding function and signal transduction events.[346]

Spectrin Self-Association. Self-association of spectrin dimers into tetramers and higher-order oligomers is perhaps the best characterized interaction of the spectrin proteins, allowing the erythrocyte membrane to acquire its mechanical properties. Disruption of spectrin self-association has been shown to lead to abnormally shaped erythrocytes and, in a number of cases, hemolytic anemia. The study of spectrin mutants reveals that defects of either the NH_2-terminal end of the α chain or the COOH-terminal end of the β chain (the "head" end of the molecule) may lead to impaired spectrin self-association.

Spectrin heterodimers ($\alpha\beta$) associate at the head end to form heterotetramers ($\alpha_2\beta_2$) and higher oligomers.[308, 309, 347–352] Both tetramers and oligomers exist on the membrane, but tetramers predominate, probably because the association constant for formation of tetramers is substantially higher than that for the larger species. At low ionic strength and physiologic temperature (37°C), spectrin dissociates into dimers, whereas physiologic ionic

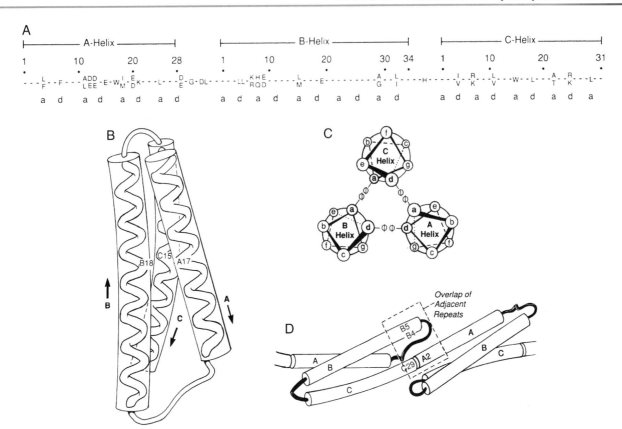

FIGURE 15–10. Structure of spectrin repeats. *A,* Consensus sequence of human erythrocyte spectrin phased according to crystallographic data, which defines three α helices that encompass the amino acids shown. Less conserved residues are marked with a dash. Residues a and d are the major contact points between helices. They tend to be hydrophobic and are conserved in most spectrins. *B,* Model of a single repeat based on the crystal structure of *Drosophila* α-fodrin. The positions of the nearly invariant tryptophans at A17 and C15 are shown. They interact with surrounding residues, including B18, at the central junction where the A helix crosses over from B to C. *C,* Cross-section of a typical repeat. The A, B, and C helices are in a triangular array, and the a and d residues lie on one face of each helix. The side chains of these amino acids are usually hydrophobic (Φ) and interact with each other to stabilize the triple-helical configuration. Salt bonds between the typically polar amino acids at positions e and g also help attach the B-C and A-C helices to each other. *D,* Interconnection of two adjacent repeats. The A and C helices are directly connected, forming one long helix. The distal repeat of each pair is rotated 60° (right-handed). The B helix of the proximal repeat *(black and white)* overlaps the A helix of the following repeat *(dashed box).* Interactions in the overlap region among conserved hydrophobic residues such as C29, B4, and B5 and the mostly hydrophobic residues at A2 probably stabilize the connection and limit mobility at the repeat junction. (From Lux SE, Palek J: Disorders of the red cell membrane. In Handin RJ, Lux SE, Stossel, TP (eds.): Blood: Principles and Practice of Hematology. Philadelphia, Lippincott-Raven, 1995, pp 1701–1818.)

strength and lower temperatures (25°C) favor the tetramer and oligomer species.[347, 348, 353, 354] At 0°C the equilibrium is kinetically frozen.[348] It is possible to extract spectrin from the membrane at such temperatures and examine its association state directly or manipulate it, *in vitro* or on the membrane, to produce any desired oligomeric species.[309, 348, 353, 355] Measurements of spectrin eluted from normal ghosts indicate that about 5 percent of the spectrin is in the dimer form and about 50 percent is tetramers. The remainder is divided between higher-order spectrin oligomers and very high-molecular-weight complexes of spectrin, actin, protein 4.1, and dematin.[309, 356] Studies of this type have contributed to our fundamental understanding of abnormalities in many patients with of hereditary elliptocytosis and pyropoikilocytosis.

The interconversion of spectrin dimers to tetramers involves a reversible opening of the dimer bond and formation of two new αβ attachments. The αβ contact closely resembles the triple-helical structure of native spectrin repeats except that in the contact site two of the helices are contributed by the COOH terminus of the β chain (helices A and B) and one (helix C) comes from the NH₂ terminus of the α chain.[307, 349, 350] Spectrin dimers exist in "open" and "closed" forms, depending on whether the ends of the α and β chains are free (open) or bound to each other (closed). The open and closed states are distinguished by their reactivity and susceptibility to proteases.[307, 357, 358] Newly assembled spectrin heterodimers open and close by interaction with each other, forming heterotetramers, or by forming an internal αβ bond. In the latter case, the longer α chain probably folds back in a hairpin structure to engage the β subunit. Opening the αβ contact (either the internal bond in closed dimers or the first αβ bond in tetramers) is the rate-limiting step in dimer-tetramer interconversion.[358] The local dissociation of spectrin tetramers into dimers appears to be an important physiologic effect that allows for accommodation of membrane distortion imposed during travel through the microvasculature.[358a]

The Nucleation Site of Spectrin. The side-to-side assembly of the α- and β-spectrin chains occurs in a zipper-like fashion, beginning with a defined nucleation site composed of four repeats from each chain, α19 to α22 and β1 to β4, respectively (see Fig. 15–5).[359–361] These are located at the tail end of the molecule, where actin binds. Two of the α repeats and one of the β repeats have eight-residue insertions that participate in the interchain interaction.[360, 362, 363] These are located between conformational segments α20/α21 and β2/β3. The model suggests that after the initial tight association of the complementary nucleation sites, a conformational change is initiated that promotes the pairing of the remaining length of the two chains.[359] Interestingly, a common polymorphism, a low expression allele called α^{LELY} or α$^{V/41}$, interferes with nucleation and effectively decreases synthesis of functionally competent α-spectrin (see later).

Ankyrin-Dependent and Ankyrin-Independent Binding of Spectrin to Membranes. The primary linkage of spectrin to the erythrocyte membrane is mediated by the binding of β-spectrin to ankyrin, which in turn binds to band 3. By functional analyses of truncated recombinant β-spectrin peptides, Kennedy and colleagues[322] showed that ankyrin binding requires almost the entire 15th repeat segment of β-spectrin and a small portion of the 16th. A similar ankyrin-binding site exists in nonerythroid β-spectrin (β-fodrin). As expected, abnormalities of the spectrin/ankyrin-binding site lead to abnormally shaped erythrocytes with unstable membranes (see later).

β-Spectrin and β-fodrin also contain an ankyrin-*independent* site in the NH$_2$-terminal half (tail half) of each molecule, which binds to brain membranes that have been stripped of peripheral membrane proteins[364, 365] and possibly to stripped erythrocyte membranes. Binding is inhibited by Ca^{2+}/calmodulin.[364] This site is called membrane association domain 1 (MAD1). β-Fodrin and the muscle/brain isoform of erythrocyte β-spectrin (see later) have a second, Ca^{2+}/calmodulin-independent site (MAD2), near the COOH terminus.[364, 365] MAD2 contains a sequence motif called the pleckstrin homology domain,[366, 367] that binds to the phospholipid PI-4,5-bisphosphate, and to the intracellular messenger IP$_3$.[366–368]

Cooperativity appears to exist between spectrin self-association and spectrin-ankyrin binding.[369] Three types of mutations disrupt the cooperative coupling of self-association and ankyrin binding: mutations of linker sequences that join helices C and A in repeat units between the two functional sites, mutations in α-spectrin repeats 4 to 6 that disrupt the ability to *trans*-regulate ankyrin binding by the adjacent β-spectrin repeats 14 and 15, and deletional mutants that force repeats 4 to 6 to fall out of register with the ankyrin-binding domain of β spectrin.

The Junctional Complex of the Erythrocyte Membrane Skeleton. A second linkage of spectrin to the plasma membrane is mediated by its association with the junctional complex that includes spectrin, actin, and protein 4.1.[343, 370] Spectrin, protein 4.1, and actin form a ternary or higher-order complex that links spectrin tetramers to one another in a tail-to-tail fashion. The spectrin/actin-binding site has been mapped to a region near the NH$_2$ terminus of β-spectrin[325] that contains a 27-amino acid sequence that is highly conserved between a number of actin-binding proteins, including α actinin, dystrophin, filamin, fimbrin, and ABP-120.[326] This site

was identified as the actin-binding site in ABP-120 and is presumed to be the actin-binding site of these proteins, including β-spectrin. Protein 4.1 is also thought to bind β-spectrin near its NH$_2$ terminus, as demonstrated by electron microscopy; however, the precise site of this interaction is unknown. A mutation in this region of β-spectrin has been described in a spherocytosis kindred whose erythrocyte membranes demonstrated impaired spectrin/protein 4.1 binding (see later). Intact spectrin dimers appear to be required for formation of the spectrin-protein 4.1 complex.

Nonerythroid Spectrins (Fodrins). Spectrin-related proteins exist in a wide variety of tissues and species.[343, 345] Two closely related, yet distinct mammalian α-spectrin subunits have been identified to date. One, α-spectrin, is expressed in mature erythroid cells; the other, α-fodrin, is expressed in all other tissues.[371, 372] Birds have a single α-spectrin subunit that is expressed in all tissues, including erythrocytes. There are a number of β subunits in mammals.[372–380] With a few exceptions, nonerythroid spectrins are composed of two nonidentical, high-molecular-weight subunits, α and β, which, like spectrin, are composed primarily of homologous repeat units of 106 amino acids. The β subunits also contain an NH$_2$-terminal actin-binding domain and a COOH-terminal pleckstrin homology domain.

Fodrin (also called tissue spectrin, brain spectrin, β-spectrin II, or spectrin G) is a heterodimer of α- and β-fodrin chains.[373, 374] It shares a number of common biologic functions with erythrocyte spectrin (spectrin I or spectrin R), including binding to actin, ankyrin, and adducin.[345, 372] Other features differ. For example, the α-fodrin contains a calmodulin-binding site that is lacking in α-spectrin, and β-fodrin contains a pleckstrin homology domain (see earlier) that is not present in erythrocyte spectrin. Other spectrins participate in skeletal networks in intracellular organelles such as lysosomes, the Golgi apparatus, or the nucleus.[343, 344, 381]

There is great variability in subcellular localization or subunit composition of erythroid and nonerythroid spectrins. Although typically thought to be localized in the membrane skeleton of the mammalian erythrocyte, spectrin exhibits developmentally regulated patterns of expression and differences in cellular distribution between various tissues.[345, 372, 382, 383] This is observed in diverse processes, such as neural development, *Drosophila* oogenesis, epithelial cell polarity, and sea urchin embryogenesis. Nonerythroid spectrins have been shown to redistribute with some types of cellular activation such as the binding of ligands or IgG to cell surface receptors, dimethyl sulfoxide–induced differentiation, cell polarization, and viral transformation. Proteolysis of fodrin is an early event in apoptosis and may contribute to the membrane blebbing in apoptotic cells. A β-fodrin homologue has even been identified in tomatoes.

Winkelmann and co-workers[384] showed that tissue-specific differential processing of the 3′ end of β-spectrin pre-mRNA generates a β-spectrin cDNA isoform in human skeletal muscle and brain encoding a COOH terminus different from that present in erythrocyte β-spectrin.[384] The encoded isoform replaces the last 22 amino acids of erythrocyte β-spectrin, a region that contains a casein kinase I consensus sequence, with a new sequence of 213 amino acids that includes the pleckstrin homology domain. The identification of frameshift mutations in the region of the β-spectrin gene 5′ to this tissue-specific splice site in the DNA of patients with membrane-related hemolytic anemias raises interesting questions regarding the expression and function of this β-spectrin isoform in muscle and brain. This pattern of splicing at the 3′ end of the β spectrin cDNA is also found in mouse. However, in *Danio rerio*, the zebrafish, the short isoform is not found.[385] In zebrafish, only the pleckstrin-homology domain–containing β-spectrin isoform is found, present in both erythroid and nonerythroid tissues. This observation suggests that distinct mammalian isoforms have evolved from modifications of β-spectrin structure and function.[385]

The Spectrin Superfamily of Proteins. The spectrin superfamily of proteins includes the erythroid and nonerythroid spectrins, dystrophin and three homologs, utrophin, DRP2, dystobrevin, and the actinins. These proteins share a number of structural properties including flexible, rod-like shapes of side-to-side subunits arranged in an antiparallel manner. Members of the spectrin superfamily are composed of homologous amino acid repeats of 106, 109, and 120 residues for spectrin, dystrophin, and α-actinin, respectively.[337, 339, 340, 371, 372] Members of this family are actin-binding proteins. Sequence comparison reveals a number of similarities between members of the spectrin superfamily of proteins.[371] There is homology in the sequence of the triple-helical repeats of spectrin, dystrophin, and actinin across species, with conservation of the invariant tryptophan at position 45 or 46. The repeats of dystrophin and spectrin are most homologous, whereas the actinin repeat is more distantly related. The COOH-terminal regions of α-spectrin, α-actinin, and dystrophin are homologous, containing potential Ca^{2+}-binding, EF-hand structures. The NH_2 termini of β-spectrin, dystrophin, and α-actinin are also homologous, encoding a potential actin-binding site. The

similarities in both structure and function suggest a common ancestral origin for the genes of this group of proteins.

Ankyrin (Bands 2.1, 2.2, 2.3, and 2.6)

Ankyrin is a large, 206-kD, 8.3×10 nm protein (see Fig. 15–3)[386] that provides the primary linkage between the spectrin/actin-based erythrocyte membrane skeleton and the plasma membrane.[343, 344, 387–389] Ankyrin is composed of an NH_2-terminal 89-kD membrane (band 3)-binding domain, a 62-kD spectrin-binding domain, and a COOH-terminal 55-kD regulatory region (Fig. 15–11).[390–402] In the red cell, ankyrin makes up approximately 5 percent of total membrane protein.[343, 387] It provides the connection between spectrin and band 3 through a high-affinity linkage ($K_d = \approx 10^{-7}$ mol/L) with β spectrin[396] and a high-affinity linkage ($K_d = \approx 10^{-7}$ to 10^{-8} mol/L) with the cytoplasmic domain of band 3.[220, 237] Selective disruption of the ankyrin–band 3 interaction in *intact* red cells, at slightly alkaline pH,[397] markedly decreases membrane stability, emphasizing the importance of the interaction.

Ankyrin appears to be involved in the local segregation of integral membrane proteins within functional domains on the plasma membrane.[343, 345, 387] This important polarization of membrane proteins may be generated by the relative affinities of the different isoforms of ankyrins for target proteins. The composition and specialized functions of membrane skeletons differ in erythroid and nonerythroid cells. This specialization appears to have evolved through the tissue-specific, developmentally regulated expression of multiple protein isoforms, including ankyrin isoforms.

Ankyrin Structure and Functions.

The Membrane Domain (or Repeat Domain) of Ankyrin. The 89-kD NH_2-terminal domain is almost entirely composed of 24 consecutive 33-amino acid repeats called cdc10/ankyrin repeats or just ankyrin repeats.[388] Binding sites for band 3[390, 391] and at least six other families of integral membrane proteins are located

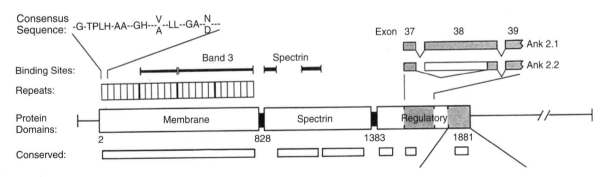

FIGURE 15–11. Structure of erythrocyte ankyrin, ANK1. The membrane domain (89 kD) contains 24 repeats (33 amino acids each), grouped in folding units of 6. Their consensus sequence is shown at the *top left* in single-letter amino acid code. *Dashes* indicate less conserved residues. The last 12 repeats form the band 3 binding site, especially repeats 22 and 23. The spectrin domain (62 kDa) contains the binding site or sites for spectrin. These two domains are the most conserved. The regulatory domain (55 kD) is thought to modulate the binding functions of the other two domains. In the middle of the domain, a highly acidic inhibitory region in exon 38 is spliced out of full-length ankyrin (ANK 2.1) to make ANK 2.2. At least eight isoforms of the last three exons exist. The last three isoforms contain a basic sequence (*open area*) that is common in brain ANK1 but rare in the red cell protein. In addition, isoforms lacking exons 38 and 39, 36 through 39, and 36 through 41 have been detected. The *asterisk* indicates the location of the translation terminator codon. (From Lux SE, Palek J.: Disorders of the red cell membrane. In Handin RJ, Lux SE, Stossel, TP (eds.): Blood: Principles and Practice of Hematology. Philadelphia, Lippincott-Raven, 1995, pp 1701–1818.)

in this domain. Repeats 7 through 12 (folding unit 2) and repeats 13 through 24 (folding units 3 and 4) form two distinct but cooperative binding sites for band 3.[398] In the red cell membrane, band 3 exists as a tetramer tightly associated with the actin-spectrin membrane skeleton via linkage with ankyrin or laterally mobile in the plane of the membrane. The presence of two binding sites potentially allows ankyrin to interact with four band 3 molecules simultaneously, which is the normal stoichiometry of ankyrin-band 3 complexes.[399, 400] Whether ankyrin actually binds to different band 3 molecules in the tetrameric complex is unknown. Red cell membranes from ankyrin-deficient *nb/nb* mice contain normal membrane skeletons but completely lack band 3 tetramers.[401] Alternatively, ankyrin may bind to two different sites on one band 3 molecule but prefer the conformation these sites assume in the band 3 tetramer. Selective disruption of the ankyrin–band 3 interaction, at slightly alkaline pH, markedly decreases membrane stability, emphasizing the importance of the interaction.[402]

Ankyrin repeats are some of the most common sequence motifs, found in more than 150 proteins with a diverse array of functions.[403] These include proteins involved in cytoskeleton organization, cell cycle control, signal transduction, toxins, and regulators of transcription and development. In most proteins, the repeats play an important role in protein-protein interactions and are usually found in multiples, from 2 in plutonium, a *Drosophila* protein involved in DNA replication early in development, to 24 in the erythrocyte membrane protein ankyrin 1. Determination of the three-dimensional structure of ankyrin repeats by x-ray crystallography and nuclear magnetic resonance studies[404–408] reveals that ankyrin repeats are L-shaped structures composed of a pair of α helices that form an antiparallel coiled-coil, followed by an extended loop perpendicular to the helices and a β hairpin. Interacting proteins may contact the β-hairpin loops, the α helices, or the outer helices of the repeat.[404, 409] The β-hairpin loops are the most common sites of repeat-protein interaction because the inner two residues of this highly exposed region are highly variable, providing the specificity required for different interacting proteins. In some interactions, the proteins contact only one of the β-hairpin loops; other proteins contact a series of the β-hairpin loops in a stack of ankyrin repeats. The other primary region of the ankyrin repeat that is not conserved and provides a site for repeat-protein interaction is along the exposed face of the α helices in the ankyrin groove. Many ankyrin repeats are capable of binding multiple protein partners. I-κB, the inhibitor of the transcription factor NF-κB, contains six ankyrin repeats, which can interact with NF-κB, p50, and two different domains of p65.[407]

The Spectrin-Binding Domain. The spectrin-binding site is located within a 62-kD globular, central domain of ankyrin (also called the 72-kD domain) and appears to involve regions in the NH_2 terminus and middle of the domain.[390, 393] The complementary binding site for ankyrin on spectrin is formed by spectrin repeats 15 and 16 near the end of the molecule involved in dimer-tetramer self-association.[322] Each spectrin tetramer apparently binds only one ankyrin molecule, even though two binding sites are available. This is probably because ankyrin binds about 10 times more avidly to spectrin tetramer than to spectrin dimer.[397]

The Regulatory Domain. The 55-kD, proteolytically sensitive, COOH-terminal domain contains regulatory sequences that enhance and diminish the binding of ankyrin to spectrin and the anion-exchange protein.[394, 410–413] Some of these are alternatively spliced, creating ankyrin isoforms of different sizes and functions. For example, ankyrin 2.2 (band 2.2) lacks an acidic 162-amino acid sequence from exon 38 that is found in full-sized ankyrin (band 2.1).[409, 411] The smaller isoform functions like an activated ankyrin, with enhanced binding to band 3 and spectrin and the ability to bind to new sites on some other plasma membranes. The 162-amino acid "repressor sequence," expressed as a separate protein, binds to ankyrin 2.2 and inhibits its interaction with band 3.[409] Over 20 alternatively spliced isoforms of the six COOH-terminal exons have been identified.[411] Some of these shortened RNAs probably form the smallest ankyrin isoforms (e.g., bands 2.3, 2.6, and 2.7). The COOH-terminal exons are highly conserved, unlike most of the 55-kD domain, which suggests that they also encode regulatory sequences. These may be activating sequences because proteolytic removal of the last 196 amino acids partially deactivates ankyrin, muting its affinity for band 3.[412]

A truncated, muscle-specific isoform of ankyrin 1 that lacks the membrane- and spectrin-binding domains, that is localized to the Z and M lines of internal myofibrils, and that is highly enriched in the sarcoplasmic reticulum has been identified.[414] This isoform, which has its own alternate promoter, consists of a highly hydrophobic 72-amino acid NH_2 terminus encoded by a muscle-specific exon that joins the COOH-terminal region of the regulatory domain.[414–416] The hydrophobic NH_2 terminus of this isoform could insert into the membrane of the sarcoplasmic reticulum, with the COOH terminus serving as a ligand for myoplasmic proteins. The specificity of the truncated ankyrin 1 for different protein ligands could be provided by the isoforms generated by alternative splicing. The sequence of the NH_2 terminus does not match that of any others in available databases, suggesting that this isoform may represent a novel class of proteins.

The regulatory domain also contains a "death domain" near its NH_2-terminal end.[417, 418] Other proteins that carry this lethal motif are part of a pathway or pathways that trigger apoptosis.[417–419] Examples include the tumor necrosis factor receptor and the proteins Fas/APO1, TRADD, RIP, FADD/MORT1, WSL-1, and *Drosophila* reaper. There is no evidence that ankyrin is involved in apoptosis, but this possibility should be investigated, especially because fodrin (tissue spectrin) is cleaved at a specific site in the α chain by a protease generated during apoptosis,[420, 421] a process that is thought to be related to the characteristic membrane blebbing observed in apoptotic cells.

The function of ankyrin is also regulated by phosphorylation.[410, 422, 423] *In vitro*, up to seven phosphates are added to ankyrin by the red cell membrane casein kinase I.[422] Unphosphorylated ankyrin binds preferentially to spectrin tetramers and oligomers rather than to spectrin dimers.[410, 422] This preference is abolished by phosphorylation, which also reduces the capacity of ankyrin to bind band 3.[423] Ankyrin is also phosphorylated by protein kinase A, but the functional effect of the modification has not been studied.

The Ankyrin Gene Family. Ankyrins, like spectrins, are members of a family of proteins.[343, 344, 387–389] Ankyrin-like molecules have a wide distribution, with immunoreactive forms found in almost all tissues. Nonerythroid ankyrins bind a variety of integral membrane proteins other than band 3, including Na^+,K^+-ATPase, the voltage-dependent axonal Na^+ channel, the amiloride-sensitive epithelial Na^+ channel, the cardiac Na^+/Ca^{2+} exchanger, H^+,K^+-ATPase, the IP_3 receptor, CD44, and a group of neurofascin-related brain adhesive proteins. The available data suggest that ankyrins localize these proteins to particular membrane domains, presumably by local interactions with cytoskeletal proteins. In addition to serving as plasma membrane linker/adaptor molecules, ankyrins have many other roles such as targeting a wide variety of proteins including ion channels and pumps and cell adhesion molecules to their proper location within the cell. Like spectrin, ankyrin appears to play a major role in the secretory pathway.

ANK1, erythrocyte ankyrin, is also found in myocytes[414–416, 424] and brain, particularly in the Purkinje cells of the cerebellum.[425, 426] ANK2, originally described as a neural form localized to neuronal cell bodies and dendrites, has been found in a variety of tissues including heart.[427–429] A mutation in ANK2 has been found to cause long QT syndrome in human.[430,★] ANK3 is the most widely distributed, particularly in epithelia and axons.[430–434] It is also expressed in megakaryocytes, macrophages, myocytes, melanocytes, hepatocytes, testicular Leydig cells, and the skin.[435]

Protein 4.1

Protein 4.1 is a member of the erythrocyte membrane skeleton that interacts with spectrin and actin, as well as proteins in the overlying lipid bilayer (see Fig. 15–3).[436, 437] The cloned protein is globular (5.7 nm diameter) and has a molecular weight of 66 kD but migrates as a 78- to 80-kD protein on SDS polyacrylamide gels. The reason for this difference is unknown. There are approximately 2×10^5 copies of protein 4.1 per cell. Chymotryptic digestion and limited sequencing have divided protein 4.1 into four domains (Fig. 15–12).[438] Beginning at the NH_2-terminal end they are a 30-kD domain (residues 1 to ≈300), a 16-kD domain (residues ≈300 to 404), a 10-kD domain (residues 405 to 471), and a 22- to 24-kD domain (residues 472 to 622). Two forms of the intact protein, designated 4.1a (80 kD) and 4.1b (78 kD), are separated on high-resolution SDS gels. Protein 4.1a is derived from protein 4.1b by gradual deamidation of Asn^{502} within the 22- to 24-kD domain,[439] leading to a predominance of protein 4.1a in older erythrocytes.[440]

Proteins That Interact with Protein 4.1. The 30-kD domain of protein 4.1 (also called the FERM domain) binds to band 3, glycophorin C, p55, calmodulin, importin-α, CD44, pIC1n, CASK, mature parasite-

infected antigen, and PS. The 10-kD domain binds spectrin, actin, importin-α, and U2AF. The COOH-terminal 22/24-kDa domain binds to the nuclear mitotic apparatus protein and FK-506 binding protein 13 and in nonerythroid cells to tight junction proteins occludin, ZO-1, and ZO-2 and eukaryotic translation initiation factor 3.[436]

Protein 4.1 binds to β-spectrin,[324, 327, 441] ($K_d = ≈10^{-7}$ mol/L) very near the actin-binding site,[323, 386] and greatly amplifies the otherwise weak spectrin-actin interaction.[442, 443] This activity can be traced to the 10-kD domain[444, 445] and, at least partly, to a 21-amino acid peptide within the domain.[446–449] Protein 4.1 also binds directly to F-actin ($K_d = ≈10^{-7}$ mol/L),[450] suggesting that it works by bridging spectrin and actin, although other mechanisms have not been excluded. The interaction of protein 4.1 with spectrin and actin is blocked by protein kinase A phosphorylation, which labels residues in the 16-kD (Ser^{331}) and 10-kD (Ser^{467}) domains,[451, 452] and by tyrosine kinase phosphorylation, which labels a site (Tyr^{418}) in the 10-kD domain.[453] The ternary complex also appears to be regulated by Ca^{2+} and calmodulin.[454–456] Calmodulin binds to protein 4.1 in a Ca^{2+}-independent manner ($K_d = ≈5 \times 10^{-7}$ mol/L) but, once bound, the calmodulin-protein 4.1 complex confers Ca^{2+} sensitivity on the viscosity increase produced by spectrin/actin/protein 4.1 binding.[456] The calmodulin-binding site is located within the 30-kD domain.[456]

Protein 4.1 also binds to the membrane and serves as a secondary attachment site for spectrin. The binding involves the 30-kD domain of protein 4.1[457, 458] and is blocked by Ca^{2+} and calmodulin[459] or by phosphorylation of protein 4.1 with protein kinase C (but not protein kinase A).[460] The identity of the membrane attachment site has been determined to be GpC,[461] but much remains to be learned about the specifics of this attachment site.[167, 462] Determination of the crystal structure demonstrates that the 30-kD domain of protein 4.1 is essentially a cloverleaf with separate binding sites for band 3, GpC, and p55.[463] Calcium-sensitive and -insensitive calmodulin-binding sites are located between the lobes.[463, 464] The interaction with band 3 has a high capacity but relatively low affinity.[241, 457] Dissociation of protein 4.1 from band 3 induces a marked decrease in membrane deformability and a marked increase in membrane mechanical stability due to increased band 3–ankyrin interactions.[465] Protein 4.1 binds directly to GpC and to p55.[457, 466] The affinity of p55 binding to GpC is increased by protein 4.1, and calmodulin binding to protein 4.1 decreases the affinity of 4.1 interactions with both GpC and p55 in a calcium-dependent manner.[466]

The major question is whether one or all of these protein-protein interactions occurs *in vivo*. Although there is evidence that all three *can* occur, the interaction with GpC is the only one that has been shown to have functional consequences in intact red cells[202]: (1) protein 4.1-deficient red cells are also deficient in GpC but not in GpA or band 3[467–469]; (2) the residual GpC is only loosely bound to the skeleton but becomes tightly bound if the deficient cells are reconstituted with protein 4.1[468]; and (3) GpC-deficient red cells are structurally unstable, whereas GpA-deficient cells are mechanically normal.[124, 202] In addition, both protein 4.1 and GpC bind p55, which may augment

---

★Bennett V: Personal communication. 2002

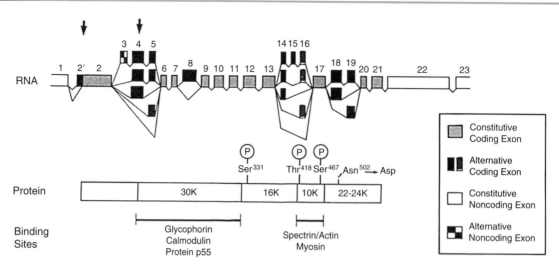

FIGURE 15–12. Protein 4.1. Top, Alternative splicing map of protein 4.1 mRNA. Reticulocyte 4.1 is translated from the downstream AUG (*arrow* over exon 4) and includes a 63-bp (21-amino acid) erythroid-specific sequence within exon 16 that is critical for spectrin-actin interactions. Many combinations of exons are expressed, although some are observed only in nonerythroid tissues. *Middle and Bottom,* Domain map of the 80-kD (erythroid) form of protein 4.1, indicating binding sites, phosphorylation sites, and the location of a COOH-terminal asparagine that is deamidated in aged red cells. (From Conboy JG: Structure, function, and molecular genetics of erythroid membrane skeletal protein 4.1 in normal and abnormal red blood cells. Semin Hematol 30:138, 1993.)

or regulate their interaction.[206, 466, 470–472] These effects are probably due to protein 4.1 deficiency rather than protein 4.1–GpC or protein 4.1–protein p55 interactions, because the mechanical weakness of GpC-deficient membranes is fully restored by reconstitution with protein 4.1 or its spectrin/actin-binding domain. In one study it was concluded that, *in vivo,* approximately 40 percent of protein 4.1 is bound directly to GpC, 40 percent is bound indirectly through protein p55, and 20 percent is bound to band 3.[457]

Protein 4.1 also interacts with PS,[473–475] CD44,[464] myosin,[476] and tubulin.[477] The protein 4.1-PS interaction may play an important role in the cellular sorting of 4.1,[475] whereas the interaction of protein 4.1 with CD44 may decrease the interaction between ankyrin and CD44.[464] The interaction with myosin ($K_d = 1.4 \times 10^{-7}$ mol/L) is interesting because the myosin-binding site lies within the 10-kD domain that regulates spectrin–actin–protein 4.1 complex formation and because protein 4.1 inhibits the actin-activated Mg^{2+}-ATPase activity of myosin.[476]

Mice with targeted deletion of protein 4.1R are viable and experience a moderate hemolytic anemia. Erythrocyte membranes from these mice have decreased amounts of spectrin and ankyrin and decreased membrane stability.[478] The mice also demonstrated defects in movement, balance, coordination, and learning.[479]

Alternatively Spliced Isoforms of Protein 4.1. Protein 4.1 is expressed as many alternatively spliced forms.[480, 481] The protein 4.1 gene is more than 90 kb in length and encodes at least 23 exons, including 10 alternatively spliced exons or "motifs" (Fig.15–12).[482] This leads to a remarkably diverse collection of protein 4.1 isoforms in both erythroid and nonerythroid cells.[482–487] Both tissue- and stage-specific isoforms have been observed. Protein 4.1 utilizes two different initiation codons, termed *upstream* and *downstream* initiation codons, which translate to isoforms of 135 and 80 kD,

respectively.[488] The 80-kD isoform, which encodes the mature erythroid isoform, is created by the splicing out of a 17-nucleotide motif that contains the upstream translation initiator. In most tissues this sequence is spliced in and a downstream 80-bp motif is spliced out. This gives rise to the elongated, 135-kD isoform that contains an additional 209 amino acids attached to the NH_2 terminus of erythroid protein 4.1. During erythropoiesis, this splicing is developmentally regulated.[488] Another important protein 4.1 isoform is created by the splicing in/out of a 63-bp motif within the 10-kD domain. This motif is expressed primarily in erythroid cells and muscle and contains the 21-amino acid spectrin/actin-binding site. Expression of this motif is linked to terminal erythroid differentiation,[486] and is regulated by the interaction of a conserved exonic splicing silencer element and hnRNP A/B proteins.[486a]

Protein 4.1 is expressed in most tissues. It appears as a variety of isoforms that are related to the 80- and 135-kD species. Protein 4.1 is not limited to the plasma membrane in nonerythroid cells but is also found in the nucleus and at cell-cell junctions.[489] At least four protein 4.1 homologs have been identified in mammalian cells.[489–494] Protein 4.1 and its homologs are members of a superfamily of proteins that includes talin, ezrin, moesin, radixin, merlin/schwannomin, and the human protein tyrosine phosphatases PTP-H1 and PTP-MEG. These proteins, which share homology to the NH_2-terminal (30 kD) domain of protein 4.1, appear to be involved in the linkage of cytoplasmic proteins to the plasma membrane.[495]

Protein 4.2

Protein 4.2 is a 78-kD peripheral membrane protein that helps link the skeleton to the lipid bilayer.[496, 497] It binds to band 3 (AE1)[498] and probably binds to ankyrin, possibly promoting their interaction,[499] and to spectrin.[499a] Protein 4.2 binds to ankyrin in solution,[244] but it has been difficult to prove that it binds ankyrin when ankyrin is attached to band 3. It is possible that protein 4.2 and ankyrin can only bind to different band 3 molecules. In *nb/nb* mice, which lack ankyrin, and in a child with hereditary spherocytosis and deletion of one ankyrin gene, a considerable reduction in protein 4.2 is observed in erythrocyte membranes.[500, 501] In addition, ankyrin elutes more easily from the red cell membranes of some humans with protein 4.2 deficiency.[502, 503] These observations strongly suggest that the two proteins sometimes interact *in vivo*. Protein 4.2 also participates in the attachment of the membrane skeleton to the Rh complex (see later in this chapter). Protein 4.2 is myristylated[504, 505] and palmitoylated.[506, 507] N-myristylation may play a role in targeting protein 4.2 to specific intracellular locations in nonerythroid cells.[505] Palmitoylation may serve as a positive modulator of band 3–protein 4.2 interaction.[507] Protein 4.2 also binds ATP,[508] conceivably supplying a membrane pool of ATP for transporters, kinases, flippases, and other local needs.

Protein 4.2 is homologous to transglutaminases,[509, 510] although it possesses no transglutaminase activity. A critical residue in the active site of transglutaminases is not conserved in protein 4.2. Perhaps some other common property, as yet unknown, of these proteins maintains their structural homology. The protein 4.2 gene resembles transglutaminases in its intron-exon organization.[511] Four isoforms exist owing to alternative splicing of 90-bp and 234-bp exons in the region corresponding to the NH_2-terminal end of the protein.[512] The respective proteins are 80 kD (both exons present), 78 kD (small exon absent), 71 kD (large exon absent), and 69 kD (both exons absent). The 78-kD protein is the predominant species (97 percent) in normal red cells[509]; isoforms lacking the 234-bp exon are rare. Protein 4.2 is expressed late in erythroid maturation after the cytoskeletal network has been assembled.[513]

Similar to patients with homozygous defects of protein 4.2, mice with targeted deletion of protein 4.2 demonstrate mild spherocytosis and alterations in red cell ion transport.[514]

Protein p55

Protein p55 is the human homologue of *dlg*, a *Drosophila* tumor suppressor gene.[515, 516] It contains three domains: an NH_2-terminal domain of unknown function that is also present in *dlg*, a central SH3 domain that may be a binding site for other proteins, and a COOH-terminal guanylate kinase domain.[472, 517] There are 80,000 copies of p55 per red cell, probably assembled into dimers. The protein is extensively palmitoylated[504] and is tightly bound to the membrane. The p55 gene is located on the long arm of the X chromosome, at Xq28, just beyond the factor VIII gene.[518] It is expressed throughout erythroid differentiation and is widely expressed in nonerythroid tissues. p55 interacts with protein 4.1 and GpC, linking them together in a ternary complex.[457, 458, 466, 470, 519] Patients who lack either protein 4.1 or GpC also lack p55,[471] and direct binding studies show that p55 binds to the 30-kD domain of protein 4.1 ($K_d = \approx 2 \times 10^{-9}$ mol/L) and to the cytoplasmic domain of GpC ($K_d = \approx 7 \times 10^{-9}$ mol/L).[457, 458, 471, 472] Considering the wide tissue distribution of all three proteins, it is likely that this interaction or interactions of p55

with other members of the protein 4.1 superfamily have a large variety of important cellular functions.

Truncation of the PDZ domain of p55 has been described in a patient with chronic myeloid leukemia in acute megakaryocytic blast crisis.[520] The biologic significance of this observation is unknown.

Actin

Red cell actin is structurally and functionally similar to other actins.[521–523] It is the β subtype, which is found in a variety of other nonmuscle cells.[523] However, unlike other nonmuscle actins, red cell actin is organized as short, double-helical F-actin "protofilaments" 12 to 13 monomers long.[524–526] These short filaments appear to be stabilized by their interactions with spectrin, adducin, protein 4.1, and tropomyosin and by capping of the slow growing or "pointed" end of the actin filament by tropomodulin[527] and the rapidly growing, "barbed" end by adducin (see later).

The state of actin polymerization appears to be functionally important to the red cell because compounds that inhibit actin polymerization increase membrane flexibility, whereas compounds that promote its polymerization make the membrane rigid.[528] Spectrin dimers bind to the side of actin filaments at a site near the tail end of the spectrin molecule.[323, 325, 524, 525] Spectrin tetramers are therefore bivalent and can cross-link actin filaments; however, binding is weak ($K_d = \approx 10^{-3}$ mol/L) and ineffectual in the absence of protein 4.1.[443, 529] Biophysical studies have demonstrated that actin protofilaments are essentially tangent to the membrane[529] and maintain this orientation during membrane skeleton deformation.[530]

Adducin

Adducin is a heteromer of structurally related proteins of ~80kD molecular mass,[531–533] α-adducin, β-adducin, or γ-adducin, encoded by separate genes.[534] The adducins are composed of three domains: an NH_2-terminal 39-kD, globular "head"; a 9-kD, connecting "neck"; and a 33-kD, protease-sensitive, extended, COOH-terminal "tail."[533] The last domain contains mostly hydrophilic residues and a highly conserved 22-amino acid *m*yristolated *a*lanine-*r*ich *C k*inase (MARCKS) domain with homology to the MARCKS protein. This domain is the site of calmodulin binding and phosphorylation by protein kinases A and C.[535] In solution, adducin is a mixture of heterodimers and heterotetramers.[536] Models suggest that the four head domains cluster in a globular core, whereas the tail domains extend to interact with spectrin and actin.[536] Alternatively, spliced isoforms of both adducin subunits have been described[537–539]; the function or functions of these isoforms are unknown. It has been estimated that there are approximately 30,000 copies of adducin per cell or one adducin per actin protofilament. Adducin is present at the erythroblast stage but is not incorporated into the red cell membrane until late in erythroid development.[540]

Adducin plays a role in the early assembly of the spectrin-actin complex by capping the ends of fast-growing actin filaments and by recruiting spectrin to the ends of actin filaments.[532, 541, 542] Phosphorylation inhibits actin capping and abolishes the recruitment of spectrin to actin filaments,[535, 543] as does calcium-calmodulin activity.[541]

Adducin is present in a number of nonerythroid cells and is concentrated at sites of cell-to-cell contact, particularly in epithelial tissues and at dendritic spines and growth cones of cultured neurons.[534, 544] The protein assembles at these sites in response to extra cellular Ca^{2+} and dissociates after treatment of the cells with phorbol esters, which stimulate phosphorylation of the protein by protein kinase C.[544, 545] Recent studies have suggested a role for adducin in cell motility and as a target for Rho-dependent, calcium-dependent, and Fyn-related pathways.[534, 546]

In humans, defects of adducin with a red cell phenotype have not been identified. Targeted disruption of the beta adducin gene in mice causes mild ellipto-spherocytosis with decreased levels of alpha adducin and increased amounts of γ-adducin in the red cell membrane.[547, 548] These mice also suffer from hypertension.[549] In certain populations, both α- and β-adducin have been implicated in the pathogenesis of essential hypertension and stroke.[550-554]

Dematin (Protein 4.9)

Human erythrocyte dematin consists of two chains of 48 and 52 kD, present in a ratio of 3:1 (48 kD:52 kD).[555-557] The native protein is a trimer. It binds to F-actin and bundles actin filaments into cables, probably in a ratio of one dematin trimer to one actin oligomer.[557, 558] This action is abolished by protein kinase A phosphorylation[555] but is not affected by protein kinase C. The COOH-terminal half of the 48-kD subunit is similar to villin,[559] an actin-binding protein that induces growth of microvilli and reorganizes actin filaments in brush borders. In contrast to villin, dematin is widely distributed, which raises the possibility that it may substitute for villin and regulate actin organization, under phosphorylation control, in tissues that lack villin. The 52-kD subunit differs from the 48-kD subunit by insertion of a 22-amino acid sequence in the COOH-terminal domain that resembles a sequence in protein 4.2[558] and contains an ATP-binding site.[560] The function of this site is unknown. Additional dematin isoforms created by alternative splicing have been identified in brain.[560] Dematin must also attach to a lipid or integral membrane protein, because it remains associated with the membrane when the other skeletal proteins are extracted; however, this site has not been identified.

Deletion of the headpiece domain of dematin by gene targeting in mice leads to a compensated spherocytic anemia.[561] Erythrocytes from these mice demonstrate decreased deformability and increased fragmentation. Loss of heterozygosity at the dematin locus, 8p21.1, has been demonstrated in prostate cancer, suggesting a role for dematin in the pathobiology of prostate tumorigenesis.[562]

Tropomyosin

Erythrocyte tropomyosin is a heterodimer of 27- and 29-kD subunits that runs on SDS gels in the region of band 7.[563] The red cell analog is similar to those of other nonmuscle tropomyosins by many criteria, except that it polymerizes poorly.[563, 564] This makes sense in the red cell where the double-helical actin filaments are short (two chains, each containing six to seven monomers). There is one copy of tropomyosin for each six to eight actin monomers, which is just enough to line both grooves of the actin protofilament. The binding of tropomyosin to actin is not affected by spectrin, but spectrin-actin interactions are inhibited by saturating concentrations of tropomyosin.[564] Possible functions of tropomyosin include stabilizing the short erythroid actin filaments and helping determine the sites of spectrin-actin interactions.

The primary tropomyosin isoforms expressed in erythrocytes are isoform 5 (hTM5), a product of the γ-tropomyosin gene,[565] and isoform 5b, a product of the α-tropomyosin gene.[566] Both isoforms have 248 residues, are approximately 33 to 35 nm long, and have high affinities toward F-actin and tropomodulin.

Tropomodulin

Tropomodulin is a 41-kD protein that binds to tropomyosin in a 2:1 molar ratio with a K_d of 5×10^{-7} mol/L.[567–569] Each protein binds to the NH_2-terminal region of the other.[565, 570–572] Tropomodulin also binds to actin.[573] It associates with the slowly growing, pointed end of actin filaments, after tropomyosin binds,[574] and blocks elongation and depolymerization of the actin filaments at the pointed end.[527, 575, 576] It does this by lowering the apparent affinity of pointed ends for actin monomers by conversion of pointed end adenosine diphosphate (ADP)• P_i-actin to ADP-actin at all pointed filament ends.[577] Capping is enhanced if the grooves of the actin filament are lined with tropomyosin.[578] Tropomodulin remains attached to the membrane when spectrin, actin, and tropomyosin are removed. Its binding site has not yet been identified.

Myosin

Red cells contain a nonmuscle myosin composed of two light chains of 19 and 25 kD associated with a 200-kD heavy chain.[579, 580] The protein forms bipolar filaments and has typical ATPase activities. Myosin bipolar minifilaments may play a role in local repair of the membrane skeleton after mechanical or chemical stress.[581] There are about 4300 copies of myosin in adult red cells and 2.5 times as many in neonatal erythrocytes[582] or about 1 myosin per 50 to 100 actin monomers, which may explain the greater motility of neonatal reticulocytes.

Membrane Physiology

Studies of the evolution of the red cell suggest that the sequestration of hemoglobin inside a cell membrane was necessary to protect it from oxidative threats and to permit its concentrations to rise to levels that would support mammalian metabolism. Metabolism, in turn, places certain constraints on the red cell membrane. In humans, the red cell must be flexible enough to negotiate splenic and capillary channels and still be durable enough to survive the turbulent journey through the circulatory system approximately half a million times during its 120-day life span. In addition, for blood to flow at reasonable rates, the red cell membrane must behave as a fluid in its interactions with other cells and plasma. In this section, some of the characteristics of the red cell membrane that allow the red cell to achieve these goals are described.

RED CELL DEFORMABILITY

The material properties of the membrane reflect the properties of both the lipid bilayer and the skeleton. During deformation of the red cell membrane, bending is restricted by the incompressibility of the lipid bilayer and is facilitated by rapid translocation of cholesterol from the inner to the outer one half of the bilayer.[16] The lipid bilayer cannot expand its surface area more than 3 to 4 percent. Consequently, when red cells are suspended in hypotonic solutions, such as during osmotic fragility testing, they swell to a spherical shape and then rupture, discharging their hemoglobin into the supernatant.[583]

The membrane skeleton determines both the solid and semisolid properties of the membrane.[584, 585] The solid properties are exemplified by the elastic extension of red cells, which completely restore their normal shape after the applied force has been removed.[585–587] An example is red cells that have been deformed when passing through fenestrations of the splenic sinus wall. This elastic recovery of the biconcave shape is facilitated by the unique molecular anatomy of the skeletal lattice. In normal red cells, individual spectrin molecules are arranged in a hexagonal array and are folded in a compact configuration. The junctional complexes are close to each other and are linked by shortened spectrin tetramers, thus allowing large unidirectional extensions without disruption of the lattice. The skeletal connections are unperturbed during such deformations. On the other hand, application of large or prolonged forces allows the skeletal elements to reorganize and make new connections.[588–591] This produces a permanent "plastic" deformation. When the force is excessive, membrane fragmentation or vesiculation ensues.[591] An example is the poikilocytosis produced in microangiopathic blood vessels where red cells may adhere to damaged endothelium and be stretched by the vascular torrent or may be clotheslined by fibrin strands.[592] After release, many of the cells are either permanently deformed or fragmented.

The need to undergo large deformations is best exemplified in the wall of the splenic sinus where red cells have to squeeze through narrow slits between the endothelial cells that line the splenic sinus wall. This "whole cell deformability" is determined by three factors: (1) cell geometry, that is, a large cell surface-to-volume ratio, which allows cells to undergo large deformations at a constant volume; (2) viscosity of the cell contents, which is principally determined by the properties and the concentration of hemoglobin in the cells; and (3) intrinsic viscoelastic properties of the red cell membrane.[584] Among these factors, the contribution of the surface-to-volume ratio and the viscosity of the cell contents are the most important, as exemplified by the cellular lesion of hereditary spherocytosis and other red cell disorders, discussed later in this chapter. On the other hand, the intrinsic deformability of the red cell membrane has a relatively small effect on red cell survival. This is best illustrated by the red cell membrane properties of Southeast Asian ovalocytes (SAO), which carry a mutant band 3 protein. Both the intact SAO red cells and their membranes are extremely rigid, yet the SAO red cells have a nearly normal survival *in vivo*.[584, 593]

STRUCTURAL INTEGRITY OF THE MEMBRANE

The skeleton is the principal determinant of membrane stability.[594, 595] As noted earlier, it is possible to manipulate the proportion of spectrin dimers and tetramers *in situ* by exposing ghosts to temperatures and salt concentrations that favor or discourage self-association. Ghosts enriched in spectrin dimers are strikingly fragile.[355] Similarly, hereditary elliptocytosis and pyropoikilocytosis are often due to α- or β-spectrin mutations that weaken spectrin self-association (see later). In such cells the hexagonal skeletal lattice is disrupted,[596] usually in association with red cell fragmentation and poikilocytosis.

The fluid lipid bilayer is stabilized both by the underlying membrane skeleton and the transmembrane proteins.[585] *In vitro*, the bilayer can be uncoupled from the skeleton at the tips of spiculated red cells by various treatments.[597] The lipids are released in the form of microvesicles, which contain integral proteins but lack skeletal components.[584] Such loss of membrane material may underlie the surface area deficiency of red cells subjected to prolonged storage[598,599] or of ATP-depleted red cells.[600] Aggregation of the band 3-containing intramembrane particles in the membrane also destabilizes the lipid bilayer.[601] In ghosts, such aggregation can be induced by treatment with Ca^{2+}, magnesium, polylysine, or basic proteins.[601] The particle-free regions bleb and release lipid microvesicles. As discussed later, all these pathways may contribute to the surface deficiency of hereditary spherocytes.

The role of the membrane skeleton in red cell shape is best illustrated by irreversibly sickled cells or hereditary elliptocytes, in which the abnormal shape is retained in the ghosts and membrane skeletons.[602, 603] This process is probably an example of "plastic deformation," the result of prolonged exposure of red cells to deforming forces, when the proteins of the deformed skeleton undergo active rearrangement that permanently stabilizes the cells in the deformed shape.[584, 588–590] Existing protein-protein contacts disconnect, and new associations form. In hereditary elliptocytosis, shape transformations may be facilitated by the weakened skeletal protein interactions.

In addition, both normal and abnormal red cell shapes can be stabilized by intermolecular cross-linking of membrane proteins, either due to formation of intermolecular disulfide bridges induced by oxidants or by transamidative protein cross-linking catalyzed by a Ca^{2+}-activated cytosolic transglutaminase.[604] These protein modifications are like endogenous fixatives and permanently stabilize cell shape *in vitro*.

THE RED CELL SURFACE

The red cell surface is rich in sialic acid residues, accounting for the negative surface charge. The majority of these residues reside on glycophorin A; the remainder are shared by other glycophorins, the anion-exchange protein, and glycolipids.[124, 125, 127] Alterations in surface charge distribution are deleterious. For example, surface charge clustering may contribute to the adhesion of sickle red cells to the surface of endothelial cells via complement-mediated mechanisms.[605, 606]

Several proteins are removed from the surface of reticulocytes that participate in cell-cell and cell-matrix interactions during erythroid differentiation.[607–610] Examples include $\alpha_4\beta_1$ integrin, which interacts with VCAM-1, an endothelial cell adhesion molecule and may contribute to attachment of sickle cells to the endothelium[608] (see Chapter 19), and Emp, a protein that has been postulated to mediate contact between erythroblasts and macrophages, promoting terminal differentiation by suppressing apoptosis.[611]

The structure and the genetic origins of red cell surface antigens, residing either on glycolipids, on externally exposed portions of transmembrane proteins or their carbohydrate side chains, or on the proteins linked by a glycosylphosphatidylinositol anchor, are discussed in Chapter 48. Furthermore, several surface receptors are involved in attachment of malarial parasites to the cells, including glycophorins, band 3 protein, and the Duffy blood group antigen.[612, 613]

Glycosylphosphatidylinositol-Anchored Membrane Proteins

A hydrophobic glycosylphosphatidylinositol (GPI) anchor is embedded in the outer leaflet of the bilayer to connect externally exposed hydrophilic proteins with the hydrophobic lipid bilayer. Among the large number of GPI-linked surface proteins, a group of complement-regulatory proteins are clinically the most important. Defective biosynthesis of the GPI anchor precludes attachment of these proteins to the membrane, causing increased susceptibility to hemolysis by complement, as clinically manifest by paroxysmal nocturnal hemoglobinuria (see Chapter 14).[614] Because this glycolipid anchor is embedded only in the outer leaflet of the bilayer, anchored surface proteins are not restricted by the membrane skeleton, in contrast to most transmembrane proteins, and are much more laterally mobile. This high mobility may be important in recruiting complement regulatory proteins to sites of complement activation. These regulatory proteins are preferentially enriched in the lipid vesicles that are released from abnormal red cells, such as vesicles derived from spicules of deoxygenated sickle cells. Consequently, GPI-linked proteins are diminished in the densest fraction of sickle cells, rendering them more susceptible to complement-mediated injury.[615]

GPI-linked proteins are found in detergent-resistant lipid rafts, which are composed of sphingolipids, cholesterol, and various proteins, including GPI-linked proteins. Lipid rafts appear to participate in signal transduction, sorting and trafficking through the secretory and endocytic pathways, and in hematopoietic cells, signaling through proteins anchored by GPI.[616] The integral membrane proteins stomatin, flotillin-1, and flotillin-2 are found in lipid rafts from mature erythrocytes.[617] Cholesterol and GPI-anchored proteins of lipid rafts may play a role in malaria infection.[618, 619]

Lateral Mobility of Transmembrane and Surface Proteins

The mobilities of membrane surface molecules influence the interaction of red cells with the outside environment. For example, cell agglutination requires rapid lateral movements of surface antigens. Their immobilization (e.g., by glutaraldehyde) inhibits agglutination.[620] The lateral mobility of proteins that are anchored exclusively in the outer leaflet of the bilayer (e.g., GPI-linked proteins) is very fast. Conversely, transmembrane proteins, such as band 3, are much less mobile. In the case of band 3, this occurs because of specific binding to ankyrin and the skeleton, steric hindrance by spectrin strands, which entangle the internal portions of band 3, self-association of band 3 into tetramers and higher oligomers, and interaction of band 3 with other transmembrane proteins, such as the glycophorins.[621–623]

ORGANIZATION OF THE MEMBRANE SKELETON

Nodes and individual filaments of the membrane skeleton are visible when stretched but not when collapsed. Stretched skeletons reveal complexes of F-actin (the nodes) cross-linked by molecular filaments of spectrin when viewed by high-resolution, negative-stain electron microscopy.[143, 524, 525, 624] Dematin, adducin, and protein 4.1 co-localize with these complexes on immunoelectron microscopy.[624] Most of the complexes are connected by spectrin tetramers (85 percent) and three-armed hexamers (10 percent).[525] Ankyrin– and band 3–containing globular complexes attach to spectrin near the site of self-association. The average thickness of the skeletal protein layer has been estimated to be 3 to 6 nm from x-ray diffraction data[625] and 7 to 10 nm from electron micrographs.[626] These dimensions suggest that the skeleton is only one or two molecules thick on average, which means it must cover 25 to 50 percent of the inner membrane surface area. This corresponds reasonably to micrographs of unspread skeletons, where the contracted, collapsed spectrin filaments appear to cover much but not all of the inner membrane surface.

A model of the membrane skeleton based on this is shown in Figure 15–3. Spectrin dimers are depicted as twisted, flexible polymers joined head to head to form tetramers and higher-order oligomers. Self-association occurs between the NH_2-terminal end of the spectrin α chain and the COOH-terminal end of the β chain, as described in detail in the earlier section on spectrin. Spectrin molecules are linked into a two-dimensional network by interactions with a complex of actin protofilaments, protein 4.1, dematin, adducin, and tropomyosin.[370] These associations occur at the tail ends of the bifunctional spectrin tetramer. The predicted complexes are morphologically similar to isolated spectrin–actin–protein 4.1 complexes and to structures observed *in situ* in normal ghosts. They serve as branch points in skeletal construction. On average, six spectrin molecules emanate from each complex, although there is some variation. This leads to a hexagonal arrangement of spectrin in spread skeletons. In unperturbed skeletons, most spectrin molecules probably fold up to about one third their length and do not extensively overlap or intertwine.[312]

Individual spectrin tetramers and oligomers are attached to the overlying lipid bilayer through high-affinity interactions with ankyrin and band 3, probably with the assistance of protein 4.2. Current evidence suggests that band 3 is a mixture of dimers and tetramers in the membrane[246, 278] and that the tetramer probably binds only one molecule of ankyrin.[240, 277] If so, about 40 percent of the band 3 molecules are involved in anchoring the membrane skeleton. Although the spectrin tetramer contains two ankyrin-binding sites, there is only enough ankyrin to fill one, and, on average, only one is filled *in situ*. Interactions between protein 4.1, protein p55, and GpC or between protein 4.1 and band 3 provide secondary sites of attachment.

Recent work has identified an additional site of membrane attachment between the Rh complex and the membrane skeleton mediated by CD47 and protein 4.2.[626a,626b,626c]

MODULATION OF MEMBRANE SKELETAL STRUCTURE

Red cell membrane proteins are subject to a large number of post-translational modifications or other regulatory effects, including phosphorylation, fatty acid acylation, methylation, glycosylation, deamidation, calpain cleavage, polyphosphoinositide and calmodulin regulation, oxidation, and modification by polyanions.[627]

Phosphorylation

Almost all of the membrane skeletal proteins are phosphorylated by one or more protein kinases. These include casein kinases (spectrin, ankyrin, band 3, protein 4.1, and dematin); protein kinase A (ankyrin, adducin, protein 4.1, and dematin); protein kinase C (adducin, protein 4.1, and dematin); and tyrosine kinases (band 3 and protein 4.1).[627] In all cases studied so far, phosphorylation inhibits membrane protein interactions. Ankyrin phosphorylation (casein kinase) abolishes the preference of ankyrin for spectrin tetramer[402, 421] and decreases binding to band 3.[422] Phosphorylation of protein 4.1 (several kinases) diminishes its binding to spectrin and its ability to promote spectrin/actin binding[452, 453, 628] and decreases its attachment to the membrane.[629] Phosphorylation by protein kinase C also inhibits binding of protein 4.1 to band 3.[460] Phosphorylation of protein 4.9 by protein kinase A prevents actin bundling.[555] Phosphorylation of Tyr[8] at the NH_2 terminus of band 3 blocks the binding of glycolytic enzymes[227] and presumably hemoglobin and results in increased glycolysis.[230, 630] Many studies have failed to identify a functional effect of spectrin phosphorylation; however, evidence shows that membrane mechanical stability is very sensitive to the state of phosphorylation.[330] Increased phosphorylation decreases and decreased phosphorylation increases membrane stability.

Polyanions

Physiologic concentrations of organic polyanions such as 2,3-DPG and ATP weaken and dissociate the membrane skeleton[573] and increase the lateral mobility of band 3 in ghosts.[631] *In vitro* these compounds dramatically inhibit spectrin-actin interactions, even in the presence of protein 4.1.[632] However, it is still not clear whether these or other polyanions (e.g., polyphosphorylated phosphoinositides) are "physiologic" mediators *in vivo*. Some studies suggest

that even supraphysiologic concentrations of 2,3-DPG have little or no effect on intact erythrocytes.[633, 634]

Calcium and Calmodulin

There is good evidence that calmodulin modifies the membrane properties of the red cell.[455] Physiologic concentrations of calmodulin, sealed in red cell ghosts, destabilize membranes in the presence of micromolar concentrations of Ca^{2+}. Studies suggest the effect may result from interactions of calmodulin with protein 4.1.[456] Submicromolar concentrations of calmodulin, even lower than those that exist in the red cell (approximately 3 to 6 µmol/L), block protein 4.1-induced gelation of actin in the presence of spectrin.[456] The effect is Ca^{2+} dependent. It begins at a Ca^{2+} concentration of 10^{-6} to 10^{-7} mmol/L, which is relatively low but still higher than the free Ca^{2+} concentration in the erythrocyte (20 to 40 nmol/L). Surprisingly, Ca^{2+}-calmodulin does not block spectrin–actin–protein 4.1 complex formation under these conditions,[456] only the extensive cross-linking needed to cause gelation. Calmodulin also binds to the spectrin β chain in a Ca^{2+}-dependent manner[454]; however, the affinity of spectrin for calmodulin is not great and it is unclear whether this effect occurs at the concentrations of calmodulin that exist in erythrocytes. β-Adducin also binds calmodulin ($K_d = 2.3 \times 10^{-7}$ mol/L).[635] Adducin that is bound to spectrin and actin fosters the attachment of a second, neighboring spectrin. This reaction is blocked by calmodulin in the presence of Ca^{2+} (>10^{-7} mol/L).[532, 636] The physiologic consequences of this effect are unclear.

Several other Ca^{2+}-dependent events do not require the presence of calmodulin. One of them is membrane protein cross-linking, catalyzed by Ca^{2+}-dependent transglutaminase.[637] This cross-linking acts as an endogenous fixative, stabilizing red cell shape.[636] However, the Ca^{2+} concentration required by this reaction is more than 100-fold greater than the normal red cell Ca^{2+} concentration, making it unlikely that transglutaminase permanently stabilizes red cell shape *in vivo*.[636] A second calmodulin-independent effect of Ca^{2+} is the so-called Gardos phenomenon, a unidirectional potassium (K^+) and water loss, producing cellular dehydration (see later). In contrast to transamidative cross-linking, the Ca^{2+} concentration required to trigger the Gardos channel is low (in the micromolar range) and thus physiologically significant. This pathway contributes to cellular dehydration of sickle red cells. A third calmodulin-independent Ca^{2+} effect involves calpain, one of a family of Ca^{2+}-stimulated neutral proteases, which are present in a variety of tissues, including red cells.[627] Susceptible membrane substrates include band 3, ankyrin, protein 4.1, and, to a lesser extent, spectrin. A fourth category of calcium effects is stimulation of phospholipases A and C and activation of various protein kinases and phosphates, controlled by a P/Q-type calcium channel.[637a] A fifth effect is calcium-dependent vesicle release.[637b] Finally, Ca^{2+} also induces phospholipid scrambling (see earlier).

Thus, increases in intracellular Ca^{2+} produce a wide range of deleterious effects. Although these phenomena are well studied *in vitro*, their role in erythrocyte pathologic changes, particularly in acquired disorders associated with abnormal red cell shape, is not well understood.

MEMBRANE PERMEABILITY

Normally the red cell membrane is nearly impermeable to monovalent and divalent cations, thereby maintaining a high K^+, low Na^+, and very low Ca^{2+} content. In contrast, the red cell is highly permeable to water and anions, which are readily exchanged by the water channel and the anion transport protein, respectively. Glucose is taken up by the glucose transporter,[637, 638] whereas larger charged molecules, such as ATP and related compounds, do not cross the normal red cell membrane.

The transport pathways for cations and anions in the human red cell membrane (Table 15–4) can be divided into five categories: (1) exchangers, such as the Na^+/H^+ exchanger and anion exchanger discussed earlier; (2) cotransporters, in which the transmembrane movements of more than one solute are coupled in the same direction (e.g., the K^+/Cl^- cotransporter and the $Na^+/K^+/Cl^-$ cotransporter); (3) the Ca^{2+}-activated K^+ channel (Gardos channel), discussed later; (4) the cation "leak" pathways, which allow Na^+ and K^+ to move in the direction of their concentration gradients; and (5) membrane pumps, such as the ouabain-inhibitable Na^+-K^+ pump and the Ca^{2+} pump, respectively. Detailed reviews of these pathways are available.[639, 640]

An important feature of the normal red cell is its ability to maintain a constant volume. One of the very intriguing, yet unanswered, questions is how cells "sense" changes in volume and activate appropriate volume regulatory pathways. One possibility is that they sense mechanical events, such as membrane stretching.[641] Such a mechanism is unlikely to operate in red cells that, by virtue of their large surface area, can undergo a substantial volume increase without stretching. Another possibility is that cell volume is controlled by the crowding of cytoplasmic macromolecules.[641] According to this theory, cell shrinkage stimulates and swelling inhibits a putative protein kinase, which, in turn, changes the activity of a volume regulatory cation transporter, such as the K^+/Cl^- cotransporter.

WATER PERMEABILITY

Water diffusion occurs through the lipid bilayer across transient defects in the lipid matrix and through specialized aqueous pores called aquaporins.[642] Aquaporins, which serve as selective pores through which water crosses the plasma membranes of many cell types, have been found in diverse species from bacteria to humans.

TABLE 15-4. Properties and Capacities of Major Cation Transporters Identified in the Normal Human Red Cell Membrane

System	Inhibitor	Capacity (mmol/ L cells per/hr)	Potential Maximum Capacity (mmol/L cells per/hr)	Activator*	Role
Na^+-K^+ pump	Oubain	1–2	No further activation possible		Long-term volume regulation, with passive leak
Passive leak	No specific	1–2	Unknown	Various	
Na^+-K^+ $2Cl^-$ cotransport	Loop diuretics Cl^- dependent[†‡]	0.1–1.2[†]	No further activation possible	Cyclic AMP, cell shrinkage in other cell types	Volume-regulatory increase in other cell types
K^+ Cl^- cotransport	DHIOA, others Cl^- dependent	0–0.2[†§]	0.5	Cell swelling N-Ethyl-malemide	Small role in short-term volume regulation
Na^+ Na^+ exchange		~0.5[†]	10		
			No further activation possible		
Ca^{2+}-activated K^+ channel	Charybdotoxin quinidine	0	50	Internal Ca^{2+}	Role in human RBC unknown; related to Ca^{2+}-activated channel in nerve
Band 3 (anion exchanger-1)	SITS, DIDS	Cations: zero, in HCO_3–free media Anions: > 1000	No further activation possible		Anion exchange services carbonic anhydrase
Na^+-linked amino acid transporters		Zero in the absence of amino acids	No further activation possible		Amino acid supply to (e.g., glutathione synthesis)

DHIOA = (dihydroinenyloxy) alkanoic acid; DIDS = 4,4′-diisothiocyanostilbene-2,2-disulfonic acid; SITS = 4-acetamido-4′-isothiocyanostilbene-2,2-′-disulfonic acid.

*Activator implies physical or pharmacologic maneuver aside from manipulation of substrate concentration.

†Shows major interindividual variation within normal population.

‡Cl⁻ dependent implies that the cation flux is inhibited by the replacement of Cl⁻ by an "inert" cation such as nitrate.

§Enhanced in capacity in reticulocytes.

From Stewart GW, Argent AC, Dash BCJ: Stomatin: A putative cation transport regulator in the red cell membrane. Biochim Biophys Acta 1993; 1225:15–25. Copyright 1993 with permission of Elsevier Science, NL, Amsterdam, The Netherlands.

Aquaporin-1, the founding member of this family of channel proteins,[643] is expressed in many tissues, including erythrocytes and may contribute to the ability of the red cell to adjust rapidly to changes in osmolality. Aquaporin 3 has been reported to be expressed in erythrocytes, with a role in water and glycerol transport.[644] This observation has been disputed, and studies using mice with targeted deletion of both aquaporin 1 and 3 suggest that this is not true.[645] Structural studies demonstrate that aquaporin 1 is composed of extracellular and cytoplasmic domains connected by a narrow pore, arranged as a homotetramer with four discrete water channels.[646–648] It has been suggested that aquaporins play a role in carbon dioxide and ion permeability.[649] If they do, the contribution by aquaporin to these functions appears small.[645, 650]

The epitope for the Colton blood group system is located in the extracellular region of aquaporin 1.[642, 651] Mutations in aquaporin 1 have been identified in patients with the rare Colton null phenotype, including one in the highly conserved NPA motif of aquaporin 1 essential for channel function.[652–655] Patients with the Colton null phenotype have no demonstrable clinical abnormalities, but mice with targeted inactivation of aquaporin 1 become hyperosmolar after fluid restriction.[656]

Transport Pathways

Two pathways exert a critical volume regulatory effect (Fig. 15–13). One is via the K^+/Cl^- cotransporter, a typical carrier-mediated cotransport pathway, which is particularly active in reticulocytes. It is activated by cell swelling, acidification, depletion of intracellular magnesium, thiol oxidation, and deoxygenation.[657, 658] The primary K^+/Cl^- cotransporter in the erythrocyte appears to be KCC1, which was the first member of a related family of K^+/Cl^- cotransporters to be cloned.[659–661] KCC3 is also present in erythrocytes.[662] The regulation of K^+/Cl^- cotransport is complex. The Src-family kinases Fgr and Hck are negative regulators of K^+/Cl^- cotransport[663] and the serine-threonine protein phosphatases PP1 and PP2A activate K^+/Cl^- cotransport.[664] Increased activity of the transporter in sickle cells and hemoglobin C erythrocytes accounts, in part, for cellular dehydration of these cells.[657, 658]

The second transporter is the Gardos channel, which causes selective loss of K^+ in response to an increase in intracellular ionized Ca^{2+}.[665–669] This channel is tightly linked at its COOH terminus to calmodulin, which opens the channel in the presence of intracellular calcium.[670, 671] Calmodulin also regulates channel assembly and trafficking.[672] The channel appears to be regulated by the cytoplasmic protein calpromotin, by cyclic adenosine monophosphate (AMP), and in sickle red cells by endothelins and cytokines.[673, 674] The channel is inhibited by insect toxins, such as charybdotoxin, and by the calcium channel blockers nitrendipine and nifedipine.[639] In sickle cells, the combination of the Gardos pathway and the K^+/Cl^- cotransporter account for the net loss of K^+ and water, leading to cellular dehydration.

Disruption of the Permeability Barrier in Abnormal Erythrocytes. The effects of breaching the red cell permeability barrier are well illustrated by complement hemolysis. Complement activation on the red cell surface leads to formation of the membrane attack

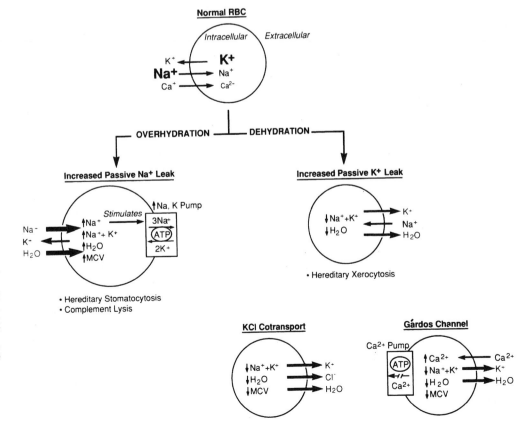

FIGURE 15–13. Cation changes leading to dehydration or overhydration of red cells. *Left,* Overhydration is caused by a massive unbalanced influx of Na^+, which overwhelms the Na^+-K^+ pump and leads to an increase in total monovalent cations ($Na^+ + K^+$) and cell water. *Right,* Dehydration is caused by excess, unbalanced K^+ leakage or by activation of K^+ losing channels such as the K^+/Cl^- cotransport channel or the Ca^{2+}-activated Gardos pathway. Dehydration is associated with a decline in total monovalent cations ($Na^+ + K^+$) and cell water. (From Lux SE, Palek J: Disorders of the red cell membrane. In Handin RJ, Lux SE, Stossel, TP (eds.): Blood: Principles and Practice of Hematology. Philadelphia, Lippincott-Raven, 1995, pp 1701–1818.)

complex, composed of the terminal complement components embedded in the lipid bilayer. This multimolecular complex acts as a cation channel, allowing passive movements of Na^+, K^+, and Ca^{2+} across the membrane according to their concentration gradients. Attracted by fixed anions, such as hemoglobin, ATP, and 2,3-DPG, Na^+ accumulates in the cells in excess of K^+ loss and in excess of the compensatory efforts of the Na^+-K^+ pump. The resulting increase in intracellular monovalent cations and water is followed by cell swelling and, ultimately, colloid osmotic hemolysis.

An alternate leak pathway in sickle cells involves an influx of Na^+ and Ca^{2+} and an efflux of K^+ during deoxygenation and sickling.[675–677] Although the molecular basis of this diffusional pathway is unknown, the magnitude of the Na^+ and K^+ leaks correlates with the degree of morphologic sickling and with lipid bilayer/skeleton uncoupling, suggesting it is caused by mechanical events.[678] This conclusion is further supported by the observation that Ca^{2+} permeability is increased by mechanical stress.[678] Such permeability pathways may be related to stretch-activated channels, described in various tissues, including endothelial, epithelial, and muscle cells.[679] The mechanism of activation of these channels is unknown, but one of the possibilities involves deformation of the submembrane skeleton.[679]

Membrane Pumps

To maintain low intracellular concentrations of Na^+ and Ca^{2+} and a high K^+ concentration, the membrane is endowed with two cation pumps, both utilizing intracellular ATP as an energy source. The ouabain-inhibitable Na^+-K^+ pump extrudes Na^+ and takes up K^+, with a stoichiometry of three Na^+ ions pumped outward for two K^+ ions pumped inward.[680] This exactly balances the normal passive leaks (Na^+ = 1.0 to 2.0 mEq/LRBC; K^+ efflux = 0.8 to 1.5 mEq/L of RBCs/hr). The enzyme is activated by intracellular Na^+ (K_M = 25 mmol/L) and extracellular K^+ (K_M = 2.5 mmol/L).[681] Because the plasma K^+ concentration is high enough to saturate the extracellular K^+ site, Na^+ and K^+ transport is primarily regulated by increases in red cell Na^+ concentration, and cell K^+ losses are rectified only if there is a concomitant Na^+ gain to stimulate active transport. Even then the ratio between the inward Na^+ leak and outward K^+ leak must not be less than the physiologic ratio of 3:2. At lower ratios, the Na^+-K^+ pump, driven by the Na^+ leak and internal Na^+ concentration will not balance the leaks and will actually exacerbate K^+ loss.[682, 683] Consequently, conditions in which K^+ loss approaches or exceeds Na^+ gain lead to irreversible K^+ depletion and cell dehydration such as hereditary spherocytosis and sickle cell anemia.

The calmodulin-activated, Mg^{2+}-dependent Ca^{2+} pump extrudes Ca^{2+} and maintains a very low intracellular free Ca^{2+} concentration ($\approx$20 to 40 nmol/L). It protects red cells from the multiple deleterious effects of Ca^{2+} (echinocytosis, membrane vesiculation, calpain activation, membrane proteolysis, and cell dehydration) described earlier in the chapter. The structure and function of the Na^+/K^+ and Ca^{2+} pumps has been reviewed.[680, 684, 685]

MEMBRANE DEVELOPMENT AND AGING

Assembly of a Stable Membrane Skeleton

Spectrin and ankyrin synthesis is detectable at very early stages of erythroid development in avian and mammalian erythroid cells.[686–688] However, these proteins turn over rapidly and do not assemble into a permanent network. Synthesis of band 3 and protein 4.1 begins at the proerythroblast stage and increases throughout terminal erythroid maturation, up to the late erythroblast stage. During the same time, the mRNA levels and synthesis of spectrin and ankyrin decline. Even so, the proportion of newly assembled spectrin and ankyrin on the membrane progressively increases, and these proteins become more stable, as indicated by their slower turnover. This increased recruitment and stabilization of spectrin and ankyrin, despite declining synthesis, is thought to be related to the progressive increase in the synthesis of band 3 and protein 4.1, because these proteins are the principal sites for attachment of the skeleton to the membrane.[688] However, mice that lack band 3, owing to a targeted gene disruption, have a normal or near-normal membrane skeleton,[689] indicating that band 3 is not required or can be adequately compensated for.

Skeletal Proteins Synthesized in Excess. The synthesis of membrane skeletal proteins is wasteful. Only fractions of newly synthesized spectrin, ankyrin, band 3, and protein 4.1 is assembled into the permanent skeletal network. The excess proteins are rapidly catabolized.[686, 690, 691] Furthermore, skeletal protein synthesis is highly asymmetric. This is most striking in the case of spectrin, for which twofold to threefold more α-spectrin is produced than β-spectrin. Yet, the two chains are assembled into the membrane skeleton in equimolar amounts as mixed heterodimers. Because of this high α-spectrin-to-β-spectrin synthetic ratio, heterozygotes for a deleted or synthetically inactive α-spectrin allele should be asymptomatic, because sufficient α-spectrin should still be made to pair with all the β-spectrin.

Rate-Limiting Steps of Membrane Skeletal Assembly. The principal rate-limiting step in membrane skeletal assembly has traditionally been considered the synthesis of band 3, which contains a high-affinity ankyrin-binding site that recruits and stabilizes spectrin and ankyrin on the membrane.[692] This view, however, has to be reconciled with observations that some patients with dominantly inherited hereditary spherocytosis and partial band 3 deficiency (see later) and mice lacking band 3[689] do not have a proportional decrease in the amounts of spectrin and ankyrin in their membranes.

The second rate-limiting step is the availability of ankyrin, which provides the high-affinity binding sites for β-spectrin. This is best illustrated by studies of membrane skeletal synthesis in *nb/nb* spherocytic mice[424, 693] and in a severe form of human hereditary spherocytosis associated with combined deficiency of spectrin and ankyrin.[694] In both disorders, ankyrin synthesis is markedly reduced, which leads to decreased assembly of spectrin and ankyrin on the membrane, despite normal spectrin synthesis.[694]

The third rate-limiting step involves synthesis of β-spectrin. Because α- and β-spectrin polypeptides are assembled on the membrane in equimolar amounts, and because β-spectrin binds to ankyrin with high affinity, the availability of β-spectrin seems to regulate the amounts of membrane-assembled αβ-spectrin heterodimers. This regulatory role of β-spectrin is illustrated by the effects of erythropoietin on membrane protein assembly. Erythropoietin stimulates the synthesis of β-spectrin and increases assembly of αβ-spectrin heterodimers on the membrane.[695] In contrast, α-spectrin, which is made in excess, does not seem to have a limiting role in the skeletal assembly. α-Spectrin becomes rate limiting only when its synthesis is markedly reduced, as it is in some patients with nondominant hereditary spherocytosis or hereditary pyropoikilocytosis.

Membrane Remodeling during Enucleation and Reticulocyte Maturation

At the orthochromic erythroblast stage, when membrane biogenesis is nearly complete, the cell membrane undergoes a series of critical remodeling steps. The cell nucleus is surrounded by an actin ring, which probably participates in the expulsion of the nucleus from the erythroblast.[696] At the same time, the spectrin skeleton segregates into the incipient reticulocyte, whereas some surface receptors cluster in the membrane surrounding the soon to be extruded nucleus. Further membrane remodeling takes place as the young multilobular reticulocyte attains the biconcave shape.[609, 697] This involves a loss of lipids and certain surface proteins, including receptors for transferrin and fibronectin. During the remodeling process, membrane mechanical stability is not completely established until the very last stages of erythrocyte maturation.[698] Autophagocytosis and phagolysosome expulsion are essential steps in erythroid maturation. These processes are inhibited in the presence of markedly elevated erythrocyte cholesterol.[698a]

Interestingly, DNase II is required for definitive erythropoiesis in the murine fetal liver.[699] Macrophages appear to supply the DNase II, which then destroys the nuclear DNA expelled from erythroid precursor cells. The extruded nuclei are probably then bound and phagocytosed by a macrophage receptor.[700]

Fetal Red Cells

Fetal erythrocytes are different from adult erythrocytes in many ways. There are differences in carbohydrate metabolism, activity of both glycolytic and nonglycolytic enzymes, altered ATP and phosphate metabolism, differences in methemoglobin content and oxygen affinity, and altered storage characteristics.[701] There are also differences in the membranes of fetal and adult erythrocytes. ABO and I antigens and the receptors for the adsorbed serum antigens of the Lewis system are incompletely expressed.

Band 3 and the Ii Blood Group. A single *N*-glycan chain is attached at Asn in the COOH-terminal membrane domain of band 3.[702] This chain is composed of a number of *N*-acetyllactosamine units of variable length arranged in an unbranched, linear fashion (i antigen) in fetal erythrocytes and has i reactivity.[703–705] In adult erythrocytes, it exists in a branched fashion (I antigen) and has I reactivity.[704, 705] Removal of the carbohydrate does not affect anion exchange. The rare absence of the I antigen in adult cells apparently results from the lack of the branching enzyme.[705]

Fetal membranes are more permeable to monovalent cations[706] and contain less or equivalent amounts of the Na^+,K^+-ATPase activity required for monovalent cation removal.[707, 708] They contain more phospholipid and cholesterol per cell[709] and, as a consequence, have a larger surface-to-volume ratio and are slightly more osmotically resistant than adult cells.[710] The ratio of SM to PC is increased in fetal membranes and differences in fatty acid composition exist, but these changes evidently tend to balance each other, because membrane fluidity is normal.[709, 711] The protein composition of fetal red cell membrane is quantitatively normal[712]; however, most of the major membrane proteins of fetal cells have not been purified and characterized, so it is uncertain whether they are all genetically and functionally identical to their counterparts in adult red cells. The fact that hereditary spherocytosis and elliptocytosis are expressed in the neonatal period indicates that the fetal and adult forms of the involved proteins—spectrin, ankyrin, band 3, protein 4.1, and protein 4.2—probably arise from the same gene. There is some evidence that band 3 may be functionally different from its adult counterpart[713] and that fetal red cells may contain more myosin[714]; however, neither of these differences is well proved.

Nothing is known about the arrangement of membrane proteins in fetal red cells compared with that in adult red cells, but there are indications that subtle differences may exist. For example, clustering and endocytosis of concanavalin A receptors can be induced in fetal but not adult human erythrocytes.[715] This endocytosis occurs through spectrin-free regions of fetal membranes.[716] Similar regions exist on adult rabbit reticulocytes and probably on adult human reticulocytes but are eliminated on maturation of these cells.[716, 717] This suggests that fetal and adult membrane skeletons differ in organization, at least in certain membrane domains. If so, this different organization might help to explain the increased rigidity,[717] increased mechanical fragility,[710] and decreased life span (average 45 to 70 days)[718] of fetal red cells. It also offers a potential explanation for the observation that fetal red cells contain numerous surface pits and vacuoles not found in adult cells,[719, 720] a fact that has generally been used as evidence for immaturity of the fetal and neonatal spleen. It is possible, however, that the apparent cause and effect are reversed and that splenic immaturity is responsible for the persistence of the spectrin-free domains, particularly because adult red cells of splenectomized persons are excessively vacuolated[719] and because it is known that the spleen normally pares lipids and some proteins from reticulocytes.[721–723]

Membrane Alterations in Senescent Red Cells

The removal of senescent red cells from the circulation is a subject of longstanding interest. The concept of red cell senescence is based on results of radioactive labeling of a cohort of reticulocytes and bone marrow erythroblasts.[724] In many species, including humans, the fraction of labeled cells remains constant for a defined time period, followed by a rapid decline of radioactivity, suggesting that the red cells are removed from the circulation in an age-dependent manner. Many techniques have been used to isolate senescent red cells, including methods based on differences in cell density, osmotic fragility, and cell size.[724–726] Density separation is most widely used, but the results obtained by this technique must be interpreted with caution. Although red cells exhibit a progressive increase in density as they age *in vivo*, not all dense red cells are senescent.[724, 726, 727]

In addition to *in vitro* separation techniques, various *in vivo* animal models have been used to study red cell aging.[724] Red cells can be labeled with biotin and then removed at defined times with avidin, which complexes tightly to biotin.[728] The senescent cells defined by these techniques exhibit numerous membrane abnormalities.[724, 726, 729, 730] Of particular note is the loss of K+ and water, leading to cell dehydration and increased cell density, and the loss of surface area, presumably due to gradual release of membrane microvesicles.[724, 725, 730, 731] The latter phenomenon is probably caused by constant exposure of red cells to the shearing forces of the microcirculation. In addition, red cell membrane proteins and lipids experience oxidative damage, as shown by high-molecular-weight aggregates containing hemoglobin, spectrin, and band 3[732, 733] and by adducts of proteins and malonylaldehyde, a product of lipid peroxidation.[734]

Early results suggested that loss of red cell surface charge,[735] due to *in vivo* loss of sialic acid residues, and exposure of the penultimate β-galactose residues[736] of the carbohydrate side chains were important factors in the recognition and removal of aged erythrocytes. Later studies revealed that the mild surface charge loss can be entirely explained by the loss of cell surface area[737] and that the surface charge density and the number of sialic acid residues per sialoglycoprotein in senescent red cells is normal.[738, 739]

In addition to red cell membrane abnormalities, red cell aging is associated with a decline of many red cell enzyme activities.[740] However, red cell ATP concentration is normal.[724] Likewise no major abnormalities have been detected in Ca2+ transport and there is no compelling evidence that Ca2+ accumulates in senescent cells.[724]

Targeting Senescent Red Cells for Destruction. Although some of the above alterations may compromise red cell microcirculatory flow, none is likely to destroy old cells. In a series of studies, senescent red cells were shown to have small amounts (a few hundred molecules per cell) of autologous immunoglobulin G (IgG) on their surface that target the cells for destruction by macrophages.[741] There is considerable evidence that antibodies are bound to band 3 in aged red cells and red cells with pathologic changes.[235, 742–745] One explanation for this phenomenon is that denatured or oxidized hemoglobin (hemichromes) induces clustering of band 3 to which antibodies to senescent antigen bind.[732, 743, 744] Band 3 clusters have been visualized by immunofluorescence microscopy and detected by biochemical methods in aged red cells. Band 3 clustering probably results from cumulative oxidative damage because similar damage, including the binding of autologous IgG, takes place on oxidized red cells or red cells containing Heinz bodies, a product of oxidative denaturation of hemoglobin[235, 746–749] and, in a canine model of erythrocyte senescence, aged erythrocytes had compromised reducing power.[750] The senescent antigen is also exposed on red cells infected with the knobby variant of *P. falciparum*.[751]

In addition to targeting senescent red cells for macrophage destruction, band 3 antibodies also trigger complement deposition on senescent cells.[747] As noted earlier, this process may be facilitated by loss of GPI-linked complement regulatory proteins from old cells through microvesiculation. Although the role of autologous IgG in the destruction of senescent erythrocytes is widely accepted, two observations suggest that other mechanisms must be considered.[729] First, blockade of the Fc portion of autologous "senescent" IgG with protein G fails to inhibit red cell phagocytosis. Second, red cell survival is the same in agammaglobulinemic mice as in controls. However, this may not be applicable to humans, because the removal of mouse red cells from the circulation is random.[724]

Altered phospholipid asymmetry also contributes to the removal of senescent erythrocytes.[752] This could occur from damage to the aminophospholipid translocase by products of lipid peroxidation.[753] Disordered phospholipid asymmetry reportedly activates the alternate complement pathway[754] and targets red cells for destruction by macrophages.[755]

Other alterations of possible pathologic significance include postsynthetic modification of red cell proteins by nonenzymatic glycosylation,[756, 757, 757a] carboxymethylation,[758, 759] or membrane damage induced by proteases.[760] Glycosylation of proteins, such as hemoglobin (to form hemoglobin A_{1c}), occurs gradually over the life of the cell and is proportional to the glucose concentration. Methylation of membrane proteins occurs primarily in older red cells with ankyrin and protein 4.1 being the principal substrates.

SURFACE-TO-VOLUME RATIO

From both a diagnostic and pathophysiologic point of view, it is useful to consider red cell morphology and membrane disorders in terms of changes in membrane surface area or cell volume. These parameters reflect two of the membrane's major functions discussed earlier: maintenance of structural integrity and control of cation permeability. Surface loss occurs by membrane fragmentation due either to inherent skeletal weakness or to acquired membrane damage and leads eventually to microspherocytosis. Some microspherocytes are usually present in patients with "surface loss disorders" whose red cells are hemolyzing; often, however, other morphologic forms predominate (e.g., bizarre poikilocytes, spiculated red cells, "bite cells," or elliptocytes), which may be viewed as intermediates in the surface loss pathway. Volume gain occurs because of changes in membrane permeability that permit cations and water to accumulate and lead to the formation of stomatocytes. Surface gain is caused by the accretion of membrane lipid; volume loss results from failure of hemoglobin synthesis or from the loss of cations and water. Both result in the formation of target cells.

These processes are all related by the surface-to-volume ratio. This ratio is indirectly measured by the unincubated osmotic fragility test, which assesses the ability of red cells to swell in increasingly hypotonic salt solutions. Cells with a decreased surface-to-volume ratio (spherocytes and stomatocytes) can tolerate less swelling than normal cells before they burst and are termed *osmotically fragile*. Target cells, with their increased surface-to-volume ratio, are relatively osmotically resistant.

In general, a decrease in surface-to-volume ratio is deleterious to the red cell, because the cell's ability to negotiate the narrow passageways separating the splenic cords and sinuses is seriously compromised as its surface-to-volume ratio approaches the limiting spherical form. In contrast, an increase in surface-to-volume ratio is usually innocuous, except in those cells that lose cations and water and become dehydrated. A summary of the major abnormalities of red cell surface area, volume, and shape is presented diagrammatically in Figure 15–14. This diagram attempts to correlate pathophysiologic processes with morphologic characteristics. Some of these processes are due to alterations in membrane structure and are discussed in the remainder of this chapter. Others are discussed more fully in other chapters in this text.

INHERITED ABNORMALITIES OF THE ERYTHROCYTE MEMBRANE

Hereditary Spherocytosis

Hereditary spherocytosis (HS) (Table 15–5) is a common, inherited hemolytic anemia in which defects of spec-

trin or proteins that participate in the attachment of spectrin to the membrane, ankyrin, protein 4.2, or band 3 lead to spheroidal, osmotically fragile cells that are selectively trapped in the spleen, resulting in a shortened red cell life span.

HISTORY

HS was first recognized more than 100 years ago by two Belgian physicians, Vanlair and Masius,[761] who gave a remarkably thorough account of the disease. They described a woman who suffered from anemia, jaundice, splenomegaly, and recurrent abdominal pain. The authors noted that most of the woman's red cells were spherical and hypothesized that a combination of splenic enlargement and liver atrophy led to their rapid destruction and their patient's anemia. They also noted that the patient's sister had suffered from an identical illness and that her mother was also subject to jaundice. In the 1890s, the British physicians Wilson and Stanley recognized the hereditary nature of the disease and were the first to recognize the characteristic pathologic appearance of the spleen engorged with red cells.[762, 763] However, a report by Minkowski in 1900, in the German literature,[764] received wide attention, and many additional papers soon appeared, including Chauffard's classic description of

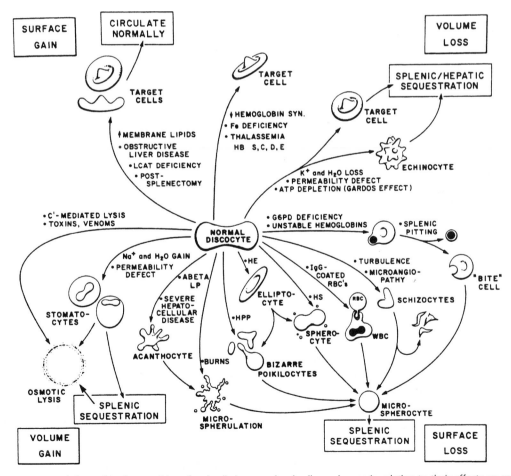

FIGURE 15–14. A summary of the major abnormalities of red cell shape and red cell membranes in relation to their effects on red cell volume and surface area. Fe, iron; HB, hemoglobin; ATP, adenosine triphosphate; G6PD, glucose-6-phosphate dehydrogenase; IgG, immunoglobulin G; ABETA LP, abetalipoprotenemia; HE, hereditary elliptocytosis; HS, hereditary spherocytosis; WBC, white blood cell. (Adapted from Lux SE, Glader BE: Hemolytic anemias III. Membrane and metabolic disorders. In Beck WS (ed): Hematology. Cambridge, MA, MIT Press, 1977, pp 269–298.)

TABLE 15–5. Classification of Red Cell Hemolytic Disorders by Predominant Morphology*

SPHEROCYTES

Hereditary spherocytosis
ABO incompatibility in neonates
Immunohemolytic anemias with IgG- or C3-coated red cells†
Acute oxidant injury (hexose monophosphate shunt defects during hemolytic crisis, oxidant drugs, and chemical reactions)
Hemolytic transfusion reactions†
Clostridial sepsis
Severe burns, other red cell thermal injuries
Spider, bee, and snake venoms
Severe hypophosphatemia
Hypersplenism‡

BIZARRE POIKILOCYTES

Red cell fragmentation syndromes (microangiopathic and macroangiopathic hemolytic anemias)
Acute oxidant injury‡
Hereditary elliptocytosis in neonates
Hereditary pyropoikilocytosis
Homozygous hereditary elliptocytosis

ELLIPTOCYTES

Hereditary elliptocytosis
Thalassemias
(Other hypochromic-microcytic anemias)
(Megaloblastic anemias)

STOMATOCYTES

Hereditary stomatocytosis
Rh_{null} or Rh_{mod} blood group
Cryohydrocytosis
Adenosine deaminase hyperactivity with low red cell ATP‡
(Liver diseases, especially acute alcoholism)
(Mediterranean stomatocytosis)
(Duchenne muscular dystrophy)‡
(Marathon running)‡
(Various medications)

IRREVERSIBLY SICKLED CELLS

Sickle cell anemia
Symptomatic sickle syndromes

INTRAERYTHROCYTIC PARASITES

Malaria
Bartonellosis
Babesiosis

PROMINENT BASOPHILIC STIPPLING

Thalassemias
Unstable hemoglobinopathies
Lead poisoning‡
Pyridine-5′-nucleotidase deficiency

SPICULATED OR CRENATED RED CELLS

Acute hepatic necrosis (spur cell anemia)
Uremia
Red cell fragmentation syndromes‡
Infantile pyknocytosis
Embden-Meyerhof pathway defects‡
Vitamin E deficiency‡
Abetalipoproteinemia
Heat stroke‡
McLeod blood group
(Postsplenectomy)
(Transiently after massive transfusion of stored blood)
(Anorexia nervosa)‡
(Decompression from hyperbaric exposure)‡
(Woronet's trait)

TARGET CELLS

Hemoglobins S, C, D and E
Hereditary xerocytosis
Thalassemias
(Lecithin: cholesterol acyltransferase deficiency)
(Other hypochromic-microcytic anemias)
(Obstructive liver disease)
(Postsplenectomy)

NONSPECIFIC OR NORMAL MORPHOLOGY

Embden-Meyerhof pathway defects‡
Hexose monophosphate shunt defects‡
Adenosine deaminase hyperactivity with low red cell ATP‡
Unstable hemoglobinopathies‡
Paroxysmal nocturnal hemoglobinuria
Dyserythropoietic anemias‡
Copper toxicity (Wilson's disease)
Cation permeability defects‡
Erythropoietic porphyria
Vitamin E deficiency
Hemolysis with infections‡
Rh hemolytic disease in neonates†
Paraxysmal cold hemoglobinuria‡
Cold hemagglutinin disease†
Hypersplenism
Immunohemolytic anemia†‡

*Nonhemolytic disorders of similar morphology are enclosed in parentheses for reference.
  †Usually associated with positive Coombs' test.
  ‡Disease or condition sometimes associated with this morphology.

osmotic fragility[765] and reticulocytosis[766] as hallmarks of the disease. The use of splenectomy was advocated and its success led to rapid acceptance of the procedure. The first successful splenectomy for HS was unintentionally performed by Wells in England 20 years before,[767] 3 years before Wilson's description of HS. While operating on a jaundiced woman for a supposed uterine fibroid, he encountered and removed an enormous spleen. The patient recovered and her jaundice disappeared. The events were reconstructed 40 years later by Dawson,[767] who found the abnormal erythrocyte osmotic fragility during an examination of the woman and her son. Thus,

the major clinical features of HS were defined by the 1920s, although nothing was known about the pathophysiology of the disease. Readers interested in more details about these and other aspects of the history of HS should consult the chapters by Dacie, Crosby, and Wintrobe in *Blood, Pure and Eloquent.*[768]

PREVALENCE AND GENETICS

HS occurs in all racial and ethnic groups. It is particularly common in Northern European peoples, where it affects approximately 1 person in 5000.[769] This is probably an underestimate, as surveys of red cell osmotic fragility suggest that mild forms of the disease may be four or five times more common than believed.[770, 771] There are no good estimates of the prevalence in other populations, but clinical experience suggests it is less common in African-Americans and Southeast Asians.

HS exhibits both dominant and nondominant phenotypes. About two thirds of patients have typical autosomal dominant disease,[769, 772, 773] with the remaining patients exhibiting nondominant inheritance.[774–780] In many patients with nondominant disease, HS is due to a *de novo* mutation, which tends to occur at CpG dinucleotides, and is associated with small insertions or deletions.[774, 775] In the remaining patients with nondominant inheritance, both parents are clinically normal but may exhibit subtle laboratory abnormalities that suggest a carrier state.[772, 775, 780] These patients probably have an autosomal recessive form of the disease, although it is not always possible to exclude dominant HS with reduced penetrance or dominant HS due to a new mutation.[772]

ETIOLOGY

The primary molecular defects in HS reside in membrane skeletal proteins, particularly the proteins whose vertical interactions connect the membrane skeleton to the lipid bilayer: spectrin, ankyrin, protein 4.2, and band 3 (Table 15–6). Red cells from the majority of European and American patients with HS have deficiencies of spectrin and ankyrin, including those with both the dominant and nondominant forms.[780, 828–830] The degree of spectrin deficiency (and by deduction ankyrin deficiency) correlates well with the spheroidicity of HS red cells, the severity of hemolysis, and the response of patients to splenectomy (Fig. 15–15).[772, 780, 831] The mechanical properties of the cells, particularly their ability to withstand shear stress, also correlate with their spectrin content.[831, 832] Microscopically, HS red cells show fewer spectrin filaments interconnecting spectrin–actin–protein 4.1 junctional complexes, but overall skeletal architecture is preserved,[596] except in the most severe forms of the disease. A minority of European and American patients with HS have deficiencies of band 3 and protein 4.2 (dominant HS) or protein 4.2 alone (recessive HS).[497, 775, 828, 833–836] In contrast, these are the most common forms of HS in Japan.[790] In Koreans, ankyrin and spectrin deficiency was most commonly observed, but protein 4.2 deficiency occurred more commonly than in whites.[837]

α-Spectrin Defects

In humans, α-spectrin synthesis exceeds β-spectrin synthesis by 3 or 4 to 1.[688] Heterozygotes for α-spectrin synthetic defects produce enough normal α-spectrin chains to pair with all, or nearly all, of the β chains that are made. Thus, α-spectrin defects are apparent in the homozygous or compound heterozygous state and are associated with recessive inheritance. In affected patients, clinical severity is often severe.[780, 829, 838]

Patients who are homozygotes or compound heterozygotes for α-spectrin defects will suffer from severe HS. Wichterle et al[819] described a patient with severe HS who

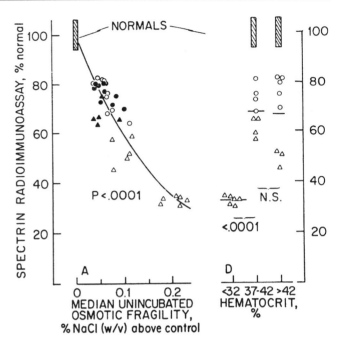

FIGURE 15–15. Correlation between spectrin deficiency and unincubated osmotic fragility in hereditary spherocytosis. Spectrin content, as measured by radioimmunoassay, is shown on the vertical axis and osmotic fragility, as measured by NaCl concentration producing 50 percent hemolysis of erythrocytes, is shown on the horizontal axis. *Circles* represent patients with typical autosomal dominant HS, and *triangles* represent patients with atypical, nondominant spherocytosis. *Open symbols* represent patients who have undergone splenectomy. The *right panel* shows the hematocrit of each patient at least 4 months after splenectomy. N.S., nonsignificant. (From Agre P, Asimos A, Casella JF, et al: Inheritance pattern and clinical response to splenectomy as a reflection of erythrocyte spectrin deficiency in hereditary spherocytosis. N Engl J Med 1986; 315:1579. Copyright 1986, Massachusetts Medical Society.)

was a compound heterozygote for two different α-spectrin gene defects: in one allele, there was a splicing defect associated with an upstream intronic mutation, α^{LEPRA}; in the other allele there was another mutation, α^{PRAGUE}. The α^{LEPRA} allele produces six times less of the correctly spliced α-spectrin transcript than the normal allele. Further studies have shown that in many patients with nondominant HS and spectrin deficiency, including a number of the patients originally described by Agre et al,[780, 829, 838] α^{LEPRA} is in linkage dysequilibrium with α$^{Bug Hill}$, an amino acid substitution in the αII domain.[839] Thus, it appears that the combination of the α^{LEPRA} allele with other defects of α spectrin in *trans*, leads to significant, spectrin-deficient spherocytic anemia. Interestingly, even in the most severe forms of α-spectrin-linked recessive HS, obligate heterozygotes show little or no spectrin deficiency.[780, 829, 838]

In a report of a lethal and near-lethal HS associated with dramatic (26 percent of normal) spectrin deficiency, pulse-labeling studies of burst-forming unit-erythroid–derived erythroblasts revealed a marked decrease in α-spectrin synthesis.[776] Although the underlying molecular basis of this defect is unknown, a family history of a mild dominantly inherited HS in the mother and the finding of slightly increased osmotic fragility in the hematologically normal father suggest that the proband inherited at least two genetic defects that in a simple heterozygote have either minimal or no adverse consequences.

TABLE 15–6. Mutations Associated with Hereditary Spherocytosis

Variant	Inheritance	Type	Gene	Location	Protein	Reference
ANKYRIN						
Unnamed	AD	Substitution	C→G	Promoter, −204	—	780
Campinas	AR	Substitution	G→A	Promoter, −153	—	781
Unnamed	AR	Substitution	T→C	Promoter, −108	—	780
Unnamed	AR	Deletion	−TG	5′- UTR, −72/−73	—	782
Chiba II	AD	Deletion, frameshift	−CCCTATTCTG	Exon 1	2–4→frameshift	783
Nara II	AD	Substitution, splicing, frameshift	G→C	ivs 1, +5	9→frameshift	783
Saitama	De novo	Deletion, frameshift	−T	Exon 5	112→frameshift	783
Shiga	De novo	Insertion, splicing, frameshift	+A	ivs 5, +3/+4	142→frameshift	783
Bugey	De novo	Deletion, frameshift	−C	Exon 6	146→frameshift	784
Osterholz	—	Deletion, frameshift	20 nt deletion	Exon 6	173→frameshift	780
Tokyo II	De novo	Deletion, frameshift	−CACGGCTGCG	Exon 6	187→frameshift	783
Limeira	AD	Missense	CAC→CGC	Exon 9	276 His→Arg	781
Stuttgart	AD	Deletion, frameshift	−GC	Exon 10	329→frameshift	780
Bari	De novo	Deletion, frameshift	−G	Exon 12	426→frameshift	785
Walsrode	AR	Missense	GTC→ATC	Exon 13	463 Val→Ile	780
Florianopolis	AD	Insertion, frameshift	+C	Exon 14	506→frameshift	786
Duisburg	AD	Missense, splicing, frameshift	C→A	ivs 16, −18	601→frameshift	780
Tokyo III	De novo	Deletion	−C	Exon 16	571→frameshift	783
Einbeck	AD	Deletion, frameshift	+C	Exon 16	572→frameshift	780
Napoli	De novo	Deletion, frameshift	−T	Exon 20	573→frameshift	787
Unnamed	—	Deletion, frameshift	−C	Exon 16	596→frameshift	788
Osaka II	De novo	Nonsense	CAG→TAG	Exon 17	612 Gln→stop	783
Bruggen	—	Missense	CGT→CAT	Exon 17	619 Arg→His	789
Unnamed	—	Nonsense	GAG→TAG	Exon 17	631 Glu→stop	790
Osaka I	De novo	Insertion, frameshift	+C	Exon 17	637→frameshift	783
Unnamed	—	Nonsense	TCG→TAG	Exon 20	765 Ser→stop	790
Marburg	AD	Deletion, frameshift	−TAGT	Exon 22	797–798→frameshift	780
Kagoshima	De novo	Deletion, frameshift	−CAGT	Exon 22	798–799→frameshift	783
Yamagata	De novo	Splicing, frameshift	GT→CT	ivs 22, +1	821→frameshift	783
Unnamed	—	Deletion, frameshift	−G	Exon 25	907→frameshift	790
Napoli II	De novo	Deletion, frameshift	−C	Exon 26	933→frameshift	785
Mie	De novo	Deletion, frameshift	−GCCGCCT	Exon 26	951–953→frameshift	783
Anzio	De novo	Deletion, frameshift	−CA	Exon 26	983→frameshift	785
Nara I	—	Missense	CTA→CCA	Exon 28	1046 Leu→Pro	783, 789
Unnamed	—	Nonsense	CGA→TGA	Exon 28	1053 Arg→stop	790
Jaguariuna	AD	Missense	ATC→ACC	Exon 28	1054 Ile→Thr	781
Chiba I	De novo	Substitution, splicing, frameshift	GT→CT	ivs 28, +1	1109→frameshift	783
Porta Westfalica	—	Deletion, frameshift	−C	Exon 29	1127→frameshift	780
Chiba III	De novo	Nonsense	TAC→TAG	Exon 31	1230 Tyr→stop	783
Tokyo I	AD	Nonsense	CGA→TGA	Exon 31	1252 Arg→stop	783
Bovendem	AD	Nonsense	CGA→TAG	Exon 36	1436 Arg→stop	780
Unnamed	—	Nonsense	CGA→TGA	Exon 37	1488 Arg→stop	790
Prague	AD	Insertion	201 nt insertion	Exon 37/38	1512–1513 67AA insertion	791
Dusseldorf	AR	Missense	GAC→AAC	Exon 38	1592 Asp→Asn	780
Toyama	AD	Nonsense	CAG→TAG	Exon 38	1640 Gln→stop	783
Saint-Etienne 1	AD	Nonsense	TGG→TGA	Exon 39	1721 Trp→stop	792

Variant	Inheritance	Type	DNA change	Location	Amino acid change	Reference
Saint-Etienne 2	AD	Nonsense	CGA→TGA	Exon 41	1833 Arg→stop	792
Bocholt	AR	Missense	CGG→TGG	Exon 41	1879 Arg→Trp	780
Rakovnik	AD	Nonsense	GAA→TAA	Exon 38	1669 Glu→stop	793
Unnamed	AD	Missense, splicing, frameshift	C→T	ivs 38, −34	1699→frameshift	780
BAND 3						
Montefiore	?AR	Missense	GAG→AAG	Exon 10	40 Glu→Lys	498
Foggia	AD	Deletion, frameshift	−C	Exon 4	54–55→frameshift	794
Kagoshima	De novo	Deletion, frameshift	TGG→TGA	Exon 4	56→frameshift	789
Hodonin	AD	Nonsense	TGG→TGA	Exon 5	81 Trp→Stop	795
Cape Town	—	Missense	GAG→AAG	Exon 5	90 Arg→Trp	796
Napoli I	AD	Insertion, frameshift	+T	Exon 5	99–100→frameshift	794
Fukayama I	AD	Deletion, frameshift	−AC	Exon 5	112–113→frameshift	789
Nachod	AD	Substitution, splicing	C→A	ivs 5, −3	117–121 GTVLL deleted	795
Fukuoka	AR	Missense	GGA→AGA	Exon 6	130 Gly→Arg	789, 874
Osnabruck I	AD	Nonsense	CGA→TGA	Exon 6	150 Arg→stop	780, 797
Lyon	AD	Nonsense	CGA→TGA	Exon 6	150 Arg→stop	781
Worcester	AD	Insertion, frameshift	+G	Exon 7	170–172→frameshift	795
Wilson	AD	Deletion, frameshift	−G	Exon 7	171→frameshift	789
Fukuyama II	AD	Insertion, frameshift, substitution,	+A	Exon 7	183→frameshift	798
Campinas	AD	Splicing, frameshift	G→T	ivs 8, +1	203→frameshift	799
Bohain	AD	Deletion, frameshift	−T	Exon 9	241→frameshift	799
Princeton	AD	Insertion, frameshift	+C	Exon 9	273–275→frameshift	795
Boston	AD	Missense	GCT→GAT	Exon 9	285 Ala→Asp	795
Tuscaloosa	?AD	Missense	CCG→CGC	Exon 10	327 Pro→Arg	800
Noirterre	AD	Nonsense	CAG→TAG	Exon 10	330 Gln→stop	801
Bruggen	AD	Deletion, frameshift	−C	Exon 11	419→frameshift	780
Benesov	AD	Missense	GGG→GAG	Exon 12	455 Gly→Glu	795
Bicetre II	AD	Deletion, frameshift	−G	Exon 12	456→frameshift	799
Pribram	AD	Substitution, splicing, frameshift	G→A	ivs 12, −1	477→frameshift	795
Coimbra	AD	Missense	CTG→ATG	Exon 13	488 Val→Met	802, 803
Bicetre I	AD	Missense	CGC→TGC	Exon 13	490 Arg→Cys	799
Evry	AD	Deletion, frameshift	−T	Exon 13	492→frameshift	799
Milano	AD	In-frame duplication	69 bp duplication	Exon 13	498–23 AA insertion	804
Dresden	AD	Missense	CGC→TGC	Exon 13	518 Arg→Cys	780
Smichov	AD	Deletion, frameshift	−C	Exon 15	616→frameshift	795
Trutnov	AD	Nonsense	TAC→TAA	Exon 15	628 Tyr→stop	795
Hobart	AD	Deletion, frameshift	−G	Exon 16	646–647→frameshift	795
Osnabruck II	AD	Inframe deletion	−ATG	Exon 16	663–664→frameshift	780
Tochigi II	De novo	Deletion/splicing	−A	ivs 16, −5	→frameshift	789
Most	AD	Missense	CTG→CCG	Exon 17	707 Leu→Pro	795
Okinawa	AD	Missense	GGG→AGG	Exon 17	714 Gly→Arg	789, 874
Prague II	AD	Missense	CGG→CAG	Exon 17	760 Arg→Gln	805
Hradec Kralove	AD	Missense	CGG→TGG	Exon 17	760 Arg→Trp	805
Chur	AD	Missense	GGC→GAC	Exon 18	771 Gly→Asp	806
Napoli II	AD	Missense	ATC→AAC	Exon 18	783 Ile→Asn	794
Jablonec	AD	Missense	CGC→TGC	Exon 18	808 Arg→Cys	805
Nara	De novo	Missense	CGC→CAC	Exon 18	808 Arg→His	789
Prague I	AD	Insertion, frameshift	+CACCCAGATC	Exon 18	819–822→frameshift	807
Birmingham	AD	Missense	CAC→CCC	Exon 19	834 His→Pro	795
Philadelphia	AD	Missense	ACG→ATG	Exon 19	837 Thr→Met	795

TABLE 15–6. Mutations Associated with Hereditary Spherocytosis (*Continued*)

Variant	Inheritance	Type	Gene	Location	Protein	Reference
Tokyo	—	Missense	ACG→GCG	Exon 19	837 Thr→Ala	808
Prague III	AD	Missense	CGG→TGG	Exon 19	870 Arg→Trp	795
Vesuvio	—	Deletion, frameshift	–C	Exon 20	894→frameshift	809
PROTEIN 4.2						
Lisboa	AR	Deletion, frameshift	–C	Exon 3	89→frameshift	810
Fukuoka	AR	Missense	TGG→TGA	Exon 3	119 Trp→Stop	811
Nippon	AR	Missense	GCT→ACT	Exon 3	142 Ala→Thr	812
Komatsu	AR	Missense	GAT→TAT	Exon 4	175 Asp→Tyr	813
Notame	AR	Splicing, frameshift	G→A	ivs 6, +1	308→frameshift	814
Tozeur	AR	Missense	CGA→CAA	Exon 7	310 Arg→Gln	815
Shiga	AR	Missense	CGC→TGC	Exon 7	317 Arg→Cys	816
Nancy	—	Deletion, frameshift	–G	Exon 7	317→frameshift	817
α-SPECTRIN						
Prague		Substitution, splicing, frameshift	A→G	ivs 36, –1	1729→frameshift	818
LEPRA		Substitution, splicing, frameshift	C→T	ivs 30, –70	1446→frameshift	818
β-SPECTRIN						
Promissão	AD	Missense/translation	ATG→GTG	Exon 2	1 Met→Val	819
Guemene-Penfao	AD	Substitution, splicing, frameshift	–1, G→C (ivs 3)	Exon 3	100→frameshift	820
Atlanta	AD	Missense	TGG→GGG	Exon 5	182 Trp→Gly	821
Unnamed	AD	Missense/splicing?	CTG→CTC	Exon 5	189 Gly→Ala	822
Ostrava	AD	Deletion, frameshift	–T	Exon 6	202→frameshift	821
Kissimmee	*De novo*	Missense	TGG→CGG	Exon 6	202 Trp→Arg	327
Oakland	AD	Missense	ATC→GTC	Exon 7	220 Ile→Val	821
Bicetre	AD	Deletion, frameshift	–TCGTGGC or –CCTCGTGG	Exon 11	443 or 444→frameshift	822
Alger	AD	Nonsense	CAG→TAG	Exon 12	514→Stop	822
Philadelphia	AD	Insertion, frameshift	+A	Exon 13	589→frameshift	821
St. Barbara	? Mosaic	Deletion, frameshift	–C	Exon 14	638→frameshift	823
Bergen	AD	Insertion	+A	Exon 14	783→frameshift	821
Baltimore	AD	Nonsense	CAG→TAG	Exon 14	845 Gln→Stop	821
Houston	AD	Deletion, frameshift	–A	Exon 15	926→frameshift	821
Winston-Salem	*De novo*	Substitution, Splicing, in-frame deletion	G→A	ivs 17, +1	935→frameshift	824
Columbus	AD	Missense	CCT→TCT	Exon 17	1227 Pro→Ser	821
Sao Paolo II	AD	Deletion, frameshift	–C	Exon 20	1392→frameshift	824a
Durham	*De novo*	In-frame deletion	Exons 22 & 23 deleted	deleted	1492→1614 123 AA deletion	825
Birmingham	AR	Missense	CGC→TGC	Exon 25	1684 Arg→Cys	821
Sao Paulo I	—	Missense	GCG→GTG	Exon 28	1884 A→Val	826
Tabor	AD	Nonsense	CAG→TAG	Exon 28	1946 Gln→Stop	821

AD = autosomal dominant; AR = autosomal recessive; UTR = untranslated region; nt = nucleotide; ivs = intervening sequence; AA = amino acid.

β-Spectrin Defects

Deficiency of the limiting β-spectrin chains limits formation of αβ-spectrin heterodimers. Thus, defects in β-spectrin are apparent in the heterozygous state, associated with dominant inheritance.

Initially, cytogenetic studies supported the hypothesis that some patients with dominant HS have defects in β-spectrin. Kimberling and colleagues[840] detected a loose linkage between polymorphisms of the immunoglobulin heavy chains (IgH) and an HS locus (now called SPH1) by combining observations on 70 patients in 11 informative families. IgH was subsequently localized to chromosome 14q32.3, reasonably close to β-spectrin (14q23-q24.2).[841]

Cloning of the β-spectrin gene, a large gene spanning over 200 kb, preceded the identification of heterozygous point mutations in a number of unrelated families with dominant HS. Spectrin[Kissimmee] is an unstable β-spectrin that lacks the ability to bind protein 4.1 and, as a consequence, binds poorly to actin.[327, 842–844] This variant is due to a point mutation, $Trp^{202} \rightarrow Arg^{364}$, in a conserved region near the NH_2 terminus of β-spectrin, which probably forms part of the protein 4.1–binding site.[327, 845] Truncated β-spectrin mutations due to a large genomic deletion that leads to exon skipping of exons 22 and 23, β-spectrin[Durham], or to splicing mutations, β-spectrin[Winston-Salem] and β-spectrin[Guemene-Penfao], have been described.[821, 825, 826] Screening of the β-spectrin gene of additional patients with HS with spectrin deficiency has identified a number of nonsense and frameshift mutations.[822, 823, 827] One of these, spectrin[Houston], a frameshift mutation due to a single nucleotide deletion, was found in patients from several unrelated kindreds[822] and may be a common β-spectrin mutation associated with dominant HS. Finally, a β-spectrin translation initiation codon mutation was identified in one family with HS and spectrin deficiency.[820] Interestingly, in many of the patients in which peripheral blood morphology has been described, those with β-spectrin mutations have had prominent acanthocytes or spiculated spherocytes as well as spherocytes.

Ankyrin Defects

Spectrin heterodimers are only stable when bound to the membrane[846] and ankyrin, the high-affinity binding site, is normally present in limiting amounts. As a result, ankyrin defects are typically expressed as a dominant defect.

Evidence implicating defects of ankyrin in HS comes from a variety of sources, including biochemical analyses, genetic studies, and study of a murine model of HS. Initially, biochemical studies suggested a defect of ankyrin in two patients with an atypical, unusually severe form of HS characterized by bizarre-shaped microspherocytes.[694] Red cell spectrin and ankyrin levels were approximately one half normal, apparently owing to failure of ankyrin synthesis or to synthesis of an unstable molecule.[847] Ankyrin mRNA concentrations were also one-half normal, and pulse-chase studies showed that newly synthesized ankyrin did not accumulate in the cytoplasm and only reached one-half normal levels on the membrane. In contrast, spectrin mRNA concentrations were normal, although only one-half of the synthesized spectrin attached to the membrane, presumably owing to the lack of ankyrin sites. Spectrin synthesis was either normal or increased; however, spectrin incorporation into the membrane skeleton was diminished owing to a marked deficiency of membrane-associated ankyrin. These studies supported the hypothesis that ankyrin deficiency or dysfunction leads to spectrin deficiency in HS.

Additional biochemical studies provided evidence that ankyrin deficiency is present in the erythrocytes of many patients with typical, dominant HS. Savvides and colleagues[828] measured red cell spectrin and ankyrin levels by radioimmunoassay in the erythrocyte membranes of 39 patients from 20 typical kindreds with dominant HS. The values ranged from 40 to 100 percent of the normal cellular levels of 242,000 ± 20,500 spectrin heterodimers and 124,500 ± 11,000 ankyrin heterodimers. Both spectrin and ankyrin levels were less than the normal range in 75 to 80 percent of kindreds. The degree of spectrin and ankyrin deficiency was very similar in 19 of the 20 kindreds studied. Similar data have been observed in other studies.[830, 833–837, 848, 849] The finding of concomitant spectrin and ankyrin deficiencies is not unexpected. Decreased ankyrin synthesis or accumulation on the erythrocyte membrane could lead to decreased assembly of spectrin on the membrane because spectrin-binding sites in ankyrin may be absent or defective.

Genetic studies supported the hypothesis that a defect of the ankyrin gene can be associated with HS. Initially, studies of atypical patients with HS and karyotypic abnormalities including translocations and interstitial deletions defined a locus for HS at chromosomal segments 8p11.2-21.1.[501, 850–854] After the ankyrin gene was cloned, it was localized to this same region, 8p11.2.[501] Fluorescence-based *in situ* hybridization of lymphocyte metaphase spreads from a patient with HS and mental retardation and an interstitial deletion of chromosome 8, band p11.1-p21 with an ankyrin genomic probe provided direct evidence that one copy of the erythrocyte ankyrin gene was deleted.[501] Ankyrin content in the patient's red blood cell membranes was reduced by 50 percent. These results demonstrated that a deficiency of ankyrin due to a gene deletion can be a cause of HS. A similar phenotype has been reported in another patient with an 8p11.1-p21.3 deletion.[853] These combined observations suggested that ankyrin deficiency was the primary defect in the majority of patients with dominant HS and that spectrin deficiency is secondary to the loss of ankyrin attachment sites.

A series of genetic studies then solidified the hypothesis that a defect in the ankyrin gene is the most common cause of dominant HS. The linkage between HS and the ankyrin gene was demonstrated in a large family with typical dominant HS using restriction fragment length polymorphisms.[855] Studies of ankyrin cDNA revealed that one third of patients with dominant HS and spectrin and ankyrin deficiencies expressed only one of their two ankyrin alleles in reticulocyte RNA, demonstrating reduced ankyrin expression from one, presumably mutant, allele.[856] A series of reports then demonstrated the precise defects in the ankyrin gene that cause HS (Table 15–6). These defects have been detected primarily by mutation screening using polymerase chain reaction (PCR)–based single-stranded conformational polymorphism (SSCP) techniques.[781] Analysis of these mutations revealed the following: (1) ankyrin mutations are common, affecting patients with both dominant and nondominant HS; (2) mutations that abolish the normal ankyrin product are common in dominant HS (e.g., frameshift and nonsense mutations); and (3) defects upstream of the coding region in the ankyrin gene erythroid promoter are common in nondominant HS. The most common variant is a T→C nucleotide substitution in the ankyrin gene promoter −108 bp from the translation start site. The allele occurrence of this variant is 29 percent in a German HS population and 2 percent in normal individuals.[781] It has also been associated with nondominant HS with ankyrin deficiency in Italy.[775] The −108 sequence variant is usually in *cis* with a G→A nucleotide substitution 153 bp from the start site.[782] These defects are silent in obligate heterozygotes; thus, patients with nondominant HS must have a second mutation. This has been discovered in two patients: a man with mild HS who carries the −108 mutation and a silent defect in *trans*, ankyrin[Walsrode] (Val[463]→Ile), and a man with moderate HS, the −108 mutation, and ankyrin[Bocholt], an Arg→Trp mutation in an alternatively spliced region near the COOH terminus.[781] Function defects associated with these promoter mutations have been demonstrated in a transgenic animal model.[857] Another promoter mutation, a deletion of the dinucleotide TG at −72/−73 has recently been shown to cause significant abnormalities in ankyrin expression *in vitro* and *in vivo*.[783]

Variations in the clinical severity and red cell ankyrin content of similar mutations indicate that other factors modify the expression of the primary ankyrin defects. For example, ankyrin[Marburg] and ankyrin[Einbeck] are frameshift mutations that occur in the NH$_2$-terminal (membrane) domain and do not produce a detectable product in mature red cells. They would be expected to have a similar phenotype, but patients with ankyrin[Marburg] have moderate to severe HS and moderate ankyrin deficiency (64 percent of normal), whereas patients with ankyrin[Einbeck] have very mild disease and normal ankyrin levels. Understanding this and similar phenotypic variations will be one of the critical problems in HS research in the next few years.

The majority of ankyrin mutations are private; that is, each individual kindred has a unique mutation. One frameshift mutation associated with severe dominant HS, ankyrin[Florianopolis], has been identified in patients with HS from three different kindreds from different genetic backgrounds.[787] Analysis of an ankyrin gene polymorphism in these individuals demonstrated that this mutation is found on different ankyrin alleles, suggesting that the ankyrin[Florianopolis] mutation has occurred more than once.

Band 3 Defects

Band 3 defects are expressed as a dominant trait because ankyrin links the membrane skeleton to band 3 and only a fraction of the band 3 molecules in the membrane are available to bind ankyrin. A primary defect in band 3 is present in approximately one third of patients with dominant HS.[806] Erythrocyte membranes from these patients are deficient in band 3 with concomitant deficiency of protein 4.2.[207]

Initially, biochemical studies suggested an association between band 3 and dominant HS, with some patients with mild to moderate HS exhibiting a 20 to 40 percent deficiency of band 3 and protein 4.2 in their erythrocyte membranes. Membrane spectrin content was normal.

Genetic linkage of HS to the band 3 gene was then described,[808] followed by the identification of mutations of the band 3 gene in a number of HS kindreds (Table 15–6). A variety of band 3 mutations have been described, and these mutations are spread out throughout the band 3 gene, occurring in both the cytoplasmic and membrane-spanning domains. They generally fall into two groups. One group affects protein 4.2 or ankyrin binding and is associated with mild band 3 deficiency. The other group is associated with more severe band 3 deficiency due to a mutation that causes mRNA instability or a mutant band 3 protein that is degraded or not otherwise inserted into the membrane.[207]

One of the initial band 3 mutants associated with HS was band 3[Prague].[808] This mutant is due to a 10-nucleotide duplication in the band 3 gene that leads to a shift in the reading frame and results in premature chain termination. The mutation occurs in a region encoding the COOH terminus of the protein, leading to an altered COOH terminus after amino acid 821 (70 new amino acids). The mutation affects the last transmembrane helix and probably alters insertion of band 3 into the membrane because the mutant protein is not detectable in mature red cells. *In vitro*, overexpression of band 3[Prague] inhibits wild-type band 3 trafficking in *Xenopus* oocytes.[858]

A group of band 3 mutations that cluster near the COOH terminus and replace a conserved arginine with another amino acid have been described (Table 15–6), with arginine 490 being a particular hot spot for HS-related band 3 mutations.[800, 859] These arginines are all located at the cytoplasmic end of a predicted transmembrane helix. Arginine residues are located in the same position in most transmembrane proteins and are thought to help orient the membrane-spanning segments. Thus, as predicted, *in vitro* studies have demonstrated that these arginine substitutions, as well as several other HS-associated band 3 missense mutations, exhibit defective cellular trafficking from the endoplasmic reticulum to the plasma membrane,[860, 861] perhaps due to misfolding.

Other band 3 mutations have been described. In two French families with dominant HS, nonsense mutations (band 3[Noirterre] and band 3[Lyon]) led to markedly decreased mRNA accumulation, presumably due to mRNA instability[781, 802]; a similar mechanism is hypothesized in other band 3 nonsense mutations. There have been several reports of severe HS in patients who are compound heterozygotes for band 3 defects.[797, 798, 804] Homozygosity for band 3 defects has been described in two kindreds. Band 3[Coimbra] was associated with nonimmune hydrops fetalis, transfusion-dependent anemia with complete absence of band 3, and distal renal tubular acidosis in the homozygous state.[803] Band 3[Neapolis] was associated with life-threatening anemia but no renal acidosis because the mutation occurred in a region of band 3 not included in the renal isoform.[862]

Frameshift mutations other than band 3[Prague] have been described (Table 15–6). One example is band

3[Milano], a 23-amino acid, in-frame duplication in transmembrane domain 4 that is probably not incorporated into the erythrocyte membrane.[805] This duplication is present in the genomic DNA and is thought to have arisen from an unequal recombination of the anti-Lepore type.

Additional band 3 gene missense mutations associated with dominant HS have also been described. Determination of the crystal structure of the cytoplasmic domain of band 3 is beginning to provide insights into the biologic significance of these mutations.[221, 863] A few of these missense mutations in band 3 have been associated with significant protein 4.2 deficiency and HS or with acanthocytosis alone (see later).

Interestingly, a number of missense mutations in band 3 have been identified in patients with dominant and recessive renal tubular acidosis (RTA) without HS.[864–867] The exceptions to this observation are patients who are homozygous for band 3 defects, such as band 3[Coimbra] described above[803] or patients with defects in band 3 mRNA processing, band 3[Pribram] or band 3[Campinas],[796, 799] who suffer from hemolytic anemia and tubular acidosis. The dominant RTA mutants are successfully incorporated into the erythrocyte membrane and thus do not cause HS, whereas most dominant HS mutations with normal mRNA stability are misfolded and do not insert into the erythrocyte membrane. The lack of RTA in patients with dominant HS and band 3 mutants supports the hypothesis that dominant RTA results from the association of mutant band 3 with wild-type band 3 into heterooligomers in the kidney, but not in erythroid cells, leading to intracellular retention or mistargeting of both proteins.[207] Why some residues are critical in the kidney but not the red cell with mutation leading to the phenotype of RTA but not HS, and, conversely, why some residues are critical in the erythrocyte but not the kidney, leading to the phenotype of HS but not RTA, are important questions to be addressed in future studies.

Finally, most patients with HS and band 3 deficiencies have a small number of mushroom-shaped or "pincered" erythrocytes, in addition to spherocytes, on peripheral blood smears. This morphologic characteristic is not observed in the other membrane protein defects.

In cows, homozygosity for a nonsense mutation in the band 3 gene leads to absence of band 3 and protein 4.2.[868] Red cell membranes are unstable and show surface area loss, as demonstrated by invagination, vesiculation, and extrusion of microvesicles. There is defective anion transport and a mild acidosis. In mice, targeted disruption of the band 3 gene causes a severe spherocytic hemolytic anemia, with exuberant loss of the membrane surface as vesicles, tubules, and myelin forms.[689] Red cell membranes also lack protein 4.2 and glycophorin A.[869] Surprisingly, the content of membrane skeletal proteins and the architecture of negative-stained, spread skeletons is normal or nearly normal.[603] For unknown reasons, these band 3-deficient mice have a significant propensity for thrombosis.[870] Finally, zebrafish with band 3 mutations, associated with the retsina phenotype, suffer from severe anemia with a complete arrest in erythroid maturation at the late erythroblast stage.[871] Many of these arrested erythroblasts have bilobed nuclei reminiscent of those seen in congenital dyserythropoietic anemia and demonstrate defects in cytokinesis.

Protein 4.2 Defects

Investigators from Asia have described families with recessive HS in which erythrocytes from affected homozygous patients lack protein 4.2 (Table 15–6), although a few patients have been described in other populations.[497, 790, 818, 872] Protein 4.2-deficient erythrocytes may also be deficient in ankyrin and band 3 protein. In the most common variant, 4.2[Nippon], the red cells contain only a small quantity of a 74/72-kD doublet of protein 4.2 instead of the usual 72-kD species, because of a Ala[142]→Thr mutation that affects the processing of the protein 4.2 mRNA.[512] Protein 4.2[Nippon]–deficient membranes lose 70 percent of their ankyrin with low ionic strength extraction, and the ankyrin loss is blocked by preincubation of the membranes with purified 4.2, which suggests that protein 4.2 stabilizes ankyrin on the membrane.[502, 503] This hypothesis is supported by the observations that the amount of protein 4.2 is low in the red cell membranes of ankyrin-deficient *nb/nb* mice and in patients with HS who lack one ankyrin gene. In addition, red cells from patients homozygous for 4.2[Nippon] are fragile and have heat-sensitive skeletons, clumped intramembranous particles (probably band 3 molecules), and increased lateral mobility of band 3.[503] However, ankyrin lability is not evident in other patients with protein 4.2 deficiency,[873, 874] some of whom have normal morphology, acanthopoikilocytosis,[874] or ovalostomatocytosis instead of spherocytosis. Presumably, these differences are examples of allelic variation.

Erythrocyte protein 4.2 deficiency has also been associated with mutations of band 3.[499, 502, 797, 801] Presumably, these mutations involve sites of band 3–protein 4.2 interactions. In one report, there was partial band 3 deficiency and total protein 4.2 deficiency in the erythrocyte membranes of a patient with HS who was a compound heterozygote for two different band 3 defects. Presumably, one mutant band 3 protein, band 3[Okinawa], binds all the available protein 4.2 in erythrocyte precursors because the other mutant band 3 protein, band 3[Fukuoka], contains a mutation in a region of the band 3–protein 4.2 interaction. Because band 3[Okinawa] cannot be inserted into the membrane, the band 3[Okinawa]–protein 4.2 complex is degraded, leading to the observed phenotype.[875]

Other Membrane Protein Defects

Inextractable spectrin was first observed some years ago in 2 of 12 patients with HS in whom spectrin failed to elute from the membrane after exposure to a low ionic strength buffer for 72 hours.[876] These are conditions that generally produce greater than 90 percent spectrin extraction. A third patient was subsequently discovered.[877] The molecular basis of this phenomenon has not been investigated, although the possibility that it might be secondary to a defect in ankyrin or β-spectrin seems obvious. In addition, some tightly bound spectrin is palmitoylated, and this fraction might be increased.[878] HS membranes contain increased amounts of hemoglobin and catalase.[879] This is a relatively nonspecific finding that is observed in a number of hemolytic anemias, particularly if red cell dehydration occurs. Its molecular basis is not understood. Two reports of apparent HS combined with partial enolase deficiency (≈50 percent) have appeared.[880, 881] In the first patient, a French woman, results of red cell osmotic fragility and autohemolysis tests were typical for HS, although spherocytes were not apparent on the blood smear. Dominant inheritance was suggested by history but could not be established because the affected father was deceased. However, dominant inheritance of both HS and partial enolase deficiency was clearly evident in the second family when both diseases could be traced through four generations. In this kindred, the enolase-deficient spherocytes resisted lysis in the acidified glycerol lysis test, another characteristic of typical HS (see later). The similarity of these two patients suggests that they may represent a unique subgroup of HS. In particular, the combination of dominant inheritance and one-half normal levels of enolase raises the possibility that the primary defect could lie in an enolase-binding membrane protein, assuming such a protein exists.

The discovery that red cell membrane proteins are phosphorylated was followed by numerous reports that phosphorylation was defective in HS. These reports are summarized and analyzed in previous editions of this book.[882] Overall, the effects were variable and generally were only demonstrable in ghosts incubated in low ionic strength buffers for relatively long periods. Initial rates of phosphorylation in HS ghosts were normal[883–885] as was membrane protein phosphorylation of intact spherocytes from splenectomized individuals.[885] It appears that the phosphorylation defects were probably secondary effects.

Secondary Membrane Effects

A large number of secondary abnormalities have been identified over the years. These are catalogued and discussed in detail in previous editions[882] and are briefly summarized later.

Membrane Lipids. The principal lipid abnormality of hereditary spherocytes is a symmetric loss of membrane lipids as part of the overall loss of membrane surface, the hallmark of the pathobiology of HS. The relative proportions of cholesterol and the various phospholipids are normal,[886] and the phospholipids show the usual transmembrane asymmetry, even in severe instances.[44, 887] It has been reported that very long chain fatty acids are missing from certain classes of phospholipids,[888] but this has not been confirmed.[889] It is unclear whether this difference is due to technical factors or to genetic heterogeneity of the disease. Even if real, it seems likely that the changes in fatty acid composition would be secondary to the underlying membrane protein defects.

Cations and Transport. It has been known for many years that HS red cells are intrinsically more leaky to Na^+ and K^+ ions than normal cells.[890–893] A similar defect exists in the erythrocytes of mice with HS.[894] The excessive Na^+ influx activates Na^+,K^+-ATPase and the monovalent cation pump, and the accelerated pumping,[895] in turn, increases ATP turnover and glycolysis. Interestingly, protein 4.2-deficient erythrocytes have increased ion transport, whereas erythrocytes deficient in spectrin, ankyrin, or band 3 have normal or increased anion transport.[896] At one time, it was believed that this modest Na^+

leak was responsible for the hemolysis of hereditary spherocytes,[892] particularly those cells trapped in the unfavorable metabolic environment of the spleen, but it now is clear that this is incorrect, because the magnitude of the Na^+ flux does not correlate with the extent of hemolysis in HS.[897] In addition, patients with hereditary stomatocytosis (see later) and a much greater defect in Na^+ permeability do not develop microspherocytes and sometimes have very little hemolysis. The leak of Na^+ into red cells in hereditary stomatocytosis is accompanied by the entry of water and cell swelling, a finding that contrasts with the well-established dehydration of hereditary spherocytes.

The dehydration of HS red cells is likely to be inflicted, at least in part, by the adverse environment of the spleen, because spherocytes from surgically removed spleens are the most dehydrated.[898] The pathways causing HS red cell dehydration have not been clearly defined. One likely candidate is increased K^+/Cl^- cotransport, which is activated by acid pH.[657] HS red cells, particularly from unsplenectomized subjects, have a low intracellular pH,[899] reflecting the low pH of the splenic environment (see later). The K^+/Cl^- cotransport pathway is also activated by oxidation,[900] which is likely to be inflicted by splenic macrophages. Lastly, hyperactivity of the Na^+-K^+ pump, triggered by increased intracellular Na^+, can dehydrate red cells directly, because three Na^+ ions are extruded in exchange for only two K^+ ions.[895] The loss of monovalent cations is accompanied by water.

Glycolysis. In general, glycolysis is mildly accelerated in HS red cells,[892, 901, 902] mostly to support increased cation pumping, and 2,3-DPG concentrations are slightly depressed,[899, 903, 904] probably because of activation of 2,3-DPG phosphatase by the acidic intracellular pH of the cell. The latter abnormalities are at least partly due to splenic detention, because the acidosis and 2,3-DPG deficiency both improve after splenectomy.[899, 903]

An apparently specific decrease in carrier-mediated transport of phosphoenolpyruvate has been noted in red cells of some patients with HS.[905] Unfortunately, only unsplenectomized patients were studied, so it is possible that the defect is caused by the metabolic derangements these cells acquire during their detention in the spleen. More likely it is caused by diminished anion exchange. Band 3 transports pyruvate and probably phosphoenolpyruvate. If so, reduced phosphoenolpyruvate transport would be expected in patients with HS and band 3 deficiency. Surprisingly, anion transport is also suppressed (30 to 35 percent) in patients with known ankyrin defects.[906] The molecular explanation is unknown.

Murine Models

A number of autosomal recessive, spherocytic hereditary hemolytic anemias have been described in the common house mouse, *Mus musculus*.[907] These are designated *sph* (spherocytosis), *ja* (jaundiced), and *nb* (normoblastosis), representing α-spectrin, β-spectrin, and ankyrin alleles. Additional alleles of *sph* have been described: *sph^1J* (formerly *sph^ha*, hemolytic anemia), *sph^2BC*, *sph^2J* (now lost), and *sph^Dem*. All of the mutants have severe hemolytic anemia, bilirubin gallstones, massive hepatosplenomegaly, and reticulocyte counts that approach 100 percent.[693]

Anemia is observed only in the homozygous state and is associated with decreased viability. Erythrocytes in homozygous, mutant animals are spectrin or spectrin/ankyrin deficient and have extremely fragile red cells. Red cells spontaneously vesiculate and ghosts disintegrate during preparation.

The *ja/ja* mutant has a defect in the spectrin β chain (Arg^{1160}→stop) and no detectable spectrin.[908] The *sph/sph* variants lack α chains, either due to decreased synthesis (*sph*, *sph^{2BC}*, and *sph^{2J}*) or to synthesis of an unstable chain (*sph^{ha}*) but have small amounts of β-spectrin. α-Spectrin gene mutations have been identified for each *sph* allele.[907, 909, 910] *sph* is a single nucleotide deletion in repeat 5 of the α-spectrin chain, leading to a frameshift and a premature chain termination. *sph^{Dem}* is a deletion of exon 11 that removes 46 amino acids near the NH$_2$ terminus of repeat 5. *sph^{2BC}* is a slicing mutation in intron 41 that leads to skipping of exon 41. *sph^{1J}* is a nonsense mutation in the extreme COOH terminus of the α-spectrin chain.

Mice with the *nb* mutation have a primary defect in ankyrin. This is due to a single nucleotide deletion leading to a frameshift and premature chain termination in the regulatory region of ankyrin.[911, 912] *nb/nb* red cells have only a trace of ankyrin mRNA and protein[424, 693] but only a partial deficiency of spectrin (50 to 70 percent of normal). This is different than ankyrin defects in human HS, in which ankyrin and spectrin levels are comparably depressed.[828, 830] *nb/nb* mice also lack ankyrin in cerebellar Purkinje cells.[424, 425] This leads to an age-related loss of Purkinje cells during the first 5 to 7 months of life and the emergence of cerebellar ataxia.[424] Spinocerebellar degeneration and related syndromes have also been reported in a few adult humans with HS,[913-921] although it is not yet known whether ankyrin is affected. Fetal *nb/nb* mice have no anemia and normal reticulocyte counts at birth,[922] possibly due to expression of ankyrin-related proteins *in utero*.[923] Humans may also be protected *in utero*, at least partially, because hydrops fetalis has not been reported in patients with probable ankyrin defects (i.e., combined spectrin/ankyrin deficiency), even in patients who become transfusion dependent after birth.

Another recessive spherocytic hemolytic anemia has been described in the deer mouse, *Peromyscus maniculatus*.[924] This disorder is less severe and closely resembles the autosomal dominant form of human HS. The spectrin content of deer mouse erythrocytes is reduced by about 20 percent.

PATHOPHYSIOLOGY

Mechanisms of Membrane Surface Loss

Vesiculation. The primary membrane lesions described earlier, all involving vertical interactions between the skeleton and the bilayer, fit the theory that HS is caused by local disconnection of the skeleton and bilayer, followed by vesiculation of the unsupported surface components. This, in turn, leads to progressive reduction in membrane surface area and to a shape called a spherocyte, although it usually ranges between a thickened discocyte and a spherostomatocyte.[925] The phospholipid and cholesterol contents of isolated spherocytes are decreased by 15 to 20 percent, consistent with the loss of surface area.[926-929] Biomechanical measurements show that HS membranes are fragile. The force required to fragment the membrane is diminished and is proportional to the density of spectrin on the membrane.[831, 832] Membrane elasticity and bending stiffness are also reduced and are proportional to spectrin density.[832, 930] In addition, HS red cells lose membrane more readily than normal red cells when metabolically deprived or when their ghosts are subjected to conditions facilitating vesiculation.[929, 930-933] However, this has not been shown to occur in metabolically healthy spherocytes, perhaps because it occurs slowly (1 to 2 percent/day) under such conditions. Because budding red cells are rarely observed in typical blood smears from patients with HS, the postulated vesiculation must either involve microscopic vesicles or occur in the reticuloendothelial system. When membrane vesicles are induced in normal red cells, they originate at the tips of spicules, where the lipid bilayer uncouples from the underlying skeleton.[597] The vesicles are small (about 100 nm) and devoid of hemoglobin and skeletal proteins, so that they are invisible during a conventional examination of stained blood films. Tiny (50 to 80 nm) bumps have been detected in studies with an atomic force microscope, on the surface of red cells obtained from patients with HS whose red cells are actively hemolyzing.[934] The bumps could be microvesicles, although this needs to be proven using more conventional microscopic techniques. They are less than the length of a spectrin molecule (100 nm) and are not present on red cells from splenectomized patients.

Models Relating Membrane Defects and Surface Loss. The observation that spectrin or spectrin/ankyrin deficiencies are common in HS has led to the suggestion that they are the primary cause of spherocytosis. According to this hypothesis, interactions of spectrin with bilayer lipids or proteins are required to stabilize the membrane. Spectrin-deficient areas would tend to bud off, leading to spherocytosis. However, this conjecture does not explain how spherocytes develop in patients whose red cells are deficient in band 3 or protein 4.2 but have normal amounts of spectrin.[502, 828] An alternate hypothesis argues that the bilayer is stabilized by interactions between lipids and the abundant band 3 molecules (Fig. 15–16). Each band 3 molecule about 14 hydrophobic transmembrane helices, many of which must interact with lipids. Such interactions presumably spread beyond the first layer of lipids and influence the mobility of lipids in successive layers. In deficient red cells the area between band 3 molecules would increase, on average, and the stabilizing effect would diminish. Transient fluctuations in the local density of band 3 could aggravate this situation and allow unsupported lipids to be lost, resulting in spherocytosis. This hypothesis is supported by targeted disruption of the band 3 gene in mice. Erythrocytes from these mice lose massive amounts of membrane surface despite a normal membrane skeleton.[689] This concept is also consistent with early studies of intramembrane particle aggregation, which leads to particle-free domains, as discussed earlier in the chapter. These domains are unstable, giving rise to surface blebs that are subsequently released from the cells as vesicles.[601] Additionally, in a

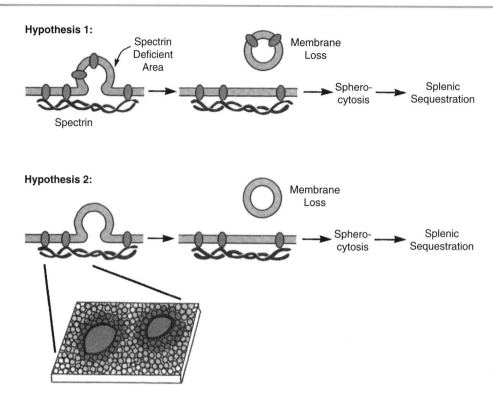

FIGURE 15–16. Two hypotheses concerning the mechanism of membrane loss in hereditary spherocytosis. *Hypothesis 1* assumes that the "membrane" (i.e., the lipid bilayer and integral membrane proteins) is directly stabilized by interactions with spectin or other elements of the membrane skeleton. Spectrin-deficient areas, lacking support, bud off, leading to spherocytosis. *Hypothesis 2* assumes the membrane is stabilized by interactions of band 3 with neighboring lipids. The influence of band 3 extends into the lipid milieu because the first layer of immobilized lipids slows the lipids in the next layer and so on. In band 3–deficient cells the area between lipid molecules increases and unsupported lipids are lost. Spectrin/ankyrin deficiency allows band 3 molecules to diffuse and transiently cluster, with the same consequences. This hypothesis is supportd by the fact that mice that lack band 3, owing to a targeted gene disruption, have marked membrane vesiculation and spherocytosis despite a nearly intact membrane skeleton.[603] (From Lux SE, Palek J: Disorders of the red cell membrane. In Handin RJ, Lux SE, Stossel TP (eds): Blood: Principles and Practice of Hematology. Philadelphia, Lippincott-Raven, 1995, pp 1701–1818.)

subset of patients with band 3 deficiency, the protein appears to be lost from the cells during their residence in the circulation. The concomitant loss of the "boundary" lipids may contribute to the deficiency of surface area. Spectrin- and ankyrin-deficient red cells could become spherocytic by a similar mechanism. Because spectrin filaments corral band 3 molecules and limit their lateral movement, a decrease in spectrin would allow band 3 molecules to diffuse and transiently cluster, fostering vesiculation.

Loss of Cellular Deformability. Hereditary spherocytes hemolyze because of the rheologic consequences of their decreased surface-to-volume ratio. The red cell membrane is very flexible, but it can only expand its surface area about 3 percent before rupturing.[935] Thus, erythrocyte becomes less and less deformable as surface area is lost. For HS red cells, poor deformability is only a hindrance in the spleen, because the cells have a nearly normal life span after splenectomy.[936, 937]

Splenic Sequestration and Conditioning

In the spleen most of the arterial blood empties directly into the splenic cords, a tortuous maze of interconnecting narrow passages formed by reticular cells and lined with phagocytes.[938–943] Histologically, this is an "open" circulation, but apparently most of the blood that enters the cords normally travels by fairly direct (i.e., functionally

closed) pathways.[828, 829] If passage through these channels is impeded, red cells are diverted deeper into the labyrinthine portions of the cords where blood flow is slow and the cells may be detained for minutes to hours. Whichever route is taken, to reenter the circulation red cells must squeeze through spaces between the endothelial cells that form the walls of the venous sinuses. Even when maximally distended, these narrow slits are always much smaller than red cells, which are greatly distorted during their passage.[940, 941] Experiments have shown that spherocytes are selectively sequestered at this cord-sinus juncture.[944–946] As a consequence, spleens from patients with HS have massively congested cords and relatively empty sinuses.[938, 947–949] In electron micrographs, few spherocytes are seen in transit through the sinus wall,[938, 948, 950] which contrasts to the situation in normal spleens where cells in transit are readily found.[942]

During detention in the spleen, HS red cells undergo additional damage marked by further loss of surface area and an increase in cell density. Many of these "conditioned" red cells escape the hostile environment of the spleen and reenter the circulation. In unsplenectomized patients with HS, two populations of spherocytes are detectable: a minor population of hyperchromic "microspherocytes" that form the "tail" of very fragile cells in the unincubated osmotic fragility test and a major population that may be only slightly more spheroidal than normal. It was known by 1913 that red cells obtained from the splenic vein were more osmotically fragile than those in the peripheral circulation,[951] and this fact was confirmed by other hematologists of the time[767, 952]; however, its significance was not clear until the classic studies of Emerson and Young in the 1950s.[946, 953] These investigators showed that osmotically fragile microspherocytes are concentrated in and emanate from the splenic pulp. After splenectomy, spherocytosis persists, but the tail of hyperfragile red cells is no longer evident on osmotic fragility testing. These and other data led to the conclusion that the spleen detains and "conditions" circulating HS red cells in a way that increases their spheroidicity and hastens their demise.[946, 954, 955] The kinetics of this process were illustrated *in vivo* by Griggs, who found that a cohort of ^{59}Fe-labeled HS red cells gradually shifted from the major, less fragile population to the more fragile, conditioned population 7 to 11 days after their release into the circulation.[955] Although most conditioned HS red cells that escape the spleen are probably recaptured and destroyed, the damage incurred is sufficient to permit extrasplenic recognition and removal, because conditioned spherocytes, isolated from the spleen and reinfused postoperatively, are rapidly eliminated.[955, 956]

The mechanism of splenic conditioning is less certain. It is difficult to obtain accurate information about the cordal environment, but the existing data suggest it is metabolically inhospitable,[945, 954, 957, 958] although perhaps less so than originally believed.[943] Crowded red cells must compete for limited supplies of glucose[957] in acidic surroundings (pH ≈ 6.6–7.2)[943, 945, 954, 958] where glycolysis is inhibited.[959, 960] The acidic environment also induces Cl^- and water entry and cell swelling[961] but, as discussed earlier, it also stimulates the K^+/Cl^- cotransporter, which produces a net loss of K^+ and water from the cells. The adverse effects of the cordal environment are further compounded by the presence of oxidant-producing macrophages. It has also been suggested that methylation of erythrocyte membrane proteins could contribute to the splenic conditioning of spectrin-deficient HS red cells.[962] Hence, the spherocyte, detained in the splenic cords because of its surface deficiency, is stressed by erythrostasis in a metabolically threatening environment.

Erythrostasis. The spherocyte is particularly vulnerable to erythrostasis. This is the basis of the well-known autohemolysis test.[963] During prolonged sterile incubation in the absence of supplemental glucose, red cells undergo a series of changes that culminate in hemolysis. The sequence of the changes is the same for HS and normal red cells; however, because HS cells are abnormally leaky and bear unstable membranes, their degeneration is accelerated. HS red cells are initially jeopardized because their membrane permeability to Na^+ is mildly increased.[891, 892] Their propensity to accumulate Na^+ and water is normally balanced by increased Na^+ pumping; however, the increased dependence on glycolysis is detrimental in erythrostasis where substrate is limited.[892] HS red cells exhaust serum glucose and become ATP depleted more rapidly than normal red cells. As ATP levels fall, ATP-dependent Na^+-K^+ and Ca^{2+} pumps fail, and the

cells gain Na^+ and water and swell. Later, when the Ca^{2+}-dependent K^+ (Gardos) pathway is activated, K^+ loss predominates and the cells lose water and shrink. The Na^+ gain is accelerated in HS red cells but is insufficient by itself to induce hemolysis. However, HS red cells are doubly jeopardized. As noted earlier, they are inherently unstable and fragment excessively during metabolic depletion.[929–933] Membrane lipids (and probably integral membrane proteins) are lost at more than twice the normal rate.[931] At first this surface loss is balanced by cell dehydration, but eventually (30 to 48 hours) membrane loss predominates, the cells exceed their critical hemolytic volume, and autohemolysis ensues.

Splenic Trapping. Calculations indicate the average normal red cell passes through the splenic cords about 14,000 times during its lifetime[149] and has an average transit time of 30 to 40 seconds, surprisingly close to measured transient times in normal human spleens *in vivo*.[964] The calculated residence time of the average HS red cell in the splenic cords is much longer, perhaps as long as 15 to 150 minutes, but still far short of the time required for metabolic depletion to occur. This conclusion is supported by direct analysis of splenic red cells. HS red cells obtained from the splenic pulp and containing 80 to 100 percent conditioned cells are moderately cation depleted and show changes in ADP and 2,3-DPG concentrations consistent with metabolism in an acidic environment, but their ATP levels are normal.[898] Others have reported similar results.[965, 966]

The data suggest that splenic conditioning is caused by mechanisms other than ATP depletion. For example, K^+ loss and membrane instability may be exacerbated by the high concentrations of acids and oxidants that must exist in a spleen filled with activated macrophages lunching on trapped HS red cells. *In vitro,* oxidants from activated phagocytes can diffuse across the membranes of bystander red cells and damage intracellular proteins within minutes. Red cells moving through the rapid transit pathways in the spleen might escape damage, but those caught in cordal traffic would be vulnerable. Oxidants, even in relatively low concentrations, cause selective K^+ loss by a variety of mechanisms[967–970] and also damage membrane skeletal proteins.[733, 745, 747, 971–974] Finally, there is preliminary evidence that HS red cells may be abnormally sensitive to oxidants.[975] When exposed to peroxides they undergo remarkable blebbing and, presumably, vesiculation.[975] If a similar process occurs in the spleen, it could be responsible for the excessive surface loss observed in conditioned cells.

Residence in the spleen may also activate proteolytic enzymes in the red cell membrane. Membrane proteins of red cells from patients with HS and splenomegaly are excessively digested during *in vitro* incubations and the degree of proteolysis correlates with splenic size.[976] Whether this occurs *in vivo* is uncertain, but if so it could contribute to skeletal weakness and membrane loss. The possibility that macrophages may directly condition HS red cells should also be considered. It is well known that spherocytosis often results from the interaction of IgG-coated red cells with macrophages, but HS red cells do not have abnormal levels of surface IgG.[977] Macrophages also bear receptors for oxidized lipids (scavenger receptor) and PS, but there is no evidence at present that HS red cells expose the relevant ligands. The involvement of macrophages is supported by observations that large doses of corticosteroids markedly ameliorate HS in unsplenectomized patients.[978, 979] The effects are similar to those produced by splenectomy; hemoglobin production, reticulocytosis, and fecal urobilinogen level declined; red cell life span doubled; and hyperspheroidal, conditioned red cells disappeared from the circulation. It is well known that similar doses of corticosteroids inhibit splenic processing and destruction of IgG- or C3b-coated red cells in patients with immunohemolytic anemias, probably by suppressing macrophage-induced red cell sphering and phagocytosis.[980, 981] Electron microscopy shows that splenic erythrophagocytosis is common in HS, particularly in the splenic cords.[948, 950, 982] In addition, phagocytes expressed from the cords of patients with HS contain bits of ghostlike "debris,"[983] presumably resulting from membrane fragmentation.

In summary, it is clear that HS red cells are selectively detained by the spleen and that this custody is detrimental, leading to a loss of membrane surface that fosters further splenic trapping and eventual destruction. It appears that the primary membrane defects involve deficiencies or defects of spectrin, ankyrin, protein 4.2, or band 3, but much remains to be learned about why these proteins are defective and how this causes surface loss. Obvious membrane budding and fragmentation are rare in patients with HS. It appears that the HS skeleton (including band 3) may not adequately support all regions of the lipid bilayer, leading to the loss of small areas of untethered lipids and integral membrane proteins (Fig. 15–16). It is not clear whether this is due directly to deficiency of spectrin and ankyrin or whether spectrin/ankyrin deficiency operates indirectly by increasing the lateral mobility of band 3 molecules and decreasing their stabilization of the lipid bilayer. The mechanisms of splenic conditioning and red cell destruction are also uncertain. Kinetic considerations make it unlikely that HS red cells are continuously trapped in the cords for the long periods required to induce passive sphering and autohemolysis by metabolic depletion; however, repetitious accrual of metabolic damage remains a possibility. A unique susceptibility of the HS red cell to the acidic, oxidant-rich environment of the spleen and active intervention of macrophages in the processing of erythrostatically damaged spherocytes must also be considered.

CLINICAL AND LABORATORY CHARACTERISTICS

Clinical Characteristics

Classification

Typical Hereditary Spherocytosis. The typical clinical picture of HS combines evidence of hemolysis (anemia, jaundice, reticulocytosis, gallstones, and splenomegaly) with spherocytosis (spherocytes on a peripheral blood smear and positive osmotic fragility or acidified glycerol lysis test results), and a positive family history (Table 15–7). Mild, moderate, and severe forms of HS have been defined according to differences in the hemoglobin and bilirubin concentrations and the reticulocyte count (Table 15–8).[772, 830] Typical HS is associated

TABLE 15–7. Characteristics of Hereditary Spherocytosis

CLINICAL MANIFESTATIONS

Anemia
Splenomegaly
Intermittent jaundice
    From hemolysis
    From biliary obstruction
Aplastic crises
Inheritance
    Dominant ≈ 2/3
    Nondominant ≈ 1/3 *de novo* or recessive
Rare manifestations
    Leg ulcers
    Extramedullary hematopoietic tumors
    Cardiomyopathy
    Spinocerebellar ataxia
    Myopathy
Excellent response to splenectomy

LABORATORY CHARACTERISTICS

Reticulocytosis
Spherocytosis
Elevated mean corpuscular hemoglobin concentration
Increased osmotic fragility
Normal direct antiglobulin test

with both dominant and nondominant inheritance. In many patients, the nondominant disease is more severe, but there is considerable overlap.[772, 775, 780] Clinical severity and the response to splenectomy roughly parallel the degree of spectrin (or ankyrin) deficiency in patients with defects in either protein.[772, 780, 830, 838, 847] It is not known whether analogous correlations are true for patients with other HS-related mutations.

HS typically presents in infancy or childhood but may present at any age.[984] In children, anemia is the most usual presenting complaint (50 percent), followed by splenomegaly, jaundice, or a positive family history.[985] No comparable data exist for adults. Two thirds to three fourths of patients with HS have incompletely compensated hemolysis and mild to moderate anemia. The anemia is often asymptomatic except for fatigue and mild pallor or, in children, nonspecific parental complaints such as irritability. Jaundice is seen at some time in about one half of patients, usually in association with viral infections. When jaundice is present it is acholuric (i.e., unconjugated [indirect] hyperbilirubinemia without detectable direct bilirubinuria). Palpable splenomegaly is detectable in about one half of infants and most (75 to 95 percent) older children and adults.[985–987] Typically, the spleen is modestly enlarged (2 to 6 cm), but it may be massive.[988, 989] There is no proven correlation between the size of the spleen and the severity of HS, although, given the pathophysiology and the response of the disease to splenectomy, such a correlation probably exists.

Silent Carrier State. The parents of patients with "nondominant" HS are clinically asymptomatic and do not have anemia, splenomegaly, hyperbilirubinemia, or spherocytosis on peripheral blood smears.[780] However, most do have subtle laboratory signs of HS, including slight reticulocytosis (average, 2.1±0.8 percent), diminished haptoglobin levels, slightly elevated osmotic fragility,

TABLE 15–8. Clinical Classification of Hereditary Spherocytosis

Trait	Trait	Mild Spherocytosis	Moderate Spherocytosis	Moderately Severe Spherocytosis*	Severe Spherocytosis†
Hemoglobin (g/dL)	Normal	11–15	8–12	6–8	<6
Reticulocytes (%)	1–3	3–8	≥8	≥10	≥10
Bilirubin (mg/dL)	0–1	1–2	≥2	2–3	≥3
Spectrin content (% of normal)‡	100	80–100	50–80	40–80§	20–50
Peripheral smear	Normal	Mild spherocytosis	Spherocytosis	Spherocytosis	Spherocytosis and poikilocytosis
Osmotic fragility					
Fresh blood	Normal	Normal or slightly increased	Distinctly increased	Distinctly increased	Distinctly increased
Incubated blood	Slightly increased	Distinctly increased	Distinctly increased	Distinctly increased	Markedly increased

*Values in untransfused patients.

†By definition, patients with severe spherocytosis are transfusion dependent.

‡Normal (± SD) = 245 ± 27 × 10⁵ spectrin dimers per erythrocyte. In most patients ankyrin content is decreased to a comparable degree. A minority of HS patients lack band 3 or protein 4.2 and may have mild to moderate spherocytosis with normal amounts of spectrin and ankyrin.

§The spectrin content is variable in this group of patients, presumably reflecting heterogeneity of the underlying pathophysiology.

Adapted from Eber SW, Armbrust R, Schröter W: Variable clinical severity of hereditary spherocytosis: relation to erythrocytic spectrin concentration, osmotic fragility and autohemolysis. J Pediatr 1990; 177: 409; Pekrun A, Eber SW, et al: Combined ankyrin and spectrin deficiency in hereditary spherocytosis. Ann Hematol 1993; 67: 89; and Lux SE, J Palek: Disorders of the red cell membrane. In Handin RI, Lux SE, Stossel TP (eds): Blood: Principles and Practice of Hematology, Philadelphia, J.B. Lippincott Co., 1995, pp 1701–1818.

shortened acidified glycerol lysis time, or elevated autohemolysis. The incubated osmotic fragility test is probably the most sensitive measure of this condition, particularly the 100 percent lysis point, which is significantly elevated in carriers (0.43±0.05 g NaCl/dL) compared with that in normal subjects (0.23±0.07 g NaCl/dL).[772] However, no single test is sufficient. Carriers can only be detected reliably by considering the results of a battery of tests. From the incidence of recessive HS (1 in 20,000; that is, ≈25 percent of all occurrences of HS, which is 1 in 5000 in the United States)[769] one can estimate that roughly 1.4 percent of the population should be silent carriers. Interestingly, screening of normal Norwegian[770] or German[771] blood donors with osmotic fragility or acidified glycerol lysis tests shows a 0.9 to 1.1 percent incidence of previously unsuspected "very mild" HS. Presumably, many of these individuals are silent carriers.

Mild Hereditary Spherocytosis. Red cell production and destruction are balanced or nearly balanced in 20 to 30 percent of patients with HS.[986, 990] These persons are considered to have "compensated hemolysis." Such patients are not anemic and are usually asymptomatic. In some patients, diagnosis may be difficult because hemolysis, splenomegaly, and spherocytosis are unusually mild. For example, in this group of patients, reticulocyte counts are generally less than 6 percent and only 60 percent have significant spherocytosis on peripheral blood smears[772]; red cell spectrin and ankyrin levels are typically more than 80 percent of normal.[772] Hemolysis may become severe with illnesses that cause splenomegaly, such as infectious mononucleosis.[991] Hemolysis may also be exacerbated by pregnancy[992, 993] or exercise,[993] to the point where it may impair athletic performance in endurance sports, even in patients with mild disease. In many of these patients HS is diagnosed during family studies or discovered as when they are adults and splenomegaly or gallstones appear. Although mild HS is usually familial, it develops sporadically in families with more severe disease.[994] Presumably this is due to the coinheritance of modifying genes, such as those affecting spectrin or ankyrin synthesis or splenic function.

One of the interesting mysteries about HS is why patients with compensated hemolysis continue to have erythroid hyperplasia when their hemoglobin levels are normal. It is difficult to reconcile this phenomenon with the generally accepted theory that erythropoiesis is regulated by tissue hypoxia. One possibility is the concentration of 2,3-DPG, which reportedly is low in hereditary spherocytes before splenectomy (although the oxygen half-saturation pressure of hemoglobin P_{50} of blood from HS patients is normal).[899, 903] Another possibility is that the dehydrated HS red cells are rheologically impaired and do not perfuse the juxtaglomerular renal vessels, the site or erythropoietin production, normally, even when the hematocrit is normal. In fact, recent measurements showing that erythropoietin is overproduced and serum erythropoietin is inappropriately elevated (up to eight times normal) in HS[995] are compatible with either possibility.

Moderate and Severe Hereditary Spherocytosis. A small fraction of patients with HS (5 to 10 percent) have moderately severe to severe anemia. Patients with "moderately severe" disease typically have a hemoglobin value of 6 to 8 g/dL, a reticulocyte count of about 10 percent, a bilirubin level of 2 to 3 mg/dL, and 40 to 80 percent of the normal red cell spectrin content. This category includes patients with both dominant and recessive HS and a variety of molecular defects. Patients with "severe" disease, by definition, have life-threatening anemia and are transfusion dependent. They almost always have recessive HS. Most probably have isolated, severe spectrin deficiency (<40 percent of normal), which is thought to be due to a defect in α-spectrin.[839] Some may have ankyrin defects.[694] Patients with severe HS are also distinguished by red cell morphology. They often have some irregularly contoured or budding spherocytes or bizarre poikilocytes in addition to typical spherocytes.[694, 829] Such cells are rare before splenectomy in patients with moderately severe disease, although some may be seen after splenectomy. In addition to the risks of recurrent transfusions, these patients often suffer from an aplastic crisis and those with severe HS may develop growth retardation, delayed sexual maturation, or aspects of thalassemic facies.[829, 988, 989]

Hereditary Spherocytosis in Pregnancy. In general, unsplenectomized patients with HS have no significant complications during pregnancy except for anemia, which worsens due to plasma volume expansion[996] and sometimes due to increased hemolysis.[992, 993] Hemolytic crises during pregnancy requiring transfusion have been reported.[993] Folic acid deficiency is also a risk.[997, 998] One group reported that 20 percent of patients with HS received transfusions during pregnancy,[993] but in the authors' experience, pregnant patients with HS rarely need transfusion.

Hereditary Spherocytosis in the Neonate. HS often presents as jaundice in the first few days of life.[999–1001] Perhaps as many as one half of all patients with HS have a history of neonatal jaundice[1002] and 91 percent of infants discovered to have HS in the first week of life are jaundiced (bilirubin level >10 mg/dL).[1000] Hyperbilirubinemia usually appears in the first 2 days of life and bilirubin levels may rise rapidly,[999, 1001, 1002] driven by the combination of hemolysis and the reduced capacity of the neonatal liver to conjugate bilirubin. Kernicterus is a risk[999]; thus, exchange transfusions are sometimes necessary, but in most patients the jaundice is controlled with phototherapy. Homozygosity for a common polymorphism in the promoter region of the uridine diphosphate–glucuronsyltransferase gene associated with Gilbert syndrome has been associated with aggravation of neonatal anemia in HS.[1003]

Only 43 percent of neonates with HS are anemic at birth (hemoglobin level <15 g/dL), and severe anemia is rare.[1000] In fact, in most patients hemoglobin levels are normal at birth, then decrease sharply over the first 3 weeks of life, leading to a transient, severe anemia.[1004] In up to three fourths of infants, the anemia is severe enough to warrant transfusion. This anemia appears to be aggravated by an inability of the infant's red cells to mount an appropriate erythropoietic response to anemia and to the development of splenic function. Most infants will outgrow the need for transfusion by the end of the first year of life.[1004]

Hydrops fetalis has been reported in a few rare patients and is associated with homozygosity or compound heterozygosity for spectrin or band 3 defects.[776, 803, 862] If hydrops fetalis is detected *in utero*, these infants may require intrauterine transfusions. No instances of hydrops fetalis have been associated with ankyrin deficiency. It is possible that infants with ankyrin defects, similar to ankyrin-deficient *nb/nb* mice,[922, 923] are partially protected *in utero* by the expression of ankyrin-related proteins in embryonic and fetal erythroblasts.

The diagnosis of HS is often more difficult in the neonatal period than later in life. Splenomegaly is uncommon; at most the spleen tip is palpable, and reticulocytosis

is variable and usually not severe.[1001, 1002] Only 35 percent of affected neonates have a reticulocyte count greater than 10 percent.[1000] In addition, the haptoglobin level is not a reliable indicator of hemolysis during the first few months of life.[1005] An even greater problem is that 33 percent of neonates with HS do not have significant numbers of spherocytes on their peripheral blood smears.[1000] Moreover, because fetal red cells are more osmotically resistant than adult cells when fresh, and more osmotically sensitive after incubation at 37°C for 24 hours,[1000, 1006] the osmotic fragility test may give false-positive (incubated) or false-negative (unincubated) results unless fetal controls are used. Fortunately, these results have been published,[1000] and they appear to reliably differentiate neonates with HS, particularly when the incubated osmotic fragility test is used.[1000–1002] Studying the erythrocytes from the parents often provides a clue to the diagnosis of HS, particularly if the infant has received a transfusion.[1007]

No evidence exists that patients with HS who show symptoms as neonates have a more severe form of the disease, even those infants who become progressively more anemic and require transfusion. This transient anemia usually happens because the marrow response to anemia is more sluggish than normal. The reticulocyte count is relatively low for the degree of anemia. Fortunately, the problem is transient, except in rare patients with severe HS, and usually remits after one or two transfusions. Administration of recombinant human erythropoietin to infants with HS was shown to be beneficial in reducing blood transfusions in an uncontrolled, open label study.[1008] In the author's experience, erythropoietin administration has not been beneficial for these patients, and in fact hemolysis worsened in two of them. If the child is otherwise well, the authors allow the hemoglobin level to fall to 5.5 to 6.5 g/dL before giving transfusions to try to stimulate the marrow, and they only raise the hemoglobin level to 9 to 11 g/dL after transfusion to avoid suppressing the desired marrow response. After the bone marrow responds, the course of the disease depends on the equilibrium between the rates of red cell production and destruction.

Laboratory Features

Peripheral Blood Smear. Spherocytes (Fig. 15–17) are the hallmark of HS. They are dense, round, and hyperchromic; lack central pallor; and have a decreased mean cell diameter. They are almost uniformly present (up to 97 percent) on blood smears from patients with moderate or moderately severe HS but are present in only 25 to 35 percent of patients with mild HS.[772, 985, 986] Hereditary spherocytes are technically misnamed; they range in shape from thickened discocytes to spherostomatocytes.[925]

In most patients with HS, spherocytes and microspherocytes are the only abnormal cells on the peripheral smear (other than polychromatophils). Rarely, a few stomatospherocytes may be seen. In severe HS, dense, irregular, contracted, or budding spherocytes may appear, and in the most severe occurrences, these abnormal forms may dominate the blood smear.

Specific morphologic abnormalities have been described in association with some membrane defects in HS. Before splenectomy, patients with band 3-deficient HS may have a

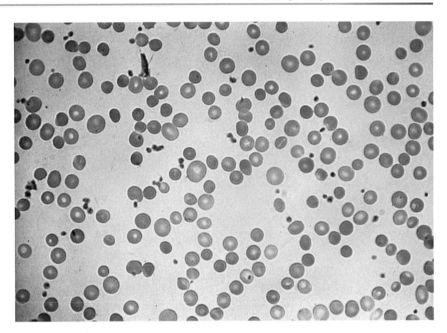

FIGURE 15–17. Peripheral blood smear from a patient with typical hereditary spherocytosis. Small, dense round spherocytes are visible throughout the smear.

small number of mushroom-shaped red cells or pincered cells on peripheral blood films.[1009] Acanthocytes or hyperchromic echinocytes are present in many patients with β-spectrin defects[842] before splenectomy, and their numbers increase after the operation. Other patients with β-spectrin defects, especially truncated β chains, have spherocytic elliptocytosis (see later). Acanthopoikilocytes[874] and oval-ostomatocytes[816] have been observed in some patients with protein 4.2 deficiency. Other patients have typical spherocytosis.[502] No specific morphologic abnormality other than spherocytosis has been identified in patients with ankyrin defects, probably the most common subgroup.[781] Bone marrow erythroblasts are morphologically normal[1010] and reticulocytes are only slightly spheroidal[1011] in typical HS, because erythrocytes gradually acquire the spherocytic shape in the circulation. Nucleated red cells are uncommon in blood smears[985] except in the most severe forms of HS.[829] Howell-Jolly bodies are also uncommon before splenectomy (4 percent of patients)[985] and suggest reticuloendothelial blockade. When a smear from a patient with suspected spherocytosis is examined, it is important that it be a high-quality smear with the erythrocytes well separated and some cells with central pallor in the field of examination, because spherocytes are a common artifact on peripheral blood smears.

Red Cell Indices. Most patients have mild to moderate HS with mild anemia (hemoglobin level of 9 to 12 g/dL) or no anemia at all (so-called compensated hemolysis). In moderate to severe HS, the hemoglobin concentration ranges from 6 to 9 g/dL. In patients with the most severe disease, the hemoglobin concentration may drop to as low as 4 to 5 g/dL. The mean corpuscular hemoglobin concentration (MCHC) of HS red cells is increased, owing to relative cellular dehydration.[986] Spherocyte Na^+ concentrations are normal or slightly increased, but K^+ concentration and water content are low, particularly in cells harvested from the splenic pulp.[898, 1012–1014]

The average MCHC exceeds the upper limit of normal (36 percent) in about one half of patients with HS, but all

patients have some dehydrated cells.[986] An MCHC greater than 35 g/dL has a sensitivity of 70 percent and a specificity of 86 percent.[1015] Combining the MCHC with the erythrocyte distribution width may lead to a specificity approaching 100 percent.[1015] The Technicon H1 blood counter and its successors (Technicon Corp., Tarrytown, NY), which measure mean corpuscular volume (MCV) by light scattering, provide a histogram of MCHCs that has been claimed to be accurate enough to identify nearly all patients with HS.[1014, 1016, 1017] This may be one of the easiest and most accurate ways to diagnose HS, particularly when one member of a family is already known to have HS and an inexpensive method of screening other family members is desired. Similar techniques, such as dual-angle laser scattering cytometry, have been evaluated in small numbers of patients as a rapid technique to assess the severity of HS.[1018] The MCHC and MCV fall within the normal range in HS,[873] except in severe HS in which the MCV may be slightly low.[829] However, the MCV is relatively low for the age of the cells (reticulocytes have a high MCV) in all patients with HS, reflecting the dehydrated state of HS red cells.

Osmotic Fragility Test. In the normal erythrocyte, a redundancy of cell membrane gives the cell its characteristic discoid shape and provides it with abundant surface area relative to cell volume. In spherocytes, there is a decrease in surface area relative to cell volume, resulting in the characteristic osmotic fragility. Osmotic fragility testing (Fig. 15–18) is performed by suspending red cells in increasingly hypotonic buffered NaCl.[954, 1019–1022] In hypotonic solutions, normal erythrocytes are able to increase their volume by swelling until they become spherical and burst, releasing hemoglobin into the supernatant. Cells that begin with a decreased surface-to-volume ratio, like spherocytes or stomatocytes, reach the spherical limit at a higher NaCl concentration than normal cells and are termed *osmotically fragile*. Freshly drawn red cells from approximately one fourth of individuals with HS will have a normal osmotic fragility, with the osmotic fragility curve

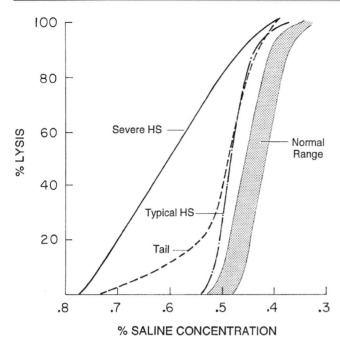

FIGURE 15–18. Osmotic fragility curves in hereditary spherocytosis. The *shaded area* is the normal range. Results representative of both typical and severe spherocytosis are shown. A "tail," representing very fragile erythrocytes that have been conditioned by the spleen, is commonly seen in many patients with HS before splenectomy.

approximating the number of spherocytes seen on peripheral smear.[987, 1021] However, after incubation at 37°C for 24 hours, HS red cells lose membrane surface area more readily than normal red cells because their membranes are leaky and unstable. This incubation accentuates the defect in HS erythrocytes and brings out the defect on osmotic fragility, making osmotic fragility testing the most sensitive test routinely available for diagnosing HS.[904] This is surprising because osmotic fragility reflects a secondary property of HS red cells, the loss of surface area, instead of the primary molecular defect. When the spleen is present, a subpopulation of very fragile erythrocytes that have been conditioned by the spleen form the "tail" of the osmotic fragility curve. This tail disappears after splenectomy.

Modifications of the osmotic fragility test have been proposed. Some have suggested that addition of 3 µmol/L ouabain during the 24-hour preincubation increases the sensitivity of the incubated osmotic fragility test, particularly for mildly affected subjects.[1023, 1024] However, this has not been confirmed.[1025] Another group has used logarithmic transforms of the osmotic fragility curve to simplify calculation of the 50 percent hemolysis point[1026]; however, this de-emphasizes the beginning and endpoints of hemolysis, which can be diagnostically useful in some patients and in silent carriers.[772] The best method for demonstrating the low surface-to-volume ratio of hereditary spherocytes is osmotic gradient ektacytometry.[1027, 1028] However, only a few laboratories are equipped with the instrument for this test.

Additional Diagnostic Tests.

Acidified Glycerol Lysis Test and Pink Test. The glycerol lysis test, in which glycerol is used to retard the osmotic swelling of red cells, was developed as an alterna-

tive to the osmotic fragility test. It is based on the rate rather than on the extent of hemolysis. The original glycerol lysis test lacked sensitivity and specificity.[1029] An acidified version, the acidified glycerol lysis test (AGLT), was more sensitive for some researchers[1030] but was not completely specific.[1031] For unknown reasons, the accuracy of the standard AGLT is greatly improved if the samples are preincubated at room temperature for 24 hours (incubated AGLT).[1032–1034] Under these conditions, for some investigators the sensitivity and specificity of the test approach 100 percent, similar to those for the incubated osmotic fragility test. Eber and associates[771] found that changing the concentration of the sodium phosphate buffer from 5.3 to 9.3 mmol/L gives 100 percent sensitivity and specificity without the need for preincubation. The modified test is easy to perform and requires very little blood. Ethylenediamine-tetraacetic acid (EDTA)–anticoagulated blood (20 µL) is diluted into a solution of 9.3 mmol/L sodium phosphate and buffered 2 mol/L glycerol–saline (pH 6.90), and the fall in absorbance at 625 nm (largely turbidity) is measured as the red cells hemolyze. The halftime for AGLT lysis is more than 30 minutes for normal samples and less than 5 minutes for HS samples. Another adaptation of the original glycerol lysis test, called the Pink test, is more reproducible and accurate than the original[1035] but requires a 1-day preincubation.[1036] Modifications of the test have made it adaptable to micro size samples (e.g., fingerstick blood samples).[1036, 1037] However, direct comparisons suggest that it is less specific than the osmotic fragility or incubated AGLT tests.[1032] Because the modified AGLT test has also been adapted to micro samples,[687] it would appear to be the test of choice if osmotic fragility testing is not available.

Hypertonic Cryohemolysis Test. This method is based on the fact that HS red cells are particularly sensitive to cooling at 0°C in hypertonic solutions.[1038–1040] It has been claimed that this test is 94 to 100 percent sensitive for HS, but the specificity is only 94 percent for normal individuals and 86 percent for patients with autoimmune hemolytic anemia. The test is independent of the surface-to-volume ratio of the cells, which is an advantage compared with other diagnostic tests.

Autohemolysis Test. The autohemolysis of erythrocytes after 48 hours at 37°C is normally less than 5 percent in the absence of glucose or less than 1 percent in the presence of glucose. Autohemolysis of spherocytes is increased to 15 to 45 percent in the absence of glucose.[963, 987, 1041] In HS, the degree of autohemolysis is reduced by the addition of glucose,[987, 1013, 1041] whereas in acquired disorders such as immune-mediated anemias, the degree of autohemolysis is not reduced. Thus, if positive results on the autohemolysis test suggest an intrinsic red cell abnormality whereas negative test results are noncontributory. Although this differentiation may be helpful, the autohemolysis test is time consuming and cumbersome, gives variable results, and is only rarely performed.

Membrane Protein Analysis. Specialized testing is available to study patients with complicated disease or those for whom additional information is desired. Useful tests for these purposes include structural and functional studies of erythrocyte membrane proteins such as protein quantitation (see later), limited tryptic digestion of spectrin, membrane protein synthesis and assembly, or ion transport studies. Membrane rigidity and fragility may be examined using an ektacytometer.

Membrane Protein Quantitation. Membrane protein concentrations are usually assessed using SDS gels. Individual stained bands are quantified by densitometry or by eluting the dye from an excised band and measuring its concentration spectrophotometrically. This technique is satisfactory for detecting spectrin deficiency (expressed as a spectrin-to-band 3 ratio),[1042] although it is not as accurate as a radioimmunoassay[828, 829] or enzyme-linked immunoassay.[830] With densitometry spectrin and ankyrin deficiencies may be underestimated because it normalizes them to band 3, which is partially lost along with membrane lipids as spherocytes circulate. As a result, the spectrin-to-band 3 ratio is lower after splenectomy. This is even more so for ankyrin, which is present in smaller amounts and migrates close to β-spectrin on gels. SDS gels do not routinely give reliable results even with a gel system that optimizes the spectrin/ankyrin separation.[829] The popular Laemmli gels are unsatisfactory because ankyrin migrates between the spectrin bands in this system. Immunoassays, on the other hand, work well.[830, 847] SDS gels are satisfactory for detecting band 3 deficiency (elevated spectrin-to-band 3 ratio) or protein 4.2 deficiency and are useful in combination with antibody staining (Western blots) for detecting mutant proteins of altered size. However, in the authors' experience direct quantitation of membrane proteins rarely detects HS if it is missed by the incubated osmotic fragility test and is a lot more difficult and expensive to perform. Recently, a rapid flow cytometric test has been introduced for the study of membrane protein deficiency.[1043] The usefulness of this test awaits further validation.

Determination of the Molecular Defect. In patients in whom molecular diagnosis is desired, studies of membrane proteins, as described earlier, may identify a defect in a specific membrane protein. In other patients there is no clue to the underlying molecular defect. For these patients, linkage analysis has been performed to include or exclude the candidate genes. Various mutation detection screening techniques have been used, the most popular of which is SSCP analysis. Mutation can be detected using direct nucleotide sequence analysis of PCR-amplified cDNA or genomic DNA.

Other Laboratory Findings. Other features of HS identified by laboratory tests are manifestations of ongoing hemolysis and reflect increased erythrocyte destruction and production. These include reticulocytosis, erythroid hyperplasia of the bone marrow, indirect hyperbilirubinemia, and increased fecal urobilinogens.[985, 986, 1044] The plasma hemoglobin level is often normal,[1045] and the haptoglobin value is only variably reduced,[1046] because most of the hemoglobin that is released when hereditary spherocytes are destroyed is catabolized at the site of destruction, so-called extravascular hemolysis. Haptoglobin may be decreased or absent in neonates and thus is an unreliable marker of hemolysis in the newborn.

Complications

Most patients with HS have well-compensated hemolysis and are rarely symptomatic. These patients only seek medical attention when complications occur. Complications are generally related to chronic hemolysis and anemia.

Gallstones. The formation of bilirubinate gallstones is one of the most common complications of HS and is a major impetus for splenectomy in many patients. Instances of gallstones occurring in infancy[1047] have been reported, but most appear in adolescents and young adults. In a retrospective study of 152 consecutive patients with HS, conducted before the development of ultrasonography, approximately one half of patients with HS developed detectable gallstones between 10 and 30 years of age.[1048] Gallstones were detected in only 5 percent of children younger than 10 years old who were adequately examined. The increase in the incidence of gallstones after age 30 paralleled the incidence in the general population,[1048] which suggests that cholelithiasis owing to HS is primarily manifest in the second and third decades.

Unfortunately, longitudinal studies using modern techniques (i.e., liver and biliary tree ultrasonography) are not available, making the true incidence and natural history of gallstones in this population unknown. Indeed, many patients with gallstones are asymptomatic, and it is unclear how many will develop symptomatic gallbladder disease or biliary obstruction. Anecdotal reports in the old HS literature suggested that 40 to 50 percent of HS patients with cholelithiasis had symptoms and that a high proportion of patients with stone-containing gallbladders had histologic evidence of cholecystitis.[1049] However, studies that include large numbers of patients with mild HS show a much lower incidence of symptomatic gallbladder disease.[1050] Clearly, more accurate data about the long-term complications of pigment stone disease are needed to assess the risk-to-benefit ratio of splenectomy in HS and the need for cholecystectomy in the asymptomatic patient with cholelithiasis. Because the pigment stones typical of HS are easily detected by ultrasonography, all patients with HS should have ultrasound examinations about every 5 years and before splenectomy.

Recent studies have clearly demonstrated that coinheritance of Gilbert syndrome with HS increases the risk for cholelithiasis.[1051–1053]

Crises.

Hemolytic Crises. Patients with HS, like patients with other hemolytic diseases such as sickle cell disease, face a number of potential "crises." Hemolytic crises are probably the most common of these, particularly mild hemolytic crises. These usually occur with viral syndromes, particularly in children younger than age 6.[1054] They are characterized by a mild transient increase in jaundice, splenomegaly, anemia, and reticulocytosis. No medical intervention is usually required. Some of these patients may actually be in the recovery phase of an aplastic crisis. Severe hemolytic crises occur rarely. Characteristic features include jaundice, anemia, vomiting, abdominal pain, and tender splenomegaly. Hospitalization, erythrocyte transfusion, and careful monitoring may be required.

Aplastic Crises, Parvovirus B19. Aplastic crises are less common than hemolytic crises but are more serious and may lead to severe anemia, resulting in congestive heart failure or even death.[767, 988] They are usually caused by parvovirus B19, the cause of erythema infectiosum (fifth disease).[1055] Parvovirus B19 infection may present as fever, chills, lethargy, vomiting, diarrhea, myalgias, and a maculopapular rash on the face (slapped cheek syndrome), trunk, and extremities.[1056] In addition, the patient with HS having an aplastic crisis may experience anemia, jaundice, pallor, and weakness.[1057, 1058] Parvovirus B19 selectively infects erythropoietic precursors and inhibits their growth by inducing cell cycle arrest at G_2 and apoptosis.[1059–1062] Parvovirus infections are often associated with mild neutropenia or thrombocytopenia, and instances of transient pancytopenia have been reported.[1055, 1063–1065] Infection with parvovirus B19 is a particular danger to susceptible pregnant women, because it can infect the fetus, leading to fetal anemia, nonimmune hydrops fetalis, and fetal demise.[1066–1068] The risk of nonimmune hydrops fetalis to the fetuses of women who become infected with B19 during pregnancy is probably low. Nevertheless, because the virus is highly contagious and is easily transmitted to patients and staff[1069, 1070] and because only one half to two thirds of pregnant women have acquired protective antibodies,[1071] it has been suggested that patients who have or are suspected of having an aplastic crisis should receive precaution therapy while hospitalized and IgG-negative contacts who are pregnant should be tested for evidence of seroconversion. Nonimmune hydrops fetalis can be detected by ultrasonography and treated with intrauterine transfusions.[1072] Parvovirus may infect several members of a family simultaneously.[1065, 1073–1076]

The sequence of events in an aplastic crisis is well described in the classic article of Owren[1057] and is illustrated in Figure 15–19. During the aplastic phase, the hematocrit level and reticulocyte count fall, marrow erythroblasts disappear, and unused iron accumulates in the serum. Giant pronormoblasts often appear and are a hallmark of the cytopathic effects of parvovirus B19.[1077, 1078] As production of new red cells declines, the cells that remain age and microspherocytosis and osmotic fragility increase. Bilirubin levels may decrease as the number of abnormal red cells that can be destroyed declines. The return of marrow function is heralded by a fall in the serum iron concentration and the emergence of granulocytes, platelets, and, finally, reticulocytes. The lack of reticulocytes early in the recovery phase should not eliminate hemolytic anemias from diagnostic consideration.

During an aplastic crisis many asymptomatic patients with HS and compensated hemolysis receive medical attention.[1079–1082] As would be expected, many family members with undiagnosed HS who are infected with parvovirus B19 have developed aplastic crises at the same time.[1065, 1073, 1083] This phenomenon has led to reports of "epidemics" or "outbreaks" of HS. Diagnostic confusion may arise during reemergence of marrow function, when the physician may mistake an aplastic crisis for a hemolytic one. Because aplastic crises usually last 10 to 14 days[1057] (about one half the life span of HS red cells),[964, 1084] the hemoglobin value typically falls to about one half its usual level before recovery occurs. Thus, aplastic crises are a serious threat to young children with HS, particularly children with more severe forms of the disease. Intensive medical management is required in these cases. The

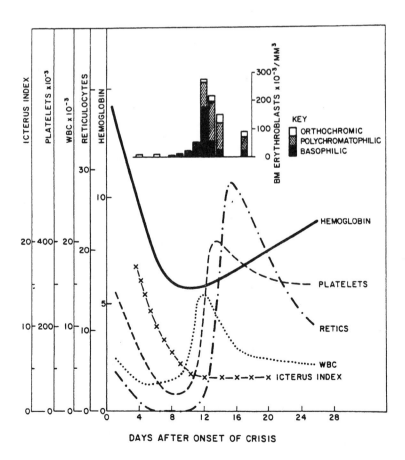

FIGURE 15–19. The temporal sequence of a severe aplastic crisis in a patient with hereditary spherocytosis who previously had well-compensated hemolysis. Note the profound reticulocytopenia and mild leukopenia and thrombocytopenia in the early phases of the reaction. Note also that the reemergence of reticulocytes is heralded by the sequential return of peripheral blood granulocytes and platelets and bone marrow normoblasts. As in this patient, jaundice frequently declines during an aplastic crisis because of a decrease in the total number of abnormal red cells that have to be destroyed. (Data from Owren PA: Congenital hemolytic jaundice. The pathogenesis of the "hemolytic crisis." Blood 1948;3: 231, 1948.)

alert clinician will recognize the signs and symptoms of an aplastic crisis and be prepared for its management. A phase I vaccine trial with recombinant parvovirus B19–like particles is underway.

Megaloblastic Crises. Rarely, patients may be seen with megaloblastic crises due to folate deficiency. These typically occurs in patients with HS who are recovering from an aplastic crisis or in patients with HS who are pregnant.[997, 998] In these patients, the dietary intake of folic acid is inadequate for the increased needs of the erythroid HS bone marrow. A megaloblastic crisis in pregnancy has been reported as the first manifestation of HS. All patients with hemolytic anemias, including HS, should routinely receive folic acid supplements ($\approx$1 mg/day) to prevent this complication.

Other Complications.

Gout and Leg Ulcers. Rarely, adults with HS develop gout,[1085, 1086] indolent leg ulcers,[1087, 1088] or a chronic erythematous dermatitis on the legs.[1089] Splenectomy appears to be curative.

Extramedullary Hematopoiesis. Adults with HS may also develop extramedullary masses of hematopoietic tissue, particularly alongside the posterior thoracic or lumbar spine[767, 1086, 1090–1095] or in the hila of the kidneys.[767] These masses may spontaneously bleed, leading to hemothorax.[1095] In one unusual instance, extramedullary hematopoiesis simulated an adrenal mass in a 9-year-old boy with HS.[1096] Surprisingly, these tumors often arise in patients with mild HS, perhaps because they often do not undergo splenectomy, and are the first manifestations of HS. The masses gradually enlarge and may be mistaken for neoplasms.[1086] Biopsy may lead to extensive bleeding. If necessary, an open biopsy should be performed. These bone marrow tumors can be diagnosed by magnetic resonance imaging,[1093] which may make biopsies unnecessary. The masses stop growing and undergo fatty metamorphosis after splenectomy, but they do not shrink in size.[1090, 1091]

Hematologic Malignancy. Over a dozen occurrences of HS and hematologic malignancy, including myeloproliferative disorders and particularly multiple myeloma and leukemia, have been reported.[1097–1101] It has been suggested that this association is due to long-standing hematopoietic stress or chronic reticuloendothelial stimulation, because splenic clearance of abnormal red cells induces proliferation of lymphocytes and plasma cells as well as macrophages.[1102] Patients with HS have a mild, polyclonal hypergammaglobulinemia,[1097–1099, 1102] and there is some evidence favoring the association of myeloma and chronic gallbladder disease.[1097, 1103] Untreated HS may also exacerbate hemochromatosis in patients who are heterozygous for the hereditary disease.[1104–1107] Several patients with HS subsequently died of liver failure or hepatoma.

Heart Disease. Untreated HS may aggravate underlying heart disease and precipitate heart failure.[1108] Gradually worsening congestive heart failure may rarely be the presenting complaint in an elderly patient with HS who has developed progressively worsening anemia as marrow senescence evolves.

Angioid Streaks. These brownish or gray streaks resembling veins in the optic fundus have been described in adult members of several HS kindreds.[1109, 1110] The rate of occurrence of this association is unknown. Angioid streaks are relatively common in some other hematologic disorders, notably sickle cell disease and thalassemia,[1109, 1111] and may be complicated by retinal vascular proliferation that requires treatment.[1112]

Diagnostic Problems

In general, HS is easily diagnosed and differentiated from other causes of spherocytosis, but there are several situations in which diagnosis can be difficult. In the neonatal period it may be hard to differentiate HS from ABO incompatibility.[1113] Anemia, hyperbilirubinemia, circulating microspherocytes, and altered osmotic fragility are found in both conditions and results of the direct antiglobulin test are sometimes negative in ABO incompatibility. However, in most affected infants with ABO incompatibility, anti-A (or -B) antibodies can be eluted from the red cells, and free anti-A (or -B) IgG antibodies can be detected in the infant's serum. Occasionally, older patients with immunohemolytic anemias and spherocytosis also have so few antibody molecules attached to their red cells that results of the direct antiglobulin test are negative and differentiation of the disease from HS is possible only with the use of radioactive antiglobulin reagents.[1114]

Spherocytosis is also seen in Heinz body hemolytic anemias during an acute hemolytic crisis and occasionally in the steady state. The diagnosis of Heinz body anemia is suggested by the presence of bite cells and blister cells on peripheral blood films and by detection of Heinz bodies in red cells stained with methyl violet.

As noted earlier, diagnostic difficulties also arise in patients who are seen during an aplastic crisis. Early in the crisis, the acute nature of the symptoms may suggest an acquired process and the absence of reticulocytes may divert the physician from a diagnosis of hemolytic anemia. Later, as marrow function returns, physicians may occasionally be misled by the properties of the emerging young HS red cells, which are less spherocytic and osmotically fragile than usual.[1011]

HS may be camouflaged by disorders that increase the surface-to-volume ratio of the red cells, such as obstructive jaundice,[926] iron deficiency,[1115] β-thalassemia,[1116] vitamin B_{12} or folate deficiency,[1117] or hemoglobin SC disease.[1118] Spherocytosis is transiently improved and results of both the osmotic fragility test and hemolysis normalize when obstructive jaundice develops.[926] This is due to the expansion of red cell membrane surface area that follows the increased uptake of cholesterol and phospholipids from the abnormal plasma lipoproteins. In normal cells, this increase in surface area leads to the formation of target cells (see later), but, in spherocytes, it leads to the appearance of discocytes. For example, we have seen a young girl who developed jaundice and symptoms of biliary obstruction at 6 years of age. She had a palpable spleen tip, evidence of mild compensated hemolysis (hemoglobin concentration of 14 g/dL; reticulocyte count of 3.3 percent), a normal peripheral blood smear, and normal results for an osmotic fragility test (fresh and incubated cells). Abdominal radiographic studies showed calcified stones in the gallbladder and common bile duct. After cholecystectomy and relief of the partial biliary obstruction, the child's hemolysis worsened (reticulocyte count of 10.8 percent) and she developed anemia (hemoglobin concentration of 10.2 g/dL), spherocytosis, and definitely abnormal results on an incubated osmotic fragility test. She subsequently underwent splenectomy with a positive response.

In a similar manner, iron deficiency corrects the abnormal shape, fragility, and high MCHC of hereditary spherocytes but does not improve their life span.[1115] Megaloblastic anemia can also mask HS, at least the morphologic characteristics of the disease.[1117] Osmotic fragility is also improved. The masking effect is observed in both vitamin B_{12} and folate deficiencies and is rapidly reversed after correction of the nutritional deficit.

The coexistence of HS and β-thalassemia trait has been described in a few case reports. It has been reported to worsen,[1119, 1120] ameliorate,[1116, 1121] or have no effect on the clinical status of the patient. In a large French family with independently segregating HS and β-thalassemia trait, patients with both traits had signs of both diseases: small, hemoglobin A_2-rich, osmotically fragile cells and some spherocytes on peripheral blood smears. However, the HS phenotype in these patients was less severe than that of family members with HS but without β-thalassemia trait.[1116]

Coinheritance of hemoglobin Q-Thailand in a Chinese family with HS had no modulating effect on HS.[1122]

Coinheritance of HS and hemoglobin SC disease may exacerbate the hemoglobinopathy.[1118] A 15-year-old boy with both diseases was much more anemic than his siblings with SC hemoglobin disease and had experienced five splenic sequestration crises. However, the two diseases may also disguise each other, at least partially. Only a few spherocytes or target cells were evident on the boy's blood smear and the surface-to-volume ratio of his red cells (and probably their osmotic fragility) was normal. Presumably this is due to the balancing effects of HS (loss of surface area) and hemoglobin SC (loss of cell volume) on red cells. Even sickle trait may be worsened by HS. Yang and colleagues[1123] reported two patients with the combination who suffered multiple splenic sequestration crises. On the other hand, spontaneous regression of HS, presumably due to development of a hyposplenic state, has been observed in two family members who had HS and sickle cell trait.[1124]

Nonerythroid Manifestations

Kindreds with HS and neurologic or muscular manifestations have been described. Patients with interstitial gene deletions (chromosome 8p11.1-8p21.1) that include ankyrin and many neighboring genes have psychomotor retardation and hypogonadism.[501, 850–853] Coetzer and co-workers[694] described a patient with ankyrin-deficient atypical HS and various neurologic manifestations. Two patients with HS and slowly progressive spinocerebellar degenerative disease were reported by McCann and Jacob.[914] Two brothers with HS, a movement disorder, and myopathy have also been described.[921] A three-generation Russian family with co-segregating HS and hypertrophic cardiomyopathy has been reported.[1125] Additional case reports in the older literature describe patients with HS and various neurologic abnormalities

such as Friedreich-like disease, cerebellar disturbances, muscle atrophy, and a tabes-like syndrome.[913–917]

The observation that erythrocyte ankyrin and erythrocyte β-spectrin are also expressed in muscle, brain, and the spinal cord raises the possibility that these patients with HS may have defects in one of these proteins.[372, 422–424, 430] This hypothesis is further supported by studies of ankyrin-deficient *nb/nb* mice. These mice have almost no detectable ankyrin-1 and have a severe, spherocytic hemolytic anemia and a late-onset cerebellar ataxia that parallels a gradual loss of Purkinje cells.[424]

TREATMENT AND OUTCOME

Splenectomy

Splenectomy cures almost all patients with typical HS, eliminating anemia and hyperbilirubinemia, and reducing the reticulocyte count to near-normal levels (1 to 3 percent). In most patients, red cell survival becomes normal or remains only slightly shortened. Spherocytosis and altered osmotic fragility persist, but the "tail" of the osmotic fragility curve, created by conditioning of a subpopulation of spherocytes by the spleen, disappears. After splenectomy, patients with the most severe forms of HS still show shortened erythrocyte survival and hemolysis, but their clinical improvement is striking.[780, 829] Interestingly, splenectomy appears to have a more beneficial effect on spectrin/ankyrin-deficient erythrocytes than band 3-deficient erythrocytes.[1125a]

Early complications of splenectomy include local infection or bleeding and pancreatitis, presumably due to injury to the tail of the pancreas incurred during removal of the spleen.[1126] In general, the morbidity of splenectomy for HS is lower than that of other hematologic disorders. However, the indications for splenectomy should be weighed carefully, because a small fraction of patients will die of overwhelming postsplenectomy infections.[1127–1131] Because the risk of postsplenectomy sepsis is very high in infancy and early childhood, splenectomy should be delayed until the age of 5 to 9 if possible and to at least 3 in all children, even if transfusions are required chronically in the interim. There is no evidence that further delay is useful, and it may be harmful, because the risk of cholelithiasis increases dramatically in children after age 10.[1048]

Risks.

Postsplenectomy Sepsis. It is difficult to estimate the risk of postsplenectomy infections after infancy.[1132] The surveys of Schwartz and colleagues[1130] and Green and co-workers[1127] are limited to adults and largely predate immunization for *Streptococcus pneumoniae* and other bacteria. They show an incidence of fulminant sepsis of 0.2 to 0.5/100 person-years of follow-up and a death rate of 0.1/100 person-years. In addition, other serious bacterial infections (e.g., pneumonia, meningitis, peritonitis, and bacteremia) were much more common (4.5/100 person-years) than normal, particularly in the first few years after the operation. More recently, Schilling[1131] reported a postsplenectomy mortality rate of 0.073/100 person-years, which is substantially better than the risk reported in the earlier studies.[1127, 1130] There was no significant difference in the risk of fatal sepsis for splenectomies performed before or after age 6 in the Schilling study, and three of the four deaths occurred 18 years or more after the operation. None of the patients who died had received pneumococcal vaccine, and none was taking prophylactic penicillin. The risk of infection would presumably be lower today, when pneumococcal immunization is routine, because 50 to 70 percent of postsplenectomy sepsis is due to *S. pneumoniae* and about 80 percent of pneumococcal disease is due to strains contained in the vaccine. Further risk reduction would be anticipated from the chronic use of prophylactic penicillin. In fact, Danish researchers have shown that the incidence of pneumococcal infection after splenectomy is dramatically lower since the introduction of pneumococcal vaccine and the promotion of early antibiotic therapy for febrile children who have had a splenectomy.[1133] Nevertheless, the risk cannot be reduced to zero. Postsplenectomy infections occur occasionally in successfully immunized patients,[1134–1136] and compliance with prophylactic medication regimens is a problem, particularly in teenagers.[1137] One report documented insufficient antibody response to pneumococcal vaccination in splenectomized patients with HS who developed postsplenectomy infection, suggesting that patients who do not have a response to the vaccine have a lifelong risk of severe postsplenectomy infection.[1138]

Penicillin-Resistant Pneumococci. The occurrence of penicillin-resistant pneumococci is increasing very rapidly all over the world.[1139–1141] In some countries, more than one half of all isolates are resistant.[1142] In the United States, the prevalence is approximately 35 percent, but it is much higher in some localities and is rising.[1139, 1141, 1143] Risk factors for the development of resistant strains include previous antibiotic use, repeat hospitalizations, and attendance in day-care facilities. Although most of the strains show some sensitivity to penicillin, some are highly resistant and others are multiply resistant.[1143–1146] The emergence of these strains will greatly complicate the use of antibiotics for pneumococcal prophylaxis during the next decade. Already, multidrug-resistant strains have been isolated from pediatric patients in the United States with sickle cell anemia.[1145, 1147, 1148] For patients in selected parts of the world, consideration must also be given to the greater risk of red cell parasitic diseases, such as malaria caused by *P. falciparum* and babesiosis, in splenectomized hosts.[1149–1150]

Cardiovascular Disease, Pulmonary Hypertension, and Thrombosis. The risk of ischemic heart disease and stroke may also increase after splenectomy for HS. In one study, Robinette and Fraumeni[1151] observed that death from ischemic heart disease occurred 1.86 times more often in splenectomized young men as in matched control subjects during a 28-year period of follow-up, a significant difference. These findings have been corroborated by others.[1152] There are several reasons that explain why splenectomy in HS increases the risk of stroke and myocardial infarction. After splenectomy, hemoglobin rises to a higher concentration than that in unaffected family members.[1153] In the Framingham study, the incidence of stroke was two times higher in patients with high versus low hemoglobin.[1154] Cholesterol levels increase after splenectomy. Finally, the chronically higher platelet count observed after splenectomy has been implicated in the pathogenesis of increased cardiovascular disease.

There is increasing evidence that splenectomy in childhood may predispose these children to pulmonary hypertension later in life.[1155–1157] This association has not only been noted for splenectomy for HS, but also for splenectomy for other hematologic disorders such as thalassemia and hereditary stomatocytosis.[1158–1160] The etiology of this association appears to be complex. Chronic postsplenectomy thrombocytosis with platelet aggregation, microthrombosis, stasis, and possible vasoconstrictive effects leading to pulmonary capillary obstruction has been suggested as a cause.[1157, 1161, 1162] The loss of the filter function of the spleen, thus allowing abnormal erythrocytes to remain in the circulation, which triggers platelet activation with subsequent trapping of these activated platelets in the pulmonary bed has been implicated. An animal model supporting this hypothesis has been described.[1163] Rabbits injected with hemolysate develop platelet-rich microthrombi in the pulmonary vascular bed after ligation of the splenic artery. Thrombi did not form in animals without ligation of the splenic artery. Finally, the development of postsplenectomy portal hypertension may contribute to the development of pulmonary hypertension.[1164–1167] In this scenario, portal hypertension leads to intrapulmonary shunting and hypoxic pulmonary vasoconstriction, which is then implicated in the pathogenesis of pulmonary hypertension.[1167]

A small subset of patients with HS have been observed to develop thrombosis.[1168] Whether thrombosis is due to an active role of pathologic erythrocytes[1169] or is due to other factors, such as associated diseases, nutritional status, genetic modifiers, infection, environment, or treatment modalities, is unknown.[1168] Major large vessel and organ thrombosis is a common finding in murine models of HS.[1170] Unlike other pathologic red cell states associated with increased thrombosis, such as thalassemic erythrocytes, erythrocytes from patients with hereditary spherocytosis and elliptocytosis do not demonstrate increased exposure of phosphatidylserine on their outer surfaces.[56]

Indications. In consideration of the risks and benefits of splenectomy, the following approach is recommended:

1. All patients with severe spherocytosis, including those with growth failure or skeletal changes, should undergo splenectomy.
2. Splenectomy is usually recommended for patients with moderate HS if they suffer from reduced vitality or physical stamina due to anemia; if, later in life, anemia compromises vascular perfusion of vital organs; or if leg ulcers or extramedullary hematopoietic tumors develop.
3. Whether patients with moderate HS and asymptomatic anemia should have a splenectomy remains controversial.
4. Splenectomy can be deferred, probably indefinitely, in patients with mild HS and compensated hemolysis.
5. The treatment of patients with mild to moderate HS and gallstones is also debatable, particularly because new treatments for gallstones such as laparoscopic cholecystectomy, endoscopic sphincterotomy, and

extracorporal choletripsy, lower the risk of this complication.[1171, 1172] If such patients have symptomatic gallstones, the authors and others favor combined cholecystectomy and splenectomy,[1173, 1174] particularly if acute cholecystitis or biliary obstruction has occurred. Prophylactic cholecystectomy at the time of splenectomy is not indicated in patients who do have cholelithiasis.[1175] There is no evidence that staging cholecystectomy and splenectomy, as was done in the past, is of any benefit.

Laparoscopic Splenectomy. When splenectomy is warranted, laparoscopic splenectomy has become the method of choice in many centers.[1176–1185] The procedure can be combined with laparoscopic cholecystectomy if desired.[1173, 1174, 1177, 1181] Although laparoscopic splenectomy requires a longer operative time than does open splenectomy,[1176, 1181, 1182] it results in less postoperative discomfort, a quicker return to preoperative diet and activities, shorter hospitalization, decreased costs, and smaller scars.[1179, 1180, 1181] The longer operative times required for the procedure undoubtedly decrease with experience. Rarely, a laparoscopic operation may have to be converted to a standard splenectomy.[1177, 1184, 1186] Even enormous spleens (>600 g) can be removed laparoscopically,[1178, 1187] because the spleen is either placed in a large nylon bag, diced, and eliminated by suction catheters or intracorporeal coring of splenic tissue is performed. Some surgeons, however, believe the risk of blood loss is greater when large spleens are removed and recommend that use of the laparoscopic technique be limited to small spleens.[1186] It is also not clear whether accessory spleens are more easily missed during laparoscopic splenectomies.[1182, 1188] One patient developed pain and a palpable nodule at a port site after laparoscopic splenectomy due to splenosis.[1189]

Partial (Subtotal) Splenectomy. The emergence of antibiotic-resistant pneumococci has led to reexamination of the role of alternate treatment modalities. Partial splenectomy has been suggested for selected patients with HS, especially those with moderate to severe disease. The goal of this operation is to decrease hemolysis while maintaining residual splenic phagocytic function. In practice, at least 90 percent of the enlarged organ is removed (Fig. 15–20). In an initial study by Tchernia and colleagues,[1190]

complications of partial splenectomy were low and regrowth of the splenic remnant was not observed during a 4-year follow-up period. Long-term follow-up (1 to 14 years) of patients with HS treated with subtotal splenectomy revealed that the decrease in hemolysis was sustained in many, but not all, patients and phagocytic function of the splenic remnant persisted.[1191] Splenic tissue has tremendous regeneration potential, as attested to by reports of previously splenectomized individuals with HS who developed enlarged accessory spleens or ectopic splenic tissue together with recurrent hemolysis later in life.[1192, 1193] Thus it is not surprising that splenic regrowth has been a problem, necessitating reoperation.[1193a] More experience and longer follow-up are needed before partial splenectomy can be recommended as a routine procedure for the majority of patients with HS.

Embolization. A case report detailing partial splenic arterial embolization in a child with HS has been published.[1194] The technique has also been used to decrease operative blood loss in patients with very large spleens before laparoscopic splenectomy.[1178] There are no additional data on this treatment in pediatric patients with HS.

Prophylaxis. All candidates for splenectomy should receive the complete series of pneumococcal and *Haemophiles influenzae* vaccines preoperatively. In some countries, immunization with meningococcal vaccine is also recommended, particularly in children. We advocate use of prophylactic antibiotics after splenectomy, with emphasis on protection against pneumococcal sepsis (i.e., penicillin V or equivalent, 125 mg orally twice daily in young children [younger than 5 years of age] and 250 mg twice daily in older children and adults), at least for the first 5 years after surgery. Previously, some recommended the use of life-long penicillin prophylaxis for splenectomized patients. The emergence of penicillin-resistant pneumococci (5 percent in 1989 to ≥35 percent in 1997) has led many to reconsider this recommendation, particularly because prior antibiotic use is a risk factor for the development of penicillin resistance in pneumococci.[1147] Patients with HS, like patients with other hemolytic disorders, should take folic acid (0.5 to 1 mg/day orally), to prevent folate deficiency.

Postsplenectomy Changes. After splenectomy, spherocytosis persists but conditioned microspherocytes

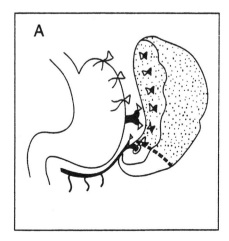

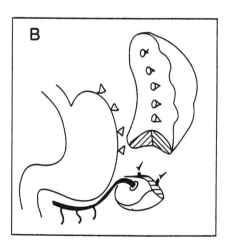

FIGURE 15–20. Surgical technique used for partial (about 80 percent) splenectomy. *A,* All vascular pedicles supplying the spleen are divided except those arising from the left gastroepiploic vessels. *B,* The upper pole of the spleen is removed at the boundary between the well-perfused and poorly perfused tissue. (From Tchernia G, Gauthier F, Mielot F, et al: Initial assessment of the beneficial effect of partial splenectomy in hereditary spherocytosis. Blood 1993; 81:2014.)

disappear; and changes typical of the postsplenectomy state, including Howell-Jolly bodies, target cells, siderocytes, and acanthocytes, become evident in the peripheral blood smear. On average, the MCV and mean red cell surface area increase and the MCHC and osmotic fragility decrease, but the effects are modest (5 to 10 percent).[1195] In typical dominant HS, reticulocyte counts fall to normal or near-normal levels,[847] although red cell life span, if carefully measured, remains slightly shortened (96 ± 13 days).[937] In all but the most severe occurrences, anemia and jaundice remit and do not recur.

Splenectomy Failure. The rare splenectomy failure (i.e., recurrence of hemolysis) is usually caused by an accessory spleen that was missed during surgery[1192, 1193] or by another red cell disorder, such as pyruvate kinase deficiency.[1196, 1197] Accessory spleens occur in 15 to 40 percent of patients and must always be sought.[1049, 1126, 1198] Recurrence of hemolytic anemia years or even decades[1193] after splenectomy should raise suspicion of an accessory spleen, particularly if Howell-Jolly bodies are no longer evident on peripheral blood smears. The absence of "pitted" red cells with crater-like surface indentations, readily seen by interference contrast microscopy, is also a sensitive measure of recrudescent splenic function.[1199, 1200] The ectopic splenic tissue can be confirmed by a radiocolloid

liver/spleen scan or a scan using ^{51}Cr-labeled, heat-damaged red cells.[1192, 1201]

Hereditary Elliptocytosis, Hereditary Pyropoikilocytosis, and Related Disorders

Hereditary elliptocytosis (HE) is characterized by the presence of elliptical or oval erythrocytes on peripheral blood smears (Fig. 15–21). Although oval or elliptical erythrocytes are normally found in camels, llamas, birds, and reptiles, in humans the presence of elliptocytes indicates a defect in the erythrocyte membrane skeleton. HE and the related disorder hereditary pyropoikilocytosis (HPP) are characterized by clinical, biochemical, and genetic heterogeneity. Clinically, these disorders range from the asymptomatic carrier state to severe hemolysis and even death *in utero* due to hydrops fetalis. Erythrocyte biochemical defects range from none to severe. To date, four different genetic loci have been defined in the pathogenesis of these disorders, and other loci have been implicated.

In the past, hereditary elliptocytic disorders have simply been considered to be variants of HS and worthy of little further attention. However, the membrane defects and their pathophysiologic consequences in HE differ fundamentally from those of HS, leading to the difference in erythrocyte shape.

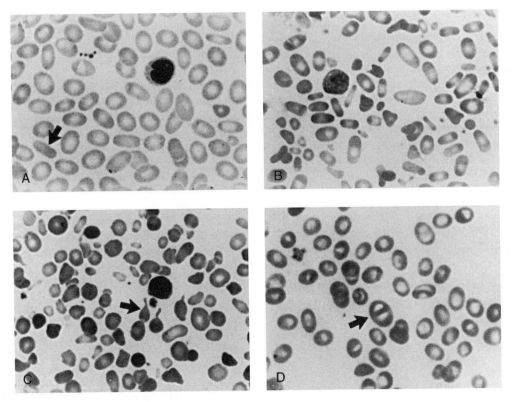

FIGURE 15–21. Peripheral blood smears from subjects with various forms of HE. *A,* Simple heterozygote with mild common HE associated with an elliptogenic spectrin mutation. Note the predominant elliptocytosis with some rod-shaped cells *(arrow)* and virtual absence of poikilocytes. *B,* "Homozygous" common HE due to a doubly heterozygous state for two α-spectrin mutations. Both parents have mild HE. There are many elliptocytes as well as numerous fragments and poikilocytes. *C,* Hereditary pyropoikilocytosis (HPP). The patient is a double heterozygote for mutant α-spectrin and a defect characterized by reduced synthesis of this protein. Note prominent microspherocytosis, micropoikilocytosis, and fragmentation. Only a few elliptocytes are present. Some poikilocytes are in the process of budding *(arrow). D,* Southeast Asian (Melanesian) ovalocytosis. The majority of cells are oval; some contain either a longitudinal slit or a transverse ridge *(arrow).* (From Palek J, Jarolim P: Clinical expression and laboratory detection of red blood cell membrane protein mutations. Semin Hematol 1993; 30:266.)

HISTORY

HE was first reported in 1904 by Dresbach,[1202] a physiologist at Ohio State University in Columbus, who discovered the condition in one of his histology students during a laboratory exercise in which the students were examining their own blood. This report elicited some controversy, because the student died soon thereafter, leading to speculation that the student actually suffered from incipient pernicious anemia.[1203] A number of famous pathologists supported Dresbach's view that the elliptocytosis was a primary disorder,[1204] and this view was substantiated during the next two decades by the reports of Bishop[1205] and Huck and Bigalow.[1206] The demonstration of the disease in three generations of one family clearly established the hereditary nature of this disorder.[1207, 1208]

In the 1930s and 1940s there was some debate about whether HE was a disease or simply a morphologic curiosity.[1207–1212] Early on, some confusion also existed in the differentiation of HE from sickle cell anemia, from hypochromic elliptocytosis (probably thalassemia), and later, from HS.[1210] These reports emphasize an important fact: the manifestation of HE and its hemolytic variants can sometimes be morphologically deceptive. Additional historical and clinical features of the disease are found in the reports of Wyandt and associates,[1211] Wolman and Ozge,[1212] and Dacie.[1213]

HE is common in people of African and Mediterranean ancestry.[1214–1222] In the United States, HE has been estimated to occur in 1 in 2000 to 4000 of the population.[1211, 1214] The true incidence of HE is unknown because its clinical severity is heterogeneous, and many patients are asymptomatic and do not have anemia. In a study of HE in Benin, an incidence of 1.6 percent was observed.[1215] The incidence of one common elliptocytic mutation of α-spectrin, α$^{I/65–68}$, approaches 1 percent in Central Africa. It has a worldwide distribution in people of African ancestry. Genetic haplotyping studies suggest that this mutation may have a "founder affect" with origins of this mutation in central Africa similar to that attributed to hemoglobin S Benin-type.[1215]

HE variants are inherited predominantly in an autosomal dominant manner. Typically, individuals who are heterozygous for an elliptocytic variant have asymptomatic elliptocytosis without anemia. Individuals who are homozygotes or compound heterozygotes for HE variants may suffer from mild to severe hemolysis with moderate to marked anemia. Spontaneous elliptocytogenic mutations have been reported. Presumably, they will also be inherited in an autosomal dominant fashion. In one kindred with Alport syndrome, mental retardation, midface hypoplasia, and elliptocytosis, inheritance was X-linked and associated with a submicroscopic chromosome X deletion, suggesting the occurrence of a contiguous gene syndrome.[1223]

CLINICAL AND LABORATORY CHARACTERISTICS OF HEREDITARY ELLIPTOCYTOSIS AND RELATED DISORDERS

Classification

Most of the reported patients with of HE can be classified into one of three clinical categories: common HE, sphero-

cytic HE, and SAO. With the exception of SAO, which is homogeneous in molecular genetic terms (see later), these classifications denote clinical phenotypes and not specific molecular etiologies, although correlations between the two exist. Numerous molecular defects in the membrane proteins of patients with HE have been identified, and HE can also be classified based on these defects (see later).

Heterozygous Common Hereditary Elliptocytosis. Common HE is, by far, the most prevalent form of HE, particularly in African populations.[1215, 1216] It is usually classified into several subtypes. The clinical characteristics of the common HE trait vary enormously, defining several clinical subtypes. It is important to note that different clinical patterns may be seen in members of the same family, and even the clinical presentation in single individuals may exhibit variability over time. Thus, the clinical patterns defined later are probably more useful for illustrating the spectrum of common HE than for classifying the disease.

Silent Carrier State. This condition was identified by analyzing asymptomatic members of kindreds with HE or HPP. The affected persons have red cells with normal morphologic characteristics and no evidence of hemolysis, but detailed investigations show a subtle defect in their membrane skeletons, with decreased red cell thermal stability, decreased mechanical stability of isolated skeletons, an increased fraction of spectrin dimers in 0°C spectrin extracts, abnormal tryptic peptide maps of spectrin, or various combinations of these defects.[1218–1222, 1234, 1225] It is notable that some patients classified as "silent carriers" have the same molecular defect as patients with mild common HE,[1221, 1222, 1224, 1225] emphasizing the variability of clinical expression.

Mild Hereditary Elliptocytosis. This is the most common clinical form of HE.[1226–1241] Patients are asymptomatic, and HE is often diagnosed incidentally when individuals are undergoing screening for an unrelated condition. These persons are not anemic and only very rarely exhibit splenomegaly. Red cell survival may be normal,[1076] but more often there is very mild, compensated hemolysis with a slight reticulocytosis and a decreased haptoglobin level.[1231, 1233, 1238, 1242] In these patients HE is hardly more than a morphologic curiosity. The peripheral blood smear shows prominent elliptocytosis with little red cell budding or fragmentation and no spherocytosis. Elliptocytes (by definition) usually exceed 30 percent of the red cells and in some instances approach 100 percent.[1211, 1224, 1225, 1238, 1242] Very elongated elliptocytes are common (>10 percent). These patients are easily separated from normal individuals, who have less than 2 to 5 percent elliptocytes.[1225, 1236, 1242] Somewhat higher proportions of elliptocytes are seen in patients with anemia, particularly megaloblastic anemias, hypochromic-microcytic anemias, myelodysplastic syndromes, and myelofibrosis,[1243] but even in these individuals elliptocytes do not exceed 35 percent.[1236] Thus, the diagnosis of common HE is rarely difficult.

Common Hereditary Elliptocytosis with Chronic Hemolysis. More severe variants of common HE occur often, even within members of the same kindred.[1230, 1244–1247] In general, the hemolysis is accompanied by evidence of membrane instability on the peripheral blood smear: budding red cells, fragments, and other bizarre poikilocytes. In patients with α-spectrin mutations, significant hemolysis is often due to coinheritance of a spectrin allele that leads to decreased α-spectrin expression, such as the α^{LELY} allele, and one of the more deleterious HE alleles affecting α-spectrin (see later).[1231, 1248–1253] Of the common mutations, $\alpha^{I/74}$-spectrin is more severe than $\alpha^{I/46-50a}$-spectrin and much more severe than $\alpha^{I/65-68}$-spectrin. Patients with α^{LELY} in *trans* to $\alpha^{I/74}$ have marked hemolysis and elliptopoikilocytosis compared with their siblings with wild-type α-spectrin and $\alpha^{I/74}$ ($+/\alpha^{I/74}$), whereas patients with $\alpha^{LELY}/\alpha^{I/65-68}$ have more elliptocytes than their siblings with $+/\alpha^{I/65-68}$ but no significant hemolysis.[1251] Less often hemolysis is caused by inheritance of a mutant spectrin that is grossly dysfunctional.[1244] This is indicated by dominant transmission of the hemolytic syndrome and by an unusually high fraction of spectrin dimers in 0°C spectrin extracts.

Common Hereditary Elliptocytosis with Sporadic Hemolysis. Patients with common HE may also develop uncompensated hemolysis in response to stimuli that cause hyperplasia of the reticuloendothelial system, particularly if the spleen is involved. Examples include viral hepatitis, cirrhosis, infectious mononucleosis, bacterial infections, and malaria.[1239, 1254–1256] Hemolysis has also been observed with thrombotic thrombocytopenic purpura and during renal transplant rejection complicated by disseminated intravascular coagulation, which suggests that elliptocytes may be especially susceptible to microangiopathic damage.[1257] For unknown reasons pregnancy and cobalamin (vitamin B_{12}) deficiency may also transiently aggravate the disease.[993, 1258]

Hereditary Elliptocytosis with Infantile Poikilocytosis. Infants with mild common HE often begin life with moderately severe hemolytic anemia, characterized by marked red cell budding, fragmentation, and poikilocytosis and by neonatal jaundice, which may require an exchange transfusion.[1219, 1232, 1242, 1259–1264] In most patients, enough elliptocytes are present to suggest the diagnosis, but sometimes this is not so and the disorder is mistaken for sepsis, infantile pyknocytosis, or a microangiopathic or oxidant-induced hemolytic anemia.[1261, 1262] Neonatal HE can easily be distinguished from these conditions if the parents' blood smears are examined, because one will show common HE. However, it is more difficult to distinguish HE with neonatal poikilocytosis from HPP (see later). Most α-spectrin variants have been associated with the neonatal poikilocytosis syndrome. The factors that determine susceptibility are unknown. With time, fragmentation and hemolysis decline, and the clinical picture of mild common HE emerges.[1265] This transition requires 4 months to 2 years. Subsequently, the disease is clinically indistinguishable from typical mild common HE. The prevalence is unknown, but in the authors' experience it is not rare.

The fragmenting neonatal red cells are very sensitive to heat, like hereditary pyropoikilocytes (see later), but unlike pyropoikilocytes, this sensitivity lessens over time.[1264] During the conversion, the poikilocytic red cells are dense and rich in hemoglobin F whereas the smooth elliptocytes are light and enriched in hemoglobin A. This finding suggests that the change in the disease corresponds to the change from fetal to adult erythropoiesis. No variations in the primary α-spectrin defect or its functional effects on spectrin self-association occur during the conversion, so other skeletal interactions must differ in fetal and adult red cells. Mentzer and associates[1266] made the interesting suggestion that 2,3-DPG is the critical agent. Because it is not bound by hemoglobin F, the concentration of 2,3-DPG is elevated in fetal red cells. The free anion is known to weaken spectrin-actin-protein 4.1 interactions[330, 631, 632] and to increase the fragility of isolated ghosts at physiologic concentrations *in vitro*.[1258] Whether this occurs in intact red cells is unclear.[633, 634] If it does, the underlying defect in spectrin self-association would certainly be aggravated.

Herediary Elliptocytosis with Dyserythropoiesis. In a small number of families with otherwise typical common HE, the sporadic occurrence of hemolysis and anemia is at least partially due to the development of dysplastic and ineffective erythropoiesis. All the reported patients with this rare syndrome are from Italy, have somewhat less elongated red cells than is typical for common HE, and show the characteristic findings of ineffective erythropoiesis, relatively low reticulocyte counts, indirect hyperbilirubinemia, high serum iron and ferritin concentrations, and rapid clearance of ^{59}Fe combined with poor incorporation of ^{59}Fe into new erythrocytes.[1267, 1268] Erythrocytes from some patients exhibit macrocytic changes. Other patients have a few spherocytes, but these are probably an artifact because osmotic fragility test results are normal.[1267] The patient's bone marrow is hyperplastic, with decreased late erythroblasts and dysplastic features (asynchrony of nuclear-cytoplasmic maturation, binuclearity, internuclear bridges, and small numbers of ringed sideroblasts). Anemia and, presumably, erythroid dysplasia usually commence during adolescence or early adult life and advance gradually over years. Because dysplasia persists after splenectomy, response to the operation is incomplete. The available data suggest that dysplasia and elliptocytosis co-segregate because no individuals with dysplasia have been observed who did not have elliptocytosis.[1267, 1268] If so, these families must represent the occurrence of a unique subtype of mild common HE. This suggestion is supported by the fact that none of the typical HE protein defects were observed in one well-studied family. Spectrin self-association, spectrin peptide maps, and the concentration of protein 4.1 and other major membrane proteins were normal.

Homozygous Common Hereditary Elliptocytosis. A number of patients who are homozygotes or compound heterozygotes for common HE have been reported.[1226, 1242, 1269–1281] Some have had very severe, even fatal, transfusion-dependent hemolytic anemia (hemoglobin level of 2 to 6 g/dL) with marked fragmentation, poikilocytosis, spherocytosis, and elliptocytosis. Others experience hemolysis to a lesser degree (hemoglobin level of 7 to 11 g/dL). It appears that these differences reflect variations in the severity of the many α-spectrin mutations that produce HE.[1242, 1282] In one interesting patient, a proband with moderate HE inherited an α-spectrin self-association site mutation from his mother and a β-spectrin self-association site mutation from his father.[1283]

Clinically, the disease resembles HPP,[1242, 1282] except for the mildest forms. Patients have an excellent response to splenectomy.

Hereditary Pyropoikilocytosis. This uncommon disorder presents in infancy or early childhood as a severe hemolytic anemia (hemoglobin level of 4 to 8 g/dL)[1242] characterized by extreme poikilocytosis with budding red cells, fragments, spherocytes, triangulocytes, and other bizarre-shaped cells and, in some patients, few or no elliptocytes (Fig. 15–22).[1221, 1284–1288] This morphologic picture is similar to that seen in patients who have severe thermal burns. It is also similar to that observed in homozygous common HE and common HE with neonatal poikilocytosis. Most of the patients are individuals of African origin. Patients typically exhibit hyperbilirubinemia in the neonatal period or marked anemia in the first few months of life.[1288] Red cell fragmentation, erythroblastosis, and splenomegaly are also seen.[1288, 1289] Complications of severe anemia including growth retardation, frontal bossing, and early gallbladder disease have been reported.[1286, 1287] Results of osmotic fragility tests are very abnormal, particularly after incubation,[1270, 1285–1287] and autohemolysis is greatly elevated.[1285–1287] A significant characteristic, microcytosis, is reflected by very low MCVs (25 to 75 fL) because of the large number of fragmented red cells.[1222–1224, 1242, 1285, 1286] Another characteristic feature of these cells is their remarkable thermal sensitivity. Hereditary pyropoikilocytes fragment at 45 to 46°C (normal 49°C) after short periods of heating (10 to 15 minutes).[1287] After splenectomy, hemolysis is markedly decreased, but not eliminated.[1286, 1287] After splenectomy, the hemoglobin level typically ranges from 10 to 14 g/dL with 3 to 10 percent reticulocytes.[1242]

Although HPP was initially considered to be a separate disease, there is convincing evidence that it is related to HE. As noted earlier, HPP is clinically and morphologically similar to the more severe forms of hemolytic elliptocytosis. In addition, for many patients, one parent or sibling has typical mild common HE, and in some of these kindreds an identical molecular defect is observed in siblings with phenotypically different diseases (i.e., HPP and common HE). In other families, all the first-degree relatives have normal phenotypes. A number of biochemical and molecular defects are shared between HE and HPP. However, HPP red cells, but not hereditary elliptocytes, are usually markedly deficient in spectrin.[1242, 1289, 1290] Typically, one parent of the HPP offspring carries an α-spectrin mutation whereas the other parent is fully asymptomatic and has no detectable biochemical abnormality.[1290] Studies of spectrin synthesis and mRNA levels reveal that such asymptomatic parents carry a silent "thalassemia-like" defect of spectrin synthesis. When coinherited with the elliptocytogenic spectrin mutation in the offspring with HPP, this thalassemia-like defect enhances the expression of the mutant spectrin in the cells and leads to a superimposed spectrin deficiency. The spectrin deficiency is thought to be responsible for the large number of spherocytes and relative paucity of elliptocytes in some patients. Other patients with HPP are homozygotes or compound heterozygotes for structural defects of spectrin.

Spherocytic Hereditary Elliptocytosis. This dominant disorder is a phenotypic hybrid of common HE and HS. It has been reported only in white families of European descent, is not linked to the Rh gene, and appears to be a unique subtype.[1209, 1239, 1291–1294] Its prevalence is unknown, but, judging from the number of published reports, it is relatively rare, probably accounting for no more than 5 percent of HE in patients of European ancestry. Unlike in mild common HE, almost all affected patients have some hemolysis. This is usually mild to moderate and is often incompletely compensated. The elliptocytes are fewer and plumper than in mild common HE, and some spherocytes, microspherocytes, and microelliptocytes are usually present. Poikilocytes and red cell fragments are uncommon, which distinguishes this disorder from common HE with hemolysis. Red cell morphology may vary, even within the same family. Some family members may

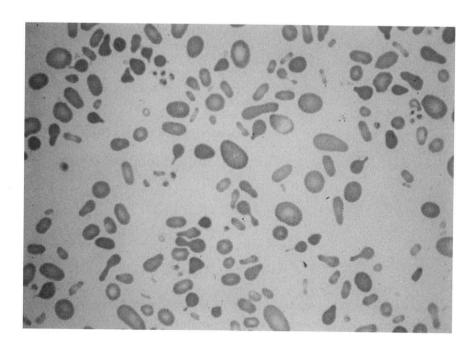

FIGURE 15–22. Peripheral blood smear from a patient with hereditary pyropoikilocytosis. Poikilocytes, budding and fragmented erythrocytes, spherocytes, and a few elliptocytes are seen.

have relatively prominent spherocytes and as few as 10 to 20 percent elliptocytes, whereas in others elliptocytes predominate and spherocytes are rare.[1209, 1291] This may cause diagnostic confusion initially, particularly if the propositus has few elliptocytes. Family studies almost always reveal some members with obvious elliptocytosis.

Spherocytic elliptocytes are osmotically fragile,[1209, 1291, 1293, 1294] particularly after incubation. Excessive mechanical fragility and increased autohemolysis that responds to glucose are also characteristic. Gallbladder disease is common, and aplastic crises are a risk.[1291, 1293] The splenic pathologic course of spherocytic HE mimics that of HS.[1295, 1296] Splenic sequestration is evident, red cells are conditioned during splenic passage, and hemolysis abates after splenectomy.[1291, 1293, 1296]

The molecular pathologic characteristics of classic spherocytic HE is unknown. However, patients with COOH-terminal truncations of β-spectrin (see later) have many of the clinical features of spherocytic HE and probably represent an example of the disorder.[1297–1306] A number of such truncations have been identified. The affected patients typically have moderate hemolysis and anemia, punctuated by recurrent, severe hemolytic crises.[1298, 1299, 1302] Blood smears show plump and usually smooth elliptocytes; although in a few instances, poikilocytosis was prominent.[1298, 1299, 1301] In all but one instance the HE red cells were mildly heat sensitive.[1298] All patients have positive osmotic fragility test results or an osmotic gradient ektacytometry pattern that resembles the pattern in HS. As with HS, the spleen is enlarged and selectively destroys labeled elliptocytes (half-life, 11 days; normal, 24 to 34 days),[1304] and splenectomy is effective.

Patients who lack GpC (see later) also have positive osmotic fragility test results and rounded, smooth elliptocytes.[1307, 1308] They should probably also be classified as having a recessive (and unusually mild) variant of spherocytic HE. Patients who lack protein 4.2 (another recessive condition) sometimes display features of spherocytic HE, such as ovalostomatocytosis[497, 816]; however, protein 4.2 deficiency more often resembles that in HS, morphologically and pathophysiologically, and is better classified as a variant of that disorder.

Rare patients appear to be compound heterozygotes for HS and HE. One Turkish girl is a particularly good candidate.[1309] Her mother and father had mild HS and very mild common HE (probably), respectively, whereas she suffered from a moderately severe hemolytic anemia (hemoglobin level, 8.4; reticulocyte count, 24 percent; bilirubin level, 1.6 mg/dL) with frontal bossing, osteoporosis, splenomegaly (10 cm), and a mixture of microspherocytes and rounded elliptocytes.

Southeast Asian Ovalocytosis. This condition, which has a unique phenotype, a unique molecular defect, and a unique geographic distribution, is discussed later in this chapter.

Analysis of Membrane Structure and Function

Thermal Sensitivity of Red Cells and Spectrin. Red cells heated to temperatures approaching 50°C for short periods of time become unstable and fragment spontaneously (Fig. 15–23),[1310–1312] probably owing to denaturation of spectrin.[1313] Normal spectrin denatures at 49°C (10-minute exposure),[603, 1313] and normal red cells fragment at the same temperature.[1287, 1314] As noted earlier, almost all patients with HPP and some patients with other forms of HE have thermally sensitive red cells. Hereditary pyropoikilocytes and red cells from infants with common HE and neonatal poikilocytosis fragment after 10 minutes at 44 to 46°C.[1264, 1287] Red cells from some but not all patients with common HE fragment at 47 to 48°C.[603, 1287] As expected, purified spectrin from these red cells is also heat sensitive.[603, 1313] This test is limited because we do not understand, in molecular terms, why specific mutations are thermally sensitive. However, it remains one of the simplest tests available for assessing HPP in laboratories that do not specialize in membrane protein analysis.

Abnormal Spectrin Oligomerization. In many patients with HE and all patients with HPP spectrin dimers are not properly converted to tetramers and higher oligomers *in vitro* or on the membrane. This important functional property is easily assessed in low-temperature spectrin extracts (Fig. 15–24). At 0°C the equilibrium between spectrin dimer and tetramer is greatly slowed. If spectrin is extracted from the membrane at 0°C and carefully protected from warming during separation of dimers, tetramers, and oligomers (usually on nondenaturing polyacrylamide gels), the proportion of each spectrin species reflects its relative proportion on the membrane.[309] Patients with defects in spectrin self-association have abnormally high proportions of spectrin dimer in 0°C spectrin extracts (i.e., more than 10 percent of total

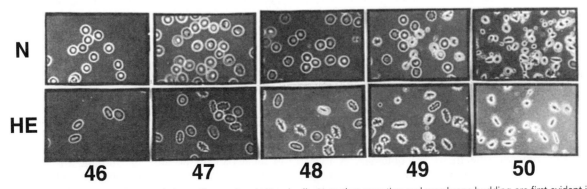

FIGURE 15–23. Effects of heat on the morphology of normal and HE red cells. Note that crenation and membrane budding are first evident in HE red cells at 47 to 48°C but do not appear in normal cells until they are heated to 49°C.

mg/ml

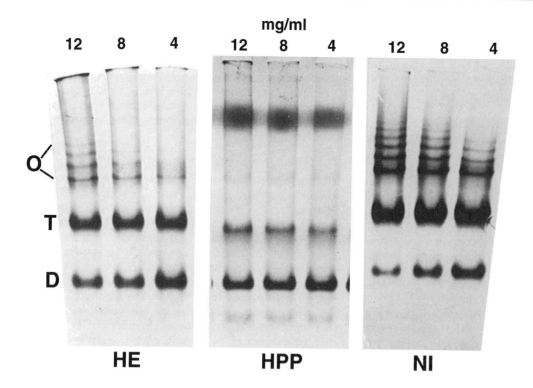

FIGURE 15–24. Nondenaturing gel electrophoresis of spectrin dimers and oligomers from normal individuals (NI) and patients with HE and HPP. Low ionic strength spectrin extracts were concentrated to 12.5, 8, and 4 mg/mL and equilibrated at 30°C for 3 hours. Note the reduced tetramer (T) and oligomer (O) formation at each concentration of spectrin from a patient with HPP. Spectrin from a patient with HE shows intermediate behavior compared with the normal control individual. The diffuse band at the top of the lanes from the patient with HPP is hemoglobin. (From Knowles WJ, Morrow JS, Speicher DW, et al: Molecular and functional changes in spectrin from patients with hereditary pyropoikilocytosis. J Clin Invest 1983; 71:1867.)

spectrin dimers and tetramers).[1246, 1314, 1315] The fraction of spectrin dimers is an important functional assessment in patients with α-spectrin defects. It correlates well with clinical severity and accurately predicts unusually severe mutations.[1252] Conversely, discordance between the degree of hemolysis and fraction of spectrin dimers may alert the physician to an underlying, secondary complication (see earlier section on common HE with chronic hemolysis).

Ektacytometry. The ektacytometer can be used to assess red cell membrane deformability and stability in patients with hemolytic disorders.[1316–1318] Isolated red cell ghosts are subjected to high shear stress in a laser diffraction viscometer, and the "deformability index" (a measure of the average elongation of the sheared ghosts) is recorded as a function of time. Fragile ghosts fragment more quickly than normal, causing their "deformability" to fall. The technique is a useful screening test because membrane stability is reduced in almost all membrane skeletal diseases. In addition, the ektacytometer can be modified to measure cellular deformability at different osmolalities, a technique termed *osmotic gradient ektacytometry*.[1027] The resulting curves depend on both membrane surface area and cell volume and are a sensitive measure of the surface loss that characterizes many skeletal defects.

Tryptic Maps of Spectrin. Limited tryptic digestion of spectrin extracted from erythrocytes, performed at 0°C, followed by SDS-PAGE or isoelectric focusing combined with SDS-PAGE (two-dimensional gels) separates the resulting trypsin-resistant domains of α- and β-spectrin.[308, 331] The gels are stained with Coomassie blue, and characteristic, reproducible maps are obtained. A two-dimensional separation of normal spectrin domains is shown in Figure 15–9. Among these peptides, the 80-kD α-I domain peptide, which contains the self-association

site of normal α-spectrin, is the most prominent. Many of the known elliptocytogenic α-spectrin mutations affect the 80-kD domain and yield peptide maps containing one or more fragments of the domain. One-dimensional maps of spectrin domains from patients with some of these HE defects are shown in Figure 15–25. In most of the defects, tryptic cleavage occurs in the third helix of the triple-helical spectrin repeats.[1319] The reported mutations reside in the vicinity of these cleavage sites either in the same helix or, less commonly, at neighboring sites in the first and second helices. Interestingly, HE mutations near the COOH terminus of β-spectrin may also alter tryptic cleavage of the neighboring 80-kD α-spectrin domain (to be discussed later). Thus, tryptic peptide mapping is a useful tool to map the approximate sites of the underlying spectrin mutations; the mutations can subsequently be defined by examination of the corresponding region at the cDNA or genomic DNA level.

Genetic Analyses. Genomic DNA isolated from peripheral blood leukocytes or reverse-transcribed reticulocyte or bone marrow mRNA can be amplified by PCR using specific DNA oligonucleotide primers flanking the region suspected to contain a mutation. The amplification product is then subjected to nucleic acid sequencing or other forms of analysis. There are many individual variations of this technique that have been used to identify the mutations described in the following sections. Screening techniques can be used when there are no biochemical clues to the location of the mutation. These techniques are particularly advantageous when the genes of large proteins, such as spectrin or ankyrin, are analyzed. Genomic DNA is tested in most patients because the mutant mRNA species may not accumulate in significant amounts. The SSCP method is a simple, sensitive, and appropriately popular example of such a screening test. Labeled, PCR-amplified DNA

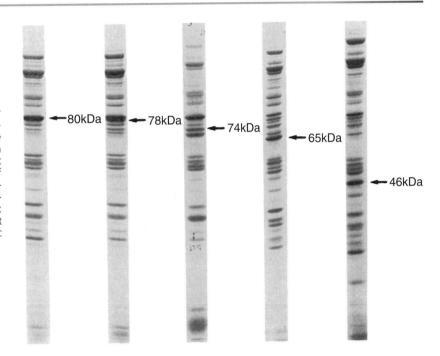

FIGURE 15–25. One-dimensional peptide maps after partial trypsin digestion of spectrin variants. In a control subject, the α-I domain appears basically in the form of a 80-kD fragment. In spectrin mutants with various alterations of the α-chain, the main fragment representing the α-I domain is shorter, because of abnormal cleavages that reflect, in turn, local conformational changes. The $\alpha^{I/78}$, $\alpha^{I/74}$, $\alpha^{I/65}$, and $\alpha^{I/46}$ phenotypes are shown. (From Delaunay J, Dhermy D: Mutations involving the spectrin heterodimer contact site: Clinical expression and; alterations in specific function. Semin Hematol 1993l; 30:21.)

fragments (100 to 400 bp) are denatured, and the single strands are refolded before running on a nondenaturing gel.[1320, 1321] Even a single nucleotide change usually alters the folding pattern enough to allow mutant and normal fragments to separate on the gel (70 to 90 percent of mutations). Abnormal fragments are sequenced. In some regions where common elliptocytogenic mutations have been identified, multiplex PCR techniques or simple restriction endonuclease digestion of amplified DNA can be used to screen rapidly for these mutations.

ETIOLOGY OF COMMON HEREDITARY ELLIPTOCYTOSIS AND RELATED DISORDERS

Spectrin Defects

Abnormalities of either α- or β-spectrin are associated with many occurrences of HE and HPP. The majority are due to mutations in the spectrin heterodimer self-association site (Fig. 15–26) with defective ability of spectrin dimers to form tetramers, resulting in destabilization of the erythrocyte membrane skeleton.

Alpha-Spectrin Defects. Most of the HE defects are in the 80-kD α-I domain at the NH_2 terminus of the α-spectrin chain. Nine tryptic cleavage defects of the normal 80-kD α-I domain peptide have been identified by tryptic mapping, characterized by loss of the normal 80-kD peptide and the appearance of one of the following: a new 78-kD peptide ($\alpha^{I/78}$), a new 74-kD peptide ($\alpha^{I/74}$), a new 65- or 68-kD peptide ($\alpha^{I/65-68}$), a new 61-kD peptide ($\alpha^{I/61}$), a new 46-kD peptide ($\alpha^{I/46}$), a new 50- or 46-kD peptide ($\alpha^{I/46-50a}$), a new 50-kD peptide with a more basic isoelectric point than $\alpha^{I/46-50a}$ ($\alpha^{I/50b}$), two new peptides of 43 and 42 kD ($\alpha^{I/43}$), or two new peptides of 36 and 33 kD ($\alpha^{I/36-33}$). In general, these defects produce decreased spectrin self-association, reflected in an increased proportion of spectrin dimers in 0°C low ionic strength extracts of spectrin and decreased conversion of spectrin dimers to tetramers in solution, in ghosts, and on inside-out vesicles. The fragile spectrin-spectrin links weaken the membrane skeleton and diminish the resistance of the isolated membrane or skeleton to shear stress.[1027, 1266, 1317] Surprisingly, this results in a stiff membrane[1343] (elevated elastic shear modulus) rather than a lax

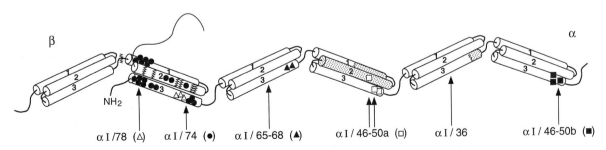

FIGURE 15–26. Triple-helical model of mutations in the αβ spectrin self-association site associated with HE and HPP. The abnormal tryptic cleavage sites in spectrin associated with different forms of HE and HPP are denoted by the *arrows*. The *open symbols* and *filled symbols* denote positions of various molecular defects found to be associated with the abnormal cleavage sites. Note that in most instances, the mutation found is adjacent to the abnormal cleavage site, either in the same helical coil or in helical coils juxtaposed next to each other in the triple-helical model. The *hashed lines* denote the location of spectrin chain truncations. (From Gallagher PG, Tse WT, Forget BG: Clinical and molecular aspects of disorders of the erythrocyte membrane skeleton. Semin Perinatol 1990; 14: 351.)

one. The dependence of the pathophysiology on spectrin/spectrin attachments fits with the observation that the severity of an α-spectrin mutation is inversely proportional to its distance from the contact site of self-association. There are exceptions to this observation: $\alpha^{I/65-68}$ is usually mild given its relative proximity to the contact site, and $\alpha^{I/50a}$ and $\alpha^{I/50b}$ are unusually severe relative to their positions. Most α-spectrin defects occur in helix C of the proposed model of triple-helical repeats. The precise mutations responsible for HE and HPP have been identified in most of these tryptic variants (Fig. 15–26; Tables 15–9 and 15–10).

Spectrin Alpha$^{I/74}$. This is a heterogeneous collection of defects that result in enhanced tryptic cleavage following Arg[45] or Lys[48] in an extrahelical segment (helix C in the crystallographic structure of the repeat) that juts out from the NH_2-terminal end of the α-spectrin chain. This is the end that participates in the formation of the spectrin self-association contact site. The corresponding (COOH-terminal) end of the β chain also contains extra helices (helices A and B) in repeat 17, followed by a phosphorylated segment. Tse and colleagues[1218] and Speicher and colleagues[306] proposed that these three helices pair up, as they do all along the spectrin chain, and that this is the bond responsible for spectrin self-association. Confirmation of the existence and functional importance of this "atypical repeat" has been provided by the study of

human mutants, biochemical studies of wild-type and mutant recombinant peptides,[350–352] and molecular modeling.[349, 1338, 1344, 1344a]

Spectrin $\alpha^{I/74}$ mutations disrupt one of the three interacting terminal helices of the contact site and markedly disrupt spectrin self-association. As a result, they are generally the most severe of the common α-spectrin mutations that cause HE and HPP. Patients who are homozygous for $\alpha^{I/74}$ defects usually have life-threatening hemolysis and an HPP-like syndrome.[1242, 1252] Patients who are compound heterozygotes for an $\alpha^{I/74}$ mutation and an $\alpha^{I/46-50a}$ or $\alpha^{I/61}$ defect also have severe hemolysis. Both groups of patients have partial (about 30 percent) spectrin deficiency,[1289] similar to that seen in HS. Spectrin deficiency and the appearance of spherocytes along with elliptocytes and poikilocytes are common features of the most severe forms of HE and HPP. Sometimes patients with $\alpha^{I/74}$ defects have so many microspherocytes and so few elliptocytes on their blood smears that the diagnosis of HE is not considered until smears from family members are examined.

In most instances, the primary defect in spectrin $\alpha^{I/74}$ variants is an amino acid substitution near the site of enhanced tryptic cleavage in the α chain.[1319, 1345] Codon 28, a CpG dinucleotide, is a "hot spot" for mutation and has been associated with four different sequence variations.

TABLE 15–9. α-Spectrin Mutations Associated with Hereditary Elliptocytosis and Hereditary Pyropoikilocytosis*

| Variant | Tryptic Phenotype | Mutation | | | Exon | Repeat Segment | α Helix | Reference |
		Codon	Gene	Protein				
Lograno	$\alpha^{I/74}$	24	ATC→AGC	Ile→Ser	2	α1	3	1321
Corbeil	$\alpha^{I/74}$	28	CGT→CAT	Arg→His	2	α1	3	1244
Unnamed	$\alpha^{I/74}$	28	CGT→CTT	Arg→Leu	2	α1	3	1243, 1283
Unnamed	$\alpha^{I/74}$	28	CGT→AGT	Arg→Ser	2	α1	3	1243, 1283
Unnamed	$\alpha^{I/74}$	28	CGT→TGT	Arg→Cys	2	α1	3	1243
Marseille	$\alpha^{I/74}$	31	GTG→GCG	Val→Ala	2	α1	3	1322
Genova	$\alpha^{I/74}$	34	CGG→TGG	Arg→Trp	2	α1	3	1323
Tunis	$\alpha^{I/78}$	41	CGG→TGG	Arg→Trp	2	α1	3	1226, 1227
Clichy	$\alpha^{I/78}$	45	AGG→AGT	Arg→Ser	2	α1	3	1258
Anastasia	$\alpha^{I/78}$	45	AGG→ACG	Arg→Thr	2	α1	3	1324
Culoz	$\alpha^{I/74}$	46	GGT→GTT	Gly→Val	2	α1	3	1325
Unnamed	$\alpha^{I/74}$	48	AAG→AGG	Lys→Arg	2	α1	3	1283
Lyon	$\alpha^{I/74}$	49	CTT→TTT	Leu→Phe	2	α1	3	1325
Ponte de Sôr	$\alpha^{I/65}$	151	GGT→GAT	Gly→Asp	4	α2	3	1326
Unnamed	$\alpha^{I/65}$	154	+TTG	+Leu	4	α2	3	1327
Dayton	$\alpha^{I/50-46}$	178–226	Insertion in intron 4†	−48 residues	5	α2	—	1328
Saint-Louis	$\alpha^{I/50-46}$	207	CTG→CCG	Leu→Pro	5	α2	2	1329
Nigerian	$\alpha^{I/50-46}$	260	CTG→CCG	Leu→Pro	6	α3	3	1330
Unnamed	$\alpha^{I/50-46}$	261	TCC→CCC	Ser→Pro	6	α3	3	1330
Sfax	$\alpha^{I/36}$	362–371	AGAT→AG/gt‡	−9 residues	8	α4	3	1248
Alexandria	$\alpha^{I/50-46b}$	469	CAT→Del	His→Del	11	α5	3	1331
Barcelona	$\alpha^{I/50-46b}$	469	CAT→CCT	His→Pro	11	α5	3	1249
Unnamed	$\alpha^{I/50-46b}$	471	CAG→CCG	G1n→Pro	11	α5	3	1330
Jendouba	$\alpha^{II/31}$	791	GAC→GAA	Asp→Glu	17	α7	3	1332
Oran	$\alpha^{II/21}$	822–863	ivs 17–1 g→a§	−41 residues	18	α8	—	1271, 1274
St. Claude	$\alpha^{II/46}$	935–965	ivs 19–13, at→ag	−31 residues	20	α9	2	1333, 1334

*References are limited to the first description of the genomic mutation. In some cases, the names of the variants has been coined subsequently. The protein phenotype is based on an initial terminology after mild trypsin digestion and peptide mapping.
†Skipping of exon 5.
‡Creation of cryptic splice site, partial in-frame skipping of exon 8.
§Skipping of exon 18.

TABLE 15–10. β-Spectrin Mutations Associated with Hereditary Elliptocytosis and Hereditary Pyropoikilocytosis

Variant	Tryptic Phenotype	Mutation		Protein	Exon	Repeat Segment	β Helix	Reference
		Codon	Gene					
Cagliari	$\alpha^{I/74}$	2018	GCC→GGC	Ala→Gly	30	β17	1	1335
Kuwaitino	$\alpha^{I/74}$	2018	GCC→GAC	Ala→Asp	30	β17	1	1282
Providence	$\alpha^{I/74}$	2019	TCT→CCT	Ser→Pro	30	β17	1	1336
Paris	$\alpha^{I/74}$	2023	GCG→GTG	Ala→Val	30	β17	1	1321
Linguere	$\alpha^{I/74}$	2024	TGG→AGG	Trp→Arg	30	β17	1	1321
Buffalo	$\alpha^{I/74}$	2025	CTG→CGG	Leu→Arg	30	β17	1	1337
Tandil★	$\alpha^{I/74}$	2041	−7 nt;GGACAGTGT→GT	PCT	30	β17	2	1300
Nice★	$\alpha^{I/74}$	2046	+2 nt;GAAG→GAGAAG	PCT	30	β17	2	1298, 1299
Kayes	$\alpha^{I/74}$	2053	GCT→CCT	Ala→Pro	30	β17	2	1217
Napoli★	$\alpha^{I/74}$	2053	−8 nt;TTTTGAGAAG→TG	PCT	30	β17	2	1338
Tokyo★	$\alpha^{I/74}$	2059	−1 nt;GCCAGC→GCAGC	PCT	30	β17	2	1339
Cotonou	$\alpha^{I/74}$	2061	TGG→AGG	Trp→Arg	30	β17	2	1214
Cosenza	$\alpha^{I/74}$	2064	CGC→CCC	Arg→Pro	30	β17	2	1340
Nagoya★	$\alpha^{I/74}$	2069	GAG→TAG	Glu→Stop	30	β17	2	1341
Prague	$\alpha^{I/74}$	Intron 29	ivs 29 −1 g→c	PCT	30	β17	2	1305
Göttingen★	$\alpha^{I/74}$	Intron 30	ivs 30 −2 t→a†	PCT	30	β17	2	1301, 1302
Le Puy★	$\alpha^{I/74}$	Intron 30	ivs 30 −4 a→g†	PCT	30	β17	2	1303, 1304
Rouen★	$\alpha^{I/74}$	Intron 31	ivs 31 −3 g→t‡	PCT	31	β17	2	1296, 1297
Campinas★	$\alpha^{I/74}$	Intron 30	ivs 30 + 1 g→a†	PCT	30	β17	2	1342

PCT-premature chain termination due to a frameshift.
★Truncated β-chain detectable on gel.
†Skipping of exon 30.
‡Skipping of exon 31.

In addition, in an increasing number of HE and HPP kindreds with $\alpha^{I/74}$ mutations, the primary defect occurs in helices A or B of repeat 17 of β-spectrin (see later). These two helices are adjacent to the $\alpha^{I/74}$ cleavage site in helix C at the NH$_2$ terminus of the β chain. These mutations support the self-association model of Speicher and colleagues[307] and Tse and colleagues.[1218]

Spectrin Alpha$^{I/46–50a}$. This disorder is also heterogeneous and variable in severity. Generally it is less severe than the disorder caused by spectrin $\alpha^{I/74}$ and more severe than that associated with spectrin $\alpha^{I/65-68}$.[1346, 1347] It is particularly common in black populations. Mutations cluster around the site of abnormal tryptic cleavage in helix C of α-spectrin repeat 2, with one informative exception,[1330] which occurs at an adjacent site in helix B of repeat 2.

Spectrin Alpha$^{I/65–68}$. This common α-spectrin mutation is widely distributed in blacks in West Africa (where the prevalence of HE is 0.67 percent),[1337] in blacks in Central Africa,[1346] and in their descendants in the West Indies and North America.[1327, 1328, 1348–1352] It is also seen in Arab populations and is the most common cause of HE in North Africa. The disorder is quite mild. It causes mild common HE in blacks, which is even milder in North Africans, who sometimes have little or no elliptocytosis (i.e., are silent carriers). Even homozygotes have only mild to moderate hemolysis. Studies indicate that, with one exception,[1327] all patients have an extra leucine inserted between codons 154 and 155, probably due to duplication of codon 154.[1328, 1331] The high rate of occurrence of $\alpha^{I/65–68}$ and its homogeneous expression strongly suggest that it has experienced genetic selection.[1215] This has led to the hypothesis that it may provide some protection from malaria or other tropical diseases caused by blood-borne parasites. This has not yet been systemati-

cally tested, although there is preliminary evidence that growth of *P. falciparum* is inhibited in $\alpha^{I/65–68}$ erythrocytes.[1353]

Spectrin Alpha$^{I/78}$. This defect has been observed mostly in North Africans.[1227, 1228, 1259] Symptoms vary greatly, ranging from asymptomatic to moderately severe hemolysis, perhaps related to coinheritance of spectrin α^{LELY} (see later). The primary mutations are located amid those that cause spectrin $\alpha^{I/74}$ defects but, for unknown reasons, they cause tryptic cleavage at a more proximal site (Lys^{16}).

Spectrin Alpha$^{I/50b}$. This defect has been observed primarily in patients of African ancestry. The clinical phenotype ranges from asymptomatic elliptocytosis to poikilocytic elliptocytosis with hemolysis.[1250, 1331, 1332, 1340] Two point mutations and a single amino acid substitution have been associated with this disorder.

Spectrin Alpha$^{I/36}$. A truncated α-spectrin with the protein phenotype of $\alpha^{I/36}$ is spectrin^{Sfax}. This mutant spectrin is shortened by nine amino acids owing to a point mutation that creates an alternate splice junction.[1249]

Beta-Spectrin Defects. β Chain abnormalities have been identified in patients with HE, defective spectrin self-association, and $\alpha^{I/74}$-spectrin on tryptic digests. All mutants described occur in repeat 17, the region involved in spectrin self-association (Fig. 15–26). A variety of mutations have been described that are either associated with a structurally abnormal β-spectrin chain or a β chain with a truncated COOH terminus. Truncated β chains have been reported in a number of kindreds with HE and chronic hemolysis.[1297, 1302–1307, 1343] SDS gels show two spectrin β bands: β and β′. The β component co-migrates with the normal spectrin β chain (220 kD), whereas β′ moves faster, consistent with loss of a portion of the peptide chain. The size of the β′ band varies from 210 to 218 kD. This end of β-spectrin contains at least four phosphorylation sites within 10 kD of the COOH terminus.[1354] In most patients the β′ component is not phosphorylated, which localizes the deletion to the COOH-terminal end of the β chain. Spectrin^{Rouen} (218 kD) is an exception; it has the shortest deletion and retains at least one phosphorylation site.[1297, 1298] Low temperature extracts of truncated β-spectrin variants contain increased spectrin dimer (approximately 50 percent of the spectrin dimer plus tetramer pool), and nearly all of the mutant β-spectrin is found in the dimer fraction, proving that it is responsible for the functional defect.

The primary genetic defect in the β-spectrin gene has been identified in several HE kindreds. In instances associated with truncated β-spectrin chains, the coding sequence terminates because of a frameshift. In several instances a splice site mutation causes the adjacent exon to be skipped.[1297, 1302–1307, 1343] In the other instances, insertions or deletions in the coding region alter the reading frame[1299–1301, 1339, 1340] or there is a nonsense mutation[1342] that leads to a shortened β-spectrin chain. The other variants probably induce conformational changes that alter the ability of spectrin to self-associate.

Spectrin Defects Outside the Heterodimer Self-Association Site. A few instances of mutant spectrins outside the heterodimer self-association site have been described in patients with HE and HPP. Some of these variants have an effect on spectrin dimer self-association, the basis of which is largely unknown. Lane and colleagues[1260] reported a truncated α-spectrin chain variant associated with HE in three generations of a family. The affected red cells had decreased stability and impaired spectrin self-association. Truncated α-spectrin varied from 10 to 45 percent of total α-spectrin. Two-dimensional tryptic peptide maps were qualitatively normal but showed a decrease in the quantity of one of the α-IV domain peptides. The genetic defect underlying this variant α-spectrin chain remains unknown.

A severe neonatal poikilocytic anemia associated with impaired spectrin dimer self-association was observed in an infant whose parents were clinically and biochemically normal.[1273] There was increased tryptic cleavage at the junction of the α-II and α-III domains and a slight modification of the molecular weights of the two major peptides of the α-II domain. The proband is homozygous for a splice junction mutation that leads to two variant mRNA species: One species encodes a truncated α-spectrin chain that is not assembled on the membrane. The other species encodes a protein that lacks exon 20 but is attached to the membrane[1334] and exhibits reduced spectrin-ankyrin binding.[1335] Because α-spectrin is produced in excess, the heterozygous parents are clinically and biochemically asymptomatic. This variant, spectrin$^{St. Claude}$, was identified in 3 percent of asymptomatic individuals from Benin, Africa[1334] and in a white family of Afrikaans origin in South Africa.[1335]

Spectrin^{Oran} is a variant of the α-II domain that is expressed at low levels.[1272] It causes no symptoms in the heterozygous state but causes severe HE in the homozygous state. Tryptic peptide mapping and amino acid sequencing of a variant peptide reveals an abnormal cleavage after Arg890,[1272, 1275] owing to a mutation of the acceptor splice site upstream of exon 18 (−1, a→g) that causes exon 18 to be skipped. A minor mRNA species utilizes an alternative acceptor site 1 base downstream from the mutated intron/exon boundary. The skipping of exon 18 probably changes the conformation of the α-II domain of spectrin, leading to its abnormal pattern of tryptic digestion.

Spectrin^{Jendouba} ($\alpha^{II/31}$) is a variant associated with asymptomatic HE, a mild defect in spectrin self-association,[1333] and abnormal tryptic cleavage after Lys^{788} owing to an Asp→Glu mutation at codon 791. This mutation apparently has a long-range effect on the self-association of spectrin dimers.

A large β-spectrin chain variant, spectrin^{Detroit}, with an estimated molecular mass of 330 kD, was isolated from a child with HE.[1355] Further study of this patient and his family members demonstrated that HE was caused by coinheritance of an α-spectrin chain variant (the $\alpha^{I/6–68}$ abnormality) rather than by the elongated β-spectrin chain. Family members with normal α-spectrin and heterozygous for the elongated β-chain variant had normal red cell morphology and no clinical abnormalities, but their erythrocyte membranes were more rigid and fragile than normal. The fragility is probably a consequence of both weaker spectrin dimer association and spectrin deficiency (total spectrin was about 80 percent of normal). A similar kindred has been reported from Brazil.[1356] The underlying molecular defect of the elongated β-spectrin chain is unknown.

Low Expression Alpha-Spectrin Allele: Alpha^{LELY}. Some patients with HE and HPP are *heterozygous* for a structural variant of spectrin involving the self-association site but have a more severe phenotype than expected, including marked hemolysis and anemia and require blood transfusions or splenectomy. These patients also have spectrin deficiency. They are usually categorized as having hemolytic HE, poikilocytic HE, or HPP. It has been postulated that they possess a second defect of α-spectrin that affects spectrin production or accumulation. The parents who transmit the postulated defect are clinically and biochemically normal. Studies of patients have focused on associated α-spectrin polymorphisms, studies of α-spectrin chain synthesis *in vitro*, and PCR-based analyses.

The best-characterized low expression allele of α-spectrin is the α^{LELY} allele. In initial studies, a polymorphism of the α domain, referred to as $\alpha^{V/41}$ and associated with increased proteolytic susceptibility of the junction between the α-IV and α domains, was identified in tryptic digests of spectrin.[1251] Patients with HE who were heterozygous for various mutant α spectrins and who possessed the $\alpha^{V/41}$ polymorphism in *trans* had a more severe form of the condition than expected.[1319] However, the polymorphism itself was asymptomatic in either the heterozygous or homozygous state. Molecular studies identified two linked abnormalities: (1) a C→T substitution at position −12 of intron 45, immediately upstream of exon 46, which causes the six amino acids encoded by exon 46 to be skipped and (2) an amino acid substitution, Leu→Val at codon 1857 in exon 40, due to a C→G substitution.[1357, 1358] Together, these changes identify the

α^{LELY} allele, which has a wide ethnic distribution and is *very common* (gene occurrences of 31 percent in whites, 21 percent in African blacks, 20 percent in Japanese, and 22 percent in Chinese).[1359] In patients who are heterozygous for α^{LELY} and an α-spectrin mutation causing HE, the limited synthesis of α^{LELY} protein decreases the amount of spectrin containing α^{LELY} that is incorporated into the membrane by approximately 50 percent and increases the relative incorporation of spectrin containing the HE α chain. α^{LELY} is poorly expressed owing to defective spectrin nucleation because the six deleted amino acids encoded by exon 46 lie within the nucleation site that joins the α- and β-spectrin chains[342, 1360] (see earlier discussion). α Chains that lack exon 46 fail to assemble into stable spectrin dimers and are degraded.

The α^{LELY} allele is clinically silent by itself, even when in the homozygous state, probably because α-spectrin is normally synthesized in a threefold or fourfold excess.[690] As explained earlier, when spectrin α^{LELY} is inherited in *trans* to an α-spectrin mutation, it has the effect of increasing the concentration of the mutant spectrin and the severity of the associated disease. The effect can be quite dramatic. For example, in one family a patient who was heterozygous for the $\alpha^{\text{I/74}}$ mutation $(+/\alpha^{\text{I/74}})$ had very mild disease and almost no morphologic abnormality, whereas a relative who had also inherited the α^{LELY} allele $(\alpha^{\text{I/74}}\ \alpha^{\text{LELY}})$ had severe elliptocytosis.[1251] Similarly, in another family the α^{LELY} allele increased the proportion of spectrin $\alpha^{\text{I/65-68}}$ in heterozygotes from 45 to 65 percent of the total spectrin.[1251] This is associated with an increase in the proportion of elliptocytes from none or only a few to nearly 100 percent.[1361, 1362] All α-spectrin mutations seem to be similarly affected (Fig. 15–27). Conversely, when the α^{LELY} allele is on the same chromosome as an α-spectrin mutation it mutes the elliptocytic phenotype.

Although the synthesis of α^{LELY} subunits is decreased, owing to poor incorporation of the peptide lacking exon 46, the production of α^{LELY} mRNA is normal. In particular, spectrin α^{LELY} should be distinguished from thalassemia-like defects of α-spectrin synthesis that, when coinherited with some of the α-spectrin mutations, also produce a phenotype of HPP. The latter defects are characterized by reduced α-spectrin mRNA levels and diminished α-spectrin synthesis. None is well characterized. Preliminary studies in an patient with HPP who was heterozygous for the $\alpha^{\text{I/50a}}$-spectrin variant and an asymptomatic parent show that α-spectrin protein synthesis is decreased, as measured by pulse labeling of late erythroblasts.[1290] Competitive PCR studies in the same patient show that α-spectrin mRNA is decreased compared with that in control subjects. In another example, three patients who are heterozygous for distinct mutations of the α-I domain of spectrin, had markedly decreased amounts of α-spectrin mRNA derived from the companion allele, leading to a phenotype of HPP.[1363] In these patients, the structural mutation either created or abolished a restriction enzyme site, producing a marker for the production-defective allele.

Molecular Determinants of the Clinical Severity of Hereditary Elliptocytosis and Hereditary Pyropoikilocytosis Spectrin Mutations. The principal determinants of clinical severity are the degree of decreased cellular deformability, the spectrin content of

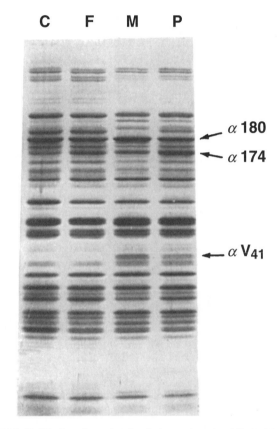

FIGURE 15–27. One-dimensional gel electrophoresis of limited tryptic digests of spectrin. Lane C contains spectrin of a normal control subject. Lane F contains spectrin of the proband's father, who is heterozygous for the αI/74 variant and lacks the $\alpha^{\text{V/41}}$ polymorphism. Lane M contains spectrin of the proband's mother, who lacks the αI/74 variant and is homozygous for the $\alpha^{\text{V/41}}$ polymorphism. Lane P contains spectrin from an HE proband doubly heterozygous for the αI/74-kDa variant and the $\alpha^{\text{V/41}}$ polymorphism. (From Baklouti F, Maréchal J, Morle L, et al: Occurrence of the α-I 22 Arg→His (CGT→CAT) spectrin mutation in Tunisia: Potential association with severe elliptocytosis. Br J Haematol 1991; 78:108.)

the cells, and the percentage of dimeric spectrin in crude spectrin extracts.[1252, 1346, 1364] The fraction of dimeric spectrin, in turn, depends principally on two factors. The first is the dysfunction of the mutant spectrin. Mutations within or near the site of self-association produce a more profound defect of spectrin function and a more severe clinical phenotype than point mutations in more distant triple-helical repeats.[1319] Molecular modeling has demonstrated that mutations of key residues in α and β spectrin, including seemingly conservative amino acid substitutions, lead to conformational rearrangements in the predicted structure and that the degree of structural disruption correlates strongly with the severity of clinical disease associated with each mutation (Fig. 15–28).

The second factor is the fraction of the mutant spectrin in the cells. This is determined by the gene dose (i.e., simple heterozygote versus homozygote or double heterozygote) and by other genetic defects such as the presence of α^{LELY}-spectrin or another defect leading to reduced synthesis of α-spectrin.[1251, 1357]

Polymorphisms of Spectrin. Spectrin polymorphisms are useful markers in genetic studies of erythrocyte

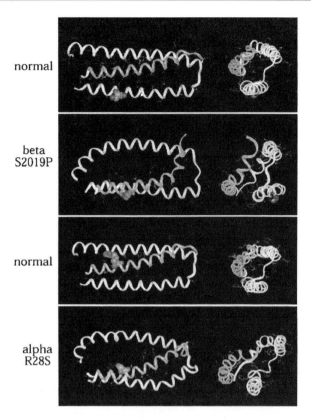

FIGURE 15–28. Molecular modeling of mutations of the spectrin self-association domain. (Top pair) Structure of normal spectrin versus spectrin^Providence, showing the position of the serine to proline amino acid replacement at codon 2019 of β-spectrin (position 12 in the A helix). Note the severe distortion of this helix, with loss of the β-spectrin pocket into which the C helix of a spectrin docks. (Bottom pair) A similar analysis of a mutation in codon 28 of α spectrin. Even though the serine in this mutation is hydrophilic like the arginine residue it replaces, the loss of two putative salt bridges formed by the lost arginine destabilizes the self-association binding site. In each model, longitudinal and end-on views are shown. (Reprinted with permission from Zhang Z, Weed SA, Gallagher PG, Morrow JS. Dynamic molecular modeling of pathogenic mutations in the spectrin self-association site. Blood 98:1645, 2001)

membrane defects. A number of protein polymorphisms have been identified by tryptic mapping of spectrin. Variant peptides have been identified in the α-II and α-III domains.[1215, 1365, 1366] Four polymorphisms of the α-II domain occur primarily in people of African origin and have been characterized at the levels of protein and DNA sequence.[1365, 1366] All four polymorphisms involve various combinations of amino acids at residues 701, 809, and 853: type 1—normal, Arg/Ile/Thr; type 2—apparent increase in molecular weight and basic shift in isoelectric point, His/Val/Arg; type 3—apparent increase in molecular weight, His/Ile/Thr; and type 4—basic shift in isoelectric point, Arg/Val/Arg. All of the amino acid variations are due to single base substitutions. These polymorphisms occur in distinct haplotypes and have been correlated with specific HE and HPP α-spectrin mutations.[1366] The α-III domain protein polymorphism is also a point mutation.[1215]

Murine Model of Hereditary Elliptocytosis. A murine model of HE, *sph*^Dem, has been described.[1367] *sph*^Dem mice suffer from severe elliptocytic hemolytic anemia due to a mutation in the self-association region of α-

spectrin. Erythrocytes are spectrin deficient and spectrin dimer-tetramer self-association is abnormal.

Protein 4.1 Defects

The link between protein 4.1 deficiency and elliptocytosis was first described in a consanguineous Algerian family.[1226, 1274] Partial absence of the protein is found in the 4.1(—) trait, which appears to be a common cause of elliptocytosis, accounting for 30 to 40 percent of occurrences in some Arab and European populations.[1233–1235, 1282, 1368] It is not observed in individuals of African ancestry.[1216]

Heterozygous Protein 4.1 Deficiency. Protein 4.1(–) heterozygotes have clinically mild HE with little or no hemolysis, prominent elliptocytosis, often approaching 100 percent, and minimal red cell fragmentation.[1369]

Homozygous Protein 4.1 Deficiency. Erythrocytes from patients homozygous for the protein 4.1(–) trait (i.e., complete protein 4.1 deficiency) are elliptical, fragmented, and poikilocytic.[1226, 1274, 1370] They are very osmotically fragile and possess normal thermal stability. Membranes from homozygous protein 4.1(–) red cells fragment much more rapidly than normal at moderate sheer stresses, an indication of their intrinsic instability.[1317] Membrane mechanical stability can be completely restored by reconstituting the deficient red cells with normal protein 4.1 or the protein 4.1/spectrin/actin-binding site.[1371, 1372] In addition to complete deficiency of protein 4.1, erythrocytes from protein 4.1(–) homozygotes lack protein p55[471, 1373] and have only 30 percent of the normal content of GpC and GpD.[469, 1274, 1373, 1374] This adds evidence to the hypothesis that GpC is one of the membrane attachment sites for protein 4.1.[468] In addition, protein 4.9 is absent from isolated membrane skeletons but not from intact red cell membranes, and membrane phospholipid asymmetry is perturbed.[473, 1226] Electron microscopic studies of homozygous 4.1(–) erythrocyte membranes have revealed a markedly disrupted skeletal network with disruption of the intramembrane particles, suggesting that protein 4.1 plays an important role in maintenance of not only the skeletal network, but also of the integral proteins of the membrane structure.[1375] Homozygous patients have a severe hemolytic anemia, requiring transfusions and splenectomy.[1226, 1274, 1370] There appears to be a good response to splenectomy.

In the original Algerian kindred,[1226] protein 4.1(–) mRNA is not translated,[1376] owing to a 318-bp deletion, which includes the downstream translation initiation site that is utilized in reticulocytes (Fig. 15–29).[435] In other patients, point mutations of the downstream initiator codon (AUG→AGG[1274] and AUG→ACG[1377]) have been identified. Interestingly (and probably fortunately), expression of protein 4.1 is relatively unimpaired in non-erythroid tissues and early erythroblasts[484–486, 1378] because most of the protein 4.1 isoforms in these tissues initiate translation at the alternatively spliced, upstream translation initiation site.

Protein 4.1 Structural Defects. Variants with abnormal molecular weights have also been described in association with HE.[1235, 1379–1382] A shortened protein 4.1 was discovered in an Italian family with very mild common HE and mechanically unstable red cells. The patients are heterozygous for a protein 4.1 variant that has lost the

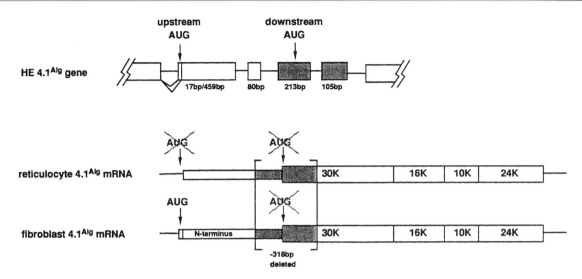

FIGURE 15–29. Genetic model of the Algerian 4.1(–) HE. Model of the isoform-specific deficiency encoded by the aberrant 4.1 gene. The upper panel shows a 5′ portion of the 4.1 gene, including the exons encoding the upstream and downstream AUGs. In the mutant gene, exons in *gray* are not spliced into 4.1 mRNAs. Reticulocyte 4.1 mRNA thus lacks any functional translation initiation site and cannot make any protein 4.1. Fibroblast 4.1 mRNA retains the upstream AUG and can therefore synthesize high molecular weight 4.1 isoforms with the NH$_2$-terminal extension. (From Conboy JG: Structure, function, and molecular genetics of erythroid membrane skeletal protein 4.1 in normal and abnormal red blood cells. Semin Hematol 1993; 30:138.)

two exons encoding the spectrin/actin-binding domain. The mutant protein runs as a doublet of 65 and 68 kD on SDS gels and seems to be present in nearly normal amounts. It is presumed, but not proven, to be functionally inept. A high-molecular-weight variant, protein 4.1[95] or protein 4.1[Hurdle-Mills],[1235] was discovered in a family of Scottish-Irish ancestry with very mild common HE. The patients are heterozygous for a duplication of three exons that include the spectrin/actin-binding domain.[1379, 1380] Membrane function appears to be preserved because red cell membranes have normal mechanical stability.[435] It is not clear how this variant causes HE.

A series of protein 4.1 variants due to mutations in the 22/24 kD COOH-terminal domain have been described in patients with HE. These mutants are characterized by heterogeneity in clinical phenotype and degree of protein 4.1 deficiency.[1381] When the mutant mRNA was stable, it produced a truncated protein that was assembled on the membrane, suggesting that this region is not required for protein 4.1 membrane assembly in mature red cells.

A large genomic deletion was identified in a kindred with HE and protein 4.1 deficiency.[1382] Differential splicing of the exons in the undeleted region was unperturbed.

Glycophorin C Defects

Elliptocytes are noted on peripheral blood smears of patients whose erythrocytes carry the Leach phenotype (i.e., lacking the Gerbich antigens, Ge: –1, –2, –3, –4).[199–201, 1307, 1308, 1381–1383] These erythrocytes are devoid of GpC and GpD and, presumably secondarily, lack protein p55 and are deficient in protein 4.1. It has been speculated that the protein 4.1 deficiency in Leach erythrocytes is the cause of their elliptocytic shape. Interestingly, the relative deficiency of protein 4.1 in Leach erythrocytes is less than the degree of GpC deficiency in homozygous protein 4.1(–) erythrocytes. These findings add supportive evidence to the hypothesis that GpC and protein p55 provide a binding site for protein 4.1 in the red cell.[471]

The Leach phenotype is usually due to a deletion of 7 kb of genomic DNA that removes exons 3 and 4 from the *GpC/GpD* locus.[1382–1384] One individual has a single nucleotide deletion preceded by a missense mutation, TGGCCG→TTGCG, leading to a frameshift with premature chain termination. Patients carrying the Leach phenotype suffer from a mild spherocytic HE with increased erythrocyte osmotic fragility.[197, 200, 201, 1307] In some individuals, no elliptocytes are detected on peripheral smear.[469] In one patient, transient elliptocytosis and GpC deficiency were associated with development of an autoantibody to GpC.[1310]

Individuals whose erythrocytes lack several of the Gerbich antigens, that is, the Yusef type (–1, –2, –3, and 4) and Gerbich type (–1, –2, –3, and 4), owing to large deletions of genomic DNA, lack GpC and GpD. Instead, these erythrocytes possess a single structurally related functional protein of molecular weight intermediate between that of GpC and GpD.[1385] These erythrocytes are not elliptocytic and have normal amounts of protein 4.1 and protein p55, suggesting that the hybrid protein is functionally active and fully capable of interacting with the two skeletal proteins. Individuals whose erythrocytes lack GpA, GpB, or both, are asymptomatic and have erythrocytes of normal shape and mechanical stability.

PATHOPHYSIOLOGY OF HEREDITARY ELLIPTOCYTOSIS/HEREDITARY PYROPOIKILOCYTOSIS

Spectrin Mutations

The principal functional consequence of the elliptocytogenic spectrin mutations is a weakening or even disruption of the spectrin dimer-tetramer contact, and, consequently, the two-dimensional integrity of the membrane skeleton. These horizontal defects are readily detected by ultrastructural examination of membrane skeletons, which reveals disruption of the normally uniform hexagonal lattice. Consequently, membrane skeletons, cell membranes, and the red cells are mechanically unstable. In patients who have severely dysfunctional spectrin mutations or in subjects who are homozygous or compound heterozygous for such mutant proteins, this membrane instability is sufficient to cause hemolytic anemia with red cell fragmentation.

How elliptocytes are formed is less clear. In common HE, red cell precursors are round and the cells become progressively more elliptical as they age *in vivo*.[1211, 1236, 1386] Red cells distorted by shear stress *in vitro* or flowing through the microcirculation *in vivo* have elliptical or parachute-like shapes, respectively.[584] Perhaps the abnormal shapes of elliptocytes and poikilocytes are permanently stabilized because the weakened skeletal interactions facilitate skeletal reorganization after prolonged or repetitive cellular deformation. Skeletal reorganization is likely to involve breakage of the unidirectionally stretched protein connections and formation of new contacts that reduce stress on the skeleton and stabilize the deformed shape.[584] This process, first proposed in 1978, has been shown to account for permanent deformation of irreversibly sickled cells.[1387]

HPP red cells have two abnormalities: they contain a mutant spectrin that disrupts spectrin self-association and they are partially deficient in spectrin.[1289, 1290] This is either due to an elliptocytogenic α-spectrin mutation and a defect involving reduced α-spectrin synthesis or to two elliptocytogenic spectrin alleles. In the latter situation, spectrin deficiency might be a consequence of spectrin instability, which would reduce the amount of spectrin available for membrane assembly. In red cells carrying a lot of unassembled spectrin dimers, the fact that one ankyrin is bound per one spectrin tetramer (i.e., two spectrin heterodimers) may also contribute to spectrin deficiency. At best only about one half of the spectrin dimers could succeed in attaching to the available ankyrin-binding sites. Probably this attachment would be less because unphosphorylated ankyrin binds spectrin dimers about 10 times less avidly than do spectrin tetramers.[412, 422]

The phenotype of HPP, characterized by the presence of fragments and elliptocytes, together with evidence of red cell surface area deficiency (i.e., microspherocytes), suggests that the membrane dysfunction involves both vertical interactions (a consequence of the spectrin deficiency) and horizontal interactions (a consequence of the elliptocytogenic spectrin mutations).

Protein 4.1 Variants

Hereditary elliptocytes that are deficient in protein 4.1 are similar in shape and membrane instability to elliptocytes that result from spectrin mutations.[584] This suggests that protein 4.1 deficiency principally affects the spectrin/actin contact (i.e., a horizontal interaction) rather than the skeletal attachment to GpC (a vertical interaction).

Permeability of Hereditary Elliptocytosis Red Cells

Red cells in HE consume more ATP and 2,3-DPG than normal erythrocytes,[1388] probably owing to increased

transmembrane Na^+ movements.[1389] As a result of the underlying skeletal defect, HE and HPP red cells are abnormally permeable to Na^+, K^+, and Ca^{2+} ions.[1286, 1389] The excessive Ca^{2+} leak was originally thought to be the primary molecular lesion in a patient with a severe microcytic hemolytic anemia and red cell thermal instability,[1286] who was subsequently shown to have a spectrin mutation and probably HPP.[1347]

Common Hereditary Elliptocytosis and Malaria

Epidemiologic studies of the elliptocytogenic mutations of spectrin in Central Western Africa suggest that their prevalence is considerably greater than would be expected for sporadic mutations. For example, the prevalence of the spectrin $\alpha^{I/65-68}$ mutation approaches 1 percent[1216] and the mutation is always associated with the same α-spectrin haplotype.[1366] Similar findings were reported for two α-spectrin mutations producing the spectrin $\alpha^{I/46-50a}$ phenotype ($Leu^{207} \rightarrow Pro$ and $Leu^{260} \rightarrow Pro$). These data are of considerable interest in light of recent *in vitro* studies, demonstrating diminished malarial parasite entry or growth in red cells that contain some of the elliptocytogenic spectrin mutants or are deficient in protein 4.1.[1353, 1390, 1391]

TREATMENT

In typical HE, the condition is mild and splenectomy is rarely required. Splenectomy to decrease hemolysis, ameliorate anemia, and avoid the formation of bilirubinate gallstones has been the cornerstone of therapy for patients with severe hemolytic HE and HPP. Most practitioners believe that the indications for splenectomy in HS should also be applied to patients with symptomatic HE and HPP. Patients with HE and HPP who have been splenectomized have experienced increased hematocrit values, decreased reticulocytosis, and improvement in clinical symptoms. If hemolysis is still active after splenectomy, folate should be administered daily. Recommendations for antibiotic prophylaxis, immunization, and monitoring during intercurrent illnesses are similar to those noted for HS patients before and after splenectomy. Serial interval ultrasound examinations, beginning at approximately 6 years of age, to detect gallstones should be performed in patients with brisk hemolysis.

Neonates should be treated as any patient with hemolytic anemia. Phototherapy and exchange transfusions are warranted in neonates with severe anemia and pathologic hyperbilirubinemia. Splenectomy is rarely necessary in the neonatal period.

SOUTHEAST ASIAN OVALOCYTOSIS

This condition, also known as Melanesian elliptocytosis or stomatocytic elliptocytosis, is inherited in an autosomal dominant pattern.[1392–1397] It is observed in the aboriginal populations of Melanesia and Malaysia and in portions of Indonesia and the Philippines.[1392–1395, 1398–1400] The abnormality is very common in Melanesia, particularly in lowland tribes in whom malaria is endemic.[1393, 1397, 1400, 1401] In these tribes, 5 to 25 percent of the population are affected. SAO has been detected rarely in white and

African-American individuals.[1402–1404] *In vivo*, there is evidence that SAO provides some protection against all forms of malaria, particularly against heavy infections and cerebral malaria.[1393, 1394, 1397, 1401, 1405–1408] The prevalence of SAO increases with age in populations challenged by malaria, suggesting that individuals with SAO have a selective advantage.[1405] *In vitro*, SAO red cells are resistant to invasion by malarial parasites,[1409–1411] apparently because the membrane is 10 to 20 times more rigid than normal.[1314, 1412–1415] Other membrane characteristics reflect this property, including unusually high heat resistance, lack of endocytosis in response to drugs that produce dramatic endocytosis in normal cells, and strong resistance to crenation, even after several days' storage in plasma or buffered salt solutions.[1314] The latter property, combined with distinctive red cell morphology (see later), provides a simple means of diagnosing the disease.

Most of the cells are rounded elliptocytes, but a few are traversed by one or two transverse bars that divide the central clear space (see Fig. 15–21*D*).[1392, 1396, 1398–1400, 1416] These "elliptical knizocytes" or "stomatocytic elliptocytes" are not seen in any other condition. Hemolysis is apparently mild or absent,[1221, 1222, 1392, 1394, 1398, 1399] although neonatal hyperbilirubinemia has been described.[1417] One patient had compensated hemolysis (no anemia), with mild splenomegaly, an absolute reticulocyte count of 150 to 300×10^{-3} (normal 10 to 100×10^{-3}), mild hyperbilirubinemia, and gallstones.[1418] This indicates that membrane rigidity is not a major determinant of red cell survival. In another well-studied patient,[1399] red cell Na^+ and K^+ permeability was increased, glucose consumption was elevated to compensate for increased cation pumping, autohemolysis was increased, and the cells were osmotically resistant. Curiously, many blood group antigens are poorly expressed on the surface of SAO red cells,[1400] possibly because the rigid membrane inhibits their clustering and impedes agglutination.

Etiology

The finding of tight linkage between an abnormal proteolytic digest of band 3 protein and the SAO phenotype led to detection of the underlying molecular defect.[1396] All carriers of the SAO phenotype are heterozygotes. One band 3 allele is normal, and the other contains two mutations in *cis*: a deletion of nine codons encoding amino acids 400 through 408, located at the boundary of the cytoplasmic and membrane domains and the replacement of Lys^{56} by Glu.[1414, 1415, 1419–1422] The $Lys^{56} \rightarrow Glu$ substitution is an asymptomatic polymorphism known as band 3 Memphis. The mutant SAO band 3 exhibits tight binding to ankyrin,[1396] increased tyrosine phosphorylation,[1423–1425] inability to transport anions,[1426, 1427] and markedly restricted lateral and rotational mobility in the membrane.[1396, 1414] Because SAO is caused by deletion of 27 bases from the band 3 gene, amplification of the deleted region in genomic DNA or reticulocyte cDNA is the most specific diagnostic test. This produces a single band in control red cells and a doublet with the second band shorter by 27 bp in SAO cells.[1414, 1419, 1428] In screening of large populations with SAO, no homozygotes have

been identified.[1429, 1430] It has been hypothesized that this would lead to embryonic or fetal lethality.

Molecular Basis of Membrane Rigidity and Malaria Resistance

SAO red cells are unique among elliptocytes in that they are rigid and hyperstable rather than unstable.[1413] The SAO band 3 mutation is the first example of a defect of an integral membrane protein leading to red cell membrane rigidity, a property that had previously been attributed to the membrane skeleton.[1431] The explanation of the rigidity is presently not clear. One hypothesis proposes that conformational changes of the cytoplasmic domain of SAO band 3 preclude lateral movement (extension) of the skeletal network during deformation.[1314, 1415, 1432] A second possibility is that SAO band 3 binds abnormally tightly to ankyrin and thus to the underlying skeleton.[1396] The increased propensity of SAO band 3 to aggregate into higher oligomers may be important because the oligomers can strengthen band 3 attachment to ankyrin.[1433] The tendency of SAO band 3 to form linear arrays would also decrease its mobility within the bilayer.[1434] Finally, SAO band 3 may adhere to the skeleton in a nonspecific manner, possibly due to denaturation of the membrane spanning domain.[1435] Solution-state NMR of the first transmembrane span of wild-type and SAO band 3 demonstrated that a bend between the cytoplasmic domain and the first transmembrane domain was absent in SAO cells, leading to formation of a stable helix in the region.[1436]

The resistance of SAO red cells to malaria is presumably related to the altered properties of SAO band 3. Band 3 serves as one of the malaria receptors, because invasion by the parasite *in vitro* is inhibited by band 3–containing liposomes.[1437] In normal red cells, parasite invasion is associated with marked membrane remodeling and redistribution of band 3–containing intramembrane particles.[1438] Intramembrane particles cluster at the site of parasite invasion, forming a ring around the orifice through which the parasite enters the cell. The invaginated red cell membrane, which surrounds the invading parasite, is free from intramembrane particles. The reduced lateral mobility of band 3 protein in SAO red cells may preclude band 3 receptor clustering and thus prevent attachment or entry of the parasites.[1396, 1414] Resistance to malaria has also been attributed to diminished anion exchange, owing to the inability of SAO band 3 to transport anions.[1427, 1427] In addition, SAO red cells consume ATP at a higher rate than that of normal cells; the ensuing partial depletion of ATP levels in ovalocytes has been proposed to account, at least in part, for the resistance of these cells to malaria invasion *in vitro*.[1412] However, diminished anion transport and ATP depletion do not appear to play a critical role in malaria resistance of SAO erythrocytes *in vivo*. This is evidenced by the fact that band 3–deficient HS red cells are considerably less resistant to malaria invasion than are SAO red cells, although both cell types have a similar decrease of anion transport, and by the fact that malaria resistance of SAO red cells is detected *in vitro* even when red cell ATP levels are maintained.

HYDROPS FETALIS SYNDROMES AND DISORDERS OF THE ERYTHROCYTE MEMBRANE

Defects of the erythrocyte membrane have been well characterized in patients with severe neonatal hemolytic anemia due to recessive HS and homozygous HE and HPP. Several well-documented kindreds with fatal or near-fatal anemia and hydrops fetalis associated with erythrocyte membrane defects have been described. In several patients, defects were identified in spectrin, the principal structural protein of the erythrocyte membrane (see later). In the other patients, homozygosity for a band 3 defect, band 3[Coimbra] or band 3[Neapolis], was discovered (see earlier). Based on the authors' experience, membrane defects have been suspected, but not proven, in numerous other patients with nonimmune hydrops fetalis with severe hemolytic anemia.

An infant who had hydrops fetalis, severe spherocytic anemia, extremely abnormal red blood cell osmotic fragility, and transfusion-dependent anemia that failed to respond to splenectomy has been described.[776] The patient's mother had typical autosomal dominant HS and her father, although clinically and hematologically normal, had red cells with slightly abnormal osmotic fragility. Cultured progenitor-derived erythroblasts from this patient showed a decrease in total cell spectrin content to 26 percent of normal. Metabolic labeling studies of cultured erythroblasts using ^{35}S-methionine revealed markedly decreased α-spectrin synthesis and absence of α-spectrin chain degradation products. It was thought that two different genetic defects caused the severe reduction of α-spectrin synthesis in the affected child's erythroid cells and that the profound spectrin deficiency resulted in cell destruction during egress of reticulocytes from the marrow or during enucleation of normoblasts. The precise genetic defect or defects in this family have not been characterized.

In another kindred,[1337] four third-trimester fetal losses that were associated with hemolytic anemia and hydrops fetalis occurred. Studies of erythrocytes and erythrocyte membranes from the parents showed abnormal membrane stability as well as structural and functional abnormalities of spectrin. A point mutation in the β-spectrin gene, Ser[2019]→Pro, spectrin[Providence], was identified in the heterozygous state in the parents and two living children and in the homozygous state in the three deceased infants studied.

A Laotian infant was born with severe hemolytic anemia (hemoglobin level of 2.7 g/dL) that produced negative Coombs test results and gross hydrops fetalis at birth.[1338] His neonatal course was marked by ongoing hemolytic anemia requiring erythrocyte transfusions. He has remained transfusion dependent for 2 years; his blood smears reveal only normal erythrocytes, which represent transfused cells and nucleated erythrocytes. His family history shows a previous sibling born with hemolytic anemia and hydrops fetalis who died on the second day of life. At autopsy it was revealed that she had diffuse tissue anoxia and marked extramedullary erythropoiesis. The parents had very rare elliptocytes and fragile erythrocyte membranes. Their spectrin exhibited weak self-association *in vitro* and displayed the mutant α[I/74] peptide on two-dimensional peptide maps. The proband and his deceased sister were homozygous for a point mutation of β-spectrin, Leu[2025]→Arg, spectrin[Buffalo], in the region of spectrin that participates in spectrin self-association. The parents were heterozygous for this mutation.

Stomatocytosis and Xerocytosis

Red cell hydration is largely determined by the intracellular concentration of monovalent cations. A net increase in Na[+] and K[+] ions causes water to enter, forming "stomatocytes" or "hydrocytes," whereas a net loss of monovalent cations produces dehydrated red cells or "xerocytes" (see Fig. 15–13).[1439–1441] In the past 35 years, numerous descriptions of congenital or familial hemolytic anemias associated with abnormal cation permeability and, in some cases, disturbed red cell hydration have been reported.[1160, 1441–1481] These span the range from severe stomatocytosis to severe xerocytosis. They can be divided into six provisional categories based on differences of severity, morphology, cation content, lipid and protein composition, genetics, and response to splenectomy (Table 15–11). It is unknown if these categories are unique entities. Indeed, none of these apparent disorders is precisely defined in either clinical or molecular terms.

HEREDITARY STOMATOCYTOSIS

Hereditary stomatocytosis, the name given by Lock and co-workers[1442] to the first reported instance, is characterized by erythrocytes with a mouth-shaped (stoma) area of central pallor on peripheral blood smears (Fig. 15–30). The clinical severity of hereditary stomatocytosis is variable; some patients experience hemolysis and anemia whereas others are asymptomatic.[1440, 1441]

Stomatocyte membranes are remarkably permeable to K[+] ions and particularly to Na[+] ions. Intracellular Na[+] is increased and K[+] is decreased, but the total monovalent cation content (Na[+] + K[+]) is high, which leads to an increase in cell water and cell volume. As a consequence, the "edematous cells" are sometimes called hydrocytes or overhydrated stomatocytes.

Pathophysiology

The major detectable defect in hereditary stomatocytosis is a marked asymmetric increase in passive Na[+] and K[+] permeability (the amount of Na[+] in is greater than the amount of K[+] out). Permeabilities as great as 15 to 40 times normal are observed.[1467, 1480] Because the influx of Na[+] exceeds the loss of K[+], stomatocytic red cells progressively gain cations and water and swell. As a result, their average density is less than normal and the swollen stomatocytes are osmotically fragile. Unlike normal cells, aged stomatocytes are less dense and more stomatocytic than stomatocytic reticulocytes.[1439, 1481]

The transporters of the red cell are similar to those of other cells in many respects.[639, 640] However, the rate of cation transport is less in the erythrocyte than in any other cell. In addition, the erythrocyte is relatively sluggish in responding to pharmacologic or other stimuli with changes in Na[+] or K[+] transport. Finally, the red cell is equipped with a high-capacity anion exchanger to service

TABLE 15–11. Clinical Heterogeneity of Hereditary Hydrocytosis-Xerocytosis Syndromes

	Stomatocytosis (Hydrocytosis)			Intermediate Syndromes		
	Severe Hemolysis	Mild Hemolysis	Cryohydrocytosis	Stomatocytic Xerocytosis	Xerocytosis with High PC	Xerocytosis
Hemolysis	Severe	Mild-moderate	Moderate	Mild	Moderate	Moderate
Anemia	Severe	Mild-moderate	Mild-Moderate	None	Mild	Moderate
Blood smear	Stomatocytes	Stomatocytes	Stomatocytes	Stomatocytes	Targets	Targets, echinocytes
MCV (80–100 fL³)*	110–150	95–130	90–105	91–98	84–92	100–110
MCHC (32%–36%)	24–30	26–29	34–40	33–39	34–38	34–38
Unincubated osmotic fragility	Very increased	Increased	Normal	Decreased	Very decreased	Very decreased
RBC Na$^+$ (5–12 mEq/LRBC)	60–100	30–60	40–50	10–20	10–15	10–20
RBC K$^+$ (90–103 mEq/LRBC)	20–55	40–85	55–65	75–85	75–90	60–80
RBC Na$^+$ + K$^+$ (95–110 mEq/LRBC)	110–140	115–145	100–105	87–103	93–99	75–90
PC content	Normal	±Increased	Normal	Normal	Increased	Normal
Cold autohemolysis	No	No	Yes	No	No	?
Effect of splenectomy	Good	Good	Fair	?	?	?Poor
Genetics	AD, ?AR	AD	AD	AD	AD	AD

PC=phosphatidylcholine; MCV=mean corpuscular volume; MCHC=mean corpuscular hemoglobin concentration; LRBC=liter of red blood cells.
*Values in parentheses are the normal range.

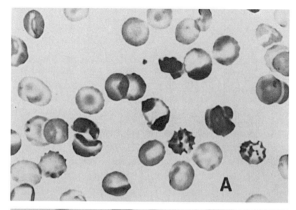

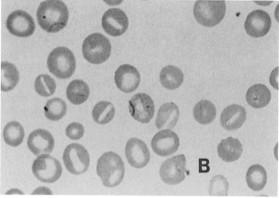

FIGURE 15–30. Peripheral blood morphology in hereditary xerocytosis and hereditary hydrocytosis. *A,* Hereditary xerocytosis: Note the presence of target cells, echinocytes, and some dense cells in which the hemoglobin is puddled at the periphery. It should be emphasized that red cell morphology is usually much less dramatic in this disease, especially before splenectomy. Often, modest targeting is the only detectable abnormality. *B,* Hereditary hydrocytosis: Many stomatocytes and occasional target cells are seen. (From Lande WM, Mentzer WC: Haemolytic anaemia associated with increased cation permeability. Clin Haematol 1985; 14:89.)

carbonic anhydrase, an intracellular respiratory enzyme, making red cell chloride transport much faster than that in other cells. The different transporters identified in the red cell are described in Table 15–4.

In stomatocytosis, monovalent cation transporters are stimulated by the influx of Na^+, particularly the Na^+-K^+-pump and K^+/Cl^- cotransporter,[1458] but are unable to keep up with the exaggerated cation leaks. There is no convincing evidence that Na^+/K^+ pumping is defective. Pump kinetics are normal[1481] and the number of pumps is increased severalfold,[1439, 1469] even after corrections for red cell age.[1482] Some authors have observed that Na^+ and K^+ are not transported in the usual ratio, 3 Na^+:2 K^+[1481, 1453, 1459] and have argued that the Na^+-K^+ pump is "decoupled."[1459] Other work suggests that this is, at least partly, an artifact of the methods used to measure cation permeability.[1483]

Bifunctional imidoesters, which cross-link proteins, reverse the abnormal shape and permeability of hereditary stomatocytes and normalize their survival in the circulation.[1484] The critical proteins involved have not been identified using these agents because many red cell membrane proteins are cross-linked at the concentrations required to achieve this effect. Stomatocytes are relatively

rigid[1455] and expend extraordinary amounts of ATP pumping Na^+ and K^+, attempting to maintain homeostasis. They are vulnerable to splenic sequestration and, predictably, splenectomy has been beneficial in some patients with severe hemolysis[1439, 1454, 1458, 1459, 1461] but not without risk (see later).[1160]

Stomatin

The red cell membranes of all or almost all patients with the classic overhydrated form of stomatocytosis, described earlier, lack a 31-kD protein called stomatin or band 7.2b (Fig. 15–31).[1444, 1447, 1448, 1458, 1485, 1486] Stomatin, a member of a related family of proteins, is an integral membrane phosphoprotein whose function is not completely understood.[1486, 1487–1494] Its importance, however, is underscored by its wide tissue and species distribution. In humans, stomatin mRNA has been detected in every tissue and cell tested. Reactivity to a monoclonal antibody directed against human erythrocyte stomatin has been observed in the erythrocyte membranes of a wide variety of species, including frog, rat, chicken, rabbit, pig, cow, and sheep.[1489] It has been hypothesized that stomatin may support, activate, or regulate an unidentified ion channel.[1486, 1490, 1491] Evidence showing a potential interaction between stomatin and the membrane skeleton protein adducin[1495] suggests that stomatin may also be a part of the junctional complex of the membrane skeleton.[370] In this capacity, it may participate in a variety of specialized cellular functions. A homologue of stomatin, *mec2*, a protein involved in mechanosensation that is linked to a Na^+ channel, has been cloned from *C. elegans*.[1496–1499] Compared to the human protein, it has extended NH_2- and COOH-terminal extensions. However, the proteins are very homologous, particularly in a region encoding glutamate and alanine residues. This region has been suggested to be an adducin-binding site.

Although hereditary stomatocytosis appears to be a dominantly inherited condition and affected individuals are presumably heterozygotes, stomatin protein is completely absent (mRNA levels are normal).[1490] This suggests a dominant-negative effect, where a mutant stomatin interacts with the wild-type protein, forming an unstable oligomeric protein complex. Stomatin protein does appear to form oligomers; however, several groups have cloned and sequenced cDNAs from patients with stomatocytosis and stomatin deficiency,[1500–1502,*] including the most severely affected patient reported,[1439,*] and all four found that the coding sequence is normal. Mice with targeted disruption of stomatin are clinically and hematologically normal.[1503] Thus, it seems more likely that the defect resides in a protein that interacts with stomatin and causes its destruction secondarily. For example, the defect could activate a protein that modifies stomatin (e.g., a kinase, phosphatase, or ubiquitinating enzyme) so that it is recognized and destroyed, that destroys stomatin directly (e.g., a protease), or that directs it to be lost along with other proteins and organelles during reticulocyte maturation.

Finally, patients with stomatin deficiency apparently do not exhibit any nonhematologic symptoms,[1500] which

---

*Lux SE, John KM: Unpublished observations, 1996.

Normal

basic   acidic

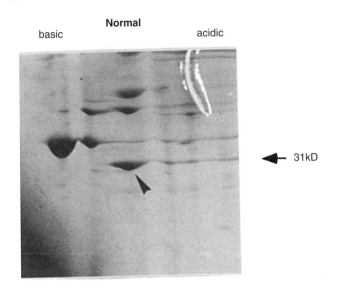

◀── 31kD

Stomatocytic

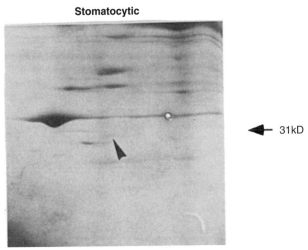

◀── 31kD

FIGURE 15–31. Two-dimensional analysis of normal and stomatocytic red cell membranes. Membranes were prepared by hypotonic lysis, stripped of peripheral proteins, and subjected to nonequilibrium pH gradient electrophoresis followed by SDS-PAGE and Coomassie blue staining. The location of the basic 31-kD protein (band 7.2b or stomatin), which is deficient in the stomatocytic cells, is noted by the arrow. (From Stewart GW, Argent AC, Dash BCJ: Stomatin: A putative cation transport regulator in the red cell membrane. Biochim Biophys Acta 1993; 1225:15.)

suggests that either the deficiency is confined to erythrocytes or stomatin is not essential for the function of other tissues.

Clinical Features

Typical Stomatin-Deficient Stomatocytosis. The diagnostic features of the classic type of hereditary stomatocytosis include the unique red cell morphology (5 to 50 percent stomatocytes), severe hemolysis, macrocytosis (110 to 150 fL), elevated erythrocyte Na^+ concentration of 60 to 100 mEq/L (normal range, 5 to 12 mEq/L), reduced K^+ concentration of 20 to 55 mEq/L (normal range, 90 to 103 mEq/L), and increased total $Na^+ + K^+$ content of 110 to 140 mEq/L (normal range, 95 to 110 mEq/L). The excess cations elevate cell water, producing large, osmotically frag-

ile cells with a low MCHC (24 to 30 percent). In many patients, hereditary stomatocytes are also moderately deficient in 2,3-DPG.[1439, 1455, 1469] Perhaps a portion of the 1,3-DPG normally used for 2,3-DPG synthesis is diverted through phosphoglycerate kinase to provide extra ATP for cation transport.[1469] The 2,3-DPG deficiency mildly enhances oxygen affinity and causes additional water entry and cell swelling. Some patients[1452, 1457] and dogs[1504, 1505] with hereditary stomatocytosis have an unexplained decrease in red cell glutathione; however, it is unlikely that this is pathophysiologically significant.

Hereditary Stomatocytosis Variants. Hereditary stomatocytosis is probably more heterogeneous than suggested earlier. Some patients with severe permeability defects have little or no hemolysis.[1481] In addition, studies of 44 Japanese patients with stomatocytosis show that the proportion of stomatocytes and the degree of Na^+ influx do not correlate with each other, and neither correlates with the amount of hemolysis or anemia.[1447] Furthermore, stomatin deficiency was not observed in Japanese patients with the most severe permeability defects and was only present to a mild degree in 5 of 9 patients with more moderate Na^+ leaks. This suggests that hereditary stomatocytosis is a complex mixture of diseases or that factors other than Na^+ leak and stomatin content are critical to the demise of the stomatocyte.

Treatment

Splenectomy reduces the hemolytic rate in patients with severe hereditary stomatocytosis[1439, 1443, 1445, 1458, 1459, 1461] and can be beneficial; however, a high proportion of patients have experienced thrombotic complications, sometimes with disastrous results.[1160] *In vitro,* stomatocytic erythrocytes from a splenectomized individual with xerocytosis and hypercoagulability demonstrated increased endothelial adherence compared with stomatocytic erythrocytes from unsplenectomized family members without hypercoagulability.[1506] *In vivo,* venous thromboemboli predominate, sometimes with the complications of pulmonary or portal hypertension.[1160] Thrombotic episodes have not occurred before splenectomy.

HEREDITARY XEROCYTOSIS (HIGH PHOSPHATIDYLCHOLINE HEMOLYTIC ANEMIA)

Several families with a hemolytic anemia in which the red cells are markedly dehydrated, as manifested by an elevated MCHC, have been described.[932, 1451, 1460, 1463, 1466–1469, 1507] Physiologically, the major red cell abnormality is a change in the relative membrane permeability to K^+. Efflux of K^+ is increased twofold to fourfold and approximates Na^+ influx. There is no metabolic or hemoglobin abnormality to account for this permeability lesion, and red cell Ca^{2+} content is not increased. The nature of the permeability defect is unknown. Monovalent cation pump activity is increased appropriately for the slightly elevated Na^+ content, but the Na^+/K^+ pump cannot compensate for K^+ losses in excess of Na^+ gain. In fact, the action of the pump significantly exacerbates the rate of K^+ loss because three Na^+ ions are pumped out for every two K^+ ions returned.[640, 680] As a consequence, xerocytes gradually become cation depleted and lose water in response to decreased intracellular osmolality. This is easily detected by centrifugation on Stractan gradients (Fig. 15–32). Little is known about the molecular pathology of this rare disease. When measured, the proportion of red cell membrane PC is increased (12 to 20 fmol/cell; normal range, 10 to 12 fmol/cell).[1463] The combination of hereditary xerocytosis and high PC is sometimes given the name high PC hemolytic anemia (HPCHA),[1450, 1463, 1464, 1467, 1469, 1508] but there appears to be little reason to distinguish HPCHA from hereditary xerocytosis.[1463] Early studies suggested that the excess PC was due to diminished transfer of PC fatty acids to PC,[1464] a pathway that is normally stimulated by cellular dehydration.[1509] It is not clear why this pathway is inhibited in hereditary xerocytosis or how it relates to the underlying membrane leakiness and hemolysis.

Xerocytic red cells are also shear sensitive[1468] and are exceptionally prone to membrane fragmentation in response to metabolic stress.[932] This finding suggests a membrane skeletal defect, but no systematic studies of xerocytic skeletons have been conducted. Results of conventional analyses of red cell membrane proteins have been normal,[932] except for an increase in the proportion of membrane-associated G3PD in one family.[1510] Quantitatively, all membrane components are increased, because, for unknown reasons, xerocytes have 15 to 25 percent more surface area than normal. Xerocytes are relatively rigid cells[1449] and probably develop a dehydration-induced membrane injury.[1468] This poorly defined lesion is also found in irreversibly sickled cells[1511] and presumably is important in the pathophysiology of hemolysis. Hereditary xerocytes are unusually sensitive to oxidants.[1512–1513] Exposure of xerocytes to concentrations of

H_2O_2 that do not affect normal cells causes a rapid loss of intracellular K^+, conversion of hemoglobin to methemoglobin, and cross-linking of hemoglobin to spectrin.[1513, 1514] Similar sensitivity occurs in dehydrated normal red cells. Conversely, rehydrated xerocytes exhibit a normal reaction to H_2O_2. Native xerocytes contain the abnormal spectrin-globin complex, and the amount correlates with the extent of dehydration in various cellular fractions and with membrane rigidity.[1515] Oxidation of normal erythrocytes with peroxide generates the spectrin/globin complex and rigid membranes.[733] Complex formation is blocked by carbon monoxide, which prevents hemoglobin oxidation, but is not blocked by lipid antioxidants. This implies a direct role for hemoglobin in cross-linking spectrin.

Clinical Features

In all families with hereditary xerocytosis that were studied, inheritance appears to be autosomal dominant. Red cell features used for diagnosis include an increased MCHC and decreased osmotic fragility (i.e., resistance to osmotic lysis). In the most severely affected patients,[1445] blood smears display contracted and spiculated red cells in which the hemoglobin appears to be aggregated in one portion of the cell. Most patients, however, have nearly normal erythrocyte morphology, with only a few target cells and an occasional echinocyte or stomatocyte. The characteristic biochemical abnormalities are reduced K^+ concentration and total monovalent cation content. In older erythrocytes, K^+ levels approach one half normal.[1463] Red cell 2,3-DPG concentrations are moderately decreased in hereditary xerocytosis,[932, 1445, 1453, 1460, 1516] as well as in hereditary stomatocytosis. The reasons are

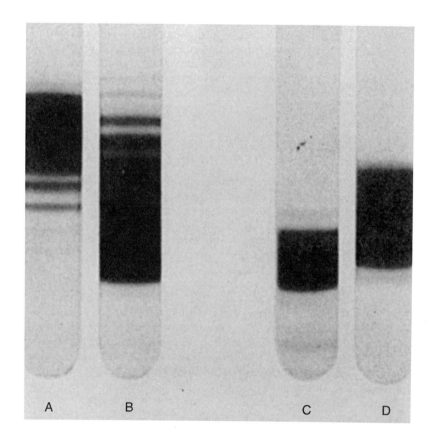

FIGURE 15–32. Separation of hydrocytes and xerocytes by density. *Left,* Control (A) and hereditary xerocytosis (B) samples. The cells were separated on Stractan density gradients. The xerocytes extend to higher densities than normal red cells. *Right,* Control (C) and hereditary stomatocytosis (D) samples. Many of the stomatocytes are lighter than the control red cells. (From Lande WM, Mentzer WC: Haemolytic anaemia associated with increased cation permeability. Clin Haematol 1985; 14:89.)

unknown. Because loss of the polyvalent DPG is compensated for by an influx of monovalent chloride ions and water, patients with xerocytosis and unusually low DPG levels have fewer dehydrated red cells than expected for the degree of cation loss and in rare cases have no dehydration at all.[1516] Patients with low DPG levels also have increased whole blood oxygen affinity and, consequently, may have little apparent anemia.[1507, 1516] Autohemolysis is increased and responds to glucose, similar to the pattern seen in HS.[932, 1453, 1466, 1469]

Hereditary xerocytes appear to be macrocytic, despite their dehydration. This, however, is partially an artifact of cellular stiffness. In Coulter-type electronic counters, the conversion of pulse height (from the resistance of a cell passing through an electric field) to a cellular volume depends on cell shape. Xerocytes do not deform to the same degree as normal cells, which causes the electronically measured MCV to be about 10 too high.[1517] This behavior also affects the hematocrit value, which is calculated from the MCV.

Splenectomy is probably not beneficial for hereditary xerocytosis. The limited experience available suggests that removing the spleen does not significantly reduce hemolysis.[1445, 1450] Presumably, xerocytes are so functionally compromised that they are easily detected and eliminated in other areas of the reticuloendothelial system. Splenectomy may even be contraindicated.[1160] One 46-year-old patient with xerocytosis had fatal pulmonary emboli after splenectomy.[1450] Fortunately, a hemoglobin level of at least 9 g/dL is maintained in most patients, so that splenectomy is not required.

The gene for xerocytosis has been mapped to 16q23-q24.[1474, 1518, 1519] A constellation of clinical findings including xerocytosis, perinatal ascites, and pseudohyperkalemia has been described.[1441, 1471, 1474, 1478] Genetic studies of patients with this constellation of disorders also shows linkage to 16q23-q24.[1474]

INTERMEDIATE SYNDROMES

Hydrocytosis and xerocytosis represent the extremes of a spectrum of red cell permeability defects. A number of families with features of both conditions have been reported. The reported patients seem to fall into three groups whose red cells differ principally in morphology, osmotic fragility, and sensitivity to cold.

Cryohydrocytosis

Patients with this disorder have a mild congenital hemolytic anemia characterized by marked autohemolysis that is greater at 4°C than at 37°C.[1456, 1472, 1475, 1520] The cold autohemolysis is sensitive to the method of anticoagulation. It is increased in the cold in heparin, EDTA, and defibrinated plasma but not in acid citrate dextrose.[1456] This may reflect unusual pH sensitivity of the abnormal red cells, because cold hemolysis is accentuated at pH 8 (the pH of blood in the first three anticoagulants at 4°C) compared with pH 7.6 (the pH of acid citrate dextrose plasma at 4°C).[1456] Blood smears show stomatocytes, some of which have an eccentric or curvilinear slit or a transverse bar bisecting the area of central pallor.[1519, 1520] Fresh erythrocytes are Na+ loaded and K+ depleted,

but the total concentration of Na+ and K+ is normal. In the cold, Na+ and K+ permeabilities are markedly increased; however, because Na+ entry greatly predominates, the red cells rapidly swell and lyse. The primary molecular lesion of these erythrocytes is unknown. Membrane lipids are quantitatively normal, and with the exception of a mild decrease in red cell glutathione, no defects in metabolism have been detected.[1456] In one patient, stomatin was missing when red cell membrane proteins were analyzed,[1448] but this defect was not observed in the authors' patients.*

Pseudohyperkalemia

Stewart and co-workers[1521, 1522] reported a family with a dominantly inherited disorder characterized by erythrocyte K+ loss that is exaggerated in the cold. Electrolyte analyses of plasma obtained from blood samples stored for just a few hours at room temperature or below may falsely suggest that affected individuals are hyperkalemic. The disorder resembles cryohydrocytosis except that K+ loss and dehydration predominate (? cryoxerocytosis) instead of Na+ gain and cryohemolysis. Studies of patients with hereditary stomatocytosis and particularly of those with xerocytosis have shown that many of these variants also cause pseudohyperkalemia.[1473, 1474, 1476, 1479, 1520] Further evidence for overlap between these syndromes is provided by linkage to the same locus as that of xerocytosis at 16q23-q24.[1474, 1476, 1518]

Stomatocytic Xerocytosis

In 1971, Miller and colleagues[1457] reported on 54 patients with dominantly inherited stomatocytosis in a large Swiss-German family. Apparent heterozygotes (51 of 54 patients) had mild hemolysis, 1 to 25 percent stomatocytes on their peripheral blood smears, and no anemia. Intracellular K+ and total monovalent cation levels were mildly decreased, and fresh red cells were osmotically resistant. Three probable homozygotes from a consanguineous mating had mild anemia, moderately severe hemolysis, marked stomatocytosis (20 to 35 percent), and greater cation permeability[1456, 1482]; however, because net Na+ and K+ levels were relatively balanced, cell hydration was not seriously deranged. The molecular defect in this kindred is unknown.

OTHER DISORDERS CHARACTERIZED BY STOMATOCYTOSIS

Acquired Stomatocytosis

In normal individuals, 3 percent or less of the red cells on peripheral blood smears are stomatocytic,[1523, 1524] although more stomatocytic forms are evident (up to 10 percent) if sensitive techniques such as scanning electron microscopy are used.[1525] Because stomatocytes may occasionally occur as a drying artifact in limited areas of the smear, one must take care to examine multiple areas on several smears before diagnosing stomatocytosis. In wet preparations, stomatocytes are bowl shaped (uniconcave). Such preparations are useful in excluding artifactual

---

*Lux SE, John KM, Landrigan P: Unpublished observations, 1996.

stomatocytes, but the presence of bowl-shaped cells cannot be used as proof of stomatocytes because target cells are also bowl shaped in solution.[1526]

Drugs. In a prospective study of 4291 peripheral blood smears, Davidson and co-workers[1527] found increased numbers of stomatocytes in 2.3 percent of the preparations. Fifty-nine percent of these smears had 5 to 20 percent stomatocytes, 35 percent had 20 to 50 percent stomatocytes, and 6 percent had more than 50 percent stomatocytes. In this and other studies, a wide variety of drugs and diagnoses were associated with stomatocytosis.[1449, 1457, 1527–1530] Further studies are needed to determine which associations are specific and reproducible. As discussed earlier in the chapter in the section on the bilayer couple hypothesis, amphophilic, lipid-soluble drugs can cause red cells to assume a stomatocytic shape if the drug partitions preferentially into the inner one half of the lipid bilayer. The affected red cells are misshapen but are not cation loaded or hydrocytic and do not usually hemolyze. Vinca alkaloids (e.g., vincristine and vinblastine) often induce hemolysis, sometimes with increased membrane Na$^+$ permeability and stomatocytosis, in the doses used for chemotherapy of leukemias and lymphomas.[1529] This is a particular problem in the rare instances in which these drugs must be given to patients with cancer who also have HS. We have seen two such patients and in both cases very severe hemolysis occurred. Presumably the explanation is that spherocytes and stomatocytes both have a decreased surface-to-volume ratio. Imposing a stomatocytic stress on HS red cells will make them even more spheroidal and hasten their demise.

Alcoholism. Acquired stomatocytosis is common in alcoholics, particularly in those with acute alcoholism (Fig. 15–33) and may be associated with moderate hemolysis.[1523, 1524] Red cell cation measurements have not been reported; however, severe hydrocytosis is unlikely, because results of osmotic fragility tests have been normal.[1523]

Rh Null Disease

The Rh(D) antigen and the other antigens of the Rh group (cCeE) are part of two minor red cell membrane proteins encoded by two closely linked genes, one encoding the D polypeptide and the other encoding the Cc/Ee proteins, the antigenic expression of which is a consequence of alternate splicing of their pre-mRNA.[1530, 1531] Patients who lack all Rh antigens (Rh$_{null}$)[1532] have a moderately severe hemolytic anemia (^{51}Cr-labeled red cell half-life of 10 to 14 days)[1533–1536] characterized by stomatocytosis and spherocytosis. Osmotic fragility is only mildly increased,[1533, 1536] but ektacytometry analysis shows a significant loss of membrane surface, particularly in denser (and presumably older) cells.[1533] Red cell membrane K$^+$ or Rb$^+$ (a K$^+$ analog) permeability is about twice normal, which is compatible with the presence of a mild xerocytosis syndrome.[1533, 1537] Stomatocytosis and hemolysis are also features of Rh$_{mod}$ disease, a related anomaly, in which the expression of Rh antigens is suppressed but not absent, owing to the influence of a suppressor gene.[1538, 1539]

The genetic bases of the Rh$_{null}$ and Rh$_{mod}$ deficiency syndromes are heterogeneous, and at least two groups can be defined. The "amorph type" has been related to defects involving the *RH30* locus encoding the RhD and RhE polypeptides, and the "regulatory type," result from mutations of a suppressor or "modifier" that modulates Rh expression, identified as *RHAG* or the Rh50 gene. Most instances of Rh$_{null}$ disease are of the "regulatory type" and are due to missense mutations, deletions, or splicing mutations leading to frameshift and premature chain termination.[1540–1544] Rh$_{null}$ disease of the amorph type due to homozygous or compound heterozygous mutations at the *RH30* locus have been reported.[1545–1547] A mutation

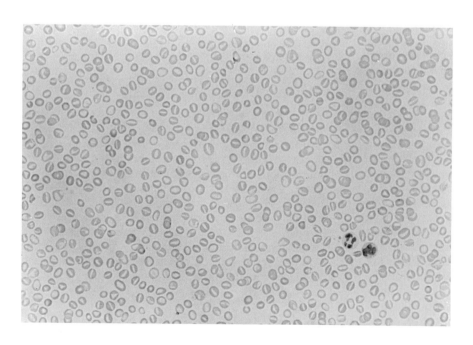

FIGURE 15–33. Peripheral blood smear from a patient with acute alcoholism. Acquired stomatocytic morphologic features are seen in almost all erythrocytes.

of the initiation codon of Rh50 has been identified in a case of Rh$_{mod}$ disease.[1548]

Tangier Disease

Tangier disease, caused by mutations in the gene encoding ATP-binding cassette 1 (ABCA1), is a rare autosomal recessive condition in which homozygotes have splenomegaly, no or very low levels of high-density lipoproteins (HDLs), reduced levels of low-density lipoproteins (LDLs) (typically 40 percent of normal), hypertriglyceridemia, mild corneal clouding, peripheral neuropathy, bone marrow foam cells (70 percent of patients), and characteristic orange-colored, cholesterol ester–laden tonsils.[1549] ABCA1 is a major determinant of plasma HDL cholesterol and is critically involved in cellular trafficking of cholesterol and choline phospholipids by mediating the first step in reverse cholesterol transport, the transfer of cholesterol and phospholipids to lipid-poor apoproteins.[1550, 1551] Cholesterol ester levels are greatly elevated in tissue macrophages in Tangier disease owing to the lack of HDLs, which normally return cholesterol esters to the liver. The HDL deficiency is caused by hypercatabolism of the lipoprotein. Normally, HDLs bind to specific receptors on macrophages, are internalized (presumably to load up on cholesterol esters), and then recycle to the membrane surface. In Tangier disease, HDLs are misrouted to macrophage lysosomes and destroyed.

Hematologic examination of one patient with Tangier disease disclosed stomatocytosis, hemolysis (hemoglobin concentration of 8.5 g/dL; reticulocyte count of 6 to 9 percent), and osmotically sensitive red cells.[1552] The membrane cholesterol level was low, the cholesterol-to-phospholipid ratio was decreased, and phospholipid analysis showed high PC and low SM levels. Red cell cation concentrations and permeabilities were not investigated. Because hematologic data have rarely been reported in patients with Tangier disease, it is difficult to be certain that this patient's data are not exceptional. However, previous reports of unexplained hemolysis in three patients suggest that they are not.[1553–1555]

Other Disorders

Stomatocytosis is also observed in at least some patients with the hemolytic anemia that results from adenosine deaminase overproduction.[1556] Dejeure-Sotos syndrome causes stomatocytosis.[1557]

OTHER DISORDERS CHARACTERIZED BY XEROCYTOSIS

ATP Depletion

When red cell ATP concentrations decrease to less than 5 to 15 percent of normal, the cells leak cations and become rigid and echinocytic.[1558] In plasma or other Ca^{2+}-containing media, a specific K^+ permeability lesion (the Gardos phenomenon) is superimposed on the unchecked normal leak of Na^+ and K^+ and leads to cation depletion and dehydration.[1559] Coincidentally, poorly defined changes occur in membrane skeletal structure.[1560, 1561]

Presumably these phenomena are involved in the hemolysis that occurs in inherited defects of glycolysis such as pyruvate kinase (PK) deficiency. Studies by Nathan and co-workers,[1562] Mentzer and Baehner,[1563] and Glader[1564] showed that PK-deficient red cells rapidly lose ATP and K^+ and become dehydrated, spiculated, and viscous when incubated *in vitro*, particularly under conditions in which residual mitochondrial production of ATP is curtailed. Contracted, crenated red cells are observed in PK deficiency[1565, 1566] and other disorders of red cell glycolysis. These "deflated echinocytes" are more rigid than normal[1567] and are relatively scarce in unsplenectomized patients,[1565, 1566] which implies that they are premorbid cells given temporary reprieve by removal of the spleen.

Little is known about the status of membrane proteins in red cells with compromised ATP production.[1559] Small amounts of disulfide-linked spectrin complexes and marked diminution of spectrin extractability were detected in a patient with glucose phosphate isomerase deficiency,[1568] which suggests that membrane protein damage may be pathologically relevant in these disorders.

Irreversibly Sickled Cells

Irreversibly sickled cells are circulating erythrocytes from patients with sickle cell anemia that retain a sickled shape when oxygenated because of an acquired defect in the membrane skeleton.[602] Biochemically, irreversibly sickled cells are deficient in total monovalent cations and water.[1569, 1570] The mechanism of their formation and the nature of the acquired membrane defects responsible for their abnormal shape, cation content, and surface topography are discussed in Chapter 19.

MISCELLANEOUS DISORDERS AFFECTING THE ERYTHROCYTE MEMBRANE

Other Causes of Decreased Erythrocyte Membrane Surface

Excluding HS, only a few conditions cause decreased membrane surface area, leading to spherocytosis on the peripheral blood smear.

IMMUNE ADHERENCE

Immunohemolytic anemias are the most common cause of acquired spherocytosis in infants and children: AB(H)-related hemolysis in neonates and warm antibody-type autoimmune (or drug-related) hemolytic anemias in older children and adults. (For unknown reasons Rh-related hemolysis in neonates rarely causes spherocytosis, whereas it does so readily later in life.) Patients who suffer from severe transfusion reactions with immunohemolysis may also have spherocytes on their peripheral blood smears. The pathophysiology of these disorders is discussed in Chapter 14.

THERMAL INJURY

More than 130 years ago Schultze[1571] observed that red cells heated to temperatures approaching 50°C for short periods developed membrane budding, fragmentation, and microspherocytosis. This phenomenon was further defined by the careful studies of Ham and co-workers and others[1310–1312] and is now believed to be due to heat denaturation of spectrin or other membrane proteins.[1313] Similar changes are observed acutely in patients with major cutaneous burns, presumably because of heat exposure of red cells in the skin and subcutaneous tissues. Other changes in erythrocytes after thermal burns include decreased deformability due to oxidative stress with activated lipid peroxidation, reduced glutathione levels, and reduced α-tocopherol levels.[1572–1574] During the first 24 to 48 hours after the burn, intravascular hemolysis develops, which is associated with red cell fragmentation and spherocytosis.[1575, 1576] The severity of the reaction is related to the extent and degree of the burn. Generally, hemolysis is evident in patients with third-degree burns involving 15 to 20 percent or more of the body surface area.[1575, 1577] In severely burned patients, up to 30 percent of the red cell mass may be destroyed. This acute hemolytic process is usually complete by the third day after the burn and is followed by a chronic anemia resembling that seen in various chronic disorders.[1578, 1579] An unusual variant of this disorder has been reported after infusion of red cells that were inadvertently overheated in a blood warmer.[1580, 1581]

MECHANICAL INJURY

Hemolysis can be caused by direct physical trauma to the red cell membrane. This occurs in a variety of disorders, which are grouped under the terms *microangiopathic* and *macroangiopathic hemolytic anemias*. Membrane damage leading to intravascular hemolysis is apparently inflicted by the interaction of red cells (flowing at arterial speeds) with prosthetic materials, damaged endothelial surfaces, or intravascular fibrin strands.[592, 1582, 1583] Dense microspherocytes are almost always produced by this process, but usually bizarre-shaped schizocytes and red cell fragments dominate the morphology. How such cells form is still not completely clear, because simple fragmentation of red cells generates spherocytes but not schizocytes. Perhaps red cells draped over fibrin strands or attached to abnormal surfaces not only are distorted by shear but also are held in the distorted position for some time, permitting rearrangement of the stressed membrane skeleton and assumption of a new, irreversibly misshapen form. This concept is strengthened by the observation that fragmentation is worsened by the presence of underlying skeletal weakness.[1257]

HYPOPHOSPHATEMIA

Red cell glucose metabolism is compromised in patients with severe hypophosphatemia (serum phosphorus level less than 0. to 0.3 mg/dL).[1584, 1585] ATP and DPG levels decline and hemoglobin oxygen affinity increases.[1586, 1587] If the red cell ATP concentration falls to very low levels (10 to 20 percent of normal), a severe hemolytic anemia characterized by marked microspherocytosis, spheroacanthocytosis, and red cell rigidity results.[1584] Hemolysis is reversible after phosphate repletion and ATP regeneration.

TOXINS AND VENOMS

Clostridial Sepsis. *Clostridium welchii* and *Clostridium perfringens* septicemias are seen in a variety of clinical situations but must particularly be considered in patients with penetrating wounds, septic abortions, peritonitis after a perforated viscus, or cholecystitis or cholangitis and in immunosuppressed patients with gastrointestinal or hematologic malignancies or neonates with necrotizing enterocolitis.[1588–1601] In patients with clostridial sepsis, severe, rapidly progressive intravascular hemolysis and microspherocytosis may occur.[1589, 1596] Hemolysis of the entire red cell mass has been reported.[1588, 1595, 1598, 1602, 1603] Complications include shock, acute renal failure, and death. Transfusion therapy may be ineffective. Antibiotics and hyperbaric oxygen have occasionally been used successfully to treat clostridial infections.[1592, 1597, 1598]

The mechanism of red cell damage is uncertain and may vary between patients. The bacteria produce several hemolytic toxins including α toxin, a 43-kD protein that contains an NH_2-terminal phospholipase domain and a COOH-terminal domain required for hemolysis,[1597, 1604–1605] and θ toxin, a 54-kD cholesterol-binding protein[1607–1609] that aggregates and forms membrane pores[1608, 1610] leading to colloid osmotic hemolysis. *C. perfringens* contains a neuraminidase that cleaves terminal sialic acids from red cell glycoproteins in some patients.[1611] The underlying galactose residues form the Thomsen-Friedenreich cryptoantigen (or T antigen). The antigen is easily detected because affected erythrocytes are agglutinated by peanut lectin.[1591] Anti-T antibodies are present in almost all adult plasma; thus, T-antigen activation can lead to significant hemolysis.[1596, 1597, 1599, 1612] In infected infants and children who lack T antibodies, transfusion may lead to massive hemolysis and death. Rarely, T-antigen activation may precede the intravascular hemolysis, leading to early detection of clostridial sepsis and life-saving therapeutic intervention.[1591]

In one patient with severe hemolysis, red cells showed profound proteolytic damage to membrane proteins, particularly spectrin, and no significant lipid alterations.[1613] This suggests that proteolytic rather than lipolytic bacterial toxins are primarily responsible for red cell destruction.

Venoms. The venoms of cobras and certain vipers and rattlesnakes may produce severe hemolysis and spherocytosis.[1614–1618] Spherocytic hemolytic anemia may also be seen in patients bitten by the common brown spiders (*Loxosceles reclusus* and *Loxosceles lata*) of South America and the central and southern sections of the United States[1619, 1621] and in individuals with massive numbers of stings of honeybees, wasps, or yellow jackets.[1621–1624] Hemolysis in a child stung by a Portuguese man-of-war jellyfish has also been reported.[1625]

A full description of the numerous toxins in these venoms and their mechanisms of action is beyond the scope of this chapter. In general, the mechanisms of hemolysis after envenomation are not fully understood. The venoms of snakes and insects often contain phospholipases (particularly phospholipase A_2)[1626] and protein toxins that enhance their action. Examples of toxins include the mastoparans of wasp and hornet venoms[1627–1629] and melittin, a polypeptide contained in honeybee (*Apis mellifera*) venom[1630–1633] that immobilizes and clusters erythrocyte protein 3, producing protein-free areas of the lipid bilayer that are susceptible to phospholipase action.[1632]

Hemolysis after brown recluse spider bites is characteristically delayed from 1 to 5 days and is caused by a different mechanism.[1620] Affected patients develop a transient, spherocytic, hemolytic anemia that produces positive Coombs test results[1634–1637] with erythrophagocytosis and IgG[1413] and C3[14112] deposition on the red cell surface. Venom from the brown recluse spider induces activation of an endogenous metalloproteinase, resulting in glycophorin cleavage from the erythrocyte membrane that facilitates the complement-mediated hemolysis.[1638–1640] The hemolysis usually subsides within a week, but it may be fatal.[1620, 1641, 1642] Complement appears to play a critical role because complement-deficient guinea pigs are resistant to the venom.[1643] The glycoprotein CD59 may play a previously unrecognized role in membrane protection from venom-induced injury.[1644] The venom also contains a phospholipase D that may contribute to the hemolysis.[1645]

Except for spider bites, which may be clinically deceptive initially, the potential for a hemolytic catastrophe should be obvious in patients who have been bitten or stung.[1620] An early sign of impending hemolysis may be a rapid rise in the serum K^+ level caused by the prelytic leak of this ion from the red cells. Once hemolysis is established, therapy other than transfusions is usually of little use. In patients with snake bites, localization or drainage of the venom and prompt administration of antivenom can be lifesaving.

HYPERSPLENISM

Occasionally, patients with infections associated with splenomegaly develop transient hemolysis associated with spherocytosis and splenic sequestration of red cells.[1646–1648] In some instances, this may be attributed to latent red cell defects such as HS; but in others, no red cell abnormalities can be identified. Typically, the latter patients have subacute infections with persistent fever, splenomegaly, and numerous cells of lymphocytic or reticuloendothelial derivation (atypical lymphocytes, monocytes, histiocytes, or plasma cells) in the peripheral blood. Only a minor population of the red cells (10 to 50 percent) are spherical on peripheral blood smears or unincubated osmotic fragility tests. Presumably the combination of delayed splenic passage caused by splenomegaly and pyrogenic stimulation of the reticuloendothelial system is sufficient to permit detention and conditioning of even normal red cells—a form of hypersplenism.

Disorders Associated with Increased Membrane Surface

TARGET CELLS

Red cells increase their surface area by an increase in membrane lipids. In dried smears the excess surface accumulates and bulges outward in the red cell's central clearing, producing the characteristic target cell morphology. Target cells are also seen when red cell volume is diminished, owing to decreased hemoglobin synthesis (e.g., thalassemia or iron deficiency), abnormal hemoglobin charge or aggregation (e.g., hemoglobins S, C, D, and E), or decreased cell cations and water. In these instances there is a relative increase in the surface-to-volume ratio. With the exception of dehydrated red cells, an increase in membrane surface, whether relative or absolute, has little effect on red cell deformability or life span and hence is usually innocuous.

Liver Disease. Target cells are particularly characteristic of biliary obstruction[1526, 1649] but also occur in other forms of liver disease. Like spur cells (see later), they form when red cells accumulate excess lipids from abnormal lipoproteins. However, unlike spur cells, target cells are characterized by a balanced increase in both free cholesterol and phospholipids.[1650–1652] The phospholipid increase is confined to PC.[1650]

The pathogenesis of lipid accumulation in target cells is relatively clear. The process is extracorpuscular and reversible and is due to an abnormal serum component. Normal cells acquire target cell surface area, morphologic characteristics, and osmotic resistance when transfused into patients with obstructive jaundice or incubated in their serum, whereas target cells from such patients lose their excess lipids and revert to biconcave discs in normal persons or their sera.[1649] Cooper and co-workers[1650] found a close relationship between the cholesterol-to-phospholipid ratios of target cells and serum lipoproteins, particularly LDLs. It is known that in obstructive jaundice a unique, abnormal lipoprotein called LP-X accumulates in the LDL density class,[1653, 1654] possibly caused, at least in part, by an acquired deficiency of the hepatic enzyme LCAT. LP-X contains approximately equal amounts of free cholesterol and PC, plus a small amount of protein, cholesterol esters, triglycerides, and lithocholic acid.[1428] Normal red cells rapidly acquire excess cholesterol, PC, and surface area when incubated with LP-X *in vitro*,[1652] and it seems likely that this may be the source of lipids for membrane expansion and targeting *in vivo*.

Membrane proteins may also be abnormal in these cells. Iida and co-workers[1655] found that protein 4.2 was diminished or absent in 11 Japanese patients with obstructive jaundice and typical lipid-laden target cells. Red cell morphology, membrane lipids, and protein 4.2 content returned to normal in 1 patient after surgical relief of the biliary obstruction. This curious observation has been neither confirmed nor denied, and its relevance, if any, to the pathophysiology of targeting remains obscure.

Familial Lecithin:Cholesterol Acyltransferase Deficiency. Familial LCAT deficiency is a rare autosomal recessive disorder characterized by anemia, corneal opacities, hyperlipemia, proteinuria, chronic nephritis, and premature atherosclerosis.[111] LCAT deficiency is relatively asymptomatic during childhood. Proteinuria and corneal opacities are among the earliest manifestations. The latter consist of minute grayish dots that concentrate near the edge of the cornea, resembling arcus senilis. Almost all of the reported patients have had a moderate normochromic anemia (hemoglobin level of 8 to 11 g/dL) characterized by prominent target cell formation and decreased osmotic fragility.[1656–1658,1658a] Hematologic studies suggest that the anemia is due to a combination of moderate hemolysis and decreased erythropoietic compensation, but interpretation of the evidence is complicated by the coexisting renal disease. Other studies have shown that the red cells are abnormally susceptible to peroxidative threat and have mechanically fragile membranes.[1657] There is no obvious explanation for these changes, but it is possible that they contribute to the shortened red cell life span.

LCAT deficiency is caused by a variety of mutations in the LCAT gene; affected individuals are either homozygotes or compound heterozygotes for these mutations.[1659, 1660] Modeling of the mutations has provided insight into LCAT structure and function.[1661] As expected from the absence of LCAT activity, there is a pronounced decrease in cholesteryl esters and an increase in free cholesterol and PC in plasma lipoproteins. Because LCAT is required for normal lipoprotein formation and catabolism, nascent lipoproteins and abnormal lipoprotein remnants accumulate in the plasma. One of the latter is LP-X.[1662] As discussed in the previous section, this lipoprotein is believed to be responsible for target cell formation in patients with the acquired LCAT deficiency of obstructive liver disease.[1652] Free cholesterol and PC levels are markedly elevated in the red cell membranes of patients with LCAT deficiency[111]; however, total red cell phospholipid levels are normal because the increase in PC is balanced by a decrease in PC and SM. As with liver disease, red cell targeting and lipid abnormalities can be induced by incubation of normal red cells in LCAT-deficient lipoproteins and reversed by incubation in normal serum.[1663] Other plasma membranes are also probably affected by the abnormal LCAT-deficient lipoproteins. For example, accumulations of lipid in endothelial membranes may underlie the atherosclerotic and nephritic complications seen in some patients. Phagocytosis of abnormal lipoproteins by reticuloendothelial cells leads to the appearance of foam cells and sea-blue histiocytes in the bone marrow, spleen, and other organs.[1656, 1664] Serum and red cell lipids are improved *in vivo* when LCAT is supplied by infusions of normal plasma; however, the short half-life of this protein, 4 to 5 days, and the large amounts of plasma required make chronic replacement therapy impractical. As would be expected, mice with targeted inactivation of the LCAT gene experience mild normocytic, normochromic anemia.[1665] Many target cells are found, and erythrocyte osmotic fragility is altered.

Fish-eye disease is caused by partial deficiency of LCAT and is also associated with mutations in the LCAT gene.[111, 1659] It is characterized by corneal opacities (which give the disease its name), hypertriglyceridemia, and very low levels of HDLs. One report noted increased target cells and decreased osmotic fragility.[1666]

After Splenectomy. In the first several weeks after splenectomy, the number of target cells gradually increases,[1526, 1667–1669] eventually (in otherwise normal persons) reaching levels of 2 to 10 percent. This change is associated with increases in osmotic resistance, membrane lipid content, and mean surface area relative to volume, indicating expansion of the red cell membrane surface. By deduction, the spleen must normally remove surplus membrane

from such cells, a process referred to as "surface remodeling."[721, 1670] Experimental studies have clearly documented that the stress reticulocytes induced by acute blood loss or hemolysis undergo extensive surface remodeling and suggest that normal reticulocytes are remodeled to a lesser degree. In addition to membrane lipids, transferrin receptors, fibronectin receptors, and a high-molecular-weight membrane protein complex[722] are also removed during the remodeling process. Postsplenectomy blood smears also show increased numbers of acanthocytes, poikilocytes, and red cells burdened with useless or potentially harmful inclusions (e.g., Heinz bodies, Howell-Jolly bodies, siderotic granules, and endocytic vesicles).[1199, 1200, 1671, 1672] The presence of these inclusions attest to the "culling" and "pitting" functions of the spleen.[1672]

Spiculated Red Cells: Echinocytes and Acanthocytes

There are two basic types of spiculated red cells—echinocytes and acanthocytes. Echinocytes typically have a serrated outline with small, uniform projections more or less evenly spread over the circumference of the cell, whereas acanthocytes have a few spicules of varying size that project irregularly from the red cell surface. These differences are easily detected in scanning electron micrographs and can usually be discerned in wet preparations, but it is often quite difficult to make the distinction in dried smears. In general, echinocytes appear crenated in smears, that is, as cells with relatively uniform scalloped edges, whereas acanthocytes appear contracted, dense, and irregular.

Echinocytes are readily produced *in vitro* by washing red cells in saline,[1673] by the interaction of red cells with glass surfaces,[1673–1675] by amphipathic molecules that partition into and expand the outer one half of the lipid bilayer,[1676] and by molecules that inhibit band 3 transport.[1677] High pH values, ATP depletion, and Ca^{2+} accumulation also cause echinocytosis.[1678–1680] *In vivo*, echinocytes are most often found in patients with advanced uremia[1680, 1681] or with defects of glycolytic metabolism,[1565] after splenectomy[1673] and in some patients with microangiopathic hemolytic anemias. Echinocytes are also commonly seen in neonates, especially those who are premature,[1682, 1683] and in divers after decompression from pressures of more than 3 to 4 bar.[1684] They are seen transiently after transfusions with large amounts of stored blood, because red cells become echinocytic after a few days of storage. Acanthocytes and echinocytes may be found in patients with severe hepatocellular damage,[1685] abetalipoproteinemia,[1686] infantile pyknocytosis,[1687] anorexia nervosa,[1688,1689] McLeod[1690] and In(Lu)[1691] blood groups, and hypothyroidism.[1692] Occasionally, they are the predominant morphologic feature in patients with myelodysplasia.[1693, 1694]

ABETALIPOPROTEINEMIA

Abetalipoproteinemia (Bassen-Kornzweig syndrome) is the paradigm of the disorders associated with acanthocytosis.[1686, 1695] Progressive ataxic neurologic disease, retinitis pigmentosa, celiac syndrome, and acanthocytosis are the primary manifestations of this disorder.[1696–1698] Intestinal absorption of lipids is defective, the serum cholesterol level is extremely low, and serum β-lipoprotein is absent. The disease is caused by failure to synthesize or secrete lipoproteins containing products of the apolipoprotein B gene. In some patients, this is due to lack of microsomal triglyceride transfer protein (MTP), which catalyzes the transport of triglyceride, cholesterol ester, and phospholipid from phospholipid surfaces.[1699–1701] MTP is a heterodimer of protein disulfide isomerase and a unique large subunit with apparent molecular mass of 88 kD. It is located in the lumen of hepatic microsomes and intestinal epithelia, the sites of lipoprotein synthesis,[1701–1703] and is the only tissue-specific component, other than apolipoprotein B, required for secretion of apolipoprotein B–containing lipoproteins.[1704] Mutations in the MTP subunits have been described.[1696, 1697]

Related entities (hypobetalipoproteinemia, normotriglyceridemic abetalipoproteinemia, and chylomicron retention disease) exist that are associated with partial production of apolipoprotein B–containing lipoproteins or with secretion of lipoproteins containing truncated forms of apolipoprotein B.[1696] Patients with these diseases may also manifest acanthocytosis and neurologic disease, depending on the severity of the lipoprotein defect. Even patients with heterozygous hypobetalipoproteinemia may have acanthocytosis, although often they do not.

Characteristically, 50 to 90 percent of the red cells are acanthocytes.[1705] The shape defect is not evident in nucleated red cells or reticulocytes and worsens as the erythrocytes age. Membrane protein composition is normal, but membrane lipid composition is not. Phosphatidylcholine concentration is decreased by about 20 percent, and the amount of sphingomyelin is correspondingly increased. The cholesterol-to-phospholipid ratio is normal to mildly elevated.[1706–1708] These changes reflect abnormalities in the distribution of plasma phospholipids and a decrease in LCAT activity.[1709] The relative increases in cholesterol and sphingomyelin concentration both decrease lipid fluidity,[1707] particularly in the outer one half of the bilayer,[1710] and presumably contribute to the acanthocytic shape. They probably do so by expanding the outer bilayer relative to the inner bilayer, because drugs that selectively intercalate into the inner bilayer convert acanthocytes to biconcave disks.[86] However, this is almost impossible to prove, because the difference in the surface areas of the outer bilayers of an acanthocyte and a discocyte is less than 0.4 percent.

Because of fat malabsorption and the absence of LDLs, which transport vitamin E,[1711] the red cells of these patients are markedly deficient in vitamin E.[1712] Exposure to lipid-soluble oxidants such as H_2O_2 leads to an increase in lipid peroxides, a decrease in phospholipids rich in unsaturated fatty acids such as PE and PS, damage to membrane proteins, and hemolysis. Oxidant sensitivity can be prevented by treatment with a water-soluble form of vitamin E (e.g., D-α-tocopherol polyethylene glycol succinate).[1712] The role of vitamin E deficiency in the pathophysiology of the disease is uncertain. It is widely believed that such deficiency may be the primary stimulus for secondary manifestations of the disease, such as neuropathy, because a similar neuropathy is observed in rare patients with chronic cholestasis[1713–1715] or selective malabsorption of vitamin E.[1716] In these latter defects[1717] and probably in abetalipoproteinemia,[1718] the neurologic disease can be delayed or prevented by chronic vitamin E administration.[1719]

Despite increased lipid viscosity and vitamin E deficiency, the hemolysis experienced by these patients is mild.[1706] This is in striking contrast to spur cell anemia (see later), in which hemolysis of similarly shaped cells is often quite severe. It has been suggested that the difference is explained by the fact that the spleen is normal in abetalipoproteinemia, whereas it is enlarged and congested by portal hypertension in spur cell anemia. Whether this is a sufficient explanation is unknown.

ACANTHOCYTOSIS WITH NEUROLOGIC DISEASE AND NORMAL LIPOPROTEINS (AMYOTROPHIC CHOREA-ACANTHOCYTOSIS)

This syndrome was first described by Estes and co-workers.[1720, 1721] Since then, additional reports have appeared, particularly from Japan.[1722–1734] The disorder is characterized by acanthocytosis, normolipoproteinemia, and progressive neurologic disease beginning in adolescence or adult life (8 to 62 years), including orofacial dyskinesia, lip and tongue biting, limb chorea, axonal sensorimotor polyneuropathy, decreased or absent tendon reflexes, muscle hypotonia, distal muscle wasting, and increased creatine phosphokinase. The extent of mental deterioration varies.[1729] Magnetic resonance imaging and pathologic examinations show atrophy of the basal ganglia, particularly the caudate and putamen. In some patients, little or no hemolysis occurs; in others, acanthocytosis precedes the onset of neurologic symptoms.[1729] In others, acanthocytes do not appear until late in the disease course.[1735] The mutant protein in chorea-acanthocytosis, chorein, has been identified and a number of mutations have been identified in affected patients.[1736, 1737] The function of chorein is unknown, but it may be involved in protein sorting.

It is likely that more than one disorder is represented by these reports, because both dominant and recessive inheritance has been recorded.[1738] In addition, variant syndromes with chorea-acanthocytosis and myopathy[1739] and with chorea-acanthocytosis, spherocytosis, and hemolysis[921] have been observed. Acanthocytosis is also associated with other unusual hereditary neurologic syndromes. One of these appears to be recessively inherited and features acanthocytosis, tics, and parkinsonism and is sometimes associated with motor neuron disease or diurnal dystonia.[1740, 1741] A second syndrome combines acanthocytosis, mitochondrial myopathy, encephalopathy, lactic acidosis, and stroke-like symptoms.[1740] A third is characterized by acanthocytosis and Hallervorden-Spatz disease (progressive dementia, dystonia, spasticity, pallidal degeneration with iron deposition, and often retinal degeneration).[1742–1744] A fourth syndrome combines acanthocytosis with abnormal lipoproteins and a Hallervorden-Spatz-like disorder (HARP syndrome—hypoprebetalipoproteinemia, acanthocytosis, retinitis pigmentosa, and pallidal degeneration with iron deposition).[1745, 1746]

Except for typical chorea-acanthocytosis, the cause or causes of these disorders are unknown, but there is evidence that the red cell membrane is defective. The red cells from patients with chorea-acanthocytosis are dense, owing to excessive K^+ loss,[1725] and may or may not have an increased proportion of SM.[1725, 1733] Ankyrin, band 3, and protein 4.2 self-digest more rapidly than normal in the red cells of these patients, suggesting a defect in the vertical connections between the membrane skeleton and the lipid bilayer.[1734] Intramembranous particles are more clustered in the chorea-acanthocytosis red cells, which is compatible with this type of defect. A defect near the COOH-terminal end of band 3, Pro[868]→Leu, has been identified in one family with chorea-acanthocytosis.[283] Hematologically, affected individuals of the latter kindred have 20 to 25 percent acanthocytes and mild anemia with reticulocytosis. Finally, abnormal cyclic AMP phosphorylation of red cell dematin has been observed in a kindred with mild spheroacanthocytosis and a choreiform movement disorder or dementia.[1745, 1747]

ANOREXIA NERVOSA

Acanthocytosis is common in many patients with severe anorexia nervosa.[1688, 1689] The cause of the acanthocytosis is unknown. Plasma lipid and LDL levels are normal or slightly decreased; however, even in those patients with low levels of LDLs,[1748] acanthocytosis may not be due solely to the lipoprotein deficiency, because patients with much lower concentrations of LDLs (e.g., those with hypobetalipoproteinemia) usually have normal red cell morphology. Severe starvation or malnutrition due to causes other than anorexia nervosa can also produce acanthocytosis[1749–1751] or target cells and hypobetalipoproteinemia.[1752]

Despite the acanthocytosis, only a small fraction of these patients experience significant anemia.[1753] Red cell life span is normal or only slightly shortened. Leukopenia and neutropenia are common, and mild thrombocytopenia is not rare.[1688, 1689, 1754] Based on morphology, these cytopenias are due to a hypoproliferative bone marrow[1688] and their severity correlates with weight.[1755] The hypoplastic marrow is also deficient in fat, which is replaced by an amorphous ground substance, perhaps acid mucopolysaccharide.[1689]

HEPATOCELLULAR DAMAGE (SPUR CELL ANEMIA)

The anemia seen in patients with liver disease has a complex etiology. Common causes include blood loss, hypersplenism, iron deficiency, folic acid deficiency, and marrow suppression from alcohol ingestion, hepatitis virus infection, and other poorly understood factors.[1756, 1757] In addition, in some patients, acquired abnormalities of the red cell membrane may contribute to anemia. Two morphologic syndromes are recognized. In one, target cells predominate. In the other, a syndrome of brisk hemolysis develops in association with acanthocytes or "spur" cells, so-called spur cell anemia.[1684, 1757–1778]

Typically, target cells are associated with obstructive liver disease and acanthocytes are associated with hepatocellular disease. In practice, the situation is more complex.

It is not uncommon for both cell morphologies to coexist, and some experimental data suggest that they are different stages of the same process. For example, when the bile duct is ligated in a rat, acanthocytes appear within 8 hours, but they convert to target cells if the obstruction persists for 7 days or more.[1779] Nevertheless, acanthocytes (spur cells) and target cells differ in many important respects, and they are considered separately in this chapter.

Spur cell anemia has most often been described in patients with alcoholic cirrhosis.[1685, 1759–1761, 1775, 1776] However, it is also reported in those with cardiac cirrhosis,[1760] metastatic liver disease,[1764] hemochromatosis,[1763] neonatal hepatitis,[1780] cholestasis,[1757, 1758, 1777] Wilson disease, and severe acute hepatitis. This suggests that it may occur in any disease in which damage to hepatocytes is severe.

Typically, patients have moderately severe hemolysis (hematocrit of 20 to 30 percent), marked indirect hyperbilirubinemia, splenomegaly, and clinical and laboratory evidence of severe hepatic dysfunction. By definition, more than 20 percent acanthocytes are evident in multiple areas on several peripheral blood smears. Because crenated and spiculated cells are a commonly seen artifact of improperly dried smears, it is useful to demonstrate that such cells are also present in wet preparations. (The freshly drawn cells should either be fixed or be examined immediately after dilution in their own plasma.) Morphologically, the acanthocytes of spur cell anemia are indistinguishable from those seen in patients with abetalipoproteinemia. In some patients significant numbers of echinocytes and target cells may be present, and spherocytes may develop, presumably as a result of microspherulation. Occasionally, this may cause some diagnostic confusion. In our experience, however, many of these "spherocytes" have fine spicules, evident on close examination, which distinguish them from true microspherocytes.

The red cell life span of spur cells is markedly shortened because of splenic sequestration,[1685, 1760, 1765, 1771] and, as expected, hemolysis abates after splenectomy.[1771] Unfortunately, splenectomy is a dangerous and often fatal procedure in these very sick patients and is not generally recommended.[1771] In addition, spur cell anemia has been reported in a splenectomized patient.[1762] Some success has been reported in treating the anemia of these patients with either phospholipid infusions[1772] or flunarizine[1773]; however, these approaches are still experimental.

The clinical syndrome of spur cell anemia can be produced by at least two different pathogenic mechanisms. In one group, typically consisting of patients with alcoholic cirrhosis,[1685, 1761, 1766] the disorder is due to an acquired abnormality of red cell lipids. The pathophysiology of spurring in these patients has been defined and reviewed by Cooper and associates[1650, 1685, 1771, 1774, 1775] and is illustrated in Figure 15–34. It occurs in two stages: cholesterol loading and splenic remodeling. In the first stage, abnormal, cholesterol-laden, apolipoprotein A-II–deficient lipoproteins, produced by the patient's diseased liver, transfer their excess cholesterol to circulating erythrocytes and increase the membrane cholesterol concentration, the cholesterol-to-phospholipid ratio, and the membrane

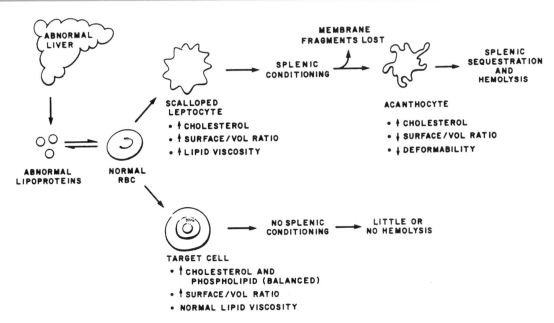

FIGURE 15–34. Schematic illustration of the pathophysiologic course of acanthocyte ("spur cell") and target cell formation in liver disease.

surface area (Fig. 15–35).[1650, 1776] This is an acquired process and can be mimicked *in vitro* by incubation of normal red cells in spur cell plasma[1685, 1771] or in artificial media containing cholesterol-phospholipid dispersions with a cholesterol-to-phospholipid ratio greater than 1.0.[1774] It can be reproduced *in vivo* in dogs fed a high cholesterol diet.[1775] In scanning electron micrographs, these cholesterol-laden cells are flattened and often folded, with an undulating periphery.[1775] They appear scalloped or crenated on dried smears.[1685, 1771] *In vivo*, in the second stage, scalloped cells are converted into spur cells by a process of splenic conditioning. Over a period of 1 to 7 days, membrane lipids and surface area are lost, cellular rigidity increases, presumably because of the decline in surface-to-volume ratio, and the cell assumes a typical acanthocytic form.[1685, 1771]

Splenectomy prevents both the formation of spur cells and their premature destruction; however, as noted earlier, it is a high-risk procedure and is seldom indicated. One alcoholic patient with spur cell anemia treated with flunarizine, pentoxifylline, and cholestyramine had a reduction in anemia, hyperbilirubinemia, and hypercholesterolemia after splenectomy.[1777]

The cholesterol-laden, incipient spur cell is presumably detained and remodeled by the spleen because it is less remodeled deformable than normal. The molecular explanation for this change in deformability is unknown. There is evidence that cholesterol affects the function of band 3.[1778] Perhaps it also influences band 3 oligomerization or its interaction with other membrane proteins. A slight increase in the cholesterol-to-phospholipid ratio to above normal markedly alters cholesterol organization in the membrane[1779] and increases the helical content of one or more of the major membrane proteins.[1780, 1781] There is also evidence that membrane proteolytic activity is increased in spur cells and that spur cell plasma can stimulate membrane degradation in normal erythrocytes.

Other studies have identified a defect in phospholipid repair.[1782] Spur cells and cholesterol-laden normal red cells readily incorporate arachidonic acid, a polyunsaturated fatty acid, into acylcarnitine, a fatty acid membrane repair intermediate, but further incorporation of arachidonate into phospholipids is slowed, and activity of the involved enzyme, lysophosphocholine acyl transferase (or arachidonoyl-CoA:1-palmitoyl-*sn*-glycero-3-phosphocholine acyl transferase), is decreased. Inhibition of this pathway, caused by cholesterol loading of the erythrocyte, impairs the red cell's ability to replace peroxidized fatty acyl side chains of phospholipids. The role of this defect in the pathophysiology of spur cell anemia is not yet clear.

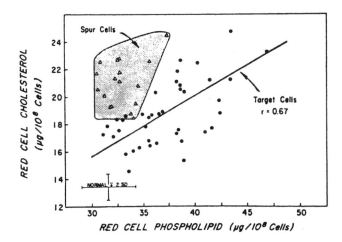

FIGURE 15–35. The cholesterol and phospholipid content of target cells (*solid circles*) and spur cells (*solid triangles*). Note that target cells tend to have a balanced increase in cholesterol and phospholipid, whereas spur cells are usually selectively enriched in cholesterol. (From Cooper RA, Diloy-Puray M, et al: An analysis of lipoproteins, bile acids, and red cell membranes associated with target cells and spur cells in patients with liver disease. J Clin Invest 1972;51: 3182.)

The second group of patients with liver disease and spur cell anemia differs in that red cell membrane lipids are normal and incubation of normal red cells in the patients' plasma does not induce spurring.[1760, 1764, 1765] The pathophysiology of this condition is unknown and largely unstudied. It has been reported in patients with alcoholic cirrhosis[1760, 1765] and metastatic liver disease,[1764] and this is the form of the disease most often seen in children with spur cells and severe hepatocellular dysfunction.

VITAMIN E DEFICIENCY

Premature infants (<36 weeks' gestation or weighing <2000 g) and children or adults with steatorrhea are susceptible to vitamin E deficiency because of decreased absorption of the vitamin.[1783–1785] Discussion of this disorder in preterm infants is now primarily only of historical interest.[1786] Infants described with this syndrome were being fed formulas that were very low in vitamin E and very high in polyunsaturated fatty acids. As the interactions among dietary iron, polyunsaturated fatty acids, and vitamin E were elucidated, infant formulas were altered so that this condition has virtually disappeared in most nurseries. However, vitamin E deficiency may cause a hemolytic anemia in infancy in patients with disorders that cause fat malabsorption such as cystic fibrosis or abetalipoproteinemia.[1787, 1788]

The features of severe vitamin E deficiency in infants are hemolysis, thrombocytosis, and a generalized edema.[1789–1791] Peripheral blood smears are often normal but sometimes show variable numbers of irregularly contracted, spiculated cells (acanthocytes or pyknocytes) and small numbers of spherocytes and fragmented red cells.[1788, 1790] The mechanism of hemolysis is uncertain. Vitamin E is a lipid-soluble antioxidant, and in its absence lipid peroxidation occurs, with damage to the double bonds of unsaturated fatty acids. Phospholipids rich in unsaturated acyl chains, such as PE, are particularly susceptible.[1708, 1712, 1792] However, there is some evidence that damage to the sulfhydryl groups of membrane proteins may also contribute to hemolysis.[1793]

Kay and co-workers[1794] found that vitamin E–deficient rat erythrocytes have many of the characteristics of aged normal red cells, especially exposure of the so-called senescent antigen. This "neoantigen," described in detail earlier in the chapter, apparently results from proteolysis, clustering, or oxidation of protein 3. It is recognized by an IgG, anti–band 3 autoantibody that initiates removal of the cells by macrophages. Autoantibody attachment is blocked by vitamin E and reversed by thiol-reducing agents in experimental situations, which suggests that membrane lipid oxidation occurs first and leads to the oxidation of band 3 thiols. Presumably, similar processes accelerate red cell destruction *in vivo* in vitamin E deficiency.

INFANTILE PYKNOCYTOSIS

In 1959, Tuffy and colleagues[1687] described a syndrome of neonatal jaundice and hemolysis associated with variable numbers of distorted, irregularly contracted, spiculated cells, which they called pyknocytes.

Morphologically, these cells are very similar (and possibly identical) to acanthocytes. Normal full-term infants have 0.3 to 1.9 percent pyknocytes/acanthocytes on peripheral blood smears. In premature infants the normal range is 0.3 to 5.6 percent. The affected infants typically are seen jaundice and slight hepatosplenomegaly in the first few days of life. Pyknocytosis and hemolytic anemia peak at 3 to 4 weeks of age and then decline spontaneously. Clinical severity is variable; however, some infants are severely affected (hemoglobin level of 4.6 g/dL; 15 to 20 percent reticulocytes; 25 to 50 percent pyknocytes), and some require exchange transfusions. Transfused erythrocytes become pyknocytic and survive poorly,[1687, 1795, 1796] indicating an extracorpuscular defect. The syndrome is seen in both premature and term infants. The only consistent chemical abnormality is a mild elevation in serum aspartate transaminase (50 to 250 IU). Parents and siblings are normal.

The cause of this syndrome has not been clearly defined, and, for unknown reasons, the diagnosis is seldom made today. Infants with severe G6PD deficiency,[1797] neonatal Heinz body hemolytic anemias,[1687, 1798] vitamin E deficiency,[1788, 1790] glycolytic enzyme deficiencies,[1565] neonatal hepatitis,[1770] HE,[1376, 1377] and microangiopathic hemolytic anemias may be seen with hemolysis and pyknocytes, and in these infants infantile pyknocytosis is sometimes misdiagnosed. However, in most of the original case reports, evidence is sufficient to exclude those disorders, which suggests that infantile pyknocytosis may be a valid entity. The transient nature, mild transaminase elevation, morphologic features, and extracorpuscular etiology suggest a metabolic defect, possibly involving a circulating oxidant; however, other hypotheses are equally tenable.

McLEOD SYNDROME

McLeod syndrome is a multisystemic disorder with acanthocytosis and, in some patients, late-onset myopathy or chorea.[1799] The McLeod blood group phenotype, first discovered in a blood donor named Hugh McLeod, is an X-linked anomaly of the Kell blood group system in which either red cells, white cells, or both react poorly with Kell antisera but behave normally in other blood group reactions. The affected cells lack Kx, the product of the *XK* gene, which has structural features that suggest a transport protein and may be a membrane precursor of the Kell antigens.[1799–1802] The relevant gene has been cloned and encodes a novel 444–amino acid integral membrane protein that has some of the features of a membrane transporter.[1802] As expected, Kx is defective in patients with McLeod syndrome.[1799, 1802–1807] Male hemizygotes who lack Kx on their red cells have variable acanthocytosis (8 to 85 percent) and mild, compensated hemolysis (3 to 7 percent reticulocytes).[1690, 1808, 1809] Some teardrop erythrocytes and bizarre poikilocytes are also present. Female heterozygotes have occasional acanthocytes (as expected by the Lyon hypothesis) and very mild hemolysis,[1690, 1808] although some of these women have more severe symptoms.[1803]

Some patients with McLeod syndrome also develop a neuropathy or myopathy. This first manifests as areflexia or an elevated creatine phosphokinase level.[1810] Later in adult life, a cardiomyopathy or slowly progressive neuropathy may appear.[1811–1816] The neuropathy is characterized by various combinations of dystonic or choreiform movements, orofacial dyskinesia, dysarthria, tongue biting, and caudate atrophy on cerebral imaging. Psychiatric symptoms, seizures, and peripheral neuropathy with muscle denervation have also been reported. These features, combined with acanthocytosis, can mimic the chorea-acanthocytosis syndromes described in a earlier section.

The *XK* gene is less than 500 kb beyond the chronic granulomatous disease locus on the short arm of the X chromosome (p21.1).[1817] Consequently, males with deletions encompassing both loci have both chronic granulomatous disease and McLeod syndrome.[1818] It is important to recognize patients with McLeod syndrome because, if they receive transfusions, they may develop antibodies that are only compatible with McLeod syndrome red cells.[1819, 1820]

UREMIA

Red cell survival is reduced in patients with advanced renal failure.[1821–1823] An extracorporeal factor is involved, because red cells from uremic patients survive normally when infused into normal persons, whereas normal red cells survive poorly in uremic patients.[1822] The factor is nondialyzable, and some studies suggest that it is parathyroid hormone (PTH).[1824–1826] PTH levels are elevated in renal failure, owing to hyperphosphatemia and secondary hyperparathyroidism. PTH levels correlate closely with red cell survival in patients with chronic renal failure who are receiving dialysis,[1826] and parathyroidectomy abolishes hemolysis in dogs with uremia.[1824] *In vitro*, relevant levels of PTH or its bioactive NH_2-terminal peptide augment Ca^{2+} entry into red cells through a cyclic AMP–independent pathway and cause the cells to develop filamentous extensions and lose membrane surface, presumably by vesiculation.[1825] These effects are largely blocked by the Ca^{2+} channel blocker verapamil. It is possible that they are responsible for the increased numbers of echinocytes observed in some uremic patients, because increased intracellular Ca^{2+} is markedly echinocytogenic.[1827]

IN(LU) GENE

The major antigens of the Lutheran blood group system are Lu^a and Lu^b. They are located on two low-abundance glycoproteins of 80 and 85 kD.[1828] About 1 person in 5000 inherits a dominantly acting inhibitor, called In(Lu),[1691, 1829] which partially suppresses expression of Lu^a and Lu^b such that they are undetectable by standard agglutination tests. This inhibition is the most common cause of the null Lutheran phenotype, Lu(a–b–). The In(Lu) gene product inhibits expression of CD44, an adhesive protein; MER2, a common red cell antigen; CR1, the C3b/C4b complement receptor; AnWj, the erythroid *H. influenzae* receptor; and the glycolipid antigens P1 and i as well as the Lu antigens.[1830] Although several of these proteins are widely expressed, the action of In(Lu) is limited only to red cells.[1830] Patients with the

In(Lu) Lu(a–b–) phenotype have abnormally shaped red cells but no hemolysis.[1691] The morphology varies from normal or mild poikilocytosis to acanthocytosis. Osmotic fragility of fresh In(Lu) Lu(a–b–) red cells is normal but during *in vitro* incubation the cells lose K^+ and become osmotically resistant.

HYPOTHYROIDISM

Patients with hypothyroidism often (20 to 65 percent) have a small number (0.5 to 2 percent) of acanthocytes on peripheral blood smears.[1692, 1831, 1832] Given the high incidence of hypothyroidism relative to other disorders that cause acanthocytosis, it has been suggested that the presence of acanthocytes should prompt physicians to consider thyroid testing, especially in adults. This approach has led to the diagnosis of previously unsuspected hypothyroidism.[1833] Infants with congenital hypothyroidism may suffer from anemia more often than is commonly recognized.[1834]

Other Membrane Disorders

OXIDANT HEMOLYSIS

Oxidant damage is incurred by the red cell membrane in a variety of inherited disorders involving abnormal hemoglobins of defects in the cells' endogenous system for detoxification of oxidants. These include sickle cell disease, thalassemias, unstable hemoglobinopathies, G6PD deficiency, and disorders of glutathione metabolism. Membrane oxidant damage may also result from encounters with exogenous oxidants, one of the most important of these being copper.

COPPER TOXICITY

Acute copper-induced hemolysis has been reported in humans after accidental or suicidal ingestion of copper or copper-containing compounds, copper sulfate therapy for burns, copper contamination of hemodialysis units, and Wilson disease.[1835–1840] In the first three instances, acute intoxication is characterized by flushing, chills, nausea and vomiting, diarrhea, abdominal pain, a metallic taste in the mouth, excessive salivation, headache, weakness, and acute intravascular hemolysis.[1835–1841]

WILSON DISEASE (HEPATOLENTICULAR DEGENERATION)

Wilson disease is an autosomal recessive disorder of copper metabolism characterized by defective biliary excretion of copper, low plasma levels of ceruloplasmin, and toxic accumulation of copper in liver, erythrocytes, kidneys, cornea, and brain.[1842, 1843] Consequences include cirrhosis, hemolysis, corneal Kayser-Fleischer rings, and a progressive neurologic syndrome.[1844–1857] The Wilson disease gene, the copper-transporting ATPase *ATP7B*, and the Wilson disease protein, WNDP, belong to the large family of cation-transporting P-type ATPases.[1858–1863] A wide variety of mutations have been described in this gene in patients with Wilson disease.[1864–1867]

Hemolysis is an early feature of Wilson disease; it is seen in 20 percent of patients who have with liver disease[1844] and may be the presenting manifestation of the disorder.[1845–1852, 1868] Because the disease is treatable and because hemolysis may presage fulminant liver disease by days to years,[1848, 1850, 1851] the clinician must always consider Wilson disease in children and young adults with hemolytic anemia that produces negative Coombs test results. Typically, these previously well children have chemical evidence of liver disease, mild hepatosplenomegaly, a low ceruloplasmin concentration, increased erythrocyte and hepatic copper levels, and increased urinary copper excretion. Jaundice is often seen and may be severe. The hemolysis observed in Wilson disease is also acute, but the clinical features, although similar to those of acute copper poisoning, are usually more subtle. Hemoglobin may be detected on urinalysis, but gross hemoglobinuria is unusual. Peripheral blood smears do not usually show characteristic changes, although we have seen one child in whom spur cells and target cells were prominent.

The belief is that in Wilson disease copper initially accumulates in the liver, where it eventually reaches a toxic level and is released into the bloodstream by hepatocellular necrosis.[1850] Plasma copper is rapidly taken up by red cells.[1869] Intravascular hemolysis occurs as a consequence of oxidative damage. The oxidative effects of copper are manifold. *In vitro*, copper inactivates numerous red cell glycolytic and hexose monophosphate shunt enzymes; directly oxidizes reduced nicotinamide adenine nucleotide phosphate (NADPH) and glutathione; oxidizes and denatures hemoglobin; damages membrane ATPases, fatty acid acylase, and probably other membrane enzymes; generates lipid peroxides; and cross-links membrane skeletal proteins into disulfide-bonded high-molecular-weight complexes, increasing membrane permeability and rigidity.[1851, 1870] However, many of these effects have not been demonstrated at concentrations of copper observed in hemolyzing erythrocytes (150 to 400 mg/dL of red cells = 2.4×10^{-5} to 6.3×10^{-5} mol/L).[1852, 1856] It is likely that oxidation results from the reaction of copper with protein thiols to yield superoxide and its subsequent conversion to peroxide and other forms of activated oxygen. So far it has not been possible to determine the exact cause of the demise of the red cells.

REFERENCES

1. Singer SJ, Nicolson GL: The fluid mosaic model of the structure of cell membranes. Science 1972; 175:720.
2. Jacobson K, Sheets ED, Simson R: Revisiting the fluid mosaic model of membranes. Science 1995; 268:1441.
3. Leitner DM, Brown FL, Wilson KR: Regulation of protein mobility in cell membranes: A dynamic corral model. Biophys J 2000; 78:125.
4. White SH, Ladokhin AS, et al: How membranes shape protein structure. J Biol Chem 2001; 276:32395.
5. Sweeley CC, Dawson G: Lipids of the erythrocyte. In Jamieson GA, Greenwalt TJ (eds): Red Cell Membrane Structure and Function. Philadelphia, JB Lippincott, 1969, p 172.
6. Turner JD, Rouser G: Precise quantitative determination of human blood lipids by thin-layer and triethylaminoethylcellulose column chromatography. II. Plasma lipids. Anal Biochem 1970; 38:437.
7. Ways P, Hanahan DJ: Characterization and quantification of red cell lipids in normal man. J Lipid Res 1964; 5:318.
8. Marchesi VT, Tillack TW, et al: Chemical characterization and surface orientation of the major glycoprotein of the human erythrocyte membrane. Proc Natl Acad Sci USA 1972; 69:1445.
9. Weinstein RS: The morphology of adult red cells. In Surgenor DM (ed): The Red Blood Cell, 2nd ed. New York, Academic Press, 1974, Vol 1, p 214.
10. Van Deenen LL, De Gier J: Lipids of the red blood cell membrane. In Surgenor DM (ed): The Red Blood Cell. 2nd ed. Vol. 1. New York, Academic Press, 1974, p 148.
11. Virtanen JA, Cheng KH, Somerharju P: Phospholipid composition of the mammalian red cell membrane can be rationalized by a super-lattice model. Proc Natl Acad Sci USA 1998; 95:4964.
12. Blau L, Bittman R: Cholesterol distribution between the two halves of the lipid bilayer of human erythrocyte ghost membranes. J Biol Chem 1978; 253:8366.
13. Hale JE, Schroeder F: Asymmetric transbilayer distribution of sterol across plasma membranes determined by fluorescence quenching of dehydroergosterol. Eur J Biochem 1982; 122:649.
14. Fisher KA: Analysis of membrane halves: Cholesterol. Proc Natl Acad Sci USA 1976; 73:173.
15. Hubbell WL, McConnell HM: Orientation and motion of amphiphilic spin labels in membranes. Proc Natl Acad Sci USA 1969; 64:20.
16. Lange Y, Dolde J, Steck TL: The rate of transmembrane movement of cholesterol in the human erythrocyte. J Biol Chem 1981; 256:5321.
17. Huang CH: A structural model for the cholesterol-phosphatidylcholine complexes in bilayer membranes. Lipids 1977; 12:348.
18. Bergelson LD, Barsukov LI: Topological asymmetry of phospholipids in membranes. Science 1977; 197:224.
19. Fujimoto K, Umeda M, Fujimoto T: Transmembrane phospholipid distribution revealed by freeze-fracture replica labeling. J Cell Sci 1996; 109(Pt 10):2453.
20. Heinrich R, Brumen M, et al: Modelling of phospholipid translocation in the erythrocyte membrane: A combined kinetic and thermodynamic approach. J Theor Biol 1997; 185:295.
21. Haest CW, Oslender A, Kamp D: Nonmediated flip-flop of anionic phospholipids and long-chain amphiphiles in the erythrocyte membrane depends on membrane potential. Biochemistry 1997; 36:10885.
22. Devaux PF: Protein involvement in transmembrane lipid asymmetry. Annu Rev Biophys Biomol Struct 1992; 21:417.
23. Boon JM, Smith BD: Facilitated phosphatidylcholine flip-flop across erythrocyte membranes using low molecular weight synthetic translocases. J Am Chem Soc 2001; 123:6221.
24. Daleke DL, Lyles JV: Identification and purification of aminophospholipid flippases. Biochim Biophys Acta 2000; 1486:108.
25. Zhou Y, Gottesman MM, Pastan I: Studies of human MDR1-MDR2 chimeras demonstrate the functional exchangeability of a major transmembrane segment of the multidrug transporter and phosphatidylcholine flippase. Mol Cell Biol 1999; 19:1450.
26. Romsicki Y, Sharom FJ: Phospholipid flippase activity of the reconstituted P-glycoprotein multidrug transporter. Biochemistry 2001; 40:6937.
27. Morrot G, Hervé P, et al: Aminophospholipid translocase of human erythrocytes: Phospholipid substrate specificity and effect of cholesterol. Biochemistry 1989; 28:3456.
28. Tang X, Halleck MS, et al: A subfamily of P-type ATPases with aminophospholipid transporting activity. Science 1996; 272:1495.
29. Abraham EH, Shrivastav B, et al: Cellular and biophysical evidence for interactions between adenosine triphosphate and P-glycoprotein substrates: Functional implications for adenosine triphosphate/drug cotransport in P-glycoprotein overexpressing tumor cells and in P-glycoprotein low-level expressing erythrocytes. Blood Cells Mol Dis 2001; 27:181.
30. Seigneuret M, Devaux PF: ATP-dependent asymmetric distribution of spin-labeled phospholipids in the erythrocyte membrane: Relation to shape changes. Proc Natl Acad Sci USA 1984; 81:3751.
31. Dekkers DW, Comfurius P, et al: Transbilayer movement of NBD-labeled phospholipids in red blood cell membranes: Outward-directed transport by the multidrug resistance protein 1 (MRP1). Biochemistry 1998; 37:14833.

32. Kamp D, Haest CW: Evidence for a role of the multidrug resistance protein (MRP) in the outward translocation of NBD-phospholipids in the erythrocyte membrane. Biochim Biophys Acta 1998; 1372:91.

33. Dekkers DW, Comfurius P, et al: Multidrug resistance protein 1 regulates lipid asymmetry in erythrocyte membranes. Biochem J 2000; 350 Pt 2:531.

34. Rappa G, Finch RA, et al: New insights into the biology and pharmacology of the multidrug resistance protein (MRP) from gene knockout models. Biochem Pharmacol 1999; 58:557.

35. Cohen AM, Liu SC, et al: Ultrastructural studies of the interaction of spectrin with phosphatidylserine liposomes. Blood 1986; 68:920.

36. Maksymiw R, Sui SF, et al: Electrostatic coupling of spectrin dimers to phosphatidylserine containing lipid lamellae. Biochemistry 1987; 26:2983.

37. Mombers C, de Gier J, et al: Spectrin-phospholipid interaction. A monolayer study. Biochim Biophys Acta 1980; 603:52.

38. Bergmann WL, Dressler V, et al: Cross-linking of SH-groups in the erythrocyte membrane enhances transbilayer reorientation of phospholipids. Evidence for a limited access of phospholipids to the reorientation sites. Biochim Biophys Acta 1984; 769:390.

39. Dressler V, Haest CW, et al: Stabilizing factors of phospholipid asymmetry in the erythrocyte membrane. Biochim Biophys Acta 1984; 775:189.

40. Franck PF, Roelofsen B, Op den Kamp JA: Complete exchange of phosphatidylcholine from intact erythrocytes after protein crosslinking. Biochim Biophys Acta 1982; 687:105.

41. Haest CW, Plasa G, et al: Spectrin as a stabilizer of the phospholipid asymmetry in the human erythrocyte membrane. Biochim Biophys Acta 1978; 509:21.

42. Devaux PF: Static and dynamic lipid asymmetry in cell membranes. Biochemistry 1991; 30:1163.

43. Calvez JY, Zachowski A, et al: Asymmetric distribution of phospholipids in spectrin-poor erythrocyte vesicles. Biochemistry 1988; 27:5666.

44. Kuypers FA, Lubin BH, et al: The distribution of erythrocyte phospholipids in hereditary spherocytosis demonstrates a minimal role for erythrocyte spectrin on phospholipid diffusion and asymmetry. Blood 1993; 81:1051.

45. Williamson P, Kulick A, et al: Ca^{2+} induces transbilayer redistribution of all major phospholipids in human erythrocytes. Biochemistry 1992; 31:6355.

46. Bevers EM, Comfurius P, et al: Lipid translocation across the plasma membrane of mammalian cells. Biochim Biophys Acta 1999; 1439:317.

47. Bucki R, Bachelot-Loza C, et al: Calcium induces phospholipid redistribution and microvesicle release in human erythrocyte membranes by independent pathways. Biochemistry 1998; 37:15383.

48. Basse F, Stout JG, et al: Isolation of an erythrocyte membrane protein that mediates Ca^{2+}-dependent transbilayer movement of phospholipid. J Biol Chem 1996; 271:17205.

49. Zhou Q, Zhao J, et al: Molecular cloning of human plasma membrane phospholipid scramblase. A protein mediating transbilayer movement of plasma membrane phospholipids. J Biol Chem 1997; 272:18240.

50. Zhao J, Zhou Q, et al: Level of expression of phospholipid scramblase regulates induced movement of phosphatidylserine to the cell surface. J Biol Chem 1998; 273:6603.

51. Zhou Q, Sims PJ, Wiedmer T: Identity of a conserved motif in phospholipid scramblase that is required for Ca^{2+}-accelerated transbilayer movement of membrane phospholipids. Biochemistry 1998; 37:2356.

52. Stout JG, Zhou Q, et al: Change in conformation of plasma membrane phospholipid scramblase induced by occupancy of its Ca^{2+} binding site. Biochemistry 1998; 37:14860.

53. Kamp D, Sieberg T, Haest CW: Inhibition and stimulation of phospholipid scrambling activity. Consequences for lipid asymmetry, echinocytosis, and microvesiculation of erythrocytes. Biochemistry 2001; 40:9438.

54. Stout JG, Basse F, et al: Scott syndrome erythrocytes contain a membrane protein capable of mediating Ca^{2+}-dependent transbilayer migration of membrane phospholipids. J Clin Invest 1997; 99:2232.

55. Dekkers DW, Comfurius P, et al: Impaired Ca^{2+}-induced tyrosine phosphorylation and defective lipid scrambling in erythrocytes from a patient with Scott syndrome: A study using an inhibitor for scramblase that mimics the defect in Scott syndrome. Blood 1998; 91:2133.

56. Kuypers FA: Phospholipid asymmetry in health and disease. Curr Opin Hematol 1998; 5:122.

57. Zwaal RF, Schroit AJ: Pathophysiologic implications of membrane phospholipid asymmetry in blood cells. Blood 1997; 89:1121.

58. de Jong K, Larkin SK, et al: Characterization of the phosphatidylserine-exposing subpopulation of sickle cells. Blood 2001; 98:860.

59. Bonomini M, Sirolli V, et al: Increased erythrocyte phosphatidylserine exposure in chronic renal failure. J Am Soc Nephrol 1999; 10:1982.

59a. Bonomini M, Sirolli V, et al: Enhanced adherence of human uremic erythrocytes to vascular endothelium: Role of phosphatidylserine exposure. Kidney Int 2002; 62:1358.

60. Setty BN, Kulkarni S, Stuart MJ: Role of erythrocyte phosphatidylserine in sickle red cell-endothelial adhesion. Blood 2002; 99:1564.

61. de Jong K, Larkin SK, et al: Hereditary spherocytosis and elliptocytosis erythrocytes show a normal transbilayer phospholipid distribution. Blood 1999; 94:319.

62. Geldwerth D, Cherif-Zahar B, et al: Phosphatidylserine exposure and aminophospholipid translocase activity in Rh-deficient erythrocytes. Mol Membr Biol 1997; 14:125.

63. Chang SH, Gallagher PG, et al: Altered erythrocyte endothelial adherence and membrane phospholipid asymmetry in hereditary hydrocytosis. Blood 2001; 98:12a.

64. Manno S, Takakuwa Y, Mohandas N: Identification of a functional role for lipid asymmetry in biological membranes: Phosphatidylserine-skeletal protein interactions modulate membrane stability. Proc Natl Acad Sci USA 2002; 99:1943.

65. Test ST, Mitsuyoshi J: Activation of the alternative pathway of complement by calcium-loaded erythrocytes resulting from loss of membrane phospholipid asymmetry. J Lab Clin Med 1997; 130:169.

66. Tanaka Y, Schroit AJ: Insertion of fluorescent phosphatidylserine into the plasma membrane of red blood cells. Recognition by autologous macrophages. J Biol Chem 1983; 258:11335.

67. McEvoy L, Williamson P, Schlegel RA: Membrane phospholipid asymmetry as a determinant of erythrocyte recognition by macrophages. Proc Natl Acad Sci USA 1986; 83:3311.

68. Fadok VA, Bratton DL, et al: A receptor for phosphatidylserine-specific clearance of apoptotic cells. Nature 2000; 405:85.

69. Hoffmann PR, deCathelineau AM, et al: Phosphatidylserine (PS) induces PS receptor-mediated macropinocytosis and promotes clearance of apoptotic cells. J Cell Biol 2001; 155:649.

70. Henson PM, Bratton DL, Fadok VA: The phosphatidylserine receptor: A crucial molecular switch? Nat Rev Mol Cell Biol 2001; 2:627.

71. Somersan S, Bhardwaj N: Tethering and tickling: A new role for the phosphatidylserine receptor. J Cell Biol 2001; 155:501.

72. Bratosin D, Estaquier J, et al: Programmed cell death in mature erythrocytes: A model for investigating death effector pathways operating in the absence of mitochondria. Cell Death Differ 2001; 8:1143.

73. Mandal D, Moitra PK, et al: Caspase 3 regulates phosphatidylserine externalization and phagocytosis of oxidatively stressed erythrocytes. FEBS Lett 2002; 513:184.

74. Rodgers W, Glaser M: Characterization of lipid domains in erythrocyte membranes. Proc Natl Acad Sci USA 1991; 88:1364.

75. Zuvic-Butorac M, Muller P, et al: Lipid domains in the exoplasmic and cytoplasmic leaflet of the human erythrocyte membrane: A spin label approach. Eur Biophys J 1999; 28:302.

76. Jost PC, Nadakavukaren KK, Griffith OH: Phosphatidylcholine exchange between the boundary lipid and bilayer domains in cytochrome oxidase containing membranes. Biochemistry 1977; 16:3110.

77. Smith RL, Oldfield E: Dynamic structure of membranes by deuterium NMR. Science 1984; 225:280.

78. Parks GD, Lamb RA: Topology of eukaryotic type II membrane proteins: Importance of N-terminal positively charged residues flanking the hydrophobic domain. Cell 1991; 64:777.

79. Yamane K, Akiyama Y, et al: A positively charged region is a determinant of the orientation of cytoplasmic membrane proteins in *Escherichia coli*. J Biol Chem 1990; 265:21166.

80. Beck JS: Relations between membrane monolayers in some red cell shape transformations. J Theor Biol 1978; 75:487.

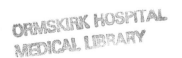

81. Ferrell JE Jr, Lee KJ, Huestis WH: Membrane bilayer balance and erythrocyte shape: A quantitative assessment. Biochemistry 1985; 24:2849.

82. Sheetz MP, Singer SJ: Biological membranes as bilayer couples. A molecular mechanism of drug-erythrocyte interactions. Proc Natl Acad Sci USA 1974; 71:4457.

83. Christiansson A, Kuypers FA, et al: Lipid molecular shape affects erythrocyte morphology: A study involving replacement of native phosphatidylcholine with different species followed by treatment of cells with sphingomyelinase C or phospholipase A2. J Cell Biol 1985; 101:1455.

84. Isomaa B, Hagerstrand H, Paatero G: Shape transformations induced by amphiphiles in erythrocytes. Biochim Biophys Acta 1987; 899:93.

85. Sheetz MP, Painter RG, Singer SJ: Biological membranes as bilayer couples. III. Compensatory shape changes induced in membranes. J Cell Biol 1976; 70:193.

86. Lange Y, Steck TL: Mechanism of red blood cell acanthocytosis and echinocytosis *in vivo*. J Membr Biol 1984; 77:153.

87. Nakao M: New insights into regulation of erythrocyte shape. Curr Opin Hematol 2002; 9:127.

88. Gedde MM, Yang E, Huestis WH: Resolution of the paradox of red cell shape changes in low and high pH. Biochim Biophys Acta 1999; 1417:246.

89. Schwarz S, Deuticke B, Haest CW: Passive transmembrane redistributions of phospholipids as a determinant of erythrocyte shape change. Studies on electroporated cells. Mol Membr Biol 1999; 16:247.

90. Henszen MM, Weske M, et al: Electric field pulses induce reversible shape transformation of human erythrocytes. Mol Membr Biol 1997; 14:195.

91. Geldwerth D, Kuypers FA, et al: Transbilayer mobility and distribution of red cell phospholipids during storage. J Clin Invest 1993; 92:308.

92. Brown KE, Anderson SM, Young NS: Erythrocyte P antigen: Cellular receptor for B19 parvovirus. Science 1993; 262:114.

93. Lange Y, Slayton JM: Interaction of cholesterol and lysophosphatidylcholine in determining red cell shape. J Lipid Res 1982; 23:1121.

94. Berridge MJ: Inositol trisphosphate and calcium signalling. Nature 1993; 361:315.

95. York JD, Guo S, et al: An expanded view of inositol signaling. Adv Enzyme Regul 2001; 41:57.

96. Levine YK, Birdsall NJ, et al: ^{13}C nuclear magnetic resonance relaxation measurements of synthetic lecithins and the effect of spin-labeled lipids. Biochemistry 1972; 11:1416.

97. McConnell HM, McFarland BG: The flexibility gradient in biological membranes. Ann NY Acad Sci 1972; 195:207.

98. Barton PG, Gunstone FD: Hydrocarbon chain packing and molecular motion in phospholipid bilayers formed from unsaturated lecithins. Synthesis and properties of sixteen positional isomers of 1,2-dioctadecenoyl-*sn*-glycero-3-phosphorylcholine. J Biol Chem 1975; 250:4470.

99. Seelig A, Seelig J: Effect of a single *cis* double bond on the structures of a phospholipid bilayer. Biochemistry 1977; 16:45.

100. Oldfield E, Chapman D: Effects of cholesterol and cholesterol derivatives on hydrocarbon chain mobility in lipids. Biochem Biophys Res Commun 1971; 43:610.

101. Lee AG, Birdsall NJ, Metcalfe JC: Measurement of fast lateral diffusion of lipids in vesicles and in biological membranes by ^{1}H nuclear magnetic resonance. Biochemistry 1973; 12:1650.

102. Cooper RA, Durocher JR, Leslie MH: Decreased fluidity of red cell membrane lipids in abetalipoproteinemia. J Clin Invest 1977; 60:115.

103. Cooper RA: Abnormalities of cell-membrane fluidity in the pathogenesis of disease. N Engl J Med 1977; 297:371.

104. Vanderkooi J, Fischkoff S, et al: Fluorescent probe analysis of the lipid architecture of natural and experimental cholesterol-rich membranes. Biochemistry 1974; 13:1589.

105. Devaux P, McConnell HM: Lateral diffusion in spin-labeled phosphatidylcholine multilayers. J Am Chem Soc 1972; 94:4475.

106. Wu ES, Jacobson K, Papahadjopoulos D: Lateral diffusion in phospholipid multibilayers measured by fluorescence recovery after photobleaching. Biochemistry 1977; 16:3836.

107. Koppel DE, Sheetz MP, Schindler M: Matrix control of protein diffusion in biological membranes. Proc Natl Acad Sci USA 1981; 78:3576.

107a. Fujiwara T, Ritchie K, et al: Phospholipids undergo hop diffusion in compartmentalized cell membrane. J Cell Biol 2002; 157:1071.

108. Reed CF: Incorporation of orthophosphate-^{32}P into erythrocyte phospholipids in normal subjects and in patients with hereditary spherocytosis. J Clin Invest 1968; 47:2630.

109. Renooij W, Van Golde LM: The transposition of molecular classes of phosphatidylcholine across the rat erythrocyte membrane and their exchange between the red cell membrane and plasma lipoproteins. Biochim Biophys Acta 1977; 470:465.

110. Shohet SB: Release of phospholipid fatty acid from human erythrocytes. J Clin Invest 1970; 49:1668.

111. Glomset JA, Assmann G, et al: Lecithin:cholesterol acyltransferase deficiency and fish eye disease. In Scriver CS, Beuadet AL, et al (eds): The Metabolic and Molecular Bases of Inherited Disease. New York, McGraw-Hill, 1995, p 1933.

112. Mulder E, van Deenen LL: Metabolism of red-cell lipids. I. Incorporation in vitro of fatty acids into phospholipids from mature erythrocytes. Biochim Biophys Acta 1965; 106:106.

113. Oliveria MM, Vaughan M: Incorporation of fatty acids into phospholipids of erythrocyte membranes. J Lipid Res 1964; 5:156.

114. Shohet SB, Nathan DG, Karnovsky ML: Stages in the incorporation of fatty acids into red blood cells. J Clin Invest 1968; 47:1096.

115. Renooij W, Van Golde LM, et al: Preferential incorporation of fatty acids at the inside of human erythrocyte membranes. Biochim Biophys Acta 1974; 363:287.

116. Fairbanks G, Steck TL, Wallach DF: Electrophoretic analysis of the major polypeptides of the human erythrocyte membrane. Biochemistry 1971; 10:2606.

117. Rubin RW, Milikowski C: Over two hundred polypeptides resolved from the human erythrocyte membrane. Biochim Biophys Acta 1978; 509:100.

118. Iolascon A, Miraglia del Giudice E, et al: Hereditary spherocytosis: From clinical to molecular defects. Haematologica 1998; 83:240.

119. Tse WT, Lux SE: Red blood cell membrane disorders. Br J Haematol 1999; 104:2.

120. Gallagher PG, Ferriera JD: Molecular basis of erythrocyte membrane disorders. Curr Opin Hematol 1997; 4:128.

121. Dodge JT, Mitchell C, et al: The preparation and chemical characteristics of hemoglobin-free ghosts of human erythrocytes. Arch Biochem Biophys 1963; 100:119.

122. Laemmli UK: Cleavage of structural proteins during the assembly of the head of bacteriophage T4. Nature 1970; 227:680.

123. Steck TL: Cross-linking the major proteins of the isolated erythrocyte membrane. J Mol Biol 1972; 66:295.

124. Chasis JA, Mohandas N: Red cell biconcave glycophorins. Blood 1992; 80:1869.

125. Fukuda M: Molecular genetics of the glycophorin A gene cluster. Semin Hematol 1993; 30:138.

126. Cartron JP, Bailly P, et al: Insights into the structure and function of membrane polypeptides carrying blood group antigens. Vox Sang 1998; 74(Suppl 2):29.

127. Cartron JP, Colin Y: Structural and functional diversity of blood group antigens. Transfus Clin Biol 2001; 8:163.

128. Anstee DJ: Antigens on red cells. Vox Sang 1998; 74(Suppl 2):255.

129. Reid ME, Yahalom V: Blood groups and their function. Baillieres Best Pract Res Clin Haematol 2000; 13:485.

130. Furthmayr H: Structural comparison of glycophorins and immunochemical analysis of genetic variants. Nature 1978; 271:519.

131. Siebert PD, Fukuda M: Isolation and characterization of human glycophorin A cDNA clones by a synthetic oligonucleotide approach: Nucleotide sequence and mRNA structure. Proc Natl Acad Sci USA 1986; 83:1665.

132. Rahuel C, London J, et al: Characterization of cDNA clones for human glycophorin A. Use for gene localization and for analysis of normal of glycophorin-A-deficient (Finnish type) genomic DNA. Eur J Biochem 1988; 172:147.

133. Irimura T, Tsuji T, et al: Structure of a complex-type sugar chain of human glycophorin A. Biochemistry 1981; 20:560.

134. Armitage IM, Shapiro DL, et al: ^{31}P nuclear magnetic resonance evidence for polyphosphoinositide associated with the hydrophobic segment of glycophorin A. Biochemistry 1977; 16:1317.

135. Mendelsohn R, Dluhy RA, et al: Interaction of glycophorin with phosphatidylserine: A Fourier transform infrared investigation. Biochemistry 1984; 23:1498.

136. Ong RL: ^{31}P and ^{19}F NMR studies of glycophorin-reconstituted membranes: Preferential interaction of glycophorin with phosphatidylserine. J Membr Biol 1984; 78:1.

137. Yeagle PL, Kelsey D: Phosphorus nuclear magnetic resonance studies of lipid-protein interactions: Human erythrocyte glycophorin and phospholipids. Biochemistry 1989; 28:2210.

138. Petrache HI, Grossfield A, et al: Modulation of glycophorin A transmembrane helix interactions by lipid bilayers: Molecular dynamics calculations. J Mol Biol 2000; 302:727.

139. Gerber D, Shai Y: In vivo detection of hetero-association of glycophorin-A and its mutants within the membrane. J Biol Chem 2001; 276:31229.

140. Smith SO, Song D, et al: Structure of the transmembrane dimer interface of glycophorin A in membrane bilayers. Biochemistry 2001; 40:6553.

141. Segrest JP, Jackson RL, et al: Human erythrocyte membrane glycoprotein: A re-evaluation of the molecular weight as determined by SDS polyacrylamide gel electrophoresis. Biochem Biophys Res Commun 1971; 44:390.

142. Gahmberg CG, Jokinen M, Andersson LC: Expression of the major sialoglycoprotein (glycophorin) on erythroid cells in human bone marrow. Blood 1978; 52:379.

143. Liu S-C, Derick LH: Molecular anatomy of the red blood cell membrane skeleton: Structure-function relationships. Semin Hematol 1992; 29:231.

144. Dahr W, Gielen W, et al: Structure of the Ss blood group antigens. I. Isolation of Ss-active glycopeptides and differentiation of the antigens by modification of methionine. Hoppe Seylers Z Physiol Chem 1980; 361:145.

145. Dahr W, Kordowicz M, et al: Structural analysis of the Ss sialoglycoprotein specific for Henshaw blood group from human erythrocyte membranes. Eur J Biochem 1984; 141:51.

146. Dahr W, Moulds JJ: High-frequency antigens of human erythrocyte membrane sialoglycoproteins, IV. Molecular properties of the U antigen. Biol Chem Hoppe Seyler 1987; 368:659.

147. Suyama K, Lunn R, et al: Expression of the Rh-related glycoprotein (Rh50). Acta Haematol 1998; 100:181.

148. Suyama K, Li H, Zhu A: Surface expression of Rh-associated glycoprotein (RhAG) in nonerythroid COS-1 cells. Blood 2000; 95:336.

149. Cartron JP: Defining the Rh blood group antigens. Biochemistry and molecular genetics. Blood Rev 1994; 8:199.

150. Ridgwell K, Eyers SA, et al: Studies on the glycoprotein associated with Rh (rhesus) blood group antigen expression in the human red blood cell membrane. J Biol Chem 1994; 269:6410.

151. Kudo S, Fukuda M: Identification of a novel human glycophorin, glycophorin E, by isolation of genomic clones and complementary DNA clones utilizing polymerase chain reaction. J Biol Chem 1990; 265:1102.

152. Vignal A, London J, et al: Promoter sequence and chromosomal organization of the genes encoding glycophorins A, B and E. Gene 1990; 95:289.

153. Anstee DJ: The nature and abundance of human red cell surface glycoproteins. J Immunogenet 1990; 17:219.

154. King MJ, Holmes CH, et al: Reactivity with erythroid and non-erythroid tissues of a murine monoclonal antibody to a synthetic peptide having amino acid sequence common to cytoplasmic domain of human glycophorins C and D. Br J Haematol 1995; 89:440.

155. Villeval JL, Le Van Kim C, et al: Early expression of glycophorin C during normal and leukemic human erythroid differentiation. Cancer Res 1989; 49:2626.

156. Cartron JP, Le Van Kim C, Colin Y: Glycophorin C and related glycoproteins: Structure, function, and regulation. Semin Hematol 1993; 30:152.

157. Chasis JA, Mohandas N, Shohet SB: Erythrocyte membrane rigidity induced by glycophorin A-ligand interaction. Evidence for a lig-and-induced association between glycophorin A and skeletal proteins. J Clin Invest 1985; 75:1919.

158. Smythe J, Gardner B, Anstee DJ: Quantitation of the number of molecules of glycophorins C and D on normal red blood cells using radioiodinated Fab fragments of monoclonal antibodies. Blood 1994; 83:1668.

159. Auffray I, Marfatia S, et al: Glycophorin A dimerization and band 3 interaction during erythroid membrane biogenesis: In vivo studies in human glycophorin A transgenic mice. Blood 2001; 97:2872.

160. Huang CH, Reid ME, et al: Human red blood cell Wright antigens: A genetic and evolutionary perspective on glycophorin A-band 3 interaction. Blood 1996; 87:3942.

161. Bruce LJ, Ring SM, et al: Changes in the blood group Wright antigens are associated with a mutation at amino acid 658 in human erythrocyte band 3: A site of interaction between band 3 and glycophorin A under certain conditions. Blood 1995; 85:541.

162. Leddy JP, Wilkinson SL, et al: Erythrocyte membrane proteins reactive with IgG (warm-reacting) anti-red blood cell autoantibodies: II. Antibodies coprecipitating band 3 and glycophorin A. Blood 1994; 84:650.

163. Telen MJ, Chasis JA: Relationship of the human erythrocyte Wr^{b} antigen to an interaction between glycophorin A and band 3. Blood 1990; 76:842.

164. Knowles DW, Chasis JA, et al: Cooperative action between band 3 and glycophorin A in human erythrocytes: Immobilization of band 3 induced by antibodies to glycophorin A. Biophys J 1994; 66:1726.

165. Che A, Cherry RJ: Loss of rotational mobility of band 3 proteins in human erythrocyte membranes induced by antibodies to glycophorin A. Biophys J 1995; 68:1881.

166. Groves JD, Tanner MJ: Glycophorin A facilitates the expression of human band 3-mediated anion transport in *Xenopus* oocytes. J Biol Chem 1992; 267:22163.

167. Chang SH, Low PS: Regulation of the glycophorin C-protein 4.1 membrane-to-skeleton bridge and evaluation of its contribution to erythrocyte membrane stability. J Biol Chem 2001; 276:22223.

168. Zhang D, Takahashi J, et al: Analysis of receptor for *Vibrio cholerae* El tor hemolysin with a monoclonal antibody that recognizes glycophorin B of human erythrocyte membrane. Infect Immun 1999; 67:5332.

169. Cortajarena AL, Goni FM, Ostolaza H: Glycophorin as a receptor for *Escherichia coli* α-hemolysin in erythrocytes. J Biol Chem 2001; 276:12513.

170. Chasis JA, Reid ME, et al: Signal transduction by glycophorin A: Role of extracellular and cytoplasmic domains in a modulatable process. J Cell Biol 1988; 107:1351.

171. Paulitschke M, Nash GB, et al: Perturbation of red blood cell membrane rigidity by extracellular ligands. Blood 1995; 86:342.

172. Perkins M: Inhibitory effects of erythrocyte membrane proteins on the in vitro invasion of the human malarial parasite (*Plasmodium falciparum*) into its host cell. J Cell Biol 1981; 90:563.

173. Pasvol G, Wainscoat JS, Weatherall DJ: Erythrocytes deficiency in glycophorin resist invasion by the malarial parasite *Plasmodium falciparum*. Nature 1982; 297:64.

174. Cartron JP, Prou O, et al: Susceptibility to invasion by *Plasmodium falciparum* of some human erythrocytes carrying rare blood group antigens. Br J Haematol 1983; 55:639.

175. Hadley TJ, Klotz FW, et al: Falciparum malaria parasites invade erythrocytes that lack glycophorin A and B (M^{k}M^{k}). Strain differences indicate receptor heterogeneity and two pathways for invasion. J Clin Invest 1987; 80:1190.

176. Orlandi PA, Klotz FW, Haynes JD: A malaria invasion receptor, the 175-kilodalton erythrocyte binding antigen of *Plasmodium falciparum* recognizes the terminal Neu5Acα(2-3)Gal-sequences of glycophorin A. J Cell Biol 1992; 116:901.

177. Sim BK, Chitnis CE, et al: Receptor and ligand domains for invasion of erythrocytes by *Plasmodium falciparum*. Science 1994; 264:1941.

178. Tanner MJA, Anstee DJ: The membrane change in En(a−) human erythrocytes. Biochem J 1976; 153:271.

179. Tanner MJA, Jenkins RE, Anstee DJ: Abnormal carbohydrate composition of the major penetrating membrane protein of En(a−) human erythrocytes. Biochem J 1976; 155:701.

180. Gahmberg CG, Myllyla G, Leikola J: Absence of the major sialo-glycoprotein in the membrane of human En(a−) erythrocytes

and increased glycosylation of band 3. J Biol Chem 1976; 251:6108.

181. Dahr W, Uhlenbruck G, Leikola J: Studies on the membrane glycoprotein defect of En(a–) erythrocytes. I. Biochemical aspects. J Immunogenet 1976; 3:329.

182. Tokunaga E, Sasakawa S, et al: Two apparently healthy Japanese individuals of type M^{k}M^k have erythrocytes which lack both the blood group MN and Ss-active sialoglycoproteins. J Immunogenet 1979; 6:383.

183. Lowe RF, Moores PP: S–s–U–red cell factor in Africans of Rhodesia, Malawi, Mozambique and Natal. Hum Hered 1972; 22:344.

184. Tanner MJ, Anstee DJ, Judson PA: A carbohydrate-deficient membrane glycoprotein in human erythrocytes of phenotype S–s–. Biochem J 1977; 165:151.

185. Dahr W, Uhlenbruck G, et al: SDS-polyacrylamide gel electrophoretic analysis of the membrane glycoproteins from S–s–U– erythrocytes. J Immunogenet 1975; 2:249.

186. Huang CH, Johe K, et al: Delta glycophorin (glycophorin B) gene deletion in two individuals homozygous for the S–s–U– blood group phenotype. Blood 1987; 70:1830.

187. Rahuel C, London J, et al: Erythrocyte glycophorin B deficiency may occur by two distinct gene alterations. Am J Hematol 1991; 37:57.

188. Anstee DJ: The blood group MNSs-active sialoglycoproteins. Semin Hematol 1981; 15:13.

189. Huang C-H, Skov F, et al: Molecular analysis of human glycophorin MiIX gene shows a silent segment transfer and untemplated mutation resulting from gene conversion via sequence repeats. Blood 1992; 80:2379.

190. Huang CH, Blumenfeld OO: Molecular genetics of human erythrocyte MiIII and MiVI glycophorins. Use of a pseudoexon in construction of two δ-α-δ hybrid genes resulting in antigenic diversification. J Biol Chem 1991; 266:7248.

191. Huang CH, Blumenfeld OO: Characterization of a genomic hybrid specifying the human erythrocyte antigen Dantu: Dantu gene is duplicated and linked to a δ glycophorin gene deletion. Proc Natl Acad Sci USA 1988; 85:9640.

192. Kudo S, Fukuda M: Structural organization of glycophorin A and B genes: Glycophorin B gene evolved by homologous recombination at Alu repeat sequences. Proc Natl Acad Sci USA 1989; 86:4619.

193. Johe KK, Smith AJ, et al: Amino acid sequence of an α-δ-glycophorin hybrid. A structure reciprocal to St^a δ-α-glycophorin hybrid. J Biol Chem 1989; 264:17486.

194. Huang CH, Guizzo ML, et al: Molecular genetic analysis of a hybrid gene encoding St^a glycophorin of the human erythrocyte membrane. Blood 1989; 74:836.

195. Huang CH, Blumenfeld OO: Identification of recombination events resulting in three hybrid genes encoding human MiV, MiV(J.L.), and St^a glycophorins. Blood 1991; 77:1813.

196. Chang S, Reid ME, et al: Molecular characterization of erythrocyte glycophorin C variants. Blood 1991; 77:644.

197. Anstee DJ, Ridgwell K, et al: Individuals lacking the Gerbich blood-group antigen have alterations in the human erythrocyte membrane sialoglycoproteins beta and gamma. Biochem J 1984; 221:97.

198. High S, Tanner MJ, et al: Rearrangements of the red-cell membrane glycophorin C (sialoglycoprotein beta) gene. A further study of alterations in the glycophorin C gene. Biochem J 1989; 262:47.

199. Telen MJ, Le Van Kim C, et al: Molecular basis for elliptocytosis associated with glycophorin C and D deficiency in the Leach phenotype. Blood 1991; 78:1603.

200. Anstee DJ, Parsons SF, et al: Two individuals with elliptocytic red cells apparently lack three minor erythrocyte membrane sialoglycoproteins. Biochem J 1984; 218:615.

201. Daniels GL, Shaw MA, et al: A family demonstrating inheritance of the Leach phenotype: A Gerbich-negative phenotype associated with elliptocytosis. Vox Sang 1986; 50:117.

202. Reid ME, Chasis JA, Mohandas N: Identification of a functional role for human erythrocyte sialoglycoproteins β and γ. Blood 1987; 69:1068.

203. Nash GB, Parmar J, Reid ME: Effects of deficiencies of glycophorins C and D on the physical properties of the red cell. Br J Haematol 1990; 76:282.

204. Reid ME, Anstee DJ, et al: Normal membrane function of abnormal β-related erythrocyte sialoglycoproteins. Br J Haematol 1987; 67:467.

205. Discher D, Knowles D, et al: Mechanical linkage between red cell skeleton and plasma membrane is *not* a demonstrated function of protein 4.1. Blood 1993; 82(Suppl 1):309a.

206. Marfatia SM, Lue RA, et al: In vitro binding studies suggest a membrane-associated complex between erythroid p55, protein 4.1, and glycophorin C. J Biol Chem 1994; 269:8631.

207. Tanner MJ: Band 3 anion exchanger and its involvement in erythrocyte and kidney disorders. Curr Opin Hematol 2002; 9:133.

208. Lux SE, John KM, et al: Cloning and characterization of band 3, the human erythrocyte anion-exchange protein (AE1). Proc Natl Acad Sci USA 1989; 86:9089.

209. Tanner MJ, Martin PG, High S: The complete amino acid sequence of the human erythrocyte membrane anion-transport protein deduced from the cDNA sequence. Biochem J 1988; 256:703.

210. Bar-Noy S, Cabantchik ZI: Transport domain of the erythrocyte anion exchange protein. J Membr Biol 1990; 115:217.

211. Bartel D, Hans H, Passow H: Identification by site-directed mutagenesis of Lys-558 as the covalent attachment site of H$_2$DIDS in the mouse erythroid band 3 protein. Biochim Biophys Acta 1989; 985:355.

212. Cabantchik ZI, Rothstein A: Membrane proteins related to anion permeability of human red blood cells. I. Localization of disulfonic stilbene binding sites in proteins involved in permeation. J Membr Biol 1974; 15:207.

213. Ho MK, Guidotti G: A membrane protein from human erythrocytes involved in anion exchange. J Biol Chem 1975; 250:675.

214. Jennings ML: Topography of membrane proteins. Annu Rev Biochem 1989; 58:999.

215. Kleinhorst A, Oslender A, et al: Band 3-mediated flip-flop and phosphatase-catalyzed cleavage of a long-chain alkyl phosphate anion in the human erythrocyte membrane. J Membr Biol 1998; 165:111.

216. Gimsa J, Ried C: Do band 3 protein conformational changes mediate shape changes of human erythrocytes? Mol Membr Biol 1995; 12:247.

217. Blackman SM, Hustedt EJ, et al: Flexibility of the cytoplasmic domain of the anion exchange protein, band 3, in human erythrocytes. Biophys J 2001; 81:3363.

218. Low PS, Westfall MA, et al: Characterization of the reversible conformational equilibrium of the cytoplasmic domain of erythrocyte membrane band 3. J Biol Chem 1984; 259:13070.

219. Low PS: Structure and function of the cytoplasmic domain of band 3: Center of erythrocyte membrane-peripheral protein interactions. Biochim Biophys Acta 1986; 864:145.

220. Bennett V, Stenbuck PJ: Association between ankyrin and the cytoplasmic domain of band 3 isolated from the human erythrocyte membrane. J Biol Chem 1980; 255:6424.

221. Zhang D, Kiyatkin A, et al: Crystallographic structure and functional interpretation of the cytoplasmic domain of erythrocyte membrane band 3. Blood 2000; 96:2925.

222. Kliman HJ, Steck TL: Association of glyceraldehyde-3-phosphate dehydrogenase with the human red cell membrane. A kinetic analysis. J Biol Chem 1980; 255:6314.

223. Tsai IH, Murthy SN, Steck TL: Effect of red cell membrane binding on the catalytic activity of glyceraldehyde-3-phosphate dehydrogenase. J Biol Chem 1982; 257:1438.

224. De BK, Kirtley ME: Interaction of phosphoglycerate kinase with human erythrocyte membranes. J Biol Chem 1977; 252:6715.

225. Jenkins JD, Madden DP, Steck TL: Association of phosphofructokinase and aldolase with the membrane of the intact erythrocyte. J Biol Chem 1984; 259:9374.

226. Murthy SN, Liu T, et al: The aldolase-binding site of the human erythrocyte membrane is at the NH$_2$ terminus of band 3. J Biol Chem 1981; 256:11203.

227. Low PS, Allen DP, et al: Tyrosine phosphorylation of band 3 inhibits peripheral protein binding. J Biol Chem 1987; 262:4592.

228. Brunati AM, Bordin L, et al: Sequential phosphorylation of protein band 3 by Syk and Lyn tyrosine kinases in intact human erythrocytes: Identification of primary and secondary phosphorylation sites. Blood 2000; 96:1550.

228a. Bordin L, Brunati AM, et al: Band 3 is an anchor protein and a target for SHP-2 tyrosine phosphatase in human erythrocytes. Blood 2002; 100:276.

229. Zipser Y, Kosower NS: Phosphotyrosine phosphatase associated with band 3 protein in the human erythrocyte membrane. Biochem J 1996; 314:881.

229a. Zipser Y, Piade A, et al: Ca2+ promotes erythrocyte band 3 trysine phosphorylation via dissociation of phosphotyrosine phosphatase from band 3. Biochem J 2002; 368:137.

230. Harrison ML, Rathinavelu P, et al: Role of band 3 tyrosine phosphorylation in the regulation of erythrocyte glycolysis. J Biol Chem 1991; 266:4106.

231. Wang CC, Tao M, et al: Identification of the major casein kinase I phosphorylation sites on erythrocyte band 3. Blood 1997; 89:3019.

232. Chétrite G, Cassoly R: Affinity of hemoglobin for the cytoplasmic fragment of human erythrocyte membrane band 3. Equilibrium measurements at physiological pH using matrix-bound proteins: The effects of ionic strength, deoxygenation and of 2,3-diphosphoglycerate. J Mol Biol 1985; 185:639.

233. Walder JA, Chatterjee R, et al: The interaction of hemoglobin with the cytoplasmic domain of band 3 of the human erythrocyte membrane. J Biol Chem 1984; 259:10238.

234. Waugh SM, Walder JA, Low PS: Partial characterization of the copolymerization reaction of erythrocyte membrane band 3 with hemichromes. Biochemistry 1987; 26:1777.

235. Kannan R, Labotka R, Low PS: Isolation and characterization of the hemichrome-stabilized membrane protein aggregates from sickle erythrocytes. Major site of autologous antibody binding. J Biol Chem 1988; 263:13766.

236. McPherson RA, Sawyer WH, Tilley L: Rotational diffusion of the erythrocyte integral membrane protein band 3: Effect of hemichrome binding. Biochemistry 1992; 31:512.

237. Bennett V, Stenbuck PJ: The membrane attachment protein for spectrin is associated with band 3 in human erythrocyte membranes. Nature 1979; 280:468.

238. Davis L, Lux SE, Bennett V: Mapping the ankyrin-binding site of the human erythrocyte anion exchanger. J Biol Chem 1989; 264:9665.

239. Willardson BM, Thevenin BJ, et al: Localization of the ankyrin-binding site on erythrocyte membrane protein, band 3. J Biol Chem 1989; 264:15893.

240. Thevenin BJ, Low PS: Kinetics and regulation of the ankyrin-band 3 interaction of the human red blood cell membrane. J Biol Chem 1990; 265:16166.

241. Pasternack GR, Anderson RA, et al: Interactions between protein 4.1 and band 3. An alternative binding site for an element of the membrane skeleton. J Biol Chem 1985; 260:3676.

242. Lombardo CR, Willardson BM, Low PS: Localization of the protein 4.1-binding site on the cytoplasmic domain of erythrocyte membrane band 3. J Biol Chem 1992; 267:9540.

243. Korsgren C, Cohen CM: Purification and properties of human erythrocyte band 4.2. Association with the cytoplasmic domain of band 3. J Biol Chem 1986; 261:5536.

244. Korsgren C, Cohen CM: Associations of human erythrocyte band 4.2. Binding to ankyrin and to the cytoplasmic domain of band 3. J Biol Chem 1988; 263:10212.

245. Thevenin BJ, Willardson BM, Low PS: The redox state of cysteines 201 and 317 of the erythrocyte anion exchanger is critical for ankyrin binding. J Biol Chem 1989; 264:15886.

246. Zhou J, Low PS: Characterization of the reversible conformational equilibrium in the cytoplasmic domain of human erythrocyte membrane band 3. J Biol Chem 2001; 276:38147.

247. Van Dort HM, Moriyama R, Low PS: Effect of band 3 subunit equilibrium on the kinetics and affinity of ankyrin binding to erythrocyte membrane vesicles. J Biol Chem 1998; 273:14819.

248. von Ruckmann B, Jons T, et al: Cytoskeleton-membrane connections in the human erythrocyte membrane: Band 4.1 binds to tetrameric band 3 protein. Biochim Biophys Acta 1997; 1325:226.

249. Jöns T, Drenckhahn D: Identification of the binding interface involved in linkage of cytoskeletal protein 4.1 to the erythrocyte anion exchanger. EMBO J 1992; 11:2863.

250. Bhattacharyya R, Das AK, et al: Mapping of a palmitoylatable band 3-binding domain of human erythrocyte membrane protein 4.2. Biochem J 1999; 340:505.

251. Wieth JO, Andersen OS, et al: Chloride-bicarbonate exchange in red blood cells: Physiology of transport and chemical modification of binding sites. Philos Trans R Soc Lond B Biol Sci 1982; 299:383.

252. Popov M, Li J, Reithmeier RA: Transmembrane folding of the human erythrocyte anion exchanger (AE1, Band 3) determined by scanning and insertional N-glycosylation mutagenesis. Biochem J 1999; 339(Pt 2):269.

253. St Vostwinkel, Haest CW, Deuticke B: Complex effects of papain on function and inhibitor sensitivity of the red cell anion exchanger AE1 suggest the presence of different transport subsites. J Membr Biol 2001; 179:205.

254. Ota K, Sakaguchi M, et al: Membrane integration of the second transmembrane segment of band 3 requires a closely apposed preceding signal-anchor sequence. J Biol Chem 2000; 275:29743.

255. Groves JD, Wang L, Tanner MJ: Complementation studies with co-expressed fragments of human red cell band 3 (AE1): The assembly of the anion-transport domain in *Xenopus* oocytes and a cell-free translation system. Biochem J 1998; 332(Pt 1):161.

256. Groves JD, Tanner MJ: Structural model for the organization of the transmembrane spans of the human red-cell anion exchanger (band 3; AE1). Biochem J 1999; 344 Pt 3:699.

257. Groves JD, Tanner MJ: Topology studies with biosynthetic fragments identify interacting transmembrane regions of the human red-cell anion exchanger (band 3; AE1). Biochem J 1999; 344 Pt 3:687.

258. Wang DN, Kuhlbrandt W, et al: Two-dimensional structure of the membrane domain of human band 3, the anion transport protein of the erythrocyte membrane. EMBO J 1993; 12:2233.

259. Askin D, Bloomberg GB, et al: NMR solution structure of a cytoplasmic surface loop of the human red cell anion transporter, band 3. Biochemistry 1998; 37:11670.

260. Jennings ML: Oligomeric structure and the anion transport function of human erythrocyte band 3 protein. J Membr Biol 1984; 80:105.

261. Lindenthal S, Schubert D: Monomeric erythrocyte band 3 protein transports anions. Proc Natl Acad Sci USA 1991; 88:6540.

262. Salhany JM, Sloan RL, Cordes KA: In situ cross-linking of human erythrocyte band 3 by bis(sulfosuccinimidyl)suberate. Evidence for ligand modulation of two alternate quaternary forms: Covalent band 3 dimers and noncovalent tetramers formed by the association of two covalent dimers. J Biol Chem 1990; 265:17688.

263. Salhany JM, Sloan RL, Cordes KA: Evidence for the development of an intermonomeric asymmetry in the covalent binding of 4,4'-diisothiocyanatostilbene-2,2'-disulfonate to human erythrocyte band 3. Biochemistry 1991; 30:4097.

264. Falke JJ, Pace RJ, Chan SI: Direct observation of the transmembrane recruitment of band 3 transport sites by competitive inhibitors. A ^{35}Cl NMR study. J Biol Chem 1984; 259:6481.

265. Gunn RB, Frohlich O: Asymmetry in the mechanism for anion exchange in human red blood cell membranes. Evidence for reciprocating sites that react with one transported anion at a time. J Gen Physiol 1979; 74:351.

266. Canfield VA, Macey RI: Anion exchange in human erythrocytes has a large activation volume. Biochim Biophys Acta 1984; 778:379.

267. Dalmark M, Wieth JO: Temperature dependence of chloride, bromide, iodide, thiocyanate and salicylate transport in human red cells. J Physiol 1972; 224:583.

268. Sekler I, Lo RS, Kopito RR: A conserved glutamate is responsible for ion selectivity and pH dependence of the mammalian anion exchangers AE1 and AE2. J Biol Chem 1995; 270:28751.

269. Muller-Berger S, Karbach D, et al: Roles of histidine 752 and glutamate 699 in the pH dependence of mouse band 3 protein-mediated anion transport. Biochemistry 1995; 34:9325.

270. Bohm R, Zaki L: Towards the localization of the essential arginine residues in the band 3 protein of human red blood cell membranes. Biochim Biophys Acta 1996; 1280:238.

271. Salhany JM: Stilbenedisulfonate binding kinetics to band 3 (AE 1): Relationship between transport and stilbenedisulfonate binding sites and role of subunit interactions in transport. Blood Cells Mol Dis 2001; 27:127.

272. Salhany JM, Schopfer LM: Kinetic mechanism of DIDS binding to band 3 (AE1) in human erythrocyte membranes. Blood Cells Mol Dis 2001; 27:844.

273. Ranney HM, Rosenberg GH, et al: Frequencies of band 3 variants of human red cell membranes in some different populations. Br J Haematol 1990; 75:262.

274. Bruce LJ, Anstee DJ, et al: Band 3 Memphis variant II. Altered stilbene disulfonate binding and the Diego (Dia) blood group antigen are associated with the human erythrocyte band 3 mutation Pro854→Leu. J Biol Chem 1994; 269:16155.

275. Jarolim P, Rubin HL, et al: Characterization of seven low incidence blood group antigens carried by erythrocyte band 3 protein. Blood 1998; 92:4836.

276. Poole J: Red cell antigens on band 3 and glycophorin A. Blood Rev 2000; 14:31.

277. Mulzer K, Kampmann L, et al: Complex associations between membrane proteins analyzed by analytical ultracentrifugation: Studies on the erythrocyte membrane proteins band 3 and ankyrin. Colloid Polym Sci 1990; 268:60.

278. Casey JR, Reithmeier RA: Analysis of the oligomeric state of band 3, the anion transport protein of the human erythrocyte membrane, by size exclusion high performance liquid chromatography. Oligomeric stability and origin of heterogeneity. J Biol Chem 1991; 266:15726.

279. Young MT, Beckmann R, et al: Red-cell glycophorin A-band 3 interactions associated with the movement of band 3 to the cell surface. Biochem J 2000; 350(Pt 1):53.

280. Bruce LJ, Groves JD, et al: Altered band 3 structure and function in glycophorin A- and B-deficient (MkMk) red blood cells. Blood 1994; 84:916.

281. Edwards HH, Mueller TJ, Morrison M: Distribution of transmembrane polypeptides in freeze fracture. Science 1979; 203:1343.

282. da Silva PP, Torrisi MR: Freeze-fracture cytochemistry: Partition of glycophorin in freeze-fractured human erythrocyte membranes. J Cell Biol 1982; 93:463.

283. Bruce LJ, Kay MM, et al: Band 3 HT, a human red-cell variant associated with acanthocytosis and increased anion transport, carries the mutation Pro-868→Leu in the membrane domain of band 3. Biochem J 1993; 293:317.

284. Kay MM, Bosman GJ, Lawrence C: Functional topography of band 3: Specific structural alteration linked to functional aberrations in human erythrocytes. Proc Natl Acad Sci USA 1988; 85:492.

285. Wickramasinghe SN: Congenital dyserythropoietic anemias. Curr Opin Hematol 2000; 7:71.

286. Zdebska E, Wozniewicz B, et al: Short report: Erythrocyte membranes from a patient with congenital dyserythropoietic anaemia type I (CDA-I) show identical, although less pronounced, glycoconjugate abnormalities to those from patients with CDA-II (HEMPAS). Br J Haematol 2000; 110:998.

287. Zdebska E, Golaszewska E, et al: Glycoconjugate abnormalities in patients with congenital dyserythropoietic anaemia type I, II and III. Br J Haematol 2001; 114:907.

288. Alper SL: The band 3-related anion exchanger (AE) gene family. Annu Rev Physiol 1991; 53:549.

289. Alper SL, Kopito RR, et al: Cloning and characterization of a murine band 3-related cDNA from kidney and from a lymphoid cell line. J Biol Chem 1988; 263:17092.

290. Demuth DR, Showe LC, et al: Cloning and structural characterization of a human non-erythroid band 3-like protein. EMBO J 1986; 5:1205.

291. Kopito RR, Lee BS, et al: Regulation of intracellular pH by a neuronal homologue of the erythrocyte anion exchanger. Cell 1989; 59:927.

292. Alper SL, Chernova MN, Stewart AK: Regulation of Na+-independent Cl−/HCO3− exchangers by pH. JOP 2001; 2:171.

293. Brosius FC, 3rd, Alper SL, et al: The major kidney band 3 gene transcript predicts an amino-terminal truncated band 3 polypeptide. J Biol Chem 1989; 264:7784.

294. Casey JR, Reithmeier RA: Anion exchangers in the red cell and beyond. Biochem Cell Biol 1998; 76:709.

295. Kudrycki KE, Newman PR, Shull GE: cDNA cloning and tissue distribution of mRNAs for two proteins that are related to the band 3 Cl−/HCO3− exchanger. J Biol Chem 1990; 265:462.

296. Drenckhahn D, Schluter K, et al: Colocalization of band 3 with ankyrin and spectrin at the basal membrane of intercalated cells in the rat kidney. Science 1985; 230:1287.

297. Alper SL, Natale J, et al: Subtypes of intercalated cells in rat kidney collecting duct defined by antibodies against erythroid band 3 and renal vacuolar H+-ATPase. Proc Natl Acad Sci USA 1989; 86:5429.

298. Richards SM, Jaconi ME, et al: A spliced variant of AE1 gene encodes a truncated form of band 3 in heart: The predominant anion exchanger in ventricular myocytes. J Cell Sci 1999; 112(Pt 10):1519.

299. Puceat M, Korichneva I, et al: Identification of band 3-like proteins and Cl−/HCO3− exchange in isolated cardiomyocytes. J Biol Chem 1995; 270:1315.

300. Ding Y, Casey JR, Kopito RR: The major kidney AE1 isoform does not bind ankyrin (Ank1) in vitro. An essential role for the 79 NH2-terminal amino acid residues of band 3. J Biol Chem 1994; 269:32201.

301. Wang CC, Moriyama R, et al: Partial characterization of the cytoplasmic domain of human kidney band 3. J Biol Chem 1995; 270:17892.

302. Sheetz MP: Integral membrane protein interaction with Triton cytoskeletons of erythrocytes. Biochim Biophys Acta 1979; 557:122.

303. Yu J, Fischman DA, Steck TL: Selective solubilization of proteins and phospholipids from red blood cell membranes by nonionic detergents. J Supramol Struct 1973; 1:233.

304. Sahr KE, Laurila P, et al: The complete cDNA and polypeptide sequences of human erythroid α-spectrin. J Biol Chem 1990; 265:4434.

305. Winkelmann JC, Chang JG, et al: Full-length sequence of the cDNA for human erythroid β-spectrin. J Biol Chem 1990; 265:11827.

306. Speicher DW, Morrow JS, et al: A structural model of human erythrocyte spectrin: Alignment of chemical and functional domains. J Biol Chem 1982; 257:9093.

307. Speicher DW, DeSilva TM, et al: Location of the human red cell spectrin tetramer binding site and detection of a related "closed" hairpin loop dimer using proteolytic footprinting. J Biol Chem 1993; 268:4227.

308. Shotton DM, Burke BE, Branton D: The molecular structure of human erythrocyte spectrin. Biophysical and electron microscopic studies. J Mol Biol 1979; 131:303.

309. Liu SC, Windisch P, et al: Oligomeric states of spectrin in normal erythrocyte membranes: Biochemical and electron microscopic studies. Cell 1984; 37:587.

310. Grum VL, Li D, et al: Structures of two repeats of spectrin suggest models of flexibility. Cell 1999; 98:523.

311. Vertessy BG, Steck TL: Elasticity of the human red cell membrane skeleton. Effects of temperature and denaturants. Biophys J 1989; 55:255.

312. McGough AM, Josephs R: On the structure of erythrocyte spectrin in partially expanded membrane skeletons. Proc Natl Acad Sci USA 1990; 87:5208.

313. Yan Y, Winograd E, et al: Crystal structure of the repetitive segments of spectrin. Science 1993; 262:2027.

314. Ziemnicka-Kotula D, Xu J, et al: Identification of a candidate human spectrin Src homology 3 domain-binding protein suggests a general mechanism of association of tyrosine kinases with the spectrin-based membrane skeleton. J Biol Chem 1998; 273:13681.

315. Noegel A, Witke W, Schleicher M: Calcium-sensitive non-muscle α-actinin contains EF-hand structures and highly conserved regions. FEBS Lett 1987; 221:391.

316. Waites GT, Graham IR, et al: Mutually exclusive splicing of calcium-binding domain exons in chick α-actinin. J Biol Chem 1992; 267:6263.

317. Fishkind DJ, Bonder EM, Begg DA: Isolation and characterization of sea urchin egg spectrin: Calcium modulation of the spectrin-actin interaction. Cell Motil Cytoskeleton 1987; 7:304.

318. Wallis CJ, Wenegieme EF, Babitch JA: Characterization of calcium binding to brain spectrin. J Biol Chem 1992; 267:4333.

319. Trave G, Lacombe PJ, et al: Molecular mechanism of the calcium-induced conformational change in the spectrin EF-hands. EMBO J 1995; 14:4922.

320. Lundberg S, Bjork J, et al: Cloning, expression and characterization of two putative calcium-binding sites in human non-erythroid α-spectrin. Eur J Biochem 1995; 230:658.

321. Trave G, Pastore A, et al: The C-terminal domain of α-spectrin is structurally related to calmodulin. Eur J Biochem 1995; 227:35.

322. Kennedy SP, Warren SL, et al: Ankyrin binds to the 15th repetitive unit of erythroid and nonerythroid beta-spectrin. J Cell Biol 1991; 115:267.

323. Cohen CM, Tyler JM, Branton D: Spectrin-actin associations studied by electron microscopy of shadowed preparations. Cell 1980; 21:875.

324. Becker PS, Schwartz MA, et al: Radiolabel-transfer cross-linking demonstrates that protein 4.1 binds to the N-terminal region of beta spectrin and to actin in binary interactions. Eur J Biochem 1990; 193:827.

325. Karinch AM, Zimmer WE, Goodman SR: The identification and sequence of the actin-binding domain of human red blood cell beta-spectrin. J Biol Chem 1990; 265:11833.

326. Bresnick AR, Janmey PA, Condeelis J: Evidence that a 27-residue sequence is the actin-binding site of ABP- 120. J Biol Chem 1991; 266:12989.

327. Becker PS, Tse WT, et al: Beta Spectrin Kissimmee: A spectrin variant associated with autosomal dominant hereditary spherocytosis and defective binding to protein 4.1. J Clin Invest 1993; 92:612.

328. Harris HW Jr, Lux SE: Structural characterization of the phosphorylation sites of human erythrocyte spectrin. J Biol Chem 1980; 255:11512.

329. Tao M, Conway R, Cheta S: Purification and characterization of a membrane-bound protein kinase from human erythrocytes. J Biol Chem 1980; 255:2563.

330. Manno S, Takakuwa Y, et al: Modulation of erythrocyte membrane mechanical function by beta-spectrin phosphorylation and dephosphorylation. J Biol Chem 1995; 270:5659.

331. Speicher DW, Morrow JS, et al: Identification of proteolytically resistant domains of human erythrocyte spectrin. Proc Natl Acad Sci USA 1980; 77:5673.

332. Winograd E, Hume D, Branton D: Phasing the conformational unit of spectrin. Proc Natl Acad Sci USA 1991; 88:10788.

333. Speicher DW, Marchesi VT: Erythrocyte spectrin is comprised of many homologous triple helical segments. Nature 1984; 311:177.

334. Pascual J, Pfuhl M, et al: Solution structure of the spectrin repeat: A left-handed antiparallel triple-helical coiled-coil. J Mol Biol 1997; 273:740.

335. Lenne PF, Raae AJ, et al: States and transitions during forced unfolding of a single spectrin repeat. FEBS Lett 2000; 476:124.

336. Rief M, Pascual J, et al: Single molecule force spectroscopy of spectrin repeats: Low unfolding forces in helix bundles. J Mol Biol 1999; 286:553.

337. Thomas GH, Newbern EC, et al: Intragenic duplication and divergence in the spectrin superfamily of proteins. Mol Biol Evol 1997; 14:1285.

338. Muse SV, Clark AG, Thomas GH: Comparisons of the nucleotide substitution process among repetitive segments of the α- and β-spectrin genes. J Mol Evol 1997; 44:492.

339. Pascual J, Castresana J, Saraste M: Evolution of the spectrin repeat. Bioessays 1997; 19:811.

340. Viel A: α-Actinin and spectrin structures: An unfolding family story. FEBS Lett 1999; 460:391.

341. Kotula L, Laury-Kleintop LD, et al: The exon-intron organization of the human erythrocyte α-spectrin gene. Genomics 1991; 9:131

342. Amin KM, Scarpa AL, et al: The exon-intron organization of the human erythroid β-spectrin gene. Genomics 1993; 18:118.

343. Bennett V, Baines AJ: Spectrin and ankyrin-based pathways: Metazoan inventions for integrating cells into tissues. Physiol Rev 2001; 81:1353.

344. De Matteis MA, Morrow JS: Spectrin tethers and mesh in the biosynthetic pathway. J Cell Sci 2000; 113(Pt 13):2331.

345. Morrow JS, Rimm DL, et al: Of membrane stability and mosaics: The spectrin cytoskeleton. In Hoffman J, Jamieson J (eds): Handbook of Physiology. London, Oxford, 1997, p 485.

346. Djinovic-Carugo K, Gautel M, et al: The spectrin repeat: A structural platform for cytoskeletal protein assemblies. FEBS Lett 2002; 513:119.

347. Morrow JS, Marchesi VT: Self-assembly of spectrin oligomers in vitro: A basis for a dynamic cytoskeleton. J Cell Biol 1981; 88:463.

348. Ungewickell E, Gratzer W: Self-association of human spectrin. A thermodynamic and kinetic study. Eur J Biochem 1978; 88:379.

349. Park S, Mehboob S, et al: Studies of the erythrocyte spectrin tetramerization region. Cell Mol Biol Lett 2001; 6:571.

350. Kotula L, DeSilva TM, et al: Functional characterization of recombinant human red cell α-spectrin polypeptides containing the tetramer binding site. J Biol Chem 1993; 268:14788.

351. Lecomte MC, Nicolas G, et al: Properties of normal and mutant polypeptide fragments from the dimer self-association sites of human red cell spectrin. Eur Biophys J 1999; 28:208.

352. Nicolas G, Pedroni S, et al: Spectrin self-association site: Characterization and study of β-spectrin mutations associated with hereditary elliptocytosis. Biochem J 1998; 332 (Pt 1):81.

353. Shahbakhti F, Gratzer WB: Analysis of the self-association of human red cell spectrin. Biochemistry 1986; 25:5969.

354. Ralston G, Dunbar J, White M: The temperature-dependent dissociation of spectrin. Biochim Biophys Acta 1977; 491:345.

355. Liu SC, Palek J: Spectrin tetramer-dimer equilibrium and the stability of erythrocyte membrane skeletons. Nature 1980; 285:586.

356. Beaven GH, Jean-Baptiste L, et al: An examination of the soluble oligomeric complexes extracted from the red cell membrane and their relation to the membrane cytoskeleton. Eur J Cell Biol 1985; 36:299.

357. Morris SA, Eber SW, Gratzer WB: Structural basis for the high activation energy of spectrin self-association. FEBS Lett 1989; 244:68.

358. DeSilva TM, Peng KC, et al: Analysis of human red cell spectrin tetramer (head-to-head) assembly using complementary univalent peptides. Biochemistry 1992; 31:10872.

358a.An X, Lecomte MC, et al: Shear-response of the spectrin dimer-tetramer equilibrium in the red blood cell membrane. J Biol Chem 2002; 277:31796.

359. Speicher DW, Weglarz L, DeSilva TM: Properties of human red cell spectrin heterodimer (side-to-side) assembly and identification of an essential nucleation site. J Biol Chem 1992; 267:14775.

360. Ursitti JA, Kotula L, et al: Mapping the human erythrocyte β-spectrin dimer initiation site using recombinant peptides and correlation of its phasing with the α-actinin dimer site. J Biol Chem 1996; 271:6636.

361. Cherry L, Menhart N, Fung LW: Interactions of the α-spectrin N-terminal region with β-spectrin. Implications for the spectrin tetramerization reaction. J Biol Chem 1999; 274:2077.

362. Viel A, Branton D: Interchain binding at the tail end of the *Drosophila* spectrin molecule. Proc Natl Acad Sci USA 1994; 91:10839.

363. Harper SL, Begg GE, Speicher DW: Role of terminal nonhomologous domains in initiation of human red cell spectrin dimerization. Biochemistry 2001; 40:9935.

364. Davis LH, Bennett V: Identification of two regions of β G spectrin that bind to distinct sites in brain membranes. J Biol Chem 1994; 269:4409.

365. Lombardo CR, Weed SA, et al: βII-Spectrin (fodrin) and βIε2-spectrin (muscle) contain NH_2- and COOH-terminal membrane association domains (MAD1 and MAD2). J Biol Chem 1994; 269:29212.

366. Maffucci T, Falasca M: Specificity in pleckstrin homology (PH) domain membrane targeting: A role for a phosphoinositide-protein co-operative mechanism. FEBS Lett 2001; 506:173.

367. Lemmon MA, Ferguson KM, Abrams CS: Pleckstrin homology domains and the cytoskeleton. FEBS Lett 2002; 513:71.

368. Rebecchi MJ, Scarlata S: Pleckstrin homology domains: A common fold with diverse functions. Annu Rev Biophys Biomol Struct 1998; 27:503.

369. Giorgi M, Cianci CD, et al: Spectrin oligomerization is cooperatively coupled to membrane assembly: A linkage targeted by many hereditary hemolytic anemias? Exp Mol Pathol 2001; 70:215.

370. Gilligan DM, Bennett V: The junctional complex of the membrane skeleton. Semin Hematol 1993; 30:74.

371. Gallagher PG, Forget BG: Spectrin genes in health and disease. Semin Hematol 1993; 30:4.

372. Winkelmann JC, Forget BG: Erythroid and nonerythroid spectrins. Blood 1993; 81:3173.

373. Hu RJ, Watanabe M, Bennett V: Characterization of human brain cDNA encoding the general isoform of β-spectrin. J Biol Chem 1992; 267:18715.

374. Chang JG, Scarpa A, et al: Cloning of a portion of the chromosomal gene and cDNA for human β-fodrin, the nonerythroid form of β-spectrin. Genomics 1993; 17:287.

375. Sakaguchi G, Orita S, et al: A novel brain-specific isoform of β spectrin: Isolation and its interaction with Munc13. Biochem Biophys Res Commun 1998; 248:846.

376. Ohara O, Ohara R, et al: Characterization of a new β-spectrin gene which is predominantly expressed in brain. Brain Res Mol Brain Res 1998; 57:181.

377. Stankewich MC, Tse WT, et al: A widely expressed βIII spectrin associated with Golgi and cytoplasmic vesicles. Proc Natl Acad Sci USA 1998; 95:14158.

378. Tse WT, Tang J, et al: A new spectrin, β IV, has a major truncated isoform that associates with promyelocytic leukemia protein nuclear bodies and the nuclear matrix. J Biol Chem 2001; 276:23974.

379. Berghs S, Aggujaro D, et al: β IV spectrin, a new spectrin localized at axon initial segments and nodes of Ranvier in the central and peripheral nervous system. J Cell Biol 2000; 151:985.

380. Stabach PR, Morrow JS: Identification and characterization of β V spectrin, a mammalian ortholog of Drosophila β H spectrin. J Biol Chem 2000; 275:21385.

381. Gascard P, Mohandas N: New insights into functions of erythroid proteins in nonerythroid cells. Curr Opin Hematol 2000; 7:123.

382. Porter GA, Scher MG, et al: Two populations of β-spectrin in rat skeletal muscle. Cell Motil Cytoskeleton 1997; 37:7.

383. Coleman TR, Fishkind DJ, et al: Contributions of the β-subunit to spectrin structure and function. Cell Motil Cytoskeleton 1989; 12:248.

384. Winkelmann JC, Costa FF, et al: β spectrin in human skeletal muscle: Tissue-specific differential processing of 3′ β spectrin pre-mRNA generates a β spectrin isoform with a unique carboxyl terminus. J Biol Chem 1990; 265:20449.

385. Liao EC, Paw BH, et al: Hereditary spherocytosis in zebrafish Riesling illustrates evolution of erythroid β-spectrin structure, and function in red cell morphogenesis and membrane stability. Development 2000; 127:5123.

386. Tyler JM, Reinhardt BN, Branton D: Associations of erythrocyte membrane proteins: Binding of purified bands 2.1 and 4.1 to spectrin. J Biol Chem 1980; 255:7034.

387. Bennett V, Chen L: Ankyrins and cellular targeting of diverse membrane proteins to physiological sites. Curr Opin Cell Biol 2001; 13:61.

388. Peters LL, Lux SE: Ankyrins: Structure and function in normal cells and hereditary spherocytes. Semin Hematol 1993; 30:85.

389. Rubtsov AM, Lopina OD: Ankyrins. FEBS Lett 2000; 482:1.

390. Davis LH, Bennett V: Mapping the binding sites of human erythrocyte ankyrin for the anion exchanger and spectrin. J Biol Chem 1990; 265:10589.

391. Davis LH, Otto E, Bennett V: Specific 33-residue repeat(s) of erythrocyte ankyrin associate with the anion exchanger. J Biol Chem 1991; 266:11163.

392. Michaely P, Bennett V: The membrane-binding domain of ankyrin contains four independently folded subdomains, each comprised of six ankyrin repeats. J Biol Chem 1993; 268:22703.

393. Platt OS, Lux SE, Falcone JF: A highly conserved region of human erythrocyte ankyrin contains the capacity to bind spectrin. J Biol Chem 1993; 268:24421.

394. Lux SE, John KM, Bennett V: Analysis of cDNA for human erythrocyte ankyrin indicates a repeated structure with homology to tissue-differentiation and cell-cycle control proteins. Nature 1990; 344:36.

395. Lambert S, Yu H, et al: cDNA sequence for human erythrocyte ankyrin. Proc Natl Acad Sci USA 1990; 87:1730.

396. Yu J, Goodman SR: Syndeins: The spectrin-binding protein(s) of the human erythrocyte membrane. Proc Natl Acad Sci USA 1979; 76:2340.

397. Weaver DC, Pasternack GR, Marchesi VT: The structural basis of ankyrin function. II. Identification of two functional domains. J Biol Chem 1984; 259:6170.

398. Wallin R, Culp EN, et al: A structural model of human erythrocyte band 2.1: Alignment of chemical and functional domains. Proc Natl Acad Sci USA 1984; 81:4095.

399. Michaely P, Bennett V: The ANK repeats of erythrocyte ankyrin form two distinct but cooperative binding sites for the erythrocyte anion exchanger. J Biol Chem 1995; 270:22050.

400. Mulzer K, Kampmann L, et al: Complex associations between membrane proteins analyzed by analytical ultracentrifugation: Studies on the erythrocyte membrane proteins band 3 and ankyrin. Colloid Polym Sci 1990; 268:60.

401. Yi SJ, Liu SC, et al: Red cell membranes of ankyrin-deficient nb/nb mice lack band 3 tetramers but contain normal membrane skeletons. Biochemistry 1997; 36:9596.

402. Low PS, Willardson BM, et al: Contribution of the band 3-ankyrin interaction to erythrocyte membrane mechanical stability. Blood 1991; 77:1581.

403. Sedgwick SG, Smerdon SJ: The ankyrin repeat: A diversity of interactions on a common structural framework. Trends Biochem Sci 1999; 24:311.

404. Huxford T, Huang DB, et al: The crystal structure of the IκBα/NF-κB complex reveals mechanisms of NF-κB inactivation. Cell 1998; 95:759.

405. Gorina S, Pavletich NP: Structure of the p53 tumor suppressor bound to the ankyrin and SH3 domains of 53BP2. Science 1996; 274:1001.

406. Batchelor AH, Piper DE, et al: The structure of GABPα/β: An ETS domain-ankyrin repeat heterodimer bound to DNA. Science 1998; 279:1037.

407. Jacobs MD, Harrison SC: Structure of an IκBα/NF-κB complex. Cell 1998; 95:749.

408. Michaely P, Tomchick DR, et al: Crystal structure of a 12 ANK repeat stack from human ankyrinR. Embo J (England) 2002; 21:6387.

409. Andrade MA, Perez-Iratxeta C, Ponting CP: Protein repeats: Structures, functions, and evolution. J Struct Biol 2001; 134:117.

410. Davis LH, Davis JQ, Bennett V: Ankyrin regulation: An alternatively spliced segment of the regulatory domain functions as an intramolecular modulator. J Biol Chem 1992; 267:18966.

411. Cianci CD, Giorgi M, Morrow JS: Phosphorylation of ankyrin down-regulates its cooperative interaction with spectrin and protein 3. J Cell Biochem 1988; 37:301.

412. Gallagher PG, Tse WT, et al: Structure and organization of the human ankyrin-1 gene. Basis for complexity of pre-mRNA processing. J Biol Chem 1997; 272:19220.

413. Hall TG, Bennett V: Regulatory domains of erythrocyte ankyrin. J Biol Chem 1987; 262:10537.

414. Zhou D, Birkenmeier CS, et al: Small, membrane-bound, alternatively spliced forms of ankyrin 1 associated with the sarcoplasmic reticulum of mammalian skeletal muscle. J Cell Biol 1997; 136:621.

415. Gallagher PG, Forget BG: An alternate promoter directs expression of a truncated, muscle-specific isoform of the human ankyrin 1 gene. J Biol Chem 1998; 273:1339.

416. Birkenmeier CS, Sharp JJ, et al: An alternative first exon in the distal end of the erythroid ankyrin gene leads to production of a small isoform containing an NH2-terminal membrane anchor. Genomics 1998; 50:79.

417. Denecker G, Vercammen D, et al: Apoptotic and necrotic cell death induced by death domain receptors. Cell Mol Life Sci 2001; 58:356.

418. Weber CH, Vincenz C: The death domain superfamily: A tale of two interfaces? Trends Biochem Sci 2001; 26:475.

419. Vander Heiden MG, Thompson CB: BCl−2 proteins: Regulators of apoptosis or of mitochondrial homeostasis? Nat Cell Biol 1999; 1:E209.

420. Martin SJ, O'Brien GA, et al: Proteolysis of fodrin (non-erythroid spectrin) during apoptosis. J Biol Chem 1995; 270:6425.

421. Cryns VL, Bergeron L, et al: Specific cleavage of α-fodrin during Fas- and tumor necrosis factor-induced apoptosis is mediated by an interleukin-1 converting enzyme/Ced-3 protease distinct from the poly(ADP-ribose) polymerase protease. J Biol Chem 1996; 271:31277.

422. Lu P-W, Soong C-J, Tao M: Phosphorylation of ankyrin decreases its affinity for spectrin tetramer. J Biol Chem 1985; 260:14958.

423. Soong CJ, Lu PW, Tao M: Analysis of band 3 cytoplasmic domain phosphorylation and association with ankyrin. Arch Biochem Biophys 1987; 254:509.

424. Moon RT, Ngai J, et al: Tissue-specific expression of distinct spectrin and ankyrin transcripts in erythroid and nonerythroid cells. J Cell Biol 1985; 100:152.

425. Peters LL, Birkenmeier CS, et al: Purkinje cell degeneration associated with erythroid ankyrin deficiency in nb/nb mice. J Cell Biol 1991; 114:1233.

426. Kordeli E, Bennett V: Distinct ankyrin isoforms at neuron cell bodies and nodes of Ranvier resolved using erythrocyte ankyrin-deficient mice. J Cell Biol 1991; 114:1243.

427. Otto E, Kunimoto M, et al: Isolation and characterization of cDNAs encoding human brain ankyrins reveal a family of alternatively spliced genes. J Cell Biol 1991; 114:241.

428. Chan W, Kordeli E, Bennett V: 440-kD ankyrin$_B$: Structure of the major developmentally regulated domain and selective localization in unmyelinated axons. J Cell Biol 1993; 123:1463.

429. Kunimoto M, Otto E, Bennett V: A new 440-kD isoform is the major ankyrin in neonatal rat brain. J Cell Biol 1991; 115:1319.

430. Chauhan VS, Tuvia S, et al: Abnormal cardiac Na$^+$ channel properties and QT heart rate adaptation in neonatal ankyrin$_B$ knockout mice. Circ Res 2000; 86:441.

431. Kordeli E, Lambert S, Bennett V: Ankyrin$_G$: A new ankyrin gene with neural-specific isoforms localized at the axonal initial segment and node of Ranvier. J Biol Chem 1995; 270:2352.

432. Peters LL, John KM, et al: Ank3 (epithelial ankyrin), a widely distributed new member of the ankyrin gene family and the major ankyrin in kidney, is expressed in alternatively spliced forms, including forms that lack the repeat domain. J Cell Biol 1995; 130:313.

433. Devarajan P, Stabach PR, et al: Identification of a small cytoplasmic ankyrin (Ank$_G$119) in kidney and muscle that binds I spectrin and associated with the Golgi apparatus. J Cell Biol 1996; 133:819.

434. Hoock TC, Peters LL, Lux SE: Isoforms of ankyrin-3 that lack the NH$_2$-terminal repeats associate with mouse macrophage lysosomes. J Cell Biol 1997; 136:1059.

435. Peters B, Kaiser HW, Magin TM: Skin-specific expression of ank-3^{93}, a novel ankyrin-3 splice variant. J Invest Dermatol 2001; 116:216.

436. Conboy JG: Structure, function, and molecular genetics of erythroid membrane skeletal protein 4.1 in normal and abnormal red blood cells. Semin Hematol 1993; 30:58.

437. Takakuwa Y: Regulation of red cell membrane protein interactions: Implications for red cell function. Curr Opin Hematol 2001; 8:80.

438. Leto TL, Marchesi VT: A structural model of human erythrocyte protein 4.1. J Biol Chem 1984; 259:4603.

439. Inaba M, Gupta KC, et al: Deamidation of human erythrocyte membrane protein 4.1: Possible role in aging. Blood 1992; 79:3355.

440. Mueller TJ, Jackson CW, et al: Membrane skeletal alterations during *in vivo* mouse red cell aging: Increase in the band 4.1a:4.1b ratio. J Clin Invest 1987; 79:492.

441. Coleman TR, Harris AS, et al: β spectrin bestows protein 4.1 sensitivity on spectrin-actin interactions. J Cell Biol 1987; 104:519.

442. Ungewickell E, Bennett PM, et al: *In vitro* formation of a complex between cytoskeletal proteins of the human erythrocyte. Nature 1979; 280:811.

443. Ohanian V, Wolfe LC, et al: Analysis of the ternary interaction of the red cell membrane skeletal proteins spectrin, actin, and 4.1. Biochemistry 1984; 23:4416.

444. Correas I, Leto TL, et al: Identification of the functional site of erythrocyte protein 4.1 involved in spectrin-actin associations. J Biol Chem 1986; 261:3310.

445. Correas I, Speicher DW, Marchesi VT: Structure of the spectrin-actin binding site of erythrocyte protein 4.1. J Biol Chem 1986; 261:13362.

446. Conboy JG, Shitamoto R, et al: Hereditary elliptocytosis due to both qualitative and quantitative defects in membrane skeletal protein 4.1. Blood 1991; 78:2438.

447. Discher D, Parra M, et al: Mechanochemistry of the alternatively spliced spectrin-actin binding domain in membrane skeletal protein 4.1. J Biol Chem 1993; 268:7186.

448. Discher DE, Winardi R, et al: Mechanochemistry of protein 4.1's spectrin-actin-binding domain: Ternary complex interactions, membrane binding, network integration, structural strengthening. J Cell Biol 1995; 130:897.

449. Schischmanoff P, Winardi R, et al: Defining the minimal domain of protein 4.1 involved in spectrin-actin binding. J Biol Chem 1995; 270:21243.

450. Morris MB, Lux SE: Characterization of the binary interaction between human erythrocyte protein 4.1 and actin. Eur J Biochem 1995; 231:644.

451. Horne WC, Prinz WC, Tang EK-Y: Identification of two cAMP-dependent phosphorylation sites on erythrocyte protein 4.1. Biochim Biophys Acta 1990; 1055:87.

452. Ling E, Danilov YN, Cohen CM: Modulation of red cell band 4.1 function by cAMP-dependent kinase and protein kinase C phosphorylation. J Biol Chem 1988; 263:2209.

453. Subrahmanyam G, Bertics PJ, Anderson RA: Phosphorylation of protein 4.1 on tyrosine-418 modulates its function *in vitro*. Proc Natl Acad Sci USA 1991; 88:5222.

454. Anderson JP, Morrow JS: The interaction of calmodulin with erythrocyte spectrin. Inhibition of protein 4.1-stimulated actin binding. J Biol Chem 1987; 262:6365.

455. Takakuwa Y, Mohandas N: Modulation of erythrocyte membrane material properties by Ca^{2+} and calmodulin. Implications for their role in regulation of skeletal protein interactions. J Clin Invest 1988; 78:80.

456. Tanaka T, Kadowaki K, et al: Ca^{2+}-dependent regulation of the spectrin/actin interaction by calmodulin and protein 4.1. J Biol Chem 1991; 266:1134.

457. Hemming NJ, Anstee DJ, et al: Identification of the membrane attachment sites for protein 4.1 in the human erythrocyte. J Biol Chem 1995; 270:5360.

458. Marfatia SM, Leu RA, et al: Identification of the protein 4.1 binding interface on glycophorin C and p55, a homologue of the *Drosophila* discs-large tumor suppressor protein. J Biol Chem 1995; 270:715.

459. Lombardo CR, Low PS: Calmodulin modulates protein 4.1 binding to human erythrocyte membranes. Biochim Biophys Acta 1994; 1196:139.

460. Danilov YN, Fennell R, et al: Selective modulation of band 4.1 binding to erythrocyte membranes by protein kinase C. J Biol Chem 1990; 265:2556.

461. Workman RF, Low PS: Biochemical analysis of potential sites for protein 4.1-mediated anchoring of the spectrin-actin skeleton to the erythrocyte membrane. J Biol Chem 1998; 273:6171.

462. Pinder JC, Chung A, et al: Membrane attachment sites for the membrane cytoskeletal protein 4.1 of the red blood cell. Blood 1993; 82:3482.

463. Han BG, Nunomura W, et al: Protein 4.1R core domain structure and insights into regulation of cytoskeletal organization. Nat Struct Biol 2000; 7:871.

464. Nunomura W, Takakuwa Y, et al: Regulation of CD44-protein 4.1 interaction by Ca2+ and calmodulin. Implications for modulation of CD44-ankyrin interaction. J Biol Chem 1997; 272:30322.

465. An XL, Takakuwa Y, et al: Structural and functional characterization of protein 4.1R-phosphatidylserine interaction: Potential role in 4.1R sorting within cells. J Biol Chem 2001; 276:35778.

466. Nunomura W, Takakuwa Y, et al: Regulation of protein 4.1R, p55, and glycophorin C ternary complex in human erythrocyte membrane. J Biol Chem 2000; 275:24540.

467. Mueller T, Manson M: Glycoconnectin (PAS2) a membrane attachment site for the human erythrocyte cytoskeleton. In Kruckeberg W, Eaton J, Greuner G (eds): Erythrocyte Membranes 2: Recent Clinical and Experimental Advances. New York, Alan R. Liss, 1981, p 95.

468. Reid ME, Takakuwa Y, et al: Glycophorin C content of human erythrocyte membrane is regulated by protein 4.1. Blood 1990; 75:2229.

469. Sondag D, Alloisio N, et al: Gerbich reactivity in 4.1(−) hereditary elliptocytosis and protein 4.1 level in blood group Gerbich deficiency. Br J Haematol 1987; 65:43.

470. Pinder JC, Gardner B, Gratzer WB: Interaction of protein 4.1 with the red cell membrane: Effects of phosphorylation by protein kinase C. Biochem Biophys Res Commun 1995; 210:478.

471. Alloisio N, Dalla Venezia N, et al: Evidence that red blood cell protein p55 may participate in the skeleton-membrane linkage that involves protein 4.1 and glycophorin C. Blood 1993; 82:1323.

472. Lue RA, Marfatia SM, et al: Cloning and characterization of hdlg: The human homologue of the *Drosophila* discs large tumor suppressor binds to protein 4.1. Proc Natl Acad Sci USA1994; 91:9818.

473. Rybicki AC, Heath R, et al: Human erythrocyte protein 4.1 is a phosphatidylserine binding protein. J Clin Invest 1988; 81:255.

474. Sato SB, Ohnishi S: Interaction of a peripheral protein of the erythrocyte membrane, band 4.1, with phosphatidylserine-containing liposomes and erythrocyte inside-out vesicles. Eur J Biochem 1983; 130:19.

475. An XL, Takakuwa Y, et al: Modulation of band 3-ankyrin interaction by protein 4.1. Functional implications in regulation of erythrocyte membrane mechanical properties. J Biol Chem 1996; 271:33187.

476. Pasternack GR, Racusen RH: Erythrocyte protein 4.1 binds and regulates myosin. Proc Natl Acad Sci USA1989; 86:9712.

477. Correas I, Avila J: Erythrocyte protein 4.1 associates with tubulin. Biochem J 1988; 255:217.

478. Shi ZT, Afzal V, et al: Protein 4.1R-deficient mice are viable but have erythroid membrane skeleton abnormalities. J Clin Invest 1999; 103:331.

479. Walensky LD, Shi ZT, et al: Neurobehavioral deficits in mice lacking the erythrocyte membrane cytoskeletal protein 4.1. Curr Biol 1998; 8:1269.

480. Gascard P, Lee G, et al: Characterization of multiple isoforms of protein 4.1R expressed during erythroid terminal differentiation. Blood 1998; 92:4404.

481. Hou VC, Conboy JG: Regulation of alternative pre-mRNA splicing during erythroid differentiation. Curr Opin Hematol 2001; 8:74.

482. Huang J-P, Tang C-JC, et al: Genomic structure of the locus encoding protein 4.1. Structural basis for complex combinational patterns of tissue-specific alternative RNA splicing. J Biol Chem 1993; 268:3758.

483. Conboy JG, Chan J, et al: Multiple protein 4.1 isoforms produced by alternative splicing in human erythroid cells. Proc Natl Acad Sci USA1988; 85:9062.

484. Conboy JG, Chan JY, et al: Tissue- and development-specific alternative RNA splicing regulates expression of multiple isoforms of erythroid membrane protein 4.1. J Biol Chem 1991; 266:8273.

485. Tang TK, Qin Z, et al: Heterogeneity of mRNA and protein products arising from the protein 4.1 gene in erythroid and nonerythroid tissues. J Cell Biol 1990; 110:617.

486. Chasis JA, Coulombel L, et al: Differentiation-associated switches in protein 4.1 expression: Synthesis of multiple structural isoforms during normal human erythropoiesis. J Clin Invest 1993; 91:329.

486a.Hou VC, Lersch R, et al: Decrease in hnRNP A/B expression during erythropoiesis mediates a pre-mRNA splicing switch. EMBO J 2002; 21:6195.

487. Winardi R, Discher D, et al: Evolutionarily conserved alternative pre-mRNA splicing regulates structure and function of the spectrin-actin binding domain of erythroid protein 4.1. Blood 1995; 86:4315.

488. Chasis JA, Coulombel L, et al: Differential use of protein 4.1 translation initiation sites during erythropoiesis: Implications for a mutation-induced stage-specific deficiency of protein 4.1 during erythroid development. Blood 1996; 87:5324.

489. Hoover KB, Bryant PJ: The genetics of the protein 4.1 family: Organizers of the membrane and cytoskeleton. Curr Opin Cell Biol 2000; 12:229.

490. Walensky LD, Gascard P, et al: The 13-kD FK506 binding protein, FKBP13, interacts with a novel homologue of the erythrocyte membrane cytoskeletal protein 4.1. J Cell Biol 1998; 141:143.

491. Walensky LD, Blackshaw S, et al: A novel neuron-enriched homolog of the erythrocyte membrane cytoskeletal protein 4.1. J Neurosci 1999; 19:6457.

492. Peters LL, Weier HU, et al: Four paralogous protein 4.1 genes map to distinct chromosomes in mouse and human. Genomics 1998; 54:348.

493. Parra M, Gascard P, et al: Cloning and characterization of 4.1G (EPB41L2), a new member of the skeletal protein 4.1 (EPB41) gene family. Genomics 1998; 49:298.

494. Parra M, Gascard P, et al: Molecular and functional characterization of protein 4.1B, a novel member of the protein 4.1 family with high level, focal expression in brain. J Biol Chem 2000; 275:3247.

495. Chishti AH, Kim AC, et al: The FERM domain: A unique module involved in the linkage of cytoplasmic proteins to the membrane. Trends Biochem Sci 1998; 23:281.

496. Cohen CM, Dotimas E, Korsgren C: Human erythrocyte membrane protein band 4.2 (pallidin). Semin Hematol 1993; 30:119.

497. Yawata Y, Kanzaki A, Yawata A: Genotypic and phenotypic expressions of protein 4.2 in human erythroid cells. Gene Funct Dis 2000; 2:61.

498. Rybicki AC, Musto S, Schwartz RS: Identification of a band-3 binding site near the N-terminus of erythrocyte membrane protein 4.2. Biochem J 1995; 309 (Pt 2):677.

499. Rybicki AC, Qiu JJ, et al: Human erythrocyte protein 4.2 deficiency associated with hemolytic anemia and a homozygous ⁴⁰glutamic acid→lysine substitution in the cytoplasmic domain of band 3 (band 3^Montefiore). Blood 1993; 81:2155.

499a.Mandal D, Moitra PK, Basu J: Mapping of a spectrin-binding domain of human erythrocyte membrane protein 4.2. Biochem J 2002; 364:841.

500. Rybicki AC, Musto S, Schwartz RS: Decreased content of protein 4.2 in ankyrin-deficient normoblastosis (nb/nb) mouse red blood cells: Evidence for ankyrin enhancement of protein 4.2 membrane binding. Blood 1995; 86:3583.

501. Lux SE, Tse WT, et al: Hereditary spherocytosis associated with deletion of the human erythrocyte ankyrin gene on chromosome 8. Nature 1990; 345:736.

502. Rybicki AC, Heath R, et al: Deficiency of protein 4.2 in erythrocytes from a patient with a Coombs negative hemolytic anemia: Evidence for a role of protein 4.2 in stabilizing ankyrin on the membrane. J Clin Invest 1988; 81:893.

503. Inoue T, Kanzaki A, et al: Electron microscopic and physicochemical studies on disorganization of the cytoskeletal network and integral protein (band 3) in red cells of band 4.2 deficiency with a mutation (codon 142:GCT→ACT). Int J Hematol 1994; 59:157.

504. Risinger M, Dotimas E, Cohen CM: Human erythrocyte protein 4.2, a high copy number membrane protein, is N-myristylated. J Biol Chem 1992; 267:5680.

505. Risinger MA, Korsgren C, Cohen CM: Role of N-myristylation in targeting of band 4.2 (pallidin) in nonerythroid cells. Exp Cell Res 1996; 229:421.

506. Das AK, Bhattacharya R, et al: Human erythrocyte membrane protein 4.2 in palmitoylated. Eur J Biochem 1994; 224:575.

507. Bhattacharyya R, Das AK, et al: Mapping of a palmitoylatable band 3-binding domain of human erythrocyte membrane protein 4.2. Biochem J 1999; 340:505.

508. Azim AC, Marfatia SM, et al: Human erythrocyte dematin and protein 4.2 (pallidin) are ATP binding proteins. Biochemistry 1996; 35:3001.

509. Korsgren C, Lawler J, et al: Complete amino acid sequence and homologies of human erythrocyte membrane protein band 4.2. Proc Natl Acad Sci USA 1990; 87:613.

510. Sung LA, Chien S, et al: Molecular cloning of human protein 4.2: A major component of the erythrocyte membrane. Proc Natl Acad Sci USA 1990; 87:955.

511. Korsgren C, Cohen CM: Organization of the gene for human erythrocyte membrane protein 4.2: Structural similarities with the gene for the subunit of factor XIII. Proc Natl Acad Sci USA 1991; 88:4840.

512. Bouhassira EE, Schwartz RS, et al: An alanine to threonine substitution in protein 4.2 cDNA is associated with a Japanese form of hereditary hemolytic anemia (protein 4.2^Nippon). Blood 1992; 79:1846.

513. Wada H, Kanzaki A, et al: Late expression of red cell membrane protein 4.2 in normal human erythroid maturation with seven isoforms of the protein 4.2 gene. Exp Hematol 1999; 27:54.

514. Peters LL, Jindel HK, et al: Mild spherocytosis and altered red cell ion transport in protein 4. 2-null mice. J Clin Invest 1999; 103:1527.

515. Bryant PJ, Woods DF: A major palmitoylated membrane protein of human erythrocytes shows homology to yeast guanylate kinase and to the product of a Drosophila tumor suppressor gene. Cell 1992; 68:621.

516. Chishti AH: Function of p55 and its nonerythroid homologues. Curr Opin Hematol 1998; 5:116.

517. Ruff P, Speicher DW, Husain-Chishti A: Molecular identification of a major palmitoylated erythrocyte membrane protein containing the src homology 3 motif. Proc Natl Acad Sci USA 1991; 88:6595.

518. Metzenberg AB, Gitschier J: The gene encoding the palmitoylated erythrocyte membrane protein, p55, originates at the CpG island 3′ to the factor VIII gene. Hum Mol Genet 1992; 1:97.

519. Marfatia SM, Morais-Cabral JH, et al: The PDZ domain of human erythrocyte p55 mediates its binding to the cytoplasmic carboxyl terminus of glycophorin C. Analysis of the binding interface by in vitro mutagenesis. J Biol Chem 1997; 272: 24191.

520. Ruff P, Chishti AH, et al: Exon skipping truncates the PDZ domain of human erythroid p55 in a patient with chronic myeloid leukemia in acute megakaryoblastic blast crisis. Leuk Res 1999; 23:247.

521. Tilney LG, Detmers P: Actin in erythrocyte ghosts in its association with spectrin: Evidence for a nonfilamentous form of these two molecules *in situ*. J Cell Biol 1975; 66:508.

522. Pinder JC, Sleep JA, et al: Concentrated Tris solutions for the preparation, depolymerization, and assay of actin: Application to erythroid actin. Anal Biochem 1995; 225:291.

523. Pinder JC, Gratzer WB: Structural and dynamic states of actin in the erythrocyte. J Cell Biol 1983; 96:768.

524. Byers T, Branton D: Visualization of the protein associations in the erythrocyte membrane skeleton. Proc Natl Acad Sci USA 1985; 82:6153.

525. Liu S-C, Derick LH, Palek J: Visualization of the hexagonal lattice in the erythrocyte membrane skeleton. J Cell Biol 1987; 104:527.

526. Fowler VM: Regulation of actin filament length in erythrocytes and striated muscle. Curr Opin Cell Biol 1996; 8:86.

527. Fowler VM, Sussmann MA, et al: Tropomodulin is associated with the free (pointed) ends of the thin filaments in rat skeletal muscle. J Cell Biol 1993; 120:411.

528. Nakashima K, Beutler E: Comparison of structure and function of human erythrocyte and human muscle actin. Proc Natl Acad Sci USA 1979; 76:935.

529. Ohanian V, Wolfe LC, et al: Analysis of the ternary interaction of the red cell membrane skeletal proteins spectrin, actin, and 4.1. Biochemistry 1984; 23:4416.

529. Picart C, Discher DE: Actin protofilament orientation at the erythrocyte membrane. Biophys J 1999; 77:865.

530. Picart C, Dalhaimer P, Discher DE: Actin protofilament orientation in deformation of the erythrocyte membrane skeleton. Biophys J 2000; 79:2987.

531. Goldberg YP, Lin BY, et al: Cloning and mapping of the α-adducin gene close to D4S95 and assessment of its relationship to Huntington disease. Hum Mol Genet 1992; 1:669.

532. Gardner K, Bennett V: Modulation of spectrin-actin assembly by erythrocyte adducin. Nature 1987; 328:359.

533. Joshi R, Gilligan DM, et al: Primary structure and domain organization of human α and β adducin. J Cell Biol 1991; 115:665.

534. Matsuoka Y, Li X, Bennett V: Adducin: Structure, function and regulation. Cell Mol Life Sci 2000; 57:884.

535. Matsuoka Y, Hughes CA, Bennett V: Adducin regulation. Definition of the calmodulin-binding domain and sites of phosphorylation by protein kinases A and C. J Biol Chem 1996; 271:25157.

536. Hughes CA, Bennett V: Adducin: A physical model with implications for function in assembly of spectrin-actin complexes. J Biol Chem 1995; 270:18990.

537. Lin B, Nasir J, et al: Genomic organization of the human α-adducin gene and its alternately spliced isoforms. Genomics 1995; 25:93.

538. Tisminetzky S, Devescovi G, et al: Genomic organization and chromosomal localization of the gene encoding human β adducin. Gene 1995; 167:313.

539. Sinard JH, Stewart GW, et al: Utilization of an 86 bp exon generates a novel adducin isoform (β 4) lacking the MARCKS homology domain. Biochim Biophys Acta 1998; 1396:57.

540. Nehls V, Drenckhahn D, et al: Adducin in erythrocyte precursor cells of rats and humans: Expression and compartmentalization. Blood 1991; 78:1692.

541. Kuhlman PA, Hughes CA, et al: A new function for adducin. Calcium/calmodulin-regulated capping of the barbed ends of actin filaments. J Biol Chem 1996; 271:7986.

542. Kuhlman PA, Fowler VM: Purification and characterization of an α 1 β 2 isoform of CapZ from human erythrocytes: Cytosolic location and inability to bind to Mg^{2+} ghosts suggest that erythrocyte actin filaments are capped by adducin. Biochemistry 1997; 36:13461.

543. Matsuoka Y, Li X, Bennett V: Adducin is an in vivo substrate for protein kinase C: Phosphorylation in the MARCKS-related domain inhibits activity in promoting spectrin-actin complexes and occurs in many cells, including dendritic spines of neurons. J Cell Biol 1998; 142:485.

544. Kaiser HW, O'Keefe E, Bennett V: Adducin: Ca^{++}-dependent association with sites of cell-cell contact. J Cell Biol 1989; 109:557.

545. Ling E, Gardner K, Bennett V: Protein kinase C phosphorylates a recently identified membrane skeleton-associated calmodulin-binding protein in human erythrocytes. J Biol Chem 1986; 261:13875.

546. Shima T, Okumura N, et al: Interaction of the SH2 domain of Fyn with a cytoskeletal protein, β-adducin. J Biol Chem 2001; 276:42233.

547. Gilligan DM, Lozovatsky L, et al: Targeted disruption of the β-adducin gene (Add2) causes red blood cell spherocytosis in mice. Proc Natl Acad Sci USA 1999; 96:10717.

548. Muro AF, Marro ML, et al: Mild spherocytic hereditary elliptocytosis and altered levels of α- and γ-adducins in β-adducin-deficient mice. Blood 2000; 95:3978.

549. Marro ML, Scremin OU, et al: Hypertension in β-adducin-deficient mice. Hypertension 2000; 36:449.

550. Manunta P, Barlassina C, Bianchi G: Adducin in essential hypertension. FEBS Lett 1998; 430:41.

551. Beeks E, Janssen RG, et al: Association between the α-adducin $Gly^{460}Trp$ polymorphism and systolic blood pressure in familial combined hyperlipidemia. Am J Hypertens 2001; 14:1185.

552. Province MA, Arnett DK, et al: Association between the α-adducin gene and hypertension in the HyperGEN Study. Am J Hypertens 2000; 13:710.

553. Morrison AC, Doris PA, et al: G-protein β3 subunit and α-adducin polymorphisms and risk of subclinical and clinical stroke. Stroke 2001; 32:822.

554. Grant FD, Romero JR, et al: Low-renin hypertension, altered sodium homeostasis, and an α-adducin polymorphism. Hypertension 2002; 39:191.

555. Husain-Chishti A, Levin A, Branton D: Abolition of actin-bundling by phosphorylation of human erythrocyte protein 4.9. Nature 1988; 334:718.

556. Husain-Chishti A, Faquin W, et al: Purification of erythrocyte dematin (protein 4.9) reveals an endogenous protein kinase that modulates actin-bundling activity. J Biol Chem 1989; 264:8985.

557. Siegel DL, Branton D: Partial purification and characterization of an actin-binding protein, band 4.9, from human erythrocytes. J Cell Biol 1985; 100:775.

558. Azim AC, Knoll JH, et al: Isoform cloning, actin binding, and chromosomal localization of human erythroid dematin, a member of the villin superfamily. J Biol Chem 1995; 270:17407.

559. Rana AP, Ruff P, et al: Cloning of human erythroid dematin reveals another member of the villin family. Proc Natl Acad Sci USA 1993; 90:6651.

560. Kim AC, Azim AC, Chishti AH: Alternative splicing and structure of the human erythroid dematin gene. Biochim Biophys Acta 1998; 1398:382.

561. Khanna R, Chang SH, et al: Headpiece domain of dematin is required for the stability of the erythrocyte membrane. Proc Natl Acad Sci USA 2002; 99:6637.

562. Lutchman M, Pack S, et al: Loss of heterozygosity on 8p in prostate cancer implicates a role for dematin in tumor progression. Cancer Genet Cytogenet 1999; 115:65.

563. Fowler VM, Bennett V: Erythrocyte membrane tropomyosin: Purification and properties. J Biol Chem 1984; 259:5978.

564. Mak AS, Roseborough G, Baker H: Tropomyosin from human erythrocyte membrane polymerizes poorly but binds F-actin effectively in the presence and absence of spectrin. Biochim Biophys Acta 1987; 912:157.

565. Sung LA, Lin JJ: Erythrocyte tropomodulin binds to the N-terminus of hTM5, a tropomyosin isoform encoded by the γ-tropomyosin gene. Biochem Biophys Res Commun 1994; 201:627.

566. Sung LA, Gao KM, et al: Tropomyosin isoform 5b is expressed in human erythrocytes: Implications of tropomodulin-TM5 or tropomodulin-TM5b complexes in the protofilament and hexagonal organization of membrane skeletons. Blood 2000; 95:1473.

567. Fowler VM: Identification and purification of a novel M_r 43,000 tropomyosin-binding protein from human erythrocyte membranes. J Biol Chem 1987; 262:12792.

568. Fowler VM: Tropomodulin: A cytoskeletal protein that binds to the end of erythrocyte tropomyosin and inhibits tropomyosin binding to actin. J Cell Biol 1990; 111:471.

569. Chu X, Thompson D, et al: Genomic organization of mouse and human erythrocyte tropomodulin genes encoding the pointed end capping protein for the actin filaments. Gene 2000; 256:271.

570. Babcock GG, Fowler VM: Isoform-specific interaction of tropomodulin with skeletal muscle and erythrocyte tropomyosins. J Biol Chem 1994; 269:27510.

571. Greenfield NJ, Fowler VM: Tropomyosin requires an intact N-terminal coiled coil to interact with tropomodulin. Biophys J 2002; 82:2580.

572. Vera C, Sood A, et al: Tropomodulin-binding site mapped to residues 7–14 at the N-terminal heptad repeats of tropomyosin isoform 5. Arch Biochem Biophys 2000; 378:16.

573. Ursitti JA, Fowler VM: Immunolocalization of tropomodulin, tropomyosin and actin in spread human erythrocyte skeletons. J Cell Sci 1994; 107:1633.

574. Gregorio CC, Fowler VM: Mechanisms of thin filament assembly in embryonic chick cardiac myocytes: Tropomodulin requires tropomyosin for assembly. J Cell Biol 1995; 129:683.

575. Gregorio CC, Weber A, et al: Requirement of pointed-end capping by tropomodulin to maintain actin filament length in embryonic chick cardiac myocytes. Nature 1995; 376:83.

576. Fowler VM: Capping actin filament growth: Tropomodulin in muscle and nonmuscle cells. Soc Gen Physiol Ser 1997; 52:79.

577. Weber A, Pennise CR, Fowler VM: Tropomodulin increases the critical concentration of barbed end-capped actin filaments by converting ADP•P$_i$-actin to ADP-actin at all pointed filament ends. J Biol Chem 1999; 274:34637.

578. Weber A, Pennise CR, et al: Tropomodulin caps the pointed ends of actin filaments. J Cell Biol 1994; 127:1627.

579. Fowler VM, Davis JP, Bennett V: Human erythrocyte myosin. Identification and purification. J Cell Biol 1985; 100:47.

580. Wong AJ, Kiehart DP, Pollard TD: Myosin from human erythrocytes. J Biol Chem 1984; 260:46.

581. Cibert C, Pruliere G, et al: Calculation of a Gap restoration in the membrane skeleton of the red blood cell: Possible role for myosin II in local repair. Biophys J 1999; 76:1153.

582. Colin FC, Schrier SL: Myosin content and distribution in human neonatal erythrocytes are different from adult erythrocytes. Blood 1991; 78:3052.

583. Rand RP, Burton AC: Area and volume changes in hemolysis of single erythrocytes. J Cell Comp Physiol 1963; 61:245.

584. Mohandas N, Chasis JA: Red cell deformability, membrane material properties, and shape: Regulation by transmembrane, skeletal, and cytosolic proteins and lipids. Semin Hematol 1993; 30:171.

585. Van Dort HM, Knowles DW, et al: Analysis of integral membrane protein contributions to the deformability and stability of the human erythrocyte membrane. J Biol Chem 2001; 276:46968.

586. Lee JC, Discher DE: Deformation-enhanced fluctuations in the red cell skeleton with theoretical relations to elasticity, connectivity, and spectrin unfolding. Biophys J 2001; 81:3178.

587. Discher DE, Carl P: New insights into red cell network structure, elasticity, and spectrin unfolding—A current review. Cell Mol Biol Lett 2001; 6:593.

588. Discher DE, Mohandas N: Kinematics of red cell aspiration by fluorescence-imaged microdeformation. Biophys J 1996; 71:1680.

589. Lee JC, Wong DT, Discher DE: Direct measures of large, anisotropic strains in deformation of the erythrocyte cytoskeleton. Biophys J 1999; 77:853.

590. Heinrich V, Ritchie K, et al: Elastic thickness compressibility of the red cell membrane. Biophys J 2001; 81:1452.

591. Knowles DW, Tilley L, et al: Erythrocyte membrane vesiculation: Model for the molecular mechanism of protein sorting. Proc Natl Acad Sci USA 1997; 94:12969.

592. Bull BS, Kuhn IN: The production of schistocytes by fibrin strands (a scanning electron microscope study). Blood 1970; 35:104.

593. Palek J, Jarolim P: Clinical expression and laboratory detection of red cell membrane protein mutations. Semin Hematol 1993; 30:249.

594. Hansen JC, Skalak R, et al: Influence of network topology on the elasticity of the red blood cell membrane skeleton. Biophys J 1997; 72:2369.

595. Discher DE: New insights into erythrocyte membrane organization and microelasticity. Curr Opin Hematol 2000; 7:117.

596. Liu S-C, Derick LH, et al: Alteration of the erythrocyte membrane skeletal ultrastructure in hereditary spherocytosis, hereditary elliptocytosis, and pyropoikilocytosis. Blood 1990; 76:198.

597. Liu S-C, Derick LH, et al: Separation of the lipid bilayer from the membrane skeleton during discocyte-echinocyte transformation of human erythrocyte ghosts. Eur J Cell Biol 1989; 49:358.

598. Wagner GM, Chiu DT-Y, et al: Spectrin oxidation correlates with membrane vesiculation in stored RBC's. Blood 1987; 69:1777.

599. Wolfe LC: The membrane and the lesions of storage in preserved red cells. Transfusion 1985; 25:185.

600. Lutz HU, Liu S-C, Palek J: Release of spectrin-free vesicles from human erythrocytes during ATP depletion. Characterization of spectrin-free vesicles. J Cell Biol 1977; 73:548.

601. Elgsaeter A, Shotton DM, Branton D: Intramembrane particle aggregation in erythrocyte ghosts: II. The influence of spectrin aggregation. Biochim Biophys Acta 1976; 426:101.

602. Lux SE, John KM, Karnovsky MJ: Irreversible deformation of the spectrin-actin lattice in irreversibly sickled cells. J Clin Invest 1976; 58:955.

603. Tomaselli MB, John KM, Lux SE: Elliptical erythrocyte membrane skeletons and heat-sensitive spectrin in hereditary elliptocytosis. Proc Natl Acad Sci USA 1981; 78:1911.

604. Haest CWM, Fischer TM, et al: Stabilization of erythrocyte shape by a chemical increase in membrane shear stiffness. Blood Cells 1980; 6:539.

605. Hebbel RP: Beyond hemoglobin polymerization: The red blood cell membrane and sickle cell disease pathophysiology. Blood 1991; 77:214.

606. Liu C, Marshall P, et al: Interaction between terminal complement proteins C5b-7 and anionic phospholipids. Blood 1999; 93:2297.

607. Patel VP, Lodish HF: A fibronectin matrix is required for differentiation of murine erythroleukemia cells into reticulocytes. J Cell Biol 1987; 105:3105.

608. Swerlick RA, Eckman JR, et al: α4β1-integrin expression on sickle reticulocytes: Vascular cell adhesion molecule-1-dependent binding to endothelium. Blood 1993; 82:1891.

609. Patel VP, Lodish HF: The fibronectin receptor on mammalian erythroid precursor cells: Characterization and developmental regulation. J Cell Biol 1986; 102:449.

610. Jakubowska-Solarska B, Solski J: Sialic acids of young and old red blood cells in healthy subjects. Med Sci Monit 2000; 6:871.

611. Hanspal M, Smockova Y, Uong Q: Molecular identification and functional characterization of a novel protein that mediates the attachment of erythroblasts to macrophages. Blood 1998; 92:2940.

612. Telen MJ: Red blood cell surface adhesion molecules: Their possible roles in normal human physiology and disease. Semin Hematol 2000; 37:130.

613. Chitnis CE: Molecular insights into receptors used by malaria parasites for erythrocyte invasion. Curr Opin Hematol 2001; 8:85.

614. Bessler M, Schaefer A, Keller P: Paroxysmal nocturnal hemoglobinuria: Insights from recent advances in molecular biology. Transfus Med Rev 2001; 15:255.

615. Test ST, Butikofer P, et al: Characterization of the complement sensitivity of calcium-loaded human erythrocytes. Blood 1991; 78:3056.

616. Brown DA, London E: Functions of lipid rafts in biological membranes. Annu Rev Cell Dev Biol 1998; 14:111.

617. Salzer U, Prohaska R: Stomatin, flotillin-1, and flotillin-2 are major integral proteins of erythrocyte lipid rafts. Blood 2001; 97:1141.

618. Naik RS, Davidson EA, Gowda DC: Developmental stage-specific biosynthesis of glycosylphosphatidylinositol anchors in intraerythrocytic *Plasmodium falciparum* and its inhibition in a novel manner by mannosamine. J Biol Chem 2000; 275:24506.

619. Samuel BU, Mohandas N, et al: The role of cholesterol and glycosylphosphatidylinositol-anchored proteins of erythrocyte rafts in regulating raft protein content and malarial infection. J Biol Chem 2001; 276:29319.

620. Victoria EJ, Muchmore EA, et al: The role of antigen mobility in anti-Rh^D-induced agglutination. J Clin Invest 1975; 56:292.

621. Cho MR, Eber SW, et al: Regulation of band 3 rotational mobility by ankyrin in intact human red cells. Biochemistry 1998; 37:17828.

622. Che A, Morrison IE, et al: Restriction by ankyrin of band 3 rotational mobility in human erythrocyte membranes and reconstituted lipid vesicles. Biochemistry 1997; 36:9588.

623. Tomishige M, Sako Y, Kusumi A: Regulation mechanism of the lateral diffusion of band 3 in erythrocyte membranes by the membrane skeleton. J Cell Biol 1998; 142:989.

624. Terada N, Fujii Y, et al: An immunocytochemical study of changes in the human erythrocyte membrane skeleton produced by stretching examined by the quick-freezing and deep-etching method. J Anat 1997; 190:397.

625. McCaughan L, Krimm S: X-ray and neutron scattering density profiles of the intact human red blood cell membrane. Science 1980; 207:1481.

626. Tsukita S, Tsukita S, Ishikawa H: Cytoskeletal network underlying the human erythrocyte membrane. Thin-section electron microscopy. J Cell Biol 1980; 85:567.

626a. Bruce LJ, Ghosh S, et al: Absence of CD47 in protein 4.2-deficient hereditary spherocytosis in man: an interaction between the Rh complex and the band 3 complex. Blood 2002; 100:1878.

626b. Dahl KN, Westhoff CM, Discher DE: Fractional attachment of CD47 (IAP) to the erythrocyte cytoskeleton and visual colocalization with Rh protein complexes. Blood 2003; In press.

626c. Mouro-Chanteloup I, Delaunay J, et al: Evidence that the red cell skeleton protein 4.2 interacts with the Rh membrane complex member CD47. Blood 2003; 101:338.

627. Cohen CM, Gascard P: Regulation and post-translational modification of the erythrocyte membrane and membrane-skeletal proteins. Semin Hematol 1992; 29:244.

628. Eder PS, Soong CJ, Tao M: Phosphorylation reduces the affinity of protein 4.1 for spectrin. Biochemistry 1986; 25:1764.

629. Chao T-S, Tao M: Modulation of protein 4.1 binding to inside-out membrane vesicles by phosphorylation. Biochemistry 1991; 30:10529.

630. Low PS, Geahlen RL, et al: Extracellular control of erythrocyte metabolism mediated by a cytoplasmic tyrosine kinase. Biomed Biochim Acta 1990; 49:S135.

631. Schindler M, Koppel D, Sheetz MP: Modulation of membrane protein lateral mobility by polyphosphates and polyamines. Proc Natl Acad Sci USA 1980; 77:1457.

632. Wolfe LC, Lux SE, Ohanian V: Spectrin-actin binding in vitro; effect of protein 4.1 and polyphosphates. J Supramol Struct Cell Biochem 1981; 5(Suppl 5):123.

633. Suzuki Y, Nakajima T, et al: Influence of 2,3-diphosphoglycerate on the deformability of human erythrocytes. Biochim Biophys Acta 1990; 1029:85.

634. Waugh RE: Effects of 2,3-diphosphoglycerate on the mechanical properties of erythrocyte membrane. Blood 1986; 68:231.

635. Gardner K, Bennett V: A new erythrocyte membrane-associated protein with calmodulin binding activity. Identification and purification. J Biol Chem 1986; 261:1339.

636. Palek J, Liu PA, Liu SC: Polymerization of red cell membrane protein contributes to spheroechinocyte shape irreversibility. Nature 1978; 274:505.

637. Lorand L, Siefring GE Jr, Lowe-Krentz L: Enzymatic basis of membrane stiffening in human erythrocytes. Semin Hematol 1979; 16:65.

637a. Andrews DA, Yang L, Low PS: Phorbol ester stimulates a protein kinase C-mediated agatoxin-TK-sensitive calcium permeability pathway in human red blood cells. Blood 2002; 100:3392.

637b. Salzer U, Hinterdorfer P, et al: Ca(++)-dependent vesicle release from erythrocytes involves stomatin-specific lipid rafts, synexin (annexin VII), and sorcin. Blood 2002; 99:2569.

638. Brown GK: Glucose transporters: Structure, function and consequences of deficiency. J Inherit Metab Dis 2000; 23:237.

639. Brugnara C: Erythrocyte membrane transport physiology. Curr Opin Hematol 1997; 4:122.

640. Ellory JC, Gibson JS, Stewart GW: Pathophysiology of abnormal cell volume in human red cells. Contrib Nephrol 1998; 123:220.

641. Parker JC: In defense of cell volume? Am J Physiol 1993; 265:1191.

642. Agre P, Bonhivers M, Borgnia MJ: The aquaporins, blueprints for cellular plumbing systems. J Biol Chem 1998; 273:14659.

643. Preston GM, Agre P: Isolation of the cDNA for erythrocyte integral membrane protein of 28 kilodaltons: Member of an ancient channel family. Proc Natl Acad Sci USA 1991; 88:11110.

644. Roudier N, Verbavatz JM, et al: Evidence for the presence of aquaporin-3 in human red blood cells. J Biol Chem 1998; 273:8407.

645. Yang B, Ma T, Verkman AS: Erythrocyte water permeability and renal function in double knockout mice lacking aquaporin-1 and aquaporin-3. J Biol Chem 2001; 276:624.

646. Walz T, Hirai T, et al: The three-dimensional structure of aquaporin-1. Nature 1997; 387:624.

647. Cheng A, van Hoek AN, et al: Three-dimensional organization of a human water channel. Nature 1997; 387:627.

648. Sui H, Han BG, et al: Structural basis of water-specific transport through the AQP1 water channel. Nature 2001; 414:872.

649. Prasad GV, Coury LA, et al: Reconstituted aquaporin 1 water channels transport CO_2 across membranes. J Biol Chem 1998; 273:33123.

650. Saparov SM, Kozono D, et al: Water and ion permeation of aquaporin-1 in planar lipid bilayers. Major differences in struc-tural determinants and stoichiometry. J Biol Chem 2001; 276:31515.

651. Smith BL, Preston GM, et al: Human red cell aquaporin CHIP. I. Molecular characterization of ABH and Colton blood group antigens. J Clin Invest 1994; 94:1043.

652. Preston GM, Smith BL, et al: Mutations in aquaporin-1 in phenotypically normal humans without functional CHIP water channels. Science 1994; 265:1585.

653. Mathai JC, Mori S, et al: Functional analysis of aquaporin-1 deficient red cells. The Colton-null phenotype. J Biol Chem 1996; 271:1309.

654. Chretien S, Catron JP: A single mutation inside the NPA motif of aquaporin-1 found in a Colton-null phenotype. Blood 1999; 93:4021.

655. Joshi SR, Wagner FF, et al: An AQP1 null allele in an Indian woman with Co(a–b–) phenotype and high-titer anti-Co3 associated with mild HDN. Transfusion 2001; 41:1273.

656. Ma T, Yang B, et al: Severely impaired urinary concentrating ability in transgenic mice lacking aquaporin-1 water channels. J Biol Chem 1998; 273:4296.

657. Lauf PK, Adragna NC: K-Cl cotransport: Properties and molecular mechanism. Cell Physiol Biochem 2000; 10:341.

658. Joiner CH, Franco RS: The activation of KCl cotransport by deoxygenation and its role in sickle cell dehydration. Blood Cells Mol Dis 2001; 27:158.

659. Gillen CM, Brill S, et al: Molecular cloning and functional expression of the K-Cl cotransporter from rabbit, rat, and human. A new member of the cation-chloride cotransporter family. J Biol Chem 1996; 271:16237.

660. Pellegrino CM, Rybicki AC, et al: Molecular identification and expression of erythroid K:Cl cotransporter in human and mouse erythroleukemic cells. Blood Cells Mol Dis 1998; 24:31.

661. Su W, Shmukler BE, et al: Mouse K-Cl cotransporter KCC1: Cloning, mapping, pathological expression, and functional regulation. Am J Physiol 1999; 277:C899.

662. Lauf PK, Zhang J, et al: K-Cl co-transport: Immunocytochemical and functional evidence for more than one KCC isoform in high K and low K sheep erythrocytes. Comp Biochem Physiol A Mol Integr Physiol 2001; 130:499.

663. De Franceschi L, Fumagalli L, et al: Deficiency of Src family kinases Fgr and Hck results in activation of erythrocyte K/Cl cotransport. J Clin Invest 1997; 99:220.

664. Bize I, Guvenc B, et al: Serine/threonine protein phosphatases and regulation of K-Cl cotransport in human erythrocytes. Am J Physiol 1999; 277:C926.

665. Joiner WJ, Wang LY, et al: hSK4, a member of a novel subfamily of calcium-activated potassium channels. Proc Natl Acad Sci USA 1997; 94:11013.

666. Ishii TM, Silvia C, et al: A human intermediate conductance calcium-activated potassium channel. Proc Natl Acad Sci USA 1997; 94:11651.

667. Logsdon NJ, Kang J, et al: A novel gene, *hKCa4*, encodes the calcium-activated potassium channel in human T lymphocytes. J Biol Chem 1997; 272:32723.

668. Jensen BS, Strobaek D, et al: Characterization of the cloned human intermediate-conductance Ca^{2+}-activated K+ channel. Am J Physiol 1998; 275:C848.

669. Vandorpe DH, Shmukler BE, et al: cDNA cloning and functional characterization of the mouse Ca^{2+}-gated K+ channel, mIK1. Roles in regulatory volume decrease and erythroid differentiation. J Biol Chem 1998; 273:21542.

670. Khanna R, Chang MC, et al: hSK4/hIK1, a calmodulin-binding KCa channel in human T lymphocytes. Roles in proliferation and volume regulation. J Biol Chem 1999; 274:14838.

671. Xia XM, Fakler B, et al: Mechanism of calcium gating in small-conductance calcium-activated potassium channels. Nature 1998; 395:503.

672. Joiner WJ, Khanna R, et al: Calmodulin regulates assembly and trafficking of SK4/IK1 Ca²⁺-activated K+ channels. J Biol Chem 2001; 276:37980.

673. Rivera A, Rotter MA, Brugnara C: Endothelins activate Ca²⁺-gated K⁺ channels via endothelin B receptors in CD-1 mouse erythrocytes. Am J Physiol 1999; 277:C746.

674. Rivera A, Jarolim P, Brugnara C: Modulation of Gardos channel activity by cytokines in sickle erythrocytes. Blood 2002; 99:357.

675. Lew VL, Ortiz OE, Bookchin RM: Stochastic nature and red cell population distribution of the sickling-induced Ca²⁺ permeability. J Clin Invest 1997; 99:2727.

676. Lew VL, Etzion Z, Bookchin RM: Dehydration response of sickle cells to sickling-induced Ca⁺⁺ permeabilization. Blood 2002; 99:2578.

677. Bookchin RM, Lew VL: Sickle red cell dehydration: Mechanisms and interventions. Curr Opin Hematol 2002; 9:107.

678. Johnson RM, Gannon SA: Erythrocyte cation permeability induced by mechanical stress: A model for sickle cell cation loss. Am J Physiol 1990; 259:C746.

679. Garcia-Anoveros J, Corey DP: The molecules of mechanosensation. Annu Rev Neurosci 1997; 20:567.

680. Kaplan JH: Biochemistry of Na,K-ATPase. Annu Rev Biochem 2002; 71:511.

681. Garrahan PJ, Glynn IM: Factors affecting the relative magnitude of the sodium:potassium and sodium:sodium exchanges catalyzed by the sodium pump. J Physiol 1967; 192:189.

682. Clark MR, Guatelli JC, et al: Study of dehydrating effect of the red cell Na⁺/K⁺ pump in nystatin-treated cells with varying Na⁺ and water content. Biochim Biophys Acta 1981; 646:422.

683. Joiner CH, Platt OS, Lux SE: Cation depletion by the sodium pump in red cells with pathologic cation leaks. J Clin Invest 1986; 78:1487.

684. Strehler EE, Zacharias DA: Role of alternative splicing in generating isoform diversity among plasma membrane calcium pumps. Physiol Rev 2001; 81:21.

685. Penniston JT, Enyedi A: Modulation of the plasma membrane Ca²⁺ pump. J Membr Biol 1998; 165:101.

686. Lazarides E: From genes to structural morphogenesis: The genesis and epigenesis of a red blood cell. Cell 1987; 51:345.

687. Lazarides E, Woods C: Biogenesis of the red blood cell membrane-skeleton and the control of erythroid morphogenesis. Annu Rev Cell Biol 1989; 5:427.

688. Hanspal M, Palek J: Biogenesis of normal and abnormal red blood cell membrane skeletons. Semin Hematol 1992; 29:305.

689. Peters LL, Shivdasani RA, et al: Anion exchanger 1 (band 3) is required to prevent erythrocyte membrane surface loss but not to form the membrane skeleton. Cell 1996; 86:917.

690. Hanspal M, Palek J: Synthesis and assembly of membrane skeletal proteins in mammalian red cell precursors. J Cell Biol 1987; 105:1417.

691. Hanspal M, Hanspal J, Kalraiya R: Asynchronous synthesis of membrane skeletal proteins during terminal maturation of murine erythroblasts. Blood 1992; 80:530.

692. Woods CM, Boyer B, et al: Control of erythroid differentiation: Asynchronous expression of the anion transporter and the peripheral components of the membrane skeleton in AEV- and S13-transformed cells. J Cell Biol 1986; 103:1789.

693. Bodine DM, Birkenmeier CS, Barker JE: Spectrin deficient inherited hemolytic anemias in the mouse: Characterization by spectrin synthesis and mRNA activity in reticulocytes. Cell 1984; 37:721.

694. Coetzer TL, Lawler J, et al: Partial ankyrin and spectrin deficiency in severe, atypical hereditary spherocytosis. N Engl J Med 1988; 318:230.

695. Hanspal M, Kalraiya R, et al: Erythropoietin enhances the assembly of β spectrin heterodimers on the murine erythroblast membranes by increasing spectrin synthesis. J Biol Chem 1991; 266:15626.

696. Takano-Ohmuro H, Mukaida M, Morioka K: Distribution of actin, myosin, and spectrin during enucleation in erythroid cells of hamster embryo. Cell Motil Cytoskeleton 1996; 34:95.

697. Chasis JA, Prenant M, et al: Membrane assembly and remodeling during reticulocyte maturation. Blood 1989; 74:1112.

698. Waugh RE, Mantalaris A, et al: Membrane instability in late-stage erythropoiesis. Blood 2001; 97:1869.

698a. Holm TM, Braun A, et al: Failure of red blood cell maturation in mice with defects in the high-density lipoprotein receptor SR-BI. Blood 2002; 99:1817.

699. Kawane K, Fukuyama H, et al: Requirement of DNase II for definitive erythropoiesis in the mouse fetal liver. Science 2001; 292:1546.

700. Qiu LB, Dickson H, et al: Extruded erythroblast nuclei are bound and phagocytosed by a novel macrophage receptor. Blood 1995; 85:1630.

701. Gallagher PG: Disorders of erythrocyte metabolism and shape. In Christensen RD (ed): Hematologic Problems in the Neonate. Philadelphia, WB Saunders, 1999, p 209.

702. Jay DG: Glycosylation site of band 3, the human erythrocyte anion-exchange protein. Biochemistry 1986; 25:554.

703. Fukuda M, Dell A, Fukuda MN: Structure of fetal lactosaminoglycan: The carbohydrate moiety of band 3 isolated from human umbilical cord erythrocytes. J Biol Chem 1984; 259:4782.

704. Fukuda M, Dell A, et al: Structure of branched lactosaminoglycan, the carbohydrate moiety of band 3 isolated from adult erythrocytes. J Biol Chem 1984; 259:8260.

705. Fukuda M, Fukuda MN, Hakomori S: Developmental change and genetic defect in the carbohydrate structure of band 3 glycoprotein of human erythrocyte membrane. J Biol Chem 1979; 254:3700.

706. Zipursky A, LaRue T, Israels LG: The in vitro metabolism of erythrocytes from newborn infants. Can J Biochem 1960; 38:727.

707. Whaun JM, Oski FA: Red cell stromal adenosine triphosphatase (ATPase) of newborn infants. Pediatr Res 1969; 3:105.

708. Gibson JS, Speake PF, et al: K⁺ transport in red blood cells from human umbilical cord. Biochim Biophys Acta 2001; 1512:231.

709. Neerhout RC: Erythrocyte lipids in the neonate. Pediatr Res 1968; 2:172.

710. Sjolin S: The resistance of red cell in vitro: A study of the osmotic properties, the mechanical resistance and the storage behavior of red cells of fetuses, children and adults. Acta Paediatr 1954; 43:1.

711. Kehry M, Yguerabide J, Singer SJ: Fluidity in the membranes of adult and neonatal human erythrocytes. Science 1977; 195:486.

712. Shapiro DL, Pasqualini P: Erythrocyte membrane proteins of premature and full-term newborn infants. Pediatr Res 1978; 12:176.

713. Chow EI, Chen D: Kinetic characteristics of bicarbonate-chloride exchange across the neonatal human red cell membrane. Biochim Biophys Acta 1982; 685:196.

714. Matovick LM, Groschel-Stewart U, et al: Myosin is a component of the erythrocyte membrane. J Cell Biol 1984; 99:2a.

715. Schekman R, Singer SJ: Clustering and endocytosis of membrane receptors can be induced in mature erythrocytes of neonatal but not adult humans. Proc Natl Acad Sci USA 1976; 73:4075.

716. Zweig S, Singer SJ: Concanavalin A–induced endocytosis in rabbit reticulocytes, and its decrease with reticulocyte maturation. J Cell Biol 1979; 80:487.

717. Gross GP, Hathaway WE: Fetal erythrocyte deformability. Pediatr Res 1972; 6:593.

718. Bratteby LE, Garby L, et al: Studies on erythrokinetics in infancy: 13. The mean life span and the life span frequency function of red blood cells formed during foetal life. Acta Paediatr Scand 1968; 57:311.

719. Holroyde CP, Oski FA, Gardner FH: The "pocked" erythrocyte: Red-cell surface alterations in reticuloendothelial immaturity of the neonate. N Engl J Med 1969; 281:516.

720. Tsukada M, Hanamura K, et al: Scanning electron microscopic study on red blood cells in several diseases of newborns and infants. Acta Paediatr Jpn 1976; 18:4.

721. Shattil SJ, Cooper RA: Maturation of macroreticulocyte membranes in vivo. J Lab Clin Med 1972; 79:215.

722. Lux SE, John KM: Isolation and partial characterization of a high molecular weight red cell membrane protein complex normally removed by the spleen. Blood 1977; 50:625.

723. Patel VP, Ciechanover A, et al: Mammalian reticulocytes lose adhesion to fibronectin during maturation to erythrocytes. Proc Natl Acad Sci USA 1985; 82:440.

724. Clark MR: Senescence of red blood cells: Progress and problems. Physiol Rev 1988; 68:503.

725. Clark MR, Shohet SB: Red cell senescence. Clin Haematol 1985; 14:223.

726. Beutler E: Isolation of the aged. Blood Cells 1988; 14:1.
727. Dale GL, Norenberg SL: Density fractionation of erythrocytes by Percoll/Hypaque results in only a slight enrichment for aged cells. Biochim Biophys Acta 1990; 1036:183.
728. Suzuki T, Dale GL: Senescent erythrocytes: Isolation of *in vivo* aged cells and their biochemical characteristics. Proc Natl Acad Sci USA 1988; 85:1647.
729. Gershon H: Is the sequestration of aged erythrocytes mediated by natural autoantibodies? Isr J Med Sci 1992; 28:818.
730. Lutz HU: Erythrocyte clearance. In Harris JR (ed): Blood Cell Biochemistry, Erythroid Cells. New York, Plenum Press, 1990, Vol I, p 81.
731. Waugh RE, Mohandas N, et al: Rheologic properties of senescent erythrocytes: Loss of surface area and volume with red blood cell age. Blood 1992; 79:1351.
732. Jain SK, Hochstein P: Polymerization of membrane components in aging red blood cells. Biochem Biophys Res Commun 1980; 92:247.
733. Snyder LM, Fortier NL, et al: Effect of hydrogen peroxide exposure on normal human erythrocyte deformability, morphology, surface characteristics and spectrin hemoglobin crosslinking. J Clin Invest 1985; 76:1971.
734. Jain SK: Evidence for membrane lipid peroxidation during the *in vivo* aging of human erythrocytes. Biochim Biophys Acta 1988; 937:205.
735. Danon D, Marikovsky Y: The aging of the red blood cell: A multifactor process. Blood Cells 1988; 14:7.
736. Aminoff D, Ghalambor MA, Henrich CJ: GOST, galactose oxidase and sialyl transferase: Substrate and receptor sites in erythrocyte senescence. In Eaton JW (ed): Erythrocyte Membranes: 2. Recent Clinical and Experimental Advances. New York, Alan R Liss, 1981, p 269.
737. Gattegno L, Bladier D, Garnier M: Changes in carbohydrate content of surface membranes of human erythrocytes during aging. Carbohydr Res 1976; 52:197.
738. Lutz HU, Fehr J: Total sialic acid content of glycophorins during senescence of human red blood cells. J Biol Chem 1979; 254:11177.
739. Seaman GV, Knox RJ, Nordt FJ: Red cell aging: I. Surface charge density and sialic acid content of density-fractionated human erythrocytes. Blood 1977; 50:1001.
740. Beutler E: Biphasic loss of red cell enzyme activity during *in vivo* aging. Prog Clin Biol Res 1985; 95:317.
741. Kay MM: Mechanism of removal of senescent cells by human macrophages *in situ*. Proc Natl Acad Sci USA 1975; 72:3521.
742. Kay MM, Marchalonis JJ, et al: Human erythrocyte aging: Cellular and molecular biology. Transfus Med Rev 1991; 5:173.
743. Schlüter K, Drenckhahn D: Co-clustering of denatured hemoglobin with band 3: Its role in binding of autoantibodies against band 3 to abnormal and aged erythrocytes. Proc Natl Acad Sci USA 1986; 83:6137.
744. Turrini F, Arese P, et al: Clustering of integral membrane proteins of the human erythrocyte membrane stimulates autologous IgG binding, complement deposition, and phagocytosis. J Biol Chem 1991; 266:23611.
745. Beppu M, Mizukami A, et al: Binding of anti-band 3 autoantibody to oxidatively damaged erythrocytes: Formation of senescent antigen on erythrocyte surface by an oxidative mechanism. J Biol Chem 1990; 265:3226.
746. Kay MM, Marchalonis JJ, et al: Definition of a physiologic aging autoantigen by using synthetic peptides of membrane protein band 3: Localization of the active antigenic sites. Proc Natl Acad Sci USA 1990; 87:5734.
747. Lutz HU, Bussolino F, et al: Naturally occurring anti-band-3 antibodies and complement together mediate phagocytosis of oxidatively stressed human erythrocytes. Proc Natl Acad Sci USA 1987; 84:7368.
748. Waugh SM, Willardson BM, et al: Heinz bodies induce clustering of band 3, glycophorin, and ankyrin in sickle cell erythrocytes. J Clin Invest 1986; 78:1155.
749. Kiefer CR, Snyder LM: Oxidation and erythrocyte senescence. Curr Opin Hematol 2000; 7:113.
750. Rettig MP, Low PS, et al: Evaluation of biochemical changes during in vivo erythrocyte senescence in the dog. Blood 1999; 93:376.
751. Winograd E, Greenan JR, Sherman IW: Expression of senescent antigen on erythrocytes infected with a knobby variant of the human malaria parasite *Plasmodium falciparum*. Proc Natl Acad Sci USA 1987; 84:1931.
752. Boas FE, Forman L, Beutler E: Phosphatidylserine exposure and red cell viability in red cell aging and in hemolytic anemia. Proc Natl Acad Sci USA 1998; 95:3077.
753. Herrmann A, Devaux PF: Alteration of the aminophospholipid translocase activity during *in vivo* and artificial aging of human erythrocytes. Biochim Biophys Acta 1990; 1027:41.
754. Wang RH, Phillips G Jr, et al: Activation of the alternative complement pathway by exposure of phosphatidylethanolamine and phosphatidylserine on erythrocytes from sickle cell disease patients. J Clin Invest 1993; 92:1326.
755. Schroit AJ, Madsen JW, Tanaka Y: *In vivo* recognition and clearance of red blood cells containing phosphatidylserine in their plasma membranes. J Biol Chem 1985; 260:5131.
756. Vlassara H, Valinsky J, et al: Advanced glycosylation end products on erythrocyte cell surface induce receptor-mediated phagocytosis by macrophages. A model for turnover of aging cells. J Exp Med 1987; 166:539.
757. Ando K, Beppu M, et al: Membrane proteins of human erythrocytes are modified by advanced glycation end products during aging in the circulation. Biochem Biophys Res Commun 1999; 258:123.
757a. Umudum F, Yucel O, et al: Erythrocyte membrane glycation and NA(+)-K(+) levels in NIDDM. J Diabetes Complications 2002; 16:359.
758. Barber JR, Clarke S: Membrane protein carboxyl methylation increases with human erythrocyte age. J Biol Chem 1983; 258:1189.
759. Galletti P, Ingrosso D, et al: Increased methyl esterification of membrane proteins in aged red-blood cells: Preferential esterification of ankyrin and band-4.1 cytoskeletal proteins. Eur J Biochem 1983; 135:25.
760. Fossati-Jimack L, Azeredo da Silveira S, et al: Selective increase of autoimmune epitope expression on aged erythrocytes in mice: Implications in anti-erythrocyte autoimmune responses. J Autoimmun 2002; 18:17.
761. Vanlair CF, Masius JB: De la microcythemie. Bull R Acad Med Belg 1871; 5:515.
762. Wilson C: Some cases showing hereditary enlargement of the spleen. Trans Clin Soc (London) 1890; 23:162.
763. Wilson C, Stanley D: A sequel to some cases showing hereditary enlargement of the spleen. Trans Clin Soc (London) 1893; 26:163.
764. Minkowski O: Über eine hereditäre, unter dem Bilde eines chronischen Ikterus mit Urobilinurie, Splenomegalie und Nierensiderosis verlaufende Affektion. Verh Dtsch Kongr Med 1900; 18:316.
765. Chauffard MA: Pathogénie de l'ictère congénital de l'adulte. Semaine Méd (Paris) 1907; 27:25.
766. Chauffard MA: Les ictères hémolytiques. Semaine Méd (Paris) 1908; 28:49.
767. Dawson of Penn. The Hume Lectures on haemolytic icterus. BMJ 1931; 1:921, 963.
768. Wintrobe MM: Blood, Pure and Eloquent. New York, McGraw-Hill, 1980.
769. Morton NE, MacKinney AA, et al: Genetics of spherocytosis. Am J Hum Genet 1962; 14:170.
770. Godal HC, Heist H: High prevalence of increased osmotic fragility of red blood cells among Norwegian donors. Scand J Haematol 1981; 27:30.
771. Eber SW, Pekrun A, et al: Prevalence of increased osmotic fragility of erythrocytes in German blood donors: Screening using a modified glycerol lysis test. Ann Hematol 1992; 64:88.
772. Eber SW, Armbrust R, Schröter W: Variable clinical severity of hereditary spherocytosis: Relation to erythrocytic spectrin concentration, osmotic fragility and autohemolysis. J Pediatr 1990; 177:409.
773. Race RR: On the inheritance and linkage relations of acholuric jaundice. Ann Eugenics 1942; 11:365.
774. Miraglia del Giudice E, Lombardi C, et al: Frequent de novo monoallelic expression of β-spectrin gene (SPTB) in children with hereditary spherocytosis and isolated spectrin deficiency. Br J Haematol 1998; 101:251.

775. Miraglia del Giudice E, Nobili B, et al: Clinical and molecular evaluation of non-dominant hereditary spherocytosis. Br J Haematol 2001; 112:42.

776. Whitfield CF, Follweiler JB, et al: Deficiency of α spectrin synthesis in burst-forming units-erythroid in lethal hereditary spherocytosis. Blood 1991; 78:3043.

777. Olim G, Marques S, et al: Red cell abnormalities in a kindred with an uncommon form of hereditary spherocytosis. Acta Méd Portug 1984; 6:137.

778. Bernard J, Boiron M, Estager J: Une grand famille hémolytique: Trieze cas de maladie de Minkowski-Chauffard observés dans la même fratrie. Semaine Hôp Paris 1952; 28:3741.

779. Duru F, Gurgey, A, et al: Homozygosity for dominant form of hereditary spherocytosis. Br J Haematol 1992; 82:596.

780. Agre P, Asimos A, et al: Inheritance pattern and clinical response to splenectomy as a reflection of erythrocyte spectrin deficiency in hereditary spherocytosis. N Engl J Med 1986; 315:1579.

781. Eber SW, Gonzalez JM, et al: Ankyrin-1 mutations are a major cause of dominant and recessive hereditary spherocytosis. Nat Genet 1996; 13:214.

782. Leite RC, Basseres DS, et al: Low frequency of ankyrin mutations in hereditary spherocytosis: Identification of three novel mutations. Hum Mutat 2000; 16:529.

783. Nilson DG, Wong C, et al: A dinucleotide deletion in the downstream promoter element of the ankyrin gene associated with hereditary spherocytosis disrupts promoter function in transgenic mice. Blood 2001; 98:8a.

784. Nakanishi H, Kanzaki A, et al: Ankyrin gene mutations in Japanese patients with hereditary spherocytosis. Int J Hematol 2001; 73:54.

785. Morlé L, Bozon M, et al: Allele Bugey: A de novo deletional frameshift variant in exon 6 of the ankyrin gene associated with spherocytosis. Am J Hematol 1997; 54:242.

786. Randon J, Miraglia del Giudice E, et al: Frequent de novo mutations of the ANK1 gene mimic a recessive mode of transmission in hereditary spherocytosis. Three new ANK1 variants: Ankyrins Bari, Napoli II and Anzio. Br J Haematol 1997; 96:500.

787. Gallagher PG, Ferreira JD, et al: A recurrent frameshift mutation of the ankyrin gene associated with severe hereditary spherocytosis. Br J Haematol 2000; 111:1190.

788. Miraglia del Giudice E, Hayette S, et al: Ankyrin Napoli: A de novo deletional frameshift mutation in exon 16 of ankyrin gene (ANK1) associated with spherocytosis. Br J Haematol 1996; 93:828.

789. Ozcan R, Jarolim P, et al: High frequency of frameshift/nonsense mutations of ankyrin-1 in Czech patients with dominant hereditary spherocytosis (DHS). Blood 1996; 88:5a.

790. Yawata Y, Kanzaki A, et al: Characteristic features of the genotype and phenotype of hereditary spherocytosis in the Japanese population. Int J Hematol 2000; 71:118.

791. Ozcan R, Jarolim P, et al: High frequency of frameshift/nonsense mutations of ankyrin-1 in Czech patients with dominant hereditary spherocytosis. Blood 1996; 88(Suppl 1):10a.

792. Jarolim P, Brabec V, et al: Ankyrin Prague: A dominantly inherited mutation of the regulatory domain of ankyrin associated with hereditary spherocytosis. Blood 1990; 76(Suppl 1):37a.

793. Hayette S, Carre G, et al: Two distinct truncated variants of ankyrin associated with hereditary spherocytosis. Am J Hematol 1998; 58:36.

794. Jarolim P, Rubin HL, et al: A nonsense mutation 1669Glu→Ter within the regulatory domain of human erythroid ankyrin leads to a selective deficiency of the major ankyrin isoform (band 2.1) and a phenotype of autosomal dominant hereditary spherocytosis. J Clin Invest 1995; 95:941.

795. Miraglia del Giudice E, Vallier A, et al: Novel band 3 variants (bands 3 Foggia, Napoli I and Napoli II) associated with hereditary spherocytosis and band 3 deficiency: Status of the D38A polymorphism within the EPB3 locus. Br J Haematol 1997; 96:70.

796. Jarolim P, Murray JL, et al: Characterization of 13 novel band 3 gene defects in hereditary spherocytosis with band 3 deficiency. Blood 1996; 88:4366.

797. Bracher NA, Lyons CA, et al: Band 3 Cape Town (E90K) causes severe hereditary spherocytosis in combination with band 3 Prague III. Br J Haematol 2001; 113:689.

798. Alloisio N, Maillet P, et al: Hereditary spherocytosis with band 3 deficiency. Association with a nonsense mutation of the band 3 gene (allele Lyon), and aggravation by a low-expression allele occurring in trans (allele Genas). Blood 1996; 88:1062.

799. Lima PR, Gontijo JA, et al: Band 3 Campinas: A novel splicing mutation in the band 3 gene (AE1) associated with hereditary spherocytosis, hyperactivity of Na+/Li+ countertransport and an abnormal renal bicarbonate handling. Blood 1997; 90:2810.

800. Dhermy D, Galand C, et al: Heterogenous band 3 deficiency in hereditary spherocytosis related to different band 3 gene defects. Br J Haematol 1997; 98:32.

801. Jarolim P, Palek J, et al: Band 3 Tuscaloosa: Pro^{327}→Arg^{327} substitution in the cytoplasmic domain of erythrocyte band 3 protein associated with spherocytic hemolytic anemia and partial deficiency of protein 4.2. Blood 1992; 80:523.

802. Jenkins PB, Abou-Alfa GK, et al: A nonsense mutation in the erythrocyte band 3 gene associated with decreased mRNA accumulation in a kindred with dominant hereditary spherocytosis. J Clin Invest 1996; 97:373.

803. Ribeiro ML, Alloisio N, et al: Severe hereditary spherocytosis and distal renal tubular acidosis associated with the total absence of band 3. Blood 2000; 96:1602.

804. Alloisio N, Texier P, et al: Modulation of clinical expression and band 3 deficiency in hereditary spherocytosis. Blood 1997; 90:414.

805. Bianchi P, Zanella A, et al: A variant of the EPB3 gene of the anti-Lepore type in hereditary spherocytosis. Br J Haematol 1997; 98:283.

806. Jarolim P, Rubin HL, et al: Mutations of conserved arginines in the membrane domain of erythroid band 3 lead to a decrease in membrane-associated band 3 and to the phenotype of hereditary spherocytosis. Blood 1995; 85:634.

807. Maillet P, Vallier A, et al: Band 3 Chur: A variant associated with band 3-deficient hereditary spherocytosis and substitution in a highly conserved position of transmembrane segment 11. Br J Haematol 1995; 91:804.

808. Jarolim P, Rubin HL, et al: Duplication of 10 nucleotides in the erythroid band 3 (AE1) gene in a kindred with hereditary spherocytosis and band 3 protein deficiency (band 3^{PRAGUE}). J Clin Invest 1994; 93:121.

809. Iwase S, Ideguchi H, et al: Band 3 Tokyo: Thr^{837}→Ala^{837} substitution in erythrocyte band 3 protein associated with spherocytic hemolysis. Acta Haematol 1998; 100:200.

810. Perrotta S, Polito F, et al: Hereditary spherocytosis due to a novel frameshift mutation in AE1 cytoplasmic COOH terminal tail: Band 3 Vesuvio. Blood 1999; 93:2131.

811. Hayette S, Dhermy D, et al: A deletional frameshift mutation in protein 4.2 gene (allele 4.2 Lisboa) associated with hereditary hemolytic anemia. Blood 1995; 85:250.

812. Takaoka Y, Ideguchi H, et al: A novel mutation in the erythrocyte protein 4.2 gene of Japanese patients with hereditary spherocytosis (protein 4.2 Fukuoda). Br J Haematol 1994; 88:527.

813. Bouhassira EE, Schwartz RS, et al: An alanine-to-threonine substitution in protein 4.2 cDNA is associated with a Japanese form of hereditary hemolytic anemia (protein 4.2^{NIPPON}). Blood 1992; 79:1846.

814. Kanzaki A, Yawata Y, et al: Band 4.2 Komatsu: 523 GAT→TAT (175 Asp→Tyr) in exon 4 of the band 4.2 gene associated with total deficiency of band 4.2, hemolytic anemia with ovalostomatocytosis and marked disruption of the cytoskeletal network. Int J Hematol 1995; 61:165.

815. Matsuda M, Hatano N, et al: A novel mutation causing an aberrant splicing in the protein 4.2 gene associated with hereditary spherocytosis (protein 4.2 Notame). Hum Mol Genet 1995; 4:1187.

816. Hayette S, Morle L, et al: A point mutation in the protein 4.2 gene (allele 4.2 Tozeur) associated with hereditary haemolytic anaemia. Br J Haematol 1995; 89:762.

817. Kanzaki A, Yasunaga M, et al: Band 4.2 Shiga: 317 CGC→TGC in compound heterozygotes with 142 GCT→ACT results in band 4.2 deficiency and microspherocytosis. Br J Haematol 1995; 91:333.

818. Beauchamp-Nicoud A, Morle L, et al: Heavy transfusions and presence of an anti-protein 4.2 antibody in 4.2(−) hereditary spherocytosis (949delG). Haematologica 2000; 85:19.

819. Wichterle H, Hanspal M, et al: Combination of two mutant α spectrin alleles underlies a severe spherocytic hemolytic anemia. J Clin Invest 1996; 98:2300.

820. Basseres DS, Vicentim DL, et al: β-Spectrin Promiss-ao: A translation initiation codon mutation of the β-spectrin gene (ATG→GTG) associated with hereditary spherocytosis and spectrin deficiency in a Brazilian family. Blood 1998; 91:368.

821. Garbarz M, Galand C, et al: A 5′ splice region G→C mutation in exon 3 of the human β-spectrin gene leads to decreased levels of β-spectrin mRNA and is responsible for dominant hereditary spherocytosis (spectrin Guemene-Penfao). Br J Haematol 1998; 100:90.

822. Hassoun H, Vassiliadis JN, et al: Characterization of the underlying molecular defect in hereditary spherocytosis associated with spectrin deficiency. Blood 1997; 90:398.

823. Dhermy D, Galand C, et al: Hereditary spherocytosis with spectrin deficiency related to null mutations of the β-spectrin gene. Blood Cells Mol Dis 1998; 24:251.

824. Basseres DS, Duarte AS, et al: β-Spectrin Sta Barbara: A novel frameshift mutation in hereditary spherocytosis associated with detectable levels of mRNA and a germ cell line mosaicism. Br J Haematol 2001; 115:347.

824a. Basseres DS, Tavares AC, et al: beta-Spectrin Sao PauloII, a novel frameshift mutation of the beta-spectrin gene associated with hereditary spherocytosis and instability of the mutant mRNA. Braz J Med Biol Res 2002; 35:921.

825. Hassoun H, Vassiliadis JN, et al: Hereditary spherocytosis with spectrin deficiency due to an unstable truncated β spectrin. Blood 1996; 87:2538.

826. Hassoun H, Vassiliadis JN, et al: Molecular basis of spectrin deficiency in β spectrin Durham. A deletion within β spectrin adjacent to the ankyrin-binding site precludes spectrin attachment to the membrane in hereditary spherocytosis. J Clin Invest 1995; 96:2623.

827. Basseres DS, Tavares AC, et al: Novel β-spectrin variants associated with hereditary spherocytosis. Blood 1997; 90:4b.

828. Savvides P, Shalev O, et al: Combined spectrin and ankyrin deficiency is common in autosomal dominant hereditary spherocytosis. Blood 1993; 82:2953.

829. Agre P, Orringer EP, Bennett V: Deficient red-cell spectrin in severe, recessively inherited spherocytosis. N Engl J Med 1982; 306:1155.

830. Pekrun A, Eber SW, et al: Combined ankyrin and spectrin deficiency in hereditary spherocytosis. Ann Hematol 1993; 67:89.

831. Chasis JA, Agre PA, Mohandas N: Decreased membrane mechanical stability and *in vivo* loss of surface area reflect spectrin deficiencies in hereditary spherocytosis. J Clin Invest 1988; 82:617.

832. Waugh RE, Agre P: Reductions of erythrocyte membrane viscoelastic coefficients reflect spectrin deficiencies in hereditary spherocytosis. J Clin Invest 1988; 81:133.

833. Premetis E, Stamoulakatou A, Loukopoulos D: Erythropoiesis: Hereditary spherocytosis in Greece: Collective data on a large number of patients. Hematology 1999; 4:361.

834. Ricard MP, Gilsanz F, Millan I: Erythroid membrane protein defects in hereditary spherocytosis. A study of 62 Spanish cases. Haematologica 2000; 85:994.

835. Lanciotti M, Perutelli P, et al: Ankyrin deficiency is the most common defect in dominant and non dominant hereditary spherocytosis. Haematologica 1997; 82:460.

836. Miraglia del Giudice E, Iolascon A, et al: Erythrocyte membrane protein alterations underlying clinical heterogeneity in hereditary spherocytosis. Br J Haematol 1994; 88:52.

837. Lee YK, Cho HI, et al: Abnormalities of erythrocyte membrane proteins in Korean patients with hereditary spherocytosis. J Korean Med Sci 2000; 15:284.

838. Agre P, Casella JF, et al: Partial deficiency of erythrocyte spectrin in hereditary spherocytosis. Nature 1985; 314:380.

839. Tse WT, Gallagher PG, et al: Amino-acid substitution in α-spectrin commonly coinherited with nondominant hereditary spherocytosis. Am J Hematol 1997; 54:233.

840. Kimberling WJ, Taylor RA, et al: Linkage and gene localization of hereditary spherocytosis (HS). Blood 1978; 52:859.

841. Fukushima Y, Byers MG, et al: Assignment of the gene for β-spectrin (SPTB) to chromosome 14q23–q24.2 by in situ hybridization. Cytogenet Cell Genet 1990; 53:232.

842. Goodman SR, Shiffer KA, et al: Identification of the molecular defect in the erythrocyte membrane skeleton of some kindreds with hereditary spherocytosis. Blood 1982; 60:772.

843. Wolfe LC, John KM, et al: A genetic defect in the binding of protein 4.1 to spectrin in a kindred with hereditary spherocytosis. N Engl J Med 1982; 307:1367.

844. Becker PS, Morrow JS, Lux SE: Abnormal oxidant sensitivity and β-chain structure of spectrin in hereditary spherocytosis associated with defective spectrin-protein 4.1 binding. J Clin Invest 1987; 80:557.

845. Tyler JM, Hargreaves WR, Branton D: Purification of two spectrin-binding proteins: Biochemical and electron microscopical evidence for site specific reassociation between spectrin bands 2.1 and 4.1. Proc Natl Acad Sci USA 1979; 76:5192.

846. Woods CM, Lazarides E: Spectrin assembly in avian erythroid development is determined by competing reactions of subunit homo- and hetero-oligomerization. Nature 1986; 321:85.

847. Hanspal M, Yoon SH, et al: Molecular basis of spectrin and ankyrin deficiencies in severe hereditary spherocytosis: Evidence implicating a primary defect of ankyrin. Blood 1991; 77:165.

848. Saad ST, Costa FF, et al: Red cell membrane protein abnormalities in hereditary spherocytosis in Brazil. Br J Haematol 1994; 88:295.

849. Rizk SH, Ibrahim AM, et al: Red cell membrane defects and inheritance in 20 Egyptian families with hereditary spherocytosis: Correlation with clinical severity. Cell Vision 1996; 3:137.

850. Chilcote RR, Le Beau MM, et al: Association of red cell spherocytosis with deletion of the short arm of chromosome 8. Blood 1987; 69:156.

851. Cohen H, Walker H, et al: Congenital spherocytosis, B19 parvovirus infection and inherited deletion of the short arm of chromosome 8. Br J Haematol 1991; 78:251.

852. Kitatani M, Chiyo H, et al: Localization of the spherocytosis gene to chromosome segment 8p11.22-8p21.1. Hum Genet 1988; 78:94.

853. Okamoto N, Wada Y, et al: Hereditary spherocytic anemia with deletion of the short arm of chromosome 8. Am J Med Genet 1995; 58:225.

854. Kimberling WJ, Fulbeck T, et al: Localization of spherocytosis to chromosome 8 or 12 and report of a family with spherocytosis and a reciprocal translocation. Am J Hum Genet 1975; 27:586.

855. Costa FF, Agre P, et al: Linkage of dominant hereditary spherocytosis to the gene for the erythrocyte membrane-skeleton protein ankyrin. N Engl J Med 1990; 323:1046.

856. Jarolim P, Rubin HL, et al: Comparison of the ankyrin (AC)$_n$ microsatellites in genomic DNA and mRNA reveals absence of one ankyrin mRNA allele in 20 percent of patients with hereditary spherocytosis. Blood 1995; 85:3278.

857. Gallagher PG, Sabatino DE, et al: Erythrocyte ankyrin promoter mutations associated with recessive hereditary spherocytosis cause significant abnormalities in ankyrin expression. J Biol Chem 2001; 276:41683.

858. Chernova MN, Jarolim P, et al: Overexpression of AE1 Prague, but not of AE1 SAO, inhibits wild-type AE1 trafficking in *Xenopus* oocytes. J Membr Biol 1995; 148:203.

859. Lima PR, Sales TS, et al: Arginine 490 is a hot spot for mutation in the band 3 gene in hereditary spherocytosis. Eur J Haematol 1999; 63:360.

860. Dhermy D, Burnier O, et al: The red blood cell band 3 variant (band 3–iceetrel:R490C) associated with dominant hereditary spherocytosis causes defective membrane targeting of the molecule and a dominant negative effect. Mol Membr Biol 1999; 16:305.

861. Quilty JA, Reithmeier RA: Trafficking and folding defects in hereditary spherocytosis mutants of the human red cell anion exchanger. Traffic 2000; 1:987.

862. Perrotta S, Nigro V, et al: Dominant hereditary spherocytosis due to band 3 Neapolis produces a life-threatening anemia at the homozygous state. Blood 1998; 92:9a.

863. Low PS, Zhang D, Bolin JT: Localization of mutations leading to altered cell shape and anion transport in the crystal structure of the cytoplasmic domain of band 3. Blood Cells Mol Dis 2001; 27:81.

864. Bruce LJ, Cope DL, et al: Familial distal renal tubular acidosis is associated with mutations in the red cell anion exchanger (band 3, AE1) gene. J Clin Invest 1997; 100:1693.

865. Jarolim P, Shayakul C, et al: Autosomal dominant distal renal tubular acidosis is associated in three families with heterozygosity for the R589H mutation in the AE1 (band 3) Cl$^-$/HCO$_3^-$exchanger. J Biol Chem 1998; 273:6380.

866. Karet FE, Gainza FJ, et al: Mutations in the chloride-bicarbonate exchanger gene AE1 cause autosomal dominant but not autosomal recessive distal renal tubular acidosis. Proc Natl Acad Sci USA 1998; 95:6337.

867. Toye AM, Bruce LJ, et al: Band 3 Walton, a C-terminal deletion associated with distal renal tubular acidosis, is expressed in the red cell membrane but retained internally in kidney cells. Blood 2002; 99:342.

868. Inaba M, Yawata A, et al: Defective anion transport and marked spherocytosis with membrane instability caused by hereditary total deficiency of red cell band 3 in cattle due to a nonsense mutation. J Clin Invest 1996; 97:1804.

869. Hassoun H, Hanada T, et al: Complete deficiency of glycophorin A in red blood cells from mice with targeted inactivation of the band 3 (AE1) gene. Blood 1998; 91:2146.

870. Hassoun H, Wang Y, et al: Targeted inactivation of murine band 3 (AE1) gene produces a hypercoagulable state causing widespread thrombosis in vivo. Blood 1998; 92:1785.

871. Paw BH: Cloning of the zebrafish retsina blood mutation: A genetic model for dyserythropoiesis and erythroid cytokinesis. Blood Cells Mol Dis 2001; 27:62.

872. Perrotta S, Iolascon A, et al: 4.2 Nippon mutation in a non-Japanese patient with hereditary spherocytosis. Haematologica 1999; 84:660.

873. Ideguchi H, Nishimura J, et al: A genetic defect of erythrocyte band 4.2 protein associated with hereditary spherocytosis. Br J Haematol 1990; 74:347.

874. Ghanem A, Pothier B, et al: A haemolytic syndrome associated with the complete absence of red cell membrane protein 4.2 in two Tunisian siblings. Br J Haematol 1990; 75:414.

875. Inoue T, Kanzaki A, et al: Homozygous missense mutation (band 3 Fukuoka: G130R): A mild form of hereditary spherocytosis with near-normal band 3 content and minimal changes of membrane ultrastructure despite moderate protein 4.2 deficiency. Br J Haematol 1998; 102:932.

876. Sheehy R, Ralston GB: Abnormal binding of spectrin to the membrane of erythrocytes in some cases of hereditary spherocytosis. Blut 1978; 36:145.

877. Price Evans DA, Mackie MJ, Anand R: Diminished extractable spectrin in the erythrocytes of a patient with 'sporadic' hereditary spherocytosis. Acta Haematol 1986; 76:136.

878. Mariani M, Maretzki D, Lutz HU: A tightly membrane-associated subpopulation of spectrin is ^{3}H palmitoylated. J Biol Chem 1993; 268:12996.

879. Allen DW, Cadman S, et al: Increased membrane binding of erythrocyte catalase in hereditary spherocytosis and in metabolically stressed normal cells. Blood 1977; 49:113.

880. Boulard-Heitzmann P, Boulard M, et al: Decreased red cell enolase activity in a 40-year-old woman with compensated hemolysis. Scand J Haematol 1984; 33:401.

881. Lachant NA, Jennings MA, Tanaka KR: Partial erythrocyte enolase deficiency: A hereditary disorder with variable clinical expression. Blood 1986; 68(Suppl 1):55a.

882. Lux SE: Disorders of the red cell membrane. In Nathan DG, Oski FA (eds): Hematology of Infancy and Childhood, 3rd ed. Philadelphia, WB Saunders, 1987, p 444.

883. Beutler E, Guinto E, Johnson C: Human red cell protein kinase in normal subjects and patients with hereditary spherocytosis, sickle cell disease, and autoimmune hemolytic anemia. Blood 1976; 48:887.

884. Boivin P, Delaunay J, Galand C: Altered erythrocyte membrane protein phosphorylation in an unusual case of hereditary spherocytosis. Scand J Haematol 1979; 23:251.

885. Wolfe LC, Lux SE: Membrane protein phosphorylation of intact normal and hereditary spherocytic erythrocytes. J Biol Chem 1978; 253:3336.

886. De Gier J, Van Deenen LLM: Phospholipid and fatty acid characteristics of erythrocytes in some cases of anaemia. Br J Haematol 1964; 10:2546.

887. Vermeulen WP, Briede JJ, et al: Enhanced Mg^{2+}-ATPase activity in ghosts from HS erythrocytes and in normal ghosts stripped of membrane skeletal proteins may reflect enhanced aminophospholipid translocase activity. Br J Haematol 1995; 90:56.

888. Kuiper PJ, Livne A: Differences in fatty acid composition between normal erythrocytes and hereditary spherocytosis affected cells. Biochim Biophys Acta 1972; 260:755.

889. Zail SS, Pickering A: Fatty acid composition of erythrocytes in hereditary spherocytosis. Br J Haematol 1979; 42:399.

890. Kanzake A, Ikeda A, Yawata Y: Membrane studies on rod-shaped red cells in hereditary elliptocytosis: Least hemolysis and normal sodium influx with decreased membrane lipids. Br J Haematol 1988; 70:105.

891. Bertles JE: Sodium transport across the surface of red blood cells in hereditary spherocytosis. J Clin Invest 1957; 36:816.

892. Jacob HS, Jandl JH: Cell membrane permeability in the pathogenesis of hereditary spherocytosis (HS). J Clin Invest 1964; 43:1704.

893. Zipursky A, Israels LG: Significance of erythrocyte sodium flux in the pathophysiology and genetic expression of hereditary spherocytosis. Pediatr Res 1971; 5:614.

894. Joiner CH, Franco RS, et al: Increased cation permeability in mutant mouse red cells with defective membrane skeletons. Blood 1994; 86:4307.

895. Wiley JS: Red cell survival in hereditary spherocytosis. J Clin Invest 1970; 49:666.

896. De Franceschi L, Olivieri O, et al: Membrane cation and anion transport activities in erythrocytes of hereditary spherocytosis: Effects of different membrane protein defects. Am J Hematol 1997; 55:121.

897. Vives Corrons JL, Besson I: Red cell membrane Na^+ transport systems in hereditary spherocytosis: Relevance to understanding the increased Na^+ permeability. Ann Hematol 2001; 80:535.

898. Mayman D, Zipursky A: Hereditary spherocytosis: The metabolism of erythrocytes in the peripheral blood and in the splenic pulp. Br J Haematol 1974; 27:201.

899. Palek J, Mirevova L, Brabec V: 2,3-Diphosphoglycerate metabolism in hereditary spherocytosis. Br J Haematol 1969; 17:59.

900. Olivieri O, Bonollo M, et al: Activation of K^+/Cl^- cotransport in human erythrocytes exposed to oxidative agents. Biochim Biophys Acta 1993; 1176:37.

901. Loder PB, Babarczy G, de Gruchy GC: Red cell metabolism in hereditary spherocytosis. Br J Haematol 1967; 13:95.

902. Mohler DN: Adenosine triphosphate metabolism in hereditary spherocytosis. J Clin Invest 1965; 44:1417.

903. Fernandez LA, Erslev AJ: Oxygen affinity and compensated hemolysis in hereditary spherocytosis. J Lab Clin Med 1972; 80:780.

904. Kagimoto T, Hayashi F, et al: Phosphorus ^{31}NMR study on nucleotides and intracellular pH of hereditary spherocytes. Experientia (Basel) 1978; 34:1092.

905. Ideguchi H, Hamasaki N, Ikehara Y: Abnormal phosphoenolpyruvate transport in erythrocytes of hereditary spherocytosis. Blood 1981; 58:426.

906. Eber SW, Cho M, et al: Increased band 3 mobility and decreased anion transport in ankyrin deficient hereditary spherocytes. Blood 1993; 82(Suppl 1):175a.

907. Peters LL, Barker JE: Spontaneous and targeted mutations in erythrocyte membrane skeleton genes: Mouse models of hereditary spherocytosis. In Zon LI (ed): Hematopoiesis. New York, Oxford University Press, 1999.

908. Bloom ML, Kaysser TM, et al: The murine mutation jaundiced is caused by replacement of an arginine with a stop codon in the mRNA encoding the ninth repeat of β-spectrin. Proc Natl Acad Sci USA 1994; 91:10099.

909. Wandersee NJ, Birkenmeier CS, et al: Murine recessive hereditary spherocytosis, *sph/sph*, is caused by a mutation in the erythroid α-spectrin gene. Hematol. J. 2000; 1:235.

910. Wandersee NJ, Birkenmeier CS, et al: Identification of three mutations in the murine erythroid α-spectrin gene causing hereditary spherocytosis in mice. Blood 1998; 92:8a.

911. White RA, Birkenmeier CS, et al: Ankyrin and the hemolytic anemia mutation, *nb*, map to mouse chromosome 8: Presence of the *nb* allele is associated with a truncated erythrocyte ankyrin. Proc Natl Acad Sci USA 1990; 87:3117.

912. Birkenmeier CS, Gifford EJ, et al: Mutations of the erythroid ankyrin gene: A hypomorph and a null. Blood 2000; 96:594a.

913. d'Ermao N, Levi M: Neurological symptoms in anemia. In Neurological Symptoms in Blood Diseases. Baltimore, University Park Press, 1972, p 1.

914. McCann SR, Jacob HS: Spinal cord disease in hereditary spherocytosis: Report of two cases with a hypothesized common mechanism for neurologic and red cell abnormalities. Blood 1976; 48:259.

915. Curshmann H: Über funikuläre Myelose bei hämolytischem Ikterus. Dtsch A Nervenheilkd 1931; 122:119.

916. Dumolard C, Sarrovy C, Portier A: Ataxie cerebelleuse assoc iée à un syndrome de splenomegalie chronique avec anemie. Bull Soc Med Hop (Paris) 1938; 54:71.

917. Lemaire A, Dumolard A, Portici A: Deux cas familiaux de maladie de Friedreich avec maladie hemolytique chez des indigenes Algeriens. Bull Soc Med Hop (Paris) 1937; 53:1084.

918. Michelazzi AM: Anemia emolitica familiare con sinomatoligia nervosa. Rass Fisiopat Clin Ter 1940; 12:145.

919. Percorella F: Sindrome neuroanemica in soggetto con ittero imolitico familiare. Riv Clin Pediatr 1946; 44:690.

920. Salmon H: Hämolytischer Ikterus und Degeneration der Hinterstränge. Med Klin 1914; 10:312c.

921. Spencer SE, Walker FO, Moore SA: Chorea-amyotrophy with chronic hemolytic anemia: A variant of chorea-amyotrophy with acanthocytosis. Neurology 1987; 37:645.

922. Peters LL, White RA, et al: Changes in cytoskeletal mRNA expression and protein synthesis during murine erythropoiesis *in vivo*. Proc Natl Acad Sci USA 1992; 89:5749.

923. Peters LL, Turtzo C, et al: Distinct fetal *Ank-1* and *Ank-2* related proteins and mRNAs in normal and *nb/nb* mice. Blood 1993; 81:2144.

924. Anderson R, Huestis RR, Motulsky AG: Hereditary spherocytosis in the deer mouse. Its similarity to the human disease. Blood 1960; 15:491.

925. LeBlond PF, De Boisfleury A, Bessis M: Erythrocytes shape in hereditary spherocytosis. A scanning electron microscopic study and relationship to deformability. Nouv Rev Fr Hematol 1973; 13:873.

926. Cooper RA, Jandl JH: The role of membrane lipids in the survival of red cells in hereditary spherocytosis. J Clin Invest 1969; 48:736.

927. Johnsson R: Red cell membrane proteins and lipids in spherocytosis. Scand J Haematol 1978; 20:341.

928. Langley GR, Feldherhof CH: Atypical autohemolysis in hereditary spherocytosis as a reflection of two cell populations: Relationship of cell lipids to conditioning by the spleen. Blood 1968; 32:569.

929. Reed CF, Swisher SN: Erythrocyte lipid loss in hereditary spherocytosis. J Clin Invest 1966; 45:777.

930. Waugh RE: Effects of inherited membrane abnormalities on the viscoelastic properties of erythrocyte membranes. Biophys J 1987; 51:363.

931. Cooper RA, Jandl JH: The selective and conjoint loss of red cell lipids. J Clin Invest 1969; 48:906.

932. Snyder LM, Lutz HU, et al: Fragmentation and myelin formation in hereditary xerocytosis and other hemolytic anemias. Blood 1978; 52:750.

933. Weed RI, Bowdler AJ: Metabolic dependence of the critical hemolytic volume of human erythrocytes: Relationship to osmotic fragility and autohemolysis in hereditary spherocytosis and normal red cells. J Clin Invest 1966; 45:1137.

934. Zachée P, Boogaerts MA, et al: Adverse role of the spleen in hereditary spherocytosis: Evidence by the use of the atomic force microscope. Br J Haematol 1992; 80:264.

935. Evans EA, Waugh R, Melnik C: Elastic area compressibility modulus of red cell membranes. Biophys J 1976; 16:585.

936. Baird R, McPherson AI, Richmond J: Red blood cell survival after splenectomy in congenital spherocytosis. Lancet 1971; 2:1060.

937. Chapman RG: Red cell life span after splenectomy in hereditary spherocytosis. J Clin Invest 1968; 47:2263.

938. Barnhart MI, Lusher JM: The human spleen as revealed by scanning electron microscopy. Am J Hematol 1976; 1:243.

939. Chen L-T, Weiss L: Electron microscopy of red pulp of human spleen. Am J Anat 1972; 134:425.

940. Chen L-T, Weiss L: The role of the sinus wall in the passage of erythrocytes through the spleen. Blood 1973; 41:529.

941. Weiss L, Tavassoli M: Anatomical hazards to the passage of erythrocytes through the spleen. Semin Hematol 1970; 7:372.

942. Weiss L: A scanning electron microscopic study of the spleen. Blood 1974; 43:665.

943. Groom AC: Microcirculation of the spleen: New concepts, new challenges. Microvasc Res 1987; 34:269.

944. Johnsson R, Vuopio P: Studies on red cell flexibility in spherocytosis using a polycarbonate membrane filtration method. Acta Haematol 1978; 60:329.

945. Murphy JR: The influence of pH and temperature on some physical properties of normal erythrocytes and erythrocytes from patients with hereditary spherocytosis. J Lab Clin Med 1967; 69:758.

946. Young LE, Platzer RF, et al: Hereditary spherocytosis: II. Observations on the role of the spleen. Blood 1951; 6:1099.

947. Ferreira JA, Feliu E, et al: Morphologic and morphometric light and electron microscopic studies of the spleen in patients with hereditary spherocytosis and autoimmune haemolytic anaemia. Br J Haematol 1989; 72:246.

948. Molnar Z, Rappaport H: Fine structure of the red pulp of the spleen in hereditary spherocytosis. Blood 1972; 39:81.

949. Wiland OK, Smith EB: The morphology of the spleen in congenital hemolytic anemia (hereditary spherocytosis). Am J Clin Pathol 1956; 26:619.

950. Fujita T, Kashimura M, Adachi K: Scanning electron microscopy (SEM) studies of the spleen-normal and pathological. Scan Electron Microsc 1982; 1:435.

951. Banti G: Splenomegalie hemolytique au hemopoietique: Le role de la rate dans l'hemolyse. Sémaine Med 1913; 33:313.

952. MacAdam W, Shiskin C: The cholesterol content of the blood in anaemia and its relation to splenic function. Q J Med 1922; 16:193.

953. Emerson CP Jr, Shen SC, et al: Studies on the destruction of red blood cells: IX. Quantitative methods for determining the osmotic and mechanical fragility of red cells in the peripheral blood and splenic pulp; the mechanism of increased hemolysis in hereditary spherocytosis (congenital hemolytic jaundice) as related to the function of the spleen. Arch Intern Med 1956; 97:1.

954. Dacie JV: Familial haemolytic anaemia (acholuric jaundice), with particular reference to changes in fragility produced by splenectomy. Q J Med (New Series) 1943; 12:101.

955. Griggs RC, Weisman R Jr, Harris JW: Alterations in osmotic and mechanical fragility related to *in vivo* erythrocyte aging and splenic sequestration in hereditary spherocytosis. J Clin Invest 1960; 39:89.

956. MacPherson AIS, Richmond J, et al: The role of the spleen in congenital spherocytosis. Am J Med 1971; 50:35.

957. Jandl JH, Aster RH: Increased splenic pooling and the pathogenesis of hypersplenism. Am J Med Sci 1967; 253:383.

958. LaCelle PL: pH in the mouse spleen and its effect on erythrocyte flow properties. Blood 1974; 44(Suppl 1):910.

959. Minakami S, Yoshikawa HL: Studies on erythrocyte glycolysis: III. The effects of active cation transport, pH and inorganic phosphate concentration on erythrocyte glycolysis. J Biochem (Tokyo) 1966; 59:145.

960. Rakitzis ET, Mills GC: Relation of red cell hexokinase activity to extracellular pH. Biochim Biophys Acta 1967; 141:439.

961. Parker JC: Ouabain-insensitive effects of metabolism on ion and water content in red blood cells. Am J Physiol 1971; 221:338.

962. Ingrosso D, D'Angelo S, et al: Cytoskeletal behaviour in spectrin and in band 3 deficient spherocytic red cells: Evidence for differentiated splenic conditioning role. Br J Haematol 1996; 93:38.

963. Dacie JV: Observations on autohemolysis in familial acholuric jaundice. J Pathol Bacteriol 1941; 52:331.

964. Ferrant A, Leners N, et al: The spleen and haemolysis: Evaluation of the intrasplenic transit time. Br J Haematol 1987; 65:331.

965. Motulsky AG, Casserd F, et al: Anemia and the spleen. N Engl J Med 1958; 259:1164, 1212.

966. Prankerd TAJ: Studies on the pathogenesis of haemolysis in hereditary spherocytosis. Q J Med 1960; 24:199.

967. Maridonneau I, Braquet P, Garay RP: Na⁺ and K⁺ transport damage induced by oxygen free radicals in human red cell membranes. J Biol Chem 1983; 258:3107.

968. Orringer EP, Parker JC: Selective increase of potassium permeability in red blood cells exposed to acetylphenylhydrazine. Blood 1977; 50:1013.

969. Orringer EP: A further characterization of the selective K movements observed in human red blood cells following acetylphenylhydrazine exposure. Am J Hematol 1984; 16:355.

970. Wiater LA, Dunham PB: Passive transport of K⁺ and Na⁺ in human red blood cells: Sulfhydryl binding agents and furosemide. Am J Physiol 1983; 245:C348.

971. Becker PS, Cohen CM, Lux SE: The effect of mild diamide oxidation on the structure and function of human erythrocyte spectrin. J Biol Chem 1986; 261:4620.

972. Caprari P, Bozzi A, et al: Oxidative erythrocyte membrane damage in hereditary spherocytosis. Biochem Int 1992; 26:265.

973. Platt OS, Falcone JF: Membrane protein lesions in erythrocytes with Heinz bodies. J Clin Invest 1988; 82:1051.

974. Schwartz RS, Rybicki AC, et al: Protein 4.1 in sickle erythrocytes. Evidence for oxidative damage. J Biol Chem 1987; 62:15666.

975. Malorni W, Iosi F, et al: A new, striking morphologic feature for the human erythrocyte in hereditary spherocytosis: The blebbing pattern. Blood 1993; 81:2821.

976. De Matteis MC, De Angelis V, et al: Role of spleen in hereditary spherocytosis: Evidence for increased in vitro proteolysis of red cell membrane. Br J Haematol 1991; 79:108.

977. Szymanski IO, Odgren PR, et al: Red blood cell associated IgG in normal and pathologic states. Blood 1980; 55:48.

978. Coleman DH, Finch CA: Effect of adrenal steroids in hereditary spherocytic anemia. J Lab Clin Med 1956; 47:602.

979. Duru F, Gürgey A: Effect of corticosteroids in hereditary spherocytosis. Acta Paediatr Jpn 1994; 36:666.

980. Atkinson JP, Schreiber AS, Frank MM: Effects of corticosteroids and splenectomy on the immune clearance and destruction of erythrocytes. J Clin Invest 1973; 52:1509.

981. Schreiber AD, Parsons J, et al: Effect of corticosteroids on the human monocyte IgG and complement receptors. J Clin Invest 1975; 56:1189.

982. Matsumoto N, Ishihara T, et al: Electron microscopic studies of the spleen and liver in hereditary spherocytosis. Acta Pathol Jpn 1973; 23:507.

983. Bowman HS, Oski FA: Splenic macrophage interaction with red cells in pyruvate kinase deficiency and hereditary spherocytosis. Vox Sang 1970; 19:168.

984. Friedman EW, Williams JC, Van Hook L: Hereditary spherocytosis in the elderly. Am J Med 1988; 84:513.

985. Krueger HC, Burgert EO Jr: Hereditary spherocytosis in 100 children. Mayo Clin Proc 1966; 41:821.

986. MacKinney AA Jr, Morton NE, et al: Ascertaining genetic carriers of hereditary spherocytosis by statistical analysis of multiple laboratory tests. J Clin Invest 1962; 41:554.

987. Young LE, Izzo MJ, Platzer RF: Hereditary spherocytosis: I. Clinical, hematologic and genetic features in 28 cases, with particular reference to the osmotic and mechanical fragility of incubated erythrocytes. Blood 1951; 6:1073.

988. Debre R, Lamy M, et al: Congenital and familial hemolytic disease in children. Am J Dis Child 1938; 56:1189.

989. Diamond LK: Indications for splenectomy in childhood: Results in fifty-two operated cases. Am J Surg 1938; 39:400.

990. Jensson O, Jonasson JL, et al: Studies on hereditary spherocytosis in Iceland. Acta Med Scand 1977; 201:187.

991. Gehlbach SH, Cooper BA: Haemolytic anaemia in infectious mononucleosis due to inapparent congenital spherocytosis. Scand J Haematol 1970; 7:141.

992. Ho-Yen DO: Hereditary spherocytosis presenting in pregnancy. Acta Haematol (Basel) 1984; 72:29.

993. Pajor A, Lehoczky D, Szakacs Z: Pregnancy and hereditary spherocytosis: Report of 8 patients and a review. Arch Gynecol Obstet 1993; 253:37.

994. Garwicz S: Atypical spherocytosis, a disease of spleen as well as of red blood cells. Lancet 1975; 1:956.

995. Guarnone R, Centenara E, et al: Erythropoietin production and erythropoiesis in compensated and anaemic states of hereditary spherocytosis. Br J Haematol 1996; 92:150.

996. Maberry MC, Mason RA, et al: Pregnancy complicated by hereditary spherocytosis. Obstet Gynecol 1992; 79:735.

997. Delamore IW, Richmond J, Davies SH: Megaloblastic anaemia in congenital spherocytosis. BMJ 1961; 1:543.

998. Kohler HG, Meynell MJ, Cooke WT: Spherocytic anaemia, complicated by megaloblastic anaemia of pregnancy. BMJ 1960; 1:779.

999. Burman D: Congenital spherocytosis in infancy. Arch Dis Child 1958; 33:335.

1000. Schröter W, Kahsnitz E: Diagnosis of hereditary spherocytosis in newborn infants. J Pediatr 1983; 103:460.

1001. Trucco JI, Brown AK: Neonatal manifestations of hereditary spherocytosis. Am J Dis Child 1967; 113:263.

1002. Stamey CC, Diamond LK: Congenital hemolytic anemia in the newborn. Am J Dis Child 1957; 94:616.

1003. Iolascon A, Faienza MF, et al: UGT1 promoter polymorphism accounts for increased neonatal appearance of hereditary spherocytosis. Blood 1998; 91:1093.

1004. Delhommeau F, Cynober T, et al: Natural history of hereditary spherocytosis during the first year of life. Blood 2000; 95:393.

1005. Bergstrand CG, Czar B: Serum haptoglobin in infancy. J Clin Lab Invest 1961; 13:576.

1006. Erlandson ME, Hilgartner M: Hemolytic disease in the neonatal period and early infancy. J Pediatr 1959; 54:566.

1007. Miraglia del Giudice E, Perrotta S, et al: Decision making at the bedside: Diagnosis of hereditary spherocytosis in a transfused infant. Haematologica 1998; 83:347.

1008. Tchernia G, Delhommeau F, et al: Recombinant erythropoietin therapy as an alternative to blood transfusions in infants with hereditary spherocytosis. Hematol J 2000; 1:146.

1009. Palek J, Sahr KE: Mutations of the red blood cell membrane proteins: From clinical evaluation to detection of the underlying genetic defect. Blood 1992; 80:308.

1010. LeBlond PF, LaCelle PL, Weed RI: Rheological properties of erythroblasts and erythrocytes in congenital spherocytosis. Nouv Rev Fr Hematol 1971; 11:537.

1011. Wiley JS, Firkin BG: An unusual variant of hereditary spherocytosis. Am J Med 1970; 48:63.

1012. Maizels M: The anion and cation content of normal and anaemic bloods. Biochem J 1936; 30:821.

1013. Selwyn JG, Dacie JV: Autohemolysis and other changes resulting from the incubation in vitro of red cells from patients with congenital hemolytic anemia. Blood 1954; 9:414.

1014. Mohandas N, Kim YR, et al: Accurate and independent measurement of volume and hemoglobin concentration of individual red cells by laser light scattering. Blood 1986; 68:506.

1015. Michaels LA, Cohen AR, et al: Screening for hereditary spherocytosis by use of automated erythrocyte indexes. J Pediatr 1997; 130:957.

1016. Gilsanz F, Ricard MP, Millan I: Diagnosis of hereditary spherocytosis with dual-angle differential light scattering. Am J Clin Pathol 1993; 100:119.

1017. Pati AR, Patton WN, Harris RI: The use of the Technicon H1 in the diagnosis of hereditary spherocytosis. Clin Lab Haematol 1989; 11:27.

1018. Ricard MP, Gilsanz F: Assessment of the severity of hereditary spherocytosis using routine haematological data obtained with dual angle laser scattering cytometry. Clin Lab Haematol 1996; 18:75.

1019. Parpart AK, Lorenz PB, et al: The osmotic resistance (fragility) of human red cells. J Clin Invest 1947; 26:636.

1020. Godal HC, Nyvold N, Russtad A: The osmotic fragility of red blood cells: A re-evaluation of technical conditions. Scand J Haematol 1979; 23:55.

1021. Young LE: Observations on inheritance and heterogeneity of chronic spherocytosis. Trans Assoc Am Phys 1955; 68:141.

1022. Fernandez-Alberti A, Fink NE: Red blood cell osmotic fragility confidence intervals: A definition by application of a mathematical model. Clin Chem Lab Med 2000; 38:433.

1023. Jacob HS: Hereditary spherocytosis: A disease of the red cell membrane. Semin Hematol 1965; 2:139.

1024. Johnsson R, Salminen S: Effect of ouabain on osmotic resistance and monovalent cation transport of red cells in hereditary spherocytosis. Scand J Haematol 1980; 29:323.

1025. Godal HC, Gjonnes G, Ruyter R: Does preincubation of the red blood cells contribute to the capacity of the osmotic fragility test to detect very mild forms of hereditary spherocytosis? Scand J Haematol 1982; 29:89.

1026. Judkiewicz L, Bartosz G, et al: Modified osmotic fragility test for the laboratory diagnosis of hereditary spherocytosis. Am J Hematol 1989; 31:136.

1027. Clark MR, Mohandas N, Shohet SB: Osmotic gradient ektacytometry: Comprehensive characterization of red cell volume and surface maintenance. Blood 1983; 61:899.

1028. Johnson RM, Ravindranath Y: Osmotic scan ektacytometry in clinical diagnosis. J Pediatr Hematol Oncol 1996; 18:122.

1029. Zanella A, Milani S, et al: Diagnostic value of the glycerol lysis test. J Lab Clin Med 1983; 102:743.

1030. Zanella A, Izzo C, et al: Acidified glycerol lysis test: A screening test for spherocytosis. Br J Haematol 1980; 45:481.

1031. Rutherford CJ, Postlewaight BF, Hallowes M: An evaluation of the acidified glycerol lysis test. Br J Haematol 1986; 63:119.

1032. Bucx MJ, Breed WP, Hoffman JJ: Comparison of acidified glycerol lysis test, Pink test and osmotic fragility test in hereditary spherocytosis: Effect of incubation. Eur J Haematol 1988; 40:227.

1033. Hoffmann JJ, Swaak-Lammers N, et al: Diagnostic utility of the pre-incubated acidified glycerol lysis test in haemolytic and non-haemolytic anaemias. Eur J Haematol 1991; 47:367.

1034. Marik T, Brabec V: Acidified glycerol lysis test in various haemolytic anaemias. Folia Haematol Int Mag Klin Morphol Blutforsch 1990; 117:259.

1035. Vettore L, Zanella A, et al: A new test for the laboratory diagnosis of spherocytosis. Acta Haematol (Basel) 1984; 72:258.

1036. Sureda-Balari A, Villarrvoia-Espinosa J, Fernandez-Fuertes I: A new modification of the 'Pink test' for the diagnosis of hereditary spherocytosis. Acta Haematol 1989; 82:213.

1037. Pinto L, Iolascon A, et al: A modification of the `Pink test' may improve the diagnosis of hereditary spherocytosis. Acta Haematol 1989; 82:53.

1038. Streichman S, Gesheidt Y, Tatarsky I: Hypertonic cryohemolysis: A diagnostic test for hereditary spherocytosis. Am J Hematol 1990; 35:104.

1039. Iglauer A, Reinhardt D, et al: Cryohemolysis test as a diagnostic tool for hereditary spherocytosis. Ann Hematol 1999; 78:555.

1040. Streichman S, Gescheidt Y: Cryohemolysis for the detection of hereditary spherocytosis: Correlation studies with osmotic fragility and autohemolysis. Am J Hematol 1998; 58:206.

1041. Young LE, Izzo MJ, et al: Studies on spontaneous *in vitro* autohemolysis in hemolytic disorders. Blood 1956; 11:977.

1042. Cutillo S, Pinto L, et al: Spectrin/band 3 ratio as diagnostic tool in hereditary spherocytosis. Eur J Pediatr 1992; 151:35.

1043. King MJ, Behrens J, et al: Rapid flow cytometric test for the diagnosis of membrane cytoskeleton-associated haemolytic anaemia. Br J Haematol 2000; 111:924.

1044. Watson CJ: Studies of urobilinogen. III. The per diem excretion of urobilinogen in the common forms of jaundice and disease of the liver. Arch Intern Med 1937; 59:206.

1045. Sears DA, Anderson RP, et al: Urinary iron excretion and renal metabolism of hemoglobin in hemolytic disease. Blood 1966; 28:708.

1046. Muller-Eberhard U, Javid J, et al: Plasma concentrations of hemopexin, haptoglobin and heme in patients with various hemolytic diseases. Blood 1968; 32:811.

1047. Gairdner D: The association of gall-stones with acholuric jaundice in children. Arch Dis Child 1939; 14:109.

1048. Bates GC, Brown CH: Incidence of gallbladder disease in chronic hemolytic anemia (spherocytosis). Gastroenterology 1952; 21:104.

1049. Lawrie GM, Ham JM: The surgical treatment of hereditary spherocytosis. Surg Gynecol Obstet 1974; 139:208.

1050. MacKinney AA Jr: Hereditary spherocytosis. Clinical family studies. Arch Intern Med 1965; 116:257.

1051. del Giudice EM, Perrotta S, et al: Coinheritance of Gilbert syndrome increases the risk for developing gallstones in patients with hereditary spherocytosis. Blood 1999; 94:2259.

1052. Sharma S, Vukelja SJ, Kadakia S: Gilbert's syndrome co-existing with and masking hereditary spherocytosis. Ann Hematol 1997; 74:287.

1053. Katz ME, Weinstein IM: Extreme hyperbilirubinemia in a patient with hereditary spherocytosis, Gilbert's syndrome, and obstructive jaundice. Am J Med Sci 1978; 275:373.

1054. Tissieres P, Kernen Y, et al: Varicella zoster virus induced haemolytic crisis in a child with congenital spherocytosis. Eur J Pediatr 2000; 159:788.

1055. Brown KE: Haematological consequences of parvovirus B19 infection. Baillieres Best Pract Res Clin Haematol 2000; 13:245.

1056. Cherry JD: Parvovirus infections in children and adults. Adv Pediatr 1999; 46:245.

1057. Owren PA: Congenital hemolytic jaundice. The pathogenesis of the hemolytic crisis. Blood 1948; 3:231.

1058. Lefrére JJ, Courouce AM, et al: Human parvovirus and aplastic crisis in chronic hemolytic anemias: A study of 24 observations. Am J Hematol 1986; 23:271.

1059. Mortimer PP, Humphries RK, et al: A human parvovirus-like virus inhibits haematopoietic colony formation *in vitro*. Nature 1983; 302:426.

1060. Ozawa K, Kurtzman G, Young N: Replication of the B19 parvovirus in human bone marrow cell cultures. Science 1986; 233:883.

1061. Yaegashi N, Niinuma T, et al: Parvovirus B19 infection induces apoptosis of erythroid cells in vitro and in vivo. J Infect 1999; 39:68.

1062. Morita E, Tada K, et al: Human parvovirus B19 induces cell cycle arrest at G_2 phase with accumulation of mitotic cyclins. J Virol 2001; 75:7555.

1063. Hanada T, Koike K, et al: Human parvovirus B19-induced transient pancytopenia in a child with hereditary spherocytosis. Br J Haematol 1988; 70:113.

1064. Saunders PW, Reid MM, Cohen BJ: Human parvovirus induced cytopenias: A report of five cases. Br J Haematol 1986; 53:407.

1065. Goss GA, Szer J: Pancytopenia following infection with human parvovirus B19 as a presenting feature of hereditary spherocytosis in two siblings. Aust NZ J Med 1997; 27:86.

1066. von Kaisenberg CS, Jonat W: Fetal parvovirus B19 infection. Ultrasound Obstet Gynecol 2001; 18:280.

1067. Markenson GR, Yancey MK: Parvovirus B19 infections in pregnancy. Semin Perinatol 1998; 22:309.

1068. Rodis JF: Parvovirus infection. Clin Obstet Gynecol 1999; 42:107.

1069. Bell LM, Nasides SJ, et al: Human parvovirus B19 infection among hospital staff members after contact with infected patients. N Engl J Med 1989; 321:485.

1070. Brown KE, Young NS: Epidemiology and pathology of erythroviruses. Contrib Microbiol 2000; 4:107.

1071. Valeur-Jensen AK, Pedersen CB, et al: Risk factors for parvovirus B19 infection in pregnancy. JAMA 1999; 281:1099.

1072. Rodis JF, Borgida AF, et al: Management of parvovirus infection in pregnancy and outcomes of hydrops: A survey of members of the Society of Perinatal Obstetricians. Am J Obstet Gynecol 1998; 179:985.

1073. Robins MM: Familial crisis in hereditary spherocytosis: Report of six affected siblings. Clin Pediatr 1965; 4:210.

1074. Skinnider LF, McSheffrey BJ, et al: Congenital spherocytic hemolytic anemia in a family presenting with transient red cell aplasia from parvovirus B19 infection. Am J Hematol 1998; 58:341.

1075. Murphy PT, O'Donnell JR: B19 parvovirus infection causing aplastic crisis in 3 out of 5 family members with hereditary spherocytosis. Ir J Med Sci 1990; 159:182.

1076. Green DH, Bellingham AJ, Anderson MJ: Parvovirus infection in a family associated with aplastic crisis in an affected sibling pair with hereditary spherocytosis. J Clin Pathol 1984; 37:1144.

1077. Ozawa K, Kurtzman G, Young N: Productive infection by B19 parvovirus of human erythroid bone marrow cells *in vitro*. Blood 1987; 70:384.

1078. Koduri PR: Novel cytomorphology of the giant proerythroblasts of parvovirus B19 infection. Am J Hematol 1998; 58:95.

1079. Lefrére JJ, Courouce A-M, et al: Six cases of hereditary spherocytosis revealed by human parvovirus infection. Br J Haematol 1986; 62:653.

1080. Megason GC, Smith JC, Iyer RV: Aplastic crisis due to human parvovirus (B19) as an initial presentation of hereditary spherocytosis. J Miss State Med Assoc 1993; 34:107.

1081. Ng JP, Cumming RL, et al: Hereditary spherocytosis revealed by human parvovirus infection. Br J Haematol 1987; 65:379.

1082. Summerfield GP, Wyatt GP: Human parvovirus infection revealing hereditary spherocytosis. Lancet 1985; 2:1070.

1083. McLellan NJ, Rutter N: Hereditary spherocytosis in sisters unmasked by parvovirus infection. Postgrad Med J 1987; 63:49.

1084. Stefanelli M, Barosi G, et al: Quantitative assessment of erythropoiesis in haemolytic disease. Br J Haematol 1980; 45:297.

1085. Tileston W: Hemolytic jaundice. Medicine (Baltimore) 1922; 1:355.

1086. Hanford RB, Schneider GF, MacCarthy JD: Massive thoracic extramedullary hemopoiesis. N Engl J Med 1960; 263:120.

1087. Lawrence P, Aronson I, et al: Leg ulcers in hereditary spherocytosis. Clin Exp Dermatol 1991; 16:28.

1088. Vanscheidt W, Leder O, et al: Leg ulcers in a patient with spherocytosis: A clinicopathological report. Dermatologica 1990; 181:56.

1089. Beinhauer LG, Gruhn JG: Dermatologic aspects of congenital spherocytic anemia. Arch Dermatol 1957; 75:642.

1090. Abe T, Yachi A, et al: Thoracic extramedullary hematopoiesis associated with hereditary spherocytosis. Intern Med 1992; 31:1151.

1091. Martin J, Palacio A, et al: Fatty transformation of thoracic extramedullary hematopoiesis following splenectomy: CT features. J Comput Assist Tomogr 1990; 14:477.

1092. Pulsoni A, Ferrazza G, et al: Mediastinal extramedullary hematopoiesis as first manifestation of hereditary spherocytosis. Ann Hematol 1992; 65:196.

1093. Pietsch B, Sigmund G, Wurtemberger G: Nuclear spin tomographic findings in compensated chronic hemolysis. A case report of a hereditary spherocytosis. Aktuelle Radiol 1993; 3:266.

1094. Reman O, Carre G, et al: Extramedullary haematopoiesis in hereditary spherocytosis simulating mediastinal tumour. Eur J Haematol 1997; 58:124.

1095. Xiros N, Economopoulos T, et al: Massive hemothorax due to intrathoracic extramedullary hematopoiesis in a patient with hereditary spherocytosis. Ann Hematol 2001; 80:38.

1096. Calhoun SK, Murphy RC, et al: Extramedullary hematopoiesis in a child with hereditary spherocytosis: An uncommon cause of an adrenal mass. Pediatr Radiol 2001; 31:879.

1097. Schafer AI, Miller JB, et al: Monoclonal gammopathy in hereditary spherocytosis: A possible pathogenic relation. Ann Intern Med 1978; 88:45.

1098. Fukata S, Tamai H, et al: A patient with hereditary spherocytosis and silicosis who developed an IgA (λ) monoclonal gammopathy. Jpn J Med 1987; 26:81.

1099. Lempert KD: Gammopathy and spherocytosis. Ann Intern Med 1978; 89:145.

1100. Martinez-Climent JA, Lopez-Andreu JA, et al: Acute lymphoblastic leukaemia in a child with hereditary spherocytosis. Eur J Pediatr 1995; 154:753.

1101. Sekido N, Kawai K, et al: Adrenal myelolipoma associated with hereditary spherocytosis. Int J Urol 1996; 3:61.

1102. Jandl JH, Files NM, et al: Proliferative response of the spleen and liver to hemolysis. J Exp Med 1965; 122:299.

1103. Isobe T, Osserman EF: Pathologic conditions associated with plasma cell dyscrasias: A study of 806 cases. Ann NY Acad Sci 1971; 190:507.

1104. Blacklock HA, Meerkin M: Serum ferritin in patients with hereditary spherocytosis. Br J Haematol 1981; 49:117.

1105. Edwards CQ, Skolnick MH, et al: Iron overload in hereditary spherocytosis: Association with HLA-linked hemochromatosis. Am J Hematol 1982; 13:101.

1106. Fargion S, Cappellini MD, et al: Association of hereditary spherocytosis and idiopathic hemochromatosis: A synergistic effect in determining iron overload. Am J Clin Pathol 1986; 86:645.

1107. Mohler DN, Wheby MS: Hemochromatosis heterozygotes may have significant iron overload when they also have hereditary spherocytosis. Am J Med Sci 1986; 292:320.

1108. Morita M, Hashizume M, et al: Hereditary spherocytosis with congestive heart failure: Report of a case. Surg Today 1993; 23:458.

1109. Clarkson JG, Altman RD: Angioid streaks. Surv Ophthalmol 1982; 26:235.

1110. McLane NJ, Grizzard WS, et al: Angioid streaks associated with hereditary spherocytosis. Am J Ophthamol 1984; 97:444.

1111. Gibson JM, Chaudhuri PR, Rosenthal AR: Angioid streaks in a case of β thalassemia major. Br J Ophthalmol 1983; 67:29.

1112. Deutman AF, Kovacs B: Argon laser treatment in complications of angioid streaks. Am J Ophthalmol 1979; 88:12.

1113. Zipursky A, Chintu C, et al: The quantitation of spherocytes in ABO hemolytic disease. J Pediatr 1979; 94:965.

1114. Gilliland BC, Baxter E, Evans RS: Red cell antibodies in acquired hemolytic anemia with negative antiglobulin serum tests. N Engl J Med 1971; 85:252.

1115. Crosby WH, Conrad ME: Hereditary spherocytosis: Observations on hemolytic mechanisms and iron metabolism. Blood 1960; 15:662.

1116. Pautard B, Féo C, et al: Occurrence of hereditary spherocytosis and β thalassemia in the same family: Globin chain synthesis and viscodiffractometric studies. Br J Haematol 1988; 70:239.

1117. Blecher TE: What happens to the microspherocytosis of hereditary spherocytosis in folate deficiency? Clin Lab Haematol 1988; 10:403.

1118. Warkentin TE, Barr RD, et al: Recurrent acute splenic sequestration crisis due to interacting genetic defects: Hemoglobin SC disease and hereditary spherocytosis. Blood 1990; 75:266.

1119. Aksoy M, Erdem S: The combination of hereditary spherocytosis and heterozygous β-thalassaemia: A family study. Acta Haematol 1968; 39:183.

1120. White BP, Farver M: Coexistence of hereditary spherocytosis and β-thalassemia: Case report of severe hemolytic anemia in an American black. SD J Med 1991; 44:257.

1121. Miraglia del Giudice E, Perrotta S, et al: Coexistence of hereditary spherocytosis (HS) due to band 3 deficiency and β-thalassaemia trait: Partial correction of HS phenotype. Br J Haematol 1993; 85:553.

1122. Leung KF, Au WY, et al: Haemoglobin Q-Thailand and hereditary spherocytosis in a Chinese family. Clin Lab Haematol 2001; 23:53.

1123. Yang YM, Donnell C, et al: Splenic sequestration associated with sickle cell trait and hereditary spherocytosis. Am J Hematol 1992; 40:110.

1124. Babiker MA, El Seed FA: A family with sickle cell trait and hereditary spherocytosis. Scand J Haematol 1984; 33:54.

1125. Moiseyev VS, Korovina EA, et al: Hypertrophic cardiomyopathy associated with hereditary spherocytosis in three generations of one family. Lancet 1987; 2:853.

1125a.Reliene R, Mariani M, et al: Splenectomy prolongs in vivo survival of erythrocytes differently in spectrin/ankyrin- and band 3-deficient hereditary spherocytosis. Blood 2002; 100:2208.

1126. Eraklis AJ, Filler RM: Splenectomy in childhood: A review of 1413 cases. J Pediatr Surg 1972; 7:382.

1127. Green JB, Shackford SR, et al: Late septic complications in adults following splenectomy for trauma: A prospective analysis in 144 patients. J Trauma 1986; 26:999.

1128. Evans DI: Postsplenectomy sepsis 10 years or more after operation. J Clin Pathol 1985; 38:309.

1129. Holdsworth RJ, Irving AD, Cuschieri A: Postsplenectomy sepsis and its mortality rate: Actual versus perceived risks. Br J Surg 1991; 78:1031.

1130. Schwartz PE, Sterioff S, et al: Postsplenectomy sepsis and mortality in adults. JAMA 1982; 248:2279.

1131. Schilling RF: Estimating the risk for sepsis after splenectomy in hereditary spherocytosis. Ann Intern Med 1995; 122:187.

1132. Hansen K, Singer DB: Asplenic-hyposplenic overwhelming sepsis: Postsplenectomy sepsis revisited. Pediatr Dev Pathol 2001; 4:105.

1133. Konradsen HB, Henrichsen J: Pneumococcal infections in splenectomized children are preventable. Acta Pediatr Scand 1991; 80:423.

1134. Buchanan GR, Smith SJ: Pneumococcal septicemia despite pneumococcal vaccine and prescription of penicillin prophylaxis in patients with sickle cell anemia. Am J Dis Child 1986; 140:428.

1135. Gonzaga RA: Fatal post-splenectomy pneumococcal sepsis despite prophylaxis. Lancet 1984; 2:694.

1136. Wong WY, Overturf GD, Powers DR: Infection caused by Streptococcus pneumoniae in children with sickle cell disease: Epidemiology, immunologic mechanisms, prophylaxis and vaccination. Clin Infect Dis 1992; 14:1124.

1137. Buchanan GR, Siegel JD, et al: Oral penicillin prophylaxis in children with impaired splenic function: A study of compliance. Pediatrics 1982; 70:926.

1138. Eber SW, Langendorfer CM, et al: Frequency of very late fatal sepsis after splenectomy for hereditary spherocytosis: Impact of insufficient antibody response to pneumococcal infection. Ann Hematol 1999; 78:524.

1139. Caputo GM, Appelbaum PC, Liu HH: Infections due to penicillin-resistant pneumococci. Clinical, epidemiologic, and microbiologic features. Arch Intern Med 1993; 153:1301.

1140. Chesney PJ: The escalating problem of antimicrobial resistance in Streptococcus pneumoniae. Am J Dis Child 1992; 146:912.

1141. Tomasz A: Antibiotic resistance in Streptococcus pneumoniae. Clin Infect Dis 1997; 24(Suppl 1):S85.

1142. Marton A, Gulyas M, et al: Extremely high incidence of antibiotic resistance in clinical isolates of Streptococcus pneumoniae in Hungary. J Infect Dis 1991; 163:542.

1143. Appelbaum PC: Microbiological and pharmacodynamic considerations in the treatment of infection due to antimicrobial-resistant Streptococcus pneumoniae. Clin Infect Dis 2000; 31(Suppl 2):S29.

1144. Friedland IR, McCracken GH Jr: Management of infections caused by antibiotic-resistant *Streptococcus pneumoniae*. N Engl J Med 1994; 331:377.

1145. Wong WY, Powars DR, Hiti AL: Multi-drug resistance to *Streptococcus pneumoniae* in sickle cell anemia. Am J Hematol 1995; 48:278.

1146. Steele RW, Warrier R, et al: Colonization with antibiotic-resistant *Streptococcus pneumoniae* in children with sickle cell disease. J Pediatr 1996; 128:531.

1147. Pai VB, Nahata MC: Duration of penicillin prophylaxis in sickle cell anemia: Issues and controversies. Pharmacotherapy 2000; 20:110.

1148. Daw NC, Wilimas JA, et al: Nasopharyngeal carriage of penicillin-resistant *Streptococcus pneumoniae* in children with sickle cell disease. Pediatrics 1997; 99:E7.

1149. Golightly LM, Hirschhorn LR, Weller PF: Infectious disease rounds: Fever and headache in a splenectomized woman. Rev Infect Dis 1989; 11:629.

1150. Rosner F, Zarrabi MH, et al: Babesiosis in splenectomized adults: Review of 22 reported cases. Am J Med 1984; 76:696.

1151. Robinette CD, Fraumeni JF Jr: Splenectomy and subsequent mortality in veterans of the 1939–45 war. Lancet 1977; 2:127.

1152. Schilling RF: Hereditary spherocytosis: A study of splenectomized persons. Semin Hematol 1976; 13:169.

1153. Schilling RF: Spherocytosis, splenectomy, strokes, and heat attacks. Lancet 1997; 350:1677.

1154. Kannel WB: Current status of the epidemiology of brain infarction associated with occlusive arterial disease. Stroke 1971; 2:295.

1155. Verresen D, De Backer W, et al: Spherocytosis and pulmonary hypertension coincidental occurrence or causal relationship? Eur Respir J 1991; 4:629.

1156. Hoeper MM, Niedermeyer J, et al: Pulmonary hypertension after splenectomy? Ann Intern Med 1999; 130:506.

1157. Hayag-Barin JE, Smith RE, Tucker FC Jr: Hereditary spherocytosis, thrombocytosis, and chronic pulmonary emboli: A case report and review of the literature. Am J Hematol 1998; 57:82.

1158. Aessopos A, Stamatelos G, et al: Pulmonary hypertension and right heart failure in patients with β-thalassemia intermedia. Chest 1995; 107:50.

1159. Sonakul D, Fucharoen S: Pulmonary thromboembolism in thalassemic patients. Southeast Asian J Trop Med Public Health 1992; 23(Suppl 2):25.

1160. Stewart GW, Amess JAL, et al: Thrombo-embolic disease after splenectomy for hereditary stomatocytosis. Br J Haematol 1996; 93:303.

1161. Marvin KS, Spellberg RD: Pulmonary hypertension secondary to thrombocytosis in a patient with myeloid metaplasia. Chest 1993; 103:642.

1162. Rostagno C, Prisco D, et al: Pulmonary hypertension associated with long-standing thrombocytosis. Chest 1991; 99:1303.

1163. Kisanuki A, Kietthubthew S, et al: Intravenous injection of sonicated blood induces pulmonary microthromboembolism in rabbits with ligation of the splenic artery. Thromb Res 1997; 85:95.

1164. McGrew W, Avant GR: Hereditary spherocytosis and portal vein thrombosis. J Clin Gastroenterol 1984; 6:381.

1165. Perel Y, Dhermy D, et al: Portal vein thrombosis after splenectomy for hereditary stomatocytosis in childhood. Eur J Pediatr 1999; 158:628.

1166. Bertolotti M, Loria P, et al: Bleeding jejunal varices and portal thrombosis in a splenectomized patient with hereditary spherocytosis. Dig Dis Sci 2000; 45:373.

1167. Teramoto S, Matsuse T, Ouchi Y: Splenectomy-induced portal hypertension and pulmonary hypertension. Ann Intern Med 1999; 131:793.

1168. Barker JE, Wandersee NJ: Thrombosis in heritable hemolytic disorders. Curr Opin Hematol 1999; 6:71.

1169. Andrews DA, Low PS: Role of red blood cells in thrombosis. Curr Opin Hematol 1999; 6:76.

1170. Kaysser TM, Wandersee NJ, et al: Thrombosis and secondary hemochromatosis play major roles in the pathogenesis of jaundiced and spherocytic mice, murine models for hereditary spherocytosis. Blood 1997; 90:4610.

1171. Rescorla FJ, Breitfeld PP, et al: A case controlled comparison of open and laparoscopic splenectomy in children. Surgery 1998; 124:670.

1172. Esposito C, Gonzalez Sabin MA, et al: Results and complications of laparoscopic cholecystectomy in childhood. Surg Endosc 2001; 15:890.

1173. Patton ML, Moss BE, et al: Concomitant laparoscopic cholecystectomy and splenectomy for surgical management of hereditary spherocytosis. Am Surg 1997; 63:536.

1174. Yamagishi S, Watanabe T: Concomitant laparoscopic splenectomy and cholecystectomy for management of hereditary spherocytosis associated with gallstones. J Clin Gastroenterol 2000; 30:447.

1175. Sandler A, Winkel G, et al: The role of prophylactic cholecystectomy during splenectomy in children with hereditary spherocytosis. J Pediatr Surg 1999; 34:1077.

1176. Lobe TE, Presbury GJ, et al: Laparascopic splenectomy. Pediatr Ann 1993; 22:671.

1177. Smith BM, Schropp KP, et al: Laparoscopic splenectomy in childhood. J Pediatr Surg 1994; 29:975.

1178. Poulin EC, Thibault C: Laparoscopic splenectomy for massive splenomegaly: Operative technique and case report. Can J Surg 1995; 38:69.

1179. Farah RA, Rogers ZR, et al: Laparoscopic splenectomy in children with hematologic disorders. Blood 1995; 86(Suppl 1):135a.

1180. Silvestri F, Russo D, et al: Laparoscopic splenectomy in the management of hematological diseases. Haematologica 1995; 80:47.

1181. Yoshida K, Yamazaki Y, et al: Laparoscopic splenectomy in children. Preliminary results and comparison with the open technique. Surg Endosc 1995; 9:1279.

1182. Rescorla FJ: Cholelithiasis, cholecystitis, and common bile duct stones. Curr Opin Pediatr 1997; 9:276.

1183. Minkes RK, Lagzdins M, Langer JC: Laparoscopic versus open splenectomy in children. J Pediatr Surg 2000; 35:699.

1184. Park A, Heniford BT, et al: Pediatric laparoscopic splenectomy. Surg Endosc 2000; 14:527.

1185. Danielson PD, Shaul DB, et al: Technical advances in pediatric laparoscopy have had a beneficial impact on splenectomy. J Pediatr Surg 2000; 35:1578.

1186. Gigot JF, de Ville de Goyet J, et al: Laparoscopic splenectomy in adults and children: Experience with 31 patients. Surgery 1996; 119:384.

1187. Hebra A, Walker JD, et al: A new technique for laparoscopic splenectomy with massively enlarged spleens. Am Surg 1998; 64:1161.

1188. Esposito C, Schaarschmidt K, et al: Experience with laparoscopic splenectomy. J Pediatr Surg 2001; 36:309.

1189. Kumar RJ, Borzi PA: Splenosis in a port site after laparoscopic splenectomy. Surg Endosc 2001; 15:413.

1190. Tchernia G, Gauthier F, et al: Initial assessment of the beneficial effect of partial splenectomy in hereditary spherocytosis. Blood 1993; 81:2014.

1191. Bader-Meunier B, Gauthier F, et al: Long-term evaluation of the beneficial effect of subtotal splenectomy for management of hereditary spherocytosis. Blood 2001; 97:399.

1192. Bart JB, Appel MF: Recurrent hemolytic anemia secondary to accessory spleens. South Med J 1978; 71:608.

1193. MacKenzie FA, Elliot DH, et al: Relapse in hereditary spherocytosis with proven splenunculus. Lancet 1962; 1:1102.

1193a. De Buys Roessingh AS, De Lagausie P, et al: Follow-up of partial splenectomy in children with hereditary spherocytosis. J Pediatr Surg 2002; 37:1459.

1194. Jimenez M, Azcona C, et al: Partial splenic embolization in a child with hereditary spherocytosis. Eur J Pediatr 1995; 154:501.

1195. De Haan LD, Werre JM, et al: Alterations in size, shape and osmotic behaviour of red cells after splenectomy: A study of their age dependence. Br J Haematol 1988; 69:71.

1196. Brook J, Tanaka KR: Combination of pyruvate kinase (PK) deficiency and hereditary spherocytosis (HS). Clin Res 1970; 18:176A.

1197. Valentine WN: Hereditary spherocytosis revisited. West J Med 1978; 128:35.

1198. Rutkow IM: Twenty years of splenectomy for hereditary spherocytosis. Arch Surg 1981; 116:306.

1199. Buchanan GR, Holtkamp CA: Pocked erythrocyte counts in patients with hereditary spherocytosis before and after splenectomy. Am J Hematol 1987; 25:253.

1200. Kvindesdal BB, Jensen MK: Pitted erythrocytes in splenectomized subjects with congenital spherocytosis and in subjects splenectomized for other reasons. Scand J Haematol 1986; 37:41.

1201. Satou S, Yokota E, et al: Relapse of hereditary spherocytosis following splenectomy. Acta Haematol Jpn 1985; 48:1337.

1202. Dresbach M: Elliptical human red corpuscles. Science 1904; 19:469.

1203. Flint A: Elliptical human erythrocytes. Science 1904; 19:796.

1204. Dresbach M: Elliptical human erythrocytes. Science 1905; 21:473.

1205. Bishop FW: Elliptical human erythrocytes. Arch Intern Med 1914; 14:388.

1206. Huck JG, Bigelow RM: Poikilocytes in otherwise normal blood (elliptical human erythrocytes). Bull Johns Hopkins Hosp 1923; 34:390.

1207. Hunter WC, Adams RB: Hematologic study of three generations of a white family showing elliptical erythrocytes. Ann Intern Med 1929; 2:1162.

1208. Hunter WC: Further study of a white family showing elliptical erythrocytes. Ann Intern Med 1932; 6:775.

1209. Giffin HZ, Watkins CH: Ovalocytosis with features of hemolytic icterus. Trans Assoc Am Physicians 1939; 54:355.

1210. Penfold J, Lipscomb JM: Elliptocytosis in man, associated with hereditary haemorrhagic telangiectasis. Q J Med 1943; 12:157.

1211. Wyandt H, Bancroft PM, Winship TO: Elliptic erythrocytes in man. Arch Intern Med 1941; 68:1043.

1212. Wolman IJ, Ozge A: Studies on elliptocytosis. I. Hereditary elliptocytosis in the pediatric age period: A review of recent literature. Am J Med Sci 1957; 234:702.

1213. Dacie JV: The lifespan of the red blood cell and circumstances of its premature death. In Wintrobe MM (ed): Blood, Pure and Eloquent. New York, McGraw-Hill, 1980, p 210.

1214. McCarty SH: Elliptical red blood cells in man. A report of eleven cases. J Lab Clin Med 1934; 19:612.

1215. Glele-Kakai C, Garbarz M, et al: Epidemiological studies of spectrin mutations related to hereditary elliptocytosis and spectrin polymorphisms in Benin. Br J Haematol 1996; 95:57.

1216. Lecomte MC, Dhermy D, et al: Hereditary elliptocytosis in West Africa: Frequency and repartition of spectrin variants. C R Acad Sci Paris 1988; 306:43.

1217. Ganesan J, George R, Lie-Injo LE: Abnormal haemoglobins and hereditary ovalocytosis in the Ulu Jempul district of Kuala Pilah, West Malaysia. Southeast Asian J Trop Med Public Health 1976; 7:430.

1218. Tse WT, Lecomte MC, et al: Point mutation in the β-spectrin gene associated with $\alpha^{I/74}$ hereditary elliptocytosis. Implications for the mechanism of spectrin dimer self-association. J Clin Invest 1990; 86:909.

1219. Lawler J, Liu S-C, et al: Molecular defect of spectrin in hereditary pyropoikilocytosis: Alterations in the trypsin resistant domain involved in spectrin self-association. J Clin Invest 1982; 70:1019.

1220. Dalla Venezia N, Wilmotte R, et al: An α-spectrin mutation responsible for hereditary elliptocytosis associated in *cis* with the $\alpha^{v/41}$ polymorphism. Hum Genet 1993; 90:641.

1221. Mentzer WC, Turetsky T, et al: Identification of the hereditary pyropoikilocytosis carrier state. Blood 1984; 63:1439.

1222. Palek J, Lux SE: Red cell membrane skeletal defects in hereditary and acquired hemolytic anemias. Semin Hematol 1983; 20:189.

1223. Jonsson JJ, Renieri A, et al: Alport syndrome, mental retardation, midface hypoplasia, and elliptocytosis: A new X linked contiguous gene deletion syndrome? J Med Genet 1998; 35:273.

1224. Palek J: Hereditary elliptocytosis and related disorders. Clin Haematol 1985; 14:45.

1225. Palek J: Hereditary elliptocytosis, spherocytosis and related disorders: Consequences of a deficiency or a mutation of membrane skeletal proteins. Blood Rev 1987; 1:147.

1226. Tchernia G, Mohandas N, Shohet SB: Deficiency of cytoskeletal membrane protein band 4.1 in homozygous hereditary elliptocytosis: Implications for erythrocyte membrane stability. J Clin Invest 1981; 68:454.

1227. Morle L, Alloisio N, et al: Spectrin Tunis ($\alpha^{I/78}$): A new α I variant that causes asymptomatic hereditary elliptocytosis in the heterozygous state. Blood 1988; 71:508.

1228. Morle L, Morle F, et al: Spectrin Tunis (Sp $\alpha^{I/78}$), an elliptocytogenic variant, is due to the CGG→TGG codon change (Arg→Trp) at position 35 of the α I domain. Blood 1989; 75:828.

1229. Lecomte MC, Dhermy D, et al: Hereditary elliptocytosis with spectrin molecular defect in a white patient. Acta Haematol (Basel) 1984; 71:235.

1230. Alloisio N, Guetorni D, et al: Sp $\alpha^{I/65}$ hereditary elliptocytosis in North Africa. Am J Hematol 1986; 23:113.

1231. Guetarni D, Roux A-F, et al: Evidence that expression of Sp $\alpha^{I/65}$ hereditary elliptocytosis is compounded by a genetic factor that is linked to the homologous α-spectrin allele. Hum Genet 1990; 85:627.

1232. Marchesi SL, Knowles WT, et al: Abnormal spectrin in hereditary elliptocytosis. Blood 1986; 67:141.

1233. Feddal S, Brunet G, et al: Molecular analysis of hereditary elliptocytosis with reduced protein 4.1 in the French Northern Alps. Blood 1991; 78:2113.

1234. Lambert S, Zail S: Partial deficiency of protein 4.1 in hereditary elliptocytosis. Am J Hematol 1987; 26:263.

1235. McGuire M, Smith BL, Agre P: Distinct variants of erythrocyte protein 4.1 inherited in linkage with elliptocytosis and Rh type in three white families. Blood 1988; 72:287.

1236. Florman AL, Wintrobe MM: Human elliptical red corpuscles. Bull Johns Hopkins Hosp 1938; 63:209.

1237. Garrdo-Lacca G, Merino C, Luna G: Hereditary elliptocytosis in a Peruvian family. N Engl J Med 1957; 256:311.

1238. Geerdink RA, Helleman PW, Verloop MC: Hereditary elliptocytosis and hyperhaemolysis: A comparative study of 6 families with 145 patients. Acta Med Scand 1966; 179:715.

1239. Jensson O, Jonasson TH, Olafsson O: Hereditary elliptocytosis in Iceland. Br J Haematol 1967; 13:844.

1240. Motulsky AG, Singer K, et al: The life span of the elliptocyte: Hereditary elliptocytosis and its relationship to other familial hemolytic diseases. Blood 1954; 9:57.

1241. Pothier B, Alloisio N, et al: Assignment of spectrin $\alpha^{I/74}$ hereditary elliptocytosis to the α or β chain of spectrin through *in vitro* dimer reconstitution. Blood 1990; 75:2061.

1242. Coetzer T, Lawler J, et al: Molecular determinants of clinical expression of hereditary elliptocytosis and pyropoikilocytosis. Blood 1987; 70:766.

1243. Rummens JL, Verfaillie C, et al: Elliptocytosis and schistocytosis in myelodysplasia: Report of two cases. Acta Haematol 1986; 75:174.

1244. Coetzer T, Sahr K, et al: Four different mutations in codon 28 of α spectrin are associated with structurally and functionally abnormal spectrin $\alpha^{I/74}$ in hereditary elliptocytosis. J Clin Invest 1991; 88:743.

1245. Garbarz M, Lecomte MC, et al: Hereditary pyropoikilocytosis and elliptocytosis in a white French family with the spectrin $\alpha^{I/74}$ variant related to a CGT to CAT codon change (Arg to His) at position 22 of the spectrin α I domain. Blood 1990; 75:1691.

1246. Lawler J, Liu S-C, et al: Molecular defect of spectrin in a subgroup of patients with hereditary elliptocytosis: Alteration in the α subunit involved in spectrin self association. J Clin Invest 1984; 73:1688.

1247. Lecomte MC, Feo C, et al: Severe hereditary elliptocytosis in two related Caucasian children with a decreased amount of spectrin (Sp) α chain [abstract]. J Cell Biochem 1989; 13B:230.

1248. Baklouti F, Marechal J, et al: Occurrence of the α I 22 Arg→His (CGT→CAT) spectrin mutation in Tunisia: Potential association with severe elliptopoikilocytosis. Br J Haematol 1991; 78:108.

1249. Baklouti F, Marechal J, et al: Elliptocytogenic $\alpha^{I/36}$ spectrin Sfax lacks nine amino acids in helix 3 of repeat 4. Evidence for the activation of a cryptic 5′-splice site in exon 8 of spectrin α-gene. Blood 1992; 79:2464.

1250. Dalla Venezia N, Alloisio N, et al: Elliptopoikilocytosis associated with the α 469 His→Pro mutation in spectrin Barcelona ($\alpha^{I/50-46b}$). Blood 1993; 82:1661.

1251. Alloisio N, Morle L, et al: Sp $\alpha^{V/41}$: A common spectrin polymorphism at the $\alpha^{IV}-\alpha^{V}$ domain junction. Relevance to the expression level of hereditary elliptocytosis due to α-spectrin variants located in *trans*. J Clin Invest 1991; 87:2169.

1252. Coetzer T, Palek J, et al: Structural and functional heterogeneity of α spectrin mutations involving the spectrin heterodimer self-association site: Relationships to hematologic expression of homozygous hereditary elliptocytosis and hereditary pyropoikilocytosis. Blood 1990; 75:2235.

1253. Randon J, Boulanger L, et al: A variant of spectrin low expression allele α^{LELY} carrying a hereditary elliptocytosis mutation in codon 28. Br J Haematol 1994; 88:534.

1254. Ozer L, Mills GC: Elliptocytosis with haemolytic anaemia. Br J Haematol 1964; 10:468.

1255. Kruetrachuo M, Asawapokee N: Hereditary elliptocytosis and *Plasmodium falciparum* malaria. Ann Trop Med Parasitol 1972; 66:161.

1256. Nkrumah FK: Hereditary elliptocytosis associated with severe haemolytic anaemia and malaria. Afr J Med Sci 1972; 3:131.

1257. Jarolim P, Palek J, et al: Severe hemolysis and red cell fragmentation due to a combination of a spectrin mutation with a thrombotic microangiopathy. Am J Hematol 1989; 32:50.

1258. Schoomaker EB, Butler WM, Diehl LF: Increased heat sensitivity of red blood cells in hereditary elliptocytosis with acquired cobalamin (vitamin B$_{12}$) deficiency. Blood 1982; 59:1213.

1259. Lecomte MC, Garbarz M, et al: Sp α$^{I/78}$: A mutation of the α I spectrin domain in a white kindred with HE and HPP phenotypes. Blood 1989; 74:1126.

1260. Lane PA, Shew RL, et al: Unique α-spectrin mutant in a kindred with common hereditary elliptocytosis. J Clin Invest 1987; 79:989.

1261. Austin RF, Desforges JF: Hereditary elliptocytosis: An unusual presentation of hemolysis in the newborn associated with transient morphologic abnormalities. Pediatrics 1969; 44:196.

1262. Carpentieri U, Gustavson LP, Haggard ME: Pyknocytosis in a neonate: An unusual presentation of hereditary elliptocytosis. Clin Pediatr 1977; 16:76.

1263. Josephs HW, Avery ME: Hereditary elliptocytosis associated with increased hemolysis. Pediatrics 1965; 16:741.

1264. Zarkowsky HS: Heat-induced erythrocyte fragmentation in neonatal elliptocytosis. Br J Haematol 1979; 41:515.

1265. Prchal JT, Castleberry RP, et al: Hereditary pyropoikilocytosis and elliptocytosis: Clinical, laboratory, and ultrastructural features in infants and children. Pediatr Res 1982; 16:484.

1266. Mentzer WC Jr, Iarocci TA, et al: Modulation of erythrocyte membrane mechanical stability by 2,3- diphosphoglycerate in the neonatal poikilocytosis/elliptocytosis syndrome. J Clin Invest 1987; 79:943.

1267. Torlontano G, Fioritoni G, Salvati AM: Hereditary haemolytic ovalocytosis with defective erythropoiesis. Br J Haematol 1979; 43:435.

1268. Jankovic M, Sansone G, et al: Atypical hereditary ovalocytosis associated with defective dyserythropoietic anemia. Acta Haematol 1993; 89:35.

1269. Dhermy D, Lecomte MC, et al: Molecular defect of spectrin in the family of a child with congenital hemolytic poikilocytic anemia. Pediatr Res 1984; 18:1005.

1270. Garbarz M, Lecomte MC, et al: Double inheritance of an α$^{I/65}$ spectrin variant in a child with homozygous elliptocytosis. Blood 1986; 67:1661.

1271. Lawler J, Coetzer TL, et al: Spectrin-α$^{I/61}$: A new structural variant of α-spectrin in a double-heterozygous form of hereditary pyropoikilocytosis. Blood 1988; 72:1412.

1272. Alloisio N, Morle L, et al: Spectrin Oran (α$^{II/21}$), a new spectrin variant concerning the α II domain and causing severe elliptocytosis in the homozygous state. Blood 1988; 71:1039.

1273. Lecomte MC, Feo C, et al: Severe recessive poikilocytic anaemia with a new spectrin α chain variant. Br J Haematol 1990; 74:497.

1274. Dalla Venezia N, Gilsanz F, et al: Homozygous 4.1(−) hereditary elliptocytosis associated with a point mutation in the downstream initiation codon of protein 4.1 gene. J Clin Invest 1992; 90:1713.

1275. Alloisio N, Wilmotte R, et al: A splice site mutation of α-spectrin gene causing skipping of exon 18 in hereditary elliptocytosis. Blood 1993; 81:2791.

1276. Grech JL, Cachia EA, et al: Hereditary elliptocytosis in two Maltese families. J Clin Pathol 1961; 14:365.

1277. Haddy TB, Rana SR: Homozygous hereditary elliptocytosis with hemolytic anemia. South Med J 1984; 77:631.

1278. Iarocci TA, Wagner GM, et al: Hereditary poikilocytic anemia associated with the co-inheritance of two α spectrin abnormalities. Blood 1988; 71:1390.

1279. Lipton EL: Elliptocytosis with hemolytic anemia: The effects of splenectomy. Pediatrics 1955; 15:67.

1280. Nielsen JA, Strunk KW: Homozygous hereditary elliptocytosis as a cause of haemolytic anaemia in infancy. Scand J Haematol 1968; 5:486.

1281. Pryor DS, Pitney WR: Hereditary elliptocytosis: A report of two families from New Guinea. Br J Haematol 1967; 13:126.

1282. Dhermy D, Garbarz M, et al: Hereditary elliptocytosis: Clinical, morphological, and biochemical studies of 38 cases. Nouv Rev Fr Hematol 1986; 28:129.

1283. Dhermy D, Galand C, et al: Coinheritance of α- and β-spectrin gene mutations in a case of hereditary elliptocytosis. Blood 1998; 92:4481.

1284. Floyd PB, Gallagher PG, et al: Heterogeneity of the molecular basis of hereditary pyropoikilocytosis and hereditary elliptocytosis associated with increased levels of the spectrin α$^{I/74}$-kilodalton tryptic peptide. Blood 1991; 78:1364.

1285. Dacie JV, Mollison PL, et al: Atypical congenital haemolytic anaemia. Q J Med 1953; 22:79.

1286. Wiley JS, Gill FM: Red cell calcium leak in congenital hemolytic anemia with extreme microcytosis. Blood 1976; 47:197.

1287. Zarkowsky HS, Mohandas N, et al: A congenital haemolytic anaemia with thermal sensitivity of the erythrocyte membrane. Br J Haematol 1975; 29:537.

1288. DePalma L, Luban NL: Hereditary pyropoikilocytosis: Clinical and laboratory analysis in eight infants and young children. Am J Dis Child 1993; 147:93.

1289. Coetzer T, Palek J: Partial spectrin deficiency in hereditary pyropoikilocytosis. Blood 1986; 59:919.

1290. Hanspal M, Hanspal JS, et al: Molecular basis of spectrin deficiency in hereditary pyropoikilocytosis. Blood 1993; 82:1652.

1291. Cutting HO, McHugh WJ, et al: Autosomal dominant hemolytic anemia characterized by ovalocytosis: A family study of seven involved members. Am J Med 1965; 39:21.

1292. Dacie JV: Hereditary elliptocytosis (HE). In The Haemolytic Anaemias, 3rd ed. Edinburgh, Churchill Livingstone, 1985, Vol I, p 216.

1293. Greenberg LH, Tanaka KR Hereditary elliptocytosis with hemolytic anemia—A family study of five affected members. Calif Med 1969; 110:389.

1294. Weiss HJ: Hereditary elliptocytosis with hemolytic anemia. Am J Med 1963; 35:455.

1295. Matsumoto N, Ishihara T, et al: Fine structure of the spleen in hereditary elliptocytosis. Acta Pathol Jpn 1976; 26:533.

1296. Wilson HE, Long MJ: Hereditary ovalocytosis (elliptocytosis) with hypersplenism. Arch Intern Med 1955, 95:438.

1297. Garbarz M, Tse WT, et al: Spectrin Rouen (β$^{220−218}$), a novel shortened β-chain variant in a kindred with hereditary elliptocytosis. Characterization of the molecular defect as exon skipping due to a splice site mutation. J Clin Invest 1991; 88:76.

1298. Lecomte MC, Gautero H, et al: Elliptocytosis-associated spectrin Rouen (β$^{220/218}$) has a truncated but still phosphorylatable β chain. Br J Haematol 1992; 80:242.

1299. Pothier B, Morle L, et al: Spectrin Nice (β$^{220/216}$): A shortened β-chain variant associated with an increase of the α$^{I/74}$ fragment in a case of elliptocytosis. Blood 1987; 69:1759.

1300. Tse WT, Gallagher PG, et al: An insertional frameshift mutation of the β-spectrin gene associated with elliptocytosis in spectrin Nice (β$^{220/216}$). Blood 1991; 78:517.

1301. Garbarz M, Boulanger L, et al: Spectrin β Tandil, a novel shortened β-chain variant associated with hereditary elliptocytosis is due to a deletional frameshift mutation in the β-spectrin gene. Blood 1992; 80:1066.

1302. Eber SW, Morris SA, et al: Interactions of spectrin in hereditary elliptocytes containing truncated spectrin β-chains. J Clin Invest 1988; 81:523.

1303. Yoon SH, Yu H, et al: Molecular defect of truncated β-spectrin associated with hereditary elliptocytosis. β-Spectrin Gottingen. J Biol Chem 1991; 266:8490.

1304. Dhermy D, Lecomte MC, et al: Spectrin β-chain variant associated with hereditary elliptocytosis. J Clin Invest 1982; 70:707.

1305. Gallagher PG, Tse WT, et al: A splice site mutation of the β-spectrin gene causing exon skipping in hereditary elliptocytosis associated with a truncated β-spectrin chain. J Biol Chem 1991; 266:15154.

1306. Jarolim P, Wichterle H, et al: β spectrin PRAGUE: A truncated β spectrin producing spectrin deficiency, defective spectrin heterodimer self-association and a phenotype of spherocytic elliptocytosis. Br J Haematol 1995; 91:502.

1307. Dahr W, Moulds J, et al: Altered membrane sialoglycoproteins in human erythrocytes lacking the Gerbich blood group antigen. Biol Chem Hoppe Seyler 1985; 366:201.

1308. Daniels GL, Reid ME, et al: Transient reduction in erythrocyte membrane sialoglycoprotein β associated with the presence of elliptocytes. Br J Haematol 1988; 70:477.

1309. Aksoy M, Erdem S, et al: Combination of hereditary elliptocytosis and hereditary spherocytosis. Clin Genet 1974; 6:46.

1310. Ham TH, Shen SC, et al: Studies on the destruction of red blood cells: IV. Thermal injury: Action of heat in causing increased spheroidicity, osmotic and mechanical fragilities and hemolysis of erythrocytes: Observations on the mechanisms of destruction in such erythrocytes in dogs and in a patient with a fatal thermal burn. Blood 1948; 3:373.

1311. Ham TH, Sayre RW, et al: Physical properties of red cells as related to effects *in vivo*: II. Effect of thermal treatment on rigidity of red cells, stroma and the sickle cell. Blood 1968; 32:862.

1312. Kimber RJ, Lander H: The effect of heat on human red cell morphology, fragility and subsequent survival *in vivo*. J Lab Clin Med 1964; 64:922.

1313. Chang K, Williamson JR, Zarkowsky HS: Effect of heat on the circular dichroism of spectrin in hereditary pyropoikilocytosis. J Clin Invest 1979; 64:326.

1314. Liu S-C, Palek J, et al: Altered spectrin dimer-dimer association and instability of erythrocyte membrane skeletons in hereditary pyropoikilocytosis. J Clin Invest 1981; 68:597.

1315. Liu S-C, Palek J, Prchal J: Defective spectrin dimer-dimer association in hereditary elliptocytosis. Proc Natl Acad Sci USA 1982; 79:2072.

1316. Chasis JA, Mohandas N: Erythrocyte membrane deformability and stability: Two distinct membrane properties that are independently regulated by skeletal protein interactions. J Cell Biol 1986; 103:343.

1317. Mohandas N, Clark MR, et al: A technique to detect reduced mechanical stability of red cell membranes: Relevance to elliptocytic disorders. Blood 1982; 59:768.

1318. Mohandas N, Clark MR, et al: Analysis of factors regulating erythrocyte deformability. J Clin Invest 1980; 66:563.

1319. Delaunay J, Dhermy D: Mutations involving the spectrin heterodimer contact site: Clinical expression and alterations in specific function. Semin Hematol 1993; 30:21.

1320. Orita M, Iwahana H, et al: Detection of polymorphisms of human DNA by gel electrophoresis as single-strand conformation polymorphisms. Proc Natl Acad Sci USA 1989; 86:2766.

1321. Sarkar G, Yoon H-S, Sommer SS: Screening for mutations by RNA single-strand conformation polymorphism (rSSCP): Comparison with DNA-SSCP. Nucleic Acids Res 1992; 20:871.

1322. Parquet N, Devaux I, et al: Identification of three novel spectrin α I/74 mutations in hereditary elliptocytosis: Further support for a triple-stranded folding unit model of the spectrin heterodimer contact site. Blood 1994; 84:303.

1323. Lecomte MC, Garbarz M, et al: Molecular basis of clinical and morphological heterogeneity in hereditary elliptocytosis (HE) with spectrin α I variants. Br J Haematol 1993; 85:584.

1324. Perrotta S, Miraglia del Giudice E, et al: Mild elliptocytosis associated with the α 34 Arg→Trp mutation in spectrin Genova (α I/74). Blood 1994; 83:3346.

1325. Perrotta S, Iolascon A, et al: Spectrin Anastasia (α I/78): A new spectrin variant (α 45 Arg→Thr) with moderate elliptocytogenic potential. Br J Haematol 1995; 89:933.

1326. Morle L, Roux AF, et al: Two elliptocytogenic α I/74 variants of the spectrin α I domain. Spectrin Culoz (GGT→GTT; α I 40 Gly→Val) and spectrin Lyon (CTT→TTT; α I 43 Leu→Phe) J Clin Invest 1990; 86:548.

1327. Boulanger L, Dhermy D, et al: A second allele of spectrin α-gene associated with the α I/65 phenotype (allele α Ponte de Sor). Blood 1994; 84:2056.

1328. Roux AF, Morle F, et al: Molecular basis of Sp α I/65 hereditary elliptocytosis in North Africa: Insertion of a TTG triplet between codons 147 and 149 in the α-spectrin gene from five unrelated families. Blood 1989; 73:2196.

1329. Hassoun H, Coetzer TL, et al: A novel mobile element inserted in the α spectrin gene: Spectrin Dayton. A truncated α spectrin associated with hereditary elliptocytosis. J Clin Invest 1994; 94:643.

1330. Gallagher PG, Tse WT, et al: A common type of the spectrin α I 46–50a-kD peptide abnormality in hereditary elliptocytosis and pyropoikilocytosis is associated with a mutation distant from the proteolytic cleavage site. Evidence for the functional importance of the triple helical model of spectrin. J Clin Invest 1992; 89:892.

1331. Sahr KE, Tobe T, et al: Sequence and exon-intron organization of the DNA encoding the α I domain of human spectrin: Application to the study of mutations causing hereditary elliptocytosis. J Clin Invest 1989; 84:1243.

1332. Gallagher PG, Roberts WE, et al: Poikilocytic hereditary elliptocytosis associated with spectrin Alexandria: An α I/50b Kd variant that is caused by a single amino acid deletion. Blood 1993; 82:2210.

1333. Alloisio N, Wilmotte R, et al: Spectrin Jendouba: An α II/31 spectrin variant that is associated with elliptocytosis and carries a mutation distant from the dimer self-association site. Blood 1992; 80:809.

1334. Fournier CM, Nicolas G, et al: Spectrin St. Claude, a splicing mutation of the human α-spectrin gene associated with severe poikilocytic anemia. Blood 1997; 89:4584.

1335. Burke JP, Van Zyl D, et al: Reduced spectrin-ankyrin binding in a South African hereditary elliptocytosis kindred homozygous for spectrin St Claude. Blood 1998; 92:2591.

1336. Sahr KE, Coetzer TL, et al: Spectrin Cagliari. An Ala→Gly substitution in helix 1 of β spectrin repeat 17 that severely disrupts the structure and self-association of the erythrocyte spectrin heterodimer. J Biol Chem 1993; 268:22656.

1337. Gallagher PG, Weed SA, et al: Recurrent fatal hydrops fetalis associated with a nucleotide substitution in the erythrocyte β-spectrin gene. J Clin Invest 1995; 95:1174.

1338. Gallagher PG, Petruzzi MJ, et al: Mutation of a highly conserved residue of βI spectrin associated with fatal and near-fatal neonatal hemolytic anemia. J Clin Invest 1997; 99:267.

1339. Wilmotte R, Miraglia del Giudice E, et al: A deletional frameshift mutation in spectrin β-gene associated with hereditary elliptocytosis in spectrin Napoli. Br J Haematol 1994; 88:437.

1340. Kanzaki A, Rabodonirina M, et al: A deletional frameshift mutation of the β-spectrin gene associated with elliptocytosis in spectrin Tokyo (β$^{220/216}$). Blood 1992; 80:2115.

1341. Qualtieri A, Pasqua A, et al: Spectrin Cosenza: A novel β chain variant associated with Sp αI/74 hereditary elliptocytosis. Br J Haematol 1997; 97:273.

1342. Maillet P, Inoue T, et al: Stop codon in exon 30 (E2069X) of β-spectrin gene associated with hereditary elliptocytosis in spectrin Nagoya. Hum Mutat 1996; 8:366.

1343. Basseres DS, Pranke PH, et al: β-Spectrin Campinas: A novel shortened β-chain variant associated with skipping of exon 30 and hereditary elliptocytosis. Br J Haematol 1997; 97:579.

1344. Zhang Z, Weed SA, et al: Dynamic molecular modeling of pathogenic mutations in the spectrin self-association domain. Blood 2001; 98:1645.

1344a. Park S, Johnson ME, Fung LW: Nuclear magnetic resonance studies of mutations at the tetramerization region of human alpha spectrin. Blood 2002; 100:283.

1345. Lorenzo F, Miraglia del Giudice E, et al: Severe poikilocytosis associated with a *de novo* α 28 Arg→Cys mutation in spectrin. Br J Haematol 1993; 83:152.

1346. Palek J, Lambert S: Genetics of the red cell membrane skeleton. Semin Hematol 1990; 27:290.

1347. Lawler J, Palek J, et al: Molecular heterogeneity of a hereditary pyropoikilocytosis: Identification of a second variant of the spectrin α-subunit. Blood 1983; 62:1182.

1348. Dhermy D, Garbarz M, et al: Abnormal electrophoretic mobility of spectrin tetramers in hereditary elliptocytosis. Hum Genet 1986; 74:363.

1349. Lawler J, Coetzer TL, et al: Sp α I/65: A new variant of the α subunit of spectrin in hereditary elliptocytosis. Blood 1985; 66:706.

1350. Lecomte MC, Dhermy D, et al: Pathologic and non-pathologic variants of the spectrin molecule in two black families with hereditary elliptocytosis. Hum Genet 1985; 71:351.

1351. Lecomte MC, Dhermy D, et al: A new abnormal variant of spectrin in black patients with hereditary elliptocytosis. Blood 1985; 65:1208.

1352. del Giudice EM, Ducluzeau MT, et al: α I/65 hereditary elliptocytosis in southern Italy: Evidence for an African origin. Hum Genet 1992; 89:553.

1353. Schulman S, Roth EF Jr, et al: Growth of *Plasmodium falciparum* in human erythrocytes containing abnormal membrane proteins. Proc Natl Acad Sci USA 1990; 87:7339.

1354. Harris HW Jr, Levin N, Lux SE: Comparison of the phosphorylation of human erythrocyte spectrin in the intact red cell and in various cell-free systems. J Biol Chem 1980; 255:11521.

1355. Johnson RM, Ravindranath Y, et al: A large erythroid spectrin β-chain variant. Br J Haematol 1992; 80:6.

1356. Pranke PH, Basseres DS, et al: Expression of spectrin α I/65 hereditary elliptocytosis in patients from Brazil. Br J Haematol 1996; 94:470.

1357. Wilmotte R, Marechal J, et al: Low expression allele α LELY of red cell spectrin is associated with mutations in exon 40 (α V/41 polymorphism) and intron 45 and with partial skipping of exon 46. J Clin Invest 1993; 91:2091.

1358. Wilmotte R, Marechal J, Delaunay J: Mutation at position -12 of intron 45 (c→t) plays a prevalent role in the partial skipping of exon 46 from the transcript of allele α^{LELY} in erythroid cells. Br J Haematol 1999; 104:855.

1359. Marechal J, Wilmotte R, et al: Ethnic distribution of allele α^{LELY}, a low-expression allele of red-cell spectrin α-gene. Br J Haematol 1995; 90:553.

1360. Wilmotte R, Harper SL, et al: The exon 46-encoded sequence is essential for stability of human erythroid α-spectrin and heterodimer formation. Blood 1997; 90:4188.

1361. Basseres DS, Pranke PH, et al: Expression of spectrin α$^{I/50}$ hereditary elliptocytosis and its association with the α^{LELY} allele. Acta Haematol 1998; 100:32.

1362. Wandersee NJ, Birkenmeier CS, Bodine DM, et al: Mutations in the murine erythroid alpha-spectrin gene alter spectrin mRNA and protein levels and spectrin incorporation into the red blood cell membrane skeleton. Blood 2003; 101:325.

1363. Gallagher PG, Tse WT, et al: A defect in α-spectrin mRNA accumulation in hereditary pyropoikilocytosis. Trans Assoc Am Physicians 1991; 104:32.

1364. Silveira P, Cynober T, et al: Red blood cell abnormalities in hereditary elliptocytosis and their relevance to variable clinical expression. Am J Clin Pathol 1997; 108:391.

1365. DiPaolo BR, Speicher KD, Speicher DW: Identification of the amino acid mutations associated with human erythrocyte spectrin α II domain polymorphisms. Blood 1993; 82:284.

1366. Gallagher PG, Kotula L, et al: Molecular basis and haplotyping of the α II domain polymorphisms of spectrin: Application to the study of hereditary elliptocytosis and pyropoikilocytosis. Am J Hum Genet 1996; 59:351.

1367. Wandersee NJ, Roesch AN, et al: Defective spectrin integrity and neonatal thrombosis in the first mouse model for severe hereditary elliptocytosis. Blood 2001; 97:543.

1368. Feo CJ, Fischer S, et al: 1st instance of the absence of an erythrocyte membrane protein (band 4(1)) in a case of familial elliptocytic anemia. Nouv Rev Fr Hematol 1980; 22:315.

1369. Alloisio N, Morle L, et al: The heterozygous form of 4.1(–) hereditary elliptocytosis [the 4.1(–) trait]. Blood 1985; 65:46.

1370. Alloisio N, Dorleac E, et al: Analysis of the red cell membrane in a family with hereditary elliptocytosis—Total or partial absence of protein 4.1. Hum Genet 1981; 59:68.

1371. Takakuwa Y, Tchernia G, et al: Restoration of normal membrane stability to unstable protein 4.1-deficient erythrocyte membranes by incorporation of purified protein 4.1. J Clin Invest 1986; 78:80.

1372. Discher D, Parra M, et al: Identification of the minimal domain of protein 4.1 involved in skeletal interactions. Blood 1993; 82(Suppl 1):4a.

1373. Alloisio N, Morle L, et al: Red cell membrane sialoglycoprotein β in homozygous and heterozygous 4.1(–) hereditary elliptocytosis. Biochim Biophys Acta 1985; 816:57.

1374. Lambert S, Conboy J, Zail S: A molecular study of heterozygous protein 4.1 deficiency in hereditary elliptocytosis. Blood 1988; 72:1926.

1375. Yawata A, Kanzaki A, et al: A markedly disrupted skeletal network with abnormally distributed intramembrane particles in complete protein 4.1-deficient red blood cells (allele 4.1 Madrid): Implications regarding a critical role of protein 4.1 in maintenance of the integrity of the red blood cell membrane. Blood 1997; 90:2471.

1376. Conboy J, Mohandas N, et al: Molecular basis of hereditary elliptocytosis due to protein 4.1 deficiency. N Engl J Med 1986; 315:680.

1377. Garbarz M, Devaux I, et al: Protein 4.1 Lille, a novel mutation in the downstream initiation codon of protein 4.1 gene associated with heterozygous 4.1(–) hereditary elliptocytosis. Hum Mutat 1995; 5:339.

1378. Conboy JG, Chasis JA, et al: An isoform-specific mutation in the protein 4.1 gene results in hereditary elliptocytosis and complete deficiency of protein 4.1 in erythrocytes but not in nonerythroid cells. J Clin Invest 1993; 91:77.

1379. Conboy J, Marchesi S, et al: Molecular analysis of insertion/deletion mutations in protein 4.1 in elliptocytosis: II. Determination of molecular genetic origins of rearrangements. J Clin Invest 1990; 86:524.

1380. Marchesi S, Conboy J, et al: Molecular analysis of insertion/deletion mutations in protein 4.1 in elliptocytosis: I. Biochemical identification of rearrangements in the spectrin/actin binding domain and functional characterizations. J Clin Invest 1990; 86:515.

1381. Moriniere M, Ribeiro L, et al: Elliptocytosis in patients with C-terminal domain mutations of protein 4.1 correlates with encoded messenger RNA levels rather than with alterations in primary protein structure. Blood 2000; 95:1834.

1382. Venezia ND, Maillet P, et al: A large deletion within the protein 4.1 gene associated with a stable truncated mRNA and an unaltered tissue-specific alternative splicing. Blood 1998; 91:4361.

1383. Tanner MJ, High S, et al: Genetic variants of human red-cell membrane sialoglycoprotein β. Study of the alterations occurring in the sialoglycoprotein-β gene. Biochem J 1988; 250:407.

1384. Winardi R, Reid M, et al: Molecular analysis of glycophorin C deficiency in human erythrocytes. Blood 1993; 81:2799.

1385. Colin Y: Gerbich blood groups and minor glycophorins of human erythrocytes. Transfus Clin Biol 1995; 2:259.

1386. Rebuck JW, van Slyck EJ: An unsuspected ultrastructural fault in human elliptocytes. Am J Clin Pathol 1968; 49:19.

1387. Liu S-C, Derick LH, Palek J: Dependence of the permanent deformation of red blood cell membranes on spectrin dimer-tetramer equilibrium: Implication for permanent membrane deformation of irreversibly sickled cells. Blood 1993; 81:522.

1388. De Gruchy GC, Loder PB, Hennessy IV: Haemolysis and glycolytic metabolism in hereditary elliptocytosis. Br J Haematol 1962; 8:168.

1389. Peters JC, Rowland M, et al: Erythrocyte sodium transport in hereditary elliptocytosis. Can J Physiol Pharmacol 1966; 44:817.

1390. Facer CA: Malaria, hereditary elliptocytosis, and pyropoikilocytosis. Lancet 1989; 1:897.

1391. Chishti AH, Palek J, et al: Reduced invasion and growth of *Plasmodium falciparum* into elliptocytic red blood cells with a combined deficiency of protein 4.1, glycophorin C, and p55. Blood 1996; 87:3462.

1392. Amato D, Booth PB: Hereditary ovalocytosis in Melanesians. Papua New Guinea Med J 1977; 20:26.

1393. Castelino D, Saul A, et al: Ovalocytosis in Papua New Guinea—Dominantly inherited resistance to malaria. Southeast Asian J Trop Med Public Health 1981; 12:549.

1394. Cattani JA, Gibson FD, et al: Hereditary ovalocytosis and reduced susceptibility to malaria in Papua New Guinea. Trans R Soc Trop Med Hyg 1987; 81:705.

1395. Fix AG, Baer AS, Lie-Injo LE: The mode of inheritance of ovalocytosis/elliptocytosis in Malaysian Orang Asli families. Hum Genet 1982; 61:250.

1396. Liu S-C, Zhai S, et al: Molecular defect of the band 3 protein in Southeast Asian ovalocytosis. N Engl J Med 1990; 323:1530.

1397. Baer A, Lie-Injo LE, et al: Genetic factors and malaria in the Temuan. Am J Hum Genet 1976; 28:179.

1398. Harrison KL, Collins KA, McKenna HW: Hereditary elliptical stomatocytosis; a case report. Pathology 1976; 8:307.

1399. Honig GR, Lacson PS, Maurer HS: A new familial disorder with abnormal erythrocyte morphology and increased permeability of the erythrocytes to sodium and potassium. Pediatr Res 1971; 5:159.

1400. Booth PB, Serjeantson S, et al: Selective depression of blood group antigens associated with hereditary ovalocytosis among Melanesians. Vox Sang 1977; 32:99.

1401. Serjeantson S, Bryson K, et al: Malaria and hereditary ovalocytosis. Hum Genet 1977; 37:161.

1402. Ravindranath Y, Goyette G Jr, Johnson RM: Southeast Asian ovalocytosis in an African-American family. Blood 1994; 84:2823.

1403. Coetzer TL, Beeton L, et al: Southeast Asian ovalocytosis in a South African kindred with hemolytic anemia. Blood 1996; 87:1656.

1404. Schischmanoff PO, Cynober T, et al: Southeast Asian ovalocytosis in white persons. Hemoglobin 1999; 23:47.

1405. Foo LC, Rekhra J-V, et al: Ovalocytosis protects against severe malaria parasitemia in the Malayan aborigines. Am J Trop Med Hyg 1992; 47:271.

1406. Allen SJ, O'Donnell A, et al: Prevention of cerebral malaria in children in Papua New Guinea by southeast Asian ovalocytosis band 3. Am J Trop Med Hyg 1999; 60:1056.

1407. Bunyaratvej A, Butthep P, et al: Malaria protection in hereditary ovalocytosis: Relation to red cell deformability, red cell parameters and degree of ovalocytosis. Southeast Asian J Trop Med Public Health 1997; 28(Suppl 3):38.

1408. Genton B, al-Yaman F, et al: Ovalocytosis and cerebral malaria. Nature 1995; 378:564.

1409. Hadley T, Saul A, et al: Resistance of Melanesian elliptocytes (ovalocytes) to invasion by *Plasmodium knowlesi* and *Plasmodium falciparum* malaria parasites *in vitro*. J Clin Invest 1983; 71:780.

1410. Dluzewski AR, Nash GB, et al: Invasion of hereditary ovalocytes by *Plasmodium falciparum in vitro* and its relation to intracellular ATP concentration. Mol Biochem Parasitol 1992; 55:1.

1411. Kidson C, Lamont G, et al: Ovalocytic erythrocytes from Melanesians are resistant to invasion by malaria parasites in culture. Proc Natl Acad Sci USA 1981; 78:5829.

1412. Saul A, Lamont G, et al: Decreased membrane deformability in Melanesian ovalocytes from Papua New Guinea. J Cell Biol 1984; 98:1348.

1413. Mohandas N, Lie-Injo LE, et al: Rigid membranes of Malayan ovalocytes: A likely genetic barrier against malaria. Blood 1984; 63:1385.

1414. Mohandas N, Winardi R, et al: Molecular basis for membrane rigidity of hereditary ovalocytosis: A novel mechanism involving the cytoplasmic domain of band 3. J Clin Invest 1992; 89:686.

1415. Schofield AE, Tanner MJ, et al: Basis of unique red cell membrane properties in hereditary ovalocytosis. J Mol Biol 1992; 223:949.

1416. O'Donnell A, Allen SJ, et al: Red cell morphology and malaria anaemia in children with Southeast-Asian ovalocytosis band 3 in Papua New Guinea. Br J Haematol 1998; 101:407.

1417. Laosombat V, Dissaneevate S, et al: Neonatal hyperbilirubinemia associated with Southeast Asian ovalocytosis. Am J Hematol 1999; 60:136.

1418. Reardon DM, Seymour CA, et al: Hereditary ovalocytosis with compensated haemolysis. Br J Haematol 1993; 85:197.

1419. Jarolim P, Palek J, et al: Deletion in the band 3 gene in malaria resistant Southeast Asian ovalocytosis. Proc Natl Acad Sci USA 1991; 88:11022.

1420. Mueller TJ, Morrison M: Detection of a variant of protein 3, the major transmembrane protein of the human erythrocyte. J Biol Chem 1977; 252:6573.

1421. Jarolim P, Rubin HL, et al: Band 3 Memphis: a widespread polymorphism with abnormal electrophoretic mobility of erythrocyte band 3 protein caused by substitution AAG→GAG (Lys→Glu) in codon 56. Blood 1992; 80:1592.

1422. Yannoukakos D, Vasseur C, et al: Human erythrocyte band 3 polymorphism (band 3 Memphis): Characterization of the structural modification (Lys 56r→Glu) by protein chemistry methods. Blood 1991; 78:1117.

1423. Jones GL: Red cell membrane proteins in Melanesian ovalocytosis autophosphorylation and proteolysis. Proc Aust Biochem Soc 1984; 16:34.

1424. Jones GL, McLemore-Edmundson H, et al: Human erythrocyte band 3 has an altered N-terminus in malaria-resistant Melanesian ovalocytosis. Biochim Biophys Acta 1991; 1096:33.

1425. Husain-Chishti A, Andrabi K, et al: Altered tyrosine phosphorylation of the red cell band 3 protein in malaria resistant Southeast Asian ovalocytosis (SAO). Blood 1991; 78(Suppl 1):80a.

1426. Schofield AE, Rearden DM, Tanner MJA: Defective anion transport activity of the abnormal band 3 in hereditary ovalocytic red cells. Nature 1992; 335:836.

1427. Tanner MJ, Bruce L, et al: The defective red cell anion transporter (band 3) in hereditary Southeast Asian ovalocytosis and the role of glycophorin A in the expression of band 3 anion transport activity in *Xenopus* oocytes. Biochem Soc Trans 1992; 20:542.

1428. Tanner MJ, Bruce L, et al: Melanesian hereditary ovalocytes have a deletion in red cell band 3. Blood 1991; 78:2785.

1429. Liu SC, Jarolim P, et al: The homozygous state for the band 3 protein mutation in Southeast Asian Ovalocytosis may be lethal. Blood 1994; 84:3590.

1430. Mgone CS, Koki G, et al: Occurrence of the erythrocyte band 3 (AE1) gene deletion in relation to malaria endemicity in Papua New Guinea. Trans R Soc Trop Med Hyg 1996; 90:228.

1431. Mohandas N, Chasis JA, Shohet SB: The influence of membrane skeleton on red cell deformability, membrane material properties, and shape. Semin Hematol 1983; 20:225.

1432. Kuma H, Inoue K, et al: Secondary structures of synthetic peptides corresponding to the first membrane-contact portion of normal band 3 and its deletion mutant (Southeast Asian ovalocytosis). J Biochem (Tokyo) 1998; 124:509.

1433. Liu S-C, Palek J, et al: Molecular basis of altered red blood cell membrane properties in Southeast Asian ovalocytosis: Role of the mutant band 3 protein in band 3 oligomerization and retention by the membrane skeleton. Blood 1995; 86:349.

1434. Che A, Cherry RJ, et al: Aggregation of band 3 in hereditary ovalocytic red cell membranes. Electron microscopy and protein rotational diffusion studies. J Cell Sci 1993; 105:655.

1435. Moriyama R, Ideguchi H, et al: Structural and functional characterization of band 3 from Southeast Asian ovalocytes. J Biol Chem 1992; 267:25792.

1436. Chambers EJ, Bloomberg GB, et al: Structural studies on the effects of the deletion in the red cell anion exchanger (band 3, AE1) associated with South East Asian ovalocytosis. J Mol Biol 1999; 285:1289.

1437. Okoye VC, Bennett V: *Plasmodium falciparum* malaria. Band 3 as a possible receptor during invasion of human erythrocytes. Science 1985; 227:169.

1438. Dluzewski AR, Fryer PR, et al: Red cell membrane protein distribution during malarial invasion. J Cell Sci 1989; 92:691.

1439. Zarkowsky HS, Oski FA, Sha'afi R: Congenital hemolytic anemia with high-sodium, low-potassium red cells: I. Studies of membrane permeability. N Engl J Med 1968; 278:573.

1440. Lande WM, Mentzer WC: Haemolytic anaemia associated with increased cation permeability. Clin Haematol 1985; 14:89.

1441. Delaunay J, Stewart G, Iolascon A: Hereditary dehydrated and overhydrated stomatocytosis: Recent advances. Curr Opin Hematol 1999; 6:110.

1442. Lock SP, Smith RS, et al: Stomatocytosis: A hereditary red cell anomaly associated with haemolytic anaemia. Br J Haematol 1961; 7:303.

1443. Bienzle U, Niethammer D, et al.: Congenital stomatocytosis and chronic haemolytic anaemia. Scand J Haematol 1975; 15:339.

1444. Eber SW, Lande WM, et al: Hereditary stomatocytosis: Consistent association with an integral membrane protein deficiency. Br J Haematol 1989; 72:452.

1445. Glader BE, Fortier N, et al: Congenital hemolytic anemia associated with dehydrated erythrocytes and increased potassium loss. N Engl J Med 1974; 291:491.

1446. Huppi PS, Ott P, et al: Congenital haemolytic anaemia in a low birth weight infant due to congenital stomatocytosis. Eur J Haematol 1991; 47:1.

1447. Kanzaki A, Yawata Y: Hereditary stomatocytosis: Phenotypical expression of sodium transport and band 7 peptides in 44 cases. Br J Haematol 1992; 82:133.

1448. Lande WM, Thiemann PV, Mentzer WC Jr: Missing band 7 membrane protein in two patients with high Na, low K erythrocytes. J Clin Invest 1982; 70:1273.

1449. Clark MR, Mohandas N, et al: Effects of abnormal cation transport on deformability of desicytes. J Supramol Struct 1978; 8:521.

1450. Lane PA, Kuypers FA, et al: Excess of red cell membrane proteins in hereditary high-phosphatidylcholine hemolytic anemia. Am J Hematol 1990; 34:186.

1451. Lo SS, Hitzig WH, Marti HR: Stomatozytose. Schweiz Med Wochenschr 1970; 100:1977.

1452. Lo SS, Marti HR, Hitzig WH: Haemolytic anaemia associated with decreased concentration of reduced glutathione in red cells. Acta Haematol 1971; 46:14.

1453. McGrath KM: Dehydrated hereditary stomatocytosis—A report of two families and a review of the literature. Pathology 1984; 16:146.

1454. Meadow SR: Stomatocytosis. Proc R Soc Med 1967; 60:13.

1455. Mentzer WC Jr, Smith WB, et al: Hereditary stomatocytosis membranes and metabolism studies. Blood 1975; 46:659.

1456. Miller G, Townes PL, et al: A new congenital hemolytic anemia with deformed erythrocytes (?"stomatocytes") and remarkable susceptibility of erythrocytes to cold hemolysis *in vitro*. I. Clinical and hematologic studies. Pediatrics 1965; 35:906.

1457. Miller DR, Rickles FR, et al: A new variant of hereditary hemolytic anemia with stomatocytosis and erythrocyte cation abnormality. Blood 1971; 38:184.

1458. Morlé L, Pothier B, et al: Reduction of membrane band 7 and activation of volume stimulated (K^+, Cl^-) cotransport in a case of congenital stomatocytosis. Br J Haematol 1989; 71:141.

1459. Mutoh S, Sasaki R, et al: A family of hereditary stomatocytosis associated with normal level of Na-K-ATPase activity of red blood cells. Am J Hematol 1983; 14:113.

1460. Nolan GR: Hereditary xerocytosis: A case history and review of the literature. Pathology 1984; 16:151.

1461. Schroter W, Ungefehr K, Tillmann W: Role of the spleen in congenital stomatocytosis associated with high sodium-low potassium erythrocytes. Klin Wochenschr 1981; 59:173.

1462. Shohet SB, Nathan DG, Livermore BM: Hereditary hemolytic anemia associated with abnormal membrane lipids. II. Ion permeability and transport abnormalities. Blood 1973; 42:1.

1463. Clark MR, Shohet SB, Gottfried EL: Hereditary hemolytic disease with increased red blood cell phosphatidylcholine and dehydration: One, two, or many disorders? Am J Hematol 1993; 42:25.

1464. Shohet SB, Livermore BM, et al: Hereditary hemolytic anemia associated with abnormal membrane lipids: Mechanism of accumulation of phosphatidyl choline. Blood 1971; 38:445.

1465. Turpin F, Lortholary P, et al: A case of hemolytic anemia with stomatocytosis. Nouv Rev Fr Hematol 1971; 11:585.

1466. Wiley JS, Ellory JC, et al: Characteristics of the membrane defect in the hereditary stomatocytosis syndrome. Blood 1975; 46:337.

1467. Yawata Y, Takemoto Y, et al: The Japanese family of congenital hemolytic anemia with high red cell phosphatidyl choline and increased sodium transport. Acta Haematol Jpn 1982; 45:672.

1468. Platt OS, Lux SE, Nathan DG: Exercise-induced hemolysis in xerocytosis: Erythrocyte dehydration and shear sensitivity. J Clin Invest 1981; 68:631.

1469. Wiley JS, Cooper RA, et al: Hereditary stomatocytosis: Association of low 2,3-diphosphoglycerate with increased cation pumping by the red cell. Br J Haematol 1979; 41:133.

1470. Gore DM, Chetty MC, et al: Familial pseudohyperkalaemia Cardiff: A mild version of cryohydrocytosis. Br J Haematol 2002; 117:212.

1471. Grootenboer S, Barro C, et al: Dehydrated hereditary stomatocytosis: A cause of prenatal ascites. Prenat Diagn 2001; 21:1114.

1472. Haines PG, Jarvis HG, et al: Two further British families with the 'cryohydrocytosis' form of hereditary stomatocytosis. Br J Haematol 2001; 113:932.

1473. Haines PG, Crawley C, et al: Familial pseudohyperkalaemia Chiswick: A novel congenital thermotropic variant of K and Na transport across the human red cell membrane. Br J Haematol 2001; 112:469.

1474. Grootenboer S, Schischmanoff PO, et al: Pleiotropic syndrome of dehydrated hereditary stomatocytosis, pseudohyperkalemia, and perinatal edema maps to 16q23-q24. Blood 2000; 96:2599.

1475. Coles SE, Chetty MC, et al: Two British families with variants of the 'cryohydrocytosis' form of hereditary stomatocytosis. Br J Haematol 1999; 105:1055.

1476. Carella M, Stewart GW, et al: Genetic heterogeneity of hereditary stomatocytosis syndromes showing pseudohyperkalemia. Haematologica 1999; 84:862.

1477. Coles SE, Ho MM, et al: A variant of hereditary stomatocytosis with marked pseudohyperkalaemia. Br J Haematol 1999; 104:275.

1478. Grootenboer S, Schischmanoff PO, et al: A genetic syndrome associating dehydrated hereditary stomatocytosis, pseudohyperkalaemia and perinatal oedema. Br J Haematol 1998; 103:383.

1479. Kilpatrick ES, Burton ID: Pseudohyperkalaemia, pseudohyponatraemia and pseudohypoglycaemia in a patient with hereditary stomatocytosis. Ann Clin Biochem 1997; 34:561.

1480. Rix M, Bjerrum PJ, et al: Medfodt stomatocytose med haemolytisk anaemi—med abnorm kationpermeabilitet og defekte membranproteiner. (Congenital stomatocytosis with hemolytic anemia—with abnormal cation permeability and defective membrane proteins.) Ugeskr Laeger 1991; 153:724.

1481. Ogburn PL, Jr, Ramin KD, et al: In utero erythrocyte transfusion for fetal xerocytosis associated with severe anemia and non-immune hydrops fetalis. Am J Obstet Gynecol 2001; 185:238.

1482. Wiley JS, Shaller CC: Selective loss of calcium permeability on maturation of reticulocytes. J Clin Invest 1977; 59:1113.

1483. Dutcher PO, Segel GB, et al: Cation transport and its altered regulation in human stomatocytic erythrocytes. Pediatr Res 1975; 9:924.

1484. Mentzer WC, Lubin BH, Emmons S: Correction of the permeability defect in hereditary stomatocytosis by dimethyl adipimidate. N Engl J Med 1976; 294:1200.

1485. Olivieri O, Girelli D, et al: A case of congenital dyserythropoietic anaemia with stomatocytosis, reduced bands 7 and 8 and normal cation content. Br J Haematol 1992; 80:258.

1486. Stewart GW, Hepworth-Jones BE, et al: Isolation of cDNA coding for an ubiquitous membrane protein deficient in high Na^+, low K^+ stomatocytic erythrocytes. Blood 1992; 79:1593.

1487. Wang D, Mentzer WC, et al: Purification of band 7.2b, a 31-kDa integral membrane phosphoprotein absent in hereditary stomatocytosis. J Biol Chem 1991; 266:17826.

1488. Hiebl-Dirschmied CM, Adolf GR, Prohaska R: Isolation and partial characterization of the human erythrocyte band 7 integral membrane protein. Biochim Biophys Acta 1991; 1065:195.

1489. Hiebl-Dirschmied C, Entler B, et al: Cloning and nucleotide sequence of cDNA encoding human erythrocyte band 7 integral membrane protein. Biochim Biophys Acta 1991; 1090:123.

1490. Stewart GW, Argent AC, Dash BC: Stomatin: A putative cation transport regulator in the red cell membrane. Biochim Biophys Acta 1993; 1225:15.

1491. Gallagher PG, Forget BG: Structure, organization, and expression of the human band 7.2b gene, a candidate gene for hereditary hydrocytosis. J Biol Chem 1995; 270:26358.

1492. Seidel G, Prohaska R: Molecular cloning of hSLP-1, a novel human brain-specific member of the band 7/MEC-2 family similar to *Caenorhabditis elegans* UNC-24. Gene 1998; 225:23.

1493. Wang Y, Morrow JS: Identification and characterization of human SLP-2, a novel homologue of stomatin (band 7.2b) present in erythrocytes and other tissues. J Biol Chem 2000; 275:8062.

1494. Gilles F, Glenn M, et al: A novel gene STORP (STOmatin-Related Protein) is localized 2 kb upstream of the promyelocytic gene on chromosome 15q22. Eur J Haematol 2000; 64:104.

1495. Sinard JH, Stewart GW, et al: Stomatin binding to adducin: A novel link between transmembrane transport and the cytoskeleton. Mol Cell Biol 1994; 5:421a.

1496. Huang M, Gu G, et al: A stomatin-like protein necessary for mechanosensation in *C. elegans*. Nature 1995; 378:292.

1497. Mannsfeldt AG, Carroll P, et al: Stomatin, a MEC-2 like protein, is expressed by mammalian sensory neurons. Mol Cell Neurosci 1999; 13:391.

1498. Sedensky MM, Siefker JM, Morgan PG: Model organisms: New insights into ion channel and transporter function. Stomatin homologues interact in *Caenorhabditis elegans*. Am J Physiol Cell Physiol 2001; 280:C1340.

1499. Goodman MB, Ernstrom GG, et al: MEC-2 regulates *C. elegans* DEG/ENaC channels needed for mechanosensation. Nature 2002; 415:1039.

1500. Stewart GW, Argent AC: Integral band 7 protein of the human erythrocyte membrane. Biochem Soc Trans 1992; 20:785.

1501. Gallagher PG, Segel G, et al: The gene for erythrocyte band 7.2b in hereditary stomatocytosis. Blood 1992; 80(Suppl 1):276a.

1502. Wang D, Turetsky T, et al: Further studies on RBC membrane protein 7.2b deficiency in hereditary stomatocytosis. Blood 1992; 80(Suppl 1):275a.

1503. Zhu Y, Paszty C, et al: Stomatocytosis is absent in "stomatin"-deficient murine red blood cells. Blood 1999; 93:2404.

1504. Pinkerton PH, Fletch SM, et al: Hereditary stomatocytosis with hemolytic anemia in the dog. Blood 1974; 44:557.

1505. Smith JE, Moore K, et al: Glutathione metabolism in canine hereditary stomatocytosis with mild erythrocyte glutathione deficiency. J Lab Clin Med 1983; 101:611.

1506. Smith BD, Segel GB: Abnormal erythrocyte endothelial adherence in hereditary stomatocytosis. Blood 1997; 89:3451.

1507. Vives-Corrons JL, Besson I, et al: Hereditary xerocytosis: A report of six unrelated Spanish families with leaky red cell syndrome and increased heat stability of the erythrocyte membrane. Br J Haematol 1995; 90:817.

1508. Jaffe ER, Gottfried EL: Hereditary nonspherocytic hemolytic disease associated with an altered phospholipid composition of the erythrocytes. J Clin Invest 1968; 47:1375.

1509. Dise CA, Goodman DBP, Rasmussen H: Selective stimulation of erythrocyte membrane phospholipid fatty acid turnover associated with decreased volume. J Biol Chem 1980; 255:5201.

1510. Fairbanks G, Dino JE, et al: Membrane alterations in hereditary xerocytosis: Elevated binding of glyceraldehyde-3-phosphate dehydrogenase. In Kruckeberg WC, Eaton JW, et al (eds): Erythrocyte Membranes: Recent Clinical and Experimental Advances. New York, Alan R Liss, 1978, p 173.

1511. Platt OS: Exercise-induced hemolysis in sickle cell anemia: Shear-sensitivity and erythrocyte dehydration. Blood 1982; 59:1055.

1512. Harm W, Fortier NL, et al: Increased erythrocyte lipid peroxidation in hereditary xerocytosis. Clin Chim Acta 1979; 99:121.

1513. Sauberman N, Fortier NL, et al: Spectrin-hemoglobin crosslinkages associated with in vitro oxidant hypersensitivity in pathologic and artificially dehydrated red cells. Br J Haematol 1983; 54:15.

1514. Snyder LM, Sauberman N, et al: Red cell membrane response to hydrogen peroxide-sensitivity in hereditary xerocytosis and in other abnormal red cells. Br J Haematol 1981; 48:435.

1515. Fortier N, Snyder LM, et al: The relationship between in vivo generated hemoglobin skeletal protein complex and increased red cell membrane rigidity. Blood 1988; 71:1427.

1516. Albala MM, Fortier NL, Glader BE: Physiologic features of hemolysis associated with altered cation and 2,3-diphosphoglycerate content. Blood 1978; 52:135.

1517. Sauberman N, Fairbanks G, et al: Altered red blood cell surface area in hereditary xerocytosis. Clin Chim Med 1981; 114:149.

1518. Carella M, Stewart G, et al: Genomewide search for dehydrated hereditary stomatocytosis (hereditary xerocytosis): Mapping of locus to chromosome 16 (16q23-qter). Am J Hum Genet 1998; 63:810.

1519. Iolascon A, Stewart GW, et al: Familial pseudohyperkalemia maps to the same locus as dehydrated hereditary stomatocytosis (hereditary xerocytosis). Blood 1999; 93:3120.

1520. Chetty MC, Stewart GW: Pseudohyperkalaemia and pseudomacrocytosis caused by inherited red-cell disorders of the 'hereditary stomatocytosis' group. Br J Biomed Sci 2001; 58:48.

1521. Stewart GW, Corrall RJ, et al: Familial pseudohyperkalemia. Lancet 1979; 2:175.

1522. Stewart GW, Ellory JC: A family with mild hereditary xerocytosis showing high membrane cation permeability at low temperatures. Clin Sci 1985; 69:309.

1523. Douglass CC, Twomey JJ: Transient stomatocytosis with hemolysis: A previously unrecognized complication of alcoholism. Ann Intern Med 1970; 72:159.

1524. Wislöff F, Boman D: Acquired stomatocytosis in alcoholic liver disease. Scand J Haematol 1979; 23:43.

1525. Simpson LO: Blood from healthy animals and humans contains nondiscocytic erythrocytes. Br J Haematol 1989; 73:561.

1526. Barrett AM: A special form of erythrocyte possessing increased resistance to hypotonic saline. J Pathol Bacteriol 1938; 46:603.

1527. Davidson RJ, How J, Lessels S: Acquired stomatocytosis: Its prevalence and significance in routine haematology. Scand J Haematol 1977; 19:47.

1528. Ducrou W, Kimber RJ: Stomatocytes, haemolytic anaemia and abdominal pain in Mediterranean migrants. Some examples of a new syndrome? Med J Aust 1969; 2:1087.

1529. Ohsaka A, Kano Y, et al: A transient hemolytic reaction and stomatocytosis following Vinca alkaloid administration. Acta Haematol Jpn 1989; 52:7.

1530. Avent ND, Reid ME: The Rh blood group system: A review. Blood 2000; 95:375.

1531. Huang CH, Liu PZ, Cheng JG: Molecular biology and genetics of the Rh blood group system. Semin Hematol 2000; 37:150.

1532. Vos GH, Vos D, et al: A sample of blood with no detectable Rh antigens. Lancet 1961; 1:14.

1533. Ballas SK, Clark MR, et al: Red cell membrane and cation deficiency in Rh$_{null}$ syndrome. Blood 1984; 63:1046.

1534. Seidl S, Spielmann W, Martin H: Two siblings with Rh$_{null}$ disease. Vox Sang 1972; 23:182.

1535. Senhauser DA, Mitchell MW, et al: Another example of phenotype Rh$_{null}$. Transfusion 1970; 10:89.

1536. Sturgeon P: Hematological observations on the anemia associated with blood type Rh$_{null}$. Blood 1970; 36:310.

1537. Lauf PK, Joiner CH: Increased potassium transport and ouabain binding in human Rh$_{null}$ red blood cells. Blood 1976; 48:457.

1538. McGuire DM, Rosenfield RE, et al: Rh$_{mod}$. A second kindred (Craig). Vox Sang 1976; 30:430.

1539. Saji H, Hosoi T: A Japanese Rh$_{mod}$ family: Serological and haematological observations. Vox Sang 1979; 37:296.

1540. Cherif-Zahar B, Raynal V, et al: Candidate gene acting as a suppressor of the RH locus in most cases of Rh-deficiency. Nat Genet 1996; 12:168.

1541. Huang CH, Liu Z, et al: Rh50 glycoprotein gene and Rh$_{null}$ disease: A silent splice donor is trans to a Gly279→Glu missense mutation in the conserved transmembrane segment. Blood 1998; 92:1776.

1542. Hyland CA, Cherif-Zahar B, et al: A novel single missense mutation identified along the RH50 gene in a composite heterozygous Rh$_{null}$ blood donor of the regulator type. Blood 1998; 91:1458.

1543. Huang CH, Cheng G, et al: Molecular basis for Rh$_{null}$ syndrome: Identification of three new missense mutations in the Rh50 glycoprotein gene. Am J Hematol 1999; 62:25.

1544. Huang CH: The human Rh50 glycoprotein gene. Structural organization and associated splicing defect resulting in Rh$_{null}$ disease. J Biol Chem 1998; 273:2207.

1545. Huang CH, Chen Y, et al: Rh$_{null}$ disease: The amorph type results from a novel double mutation in RhCe gene on D-negative background. Blood 1998; 92:664.

1546. Cherif-Zahar B, Matassi G, et al: Molecular defects of the RHCE gene in Rh-deficient individuals of the amorph type. Blood 1998; 92:639.

1547. Kato-Yamazaki M, Okuda H, et al: Molecular genetic analysis of the Japanese amorph rh$_{null}$ phenotype. Transfusion 2000; 40:617.

1548. Huang C, Cheng GJ, et al: Rh$_{mod}$ syndrome: A family study of the translation-initiator mutation in the Rh50 glycoprotein gene. Am J Hum Genet 1999; 64:108.

1549. Oram JF: Tangier disease and ABCA1. Biochim Biophys Acta 2000; 1529:321.

1550. Oram JF, Lawn RM: ABCA1. The gatekeeper for eliminating excess tissue cholesterol. J Lipid Res 2001; 42:1173.

1551. Schmitz G, Langmann T: Structure, function and regulation of the ABC1 gene product. Curr Opin Lipidol 2001; 12:129.

1552. Reinhart WH, Gossi U, et al: Haemolytic anaemia in analphalipoproteinaemia (Tangier disease): Morphological, biochemical, and biophysical properties of the red blood cell. Br J Haematol 1989; 72:272.

1553. Hoffman HN, Fredrickson DS: Tangier disease (familial high density lipoprotein deficiency): Clinical and genetic features in two adults. Am J Med 1965; 39:582.

1554. Kummer H, Laissue J, et al: Familial analphalipoproteinemia (Tangier disease). Schweiz Med Wochenschr 1968; 98:406.

1555. Shaklady MM, Djardjouras EM, Lloyd JK: Red-cell lipids in familial alphalipoprotein deficiency (Tangier disease). Lancet 1968; 2:151.

1556. Miwa S, Fujii H, et al: A case of red-cell adenosine deaminase overproduction associated with hereditary hemolytic anemia found in Japan. Am J Hematol 1978; 5:107.

1557. Takashima H, Nakagawa M, et al: Germline mosaicism of MPZ gene in Dejerine-Sottas syndrome (HMSN III) associated with hereditary stomatocytosis. Neuromuscul Disord 1999; 9:232.

1558. Weed RI, LaCelle PL, Merrill EW: Metabolic dependence of red cell deformability. J Clin Invest 1969; 48:795.

1559. Hoffman JF: ATP compartmentation in human erythrocytes. Curr Opin Hematol 1997; 4:112.

1560. Lux SE, John KM, Ukena TE: Diminished spectrin extraction from ATP-depleted human erythrocytes. Evidence relating spectrin to changes in erythrocyte shape and deformability. J Clin Invest 1978; 61:815.

1561. Palek J, Liu SC, Snyder LM: Metabolic dependence of protein arrangement in human erythrocyte membranes. I. Analysis of spectrin-rich complexes in ATP-depleted red cells. Blood 1978; 51:385.

1562. Nathan DG, Oski FA, et al: Extreme hemolysis and red cell distortion in erythrocyte pyruvate kinase deficiency. II. Measurements of erythrocyte glucose consumption, potassium flux and adenosine triphosphate stability. N Engl J Med 1965; 272:118.

1563. Mentzer WC Jr, Baehner RL, et al: Selective reticulocyte destruction in erythrocyte pyruvate kinase deficiency. J Clin Invest 1971; 50:688.

1564. Glader BE: Salicylate-induced injury of pyruvate kinase deficient erythrocytes. N Engl J Med 1976; 294:916.

1565. Oski FA, Nathan DG, et al: Extreme hemolysis and red cell distortion in erythrocyte pyruvate kinase deficiency. I. Morphology, erythrokinetics and family enzyme studies. N Engl J Med 1964; 270:1023.

1566. Leblond PF, Lyonnais J, Delage JM: Erythrocyte populations in pyruvate kinase deficiency anaemia following splenectomy. I. Cell morphology. Br J Haematol 1978; 39:55.

1567. Leblond PF, Coulombe L, Lyonnais J: Erythrocyte populations in pyruvate kinase deficiency anaemia following splenectomy: II. Cell deformability. Br J Haematol 1978; 31:63.

1568. Coetzer T, Zail SS: Erythrocyte membrane proteins in hereditary glucose phosphate isomerase deficiency. J Clin Invest 1979; 63:552.

1569. Pintaudi AM, Tesoriere L, et al: Oxidative stress after moderate to extensive burning in humans. Free Radic Res 2000; 33:139.

1570. McGoron AJ, Joiner CH, et al: Dehydration of mature and immature sickle red blood cells during fast oxygenation/deoxygenation cycles: Role of KCl cotransport and extracellular calcium. Blood 2000; 95:2164.

1571. Schultze M: Ein Heizbarer objectisch und seine Verwendung bei Untersuchungen des Blutes. Arch Mikrok Anat 1865; 1:1.

1572. Schwartz RS, Musto S, et al: Two distinct pathways mediate the formation of intermediate density cells and hyperdense cells from normal density sickle red blood cells. Blood 1998; 92:4844.

1573. Bekyarova G, Yankova T, et al: Reduced erythrocyte deformability related to activated lipid peroxidation during the early post-burn period. Burns 1996; 22:291.

1574. Bekyarova G, Yankova T: α-Tocopherol and reduced glutathione deficiency and decreased deformability of erythrocytes after thermal skin injury. Acta Physiol Pharmacol Bulg 1998; 23:55.

1575. Shen SC, Ham TH, Fleming AB: Studies on the destruction of red blood cells: III. Mechanism and complication of hemoglobinuria in patients with thermal burns: Spherocytosis and increased osmotic fragility of red blood cells. N Engl J Med 1943; 229:701.

1576. Topley E: The usefulness of counting "heat-affected" red cells as a guide to the risk of the later disappearance of red cells after burns. J Clin Pathol 1961; 14:295.

1577. James GW III, Purnell OJ, et al: The anemia of thermal injury: I. Studies of pigment excretion. J Clin Invest 1951; 30:181.

1578. James GW III, Abbott LD, et al: The anemia of thermal injury: III. Erythropoiesis and hemoglobin metabolism studied with N^{15}-glycine in dog and man. J Clin Invest 1954; 33:150.

1579. Moore FD, Peacock WC, et al: The anemia of thermal burns. Ann Surg 1946; 124:811.

1580. McCollough J, Polesky HF, et al: Iatrogenic hemolysis: A complication of blood warmed by a microwave device. Anesth Analg 1972; 51:102.

1581. Staples PJ, Griner PF: Extracorporeal hemolysis of blood in a microwave blood warmer. N Engl J Med 1971; 285:317.

1582. Brain MC, Dacie JV: Microangiopathic haemolytic anaemia: The possible role of vascular lesions in pathogenesis. Br J Haematol 1962; 8:358.

1583. Nevaril CG, Lynch EC: Erythrocyte damage and destruction induced by shearing stress. J Lab Clin Med 1968; 71:784.

1584. Jacob HS, Amsden T: Acute hemolytic anemia with rigid red cells in hypophosphatemia. N Engl J Med 1971; 285:1446.

1585. Lichtman MA, Miller DR, et al: Reduced red cell glycolysis, 2,3-diphosphoglycerate and adenosine triphosphate concentration, and increased hemoglobin-oxygen affinity caused by hypophosphatemia. Ann Intern Med 1971; 74:562.

1586. Kalan G, Derganc M, Primocic J: Phosphate metabolism in red blood cells of critically ill neonates. Pflugers Arch 2000; 440:R109.

1587. Larsen VH, Waldau T, et al: Erythrocyte 2,3-diphosphoglycerate depletion associated with hypophosphatemia detected by routine arterial blood gas analysis. Scand J Clin Lab Invest Suppl 1996; 224:83.

1588. Dean HM, Decker CL, Baker LD: Temporary survival in clostridial hemolysis with absence of circulating red cells. N Engl J Med 1967; 277:700.

1589. Myers G, Ngoi SS, et al: Clostridial septicemia in an urban hospital. Surg Gynecol Obstet 1992; 174:291.

1590. Ifthikaruddin JJ, Holmes JA: *Clostridium perfringens* septicaemia and massive intravascular haemolysis as a terminal complication of autologous bone marrow transplant. Clin Lab Haematol 1992; 14:159.

1591. Batge B, Filejski W, et al: Clostridial sepsis with massive intravascular hemolysis: Rapid diagnosis and successful treatment. Intens Care Med 1992; 18:488.

1592. Tsai IK, Yen MY, et al: *Clostridium perfringens* septicemia with massive hemolysis. Scand J Infect Dis 1989; 21:467.

1593. Becker RC, Giuliani M, et al: Massive hemolysis in *Clostridium perfringens* infections. J Surg Oncol 1987; 35:13.

1594. Bennett JM, Healey PJM: Spherocytic hemolytic anemia and acute cholecystitis caused by *Clostridium welchii*. N Engl J Med 1963; 268:1070.

1595. Mera CL, Freedman MH: *Clostridium* liver abscess and massive hemolysis: Unique demise in Fanconi's aplastic anemia. Clin Pediatr 1984; 23:126.

1596. Mupanemunda RH, Kenyon CF, et al: Bacterial-induced activation of erythrocyte T-antigen complicating necrotizing enterocolitis: A case report. Eur J Pediatr 1993; 152:325.

1597. Placzek MM, Gorst DW: T activation haemolysis and death after blood transfusion. Arch Dis Child 1987; 62:743.

1598. Warren S, Schreiber JR, Epstein MF: Necrotizing enterocolitis and hemolysis associated with *Clostridium perfringens*. Am J Dis Child 1984; 138:686.

1599. Williams RA, Brown EF, et al: Transfusion of infants with activation of erythrocyte T antigen. J Pediatr 1989; 115:949.

1600. Alvarez A, Rives S, et al: Massive hemolysis in *Clostridium perfringens* infection. Haematologica 1999; 84:571.

1601. Singer AJ, Migdal PM, et al: *Clostridium perfringens* septicemia with massive hemolysis in a patient with Hodgkin's lymphoma. Am J Emerg Med 1997; 15:152.

1602. Abdominal pain, total intravascular hemolysis, and death in a 53 year old woman [clinical conference]. Am J Med 1990; 88:667.

1603. Terebelo HR, McCue RL, Lenneville MS: Implication of plasma free hemoglobin in massive clostridial hemolysis. JAMA 1982; 248:2028.

1604. Titball RW, Leslie DL, et al: Hemolytic and sphingomyelinase activities of *Clostridium perfringens* α toxin are dependent on a domain homologous to that of an enzyme from the human arachidonic acid pathway. Infect Immun 1991; 59:1872.

1605. Leslie D, Fairweather N, et al: Phospholipase C and haemolytic activities of *Clostridium perfringens* α toxin cloned in *Escherichia coli*: Sequence and homology with a *Bacillus cereus* phospholipase C. Mol Microbiol 1989; 3:383.

1606. Walker N, Holley J, et al: Identification of residues in the carboxy-terminal domain of *Clostridium perfringens* α-toxin (phospholipase C) which are required for its biological activities. Arch Biochem Biophys 2000; 384:24.

1607. Iwamoto M, Ohno-Iwashita Y, Ando S: Role of the essential thiol group in the thiol-activated cytolysin from *Clostridium perfringens*. Eur J Biochem 1987; 194:25.

1608. Iwamoto M, Ohno-Iwashita Y, Ando S: Effect of isolated C-terminal fragment of theta toxin (perfringolysin O) on toxin assembly and membrane lysis. Eur J Biochem 1990; 194:25.

1609. Tweten RK: Cloning and expression in *Escherichia coli* of the perfringolysin O (theta toxin) from *Clostridium perfringens* and characterization of the gene product. Infect Immun 1988; 56:3228.

1610. Harris RW, Sims PJ, Tweten RK: Kinetic aspects of the aggregation of *Clostridium perfringens* theta-toxin on erythrocyte membranes. A fluorescence energy transfer study. J Biol Chem 1991; 266:6936.

1611. Hubl W, Mostbeck B, et al: Investigation of the pathogenesis of massive hemolysis in a case of *Clostridium perfringens* septicemia. Ann Hematol 1993; 67:145.

1612. Ramasethu J, Luban N: T activation. Br J Haematol 2001; 112:259.

1613. Simpkins H, Kahlenberg A: Structural and compositional changes in the red cell membrane during *Clostridium welchii* infection. Br J Haematol 1971; 21:173.

1614. Iyaniwura TT: Snake venom constituents: Biochemistry and toxicology (Part 1). Vet Hum Toxicol 1991; 33:468.

1615. Perkash A, Sarup BM: Red cell abnormalities after snake bite. J Trop Med Hyg 1972; 75:85.

1616. Reid HA: Cobra-bites. BMJ 1964; 2:540.

1617. Gibly RL, Walter FG, et al: Intravascular hemolysis associated with North American crotalid envenomation. J Toxicol Clin Toxicol 1998; 36:337.

1618. Flachsenberger W, Leigh CM, Mirtschin PJ: Sphero-echinocytosis of human red blood cells caused by snake, red-back spider, bee and blue-ringed octopus venoms and its inhibition by snake sera. Toxicon 1995; 33:791.

1619. Foil LD, Norment BR: Envenomation by *Loxosceles reclusa* [review]. J Med Entomol 1979; 16:18.

1620. Nance WE: Hemolytic anemia of necrotic anachnoidism. Am J Med 1961; 31:801.

1621. Dacie JV: Haemolytic anemias due to drugs, chemicals and venoms: Glucose-6-phosphate dehydrogenase deficiency and favism. In The Haemolytic Anaemias, Congenital and Acquired, 2nd ed. New York, Grune & Stratton, 1967, Part IV, p 993.

1622. Monzon C, Miles J: Hemolytic anemia following a wasp sting. J Pediatr 1980; 96:1039.

1623. Schulte KL, Kochen MM: Haemolytic anemia in an adult after a wasp sting. Lancet 1981; 2:478.

1624. Bousquet J, Huchard G, Michel FB: Toxic reactions induced by *Hymenoptera* venom. Ann Allergy 1984; 52:371.

1625. Guess HA, Saviteer PL, Morris CR: Hemolysis and acute renal failure following a Portuguese man-of-war sting. Pediatrics 1982; 70:979.

1627. Diaz C, Leon G, et al: Modulation of the susceptibility of human erythrocytes to snake venom myotoxic phospholipases A$_2$: Role of negatively charged phospholipids as potential membrane binding sites. Arch Biochem Biophys 2001; 391:56.

1627. Argiolas A, Pisano JJ: Facilitation of phospholipase A$_2$ activity by mastoparans, a new class of mast cell degranulation peptides from wasp venom. J Biol Chem 1983; 25:13697.

1628. Ho CL, Hwang LL: Structure and biological activities of a new mastoparan isolated from the venom of the hornet *Vespa basalis*. Biochem J 1991; 274: 453.

1629. Katsu T, Kuroko M, et al: Interaction of wasp venom mastoparan with biomembranes. Biochim Biophys Acta 1990; 1027:85.

1630. Claque MJ, Cherry RJ: A comparative study of band 3 aggregation in erythrocyte membranes by melittin and other cationic agents. Biochim Biophys Acta 1989; 980:93.

1631. Dempsey CE: The actions of melittin on membranes. Biochim Biophys Acta 1990; 1031:143.

1632. Dufton MJ, Hider RC, Cherry RJ: The influence of melittin on the rotation of band 3 protein in the human erythrocyte membrane. Eur Biophys J 1984; 11:17.

1633. Hui SW, Stewart CM, Cherry RJ: Electron microscopic observation of the aggregation of membrane proteins in human erythrocyte by melittin. Biochim Biophys Acta 1990; 1023:335.

1634. Eichner ER: Spider bite hemolytic anemia: Positive Coombs' test, erythrophagocytosis, and leukoerythroblastic smear. Am J Clin Pathol 1984; 81:683.

1635. Hardman JT, Beck ML, et al: Incompatibility associated with the bite of a brown recluse spider (*Loxosceles reclusa*). Transfusion 1983; 23:233.

1636. Madrigal GC, Ercolani RL, Wenzl JE: Toxicity from a bite of the brown spider (*Loxosceles reclusus*): Skin necrosis, hemolytic anemia, and hemoglobinuria in a nine-year-old child. Clin Pediatr 1972; 11:641.

1637. Wright SW, Wrenn KD, et al: Clinical presentation and outcome of brown recluse spider bite. Ann Emerg Med 1997; 30:28.

1638. Futrell JM, Morgan PN, et al: Location of brown recluse venom attachment sites on human erythrocytes by the ferritin-labeled antibody technique. Am J Pathol 1979; 95:675.

1639. Kurpiewski G, Campbell BJ, et al: Alternate complement pathway activation by recluse spider venom. Int J Tissue React 1981; 3:39.

1640. Tambourgi DV, Morgan BP, et al: *Loxosceles intermedia* spider envenomation induces activation of an endogenous metalloproteinase, resulting in cleavage of glycophorins from the erythrocyte surface and facilitating complement-mediated lysis. Blood 2000; 95:683.

1641. Taylor EH, Denny WF: Hemolysis, renal failure and death, presumed secondary to bite of brown recluse spider. South Med J 1966, 59:1209.

1642. Vorse H, Seccareccio P, et al: Disseminated intravascular coagulopathy following fatal brown spider bite (necrotic arachnidism). J Pediatr 1972; 80:1035.

1643. Gebel HM, Finke JH, et al: Inactivation of complement by *Loxosceles reclusa* spider venom. Am J Trop Med Hyg 1979; 28:756.

1644. Holt DS, Botto M, et al: Targeted deletion of the CD59 gene causes spontaneous intravascular hemolysis and hemoglobinuria. Blood 2001; 98:442.

1645. Bernheimer AW, Campbell BJ, Forrester LJ: Comparative toxicology of *Loxosceles reclusa* and *Corynebacterium pseudotuberculosis*. Science 1985; 228:590.

1646. Jandl JH, Jacob HS: Hypersplenism due to infection: A study of five cases manifesting hemolytic anemia. N Engl J Med 1961; 264:1063.

1647. Harris IM, McAlister J, et al: Splenomegaly and the circulating red cell. Br J Haematol 1958; 4:97.

1648. Crane GG: The anemia of hyperreactive malarious splenomegaly. Rev Soc Bras Med Trop 1992; 25:1.

1649. Cooper RA, Jandl JH: Bile salts and cholesterol in the pathogenesis of target cells in obstructive jaundice. J Clin Invest 1968; 47:809.

1650. Cooper RA, Diloy-Puray M, et al: An analysis of lipoproteins, bile acids, and red cell membranes associated with target cells and spur cells in patients with liver disease. J Clin Invest 1972; 31:3182.

1651. Neerhout RC: Abnormalities of erythrocyte stromal lipids in hepatic disease: Erythrocyte stromal lipids in hyperlipemic states. J Lab Clin Med 1968; 71:438.

1652. Verkleij AJ, Nanta ICD, et al: The fusion of abnormal plasma lipoprotein (LP-X) and the erythrocyte membrane in patients with cholestasis studied by electron microscopy. Biochim Biophys Acta 1976; 436:366.

1653. Narayanan S: Biochemistry and clinical relevance of lipoprotein X. Am Clin Lab Sci 1984; 14:371.

1654. Seidel D, Alaupovic P, Furman RH: A lipoprotein characterizing obstructive jaundice: I. Method for quantitative separation and identification of lipoproteins in jaundice subjects. J Clin Invest 1969; 48:1211.

1655. Iida H, Hasegawa I, Nozawa Y: Biochemical studies on abnormal membranes: Protein abnormality of erythrocyte membrane in biliary obstruction. Biochim Biophys Acta 1976; 443:394.

1656. Gjone E, Torsvik H, Norum KR: Familial plasma cholesterol ester deficiency: A study of the erythrocytes. Scand J Clin Lab Invest 1968; 21:327.

1657. Jain SK, Mohandas N, Sensabaugh GF: Hereditary plasma lecithin-cholesterol acyl transferase deficiency: A heterozygous variant with erythrocyte membrane abnormalities. J Lab Clin Med 1982; 99:816.

1658. Murayama N, Asano Y, Hosoda S: Decreased sodium influx and abnormal red cell membrane lipids in a patient with familial plasma lecithin:cholesterol acyltransferase deficiency. Am J Hematol 1984; 16:129.

1658a. Suda T, Akamatsu A, et al: Alterations in erythrocyte membrane lipid and its fragility in a patient with familial lecithin:cholesterol acyltrasferase (LCAT) deficiency. J Med Invest 2002; 49:147.

1659. Kuivenhoven JA, Pritchard H, et al: The molecular pathology of lecithin:cholesterol acyltransferase (LCAT) deficiency syndromes. J Lipid Res 1997; 38:191.

1660. Miettinen HE, Gylling H, et al: Molecular genetic study of Finns with hypoalphalipoproteinemia and hyperalphalipoproteinemia: A novel Gly230 Arg mutation (LCAT^{Fin}) of lecithin:cholesterol acyltransferase (LCAT) accounts for 5 percent of cases with very low serum HDL cholesterol levels. Arterioscler Thromb Vasc Biol 1998; 18:591.

1661. Peelman F, Verschelde JL, et al: Effects of natural mutations in lecithin:cholesterol acyltransferase on the enzyme structure and activity. J Lipid Res 1999; 40:59.

1662. Gjone E, Javitt NB, et al: Studies of lipoprotein-X (LP-X) and bile acids in familial lecithin:cholesterol acyltransferase deficiency. Acta Med Scand 1973; 194:377.

1663. Norum KR, Gjone E: The influence of plasma from patients with familial lecithin:cholesterol acyltransferase deficiency on the lipid pattern of erythrocytes. Scand J Clin Lab Invest 1968; 22:94.

1664. Jacobsen CD, Gjone E, Hovig T: Sea-blue histiocytes in familial lecithin:cholesterol acyltransferase deficiency. Scand J Haematol 1972; 9:106.

1665. Lambert G, Sakai N, et al: Analysis of glomerulosclerosis and atherosclerosis in lecithin cholesterol acyltransferase-deficient mice. J Biol Chem 2001; 276:15090.

1666. Frohlich J, Hoag G, et al: Hypoalphalipoproteinemia resembling fish eye disease. Acta Med Scand 1987; 221:291.

1667. Singer K, Miller EB, et al: Hematologic changes following splenectomy in man, with particular reference to target cells, hemolytic index and lysolecithin. Am J Med Sci 1941; 202:171.

1668. Singer K, Weisz L: The life cycle of the erythrocyte after splenectomy and the problems of splenic hemolysis and target cell formation. Am J Med Sci 1945; 210:301.

1669. DeHaan LD, Werre JM, et al: Alterations in size, shape and osmotic behaviour of red cells after splenectomy: A study of their age dependence. Br J Haematol 1988; 69:71.

1670. Come SE, Shohet SB, Robinson SH: Surface remodeling vs whole-cell hemolysis of reticulocytes produced with erythroid stimulation or iron-deficiency anemia. Blood 1974; 44:817.

1671. Smith CH, Khakoo Y: Burr cells: Classification and effect of splenectomy. J Pediatr 1970; 76:99.

1672. Crosby WH.: Normal function of the spleen relative to red blood cells: A review. Blood 1959; 14:399.

1673. Brecher G, Haley JE, Wallerstein RO: Spiculed erythrocytes after splenectomy acanthocytes or non-specific poikilocytes? Nouv Rev Fr Hematol 1972; 12:751.

1674. Furchgott RF: Disk-sphere transformation in mammalian red cells. J Exp Biol 1940; 17:30.

1675. Artmann GM, Sung KL, et al: Micropipette aspiration of human erythrocytes induces echinocytes via membrane phospholipid translocation. Biophys J 1997; 72:1434.

1676. Iglic A, Kralj-Iglic V, Hagerstrand H: Amphiphile induced echinocyte-spheroechinocyte transformation of red blood cell shape. Eur Biophys J 1998; 27:335.

1677. Wong P: A basis of echinocytosis and stomatocytosis in the disc-sphere transformations of the erythrocyte. J Theor Biol 1999; 196:343.

1678. Nakao M, Nakao T, Yamazoe S: Adenosine triphosphate and shape of erythrocytes. J Biochem 1961; 45:487.

1679. Palek J, Stewart G, Lionetti FJ: The dependence of shape of human erythrocyte ghosts on calcium, magnesium, and adenosine triphosphate. Blood 1974; 44:583.

1680. Aherne WA: The "burr" red cell and azotaemia. J Clin Pathol 1957; 10:252.

1681. Schwartz SO, Motto SA: The diagnostic significance of "burr" red blood cells. Am J Med Sci 1949; 218:513.

1682. Feo CJ, Tchernia G, et al: Observation of echinocytosis in eight patients: A phase contrast and SEM study. Br J Haematol 1978; 40:519.

1683. Zipursky A, Brown E, et al: The erythrocyte differential count in newborn infants. Am J Pediatr Hematol 1983; 5:45.

1684. Carlyle RF, Nichols G, Rowles PM: Abnormal red cells in blood of men subjected to simulated dives. Lancet 1979; 1:1114.

1685. Cooper RA: Anemia with spur cells: A red cell defect acquired in serum and modified in the circulation. J Clin Invest 1969; 48:1820.

1686. Bassen FA, Kornzweig AL: Malformation of the erythrocytes in a case of atypical retinitis pigmentosa. Blood 1950; 5:381.

1687. Tuffy P, Brown AK, et al: Infantile pyknocytosis: A common erythrocyte abnormality of the first trimester. Am J Dis Child 1959; 98:227.

1688. Kay J, Stricker RB: Hematologic and immunologic abnormalities in anorexia nervosa. South Med J 1983 76:1008.

1689. Mant MJ, Faragher BS: The haematology of anorexia nervosa. Br J Haematol 1972; 23:737.

1690. Symmans WA, Shepard CS, et al: Hereditary acanthocytosis associated with the McLeod phenotype of the Kell blood group system. Br J Haematol 1979; 42:575.

1691. Udden MM, Umeda M, et al: New abnormalities in the morphology, cell surface receptors, and electrolyte metabolism of In(Lu) erythrocytes. Blood 1987; 69:52.

1692. Wardrop C, Hutchison HE: Red-cell shape in hypothyroidism. Lancet 1969; 1:1243.

1693. Doll DC, List AF, et al: Acanthocytosis associated with myelodysplasia. J Clin Oncol 1989; 7:1569.

1694. Ohsaka A, Yawata Y, et al: Abnormal calcium transport of acanthocytes in acute myelodysplasia with myelofibrosis. Br J Haematol 1989; 73:568.

1695. Salt HB, Wolff OH, et al: On having no β-lipoprotein. A syndrome comprising a-beta-lipoproteinaemia, acanthocytosis, and steatorrhoea. Lancet 1960; 2:326.

1696. Schonfeld G: The hypobetalipoproteinemias. Annu Rev Nutr 1995; 15:23.

1697. Gregg RE, Wetterau JR: The molecular basis of abetalipoproteinemia. Curr Opin Lipidol 1994; 5:81.

1698. Dieplinger H, Kronenberg F: Genetics and metabolism of lipoprotein$_a$ and their clinical implications (Part 1). Wien Klin Wochenschr 1999; 111:5.

1699. Wetterau JR, Aggerbeck LP, et al: Absence of microsomal triglyceride transfer protein in individuals with abetalipoproteinemia. Science 1992; 258:999.

1700. Berriot-Varoqueaux N, Aggerbeck LP, et al: The role of the microsomal triglyceride transfer protein in abetalipoproteinemia. Annu Rev Nutr 2000; 20:663.

1701. Gordon DA, Jamil H: Progress towards understanding the role of microsomal triglyceride transfer protein in apolipoprotein-B lipoprotein assembly. Biochim Biophys Acta 2000; 1486:72.

1702. Black DD, Hay RV, et al: Intestinal and hepatic apolipoprotein B gene expression in abetalipoproteinemia. Gastroenterology 1991; 101:520.

1703. Glickman RM, Glickman JN, et al: Apolipoprotein synthesis in normal and abetalipoproteinemic intestinal mucosa. Gastroenterology 1991; 101:749.

1704. Lieper JM, Bayliss JD, et al: Microsomal triglyceride transfer protein, the abetalipoproteinemia gene product, mediates the secretion of apolipoprotein B-containing lipoproteins from heterologous cells. J Biol Chem 1994; 269:21951.

1705. Gheeraert P, DeBuyzere M, et al: Plasma and erythrocyte lipids in two families with heterozygous hypobetalipoproteinemia. Clin Biochem 1988; 21:371.

1706. Simon ER, Ways P: Incubation hemolysis and red cell metabolism in acanthocytosis. J Clin Invest 1964; 43:1311.

1707. Barenholz Y, Yechiel E, et al: Importance of cholesterol-phospholipid interaction in determining dynamics of normal and abetalipoproteinemia red blood cell membrane. Cell Biophys 1981; 3:115.

1708. Iida H, Takashima Y, et al: Alterations in erythrocyte membrane lipids in abetalipoproteinemia: Phospholipid and fatty acyl composition. Biochem Med 1984; 32:79.

1709. Cooper RA, Gulbrandsen CL: The relationship between serum lipoproteins and red cell membranes in abetalipoproteinemia: Deficiency of lecithin:cholesterol acyltransferase. J Lab Clin Med 1971; 78:323.

1710. Flamm M, Schachter D: Acanthocytosis and cholesterol enrichment decrease lipid fluidity of only the outer human erythrocyte membrane leaflet. Nature 1982; 298:290.

1711. McCormick EC, Cornwell DG, et al: Studies on the distribution of tocopherol in human serum lipoproteins. J Lipid Res 1969; 1:211.

1712. Dodge JT, Cohen G, et al: Peroxidative hemolysis of red blood cells from patients with abetalipoproteinemia (acanthocytosis). J Clin Invest 1967; 46:357.

1713. Elias E, Muller DP, Scott J: Association of spinocerebellar disorders with cystic fibrosis or chronic childhood cholestasis and very low serum vitamin E. Lancet 1981; 2:1319.

1714. Alvarez F, Landrieu P, et al: Vitamin E deficiency is responsible for neurologic abnormalities in cholestatic children. J Pediatr 1985; 107:422.

1715. Sokol RJ, Guggenheim MA, et al: Frequency and clinical progression of the vitamin E deficiency neurologic disorder in children with prolonged neonatal cholestasis. Am J Dis Child 1985; 139:1211.

1716. Harding AE, Matthews S, et al: Spinocerebellar degeneration associated with a selective defect of vitamin E absorption. N Engl J Med 1985; 313:32.

1717. Sokol RJ, Guggenheim M, et al: Improved neurologic function after long-term correction of vitamin E deficiency in children with chronic cholestasis. N Engl J Med 1985; 313:1580.

1718. Muller DPR, Lloyd JK, Bird AC: Long-term management of abetalipoproteinaemia. Arch Dis Child 1977; 52:209.

1719. Chowers I, Banin E, et al: Long-term assessment of combined vitamin A and E treatment for the prevention of retinal degeneration in abetalipoproteinaemia and hypobetalipoproteinaemia patients. Eye 2001; 15:525.

1720. Estes JW, Morléy JT, et al: A new hereditary acanthocytosis syndrome. Am J Med 1967; 42:868.

1721. Levine IM, Estes JW, Looney JM: Hereditary neurological disease with acanthocytosis. Arch Neurol 1968; 19:403.

1722. Hardie RJ: Acanthocytosis and neurological impairment—A review. Q J Med 1989; 71:291.

1723. Alonso ME, Teixeira F, et al: Chorea-acanthocytosis: A report of a family and neuropathological study of two cases. Can J Neurol Sci 1989; 16:426.

1724. Asano K, Osawa Y, et al: Erythrocyte membrane abnormalities in patients with amyotrophic chorea with acanthocytosis: II. Abnormal degradation of membrane proteins. J Neurol Sci 1985; 68:161.

1725. Clark MR, Aminoff MJ, et al: Red cell deformability and lipid composition in two forms of acanthocytosis: Enrichment of acanthocytic populations by density gradient centrifugation. J Lab Clin Med 1989; 113:469.

1726. Critchley EM, Clark DB, Wikler A: Acanthocytosis and neurological disorder without abetalipoproteinemia. Arch Neurol 1968; 18:134.

1727. Faillace RT, Kingston WJ, et al: Cardiomyopathy associated with the syndrome of amyotrophic chorea and acanthocytosis. Ann Intern Med 1982; 96:616.

1728. Gross KB, Skrivanek JA, et al: Familial amyotrophic chorea with acanthocytosis: New clinical and laboratory investigations. Arch Neurol 1985; 42:753.

1729. Hardie RJ, Pullon HW, et al: Neuroacanthocytosis: A clinical, haematological and pathological study of 19 cases. Brain 1991; 114:13.

1730. Sotaniemi KA: Chorea-acanthocytosis: Neurological disease with acanthocytosis. Acta Neurol Scand 1983; 68:53.

1731. Ueno E, Oguchi K, et al: Morphological abnormalities of erythrocyte membrane in the hereditary neurological disease with chorea, areflexia and acanthocytosis. J Neurol Sci 1982; 56:89.

1732. Vance JM, Pericak-Vance MA, et al: Chorea-acanthocytosis: A report of three new families and implications for genetic counseling. Am J Med Genet 1987; 28:403.

1733. Villegas A, Moscat J, et al: A new family with choreo-acanthocytosis. Acta Haematol (Basel) 1987; 77:215.

1734. Vita G, Serra S, et al: Peripheral neuropathy in amyotrophic chorea-acanthocytosis. Ann Neurol 1989; 26:583.

1735. Sorrentino G, De Renzo A, et al: Late appearance of acanthocytes during the course of chorea-acanthocytosis. J Neurol Sci 1999; 163:175.

1736. Rampoldi L, Dobson-Stone C, et al: A conserved sorting-associated protein is mutant in chorea-acanthocytosis. Nat Genet 2001; 28:119.

1737. Ueno S, Maruki Y, et al: The gene encoding a newly discovered protein, chorein, is mutated in chorea-acanthocytosis. Nat Genet 2001; 28:121.

1738. Stevenson VL, Hardie RJ: Acanthocytosis and neurological disorders. J Neurol 2001; 248:87.

1739. Lupo I, Aragona F, et al: Choreo-acanthocytosis with myopathy: Report of a case. Acta Neurol (Napoli) 1987; 9:334.

1740. Spitz MC, Jankovic J, Killian JM: Familial tic disorder, parkinsonism, motor neuron disease, and acanthocytosis: A new syndrome. Neurology 1985; 35:366.

1741. Peppard RF, Lu CS, et al: Parkinsonism with neuroacanthocytosis. Can J Neurol Sci 1990; 17:298.

1742. Roth AM, Hepler RS, et al: Pigmentary retinal dystrophy in Hallervorden-Spatz disease: Clinicopathological report of a case. Surv Ophthalmol 1971; 16:24.

1743. Swisher CN, Menkes JH, et al: Coexistence of Hallervorden-Spatz disease with acanthocytosis. Trans Am Neurol Assoc 1972; 97:212.

1744. Luckenbach MW, Green WR, et al: Ocular clinicopathologic correlation of Hallervorden-Spatz syndrome with acanthocytosis and pigmentary retinopathy. Am J Ophthalmol 1983; 95:369.

1745. Higgins JJ, Patterson MC, et al: Hypoprebetalipoproteinemia, acanthocytosis, retinitis pigmentosa, and pallidal degeneration (HARP syndrome). Neurology 1992; 42:194.

1746. Orrell RW, Amrolia PJ, et al: Acanthocytosis, retinitis pigmentosa, and pallidal degeneration: A report of three patients with hypoprebetalipoproteinemia (HARP syndrome). Neurology 1995; 45:487.

1747. Cianci CD, Mische SM, Morrow JS: Impaired cAMP dependent phosphorylation of erythrocyte protein 4.9 in patients with hereditary spheroechinocytosis and neurodegenerative disease. J Cell Biol 1989; 107:469a.

1748. Amrein PC, Friedman R, et al: Hematologic changes in anorexia nervosa. JAMA 1979; 241:2190.

1749. Eto Y, Kitagawa T: Wolman's disease with hypobetalipoproteinemia and acanthocytosis: Clinical and biochemical observations. J Pediatr 1970; 77:862.

1750. Gracey M, Hilton HB: Acanthocytes and hypobetalipoproteinemia. Lancet 1973; 1:679.

1751. Paramathypathy K, Aw SE: Acanthocytosis with β-lipoprotein deficiency in an Indian girl. Med J Aust 1970; 2:1081.

1752. Fondu P, Mozes N, et al: The erythrocyte membrane disturbances in protein-energy malnutrition: Nature and mechanisms. Br J Haematol 1980; 44:605.

1753. Kaiser U, Barth N: Haemolytic anaemia in a patient with anorexia nervosa. Acta Haematol 2001; 106:133.

1754. Warren MP, Vande Wiele RL: Clinical and metabolic features of anorexia nervosa. Am J Obstet Gynecol 1973; 117:435.

1755. Herpertz-Dahlmann B, Remschmidt H: Weight-dependent changes in the hematology of anorexia nervosa. Monatsschr Kinderheilkd 1988; 136:739.

1756. Kimber CD, Deller J, et al: The mechanism of anaemia in chronic liver disease. Q J Med 1965; 34:33.

1757. Balistreri WF, Leslie MH, Cooper RA: Increased cholesterol and decreased fluidity of red cell membranes (spur cell anemia) in progressive intrahepatic cholestasis. Pediatrics 1981; 67:461.

1758. Cynamon HA, Isenberg JN, et al: Erythrocyte lipid alterations in pediatric cholestatic liver disease: Spur cell anemia of infancy. J Pediatr Gastroenterol Nutr 1985; 4:542.

1759. Doll DC, Doll NJ: Spur cell anemia. South Med J 1982; 75:1205.

1760. Douglass CC, McCall MS, Frenel EP: The acanthocyte in cirrhosis with hemolytic anemia. Ann Intern Med 1968; 68:390.

1761. Grahn EP, Dietz AA, et al: Burr cells, hemolytic anemia and cirrhosis. Am J Med 1968; 45:78.

1762. Greenberg MS, Choi ES: Post-splenectomy spur cell hemolytic anemia. Am J Med Sci 1975; 269:277.

1763. Hitchins R, Naughton L, et al: Spur cell anemia (acanthocytosis) complicating idiopathic hemochromatosis. Pathology 1988; 20:59.

1764. Keller JW, Majerus PW, Finke EH: An unusual type of spiculated erythrocyte in metastatic liver disease and hemolytic anemia: Report of a case. Ann Intern Med 1971; 74:732.

1765. Silber R, Amorosi E, et al: Spur-shaped erythrocytes in Laennec's cirrhosis. N Engl J Med 1966; 275:639.

1766. Smith JA, Lonergan ET, et al: Spur cell anemia: Hemolytic anemia with red cells resembling acanthocytes in alcoholic cirrhosis. N Engl J Med 1964; 276:396.

1767. Stillman AE, Giordano GF: Spur cell anemia associated with extrahepatic biliary tract obstruction. Am J Gastroenterol 1983; 78:589.

1768. Allen DW, Manning N: Cholesterol-loading of membranes of normal erythrocytes inhibits phospholipid repair and arachidonoyl-CoA:1-palmitoyl-*sn*-glycero-3-phosphocholine acyl transferase. A model of spur cell anemia. Blood 1996; 87:3489.

1769. Taniguchi M, Tanabe F, et al: Experimental biliary obstruction of rat: Initial changes in the structure and lipid content of erythrocytes. Biochim Biophys Acta 1983; 753:22.

1770. Tchernia G, Navarro J, et al: Hemolytic anemia with acanthocytosis and dyslipidemia associated with 2 neonatal hepatitis cases. Arch Fr Pediatr 1968; 25:729.

1771. Cooper RA, Kimball DB, Dorocher JR: Role of the spleen in membrane conditioning and hemolysis of spur cells in liver disease. N Engl J Med 1974; 290:1279.

1772. Salvioli G, Rioli G, et al: Membrane lipid composition of red blood cells in liver disease: Regression of spur cell anaemia after infusion of polyunsaturated phosphatidylcholine. Gut 1978; 19:844.

1773. Fossaluzza V, Rossi P: Flunarizine treatment for spur cell anaemia. Br J Haematol 1983; 55:715.

1774. Cooper RA, Leslie MH, et al: Factors influencing the lipid composition and fluidity of red cell membranes *in vitro:* Production of red cells possessing more than two cholesterols per phospholipid. Biochemistry 1978; 17:327.

1775. Cooper RA, Leslie MH, et al: Red cell cholesterol enrichment and spur cell anemia in dogs fed a cholesterol-enriched atherogenic diet. J Lipid Res 1980; 21:1082.

1776. Duhamel G, Forgez P, et al: Spur cells in patients with alcoholic liver cirrhosis are associated with reduced plasma levels of apo A-II, HDL, and LDL. J Lipid Res 1983; 24:1612.

1777. Aihara K, Azuma H, et al: Successful combination therapy—flunarizine, pentoxifylline, and cholestyramine—for spur cell anemia. Int J Hematol 2001; 73:351.

1778. Schubert D, Boss K: Band 3 protein-cholesterol interactions in erythrocyte membranes: Possible role in anion transport and dependency on membrane phospholipid. FEBS Lett 1982; 150:4.

1779. Lange Y, Cutler HB, Steck TL: The effect of cholesterol and other interrelated amphipaths on the contour and stability of the isolated red cell membrane. J Biol Chem 1980; 255:9331.

1780. Seigneuret M, Favre E, et al: Strong interactions between a spin-labeled cholesterol analog and erythrocyte proteins in the human erythrocyte membrane. Biochim Biophys Acta 1985; 813:174.

1781. Rooney MW, Lange Y, Kauffman JW: Acyl chain organization and protein secondary structure in cholesterol-modified erythrocyte membranes. J Biol Chem 1984; 259:8281.

1782. Allen DW, Manning N: Abnormal phospholipid metabolism in spur cell anemia: Decreased fatty acid incorporation into phosphatidylethanolamine and increased incorporation into acylcarnitine in spur cell anemia erythrocytes. Blood 1994; 84:1283.

1783. Melhorn DK, Gross S: Vitamin E-dependent anemia in the premature infant: II. Relationships between gestational age and absorption of vitamin E. J Pediatr 1971; 79:581.

1784. Ehrenkranz RA: Vitamin E and the neonate. Am J Dis Child 1980; 134:1157.

1785. Zipursky A: Vitamin E deficiency anemia in newborn infants. Clin Perinatol 1984; 11:393.

1786. Gallagher PG, Ehrenkranz RA: Nutritional anemias in infancy. Perinatal Hematol 1995; 22:671.

1787. Dolan TF Jr: Hemolytic anemia and edema as the initial signs in infants with cystic fibrosis. Clin Pediatr 1976; 15:597.

1788. Monzon CM, Woodruff CW: Anemia and edema as presenting signs in cystic fibrosis: A case report. J Med 1986; 17:135.

1789. Melhorn DK, Gross S: Vitamin E-dependent anemia in the premature infant: I. Effects of large doses of medicinal iron. J Pediatr 1971; 79:569.

1790. Oski FA, Barness LA: Vitamin E deficiency: A previously unrecognized cause of hemolytic anemia in the premature infant. J Pediatr 1967; 70:211.

1791. Ritchie JH, Fish MB, et al: Edema and hemolytic anemia in premature infants: A vitamin E deficiency syndrome. N Engl J Med 1968; 279:1185.

1792. Jacob HS, Lux SE: Degradation of membrane phospholipids and thiols in peroxide hemolysis: Studies in vitamin E deficiency. Blood 1968; 32:549.

1793. Brownlee NR, Huttner JJ, et al: Role of vitamin E in glutathione-induced oxidant stress: Methemoglobin, lipid peroxidation, and hemolysis. J Lipid Res 1977; 18:635.

1794. Kay MM, Bosman GJ, et al: Oxidation as a possible mechanism of cellular aging: Vitamin E deficiency causes premature aging and IgG binding to erythrocytes. Proc Natl Acad Sci USA 1986; 83:2463.

1795. Ackerman BD: Infantile pyknocytosis in Mexican-American infants. Am J Dis Child 1969; 117:417.

1796. Keimowitz R, Desforges JF: Infantile pyknocytosis. N Engl J Med 1965; 273:1152.

1797. Zannos-Mariola L, Kattamis C, et al: Infantile pyknocytosis and glucose-6-phosphate dehydrogenase deficiency. Br J Haematol 1962; 8:258.

1798. Allison AC: Acute haemolytic anaemia with distortion and fragmentation of erythrocytes in children. Br J Haematol 1957; 3:1.

1799. Redman CM, Russo D, Lee S: Kell, Kx and the McLeod syndrome. Baillieres Best Pract Res Clin Haematol 1999; 12:621.

1801. Redman CM, Marsh WL, et al: Biochemical studies on McLeod phenotype red cells and isolation of Kx antigen. Br J Haematol 1988; 68:131.

1801. Khamlichi S, Bailly P, et al: Purification and partial characterization of the erythrocyte Kx protein deficient in McLeod patients. Eur J Biochem 1995; 228:931.

1802. Russo D, Redman C, Lee S: Association of XK and Kell blood group proteins. J Biol Chem 1998; 273:13950.

1803. Ho M, Chelly J, Carter N: Isolation of the gene for McLeod syndrome that encodes a novel membrane transport protein. Cell 1994; 77:869.

1804. Ho MF, Chalmers RM, et al: A novel point mutation in the McLeod syndrome gene in neuroacanthocytosis. Ann Neurol 1996: 39:672.

1805. Danek A, Rubio JP, et al: McLeod neuroacanthocytosis: Genotype and phenotype. Ann Neurol 2001; 50:755.

1806. Lee S, Russo DC, et al: Molecular defects underlying the Kell null phenotype. J Biol Chem 2001; 276:27281.

1807. Supple SG, Iland HJ, et al: A spontaneous novel XK gene mutation in a patient with McLeod syndrome. Br J Haematol 2001; 115:369.

1808. Jung HH, Hergersberg M, et al: McLeod syndrome: A novel mutation, predominant psychiatric manifestations, and distinct striatal imaging findings. Ann Neurol 2001; 49:384.

1809. Taswell HF, Lewis JC, et al: Erythrocyte morphology in genetic defects of the Rh and Kell blood group systems. Mayo Clin Proc 1977; 52:157.

1810. Wimmer BM, Marsh WL, et al: Haematological changes associated with the McLeod phenotype of the Kell blood group system. Br J Haematol 1977; 36:219.

1811. Marsh WL, Marsh NJ, et al: Elevated serum creatine phosphokinase in subjects with McLeod syndrome. Vox Sang 1981; 40:403.

1812. Swash M, Schwartz MS, et al: Benign X-linked myopathy with acanthocytosis (McLeod syndrome): Its relationship to X-linked muscular dystrophy. Brain 1983; 106:717.

1813. Witt TN, Danek A, et al: McLeod syndrome: A distinct form of neuroacanthocytosis: Report of two cases and literature review with emphasis on neuromuscular manifestations. J Neurol 1992; 239:302.

1814. Danek A, Uttner I, et al: Cerebral involvement in McLeod syndrome. Neurology 1994; 44:117.

1815. Takashima H, Sakai T, et al: A family of McLeod syndrome, masquerading as chorea-acanthocytosis. J Neurol Sci 1994; 124:56.

1816. Malandrini A, Fabrizi GM, et al: Atypical McLeod syndrome manifested as X-linked chorea-acanthocytosis, neuromyopathy and dilated cardiomyopathy: Report of a family. J Neurol Sci 1994; 124:89.

1817. Bertelson CJ, Pogo AO, et al: Localization of the McLeod locus (XK) within Xp21 by deletion analysis. Am J Hum Genet 1988; 42:703.

1818. Francke U, Ochs HD, et al: Minor Xp21 chromosome deletion in a male associated with expression of Duchenne muscular dystrophy, chronic granulomatous disease, retinitis pigmentosa, and McLeod's syndrome. Am J Hum Genet 1985; 37:250.

1819. Giblett ER, Klebanoff SJ, et al: Kell phenotypes in chronic granulomatous disease: A potential transfusion hazard. Lancet 1971; 1:1235.

1820. Hart MVD, Szaloky A, van Loghem JJ: A "new" antibody associated with the Kell blood group system. Vox Sang 1968; 15:456.

1821. Joske RA, McAlister JM, et al: Isotope investigations of red cell production and destruction in chronic renal disease. Clin Sci (Oxford) 1956; 15:511.

1822. Loge JP, Lange RD, et al: Characterization of the anemia associated with chronic renal insufficiency. Am J Med 1958; 24:4.

1823. Nathan DG, Schupak E, et al: Erythropoiesis in anephric man. J Clin Invest 1964; 43:2158.

1824. Akmal M, Telfer N, et al: Erythrocyte survival in chronic renal failure: Role of secondary hyperparathyroidism. J Clin Invest 1985; 76:1695.

1825. Bogin E, Massry SG, et al: Effect of parathyroid hormone on osmotic fragility of human erythrocytes. J Clin Invest 1982; 69:1017.

1826. Saltissi D, Carter GD: Association of secondary hyperparathyroidism with red cell survival in chronic haemodialysis patients. Clin Sci 1985; 68:29.

1827. White JG: Effects of an ionophore A23187 on the surface morphology of normal erythrocytes. Am J Pathol 1974; 77:507.

1828. Parsons SF, Mallinson G, et al: Evidence that the Lu^b blood group antigen is located on red cell membrane glycoproteins of 85 and 78 kd. Transfusion 1987; 27:61.

1829. Shaw MA, Leak MR, et al: The rare Lutheran blood group phenotype Lu(a-b-): A genetic study. Ann Hum Genet 1984; 48:229.

1830. Telen MJ: The Lutheran antigens and proteins affected by Lutheran regulatory genes. In Agre PC, Cartron JP (eds): Protein Blood Group Antigens of the Human Red Cell: Structure, Function and Clinical Significance. Baltimore, Johns Hopkins University Press, 1992, p 70.

1831. Horton L, Coburn RJ, et al: The haematology of hypothyroidism. Q J Med 1976; 45:101.

1832. Perillie PE, Tembrevilla C: Red-cell changes in hypothyroidism. Lancet 1975; 2:1151.

1833. Betticher DC, Pugin P: Hypothyroidism and acanthocytes: Diagnostic significance of blood smear. Schweiz Med Wochenschr 1991; 121:1127.

1834. Franzese A, Salerno M, et al: Anemia in infants with congenital hypothyroidism diagnosed by neonatal screening. J Endocrinol Invest 1996; 19:613.

1835. Chuttani HK, Gupta PS, et al: Acute copper sulfate poisoning. Am J Med 1965; 39:849.

1836. Fairbanks VF: Copper sulfate induced hemolytic anemia: Inhibition of glucose-6-phosphate dehydrogenase and other possible etiologic mechanisms. Arch Intern Med 1967; 120:428.

1837. Holtzman NA, Elliott DA, Heller RH: Copper intoxication. N Engl J Med 1966; 275:347.

1838. Manzler AD, Schreiner AW: Copper-induced acute hemolytic anemia: A new complication of hemodialysis. Ann Intern Med 1970; 73:409.

1839. Roberts RH: Hemolytic anemia associated with copper sulfate poisoning. Miss Doctor 1956; 33:292.

1840. Clopton DA, Saltman P: Copper-specific damage in human erythrocytes exposed to oxidative stress. Biol Trace Elem Res 1997; 56:231.

1841. Oski FA: Chickee, the copper [editorial]. Ann Intern Med 1970; 73:485.

1842. Loudianos G, Gitlin JD: Wilson's disease. Semin Liver Dis 2000; 20:353.

1843. Sternlieb I: Wilson's disease. Clin Liver Dis 2000; 4:229.

1844. Walshe JM: Wilson's disease: The presenting symptoms. Arch Dis Child 1962; 37:253.

1845. Buchanan GR: Acute hemolytic anemia as a presenting manifestation of Wilson's disease. J Pediatr 1975; 86:245.

1846. Forman SJ, Kumar KS, et al: Hemolytic anemia in Wilson disease: Clinical findings and biochemical mechanisms. Am J Hematol 1980; 9:269.

1847. Groter W: Hamolytische Krisen als Fruhmanifestation der Wilson'schen Krankheit. Dtsch Z Nervenheilkd 1959; 179:401.

1848. Lehr H, Pauschinger M, et al: Haemolytic anaemia as initial manifestation of Wilson's disease. Blut 1988; 56:45.

1849. Robitaille GA, Piscatelli RL, et al: Hemolytic anemia in Wilson's disease. JAMA 1977; 237:2402.

1850. Roche-Sicot J, Benhamou J-P: Acute intravascular hemolysis and acute liver failure associated as a first manifestation of Wilson's disease. Ann Intern Med 1977; 86:301.

1851. Willms B, Blume KG, et al: Hemolytic anemia in Wilson's disease (hepato-lenticular degeneration). Klin Wochenschr 1972; 50:995.

1852. Deiss A, Lee GR, Cartwright GE: Hemolytic anemia in Wilson's disease. Ann Intern Med 1970; 73:413.

1853. Dobyns WB, Goldstein NP, Gordon H: Clinical spectrum of Wilson's disease (hepatolenticular degeneration). Mayo Clin Proc 1979; 54:35.

1854. Hoagland HC, Goldstein NP: Hematologic (cytopenic) manifestations of Wilson's disease. Mayo Clin Proc 1978; 53:498.

1855. Iser JH, Stevens BJ, et al: Hemolytic anemia of Wilson's disease. Gastroenterology 1974; 67:290.

1856. McIntyre N, Clink HM, Levi AJ: Hemolytic anemia in Wilson's disease. N Engl J Med 1967; 276:439.

1857. Meyer RJ, Zalusky R: The mechanisms of hemolysis in Wilson's disease: Study of a case and review of the literature. Mt Sinai J Med 1977; 44:530.

1858. Petrukhin K, Fischer SG, et al: Mapping, cloning and genetic characterization of the region containing the Wilson disease gene. Nat Genet 1993; 5:338.

1859. Bull PC, Thomas GR, et al: The Wilson disease gene is a putative copper transporting P-type ATPase similar to the Menkes gene. Nat Genet 1993; 5:327.

1860. Tanzi RE, Petrukhin K, et al: The Wilson disease gene is a copper transporting ATPase with homology to the Menkes disease gene. Nat Genet 1993; 5:344.

1861. Yamaguchi Y, Heiny ME, Gitlin JD: Isolation and characterization of a human liver cDNA as a candidate gene for Wilson disease. Biochem Biophys Res Commun 1993; 197:271.

1862. Mercer JF: The molecular basis of copper-transport diseases. Trends Mol Med 2001; 7:64.

1863. Camakaris J, Voskoboinik I, Mercer JF: Molecular mechanisms of copper homeostasis. Biochem Biophys Res Commun 1999; 261:225.

1864. Thomas GR, Forbes JR, et al: The Wilson disease gene: Spectrum of mutations and their consequences. Nat Genet 1995; 9:210.

1865. Figus A, Angius A, et al: Molecular pathology and haplotype analysis of Wilson disease in Mediterranean populations. Am J Hum Genet 1995; 57:1318.

1866. Shah AB, Chernov I, et al: Identification and analysis of mutations in the Wilson disease gene (ATP7B): Population frequencies, genotype-phenotype correlation, and functional analyses. Am J Hum Genet 1997; 61:317.

1867. Grudeva-Popova JG, Spasova MI, et al: Acute hemolytic anemia as an initial clinical manifestation of Wilson's disease. Folia Med (Plovdiv) 2000; 42:42.

1868. Michel M, Lafaurie M, et al: Hemolytic anemia disclosing Wilson's disease. Report of 2 cases. Rev Med Interne 2001; 22:280.

1869. Gubler CJ, Labey ME, et al: Studies on copper metabolism. IX. Transportation of copper in blood. J Clin Invest 1953; 32:405.

1870. Hochstein P, Kumar KS, Forman SJ: Mechanisms of copper toxicity in red cells. In Brewer GJ (ed): The Red Cell. New York, Alan R Liss, 1978.

16 | Pyruvate Kinase Deficiency and Disorders of Glycolysis

William C. Mentzer, Jr.

The mature erythrocyte, devoid of nucleus, mitochondria, ribosomes, and other organelles, has no capacity for cell replication, protein synthesis, or oxidative phosphorylation. The glycolytic production of adenosine triphosphate (ATP), the sole known energy source of such erythrocytes, is sufficient to meet their limited metabolic requirements. The discovery that hemolytic anemia may result from any of several glycolytic enzymopathies has underscored the dependence of erythrocytes upon glycolysis. In this chapter, the clinical, biochemical, and genetic features associated with abnormalities of erythrocyte glycolysis will be described in detail. Because they have been more thoroughly studied, the congenital hemolytic anemias will be discussed at length, whereas the various acquired disorders will be dealt with more briefly.

Hereditary hemolytic anemias resulting from altered erythrocyte metabolism are distinguished from hereditary spherocytosis by the absence of spherocytes on the peripheral blood smear, by normal osmotic fragility of fresh erythrocytes, by a partial therapeutic response to splenectomy, and by a recessive mode of inheritance. Hemoglobin structure and synthesis are normal. Because no specific morphologic abnormality is associated with these disorders, they have become known as congenital nonspherocytic hemolytic anemias (CNSHAs).[1] Although these anemias are usually transmitted in an autosomal recessive fashion, phosphoglycerate kinase deficiency is an X-linked abnormality, and adenosine deaminase (ADA) overproduction is an autosomal dominant disorder. Symptoms and signs may be limited to the manifestations of hemolysis or, if the enzymopathy is present in other tissues, may involve other organ systems. In the latter instance, the specific pattern of involvement of nonerythroid tissues may be of assistance in diagnosis.[2]

Initial attempts to classify these anemias were based on the autohemolysis test, in which saline-washed erythrocytes were incubated without glucose in vitro at 37°C under sterile conditions, and the percentage of hemolysis was determined after 48 hours.[3, 4] Autohemolysis was greater than normal in almost all patients with CNSHA. If glucose was added before incubation, hemolysis was reduced in control subjects and in some patients with CNSHA (type I) but was unchanged, or actually increased, in others (type II). Type II erythrocytes did not metabolize glucose well[3] and contained subnormal amounts of ATP but markedly increased amounts of 2,3-diphosphoglycerate (2,3-DPG), suggesting a defect in glycolysis below the site of 2,3-DPG synthesis. In 1961, Valentine and associates[5] identified the glycolytic defect to be a deficiency of erythrocyte pyruvate kinase (PK) in three patients with CNSHA. Subsequently, abnormalities of other glycolytic enzymes have also been associated with CNSHA, as indicated in Figure 16–1. Specific alterations in protein structure underlie many of the enzyme-deficiency states, and many of the underlying mutations have been identified.[6, 7]

The presence of a glycolytic enzymopathy should be suspected when chronic hemolysis occurs in the absence of marked abnormalities of erythrocyte morphology or osmotic fragility. An exception to the usually unremarkable red cell morphology in CNSHA is the pronounced basophilic stippling found in pyrimidine-5'-nucleotidase (P-5'-N) deficiency.[8] Hemoglobin electrophoresis, stains for inclusion bodies, hemoglobin heat stability, acid hemolysis, and appropriate studies for immune hemolysis are normal. Despite its initial usefulness in directing the attention of investigators to the glycolytic pathway, further experience with the autohemolysis test has shown that it lacks specificity and has, at best, limited value in the evaluation of CNSHA.[9] Unfortunately, no other simple, convenient laboratory screening test has been developed that will unequivocally reveal the presence of a glycolytic enzymopathy. Therefore, the appropriate diagnostic strategy for the evaluation of a suspected enzymopathy is first to eliminate easily identified causes of hemolysis, such as hemoglobinopathies or spherocytosis, before proceeding to tests for enzyme disorders.[10] Definitive diagnosis depends upon quantitative assay of the activity of the suspected enzyme or identification of a specific mutation by DNA analysis. The availability of such assays is limited, but screening tests for deficiencies of PK, triose phosphate isomerase (TPI), and glucose phosphate isomerase can be carried out in any well-equipped clinical laboratory.[11] The in vitro properties of

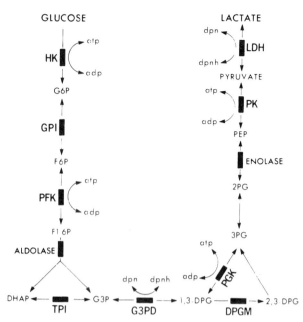

FIGURE 16–1. The Embden-Meyerhof pathway. Recognized enzyme defects are indicated by *solid bars*. HK = hexokinase; GPI = glucose phosphate isomerase; PFK = phosphofructokinase; TPI = triose phosphate isomerase; G3PD = glucose-3-phosphate dehydrogenase; DPGM = 2,3-disphosphoglycerate mutase; PK = pyruvate kinase; LDH = lactate dehydrogenase; atp =adenosine triphosphate; adp = adenosine diphosphate; G6P = glucose 6-phosphate; F6P = fructose 6-phosphate; F16P = fructose 1,6-phosphate; DHAP = dihydroxyacetone phosphate; PEP = phosphoenolpyruvate; PG = phosphoglycerate.

mutant enzyme proteins vary (Table 16–1), and characterization of such properties has improved understanding of the genetics and pathogenesis of anemias associated with defective glycolytic enzymes. Measurement of glycolytic intermediates extracted from freshly obtained erythrocytes has provided confirmation of the in vivo significance of in vitro abnormalities of enzyme function. The usual finding is an accumulation of proximal intermediates and a depletion of distal intermediates, giving rise to a characteristic transition or crossover pattern at the locus of an abnormal enzyme. Secondary crossovers

TABLE 16–1. Parameters Commonly Used *in Vitro* to Characterize Mutant Enzyme Protein

1. V_{max}	Maximal enzyme velocity obtainable with saturating substrate concentrations
2. K_m	The substrate concentration yielding half-maximal activity; an index of catalytic efficiency
3. pH optimum	The pH at which maximal enzyme activity is present
4. Heat stability	Resistance of enzyme protein to heat denaturation
5. Electrophoretic mobility	Migration of enzyme protein in an electric field
6. Specific activity	Enzyme activity per defined amount of enzyme protein (e.g., mg); enzyme protein is measured immunologically with antienzyme antibodies

are sometimes observed, reflecting the influence of altered concentrations of metabolites on key regulatory enzymes such as hexokinase (HK), phosphofructokinase (PFK), and PK. As a result of secondary crossovers, the pattern of glycolytic intermediates may become so complex that it has only limited usefulness in the identification of an enzymopathy. On the other hand, measurement of intracellular metabolites is currently the most convenient way to screen for abnormalities of nucleotide metabolism. Red cell ATP levels are below normal with overproduction of ADA, whereas P-5′-N deficiency is associated with increased concentrations of red cell ATP and reduced levels of glutathione. The apparent increase in ATP is, in fact, due to the presence of large amounts of cytidine and uridine nucleotides, which are also measured in the enzymatic assay for ATP. Spectral analysis of a deproteinized extract of red cells provides a straightforward means of identifying such nucleotides, and it is a simple method to screen patients for suspected P-5′-N deficiency.[8]

A certain amount of caution is necessary in interpreting the results of quantitative assays of enzyme activity. First, only surviving cells are available for sampling in the circulating blood, and the metabolic circumstances of these favored cells cannot necessarily be extrapolated to indicate the status of cells already hemolyzed. Second, assay *in vitro* under optimal conditions may not adequately reflect the performance of an enzyme under less favorable circumstances *in vivo*. Third, the high specific activity of certain enzymes in leukocytes may result in spurious normal values for erythrocyte enzyme activity unless contaminating leukocytes either are removed before assay or their contribution to total activity is compensated for by appropriate calculations. Fourth, transfusion therapy with normal erythrocytes within several months before assay may obscure the presence of an enzyme defect. Fifth, the mean enzyme activity that is determined fails to portray distribution of activity within individual erythrocytes. The endowment of intracellular enzymes is fixed with the disappearance of protein synthetic ability at the reticulocyte stage; thereafter, the inevitable denaturation of enzyme protein that accompanies cell aging reduces enzymatic activity at a rate characteristic of each enzyme. Transient accentuation of reticulocytosis, therefore, is often accompanied by rising mean enzyme activity. Certain glycolytic enzymes (notably HK and PK) are strikingly more active in reticulocytes than in postreticulocyte red cells, and the majority of this excess activity is rapidly lost coincident with reticulocyte maturation.[12–14] The true magnitude of an enzyme deficiency may not be apparent unless comparison is made with blood that is equally rich in reticulocytes,[13] or corrections are applied that separate out the contribution of the reticulocyte subfraction to total enzyme activity.[14]

Finally, there is evidence that reversible binding of glyceraldehyde-3-phosphate dehydrogenase (G3PD), HK, and PFK to the band 3 membrane protein is involved in the regulation of glycolysis[15] and altered binding of mutant forms of these enzymes (and perhaps others) is not assessed in conventional assays performed on hemolysates.

HEXOKINASE DEFICIENCY

$$\text{Glucose} \xrightarrow[\text{ATP} \quad \text{Mg}^{2+} \quad \text{ADP}]{\text{Hexokinase}} \text{Glucose-6-phosphate}$$

Clinical Manifestations

CNSHA in 22 patients has been attributed to deficient erythrocyte HK activity (Table 16–2). Severely affected individuals may exhibit neonatal hyperbilirubinemia and thereafter require transfusion at regular intervals for intractable anemia, but in patients with mild disease, hemolysis is fully compensated for and anemia is absent. However, jaundice, reticulocytosis, and splenomegaly are usually present in such patients. Gallstones may be evident, even in early childhood.[24] Hyperhemolytic episodes are not a feature of the disorder. Results of red cell morphologic examination are usually unremarkable, but occasional burr cells, target cells, stippled cells, and densely stained spiculated cells may be observed after splenectomy. The osmotic fragility of fresh erythrocytes is normal, but after incubation at 37°C a fragile population of cells may appear.

Deficient erythrocyte HK activity in association with macrocytic anemia has also been found in a few individuals who had the clinical features of Fanconi aplastic anemia,[34] thus differing from patients with isolated congenital hemolytic anemia. Thrombocytopenia and leukopenia were present, and both platelet and white cell HK activity were reduced. Other patients with Fanconi anemia have not had HK deficiency. In patients with Fanconi anemia, HK deficiency is probably a manifestation of dyserythropoiesis rather than a cause of the anemia.

Biochemistry

In human red cells, HK is a monomer (molecular weight 112,000).[35] It is encoded by a gene *(HK1)* located on chromosome 10q22.[19] HK activity declines as red cells age. Loss of activity is particularly striking during reticulocyte maturation. In human reticulocytes, two major isoenzymes of HK have been identified by chromatographic techniques.[36] One (HK_R) has an apparent half-life *in vivo* of only 10 days, whereas the other (HK_1) has a longer half-life of 66 days. These two proteins are the products of two closely similar messenger RNAs (mRNAs) that are transcribed from a single gene *(HK1)* by the use of alternate promotors. Exon one is unique to each mRNA species while the remaining 17 exons are identical.[37] Differential loss of these two isoenzymes appears to explain the biphasic character of the decay in HK activity during erythrocyte aging. An ATP- and ubiquitin-dependent proteolytic system, capable of degrading about 80 percent of HK activity, may explain the rapid loss of HK in rabbit reticulocytes[38] or the loss may be secondary to an intrinsic property of the HK molecule itself.[39] Prior oxidative injury appears to be necessary for recognition and destruction of HK by the ubiquitin-dependent system.[40] Because ATP- and

TABLE 16–2. Hexokinase Variants Associated with Hemolytic Anemia

	Clinical Features				Properties of RBC Hexokinase			
Reference	No. of Patients	Inheritance	Hemolytic Anemia	Other	Activity (% of Normal)	Kinetic Abnormalities	Stability *in Vitro*	Electrophoretic Mobility
16	1	—	+	Congenital malformations	13-24★	0	—	—
17	1	Recessive	++		15-20★	+	Normal	Abnormal
18	1	Recessive	++		16★	0	—	Abnormal
19	1	Recessive	+++	Hydrops fetalis	17		—	
20	1	Recessive	+		20★	0	Normal	Normal
21,22	1	Recessive	++	Low platelet and fibroblast hexokinase activity	20★	0	Low	Normal
23	1	Recessive	++	Low platelet hexokinase activity	25★	+	Normal	Abnormal
24	1	Recessive	+		25★	0	Low	Normal
25	2	Dominant	+	Spherocytes, ovalocytes	30★	0	Low	Normal
26	1	Recessive	+	Psychomotor retardation	45+	+	Normal	Normal
27	1	Recessive	+		50★	0	Normal	Normal
28	1	—	+	Congenital malformations	33★	+	—	—
29	2	Recessive	+		40-53★	+	Low	Normal
30	1	—	+		50★	+	—	—
31	1				53		—	—
32	5	Dominant	+		45-91+	+	Normal	Abnormal
33	2	Dominant	++	WBC hexokinase activity low	75★	+	Normal	Abnormal

★Maximal enzyme activity (V_{max}) compared with reticulocytosis controls.
+Maximal enzyme activity (V_{max}) compared with normal red cells

ubiquitin-dependent proteolysis is limited to reticulocytes,[38] it cannot be responsible for the loss of HK in aging human red cells.

HK is the glycolytic enzyme with the lowest activity in normal red cells, and a variety of observations indicate that it plays a rate-limiting role in erythrocyte glycolysis.[41–44] The maximal activity of erythrocyte HK from deficient patients has varied from 13 to 91 percent of normal (Table 16–2). In evaluating these findings, comparisons of enzyme activity between red cell populations of equivalent youth must be made. In the case described by Valentine and associates,[45] for example (Fig. 16–2), although HK activity was 62 percent of the normal value for mature erythrocytes; it was only 14 percent of the activity found in blood with high reticulocyte counts. A separation of young and old red cell populations by centrifugation revealed only the expected moderate diminution (to 0.11 mol/min/10^{10} red blood cells) of HK activity in older cells from this patient.[45] HK activity was even lower (0.075 mol/min/10^{10} red blood cells) in an asymptomatic brother, yet no evidence of undue hemolysis was present. However, Figure 16–2 shows that the brother's cells are actually far less deficient with respect to cell age than are the immature cells of the propositus. The impact of HK deficiency is clearly greater in energetic young erythrocytes, whereas cells that survive to an older age can meet their limited metabolic requirements even at very low HK levels.[46] As the erythrocyte ages, *in vivo* changes in stability or kinetics peculiar to mutant HK may also render older cells liable to undergo premature hemolysis. In rats and rabbits, HK from immature erythrocytes has a higher K_m (Michaelis constant) for glucose than that seen in mature cells, but such is not the case in normal human erythrocytes.[47]

In keeping with their enzymatic defect, HK-deficient erythrocytes have usually demonstrated subnormal glucose consumption and lactate production in *vivo*. Such cells also metabolize fructose poorly but utilize mannose or galactose normally[46] because these substrates are not metabolized by HK. Some HK-deficient erythrocytes are

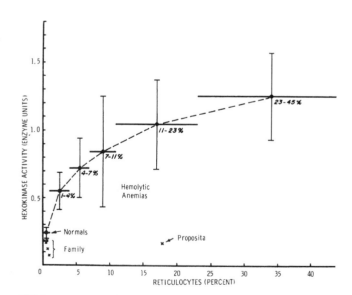

FIGURE 16–2. Hexokinase activity observed in 54 patients with hemolytic anemia of various causes plotted against reticulocyte percentages in cells assayed. Patients are grouped according to reticulocyte levels. Mean HK activity for each group is plotted against mean reticulocyte percentage in cells of that group. Standard deviations are indicated by *vertical bars*. Values for a single HK-deficient patient (proposita) and her family are designated separately. (From Valentine WN, Oski FA, et al: In Beutler E (ed): Hereditary Disorders of Erythrocyte Metabolism. New York, Grune & Stratton, 1968, p. 294.)

capable of normal glucose consumption at the glucose concentrations (5 mmol/L) customarily found in plasma but utilize glucose poorly or not at all at lower glucose concentrations, either because of an abnormally low affinity for glucose[33] or because of enzyme instability under conditions of low substrate availability.[29] Such erythrocytes may encounter a particularly unfavorable metabolic environment within the spleen. The concentration of glucose in normal splenic homogenates has been found by Necheles and co-workers[33] to be only 5 to 11 μmol/g of tissue, and in a patient with HK deficiency the concentration was even lower (1.1 μmol/g of tissue). Furthermore, because splenic tissue metabolizes glucose rapidly,[48] prolonged vascular pooling in the spleen is probably accompanied by profound local hypoglycemia. Erythrocytes with unfavorable kinetics for glucose metabolism are clearly at a disadvantage competing with reticuloendothelial cells for such a reduced glucose supply. Another disadvantage of the splenic environment is its relative acidity. The pH optimum of erythrocyte HK is approximately 8; at lower pH values, diminished enzyme activity may be expected. Possibly of greater importance, at low pH values, glucose 6-phosphate, a potent inhibitor of HK, accumulates because of phosphofructokinase inhibition.[49] An erythrocyte that has diminished HK activity under optimal pH conditions will be further compromised in the acidic environment of the spleen. The clinical improvement that follows splenectomy attests to the importance of this organ in the pathogenesis of hemolysis. Detailed isotopic studies to define red cell kinetics and sites of hemolysis have yet to be reported. Although no splenic sequestration of chromated autologous erythrocytes was noted in two patients,[24, 50] in another sequestration was present.[34] Thus, in this disorder, the red cells may be damaged by the spleen and die elsewhere.

Significant alterations in intracellular metabolites are associated with defective HK function. The erythrocyte ATP concentration is sometimes,[34,30,35] but not always,[20,23,28,32] subnormal. The glucose 6-phosphate concentration is reduced to approximately one-half normal, and the concentrations of other more distal intermediates, most notably 2,3-DPG, are also usually reduced. These metabolites may exert a significant regulatory influence upon glycolysis. For example, Brewer[49] has shown that concentrations of 2,3-DPG in the physiologic range inhibit HK so that the low 2,3-DPG levels in HK-deficient red cells may facilitate the performance of available HK. The increased hemoglobin-oxygen affinity expected to be associated with subnormal 2,3-DPG levels has been documented in one anemic patient with HK deficiency by Delivoria-Papadopoulos and co-workers[50] and by Oski and associates.[51] This patient, whose hemoglobin oxygen affinity (P_{50}) was 19 mm Hg (normal = 27 ± 1.2). was capable of only minimal exercise, despite only moderate anemia (hemoglobin = 9.8 g/dL). On exercise, her central venous partial pressure of oxygen (pO_2) promptly fell to minimal levels as oxygen consumption rose. Increased oxygen delivery was achieved primarily by an increase in cardiac output, because the unfavorable oxygen affinity curve precluded any substantial further desaturation of hemoglobin.[51] Thus, the altered concentration of intracellular metabolites induced by HK defi-

ciency may, as in this patient, accentuate symptoms associated with anemia.

Because of its reactive sulfhydryl group, HK is susceptible to oxidant inactivation in the absence of sufficient glutathione.[52] Both normal and low glutathione levels have been reported in HK deficiency, and although Lohr and co-workers[34] discovered Heinz bodies in their patients with Fanconi anemia, these have not been observed in other HK-deficient individuals. Resting hexose monophosphate (HMP) shunt activity, measured with [1-^{14}C]glucose, was quantitatively normal in one patient, despite subnormal glucose consumption, but stimulation with methylene blue was suboptimal.[45] Failure of the shunt at low glucose concentrations has also been noted in an HK mutant with a high K_m for glucose.[31] Methylene blue–stimulated methemoglobin reduction was subnormal in the single instance that it was evaluated.[16] When HK inactivating antibodies are incorporated into normal red cells by the process of hypotonic lysis and isotonic reannealing, enzyme-deficient cells exhibit a greatly impaired response to HMP shunt stimulation by methylene blue.[42] These studies, although not indicating a central role for defective shunt activity in the pathogenesis of hemolysis, do suggest that under unusual circumstances HK-deficient cells might be compromised by a limited shunt. Such circumstances, for example, might arise upon exposure to a potent oxidant in the low glucose environment of the spleen.

Genetics

Inheritance is autosomal recessive. Biochemical identification of asymptomatic carriers is not always possible, because enzyme activity often falls within the low normal range. In a few pedigrees (Table 16–2), the heterozygous state appears to be severe enough to result in hemolytic anemia. One such heterozygote appeared to be doubly heterozygous for HK and glucose-6-phosphate dehydrogenase (G6PD) deficiency.[53]

The qualitative abnormalities characteristic of variant HK (Table 16–2) may reflect either a structural or a regulatory gene mutation. On electrophoresis, mutant HK lacks one or more of the normal bands of activity, but no bands migrating in an abnormal position have been observed. The various bands represent the presence of several isozymes of HK. Diminished synthesis of one or more isozymes with predominance of the remaining isozyme(s) accounts for the electrophoretic differences observed (Table 16–2). DNA analysis has defined two separate HK mutations in a compound heterozygote who exhibited nonspherocytic hemolytic anemia.[19, 54, 55] One was a missense mutation (T^{1667}→C) and the other was a deletion of exon 5 (96 bp). Expression of each HK mutation in a bacterial system allowed recovery of sufficient purified enzyme to determine that the missense mutation completely abolished HK activity, whereas the deletion reduced activity to about 10 percent of normal.[55] In a Japanese family, a stillborn fetus with HK deficiency was found to be homozygous for a large deletion that removed exons 5 through 8 in HK mRNA and led to premature termination of translation.[19] The kinetic abnormalities noted in many other mutant forms of HK undoubtedly also reflect as yet undefined structural abnormalities of enzyme protein.[16, 17, 21, 26, 27, 31]

Studies of the tissue distribution of HK deficiency have been performed in blood cells and cultured fibroblasts. Electrophoresis of leukocyte or platelet HK reveals an anodal isozyme (Hk$_3$) distinct from those of the erythrocyte (Hk$_1$ and Hk$_2$), as well as a shared isozyme (Hk$_1$).[56, 57] Leukocyte HK activity has been normal in some patients,[29, 45] but the qualitative abnormality of leukocyte HK described by Necheles and colleagues,[33] as well as the case of generalized HK deficiency in all blood cells reported by Rijksen and co-workers,[23] indicate that to some extent the enzyme is under common genetic control in different tissues. When platelet HK activity has been low, platelet function has been normal despite subtle defects in *in vitro* energy metabolism.[58] Cultured fibroblasts from two individuals with different HK mutants contained HK with properties and activity like those found in red cells,[22] suggesting that this source of fetal tissue could be used for prenatal diagnosis.

Therapy

Treatment consists of red cell transfusion as indicated, supplemental folic acid, and close observation for cholelithiasis. Splenectomy may alleviate but does not eliminate anemia.[17, 21, 23, 29, 33, 45]

GLUCOSE PHOSPHATE ISOMERASE DEFICIENCY

$$\text{Glucose-6-phosphate} \xleftrightarrow{\text{Glucose phosphate isomerase}} \text{Fructose-6-phosphate}$$

Clinical Manifestations

A deficiency of erythrocyte GPI has been reported in more than 60 patients with congenital hemolytic anemia.[59] Hemolytic anemia usually first appears in infancy and often requires red cell transfusion therapy. Hyperbilirubinemia,[60] hydrops fetalis,[61, 62] or death[63] may occur during the neonatal period. Several patients have experienced hyperhemolytic crises after infections or drug exposure.[60, 64] In some of these individuals, G6PD, as well as GPI, has been deficient.[64, 65] Hemolytic anemia is usually the sole clinical manifestation of GPI deficiency. A subset of patients also exhibit neurologic dysfunction.[66–71] In one patient, neuromuscular abnormalities were correlated with a severe reduction in muscle and cerebrospinal fluid GPI activity.[69] Blockade of glycolysis at the GPI step may divert the flow of glucose metabolism in the direction of glycogen synthesis. Several patients with GPI deficiency have been reported to have increased hepatic glycogen stores,[72, 73] and, in one, complaints of muscular fatigue were severe enough to suggest a diagnosis of glycogen storage disease.[73] An animal model of GPI deficiency and chronic hemolytic anemia has been developed in the mouse. Clinical and biochemical features of the disease in mice closely resemble those found in humans.[74]

Red cell morphologic characteristics generally resemble those seen in other types of congenital nonspherocytic

hemolytic anemias. In severely anemic patients, dense, spiculated, or "whiskered" microspherocytes have been noted after splenectomy. In one instance, sufficient numbers of such cells were present before splenectomy to suggest the diagnosis of hereditary spherocytosis.[75] In another, the predominant morphologic abnormality was stomatocytosis.[76] Reticulocytosis may be profound. The mean corpuscular volume is elevated (97 to 139 fL). With incubation at 37°C, a variable fraction of erythrocytes may exhibit abnormally increased osmotic fragility, whereas fresh cells are usually normal. The survival of chromated autologous red cells is reduced, often,[77–79] but not invariably,[63, 77, 80] with evidence of splenic sequestration.

Biochemistry

GPI is a dimer[81] composed of two identical subunits, each with a molecular weight of approximately 60,000.[79, 81] Subunit synthesis is directed by a single genetic locus located on chromosome 19.[82] GPI is a multifunctional protein. The dimeric form exhibits glycolytic enzyme activity whereas the monomeric form functions as a cytokine. Monomeric GPI is 100 percent homologous to neuroleukin, a neurotrophic growth factor secreted by lectin-stimulated T cells[59, 83, 84]; to autocrine motility factor, which stimulates cell motility and the growth of metastases[85]; and to a differentiation and maturation mediator for human myeloid leukemia cells in tissue culture.[86] Altered neuroleukin function may explain the neurologic disorder associated with several GPI mutations.[59, 71]

The metabolic events that precede hemolysis of GPI-deficient erythrocytes are poorly understood. Erythrocyte glycolysis is impaired *in vivo*, as reflected by an increased ratio of substrate to product (i.e., of glucose 6-phosphate to fructose 6-phosphate) in freshly obtained GPI-deficient cells.[65, 75, 87–92] Paradoxically, with only occasional exceptions,[75, 93] such cells are fully capable of glycolysis *in vitro*.[65, 80, 94–97] In contrast to HK deficiency, in which 2,3-DPG levels are low, sufficient glycolysis usually occurs in GPI deficiency to maintain the 2,3-DPG concentration at or above the normal level.[85, 87, 89, 93, 96, 98] Except for three patients with diminished ATP concentrations, two of whom also exhibited reduced *in vitro* glycolysis for cell age,[65, 75, 80] the erythrocyte ATP concentration has been normal.

A profound defect in recycling of fructose 6-phosphate through the pentose phosphate pathway has been observed repeatedly in GPI-deficient red cells.[75, 97, 98] Increased formation of Heinz bodies[63, 76] as well as glutathione instability[67, 91] after exposure to acetylphenylhydrazine, an abnormal ascorbate cyanide test, and diminished concentrations of red cell glutathione[76, 80, 88, 89, 91] in fresh erythrocytes all suggest that diminished shunt activity *in vivo* may contribute to hemolysis.

With rare exceptions,[69] mutant forms of red cell GPI exhibit considerable thermal lability *in vitro*, making it likely that enzyme lability *in vivo* as red cells age will lead to premature metabolic collapse and hemolysis. Separation of red cells by centrifugation into young and old subpopulations has usually demonstrated accelerated decay of enzyme activity in the older cells.[80, 99] Arnold and co-workers[99] simulated the *in vivo* process of aging by incubating red cells *in vitro* at 37°C for 8 days, changing the incubation medium often to ensure that glucose availability and pH remained constant. GPI activity declined by 66 percent in GPI-deficient red cells during the incubation, reaching a level of only 6 percent of normal, and lactate production, normal at the onset, was reduced to 11 percent of normal. In contrast, normal reticulocyte-rich blood lost only 6 percent of the original GPI activity after 8 days, and lactate production fell only 7 percent. If mannose, rather than glucose, was used, GPI-deficient and normal red cells made equivalent amounts of lactate, and there was little or no loss in lactate production after 8 days. The normal glycolytic rate noted with mannose, which is isomerized by mannose phosphate isomerase and thus bypasses the GPI reaction, clearly pinpoints defective GPI activity as the cause of glycolytic failure in GPI-deficient cells. ATP depletion with consequent erythrocyte rigidity and reticuloendothelial entrapment would be anticipated to follow failure of glycolysis. GPI-deficient red cells are, indeed, less deformable than normal cells, particularly when comparison is made to young, reticulocyte-rich populations of cells.[86,87,100–102] Goulding[103] studied a 9-year-old patient with GPI deficiency and priapism and concluded that the priapism was the consequence of abnormal erythrocyte deformability. Studies by Coetzer and Zail[104] revealed aggregation of membrane spectrin in GPI-deficient erythrocytes. The extent of aggregation is a function of cell age.

Even reticulocytes may be severely GPI-deficient.[72] Deficient reticulocytes with limited anaerobic glycolytic capabilities may also be incapable of effective oxidative phosphorylation in the acidic, hypoglycemic splenic environment (see section on pyruvate kinase deficiency), leading to metabolic failure and hemolysis. Large numbers of reticulocytes were found when specimens from the spleen of a patient with GPI deficiency were examined by transmission electron microscopy.[72] Furthermore, the reticulocyte count often increases after splenectomy.[63, 72, 78, 80] Because hemoglobin levels also increase, this observation suggests survival of a population of reticulocytes that would otherwise be hemolyzed almost immediately after their release from the marrow.

Genetics and Inheritance

Like most other glycolytic enzymopathies, GPI deficiency is inherited as an autosomal recessive trait. Heterozygotes are hematologically normal but exhibit reduced erythrocyte GPI activity (usually to about 50 percent of normal). They inherit one mutant and one normal *GPI* allele, resulting in the synthesis of two unlike GPI subunits that may combine in one of three ways to form a normal homodimer, a mutant homodimer, or a heterodimer that contains both normal and mutant subunits. Electrophoresis of GPI from the erythrocytes of heterozygotes will demonstrate one to three bands, depending on the extent to which the charge or activity of the mutant

subunit is altered. Post-translational events, such as oxidation of enzyme protein, may alter the electrophoretic pattern and confuse its interpretation.[105, 106]

GPI mutations associated with hemolytic anemia are listed in Table 16–3. Of the 29 known mutations, 2 are splice site, 3 are nonsense, and 24 are missense, involving a single amino acid substitution.[59] The mutations are found in 12 of the 18 exons and are generally unique to one or at most a few families. The rarity of GPI deficiency and the heterogeneity of the mutations identified indicate that no selective advantage is conferred on affected individuals. One half of the homozygotes or compound heterozygotes for missense mutations have mild to moderate hemolytic anemia, and one half have severe anemia. In contrast, all compound heterozygotes for missense mutations and either splice site or nonsense mutations have severe hemolytic anemia. Hemolytic anemia occurs in individuals when GPI activity drops below about 40 percent of the normal mean activity. Substrate kinetics and the pH optimum of mutant enzymes have almost always been normal, but most mutant enzymes have exhibited varying degrees of thermal instability. Short of direct detection of the mutation at the DNA level, the most useful means of classifying the numerous GPI variants reported has been on the basis of stability, electrophoretic mobility, or residual enzyme activity in red cells and leukocytes.★ Until DNA mutation analysis has been completed on these variants it will not be clear how many are truly unique. Immunologic titration of functionally inactive enzyme protein in red cells indicates that some mutant *GPI* alleles are "silent" and produce no detectable enzyme protein, whereas others produce structurally altered protein with varying degrees of activity and stability *in vivo*.[107–109]

A single GPI isozyme is present in all human tissues.[82] GPI deficiency is usually less severe in nonerythroid tissues than in erythrocytes, because nonerythrocytic tissues retain the ability to synthesize GPI subunits. Clinical abnormalities outside the hematopoietic system are rare, and, if present, are neuromuscular in nature. Leukocytes are capable of normal phagocytosis and chemotaxis, despite a reduction in GPI activity to 25[87] to 73 percent[95] of normal, but if GPI activity is more severely depressed, granulocyte function is impaired.[69, 110] Similarly, platelet GPI may be only 20 to 30 percent of normal, but clot formation, platelet aggregation, and other clotting studies are normal.[87, 95] Prenatal diagnosis is feasible by DNA analysis if the mutations are known or by measurement of GPI activity in amniotic fluid fibroblasts[61] or chorionic villus trophoblasts.[111]

Therapy

Transfusion requirements are usually eliminated by removal of the spleen, but anemia persists.[63, 72, 78, 95] The postsplenectomy hemoglobin levels of 6.7 to 10.3 g/dL and reticulocyte counts of 36 to 73 percent observed in three siblings by Paglia and co-workers[98] reflect the magnitude of the continued hemolysis that may be present.

★References 62, 63, 65–69, 76–80, 87–95, 97, 98, and 107–110.

TABLE 16–3. Mutations Associated with Glucose Phosphate Isomerase Deficiency and Hemolytic Anemia

Variant	Ethnic Origin	Genotype	Exon	Amino Acid Change	Red Blood Cell GPI Activity (IU/g Hb)*
HOMOZYGOTES—MISSENSE MUTATIONS					
Matsumoto	Japanese	14C→T	1	Thr^{5}Ile	27
	Native American	247C→T	3	Arg^{83}Trp	16.4
Sarsina	Italian	301G→A	4	Val^{101}Met	7.2†
Iwate	Japanese	671C→T	7	Thr^{224}Met	10.2
	Turkish	970G→A	12	Gly^{324}Ser	49.7†
Morcone	Italian	1028A→G	12	Gln^{343}Arg	7.2†
Narita	Japanese	1028A→G	12	Gln^{343}Arg	32.4
Mount Scopus	Ashkenazi	1039C→T	12	Arg^{347}Cys	14.8+†
	Hispanic	1415G→A	16	Arg^{472}His	15.4
	Turkish	1415G→A	16	Arg^{472}His	24.9
	?English	1574T→C	18	Ile^{525}Thr	3†
Fukuoka	Japanese	1615G→A	18	Asp^{539}Asn	6.4
COMPOUND HETEROZYGOTES—NONSENSE/MISSENSE MUTATIONS					
Stuttgart	German	43C→T/1028A→G	1, 12	Gln^{15}stop/Gln^{343}Arg	27.9†
Elyria	Caucasian	223A→G/286C→T	3, 4	Arg^{75}Gly/Arg^{96}stop	4†
Bari	Italian	286C→T/584C→T	4, 6	Arg^{96}stop/Thr^{196}Ile	14.9†
	Russian	286C→T/1039C→T	4, 12	Arg^{96}stop/Arg^{347}Cys	19
Zwickau	German	1039C→T/1538G→A	12, 17	Arg^{347}Cys/Trp^{513}stop	21†
COMPOUND HETEROZYGOTES—SPLICE SITE/MISSENSE MUTATIONS					
Mola	Italian	584C→T/del1473-IVS16(+2)	6, 16	Thr^{195}Ile/splice site	12.9†
Nordhorn	German	1028A→G/IVS15(-2) A→C	12/IVS15	Gln^{343}Arg/splice site	11.4†
COMPOUND HETEROZYGOTES—MISSENSE/MISSENSE MUTATIONS					
Homberg	German	59A→C/1016T→C	1, 12	His^{20}Pro/Leu^{339}Pro	3.5+†
	?English	475G→A/1040G→A	5, 12	Gly^{159}Ser/Arg^{347}His	6†
	African American	671C→T/1483G→A	7, 17	Thr^{224}Met/Glu^{495}Lys	12.2
	African American	818G→A/1039C→T	10, 12	Arg^{273}His/Arg^{347}Cys	15.9
	Caucasian	833C→T/1459C→T	10, 16	Ser^{278}Leu/Leu^{487}Phe	9.8
	Hispanic	898G→C/1039C→T	11, 12	Ala^{300}Pro/Arg^{347}Cys	25.4†
Kinki	Japanese	1124C→G/1615G→A	13, 18	Thr^{375}Arg/Asp^{539}Asn	3.7†
Calden	German	1166A→G/1549C→G	13, 18	His^{389}Arg/Leu^{517}Val	12†

GPI = glucose phosphate isomerase; Hb = hemoglobin; del = deletion; IVS = intervening sequence; stop = stop codon.

*Normal: 50 ± 10.5 IU/g Hb.

†Severe disease (splenectomy, regular red cell transfusions, or reticulocyte count >15 percent).

From Kugler W, Lakomek M: Glucose-6-phosphate isomerase deficiency. Bailliere's Clin Haematol 2000:13:89 (Tables 1 and 4).

Attempts by Arnold and colleagues[95] to enhance glycolysis in a GPI-deficient patient by intravenous administration of methylene blue or inorganic phosphate (P_i) did not have a lasting benefit.

PHOSPHOFRUCTOKINASE DEFICIENCY

$$\text{Fructose 6-phosphate} \xrightleftharpoons[\text{ATP} \quad \text{Mg}^{2+} \quad \text{ADP}]{\text{Phosphofructokinase}} \text{Fructose 1,6-diphosphate}$$

Clinical Manifestations

Inherited deficiency of PFK can involve erythrocytes, muscle, or both, depending on the PFK subunit affected and the nature of the biochemical defect (Table 16–4).

Although low erythrocyte PFK activity and mild hemolytic anemia are commonly found in type VII glycogen storage disease (Tarui syndrome), the dominant clinical feature of this disorder is exertional myopathy due to deficient muscle PFK activity.[116, 117] Physical activity is limited not by anemia but by weakness, easy fatigability, and severe muscle cramps associated with the myopathy. The disease may manifest at birth and cause death during infancy from respiratory insufficiency and other complications[118] or may be so mild that it presents in old age,[119] but in most affected individuals the disorder is first detected during adolescence or young adulthood. The diagnosis may be suspected if no lactate is produced during an ischemic (anaerobic) forearm exercise test, but confirmation requires muscle biopsy for determination of PFK activity or noninvasive magnetic resonance imaging studies of muscle carbohydrate metabolism.[120]

When PFK deficiency is confined to erythrocytes, there are no symptoms of myopathy, and there is a normal blood lactate response to anoxic exercise.[121–123] Such patients may be hematologically normal[114, 124, 125] or

TABLE 16–4. Various Forms of Human Phosphofructokinase (PFK) Deficiency

Type	No. of Patients	Affected PFK Subunit	Red Blood Cell		Muscle		Other
			Hemolysis	PFK Activity*	Myopathy	PFK Activity*	
I	18	M (absent or unstable)	+	29–64	+	0–5	Hyperuricemia, arthritis
II	3	NA	NA	17	+	0–6	
III	3	M (unstable)	+	8–62	0	100†	
IVa	2	M (unstable)	0	28–50	0	78†	Asymptomatic
IVb	3	L (unstable)	0	60–65	0	NA	Asymptomatic
V	3	NA	NA	75†	++	2–6	Arthritis

NA = data not available.
*Percentage of normal value.
†Studied in only one patient.
Data are from Tani and associates[112,113] and Vora and co-workers.[114,115]
From Mentzer WC, Glader BE: Disorders of erythrocyte metabolism. In Mentzer WC, Wagner GM (eds): The Hereditary Hemolytic Anemias. New York, Churchill Livingstone, Inc., 1989, pp 267–319.

exhibit mild to moderate hemolytic anemia.[121, 125] In general, red cell morphologic characteristics are not strikingly abnormal, although prominent basophilic stippling has occasionally been present.

Biochemistry

PFK is one of several glycolytic enzymes that reversibly bind to the inner aspect of the erythrocyte membrane. Binding, which is thought to occur between the amino-terminal position of the *trans* membrane protein band 3 and the adenine nucleotide binding site, located in a cleft between the two dimers that compromise the PFK tetramer, may serve both to activate the enzyme and to protect it against proteolytic degradation during erythrocyte aging.[126]

The active form of human erythrocyte PFK is a tetramer (molecular weight 380,000) composed in varying combinations of two different subunits, one identical to the M subunit found in muscle PFK and the other identical to the L subunit found in liver PFK.[127, 128] The molecular weight of the M subunit is 85,000 and that of the L subunit is 80,000.[127] About 50 percent of the erythrocyte enzyme is formed from M subunits,[122, 127] whereas muscle PFK is composed entirely of M subunits.[122, 129] A deficiency in M subunits severely depresses muscle PFK activity, resulting in myopathy, but has a lesser effect on erythrocyte PFK because residual L subunits, under separate genetic control, combine to form an active L_4 tetramer of PFK. However, PFK formed entirely from L subunits is unstable to heat or dilution *in vitro* and is more sensitive to ATP inhibition than is muscle (M_4) PFK.[121] At the *in vivo* concentrations of ATP that are present within normal erythrocytes, the enzyme activity of L_4 PFK tetramers is severely inhibited, possibly explaining the presence of hemolytic anemia even when enzyme activity, as measured *in vitro*, is approximately 50 percent of normal. Most recognized examples of PFK deficiency are the result of either missing[110, 114, 116] or structurally altered[123] M subunits. An interesting exception was found in a clinically normal individual, fortuitously discovered when he volunteered to serve as a "control" during studies of red cell PFK carried out by Vora and colleagues.[114]

Normal M subunits but mutant, unstable L subunits were found in his red cells. There was no myopathy, and, although erythrocyte PFK was only 65 percent of normal, hemolytic anemia was not found, presumably because residual enzyme activity within the red cell was entirely due to the presence of M_4 tetramers of PFK. The relatively greater stability and lesser susceptibility to ATP inhibition of this form of PFK apparently allowed adequate enzyme activity under conditions normally found within the red cell *in vivo*.

Because of the central role of PFK in regulation of erythrocyte metabolism, it is not surprising to find that a deficiency of this important enzyme is associated with hemolysis. The mechanism of hemolysis of PFK-deficient red cells is not well understood. Erythrocyte sodium and potassium concentrations, sodium influx, and lactate production were normal in one patient.[120] Despite their normal glycolytic capabilities *in vitro*, deficient cells were incapable of maintaining normal ATP concentrations *in vivo*. The low (73 percent of normal) intracellular ATP concentration in these cells, although indicative of an abnormality of cellular metabolism, may also exert a positive influence by partially relieving the inhibitory influence of ATP on PFK.

The complex interaction between metabolites that may dictate actual PFK activity *in vivo* is illustrated by physiologic studies performed on four individuals with Tarui syndrome.[130] At usual levels of physical activity, the pattern of erythrocyte glycolytic intermediates clearly reflected inhibition at the PFK step, and the concentration of the important downstream metabolite 2,3-DPG was only 50 percent of the level found in normal red cells. After patients had 2 days of bed rest, their red cell 2,3-DPG levels sank to just one third of normal. Subsequently, ergometric exercise on a bicycle eliminated the glycolytic intermediate pattern of PFK inhibition and allowed downstream intermediates, including 2,3-DPG, to increase toward normal. Release of large amounts of inosine and ammonia from enzymopathic muscle during exercise into the plasma was observed in these patients. Ammonia is a powerful activator of PFK; inosine can be metabolized to lactate by glycolytic pathways (i.e, the HMP shunt) that bypass the PFK reaction. Thus, the muscle metabolic abnormalities created by PFK deficiency generate metabolites that alleviated the enzymopathy in erythrocytes. (Diversion of the flow of erythrocyte glycolysis through the HMP shunt by the block at PFK may also generate increased amounts of purines and pyrimidines from 5-phosphoribosylprophosphate [PRPP].) The hyperuricemia sometimes noted in individuals with PFK deficiency (Table 16–4) may be explained on this basis.[115]

An inherited deficiency of PFK found in English springer spaniels allows interesting comparisons to be made with the human condition.[131–133] As in humans, canine PFK deficiency is an autosomal recessive disorder. Red cell PFK levels are only 7 to 22 percent of normal levels in homozygotes, because the muscle subunit, which is lacking, comprises the majority of the available subunits in normal dog red cells.[134] PFK deficiency in dogs is associated with a severe hemolytic anemia. Newborn dogs are not anemic, because there is a greater abundance of L subunits and thus of functional PFK enzymes in their red cells. The hemolytic anemia appears because the normal developmental pattern of replacement of L by M subunit synthesis occurs in a setting where M subunits are either not synthesized or are defective.[135]

A unique feature of dog PFK deficiency is episodic hemolysis induced by hyperventilation during exercise, mating, barking, or other similar activities.[133] Dog red cells with high sodium levels exhibit spontaneous hemolysis at alkaline pH; even the small pH change induced by hyperventilation is sufficient to generate the effect in PFK-deficient animals. Underlying the susceptibility of PFK-deficient dog red cells to hyperventilation-induced hemolysis may be their low 2,3-DPG levels, which increase intracellular pH. Raising 2,3-DPG levels to normal *in vitro* normalizes the response to alkalinity.[136] In comparison to humans, there is less evidence of exertional myopathy, even though dog muscle PFK activity is nearly absent,[137] because dogs do not rely upon anaerobic glycolysis for energy generation during exercise.[138] During exercise, PFK-deficient dogs do exhibit less extraction of oxygen from hemoglobin than normal dogs, either because hemoglobin oxygen affinity is high (caused by low 2,3-DPG levels in their erythrocytes) or because oxidative metabolism is impaired.[139]

PFK activity in erythrocytes from newborn infants is about 50 to 60 percent of that in normal adult cells.[140] PFK deficiency is more evident in older cells made earlier in gestation, perhaps because of accelerated enzyme decay.[141] Vora and Piomelli[142] showed that 25 to 30 percent of newborn erythrocyte PFK is L_4 isozyme, with the remainder being divided equally between three hybrid isozymes of L and M subunits (L_1M_3, L_2M_2, and L_3M_1). The L_4 isozyme, not found in normal adult red cells, is unstable, presumably accounting for the reduced PFK activity of older cord red cells. The demonstration that PFK deficiency may result in hemolytic anemia in adults suggests that the enzyme deficiency characteristic of newborn red cells may contribute to their shortened survival.

Genetics and Inheritance

The gene locus for the L subunit of PFK has been assigned to chromosome 21, whereas the M subunit locus is on chromosome 1.[115] The erythrocytes, but not the leukocytes and platelets, of individuals with trisomy 21 consistently contain increased PFK activity.[143] Increased erythrocyte PFK activity is due to increased amounts of L subunit, consistent with a simple gene dosage effect.[115]

Inheritance is autosomal recessive. Type I PFK deficiency (Tarui disease), which is found predominantly in Ashkenazi Jews and in Japanese, is the result of mutations involving the *PFKM* gene.[144, 145] The 15 reported mutations[146] (5 splice site, 8 missense, 1 nonsense, and 1 frameshift) are shown in Figure 16–3. The widely scattered location of the mutations makes it difficult to correlate genotype and phenotype. In PFK-deficient dogs, a missense mutation 120 nucleotides from the 3′ end of the

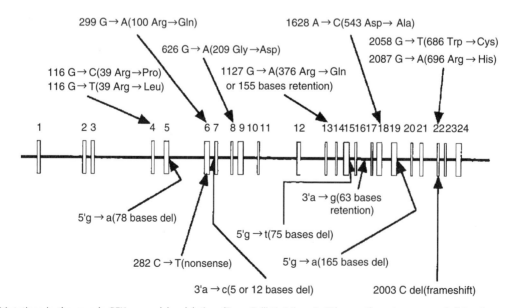

FIGURE 16–3. Mutations in the muscle *PFK* gene. del = deletion. (From Fujii H, Miwa S: Other erythrocyte enzyme deficiencies associated with non-haematological symptoms: Phosphoglycerate kinase and phosphofructokinase deficiency. *Bailliere's Clin Haematol* 2000; 13:141. By copyright permission of Harcourt Publishers Ltd.)

coding region produces a truncated mRNA and an unstable *PFKM*-subunit tetramer with altered kinetic properties.[147, 148]

Therapy

Supportive care with red cell transfusions as needed and daily folic acid supplementation are the mainstays of therapy for the hemolytic anemia.

ALDOLASE DEFICIENCY

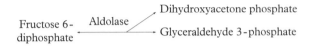

Clinical Manifestations, Biochemistry, and Genetics

Two members of a Japanese family who had a severe deficiency of red cell aldolase A (4.7 to 5.5 percent of normal activity)[149] exhibited severe chronic hemolytic anemia, sometimes exacerbated by infections. *In vitro*, red cell glycolysis and HMP shunt activity were depressed, indicating that the deficiency of aldolase was of functional significance. Both parents were hematologically normal but had intermediate reductions in red cell aldolase A activity. The mutant aldolase was strikingly thermolabile. A missense mutation (GAT→GGT), giving rise to a single amino acid substitution (Asp→Gly) at position 128, was present in the mutant enzyme.[150] Transfection of *Escherichia coli* with an expression plasmid containing normal, mutant, or modified (by site-directed mutagenesis) aldolase A complementary DNA (cDNA) generated functional aldolase molecules that were used to confirm that the amino acid substitution at position 128, a site distant from the catalytic site but within an exposed hinge region, was responsible for enzyme thermolability.[151]

In a German child, homozygosity for a point mutation at residue 206 (Glu→Lys) in the coding region of aldolase A also led to thermolability and severe enzyme deficiency in both erythrocytes and skeletal muscle.[152] Unlike the Japanese subjects, this child had a metabolic myopathy as well as mild to moderate hemolytic anemia. The mutation at residue 206 would be predicted to disrupt the main subunit interface of the aldolase tetramer, causing thermolability. Why myopathy was noted in one setting but not in the other is unknown.

Another patient with aldolase deficiency exhibited congenital nonspherocytic hemolytic anemia, mental retardation, mild glycogen storage disease, intestinal lactase deficiency, growth retardation, and peculiar facial features. Enzyme activity was approximately 15 percent of normal in erythrocytes and in cultured skin fibroblasts.[153] No structural abnormality of residual erythrocyte aldolase was detected by electrophoresis, isoelectric focusing, heat stability studies, or kinetic examination. The patient was the offspring of a consanguineous marriage, but both parents were hematologically normal and had normal red cell aldolase activity.

TRIOSE PHOSPHATE ISOMERASE DEFICIENCY

Triose phosphate isomerase

Dihydroxyacetone ——————— Glyceraldehyde 3-
phosphate phosphate

Clinical Manifestations

An association with TPI deficiency has been documented in approximately 50 patients with congenital hemolytic anemia.[154–170] In addition to chronic hemolysis, a severe neuromuscular disorder, characterized initially by spasticity and psychomotor retardation often progressing to weakness and hypotonia, has been found in nearly all patients surviving beyond the neonatal period. Increased susceptibility to bacterial infection has also been noted. The neurologic abnormalities are usually not manifest before 6 to 12 months of age and are progressive, generally leading to death before the age of 5 years. Occasionally, these abnormalities may stabilize during childhood[171] or adolescence.[155] In a Hungarian family, one son with severe TPI deficiency had extrapyramidal neurologic symptoms whereas his older brother, whose enzymopenia was equally severe, remained symptom free.[168, 172]

Anemia has ranged from severe to moderate, with most patients requiring at least occasional blood transfusions. Macrocytosis and polychromatophilia are evident on the blood smear, reflecting the presence of reticulocytosis, which may reach 50 percent on occasion. Aside from occasional small, dense, spiculated cells, no striking changes in erythrocyte morphologic characteristics are present.

Biochemistry

TPI is a homodimer whose two subunits (molecular weight 26,750)[173] are the product of a single locus on the short arm of chromosome 12.[169–175] Post-translational modification of one or both subunits may occur by deamidination of aspartines at positions 15 and 71, resulting in multiple forms of the enzyme and creating a complex multibanded pattern on electrophoresis.[176–178] The 248–amino acid sequence of human (placental) TPI has been determined directly[173] and is nearly but not completely identical to the sequence predicted by nucleotide analysis of adult human liver cDNA.[160]

TPI is a classic housekeeping gene, present in all tissues, whose amino acid sequence has been remarkably well conserved during evolution.[179] The eight-stranded αβ barrel structure of the human enzyme has been confirmed at 2.8-nm resolution by x-ray crystallography.[179] TPI has no requirement for cofactors or metal ions, and there is no evidence for cooperativity or allosteric interactions between subunits.

When measured *in vitro*, erythrocyte TPI activity is approximately 1000 times that of HK, the least active glycolytic enzyme. Even TPI-deficient erythrocytes exhibiting only 2 to 35 percent of normal TPI activity *in vitro* possess far more TPI than HK activity. Not surprisingly,

TPI-deficient erythrocytes are capable of normal glycolysis *in vitro*, even when compared with reticulocyte-rich normal blood.[155] Nonetheless, dihydroxyacetone phosphate, the substrate for TPI, accumulates to high levels in TPI-deficient erythrocytes and the ATP concentration is usually low for cell age. These results indicate the presence of a substantial impairment of glycolysis *in vivo*. Modulation of residual TPI activity in deficient cells by binding to the red cell membrane has been proposed to account for some of the differences between *in vitro* determinations of TPI activity and the evidence of a more severe impairment of enzyme function *in vivo*.[180, 181]

The defect can be partially bypassed by way of the HMP shunt, which generates glyceraldehyde 3-phosphate from glucose without the participation of TPI. Methylene blue stimulation of the shunt produces a lesser increase in glycolysis relative to baseline in TPI-deficient erythrocytes than in reticulocyte-rich control blood.[155] This has been interpreted as indicating a markedly greater "resting" shunt rate in the deficient cells, consistent with the proposed reliance of such cells on the shunt. Evidence indicates that TPI-deficient red cells are relatively deficient in antioxidant capabilities and that this may contribute to their shortened life span.[157, 182]

Rare electrophoretic variants of TPI, not associated with reduced enzyme activity or hemolysis, have been described.[178,179,183,184] In anemic patients, enzyme kinetics and electrophoretic mobility are usually normal, but evidence *in vitro* of enzyme lability after heating is often obtained,[159, 160, 161, 163] suggesting that instability and rapid loss of enzyme protein plays an important role in the pathogenesis of hemolysis *in vivo*.[159, 161] A single amino acid substitution (Glu→Asp) at position 104 has been identified in at least 17 geographically widely distributed families with clinically affected children and is the most commonly encountered mutation responsible for TPI deficiency.[165, 170] Its relative rate of occurrence is thought to be due to a founder effect. The *TPI* gene product is thermolabile.[185] Computer modeling indicates that a substituted amino acid at position 104, which is buried in a hydrophilic side pocket of the normal enzyme, will reduce the stability of the pocket, promote unfolding, and enhance thermolability[185]

A total of 14 TPI mutations have been defined at the molecular level.[165] Most clinically affected individuals are homozygous for a single mutation or compound heterozygous for two different mutations. In the Hungarian pedigree mentioned earlier,[172] a point mutation at codon 240 (Phe→Leu) produced a moderately thermolabile TPI with abnormal substrate kinetics and electrophoretic migration.[186] Phe[240] is near the active site of the enzyme and appears to be essential for maintaining its correct geometry.[179] Also inherited by both anemic brothers in this pedigree was a nonsense mutation at codon 145 that terminated TPI protein synthesis, producing a truncated protein, and also reduced the output of TPI mRNA from the affected allele by 10- to 20-fold.[187] The red cells of the brothers had less than 10 percent of the TPI activity found in normal cells.[172, 186]

The enzyme deficiency is manifest not only in red cells but also in leukocytes, platelets, muscle, serum, and cerebrospinal fluid. Histologic examination of muscle from one girl with TPI deficiency and myopathy revealed marked degenerative changes of the contractile system, altered mitochondria, and absent TPI by histochemical staining.[188] Brain and nerve tissue have not yet been analyzed, but the cerebrospinal fluid deficiency suggests that deficient TPI activity in neural tissue is responsible for the neurologic abnormalities observed in enzymopenic patients. Although increased susceptibility to infection might be the consequence of defective function by TPI-deficient leukocytes,[162] the functional studies carried out on such cells in *vitro* have often been normal.[158, 171] A functional defect in TPI-deficient platelets has been described.[189]

Genetics and Inheritance

Results of studies of several large pedigrees are consistent with an autosomal recessive mode of inheritance.[158, 161, 165] Obligate heterozygotes are clinically normal, but their erythrocytes contain only approximately one half the TPI activity of control erythrocytes. As is often the case in other glycolytic enzymopathies, no clear boundary exists between heterozygous-deficient and low normal enzyme activity. Several upstream polymorphisms are found at a high rate of occurrence in African-American populations.[165, 175] Although they may be associated with mild reductions in erythrocyte TPI activity, they do not seem to be associated with clinical abnormalities, even in homozygotes.[165] At the other extreme, in mice the homozygous state for a TPI null allele is lethal early in embryogenesis.[190] Simultaneous heterozygous inheritance of TPI deficiency and either G6PD deficiency or sickle cell trait has not altered the typical clinical pattern of the disorders when either is present alone.[157] TPI deficiency can be diagnosed prenatally by analysis of fetal blood cells,[164] cultured amniocytes,[163] or trophoblastic cells[169] with suitable precautions.[191] If the mutation is known, mutation analysis can be performed directly on fetal DNA.[169, 187]

Therapy

Transfusions and folic acid supplementation are the therapies presently available. Splenectomy in one patient did not alter the intensity of hemolysis.[158] *In vitro* studies point to the possibility of transfer of TPI enzyme protein from normal into deficient cells with transient improvement in enzyme activity and reduction in dihydroxyacetone phosphate levels.[192] There have been no attempts to deliver normal TPI enzyme to patient tissues as yet, but in other disease settings direct enzyme transfer from normal hematopoietic stem cell–derived microglial cells to enzyme-deficient nervous tissue after allogeneic stem cell transplantation has been successful.[192]

GLYCERALDEHYDE-3-PHOSPHATE DEHYDROGENASE DEFICIENCY

Glyceraldehyde-3-phosphate dehydrogenase

Glyceraldehyde 3-phosphate ⟶ 1,3-Diphosphoglycerate

NAD P_i NADH

Clinical Manifestations, Biochemistry, and Genetics

Three males in whom hemolytic anemia was associated with reduced erythrocyte G3PD activity have been briefly described.[193,194] Differences in erythrocyte osmotic fragility and in G3PD activity indicate that the disorder in one of the patients may not be identical to that in the other two. In this patient, infection and an antimalarial drug (dapsone), accelerated hemolysis, yet in all three patients the concentration and stability of reduced glutathione were normal. Changes in the pattern of glycolytic intermediates similar to those induced by iodoacetic acid, a known inhibitor of G3PD, were found in the erythrocytes of one patient. Iodoacetic acid inhibited glycolysis more in affected erythrocytes than in control erythrocytes. The disorder is probably hereditary, because both father and son were affected in one pedigree. In one patient, enzyme activity was normal in platelets and reduced in leukocytes.

Results of a study of a large kindred in which three members exhibited a reduction of erythrocyte G3PD activity to 50 percent of normal levels, yet were hematologically normal, have clearly established that G3PD deficiency need not result in hemolysis.[195] The gene for hereditary spherocytosis was also present in this kindred, and four members were found to have inherited both hereditary spherocytosis and G3PD deficiency. The clinical severity of hemolytic anemia in these individuals with spherocytosis was not altered by the simultaneous inheritance of G3PD deficiency. Thus, the relationship of G3PD deficiency to hereditary hemolytic anemia is not yet established. Affected members of this kindred were presumed to be heterozygotes, because the amounts of both G3PD enzyme activity and enzyme protein were reduced equally to about 50 percent of normal, and the amount of residual G3PD was qualitatively normal. Two of the three anemic patients with G3PD deficiency in other kindreds had even lower levels of enzyme activity (20 to 30 percent of normal) and conceivably are either homozygotes or doubly heterozygous for two mutant G3PD genes.

PHOSPHOGLYCERATE KINASE DEFICIENCY

Phosphoglycerate Kinase
1,3-Diphosphoglycerate ⟷ 3-Phosphoglycerate
ATP Mg²⁺ ADP

Clinical Manifestations

Phosphoglycerate kinase (PGK) deficiency is a sex-linked disorder that largely affects males. Nonspherocytic hemolytic anemia may occur alone or in combination with neurologic abnormalities ranging from emotional instability to seizures, movement disorders, psychomotor retardation, aphasia, or tetraplegia.[146] In a subset of individuals with PGK deficiency, myopathy is the dominant clinical manifestation (Table 16–5). Individuals with one form of

mild PGK deficiency (PGK München) exhibit no clinical abnormalities (Table 16–5). In females, erythrocyte PGK activity is less depressed than it is in males, hemolytic anemia is mild or absent, and neurologic and muscle abnormalities are not seen (Table 16–5).

Hematologic findings in anemic individuals with PGK deficiency have been those customarily associated with hemolysis, namely, jaundice and reticulocytosis. No changes in erythrocyte morphologic characteristics have been seen, and osmotic fragility has usually been normal.

Biochemistry

PGK is a monomeric enzyme with a primary structure consisting of 417 amino acids.[224] Horse muscle PGK has a primary structure that is highly homologous to that of human PGK. Crystallographic studies show that its tertiary structure consists of two lobes (the C and N domains) connected by a hingelike structure that allows considerable conformational change to occur during substrate binding (Fig. 16–4).[225] Because the nucleotide (adenosine diphosphate [ADP] and ATP) combining site is located within the C domain and the phosphoglycerate (1,3-DPG or 3-phosphoglyerate [PG]) binding site within the N domain, bending of the enzyme is required to bring into close proximity the several substrates required for the PGK reaction.[225]

PGK-deficient red cells are capable of normal glycolysis *in vitro*.[196, 222, 226] Intracellular ATP concentrations are normal or slightly low,[196, 200, 222, 226, 227] whereas the 2,3-DPG concentration is elevated, sometimes to two or three times the normal level.* These results reflect increased flow through the 2,3-DPG cycle (see Fig. 16–1) at the expense of the ATP-generating PGK reaction. Despite the availability of an alternative pathway (the Rapoport-Luebering shunt or 2,3-DPG cycle) to bypass PGK, substantial accumulation of glycolytic intermediates proximal to the enzyme defect is found in fresh red cells, indicating that the normal flow of erythrocyte glycolysis is impeded *in vivo*.

Little is known about the mechanism of hemolysis of PGK-deficient red cells. Most PGK activity is membrane associated.[228] It has been suggested that ATP for membrane adenosine triphosphatase (ATPase)-mediated cation transport is mostly (or entirely) generated by membrane-bound PGK. Indeed, ADP derived from membrane ATPase exerts an important regulatory influence on glycolysis by its participation in the PGK reaction.[229] However, the implication of a special role for PGK in cation transport has been challenged.[230] The active transport of Na⁺ and K⁺ by PGK-deficient red cells with residual PGK activity only 10 to 15 percent of normal was not impaired, even with the challenge of an increase in intracellular Na⁺ concentration.[231] Thus, it seems unlikely that hemolysis of PGK-deficient red cells is related to premature cation pump failure owing directly to inadequate PGK activity.

PGK activity in leukocytes is consistently subnormal in affected males, but white cell function is not usually compromised. In one patient, PGK-deficient leukocytes

---

*References 196, 200, 205, 209, 222, 226, and 227.

TABLE 16–5. Characteristics of Reported Patients with Phosphoglycerate Kinase Deficiency

References	Variant	Mutation	Red Blood Cell PGK Activity (% of Normal)	Stability in Vitro	Kinetic Abnormalities	Hemolytic Anemia	Neurologic Abnormalities	Myopathy
HEMIZYGOTES (MALE): HEMOLYTIC ANEMIA OR NO CLINICAL MANIFESTATIONS								
196–198	Amiens	Asp^{163}→Val	2.7	Normal		+	+	0
199	Alabama	Lys$^{190-191}$ del	4			+	0	0
200–202	Matsue	Leu^{88}→Pro	5	Low	+	+	+	0
203, 204	Uppsala	Arg^{205}→Pro	5–10	Low	+	+	+	0
205, 206	Cincinnati		8–11			+	+	0
207	Tokyo	Val^{265}→Met	10	Low	+	+	+	0
208	Michigan	Cys^{315}→Arg	10	Low	+	+	+	0
209	San Francisco		12	Normal	+	+	0	0
210, 211	München	Asp^{267}→Asn	21	Low	0	0	0	0
212	Herlev	Asp^{285}→Val	50			+	0	0
HEMIZYGOTES (MALE): MUSCLE DISEASE								
213	Shizuoka	Gly^{157}→Asp	0.7	Normal	0	+	0	+
214	North Carolina	10 a.a. insert	3	Normal	+	0	+	+
215	Creteil	Asp^{314}→Asn	3	Low	+	0	0	+
216	Trondheim		5			0	0	+
216	Antwerp	Glu^{251}→Ala★	5.6			0	0	+
217	Fukui	4 bp del, exon 6†				0	0	+
218, 219	Hammamatsu	Ile^{252}→Thr	8	Normal	0	0	+	+
220	New Jersey		18	Normal	+	0	0	+
221	Alberta		1.5 (muscle)	Normal	+	0	0	+
HETEROZYGOTES (FEMALE)								
222	Piedmont		27			+	0	0
223	Memphis		78			+	0	0
196–198	Amiens		77			+	0	0

PGK = phosphoglycerate kinase; a.a. = amino acid; del = deletion.
★This mutation also adversely affects messenger RNA splicing efficiency by reducing it to about 10 percent of normal.
†Frameshift at codon 716 to 718, resulting in stop codon to 780 to 782, truncating PGK to 231 amino acids in length.

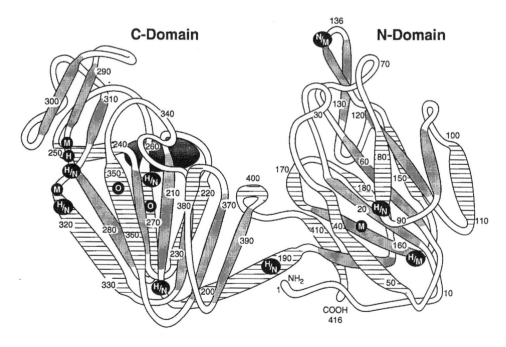

FIGURE 16–4. Three-dimensional model of human phosphoglycerate kinase. This figure is based on the three-dimensional model of horse PGK published by Banks et al.[194] Positions of the amino acid substitutions and the clinical features associated with 14 PGK point mutations are indicated by *filled circles* (O = no clinical abnormalities; M = muscle disease; H = hemolytic anemia; N = neurologic manifestations). The *shaded ellipse* in the C domain indicates the location of the adenosine triphosphate (ATP) and adenosine diphosphate (ADP) binding site. Random coil (*clear*), β strands (*solid*), and α helices (*striped*) are indicated by shading. (Modified from Fujii H, Kanno H, Hironi A, et al: A single amino acid substitution (157 Gly→Val) in a phosphoglycerate kinase variant (PGK Shizuoka) associated with chronic hemolysis and myoglobinuria. Blood 1992; 79:1582.)

exhibited increased Krebs cycle activity both at rest and during phagocytosis. Abolition of Krebs cycle metabolism with cyanide severely impaired the ingestion of bacteria by such cells but had little or no effect on normal leukocytes.[232] Thus, the PGK-deficient leukocyte appeared to compensate for its glycolytic defect by increased Krebs cycle activity. However, although ingestion of bacteria was normal, deficient leukocytes were unable to kill or iodinate ingested *Staphylococcus aureus* effectively *in vitro*. In contrast to the abnormalities observed in this single patient, white cell function has been completely normal in three other males with PGK deficiency.[206, 227] Leukocyte function *in vivo* is probably not compromised, because an increased incidence of infection has not been a feature of PGK deficiency.

Genetics and Inheritance

The major structural gene for PGK, located on the long arm of the X chromosome, is 23 kb in size and is composed of 11 exons and 10 introns.[220, 233-236] PGK-deficient male hemizygotes have very little active enzyme and are show more symptoms than heterozygous females who have higher levels of PGK activity (Table 16–5). A second functional *PGK* gene, expressed only in spermatozoa, is found on chromosome 19.[237] This autosomal *PGK* gene lacks introns but is otherwise similar to the X chromosomal *PGK* gene. A single isozyme of PGK is found in all human nonhematopoietic tissues except spermatozoa.[238] It is therefore not surprising that nonerythroid tissues may be compromised in patients with erythrocyte PGK deficiency.

In 1972, Yoshida and co-workers[239] succeeded in purifying and sequencing both normal erythrocyte PGK and a clinically normal but electrophoretically distinct human mutant PGK, the New Guinea variant. The mutant enzyme differed from normal PGK by the substitution of arginine for threonine at position 352.[224] Subsequently, the structure of 13 of the PGK mutants associated with hemolytic anemia has been determined by peptide or nucleotide sequencing.* Eleven of these involve only a single amino acid (10 missense mutations and 1 deletion). The 12th activates a cryptic splice site, leading to the insertion of 10 additional amino acids into the PGK polypeptide, and the 13th also affects splicing, producing a truncated polypeptide. The majority of the mutants are found within the C domain, as shown in Figure 16–4. It is not clear how the particular spectrum of clinical abnormalities associated with each mutation is related to its position within the molecule. For example, PGK Michigan, a point mutation at amino acid 315, is associated with hemolytic anemia and neurologic abnormalities whereas individuals with PGK Creteil, a point mutation of the adjacent amino acid at position 314, do not have anemia and neurologic abnormalities but exhibit rhabdomyolysis.[240] Both mutants are thermolabile and exhibit kinetic abnormalities *in vitro* and both have similarly reduced activity in erythrocytes (Table 16–5). Random inactivation of the mutant X chromosome may produce differing proportions of enzyme-deficient cells in female heterozygotes. Some may be anemic (Table 16–5), whereas others are clinically and hematologically normal.[200] In the latter, the population of PGK-deficient red cells may be so small that erythrocyte PGK activity will be completely normal.[200]

Therapy

In one patient, splenectomy had no beneficial effect on anemia,[223] but in several others, surgery has reduced or eliminated the need for transfusions, reduced the degree of reticulocytosis, and sometimes resulted in an increase of several grams in the hemoglobin level.

2,3-BISPHOSPHOGLYCERATE MUTASE DEFICIENCY

Clinical Manifestations

Whether deficient erythrocyte 2,3-bisphosphoglycerate mutase (BPGM) activity adversely affects red cell life span is unclear. In one pedigree, four siblings who completely lacked functional red cell BPGM had polycythemia but otherwise were clinically and hematologically normal. All three children of these individuals had about 50 percent of the normal amount of red cell BPGM and were hematologically normal except for polycythemia.[242, 243] In several other pedigrees, partial deficiency of 2,3-DPG mutase has also not been associated with evidence of hemolysis.[244, 245] In another report, compensated hemolysis was present in two patients with moderately reduced red cell BPGM activity,[246, 247] but a causal association between BPGM deficiency and hemolysis was not proven.

Biochemistry

Human red cell BPGM is a homodimer whose identical subunits (molecular weight 29,840) each consist of 258 amino acids.[248] Nearly all 2,3-bisphosphoglycerate phosphatase activity also resides in the BPGM molecule, so that 2,3-DPG metabolism is controlled by a single, multifunctional enzyme. In fact, purified BPGM is also capable of performing as a monophosphoglycerate mutase, although at a low rate of activity.[249] Considerable structural homology exists between red cell 2,3-DPG mutase and monophosphoglycerate mutase,[250, 251] and the enzymes, to some extent, exhibit overlapping functions. However, both biochemical[250] and genetic[252] evidence indicates that they are each unique and under separate genetic control.

The BPGM molecule has been modified *in vitro* by site-directed mutagenesis in an attempt to model a potential therapeutic approach to sickle cell disease.[253] Replacement of Gly[13] by Arg enhances phosphatase activity at the expense of the mutase. The effect of such an alteration *in vivo*, achieved by gene therapy or by pharmacologic means, would be to lower erythrocyte 2,3-DPG levels, increase hemoglobin oxygen affinity, and in this way retard the polymerization of hemoglobin S.

---

*References 197, 201, 203, 207, 208, 212–214, 216, 217, 219, 221, and 240–242.

BPGM deficiency results in reduced synthesis of 2,3-DPG. In complete BPGM deficiency, there is virtually no 2,3-DPG within the red cell,[242, 243] whereas when enzyme activity is less severely depressed, 2,3-DPG levels are generally about 30 to 40 percent of normal.[242, 245, 247] Whole-blood oxygen affinity is increased because of lack of 2,3-DPG, accounting for the polycythemia noted in individuals with BPGM deficiency,[242–245, 247] The pattern of glycolytic intermediates is disturbed,[242] sometimes exhibiting a crossover at PFK,[243, 245] which is consistent with relief of the inhibitory influence of 2,3-DPG on PFK. The erythrocyte ATP concentration is usually normal or slightly increased, compatible with the diversion of 2,3-DPG into the PGK reaction as a consequence of reduced flow through BPGM. Erythrocyte glycolysis[245, 247] and pentose phosphate pathway activity have been normal in vitro.[242] Probably as a consequence of the large amount of 1,3-DPG present in BPGM-deficient red cells, hemoglobin A may undergo post-translational modification by glycerylation at $\alpha82$. The modified hemoglobin, about 3 percent of the total, has a lower isoelectric-electric point than hemoglobin A_1C and is easily identified by isoelectric focusing.[254]

Genetics and Inheritance

The BPGM locus is on chromosome 7 (7q22-34).[255] The gene is fully expressed only in erythroid tissue.[256] BPGM deficiency has the expected autosomal recessive mode of inheritance.[242–245, 247]

Individuals with polycythemia and virtually no red cell BPGM activity have been shown to be compound heterozygotes for two different BPGM mutations. One, BPGM Creteil I, is a point mutation ($Arg^{89} \to CYS$) at or near the BPGM active site[257] and the other, BPGM Creteil II, is a frameshift mutation due to a deletion of nucleotide 205 or 206.[258] Only BPGM Creteil I enzyme protein is found in red cells.[259] It is catalytically inactive and thermolabile in vitro and exhibits altered electrophoretic mobility.[259] Although BPGM and 2,3-bisphosphoglycerate phosphatase activities were virtually absent in compound heterozygotes, monophosphoglycerate mutase activity was nearly normal, illustrating the complex nature of this multifunctional enzyme.[257]

Therapy

Polycythemia, if symptomatic, may require phlebotomy.[243]

ENOLASE DEFICIENCY

Enolase

2-phosphoglycerate $\longleftrightarrow$ Phosphoenol pyruvate

Clinical Manifestations, Biochemistry, Genetics, and Therapy

A woman in whom red cell enolase activity was only 6 percent of normal exhibited a modest reduction in the survival of ^{51}Cr-labeled autologous erythrocytes (half-life of 18 days; normal, 25 to 30 days) but no overt chronic anemia.[260] A severe, life-threatening acute hemolytic episode occurred when nitrofurantoin was administered for treatment of a urinary tract infection. Poikilocytosis, spherocytosis, and schistocytosis were evident on the peripheral blood smear during the episode of hemolysis, and the same morphologic abnormalities could subsequently be reproduced in vitro by incubation of enolase-deficient red cells with nitrofurantoin. Results of the ascorbate-cyanide test and the Heinz body test were positive, but enzymes of the HMP all exhibited normal or increased activity, and glutathione stability was normal. Such drug-induced hemolysis is distinctly uncommon in disorders of the Embden-Meyerhof pathway, although it is theoretically possible in enzyme-deficient reticulocytes.[261] In this patient, in whom sudden massive hemolysis involved predominantly mature red cells, no biochemical mechanism has yet been defined, and the association between enolase deficiency and hemolytic anemia may be coincidental. A sister was hematologically normal, but her red cells were as deficient in enolase activity as were those of the propositus. Leukocyte and platelet enolase activity was normal in both the patient and her sister. Data were insufficient to define the precise mechanism of inheritance.

Partial red cell enolase deficiency was inherited in an autosomal dominant manner by six members of a second pedigree that spanned four generations. With the exception of the propositus, a 13-day-old male with profound hemolytic anemia, affected family members were not anemic and had little or no evidence of hemolysis. Spherocytes were present on the peripheral blood smear, and the mean corpuscular hemoglobin concentration was usually elevated.[262]

Therapy remains undefined, but avoidance of oxidant drugs would seem prudent.

PYRUVATE KINASE DEFICIENCY

Pyruvate Kinase

Phosphoenolpyruvate $\longleftrightarrow$ Pyruvate

K^+

ADP Mg^{2+} ATP

Clinical Manifestations

PK deficiency is the most commonly encountered glycolytic enzymopathy associated with anemia. Its incidence has been estimated to be 51 cases per million in the white population.[263] Of the approximately 500 human patients thus far reported,[6] the majority have been of Northern European extraction. Sporadic instances have been seen in other ethnic groups. A hemolytic anemia resembling that seen in human PK deficiency has also been described in basenji dogs[264, 265] and in beagles[266] that have inherited a mutant, unstable form of erythrocyte PK. Anemia, jaundice, and splenomegaly are regularly present in PK deficiency. Anemia may be profound, presenting in utero[267, 268] or in early infancy[60] and requiring regular blood transfusions for survival. Conversely, the anemia may be mild enough to evade discovery until adulthood. In a few patients, anemia is absent, hemolysis is fully compensated for, and jaundice may be the sole clinical abnormality. When present, anemia is a lifelong condition and its intensity usually varies little, although it may become more severe during pregnancy.[269, 270] Exacerbations of anemia are uncommon and usually result from transient erythroid hypoplasia after infections[271] or, rarely, from increased hemolysis of unknown cause. Manifestations of PK deficiency outside the hematopoietic system are uncommon. In several pedigrees, chronic leg ulcers have been observed in family members with PK deficiency and hemolytic anemia.[272, 273]

Hyperbilirubinemia is often encountered in newborns with PK deficiency, and these infants may require exchange transfusions.[60] Serum unconjugated bilirubin levels remain elevated in later life, and gallstones are common. Unconjugated bilirubin levels greater than 6 mg/dL are occasionally seen[274]; one brother and sister regularly had levels greater than 20 mg/dL.[275] These patients have abnormal hepatic function in addition to hemolysis. Whether abnormalities of liver PK contribute to hyperbilirubinemia is unknown.[276, 277]

Macrocytosis, occasional shrunken, spiculated erythrocytes, and, rarely, acanthocytes may be observed on examination of the blood smear; these changes may be accentuated by splenectomy. More extreme alterations in erythrocyte morphologic characteristics are sometimes encountered (Fig. 16–5).[278,279] Such abnormalities in shape may result from the inadequate ATP synthesis characteristic of PK-deficient erythrocytes.[280] A paradoxical increase in the reticulocyte count often follows splenectomy, despite evidence of a beneficial reduction in the rate of hemolysis. Reticulocyte counts may exceed 90 percent, and in many patients counts of 40 to 70 percent are maintained for years. Conversely, in other patients the expected reduction in reticulocyte count is seen after splenectomy. The osmotic fragility of fresh and incubated erythrocytes is most often normal, although, in occasional patients, minor populations of fragile or resistant cells may be encountered after incubation. Results of an auto-

hemolysis test are usually, but not invariably,[281] abnormal, with hemolysis of as many as 50 percent of erythrocytes after 48 hours of incubation in saline. Prior addition of glucose may reduce hemolysis in some instances, but usually glucose has little or no effect. In fact, if the reticulocyte count exceeds 25 percent, incubation with glucose regularly accentuates hemolysis. This phenomenon has been attributed to inhibition of oxidative phosphorylation by glucose (Crabtree effect) with unfavorable consequences in PK-deficient reticulocytes because of their reliance upon oxidative phosphorylation for ATP synthesis.[282]

Biochemistry

The active form of PK is a homotetramer formed from one of four different tissue-specific subunits. The R subunit is found in red cells; the L subunit in liver; the M_1 subunit in muscle, heart, and brain; and the M_2 subunit in all early fetal tissues and most adult tissues including leukocytes and platelets.[283] R and L subunits derive from a common gene *(PKLR)* located on chromosome 1 (1q21),[284] whereas M_1 and M_2 subunits are generated by a second gene *(PKM)*, located on chromosome 15 (15q22).[285] In the rat, the *PKM* gene is 20 kb long and consists of 12 exons and 11 introns.[286] M_1 or M_2 specific mRNA is formed from a common primary transcript by alternate splicing involving the removal of either exon 9 (M_2) or exon 10 (M_1).[287] Because human and rat M_2 cDNAs are highly homologous,[285] alternative splicing probably also accounts for the differences in M_1 and M_2 mRNA in humans. The *PKLR* gene also consists of 12 exons.[288] Tissue-specific expression of one of two different promotors generates a transcript containing either an R or an L exon at the 5′ end.[289, 290] The remaining 10 exons are identical. L-type cDNA encodes a polypeptide of 543 amino acids[289] whereas R-type cDNA encodes a product that is longer by 31 amino acids.[283]

The three-dimensional structure of cat and rabbit muscle PK has been studied by x-ray crystallography.[292]

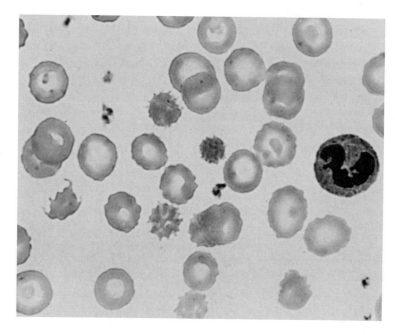

FIGURE 16–5. Postsplenectomy blood smear from a patient with severe PK deficiency. (From Nathan DG, Oski FA, et al: Extreme hemolysis and red cell distortion in erythrocyte pyruvate kinase deficiency. I. Morphology, erythrokinetics, and family enzyme studies. N Engl J Med 1964; 270:1024. Reprinted by permission of the *New England Journal of Medicine.*)

There is extensive sequence homology among species and between M and R subunits, particularly in the vicinity of the active site,[292] indicating that the enzyme structure has been conserved during evolution. As shown in Figure 16–6, each muscle PK (M_1) subunit consists of a short amino-terminal region and three distinct domains (A, B, and C). Domain A is cylindrical, formed by eight parallel strands of β sheet encased by an outer coaxial cylinder of eight α helices, domain B consists of a closed antiparallel β sheet, and domain C is a five-stranded β sheet connected by α helices. The active site lies in a pocket between domains A and B, the potassium and magnesium binding sites are in domain A, and allosteric modulation of PK function primarily involves interactions with domain C.

In erythroid cells, PK is a tetramer (molecular weight 230,000) whose subunits may vary in type. In erythroid precursors, M_2 homotetramers are the predominant PK isoenzyme. With erythroid maturation, synthesis of M_2 subunits declines and is replaced by production of R-type subunits.[293–295] The mature red cell enzyme may exist in either of two physical conformations, analogous to the R and T forms proposed by Monod and colleagues[296] for allosteric proteins. Partially purified enzyme preparations usually exhibit sigmoid kinetics in the presence of increasing concentrations of substrate (phosphoenolpyruvate). Small amounts of phosphoenolpyruvate facilitate further binding of substrate by the enzyme in a manner analogous to that seen with heme-heme interactions. Fructose 6-diphosphate (FDP) induces a transition from sigmoid to hyperbolic kinetics, probably by acting directly at the phosphoenolpyruvate binding site.[297]

A number of factors may result in post-translational modification of the enzyme. Transition between an FDP-sensitive conformation with sigmoid kinetics and an insensitive form with hyperbolic kinetics has been achieved by varying pH,[298] temperature,[298–300] and conditions of storage.[289, 301, 302] Aging of the enzyme *in vivo* appears to favor the FDP-sensitive conformation.[303] These transitions may play a significant role in modulation of PK activity *in vivo*. Post-translational modification of enzyme properties mediated by oxidation of exposed thiol groups on the surface of the molecule may explain some abnormalities previously ascribed to genetic or acquired alterations in the primary structure of the enzyme.[303–308] In several instances, with the use of sulfhydryl reagents it has been possible to restore to normal the altered stability and abnormal kinetics of mutant PK from individuals with hemolytic anemia.[304, 309] On the other hand, it has often not been possible to implicate oxidation of enzyme thiol groups as a cause of abnormal enzyme.[310, 311]

The enzyme is subject to numerous other regulatory influences. ATP is a competitive inhibitor ($K_i = 3.5 \times 10^{-4}$ mol/L)[312]; at physiologic ATP concentrations (approximately 1 mmol/L), erythrocyte PK activity should be significantly constrained by ATP. Both potassium[297, 300] and magnesium[300, 313] activate PK; rubidium (Rb+) or ammonium (NH_4^+) substitute for potassium (K+), whereas manganese (Mn^{2+}) or cobalt (Co^{2+}) can replace magnesium (Mg^{2+}).[306] Activation of purified PK by FDP has been demonstrated at concentrations normally found within the erythrocyte.[314] At a higher concentration (0.5 mmol/L), another glycolytic intermediate, glucose 6-phosphate, activates PK.[315] The glycolytic intermediate 2,3-DPG, of particular interest because of its high concentration in PK-deficient erythrocytes, has no influence upon PK in hemolysates[316] but has variously been reported to inhibit[317] or activate[318] purified PK. Phosphorylation of PK, mediated by cyclic adenosine monophosphate, alters its kinetic properties and may regulate 2,3-DPG levels and thus oxygen transport by red cells.[318, 319] It is clear that intracellular PK activity will be determined by the complex interplay of a number of regulatory factors and may bear little relation to measures of activity determined *in vitro* under optimal conditions.

When erythrocyte PK (R homotetramer) is abnormal, hepatic PK (L homotetramer) may also be affected because R and L subunits derive from a common gene. In two anemic individuals with PK deficiency, liver PK was reduced to 59[320] and 46 percent[321] of normal. Residual liver PK, measured in the latter patient, was mostly M_2 type. No disorders of hepatic function appear to result

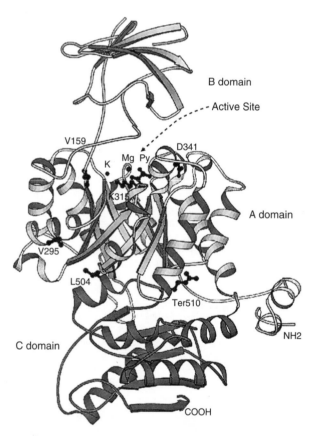

FIGURE 16–6. Ribbon representation of the structure of rabbit muscle PK. The three domains (A, B, and C), the position of potassium (K) and magnesium (Mg) ions, and the location of the active catalytic site (Py) that binds pyruvate are indicated. Six point mutations that alter a single amino acid in the primary structure of R (erythrocyte) PK are indicated. V295 is an asymptomatic heterozygote with nearly normal erythrocyte PK activity, L504 is a homozygote with severe hemolytic anemia, and the remaining four are compound heterozygotes for the indicated mutation (V159, K315, D341, or Ter510) and a second mutation at a different site. (Modified from Demina A, Varughese KI, et al: Six previously undescribed pyruvate kinase mutations causing enzyme deficiency. Blood 1998; 92:647.)

from such partial deficiency of PK.[322] In another individual, total liver PK activity was only 22 percent of normal, virtually no L-type enzyme was detectable, and there were abnormalities in serum amino transferases.[276] Paradoxically, in still another individual, liver type L PK exhibited entirely normal activity and properties, despite abnormalities in the supposedly identical isoenzyme in the red cells.[277]

The metabolic capabilities of PK-deficient erythrocytes *in vitro* vary considerably. Although resting HMP shunt activity may be slightly to moderately low for cell age,[323] no significant effect on either oxidized or reduced glutathione levels has been observed,[324–326] even after incubation with acetylphenylhydrazine.[283, 325, 327, 328] However, results of the ascorbate cyanide test are abnormal in patients with PK deficiency, and stimulated HMP shunt activity is modestly depressed.[326, 329] In many instances, glycolysis, as measured by the glucose consumption or lactate production of incubated erythrocytes, is markedly subnormal.[275, 282, 323] Such diminished glycolysis is relative, rather than absolute, because the glycolytic rate of enzymopenic cells can be increased substantially by incubation in a high P_i medium.[282, 330, 331] A reduction of residual PK activity within the erythrocyte to 10 percent of normal will still leave sufficient enzyme to support normal glycolysis if potential enzyme activity is fully utilized. Such considerations indicate that intracellular regulators of PK function must play an important role in the reduced glycolysis characteristic of enzymopenic cells. Often, particularly with kinetic variants of PK, glycolytic rates characteristic of mature normal erythrocytes are achieved.[302, 332–335] However, such rates are clearly subnormal compared with those attained by reticulocyte-rich control blood of an equivalent mean cell age.[332] Furthermore, the glucose consumption of incubated normal hemolysate is unchanged when supplemental purified PK is added, whereas addition of supplemental PK to hemolysate from PK-deficient erythrocytes produces a substantial rise in glucose consumption.[332]

Accumulation of glycolytic intermediates proximal to the enzyme defect has customarily,[299, 332, 335] although not invariably,[332] been observed.[334] Detection of elevated 2,3-DPG or 3-PG levels in red cells may help confirm a clinical diagnosis of PK deficiency[336, 337] and the degree of elevation in 2,3-DPG or glucose 6-phosphate levels is directly correlated with clinical severity.[338, 339] An alteration in the normal ratio of reduced nicotinamide adenine dinucleotide (NADH) to nicotinamide adenine dinucleotide (NAD), as well as complex changes in the substrates governing the rate of PK and 2,3-DPG mutase, appears to be responsible for triose phosphate accumulation when glycolysis is accelerated by P_i in normal red cells.[340] Such striking elevations in triose phosphate intermediates can be returned to normal in both control and in PK-deficient red cells by the addition of exogenous pyruvate or another oxidant.[331] The concentrations of both NAD and NADH are low in PK-deficient erythrocytes,[299, 322, 341] or if the level of NAD is normal in fresh cells, it falls with undue rapidity on incubation *in vitro*.[328] The concentration of 2,3-DPG in PK-deficient erythrocytes may be greater than three times normal values, leading to a rightward shift of the hemoglobin-oxygen

dissociation curve.[42, 43] The ability to extract a greater percentage of available oxygen from hemoglobin at any given pO_2 associated with such a right-shifted curve increases the exercise tolerance of patients with PK deficiency.[42] Such patients, although anemic, may exhibit none of the expected symptoms of fatigue and exercise intolerance.

The level of erythrocyte ATP and the formation of PRPP[342] are often abnormally low in PK deficiency, although patients with reticulocyte counts greater than 25 percent usually have normal ATP levels. In blood with such high reticulocyte counts, ATP is unstable on incubation with glucose in contrast to normal reticulocyte-rich blood. When incubated without glucose, however, the PK-deficient reticulocyte conserves ATP more successfully than does the normal cell.[282] The reticulocyte, able to generate ATP from substrates other than glucose via oxidative phosphorylation, can circumvent its glycolytic defect. However, in a high-glucose environment ATP levels plummet. The PK-deficient reticulocyte is, thus, exquisitely dependent upon oxidative phosphorylation for maintenance of ATP, as was first shown by Keitt.[282] The increased oxygen consumption of PK-deficient reticulocytes, compared with normal (3.75 ± 1.55 versus 0.56 ± 0.5 μL of $O_2/10^9$ reticulocytes/h) reticulocytes,[275] underscores the reliance of such cells upon oxidative phosphorylation. Reticulocyte oxygen consumption is abolished by hypoxia *in vitro* at approximately venous pO_2 levels (Fig. 16–7). When exposed to prolonged periods of hypoxia *in vivo*, therefore, or upon maturation with consequent loss of mitochondria, the PK-deficient immature erythrocyte will become reliant upon its inadequate glycolytic apparatus, with loss of cell ATP the inevitable consequence. In contrast, the reduced ATP needs of the mature erythrocyte may be marginally, but adequately, served for a time by the diminished glycolytic activity of the PK-deficient cell.

ATP depletion greatly increases the cation permeability of PK-deficient erythrocytes.[275] In part, this is the consequence of failure of the ouabain-inhibitable ATPase cation pump, which transports approximately 1 to 2 mEq of K^+ per hour per liter of erythrocytes.[343] Although adequate membrane ATPase is present,[332, 344] a net loss of from 0.2 to 6.3 mEq of K^+ per hour per liter of cells occurs in freshly obtained PK-deficient blood.[280, 332, 343] After ATP depletion, net K^+ loss may exceed 20 mEq/h/L of cells.[275] Failure of the cation pump cannot explain such large losses of K^+. The effect of ATP depletion on K^+ permeability, first described by Gardos and Straub,[345] is a feature of all metabolically depleted red cells and is not unique to PK deficiency. It is thought to be related to altered binding of membrane-associated Ca^{2+} and can be partially prevented by ethylenediaminetetraacetic acid or quinine, even though these agents have no direct influence on the rate or extent of ATP depletion.[275, 346]

Initially, in the ATP-depleted cell, potassium loss exceeds sodium gain. The resultant net loss of cations is accompanied by an obligate osmotic loss of water and a reduction in cell volume. The shrunken, crenated cells produced by ATP depletion in PK-deficient reticulocytes are shown in Figure 16–8. These spiculated cells pass, with difficulty, through 8-μ Millipore filters, and cell

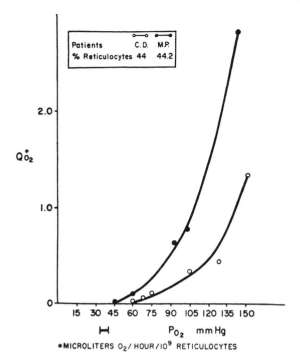

FIGURE 16–7. Influence of PO₂ on oxygen consumption by PK-deficient reticulocytes. The normal range for venous PO₂ is indicated by the *solid bar*. (From Mentzer WC, Baehner RL, et al: Selective reticulocyte destruction in erythrocyte pyruvate kinase deficiency. J Clin Invest 1971; 50:688, by copyright permission of the American Society for Clinical Investigation.)

suspensions demonstrate increased viscosity in the Wells-Brookfield viscometer.[275] The destiny of such ATP-depleted erythrocytes, then, is to become dehydrated, rigid "desicytes" or "xerocytes," whose unfavorable characteristics may well prematurely terminate their existence.[347] Membranes prepared from PK-deficient or normal ATP-depleted red cells are more dense than normal as a result of absorption of cytoplasmic components—in particular, an as yet unidentified 50,000-dalton protein—on the inner membrane surface.[348] Such changes in the cell membrane may contribute to the increased rigidity of these cells. There is evidence that membrane abnormalities not related to ATP depletion may also exist in PK-deficient red cells, but the role, if any, of such abnormalities in the hemolytic process is not established.[349] Not all workers have found abnormalities in the red cell membrane protein profile on sodium dodecyl sodium–polyacrylamine electrophoresis,[350] and results of several other types of membrane analyses (spectrin extractability and membrane fluidity) have been normal.[351]

As enzyme-deficient erythrocytes age, a progressive reduction in glycolysis should accompany the inevitable gradual degradation of enzyme protein. Such deteriorating glycolysis will eventually result in ATP depletion and, subsequently, in hemolysis. However, centrifuge studies have not revealed dramatic differences in the PK activity of enzymopenic young and old cells,[275] with the exception of one unstable PK variant[352] in which accelerated denaturation of enzyme protein was present *in vivo*, as

well as *in vitro*. Deterioration in catalytic efficiency, reported to occur in both normal[303] and variant[353] enzymes on aging *in vivo*, may also hasten the demise of enzymopenic cells.

The normal or near-normal survival of radiolabeled, severely PK-deficient erythrocytes reported by several investigators[275, 299, 333, 334] indicates that diminished PK activity need not significantly curtail the life span of affected erythrocytes. Biphasic erythrocyte survival curves are sometimes obtained[354, 355] and suggest that two populations of cells are present, one destined for almost immediate destruction and the other having a considerably better outlook for survival.

Ferrokinetic studies[275, 355] indicate that destruction of newly made erythrocytes in the bone marrow, spleen, or liver may be the major source of hemolysis in this disorder. Organ monitoring has shown that, as reticulocytes are released from the marrow, some are almost immediately sequestered in the spleen. The paradoxical reticulocytosis that follows splenectomy is probably the consequence of improved survival of this population of reticulocytes.

Spleens removed from anemic patients with PK deficiency contain an unduly large number of reticulocytes.[327, 356] Splenic histologic analysis shows the following results that contrast with those seen in hereditary spherocytosis: (1) the pulp spaces are empty rather than packed with erythrocytes; (2) erythrophagocytosis of reticulocytes and of mature red cells by reticuloendothelial histiocytes is prominent in PK deficiency but rare in spherocytosis; and (3) many more crenated, deformed cells are seen in PK deficiency.[356, 357] Studies of such cells obtained from the peripheral blood have demonstrated them to be poorly deformable.[358] The hypoxic, acidic environment of the spleen would be expected to produce just such crenation in reticulocytes through the sequence of events outlined earlier—inhibition of oxidative phosphorylation, ATP depletion, selective K⁺ leakage, loss of cell water, and resultant loss of cell volume. These rigid desicytes should negotiate only with difficulty the 3-µ fenestrations between the splenic cords and sinuses. Thus, they are doomed to a stay of uncertain duration in the metabolically unfavorable splenic environment, and further deterioration in cell capabilities would seem inevitable. Isotope studies show that the final *coup de grace* often occurs in the liver.[359, 360]

Splenic destruction of reticulocytes is a variable feature of PK deficiency; in some instances, either bone marrow or liver destruction predominates. Why some reticulocytes are destroyed whereas others survive to reach maturity and thereafter have a near-normal existence despite their enzyme defect is unclear. It is possible that chance determines which reticulocytes will be detained in unfavorable metabolic circumstances. On the other hand, there is some evidence for actual variation in PK activity among reticulocytes.[275] Those with the most PK activity would be more likely to survive.

Although cellular dehydration has been given a central mechanistic role in the destruction of PK-deficient human red cells, it appears to be unimportant in the hemolytic process in PK-deficient basenji dogs. When PK-deficient dog red cells with high sodium levels are exposed to cyanide *in vitro*, they rapidly lose ATP. However, the ensu-

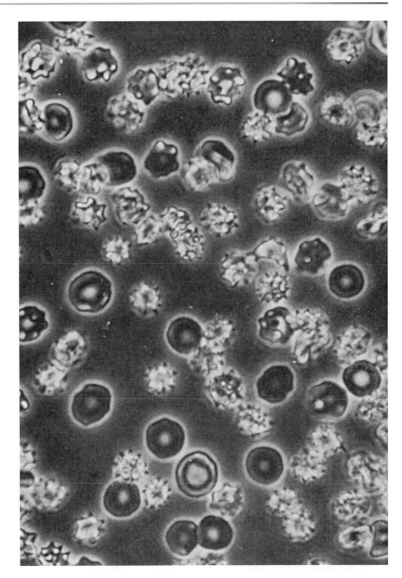

FIGURE 16–8. Phase contrast micrograph of PK-deficient blood (patient C.D., whose anemia was severe after 2-hour exposure to 5 mmol/L of cyanide to deplete ATP. The spiculated cells are, for the most part, reticulocytes. Magnification: ×6600. (From Mentzer WC, Baehner RL, et al: Selective reticulocyte destruction in erythrocyte pyruvate kinase deficiency. J Clin Invest 1971; 50:695, by copyright permission of the American Society for Clinical Investigation.)

ing K⁺ loss is balanced by an equivalent sodium (Na⁺) gain, so there is no cellular dehydration. Other mechanisms must explain hemolysis in this setting.[359]

Genetics and Inheritance

Autosomal recessive transmission of the enzyme defect is usually observed in PK deficiency. Homozygotes and compound heterozygotes exhibit hemolytic anemia. Simple heterozygotes can be distinguished from compound heterozygotes or homozygotes by the degree of reticulocytosis, the extent of accumulation of red cell glucose 6-phosphate and the *in vitro* properties of the mutant PK.[360, 362] Although simple heterozygotes usually remain clinically normal despite an approximately 50 percent reduction in erythrocyte PK activity, some may exhibit evidence of mild hemolysis.[361, 362] Population surveys based on assays of red cell PK activity have estimated the incidence of PK heterozygosity to be 6 percent in Saudi Arabia,[363] 0 to 3.4 percent in Hong Kong,[364] 2.2 percent in Canton, China,[365] 1.4 percent in Germany,[366] and only 0.14 percent in Ann Arbor, Michigan.[367] A survey based on DNA analysis reported the rate of occurrence of het-

erozygosity for the 1456T mutation, the most common PK mutation in Southern Europe, to be 3.5×10^{-3}.[263] Extension of DNA analysis to other population groups and to other common mutations should yield more accurate estimates of the rate of occurrence of PK mutant heterozygosity. There is little correlation between severity of anemia in homozygotes and the level of erythrocyte PK activity as measured by the conventional *in vitro* assay system unless enzyme activity is corrected for the degree of reticulocytosis present.[338] Variable clinical severity is explained, at least in part, by the existence of numerous mutant forms of the enzyme whose differing properties result in variable degrees of hemolysis. Mutants are distinguishable *in vitro* on the basis of maximal activity, electrophoretic mobility, substrate kinetics, stability, immunologic properties, and response to the activator FDP. In general, mutants with unfavorable kinetics are usually associated with more severe hemolysis.[338, 368, 369] Diminished thermal stability of the enzyme *in vitro* also seems important in determining clinical severity.[275]

International standards for the characterization of mutant PK phenotypes have facilitated the comparison of mutants studied in different laboratories.[370] In compound heterozygotes, full characterization is difficult because tetramers formed from varying proportions of the two different mutant subunits are present, each with unique properties.[368] The best-defined phenotypes are those found in true homozygotes, who are usually the offspring of consanguineous matings. The kinetic and electrophoretic abnormalities characteristic of each variant PK reflect underlying structural changes in the enzyme due to point mutations or deletions. At present, a total of 134 mutations in the *PKLR* gene have been defined at the nucleic acid level. Four are promotor mutations, 2 involve insertions, 4 are deletions (one large deletion of exon 11 and 3 small deletions), 12 are frameshift mutations, 13 are splice site mutations, 9 create stop codons, and 92 are single nucleotide missense mutations.[371-373] In the basenji dog, PK deficiency is attributable to a frameshift mutation (deletion of C at nucleotide 433).[374] Most PK mutations are extremely rare and are usually limited to a single family. Exceptions are the 1529G→A substitution, which is common in European patients with PK deficiency[375-377] and the 1151C→T substitution common in Japanese patients.[378] The majority of the mutations are located within exon 8 or 9 (A domain), where components of the active site and the K^+ binding site are located, or in exons 10 or 11 (C domain), a region responsible for the allosteric regulatory properties of the enzyme. Although important information about genotype/phenotype correlations has been developed,[339, 373, 379-381] detailed analysis of the way in which each mutation disturbs the function of PK and produces the clinical phenotype observed has only recently become available following ascertainment of the crystalline structure of R PK.[381a] DNA analysis has indicated that several PK variants thought to be unique because of differing enzyme properties are in fact due to a single shared mutation. For example PK Maebashi, PK Fukushima, and PK Sendai are each the consequence of a substitution of A for C at nucleotide 1261.[371] Further DNA analysis of PK mutations will clarify the true number of variant enzymes and will also make possible prenatal diagnosis of affected fetuses, as already demonstrated by Baronciani and Beutler.[382]

When kinetic abnormalities have been discovered in anemic patients, at least one parent has exhibited similar abnormalities. The other parent may also have kinetically aberrant PK[383] or is found to have a low-activity variant with normal kinetics.[384] Occasionally, it has not been possible to demonstrate an abnormality of erythrocyte PK in one[385] or both[352] parents of patients with PK activity in the homozygous deficient range. Staal and co-workers[352] have speculated that, in some heterozygotes, a compensatory increase in synthesis of enzyme protein by the normal allele may result in enzyme activity indistinguishable from normal. The "classic" form of PK deficiency is associated with severe enzyme deficiency, persistence of the M_2 isoenzyme in mature erythrocytes, and little or no R isozymes. The persistence of M_2 isoenzyme may represent an attempt to compensate for the lack of R subunit–containing forms of PK.[386] An analogy to the persistence of fetal hemoglobin synthesis in β-thalassemia has been made by Miwa.[387] When M_2 compensation is incomplete, PK activity in mature red cells is low, and hemolytic anemia ensues. When M_2 isoenzyme is

synthesized at a higher rate, greater than normal amounts of PK activity can accumulate in mature red cells.[295, 388-391] In such patients there is no hemolytic anemia and, in fact, the increased glycolytic flow through PK at the expense of the 2,3-DPG generating pathway may lower 2,3-DPG levels, increase hemoglobin oxygen affinity, and result in erythrocytosis. Similarly, mice bearing a mutant form of R PK exhibit a delayed onset of hemolytic anemia after birth that coincides with delayed switching from the M_2 isoenzyme to the mutant R isoenzyme.[392]

A kindred in whom hemolytic anemia occurred in heterozygotes for PK mutants was studied by Etiemble et al.[393] PK activity was well below (17 to 45 percent) the 50 percent activity usually encountered in the presence of one normal and one mutant PK allele. It was thought that perhaps the presence of only one mutant subunit in the PK tetramer might be sufficient to reduce its catalytic function, with greater impairment found in the presence of additional mutant subunits. Similar considerations were raised in another kindred (PK Greensboro) in which heterozygotes exhibited less than 50 percent of the normal red cell PK activity but no hemolytic anemia.[394] However, in neither kindred was the presence of multiple combinations of mutant and normal subunits (i.e., M_4, M_3N, M_2N_2, M, N_3, and N_4, where M = the mutant subunit, and N = the normal subunit) actually confirmed.

To date, no evidence suggests interaction between PK deficiency and other disorders of the erythrocyte such as β-thalassemia minor[395] or G6PD deficiency.[278] Reports of spherocytosis or paroxysmal nocturnal hematuria in heterozygotes for PK deficiency have not mentioned unusual features of either disease. Markedly increased involvement of the kidneys was noted at autopsy in a patient with Gaucher disease who also exhibited hemolytic anemia and deficiency of erythrocyte PK. It was suggested that cerebroside production was enhanced as a result of hemolysis.[396]

Therapy

Although a complete cure is not achieved by splenectomy, elimination or amelioration of transfusion requirements, a decrease in bilirubin level, and an increase in hemoglobin concentration are quite often seen. Although splenectomy may be lifesaving in individuals with severe anemia,[327, 334] the procedure may have no effect in individuals with mild anemia. When significant morbidity exists, it would seem reasonable to recommend splenectomy, bearing in mind the fact that the degree of benefit cannot be predicted with certainty.[397] Standard studies of erythrocyte survival and sequestration using ^{51}Cr-labeled cells are often not useful in selecting patients for surgery, particularly when hemolysis of newly made cells predominates. Such cells are unavailable for tagging in the circulating blood, and their presence and fate are not reflected in the results obtained. Ferrokinetic studies, with appropriate organ monitoring, may allow a better assessment of the role of the spleen in such circumstances.

Results of therapeutic intervention with agents that either circumvent the metabolic aberrations induced by the defective enzyme or directly modify enzyme activity have generally been disappointing.[261, 309, 352, 398]

Although hemolytic crises are uncommon in patients with PK deficiency and have not been associated with drug ingestion, Glader[399] demonstrated a potential hazard with the use of large doses of salicylate in patients with severe PK deficiency. Salicylates inhibit oxidative phosphorylation and thus cause ATP depletion and cellular dehydration in severely PK-deficient reticulocytes *in vitro*. The salicylate doses used by Glader were high but were equivalent to serum levels achieved with chronic salicylate therapy for disorders such as rheumatoid arthritis. It is prudent to select alternative therapy for such patients when possible or to monitor them carefully for signs of increased hemolysis.

Bone marrow transplantation has permanently corrected the hemolytic anemia seen in PK-deficient basenji dogs and in PK-deficient mice[261, 399–401] but has not yet been attempted in humans. The potential feasibility of gene therapy has been demonstrated in PK-deficient mice.[402]

LACTATE DEHYDROGENASE DEFICIENCY

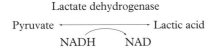

$$\text{Pyruvate} \xrightleftharpoons[\text{NADH} \quad \text{NAD}]{\text{Lactate dehydrogenase}} \text{Lactic acid}$$

Clinical Manifestations, Biochemistry, and Genetics

Partial or complete absence of the H subunit of lactate dehydrogenase (LDH) in erythrocytes, leukocytes, platelets, and serum is not associated with anemia or hemolysis.[403] M-subunit deficiency, although associated with exertional myoglobinuria and a characteristic skin eruption, also does not lead to hemolytic anemia.[404] In contrast to humans, mice homozygous for a low-activity mutation of the skeletal muscle subunit of LDH have less than 10 percent of normal enzyme activity in erythrocytes and exhibit severe lifelong hemolytic anemia.[405]

ABNORMALITIES OF ERYTHROCYTE NUCLEOTIDE METABOLISM

In individuals with congenital nonspherocytic hemolytic anemia, low erythrocyte ATP levels often play a central role in the pathogenesis of hemolysis. Hemolytic anemia associated with an unusually high erythrocyte ATP level has also been described.[406] In the affected pedigree, red cell PK levels were normal, so that the mechanism for ATP elevation would appear to differ from that found in other families with high red cell ATP levels, low 2,3-DPG, erythrocytosis, and twofold or greater elevation in PK activity.[388–390] In yet another family, two infants with hemolytic anemia, high erythrocyte ATP levels, and low 2,3-DPG levels had reduced 2,3-DPG phosphatase activity.[407] The relationship of this enzyme abnormality to the unusual elevation of the erythrocyte ATP level or to

hemolysis is uncertain. In the three disorders of erythrocyte nucleotide metabolism to be described in the text that follows, evidence of a relationship between the abnormal enzyme and hemolytic anemia is more convincing, although, even in these disorders, much remains to be learned about the pathogenesis of hemolysis.

Pyrimidine 5′-Nucleotidase Deficiency

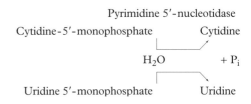

$$\text{Cytidine-5′-monophosphate} \xrightarrow{\text{Pyrimidine 5′-nucleotidase}} \text{Cytidine}$$

CLINICAL MANIFESTATIONS

Deficiency of erythrocyte P-5′-N is associated with lifelong chronic hemolytic anemia of moderate severity.[8, 408–417] The half-life survival time of ^{51}Cr-labeled autologous red cells has ranged from 9 to 23 days. Splenomegaly is usually present. Pronounced basophilic stippling, which may occur in as many as 5 percent of all erythrocytes, is an important and useful finding and is an exception to the usual lack of distinguishing morphologic abnormalities in erythroenzymopathies. Erythrocyte osmotic fragility is normal or slightly increased. Definitive diagnosis requires assay of red cell P-5′-N activity.

BIOCHEMISTRY

Reticulocyte maturation requires disposition of intraerythrocytic ribosomal RNA, which is no longer required for protein synthesis. The hydrolysis of pyrimidine nucleotides (cytidine monophosphate [CMP] and uridine monophosphate [UMP]) formed by the action of ribonucleases on ribosomal RNA, an essential step in RNA degradation, is catalyzed by P-5′-N. The cytidine and uridine formed can diffuse across the cell membrane, whereas the pyrimidine nucleotide substrates of the nucleotidase reaction are incapable of diffusion and accumulate within the cell when activity of the nucleotidase is subnormal.[8]

Hirono and associates[418] found two different isoenzymes of P-5′-N in hemolysates from normal subjects and those with P-5′-N deficiency. Only one isoenzyme, CMP-responsive, was deficient in all five subjects with P-5′-N deficiency evaluated, whereas the other, deoxythymidine monophosphate–responsive, was normal. Kinetic and thermostability abnormalities were seen in the CMP-responsive isoenzyme from subjects with P-5′-N deficiency but not in the dTMP-responsive isoenzyme. Apparently the lack of overlapping substrate sensitivities makes it impossible for the residual normal isoenzyme to substitute for its deficient partner in enzymopenic individuals.

The amount of nucleotides in P-5′-N–deficient red cells is increased by 1.3 to 5.0 times, chiefly due to an increase in pyrimidine derivatives (CMP, cytidine diphosphate [CDP], cytidine triphosphate [CTP], UMP, uridine diphosphate, and uridine triphosphate [UTP]).[8, 410, 411, 419, 420] The most abundant derivatives are the diphosphodiesters, CDP-choline and CDP-ethanolamine.[418] Accumulation of pyrimidine derivatives is undoubtedly due in part to RNA degradation[411] but may also reflect *de novo* synthesis of these compounds from uridine and orotate transported into the red cell.[421] Classification of P-5'-N deficiency as a high-ATP syndrome was based on early observations of unusually high ATP levels in cells, as measured with an enzymatic assay of ATP content that also reflected the presence of other nucleotide triphosphates, notably CTP and UTP. More specific assays have subsequently shown that cell adenine nucleotide levels are normal[8, 412, 420] or even low[412] rather than elevated.[8]

The extraordinary accumulation of pyrimidine nucleotides within P-5'-N–deficient red cells is easily detected by subjecting cellular extracts to MRI[422] or to ultraviolet spectroscopy. Extracts from normal cells exhibit an absorbance peak at 255 to 260 nm (due almost entirely to the presence of adenine nucleotides). In P-5'-N deficiency, a higher absorbance peak slightly shifted in position (266 to 270 nm) is observed, reflecting the presence of large amounts of pyrimidine nucleotides and providing a relatively simple means of screening patients for the disorder.[8, 411] The secondary effects of P-5'-N deficiency are complex. For example, the concentration of reduced glutathione (GSH) is regularly increased by a factor of 1.5 to 2.3,[411] a finding that may help to confirm the diagnosis in patient suspected of having P-5'-N deficiency. Red cell PRPP synthetase activity is markedly low (15 to 35 percent of normal) in P-5'-N–deficient red cells.[423, 424] In fact, PRPP synthetase deficiency was originally thought to be the primary defect responsible for hemolysis. It is now regarded as a secondary phenomenon.[417] Pyrimidine nucleotides have been shown to bind and sequester magnesium, a cofactor required for subunit aggregation and maximal activation of PRPP synthetase.[425] Magnesium depletion (by the addition of pyrimidine nucleotides) also inhibits PK activity and pentose phosphate pathway activity in hemolysates. On the other hand, red cell magnesium levels are normal or even elevated in P-5'-N–deficient red cells, and incubation of these cells with exogenous magnesium does not reduce their susceptibility to autohemolysis or to Heinz body formation.[426] The role of magnesium deficiency (or unavailability) in the central abnormalities that limit the life span of P-5'-N–deficient red cells is not clear.

In fact, it is not known why P-5'-N–deficient red cells are destroyed prematurely. Perhaps the pyrimidine nucleotides that accumulate interfere with the normal function of key glycolytic enzymes by competing for available binding sites with the adenine nucleotides that are the normal enzyme substrate. The possible importance of pyrimidine nucleotides in hemolysis is underscored by the report of an individual with chronic hemolysis, basophilic stippling, and normal P-5'-N activity, in whom the only biochemical abnormality detected was a striking elevation in erythrocyte CDP-choline.[427] Pyrimidine nucleotide accumulation has been shown to lower red cell pH in P-5'-N–deficient red cells as a result of shifts in the Donnan equilibrium caused by the increase in fixed intracellular anion.[415, 419] This drop of 0.1 to 0.2 pH unit is sufficient to increase red cell oxygen affinity above the normal range[419] and may also explain the slightly subnormal glycolytic rate of P-5'-N–deficient red cells.[428] Tomoda and colleagues[415] have demonstrated a moderate impairment of stimulated pentose phosphate pathway activity in P-5'N–deficient erythrocytes, which they attribute to inhibition of G6PD by pyrimidine nucleotides. This impairment in shunt activity is noted in both light and dense red cells separated by centrifugation and is accompanied by a parallel decrease in G6PD activity.[429] It is hard to visualize how pentose phosphate pathway failure could result in the unusually high levels of reduced GSH characteristic of P-5'-N deficiency, because the opposite effect, a deficiency of reduced GSH, would be predicted.[415]

Study of individuals with lead poisoning has confirmed the central role of P-5'-N deficiency in the origin of hemolytic anemia. P-5'-N is markedly inhibited *in vitro* by low concentrations of lead, and the red cells of patients with significant lead poisoning have depressed levels of P-5'-N activity.[430] The basophilic stippling that is present in some patients with lead poisoning has been attributed to nucleotidase deficiency.[431] Although accumulation of pyrimidine nucleotides within erythrocytes is not found in all patients with lead poisoning in which P-5'-N activity is reduced, it is regularly found in patients exhibiting acute lead-induced hemolytic anemia.[429–432] Perhaps because of the shorter duration or less severe character of the enzyme deficiency, the red cells of lead-poisoned individuals do not exhibit R PK deficiency.[431] GSH levels are normal[431] or elevated.[411] Despite the less than perfect homology between congenital and acquired P-5'-N deficiency, study of the latter may be expected to provide important insights into the mechanisms of hemolysis in this disorder.

GENETICS AND INHERITANCE

More than 35 unrelated families with P-5'-N deficiency and hemolytic anemia have been described.[417] The disorder has been found in whites,[8, 424] blacks,[8, 423] Ashkenazi Jews,[408] Arabs,[433] and Asians.[410, 416, 418, 434] Inheritance is autosomal recessive.[411] Heterozygotes have no clinical manifestations but exhibit a reduction of about 50 percent in red cell P-5'-N activity.[8, 411, 417] The wide range of enzyme activity encountered in normal individuals makes detection of heterozygotes difficult in some families.[435] Variation in the severity of disease is, in part, due to heterogeneity in the molecular nature of the defective enzyme. Several instances of hemolytic anemia in which red cell P-5'-N exhibited abnormal physical properties as well as reduced activity have been recognized.[409, 418, 434] P-5'-N has been found in spleen,[434] kidney, and brain.[412, 436] The presence of the enzyme in brain may be relevant to the mental retardation noted in several P-5'-N–deficient individuals with hemolytic anemia.[412] The gene for P-5'-N is located on chromosome 7 and consists of 10 exons. Alternate splicing of exon 2 leads to the production of two proteins: one is 286 amino acids long and the other is 297 amino acids long.[437] One missense, one nonsense, and one splicing mutation have been identified in three families with P-5'-N deficiency and hemolytic anemia.[437]

THERAPY

The congenital form of P-5′-N deficiency must be distinguished from the acquired form associated with lead poisoning, because specific therapy is available for the latter. The benefit of splenectomy in congenital P-5′-N deficiency is limited.[417] Investigational therapeutic use of allopurinol in one affected individual had no effect on hemolysis and actually increased erythrocyte pyrimidine nucleotide levels.[421]

Adenylate Kinase Deficiency

$$2\ \text{ADP} \xrightleftharpoons{\text{Adenylate Kinase}} \text{ATP} + \text{AMP}$$

CLINICAL MANIFESTATIONS, BIOCHEMISTRY, AND GENETICS

Controversy exists regarding the exact role of adenylate kinase (AK) deficiency in hemolytic anemia. Beutler and colleagues[438] studied two black siblings whose red cells lacked measurable AK activity. One had hemolytic anemia, but the other did not. It was suggested that in this family, hemolysis was either unrelated to AK deficiency or that another, coexistent defect was required for hemolysis to occur. The latter seemed to be the case in an Arab family in which two siblings had severe red cell AK deficiency, but only the sibling who had also inherited severe G6PD deficiency had hemolysis.[439] However, further investigation of this large pedigree disclosed six more individuals with severe AK deficiency and mental retardation.[440] All had chronic nonspherocytic hemolytic anemia. Three also had inherited G6PD deficiency and were severely anemic, requiring red cell transfusions 6 to 10 times annually. The other three, who did not have G6PD deficiency, were moderately anemic and only occasionally required transfusions. Family members who had carrier levels of red cell AK activity (50 percent of normal) either with or without G6PD deficiency and individuals with G6PD deficiency alone did not have chronic hemolytic anemia. These results suggest either that AK deficiency has a direct role in hemolysis or that the enzyme defect is a marker for another genetically linked but as yet unidentified defect that is the primary cause of anemia.[441] Lachant and colleagues[441] found no AK activity in the red cells of a Syrian girl who had chronic hemolytic anemia. Only modest impairment in the formation of ADP from adenosine monophosphate was observed in intact cells, suggesting that alternative pathways might be available to substitute for the missing AK. Alternatively, it was proposed that AK itself might be present in intact cells but somehow inactivated during the preparation of a hemolysate for assay of enzyme activity. Five additional patients with AK deficiency associated with hemolytic anemia have been reported in France,[442] Japan,[443, 444] and Italy.[445, 446] The Japanese subject inherited a point mutation (Arg[128]→Trp) in the coding region of the AK 1 gene from her mother and a normal AK 1 allele from her father. Although both mother and child were heterozygous for AK deficiency, only the child exhibited hemolytic anemia, whereas the mother was hematologically normal.[444] An Italian girl homozygous for a missense mutation at codon 164 had virtually undetectable erythrocyte AK activity and moderate hemolytic anemia.[445] Two siblings in another Italian family who were homozygous for a nonsense mutation at codon 107 (CGA→TGA) also had no detectable erythrocyte AK activity and mild to moderate chronic hemolytic anemia.[446] Both siblings also exhibited psychomotor retardation. Similar findings in other families[440, 442] suggest that AK deficiency may be shared by the red cell and the brain.

THERAPY

Splenectomy was performed in five of six Arab patients, and prompt disappearance of anemia and hemolysis was seen.[438]

Adenosine Deaminase Overproduction

$$\text{Adenosine} + \text{H}_2\text{O} \xrightleftharpoons[+\ \text{H}_2\text{O}]{\text{Adenosine deaminase}} \text{Inosine}$$

CLINICAL MANIFESTATIONS, BIOCHEMISTRY, AND GENETICS

Fourteen individuals in three families have been found to have hereditary hemolytic anemia, sharply diminished amounts of intraerythrocytic adenosine nucleotides (to less than 50 percent of normal), and a remarkable 45- to 110-fold increase in red cell ADA activity.[447–450] In contrast to virtually all other erythroenzymopathies, ADA excess is transmitted as an autosomal dominant trait. Hemolysis is apparently the consequence of diminished red cell ATP content, which is caused by the diversion of nearly all adenosine metabolism through the unusually active ADA reaction at the expense of the competing adenosine kinase reaction. The former results in irreversible loss of adenosine nucleotides, whereas the latter conserves such nucleotides and preserves cell ATP stores. Abnormalities of lesser magnitude have been found in other enzymes of nucleotide metabolism in affected individuals, suggesting that excess ADA activity may be caused by an as yet undefined primary defect. The physical properties of the mutant ADA are normal,[449, 451] indicating that the great excess of ADA activity is due to overproduction rather than to an increase in catalytic efficiency. In one subject, an increase in red cell ADA protein equivalent to the striking increase in ADA activity was demonstrated by immunoblotting.[452] Synthesis of ADA by erythroid progenitors grown from bone marrow cells was 11-fold greater in an affected individual.[453] RNase mapping techniques and Northern blotting have revealed at least a 100-fold increase over normal in the ADA mRNA content of affected reticulocytes. Sequencing of ADA cDNA showed no abnormalities in the coding region and 5′- and 3′-untranslated regions of the parent mRNA. Examination of genomic DNA by Southern blotting did not disclose evidence of gene amplification, deletion, or gross rearrangements. Thus, although the basis for ADA excess appears to be an overabundance of apparently normal mRNA, the mechanism underlying this abnormality remains obscure.[454]

Linkage analysis with a polymorphic TAAA repeat located 1.1 kb upstream from the *ADA* gene indicated strongly that the mutation was located in *cis* rather than in *trans*.[455] DNA constructs containing 10.6 kb of 5′-flanking sequences and 12.3 kb of the first intron of the normal or mutant *ADA* gene were linked to a reporter gene (chloramphenicol acyl transferase) and used to study expression in transient transfection assays and in transgenic mice. No difference in expression between wild-type and mutant alleles was found. Therefore, the mutation is thought to reside at a more distant 5′ site, within a different intron, or 3′ to the coding region.[456]

Much lesser increases in ADA activity (approximately fourfold) are seen in congenital hypoplastic anemia,[457, 458] arthrogryposis multiplex congenita,[459] acquired immunodeficiency syndrome,[460] and cartilage-hair hypoplasia.[461] The origin and implications of these increases are obscure, but they are not associated with hemolysis.

ACQUIRED DISORDERS OF ERYTHROCYTE GLYCOLYSIS

Alterations in the external chemical milieu may profoundly influence erythrocyte metabolism. The rate of glycolysis, for example, is governed by the availability of P_i. High concentrations of P_i augment and low concentrations impede the glycolytic synthesis of ATP and 2,3-DPG. Erythrocytes from uremic patients with hyperphosphatemia contain an average of 70 percent more ATP than do normal erythrocytes, and a lesser, but significant, increase in 2,3-DPG concentration is also found in the hyperphosphatemic cell.[462] Equivalent changes in organic phosphates can be induced in normal erythrocytes by incubation either in hyperphosphatemic uremic plasma or in autologous normal plasma supplemented with P_i.[462] Conversely, hypophosphatemia induced by hyperalimentation with low-phosphate nutrients[463] or by anion resin therapy for hyperphosphatemia[464] is associated with a reduction in erythrocyte organic phosphates. Organic phosphate depletion resulting from hypophosphatemia may be sufficient to displace the oxyhemoglobin dissociation curve to the left, unfavorably influencing tissue oxygenation. Profound hypophosphatemia may produce a spherocytic hemolytic anemia due to erythrocyte ATP deficiency.[465–467] Less is known about the influence of other components of the chemical environment upon erythrocyte glycolysis. Some investigators have found that experimental magnesium deficiency in the rat resembles hypophosphatemia, in that erythrocyte glycolysis is inhibited, ATP and 2,3-DPG levels are subnormal, and red cell rigidity is increased. Spherocytes are evident on the blood smear, and red cell survival is reduced.[467] Magnesium is essential for the normal function of a variety of glycolytic and nonglycolytic enzymes. However, using a different diet to induce magnesium deficiency, Piomelli and co-workers[468] showed that although a hemolytic anemia

accompanies magnesium depletion in rats, erythrocyte glycolysis and the activity of red blood cell glycolytic enzymes remain normal. Magnesium deficiency also influences other red cell components, notably the membrane,[469] and the relative contribution of such abnormalities to shortened red cell life span remains undefined. It is not known whether hematologic changes similar to those seen in the rat occur in human magnesium deficiency.

Iron deficiency not only decreases the production of red cells but also accelerates their destruction.[470] Studies of the metabolic properties of iron-deficient red cells have revealed several abnormalities that might reduce cell viability. Although erythrocyte glycolysis *in vitro* is normal for cell age,[471] cell ATP is unstable on incubation. The ATP concentration in freshly obtained red cells may either be normal[472] or low.[473] The spontaneous autohemolysis of iron-deficient red cells incubated at 37°C is increased.[474] The increased rigidity characteristic of the ATP-depleted cell is present in iron-deficient cells as well.[474] These findings suggest that a defect in energy metabolism may contribute to the shortened survival of iron-deficient red cells.

Little is known about the possible influence of hormones upon erythrocyte glycolytic enzymes. The activity of HK, phosphofructokinase, PK, G6PD is often reduced in the erythrocytes of diabetic patients.[475] The activities of the same enzymes were remarkably increased in one patient with an insulinoma before removal of the tumor. The activity of several erythrocyte enzymes is reduced in patients with hypothyroidism and becomes normal after therapy,[476] probably reflecting changes in the mean erythrocyte cell age rather than a direct influence of the hormone on the enzymes. However, Snyder and Reddy[477] have shown that 2,3-DPG synthesis *in vitro* by hemoglobin and membrane-free extracts of erythrocytes is enhanced by thyroid hormone.

Alterations in erythrocyte enzyme activity are often found during the course of either acute or chronic leukemia,[478] nonmalignant pancytopenias,[478] congenital dyserythropoietic anemia,[479] acquired dyserythropoietic anemia,[478, 480] myeloid metaplasia,[478] and polycythemia vera.[478] One, several, or many enzymes may be involved, and activity may be either increased or decreased. The unusual pattern of enzyme activities may, on occasion, be useful in diagnosis, for example, to distinguish congenital hypoplastic anemia from transient erythroblastopenia of childhood.[481]

Several quite different processes appear to be responsible for the development of acquired enzymopathies.[482] Reversion to fetal hematopoiesis may alter enzyme function.[483] Post-translational changes in normal enzyme protein have been demonstrated.[484] In such instances, incubation of affected cells in normal plasma, modification of affected hemolysate by dialysis or treatment with sulfhydryl reagents, or partial purification of the enzyme restores normal enzyme activity and functional properties. In other instances, enzyme-specific activity is normal (measured immunologically), but total activity is low and not enhanced by the measures just described.[484] In these cases, synthesis of enzyme protein by developing erythroid cells is apparently impaired, perhaps as a result of alterations in chromosome number or disorderly and dyssynchronous nuclear maturation. Although some components of the abnormal pattern of enzymes (such as low PFK or high enolase activity) may suggest a reversion to fetal erythropoiesis, others do not. The possibility that these enzyme abnormalities may be familial and antedate the onset of an acquired blood disorder has not been fully explored.

REFERENCES

1. Dacie LV, Mollison PL, et al: Atypical congenital hemolytic anemia. Q J Med 1953; 22:79.
2. Valentine WN, Paglia DE: Erythrocyte enzymopathies, hemolytic anemia, and multisystem disease. An annotated review. Blood 1984; 64:583.
3. Selwyn JG, Dacie JV: Autohemolysis and other changes resulting from the incubation in vitro of red cells from patients with congenital hemolytic anemia. Blood 1954; 9:414.
4. Robinson MA, Loder PB, et al: Red cell metabolism in nonspherocytic congenital haemolytic anaemia. Br J Haematol 1961; 7:327.
5. Valentine WN, Tanaka KR, et al: A specific erythrocyte enzyme defect (pyruvate kinase) in three subjects with congenital non-spherocytic hemolytic anemia. Trans Assoc Am Physicians 1961; 74:100.
6. Jacobasch G.: Biochemical and genetic basis of red cell enzyme deficiencies. Bailliere's Clin Haematol 2000; 13:1.
7. Miwa S, Fujii H.: Molecular basis of erythroenzymopathies associated with hereditary hemolytic anemia: Tabulation of mutant enzymes. Am J Hematol 1996; 51:122.
8. Valentine WN, Fink K, et al: Hereditary hemolytic anemia with human erythrocyte pyrimidine-5′-nucleotidase deficiency. J Clin Invest 1974; 54:866.
9. Beutler E: Why has the autohemolysis test not gone the way of the cephalin flocculation test? Blood 1978; 51:109.
10. Keitt AS: Diagnostic strategy in a suspected red cell enzymopathy. Clin Haematol 1981; 10:3.
11. Beutler E: Red Cell Metabolism: A Manual of Biochemical Methods, 3rd ed. Orlando, FL, Grune & Stratton, 1984.
12. Jansen G, Koenderman L, et al: Characteristics of hexokinase, pyruvate kinase, and glucose-6-phosphate dehydrogenase during adult and neonatal reticulocyte maturation. Am J Hematol 1985; 20:203.
13. Beutler E: Biphasic loss of red cell enzyme activity during in vivo aging. In Eaton JW, Konzen DK, White JG (eds.): Cellular and Molecular Aspects of Aging: The Red Cell as a Model. New York, Alan R Liss, 1985, p 317.
14. Lakomek M, Schroter W, et al: On the diagnosis of erythrocyte defects in the presence of high reticulocyte counts. Br J Haematol 1989; 72:445.
15. Low PS, Rathinavelu P, Harrison M L: Regulation of glycolysis via reversible enzyme binding to the membrane protein, band 3. J Biol Chem 1993; 268:14627.
16. Gilsanz F, Meyer E, et al: Congenital hemolytic anemia due to hexokinase deficiency. Am J Dis Child 1978; 132:636.
17. Rijksen G, Staal GE J.: Human erythrocyte hexokinase deficiency: Characterization of a mutant enzyme with abnormal regulatory properties. J Clin Invest 1978; 62:294.
18. Valentine WN, Oski FA, et al: Hereditary hemolytic anemia with hexokinase deficiency. N Engl J Med 1967; 276:1.
19. Kanno H: Hexokinase: Gene structure and mutations. Bailliere's Clin Haematol 2000; 13:83.
20. Paglia DE, Shende A, et al: Hexokinase "New Hyde Park": A low activity erythrocyte isozyme in a Chinese kindred. Am J Hematol 1981; 10:107.
21. Magnani M, Stocchi V, et al: Hereditary nonspherocytic hemolytic anemia due to a new hexokinase variant with reduced stability. Blood 1985; 66:690.
22. Magnani M, Chiarantini L, et al: Glucose metabolism in fibroblasts from patients with erythrocyte hexokinase deficiency. J Inherit Metab Dis 1986; 9:129.
23. Rijksen G, Akkerman JW N, et al: Generalized hexokinase deficiency in the blood cells of a patient with nonspherocytic hemolytic anemia. Blood 1986; 61:12.
24. Board PG, Trueworthy R, et al: Congenital nonspherocytic hemolytic anemia with an unstable hexokinase variant. Blood 1978; 51:111.
25. Newman P, Muir A, et al: Non-spherocytic haemolytic anaemia in mother and son associated with hexokinase deficiency. Br J Haematol 1980; 46:537.
26. Magnani M, Stocchi V, et al: Human erythrocyte hexokinase deficiency: A new variant with abnormal kinetic properties. Br J Haematol 1985; 61:41.
27. Beutler E, Dyment PG, et al: Hereditary nonspherocytic hemolytic anemia and hexokinase deficiency. Blood 1978; 51:935.
28. Goebel KM, Gassel WD, et al: Hemolytic anemia and hexokinase deficiency associated with malformations. Klin Wochenschr 1972; 50:349.
29. Keitt AS: Hemolytic anemia with impaired hexokinase activity. J Clin Invest 1969; 48:1997.
30. Moser K, Ciresa M, et al: Hexokinasemangel bei hämolytischer Anämie. Med Welt 1970; 21:1977.
31. Semenuk M, Wicks T, Toews C J, et al: Hexokinase Hamilton: An enzyme variant with abnormal K_m for adenosine triphosphate (ATP) in non-spherocytic hemolytic anemia. Clin Res 1975; 23:628a.
32. Siimes MA, Rahiala EL, et al: Hexokinase deficiency in erythrocytes: A new variant in 5 members of a Finnish family. Scand J Haematol 1979; 22:214.
33. Necheles TF, Rai US, et al: Congenital nonspherocytic hemolytic anemia associated with an unusual erythrocyte hexokinase abnormality. J Lab Clin Med 1970; 76:593.
34. Lohr GW, Waller HD, et al: Hexokinasemangel in Blutzellen bei einer Sippe mit familiärer panmyelopathie (Typ Fanconi). Klin Wochenschr 1965; 43:870.
35. Magnani M, Serafini G, et al: Hexokinase type I multiplicity in human erythrocytes. Biochem J 1988; 254:617.
36. Murakami K, Blei F, et al: An isozyme of hexokinase specific for the human red blood cell (HKg). Blood 1990; 75:770.
37. Murakami K, Kanno H, Miwa S, et al: Human HK_R isozyme: Organization of the hexokinase I gene, the erythroid-specific promoter, and transcription initiation site. Mol Genet Metab 1999; 67:118.
38. Magnani M, Stocchi V, et al: Rabbit red blood cell hexokinase. Decay mechanism during reticulocyte maturation. J Biol Chem 1986; 261:8327.
39. Murakami K, Piomelli S: The isoenzymes of mammalian hexokinase: Tissue specificity and in vivo decline. In Magnani M, De Flora A (eds.): Red Blood Cell Aging. New York, Plenum Press, 1991, p 277.
40. Thorburn DR, Beutler E: Decay of hexokinase during reticulocyte maturation: Is oxidative damage a signal for destruction? Biochem Biophys Res Commun 1989; 162:612.
41. Fornaini G, Dacha M, et al: Role of hexokinase in the regulation of glucose metabolism in human erythrocytes. Ital J Biochem 1986; 35:316.
42. Magnani M, Rossi L, et al: Role of hexokinase in the regulation of erythrocyte hexose monophosphate pathway under oxidative stress. Biochem Biophys Res Commun 1988; 155:423.
43. Magnani M, Rossi L, et al: Improved metabolic properties of hexokinase-overloaded human erythrocytes. Biochim Biophys Acta 1988; 972:1.
44. Magnani M, Rossi L, et al: Human red blood cell loading with hexokinase-inactivating antibodies. An in vitro model for enzyme deficiencies. Acta Haematol 1989; 82:27.
45. Valentine WN, Oski FA, et al: Erythrocyte hexokinase and hereditary hemolytic anemia. In Beutler E (ed.): Hereditary Disorders of Erythrocyte Metabolism. New York, Grune & Stratton, 1968, p 288.
46. Gerber GK, Schultz M, et al: Occurrence and function of a high K_m hexokinase in immature red blood cells. Eur J Biochem 1970; 17:445.
47. Jandl JH, Aster RH: Increased splenic pooling and the pathogenesis of hypersplenism. Am J Med Sci 1967; 253:282.
48. Rakitzis ET, Mills GC: Relation of red-cell hexokinase activity to extracellular pH. Biochim Biophys Acta 1967; 141:439.
49. Brewer GJ: Erythrocyte metabolism and function: Hexokinase inhibition by 2,3-diphosphoglycerate and interaction with ATP and Mg^{2+}. Biochim Biophys Acta 1969; 192:157.

50. Delivoria-Papadopoulos M, Oski FA, et al: Oxygen hemoglobin dissociation curves: Effect of inherited enzyme defects of the red cell. Science 1969; 165:601.

51. Oski FA, Marshall BE, et al: Exercise with anemia: The role of the left-shifted or right-shifted oxygen-hemoglobin equilibrium curve. Ann Intern Med 1971; 74:44.

52. Kosower NS, Vanderhoff GA, et al: Hexokinase activity in normal and glucose-6-phosphate dehydrogenase deficient erythrocytes. Nature 1964; 201:684.

53. Bethenod M, Kissin C, et al: Déficit en hexokinase intraérythrocytaire. Ann Pediatr 1967; 50:825.

54. Bianchi M, Magnani M: Hexokinase mutations that produce nonspherocytic hemolytic anemia. Blood Cells Mol Dis 1995; 21:2.

55. Bianchi M, Crinelli R, Serafini G, et al: Molecular bases of hexokinase deficiency. Biochim Biophys Acta 1997; 1360:211.

56. Rogers PA, Fisher RA, et al: An electrophoretic study of the distribution and properties of human hexokinases. Biochem Genet 1975; 13:857.

57. Povey S, Corney G, et al: Genetically determined polymorphism of a form of hexokinase, HK III, found in human leukocytes. Ann Hum Genet 1975; 38:407.

58. Akkerman JW N, Rijksen G, et al: Platelet function and energy metabolism in a patient with hexokinase deficiency. Blood 1984; 63:147.

59. Kugler W, Lakomek M: Glucose-6-phosphate isomerase deficiency. Bailliere's Clin Haematol 2000:13:89.

60. Matthay KK, Mentzer WC: Erythrocyte enzymopathies in the newborn. Clin Haematol 1981; 10:31.

61. Whitelaw AG L, Rogers PA, et al: Congenital haemolytic anaemia resulting from glucose phosphate isomerase deficiency: Genetics, clinical picture, and prenatal diagnosis. J Med Genet 1979; 16:189.

62. Ravindranath Y, Paglia DE, et al: Glucose phosphate isomerase deficiency as a cause of hydrops fetalis. N Engl J Med 1987; 316:258.

63. Hutton JJ, Chilcote RR: Glucose phosphate isomerase deficiency with hereditary nonspherocytic hemolytic anemia. J Pediatr 1974; 85:494.

64. Arnold H, Lohr GW, et al: Combined erythrocyte glucosephosphate isomerase (GPI) and glucose-6-phosphate dehydrogenase (G6PD) deficiency in an Italian family. Hum Genet 1981; 57:226.

65. Schroter W, Brittinger G, et al: Combined glucosephosphate isomerase and glucose-6-phosphate dehydrogenase deficiency of the erythrocytes: A new hemolytic syndrome. Br J Haematol 1971; 20:249.

66. Kahn A, Bue HA, et al: Molecular and functional anomalies in two new mutant glucose-phosphateisomerase variants with enzyme deficiency and chronic hemolysis. Hum Genet 1978; 40:293.

67. Van Biervliet JPGM: Glucosephosphate isomerase deficiency in a Dutch family. Acta Paediatr Scand 1975; 64:868.

68. Zanella A, Izzo C, et al: The first stable variant of erythrocyte glucose-phosphate isomerase associated with severe hemolytic anemia. Am J Hematol 1980; 9:1.

69. Schroter W, Eber SW, et al: Generalised glucosephosphate isomerase (GPI) deficiency causing haemolytic anaemia, neuromuscular symptoms and impairment of granulocytic function: A new syndrome due to a new stable GPI variant with diminished specific activity (GPI Homburg). Eur J Paediatr 1985; 144:301.

70. Beutler E, West C, Britton HA, et al: Glucosephosphate isomerase (GPI) deficiency mutations associated with hereditary nonspherocytic hemolytic anemia (HNSHA). Blood Cells Mol Dis 1997; 23:402.

71. Kugler W, Breme K, Laspe P, et al: Molecular basis of neurological dysfunction coupled with haemolytic anaemia in human glucose-6-phosphate isomerase (GPI) deficiency. Hum Genet 1998; 103:450.

72. Matsumoto N, Ishihara T, et al: Fine structure of the spleen and liver in glucosephosphate isomerase (GPI) deficiency hereditary nonspherocytic hemolytic anemia: Selective reticulocyte destruction as a mechanism of hemolysis. Acta Haematol Jpn 1973; 36:46.

73. Van Biervliet JPGM, Staal EJ: Excessive hepatic glycogen storage in glucosephosphate isomerase deficiency. Acta Paediatr Scand 1977; 66:311.

74. Merkle S, Pretsch W: Glucose-6-phosphate isomerase associated with nonspherocytic hemolytic anemia in the mouse: An animal model for the human disease. Blood. 1993; 81:206.

75. Oski FA, Fuller E: Glucose-phosphate isomerase (GPI) deficiency associated with abnormal osmotic fragility and spherocytes. Clin Res 1971; 19:427.

76. Vives-Corrons LL, Carrera A, et al: Anemia hemolitica por deficit congenito en fosfohexosaisomerasa. Sangre 1975; 20:197.

77. Blume KG, Hryniuk W, et al: Characterization of two new variants of glucose-phosphate-isomerase deficiency with hereditary nonspherocytic hemolytic anemia. J Lab Clin Med 1972; 79:942.

78. Cayanis E, Penfold GK, et al: Haemolytic anaemia associated with glucosephosphate isomerase (GPI) deficiency in a black South African child. Br J Haematol 1977; 37:363.

79. Van Biervliet JP, Vlug A, et al: A new variant of glucosephosphate isomerase deficiency. Humangenetik 1975; 30:35.

80. Schroter W, Koch HH, et al: Glucose phosphate isomerase deficiency with congenital nonspherocytic hemolytic anemia; a new variant (type Nordhorn). I. Clinical and genetic studies. Pediatr Res 1974; 8:18.

81. Tilley BE, Gracy RW: A point mutation increasing the stability of human phosphoglucose isomerase. J Biol Chem 1974; 249:4571.

82. McMorris FA, Chen TR, et al: Chromosome assignments in man of the genes from two hexosephosphate isomerases. Science 1973; 17:1129

83. Chaput M, Claes V, Portetelle D, et al: The neurotrophic factor neuroleukin is 90% homologous with phospho-hexose isomerase. Nature 1988; 332:454.

84. Faik P, Walker JIH, Redmill AAM, et al: Mouse glucose-6-phosphate isomerase and neuroleukin have identical 3′ sequences. Nature 1988; 332:455.

85. Watanabe H, Takehana K, Date M, et al: Tumor cell autocrine motility factor is the neuroleukin phosphohexose isomerase polypeptide. Cancer Res 1996; 56:2960.

86. Xu W, Seiter K, Feldman E, et al: The differentiation and maturation mediator for human myeloid leukemia cells shares homology with neuroleukin or phosphoglucose isomerase. Blood 1996; 87:4502.

87. Helleman PW, Van Biervliet JPGM: Haematological studies in a new variant of glucosephosphate isomerase deficiency (GPI Utrecht). Helv Paediatr Acta 1975; 30:525

88. Beutler E, Sigalove WH, et al: Glucosephosphateisomerase (GPI) deficiency: GPI Elyria. Ann Intern Med 1974; 80:730.

89. Miwa S, Nakashima K, et al: Three cases in two families with congenital nonspherocytic hemolytic anemia due to defective glucosephosphate isomerase: GPI Matsumoto. Acta Haematol Jpn 1975; 38:238.

90. Staal GE J, Akkerman JW N, et al: A new variant of glucosephosphate isomerase deficiency: GPI-Kortrijk. Clin Chim Acta 1977; 78:121.

91. Zanella A, Rebulla P, et al: A new mutant erythrocyte glucosephosphate isomerase associated with GSH abnormality. Am J Hematol 1978; 5:11.

92. Arnold H, Hasslinger K, et al: Glucosephosphateisomerase type Kaiserslautern: A new variant causing congenital nonspherocytic hemolytic anemia. Blut 1983; 46:271.

93. Paglia DE, Paredes R, et al: Unique phenotypic expression of glucosephosphate isomerase deficiency. Am J Hum Genet 1975; 27:62.

94. Arnold H, Engelhardt R, et al: Glucosephosphatisomerase typ Recklinghausen: Eine neue defektvariante mit hämolytischer anamie. Klin Wochenschr 1973; 51:1198.

95. Arnold H, Blume KG, et al: Klinische und biochemische Untersuchungen zur Glucosephosphatisomerase normaler menschlicher Erythrocyten und bei Glucosephosphatisosmerase Mangel. Klin Wochenschr 1970; 21:1299.

96. Cartier P, Temkine H, et al: Étude biochemique d'une anémie hémolytique avec déficit familial en phosphohexoisomerase. In Proceedings of the 7th International Congress of Clinical Chemistry, Geneva/Evian, 1969. Vol. 2: Clinical Enzymology. Basel, Karger, 1970, p 139.

97. Baughan M, Valentine WN, et al: Hereditary hemolytic anemia associated with glucosephosphate isomerase (GPI) deficiency—A new enzyme defect of human erythrocytes. Blood 1968; 32:236.

98. Paglia DE, Holland P, et al: Occurrence of defective hexosephosphate isomerization in human erythrocytes and leukocytes. N Engl J Med 1969; 280:66.

99. Arnold H, Blume KG, et al: Glucosephosphate isomerase deficiency: Evidence for in vivo instability of an enzyme variant with hemolysis. Blood 1973; 41:691.

100. Schroter W, Tillmann W: Decreased deformability of erythrocytes in haemolytic anaemia associated with glucosephosphate isomerase deficiency. Br J Haematol 1977; 36:475.

101. Chilcote RR, Baehner RL: Red cell (RBC) glucose phosphate isomerase deficiency (GPI): Clinical and laboratory evidence of increased blood viscosity. Pediatr Res 1974; 8:398.

102. Lakomek M, Winkler H: Erythrocyte pyruvate kinase-and glucose phosphate isomerase deficiency: Perturbation of glycolysis by structural defects and functional alterations of defective enzymes and its relation to the clinical severity of chronic hemolytic anemia. Biophys Chem 1997; 66:269.

103. Goulding FJ: Priapism caused by glucose phosphate isomerase deficiency. J Urol 1976; 116:819.

104. Coetzer T, Zail SS: Erythrocyte membrane proteins in hereditary glucose phosphate isomerase deficiency. J Clin Invest 1979; 63:552.

105. Hopkinson DA: The investigation of reactive sulphydryls in enzymes and their variations by starch-gel electrophoresis: Studies on the human phosphohexose isomerase variant PH15–1. Ann Hum Genet 1970; 34:79.

106. Detter JC, Ways PO, et al: Inherited variations in human phosphohexose isomerase. Ann Hum Genet 1968; 31:329.

107. Arnold H, Seiberling M, et al: Immunological studies on glucosephosphate isomerase deficiency: Instability and impaired synthesis of the defective enzyme. Klin Wochenschr 1975; 53:1135.

108. Kahn A, Vives-Corrons JL, et al: Glucosephosphate isomerase deficiency due to a new variant (GPI Barcelona) and to a silent gene: Biochemical, immunological and genetic studies. Clin Chim Acta 1976; 66:145.

109. Kahn A, Van Biervliet JPGM, et al: Genetic and molecular mechanisms of the congenital defects in glucose phosphate isomerase activity: Studies of four families. Pediatr Res 1977; 11:1123.

110. Neubauer BA, Eber SW, et al: Combination of congenital nonspherocytic haemolytic anaemia and impairment of granulocyte function in severe glucose phosphate isomerase deficiency. Acta Haematol 1990; 83:206.

111. Dallapiccola BH, Novelli G, et al: First trimester monitoring of a pregnancy at risk for glucose phosphate isomerase deficiency. Prenat Diagn 1986; 6:101.

112. Tani K, Fujii H, et al: Phosphofructokinase deficiency associated with congenital nonspherocytic hemolytic anemia and mild myopathy: Biochemical and morphological studies on muscle. Tohoku J Exp Med 1983; 141:287.

113. Tani K, Fujii H, et al: Two cases of phosphofructokinase deficiency associated with congenital hemolytic anemia found in Japan. Am J Hematol 1983; 14:165.

114. Vora S, Davidson M, et al: Heterogeneity of the molecular lesions in inherited phosphofructokinase deficiency. J Clin Invest 1983; 72:1995.

115. Vora S: Isozymes of phosphofructokinase. Isozymes. Curr Top Biol Med Res 1982; 6:119.

116. Tarui S, Okuno G, et al: Phosphofructokinase deficiency in skeletal muscle: A new type of glycogenolysis. Biochem Biophys Res Commun 1965; 19:517.

117. Layzer RB, Rowland LP, et al: Muscle phosphofructokinase deficiency. Arch Neurol 1967; 17:512.

118. Servidei S, Bonilla E, et al: Fatal infantile form of phosphofructokinase deficiency. Neurology 1986; 36:1465.

119. Danon MJ, Serenella S, et al: Late-onset muscle phosphofructokinase deficiency. Neurology 1988; 38:956.

120. Duboc D, Jehenson P, et al: Phosphorus NMR spectroscopy study of muscular enzyme deficiencies involving glycogenolysis and glycolysis. Neurology 1987; 37:663.

121. Miwa S, Sato T, et al: A new type of phosphofructokinase deficiency: Hereditary nonspherocytic hemolytic anemia. Acta Haematol Jpn 1972; 35:113.

122. Waterbury L, Frankel EP: Hereditary nonspherocytic hemolysis with erythrocyte phosphofructokinase deficiency. Blood 1972; 39:415.

123. Etiemble J, Kahn A, et al: Hereditary hemolytic anemia with erythrocyte phosphofructokinase deficiency. Hum Genet 1975; 31:83.

124. Boulard MR, Meienhofer MC, et al: Red cell phosphofructokinase deficiency. N Engl J Med 1974; 291:978.

125. Etiemble J, Picat C, et al: Inherited erythrocyte phosphofructokinase deficiency: Molecular mechanism. Hum Genet 1980; 55:383.

126. Jenkins JD, Kezdy F, et al: Mode of interaction of phosphofructokinase with the erythrocyte membrane. J Biol Chem 1985; 260:10426.

127. Karadsheh NS, Uyeda K, et al: Studies on structure of human erythrocyte phosphofructokinase. J Biol Chem 1977; 252:3515.

128. Vora S, Piomelli S: A fetal isozyme of phosphofructokinase in newborn erythrocytes. Pediatr Res 1977; 11:483.

129. Layzer RB, Rasmussen J: The molecular basis of muscle phosphofructokinase deficiency. Arch Neurol 1984; 31:411.

130. Shimizu T, Kono N, et al: Erythrocyte glycolysis and its marked alteration by muscular exercise in type VII glycogenosis. Blood 1988; 71:1130.

131. Giger U, Harvey JW: Hemolysis caused by phosphofructokinase deficiency in English springer spaniels: Seven cases (1983–1986). J Am Vet Med Assoc 1987; 191:453.

132. Giger U, Reilly MP, et al: Autosomal recessive inherited phosphofructokinase deficiency in English springer spaniel dogs. Anim Genet 1986; 17:15.

133. Giger U, Harvey JW, et al: Inherited phosphofructokinase deficiency in dogs with hyperventilation-induced hemolysis: Increased in vitro and in vivo alkaline fragility of erythrocytes. Blood 1985; 65:345.

134. Vora S, Giger U, et al: Characterization of the enzymatic lesion in inherited phosphofructokinase deficiency in the dog: An animal analogue of human glycogen storage disease type VII. Proc Natl Acad Sci USA 1985; 82:8109.

135. Harvey JW, Reddy GR: Postnatal hematologic development in phosphofructokinase-deficient dogs. Blood 1989; 74:2556.

136. Harvey JW, Sussman WA, et al: Effect of 2,3-diphosphoglycerate concentration on the alkaline fragility of phosphofructokinase-deficient canine erythrocytes. Comp Biochem Physiol 1988; 89B:105.

137. Giger U, Kelly AM, et al: Biochemical studies of canine muscle phosphofructokinase deficiency. Enzyme 1988; 40:24.

138. Giger U, Argov Z, et al: Metabolic myopathy in canine muscle-type phosphofructokinase deficiency. Muscle Nerve 1988; 11:1260.

139. McCully K, Chance B, Giger U: In vivo determination of altered hemoglobin saturation in dogs with M-type phosphofructokinase deficiency. Muscle Nerve 1999; 22:621.

140. Komazawa M, Oski FA: Biochemical characteristics of "young" and "old" erythrocytes of the newborn infant. J Pediatr 1975; 87:102.

141. Travis SF, Garvin JH: In vivo lability of red cell phosphofructokinase in term infants: The possible molecular basis of the relative phosphofructokinase deficiency in neonatal red cells. Pediatr Res 1977; 11:1159.

142. Vora S, Piomelli S: Multiple isozymes of human erythrocyte phosphofructokinase and their subunit structural characterization. Blood 1977; 50 (Suppl 1):87.

143. Layzer RB, Epstein CJ: Phosphofructokinase and chromosome I. Am J Hum Genet 1972; 24:533.

144. Sherman JB, Raben N, et al: Common mutations in the phosphofructokinase-M gene in Ashkenazi Jewish patients with glycogenesis VII and their population frequency. Am J Hum Genet 1994; 55:305.

145. Nakajima H, Kono N, et al: Genetic defect in muscle phosphofructokinase deficiency. J Biol Chem 1990; 265:9392.

146. Fujii H, Miwa SI: Other erythrocyte enzyme deficiencies associated with non-haematological symptoms: Phosphoglycerate kinase and phosphofructokinase deficiency. Bailliere's Clin Haematol 2000; 13:141.

147. Mhaskar Y, Giger U, et al: Presence of a truncated M-type subunit and altered kinetic properties of 6-phosphofructo-1-kinase isozymes in the brain of a dog affected by glycogen storage disease type VII. Enzyme 1991; 45:137.

148. Smith BF, Stedman H, et al: Molecular basis of canine muscle type phosphofructokinase deficiency. J Biol Chem 1996; 271:20070

149. Miwa S, Fujii H, et al: Two cases of red cell aldolase deficiency associated with hereditary hemolytic anemia in a Japanese family. Am J Hematol 1981; 11:425.

150. Kishi H, Mukai T, et al: Human aldolase A deficiency associated with a hemolytic anemia: Thermolabile aldolase due to a single base mutation. Proc Natl Acad Sci USA 1987; 84:8623.

151. Takasaki Y, Takahashi I, et al: Human aldolase A of a hemolytic anemia patient with Asp-128→Gly substitution: Characteristics of an

enzyme generated in *E. coli* transfected with the expression plasmid pHAAD128G. J Biochem (Tokyo) 1990; 108:153.

152. Kreuder J, Borkhardt A, et al: Brief report: Inherited metabolic myopathy and hemolysis due to a mutation in aldolase A. N Engl J Med 1996; 334:1100–1104.

153. Beutler E, Scott S, et al: Red cell aldolase deficiency and hemolytic anemia: A new syndrome. Trans Assoc Am Physicians 1973; 86:154.

154. Schneider AS, Valentine WN, et al: Triosephosphate isomerase deficiency. A multisystem inherited enzyme disorder: Clinical and genetic aspects. In Beutler E (ed.): Hereditary Disorders of Erythrocyte Metabolism. New York, Grune & Stratton, 1968, p 265.

155. Schneider AS, Dunn I, et al: Triosephosphate isomerase deficiency. B. Inherited triosephosphate isomerase deficiency. Erythrocyte carbohydrate metabolism and preliminary studies of the erythrocyte enzyme. In Beutler E (ed.): Hereditary Disorders of Erythrocyte Metabolism. New York, Grune & Stratton, 1968, p 273.

156. Harris SR, Paglia DE, et al: Triosephosphate isomerase deficiency in an adult. Clin Res 1970; 18:529.

157. Valentine WN, Schneider AS, et al: Hereditary hemolytic anemia with triosephosphate isomerase deficiency. Am J Med 1966; 41:27.

158. Schneider AS, Valentine WN, et al: Hereditary hemolytic anemia with triose phosphate isomerase deficiency. N Engl J Med 1965; 272:229.

159. Skala H, Dreyfus JC, et al: Triose phosphate isomerase deficiency. Biochem Med 1977; 18:226.

160. Maquat LE, Chilcote R, et al: Human triosephosphate isomerase cDNA and protein structure. Studies of triosephosphate isomerase deficiency in man. J Biol Chem 1985; 260:3748.

161. Rosa R, Prehu MO, et al: Hereditary triose phosphate isomerase deficiency: Seven new homozygous cases. Hum Genet 1985; 71:235.

162. Zanella A, Mariana M, et al: Triosephosphate isomerase deficiency: 2 new cases. Scand J Haematol 1985; 34:417.

163. Clark ACL, Szobolotsky MA: Triose phosphate isomerase deficiency: Report of a family. Aust Paediatr J 1987; 22:135.

164. Bellingham AJ, Lestas AN, et al: Prenatal diagnosis of a red cell enzymopathy: Triosephosphate isomerase deficiency. Lancet 1989; 2:419.

165. Schneider AS: Triosephosphate isomerase deficiency: Historical perspectives and molecular aspects. Bailliere's Clin Haematol 2000; 13:119.

166. Schneider A, Westwood B, et al: Triosephosphate isomerase deficiency: Repetitive occurrence of point mutation in amino acid 104 in multiple apparently unrelated families. Am J Hematol 1995; 50:263.

167. Pekrun A, Neubauer BA, et al: Triosephosphate isomerase deficiency: Biochemical and molecular genetic analysis for prenatal diagnosis. Clin Genet 1995; 47:175.

168. Valentin C, Pissard S, et al: Triose phosphate isomerase deficiency in 3 French families: Two novel null alleles, a frameshift mutation (TPI Alfortville) and an alteration in the initiation codon (TPI Paris). Blood 2000; 96:1130.

169. Arya R, Lalloz MRA: Prenatal diagnosis of triosephosphate isomerase deficiency. Blood 1996; 87:4507.

170. Arya R, Lalloz MRA, Bellingham AJ, et al: Evidence for founder effect of the Glu104Asp substitution and identification of new mutations in triosephosphate isomerase deficiency. Hum Mutat 1997; 10:290.

171. Eber W, Pekrun A, et al: Triosephosphate isomerase deficiency: Haemolytic anaemia, myopathy with altered mitochondria and mental retardation due to a new variant with accelerated enzyme catabolism and diminished specific activity. J Pediatr 1991; 150:761.

172. Hollan S, Fujii H, et al: Hereditary triosephosphate isomerase (TPI) deficiency: Two severely affected brothers, one with and one without neurological symptoms. Hum Genet 1993; 92:486.

173. Lu HS, Yuan PM, et al: Primary structure of human triosephosphate isomerase. J Biol Chem 1984; 259:11958.

174. Jongsma APM, Los WR T, et al: Evidence for synteny between the human loci for triose phosphate isomerase, lactate dehydrogenase-B, peptidase-B and the regional mapping of these loci on chromosome 12. Cytogenet Cell Genet 1974; 13:106.

175. Mohrenweiser HW, Fielek S: Elevated frequency of carriers for triosephosphate isomerase deficiency in newborn infants. Pediatr Res 1982; 16:960.

176. Yuan PM, Talent JM, et al: A tentative elucidation of the sequence of human triosephosphate isomerase by homology peptide mapping. Biochim Biophys Acta 1981; 671:211.

177. Yuan PM, Talent JM, et al: Molecular basis for the accumulation of acidic isozymes of triosephosphate isomerase on aging. Mech Ageing Dev 1981; 17:151.

178. Peters J, Hopkinson DA, et al: Genetic and nongenetic variation of triose phosphate isomerase isozymes in human tissues. Ann Hum Genet 1973; 36:297.

179. Mande SC, Mainfroid V, et al: Crystal structure of recombinant human triosephosphate isomerase at 2.8 A resolution. Triosephosphate isomerase-related human genetic disorders and comparison with the trypanosomal enzyme. Protein Sci 1994; 3:810.

180. Orosz F, Vertessy BG, et al: Triosephosphate isomerase deficiency: Predictions and facts. J Theor Biol 1996; 182:437.

181. Orosz F, Wagner G, et al: Enhanced association of mutant triosephosphate isomerase to red cell membranes and to brain microtubules. Proc Natl Acad Sci USA 2000; 97:1026.

182. Karg E, Nemeth I, et al: Diminished blood levels of reduced glutathione and α-tocopherol in two triosephosphate isomerase-deficient brothers. Blood Cells Mol Dis 2000; 26:91.

183. Asakawa J, Sutoh C, et al: Electrophoretic variants of blood proteins in Japanese. III. Triosephosphate isomerase. Hum Genet 1984; 68:185.

184. Perry BA, Mohrenweiser HW: Human triosephosphate isomerase: Substitution of Arg for Gly at position 122 in a thermolabile electromorph variant, TPI-Manchester. Hum Genet 1992; 88:634.

185. Daar IO, Artymuik PJ, et al: Human triosephosphate isomerase deficiency: A single amino acid substitution results in a thermolabile enzyme. Proc Natl Acad Sci USA 1986; 83:7903.

186. Chang ML, Artymiuk PJ et al: Human triosephosphate isomerase deficiency resulting from mutation of Phe-240. Am J Hum Genet 1993; 52:1260.

187. Valentin C, Cohen-Solal M, et al: Identical germ-line mutations in the triosephosphate isomerase alleles of two brothers are associated with distinct clinical phenotypes. C R Acad Sci III 2000; 323:245.

188. Bardosi A, Eber SW, et al: Myopathy with altered mitochondria due to a triosephosphate isomerase (TPI) deficiency. Acta Neuropathol 1990; 79:387.

189. Pogliani EM, Colombi M, et al: Platelet function defect in triosephosphate isomerase deficiency. Haematologica 1986; 71:349.

190. Merkle S, Pretsch W: Characterization of triosephosphate isomerase mutants with reduced enzyme activity in *Mus musculus*. Genetics 1989; 123:837.

191. Bellingham AJ, Lestas AN: Prenatal diagnosis of triose phosphate isomerase deficiency. Lancet 1990; 1:230.

192. Ationu A, Humphries A, et al: Reversal of metabolic block in glycolysis by enzyme replacement in triosephosphate isomerase-deficient cells. Blood 1999; 94:3193

193. Harkness DR: A new erythrocytic enzyme defect with hemolytic anemia: Glyceraldehyde-3-phosphate dehydrogenase deficiency. J Lab Clin Med 1966; 68:879.

194. Oski FA, Whaun J: Hemolytic anemia and red cell glyceraldehyde-3-phosphate dehydrogenase. Paper presented at the 39th Annual Meeting of the Society for Pediatric Research, 1969, Atlantic City, p 151.

195. McCann SSR, Finkel B, et al: Study of a kindred with hereditary spherocytosis and glyceralhyde-3-phosphate dehydrogenase deficiency. Blood 1976; 47:171.

196. Valentine WN, Hsieh HS, et al: Hereditary hemolytic anemia associated with phosphoglycerate kinase deficiency in erythrocytes and leukocytes. N Engl J Med 1969; 280:528.

197. Turner G, Fletcher J, Elber J, et al: Molecular defect of a phosphoglycerate kinase variant associated with haemolytic anaemia and neurological disorders in a large kindred. Br J Haematol 1995; 91:60.

198. Dogson SJ, Lee CS, et al: Erythrocyte phosphoglycerate kinase deficiency: Enzymatic and oxygen binding studies. NZ J Med 1980; 10:614.

199. Yoshida A, Twele TW, et al: Molecular abnormality of a phosphoglycerate kinase variant (PGK Alabama). Blood Cells Mol Dis 1995; 21:179.

200. Miwa S, Nakashima K, et al: Phosphoglycerate kinase (PGK) deficiency hereditary nonspherocytic hemolytic anemia: Report of a case found in Japanese family. Acta Haematol Jpn 1972; 35:571.

201. Maeda M, Yoshida A: Molecular defect of a phosphoglycerate kinase variant (PGK Matsue) associated with hemolytic anemia: Leu→Pro substitution caused by T/A→C/G transition in exon 3. Blood 1991; 77:1348.

202. Yoshida A, Miwa S: Characterization of a phosphoglycerate kinase variant associated with a hemolytic anemia. Am J Hum Genet 1974; 26:378.

203. Fujii H, Yoshida A: Molecular abnormality of phosphoglycerate kinase-Uppsala associated with chronic nonspherocytic hemolytic anemia. Proc Natl Acad Sci USA 1980; 77:5461.

204. Hjelm M, Wadam B, et al: A phosphoglycerate kinase variant, PGK Uppsala, associated with hemolytic anemia. J Lab Clin Med 1980; 96:1015.

205. Konrad PN, McCarthy DJ, et al: Erythrocyte and leukocyte phosphoglycerate kinase deficiency with neurologic disease. J. Pediatr 1973; 82:456.

206. Strauss RG, McCarthy DJ, et al: Neutrophil function in congenital phosphoglycerate kinase deficiency. J. Pediatr 1974; 854:341.

207. Fujii H, Chen SH, et al: Use of cultured lymphoblastoid cells for the study of abnormal enzymes: Molecular abnormality of a phosphoglycerate kinase variant associated with hemolytic anemia. Proc Natl Acad Sci USA 1981; 78:2587.

208. Maeda M, Bawle EV, et al: Molecular abnormalities of a phosphoglycerate kinase variant generated by spontaneous mutation. Blood 1992; 79:2759.

209. Guis MS, Karadsheh N, et al: Phosphoglycerate kinase San Francisco: A new variant associated with hemolytic anemia but not with neuromuscular manifestations. Am J Hematol 1987; 25:175.

210. Fujii H, Krietsch WK G, and Yoshida A: A single amino acid substitution (Asp-Asn) in a phosphoglycerate kinase variant (PGK Munchen) associated with enzyme deficiency. J Biol Chem 1980; 255:6421.

211. Knetsch WK G, Eber SW, et al: Characterization of a phosphoglycerate kinase deficiency variant not associated with hemolytic anemia. Am J Hum Genet 1980; 32:364.

212. Valentin C, Birgens H, Craescu CT, et al: A phosphoglycerate kinase mutant (PGK Herlev; D285V) in a Danish patient with isolated chronic hemolytic anemia: Mechanism of mutation and structure-function relationships. Hum Mutat 1998; 12:280.

213. Fujii H, Kanno H, et al: A single amino acid substitution (157 Gly→Val) in a phosphoglycerate kinase variant (PGK Shizuoka) associated with chronic hemolysis and myoglobinuria. Blood 1992; 79:1582.

214. Aasly J, van Diggelen OP, Boer AM, et al Phosphoglycerate kinase deficiency in two brothers with McArdle-like clinical symptoms. Eur J Neurol 2000; 7:111.

215. Rosa R, Geore C, et al: A new case of phosphoglycerate kinase deficiency, PGK Creteil, associated with rhabdomyolysis and lacking hemolytic anemia. Blood 1982; 60:84.

216. Ookawara T, Dave V, Willems P, et al: Retarded and aberrant splicings caused by single point mutation in a phosphoglycerate kinase variant. Arch Biochem Biophys 1996; 327:35.

217. Hamano T, Mutoh T, Sugie H, et al: Phosphoglycerate kinase deficiency: An adult myopathic form with a novel mutation. Neurology 2000; 54:1188.

218. Sugie H, Sugie Y, et al: Recurrent myoglobinuria in a child with mental retardation phosphoglycerate kinase deficiency. J Child Neurol 1989; 4:95.

219. Sugie H, Sugie Y, Ito M, et al: A novel missense mutation (837T→C) in the phosphoglycerate kinase gene of a patient with a myopathic form of phosphoglycerate kinase deficiency. J Child Neurol 1998; 13:95.

220. DiMauro S, Dalakas M, et al: Phosphoglycerate kinase deficiency: Another cause of recurrent myoglobinuria. Ann Neurol 1983; 13:11.

221. Tonin P, Shanske S, et al: Phosphoglycerate kinase deficiency: Biochemical and molecular genetic studies in a new myopathic variant (PGK Alberta). Neurology 1993; 43:387.

222. Arese P, Bosai A, et al: Red cell glycolysis in a case of 3-phosphoglycerate kinase deficiency. Eur J Clin Invest 1973; 3:86.

223. Kraus AP, Langston MF, et al: Red cell phosphoglycerate kinase deficiency. Biochem Biophys Res Commun 1968; 30:173.

224. Huang IY, Fujii H, et al: Structure and function of normal and variant human phosphoglycerate kinase. Hemoglobin 1980; 4:601.

225. Banks RD, Blake CC, et al: Sequence, structure and activity of phosphoglycerate kinase: A possible hinge-bending enzyme. Nature 1979; 279:773.

226. Cartier P, Habibi B, et al: Anémie hémolytique congénitale associée à un déficit en phosphoglyceratekinase dansles globules rouges, les polynucléaires et les Iymphocytes. Nouv Rev Fr Hematol 1971; 11:565.

227. Boivin P, Hakim J, et al: Erythrocyte and leucocyte 3-phosphoglycerate kinase deficiency. Studies of properties of the polymorphonuclear leucocytes and a review of the literature. Nouv Rev Fr Hematol 1974; 14:495.

228. Schrier SL, Ben-Bassat I, et al: Characterization of erythrocyte membrane-associated enzymes (glyceraldehyde-3-phosphate dehydrogenase and phosphoglyceric kinase). J Lab Clin Med 1975; 85:797.

229. Parker JC, Hoffman JF: The role of membrane phosphoglycerate kinase in the control of glycolytic rate by active cation transport in human red cells. J Gen Physiol 1967; 50:893.

230. Chillar RK, Beutler E: Explanation for the apparent lack of ouabain inhibition of pyruvate production in hemolysates; the "backward" PGK reaction. Blood 1976; 47:507.

231. Segel GB, Feig SA, et al: Energy metabolism in human erythrocytes: The role of phosphoglycerate kinase in cation transport. Blood 1975; 46:271.

232. Baehner RL, Feig SA, et al: Metabolic, phagocytic, and bactericidal properties of phosphoglycerate kinase deficient polymorphonuclear leukocytes. Blood 1971; 38:833.

233. Chen SH, Malcolm LA, et al: Phosphoglycerate kinase: An X-linked polymorphism in man. Am J Hum Genet 1971; 23:87.

234. Michelson AM, Blake CF, et al: Structure of the human phosphoglycerate kinase gene and the intron-mediated evolution and dispersal of the nucleotide-binding domain. Proc Natl Acad Sci USA 1985; 82:6965.

235. Peys BF, Grzeschick KH, et al: Human phosphoglycerate kinase and inactivation of the X chromosome. Science 1972; 175:1002.

236. Michelson AM, Markham AF, et al: Isolation and DNA sequence of a full-length cDNA clone for human X chromosome-encoded phosphoglycerate kinase. Proc Natl Acad Sci USA 1983; 80:472.

237. Gartler SM, Riley DE, et al: Mapping of human autosomal phosphoglycerate kinase sequence to chromosome 19. Somat Cell Mol Genet 1986; 12:395.

238. Beutler E: Electrophoresis of phosphoglycerate kinase. Biochem Genet 1969; 3:189.

239. Yoshida A, Watanabe S, et al: Human phosphoglycerate kinase II. Structure of a variant enzyme. J Biol Chem 1972; 247:446.

240. Cohen-Solal M, Valentin C, et al: Identification of new mutations in two phosphoglycerate kinase (PGK) variants expressing different clinical syndromes: PGK Créteil and PGK Amiens. Blood 1994; 84:898.

241. Tsujino S, Tonin P, Shanske S, et al: A splice junction mutation in a new myopathic variant of phosphoglycerate kinase deficiency (PGK North Carolina). Ann Neurol 1994; 35:349.

242. Galacteros F, Rosa R, et al: Deficit en diphosphoglycerate mutase: Nouveaux cas associes a une polyglobulie. Nouv Rev Fr Hematol 1984; 26:69.

243. Rosa R, Prehu MO, et al: The first case of a complete deficiency of diphosphoglycerate mutase in human erythrocytes. J Clin Invest 1978; 62:907.

244. Schroter W: Kongenitale nichtesphärocytare hämolytische Anämie bei 2,3 Diphosphoglyceratemutasemangel der Erythrocyten im frühen Säuglingsalter. Klin Wochenschr 1965; 43:1147.

245. Cartier P, Labie P, et al: Déficit familial en diphosphoglycerate mutase: Étude hématologique et biochimique. Nouv Rev Fr Hematol 1972; 12:269.

246. Koler RD, McClung MR, et al: Physiologic and genetic alterations in human red cell DPGM. Hemoglobin 1980; 4:593.

247. Travis SF, Martinez J, et al: Study of a kindred with partial deficiency of red cell 2,3-diphosphoglycerate mutase (2,3-DPGM) and compensated hemolysis. Blood 1978; 51:1107.

248. Joulin V, Peduzzi J, et al: Molecular cloning and sequencing of the human erythrocyte 2,3-bisphosphoglycerate mutase cDNA: Revised amino acid sequence. EMBO J 1986; 5:2275.

249. Kappel WK, Hass LF: The isolation and partial characterization of diphosphoglycerate mutase from human erythrocytes. Biochemistry 1976; 15:290.

250. Hass LF, Kappel WK, et al: Evidence for structural homology between human red cell phosphoglycerate mutase and 2,3-biphosphoglycerate synthase. J Biol Chem 1978; 253:77.

251. Craescu CT, Schaad O, et al: Structural modeling of the human erythrocyte bisphosphoglycerate mutase. Biochimie 1992; 74:519.

252. Chen SH, Anderson JE, et al: Human red cell 2,3-diphosphoglycerate mutase and monophosphoglycerate mutase: Genetic evidence for two separate loci. Am J Hum Genet 1977; 29:405.

253. Garel MC, Arous N, et al: A recombinant bisphosphoglycerate mutase variant with acid phosphatase homology degrades 2,3-diphosphoglycerate. Proc Natl Acad Sci USA 1994; 91:3593.

254. Blouquit Y, Rhoda MD, et al: Glycerated hemoglobin in $\alpha_2\beta_2$82 (EF6) N-ϵ-glyceryllysine: A new posttranslational modification occurring in erythrocyte bisphosphoglyceromutase deficiency. BioMed Biochim Acta 1987; 46:S202.

255. Barichard F, Joulin V, et al: Chromosomal assignment of the human 2,3-bisphosphoglycerate mutase gene (BPGM) to region 7q34→7q22. Hum Genet 1987; 77:283.

256. Joulin V, Garel MC, et al: Isolation and characterization of the human 2,3-bisphosphoglycerate mutase gene. J Biol Chem 1988; 263:15785.

257. Rosa R, Galacteros MO, et al: Inactive bisphosphoglycerate mutase variants: New data. BioMed Biochim Acta 1987; 46:S207.

258. Lemarchandel V, Joulin V, et al: Compound heterozygosity in a complete erythrocyte bisphosphoglycerate mutase deficiency. Blood 1992; 80:2643.

259. Rosa R, Blouquit Y, et al: Isolation, characterization, and structure of a mutant 89 Arg→Cys bisphosphoglycerate mutase. Implication of the active site in the mutation. J Biol Chem 1989; 264:7837.

260. Stefanini M: Chronic hemolytic anemia associated with erythrocyte enolase deficiency exacerbated by ingestion of nitrofurantoin. Am J Clin Pathol 1972; 58:408.

261. Staal GE J, Van Berkel TH, et al: Normalization of red blood cell pyruvate kinase in pyruvate kinase deficiency by riboflavin treatment. Clin Chim Acta 1975; 60:323.

262. Lanchant NA, Jennings MA, et al: Partial erythrocyte enolase deficiency: A hereditary disorder with variable clinical expression. Blood 1986; 68:55A.

263. Beutler E, Gelbart T: Estimating the prevalence of pyruvate kinase deficiency from the gene frequency in the general white population. Blood 2000; 95:3585.

264. Searcy GP, Miller DR, et al: Congenital hemolytic anemia in the basenji dog due to erythrocyte pyruvate kinase deficiency. Can J Comp Med 1971; 35:67.

265. Nakashima K, Miwa S, et al: Electrophoretic, immunologic and kinetic characterization of erythrocyte pyruvate kinase in the basenji dog with pyruvate kinase deficiency. Tohoku J Exp Med 1975; 117:179.

266. Prasse KW, Crouser D, et al: Pyruvate kinase deficiency anemia with terminal myelofibrosis and osteosclerosis in a beagle. J Am Vet Med Assoc 1975; 166:1170.

267. Ghidini A, Sirtori M, et al: Hepatosplenomegaly as the only prenatal finding in a fetus with pyruvate kinase deficiency anemia. Am J Perinatol 1991; 8:44.

268. Hennekam RC, Beemer FA, et al: Hydrops fetalis associated with red cell pyruvate kinase deficiency. Genet Couns 1990; 1:75.

269. Fanning J, Hinkle RS: Pyruvate kinase deficiency hemolytic anemia: Two successful pregnancy outcomes. Am J Obstet Gynecol 1985; 153:313.

270. Ghidini A, Korker VL: Severe pyruvate kinase deficiency anemia. A case report. J Reprod Med 1998; 43:713.

271. Duncan JR, Capellini MD, et al: Aplastic crisis due to parvovirus infection in pyruvate kinase deficiency. Lancet 1983; 2:14.

272. Muller-Soyano Z, de Roura ET, et al: Pyruvate kinase deficiency and leg ulcers. Blood 1976; 47:807.

273. Vives-Corrons JL, Marie J, et al: Hereditary erythrocyte pyruvate kinase (PK) deficiency and chronic hemolytic anemia: Clinical, genetic and molecular studies in six new Spanish patients. Hum Genet 1980; 53:401.

274. Morisaki T, Tani K, et al: Ten cases of pyruvate kinase (PK) deficiency found in Japan: Enzymatic characterization of the patients' PK. Acta Haematol Jpn 1988; 51:1080.

275. Mentzer WC, Baehner RL, et al: Selective reticulocyte destruction in erythrocyte pyruvate kinase deficiency. J Clin Invest 1971; 50:688.

276. Staal GE J, Rijksen G, et al: Extreme deficiency of L-type pyruvate kinase with moderate clinical expression. Clin Chim Acta 1982; 118:241.

277. Etiemble J, Picat C, et al: A red cell pyruvate kinase mutant with normal L-type PK in the liver. Hum Genet 1982; 61:256.

278. Oski FA, Nathan DG, et al: Extreme hemolysis and red cell distortion in erythrocyte pyruvate kinase deficiency. I. Morphology, erythrokinetics, and family enzyme studies. N Engl J Med 1964; 270:1023.

279. Leblond PF, Lyonnais J, et al: Erythrocyte populations in pyruvate kinase deficiency anemia following splenectomy. I. Cell morphology. Br J Haematol 1978; 39:55.

280. Nathan DG, Oski FA, et al: Studies of erythrocyte spicule formation in haemolytic anaemia. Br J Haematol 1966; 12:385.

281. Zanella A, Colombo MB, et al: Erythrocyte pyruvate kinase deficiency: 11 new cases. Br J Haematol 1988; 69:399.

282. Keitt AS: Pyruvate kinase deficiency and related disorders of red cell glycolysis. Am J Med 1966; 41:762.

283. Kanno H, Fujii H, et al: cDNA cloning of human R-type pyruvate kinase and identification of a single amino acid substitution (Thr→Met) affecting enzymatic stability in a pyruvate kinase variant (PK Tokyo) associated with hereditary hemolytic anemia. Proc Natl Acad Sci USA 1991; 88:8218.

284. Tani K, Fujii H, et al: Human liver type pyruvate kinase: cDNA cloning and chromosomal assignment. Biochem Biophys Res Commun 1987; 143:431.

285. Tani K, Yoshida MC, et al: Human M_2-type pyruvate kinase: cDNA cloning, chromosomal assignment and expression in hepatoma. Gene 1988; 73:509.

286. Takenaka M, Noguchi T, et al: Rat pyruvate kinase M gene. J Biol Chem 1989; 264:2363.

287. Noguchi T, Inoue H, et al: The M_1-and M_2-type isozymes of rat pyruvate kinase are produced from the same gene by alternative RNA splicing. J Biol Chem 1986; 261:13807.

288. Baronciani L, Beutler E: Analysis of pyruvate kinase deficiency mutations that produce nonspherocytic hemolytic anemia. Proc Natl Acad Sci USA 1993; 90:4324.

289. Marie J, Simon MP, et al: One gene, but two messenger RNAs encode liver L and red cell L′ pyruvate kinase subunits. Nature 1981; 292:7.

290. Noguchi T, Kazuya Y, et al: The L- and R-type isozymes of rat pyruvate kinase are produced from a single gene by use of different promoters. J Biol Chem 1987; 262:14366.

291. Tani K, Fujii H, et al: Human liver type pyruvate kinase: Complete amino acid sequence and the expression in mammalian cells. Proc Natl Acad Sci USA 1988; 85:1792.

292. Muirhead H, Clayden DA, et al: The structure of cat muscle pyruvate kinase. EMBO J 1986; 5:475.

293. Takegawa S, Fujii H, et al: Change of pyruvate kinase isozymes from M_2- to L-type during development of the red cell. Br J Haematol 1983; 54:467.

294. Takegawa S, Miwa S: Change of pyruvate kinase (PK) isozymes in classical type PK deficiency and other PK deficiency cases during red cell maturation. Am J Hematol 1984; 16:53.

295. Max-Audit I, Kechemir MT, et al: Pyruvate kinase synthesis and degradation by normal and pathologic cells during erythroid maturation. Blood 1988; 72:1039.

296. Monod J, Wyman J, et al: On the nature of allosteric transitions: A plausible model. J Mol Biol 1964; 12:88.

297. Koler RD, Vanbellinghen P: The mechanism of precursor modulation of human pyruvate kinase I by fructose diphosphate. Adv Enzyme Regul 1968; 6:127.

298. Koster JF, Staal GEJ, et al: The effect of urea and temperature on red blood cell pyruvate kinase. Biochim Biophys Acta 1971; 236:362.

299. Cartier P, Najman A, et al: Les anomalies de la glycolyse au cours de l'anémie hémolytique par déficit du globule en pyruvate kinase. Clin Chim Acta 1968; 22:165.

300. Lakomek M, Scharnetzky M, et al: On the temperature and salt-dependent conformation change in human erythrocyte pyruvate kinase. Hoppe-Seyler's Z Physiol Chem 1983; 364:787.

301. Peterson JS, Chern CJ, et al: The subunit structure of human muscle and human erythrocyte pyruvate kinase isozymes. FEBS Lett 1974; 49:73.

302. Boivin P, Galand C, et al: Coéxistence de deux types de pyruvate kinase cinétiquement différents dans les globules rouges humains normaux. Nouv Rev Fr Hematol 1972; 12:159.

303. Paglia DE, Valentine WN: Evidence of molecular alteration of pyruvate kinase as a consequence of erythrocyte aging. J Lab Clin Med 1970; 76:202.

304. Van Berkel JC, Staal GEJ, et al: On the molecular basis of pyruvate kinase deficiency. II. Role of thiol groups in pyruvate kinase from pyruvate kinase-deficient patients. Biochim Biophys Acta 1974; 334:361.

305. Valentine WN, Toohey JI, et al: Modification of erythrocyte enzyme activities by persulfides and methanethiol: Possible regulatory role. Proc Natl Acad Sci USA 1987; 84:1394.

306. Solovonuk PF, Collier HB: The pyruvic phosferase of erythrocytes. I. Properties of the enzyme and its activity in erythrocytes of various species. Can J Biochem Physiol 1955; 33:38.

307. Valentine WN, Paglia DE: Studies with human erythrocyte pyruvate kinase (PK): Effect of modification of sulfhydryl groups. Br J Haematol 1983; 53:385.

308. Badwey JA, Westhead EW: Post-translational modification of human erythrocyte pyruvate kinase. Biochem Biophys Res Commun 1977; 74:1326.

309. Zanella A, Rebulla P, et al Effects of sulphydryl compounds on abnormal red cell pyruvate kinase. Br J Haematol 1976; 32:373.

310. Nakashima K: Further evidence of molecular alteration and aberration of erythrocyte pyruvate kinase. Clin Chim Acta 1974; 55:245.

311. Blume KG, Arnold H, et al: On the molecular basis of pyruvate kinase deficiency. Biochim Biophys Acta 1974; 370:601.

312. Koler RD, Bigley RH, et al: Pyruvate kinase: Molecular differences between human red cell and leukocyte enzyme. Symp Quant Biol 1964; 29:213.

313. Munro GF, Miller DR: Mechanism of fructose diphosphate activation of a mutant pyruvate kinase from human red cells. Biochim Biophys Acta 1970; 206:87.

314. Blume KG, Hoffbauer RW, et al: Purification and properties of pyruvate kinase in normal and in pyruvate kinase-deficient human red blood cells. Biochim Biophys Acta 1971; 227:364.

315. Staal GEJ, Koster JF, et al: Human erythrocyte pyruvate kinase. Its purification and some properties. Biochim Biophys Acta 1971; 227:86.

316. Srivastava SK, Beutler E: The effect of normal red cell constituents on the activities of red cell enzymes. Arch Biochem Biophys 1972; 148:249.

317. Ponce J, Roth S, et al: Kinetic studies on the inhibition of glycolytic kinases of human erythrocytes by 2,3-diphosphoglyceric acid. Biochim Biophys Acta 1971; 250:63.

318. Westhead EW, Kiener PA, et al: Control of oxygen delivery from the erythrocyte by modification of pyruvate kinase. Curr Top Cell Regul 1984; 24:21.

319. Fujii S, Nakashima K, et al: Cyclic AMP-dependent phosphorylation of erythrocyte variant pyruvate kinase. Biochem Med 1984; 31:47.

320. Brunetti P, Puxeddu A, et al: Anemia emolitica congenita non sferocitica de carenza di piruvico-chinasi (PK). Haematol Arch 1962; 47:505.

321. Bigley RH, Koler RD: Liver pyruvate kinase (PK) isoenzymes in a PK-deficient patient. Ann Hum Genet 1968; 31:383.

322. Nakashima K, Miwa S, et al: Characterization of pyruvate kinase from the liver of a patient with aberrant erythrocyte pyruvate kinase, PK Nagasaki. J Lab Clin Med 1977; 90:1012.

323. Grimes AJ, Meisler A, et al: Hereditary nonspherocytic haemolytic anaemia. A study of red-cell carbohydrate metabolism in twelve cases of pyruvate kinase deficiency. Br J Haematol 1964; 10:403.

324. Miwa S, Nagate M: Pyruvate kinase deficiency hereditary nonspherocytic hemolytic anemia. Report of two cases in a Japanese family and review of literature. Acta Haematol Jpn 1965; 28:1.

325. Necheles TF, Finkel HE, et al: Red cell pyruvate kinase deficiency. The effect of splenectomy. Arch Intern Med 1966; 118:75.

326. Tomoda A, Lachant NA, et al: Inhibition of the pentose phosphate shunt by 2,3-diphosphoglycerate in erythrocyte pyruvate kinase deficiency. Br J Haematol 1983; 54:475.

327. Bowman HS, Procopio F: Hereditary nonspherocytic hemolytic anemia of the pyruvate-kinase deficient type. Ann Intern Med 1963; 58:567.

328. Oski FA, Diamond LK: Erythrocyte pyruvate kinase deficiency resulting in congenital nonspherocytic hemolytic anemia. N Engl J Med 1963; 269:269.

329. Glader BE: Oxidant-induced injury in pyruvate kinase (PK) deficient erythrocytes. Pediatr Res 1974; 8:401.

330. Jacobasch G, Boese C: Regulation des Kohlenhydratstoff-wechsels roter Blutzellen bei Pyruvatkinasemangel. Folia Haematol Int Mag Klin Morphol Blutforsch 1969; 91:70.

331. Rose IA, Warms JVB: Control of glycolysis in the human red blood cell. J Biol Chem 1966; 241:4848.

332. Oski FA, Bowman H: A low K_m phosphoenolpyruvate mutant in the Amish with red cell pyruvate kinase deficiency. Br J Haematol 1969; 17:289.

333. Paglia DE, Valentine WN, et al: An inherited molecular lesion of erythrocyte pyruvate kinase. Identification of a kinetically aberrant isoenzyme associated with premature hemolysis. J Clin Invest 1968; 47:1929.

334. Zuelzer WW, Robinson AR, et al: Erythrocyte pyruvate kinase deficiency in nonspherocytic hemolytic anemia: A system of multiple genetic markers? Blood 1968; 32:33.

335. Miwa S, Nishina T, et al: Studies on erythrocyte metabolism in various hemolytic anemias: With special reference to pyruvate kinase deficiency. Acta Haematol Jpn 1970; 33:501.

336. Lestas AN, Kay LA, et al: Red cell 3-phosphoglycerate level as a diagnostic aid in pyruvate kinase deficiency. Br J Haematol 1987; 67:485.

337. Colombo MB, Zanella A, et al: 2,3-Diphosphoglycerate and 3-phosphoglycerate in red cell pyruvate kinase deficiency. Br J Haematol 1987; 68:423.

338. Lakomek M, Neubauer B, et al: Erythrocyte pyruvate kinase deficiency: Relations of residual enzyme activity, altered regulation of defective enzymes and concentrations of high-energy phosphates with the severity of clinical manifestation. Eur J Haematol 1992; 49:82.

339. Lakomek M, Winkler H.: Erythrocyte pyruvate kinase- and glucose phosphate isomerase deficiency: Pertubation of glycolysis by structural defects and functional alterations of defective enzymes and its relation to the clinical severity of chronic hemolytic anemia. Biophys Chem 1997; 66:269.

340. Rose IW, Warms JV B.: Control of red cell glycolysis. The cause of triose phosphate accumulation. J Biol Chem 1970; 245:4009.

341. Zerez CR, Tanaka KR: Impaired nicotinamide adenine dinucleotide synthesis in pyruvate kinase-deficient human erythrocytes: A mechanism for decreased total NAD content and a possible secondary cause of hemolysis. Blood 1987; 69:999.

342. Zerez CR, Wong MD, et al: Impaired erythrocyte phosphoribosylpyrophosphate formation in hemolytic anemia due to pyruvate kinase deficiency. Blood 1988; 72:500.

343. Nathan DG, Oski FA, et al: Extreme hemolysis and red cell distortion in erythrocyte pyruvate kinase deficiency. II. Measurements of erythrocyte glucose consumption, potassium flux and adenosine triphosphate stability. N Engl J Med 1965; 272:118.

344. Twomey JJ, O'Neal FB, et al: ATP metabolism in pyruvate kinase deficient erythrocytes. Blood 1967; 30:576.

345. Gardos G, Strau FB: Über die rolle des adenosintriphosphor-säure (ATP) in der K-permeabilität der menschlichen roten Blutkörperchen. Acta Physiol Acad Sci Hung 1957; 12:1.

346. Koller CA, Orringer EP, et al: Quinine protects pyruvate-kinase deficient red cells from dehydration. Am J Hematol 1979; 7:193.

347. Nathan DG, Shohet SB: Erythrocyte ion transport defects and hemolytic anemia: "hydrocytosis" and "desicytosis." Semin Hematol 1970; 7:381.

348. Allen DW, Groat JD, et al: Increased adsorption of cytoplasmic proteins to the erythrocyte membrane in ATP depleted normal and pyruvate kinase-deficient mature cells and reticulocytes. J Clin Invest 1981; 70:502.

349. Zanella A, Brovelli A, et al: Membrane abnormalities of pyruvate kinase deficient red cells. Br J Haematol 1979; 42:101.

350. Marik T, Brabec V, et al: Reticulocyte-dependent labeling alterations of red cell membrane in pyruvate kinase deficiency anemia. Biomed Biochim Acta 1987; 46:S192.

351. Marik T, Brabec V, et al: Pyruvate kinase-deficiency anemia: Membrane approach. Biochem Med Metab Biol 1988; 39:55.

352. Staal GEJ, Sybesma HB, et al: Familial hemolytic anaemia due to pyruvate kinase deficiency. Folia Med Neerl 1971; 14:72.

353. Staal GEJ, Koster JF, et al: A new variant of red blood cell pyruvate kinase deficiency. Biochim Biophys Acta 1971; 258:685.

354. Nathan DG, Oski FA, et al: Life-span and organ sequestration of the red cells in pyruvate kinase deficiency. N Engl J Med 1968; 278:73.

355. Najean Y, Dresch C, et al: Étude de l'érythrocinétique dans 8 cas de déficit homozygote en pyruvate kinase. Nouv Rev Fr Hematol 1969; 9:850.

356. Bowman HS, Oski FA: Splenic macrophage interaction with red cells in pyruvate kinase deficiency and hereditary spherocytosis. Vox Sang 1970; 19:168.

357. Matsumoto N, Ishihara T, et al: Sequestration and destruction of reticulocytes in the spleen in pyruvate kinase deficiency hereditary nonspherocytic hemolytic anemia. Acta Haematol Jpn 1972; 35:525.

358. Leblond PF, Couloumbe L, et al: Erythrocyte populations in pyruvate kinase deficiency following splenectomy. II. Cell deformability. Br J Haematol 1978; 39:63.

359. Muller-Soyano A, Platt O, et al: Pyruvate kinase deficiency in dog and human erythrocytes: Effects of energy depletion on cation composition and cellular hydration. Am J Hematol 1986; 23:217.

360. Lakomek M, Winkler H, et al: Erythrocyte pyruvate kinase deficiency: A kinetic method for differentiation between heterozygosity and compound-heterozygosity. Am J Hematol 1989; 31:225.

361. Bossu M, Dacha M, et al: Neonatal hemolysis due to a transient severity of inherited pyruvate kinase deficiency. Acta Haematol 1968; 40:166.

362. Paglia DE, Valentine WN, et al: An isozyme of erythrocyte pyruvate kinase (PK-Los Angeles) with impaired kinetics corrected by fructose-1,6-diphosphate. Am J Clin Pathol 1977; 78:229.

363. el-Hazmi MAF, Al-Swailem AR, et al: Frequency of glucose-6-phosphate dehydrogenase, pyruvate kinase and hexokinase deficiency in the Saudi population. Hum Hered 1986; 36:45.

364. Feng CS, Tsang SS, et al: Prevalence of pyruvate kinase deficiency among the Chinese: Determination by the quantitative assay. Am J Hematol 1993; 43:271.

365. Wu ZL, Yu WD, et al: Frequency of erythrocyte pyruvate kinase deficiency in Chinese infants. Am J Hematol 1985; 20:139.

366. Blume KG, Lohr GW, et al: Beitrag sur Populationsgenetik der Pyruvat-kinase menshlicher Erythrocyten. Humangenetik 1968; 6:261.

367. Mohrenweiser HW: Frequency of enzyme deficiency variants in erythrocytes of newborn infants. Proc Natl Acad Sci 1981; 78:5046.

368. Ishida Y, Miwa S, et al: Thirteen cases of pyruvate kinase deficiency found in Japan. Am J Hematol 1981; 10:239.

369. Kahn A, Marie J, et al: Search for a relationship between molecular anomalies of the mutant erythrocyte pyruvate kinase variants and their pathological expression. Hum Genet 1981; 57:172.

370. Miwa S: Recommended methods for the characterization of red cell pyruvate kinase variants. Br J Haematol 1979; 43:375.

371. Bianchi P, Zanella A: Hematologically important mutations: Red cell pyruvate kinase (third update). Blood Cells Mol Dis 2000; 26:47.

372. Zanella A, Bianchi P, et al: Molecular characterization of the PK-LR gene in sixteen pyruvate kinase-deficient patients. Br J Haematol 2001; 113:43.

373. Zanella A, Bianchi P. Red cell pyruvate kinase deficiency: From genetics to clinical manifestations. Bailliere's Clin Haematol 2000; 13:57.

374. Whitney KM, Goodman SA, et al: The molecular basis of canine pyruvate kinase deficiency. Exp Hematol 1994; 22:866.

375. Lenzner C, Nurnberg P, et al: Mutations in the pyruvate kinase L-gene in patients with hereditary hemolytic anemia. Blood 1994; 83:2817.

376. Baronciani L, Beutler E: Molecular study of pyruvate kinase-deficient patients with hereditary nonspherocytic hemolytic anemia. J Clin Invest 1995; 95:1702.

377. Lakomek M, Huppke P, et al: Mutations in the R-type pyruvate kinase gene and altered enzyme kinetic properties in patients with hemolytic anemia due to pyruvate kinase deficiency. Ann Hematol 1994; 68:253.

378. Kanno H, Fujii H, et al: Identical point mutations of the R-type pyruvate kinase (PK) cDNA found in unrelated PK variants associated with hereditary hemolytic anemia. Blood 1992; 79:1347.

379. Demina A, Varughese K.I, et al: Six previously undescribed pyruvate kinase mutations causing enzyme deficiency. Blood 1998; 92:647.

380. van Solinge WW, Kraaijenhagen RJ, et al: Molecular modelling of human red blood cell pyruvate kinase: Structural implications of a novel G1091 to A mutation causing severe nonspherocytic hemolytic anemia. Blood 1997; 90:4987.

381. Pastore L, Della Morte R, et al: Novel mutations and structural implications in R-type pyruvate kinase-deficient patients from Southern Italy. Hum Mutat 1998; 11:127.

381a. Valentin G, Chiarelli LR, et al: Structure and function of human erythrocyte pyruvate kinase: Molecular basis of nonspherocytic hemolytic anemia. J Biol Chem 2002; 277:23807.

382. Baronciani L, Beutler E: Prenatal diagnosis of pyruvate kinase deficiency. Blood 1994; 84:2354.

383. Sachs JR, Wicker DJ, et al: Familial hemolytic anemia resulting from an abnormal red blood cell pyruvate kinase. J Lab Clin Med 1968; 72:359.

384. Paglia DE, Valentine, WN, et al: Defective erythrocyte pyruvate kinase with impaired kinetics and reduced optimal activity. Br J Haematol 1972; 221:651.

385. Busch D, Witt I, et al: Deficiency of pyruvate kinase in the erythrocytes of a child with hereditary nonspherocytic hemolytic anemia. Acta Paediatr Scand 1966; 55:177.

386. Takegawa S, Miwa S: Change of pyruvate kinase (PK) isozymes in classical type PK deficiency and other PK deficiency cases during red cell maturation. Am J Hematol 1984; 16:53.

387. Miwa S: Hereditary disorders of red cell enzymes in the Embden-Meyerhof pathway. Am J Hematol 1983; 14:381385.

388. Max-Audit I, Rosa R, et al: Pyruvate kinase hyperactivity genetically determined: Metabolic consequences and molecular characterization. Blood 1980; 56:5.

389. Rosa R, Max-Audit I, et al: Hereditary pyruvate kinase abnormalities associated with erythrocytosis. Am J Hematol 1981; 10:47.

390. Staal GE J, Jansen G, et al: Pyruvate kinase and the "high ATP syndrome." J Clin Invest 1984; 74:231.

391. Kechemir D, Max-Audit I, et al: Comparative study of human M_2-type pyruvate kinases isolated from human leukocytes and erythrocytes of a patient with red cell pyruvate kinase hyperactivity. Enzyme 1989; 41:121.

392. Tsujino K, Kanno H, et al: Delayed onset of hemolytic anemia in CBA-Pk-1slc/Pk1slc mice with a point mutation of the gene encoding red blood cell type pyruvate kinase. Blood 1998; 91:2169.

393. Etiemble J, Picat C, et al: Erythrocytic pyruvate kinase deficiency and hemolytic anemia inherited as a dominant trait. Am J Hematol 1984; 17:251

394. Valentine WN, Herring WB, et al: Pyruvate kinase Greensboro. A four-generation study of a high $K_{0.5s}$ (phosphoenolypyruvate) variant. Blood 1988; 72:1054.

395. Baughan MA, Paglia DE, et al: An unusual hematological syndrome with pyruvate kinase deficiency and thalassemia minor in the kindreds. Acta Haematol 1968; 39:345.

396. Eudlerink F, Cleton FS: Gaucher's disease with severe renal involvement combined with pyruvate kinase deficiency. Pathol Eur 1970; 5:409.

397. Sandoval C, Stringel G: Failure of partial splenectomy to ameliorate the anemia of pyruvate kinase deficiency. J Pediatr Surg 1997; 32:641.

398. Blume KG, Busch D, et al: The polymorphism of nucleoside effect in pyruvate kinase deficiency. Humangenetik 1970; 9:257.

399. Glader BE: Salicylate-induced injury of pyruvate-kinase deficient erythrocytes. N Engl J Med 1976; 294:916.

400. Weiden PL, Hackman RC, et al: Long-term survival and reversal of iron overload after marrow transplantation in dogs with congenital hemolytic anemia. Blood 1981; 57:66.

401. Morimoto M, Kanno H, et al: Pyruvate kinase deficiency of mice associated with nonspherocytic hemolytic anemia and cure of the anemia by marrow transplantation without host irradiation. Blood 1995; 86:4323.

402. Tani K, Yoshikubo T, et al: Retrovirus-mediated gene transfer of human pyruvate kinase (PK) cDNA into murine hematopoietic cells: Implications for gene therapy of human PK deficiency. Blood 1994; 83:2305.

403. Miwa S, Nishina T, et al: Studies on erythrocyte metabolism in a case with hereditary deficiency of H-subunit of lactate dehydrogenase. Acta Haematol Jpn 1971; 34:228.

404. Kanno T, Maekawa M: Lactate dehydrogenase M-subunit deficiencies: Clinical features, metabolic background, and genetic heterogeneities. Muscle Nerve 1995; Suppl 3: S54.

405. Kremer JP, Datta T, et al: Mechanisms of compensation of hemolytic anemia in a lactate dehydrogenase mouse mutant. Exp Hematol 1987; 15:664.

406. Brewer GJ: A new inherited abnormality of human erythrocytes: Elevated erythrocyte adenosine triphosphate. Biochem Biophys Res Commun 1965; 18:430.

407. Jacobasch G, Syllm-Rappoport I, et al: 2,3PGase-Mangel als mögliche ursache erhöhten ATP-Gehaltes. Clin Chim Acta 1964; 10:477.

408. Ben-Bassat I, Brok-Simoni F, et al: A family with red cell pyrimidine 5'-nucleotidase deficiency. Blood 1976; 47:919.

409. Rosa R, Rochant H, et al: Electrophoretic and kinetic studies of human erythrocytes deficient in pyrimidine-5'-nucleotidase. Hum Genet 1977; 38:209.

410. Miwa S, Nakashima K, et al: Three cases of hereditary hemolytic anemia with pyrimidine-5'-nucleotidase deficiency in a Japanese family. Hum Genet 1977; 37:361.

411. Paglia DE, Valentine WN: Haemolytic anaemia associated with disorders of the purine and pyrimidine salvage pathways. Clin Haematol 1981; 10:81.

412. Beutler E, Baranko PV, et al: Hemolytic anemia due to pyrimidine-5'-nucleotidase deficiency; report of eight cases in six families. Blood 1980; 56:251.

413. Miwa S, Ishida Y, Kibe A, et al: Two cases of hereditary hemolytic anemia with pyrimidine-5'nucleotidase deficiency. Acta Haematol Jpn 1981; 44:187.

414. Ozsoylu S, Gurgey A: A case of hemolytic anemia due to erythrocyte pyrimidine-5'-nucleotidase deficiency. Acta Haematol 1981; 66:56.

415. Tomoda A, Noble NA, et al: Hemolytic anemia in hereditary pyrimidine 5'-nucleotidase deficiency: Nucleotide inhibition of G6PD and the pentose phosphate shunt. Blood 1982; 60:1212.

416. Willy T, Hansen R, et al: Erythrocyte pyrimidine-5'-nucleotidase deficiency. Scand J. Haematol 1983; 31:122.

417. Vives I Corrons J-L: Chronic non-spherocytic haemolytic anaemia due to congenital pyrimidine 5' nucleotidase deficiency: 25 years later. Bailliere's Clin Haematol 2000; 13:103.

418. Hirono A, Fujii H, et al: Chromatographic analysis of human erythrocyte pyrimidine-5'-nucleotidase from five patients with pyrimidine-5'-nucleotidase deficiency. Br J Haematol 1987; 65:35.

419. Swanson MS, Angle CR, et al: ^{31}P NMR study of erythrocytes from a patient with hereditary pyrimidine-5'-nucleotidase deficiency. Proc Natl Acad Sci USA 1983; 80:169.

420. Swanson MS, Markin RS, et al: Identification of cytidine diphosphodiesters in erythrocytes from a patient with pyrimidine nucleotidase deficiency. Blood 1984; 63:665.

421. Harley EH, Heaton A, et al: Pyrimidine metabolism in hereditary erythrocyte pyrimidine-5'-nucleotidase deficiency. Metabolism 1978; 27:12.

422. Kagimoto T, Shirono K: Detection of pyrimidine-5'-nucleotidase deficiency using H- or P-nuclear magnetic resonance. Experientia 1986; 42:69.

423. Valentine WN, Anderson HM, et al: Studies on human erythrocyte nucleotide metabolism. II. Nonspherocytic hemolytic anemia, high red cell ATP, ribosephosphate pyrophosphokinase (RPK, EC 2.7.6.1) deficiency. Blood 1972; 39:674.

424. Valentine WN, Bennett JM, et al: Nonspherocytic haemolytic anaemia with increased red cell adenine nucleotides, glutathione and basophilic stippling and ribosephosphate pyrophosphokinase (RPK) deficiency: Studies on two new kindreds. Br J Haematol 1973; 24:157.

425. Lachant NA, Zerez CR, et al: Pyrimidine nucleotides impair phosphoribosylpyrophosphate (PRPP) synthetase subunit aggregation by sequestering magnesium. A mechanism for the decreased PRPP synthetase activity in hereditary erythrocyte pyrimidine-5'-nucleotidase deficiency. Biochem Biophys Acta 1989; 994:81.

426. Lachant NA, Tanaka KR: Red cell metabolism in hereditary pyrimidine-5'-nucleotidase deficiency: Effect of magnesium. Br J Haematol 1986; 63:615.

427. Paglia DE, Valentine WN, et al: Cytosol accumulation of cytidine diphosphate (CDP)-choline as an isolated erythrocyte defect in chronic hemolysis. Proc Natl Acad Sci USA 1983; 80:3081.

428. Oda S, Tanaka KR: Metabolism studies in erythrocyte pyrimidine 5'-nucleotidase deficiency. Clin Res 1976; 34:149A.

429. David O, Ramenghi U, et al: Inhibition of hexose monophosphate shunt in young erythrocytes by pyrimidine nucleotides in hereditary pyrimidine-5' nucleotidase deficiency. Eur J Haematol 1991; 47:48.

430. Paglia DE, Valentine WN, et al: Effects of low-level lead exposure on pyrimidine-5'-nucleotidase and other erythrocyte enzymes. J Clin Invest 1975; 56:1164.

431. Valentine WN, Paglia DE, et al: Lead poisoning. Association with hemolytic anemia, basophilic stippling erythrocyte pyrimidine-5'-nucleotidase deficiency, and intraerythrocytic accumulation of pyrimidines. J Clin Invest 1976; 58:926.

432. Paglia DE, Valentine WN, et al: Studies on the pathogenesis of lead induced hemolytic anemia. Blood 1977; 50:96.

433. Ghosh K, Abdulrahman HI, et al: Report of the first case of pyrimidine-5' nucleotidase deficiency from Kuwait detected by a screening test. A test report. Haematologia 1991; 24:229.

434. Li JY, Wan SD, et al: A new mutant erythrocyte pyrimidine-5'-nucleotidase characterized by fast electrophoretic mobility in a Chinese boy with chronic hemolytic anemia. Clin Chim Acta 1991; 200:43.

435. Torrance JD, Whittaker D, et al: Erythrocyte pyrimidine-5'-nucleotidase. Br J Haematol 1980; 45:585.

436. Beutler E, West C: Tissue distribution of pyrimidine-5'-nucleotidase. Biochem Med 1982; 27:334.

437. Marinaki AM, Escuredo E, et al: Genetic basis of hemolytic anemia caused by pyrimidine 5' nucleotidase deficiency. Blood 2001; 97:3327.

438. Beutler E, Carson D, et al: Metabolic compensation for profound erythrocyte adenylate kinase deficiency: A hereditary enzyme defect without hemolytic anemia. J Clin Invest 1983; 72:648.

439. Szeinberg A, Kahana D, et al: Hereditary deficiency of adenylate kinase in red blood cells. Acta Haematol 1969; 42:111.

440. Toren A, Brok-Simoni F, et al: Congenital haemolytic anaemia associated with adenylate kinase deficiency. Br J Haematol 1994; 87:376.

441. Lachant NA, Zerez CR, et al: Hereditary erythrocyte adenylate kinase deficiency: A defect of phosphotransferases. Blood 1991; 77:2774.

442. Boivin P, Galand C, et al: Anémie hémolytique congénitale non sphérocytaire et déficit héréditaire en adenylate kinase érythrocytaire. Presse Med 1971; 79:215.

443. Miwa S, Fujii H, et al: Red cell adenylate kinase deficiency associated with hereditary nonspherocytic hemolytic anemia: Clinical and biochemical studies. Am J Hematol 1983; 14:325.

444. Matsuura S, Igarashi M, et al: Human adenylate kinase deficiency associated with hemolytic anemia. A single base substitution affecting solubility and catalytic activity of the cytosolic adenylate kinase. J Biol Chem 1989; 264:10148.

445. Qualtieri A, Pedace V, et al: Severe erythrocyte adenylate kinase deficiency due to homozygous ArG substitution at codon 164 of human AK gene associated with chronic haemolytic anaemia. Br J Haematol 1997; 99:770.

446. Bianchi P, Zappa M, et al: A case of complete adenylate kinase deficiency due to a nonsense mutation in AK-1 gene (Arg 107→stop, CGA→TGA) associated with chronic haemolytic anaemia. Br J Haematol 1999; 105:75.

447. Valentine WN, Paglia DE, et al: Hereditary hemolytic anemia with increased red cell adenosine deaminase (45- to 70-fold) and decreased adenosine triphosphate. Science 1977; 195:783.

448. Miwa S, Fujii H, et al: A case of red-cell adenosine deaminase overproduction associated with hereditary hemolytic anemia found in Japan. Am J Hematol 1978; 5:107.

449. Perignon JL, Hamet M, et al: Biochemical study of a case of hemolytic anemia with increased (85-fold) cell adenosine deaminase. Clin Chim Acta 1982; 124:205.

450. Kanno H, Tani K, et al: Adenosine deaminase (ADA) overproduction associated with congenital hemolytic anemia: Case report and molecular analysis. Jpn J Exp Med 1988; 58:1.

451. Fujii H, Miwa S, et al: Purification and properties of adenosine deaminase in normal and hereditary hemolytic anemia with increased red cell activity. Hemoglobin 1980; 4:693.

452. Chottiner EG, Cloft HJ, et al: Elevated adenosine deaminase activity and hereditary hemolytic anemia. Evidence for abnormal translational control of protein synthesis. J Clin Invest 1987; 79:1001.

453. Fujii H, Miwa S, et al: Overproduction of structurally normal enzyme in man: Hereditary haemolytic anaemia with increased red cell adenosine deaminase activity. Br J Haematol 1982; 51:427. 451.

454. Chottiner EG, Ginsburg D, et al: Erythrocyte adenosine deaminase overproduction in hereditary hemolytic anemia. Blood 1989; 74:448.

455. Chen EH, Tartaglia AP, et al: Hereditary overexpression of adenosine deaminase in erythrocytes: Evidence for a *cis*-acting mutation. Am J Hum Genet 1993; 53:889.

456. Chen EH, Mitchell B: Hereditary overexpression of adenosine deaminase in erythrocytes: Studies in erythroid cell lines and transgenic mice. Blood 1994; 84:2346.

457. Glader BE, Backer K, et al: Elevated erythrocyte adenosine deaminase activity in congenital hypoplastic anemia. N Engl J Med 1983; 309:1486.

458. Glader BE, Backer K: Comparative activity of erythrocyte adenosine deaminase and orotidine decarboxylase in Diamond-Blackfan anemia. Am J Hematol 1986; 23:135.

459. Novelli G, Stocchi, et al: Increased erythrocyte adenosine deaminase activity without haemolytic anaemia. Hum Hered 1986; 36:37.

460. Cowan MJ, Brady RO, et al: Elevated erythrocyte adenosine deaminase activity in patients with acquired immunodeficiency syndrome. Proc Natl Acad Sci USA 1986; 83:1089.

461. Sanchez-Corona J, Garcia-Cruz D, et al: Increased adenosine deaminase activity in a patient with cartilage-hair hypoplasia. Ann Genet 1990; 33:99.

462. Lichtman MA, Miller DR: Erythrocyte glycolysis, 2,3-diphosphoglycerate and adenosine triphosphate concentration in uremic subjects: Relationship to extracellular phosphate concentration. J Lab Clin Med 1970; 76:267.

463. Travis SF, Sugarman HJ, et al: Red cell metabolic alterations induced by intravenous hyperalimentation. N Engl J Med 1971; 285:63.

464. Lichtman MA, Miller DR, et al: Energy metabolism in uremic red cells: Relationship of red cell adenosine triphosphate concentration to extracellular phosphate. Trans Assoc Am Physicians 1969; 82:331.

465. Jacob HS, Amsden T: Acute hemolytic anemia with rigid red cells in hypophosphatemia. N Engl J Med 1971; 285:1446.

466. Weed RI, LaCelle PL, et al: Metabolic dependence of red cell deformability. J Clin Invest 1969; 48:795.

467. Oken MM, Lichtman MA, et al: Spherocytic hemolytic disease during magnesium deprivation in the rat. Blood 1971; 38:468.

468. Piomelli S, Jansen V, et al: The hemolytic anemia of magnesium deficiency in adult rats. Blood 1973; 41:451.

469. Elin RJ, Tan HK: Erythrocyte membrane plaques from rats with magnesium deficiency. Blood 1977; 49:657.

470. MacDougall LG, Judisch JM, et al: Red cell metabolism in iron deficiency anemia. II. The relationship between red cell survival and alterations in red cell metabolism. J Pediatr 1970; 76:660.

471. MacDougall LG: Red cell metabolism in iron deficiency anemia. J. Pediatr 1968; 71:303.

472. Slawsky P, Desforge JF: Erythrocyte 2,3-diphosphoglycerate in iron deficiency. Arch Intern Med 1972; 129:914.

473. Brewer GJ: Metabolism of ATP in thalassemic and iron-deficient erythrocytes. J Lab Clin Med 1967; 7:1016.

474. Card RT, Weintraub LR: Metabolic abnormalities of erythrocytes in severe iron deficiency. Blood 1971; 37:725.

475. Kimura H, Horiuchi N, et al: Hormonal response of glycolytic key enzymes of erythrocytes in insulinoma. Metabolism 1971; 20:1119.

476. Butenandt O: Erythrocytic enzyme activities in hypothyroid children. Acta Haematol 1972; 47:335.

477. Snyder LM, Reddy WJ: Thyroid hormone control of erythrocyte 2,3-diphosphoglyceric acid. Science 1970; 169:879.

478. Boivin P, Galand C, et al: Acquired erythroenzymopathies in blood disorders: Study of 200 cases. Br J Haematol 1975; 31:531.

479. Valentine WN, Crookston JH, et al: Erythrocyte enzymatic abnormalities in HEMPAS (hereditary erythroblastic multinuclearity with a positive acidified-serum test). Br J Haematol 1972; 23:107.

480. Valentine WN, Konrad PN, et al: Dyserythropoiesis, refractory anemia, and "preleukemia": Metabolic features of the erythrocytes. Blood 1973; 41:857.

481. Wang WC, Mentzer WC: Differentiation of transient erythroblastopenia of childhood from congenital hypoplastic anemia. J. Pediatr 1976; 88:784.

482. Kahn A: Abnormalities of erythrocyte enzymes in dyserythropoiesis and malignancies. Clin Haematol 1981; 10:123.

483. Tani K, Fujii H, et al: Erythrocyte activities in myelodysplastic syndromes: Elevated pyruvate kinase activity. Am J Hematol 1989; 30:97.

484. Kahn A, Mane J, et al: Mechanisms of the acquired erythrocyte enzyme deficiencies in blood diseases. Clin Chim Acta 1976; 71:379.

17 | Glucose-6-Phosphate Dehydrogenase Deficiency and Hemolytic Anemia

Lucio Luzzatto

Most hemolytic anemias can be neatly categorized, at least in first approximation, as being either inherited or acquired, either due to intracorpuscular or to extracorpuscular causes. Hemolytic anemia associated with deficiency of glucose-6-phosphate dehydrogenase (G6PD) glaringly defies this categorization. Indeed, the majority of persons with inherited G6PD deficiency have no anemia and almost no hemolysis. They develop both only as a result of challenge by exogenous agents. Because the metabolic role of G6PD in red blood cells is primarily related to its reductive potential, the threat to G6PD-deficient red cells is that of oxidative damage. Thus, to understand hemolytic anemia associated with G6PD deficiency we need to define the physiologic role of G6PD[1-3] and to find out why the red cells are G6PD deficient,[4-6] and why proliferating cells may also be sensitive to G6PD deficiency due to oxidant damage to DNA repair enzymes[7] and AMP deaminase,[8] despite the fact that G6PD-deficient stem cells can serve effectively in bone marrow transplantation.[9]*

G6PD IN RED CELL METABOLISM

The time-honored phrase hexose monophosphate shunt, or pentose phosphate pathway, conveys a somewhat preconceived notion that this sequence of reactions, of which G6PD is the first (Fig. 17–1), is a sideline to glycolysis, contributing little (usually less than 10%) to glucose utilization.[1, 10] It is now clear that the hexose monophosphate shunt is not necessary for glucose utilization; and it is not necessary for pentose synthesis either, because this sugar can be produced through the concerted action of transketolase and transaldolase. In fact, the main role of the so-called pentose phosphate pathway is the production of the reduced form of nicotinamide adenine dinucleotide phosphate (NADPH), which, in turn, is closely related to the metabolism of glutathione (GSH). GSH is of key importance in all cells, for the preservation of sulfhydryl groups in numerous proteins and to prevent oxidative damage in general (Fig. 17–2). This role is particularly crucial in red cells because, being oxygen carriers *par excellence*, they have a literally built-in danger of damage by oxygen radicals, generated continuously in the course of methemoglobin formation.[11] The highly reactive oxygen radicals either decay spontaneously or are converted by superoxide dismutase to hydrogen peroxide (H_2O_2), which is still highly toxic. H_2O_2 detoxification to H_2O is effected by glutathione peroxidase (GSHPX);[12, 13]† one molecule of GSH is oxidized to GSSG for every molecule of H_2O_2 detoxified, and

---

*Only selected references are given in this chapter. For a more extensive bibliography the reader is referred to several reviews that have surveyed extensively the area of G6PD and G6PD deficiency.[4–6, 70, 79]

---

†An alternative to GSHPX in effecting H_2O_2 detoxification is catalase. In first approximation this alternative[195] does not seem to be important in red cells, since acatalasemia is not associated with hemolysis. However, it is interesting that NADPH is an integral constituent of catalase,[12] and it has been suggested that the contribution of catalase to H_2O_2 detoxification may become comparable to that of GSHPX in G6PD-deficient red cells.[13]

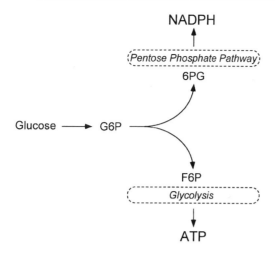

FIGURE 17–1. The role of glucose-6-phosphate dehydrogenase (G6PD) in red blood cell glucose metabolism. As a somewhat crude oversimplification, glucose can be visualized, after phosphorylation to glucose 6-phosphate (G6P), as being at the bifurcation between two major pathways: glycolysis, producing high-energy phosphate (adenosine triphosphate [ATP]), and the pentose phosphate pathway, generating reducing power (reduced nicotinamide adenine dinucleotide phosphate [NADPH]). Under "normal" conditions, probably less than 1 percent of G6P enters the pentose phosphate pathway; under maximal oxidative stress, the amount may reach 10 percent. The G6PD reaction is the first and rate-limiting step of the pentose phosphate pathway. 6PG = 6-phosphoglycerate; F6P = fructose 6-phosphate.

therefore GSH can only fulfill its functional role if it is continuously and stoichiometrically regenerated to GSH by glutathione reductase. Thus, GSH can be regarded as the key compound in preventing endogenous as well as exogenous oxidative damage (see later).

Structure and Biochemistry of G6PD

G6PD is a ubiquitous enzyme that must be quite ancient in evolution because it has been found in all organisms, from prokaryotes to yeasts, to protozoa, to plants and animals.[2, 14] In mammals, G6PD is a typical cytoplasmic enzyme, although some G6PD activity is associated with peroxisomes in liver and kidney cells.[15] This is interesting in view of the fact that these organelles are thought to have evolved as part of the need of early eukaryotes to defend

against oxygen, which is germane to the role of G6PD today.

The enzymatically active form of G6PD is either a dimer or a tetramer of a single polypeptide subunit of about 59 kd.[16] The complete primary structure of the human enzyme has been deduced from the sequence of a full-length complementary DNA clone.[17] The amino acid sequence of rat liver G6PD shows 94% homology to the human sequence and provides evidence that the N-terminal amino acid is N-acetylalanine, which must result from post-translational cleavage of the N-terminal methionine. The same is probably true of the human enzyme.[18] The tertiary structure of the molecule has been determined (Fig. 17–3).[19]

Extensive data are available on the kinetics of G6PD (Table 17–1). The coenzyme specificity is exquisite, in the sense that human G6PD has practically no activity with NAD. The substrate specificity is also very high, because activity on other hexose phosphates (e.g., mannose 6-P or galactose 6-P) is negligible.* By contrast, there is significant activity on substrate analogues, such as desamino-NADP and 2-deoxyglucose 6-P. These compounds, although artificial, have been useful in the characterization of variants (see later). The affinity for NADP is about one order of magnitude higher than the affinity for G6P. There is evidence that the G6P-binding site is near Lys[205], because this residue can be specifically labeled with pyridoxal 5-phosphate and this reaction is prevented by G6P itself.[20] The critical role of this amino acid has been confirmed by showing that its replacement with threonine (produced artificially by site-directed mutagenesis), nearly abolishes catalytic activity.[21] Moreover, by purifying to homogeneity recombinant human G6PD produced in *Escherichia coli*, it has been shown that Lys[205] is essential for electron transfer rather than for G6P binding.[22]

By contrast, biochemical labeling of the NADP-binding site has proven difficult, and therefore its location remained uncertain. The crystal structure of the G6P from the

---

*Hexose dehydrogenase, active on these compounds and also on non-phosphorylated hexose sugars, is an enzyme encoded by an autosomal gene expressed in the liver,[196] quite different from G6PD.

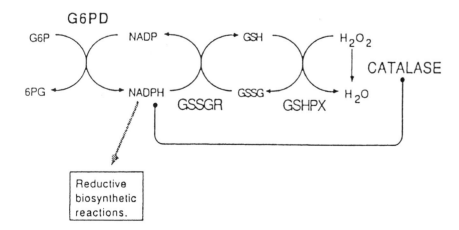

FIGURE 17–2. G6PD and the glutathione (GSH) cycle. The front-line defense against oxidative damage by hydrogen peroxide (H_2O_2) is GSH, by means of GSH peroxidase (GSHPX). GSHPX uses up GSH, and its regeneration can be effected only in the red blood cell through GSH reductase (GSSGR) by NADPH, which is ultimately provided by G6PD. NADP = nicotinamide adenine dinucleotide phosphate; GSSG = glutathione disulfide. (From Luzzatto L, Mehta A: Glucose 6-phosphate dehydrogenase deficiency. In Scriver CR, Beaudet AL, et al (eds): Molecular Basis of Inherited Disease, 7th ed. New York, McGraw-Hill, 1995, pp 3367–3398.)

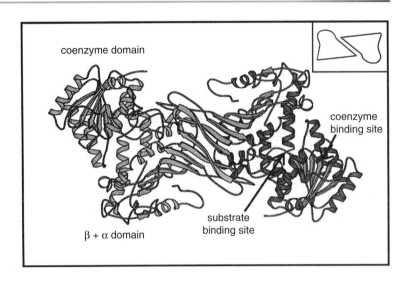

FIGURE 17–3. Model of the human dimer. In this figure, subunit P is equivalent to subunit A in published illustrations of the dimer of *Leuconostoc mesenteroides* G6PD.[6] The monomer consists of two domains—a smaller coenzyme domain encompassing residues 1 to 198 and a larger β + α domain comprising residues 199 to 515. The sequence GASGDLA (residues 38 to 44) is at the coenzyme binding site (arrow). The G6P binding site includes residues from the perfectly conserved 9-amino acid sequence RIDHYLGKE (198 to 206). Three adjacent strands of the β-sheet of the β + α domain (residues 380 to 425) are in the area of the dimer interface. (From Naylor CD, Rowland P, et al: Glucose 6-phosphate dehydrogenase mutations causing enzyme deficiency in a model of the tertiary structure of the human enzyme. Blood 1996; 87:2974.)

microorganism *Leuconostoc mesenteroides* has been solved at a resolution of 2.8 Å,[23] and, based on this structure, a model of the human G6PD dimer has been obtained.[24] This analysis has placed the NADP binding site at a fan of β-sheet structures, with a critical G-X-X-G-X-X peptide motif corresponding to amino acids 38 to 43 in exon 3.

Although many natural and non-natural substances can affect the activity of G6PD, it is not certain which ones may be important physiologically. NADPH, one product of the G6PD reaction, is a potent quasi-competitive inhibitor,[25] and because most of the coenzyme in cells is in the reduced form,[26] it can be assumed that G6PD is normally under strong inhibition. Because the K_m values for both G6P and NADP are higher than their normal respective intracellular concentrations, it is likely that these two substrates themselves are the main regulators of intracellular G6PD activity, together with NADPH. Any oxidative event affecting the cell will alter the NADPH/NADP ratio in favor of NADP. The simultaneous increase in NADP and decrease in NADPH act additively to increase G6PD activity by increasing the substrate drive on the reaction rate and decreasing product inhibition.[27] Under most conditions this may be the most important short-term regulatory signal, although it is, of course, possible that other regulatory effects play a role as well.

FEATURES OF G6PD IN RED CELLS

Biochemical evidence is in keeping with the notion that the G6PD protein in red cells is the same as in other somatic cells. This is supported by genetic evidence. Indeed, there is only one structural gene for G6PD in the human genome (see later); and when red cells are severely G6PD deficient, this deficiency is found to a greater or lesser degree also in other somatic cells.[10] However, a significant difference in the metabolism of G6PD arises from the characteristic inability of mature red cells to synthesize protein. As a result, whereas in most somatic cells G6PD is subject to turnover, in red cells any G6PD molecule undergoing denaturation or proteolytic breakdown cannot be replaced (this is true, of course, not only of G6PD but of most other red cell enzymes as well[28]). In normal red cells, the decay of G6PD approximates an exponential with a half-life of about 60 days,[29] although it has been claimed that it may approximate more closely a two-slope curve with a very fast breakdown when reticulocytes mature to erythrocytes and a much slower breakdown subsequently.[30] The age-dependence of red cell G6PD activity is so characteristic that it can be regarded almost as a marker of red cell age. In normal blood, reticulocytes have about five times more activity than the 10% oldest red cells.[31]

Genetics of G6PD

A NOTE ON TERMINOLOGY

G6PD is the accepted abbreviation for the enzyme glucose-6-phosphate dehydrogenase (E.C. 1.1.1.49). The G6PD gene is designated *Gd*.[4, 14] In this chapter, the terms *G6PD normal* and *G6PD deficient* are used to designate phenotypes of persons; G6PD(+) and G6PD(−) are used to designate the phenotype of individual cells.

TABLE 17–1. Distinctive Biochemical Properties of Individual Glucose-6-Phosphate Dehydrogenase Variants

Variant	Class	Activity (% of Normal)	Electrophoretic Mobility (% of Normal)	K_m of G6P (μmol/L)	Activity on 2 day G6P (% of Normal)
Normal (B)	IV	100	100	70	5
A⁻	III	13	110	70	5
Mediterranean	II	3	100	25	50
Harilaou	I	2	95	90	8

G6P = glucose 6-phosphate.

Because *Gd* is X-linked, males can be only normal hemizygotes (*Gd⁺*) or deficient hemizygotes (*Gd⁻*); females can be normal homozygotes (*Gd⁺/Gd⁺*), deficient homozygotes (*Gd⁻/Gd⁻*), or heterozygotes (*Gd⁺ / Gd⁻*). The phenotype of the last group is often referred to as "intermediate," because usually their overall red cell G6PD level lies in between the normal and the deficient range: however, exceptions do occur (see later). Because the majority of G6PD-deficient persons are mostly asymptomatic, their G6PD deficiency is referred to as mild, simple, or common; the minority of persons who have congenital nonspherocytic hemolytic anemia (CNSHA) are referred to as having rare, sporadic, or severe G6PD deficiency.

CYTOGENETICS AND MOLECULAR GENETICS

Because G6PD is an oligomer of a single polypeptide chain, its structure is fully specified by a single gene located in the telomeric region of the long arm of the X-chromosome[32–38] (band Xq28) (Fig. 17–4).★ The G6PD gene, *Gd*, is genetically and physically closely linked to the genes encoding factor VIII and to those encoding the retinal pigments[39] (whose mutations are responsible for colorblindness). This region of the X chromosome is one of the best mapped in the human genome,[40, 41] with several polymorphic loci being in strong linkage disequilibrium with G6PD itself;[42, 43] the entire G6PD genomic gene has been fully sequenced,[44] as well as more than 200 kb of DNA surrounding it.† A recently constructed website offers an integrated database of G6PD mutations,[45] and regional mutations continue to be reported.[46]

X-linkage of *Gd* has naturally two important consequences: (1) *Gd* mutations display the typical pattern of mendelian X-linked inheritance. (2) As a result of the phenomenon of X-chromosome inactivation, to which the *Gd* locus is subject, females heterozygous for two different alleles exhibit somatic cell mosaicism.[47] This means that, if one of the alleles entails enzyme deficiency, about one half of the cells will be G6PD(+) and the other half will be G6PD(−). Because of this, G6PD deficiency should not be regarded as a recessive, but rather as a co-dominant, trait.

At the genomic level, the *Gd* gene (Fig. 17–5) consists of 13 exons, the first one of which is noncoding.[48] The total length of the gene, which has been fully sequenced,[44] is about 18.5 kb, much of which (about 12 kb) consists of intron II. The promoter region is highly enriched in guanine and cytosine residues (i.e., GC rich), as found characteristically in other housekeeping genes analyzed so far.[33] Deletion analysis has revealed that the "essential" portion of the promoter is only about 150 bp long.[49] Within this region, two Sp1-binding sites have been identified, either of which is essential for promoter activity.[50] The significance of the large intron is unknown: it may be

*It has been claimed that a portion of the G6PD protein is encoded by an autosomal gene mapped to chromosome 6.[34] However, this latter gene turns out to encode instead guanosine monophosphate reductase,[33] and the claim has been refuted[32, 35] and subsequently retracted.[197]

†GDB accession number X55448, and Chen E: Personal communication, 1994.

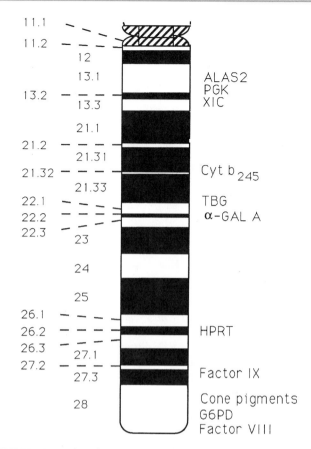

FIGURE 17–4. The telomeric region of the long arm of the X chromosome. The G6PD gene maps very close to the Xq27.3 fragile site, to colorblindness, and to the hemophilia A (factor VIII) gene. Physical linkage between the G6PD and the factor VIII genes has been established: they are only 400 kb apart from each other. ALAS2 = aminolerulinic acid synthetase 2; PGK = phosphoglycerate kinase; XIC = X inactivation center; Cyt *b* = cytochrome b; TBG = thyroid-binding globulin; α-GAL A = α-galactose A; HPRT = hypoxanthine phosphoribosyltransferase.

important for efficient transcription or for processing, because it is still the largest intron even in the compressed version of the G6PD gene found in *Fugu rubripes* (a type of puffer fish).[51]

G6PD DEFICIENCY IN HETEROZYGOTES

Gd⁺/Gd⁻ heterozygous women would be expected to have an approximately 1:1 ratio of G6PD(+) to G6PD(−) red cells, with an overall level of G6PD in a whole blood hemolysate equal to about 50% of normal. If a group of heterozygotes is analyzed, this is indeed found to be the modal value of G6PD activity; however, a wide range is observed.[52] The question of why in a heterozygote there may be a wide deviation from the theoretical 1:1 ratio of G6PD(+) to G6PD(−) red cells is incompletely solved. In first approximation it can be assumed that X-inactivation takes place completely at random, and therefore a binomial distribution would be expected: the width of this depends on the number of cells in the embryo at the time of X-inactivation. If this number is 32-64, a fraction of about 2% of women with an "extreme phenotype" is predicted, that is, with less than 5% of one of the two cell types: this is in good agreement with observation in an

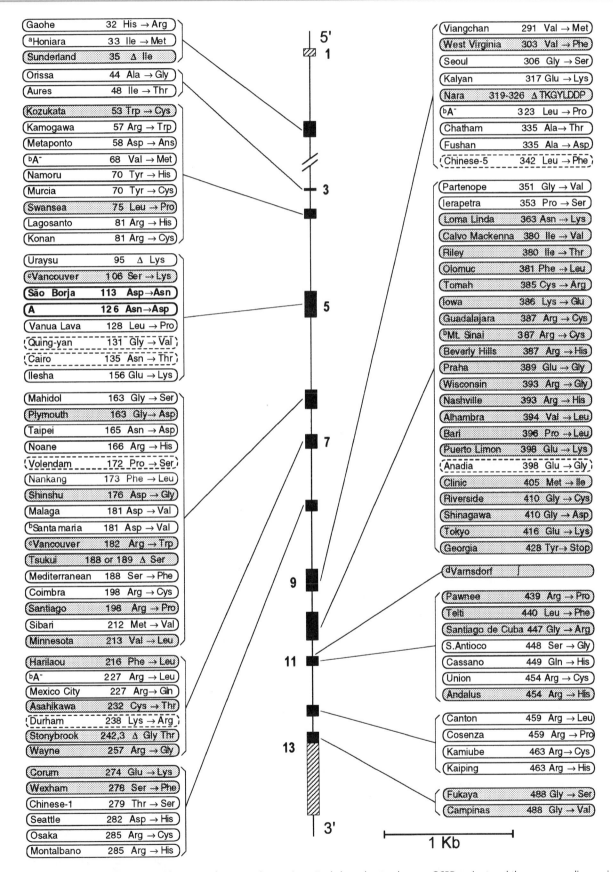

FIGURE 17–5. The human G6PD gene with a map of structural mutations. Each *boxed entry* shows a G6PD variant and the corresponding amino acid replacement. All variants shown, except G6PD A, are associated with enzyme deficiency. The *shaded boxes* indicate congenital nonspherocytic hemolytic anemia: these variants belong, by definition, to class I (see Table 17–1). The remaining variants belong to class II or III. Note that G6PD A⁻ is heterogeneous, because it can result from the combination of the Asn[126]→Asp replacement with any of three additional mutations. However, in the large majority of instances (probably more than 90 percent), the second mutation of G6PD A⁻ is Val[68]→Met. This figure includes only the variants for which the molecular basis has been elucidated. For more information see reference 53.

unselected sample of Gd^+/Gd^- heterozygotes,[53] although some studies have suggested an even larger proportion.[54] Thus, it seems likely that, in general, unbalanced phenotypes may arise simply by chance, according to the laws of statistics. However, in certain cases there is evidence of selection at the somatic cell level after X-chromosome inactivation. This is well established in women who are heterozygous for hypoxanthine phosphoribosyltransferase (HPRT) deficiency,[55] and it has been observed also in several women heterozygous for severely deficient G6PD variants.[56, 57] In these cases one has to infer that the G6PD(–) state is a selective disadvantage for hematopoietic stem cells; interestingly, this disadvantage is cell lineage specific, because it does not affect, for instance, fibroblasts.[56] Lastly, it seems reasonable to surmise that if selection can favor certain HPRT and certain G6PD alleles, the same notion can be extrapolated to alleles at other X-linked loci. Thus, heterozygotes exhibiting extreme phenotypes by analysis of G6PD may arise from selection acting on an allele at another locus (a "hitchhiking effect"), as has been suggested in a family with G6PD Ilesha.[58–61]*

Biochemical Basis of G6PD Deficiency

In principle, deficiency of G6PD, like that of any other protein, might be due to deletions or to point mutations affecting transcription, processing, or the primary structure. Careful testing of G6PD-deficient cells has uniformly revealed that the enzyme activity, even when very severely reduced (sometimes to less than 1% of normal), is never completely absent. This essentially rules out large deletions. Further analysis of enzymic properties of the residual G6PD activity has almost invariably revealed deviations from the properties of the normal enzyme,[10] suggesting that G6PD deficiency was due to structural abnormalities (i.e., mutations in the coding region) rather than merely to a decrease in number of normal molecules (as would be expected with transcriptional or processing mutants). Changes in the primary structure (i.e., substitutions of individual amino acids) can cause G6PD deficiency either by affecting its catalytic function or by decreasing the *in vivo* stability of the protein or by both of these mechanisms. It is likely that one or the other is the main factor responsible for G6PD deficiency in individual cases. For some variants, an accelerated *in vivo* breakdown has been demonstrated directly by assaying the activity of G6PD in age-fractionated red cells.[29, 62, 63] In extreme cases, G6PD deficiency can be visualized simply as resulting from a marked change in the exponential decay constant of the enzyme, whereby the half-life becomes, instead of 50 days, 10 days or even less. In such cases the G6PD activity of reticulocytes may be practically normal.

---

*The use of G6PD as a marker to analyze the clonal origin of neoplastic cell populations[58, 59, 198] is discussed elsewhere.[6] "Homogeneous with respect to G6PD" is not synonymous with "monoclonal" because this situation could arise through somatic cell selection rather than common origin from a single cell. By contrast, if a cell population does have a mixed phenotype with respect to G6PD, it cannot be monoclonal.

Molecular Basis of G6PD Deficiency

Since the cloning of the G6PD gene,[17] and especially since the introduction of polymerase chain reaction amplification of individual exons or groups of exons,[64] the analysis of G6PD mutations has been relatively easy, and there is now a database of about 100 variants characterized at the molecular level[65] (see Fig. 17–5). From this set of mutants a reasonably clear pattern is beginning to emerge for the molecular basis of G6PD deficiency. First, in nearly all the G6PD variants there is a single amino acid replacement, caused by a single missense point mutation. In a few cases (the three types of "A–" variant, G6PD Santamaria and G6PD Mount Sinai) two amino acid replacements are found, and in all of these one of the replacements is that of G6PD A. Because this variant is polymorphic in Africa, the most likely explanation is that a second point mutation has taken place in a Gd^A gene. In one case, three separate amino acid replacements have been reported (G6PD Vancouver): although this finding is thus far unique, one of these replacements is the same as that in G6PD Coimbra, which is polymorphic in the Mediterranean area. Only one mutation affecting splicing has been discovered and only three in-frame deletions—of a single amino acid (G6PD Sunderland), of two adjacent amino acids (G6PD Stonybrook), and of eight amino acids (G6PD Nara), respectively.

Thus, the predictions made by biochemical analysis have been largely validated, in that all mutations are compatible with some residual activity and all have the potential to affect the kinetic properties, the stability of the enzyme, or both. Unlike in many other inherited disorders (e.g., thalassemias, hemophilia, muscular dystrophy), large deletions or major rearrangements have been conspicuous by their absence. An important functional difference between these conditions and G6PD deficiency is that the former result from mutations in tissue-specific genes, whereas G6PD is a housekeeping gene. If a tissue-specific gene is totally inactivated by a mutation, it may not interfere with embryonic development but it may cause severe disease in the respective tissue in the adult. By contrast, at least a low level of G6PD activity may be indispensable for the majority of cells; and, therefore, complete inactivation of the gene (e.g., by a large deletion) may be lethal early in embryonic life, even though it allows the survival of embryonic stem cells.[66]

If G6PD deletions are not encountered because the gene is indispensable, can we identify any rule as to why certain point mutations are seen in preference to others? In this respect some speculations can be offered:

1. *Sporadic mutations.* These are probably the majority, and most of them have been detected because they cause clinical manifestations in the form of CNSHA, by causing sufficient loss of activity in red cells to become limiting for their *in vivo* survival. This, in turn, may result, in principle, from two (non–mutually exclusive) mechanisms: (a) severe alterations in the interaction with the substrates, particularly G6P, and (b) marked intracellular instability. Sporadic variants associated with CNSHA are not likely to spread by genetic drift. Thus, the fact that the same variant may be found recurrently and

independently in people who are almost certainly not ancestrally related is not trivial. The authors have found, for instance, G6PD Tokyo in Scotland,[67] whereas G6PD Guadalajara has been reported in Japan[68] and in Belfast.[67, 69] These observations corroborate the notion that subtle constraints make a sporadic variant have a distinctly severe clinical expression while remaining compatible with life.

2. *Polymorphic mutations.* The majority of known mutations in this category are again associated with G6PD deficiency, and there is overwhelming evidence that these have become polymorphic as a result of malaria selection (see later). For these mutations we can visualize more stringent constraints: indeed, although still causing deficiency in red cells, they must not affect them so severely as to outweigh the advantage with respect to malaria. Thus, it is not surprising that nearly all the polymorphic variants fall in classes II or III, and none of them causes CNSHA (class I). Finally, as for other protein polymorphisms, electrophoretically silent, and therefore hitherto undetected, G6PD variants are likely to exist as well.

CLINICAL MANIFESTATIONS OF G6PD DEFICIENCY

The most classic manifestation of G6PD deficiency is acute hemolytic anemia (AHA); in children, however, another syndrome of great clinical and public health importance is neonatal jaundice (NNJ). CNSHA is a much more rare manifestation of G6PD deficiency and a life-long hemolytic process. These different clinical manifestations are now discussed in turn.[1, 70, 71]

Acute Hemolytic Anemia

Clinical Picture. A child with G6PD deficiency is clinically and hematologically normal most of the time, and this can be designated as a steady-state condition.[72] What happens in a situation of "oxidative challenge" after a drug challenge or even the application of henna to the hair[73] has been best characterized after ingestion of fava beans (favism).[74] After a period of hours the child may become fractious and irritable or subdued and even lethargic. Within 24 to 48 hours there is often a moderate elevation of the temperature (up to 38°C). There may be nausea, abdominal pain, and diarrhea and rarely vomiting. In striking contrast to these relatively unspecific symptoms, the patient or a parent will observe, within 6 to 24 hours, the telltale and rather frightening event that the urine is discolored (Fig. 17–6): it will be reported as dark, or red, or brown, or black, or as "passing blood instead of water"; it will be stated, depending on experience, culture, and socio-economic background, as resembling Coca-Cola or strong tea or port wine. At about the same time jaundice will become obvious. Physical examination may reveal little more than the signs corresponding to these symptoms. The child will be invariably pale and tachycardic; in severe cases there may be evidence of hypovolemic shock or, less likely, of heart failure. The spleen is usually moderately enlarged, and the liver also may be enlarged; either or both may be tender.

Laboratory Findings. Anemia may be from moderate to extremely severe (hemoglobin values of 2.5 g/dL have been recorded). In the absence of other pre-existing hematologic abnormalities the anemia is normocytic and normochromic. The morphology of the red cells may be striking (Fig. 17–7). There is often marked anisocytosis (reflected in a wide red cell size distribution on the electronic counter), owing to the coexistence of large polychromatic cells and of "contracted" cells, some of which can be frankly classified as spherocytes. There is also marked poikilocytosis, with presence of distorted red cells, of "irregularly contracted" red cells, and of red cells with apparently uneven distribution of the hemoglobin inside them (hemighosts[75]). Although some of these appearances are probably smearing artifacts, electron micrographic evidence suggests that in some of the cells opposing surfaces of the membrane have become "crosslinked."[76] Probably the most characteristic poikilocytes are those in which the cell margin appears literally dented, as though a portion has been plucked out or bitten away ("bite cells"; see Fig. 17–7). The reticulocyte count is increased and may reach peaks of 30% or more. Careful inspection of the reticulocyte preparations may reveal inclusion bodies different from those normally seen in reticulocytes, because they are discrete, round, and 1 to 3 μm in diameter, and they usually appear to be leaning, from the interior, against the cell membrane. These inclusions are more clearly displayed by supravital staining with methyl violet, when they are referred to as Heinz bodies. They consist of precipitates of denatured hemoglobin, and they are the vivid manifestation of the oxidative insult that this protein and the cell itself has suffered. Although Heinz bodies are a classic and characteristic finding, it is important to realize that it is a very transient finding, because the Heinz bodies are "pinched off" by the spleen[77] (thus giving rise to the bite cells), and the red cells containing them are very rapidly removed from the circulation. Haptoglobin is reduced to the point of being undetectable. In severe cases it is possible to demonstrate free hemoglobin in the plasma (the somewhat incongruous term of *hemoglobinemia* is used to describe this finding in one word). The white blood cell count is usually moderately elevated, with predominance of granulocytes. The platelet count may be normal, increased, or moderately decreased. The unconjugated bilirubin level is elevated, but the "liver enzyme" levels are usually normal. The dark urine tests strongly positive for blood. It is easy to demonstrate that this is due to free hemoglobin because after centrifugation the supernatant is as dark as before and in the sediment there are few if any red cells. (Patients are not always alone in confusing hemoglobinuria with hematuria. The importance for the physician of recognizing one from the other in the differential diagnosis of a patient with dark urine cannot be overemphasized) (Table 17–2).

Clinical Course. In the majority of cases the hemolytic attack, even if severe, is self-limited and tends to resolve spontaneously.[78] In the absence of additional or pre-existing pathology the bone marrow response is prompt and effective. Depending on the proportion of red cells that have been destroyed (reflected in the severity of

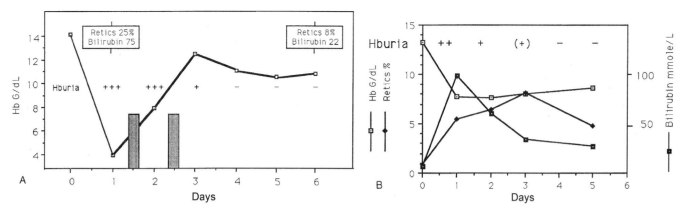

FIGURE 17–6. Clinical charts of children with acute favism. *A*, A severe attack in a 21-month-old boy, who required two blood transfusions (*hatched bars*) because of life-threatening anemia after ingestion of fava beans. The second blood transfusion was administered because of the persistent hemoglobinuria (Hburia). *B*, A milder attack in a 5-year-old boy. The mother, who is a physician and knows that she is G6PD deficient, reported that the child had eaten fava beans 2 days before admission. Both children had severe G6PD deficiency (red blood cell G6PD activity less than 3 percent of normal). The values on day 0 are presumed. Hb = hemoglobin; Retics = reticulocytes. (Courtesy of Professor Tullio Meloni, Sassari, Sardinia.)

the anemia), the hemoglobin level may be back to normal in 3 to 6 weeks. Although there may be transient elevation of the blood urea level, the development of renal failure in children is exceedingly rare, even in the presence of massive hemoglobinuria (see Fig. 17–6).

Diagnosis. With a history of fava bean ingestion and the finding of hemoglobinuria (clearly reported or directly observed), the diagnosis is almost always straightforward, and it can be made quite confidently even before obtaining the final proof that the patient is G6PD deficient (see later). The differential diagnosis of hemoglobinuria is given in Table 17–2. If hemoglobinuria has already subsided, and the history is uncertain, one is faced instead with the much wider differential diagnosis of an acute hemolytic anemia. The negative direct antiglobulin test will militate against autoimmune hemolytic anemia. In endemic areas it will be important to exclude malaria infection, or the much rarer babesiosis. In the hemolytic-uremic syndrome the red cell morphology is different and there will be evidence of impaired renal function. In all

cases the demonstration of G6PD deficiency will be conclusive, and in uncertain cases it will be crucial.

Pathophysiology. The very clinical picture of AHA associated with G6PD deficiency conveys forcefully the impression that, as stated at the beginning of this chapter, hemolysis results from the action of an exogenous factor on intrinsically abnormal red cells.[79] Hemoglobinemia and hemoglobinuria indicate unambiguously that the hemolysis is at least in part intravascular. In first approximation it is easy to visualize the following sequence of events: (1) An oxidative agent causes conversion of GSH to GSSG. (2) Owing to the limited capacity to regenerate GSH of G6PD deficient red cells, their GSH reserve is rapidly depleted. (3) Once GSH is exhausted, the sulfhydryl groups of hemoglobin and probably of other proteins are oxidized to disulfides or sulfoxides. (4) Coarse precipitates of denatured hemoglobin cause irreversible damage to the membrane and the red cells lyse.

Although GSH depletion is a classic *in vitro* finding when red cells are challenged, for instance, with

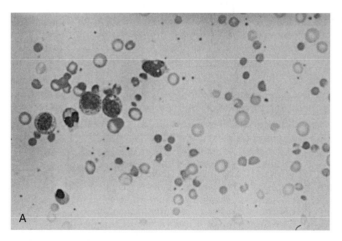
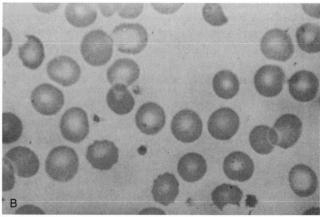

FIGURE 17–7. Blood smear in G6PD deficiency. *A*, Acute hemolytic anemia (favism). Marked morphologic abnormalities of red blood cells with anisocytosis, polychromasia, bizarre poikilocytes, "bite cells," and "hemighosts." Note the nucleated red blood cell and polymorph leukocytosis with marked shift to the left. *B*, Chronic nonspherocytic hemolytic anemia. The morphologic abnormalities are much less pronounced, but several poikilocytes and the occasional bite cells are seen.

TABLE 17–2. Hemoglobinuria in Children

Condition	Circumstances	Diagnostic Approach
G6PD deficiency	Exposure to trigger of hemolysis	Test for G6PD activity
Blackwater fever	Relatively rare complication of malaria	Blood slide for malaria parasites
Paroxysmal cold hemoglobinuria	Usually associated with viral infection	Search for Donath-Landsteiner antibody
Mismatched blood transfusion	Usually, ABO incompatibility	Repeat crossmatch
Paroxysmal nocturnal hemoglobinuria	Very rare in children	Ham's test
Clostridium welchii septicemia	Burns; severe open trauma; transfusion of contaminated blood	Culture of blood or appropriate patient material

G6PD = glucose-6-phosphate dehydrogenase.

acetylphenylhydrazine,[80] not all of these steps have been fully documented *in vivo*.[81] One major difficulty in analyzing the sequential changes that take place in a patient with AHA from the oxidative attack to the final hemolysis is that red cells sampled from the patient are obviously, at any given stage, those that have not yet hemolyzed. However, in one careful study it has been demonstrated that in the course of an episode of favism the first measurable biochemical change is a fall in NADPH, followed by a fall in GSH,[82] in keeping with stages 1 and 2 described earlier. The Heinz bodies are the visible expression of stage 3. Stage 4 is more obscure, because it is not known exactly how the membrane is damaged, although studies suggest that binding of hemichromes (arising from hemoglobin denaturation) to band 3 molecules may be one intermediate step.[83, 84] Although the diagnostic and pathophysiologic importance of intravascular hemolysis has been emphasized, it is certain that not *all* of the hemolysis is intravascular, as witnessed, for instance, by the enlargement of the spleen. It is not difficult to visualize that the most severely damaged red cells will hemolyze in the blood stream without help, whereas less severely damaged red cells will be recognized as abnormal by macrophages and will undergo extravascular hemolysis in the reticuloendothelial system. This process has been referred to as an example of an "innocent bystander" phenomenon[85] (although the red cells, by virtue of being G6PD deficient, are not that innocent). The role of complement and of immunoglobulins in extravascular hemolysis of damaged G6PD-deficient red cells mediated by macrophages has been discussed in detail.[79]

The clinical picture of AHA impresses one as a sharp transition between the normal steady state and the hemolytic attack, as though the oxidative challenge had tipped the red cell over the hump of a smooth surface leading to a catastrophe. Some chromium-51-labeled red cell survival studies that have been carried out in the *absence* of overt hemolysis in G6PD-deficient subjects have revealed a half-life of 90 to 100 days[86] with some variants but an entirely normal red cell survival with others (A⁻).[87] Because hemolysis of such a low grade, if any, is undetectable on clinical or hematologic grounds, it is reasonable to refer to these subjects as having only acute and not chronic hemolysis.

Finally, it is a very important feature of red cell destruction in AHA associated with G6PD deficiency that it is an orderly function of red cell age. The oldest red cells with the least G6PD are the first to hemolyze, and the

hemolytic process progresses upstream toward the cells with more and more G6PD.[88] As a result, there is a selective enrichment in red cells that, although genetically G6PD deficient, have relatively higher levels of G6PD. This phenomenon can be so marked with certain G6PD variants that patients in the posthemolytic state are found to be relatively resistant to further challenge. Under these circumstances,[51] Cr-labeled red cell survival studies will show that this is less than normal, demonstrating that the patient is in a state of compensated hemolysis.[78]

Triggers and Mechanism of Hemolysis. Favism has been used here as a prototypical example of AHA associated with G6PD deficiency, but fava beans are not the only exogenous agent that can cause this manifestation. Indeed, G6PD deficiency was first discovered in the course of investigations on the genetic basis for sensitivity to primaquine. Since that time, numerous other drugs have been reported as potentially dangerous in G6PD-deficient individuals (Table 17–3). There is no obvious relationship in chemical structure among all of these substances, but they have in common the ability to stimulate the pentose phosphate pathway in red cells,[89] which must mean that they are able to oxidize NADPH, directly or indirectly. Extensive studies on the components of fava beans responsible for hemolysis have led to the identification of vicine and convicine, two β-glycosides having as aglycones the substituted pyrimidines divicine and isouramil.[90] These compounds, in the course of their auto-oxidation produce free radicals, which, in turn, oxidize GSH, activating the chain reaction of events previously outlined.[91] The drugs listed in Table 17–3, or their metabolites, act in a similar way.

An intriguing feature of AHA associated with G6PD deficiency is its considerably erratic character, which is more conspicuous with certain agents than with others. For instance, it is estimated that in adults ingestion of fava beans does not trigger AHA in more than 25% of cases, and even in the same person favism may occur on one occasion but not on another.[79] Whereas this should not make us complacent, especially with respect to G6PD-deficient children, it poses the question of why this is so. One obvious factor must be the dosage, that is, the amount of fava beans ingested (in relation to body mass). Another is the quality, whereby raw fava beans are more likely to cause favism than cooked, frozen, or canned fava beans. Perhaps even more important is the finding that the glycoside content is a function of the maturity of the beans, with the young, small beans being much richer (as well as more tasty!).

TABLE 17–3. Drugs to be Avoided in Glucose-6-Phosphate Dehydrogenase Deficiency

ANTIMALARIALS
Primaquine*
Pamaquine
Chloroquine† (may be used under surveillance when required for prophylaxis or treatment of malaria)

ANALGESICS
Aspirin§
Phenacetin‖

SULFONAMIDES AND SULFONES
Sulfanilamide
Sulfapyridine
Sulfadimidine
Sulfacetamide
Sulfisoxazole (Gantrisin)
Sulfasalazine
Dapsone‡
Sulfoxone‖
Glucosulfone sodium
Septrin (Glibenclamide)

ANTHELMINTHICS
β-Naphthol
Stibophen
Niridazole

OTHER ANTIBACTERIAL COMPOUNDS
Nitrofurans

Nitrofurantoin
Furazolidone
Nitrofurazone
[Nalidixic acid]
Chloramphenicol
p-Aminosalicylic acid
[Ciprofloxacin]

MISCELLANEOUS
Vitamin K analoges¶
Naphthalene
Probenecid
Dimercaprol (BAL)
Methylene blue

*Reduced dose can be given under surveillance if necessary.
†Can be given under surveillance if necessary.
‡These drugs may cause hemolysis in normal individuals if given in large doses. Many other drugs may produce hemolysis in particular individuals.
§Paracetamol acetaminophen is a safe alternative.
‖Moderate doses probably safe for most patients.
¶Menadiol, 1 mg, parenterally is safe for the prophylaxis of hemorrhagic disease of the newborn.
Drugs in **bold** print should be avoided by people with all forms of G6PD deficiency.
Drugs in normal print should be avoided, in addition, by persons of Mediterranean, Middle Eastern, or Asian origin with G6PD deficiency.
Drugs in brackets reflect single case reports or unpublished information.
Modified from WHO Working Group: Glucose 6-phosphate dehydrogenase deficiency. Bull WHO 1989; 67:601.

Finally, it is possible that β-glycosidases, present in varying amounts both in the beans and in the intestinal mucosa of the consumer, may play an important role in determining the amount and rate of release of active aglycones.[79] As for the drugs, primaquine causes hemolysis regularly but aspirin does so only sometimes.[92] Here it can only be hypothesized that genetic or acquired factors affecting the metabolism of the drug may be responsible.

A rather neglected trigger of hemolysis is bacterial infection (e.g., from pneumococcus).[93] It has been suggested that the mechanism of this may be the release of peroxides during phagocytosis of bacteria by granulocytes.[94] From the clinical point of view it is important to be aware of this complication. Indeed, it is likely that in the past hemolysis has been sometimes attributed to drugs used for treating infection, when it should have been blamed on the infection itself. It is more difficult to imagine a mechanism by which viral infection can trigger hemolysis, but this has been documented in the course of viral hepatitis.[95]

Neonatal Jaundice

Since the elucidation of the mechanism of hemolytic disease of the newborn (HDN) due to rhesus alloimmunization, it has been inevitable that jaundice from any cause developing in the neonatal period would be measured against that yardstick. However, from the epidemiologic point of view it is worth noting that in many populations where G6PD deficiency is prevalent there is a relatively low proportion of pregnancies at risk for rhesus incompatibility.[96, 97] However, as rhesus-related HDN is disappearing thanks to the implementation of appropriate prophylaxis, one can expect G6PD-related NNJ to be generally on the increase, at least in relative terms.

The clinical picture of NNJ related to G6PD deficiency differs (Fig. 17–8) from the classic rhesus-related NNJ in two main respects: (1) It is very rarely present at birth, and the peak incidence of clinical onset is between day 2 and day 3.[98] (2) There is more jaundice than anemia, and the anemia is very rarely severe.[99] For this reason the terms *HDN* and *NNJ* cannot be regarded as interchangeable, at least in the context of G6PD deficiency.

The severity of NNJ varies enormously from being subclinical to imposing the threat of kernicterus if not treated. Thus, prompt recognition of the problem is extremely important to avoid crippling neurologic sequelae.[100–103]

Nature of the Association Between G6PD Deficiency and NNJ. It is not clear why some but not all G6PD-deficient newborns develop NNJ. Indeed, because of this erratic character, one might question whether there is a causal link at all between the two. However, several clinical studies have established beyond any possible doubt that the association is statistically much higher than could be expected by chance (Table 17–4).[104] However, because not *all* G6PD-deficient newborns have NNJ, it is likely that some factor in addition to G6PD deficiency is involved and that the same factors that cause NNJ can also, if more extreme, make it severe. There has been an active search for an "additional factor" that may cause NNJ when combined with G6PD deficiency. Several studies have been carried out in an attempt to find such an additional factor. One possibility was that, in view of the marked genetic heterogeneity of G6PD deficiency (see later), NNJ was the prerogative of some but not of others. However, the finding that NNJ is prevalent in widely remote parts of the world (e.g., Sardinia,[105] Nigeria,[104] Singapore,[106] China[107]) does not support this notion. Moreover, NNJ was found among all three different G6PD variants known to be polymorphic in Sardinia.[108]*

Another possibility was that NNJ correlated with the quantitative level of residual G6PD activity in G6PD-defi-

*In some cases, variants reported as distinct and assigned different names have turned out to be identical at the molecular level,[137, 199] illustrating the limitations of biochemical analysis or implicating the possibility of postsynthetic modifications.

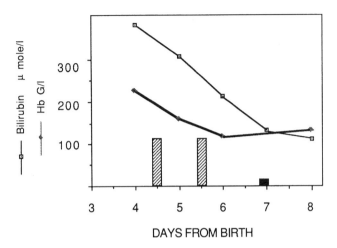

FIGURE 17–8. Clinical chart of a newborn with G6PD deficiency. The newborn was full term (weight at birth, 3200 g). The grandfather was known to have suffered from favism. Clinical jaundice was noted on day 3. The *light hatched bars* represent two full exchange blood transfusions. Red blood cell G6PD activity was less than 3 percent of normal. Notice that the newborn was not anemic before exchange blood transfusion. The subsequent anemia was corrected by a "top-up" packed cells transfusion (*solid bar*). The infant recovered fully. (Courtesy of Professor Tullio Meloni, Sassari, Sardinia.)

cient newborns, but this was also disproven.[109] Because it is known that fetal red cells differ from those produced after birth in many ways, a third possibility was that in the red cells of some newborns there might be a transient, developmentally related additional enzyme deficiency that, when superimposed on genetically determined G6PD deficiency, would cause NNJ. In this respect, studies have been carried out on glutathione peroxidase, glutathione reductase,[110] and superoxide dismutase,[111] but with negative results. Marked differences in the incidence of NNJ have been demonstrated among different Greek islands;[112] although the study was carried out in the search for an additional genetic factor, thought to be autosomal, it is possible instead that there may be an environmental factor that is different in different islands. In support of the latter possibility, work in Nigeria has revealed that G6PD-deficient newborns with NNJ had had a significantly higher rate of exposure to naphthalene (used in their beddings and clothing) than G6PD-deficient control newborns.[113]

In brief, it is not yet known why some G6PD-deficient newborns develop NNJ, nor are we able to predict which

ones will and which ones will not. This, in turn, is related to the question of pathogenesis. Because of the characteristic tendency of G6PD-deficient red cells to hemolyze, and because NNJ is classically the result of HDN, it has been almost taken for granted that NNJ in G6PD-deficient newborns is a manifestation of hemolysis. However, already for some years Meloni and co-workers[99, 105] have called attention to the remarkable dissociation between hyperbilirubinemia and anemia in these newborns; indeed, in one series there was no difference in the distribution of hematocrit values in the cord blood and on day 3 between jaundiced and nonjaundiced G6PD-deficient newborns. They have suggested, therefore, that in a majority of cases this jaundice may be not of hemolytic but of hepatic origin, a view that is still to some extent in dispute, but which has recently received further support.[114]

In summary, it may be heuristically useful to consider two different types of NNJ associated with G6PD deficiency. (1) A more common type can be best visualized as a marked exaggeration of "physiologic jaundice." This type is not greatly influenced by the environment, and it may result from G6PD deficiency being expressed in the liver. (2) A more rare, frankly hemolytic type, can be visualized as AHA occurring in a newborn because it happened to be exposed to one of the same agents that could cause AHA even in an adult.[115] Here the exogenous agent may be a drug, or infection such as viral hepatitis,[116] or some particular local habit, such as the extensive use of naphthalene ("moth balls" or "camphor balls") in looking after infants.[113] An extreme and preventable example of this type of AHA in the neonatal period, causing severe NNJ, has been reported in a girl heterozygous for G6PD deficiency whose mother had a fava beans meal before delivery. This infant has been described as having favism *in utero*.[117]

Congenital Nonspherocytic Hemolytic Anemia

As stated earlier, all G6PD-deficient individuals have a slightly reduced red cell survival. However, in the steady state the vast majority of them are clinically normal, and their low-grade hemolysis cannot be revealed by any laboratory method short of a chromium-51 study.[70, 118] By contrast, a small minority of G6PD-deficient individuals have a degree of hemolysis that is easily diagnosed by conventional methods and that is sufficiently pronounced to cause them to be anemic. This group of patients is clinically very heterogeneous, for reasons that are explained later; and, therefore, it is not possible to describe any level of expression of this condition as being "typical."

The patient is almost invariably male, and in general he presents because of unexplained jaundice. Frequently the onset is at birth, and a diagnosis is made of NNJ, which may be severe enough to require exchange transfusion. Unfortunately anemia recurs and the jaundice fails to clear completely; this is often the reason for further investigation. In many cases, however, NNJ may become forgotten and the patient is only reinvestigated much later in life (e.g., because of gallstones in a boy or in a young adult). The severity of anemia ranges in different patients from being borderline to being transfusion dependent. The anemia is usually normochromic but

TABLE 17–4. Association between Glucose-6-Phosphate Dehydrogenase Deficiency and Jaundice in Male Newborns

	No. of Newborns	G6PD Deficiency (%)
Normal	500	22.5
Mild jaundice (bilirubin 150-200 μmol/L)	38	45
Severe jaundice (bilirubin >230 μmol/L)	70	60
Admitted with kernicterus	20	78

Data collected in Ibadan, Nigeria (see reference 124 and Effiong C. Bienzle U, Luzzatto L: unpublished observations).

somewhat macrocytic, because a large proportion of reticulocytes (up to 20% or more) will cause an increased mean corpuscular volume and a shifted, wider than normal red cell size distribution curve. The red cell morphology is mostly not characteristic, and for this reason it is referred to in the negative as being "nonspherocytic." The bone marrow shows normoblastic hyperplasia, unless the increased requirement of folic acid associated with the high red cell turnover has caused it to become megaloblastic. There is chronic hyperbilirubinemia, decreased haptoglobin, and increased lactate dehydrogenase. Hemoglobinuria is rare, but hemosiderinuria may be detected sometimes. The spleen is usually moderately enlarged in small children, and subsequently it may increase in size sufficiently to cause mechanical discomfort, or hypersplenism, or both.

Pathophysiology. The clinical picture just described is obviously very different from that of AHA seen, for instance, in favism; and it is much more reminiscent of the chronic hemolysis seen in hereditary spherocytosis. Even in severe cases it is different from thalassemia major, because there is no evidence of ineffective erythropoiesis; accelerated destruction is limited to mature circulating red cells. The fact that there is no hemoglobinuria, at least in the steady state, suggests that the hemolysis is mainly extravascular and that therefore its mechanism is different from that of AHA. Indeed, studies of red cell membrane proteins have revealed the presence of high-molecular-weight aggregates,[111, 119] consisting largely of spectrin, which have not been found in asymptomatic G6PD-deficient subjects. These findings suggest that whereas in the latter the reductive potential of residual G6PD is adequate in the steady state, in the former continuous oxidation of sulfhydryl groups takes place, followed by irreversible changes in the configuration of membrane proteins.[120] Naturally this does not mean that the red cells of patients with severe G6PD deficiency are not vulnerable to acute oxidative damage of hemoglobin as well; indeed, the same agents that can cause AHA in persons with the ordinary type of G6PD deficiency will cause severe exacerbations with hemoglobinuria in persons with the severe form of G6PD deficiency. The reason why the severity of CNSHA associated with G6PD deficiency is so variable is that almost every case is due to a different mutation (see later), and each mutation will have a different effect on the stability of the enzyme, on its kinetic properties, or on both.

Diagnosis. The diagnosis of G6PD deficiency is discussed next, but a special problem in relation to CNSHA is to establish firmly the causal link between the former and the latter. If the patient is, for example, a Swede of Swedish ancestry or a Japanese of Japanese ancestry, the link will be taken for granted, and this is generally justified, given the rarity of G6PD deficiency in these populations. On the other hand, if the patient is from a population in which G6PD deficiency is common, its presence in a patient with CNSHA might be a mere coincidence, and the cause of the CNSHA might be something else altogether. In these cases, while other causes of CNSHA are being ruled out, it becomes essential to characterize the G6PD of the patient. If it is a common variant, known to be asymptomatic in other subjects, it can be

certainly exonerated, whereas if it is a new unique variant, it is likely to be the culprit.

DIAGNOSIS OF G6PD DEFICIENCY

Although the clinical picture of favism and of other forms of AHA associated with G6PD deficiency is characteristic, the final diagnosis must rely on the direct demonstration of decreased activity of this enzyme in red cells. In NNJ and CNSHA the differential diagnosis is much wider, and therefore this test is even more important. Fortunately, the enzyme assay is very easy, and numerous "screening tests" can be used as substitutes if a spectrophotometer is not available. However, a number of potential pitfalls and sources of error must be understood; and the use of commercial kits is not a substitute for such understanding. Here the value and limitations of the regular quantitative assay are discussed first, and then the use of alternatives is mentioned.

Tests for G6PD Deficiency

G6PD can be assayed by the classic method of Horecker and Smyrniotis,[121] which measures directly the rate of formation of NADPH through its characteristic absorption peak in the near ultraviolet spectrum at 340 nm. The red cell activity is expressed in International Units (micromoles of NADPH produced per minute) per gram of hemoglobin; therefore, it is best to assay the enzyme activity and the hemoglobin concentration in the same hemolysate and work out the ratio. Because G6PD activity is much higher in leukocytes (particularly in granulocytes) than in erythrocytes, for accurate measurements it is essential to remove all leukocytes by the Ficoll-Hypaque method, or by filtration through cellulose powder,[122] rather than by the cruder approach of sucking off the buffy coat: however, in most cases this is not necessary just for the purpose of diagnosing G6PD deficiency. In normal red cells the range of G6PD activity, measured at 30°C, is 7 to 10 IU/g of hemoglobin.

Several "screening tests" for G6PD deficiency are useful and reliable provided they are properly run and their limitations are understood. The most popular are the dye decolorization tests,[123] the methemoglobin reduction test,[124] and the fluorescence spot test.[125] All of these methods are semi-quantitative, and they are meant to classify a sample simply as "normal" or "deficient." The cutoff point can be set by following the appropriate instructions and by trial and error in the individual diagnostic laboratory: one should aim to classify as deficient any sample having less than 30% of the normal activity, because above this level one is unlikely to encounter clinical manifestations. Screening tests are of course especially useful for testing large numbers of samples. They are also perfectly adequate for diagnostic purposes in patients who are in the steady state but *not* for patients in the post-hemolytic period or with other complications; also, they cannot be expected to identify all heterozygotes. Finally, an ideal screening test ought not to give "false-negative" results (i.e., it should not misclassify a G6PD-deficient subject as normal), but it can be allowed to give a few "false-positive" results (i.e., a G6PD normal subject might be misclassified as G6PD deficient). Ideally, every patient found to be G6PD deficient by screening should be confirmed by the spectrophotometric assay.

Biologic and Technical Problems

The biochemical definition of G6PD deficiency is somewhat arbitrary, because different genetic variants are associated with different degrees of deficiency. However, it seems reasonable to choose as the cutoff point a level that can cause clinical manifestations. As stated earlier, in males there will be no hemolytic complications with a red cell G6PD activity greater than 30% of normal. Thus, from the clinical point of view the demarcation between G6PD-normal and G6PD-deficient males is in principle quite clear-cut. However, two problems deserve consideration (Table 17–5).

1. *The effect of red cell age.* It was mentioned earlier that G6PD decreases gradually as red cells age.[28] Therefore, any condition associated with reticulocytosis will entail an *increase* in G6PD activity. This means that if the subject is genetically G6PD normal the red cell G6PD activity will now be *above* the normal range. This does not affect diagnosis, because G6PD deficiency will be correctly ruled out. However, if the subject is genetically G6PD deficient, the red cell G6PD may now be raised to the extent of being near to or even within the normal range, and the patient might be therefore misclassified as G6PD normal.[126] However, the level may well be low at the time of an attack.[127]

2. *The effect of selective hemolysis.* After a hemolytic attack two circumstances concur to cause the risk of misdiagnosis: first, the older cells have been destroyed selectively; second, the marrow response has caused a sudden outpouring of young cells into the peripheral blood. (A third confusing factor may be admixture of G6PD-normal red cells if the patient has been transfused.) Although the reticulocyte count is a good warning to avoid this mistake, it must be realized that, because reticulocytes turn into morphologically "mature" erythrocytes within 1 to 2 days, their count is not a sensitive index of the mean red cell age: in other words, the mean red cell age may be significantly younger than normal even when the reticulocyte count is normal.

There are several ways to circumvent these problems. First, a G6PD level in the low-normal range (as opposed to higher than normal) in the presence of reticulocytosis is always suspicious. In first approximation, this finding in itself suggests that the patient is actually G6PD deficient. Second, if the patient is suffering or is recovering from AHA, the suspicion generated from the just-mentioned finding can be simply kept in store for a few weeks, when the situation will be evolving toward the steady state, and a repeat test will prove whether the patient is indeed G6PD deficient. Third, if either the urgency of some clinical decision or academic curiosity demands a more prompt solution of the problem, the presence of severely G6PD-deficient

red cells can be demonstrated either by enzyme assay of the oldest cells (fractionated by sedimentation) or by a cytochemical method.[128–130]

3. *G6PD deficiency in heterozygotes.* Heterozygote diagnosis by a quantitative test is not difficult in most cases, because the level of G6PD will be intermediate between the normal and the deficient male range: however, in about 10% of cases the G6PD level will "trespass" into either. In addition, the problems outlined for male patients will be compounded in the case of heterozygous females: they can be usually overcome by similar methodologies, particularly by the use of a cytochemical test. With good technique, even only 5% of G6PD-deficient red cells will indicate that the patient is a heterozygote. However, it must be realized that in cases of "extreme phenotypes" (sometimes referred to as arising from "imbalanced lyonization") no test can demonstrate what is not there. In such cases only a family study, if practicable, or DNA analysis, if the mutation involved is known, can prove that the woman is a heterozygote. Fortunately this is not crucial from the clinical point of view. The susceptibility of heterozygotes to develop AHA and its severity are roughly proportional to the percentage of G6PD-deficient red cells. Thus, if this percentage is so low as to be hard to detect, the patient's AHA is most unlikely to be G6PD related.

A special mention should be made of heterozygotes for G6PD variants associated with CNSHA. In the author's experience the mothers of (male) patients with this condition are often G6PD normal either because the variant in the offspring is due to a *de novo* mutation[131] or because the mother is a heterozygote but is phenotypically normal, presumably because somatic selection has favored the hematopoietic progenitor cells with normal G6PD.[57, 61]

GENETIC VARIATION AND GENETIC POLYMORPHISM OF G6PD

One of the most striking findings in the study of human G6PD has been the high rate of variation that can be revealed in many populations by electrophoretic and quantitative analysis.[14] So many variants have been described that some kind of classification became desirable.[132, 133] From the point of view of hematology, the most important criterion is, of course, clinical expression. From the biochemical point of view, a simple criterion is the amount of residual enzyme activity that is found even in G6PD-deficient red cells.* A widely accepted classification has been one that combines these two criteria[134] (Table 17–6). In general, not surprisingly, there is a good correlation between the severity of G6PD deficiency and clinical expression. However, there is overlap between the residual enzyme activity in class I variants (which, by def-

---

*There have been reports in the literature of "complete" G6PD deficiency.[200, 202] Naturally what is called complete depends on the sensitivity of the technique used. In fact, if the enzyme is concentrated from a hemolysate after removal of hemoglobin, some G6PD activity is invariably recovered. For the moment, it is safe to assume that complete G6PD deficiency does not exist and it would probably be lethal.

TABLE 17–5. Red Blood Cell Glucose-6-Phosphate Dehydrogenase Levels in Various Clinical Situations

Clinical Condition	Sex	Result of Screening Test	Result of G6PD Assay	Interpretation
Normal	M or F	Normal	8.1	Normal
Normal	M	Abnormal	0.4	G6PD deficiency, steady state
Normal	F	Abnormal	2.1	Heterozygote for G6PD deficiency
Normal	F	Normal	4.9	Heterozygote for G6PD deficiency
Acute hemolysis	M	Abnormal	1.6	Hemolytic attack in G6PD deficiency
Acute hemolysis	F	Normal	7.2	Hemolytic attack in G6PD heterozygote
Chronic hemolysis	M	Normal	15.5	Hemolysis unrelated to G6PD deficiency
Chronic hemolysis	M	Abnormal	1.4	CNSHA, probably due to G6PD deficiency

CNSHA = congenital nonspherocytic hemolytic anemia.

inition, are associated with CNSHA) and class II variants (which, by definition, are only associated with AHA). On the other hand, there is wide overlap in clinical expression between class II and class III variants, because both groups are associated with both AHA and NNJ. Class IV and class V do not entail any known clinical manifestations.

As stated in a previous section, it is reasonable to assume that most of these variants result from point mutations within the coding region of the G6PD gene. Indeed, sequence analysis has largely validated this assumption: in other words, each variant is encoded by a different allele at the G6PD structural locus.[†] An important characteristic of numerous G6PD variants is that they are so prevalent in certain populations to be regarded as "polymorphisms," rather than pathologic mutants. This distinction is to some extent arbitrary. In classic population genetics the rigorous definition of a polymorphic allele is that its frequency is higher than could be accounted for by recurrent mutation: for convenience, an allele is designated as polymorphic when its frequency is at least 1% (a very conservative approximation of the more rigorous definition). By this criterion, there are an estimated 100 or so polymorphic G6PD alleles already known.

Not surprisingly, individual variants are characteristically found in certain geographic areas. Thus, G6PD Mediterranean is the most prevalent variant in this area and in the Middle East, and it is also found as far as Iran and India.[80] G6PD A⁻ is characteristic of Africa,[135] but it has been found also in southern Italy,[131] Spain,[136] and Mexico.[137] G6PD Mahidol is characteristic of Thailand and may be quite widespread elsewhere in Southeast Asia.[138]

The ratio of subjects having G6PD deficiency associated with CNSHA to those having "simple" G6PD deficiency varies in different populations. For instance, in Japan, where G6PD deficiency is, on the whole, very rare, the majority of patients with G6PD deficiency have been

reported to have CNSHA.[139] This suggests that CNSHA, caused by rare sporadic variants, many of which may result from recent mutations, reflects the intrinsic mutation rate of the human *Gd* gene, which is likely to be uniform throughout the world, whereas "simple" G6PD deficiency results almost always from common variants, which have arisen many generations ago and spread through biologic selection.

G6PD Variants and Clinical Manifestations

The three variants mentioned previously, G6PD A⁻, G6PD Mediterranean, and G6PD Mahidol, are probably those for which the clinical expression has been best characterized.[118] It is conventionally reported that Mediterranean and Mahidol (class II variants) give more severe manifestations than A⁻ (a class III variant). Although this may be true when large series of cases are compared, there is certainly so much overlap among the groups that in an individual case the differences are, in my own view, not very relevant with respect to patient management. For instance, whether hemolysis is "self limited" or not depends on the offending agent, on its dose, and on the time course of exposure at least as much as it depends on the G6PD variant involved. Notably, favism has been unambiguously documented with A⁻ G6PD deficiency.[140, 141]

Genotype-Phenotype Correlations

In terms of clinical expression, the demarcation between class I variants and all others is, by definition, much more clear-cut. Indeed, one of the outstanding questions in the biochemical genetics of G6PD is why a particular variant can cause CNSHA, rather than just AHA. In certain cases the level of residual enzyme activity is not the whole answer: qualitative differences are important, as first suggested by Kirkman.[142] The most likely way in which a structural change can significantly alter the function of G6PD, *given the same level of deficiency*, is that it affects the binding of one of the main ligands (i.e., G6P, NADP, NADPH). For instance, G6PD Mediterranean and G6PD Coimbra both have mutations near the G6P-binding site, and both have *increased* affinity for G6P. Perhaps because of this, although they are both severely deficient, they belong to class II and not to class I. G6PD Orissa, identified very recently as the main polymorphic variant in tribal Indian populations,[143] also belongs to class II, in

---

[†]In some cases, variants reported as distinct and assigned different names have turned out to be identical at the molecular level,[120,177] illustrating the limitations of biochemical analysis or implicating the possibility of postsynthetic modifications. On the other hand, the A⁻ variant has been proven to be heterogenous[119] and the same may turn out to be true of others. Therefore, the figures in Table 17–6 are not necessarily overestimating the genetic variability of human G6PD.

TABLE 17–6. Genetic Polymorphism of Glucose-6-Phosphate Dehydrogenase

Class	Clinical Expression	Residual G6PD Activity (% of Normal)	Variants Reported*	No. of Variants†	Electrophoretically Normal (%)
I‡	Severe (CNSHA)	<20‡	94	44	35
II	Mild	<10	114	28	31
III	Mild	10–60	110	16	15
IV	None	100	52	2	10
V	None	>100	2		
Total			372	90	

*Based on biochemical characterization, before molecular analysis available.
†Based on specific mutations identified by molecular analysis.
‡Class I variants are defined by their clinical phenotype of CNSHA, regardless of the level of residual activity; partly because of reticulocytosis in these patients, they may be associated with enzyme levels higher than those for some class II variants.

spite of having a *decreased* affinity for NADP. Thus, the affinity for G6P appears to be of greater importance. Indeed, an analysis of the distribution of K_m^{G6P} values of class I variants, compared with that of class II and III variants, shows that they are significantly lower in the latter group.[10]

However, in most cases the main factor responsible for causing CNSHA is a very low level of residual activity in red cells, which, in turn, is due to marked *in vivo* instability. It is quite remarkable that, although G6PD mutations as a whole are evenly spread throughout the gene's coding sequence, the majority of class I mutations are clustered in exons 10 and 11. The three-dimensional model of the human G6PD dimer has, at long last, provided a reasonable explanation for this finding.[24] Indeed, these two exons encode the protein region that constitutes the interface between the two identical subunits of the enzyme. As a result, any mutation in this region causes the respective amino acid replacements in the two subunits to be quite near each other in the dimer structure, thus potentially increasing their deleterious effects. Even more important, because there is no covalent link between the subunits, it stands to reason that any interference with the shape of the interface surfaces may affect their mutual fit and thus dramatically destabilize the active form of the enzyme.

G6PD Polymorphism and Malaria[144]

The striking correlation between the worldwide distribution of G6PD deficiency (Fig. 17–9) and that of *Plasmodium falciparum* prompted the formulation of the "malaria hypothesis" 30 years ago.[88, 144–148] Since that time, numerous more detailed epidemiologic studies (which can be referred to as "micro-mapping"[149]), as well as clinical studies,[88, 150, 151] have provided additional evidence to support the hypothesis that malaria selects for G6PD deficiency. A more difficult question is to understand the mechanism of this phenomenon. *In vivo* studies have shown that *P. falciparum* parasitemia tends to be lower in G6PD-deficient heterozygous (*Gd⁺/Gd⁻*) girls than in G6PD normal subjects;[152] this might protect them from developing those high levels of parasitemia that become life-threatening. However, there are conflicting data on whether this is also the case for G6PD-deficient (*Gd⁻*) hemizygous boys.[152, 153] *In vitro* studies have shown that invasion by *P. falciparum* of G6PD-deficient red cells

takes place normally, but intracellular development of the parasite (i.e., schizogony) is impaired.[154, 155] This impairment is almost completely overcome after the parasite has gone through several schizogonic cycles in G6PD-deficient red cells.[27, 156] This could explain why heterozygotes, who are genetic mosaics, are relatively protected, but hemizygotes are not.[145] However, the precise mechanism whereby growth of the parasite is first inhibited, and whereby the same parasite subsequently adapts to the G6PD-deficient cellular environment remains unexplained. It has been shown conclusively that *P. falciparum* has its own G6PD,[157] with properties that are significantly different from those of the host cell enzyme,[158, 159] and it is possible that further investigations of how the parasite's G6PD synthesis is regulated might shed light on the mechanism of protection by G6PD deficiency against malaria and therefore of selection by malaria for G6PD deficiency.

In the meantime, an added strong argument in favor of malaria selection is the genetic heterogeneity of polymorphic *Gd⁻* alleles in itself. Indeed, each one of these alleles, having arisen through an independent mutational event, must have increased in frequency, on its own, in a particular geographic area where malaria was or still is endemic—a good example of convergent evolution driven by the same selective force.

MANAGEMENT OF G6PD DEFICIENCY

Preventive Medicine

Because NNJ and AHA are the most common manifestations of G6PD deficiency, it is most important to consider how they can be prevented. The first step is to identify G6PD-deficient individuals, and this is where screening is most pertinent. Of course, whether population-wide screening is both desirable and feasible depends primarily on the prevalence of G6PD deficiency in any particular community. This will determine the cost-benefit ratio (the main cost being labor, because the reagents and equipment needed are relatively very inexpensive). If screening is done at all, it is best done on cord blood; and this is already practiced, for instance, in Sardinia, in Thailand, and in Malaysia. Once a subject is known to be G6PD deficient, the two main implications are the risk of NNJ and the importance to avoid exposure to agents that can cause AHA. NNJ cannot be prevented as yet, but the

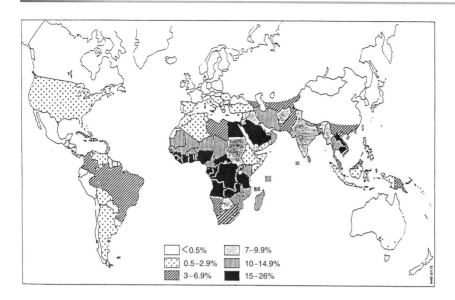

FIGURE 17–9. World map of G6PD deficiency. (From WHO Working Group: Glucose-6-phosphate dehydrogenase deficiency. Bull WHO 1989; 67:601.)

awareness of G6PD deficiency must entail surveillance for NNJ until at least day 4 and special recommendations with respect to factors, such as naphthalene, that can cause it or make it worse. By contrast, at least one type of AHA, namely, favism, is completely preventable, if the persons concerned, and their families in the first place, accept the advice to give up eating fava beans (Fig. 17–10). Prevention of infection-induced hemolysis is obviously more difficult. Prevention of drug-induced hemolysis is possible in most cases by choosing alternative drugs, but it may be difficult when there are none. The most common problem is the need to administer primaquine for the eradication of malaria due to *P. vivax* or *P. malariae*. In these cases the administration of a lower dosage for a longer time is the recommended approach. There will still be hemolysis, but under appropriate surveillance it will be of an acceptably mild degree.

A special problem in prevention is what to do about new drugs, the hemolytic potential of which is unknown. Although *in vitro* methods to test drugs in this respect do exist,[160, 161] such tests are not carried out before drugs are released on the market. This is unfortunate, especially when a new drug is introduced in an area where G6PD deficiency is common; and in practice their hemolytic potential will become apparent only from clinical observation.

Treatment

A child with AHA may be a diagnostic problem that, once solved, does not require any specific treatment at all; or he may be a medical emergency requiring immediate action. The most urgent question is whether the child needs a blood transfusion or not. It is difficult to give absolute directives, but the following guidelines may be useful[162]:

1. If the hemoglobin level is below 7 g/dL, the child should be transfused forthwith.
2. If the hemoglobin level is below 9 g/dL, and there is evidence of persistent brisk hemolysis (hemoglobinuria), immediate blood transfusion is also indicated.
3. If the hemoglobin level is above 9 g/dL but hemoglobinuria persists, or if the hemoglobin level is

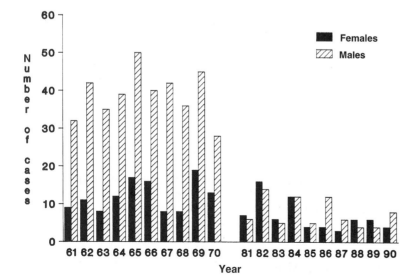

FIGURE 17–10. Control of favism in a community. The data show the decrease in the number of yearly admissions for favism in the children's department of the main city and university hospitals in Sassari, northern Sardinia. During the 10-year period intervening between the two sets of data, two preventive measures were adopted: (1) education through the media and (2) screening of all newborns for G6PD deficiency. Note the dramatic reduction in the incidence of favism in boys and the more modest decrease in girls. The data suggest that (1) preventive measures are effective, (2) the increased proportion of girls can be attributed to failure of the screening method used to pick out many of the heterozygotes, and (3) in view of (2), the dramatic reduction observed in boys can perhaps be credited to screening more than to the educational campaign. (Courtesy of Professor Tullio Meloni, Sassari, Sardinia.)

between 7 and 9 g/dL but there is no hemoglobinuria, the child is kept under close observation for at least 48 hours and transfused if either condition 1 or 2 develops.

The most important complication that may require treatment is acute renal failure, which is exceedingly rare in children. Apart from a standard renal failure regimen, hemodialysis may be necessary. It has been claimed that haptoglobin administration may help to prevent renal failure in hemolytic anemia associated with G6PD deficiency,[69] but this anecdotal report does not seem convincing.[163]

Management of NNJ. The management of NNJ due to G6PD deficiency does not differ from that recommended for other causes. Thus, mild cases do not require treatment; intermediate cases require phototherapy; and severe cases require exchange transfusion treatment, just as in NNJ due to "classic" HDN. A "gentler" approach to the management of NNJ has been advocated.[164] Although it is unquestionable that the prompt use of phototherapy has effectively reduced markedly the number of newborns needing exchange transfusion, one should be probably very cautious in avoiding the other extreme. Kernicterus is still an impending threat, especially when severe NNJ is associated with anemia, hypoxia, or infection. In addition, it is not impossible (although entirely speculative) that G6PD deficiency may be expressed in the brain, thus increasing the risk of neurologic damage. For these reasons, the guidelines for the management of NNJ associated with G6PD deficiency still stand.[162] Specifically, it is recommended that, in full-term newborns, exchange transfusion is carried out if the serum bilirubin level exceeds 15 mg/dL in the first 2 days of life, or 20 mg/dL at any time in the first week of life.

Management of CNSHA. In general terms, management of CNSHA from G6PD deficiency does not differ from that of CNSHA due to other causes (e.g., pyruvate kinase deficiency). If the anemia is not severe, regular folic acid supplements and regular hematologic surveillance suffice. It is important to avoid exposure to potentially hemolytic drugs, and blood transfusion may be indicated when exacerbations occur, mostly in concomitance with intercurrent infection. In rare patients, the anemia is so severe that it must be regarded as transfusion dependent. In these cases blood transfusion will be probably needed at approximately 2-month intervals, to keep the hemoglobin in the 8- to 10-g/dL range. A hypertransfusion regimen aiming to maintain a normal hemoglobin level is not indicated (because there is no ineffective erythropoiesis in the bone marrow). However, depending on the extent of blood transfusion requirement, appropriate iron chelation should be instituted from the age of 2 years onward and must be continued as long as transfusion treatment is necessary; sometimes the transfusion requirement may decrease after puberty.

A special problem is that of splenectomy. There is no evidence of *selective* red cell destruction in the spleen, as in hereditary spherocytosis. However, the fact that the spleen is usually enlarged suggests that its role in hemolysis is not negligible. In practice, there are three indications for splenectomy: (1) if splenomegaly becomes a physical encumbrance; (2) if there is evidence of hypersplenism;

and (3) if the anemia is severe, even in the absence of the first two indications. Splenectomy may reduce the overall rate of hemolysis just enough to make a transfusion-dependent child become transfusion independent. This is doubly important because it will make it possible to dispense with desferrioxamine. The author knows of two patients in whom splenectomy did thus benefit G6PD-deficient patients with severe CNSHA. Of course Pneumovax immunization should be given before splenectomy and penicillin prophylaxis after splenectomy.

When a diagnosis of CNSHA is made, the family must be given genetic counseling, and an effort should be made to establish whether the mother is a heterozygote (this may not be easy by conventional techniques; see earlier). If she is, the chance of recurrence is 1:2 for every subsequent male pregnancy. Prenatal diagnosis can be offered, and it can be carried out by a G6PD assay on amniotic fluid cells, although the expression of G6PD deficiency in these cells varies with each G6PD variant. Nowadays a probably better alternative is to test DNA from chorionic villi with one of the available polymorphic probes that are closely linked to G6PD, and for which the mother is heterozygous. Ideally, the mutation in the G6PD gene of the boy affected by CNSHA could be identified, which will make it possible to establish conclusively whether the mother is heterozygous. Prenatal diagnosis could then be carried out by customized allele-specific oligonucleotide hybridization or by analysis with an appropriate restriction enzyme.[165]

G6PD DEFICIENCY IN NONERYTHROID CELLS

As mentioned earlier, because nucleated somatic cells have the capability to synthesize G6PD constitutively, they are less affected than red cells by G6PD deficiency.[166] Specifically, if G6PD deficiency is due to instability of a mutant enzyme one would not expect nucleated cells to be severely affected. For instance, subjects with G6PD Mediterranean have less than 5% G6PD activity in red cells but about 30% of normal in granulocytes; subjects with G6PD A⁻ have about 12% G6PD activity in red cells but near-normal activity in granulocytes. On the other hand, if deficiency results from a drastic change in catalytic efficiency, or in substrate affinity, then deficiency may be more universal. In practice, the only well-documented pathologic effect is expressed in granulocytes. Very few of the class I G6PD variants cause not only CNSHA but also granulocyte dysfunction, mainly in the way of impaired killing of phagocytosed bacteria (an example is G6PD Barcelona[167]). Patients with these variants have increased susceptibility to bacterial infection, particularly with *Staphylococcus aureus*. The mechanism whereby G6PD deficiency impairs phagocytosis is a defect of the oxidative burst, due to a shortage in NADPH supply, similar to that observed in chronic granulomatous disease, in which one of the components of the cytochrome-b_{245} system is defective.[168]*

---

*Because chronic granulomatous disease is also X linked, it was thought initially that it was related to G6PD deficiency.[201] In fact, cytochrome-b_{245} has now been mapped to Xq21, and its relationship to G6PD is significant at the metabolic level rather than at the genetic level.

Erythrocytes are not the only non-nucleated cells in the body. Another example is in the eye lens, and juvenile cataracts have been reported occasionally in subjects with G6PD deficiency.[169, 170] Whether G6PD deficiency is more generally associated with higher frequency or earlier onset of cataracts appears to be still controversial.[171–176]

HEMATOLOGIC ASSOCIATIONS OF G6PD DEFICIENCY

Because the epidemiology of G6PD deficiency overlaps with that of other polymorphic red cell traits, it is not surprising that they may occur together in the same person. In several studies, the combination of G6PD deficiency with the sickle cell trait has been no more frequent than could be expected by chance.[177–180] The combination of G6PD deficiency with the β-thalassemia trait has been found to cause a significant increase of the mean corpuscular volume,[159, 160] which remains, however, below the normal range. From the clinical point of view, the most important association is that of G6PD deficiency with homozygous sickle cell anemia. Some earlier anecdotal reports had suggested that the former might ameliorate the latter. In fact, several studies have shown that there is no significant difference in a variety of clinical and hematologic parameters between two otherwise comparable groups of patients with sickle cell anemia, with and without G6PD deficiency;[126, 179, 183, 184] but it must be born in mind that acute intravascular hemolysis superimposed on chronic severe extravascular hemolysis is an added risk with this association.[185] Association of G6PD deficiency with thalassemia major is unlikely to be a problem, because patients with the latter condition are treated with regular blood transfusion or with bone marrow transplantation. However, the association may be significant in patients with various forms of thalassemia intermedia syndromes (e.g., E-β thalassemia[186]).

Occasionally, G6PD deficiency has been observed in association with much more rare red cell abnormalities, such as pyruvate kinase deficiency,[187, 188] congenital dyserythropoietic anemia type II,[189–191] and hereditary elliptocytosis.[192] In these cases the two abnormalities seem to produce only additive clinical effects, but in at least one family G6PD deficiency was synergistic with hereditary spherocytosis in causing a moderately severe chronic hemolytic anemia.[193, 194]

REFERENCES

1. Beutler E: Glucose 6-phosphate dehydrogenase deficiency. In Beutler E (ed): Hemolytic Anemia in Disorders of Red Cell Metabolism. New York, Plenum Medical Book Co., 1978, pp 23–167.
2. Levy HR: Glucose 6-phosphate dehydrogenase. In Meister A (ed): Advances in Enzymology. Vol. 48. New York, John Wiley & Sons, Inc., 1979, pp 97–192.
3. Arese P, Mannuzzu L, Turrini F: Pathophysiology of favism. Folia Haematol 1989; 116:745.
4. Beutler E: The genetics of glucose-6-phosphate dehydrogenase deficiency. Semin Hematol 1990; 27:137.
5. Beutler E: Glucose 6-phosphate dehydrogenase deficiency. N Engl J Med 1991; 324:169.
6. Luzzatto L, Mehta A: Glucose 6-phosphate dehydrogenase deficiency. In Scriver CR, Beaudet AL, et al (eds): The Metabolic and Molecular Basis of Inherited Disease. 7th ed. New York, McGraw-Hill Book Co., 1995, pp 3367–3398.
7. Ayene IS, Stamato TD, Mauldin SK, et al: Mutation in the glucose-6-phosphate dehydrogenase gene leads to inactivation of Ku DNA end binding during oxidative stress. J Biol Chem 2002; 277:9929–35.
8. Tavazzi B, Amorino AM, Fazzina G, et al: Oxidative stress induces impairment of human erythrocyte energy metabolism through the oxygen radical-mediated direct activation of AMP-deaminase. J Biol Chem 2001; 276:48083-92.
9. Au WY, Ma SK, Lie AK, et al: Glucose-6-phosphate dehydrogenase deficiency and hematopoietic stem cell transplantation. Bone Marrow Transplant 2002; 29:399-402.
10. Luzzatto L, Testa U: Human erythrocyte G6PD. Structure and function in normal and mutant subjects. In Piomelli S, Yachnin S (eds): Current Topics in Hematology. Vol. 1. New York, Alan R. Liss, Inc., 1978, pp 1–70.
11. Peisach J, Blumberg WE, Rachmilewicz EA: The demonstration of ferrihemochrome intermediates in Heinz body formation following the reduction of oxyhemoglobin A by acetylphenylhydrazine. Biochim Biophys Acta 1975; 393:404.
12. Kirkman HN, Gaetani GF: Catalase: a tetrameric enzyme with four tightly bound molecules of NADPH. Proc Natl Acad Sci U S A 1984; 81:4343.
13. Gaetani GF, Galiano S, et al: Catalase and glutathione peroxidase are equally active in detoxification of hydrogen peroxide in human erythrocytes. Blood 1989; 73:334.
14. Luzzatto L, Battistuzzi G: Glucose 6-phosphate dehydrogenase. Adv Hum Genet 1985; 14:217.
15. Antonenkov VD: Dehydrogenases of the pentose phosphate pathway in rat liver peroxisomes. Eur J Biochem 1989; 183:75.
16. Cohen P, Rosemeyer MA: Human glucose-6-phosphate dehydrogenase: purification of the erythrocyte enzyme and the influence of ions on its activity. Eur J Biochem 1969; 8:1.
17. Persico MG, Viglietto G, et al: Isolation of human glucose-6-phosphate dehydrogenase (G6PD) cDNA clones: primary structure of the protein and unusual 5' non-coding region. Nucleic Acids Res 1986; 14:2511.
18. Jeffery J, Soderling-Barros J, et al: Glucose 6-phosphate dehydrogenase. Characteristics revealed by the rat liver enzyme. Eur J Biochem 1989; 186:551.
19. Naylor CD, Rowland P, et al: Glucose 6-phosphate dehydrogenase mutations causing enzyme deficiency in a model of the tertiary structure of the human enzyme. Blood 1996; 87:2974.
20. Camardella L, Caruso C, et al: Human erythrocyte glucose-6-phosphate dehydrogenase. Identification of a reactive lysyl residue labelled with pyridoxal 5'-phosphate. Eur J Biochem 1988; 171:485.
21. Mason PJ, Vulliamy TJ, et al: The production of normal and variant human glucose-6-phosphate dehydrogenase in cos cells. Eur J Biochem 1988; 178:109.
22. Bautista JM, Mason PJ, Luzzatto L: Human glucose-6-phosphate dehydrogenase lysine 205 is dispensable for substrate binding but essential for catalysis. FEBS Lett 1995; 366:61.
23. Rowland P, Basak A, et al: The three-dimensional structure of glucose 6-phosphate dehydrogenase from Leuconostoc mesenteroides refined at 2.0 A resolution. Structure 1994; 2:1073.
24. Naylor CE, Rowland P, et al: Glucose 6-phosphate dehydrogenase mutations causing enzyme deficiency in a model of the tertiary structure of the human enzyme. Blood 1996; 87:2974.
25. Luzzatto L: Regulation of the activity of glucose-6-phosphate dehydrogenase by NADP+ and NADPH. Biochim Biophys Acta 1967; 146:18.
26. Kirkman HN, Gaetani GD, et al: Red cell NADP and NADPH in glucose-6-phosphate dehydrogenase deficiency. J Clin Invest 1975; 55:875.
27. Luzzatto L, Sodeinde O, Martini G: Genetic variation in the host and adaptive phenomena in Plasmodium falciparum infection. In Evered D, Whelan J (eds): Malaria and the Red Cell, Ciba Foundation Symposium 94. London, Pitman Medical Publishing Co., 1983, pp 159–173.
28. Beutler E: The red cell. In Beutler E (ed): Hemolytic Anemia in Disorders of Red Cell Metabolism. New York, Plenum Medical Book Co., 1978, pp 1–21.

29. Piomelli S, Corash LM, et al: *In vivo* lability of glucose-6-phosphate dehydrogenase in Gd A and Gd Mediterranean deficiency. J Clin Invest 1968; 47:940.

30. Beutler E: The relationship of red cell enzymes to red cell life-span. Blood Cells 1988; 14:69.

31. Marks PA, Johnson AB: Relationship between the age of human erythrocytes and their osmotic resistance: a basis for separating young and old erythrocytes. J Clin Invest 1958; 37:1542.

32. Beutler E, Gelbart T, Kuhl W: Human red cell glucose-6-phosphate dehydrogenase: all active enzyme has sequence predicted by the X chromosome-encoded cDNA. Cell 1990; 62:7.

33. Henikoff S, Smith JM: The human mRNA that provides the N-terminus of chimeric G6PD encodes GMP reductase. Cell 1989; 58:1021.

34. Kanno H, Huang I-Y, et al: Two structural genes on different chromosomes are required for encoding the major subunit of human red cell glucose-6-phosphate dehydrogenase. Cell 1989; 58:595.

35. Mason PJ, Bautista J, et al: Human red cell glucose 6-phosphate dehydrogenase is encoded only on the X-chromosome. Cell 1990; 63:9.

36. Pai GS, Sprenkle JA, et al: Localization of the loci for hypoxanthine phosphoribosyltransferase and glucose-6-phosphate dehydrogenase and biochemical evidence of non-random X-chromosome expression from studies of human X-autosome translocation. Proc Natl Acad Sci U S A 1980; 77:2810.

37. Szabo P, Purrello M, et al: Cytological mapping of the human glucose-6-phosphate dehydrogenase gene distal to the fragile-X site suggests a high rate of meiotic recombination across this site. Proc Natl Acad Sci U S A 1984; 81:7855.

38. Yoshida A, Kan YW: Origin of "fused" glucose-6-phosphate dehydrogenase. Cell 1990; 62:11.

39. Patterson M, Schwartz C, et al: Physical mapping studies on the human X chromosome in the region Xq27-Zqter. Genomics 1987; 1:297.

40. Willard HF, Cremers F, et al: Report and abstracts of the Fifth International Workshop on Human X Chromosome Mapping 1994. Heidelberg, Germany, April 24–27, 1994. Cytogenet Cell Genet 1994; 67:295.

41. Pilia G, Little RD, et al: Isochores and CpG islands in YAC contigs in human Xq26.1-qter. Genomics 1993; 17:456.

42. Vulliamy TJ, Othman A, et al: Polymorphic sites in the African population detected by sequence analysis of the glucose 6-phosphate dehydrogenase gene outline the evolution of the variants A and A –. Proc Natl Acad Sci U S A 1991; 88:8568.

43. Filosa S, Calabro V, et al: G6PD haplotypes spanning Xq28 from F8C to red/green color vision. Genomics 1993; 17:6.

44. Chen EY, Cheng A, et al: Sequence of human glucose 6-phosphate dehydrogenase cloned in plasmids and a yeast artificial chromosome. Genomics 1991; 10:792.

45. Kwok CJ, Martin AC, Au SW, et al: G6PDdb, an integrated database of glucose-6-phosphate dehydrogenase (G6PD) mutations. Hum Mutat 2002; 19:217–224.

46. Nuchprayoon I, Sanpavat S, Nuchprayoon S: Glucose-6-phosphate dehydrogenase (G6PD) mutations in Thailand: G6PD Viangchan (871G>A) is the most common deficiency variant in the Thai population. Hum Mutat 2002; 19:185.

47. Beutler E, Yeh M, Fairbanks VF: The normal human female as a mosaic of X-chromosome activity: studies using the gene for G6PD deficiency as a marker. Proc Natl Acad Sci U S A 1962; 48:9.

48. Martini G, Toniolo D, et al: Structural analysis of the X-linked gene encoding human glucose 6-phosphate dehydrogenase. EMBO J 1986; 5:1849.

49. Ursini MV, Scalera L, Martini G: High level of transcription driven by a 400 bp segment of the human G6PD promoter. Biochem Biophys Res Commun 1990; 170:1203.

50. Philippe M, Larondelle Y, et al: Promoter function of the human glucose-6-phosphate dehydrogenase gene depends on two GC boxes that are cell specifically controlled. Eur J Biochem 1994; 226:377.

51. Mason PJ, Stevens DJ, et al: Genomic structure and sequence of the *Fugu rubripes* glucose 6-phosphate dehydrogenase gene (G6PD). Genomics 1995; 26:587.

52. Nance WE: Genetic tests with a sex-linked marker: G-6-PD. Cold Spring Harbor Symp Quant Biol 1964; 29:415.

53. Rinaldi A, Filippi G, Siniscalco M: Variability of red cell phenotypes between and within individuals in an unbiased sample of 77 certain heterozygotes for G6PD deficiency in Sardinians. Am J Hum Genet 1976; 28:496.

54. Gale RE, Wheadon H, Linch DC: X-chromosome inactivation patterns using HPRT and PGK polymorphisms in haematologically normal and post-chemotherapy females. Br J Haematol 1991; 79:193.

55. Nyhan WL, Bakay B, et al: Hemixygous expression of glucose 6-phosphate dehydrogenase deficiency in erythrocytes of heterozygotes for the Lesch-Nyhan syndrome. Proc Natl Acad Sci U S A 1970; 65:214.

56. Town M, Athanasiou-Metaxa M, Luzzatto L: Intragenic interspecific complementation of glucose 6-phosphate dehydrogenase in human-hamster cell hybrids. Somatic Cell Mol Genet 1990; 16:97.

57. Filosa S, Giacometti N, et al: Somatic cell selection is a major determinant of the blood cell phenotype in heterozygotes for glucose 6-phosphate dehydrogenase mutations causing severe enzyme deficiency. Am J Hum Genet 1996; 59:887.

58. Gaetani GF, Ferraris AM: Recent developments on Mediterranean G6PD. Br J Haematol 1988; 68:1.

59. Linder D, Gartler SM: Glucose 6-phosphate dehydrogenase mosaicism. Utilization as a cell marker in the study of leiomyomas. Science 1965; 150:67.

60. Luzzatto L, Mehta A: Glucose-6-phosphate dehydrogenase deficiency. In Scriver CR, Beaudet AL, et al (eds): The Metabolic Basis of Inherited Disease. 6th ed. New York, McGraw-Hill Book Co., 1989, pp 2237–2265.

61. Luzzatto L, Usanga EA, et al: Imbalance in X-chromosome expression: evidence for a human X-linked gene affecting growth of haemopoietic cells. Science 1979; 205:1418.

62. Morelli A, Benatti U, et al: Biochemical mechanisms of glucose-6-phosphate dehydrogenase deficiency. Proc Natl Acad Sci U S A 1978; 75:1979.

63. Viglietto G, Montanaro V, et al: Common glucose 6-phosphate dehydrogenase (G6PD) variants from the Italian population: biochemical and molecular characterization. Ann Hum Genet 1990; 54:1.

64. Poggi V, Town M, et al: Identification of a single base change in the G6PD gene by PCR amplification of the entire coding region from genomic DNA. Biochem J 1990; 271:157.

65. Beutler E, Vulliamy T, Luzzatto L: Hematologically important mutations: glucose 6-phosphate dehydrogenase. Blood Cells Mol Dis 1996; 22:49.

66. Pandolfi PP, Sonati F, et al: Targeted disruption of the housekeeping gene encoding glucose 6-phosphate dehydrogenase (G6PD): G6PD is dispensable for pentose synthesis but essential for defense against oxidative stress. EMBO J 1995; 14:5209.

67. Mason PJ, Sonati MF, et al: New glucose 6-phosphate dehydrogenase mutations associated with chronic anemia. Blood 1995; 85:1377.

68. Ohga S, Higashi E, et al: Haptoglobin therapy for acute favism: a Japanese boy with glucose-6-phosphate dehydrogenase Guadalajara. Br J Haematol 1995; 89:421.

69. Mason PJ: New insights into G6PD deficiency. Br J Haematol 1996; 94:585.

70. Dacie JV: Hereditary enzyme deficiency haemolytic anaemias. III: Deficiency of glucose-6-phosphate dehydrogenase. In Dacie JV (ed): Haemolytic Anaemias. The Hereditary Haemolytic Anaemias. 3rd ed. London, Churchill Livingstone, Inc., 1985, pp 364–418.

71. Luzzatto L: Inherited haemolytic anaemias. In Hoffbrand AV, Lewis SM (eds): Postgraduate Haematology. 3rd ed. London, Heinemann, 1989, pp 146–182.

72. Sansone G, Piga AM, Segni G. Il Favismo. Torino, Minerva Medica, 1958.

73. Raupp P, Hassan JA, Varughese M, et al: Henna causes life threatening haemolysis in glucose-6-phosphate dehydrogenase deficiency. Arch Dis Child 2001; 85:411–412.

74. Fermi C, Martinetti P: Studio sul fayismo. Ann Ig Sper 1905; 15:76.

75. Chan TK, Chan WC, Weed RI: Erythrocyte hemighosts: a hallmark of severe oxidative injury *in vivo*. Br J Haematol 1982; 50:575.

76. Fischer TM, Meloni T, et al: Membrane cross bonding in red cells in favic crisis: a missing link in the mechanism of extravascular hemolysis. Br J Haematol 1985; 59:159.

77. Rifkind RA: Heinz bodies anaemia: an ultrastructural study. II. Red cell sequestration and destruction. Blood 1965; 26:433.

78. Tarlov AR, Brewer GJ, et al: Primaquine sensitivity. Glucose-6-phosphate dehydrogenase deficiency: an inborn error of metabolism of medical and biological significance. Arch Intern Med 1962; 109:209.

79. Arese P, De Flora A: Pathophysiology of hemolysis in glucose 6-phosphate dehydrogenase deficiency. Semin Hematol 1990; 27:1.

80. Beutler E, Dern RJ, Alving AS: The hemolytic effect of primaquine. VI. An *in vitro* test for sensitivity of erythrocytes to primaquine. J Lab Clin Med 1955; 45:40.

81. Jollow DJ, McMillan DC: Oxidative stress, glucose-6-phosphate dehydrogenase and the red cell. Adv Exp Med Biol 2001; 500:595–605.

82. Mareni C, Repetto L, et al: Favism: looking for a autosomal gene associated with glucose-6-phosphate dehydrogenase deficiency. J Med Genet 1984; 21:278.

83. Low PS: Structure and function of the cytoplasmic domain of band 3: center of erythrocyte membrane-peripheral protein interactions. Biochim Biophys Acta 1986; 864:145.

84. Waugh SM, Walder JA, Low PS: Partial characterization of the copolymerization reaction of erythrocyte membrane band 3 with hemichrome. Biochemistry 1987; 26:1777.

85. Kasper ML, Miller WJ, Jacob HS: G6PD deficiency infectious haemolysis: a complement dependent innocent bystander phenomenon. Br J Haematol 1986; 63:85.

86. Bernini L, Latte B, et al: Survival of ^{51}Cr-labelled red cells in subjects with thalassaemia trait, G6PD deficiency or both abnormalities. Br J Haematol 1964; 10:171.

87. McCurdy PR: Discussion. In Yoshida A, Beutler E (eds): Glucose 6-Phosphate Dehydrogenase. New York, Academic Press, 1986, pp 273–278.

88. Beutler E, Dern RJ, Alving AS: The hemolytic effect of primaquine. IV. The relationship of cell age to hemolysis. J Lab Clin Med 1954; 44:439.

89. Szeinberg A, Marks PA: Substances stimulating glucose catabolism by the oxidative reactions of the pentose phosphate pathway in human erythrocytes. J Clin Invest 1961; 40:914.

90. Chevion M, Navok T, et al: The chemistry of favism-inducing compounds. The properties of isouramil and divicine and their reaction with glutathione. Eur J Biochem 1982; 127:405.

91. Winterbourn C, Cowden WB, Sutton HC: Auto-oxidation of dialuric acid, divicine and isouramil. Superoxide dependent and independent mechanisms. Biochem Pharmacol 1989; 38:611.

92. Meloni T, Forteleoni G, et al: Aspirin-induced acute hemolytic anemia in glucose 6-phosphate dehydrogenase deficient children with systemic arthritis. Acta Haematol 1989; 81:208.

93. Tugwell P: Glucose 6-phosphate dehydrogenase deficiency in Nigerians with jaundice associated with lobar pneumonia. Lancet 1973; 1:968.

94. Baehner RL, Nathan DG, Castle WB: Oxidant injury of caucasian glucose-6-phosphate dehydrogenase deficient red blood cells by phagocytosing leukocytes during infection. J Clin Invest 1971; 50:2466.

95. Kattamis CA, Tjortjatou F: The hemolytic process of viral hepatitis in children with normal or deficient glucose 6-phosphate dehydrogenase activity. J Pediatr 1970; 77:422.

96. Valaes T: Severe neonatal jaundice associated with glucose-6-phosphate dehydrogenase deficiency: pathogenesis and global epidemiology. Acta Paediatr 1994; Suppl 394:58.

97. Worlledge S, Luzzatto L, Ogiemudia SE, et al: Rhesus immunization in Nigeria. Vox Sang 1968; 14:202.

98. Doxiadis SA, Valaes F: The clinical picture of glucose 6-phosphate dehydrogenase deficiency in early childhood. Arch Dis Child 1964; 39:545.

99. Meloni S, Costa S, Cutillo S: Haptoglobin, hemopexin, hemoglobin and hematocrit in newborns with erythrocyte glucose 6-phosphate dehydrogenase deficiency. Acta Haematol 1975; 54:284.

100. Singh A: Glucose 6-phosphate dehydrogenase deficiency: a preventable cause of mental retardation. BMJ 1986; 292:397.

101. Kaplan M, Hammerman C, Vreman HJ, et al: Acute hemolysis and severe neonatal hyperbilirubinemia in glucose 6-phosphate dehydrogenase-deficient heterozygotes. J Pediatr 2001; 139:137-140.

102. Kaplan M, Hammerman C, Renbaum P, et al: Differing pathogenesis of perinatal bilirubinemia in glucose-6-phosphate dehydrogenase-deficient versus-normal neonates. Pediatr Res 2001; 50:532-537.

103. Kaplan M, Algur N, Hammerman C: Onset of jaundice in glucose-6-phosphate dehydrogenase-deficient neonates. Pediatrics 2001; 108:956-959.

104. Bienzle U, Effiong CE, Luzzatto L: Erythrocyte glucose 6-phosphate dehydrogenase deficiency (G6PD type A⁻) and neonatal jaundice. Acta Paediatr Scand 1976; 65:701.

105. Meloni T, Cagnazzo G, et al: Phenobarbital for prevention of hyperbilirubinemia in glucose 6-phosphate dehydrogenase-deficient newborn infants. J Pediatr 1973; 82:1048.

106. Tan KL, Boey KW: Clinical experience with phototherapy. Ann Acad Med Singapore 1989; 18:43.

107. Yu MW, Hsiao KJ, Wuu KD, et al: Association between glucose-6-phosphate dehydrogenase deficiency and neonatal jaundice: interaction with multiple risk factors. Int J Epidemiol 1992; 21:947.

108. Testa U, Meloni T, et al: Genetic heterogeneity of glucose 6-phosphate dehydrogenase deficiency in Sardinia. Hum Genet 1980; 56:99.

109. Meloni T, Cutillo S, et al: Neonatal jaundice and severity of glucose 6-phosphate dehydrogenase deficiency in Sardinian babies. Early Hum Dev 1987; 15:317.

110. Bienzle U, Effiong CE, et al: Erythrocyte enzymes in neonatal jaundice. Acta Haematol 1976; 55:10.

111. Allen DW, Johnson GJ, et al: Membrane polypeptide aggregates in glucose-6-phosphate dehydrogenase deficient and *in vitro* aged red blood cells. J Lab Clin Med 1978; 91:321.

112. Doxiadis SA, Valaes T, et al: Risk of severe jaundice in glucose 6-phosphate dehydrogenase deficiency of the newborn. Differences in population groups. Lancet 1964; 2:1210.

113. Owa JA: Relationship between exposure to icterogenic agents, glucose-6-phosphate dehydrogenase deficiency and neonatal jaundice in Nigeria. Acta Paediatr Scand 1989; 78:848.

114. Kaplan M, Vreman HJ, et al: Contribution of haemolysis to jaundice in Sephardic Jewish glucose-6-phosphate dehydrogenase deficient neonates. Br J Haematol 1996; 93:822.

115. Ifekwunigwe AE, Luzzatto L: Kernicterus in G6PD deficiency. Lancet 1966; 1:667.

116. Mert A, Tabak F, Ozturk R, et al: Acute viral hepatitis with severe hyperbilirubinemia and massive hemolysis in glucose-6-phosphate dehydrogenase deficiency. J Clin Gastroenterol 2001; 32:461–462.

117. Corchia C, Balata A, et al: Favism in a female newborn infant whose mother ingested fava beans before delivery. J Pediatrics 1995; 127:807.

118. Luzzatto L: Inherited haemolytic states: glucose-6-phosphate dehydrogenase deficiency. Clin Hematol 1975; 4:83.

119. Johnson GJ, Allen DW, et al: Red cell membrane polypeptide aggregates in glucose-6-phosphate dehydrogenase mutants with chronic haemolytic disease: a clue to the mechanism of haemolysis. N Engl J Med 1979; 301:522.

120. Johnson RM, Ravindranath Y, et al: Oxidant damage to erythrocyte membrane in glucose 6-phosphate dehydrogenase deficiency: correlation with *in vivo* reduced glutathione concentration and membrane protein oxidation. Blood 1994; 83:1117.

121. Horecker BL, Smyrniotis A: Glucose 6-phosphate dehydrogenase. In Colowick N, Kaplan NO (eds): Methods in Enzymology. Vol. 1. New York, Academic Press, Inc., 1955.

122. Morelli A, Benatti U, et al: The interference of leukocytes and platelets with measurement of glucose 6-phosphate dehydrogenase activity of erythrocytes with low activity variants of the enzyme. Blood 1981; 58:642.

123. Motulsky AG, Campbell-Kraut JM: Population genetics of glucose 6-phosphate dehydrogenase deficiency of the red cell. In Blumberg BS (ed): Proceedings of Conference on Genetic Polymorphisms and Geographic Variations in Disease. New York, Grune & Stratton, Inc., 1961, pp 159–180.

124. Brewer GJ, Tarlov AR, Alving AS: The methemoglobin reduction test for primaquine-type sensitivity of erythrocytes. A simplified procedure for detecting a specific hypersusceptibility to drug hemolysis. JAMA 1962; 180:386.

125. Beutler E: Special modifications for the fluorescent screening test for glucose 6-phosphate dehydrogenase deficiency. Blood 1968; 32:816.

126. Bienzle U, Sodeinde O, et al: G6PD deficiency and sickle cell anemia: frequency and features of the association in an African community. Blood 1975; 46:591.

127. Herschel M, Beutler E: Low glucose-6-phosphate dehydrogenase enzyme activity level at the time of hemolysis in a male neonate with the African type of deficiency. Blood Cells Mol Dis 2001; 27:918–923.

128. Abd-Allah MA, Foda YH, et al: Treatment to reduce total vicine in Egyptian fava bean (Giza 2 variety). Plant Foods Hum Nutr 1988; 38:201.

129. Fairbanks VF, Lampe LT: A tetrazolium-linked cytochemical method for estimation of glucose 6-phosphate dehydrogenase activity in individual erythrocytes: applications in the study of heterozygotes for glucose 6-phosphate dehydrogenase deficiency. Blood 1968; 31:589.

130. Van Noorden CJF, Vogels IMC, et al: A sensitive cytochemical staining method for glucose 6-phosphate dehydrogenase activity in individual erythrocytes. Histochemistry 1982; 75:493.

131. Vulliamy TJ, D'Urso M, et al: Diverse point mutations in the human glucose-6-phosphate dehydrogenase gene cause enzyme deficiency and mild or severe hemolytic anemia. Proc Natl Acad Sci U S A 1988; 85:5171.

132. Betke K, Beutler E, et al: Standardisation of procedures for the study of glucose-6-phosphate dehydrogenase. Report of a WHO Scientific Group. WHO Tech Rep 1967; 366:5.

133. WHO Working Group: Glucose-6-phosphate dehydrogenase deficiency. Bull WHO 1989; 67:601.

134. Beutler E, Yoshida A: Genetic variation of glucose-6-phosphate dehydrogenase: a catalog and future prospects. Medicine 1988; 67:311.

135. Luzzatto L: Studies of polymorphic traits for the characterization of populations: African populations south of the Sahara. Isr J Med Sci 1973; 9:1181.

136. Beutler E, Kuhl W, et al: Molecular heterogeneity of glucose 6-phosphate dehydrogenase A −. Blood 1989; 74:2550.

137. Beutler E, Kuhl W, et al: Some Mexican glucose 6-phosphate dehydrogenase (G-6-PD) variants revisited. Hum Genet 1991; 86:371.

138. Panich V: Glucose 6-phosphate dehydrogenase deficiency: II. Tropical Asia. Clin Haematol 1981; 10:800.

139. Miwa S, Fujii H: Glucose 6-phosphate dehydrogenase variants in Japan. In Yoshida A, Beutler E (eds): Glucose 6-Phosphate Dehydrogenase. New York, Academic Press, Inc., 1986, pp 261–272.

140. Calabro V, Cascone A, et al: Glucose 6-phosphate dehydrogenase (G6PD) deficiency in Southern Italy: a case of G6PD A(−) associated with favism. Haematologica 1989; 74:71.

141. Galiano S, Gaetani GF, et al: Favism in the African type of glucose-6-phosphate dehydrogenase deficiency (A−). BMJ 1990; 300:236.

142. Kirkman HN, Riley HD: Congenital nonspherocytic hemolytic anemia: studies on a family with a qualitative defect in glucose-6-phosphate dehydrogenase. Am J Dis Child 1961; 102:313.

143. Kaeda JS, Chootray GP, et al: A new G6PD variant, G6PD Orissa (44 Ala→Gly), is the major polymorphic variant in tribal populations in India. Am J Hum Genet 1995; 57:1335.

144. Luzzatto L, Notaro R: Malaria. Protecting against bad air. Science 2001; 293:442–443.

145. Luzzatto L, O'Brien S, Usanga E, Wanachiwanawin W: Origin of G6PD polymorphism: malaria and G6PD deficiency. In Yoshida A, Beutler E (eds): Glucose-6-Phosphate Dehydrogenase. New York, Academic Press, Inc., 1986, pp 181–193.

146. Miller LH: Genetically determined human resistance factors. In Wernsdorfer WH, McGregor I (eds): Malaria: Principles and Practice of Malariology. Edinburgh, Churchill-Livingstone, Inc., 1988, pp 487–500.

147. Allison AC: Glucose-6-phosphate dehydrogenase deficiency in red blood cells of East Africans. Nature 1960; 186:531.

148. Motulsky AG: Metabolic polymorphisms and the role of infectious diseases in human evolution. Hum Biol 1960; 32:28.

149. Luzzatto L: Genetic factors in malaria. Bull WHO 1974; 50:195.

150. Ruwende C, Khoo SC, et al: Natural selection of hemi- and heterozygotes for G6PD deficiency in Africa by resistance to severe malaria. Nature 1995; 376:246.

151. Kar S, Seth S, Seth PK: Prevalence of malaria in Ao Nagas and its association with G6PD and HbE. Hum Biol 1992; 64:187.

152. Bienzle U, Ayeni O, et al: Glucose-6-phosphate dehydrogenase deficiency and malaria. Greater resistance of females heterozygous for enzyme deficiency and of males with non-deficient variant. Lancet 1972; 1:107.

153. Ruwende C, Khoo SC, et al: Natural selection of hemi- and heterozygotes for G6PD deficiency in Africa by resistance to severe malaria. Nature 1995; 376:246.

154. Luzzatto L: Genetics of human red cells and susceptibility to malaria. In Michal F (ed): Modern Genetic Concepts and Techniques in the Study of Parasites. Basel, Schwabe & Co., 1981, pp 257–277.

155. Roth EF Jr, Raventos-Suarez C, et al: Glucose 6-phosphate dehydrogenase deficiency inhibits *in vitro* growth of *Plasmodium falciparum*. Proc Natl Acad Sci U S A 1983; 80:298.

156. Usanga EA, Luzzatto L: Adaptation of *Plasmodium falciparum* to glucose 6-phosphate dehydrogenase deficient host red cells by production of parasite-encoded enzyme. Nature 1985; 313:793.

157. Ling IT, Wilson RJM: G6PD activity of the malarial parasite *Plasmodium falciparum*. Mol Biochem Parasitol 1988; 31:47.

158. Kurdi-Haidar B, Luzzatto L: Expression and characterization of glucose 6-phosphate dehydrogenase of *Plasmodium falciparum*. Mol Biochem Parasitol 1990; 41:83.

159. Clarke JL, Scopes DA, Sodeinde O, et al: Glucose-6-phosphate dehydrogenase-6-phosphogluconolactonas. A novel bifunctional enzyme in malaria parasites.

160. Gaetani GF, Mareni C, et al: Haemolytic effect of two sulphonamides evaluated by a new method. Br J Haematol 1976; 32:183.

161. Magon AM, Leipzig RM, et al: Interactions of glucose 6-phosphate dehydrogenase deficiency with drug acetylation and hydroxylation reactions. J Lab Clin Med 1981; 97:764.

162. Luzzatto L, Meloni T: Hemolytic anemia due to glucose 6-phosphate dehydrogenase deficiency. In Brain MC, Carbone PP (eds): Current Therapy in Hematology-Oncology: 1985–1986. Toronto, BC Decker, 1985, pp 21–24.

163. Luzzatto L, Mehta A, Meloni T: Haemoglobinuria and haptoglobin in G6PD deficiency. Br J Haematol 1995; 91:511.

164. Newman TB, Maisels MJ: Evaluation and treatment of jaundice in the term infant: a kinder, gentler approach. Pediatrics 1992; 89:809.

165. Beutler E, Kuhl W, et al: Prenatal diagnosis of glucose 6-phosphate dehydrogenase deficiency. Acta Haematol 1992; 87:103.

166. Morellini M, Colonna-Romano S, et al: Glucose 6-phosphate dehydrogenase of leukocyte sub-populations in normal and enzyme-deficient individuals. Haematologica 1985; 70:390.

167. Vives-Corrons JL, Feliu E, et al: Severe glucose-6-phosphate dehydrogenase (G6PD) deficiency associated with chronic hemolytic anaemia, granulocyte dysfunction and increased susceptibility to infections. Description of a new molecular variant (G6PD Barcelona). Blood 1982; 59:428.

168. Roos D, deBoer M, et al: Mutations in the X-linked and autosomal recessive forms of chronic granulomatous disease. Blood 1996; 87:1663.

169. Westring DN, Pisciotta AV: Anemia, cataracts and seizures in a patient with glucose-6-phosphate dehydrogenase deficiency. Arch Intern Med 1966; 118:385.

170. Harley JD, Agar NS, Yoshida A: Glucose 6-phosphate dehydrogenase variants: Gd(+) Alexandra associated with neonatal jaundice and Gd(−) Camperdown in a young man with lamellar cataracts. J Lab Clin Med 1978; 91:295.

171. Orzalesi M, Fossarello M, et al: The relationship between glucose 6-phosphate dehydrogenase deficiency and cataracts in Sardinia. An epidemiological and biochemical study. Doc Ophthalmol 1984; 57:187.

172. Moro F, Gorgone G, et al: Glucose 6-phosphate dehydrogenase deficiency and incidence of cataract in Sicily. Ophthalmic Paediatr Genet 1985; 5:197.

173. Yuregir G, Varinli I, Donma O: Glucose 6-phosphate dehydrogenase deficiency both in red blood cells and lenses of the normal and cataractous native population of Cukurova, the southern part of Turkey. Part I. Ophthalmic Res 1989; 21:155.

174. Meloni T, Carta F, et al: Glucose 6-phosphate dehydrogenase deficiency and cataract of patients in northern Sardinia. Am J Ophthalmol 1990; 110:661.

175. Chen Y, Zeng L, et al: The study of G6PD in erythrocyte and lens in senile and presenile cataract. Yen Ko Hsueh Pao 1992; 8:12.

176. Assaf AA, Tabbara KF, el-Hazmi MA: Cataracts in glucose-6-phosphate dehydrogenase deficiency. Ophthalmic Paediatr Genet 1993; 14:81.

177. Luzzatto L, Allan NC: Relationship between the genes for glucose 6-phosphate dehydrogenase and haemoglobin in a Nigerian population. Nature 1968; 219:1041.

178. Nhonoli AM, Kujwalile JM, et al: Correlation of glucose-6-phosphate dehydrogenase (G6PD) deficiency and sickle cell trait (Hb-AS). Trop Geogr Med 1978; 30:99.

179. Gibbs WN, Wardle J, Serjeant GR: Glucose 6-phosphate dehydrogenase deficiency and homozygous sickle cell disease in Jamaica. Br J Haematol 1980; 45:73.

180. Nieweunhuis F, Wolf B, et al: Haematological study in Cabo Delgado province, Mozambique; sickle cell trait and G6PD deficiency. Trop Geogr Med 1986; 38:183.

181. Piomelli S, Siniscalco M: The haematological effects of glucose 6-phosphate dehydrogenase deficiency and thalassaemia trait: interaction between the two genes at the phenotype level. Br J Haematol 1969; 16:537.

182. Sanna G, Frau F, et al: Interaction between the glucose-6-phosphate dehydrogenase deficiency and thalassaemia genes at phenotype level. Br J Haematol 1980; 44:555.

183. Steinberg MH, West MS, et al: Effects of glucose-6-phosphate dehydrogenase deficiency upon sickle cell anemia. Blood 1988; 71:748.

184. Awamy BH: Effect of G-6 PD deficiency on sickle cell disease in Saudi Arabia. Indian J Pediatr 1992; 59:331.

185. Smits HL, Oski FA, Brody JI: The hemolytic crisis of sickle cell disease: the role of glucose 6-phosphate dehydrogenase deficiency. J Pediatr 1969; 74:544.

186. Carpentieri U, Haggard ME, et al: Hb E-beta thalassemia associated with G6PD deficiency. South Med J 1980; 73:518.

187. Vives Corrons JL, Garcia AM, et al: Heterozygous pyruvate kinase deficiency and severe hemolytic anemia in a pregnant woman with concomitant, glucose-6-phosphate dehydrogenase deficiency. Ann Hematol 1991; 62:190.

188. Mahendra P, Dollery CT, et al: Pyruvate kinase deficiency: association with G6PD deficiency. BMJ 1992; 305:760.

189. Ventura A, Panizon F, et al: Congenital dyserythropoietic anaemia Type II associated with a new type of G6PD deficiency (G6PD Gabrovizza). Acta Haematol 1984; 71:227.

190. Szeto SC, Ng CS: A case of congenital dyserythropoietic anemia in a male Chinese. Pathology 1986; 18:165.

191. Gangarossa S, Romano V, et al: Congenital dyserythropoietic anemia type II associated with G6PD Seattle in a Sicilian child. Acta Haematol 1995; 93:36.

192. Panich V, Na-Nakorn S, Wasi P: Hereditary elliptocytosis (the first report in Thailand) in association with erythrocyte glucose-6-phosphate dehydrogenase deficiency and hemoglobin E. J Med Assoc Thai 1970; 53:593.

193. Alfinito F, Calabrò V, et al: Glucose 6-phosphate dehydrogenase deficiency and red cell membrane defects: additive or synergistic interaction in producing chronic haemolytic anaemia. Br J Haematol 1994; 87:148.

194. Meloni T, Forteleoni G, Meloni GF: Marked decline of favism after neonatal glucose-6-phosphate dehydrogenase screening and health education: the northern Sardinian experience. Acta Haematol 1992; 87:29.

195. Winterbourn CC, Stern A: Human red cells scavenge extracellular hydrogen peroxide and inhibit formation of hypochlorous acid and hydroxyl radical. J Clin Invest 1987; 80:1486.

196. Hori SH: Glucose-6-phosphate dehydrogenase and hexose-6-phosphate dehydrogenase: an evolutionary aspect. In Yoshida A, Beutler E (eds): Glucose-6-Phosphate Dehydrogenase. Orlando, FL, Academic Press, Inc., 1986.

197. Lux SE, Tse WT, et al: Hereditary spherocytosis associated with deletion of human erythrocyte ankyrin gene on chromosome 8. Nature 1990; 345:736.

198. Fialkow PJ: Clonal origin of human tumors. Biochim Biophys Acta 1976; 458:283.

199. DeVita G, Alcalay M, et al: Two point mutations are responsible for G6PD polymorphism in Sardinia. Am J Hum Genet 1989; 44:233.

200. Escobar MA, Heller P, Trobaugh FE Jr: "Complete" erythrocyte glucose 6-phosphate dehydrogenase deficiency. Arch Intern Med 1964; 113:428.

201. Cooper MR, De Chatelet LR, et al: Complete deficiency of leukocyte glucose 6-phosphate dehydrogenase with defective bactericidal activity. J Clin Invest 1972; 51:769.

202. Gray FR, Klebanoff SJ, et al: Neutrophil dysfunction, chronic granulomatous disease and non-spherocytic haemolytic anemia caused by complete deficiency of glucose-6-phosphate dehydrogenase. Lancet 1973; 2:530.

VI Disorders of Hemoglobin

18 | Hemoglobins: Normal and Abnormal

Ronald L. Nagel

This chapter deals with the structure and properties of hemoglobin (Hb) and the disorders stemming from structural abnormalities (mutations of the coding sequence) that lead to clinical manifestations related to alterations of the function (oxygen [O_2] affinity and electronic state of the heme iron) or stability of the Hb molecule. Not included are disorders resulting from the presence of aggregating Hb such as HbS, HbC, or the thalassemias.

At last count (mid-2002), 854 human Hb mutations have been cataloged: 214 for the $\alpha 1$ gene, 254 for the $\alpha 2$ gene, 650 for the β gene, 57 for the δ gene, 45 for the $^A\gamma$ gene, and 54 for the $^G\gamma$ gene. Of these, 80 have high affinity for O_2, 59 have low affinity, and 122 are unstable. (A list of the mutants can be found at the Globin Gene Server [http://globin.cse.psu.edu], a web site founded by Ross Hardison and initially based on Titus Huisman's database.)

NORMAL HEMOGLOBINS: STRUCTURE AND FUNCTION

Overall Hemoglobin Structure

The major Hb molecule in adults is a tetramer formed by four polypeptide chains, two α chains (141 amino acids long), and two β chains (146 amino acids long). The primary structure (amino acid sequence) is illustrated in Table 18–1. Each of these chains is attached to a prosthetic group called *heme*, formed by protoporphyrin IX complexed with an iron molecule. All globins consist of eight helices and interconnecting loops (nonhelical) except α Hb subunits which lack the D helix owing to deletion of five consecutive residues. Each chain is formed by helical regions and nonhelical regions (that allow for bending) and the product is a tightly globular protein. In the discussion of Hb we will compare the chains to myoglobin (Fig. 18–1), a single chain carrier of O_2, which allows us to understand what is critical for tetramer formation.

α Chains of Hemoglobin (Tertiary Structure)

The α *chains* have the general architecture of myoglobin, but have shorter chains, containing 141 rather than 153 amino acids, that result from the absence of six residues

from the C-terminal portion (two are the last members of the H helix and four are from the nonhelical tail of β chains). The D helix in myoglobin and in the β subunit of Hb is required for the retention of heme.[1]

The deletion of the D helix in the α chains has no explanation. The disappearance of the nonhelical C-terminal residues could be related to the important bond between Arg-$\alpha 141$ and Tyr-$\alpha 140$ and the appropriate receptor, which are important to the conformational changes involved in the transformation from oxygenated (oxy)-to-deoxygenated (deoxy) forrms (see later discussion), a central feature of the tetramer structure-function relationship. The N-terminal–added residues in myoglobin might strain these critical molecular distances and make the conformational change impossible.

The differences between α chains and myoglobin could also be derived from the need that α chains have to bind several different β like chains (γ, δ, and ϵ) with varied requirements for the generation of the quaternary structure. Specifically, the generation of a quaternary structure implies changes in the character of the residues involved in subunit contact. That is, residues that are polar in myoglobin (because they are in direct contact with the solvent) might be buried in an intersubunit contact in several of the Hbs and hence have to be replaced by hydrophobic amino acids. Two examples of this are found in residue B15, a lysine in myoglobin that becomes a leucine, and residue C1, a histidine in myoglobin, which is a phenylalanine in human α chains.[1,2]

β Chains of Hemoglobin (Tertiary Structure)

The human β *chains* are also shorter than myoglobin, containing 146 residues. The general architecture of the chain and of its secondary and tertiary structure complies closely with the myoglobin fold.[3–5]

TABLE 18–1. Primary Amino Acid Structure of the Hemoglobin Molecule

Helix	α	ζ	Helix	β	δ	γ	ϵ
NA1	1 Val	Ser	NA1	1 Val	Val	Gly	Val
			NA2	2 His	His	His	His
NA2	2 Leu	Leu	NA3	3 Leu	Leu	Phe	Phe
A1	3 Ser	Thr	A1	4 Thr	Thr	Thr	Thr
A2	4 Pro	Lys	A2	5 Pro	Pro	Glu	Ala
A3	5 Ala	Thr	A3	6 Glu	Glu	Glu	Glu
A4	6 Asp	Glu	A4	7 Glu	Glu	Asp	Glu
A5	7 Lys	Arg	A5	8 Lys	Lys	Lys	Lys
A6	8 Thr	Thr	A6	9 Ser	Thr	Ala	Ala
A7	9 Asn	lle	A7	10 Ala	Ala	Thr	Ala
A8	10 Val	lle	A8	11 Val	Val	lle	Val
A9	11 Lys	Val	A9	12 Thr	Asn	Thr	Thr
A10	12 Ala	Ser	A10	13 Ala	Ala	Ser	Ser
A11	13 Ala	Met	A11	14 Leu	Leu	Leu	Leu
A12	14 Trp	Trp	A12	15 Trp	Trp	Trp	Trp
A13	15 Gly	Ala	A13	16 Gly	Gly	Gly	Ser
A14	16 Lys	Lys	A14	17 Lys	Lys	Lys	Lys
A15	17 Val	lle	A15	18 Val	Val	Val	Met
A16	18 Gly	$$Ser					
AB1	19 Ala	Thr					
B1	20 His	Gln	B1	19 Asn	Asn	Asn	Asn

TABLE 18–1. Primary Amino Acid Structure of the Hemoglobin Molecule (*Continued*)

Helix	α	ζ
B2	21 Ala	Ala
B3	22 Gly	Asp
B4	23 Glu	Thr
B5	24 Tyr	lle
B6	25 Gly	Gly
B7	26 Ala	Thr
B8	27 Glu	Glu
B9	28 ALa	Thr
B10	29 Leu	Leu
B11	30 Glu	Glu
B12	31 Arg	Arg
B13	32 Met	Leu
B14	33 Phe	Phe
B15	34 Leu	Leu
B16	35 Ser	Ser
C1	36 Phe	His
C2	37 Pro	Pro
C3	38 Thr	Gln
C4	39 Thr	Thr
C5	40 Lys	Lys
C6	41 Thr	Thr
C7	42 Tyr	Tyr
CE1	43 Phe	Phe
CE2	44 Pro	Pro
CE3	45 His	His
CE4	46 Phe	Phe
CE5	47 Asp	Asp
CE6	48 Leu	Leu
CE7	49 Ser	His
CE8	50 His	Pro
CE9	51 Gly	Gly
E1	52 Ser	Ser
E2	53 Ala	Ala
E3	54 Gln	Gln
E4	55 Val	Leu
E5	56 Lys	Arg
E6	57 Gly	Ala
E7	58 His	His
E8	59 Gly	Gly
E9	60 Lys	Ser
E10	61 Lys	Lys
E11	62 Val	Val
E12	63 Ala	Val
E13	64 Asp	Ser
E14	65 Ala	Ala
E15	66 Leu	Val
E16	67 Thr	Gly
E17	68 Asn	Asp
E18	69 Ala	Ala
E19	70 Val	Val
E20	71 Ala	Lys
EF1	72 His	Ser
EF2	73 Val	lle
EF3	74 Asp	Asp
EF4	75 Asp	Asp
EF5	76 Met	lle
EF6	77 Pro	Gly
EF7	78 Asn	Gly
EF8	79 Ala	Ala

Helix	β	δ	γ	ε
B2	20 Val	Val	Val	Val
B3	21 Asp	Asp	Glu	Glu
B4	22 Glu	Ala	Asp	Glu
B5	23 Val	Val	Ala	Ala
B6	24 Gly	Gly	Gly	Gly
B7	25 Gly	Gly	Gly	Gly
B8	26 Glu	Glu	Glu	Glu
B9	27 Ala	Ala	Thr	Ala
B10	28 Leu	Leu	Leu	Leu
B11	29 Gly	Gly	Gly	Gly
B12	30 Arg	Arg	Arg	Arg
B13	31 Leu	Leu	Leu	Leu
B14	32 Leu	Leu	Leu	Leu
B15	33 Val	Val	Val	Val
B16	34 Val	Val	Val	Val
C1	35 Tyr	Tyr	Tyr	Tyr
C2	36 Pro	Pro	Pro	Pro
C3	37 Trp	Trp	Trp	Trp
C4	38 Thr	Thr	Thr	Thr
C5	39 Gln	Gln	Gln	Gln
C6	40 Arg	Arg	Arg	Arg
C7	41 Phe	Phe	Phe	Phe
CD1	42 Phe	Phe	Phe	Phe
CD2	43 Glu	Glu	Asp	Asp
CD3	44 Ser	Ser	Ser	Ser
CD4	45 Phe	Phe	Phe	Phe
CD5	46 Gly	Gly	Gly	Gly
CD6	47 Asp	Asp	Asn	Asn
CD7	48 Leu	Leu	Leu	Leu
CD8	49 Ser	Ser	Ser	Ser
D1	50 Thr	Ser	Ala	Pro
D2	51 Pro	Pro	Ser	Ser
D3	52 Asp	Asp	Ser	Ser
D4	53 Ala	Ala	Ala	Ala
D5	54 Val	Val	lle	lle
D6	55 Met	Met	Met	Leu
D7	56 Gly	Gly	Gly	Gly
E1	57 Asn	Asn	Asn	Asn
E2	58 Pro	Pro	Pro	Pro
E3	59 Lys	Lys	Lys	Lys
E4	60 Val	Val	Val	Val
E5	61 Lys	Lys	Lys	Lys
E6	62 Ala	Ala	Ala	Ala
E7	63 His	His	His	His
E8	64 Gly	Gly	Gly	Gly
E9	65 Lys	Lys	Lys	Lys
E10	66 Lys	Lys	Lys	Lys
E11	67 Val	Val	Val	Val
E12	68 Leu	Leu	Leu	Leu
E13	69 Gly	Gly	Thr	Thr
E14	70 Ala	Ala	Ser	Ser
E15	71 Phe	Phe	Leu	Phe
E16	72 Ser	Ser	Gly	Gly
E17	73 Asp	Asp	Asp	Asp
E18	74 Gly	Gly	Ala	Ala
E19	75 Leu	Leu	lle, Thr	lle
E20	76 Ala	Ala	Lys	Lys
EF1	77 His	His	His	Asn
EF2	78 Leu	Leu	Leu	Met
EF3	79 Asp	Asp	Asp	Asp
EF4	80 Asn	Asn	Asp	Asn
EF5	81 Leu	Leu	Leu	Leu
EF6	82 Lys	Lys	Lys	Lys
EF7	83 Gly	Gly	Gly	Pro
EF8	84 Thr	Thr	Thr	Ala

TABLE 18–1. Primary Amino Acid Structure of the Hemoglobin Molecule (*Continued*)

Helix	α	ζ	Helix	β	δ	γ	ε
F1	80 Leu	Leu	F1	85 Phe	Phe	Phe	Phe
F2	81 Ser	Ser	F2	86 Ala	Ser	Ala	Ala
F3	82 Ala	Lys	F3	87 Thr	Gln	Gln	Lys
F4	83 Leu	Leu	F4	88 Leu	Leu	Leu	Leu
F5	84 Ser	Ser	F5	89 Ser	Ser	Ser	Ser
F6	85 Asp	Glu	F6	90 Glu	Glu	Glu	Glu
F7	86 Leu	Leu	F7	91 Leu	Leu	Leu	Leu
F8	87 His	His	F8	92 His	His	His	His
F9	88 Ala	Ala	F9	93 Cys	Cys	Cys	Cys
FG1	89 His	Tyr	FG1	94 Asp	Asp	Asp	Asp
FG2	90 Lys	Ile	FG2	95 Lys	Lys	Lys	Lys
FG3	91 Leu	Leu	FG3	96 Leu	Leu	Leu	Leu
FG4	92 Arg	Arg	FG4	97 His	His	His	His
FG5	93 Val	Val	FG5	98 Val	Val	Val	Val
G1	94 Asp	Asp	G1	99 Asp	Asp	Asp	Asp
G2	95 Pro	Pro	G2	100 Pro	Pro	Pro	Pro
G3	96 Val	Val	G3	101 Glu	Glu	Glu	Glu
G4	97 Asn	Asn	G4	102 Asn	Asn	Asn	Asn
G5	98 Phe	Phe	G5	103 Phe	Phe	Phe	Phe
G6	99 Lys	Lys	G6	104 Arg	Arg	Lys	Lys
G7	100 Leu	Leu	G7	105 Leu	Leu	Leu	Leu
G8	101 Leu	Leu	G8	106 Leu	Leu	Leu	Leu
G9	102 Ser	Ser	G9	107 Gly	Gly	Gly	Gly
G10	103 His	His	G10	108 Asn	Asn	Asn	Asn
G11	104 Cys	Cys	G11	109 Val	Val	Val	Val
G12	105 Leu	Leu	G12	110 Leu	Leu	Leu	Met
G13	106 Leu	Leu	G13	111 Val	Val	Val	Val
G14	107 Val	Val	G14	112 Cys	Cys	Thr	Ile
G15	108 Thr	Thr	G15	113 Val	Val	Val	Ile
G16	109 Leu	Leu	G16	114 Leu	Leu	Leu	Leu
G17	110 Ala	Ala	G17	115 Ala	Ala	Ala	Ala
G18	111 Ala	Ala	G18	116 His	Arg	Ile	Thr
G19	112 His	Arg	G19	117 His	Asn	His	His
GH1	113 Leu	Phe	Gh1	118 Phe	Phe	Phe	Phe
GH2	114 Pro	Pro	GH2	119 Gly	Gly	Gly	Gly
GH3	115 Ala	Ala	GH3	120 Lys	Lys	Lys	Lys
GH4	116 Glu	Asp	GH4	121 Glu	Glu	Glu	Glu
GH5	117 Phe	Phe	Gh5	122 Phe	Phe	Phe	Phe
H1	118 Thr	Thr	H1	123 Thr	Thr	Thr	Thr
H2	119 Pro	Ala	H2	124 Pro	Pro	Pro	Pro
H3	120 Ala	Glu	H3	125 Pro	Gln	Glu	Glu
H4	121 Val	Ala	H4	126 Val	Met	Val	Val
H5	122 His	His	H5	127 Gln	Gln	Gln	Gln
H6	123 Ala	Ala	H6	128 Ala	Ala	Ala	Ala
H7	124 Ser	Ala	H7	129 Ala	Ala	Ser	Ala
H8	125 Leu	Trp	H8	130 Tyr	Tyr	Trp	Trp
H9	126 Asp	Asp	H9	131 Gln	Gln	Gln	Gln
H10	127 Lys	Lys	H10	132 Lys	Lys	Lys	Lys
H11	128 Phe	Phe	H11	133 Val	Val	Met	Leu
H12	129 Leu	Leu	H12	134 Val	Val	Val	Val
H13	130 Ala	Ser	H13	135 Ala	Ala	Thr	Ser
H14	131 Ser	Val	H14	136 Gly	Gly	Gly, Ala	Ala
H15	132 Val	Val	H15	137 Val	Val	Val	Val
H16	133 Ser	Ser	H16	138 Ala	Ala	Ala	Ala
H17	134 Thr	Ser	H17	139 Asn	Asn	Ser	Ile
H18	135 Val	Val	H18	140 Ala	Ala	Ala	Ala
H19	136 Leu	Leu	H19	141 Leu	Leu	Leu	Leu
H20	137 Thr	Thr	H20	142 Ala	Ala	Ser	Ala
H21	138 Ser	Glu	H21	143 His	His	Ser	His
HC1	139 Lys	Lys	HC1	144 Lys	Lys	Arg	Lys
HC2	140 Tyr	Tyr	HC2	145 Tyr	Tyr	Tyr	Tyr
HC3	141 Arg	Arg	HC3	146 His	His	His	His

*The α and α-related (δ) subunits are shown at the left. The β and β-related (δ, γ, and ε) chains are at the right. The amino acids' relationship to the eight globin helices (A to H) is also shown. Thus, A16 is the 16th amino acid in the A helix. Interhelical elbows are named for the two adjacent helices (e.g., AB1 is the first amino acid between helices A and B). The N- and C-terminal residues are labeled NA and HC, respectively. The residues are aligned to maximize the homology between subunits, which causes some gaps.

(Modified from Bunn HF, Forget BG. Hemoglobin: molecular, genetic, and clinical aspects. Philadelphia, WB Saunders, 1986)

FIGURE 18–1. The myoglobin fold. The myoglobin molecule consists of eight stretches of helix that surround the heme group forming a pocket. *Single letters* signify a helix; *double letters,* a corner or bend (nonhelical regions). The heme pocket is formed by helices E and F. Helices B, G, and H are at the *bottom,* and the CD corner closes the open end. Histidine side chains interact with the heme from both sides. (From Dickerson RE, Geis I: Hemoglobin: Structure, Function, Evolution, and Pathology. Menlo Park, CA, Benjamin/Cummings, 1983, p 26.)

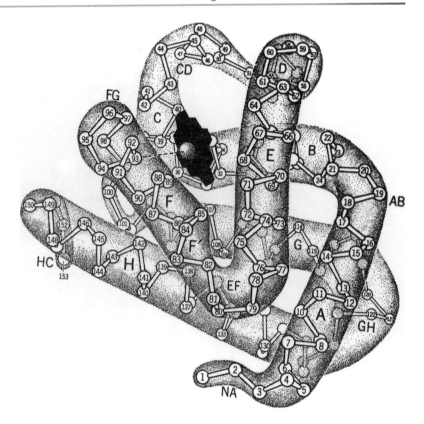

Two small structural differences with myoglobin are apparent: the disappearance of two residues from the junction of A and B helices, making the AB elbow sharper, as well as six residues missing from the C-terminal sequence (as in the α chains). The reason for the change in the AB elbow is not understood. The critical bonds involving His-β142 and Tyr-β145 might be incompatible with the presence of the nonhelical terminal residues found in myoglobin. In the β chains, changes of charged to hydrophobic residues can also be observed in the areas of the sequence involved in subunit interaction.

The Tetramer (Quaternary Structure)

The Hb molecule is a tetramer formed by two α chains and two β chains, with a total molecular mass of 64.5 kD.

How Do the Two Pairs of Chains Generate a Tetramer? The arrangement of the two types of chains in the tetramer complies with a 222 symmetry. This designation means that the structure can be characterized by three twofold axes of symmetry, perpendicular to each other (Fig. 18–2). To understand this symmetry, consider the upper half (the dark pair of chains) in the vertical axis. If you rotate these two chains by 180°, they will coincide perfectly with the light-colored pair of chains: this is called a *twofold* or *diad axis of symmetry;* hence, the three twos. Of course, α chains are not identical to β chains. Therefore, in an actual Hb molecule this symmetry is only approximate. The homotetramer of β chains (β$_4$ or HbH), observed in a severe form of α-thalassemia, exhibits the perfect 222 symmetry in the oxygenated tetramer, because all chains are truly identical.

How Do the Four Chains Interact? The tetramer α$_2$β$_2$ exhibits several types of subunit interactions, but the weakest contact occurs between identical chains, that is, in the α$_1$α$_2$ or β$_1$β$_2$ interfaces. The strong interactions are in the contacts between the dissimilar pair of chains, that is, in the interfaces α$_1$β$_1$ and or the equivalent α$_2$β$_2$.

The next level of complexity is the contact between these two pairs of unlike chains. The contact occurs in two areas in the surfaces of these dimers: the α$_1$β$_2$ contact (Fig. 18–2) and the equivalent α$_2$β$_1$ contact, which is called the *sliding contact.* Conversely, the α$_1$β$_1$ dimer has areas of interaction between the α and β chains that are called *packing contacts.* Tetramers are strong and can be broken only with very high urea concentrations and certain salts, and they remain as such throughout the conformational changes of Hb.

The sliding contact, on the other hand, is weaker and has strategically located hydrogen (H$^+$) bonds and salt bridges that can be broken and reformed elsewhere, allowing the mobility of the two surfaces, a phenomena indispensable for conformational changes (see next section). In conclusion, the interactions between like chains are weak, whereas the interactions between unlike chains are strong; hence, when the tetramer dissociates, α$_1$β$_2$ dimers are generated. About 20 percent of the surface area of the subunits is consumed in subunit-subunit interactions, of which 60 percent are involved in packing contacts and 35 percent in sliding contacts.[6]

Oxygen Binding of Hemoglobin and the Structure-Function Relationships

Hb carries O$_2$ from the lungs to the capillaries and carbon dioxide (CO$_2$) in the reverse direction. In addition, mammals need to adapt to sudden changes in oxygenation

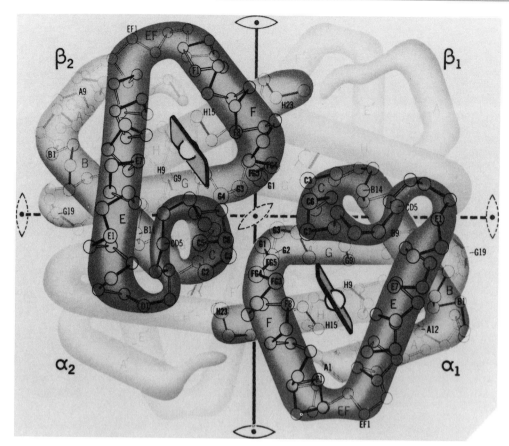

FIGURE 18–2. The four chains of hemoglobin, front view: $\alpha_1\beta_2$ contacts (the $\alpha_2\beta_1$ contacts are identical on the back side of the molecule). The perpendicular pseudoaxis is indicated by *dashes*. Only the carbons of the main chains are shown. The side chains involved in contacts between subunits are indicated by *boldface numbers in large circles*. (From Dickerson RE, Geis I: Hemoglobin: Structure, Function, Evolution, and Pathology. Menlo Park, CA, Benjamin/Cummings, 1983, p 36.)

requirements; therefore, they require modulation of its O_2 carrying capacity. The functions of Hb are summarized as follows:

1. It binds O_2 with a sigmoid curve—that is, allosterically (see later).
2. It binds CO_2 while it is delivering O_2 and releases CO_2 when it is binding O_2.
3. It binds H^+ efficiently in a low pH environment and releases it when it encounters high pH (Bohr effect).
4. Allosteric effectors, that is, 2,3-diphosphoglycerate (2,3-DPG), chloride (Cl^-), H^+, and CO_2, modulate O_2 affinity.

Hemoglobin Binds Oxygen Allosterically. The myoglobin molecule, being a monomer, binds O_2 as predicted by mass law: a plot of the partial pressure of O_2 (Po_2) versus O_2 saturation can be described by a hyperbole. On the other hand, the Hb tetramer, with four hemes, binds O_2 with a sigmoidal curve (Fig. 18–3). Myoglobin binding of O_2 can be described at equilibrium by the simple relation

$$y = K_a Po_2/1 + K_a Po_2,$$

where y is the fractional saturation of the myoglobin molecule with O_2, K_a is the association constant, and Po_2 is the partial pressure of O_2.

For the Hb molecule, the binding of O_2 is different, and at equilibrium this reaction can be described by the formula

$$y = K_a Po_2{}^n/1 + K_a Po_2{}^n.$$

The difference is the power of n to which Po_2 is elevated: n is the Hill coefficient, an empiric number that is an index of the sigmoidicity of the curve and a feature of the function that is related to the extent of cooperativity. The Hill coefficient is 2.8 for Hb, whereas it is equal to 1 for myoglobin.

What Is Cooperativity? Cooperativity is the reason for the sigmoid shape of the O_2 equilibrium curve of Hb. The initial portion of the curve has a very low slope, reflecting a low affinity for O_2 by Hb at the beginning of the loading process. That is, when Hb is totally deoxygenated, it has a rather poor avidity for O_2 (Fig. 18–3). As the loading proceeds and as the molecule binds more O_2 molecules, the slope of the reaction begins to change rapidly and becomes steep. Hence, the affinity for O_2 becomes much higher despite the initial sluggishness. In other words, the initial molecules of O_2 that bind a deoxy-Hb tetramer change the avidity of the protein for O_2. This property, called *cooperativity*, ensures that the Hb tetramer, after it begins to accept O_2, is promptly fully oxygenated. Thus, if we measure the distribution of O_2 in

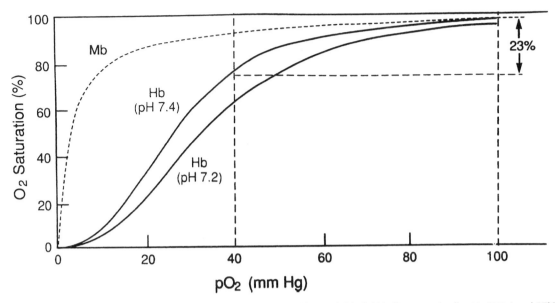

FIGURE 18–3. Oxygen equilibrium curves of sperm whale myoglobin (Mb) and hemoglobin (Hb) in human red cells. At pH 7.4 and 37°C, the oxygen saturation of the red cells is 98 percent at the arterial blood partial pressure of O_2 (pO_2) (100 mm Hg) and 75 percent at the mixed venous blood pO_2 (40 mm Hg) so that oxygen corresponding to a 23 percent saturation difference is transported by circulating red cells. (After Imai K: Allosteric effects in haemoglobin. Cambridge, UK, Cambridge University Press, 1982.)

all of the Hb molecules in a solution that contains enough O_2 to oxygenate only half of the hemes available, most Hb molecules would either not be oxygenated at all or would be entirely oxygenated, with a small compartment of partially oxygenated Hbs.

The Molecular Basis of Cooperativity. One generally accepted basis of cooperativity is the *two-state* (or *concerted*) model of Monod, Wyman, and Changeaux[7] (MWC model). The model is based on two fundamentally different conformations: one for oxygenated Hb and another for the deoxygenated molecule. In its strictest form, this model does not accept meaningful intermediate conformations, only two extreme ones. It predicts that the molecule of Hb will bind two or three molecules of O_2 at low affinity (deoxy conformation) and then, suddenly, the molecule will flip to the oxygenated conformation, drastically increasing the O_2 affinity of the molecule as a whole. Perutz and colleagues[8–10] have applied this model to Hb with great success (Fig. 18–4).

Formally, the two-state model can be defined by two quantities: *c*, which represents the difference in activity between the two enzyme states, but in the special case of Hb, corresponds to the ratio of O_2 affinity constants between the two conformation states (K_a oxy/K_a deoxy = *c*). The second quantity, the allosteric constant *L*, is the fraction of Hb molecules in the T state. The rest are R structures. *L* defines the equilibrium constant for the conformational change itself between the two states: T for tense, the nonaccepting or low-affinity state (the deoxygenated conformer in the case of Hb) and R for relaxed, the accepting or high-affinity state (the oxygenated conformer in the case of Hb). The significant switch of conformation must occur in Hb somewhere in *between the binding of two and three molecules* of O_2. Under physiologic conditions of pH, the presence of effectors and osmolarity, at full saturation, only 1 of 3,000,000 Hb molecules

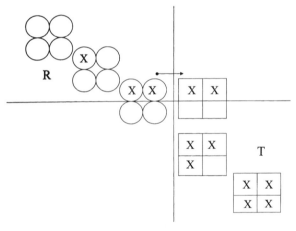

FIGURE 18–4. This diagram illustrates the two-state model of the binding of oxygen and other ligands to hemoglobin. R stands for the *relax* or high-affinity conformer, and T stands for the *tense* or low-affinity conformer. X stands for the ligand. Each chain is in the r state (sphere) or the t state (square). Notice that when the tetramer is ligaded in two of the hemes it tends to adopt (switches to) the T conformer.

has the T structure. The results of recent analyses argue convincingly that the two-state model of Perutz defines the fundamental function of Hb and, in addition, cast doubt on the interpretation of some of the experiments that seem to contradict this model.[11, 12]

Why is the Hb tetramer of higher organisms allosteric? Allosterism makes Hb a molecule with lower affinity for O_2 than for myoglobins or the isolated Hb chains. Allosteric effectors such as 2,3-DPG and Cl^- and H^+ ions modulate the reduced affinity by lowering K_T (the association constant for the T state) and raising the *L* constant. The K_R (association constant of the R state) and *L* at O_2 saturation are not modified.[8]

What Are the Structural Events Underlying Cooperativity? The critical differences between R and T conformers involve the areas of contact between the $\alpha_1\beta_2$ and $\alpha_2\beta_1$ dimers. The $\alpha_1\beta_1$ and $\alpha_2\beta_2$ areas of contact are essentially immobile during the conformational change, because these dimers move as a unit. These events are pictured in Figure 18–5.

Three regions sustain the major changes during the R to T conformational change, which is a 15° rotation of the $\alpha_1\beta_1$ dimer with respect to the $\alpha_2\beta_1$ dimer around a pivot passing through the terminal portions of the H helix in both chains. The movements involve exclusively the residues that touch each other in the $\alpha_1\beta_2$ areas of contact (Fig. 18–6). One movement involves the pivotal sliding of the two dimers with respect to each other, with the contact involving the β FG corner moving farther away from the pivotal axis. This is called the *switch region*. Another movement involves the FG corner of the α chains contacting the C helix of the β chains, but the contact is less affected because the α FG corner is much closer to the pivotal axis. This is called the *flexible joint*. In addition, a change is seen in the set of salt bridges between the H helix (C-terminal portion of the β chain) and the C helix of the α chain and between the C-terminal portion of the α chains and the C helix of the β chain. These contact points have no particular name, but they are referred to here as the *C-terminal changes*. Detailed residue interactions are depicted in Figure 18–6.

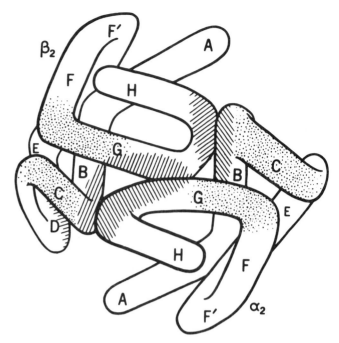

FIGURE 18–5. The $\alpha_2\beta_2$ dimer is seen in a side view. The *dotted areas* depict the packing contacts that hold the dimer together. The sliding contacts with the $\alpha_1\beta_1$ dimer are depicted by areas of *gray stippling*. (From Dickerson RE, Geis I: Hemoglobin: Structure, Function, Evolution, and Pathology. Menlo Park, CA, Benjamin/Cummings, 1983, p 38.)

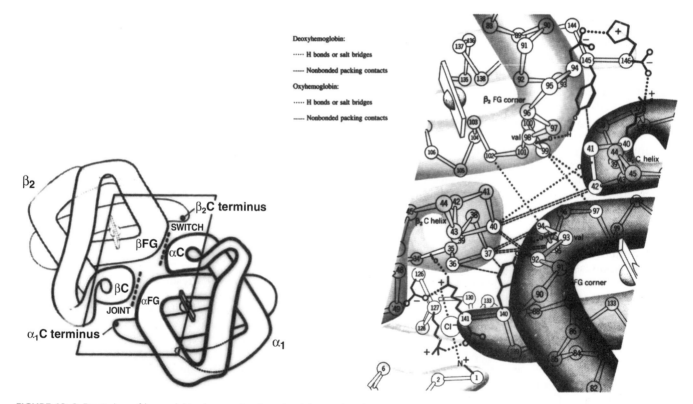

FIGURE 18–6. Front view of hemoglobin shows extensive subunit interactions between FG corners and C helices in the $\alpha_1\beta_2$ contacts. The area in *A* is enlarged in *B*. Important interaction regions from *top to bottom* are the β-chain C-terminal, the switch region, the flexible joint, and the α-chain terminal. (From Dickerson RE, Geis I: Hemoglobin: Structure, Function, Evolution, and Pathology. Menlo Park, CA, Benjamin/Cummings, 1983, p 43.)

All of these H bonds and salt bridges are broken in the *oxy conformer*, providing one of the most important sources of the difference in free energy between the T and R states in Hb.

What Triggers the Conformation Change at the Level of the Heme? The iron in deoxy-Hb is slightly out of the plane of the heme (domed configuration) because the pyrrole rings are also slightly pyramidal (Fig. 18–7). The angle between the heme plane and the iron is 8° in the α heme and 7° in the β heme. The His F8 axis is 8° off center, and the Val FG5 is in contact with the vinyl side chain of pyrrole 3 (Fig. 18–8). When the ligand binds the sixth coordinating position of the iron, significant steric stresses are introduced, particularly between the heme and the proximal histidine, the ligand and the heme, and the heme and the Val FG5. To relieve this strain, the histidine moves 8° to become perpendicular to the heme, significantly decreasing the doming of the iron (the angle between iron and the heme falls to 4°). Also, displacement of FG5 is present in the direction of His F8. The configuration around the heme has now changed to the oxygenated or R state, and a chain of events involving the critical interactions in the $\alpha_1\beta_2$ area of contact follows.

What Is the Conformational Micropath between the Heme and the Globin? In the α chain, the displacement of the His F8 to straighten up its 8° tilt in the liganded heme requires that the F helix move with it. This displacement of the F helix, along its axis, is accompanied by a shift downward, which moves closer to the heme. The heme shifts toward the interior of the heme pocket. The changes in the F helix are propagated along the E and G helices, but leave the rest of the α chain unchanged. In the β subunit, the changes are similar, except that the heme also tilts around a pyrrole 2–4 axis. In both heme niches, the Val FG5 moves closer to the vinyl side chains; this Van der Waals contact breaks the critical H bonds between Val[98] and Tyr[145] in the β chain and between Val[98] and Tyr[140] in the α chain. The rest of the H bonds and salt bridges described earlier for the C termini become weakened to the point of breakage, releasing the molecule from the T state (closed and low affinity) to the R state (open and high affinity).

These features of this micropath for the conformational changes of Hb were proposed early but with insufficient evidence.[13] Significant proof came from a mixture of analytical techniques.[14–16]

Hemoglobin Binds CO_2 While It Is Delivering O_2 and Releases CO_2 When It Is Binding O_2. The Hb is designed to bind CO_2 after delivering O_2 to the tissues, helping to dissipate the increase in concentration of CO_2 in delivery of this metabolic end product to the lung alveoli. This exchange is facilitated because CO_2 is an allosteric inhibitor of Hb, decreasing the O_2 affinity of the molecule.

CO_2 binds Hb by forming carbamates with the α amino groups of the α chains. Through this new negative charge, CO_2 can bind Arg 141 in the *absence* of Cl^- ions. This bond stabilizes the T conformer and decreases the O_2 affinity of the molecule.[17] The reaction is

$$Hb-NH_2 + CO_2 \rightarrow Hb-NH-COO^- + H^+.$$

Although CO_2 also binds the α amino groups of the β chains, helping to transport more of this end product, the reaction does not contribute to allosterism. The β chain carbamate reaction favors the deoxy conformer by the production of H^+, but this effect is counteracted by the reduction of positive charges in the central cavity, an event that favors the R state.

Hemoglobin Binds H+ Efficiently at a Low pH and Releases Protons at High pH (Bohr Effect). The Bohr effect describes the changes of O_2 affinity related to pH changes exhibited by Hb (Fig. 18–9). Within a certain range, the lower the pH is, the lower the affinity or the higher the partial pressure of O_2 at which Hb is one-half saturated (P_{50}).[14–16] That is, an increased concentration of protons favors a low-affinity state in Hb. Deoxy-Hb binds more protons than the oxy conformer, which means that in the absence of a buffer, a ligand change in Hb can be recorded by a change in the solution pH (Haldane effect).

All the features described in the previous paragraph are the consequence of H^+ ions acting as allosteric inhibitors: H^+ binds more avidly to the deoxy conformer (T state) than to the oxy conformer (R state). The so-called Bohr protons (protons released during oxygenation) originate primarily from the breakage of the C-terminal bonds during ligand binding (see Fig. 18–6).

Seventy-five percent of the Bohr effect is derived from the differences in the pK of the following residues when the molecule changes from the oxy to the deoxy conformation: (1) the two terminal histidines of the β chains (β146 His) account for 40 percent of the Bohr protons as determined by Kilmartin and associates[18]; (2) the α amino groups of the two N-terminal residues (Val[1]) of the α chains account for 25 percent of the Bohr proteins; and (3) α122 His contributes 10 percent of the Bohr protons (although no rationale for this effect has been found).[20]

Recently individual pK values of the 24 histidyl residues of HbA have been measured.[21] Among those surface histidyl residues, β146 His has the biggest contribution to the alkaline Bohr effect (63 percent at pH 7.4), and β143 His has the biggest contribution to the acid Bohr effect (71 percent at pH 5.1). The α20 His, α112 His, and β117 His residues have essentially no contribution; the α50 His, α72 His, α89 His, β92 His, and β116 His residues have moderate positive contributions; and the β2 His and β77 His residues have a moderate negative contribution to the Bohr effect. The sum of the contributions from 24 surface histidyl residues accounted for 86 percent of the alkaline Bohr effect at pH 7.4 and about 55 percent of the acid Bohr effect at pH 5.1. Results of this study support the presence of a global electrostatic network for regulation of the Bohr effect of the Hb molecule.

Other (2,3-Diphosphoglycerate and Cl^-) Allosteric Effectors Modulate the O2 Affinity of Hemoglobin. Benesch and Benesch[22] discovered the effects of 2,3-DPG on the function of Hb when they noticed, while examining tabular data in preparation for a lecture to medical students, that this intraerythrocytic organic phosphate was almost equimolar to Hb. Oxygen equilibrium measurements in the presence and absence of 2,3-DPG rapidly demonstrated that this effector drastically displaced the P_{50} of Hb to the right, making the Hb less avid for the ligand.

A

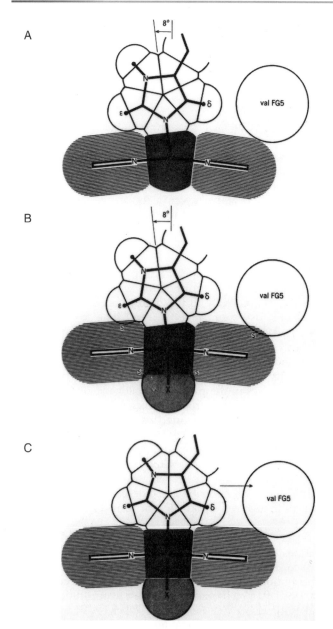

B

C

FIGURE 18–7. Ligation and strain in the heme environment. *A,* Unliganded heme in deoxyhemoglobin, with the histidine tilted, the iron out of plane, and the heme in contact with the Val FG5 side chain. *B,* Liganded heme held in its deoxy configuration before the T-to-R subunit transition. Steric strain (marked *s*) among heme, histidine, ligand (X), and valine can be relieved only after this transition. *C,* Relaxed, unstrained liganded heme after the T-to-R shift. Both His F8 and Val FG5 have shifted to the right, and the histidine now is perpendicular to the heme plane. The heme is largely undomed. (From Dickerson RE, Geis I: Hemoglobin: Structure, Function, Evolution, and Pathology. Menlo Park, CA, Benjamin/Cummings, 1983, p 43.)

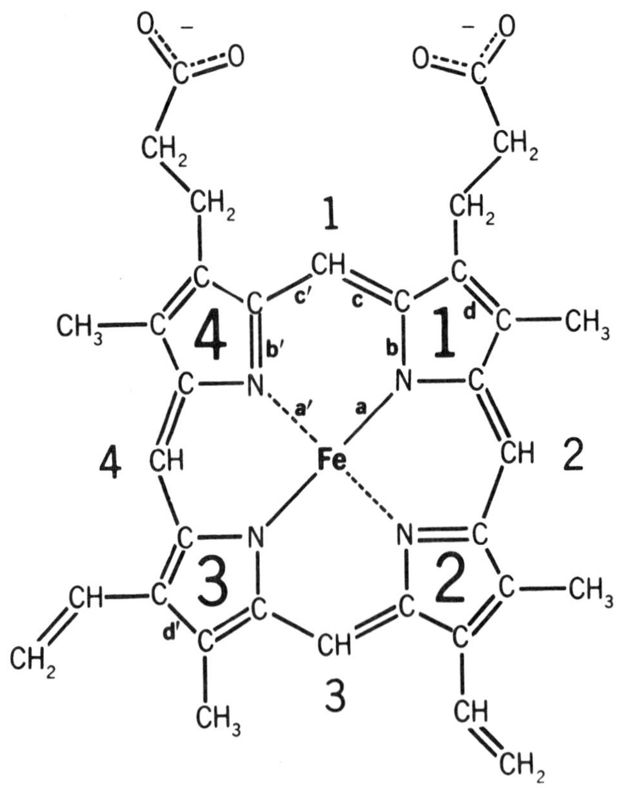

FIGURE 18–8. The protoporphyrin IX heme structure consists of four pyrrole rings with the following side-chain replacements: two methyl and two propionic acids in pyrrole 1 and 4; and two methyl and two vinyls in pyrroles 2 and 3. Iron is tetracoordinated by the nitrogens of the pyrrole rings. (From Dickerson RE, Geis I: Hemoglobin: Structure, Function, Evolution, and Pathology. Menlo Park, CA, Benjamin/Cummings, 1983, p 55.)

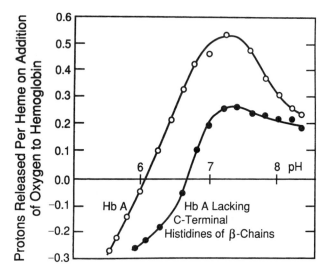

FIGURE 18–9. Discharge of protons on uptake of oxygen (Bohr effect) by normal human hemoglobin A and hemoglobin from which the C-terminal histidines of the β chains have been cleaved with carboxypeptidase B (des-His-146β hemoglobin). Note the reversal of the alkaline Bohr effect at pH 6.0 in HbA and at the pH 6.7 in des His hemoglobin and the halving of the alkaline Bohr effect in the latter. (After Kilmartin JV, Wootton JF: Inhibition of Bohr effect after removal of C-terminal histidines from hemoglobin β chains. Nature 1970; 228:766.)

Independently and simultaneously, Chanutin and Curnish[23] realized that these substances have an important biologic effect on the red blood cell. Their discoveries were followed by the finding that inositol hexaphosphate, a higher-level polyphosphate than 2,3-DPG and a more powerful effector has the same function as 2,3-DPG but at lower concentrations in the red cells of birds. Finally, in some fish, red cell adenosine triphosphate (ATP) and guanosine triphosphate seem to be the physiologic O_2 modulators.

In an allosteric model, the effector must bind differentially to each one of the conformational states. For an effector to be an inhibitor (a molecule that decreases the activity of the molecule—in this case the O_2 affinity), it must bind more strongly to the T form. Crystallographic evidence[24] has demonstrated that 2,3-DPG binds to the central cavity of Hb, that is, the space surrounding the true diad axis of symmetry between the two β chains (ββ) (Fig. 18–10). The displacement of the β chains away from each other by 7 Å in deoxy-Hb makes this single site in the tetramer capable of accommodating the highly negatively charged 2,3-DPG molecule, whereas the tighter ββ interaction in oxy-Hb does not allow the effector to penetrate the central cavity. The *five* negative charges of 2,3-DPG find proper positive charges to form salt bridges just under the edge of the ββ central cavity. The globin residues

involved in the binding are the two N-termini of the α and β chains, the two β143 histidines, and one of the two β82 lysines. The purpose of this effector is to modulate the O_2 equilibrium curve according to physiologic requirements. For example, in anemia the synthesis of 2,3-DPG increases, favoring the release of O_2 and partially coping with the decrease in the number of O_2 carriers.

Cl^- is another allosteric effector that decreases the O_2 affinity of Hb. Two mechanisms are involved. Cl^- binds preferentially to the deoxy conformer, the classic mechanism by which allosteric inhibitors operate in Hb. As noted earlier, Argα141, among its many interactions, forms a salt bridge with the N-termini of the opposite α chain across the $\alpha_1\beta_1$ area of contact through a Cl^- ion (Fig. 18–11). These bonds are broken in the oxy conformer, and the binding of Cl^- is no longer possible. The other type of Cl^- binding to Hb is less clear. Bonaventura and colleagues[25] found that anions, including Cl^-, in the

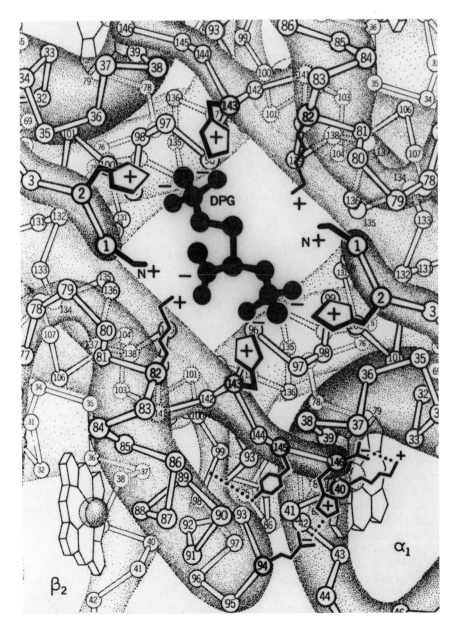

FIGURE 18–10. Amino acid side chains around the 2,3-diphosphoglycerate (DPG) binding site. This top view of the central cavity in human deoxyhemoglobin shows the positive charges lining the DPG site: two each from the N-terminal (Val-β1), from His-β2, from Lys-β82, and from His-β143. The DPG molecule with its five negative charges sits in the middle of this ring of positive charges. The fetal γ chain loses two of its eight positive charges by substituting Ser for His at β143, decreasing the affinity for DPG: Also shown are the salt bridges and the hydrogen-bonding pattern around the C terminus of the β chain (*lower part of figure*), which emphasizes their contribution to the Bohr effect. (From Dickerson RE, Geis I: Hemoglobin: Structure, Function, Evolution, and Pathology. Menlo Park, CA, Benjamin/Cummings, 1983, p 44.)

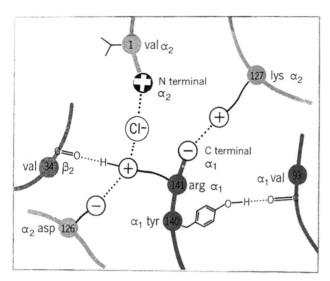

FIGURE 18–11. Chloride binding. Salt bridges and hydrogen bonds between other groups and the N-terminal and C-terminal residues in the α chains of deoxyhemoglobin. All these bonds are ruptured in oxyhemoglobin. A shift to the oxy configuration brings the C termini closer together. The side chain of Arg $\alpha_1$141(HC3) is squeezed out, rupturing all the bonds shown, an event that affects the binding of chloride (Cl^-). One of the two groups that contribute to the Bohr effect by becoming partially deprotonated in the oxy configuration is shown by a *black-encircled plus sign*. (From Dickerson RE, Geis I: Hemoglobin: Structure, Function, Evolution, and Pathology. Menlo Park, CA, Benjamin/Cummings, 1983, p 45.)

absence of 2,3-DPG can bind the positive charges available in the central cavity. This binding might not affect the O_2 affinity of Hb through the T-to-R conversion, because the same effect is observed in isolated chains. The physical basis of this effect remains unresolved.

Red Cell Oxygen Transport

RED CELL OXYGEN BINDING

The O_2 equilibrium of red cells depends on the following factors: (1) the intrinsic O_2 affinity of the Hb molecule (determined in solutions stripped of phosphate), (2) intraerythrocytic pH, (3) the intraerythrocytic concentration of 2,3-DPG, (4) temperature, and (5) the partial pressure of CO_2 (Pco_2).

Intraerythrocytic pH. The Bohr effect of whole blood is essentially identical to that of Hb in solution. For normal blood (37°C and 40 mm Hg CO_2), the log P_{50}-to-pH ratio is close to 0.5. The intracellular pH is 0.2 unit below the extracellular pH, determined by the concentration of permeant ions H^+, hydroxy (OH^-), Cl^-, and bicarbonate and the major impermeant ions, Hb itself and 2,3-DPG.

The concentrations of solutes inside and outside the red cell follow the Gibbs-Donnan relation that requires electroneutrality and due consideration to activity coefficient differences in the two compartments. As Hb and 2,3-DPG, which are negatively charged at pH 7.4, are trapped inside the red cell, the erythrocyte Cl^- concentration has to be decreased, thus, the ratio of 0.7 between intracellular and extracellular Cl^-. Calculation of the

Gibbs-Donnan equilibrium predicts the observed 0.2 pH unit difference between the inside and outside of the red cell, suggesting that no significant participant is missing in this phenomenon.

2,3-Diphosphoglyerate. The normal mean level of red cell 2,3-DPG is 12.8 mol/g of Hb for males and 13.8 mol/g of Hb for females.[26] Children younger than 5 years of age and elderly patients have increased and decreased levels, respectively.[27, 28] This amount makes organic phosphate almost equimolar with Hb in red cells, whereas in other cells it exists in very small concentrations.

Metabolically, 2,3-DPG is generated by the Rapoport-Luebering shunt from 1,3-DPG by 2,3-DPG synthase or mutase. Its level depends on the rates of synthesis and hydrolysis. The rate of synthesis is complex and depends on the amount of the substrate 1,3-DPG generated by glycolysis, which in turn increases directly with pH, and on the amount of 1,3-DPG entering the shunt. The alternative pathway for 1,3-DPG, and the most energetic, is conversion into 3-phosphoglycerate and generation of an ATP molecule. This alternative is probably greatly affected by the activity of the synthase, which is stimulated in direct proportion to the red cell pH and is under end-product inhibition by the concentration of 2,3-DPG.

Hypoxia has a tremendous impact on these relations, and the consequences of acidosis and alkalosis are described in Fig. 18–12.

Temperature. The P_{50} of blood is almost doubled by an increase of 10°C (between 20 and 30°C), an appropriate response to hypothermia and hyperthermia. Cold decreases metabolic requirements and reduces the need for O_2. During fever, metabolism is increased dramatically, and an increase in the delivery of O_2 is required.

Oxygen Transport to the Tissues

The fundamental relation that describes the delivery of O_2 to the tissues is the Fick equation:

$$Vo_2 = 0.139(Q)(Hb)(Sao_2 - Svo_2)$$

which says that the amount of O_2 delivered to the tissues (Vo_2) in liters per minute is the product of three independent variables: (1) the blood flow (Q); (2) the amount of O_2 carried by that flow, which is the product of 0.139 and the grams of Hb (1.39 is the amount of O_2, in millimeters of mercury, that a fully saturated gram of Hb is capable of carrying); and (3) the extraction of O_2 at the level of the tissues, which is the difference between the saturation of the arterial blood (Sao_2) and the saturation of the mixed venous blood (Svo_2).

The consequence of this analysis is that when regulation of O_2 release is desired, it is best done in the following areas. (1) *Blood flow* (Q)—This is affected in turn by cardiac output and by microcirculatory size and distribution. (2) *Hemoglobin concentration*—The red cell mass is the balance between erythropoiesis and red cell destruction and is actively regulated by erythropoietin as a response to hypoxia detected in the postarterial side of the renal circulation by a detection system that is described in Chapter 6. (3) *Oxygen extraction by the tissues* (Sao_2 – Svo_2)—This parameter depends on the shape of the O_2

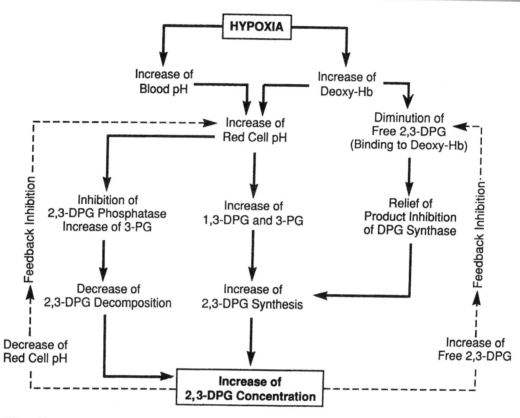

FIGURE 18–12. Effect of hypoxia on red cell pH and 2,3-DPG. (After Bunn HF, Forget BG: Hemoglobin: Molecular, Genetic, and Clinical Aspects. Philadelphia, WB Saunders, 1986.)

equilibrium curve, as discussed earlier, and on tissue Po_2. The determinants of tissue Po_2 and its regulation are poorly understood.

Nitric Oxide Binding to Hemoglobin

PHYSIOLOGY AND CHEMISTRY

Nitric oxide (NO) is the product of the action of endothelial synthases (constitutive nitric oxide synthase [cNOS] and brain nitric oxide synthase [bNOS], which is also called iNOS, for "inducible") and macrophage nitric oxide synthase (mNOS) on L-arginine, differentially stimulated by calcium (Ca^{2+})-dependent calmodulin, tumor necrosis factor, and other cytokines (Table 18–2). In addition, the NO synthases are specific for cell types,[29] including endothelium, macrophages, neutrophils, adrenal tissue, cerebellum, and others.

NO action is mediated by the activation of a soluble guanylyl cyclase to produce cyclic guanosine monophosphate (cGMP). This second messenger is involved in many cellular functions. The NO formed diffuses out of the originating cells and affects only nearby target cells (because NO has a short half-life), binding the heme group of cytosolic guanylate cyclase and activating this enzyme by breaking the iron-proximal histidine bond. A similar mechanism occurs when NO binds to the heme of Hb (see later). Nevertheless, most NO activity may involve direct cell-to-cell interactions and not be mediated by blood NO.

The steady-state level of blood NO reflects a balance between the production of NO by nitric oxide synthases and the binding or scavenging of NO by Hb (bound at the heme level). One of the main functions of NO is the maintenance of an appropriate vascular tone. The affinity of NO for Hb is 100 times higher than that for CO and 20,000 times higher than that for O_2, which explains the reputation of NO as a extremely toxic compound without physiologic or therapeutic importance.

Reports that pharmacologic concentrations of NO shift the O_2 equilibrium binding curve of sickle blood to the left but do not affect the O_2 equilibrium of normal blood[30] have not been confirmed.[31] This shift can be induced by methemoglobin (MetHb), which is formed at toxic levels of NO. When NO dissolved in buffer is used, the P_{50} of Hb correlates with the amount of MetHb generated.[31]

Other researchers have proposed that another physiologic function of red blood cell NO is related to the formation of *S*-nitrosyl-Hb (*S*-NO-Hb), which is generated by the binding of NO to the β93 cysteine of hemoglobin.[32] (For a primer on the chemistry of NO, see Fig. 18–13.) They suggest that *S*-NO-Hb is generated in the lungs, where Hb is in the R or oxygenated state and that NO is released in the microcirculation, where the transition of the R→T conformation induced by deoxygenation liberates NO from the Cys[93] site to relax subendothelial muscle and increase blood flow.

Less than 1 percent of Hb has *S*-NO in patients breathing NO at several concentrations,[31] which makes the physiologic or pathophysiologic role of *S*-NO-Hb

TABLE 18–2. Nitric Oxide Syntheses

	NOS1	NOS2	NOS3
Synonyms	Type 1 NOS (n)eural NOS (b)rain NOS	Type 2 NOS (mac)rophage NOS (i)nducible NOS	Type 3 NOS (e)ndothelial NOS
Localization	Cytosol and attached to membrane	Cytosol and vesicles	Plasmalemmal Caveolae
Synthesis	Constitutive	Cytokine induced	Constitutive
Ca^{2+} dependence	Yes	No	Yes
Regulation by cytokines	Weak	Strong	Weak
NO production	Low	High	Low
Some cell types	Neurons	Microphages	Endothelium
	Skeletal muscle	Microglia	Some epithelium
		Hepatocytes	
Key functions	Neurotransmission	Antimicrobial	Inhibition of platelet aggregation
	Neuroprotection	Immunoregulation	Vasodilation
		Tissue damage	Hypotension

NOS = nitric oxide synthase.
Modified from Bogdan C: Nitric oxide and the regulation of gene expression. Trends Cell Biol 2001; 11:66.

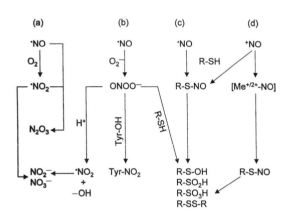

FATE OF NO AND NO RADICALS ('NO) GENERATED BY NOS OR NO DONORS

Legend:
(a) Oxygen oxidizes 'NO to NO_2^-; in turn, 'NO oxidases NO_2 to NO_3.
(b) In the presence of superoxide ($O2^-$), 'NO can result in ONOO–(peroxynitrite) which in turn results in the nitration of tyrosines.
(c) ONOO– and 'NO can nitrosylate thiols to sulfenic and sulfonic acids or the formation of NO_2^- and hydroxy (–OH) radicals.
(d) NO+ (nitrosonium ions), in the presence of trace metals (Fe, Zn or Cu) form metal-nytrosyl complexes and nitrosylate thiol groups and result in sulfenic and sulfonic acids.

FIGURE 18–13. Chemistry of nitrous oxide (NO). (Modified from Bogdan C: Nitric oxide and the regulation of gene expression. Trends Cell Biol 2001; 11:66.)

controversial. In addition, in the hypothesis of Gow and Stamler[32] the deoxy form of Hb releases NO from S-NO-Hb. Recent data[33] show that S-NO-Hb has a higher affinity for O_2 than does native Hb, implying that NO transfer from S-NO-Hb *in vivo* would be limited to regions of extremely low O_2 tension. Furthermore, the kinetics of the transnitrosation reactions between glutathione (GSH) and S-NO-Hb, another potentially physiologic important reaction,[32] is relatively slow according to others,[33] making transfer of NO^+ from S-NO-Hb to GSH less likely as a mechanism to elicit vessel relaxation. These data suggest

that O_2-dependent S-nitrosation of GSH from S-NO-Hb involves biochemical mechanisms that are not intrinsic to the Hb molecule and are presently unknown.

Yonetani[34] found no evidence that NO is liberated from the Cys^{93} site as Hb turns into the T state. Also, the nitroso compounds do not liberate NO but rather NO^+, which needs to be deprotonated before it is active. The mechanisms involved in deprotonation are not fully known or necessarily available in red cells. Finally, the process of exportation of NO^+ from the red cell needs further elucidation. Overall, the physiologic and potential pathophysiologic significance of NO binding to βCys^{92} requires further research.

Finally, whereas both O_2 and NO diffuse into red blood cells, only O_2 diffuses out. For dilatation of blood vessels to take place by red blood cell-mediated events, export of NO-related vasoactivity is indispensable. Recent data[36] have shown that S-NO-Hb generated from NO associates predominantly with the red blood cell membrane and principally with cysteine residues in the Hb-binding, cytoplasmic domain of band 3. The authors postulate that the interaction with band 3, the integral protein of the red cell membrane, promotes the deoxygenated structure in S-NO-Hb, which facilitates NO transfer to the membrane. Furthermore, they show that vasodilatory activity is released from the red cell membrane with the help of deoxygenation. If confirmed, this model would overcome the criticisms of the original postulate.

CLINICAL APPLICATIONS, TOXICITY, AND PATHOPHYSIOLOGY OF NITRIC OXIDE

For a long time NO was thought to be highly toxic until physicians began using low concentrations of the gas, generally 5 to 10 ppm, to manage the acute pulmonary hypertension seen in acute respiratory distress syndrome. The use of NO is still considered dangerous in the presence of sepsis, because production of NO is increased in this condition.[35]

Animal studies show that concentrations of 10 to 40 ppm of NO inhaled for 6 months have no ill effects and do not produce hypotension. The common explanation for this lack of effect is that rapid binding of NO by Hb mops up this dangerous vasodilator. However, the binding of NO results in a low-affinity form of Hb, so an explanation for the lack of effects of this alteration is needed.

NO binds the hemes of the α-globin chains preferentially, inducing a conformational change of Hb to a super-T state owing to the breakage of the bond between the iron and the proximal histidine.[37] The hemes that bind NO exclude O_2; hence, the two remaining hemes have a particularly low O_2 affinity and deliver O_2 to the tissues more effectively than in the normal T state. Thus, despite the fact that the NO-Hb tetramer has only two ligand-carrying oxygenated hemes, it delivers O_2 almost as well as the normal Hb tetramer.

The tetramers with hemes containing NO will, in about one-half hour, be converted to MetHbs, lose their NO, and be reduced by the MetHb reductase system of the red cell to normal Hb molecules. This is the reason why NO, within limits, is not as toxic as expected.

OTHER NORMAL HEMOGLOBINS

Hemoglobin F

In 1866, Korber[37] discovered that the red cells of newborns are resistant to alkaline denaturation, which was the first suggestion that these cells contain Hb that is different from normal adult Hb. The composition of this fetal hemoglobin (HbF) is $\alpha_2\gamma_2$.

The γ chains are different from the β chains in 39 to 40 positions in the sequence.[38] γ Chains are the product of two genes placed in tandem between the ϵ and pseudo-β genes, in the β-like globin cluster on chromosome 11. The only difference between the two gene products is the presence of glycine in position γ136 in the $^G\gamma$-gene, the left gene, and the presence of alanine in the same position in the $^A\gamma$ gene, to the right. A common polymorphism is in the $^A\gamma$ gene, in which threonine in $\gamma^A\gamma^T$ replaces isoleucine in $\gamma^A\gamma^I$.[39] The striking similarities in the protein sequences are reflected at the nucleotide level, where the homology between the two genes is high. Smithies and associates[40] were the first to point out that this is a consequence of *gene conversion*, a mutational event in which the sequences upstream replace sequences downstream, particularly in tandem genes, homogenizing them in the process. That this process is ongoing was demonstrated in the Bantu haplotype linked to the β^S gene.[41]

One interpretation of this phenomenon is that considerable selective value is placed on the sequence of γ chains and on the structure of HbF. This is not surprising because HbF is present throughout most of fetal life (although mostly during the last two trimesters), and abnormalities could easily cause fetal death.

SEQUENCE DIFFERENCES BETWEEN γ AND β CHAINS

The 39 differences are mostly on the surface of the molecule, exactly 22 of them (see Table 18–1). Four critical substitutions are in the $\alpha_1\beta_1$ area of contact (the packing contact). This is the strong contact that dissociates only under extreme conditions (e.g., a very high butylurea concentration, iodine salts, or extreme pH).

Nevertheless, two of these substitutions, Thr^{112} and Try^{130}, in the $\alpha_1\gamma_1$ contact, could be involved in the alkaline resistance of HbF, as well as in its decreased dissociation to monomers. In the β chains, position β112 is a Cys and β130 is a Tyr. Both of these residues ionize at alkaline pH, which could promote dissociation of the dimer into monomers. Thr and Tyr are polar but not ionizable. No sequence changes affect the $\alpha_1\beta_2$ area of contact (sliding contact), which is critical for the ligand-dependent conformational changes.

PROTEIN CONFORMATION

Crystallographic studies of HbF at 2.5 Å resolution show almost entire isomorphism between HbA and HbF.[42] The only difference is in the N-terminal portion. This change increases the distance of 2,3-DPG to the γ2 His, which may contribute to the reduction of the effect of 2,3-DPG on HbF.

LIGAND BINDING

Red cells of newborns (containing mostly HbF) have a higher O_2 affinity than that of adult red cells (P_{50} of 29 mm Hg versus 26 mm Hg in adults), but the O_2 affinities of neonatal and adult red cell hemolysates are indistinguishable.[43] This finding suggests that HbF and HbA have identical O_2-binding properties, but the red cells contain effectors that interact differently with HbF.

2,3-DPG has decreased binding to HbF.[44] The structural basis for this is the replacement of β143 His (phosphate binding site in the central cavity) with a serine residue at γ143. This substitution abolishes an important binding site. Secondary effects come from displacement of the N-terminal portion of the γ chains, which inhibits the binding of phosphates with γ2 His. Also, HbF molecules that are acetylated at the γ chain N-terminal are incapable of binding 2,3-DPG.[45]

The effect of Cl^- is also altered.[46] This anion binds in the 2,3-DPG site in the central cavity. At low NaCl concentrations (up to 0.05 mol/L), HbF has a lower affinity for O_2 than does HbA. At higher Cl^- concentrations, the differences disappear. This effect is not well understood but might have to do with the diminution of positive charges in the central cavity; therefore, the binding affinity for anions and the destabilizing effect on the T state are reduced. The increased stability of the T state induced by the absence of anion neutralizing positive charges would favor low ligand affinity.

The binding of CO_2 to HbF is drastically decreased.[47] Fewer carbamates are formed at the N terminus over a range of P_{CO_2} values. The γ-chain N-terminal amino acid has a pK_a of 8.1, which is much higher than the pK_a of β chains (6.6). At physiologic conditions, 90 percent of the γ sites are protonated and unable to bind CO_2.

The alkaline Bohr effect (relationship between high pH and ligand affinity) is increased by 20 percent in HbF-containing red cells.[48] This seems to be a Cl^- effect, because in isolated HbF at low anion concentrations, HbA and HbF have an identical Bohr effect, and the Bohr effect of HbF increases pari passu with the Cl⁻ concentration. A plausible explanation is that the binding of Cl⁻ at low pH to β143 His stabilizes the R state. The absence of this Cl⁻ site in γ chains would lower the low pH Bohr effect, because it is a situation that favors the T state. As a consequence, the alkaline Bohr effect is favored in HbF.

PHYSIOLOGY OF HEMOGLOBIN F–CONTAINING RED CELLS

How do the modified properties of HbF benefit the fetus and the newborn? Perhaps the main feature of fetal circulation, compared with circulation in postnatal life, is that O_2 loading is done under more difficult circumstances in the fetus (liquid-liquid interface) than in the neonate (gas-liquid interface). On the positive side, the tissues of the fetus have a high metabolic rate; therefore, the limitation may be on loading sufficient O_2 rather than on delivery of O_2, because a significant difference between the Po_2 of blood and that of tissue is likely to exist in the fetus. This analysis explains why the O_2 affinity of HbF-containing red cells is increased, a situation that favors uptake of O_2 in the placenta. It also explains why modulation of delivery of O_2 is less needed, because modulation generally consists of a decrease in the affinity of HbA for O_2. Hence, no 2,3-DPG response is found in HbF. This analysis explains why the Bohr effect is increased: fetal blood increases in pH when it passes through the intravillous spaces because of release of CO_2.

The Bohr effect accounts for 40 percent of the normal fetal gas exchange.[48] In addition, in the fetus, an increased Bohr effect can modulate delivery of O_2 to tissues (if needed), even in the absence of 2,3-DPG. About 50 percent of the delivery to tissues is accounted for by the increased Bohr effect. Finally, the increased Bohr effect could also explain the paradox observed[49] in which mothers with high-affinity Hb variants did not have pregnancy complications or fetal morbidity. The advantage of HbF is not limited to the P_{50} difference with HbA. If the affinity difference is erased, as in patients with high-affinity Hb, the enhanced Bohr effect can make up at least some of the difference.

GENETIC HETEROGENEITY

As noted earlier, γ chains are synthesized by two sequence-identifiable genes. This genetic heterogeneity is unique among globins. Additional heterogeneity arises from the 10 to 15 percent of HbF molecules of newborns who have a post-translation modification of the N-terminal glycine of the γ chains. Acetylation is common in proteins that have N-terminal alanine, serine, and, to a lesser extent, glycine residues. Hb needs to have its N terminus free for functional reasons; therefore, it is not surprising that acetylation has been excluded largely by selection. In the case of HbF, it contributes to the decrease in 2,3-DPG binding, apparently a welcome feature. Acetylation occurs after synthesis, probably early in the process, and involves catalytic transfer of the acetyl moiety from acetyl-coenzyme A to the protein by acetyltransferase. *Hb Raleigh* (β1 [NAI] Val→acetylatable alanine) is 100 percent acety-

lated. Cat Hb, in which the β1 residue is serine, is also 100 percent acetylated (and does not bind 2,3-DPG well).

GENDER-RELATED AND *TRANS*-ACTING MODULATION OF HEMOGLOBIN F LEVELS

In normal, healthy Japanese adults, the ranges of HbF concentrations (0.17 to 2.28 g/dL) and of HbF-containing erythrocytes, F-cells[50] (0.3 to 16.0 percent) were affected by gender.[51] Studies of families studies with high HbF levels and F cells suggested a dominant X-linked pattern of inheritance. In another study in patients with sickle cell anemia, there were higher HbF levels among females,[52] complementing the findings of others.[53, 54]

These results suggest that a factor linked to the X chromosome may influence the level of HbF in normal individuals and patients with sickle cell anemia. F cells are increased in females with sickle cell anemia and sickle cell trait. It has been postulated that there are two genes and theoretically three alleles (*LL, HL,* and *HH*) linked to F cell production or the *FCP* locus on the X chromosome.[55, 56] An restriction-fragment length polymerism detected by anonymous probes seems to locate this locus to the end of short arm of the X chromosome. In one study, this locus accounted for about 40 percent of HbF variability in sickle cell anemia.[56] Nevertheless, the interpretation of these results depends heavily on the still unproven accuracy of the postulated locus structure. We need to wait for the cloning, localization, and structure of the locus before this result can be properly evaluated.

Variations in HbF levels and numbers of F cells have also been linked to chromosome 6q22.3-23.2 in an Asian-Indian family.[57, 58] Evidence for another *trans*-acting quantitative trait locus unlinked to chromosome 6 or to the X chromosome has been found in an English family.[59] In studies of monozygotic and dizygotic twins, 15 percent of the variability in F-cell levels could be ascribed to the *Xmn*I restriction site polymorphism 5′ to the $^G\gamma$-globin gene, leaving more than 70 percent to be explained by other genetic modulators.[60, 61]

LABORATORY DETERMINATION OF HEMOGLOBIN F

The best methods for determining the level of HbF in the hemolysate depend on its concentration. For normal levels (0.1 to 1.5 percent) of the total Hb, the immunologic assays are best. For levels between 1.5 and 40 percent, alkaline denaturation is accurate. For levels greater than 40 percent, high-performance liquid chromatography (HPLC) is probably the best method, although it can also be used at lower concentrations. A method of enriching the HbF by chromatography or isoelectric focusing, followed by HPLC, allows this technique to be applied to all concentrations of HbFs. Disposable columns for the determination of HbF in hemolysates that contain no HbA (such as red cells from patients with Hb SS or Hb CC disease) are also available and produce reasonably accurate results.

HbF is unevenly distributed among red cells in normal subjects and in those with most medical conditions except for some forms of hereditary persistence of HbF.[50] Immunologic techniques that allow the identification of red cells containing HbF (F cells and F reticulocytes) and measurement of the average amount of HbF per cell have become powerful tools for the study of HbF expression.[62–64] About 0.5 to 7 percent of red cells are F cells in normal adults.

Agar electrophoresis at pH 6.4 (available as a kit) offers an additional method to isolate or identify HbF. Hbs are subjected to a combination of chromatography and electrophoresis in agar. The agar matrix interacts with the central cavity of Hbs,[65] and Hbs with abnormalities in that region (such as HbF) tend to migrate faster (or slower) than their electrophoretic mobility would predict at pH 6.4. Therefore, when a Hb with an anomalous electrophoretic mobility in agar is compared with cellulose acetate (pH 8.6), a mutation of the central cavity should be suspected. *Hb Hope* is an example of this phenomenon.

MEDICAL CONDITIONS OUTSIDE OF HEMOGLOBINOPATHIES ASSOCIATED WITH HIGH FETAL HEMOGLOBIN EXPRESSION IN INFANTS AND ADULTS

Newborns have between 65 and 95 percent HbF. This amount decreases progressively during the first year of life. The normal adult level is approached by 1 year of age and is achieved by 5 years. Normal subjects have a gender-determining dispersion of their HbF levels. As noted earlier,[52] a excess of high normal values in women has been reported together with evidence that this trait is inherited as an X-linked characteristic. Identification of an X-linked modulator of HbF expression is being actively pursued.

Pregnancy is associated with a modest increase in HbF in the second trimester. Hydatidiform moles are associated with particularly high HbF values. Although maternal pregnancy hormones have been implicated, the mechanism of this elevation is not clear.[52]

Some conditions (besides hemoglobinopathies) retard the down-regulation of HbF in the first 5 years of life. These conditions include prematurity, trisomy 21, and maternal diabetes.[54] Acceleration of the decrease in HbF is observed in patients with Down syndrome and those with C/D translocations.

Hemolytic anemias, acute bleeding, and treatment with hydroxyurea or arabinocytidine all can be associated with higher than normal values of HbF. This phenomenon has been interpreted to mean that under these conditions early progenitors are rushed through development while they retain their HbF program, because the reduction in the number of cell division precluded their down-regulation.

Invariably, juvenile chronic myeloid leukemia, Diamond-Blackfan anemia, and Fanconi anemia are accompanied by significant elevations of HbF. Erythroleukemia, paroxysmal nocturnal hemoglobinuria, kala azar, preleukemia, and recovery from marrow aplasia are also accompanied by variable elevations of HbF. The highest levels are found in patients with DiGuglielmo disease (erythroleukemia). Many conditions, including solid tumors, occasionally cause increased levels of HbF.[54, 55, 66]

MUTATIONS IN THE $^G\gamma$ GENES

Variants of the $^G\gamma$ Gene. Fifty-two variants with a single amino acid substitution in the $^G\gamma$ gene have been described. Of these, two are unstable: *Hb F-Poole* ($^G\gamma$130(H8) Trp→Gly), which is significantly unstable, and *Hb F-Xin Jin* ($^G\gamma$119(GH2) Gly→Arg).[67] A mutation of the same site, but not the same amino acid as Hb Poole, has also been identified in β chains (Hb Wien [β130 Try→Asp]).

Also found in HbF is the equivalent of M Hbs in the β chains: *Hb F-M-Fort Ripley*, which has a cyanotic phenotype in the newborn and corresponds to the substitution of the proximal histidine, γ92(F8) His→Tyr. It is perfectly equivalent to Hb Hyde Park. The other mutation, *Hb F-M-Osaka*,[68] involves the distal histidine, γ63(E7) His→Tyr, and is equivalent to Hb M-Saskatoon. Newborns with α-chain substitutions of the proximal or distal histidines have the same cyanotic phenotype as that of adults, with the cyanosis appearing early in the neonatal period.[70, 71]

Finally, one high-affinity variant has been described: *Hb F-Onoda*[69] ($^G\gamma$146(HC3) His→Tyr).

Variants of the $^A\gamma$ Gene and the Common Variant $^A\gamma^T$ (Hemoblobin F Sardinia). Forty-five variants of the $^A\gamma$ gene have been described so far, but none of them has a functional abnormality. Six variants of the common $^A\gamma^T$ variant have been described,[72] but only *Hb F-Xinjiang* ($^A\gamma^T$25(B7) Gly→Arg) is unstable.

Note that Hb F-Texas, Hb F-Alexandria, and Hb F-Ube have not been assigned to the corresponding γ gene.

Hemoglobin A$_2$

HbA$_2$ begins to be expressed in the neonatal period and during the rest of an individual's life and is the product of the combination of α chains with δ chains ($\alpha_2\delta_2$). The δ chains are the product of the δ gene, which transcribes a δ message at a low level. HbA$_2$ represents about 2.4 percent of the Hbs present in normal hemolysates. The δ gene resides in the cluster of β-like genes between the pseudo-β gene and the β gene.

δ GENE

The δ gene arose from a duplication of the β gene about 40 million years ago (although one cannot exclude the possibility that gene conversion could have erased differences of an older gene). The δ gene also exists and is expressed at low levels in new-world primates (1 to 6 percent). In some old-world primates, the δ gene is present but is not expressed. The δ gene is absent in other mammals. In any case, the distribution among animals suggests that this was the last globin gene to emerge in the β-like gene cluster. Its relatively recent appearance (or recent gene conversion) explains why the δ chain exhibits only 10 sequence differences from the β gene.

The low level of transcription might be the consequence of changes in the 5′-flanking region. Of the three CCAAT boxlike sequences, none is perfectly conserved. Instability of δ-mRNA may also contribute to the poor expression of the δ gene.

FUNCTIONAL AND STRUCTURAL ASPECTS

HbA and HbA$_2$ have similar ligand binding curves, although the latter has slightly higher O$_2$ affinity. The Bohr effect, cooperativity, and the response to 2,3-DPG are identical.

Among the differences are that the fact HbA$_2$ is more thermostable. This is due to a change at Arg-δ116. This Arg forms a salt bridge with Pro-α114, increasing even further the stability of the $\alpha_1\beta_1$ packing contact. Another difference is that HbA$_2$ binds to the red cell membrane better than does HbA.[73]

The low levels of HbA$_2$ and the multiple functionally abnormal mutations found in primate δ-like genes have been suggested as reasons for the lack of functional importance for this minor component. According to this view, the δ gene is condemned to the biologic trash heap of history as a pseudogene. This conclusion presupposes that the only functional role of any Hb is to carry O$_2$. If so, HbA$_2$ is clearly useless. Alternatively, the increased binding of HbA$_2$ to the membrane could indicate another role for this Hb. It is necessary to know what proteins in addition to band 3 are capable of binding this Hb and whether such binding has any functional role. The finding of HbA$_2$ at polymorphic rates in the Dogon region of the Republic of Mali (see later) stimulates this thinking.

MUTATIONAL EVENTS INVOLVING THE δ GENE

Fifty-seven amino acid substitutions, all due to single base changes, have been described in HbA$_2$. This might be the tip of the iceberg, because these substitutions are difficult to detect. Two mutations, *Hb A$_2$-Wrens* (γ98 FG4 Val$\rightarrow$Met)[74] and *HbA$_2$-Manzanares* (γ121 GH4 Glu$\rightarrow$Val),[75] are unstable. *Hb A$_2$-Canada* (γ99 G1 Asp$\rightarrow$Asn)[76] has very high affinity for O$_2$, but no erythrocytosis is present.

A common mutation, found mostly among African-Americans and Africans, is *HbA$'_2$*, also called *HbB$_2$*. In Africa, it has been described in samples from different geographic locations, one of which is Ghana. HbA$'_2$ has been found at polymorphic rates in one of the castes in the Dogon region of the Republic of Mali. Haplotype analysis of the Mali β-like gene cluster demonstrates that all unrelated persons carrying this mutation have the same haplotype. Samples from unrelated African-Americans with this mutation also demonstrate haplotype homogeneity. Hence, it is possible that HbA$'_2$ arose in Africa unicentrically and distributed itself to other regions of Africa by gene flow.

An interesting set of mutational events involves the unequal crossover between the δ gene and the β gene. This generates Hbs with portions of δ chains and portions of β chains. They are called *Lepore-type Hbs* after the first family described. The first three examples of this type of event were characterized in heterozygotes by low levels of the Lepore-type Hb (about 20 percent), electrophoretic migration similar to that of HbS, and a thalassemic phenotype (microcytosis, hypochromia, and hemolytic anemia). In homozygotes for this condition, severity varies from transfusion dependency to moderate anemia.

Groups at risk are principally Italians, Greeks, and Yugoslavians (the latter being the most severely affected), but examples have been found in Turkish Cypriots, inhabitants of Papua New Guinea, African-Americans, Indians, and Romanians.

Hb Lepore Hollandia, Hb Lepore Baltimore, and Hb Lepore Washington-Boston (the first described)[77–79] have different lengths of the δ sequence in the N-terminal portion of the hybrid chain and complementary portions of the β chains at the C-terminal end. All have a total of 146 amino acids. The more recently described Lepore-type Hb, Hb Parchman, is a patchwork in which a segment of the β sequence is located in the center of the chain. The location of the crossover is uncertain because, with only 10 amino acid differences between the δ and β chains, there are too few informative sites.

If a Lepore-type unequal crossover occurs, an anti-Lepore Hb molecule is also generated, but finding it depends on its prevalence and on luck. Hb P Nilotic is the anti-Lepore of Lepore Hollandia. Hb Lincoln Park is probably the same with an added deletion at position δ137. Hb Miyada and Hb P-Congo could be anti-Lepores of Lepore Hbs that are yet to be found. Electrophoretically, Hb P-Congo, Hb P-Nilotic, and Hb Lincoln Park migrate like HbS, whereas Hb Miyada and Hb Parchman migrate like HbC.

VARIATION OF HEMOGLOBIN A$_2$ LEVELS WITH OTHER CLINICAL CONDITIONS

The levels of HbA$_2$ are elevated in a number of conditions; in some instances, this feature is of diagnostic value. The most common clinical instance is β-thalassemia. HbA$_2$ is also elevated in sickle trait, in blood from patients with SS disease, particularly SS disease with α-thalassemia, and in acquired conditions such as megaloblastic anemias and hyperthyroidism. Controversial evidence exists that HbA$_2$ is elevated in patients with malaria. Elevation of HbA$_2$ is not due to an increase in the synthesis of δ chains but is a consequence of the preferential assemblage of δ with α chains, particularly if β chains are in short supply. Decreased levels of HbA$_2$ are found in α-thalassemia, $\delta\beta$-thalassemia, and δ-thalassemia and with the hereditary persistence of HbF, either because the δ gene is deleted or because the α chains are more avid for γ or β chains than for δ chains. A decrease of HbA$_2$ seen with iron deficiency can confuse this picture. A good suggestion to determine whether iron deficiency is present is to give the patient iron and then perform the test again.

Embryonic Hemoglobins

At 4 to 14 weeks of gestation, the human embryo synthesizes three distinct hemoglobins in yolk sac–derived primitive nucleated erythroid cells: $\zeta_2\varepsilon_2$ (Hb Gower-1), $\zeta_2\gamma_2$ (Hb Portland), and $\alpha_2\varepsilon_2$ (Hb Gower-2).[80] ζ- and ε-globin chains are expressed before the γ- and α-globin chain. After the establishment of the placenta, at 14 days of development, embryonic Hbs are replaced by HbF, but ζ- and ε-globin chains can be found in definitive fetal erythrocytes.[81] At 15 to 22 weeks of gestation, 53 percent of fetal cells contained ζ-globin chains and 5 percent had ε-globin chains. At term, cord blood contained 34 percent and 0.6 percent of ζ- and ε-globin chain positive cells, respectively. Erythrocytes from normal adults do not contain embryonic globins.

Developmental timing of the synthesis of embryonic Hbs has been studied in embryonic erythroid cells.[82] Embryonic, fetal, and adult globins are synthesized *in vivo* and in cultures of erythroid burst-forming units in the yolk sac (where primitive erythropoiesis occurs) and in liver cells (site of definitive erythropoiesis). Similarly, the adult α-globin gene and the corresponding embryonic α-like chains (ζ-globin gene) are coexpressed in the earliest murine erythrocyte progenitors.[83] From these studies and from the recent finding of embryonic Hb in cord blood, it appears that embryonic globin is expressed in both primitive and definitive erythroblasts, although in vastly different quantities. These results are compatible with the notion that the switch from embryonic to fetal globin synthesis represents a time-dependent change in programs of progenitor cells rather than a change in hemopoietic cell lineages.

Embryonic Hbs obtained from an *in vitro* expression system and in the absence of any effector of Hb function, including Cl^-, all have O_2 affinities and ligand binding rates similar to those of HbA.[84] In the presence of organic phosphates, the O_2 affinities of $\zeta_2\varepsilon_2$ and $\alpha_2\varepsilon_2$ are lowered for Hb Gower-2 to a lesser extent than for normal HbA. This demonstrates that the ζ- and ε-globin chains do bind 2,3-DPG, but differently from the way they bind HbA, which requires explanation (see later). Hb Portland does not bind organic phosphates well, which is not surprising, because its central cavity is formed by γ-globin chains (see earlier discussion).

The rates of O_2 dissociation from the embryonic Hbs appear to be responsible for the high O_2-binding affinity of the embryonic proteins.[85] The pH dependence of the O_2 dissociation rate constants also accounts for the rather unusual Bohr effects characteristic of embryonic Hbs.

A reduction in the destabilizing effect of an excess of positive charges in the central cavity[86] is indispensable for the proper functioning of Hb. Cl^- binding to oxy-Hb accomplishes that task and preserves the physiologic O_2 affinity of Hb. The Cl^- interactions with embryonic Hbs are particularly interesting.[87] Hb Portland is completely insensitive to Cl^-, whereas Hb Gower-1 has a small reaction and Hb Gower-2 has a reaction approaching that of HbA. Cl^- binding and the Bohr effect of these Hbs are in accordance with the allosteric model proposed.[86]

In $\alpha_2\varepsilon_2$ (Hb Gower2)[87] the tertiary structure of the α-globin chain is unchanged, compared with that of Hb A and HbF. It is possible that the decrease in the effect of Cl^- is the sum of small aggregated changes and not the result of a single amino acid substitution.

Crystallographic data on the CO form are available for $\alpha_2\varepsilon_2$ (Hb Gower-2)[88] (Fig. 18–14). Compared with structures of HbA and HbF, the tertiary structure of the α-globin chain is unchanged. The ε-globin chain has a structure very similar to that of the β-globin chain with small differences in the N terminus and A helix. The Cl^-—binding sites involve the 11 polar residues within

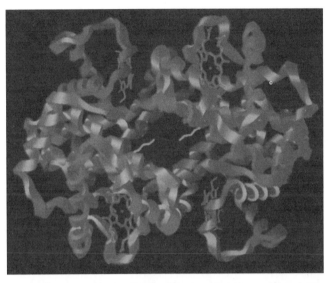

FIGURE 18–14. Crystallographic examination of Hb Gower-2 ($\alpha_2\varepsilon_2$). The figure was prepared by the GRASP software by Nichols and associates in 1991 on data by Sutherland-Smith et al.[88] The position of ε-Lys104, (the lighter, thin structures extending into the central cavity from the left and right) illustrates a difference between ε chains and β chains. (See the color plate at the front of the book.)

the central cavities. Of these, only β104 Arg is changed to a Lys in the ε-globin chain. The ε-globin Lys residue might be involved in an ionic interaction with ε101 Glu, but whether the pK of Lys is low enough to be non-ionized in physiologic conditions and whether this sequence change can explain the decrease in Cl^- binding is uncertain.

The most distinct difference in Hb Gower-2 compared with Hb A is a shift of the N terminus and the A helix, similar to that seen in HbF. The α helix moves into the central cavity as a consequence of a complex disruption of the N-terminal region. To establish definitively the mechanism of the decrease in 2,3-DPG binding, it is necessary to know the T crystal structure of Hb Gower-2, but the A helix shift remains a likely candidate.

Finally, embryonic ζ- and ε-globin subunits assemble with each other and with adult α- and β-globin subunits into Hb heterotetramers in both primitive and definitive erythrocytes. The use of complex transgenic knockout mice that express these Hbs at high levels has allowed the functional characterizations of these hybrids.[89] The exchange of ζ chains for α chains increases the P_{50} and decreases the Bohr effect, increasing O_2 transport capacity. In comparison, the exchange of ε chains for β chains has little impact on these parameters. Hb Gower-1, assembled entirely from embryonic subunits, displays an elevated P_{50}, a reduced Bohr effect, and increased 2,3-DPG binding compared with HbA. The data support the hypothesis that Hb Gower-2, assembled from reactivated ε globin in individuals with hemoglobinopathies and thalassemias, would serve as a physiologically acceptable substitute for deficient or dysfunctional HbA. In addition, the unexpected properties of Hb Gower-1 make its primary role in embryonic development unlikely.

MUTATIONS AFFECTING EMBRYONIC HEMOGLOBINS

The most common mutation producing lethal hydrops fetalis is the Southeast Asian (–/SEA) double α-globin gene deletion.[90] Erythrocytes from adults *heterozygous* for the (–/SEA) deletion have minute amounts of embryonic ζ-globin chains detectable by anti-ζ-globin monoclonal antibodies. The majority of subjects are of Filipino, Chinese, or Laotian ancestry. The (–/SEA) double α deletion was the only abnormality in two thirds of these patients. In others, this deletion was combined with α-globin or β-globin mutations or coincidental iron deficiency. Four other samples from (–/SEA) heterozygotes produced negative results by this immunologic assay. Anti-ζ–negative samples included deletions of the *total* α-globin region (–/Tot), single α-globin deletions, and a variety of β-globin mutations; normocytic samples with normal α genes also produced negative results. Benign triplicated ζ-globin genes were also detected. Anti-ζ immunobinding testing provides rapid, simple, and reliable screening for the (–/SEA) double α-globin deletion, although it does not detect the (–/Tot) total α-globin deletions.

PATHOPHYSIOLOGY OF HEMOGLOBIN ABNORMALITIES

High Ligand Affinity Hemoglobins: Erythrocytosis

STRUCTURAL DEFECTS

Mutations resulting in changes in the primary structure of the α or β chains can lead to changes in the affinity toward ligands of these Hb variants. Increases in the O_2 affinity of Hb results from various mechanisms. In most instances, the changes in O_2 affinity are in concordance with our understanding of the structure-function relationships of Hb. In a few instances, the known alterations of the primary structure are not sufficient to explain the observed effect, given the state of our knowledge.

The mutations that generate high-affinity Hbs can arise from single point substitutions, double point substitutions (although some of these could be crossover events between two mutated chains), deletions, additions, frameshift mutations, and fusion genes.

The molecular mechanisms of ligand high-affinity Hb mutants are summarized here and described in the following sections (for some high-affinity Hbs, there is no explanation for their functional behavior):

1. Alterations of the *switch region*, the *flexible joint*, or the *C termini* in the $\alpha_1\beta_2$ area of contact that favor the R (or oxy) state, either by stabilizing this conformer or by destabilizing the T (or deoxy) state;
2. Alteration of the $\alpha_1\beta_1$ *area* of contact with disruption of the overall architecture of Hb that favors the R state;
3. Reduction in the *heme-heme interaction* by restraining of the quaternary conformation due to a tendency to aggregate or polymerize;
4. Mutations that decrease the affinity of Hb for *2,3-DPG*; and
5. *Elongation* of the globin chains, disrupting the quaternary structure.

Alterations of the Switch Region, Flexible Joint, or C Termini in the $\alpha_1\beta_2$ Area of Contact. These alterations favor the R state, either by stabilizing this conformer or by destabilizing the T state (see Fig. 18–5).

Examples of α Chain Abnormalities. Hb Chesapeake (α92 (FG4) Arg→Leu),[91–93] the first high-affinity mutant, was described in a classic paper.[91] At pH 8.61, it is a fast-moving electrophoretic variant, representing about 20 percent of the hemolysate. It has a moderately high O_2 affinity (whole blood Po_2: 19 mm Hg) and normal Bohr and 2,3-DPG effects, and it produces moderate erythrocytosis. It involves a substitution of an invariant residue (a residue in most α chains analyzed regardless of species). The molecular mechanism is the stabilization of the R state at the level of the $\alpha_1\beta_2$ area of contact.

Hb Nunobiki (α141 (HC3) Arg→Cys) is one of four mutations at the same site, all of which exhibit a high affinity for O_2, significantly decreased heterotropic interactions (effect of H⁺, Cl⁻, and 2,3-DPG), and moderate to mild erythrocytosis.[94] The mutation affects an invariant residue. Hb Nunobiki is particularly interesting. At pH 8.6, it is an electrophoretically fast-moving abnormal Hb, expressed at a low level (13 percent). Most α-chain abnormalities represent 20 to 25 percent of the hemolysate, because they are produced by one of four α genes.

The consequences of the presence of the cysteine residue in position α141 are varied. First, during storage the Hb changes mobility (becomes faster), presumably through the oxidation of the cysteine residue to a negatively charged sulfoxide —SO⁻) or sulfitic acid—SOO⁻). Second, Hb Nunobiki is more resistant to autoxidation, probably because of the protection toward oxidants rendered by its high-affinity status and the addition of a new site (cysteine residue) for the consumption of the oxidants. Third, the low percentage of the α mutant is explained by the fact that it is a mutant of the α_1 gene (closest to the 3′ region of the cluster), shown to be expressed one-third to two-thirds less often than the α_2 gene. Finally, as with other mutations of the N-terminal end of the α chains, Hb Nunobiki produces little erythrocytosis despite its high affinity, because of the low percentage that is present in the red cells. The high ligand affinity is due to the breaking of the C-terminal to C-terminal salt bridge indispensable for the stabilization of the T state. Hence, the R state is greatly favored.

Examples of β Chain Abnormalities. Hb Poissy (β56(D7) Gly→Arg and β86 [F2] Ala→Pro)[95] is a double-site mutation; one mutation (Arg at the β56 site) had been described previously as *Hb Hamadan*, exhibiting no functional abnormalities. When a second instance was found, the patient had erythrocytosis and red cells with a high affinity for O_2. A discrepancy that needed explanation was apparent. Recent reexamination of the structure of the mutant Hb by HPLC revealed that the propositus carries a β chain with two mutations, one identical to Hb Hamadan and the other an electrophoretically silent mutation in the same β chain but at position 86, in which

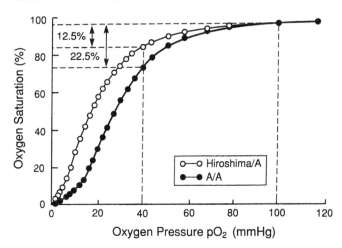

FIGURE 18–15. Oxygen equilibrium curves of red cells from a healthy person (A/A) and those from a person heterozygous for Hb Hiroshima (Hiroshima/A). Oxygen pressure is plotted against oxygen saturation. *Vertical dotted lines* mark the typical PO_2 of the lungs (100 mm Hg) and of the tissues (40 mm Hg). *Horizontal dotted lines* mark the oxygen extraction (lungs minus tissues) for normal red cells (22.5 percent) and the reduction observed for the high-affinity red cells (12.5 percent).

an alanine has been substituted by a proline. This new Hb has a threefold increase in O_2 affinity, with a low *n* coefficient and a diminished Bohr effect. It also shows a biphasic curve in the autoxidation rate, suggesting a great inequivalence in the propensity for MetHb formation of the α and β hemes. Nuclear magnetic resonance (NMR) studies in this mutant suggest that the helix-breaking proline residue displaces the F helix toward the heme, destabilizing this helix toward the critical FG corner. This interferes with the $\alpha_1\beta_2$ contact area, favors the R state, and modifies the environment of the hemes.

Four mutations are described for site β146(HC3): *Hb Hiroshima* (His→Asp)[96, 97], *Hb York* (His→Pro), *Hb Cowtown* (His→Leu), and *Hb Cochin-Port Royal* (His→Arg).[98, 99] These hemoglobins are detectable by electrophoresis. They have moderately increased O_2 affinity and a Bohr effect that is one-half normal (Fig. 18–15). In addition, Hb Cowtown has a decreased 2,3-DPG effect. These mutants disrupt a T state salt bridge and eliminate the residue from which 50 percent of the Bohr protons originate. The decrease in 2,3-DPG binding might result from the decrease of positive charges in the central cavity or the destabilization of the T state. Hb Cochin-Port Royal exhibits normal O_2 affinity and a reduced Bohr effect. These mutants disrupt a salt bridge that stabilizes the T state and the absence of the His-β146 reduces the Bohr protons by one half. Reduced 2,3-DPG binding results from the reduction of central cavity positive charges and the destabilization of T state.

Alteration of the $\alpha_1\beta_1$ Area of Contact with Disruption of the Overall Architecture of Hemoglobin That Favors the R State. Two examples follow.

Hb San Diego (β109(G11) Val→Met) is an electrophoretically silent mutation with moderately high O_2 affinity, a normal Bohr effect, and clinically apparent erythrocytosis.[100] The molecular mechanism probably involves a steric hindrance, induced by the larger bulk of

methionine compared with that of valine in the $\alpha_1\beta_1$ contact, particularly in the deoxy configuration. This biases the molecule toward the R state.

Hb Crete (β129(H7) Ala→Pro)[101] presented with a curious combination of erythrocytosis, hemolysis, splenomegaly, abnormal red cell morphology, and marked erythroid hyperplasia. The propositus was a compound heterozygote for Hb Crete and δβ-thalassemia. The red cell P_{50} was 11.3 mm Hg, whereas isolated Hb Crete had a P_{50} of 2.2 mm Hg compared with 5.4 mm Hg for HbA. This mutation has moderately decreased cooperativity and a normal Bohr effect, and is mildly unstable. Proline does not accommodate well in the α helix structure and disturbs the H helix while also having a longer-range effect on nearby residues in the $\alpha_1\beta_1$ interface, perturbing this area of subunit contact.

This mutation is instructive. Splenomegaly is not usually associated with erythrocytosis caused by high-affinity Hbs and suggests polycythemia vera. However, here it was caused by δβ-thalassemia. The high affinity of Hb Crete is complex. Another family member heterozygous for Hb Crete alone had only 38 percent of this variant and a hematocrit of 50 percent. The propositus had more erythrocytosis because the level of Hb Crete was much higher and a high level of the high ligand affinity HbF was present.

Reduction of Heme-Heme Interaction by Restraining the Quaternary Conformation Due to a Tendency to Aggregate or Polymerize. An example is *Hb Pôrto Alegre* (β9(A6) Ser→Cys), an interesting mutant with higher than normal O_2 affinity and a tendency to aggregate.[103] No erythrocytosis is apparent in the carriers. The polymerization of Hb Pôrto Alegre is based on the formation of —S—S— bonds in oxygenated samples, and thus it is different from HbS. The polymerization of this mutant diminishes the heme-heme interaction and increases the O_2 affinity.[104] This is a unique molecular mechanism.

Mutations That Decrease the Affinity of Hemoglobin for 2,3-DPG. An example is *Hb Old Dominion* (β143(H21) His→Tyr),[102] found among those of Scotch-Irish ancestry, which has a mild increase in O_2 affinity and causes no clinical abnormalities. This Hb elutes before HbA by reverse-phase HPLC and forms 50 percent of the hemolysate. Of interest is the fact that the mutation disrupts the 2,3-DPG binding site in the central cavity. Hb Old Dominion coelutes with HbA_{1C} on ion-exchange chromatography and may therefore lead to the erroneous diagnosis of diabetes or to mistreatment of a diabetic patient with this variant.

Elongation of the Globin Chains, Disrupting the Quaternary Structure. *Hb Tak* is an abnormal Hb that corresponds to an elongation of the β chains by 11 residues (157 residues total) probably due to unequal crossing-over.[105, 106] The abnormal Hb constitutes 40 percent of the hemolysate, has a high O_2 affinity with no cooperativity (*n* = 0), and has no allosteric effects with pH or 2,3-DPG, which is not a surprise because the C terminus of the β chain is actively involved in the stabilization of the T state. Hence, Hb Tak, by having these stabilizing interactions disrupted, is frozen in the R state. It is also slightly unstable. Despite these severe functional abnormalities, the heterozygous patient exhibited no erythrocytosis.

This puzzling situation could be explained by the extraordinarily biphasic O_2 affinity curve observed with mixtures of Hb Tak and HbA, suggesting that no hybrid formation is present. The top portion of the O_2 equilibrium curve of the mixture is normal and begins to be abnormal only at less than 40 percent saturation. As physiologic O_2 exchange occurs (most often above that level of saturation), the tissues might not be aware of the presence of the abnormal Hb.

Another extended chain hemoglobin, *Hb Thionville*,[107] has intrinsically high affinity due to changes in the $\alpha_1\beta_1$ contact surface, but because it affects one of 4 α genes, it is expressed only at a 21 percent level.

This abnormality illuminates another feature of Hb synthesis. In humans, globin translation is initiated by a methionine residue that is cleaved by the enzyme methionine aminopeptidase after the chain has reached about 30 amino acids. If a charged amino acid is introduced (as in Hb Thionville), the cleavage does not take place, and there is one amino acid extension at the N-terminal. In the β chain, this same phenomenon has been described in *Hb Doha*.[108] In another case, the $\beta 1$ valine is replaced by methionine (*Hb South Florida*).[109] The post-translation modification continues because a globin chain with an N-terminal methionine is acetylated when the chain reaches about 50 residues in length. As discussed later, N-terminal valine strongly inhibits acetylation, as demonstrated in normal α and β chains, whereas Met-Glu is a particularly good acceptor for complete acetylation. This is the case not only for globin but also for other proteins (such as band 3 protein in the red cell membrane). In *Hb Long Island-Marseille*,[110] the methionine is not acetylated because the second position in the β chain ($\beta 2$) is Val instead of Glu.

Finally, because it is an α chain abnormality, it identifies the allosteric interactions in which α chains participate. It shows a reduced Bohr effect and reduced Cl^- binding whereas 2,3-DPG binding, which is mainly due to an allosteric interaction of the β chains, is normal. It also illustrates how acetylation of the N-terminal interferes with the R→T transition. This demonstrates the need to keep the N-terminal nonacetylated, that is, without methionine, for the conformational changes of Hb to take place.

Some High-Affinity Hemoglobins That Lack an Explanation for Their Functional Behavior. *Hb Heathrow* ($\beta 103$(G5) Phe→Leu) is an intriguing, electrophoretically silent mutation with moderately high O_2 affinity and clinically apparent erythrocytosis.[111] This mutation affects an invariant residue that guards the entrance of the heme pocket. The molecular mechanism is not known. The smaller side chain at the bottom of the heme pocket might alter ligand micropaths or the electronic environment of the prosthetic group, but this is speculation. We might not know why this mutant has a high O_2 affinity, but nature surely does, because the mutated residue is invariant.

IDENTIFICATION OF HIGH OXYGEN AFFINITY HEMOGLOBINS

In 1966 an 81-year-old patient was seen with erythrocytosis, was found to have an abnormal band in his Hb on electrophoresis, had red cells with increased O_2 affinity, and complained of mild angina.[92] The abnormal Hb proved to be a substitution of Leu→Arg in residue 92 of the α chains. The discovery of the first carrier of Hb Chesapeake opened a new chapter in the study of hemoglobinopathies, because it demonstrated that a variant of this molecule could generate another clinical syndrome. The discovery of this abnormal Hb and others has been useful in the elucidation of the molecular mechanisms underlying the function of normal Hb.

Is the mild angina seen in the Hb Chesapeake pedigree a characteristic of the carriers of high-affinity Hbs? Other members of the same pedigree and a large number of carriers of high-affinity Hbs generally have no clinical consequences (the exception is discussed later). Their only risk is inappropriate iatrogenic interventions when the diagnosis has been ignored or polycythemia vera has been diagnosed by mistake.

Patients with high-affinity Hbs have normal white cell and platelet counts and do not have splenomegaly (except when splenomegaly is concomitant with β-thalassemia or is present from other causes). They sometimes have a family history of "thick blood," but a significant number of high-affinity Hbs are new mutations; that is, no abnormal Hb is found among parents or siblings.

The differential diagnosis of erythrocytosis is outlined in Table 18–3. Erythrocytosis should not be confused with polycythemia, in which numbers of white cells and platelets are elevated and splenomegaly is usually present. The diagnosis of the conditions in Table 18–3 requires measurement of blood erythropoietin levels. Hypoxia of pulmonary or cardiovascular origin can be excluded on the basis of values for arterial blood gases. Affected patients characteristically have low Po_2 values and low O_2 saturations. Patients with red cells that have an altered capacity to transport O_2 have a normal arterial Po_2.

Among the patients with abnormal red cells, the different subtypes can be distinguished by a strategy based on comparison of the affinity of hemolysates (those that contain only Hb at defined conditions of pH and salt) with the O_2 equilibrium of the red cells. The hemolysates identify intrinsic defects in the Hb molecule; study of intact red cells identifies other red cell factors (such as 2,3-DPG) that alter the O_2 affinity of an otherwise normal Hb. Specifically, abnormal Hbs have red cells with a high O_2 affinity, a high O_2 affinity hemolysate, and a near-normal 2,3-DPG concentration. The enzymatic defects of 2,3-DPG mutase are characterized by high O_2 affinity red cells, normal O_2 affinity of the red cell hemolysate, and a very low 2,3-DPG concentration.[112] In all of the above the absorption spectrum of hemolysates is normal.

MetHb (such as that seen in congenital methemoglobinemia) can be identified by the presence of an abnormal peak at 620 nm, and carboxy-Hb (e.g., carbon monoxide [CO] poisoning)[113] can be assayed by a three-wavelength measurement, because the spectra of carboxy-Hb and oxy-Hb differ significantly. Several gas-measuring apparatuses are available in hospitals (e.g., the IL CO oximeter), which can give an accurate reading of MetHb and carboxy-Hb concentrations in whole blood.

Finally, patients with familial erythrocytosis have a normal O_2 affinity, whether red cells or hemolysate is used.

TABLE 18–3. Differential Diagnosis of Erythrocytosis

A. Primary increase of erythropoietin (inappropriately high erythropoietin levels)
  1. Erythropoietin-producing neoplasms
  2. Erythropoietin-producing renal lesions
B. Mutations of the erythropoietin receptor
C. Secondary increase in erythropoietin (appropriately high erythropoietin levels)
  1. Hypoxemia related to
    a. Chronic pulmonary disease
    b. Right-to-left cardiac shunts
    c. Sleep apnea
    d. Massive obesity (Pickwickian syndrome)
    e. High altitude
  2. Hypoxemia related to red cell defects
    a. High oxygen affinity hemoglobins
    b. Absence or decrease in 2,3-diphosphoglycerate mutase
    c. Some case of congenital methemoglobinemia
    d. Chronic carbon monoxide poisoning (smoking and work-related exposures)
    e. Methemoglobinemia
D. Idiopathic familial erythrocytosis and Chubash erythrocytosis

The disease has a recessive inheritance pattern and is sometimes associated with clubbing.[114] Two interesting groups of patients with erythrocytosis that is not related to Hb variants nor enzyme abnormalities have been identified. They are erythropoietin receptor mutations and Chuvashian erythrocytosis.

Erythropoietin Receptor Mutations. Several patients have been have been found in whom erythrocytosis is associated with truncation of the cytosolic portion of the erythropoietin receptor, eliminating the negative regulatory domain of the receptor. The truncation does not allow the physiologically appropriate shut-off of the signaling cascade induced by erythropoietin binding and receptor dimerization. This leads to inappropriate erythropoietin signaling, increased red cell formation relative to the plasma levels of erythropoietin, and higher plasma Hb levels than would be expected for the patients' blood oxygenation.

Chuvashian Erythrocytosis. Familial and congenital erythrocytosis, not due to Hb or red cell enzyme mutations, is common in the Chuvash population of the Chuvashia Autonomous Republic of the Russian Federation, located in the European portion of Russia, southeast from Moscow.[115] Hundreds of individuals appear to be affected with an autosomal recessive and severe form of the disease with Hb concentrations of about 22 g/dL. In addition, the phenotype has features of polycythemia vera, with a high incidence of thrombosis, stroke, and occasionally splenomegaly. However, platelet and white blood cell counts are normal. The defect is not connected with the erythropoietin gene.[116] The Chuvash erythrocytosis represents a distinct disease involving a yet unknown gene that has the potential of increasing our understanding of the regulation of red cell production.

To summarize, in the identification of high-affinity Hb variants, the following points should be remembered:

1. Normal results on electrophoresis do *not* exclude the diagnosis of a high-affinity Hb.

2. A P_{50} value useful for the diagnosis of a high-affinity Hb cannot be a value "calculated" from P_{O_2} data. (One has to be able to measure directly the saturation of Hb and the P_{O_2} to obtain a useful P_{50} value. Types of apparatus such as the Hem-o-Scan are perfectly adequate for this purpose.).

3. Plasma EPO levels are useful.

PATHOPHYSIOLOGIC AND CLINICAL ASPECTS OF HIGH OXYGEN AFFINITY HEMOGLOBINS

Most patients with high-affinity Hbs and erythrocytosis have a benign clinical course and no apparent complications. Although the first high-affinity Hb was identified in the course of a workup for angina, this circumstance was probably fortuitous.

Patients with *Hb Moke* have been reported to have symptoms and to have benefited from phlebotomy and the transfusion of normal blood, but this is the exception and not the rule.[117] In a significant number of these patients erythrocytosis is diagnosed during a routine hematologic examination or when the pedigree of a propositus is examined. There are generally no physical findings, except occasionally a ruddy complexion. The Hb and hematocrit levels are only moderately increased.

The most pressing reason to identify these high-affinity Hbs early and accurately is to avoid submitting the patient to unnecessary invasive diagnostic procedures and inappropriate and often dangerous therapeutic interventions. Many of these patients have undergone expensive and unnecessary cardiac catheterization. Others have undergone several courses of radioactive phosphorus (^{32}P) treatment based on a mistaken diagnosis of polycythemia vera. As a general rule, any patient suspected of having polycythemia vera who is about to undergo a serious therapeutic intervention should have a whole blood O_2 equilibrium measurement.

The main issues still pending that concern students of this subject are the following.

Do the carriers of high-affinity Hbs have problems in the delivery of O_2 to the tissues? In patients who have had a physiologically significant high-affinity Hb all their lives reasonable compensation is probably present. The reduced delivery of O_2 to the tissues is compensated for primarily by increases in erythropoietin-induced red cell mass, and also probably by increases in blood flow and changes in perfusion patterns in selected regions (Fig. 18–16).

Erythropoietin-mediated increases in red cell mass respond to hypoxic stimuli.[118–120] Patients with several high-affinity Hbs with erythrocytosis had normal urinary erythropoietin levels that dramatically increased when they were phlebotomized to a normal red cell mass. This effect was not observed among patients with idiopathic familial erythrocytosis. Patients with high-affinity Hbs have normal O_2 consumption, normal arterial P_{O_2} values,[118] slightly reduced mixed venous P_{O_2} values in some instances, and slightly decreased resting cardiac output. More important, these numbers change significantly after phlebotomy or measured exercise, with marked increases in cardiac output and lowering of the mixed venous P_{O_2} value. The compensatory mechanisms might include

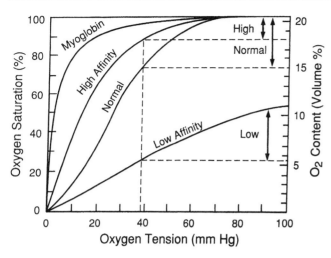

FIGURE 18–16. Oxygen equilibrium curves of myoglobin (no heme-heme interaction, hence $n = 1$) and of normal hemoglobin–containing red cells, flanked by curves of high-affinity and low-affinity hemoglobin–containing red cells. Oxygen tension (PO_2) is plotted against percentage of oxygen saturation and oxygen content as volume percent. Oxygen content takes into account the amount of hemoglobin present. The oxygen extraction is the difference in oxygen content of red cells at PO_2 of 100 mm Hg in the lungs and red cells at PO_2 of 40 mm Hg in the tissues. That subtraction renders about 5 volumes of oxygen for normal hemoglobin. High-affinity hemoglobin renders 2.5 volumes of oxygen and causes tissue hypoxia. The very low oxygen affinity hemoglobin (P_{50} of 85 mm Hg as in Hb Beth Israel) results in an extraction of a little more than 5 volumes, which is essentially normal. Nevertheless, any curve between this and the normal will have an increased oxygen extraction, and it is possible the tissues will respond to this increased oxygen delivery with a decrease in the release of erythropoietin and anemia.

increased perfusion efficiency. For example, patients with Hb Malmo have been shown to have increased myocardial blood flow, and patients with Hb Yakima have increased cerebral blood flow.

No increase in morbidity or mortality in the infant or mother is observed, suggesting that compensatory mechanisms other than the differences in O_2 affinity between HbF and HbA (the former has a lower affinity) must operate in pregnancies in which the mother's Hb has a higher O_2 affinity than that of HbF.[121]

Why do the levels of Hb vary among carriers of the same high-affinity Hb? Charache and colleagues[121] observed that carriers of Hb Osler had the same O_2 affinity as patients with Hb McKees Rocks, but Hb levels were significantly higher (by more than 4 g/dL) in male carriers of the former. When O_2 transport was assessed in these two groups, only a small decrease in mixed venous PO_2 was observed. This could be the consequence of better O_2 extraction by carriers of Hb McKees Rocks; thus they do not require as much of an increase in red cell mass as is needed for those with Hb Osler.

These results imply that epistatic (modifier) genetic effects might be operating, making the level of increase in red cell mass variable according to a person's genetic makeup. Charache and colleagues[121] have pointed out that adaptation to hypoxia at high altitude is also different in different ethnic groups. Among the Sherpas of Nepal, a lower hematocrit value, no chronic mountain sickness, and a normal O_2 equilibrium curve are found, whereas in the populations adapted to the Andes (Quechuas and Aymaras), a higher hematocrit value, chronic mountain

sickness, and right-shifted O_2 equilibrium curves are observed. These findings suggest that adaptation might involve a choice among several possible strategies (with potential differences in success) according to the different genetic background.

Should carriers of high-affinity hemoglobins receive phlebotomy? The preceding discussion suggests that patients with high-affinity Hbs have a reasonable compensation for their abnormality with correction of the delivery of O_2 to the tissues despite increases in blood viscosity; therefore, no intervention is needed. Results of exercise studies before and after phlebotomy in patients with Hb Osler showed no need for phlebotomy.[122] Nevertheless, as mentioned earlier, there are reports of individual patients who have benefited from the procedure. Perhaps, in some patients other factors interfere with the normal compensation for a high-affinity Hb and the increased viscosity may become a burden. These are exceptional patients, and prudence dictates a conservative approach and review of the patient's condition at 6-month intervals during the first few years after diagnosis. In older patients, attention to coronary status is recommended.

Conditions of low ambient PO_2 (e.g., unpressurized airplane cabins or living or climbing in mountains) do not represent a risk to patients with these high-affinity Hbs. In fact, they are better equipped than the average person to handle such situations, because their Hbs bind O_2 avidly.

Low Oxygen Affinity Hemoglobin Mutants: Cyanosis

Carriers of some low O_2 affinity Hb variants have a slate gray color of the skin and other teguments related to cyanosis. Cyanosis can be present from birth in the α-chain abnormalities and from the middle to the end of the first year of life in the β-chain mutants. This differential pattern results because α chains are expressed from the second trimester of fetal life, whereas β chains begin to be synthesized in the perinatal period and reach a significant concentration after about 6 months of age. Noncardiopulmonary cyanotic syndrome, related to abnormal Hbs, has to be distinguished from other causes of cyanosis.

Many fewer low-affinity than high-affinity Hbs are described. They can be classified as resulting from the following three conditions, which are discussed at length later:

1. Alterations of the switch region, the flexible joint, or the C termini of the $\alpha_1\beta_2$ area of contact that favor the T state, either by stabilizing this conformer or by destabilizing the R state
2. Steric hindrance to the heme, resulting in decreased affinity for ligands
3. Alteration of the $\alpha_1\beta_1$ area of contact with disruption of the overall architecture of the Hb that favors the T state

Alterations of the Switch Region, the Flexible Joint, or the C-termini in the $\alpha_1\beta_2$ Area of Contact That Favor the T State, Either by Stabilizing This Conformer or by Destabilizing the R State. *Hb Bruxelles* ($\beta42$(CD1) Phe→0)[123, 124] is a deletion of the most phylogenetically conserved amino acid residue of Hb. Phenylalanine residues at β41 and β42 are conserved in all normal mammalian non–α-globin chains and are indispensable for the structural integrity and O_2-binding functions of the molecule. DNA analysis showed that the missing codon was the TTT of β42.

The propositus for Hb Bruxelles had severe hemolytic anemia and cyanosis early in life, requiring blood transfusion on one occasion. Later, her Hb concentration stabilized at about 10 g/dL. Reasons for this "switch" of phenotype are unknown. Other mutations of β41 and β42, which are predominately unstable Hbs, are discussed later.

The striking feature of the O_2 equilibrium curve of Hb Bruxelles is that unlike the normal curve, which is roughly symmetrical with maximum cooperativity at one-half saturation, Hb Bruxelles has almost nonexistent cooperativity and a shift of the allosteric equilibrium almost entirely to the T or deoxy state. Hb Bruxelles provides a fine example of the separation of ligand affinity and allosteric effects. The shift to the T state is so large (allosteric effect) that the O_2 equilibrium/CO kinetics show essentially T-state properties. Because cooperativity is minimal in the absence of effectors, the shift in P_{50} observed with 2,3-DPG is exclusively a ligand affinity effect. The molecule is already nearly totally in the T state. In HbA, allosteric effects and ligand affinity contribute equally to the 2,3-DPG shift in O_2 affinity.

Hb Beth Israel[125] was found in a person of Italian descent, but the abnormal Hb was not detected in his parents. The propositus exhibited clinically apparent cyanosis involving his fingers, lips, and nailbeds.[125] He had been severely disciplined in the past for constantly having "dirty hands," and the abnormal skin color was not noticeable to him or his parents. The cyanosis was detected by a surgeon about to perform a herniorrhaphy. The whole blood P_{50} was 88 mm Hg (normal is 26 mm Hg), and the arterial blood was only 63 percent saturated despite a normal Po_2 of 97 mm Hg. The red cell 2,3-DPG was mildly elevated (20 mmol/L). The hemolysate showed a low O_2 affinity and a normal Bohr effect. The molecular mechanism involved here is the same as that in Hb Kansas, although the defect might be more disruptive locally since serine is shorter than threonine.

Steric Hindrance to the Heme Resulting in Decreased Affinity for Ligands. *Hb Chico* is a mutation of β66(E10), in which Lys is replaced by Thr. The interesting feature of this variant is the low affinity (P_{50} about 50 percent of normal).[125] This feature is not limited to the tetramer, but it is also present in the isolated Chico β chain, suggesting that the mutation creates conditions of decreased affinity for ligands by changes in the heme environment unrelated to the R→T transition. The best interpretation is that this effect is a consequence of the rupture of the salt bridge that Lys^{66} forms with one of the propionate side chains of the β heme. Crystallography shows hydrogen bonding of the introduced β66 Thr to the distal β63(E7) His. Nevertheless, although distal histidines are important in ligand binding in α chains, site-directed mutagenesis shows they are not significant in β chains.[126-128] Hence, the low affinity of Hb Chico must be caused by direct steric hindrance.

Alteration of the $α_1β_1$ Area of Contact with Disruption of the Overall Architecture of the Hb That Favors the T State. Two mutant Hbs have been described for site β108(G10): *Hb Yoshizuka* (Asn→Asp)[129] and *Hb Presbyterian* (Asn→Lys).[130] Hb Yoshizuka is electrophoretically distinct, amounts to 51 percent of the hemolysate, and has significantly low O_2 affinity and a decreased Bohr effect (by 30 percent). Affected carriers usually have mild anemia and no cyanosis. Asn^{108} lies in the central cavity and is hydrogen-bonded to His^{103}, a residue located in the $α_1β_1$ area of contact. In addition, this residue is linked extensively through hydrogen bonding (by water molecules) to other residues in both the α and β chains. The introduction of the carbonyl group of the Asp residue disrupts this contact severely and changes the electrostatic properties of the central cavity, resulting in destabilization of the oxy conformation.

Hb Presbyterian, in which the mutation introduces a residue with opposite charge than that in Hb Yoshizuka (Lys→Asp), amounts to 40 percent of the hemolysate, is an electrophoretically fast component, exhibits significantly low O_2 affinity, and has an abnormally high Bohr effect (increased by 30 percent) and normal interactions with 2,3-DPG. Heterozygotes are mildly anemic. The molecular mechanism involved here is probably similar to that of Hb Yoshizuka. This Hb does not dissociate in the R state, suggesting that it is abnormally biased toward the T state.[129]

These two Hbs teach us that any charge disrupts the $α_1β_1$ area of contact drastically.

PATHOPHYSIOLOGIC CONSIDERATIONS

Low-affinity Hbs deliver more O_2 to the tissues. Figure 18–17 depicts the amount of O_2 extracted from a curve situated to the right of the normal O_2 equilibrium curve. The O_2 binding at 100 mm Hg (lungs) and 40 mm Hg (tissues) in a low-affinity curve can be as high as double the difference of a normal O_2 equilibrium curve. However, the increase in extraction is not monotonic with the increase in P_{50}. Hence, patients with moderately right-shifted red cell O_2 equilibrium curves (P_{50} of 35 to 55 mm Hg) could be anemic. No anemia should be expected in patients with severely right-shifted curves ($P_{50} ≈80$ mm Hg). Findings in patients with Hb Kansas, Hb Beth Israel, Hb Titusville, and Hb Seattle confirm this analysis. Clinically apparent cyanosis is observed in carriers with significantly right-shifted curves ($P_{50} > 50$ mm Hg).

The effect of the right-shifted curve on the level of 2,3-DPG is of interest. In erythrocytes, 20 percent of the conversion of 1,3-DPG to 3-phosphoglycerate is done indirectly through the formation of 2,3-DPG. The level of red cell 2,3-DPG rises in conditions associated with hypoxia. This effect is related to the decrease in O_2 saturation of red cells and is independent of the presence of hypoxia per se; therefore, it applies to the low-affinity Hbs despite the absence of tissue hypoxia.

Desaturation increases intraerythrocytic pH as a result of deoxy-Hb binding more protons than oxy-Hb (Bohr effect). This slight red cell alkalosis stimulates two enzymes involved in 2,3-DPG synthesis: phosphofructokinase,

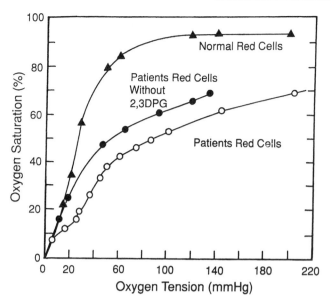

FIGURE 18–17. Oxygen equilibrium curves of normal red cells *(triangles)* and red cells from a patient heterozygous for Hb Beth Israel before *(open circles)* and after *(closed circles)* depletion of 2,3-DPG: The P_{50} for Hb Beth Israel–containing cells was 88 mm Hg (normal, 27 mm Hg). Patient's cells depleted of 2,3-DPG had a P_{50} of 55 mm Hg. Normal red cells subjected to the same procedure had a P_{50} of 16 mm Hg. The heterozygous patient's red cells have a biphasic or triphasic curve, composed of the oxygen affinity curves of normal hemoglobin (particularly the bottom portion of the composite patient curve), the abnormal hemoglobin Beth Israel (top of the composite curve), and probably hybrid molecules containing one β Beth Israel chain and one normal β chain (intermediate portion of the curve). (After Nagel RL, Joshua L, Johnson J, et al: Hemoglobin Beth Israel: A mutant causing clinically apparent cyanosis. N Engl J Med 1976; 295:125.)

which controls the overall glycolytic rate, and 2,3-DPG mutase, which directly controls the rate of 2,3-DPG synthesis. In addition, high pH inhibits 2,3-DPG phosphatase. Hence, high pH simultaneously increases the synthesis of 2,3-DPG and decreases its destruction. Finally, release of end-product inhibition may also be involved. Red cells with low-affinity Hb have an increased proportion of deoxy-Hb and will bind more 2,3-DPG, decreasing the free 2,3-DPG and thus inhibiting 2,3-DPG mutase[26] (Fig. 18–18).

IDENTIFICATION OF LOW OXYGEN AFFINITY HEMOGLOBIN VARIANTS

The presence of a low-affinity Hb should always be considered in patients with cyanosis, particularly when cardiopulmonary causes can be ruled out. In patients with cyanosis of unknown origin, it is probably advisable to obtain an electrophoresis of Hb and a whole blood P_{50} measurement before expensive or risky invasive diagnostic procedures are undertaken. The search for low-affinity Hbs as the explanation for anemia is less compelling, because the yield is probably very low and the tests are not cost-effective. Nevertheless, if other investigations prove to be fruitless, unexplained normocytic anemias should be explored with electrophoresis of Hb and a whole blood P_{50} measurement.

A simple test (even able to be performed at bedside) to distinguish low-affinity Hbs and cardiopulmonary cyanosis from methemoglobinemia, the presence of M Hbs, and sulfhemoglobinemia is to expose blood from the patient to pure O_2. This will turn the purple-greenish blood of normal persons and that of patients with low-affinity Hbs to the bright red color of fully oxygenated blood. In contrast, the blood of patients with methemoglobinemia, sulfhemoglobinemia, or M Hbs retains its abnormal color despite the exposure to pure O_2.

M Hemoglobins: Pseudocyanosis

DESCRIPTION AND PATHOPHYSIOLOGIC FEATURES OF THE M HEMOGLOBINS

Horlein and Weber[131] described a family with congenital cyanosis due to abnormal red cells 1 year before Pauling's discovery of HbS. The defect was autosomal dominant and was produced by red cells with an abnormal pigment that was similar to MetHb. The genetic defect resided in the globin and not in the heme, based on recombination experiments in which the patients' globin was bound to normal heme and the patients' heme to normal globin. The amino acid substitutions characterizing three of these M Hbs were accomplished by Gerald and Efron.[132] About the same time, the Japanese[133] solved the problem of hereditary nigremia (kuroko or "black child"), observed in the Shiden village of the Iwate prefecture for more than 160 years. They found a brownish-colored Hb in the hemolysate of a patient with this condition, which was later called Hb Iwate.

In the M Hbs, each mutated globin chain (α or β) creates an abnormal microenvironment for the heme iron, displacing the equilibrium toward the oxidized or ferric state. The combination of the iron (Fe^{3+}) and its abnormal coordination with the substituted amino acid generates an abnormal visible spectrum that resembles but is different from MetHb (oxidized heme iron in a normal globin chain). The strength by which the abnormal hemes are locked into this situation differs from one MHb to another. Figure 18–19 is a diagram of the M Hb mutations.

In four of the five known M Hbs, the distal or proximal histidine that interacts with the heme iron is replaced by tyrosine, either in the α chains or the β chains. In the fifth, *Hb M-Milwaukee-I*, Val-β67(E11) is replaced by a glutamic acid whose longer side chains can reach and perturb the heme iron.

Several molecular abnormalities are associated with the M Hbs. They can be classified into the following categories.

Weak Heme Attachment. The x-ray crystallographic studies of deoxy-*Hb M-Hyde Park* (β92(F8) His→Tyr) showed a loss of 20 to 30 percent of the heme.[134] Others detected a minor component (5 percent) in the hemolysate of these patients, which migrated between HbA₂ and Hb A-Hyde Park.[135] The α chains of the abnormal component were normal, but only one of the two $β^{HP}$ chains contained heme.

In this context the mutation in *Hb Auckland* (α97(F8) His→Asn) is particularly interesting.[136] This mutation,

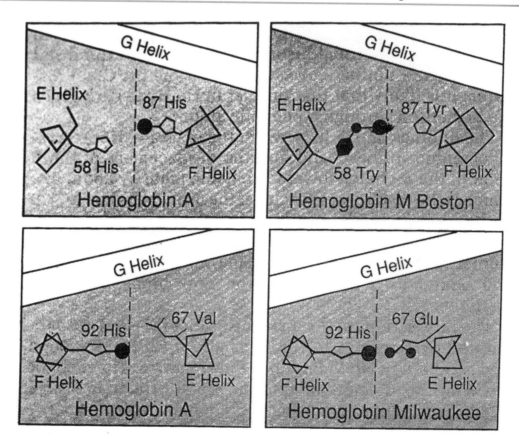

FIGURE 18–18. Schematic depiction of the crystallographic findings in Hb M-Boston (*A*, α58(E7) His→ Tyr) and Hb M-Milwaukee-I (*B*, β67 (E11) Val→ Glu) compared with those of normal hemoglobin. (*A* after Pulsinelli PD, Perutz MF, Nagel RL: Structure of hemoglobin M Boston, a variant with a five-coordinated ferric heme. Proc Natl Acad Sci USA 1973; 70:3870. *B* after Perutz MF, Pulsinelli PD, Ranney HM: Structure and subunit interaction of haemoglobin M-Milwaukee. Nature 1972; 237:259.)

involving the proximal histidine, does not lead to methemoglobinemia, as do other mutations of the proximal histidine, but to instability and accelerated heme loss. The clinical picture is a mild compensated hemolytic anemia and notmethemoglobinemia, owing to the absence of the ferric heme.

Binding of the Iron to the Remaining Histidine and to the Newly Introduced Tyrosine. The status of proximal histidine (F8) in the β^M chains (Hb Hyde Park) and α^M chains (Hb M-Iwate) is as follows. Crystallographic studies demonstrate that the Tyr must be accommodated by movements of the F helix, which appears to be largely destabilized.[134]

The findings in *Hb M-Iwate* (α87(F8) His→Tyr) are the opposite. Here, crystallographic studies[134] show that the E helix of the α chains is displaced toward the heme plate by about 2 Å, which is the distortion expected if the distal histidine (α58(E7)) moves to bind the fifth coordinating position in the heme iron.[132] To complicate matters, when the abnormal heme is reduced and bound to a ligand, the iron now binds the distal histidine.[137–139]

The interactions of the distal histidines (E7) that are substituted by tyrosines in the β^M chain of *Hb M-Saskatoon* (β63 (E7) His→Tyr) and α^M chain in *Hb M-Boston* (α58(E7) His→Tyr) are also known. The data for Hb M-Boston are more precise and are illustrated in Figure18–19. The new residue Tyr^{58} (E7) surprisingly fills

the fifth coordinating position of the heme iron despite the presence of a normal proximal histidine.[140] This bond moves the plane of the heme sufficiently to make the interaction between the proximal histidine and the heme iron impossible. No crystallographic data are available on Hb M-Saskatoon (Figure 18–19).

Finally, *Hb M-Milwaukee-I* is unique among the M Hbs because it is not a mutation of the proximal or distal histidines, but of a residue nearby (Val^{67}(E11)). When substituted by Glu, it perturbs the heme iron and generates an M Hb (defined as a variant having an abnormal MetHb-like spectrum). Other mutations of that site, such as Hb Bristol (Asp) or Hb Sidney (Ala), are unstable or have low affinity but do not generate an abnormal ferric state for the heme iron. The carboxylic group of the new glutamate occupies the sixth coordination position of the iron, and the proximal histidine maintains its role as the tenant of the fifth coordinating position.[141] This situation, of course, stabilizes the abnormal ferric state of Hb M-Milwaukee-I.

Oxygen-Binding Properties and R→T Transition of M Hemoglobins. Hb M-Milwaukee-I, Hb M Hyde Park, and Hb M-Boston all adopt deoxy or deoxy-like conformation on the deoxygenation of the two normal chains (despite the fact that the abnormal chains cannot deoxygenate). This finding helps us to understand the function of normal Hb; that is, after two hemes become

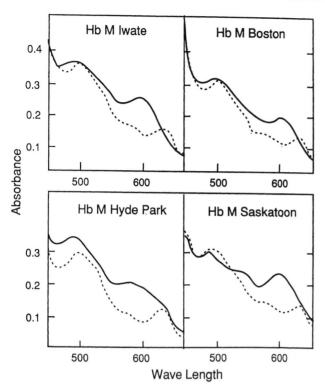

FIGURE 18–19. Spectra between 450 and 650 m of the oxidized form of four M hemoglobins are compared in each case with the normal methemoglobin spectra. In these spectra, the normal chains are met and the abnormal chains have their own particular spectral properties. (After Shibata S, Miyaji T, Iuchi I: Methemoglobin M's of the Japanese. Bull Yamaguchi Med Sch 1967; 14:141.)

deoxygenated, the molecule as a whole adopts a deoxy conformation (T state).

A Bohr effect and the P_{50} value strongly suggest that in Hb M-Milwaukee-I, Hb M-Saskatoon, and Hb M-Hyde Park the molecule adopts the R state when the two normal chains are oxygenated. NMR studies on Hb M-Milwaukee-I[142] support the theory that the conformational changes take place when the normal hemes are oxygenated. On the other hand, Hb M-Iwate is in the crystallographic T-configuration state when the normal hemes are in the ferric state. This explains its decreased affinity. The molecule does not shift to the R state when the normal hemes are liganded and remains in the low-affinity T state. Similarly in Hb M-Boston, the deoxy-Hb crystal remains intact after oxygenation, suggesting that no conformational change has occurred that would necessitate a different crystal structure.[132]

The reason Hb M-Saskatoon and Hb M-Boston have different properties (despite their common substitution of the distal histidine) is that the former does not change conformation when oxygenated and the latter does. Why β chains differ from α chains when their distal histidine is substituted has not been resolved.

Iron Oxidation and Spectral Characteristics. The fundamental characteristic of the M Hbs is that their hemes are stabilized in the abnormal ferric state. Hence, they exhibit an abnormal visible spectrum that can be easily distinguished from that of regular MetHbs (Figs. 18–20 and 18–21). This characteristic separates these

variants from Hb mutants that have a tendency to form normal MetHb, such as Hb Saint Louis,[143] Hb Bicêtre,[144] Hb I-Toulouse,[145] and Hb Seattle,[146] all of which are unstable. Column chromatography, which separates the M Hbs from HbA, dramatically shows the differences in the state of the iron in the two Hbs.

CLINICAL ASPECTS AND DIAGNOSIS

The predominant clinical feature associated with M Hb carriers is a condition similar to cyanosis, which is called *pseudocyanosis*.[147–157] The skin and mucosal membranes may be brownish or slate-colored, more like the coloration seen in methemoglobinemia, but not as blue-purple as in true cyanosis. The distinction is subtle and might not be apparent without contrasting the two conditions simultaneously. The reason for the difference is that the color of the skin is induced by Hb molecules that have an abnormal MetHb state, whereas cyanosis is caused by the presence of more than 5 g/dL of deoxy-Hb. The cyanosis is present from birth in α-chain abnormalities and from the middle of the first year in the β-chain mutants. In addition, a mixture of the abnormal pigment and true cyanosis due to Hb desaturation (of the normal chains) is observed in the low-affinity M Hb (Hb M-Boston and Hb M-Iwate).

Pseudocyanosis is not associated with dyspnea or clubbing, and affected persons apparently have a normal life expectancy. A mild hemolytic anemia (with increased reticulocyte count) has been observed in Hb M-Hyde Park and can be explained by the instability of the Hb induced by partial loss of the hemes.

The possibility of M Hb should be considered in all patients with abnormal homogeneous coloration of the skin and mucosa, particularly when pulmonary and cardiac function are normal. The diagnosis can be reinforced by observing an abnormal brown coloration of the blood in a tube. To distinguish this coloration from that due to MetHb, the addition of potassium cyanide to the hemolysate is useful. Hemolysates containing MetHb turn red; those containing M Hb often change color more slowly. The rate of color conversion varies among the M Hbs. A recording spectrophotometer is required for the next step in the diagnosis, although any spectrophotometer that is recommended for the differential diagnosis of cyanotic syndromes can be used for the overall technique (see next section). Figures 18–20 and 18–22 illustrate the differences in the spectra observed with the M Hbs, but all spectra clearly differ from the normal MetHb spectrum with its maximum at 620 nm.

Electrophoresis is of limited value because the oxy forms are not separable from normal Hb by cellulose acetate. The usefulness of agar electrophoresis is a little better. Ion-exchange chromatography (BioRex 70 equilibrated and developed with 0.196 mmol/L Na_2PO_4, pH 6.42) can separate the brown Hb from the normal Hb, rendering the diagnosis. Hemoglobin chains can be prepared by blocking the Cys thiols with *p*-chloromercuribenzoate and separating the chains chromatographically, allowing the determination of which chain has an abnormal color and hence the mutation.

Perhaps the greatest hazard for carriers of M Hb is *misdiagnosis* and the risk of expensive and hazardous

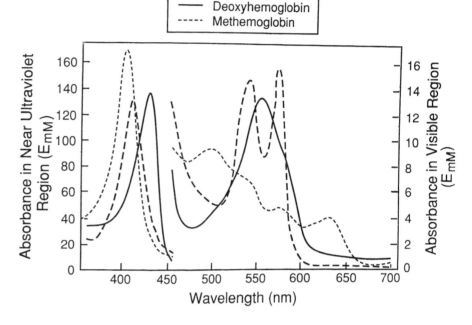

FIGURE 18–20. Light absorption spectra of oxyhemoglobin (– / – / –), deoxyhemoglobin (—), and methemoglobin (- / - / -) in the visible and near ultraviolet regions. E_{mM} is the millimolar extinction coefficient in 0.1 mol/L potassium phosphate buffer (pH 7.4). (After Imai K: Allosteric effects in haemoglobin. Cambridge, UK, Cambridge University Press, 1982.)

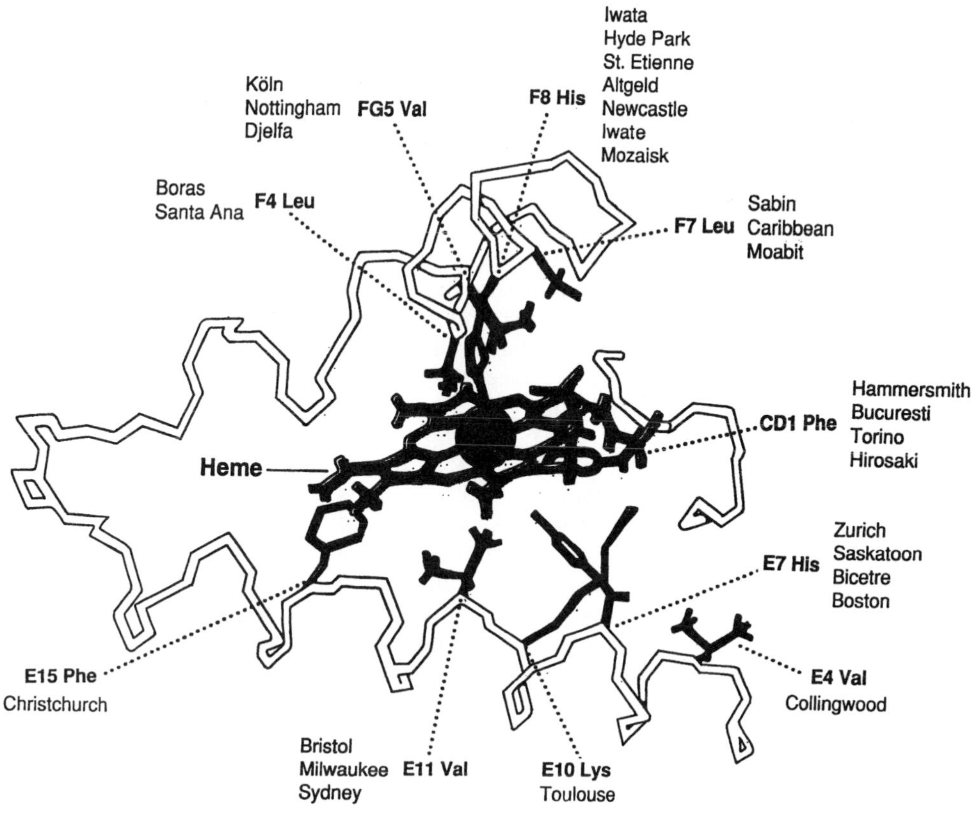

FIGURE 18–21. Diagram of the heme pocket, showing the replacement site of several of the unstable hemoglobins. Valine E4 is at the corner of the pocket, and its side chain does not make contact with the heme but does affect the placement of adjacent amino acid side chains. (After Williamson D, Brennan SO, Muir H, et al: Hemoglobin Collingwood β60 (E4) Val→Ala. A new unstable hemoglobin. Hemoglobin 1983; 7:511.)

workups. I am aware of one instance in which a 1-week-old infant underwent a Blalock procedure because of a misdiagnosis of pseudotruncus arteriosus. When the family study was completed many years later, the father was identified as a carrier of Hb M-Boston and the child was also recognized as a carrier of this abnormal Hb.

DIFFERENTIAL DIAGNOSIS OF LOW-AFFINITY HEMOGLOBINS AND PSEUDOCYANOSIS FROM METHEMOGLOBINEMIA AND SULFHEMOGLOBINEMIA

In this section, a more general problem is analyzed: the pathophysiologic and diagnostic aspects of the condition

Reversible Hemichromes	Irreversible Hemichromes

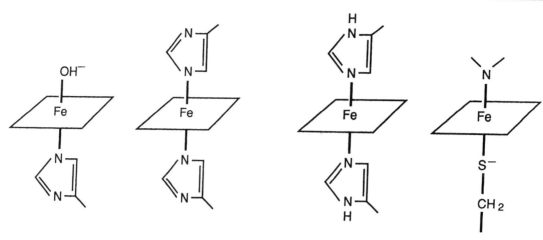

FIGURE 18–22. Diagrammatic representation of the structure of hemichromes, showing proximal histidine below the plane of the heme and distal histidine above the plane. One or both of the histidines can be substituted. (After Peisach J, Blumberg WE, Rachmilewitz EA: The demonstration of ferrihemochrome intermediates in Heinz body formation following the reduction of oxyhemoglobin A by acetylphenylhydrazine. Biochim Biophys Acta 1975; 393:404.)

of the patient with cyanosis not of cardiopulmonary origin.

Although the cardiac and pulmonary systems are major targets in the evaluation of a patient with apparent cyanosis, the differential diagnosis of this clinical sign includes two classes of hemoglobinopathies. First, the presence of an abnormal Hb with a normal visible spectrum but a markedly right-shifted P_{50} results in significant arterial desaturation.[158–159] Second, with sulfhemoglobin (sulfHb),[157, 158] MetHb, and M Hb, the altered visible spectrum of the abnormal pigments is responsible for the gray skin color. Comparing the spectral properties of sulfHb with those of MetHb shows that less of the former is needed to produce cyanosis. A patient can be markedly cyanotic with only 12 percent (1.6 g/dL) sulfHb.[160, 161]

The respiratory status of persons with cyanosis resulting from an abnormal Hb varies with the entity. There is general agreement that clinically apparent dyspnea is not associated with the mutant Hbs with right-shifted P_{50} values[158, 159] or with the M Hbs[162, 163] but can be associated with even relatively mild degrees of methemoglobinemia.[159, 164] For sulfhemoglobinemia, there is no agreement. Most case reports indicate that dyspnea is not a feature, but in others the symptoms associated with methemoglobinemia and sulfhemoglobinemia are found to be "identical."[157]

Because the altered hemes in M Hb, sulfHb, and MetHb do not transport O_2,[159] affected persons with all three entities may have normal Hb levels but exhibit the physiologic effects of an anemia simply because insufficient functional hemes remain. This effect, in isolation, would be clinically significant only in extreme instances of methemoglobinemia and sulfhemoglobinemia or when the overall Hb level was low. Severe instances of both sulfhemoglobinemia[147] and methemoglobinemia[162, 166] have been reported in which the abundance of nonfunctional hemes was the major concern. In contrast, with that seen with M Hbs, the proportion of normal to abnormal

hemes is genetically determined to be greater than 75 percent (because the carriers are heterozygotes and there are two genetically different chains), so that the decrease of O_2-binding capacity is a problem only when anemia is already present.

The clinical effects of nonfunctional hemes need not be limited to their inability to transport O_2. Small amounts of nonfunctional hemes can have clinical significance beyond that of comparable degrees of anemia if their presence in partially modified tetramers produces a physiologically dysfunctional shift in the oxygenation curve of neighboring unmodified subunits. This is the molecular basis of the left-shifted oxygenation curve, the impaired O_2 delivery to the periphery, and the resulting respiratory distress seen with relatively mild degrees of methemoglobinemia. This phenomenon, called the *Darling-Roughton effect*, occurs because the oxidized subunits in partially oxidized tetramers are held in an R-like (or liganded) conformation, which increases the O_2 affinity of the remaining subunits in those tetramers.[164] Although mixed venous blood is unusually saturated, the abnormal spectrum of the MetHb outweighs this effect and the person appears cyanotic. An analogous left shift in the oxygenation curve occurs to a more pronounced degree in CO poisoning, and here, too, the impaired O_2 delivery is thought to exacerbate dyspnea.

In the M Hbs, the presence of the abnormal nonfunctional hemes in the affected tetramers results in a marked flattening of the O_2 affinity curve. The curve is also right-shifted, especially in the most physiologically relevant P_{O_2} range.[162] This leads to normal or even enhanced ability to deliver O_2 to the periphery, which is consistent with the absence of respiratory insufficiency in these syndromes.

The following system has been suggested[157, 158] for evaluating the blood of persons with pseudocyanosis after exposure to drugs or chemicals associated with methemoglobinemia or sulfhemoglobinemia (Fig. 18–22).

Procedure: If the visible spectrum of the hemolysate reveals a peak in the 610- to 640-nm range, the following sequence of spectra should be obtained: (1) air-equilibrated sample with and without potassium cyanide; (2) sample with dithionite; and (3) sample with CO.

Interpretation: If only MetHb is present, the abnormal peak will disappear immediately after the addition of dithionite or cyanide. For M Hb, the peak disappears more slowly and can require hours. For sulfHb, the peak undergoes a very slow decrease as a result of instability.

Differentiation: To distinguish sulfHb from M Hb, compare the spectra of the air- and CO-equilibrated samples. If CO results in an augmentation and downfield shift of the peak, the sample contains sulfHb.

Unstable Hemoglobin Variants: Congenital Heinz Body Hemolytic Syndrome

Some Hb mutants have substitutions that alter the solubility of the molecule in the red cell.[165] The intraerythrocytic precipitated material derived from the unstable abnormal Hb is detectable by a supravital stain as dark globular aggregates called *Heinz bodies (HBs).* These intracellular inclusions reduce the life expectancy of the red cell and generate a hemolytic syndrome of varied severity called the *Heinz body hemolytic syndrome.* Use of the word *syndrome* is advisable because this clinical picture is not exclusive to the presence of unstable Hbs but can also be generated by congenital enzyme deficiencies.

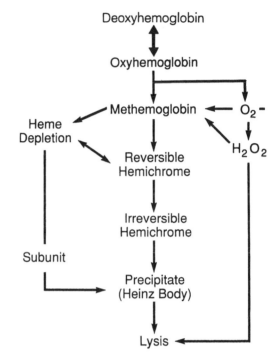

FIGURE 18–23. Scheme of the intraerythrocyte denaturation of unstable hemoglobins as proposed by Winterbourne and Carrell. (After Winterbourne CC, Carrell DW: Studies of hemoglobin denaturation and Heinz body formation in the unstable hemoglobins. J Clin Invest 1974; 54:678.)

STRUCTURAL ABNORMALITIES INVOLVED IN UNSTABLE HEMOGLOBINS

Substitutions in the primary sequence can lead to alterations in the tertiary or quaternary structure and result in a globin polypeptide chain or a Hb tetramer that is relatively unstable and tends to precipitate inside the red cell. The structural alterations leading to this event can be classified as follows.

Mutations That Weaken or Modify the Heme-Globin Interactions. The binding of the heme to the globin is important not only for the O_2-binding properties of the molecule but also for its stability and solubility. Figure 18–23 depicts several of the mutations involving residues with defined interactions with the heme group. These mutations include the following:

1. Substitutions that introduce a charged side chain into the heme pocket where a nonpolar side chain existed previously: examples are Hb Boras, Hb Bristol, Hb Olsted, Hb Himeji, and others
2. Deletions involving residues that directly interact with the heme, such as Hb Gun Hill
3. The nontyrosine substitutions of the proximal histidine (F8), such as Hb Saint Etienne (also known as Hb Istanbul), Hb J-Altgeld Gardens, Hb Mozhaisk, Hb Newcastle, Hb Iwata, and Hb Redondo (also known as Hb Ishehara)
4. Nontyrosine substitutions of the distal histidine (E7), such as Hb Zurich and Hb Bicêtre

Hb Zurich (β63 (E7) His→Arg) is an interesting mutation, which deserves special mention.[166-179] The substitution of an arginine for the distal histidine in the β chains

makes the space available for ligand binding around the iron much larger, fundamentally changing some of its interactions with ligands.

Although the extra space in the heme pocket has little effect on the O_2 molecule that binds iron at an angle, a significant difference for CO becomes apparent. The biatomic CO binds perpendicularly to the heme and because of steric constraints present in the normal heme pocket, its binding to iron is reduced with respect to that of O_2. This reduction of the binding constant is a normal adaptation to the endogenous generation of CO (one CO molecule evolves from each heme catabolized) and protects individuals from excessive accumulation of carboxy-Hb (COHb). The toxicity of CO stems from the significant reduction in the dissociation constant, compared with O_2, making COHb a particularly stable ligand species.

Carriers of Hb Zurich exhibit an increased affinity for CO owing to the increase in the binding constant. This molecular pathologic change is a protective mechanism of sorts. It does not allow the abnormal β chain to become ferric, which would increase its instability. Smokers with Hb Zurich have high levels of COHb, but carriers who are nonsmokers also have abnormal COHb levels. Because of the partially protective effect of COHb Zurich, HBs are less common among smokers than among nonsmokers with this abnormal Hb.[168]

Carriers of Hb Zurich are especially susceptible to hemolytic crises induced by sulfanilamide. The increased aperture of the heme pocket also explains this phenomenon: sulfanilamide is capable of binding to the heme and producing MetHb directly. Again, CO has a protective effect.

Mutations That Interfere with the Secondary Structure of the Subunits. As previously mentioned, Hb is composed of more than 75 percent α-helical regions, and any disruption of this secondary structure reduces the solubility of the subunit. Unstable Hb mutants can result from the introduction of proline in the helical structure or the substitution of glycine by a mutation in invariant positions in the bands. Twenty-one of the 139 mutations correspond to the introduction of a proline residue.

Hb Brockton (β138(H16) Ala→Pro)[169] is associated with moderate anemia. It cannot be separated from HbA by standard electrophoretic procedures. Crystallography showed that the tertiary structure was disrupted in the vicinity of the mutated residue. Molecular instability is probably the result of the breakage of a buried H bond, normally tying Ala-β138 with Val-β134, a task that the proline side chain cannot accomplish.

One special case does not constitute an exception. *Hb Singapore* (α141 Arg→Pro) is an abnormal Hb in which the introduction of a proline is not accompanied by instability. The reason is simple. The substituted residue is the last amino acid of the α chain, Arg^{141}, and no disruption of an α helix takes place.

Mutations That Interfere with the Tertiary Structure of the Subunits. Hemoglobin is a globular protein, quite tightly bound, which means that the α-helical regions must be folded into a solid sphere. This design introduces enormous constraints to the architecture. Substitutions of the sequence can occur with no change in solubility as long as (1) no charged residues (hydrophilic) are allowed to point inward, (2) no bulky side chains are allowed to substitute for less bulky residues inside the molecule, and (3) the loss of critical nonpolar residues from the surface of the subunit is avoided. A special case is what Fermi and Perutz called the "loss of a nonpolar plug." This is a reference to hydrophobic residues that are located on the surface and serve to prevent water from invading the interior of the molecule. This is a common cause of instability for Hb and about half of the instances of unstable Hb correspond to substitution of an Arg for a Leu.

Hb J-Biskra[170] is the result of an eight-residue deletion between either α50–57 or α52–59, clearly altering the tertiary structure by amino acid reduction. This is the longest described amino acid deletion of the Hb molecule.[180] Although the deletion includes the distal histidine and neighboring residues, the Hb is only mildly unstable *in vitro*, hemolysis is absent, and the concentration of this variant is about that expected for a variant of the α$_1$-globin gene. This mutation might appear to defy the rules stated above but it does not: Hb J-Biskra involves the removal of a string of amino acids, and it does not add inappropriate side chains to the interior of the molecule.

Mutations That Affect Subunit Interactions: Interference with Quaternary Structure. These mutations involve the introduction of charged residues in the interior or the loss of intersubunit contact hydrogen bonds or salt bridges in the α$_1$β$_1$ contact. This contact is critical for stability because it does not dissociate normally, unlike the α$_1$β$_2$ area of contact, which dissociates under conditions found in the red cell, yielding Hb dimers. Because dimerization is a first-order reaction (concentration independent) and tetramerization is a second-order reaction (concentration dependent), the proportion of dimers in the concentrated Hb milieu of the red cell is small. Nevertheless, dissociation is possible and is constantly occurring.

In contrast, the breakdown of α$_1$β$_1$ dimers normally occurs to a vanishingly small extent, but is a great threat to the molecule, because it generates methemoglobin and consequent instability. Dissociation of α$_1$β$_1$ dimers generates monomeric α and β chains, which uncoil, loosening their heme-globin interaction and favoring methemoglobin formation. Several unstable Hb mutations involve residues located in the α$_1$β$_1$ area of contact: Hb Philly,[171] Hb Peterborough,[172] Hb Stanmore,[173] Hb J-Guantanamo,[174] and Hb Khartoum.[180]

Mutations That Interfere with Heme Binding to Globin. *Hb Auckland* is a newly described unstable Hb with a mutation of α97(F8) His→Asn.[176] This substitution, involving the proximal histidine, does not lead to methemoglobinemia, but to instability, accelerated heme loss, and low O$_2$ saturation. The usual O$_2$ saturation was 92 percent. The clinical picture is a mild compensated hemolytic anemia. Results of the isopropanol stability test (see later) were positive. The abnormal Hb was further studied by electrospray ionization mass spectrometry of the total lysate: 14 percent of the α chains had a mass of 15,103.4 D, which is 23 D less than normal and is due to the Asn substitution.

Hyperunstable Hemoglobins. This term was coined by Ohba[177, 182] to characterize unstable Hbs that are either barely detectable or undetectable in hemolysates. These Hbs are presumably synthesized normally but are rapidly destroyed in the bone marrow, creating a phenotype closer to thalassemia than to the hemolytic anemia normally associated with unstable Hbs.

Hb Hirosaki (α43(CE1) Phe→Leu)[178] accounts for 1 percent of the hemolysate and is clinically silent in some carriers and expressed as a hemolytic anemia in others.

Hb Quong Sze (α125(H8) Leu→Pro)[177] is undetectable in red cells by electrophoresis, chromatography, or biosynthetic studies. It was discovered by sequencing the α$_2$ gene and confirmed by biosynthesis in a cell-free system.

Hb Toyama (α136(H19) Leu→Arg)[179] corresponds to less than 1 percent of the hemolysate and is detectable only in biosynthetic studies. Although some of the carriers have severe normocytic hemolytic anemias, others are not anemic but have microcytic red cells.

Presumably, the disappearance of these chains in the cytosol is the consequence of proteases that are particularly effective in digesting the mutated chains. The interesting variability in phenotype strongly suggests the phenomenon of epistasis (the effect of other genes besides the one affected, that is, epistatic genes [also called modifier genes] in defining the phenotype). It is possible that the level or type of proteases expressed in the red cell cytosol differs in individuals. Carriers have microcytosis and hypochromia if they express effective proteases and have hemolytic anemia if they do not.

CLINICAL CHARACTERISTICS OF THE CONGENITAL HEINZ BODY HEMOLYTIC ANEMIAS

Anemia is the centerpiece of the syndrome, but its intensity varies widely among patients, depending on the Hb variant.

Unstable Hbs are uncommon mutational events generally limited to a single pedigree. The exception is *Hb Köln*(β98(FG5) Val→Met), which has been detected in several different pedigrees and geographic locations. The time when anemia appears depends on the chain affected. One of the α-chain mutants, *Hb Hasharon* (α47(CE5) Asp→His), which is found predominantly among Ashkenazi Jews, produces significant hemolysis in newborns but is milder in adults.[183, 184] In some carriers, it produces a mild anemia, whereas no hemolysis is observed in other carriers of the same pedigree. Epistatic effects of other nonlinked genes are probably involved here.

Unstable γ-chain variants, such as Hb F Poole, cause significant hemolysis in the first 3 months life,[67] that is ameliorated with the emergence of the β chains at the end of the first year.

Patients with unstable Hb may have hemolytic crises associated with bacterial or viral infections or with exposure to oxidants. Pyrexia and transient acidosis contribute to hemolysis, because they increase Hb denaturation. Drugs (i.e., sulfonamides) have been directly implicated in hemolytic crisis associated with Hb Zurich, Hb Hasharon, Hb Shepards Bush, and Hb Peterborough. The crises are generally self-limited, and stopping the administration of all drugs is prudent. Patients are also susceptible to parvovirus B19-induced aplastic crises.

Patients with unstable Hbs can have characteristically dark urine or pigmenturia. The color change is not due to bilirubin but rather to the presence of dipyrrole methylenes of the mesobilifuscin group.[185] The origin of these fluorescent compounds is not clear. Their structure—two pyrrole rings still bound to each other by a methenyl bridge—suggests the malfunctioning of the methenyl oxygenase, the enzyme involved in the breaking of the — CH= bridges. Apparently, fluorescent dipyrroles are also present in HB.[186]

The absence of pigmenturia does not exclude the diagnosis of unstable Hb, because not all mutants exhibit pigmenturia. In addition, the extent of hemolysis does not correlate with pigmenturia, since significant pigmenturia is seen with both Hb Köln (severe hemolytic anemia) and Hb Zurich (little hemolysis).

Congenital HB hemolytic anemias related to unstable Hbs are generally mild and do not require therapy, except for supportive and preventive measures including administration of folic acid to ensure that the overworked marrow does not become deficient in this nutrient, prevention and prompt treatment of infections, avoidance of pyrexia with use of aspirin, and avoidance of oxidant drugs, including acetaminophen.

The question of splenectomy arises for patients with more severe hemolysis. There is little doubt that the spleen plays an important pathophysiologic role in the destruction of HB-containing red cells. Nevertheless, this needs to be balanced with the role of the spleen in the susceptibility to pneumococcal infections early in life and the need to use antipneumococcal vaccines after splenectomy in childhood. Splenectomy is beneficial, on balance, for patients with the most severe unstable hemoglobinopathies, and partial correction of the anemia has been achieved.[187] Nevertheless, the success of the splenectomy cannot be ensured.

IDENTIFICATION OF UNSTABLE HEMOGLOBINS

The elements for the differential diagnosis of unstable Hbs are the following:

1. HBs spontaneously present in the blood (less often) or induced by 24-hour incubation of a sterile sample on sterile saline and stained by supravital pigments
2. Positive results of Hb electrophoresis (sometimes a smeared band is observed); negative results are not diagnostically useful
3. Positive results for a heat stability test

All of these tests are useful and should be pursued because results for any one of them could be negative. The heat stability test is the least likely to result in a false-negative outcome.

Because the spleen removes HBs efficiently, many patients with unstable Hbs lack HBs before splenectomy and the differential diagnosis includes autoimmune hemolytic anemias and other disorders with nonspecific red cell morphology, such as glycolytic and other red cell enzyme defects, Wilson disease, paroxysmal nocturnal hemoglobinuria, hereditary xerocytosis, and (very rarely) erythropoietic porphyria.

The differential diagnosis of an unstable hemoglobinopathy in the adult is the same as that given for other causes of congenital HB hemolytic syndrome and acquired forms of HB hemolytic anemias (acquired methemoglobinemia, chemical and drug oxidants, and other conditions). In rare instances, several of these entities interact with each other to the detriment of the patient.[188]

Smear and Heinz Body Preparation. The blood smear is not a specific test. It reveals anisocytosis, sometimes hypochromia, and often *prominent basophilic stippling*. The latter is often the most useful clue to the diagnosis because prominent basophilic stippling is uncommon in other hemolytic anemias, except for the rare pyridine 5′-nucleotidase deficiency. Howell-Jolly bodies, normoblasts, and some microspherocytes may also be observed in the peripheral blood.

HB detection requires the use of methyl blue or crystal violet supravital stains. HBs appear as irregular pale purple inclusions, singly or a few together, that are 2 μm in diameter or less and often appear to be attached to the membrane.[185] Sometimes HBs are apparent in fresh blood, but usually sterile incubation of the blood for 24 hours in the absence of glucose is required to elicit them. A sample of normal blood should always be run as a control. After splenectomy, red cells with HBs occur more often and are easier to detect. Indeed, in occasional patients HBs can *only* be detected after splenectomy.

Electrophoresis. Electrophoresis of Hb can demonstrate an abnormal component, but many times the unstable Hb appears as a diffuse band. This alteration is probably related to the partial denaturation of Hb molecules during electrophoresis (due to heat generated) or during the manipulations of the hemolysate. Occasionally, only precipitated material at the origin is observed. Many unstable Hbs are not detectable by electrophoresis.

Heat Stability Test. The heat denaturation test, consisting of the incubation of a hemolysate for 1 or 2 hours at 50°C, is a simple and reliable procedure.[189, 190] Normal hemolysates are stable under these conditions, and the presence of an unstable Hb is signaled by the appearance of a visible precipitate. Some abnormal Hbs, such as Hb Hasharon, precipitate at higher temperatures than 50°C, but if higher temperatures are used, controls are indispensable, because normal Hb begins to precipitate at about 55°C.

Other laboratory procedures are available. The isopropanol test[191] is used in many laboratories, but it gives false-positive results when the sample contains more than 5 percent HbF. HbF does not interfere with zinc acetate precipitation.[192] The mechanical agitation procedure of Asakura and colleagues[193] can reveal the presence of unstable hemoglobins.[194]

PATHOPHYSIOLOGY OF THE HEINZ BODY HEMOLYTIC SYNDROME PRODUCED BY UNSTABLE HEMOGLOBINS

Thermostability of Hemoglobins. When heat-unstable Hbs were related to the presence of a HB hemolytic anemia,[189, 195] the conceptual framework for the understanding of this syndrome was generated. Homeothermic mammals and birds have relatively thermostable Hbs. If a hemolysate is incubated for 1 or 2 hours at 50°C, little protein precipitation occurs. This property is observed even among the reptile Hbs, although to a lesser degree. Among amphibians and fish, the thermostability of Hb decreases substantially.

The molecular basis of thermostability is not clear. Perutz[196] suggested that thermostability of proteins, including Hb, is based on electrostatic interactions and salt bridge formations. Others[197] contend that hydrophobic interactions are critical, and some claim that both electrostatic and hydrophobic interactions are contributory.[198] Most of the evidence is from structural analysis of proteins obtained from thermophilic and mesophilic bacteria[180] or from comparing amino acid sequences in Hbs of organisms living at different temperatures.[199]

Other contributions to the thermostability come from the strength of the heme-globin bonds. Heme exchanges between Hb and albumin and between Hbs decreases considerably when the MetHb heme is ligated with cyanide.[200] Presumably, cyanomethemoglobin has a stronger heme-globin attachment than MetHb and is more similar to liganded Hb. Deoxy-Hb has an even the tighter bond.

Denaturation of Hemoglobin and Hemichrome Formation. HBs, one of the hallmarks of the hemolytic syndrome generated by unstable Hbs, are the product of Hb denaturation. Initial suggestions were that HBs are composed of heme-depleted globin chains.[201, 202] The precipitated material is *hemichromes*.[181, 203–205] These are derivatives of the low-spin forms of ferric Hb that have the sixth coordination position occupied by a ligand provided by the globin: a hydroxyl group (—OH) or unprotonated histidyl (reversible hemichrome) or an protonated histidyl (irreversible hemichrome)[206] (Fig. 18–24). Irreversible hemichromes seem to be an indispensable stage in the formation of HBs, and both α and β chains are present.[207] In addition, a general scheme for the generation of HBs has been proposed.[195]

Anemia with the Unstable Hemoglobins That Generates Heinz Body Hemolytic Syndrome. The primary cause of the anemia is the reduced lifespan of the red cells that contain HBs. Evidence indicates that HBs, at least in part, adhere to the cytosolic side of the membrane[196, 208] by hydrophobic interactions and not through covalent bonds, as previously suggested.[209, 210]

The anion exchanger (AE-1 or band 3) is the most common transmembrane protein in the mature red cell. It spans the membrane with a glycosylated portion on the surface of the red cell, a hydrophobic portion across the lipid bilayer, and a cytosolic domain of about 43 kD. The N-terminal portion of the cytosolic domain is highly negatively charged. The enzymes phosphofructokinase, glyceraldehyde-3-phosphate dehydrogenase, and aldolase bind to this region of band 3. In addition, this is the portion of the molecule to which Hb and hemichromes bind.[211, 212]

The negatively charged band 3 sequence threads itself into the positively charged central cavity of Hb, which is why it binds deoxy-Hb preferentially and in a reversible way: the higher the positive charge, the higher the affinity. This is why HbA_2 and HbC (particularly the latter) attach tenaciously to the membrane. HbS is intermediate in affinity. HbC also exhibits reversible binding, and HbS has an irreversible component, which may be due to hemichrome binding to band 3. Hemichromes bind at the same site as Hb, but the binding seems to be irreversible and causes band 3 molecules (and associated membrane proteins) to aggregate.[211–218]

Unstable Hbs generate considerable amounts of hemichromes, and some of these bind to band 3. It is not surprising that these red cells exhibit decreased deformability, a characteristic that will condemn them to be preferentially trapped in the red cell quality control organ, the spleen.[219, 220] It is possible that HB-containing red cells are pitted initially. The term *pitting* refers to the mechanism by which HBs and a portion of the overlying plasma membrane are excised from the cells during their passage through the spleen. This manipulation converts red cells progressively into spherocytes through membrane loss, producing a rigid remnant that will be eliminated eventually from the circulation.

Other sources of membrane damage come from peroxidation and cross-linking of membrane proteins. These are probably related to the presence of free heme and iron and to free radicals generated during methemoglobin formation and Hb denaturation.[221–224] Other evidence of membrane alteration is the presence of abnormal potassium (K^+) efflux in some of these cells.[220, 225]

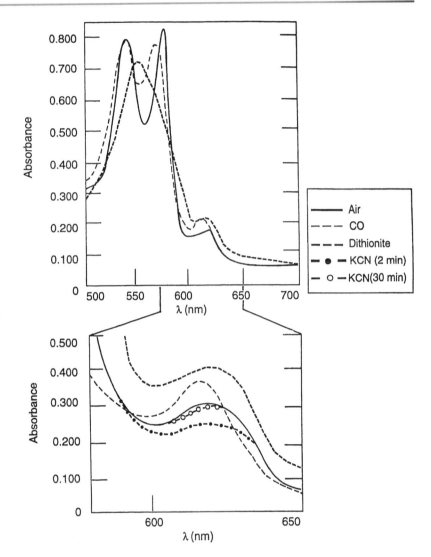

FIGURE 18–24. Visible spectra of the hemolysate of a patient with sulfhemoglobinemia. *A,* The spectrum of the air-equilibrated sample, the sample after equilibration with carbon monoxide (CO), and the sample treated with the reducing agent dithionite. *B,* The abnormal peak in the air-equilibrated sample at 2 and 30 minutes after the addition of potassium cyanide (KCN). The augmentation and shift of the peak toward lower wavelength with the addition of carbon monoxide provides the basis for the diagnostic procedure for sulfhemoglobinemia. (After Park CM, Nagel RL: Sulfhemoglobin: Clinical and molecular aspects. N Engl J Med 1984; 310:1579.

Another determinant of the anemia in patients with unstable Hbs is the O_2 equilibrium curve. The level of 2,3-DPG is generally normal,[226] but some variants have a high or low O_2 affinity. As discussed before, persons with high-affinity unstable Hbs tend to have less anemia than those with low-affinity unstable Hbs. Nevertheless, there is considerable overlapping of these abnormal properties. The question of abnormal synthesis or catabolism of the unstable Hbs is also of interest. The extreme case is that in which the Hb is so unstable that none can be detected in the red cell. This is the case for *Hb Quong Sze,* a α-chain mutant that can be identified only by DNA sequencing. *Hb Terre Haute* (β106 Leu→Arg), originally incorrectly identified as Hb Indianapolis (β112 Cys→Arg), is an extremely unstable Hb and is expressed as a dominant thalassemic syndrome (see next section), with an α-globinto-β-globin synthesis ratio of 0.4:1 (normal is 1.10:1).[227, 228]

Finally, several unstable Hbs coexist with α- or β-thalassemia: the α-chain mutants *Hb Suan-Dok* and *Hb Petah Tikva* coexist in *cis* with α-thalassemia, and the β-chain mutant *Hb Leiden* coexists in *cis* with a β-thalassemia.

Hemoglobin Structural Mutations with Abnormal Assembly: Dominant Thalassemia Syndrome

The dominant thalassemia syndrome includes mutations of the coding region of the globin genes that lead to a significant deficit in synthesis and that present clinically as autosomal dominant thalassemia.

CLINICAL PICTURE AND DIAGNOSIS

The dominant thalassemia syndrome is characterized by significant anemia, often transfusion-dependent, by splenomegaly, and by a blood smear with prominent hypochromia, microcytosis, and basophilic stippling.[229] The reticulocyte count is often high. Inclusion bodies are often observed in erythrocyte *precursors* with supravital staining, which is why some authors call this syndrome "inclusion body thalassemia." The bone marrow shows considerable erythroid hyperplasia and evidence of ineffective erythropoiesis. Finally, the full-fledged thalassemic syndrome is found in members of different generations in the same pedigree, often in one of the parents or progeny of the propositus. Although the syndrome is similar to thalassemia intermedia, an astute clinician can exclude this diagnosis when the intensity of the disease in the parents or descendants is equal to that seen in the propositus. Thalassemia intermedia usually results from homozygosity or double heterozygosity for much milder defects; hence, the parents or progeny have a much milder disease. Nevertheless, lack of parental involvement does not exclude the diagnosis because the mutation can be *de novo*. A clinical picture of thalassemia in a patient with an ethnic origin not associated with β-thalassemia should also increase the suspicion of the clinician for this syndrome.

Electrophoresis might not reveal an abnormal band because the abnormal Hb is either synthesized at an extremely low level, is rapidly catabolized, or both.

Hb Manhattan (β109 [G11] →0)[230] is a frameshift mutation produced by a single nucleotide deletion in codon 109. The mutation was discovered in a 78-year-old Lithuanian Jew with lifelong chronic hemolytic anemia and thalassemic features. Laboratory tests revealed a hemoglobin level of 8.5 g/dL, low mean corpuscular volume, marked anisocytosis with hypochromia, marked basophilic stippling, reticulocyte count of 1.2 percent, and no spontaneous or incubated HB. It leads to an abnormal globin ($\beta_{Manhattan}$) that is elongated to 156 amino acids. Synthetic studies did not reveal the abnormal chain, and the α-globin-to-β-globin synthesis ratio was 0.5:1.

Highly unstable α-globin variants, in contrast to β-globin variants, are usually only phenotypically apparent when they interact with other α-thalassemia mutations. A child with clinical and hematologic features consistent with those of β-thalassemia intermedia, nevertheless had a DNA analysis that excluded β-globin gene mutations. Instead the propositus had a novel deletion (β37 (C2) Pro→0 [*Hb Heraklion*]) in the α_1-globin gene, in *trans* to a common Mediterranean nondeletional α-thalassemia mutation.[231] This deletion results in severe instability of the variant Hb, which interacts with the α-thalassemia mutation, causing a relatively severe dyserythropoietic anemia—an alternative phenotype associated with the highly unstable α-chain variants. The diserythopoietic marrow is due to the alteration of early red cell precursors.

PATHOPHYSIOLOGY

The molecular basis of the dominant thalassemia syndrome involve two types of changes: (1) single-point mutations (substitutions and deletions) affecting, in particular, exon 3; and (2) exon 3 chain-length shortening (premature termination) or elongation (frameshift mutation leading to an altered stop codon).

What causes the *severity* of the phenotype of dominant thalassemia? The answer lies in the notion that in dominant thalassemia the abnormal chain is synthesized at a close to normal rate but is rapidly destroyed because it cannot assemble into tetramers, creating inclusions and generating free radicals (conversion of the heme groups to metheme). The reason for the lack of assembly is that all these mutations affect the residues coded in exon 3 and

involved in the $\alpha_1\beta_1$ *area of contact*, critical for stabilization and without which a tetramer cannot exist.[231] The mutations found in dominant thalassemia affect the $\alpha_1\beta_2$ area of contact, either directly (most cases) or indirectly (as in *Hb Chesterfield* [β28 (B10) Leu→Arg] or *Hb Cagliari* [β60 (E4) Val→Glu], in which an internal residue is replaced by a bulky, charged amino acid, or *Hb Korea* [β33 or β34 (B15 or B16) Val→0], in which a deletion completely destroys the tertiary structure).

Interesting Interactions among Mutant Hemoglobins: Hemoglobin S–, C–, S-Oman–, Korle-Bu–, Quebec-Chori–, and O-Arab–Containing Red Cells

HbC (β6 [A3] Glu→Lys), HbS, and HbE are the three most prevalent abnormal hemoglobins in humans. The unique pathogenetic feature of HbC is its capacity to induce erythrocyte dehydration. In CC disease (homozygous state for the HbC gene), this pathologic change results only in mild hemolytic anemia. In SC disease, in which equal levels of HbS and HbC coexist, HbC accentuates the deleterious properties of HbS and produces a clinically significant disorder, although milder than sickle cell anemia.[232]

ORIGINS, SELECTION, AND DISTRIBUTION OF THE HEMOGLOBIN C GENE

HbC is the product of the β^C-globin gene, generated by a $\underline{G}$ AG→$\underline{A}$ AG (Glu→Lys) substitution in codon 6 of the -globin gene. The β^C mutation occurred originally among ethnic groups in Burkina Faso (previously Upper Volta). HbC reaches its highest rate of occurrence in Central West Africa and gene occurrence decreases concentrically outward from this region. It is also found in West Africa, west of the Niger River, and exclusively in areas where HbS is also present.[232]

The HbC gene exists at polymorphic rates (>1 percent), suggesting that its presence confers selective advantage to the carrier. Modiano et al,[233] in a large case-control study performed in Burkina Faso on 4348 Mossi subjects, found that HbC is associated with a 29 percent reduction in the risk of clinical malaria in HbC heterozygotes (AC) (P = .0008) and of 93 percent in HbC homozygotes (CC) (P = .0011). These findings establish the fact that HbC is selected for in malaria caused by *Plasmodium falciparum*. Balanced polymorphism[234] explains the selective advantage of the HbS trait and is based on the advantage of the heterozygote and the disadvantage of the homogyzote. It seems not to apply to HbC, because both heterozygotes and homozygotes have some level of advantage, and, surprisingly, that of the homozygote is the strongest. These findings, together with the limited pathologic changes of the AC and CC genotypes compared with those of the severely affected SS and SC genotypes and the low β^S gene occurrence in the geographic epicenter of HbC, also support the hypothesis that, in the long term and in the absence of malaria control, HbC interferes with the lysis of parasitized red cells in the late schizont state, impairing the dispersion of merozoites.[235]

PROPERTIES OF HEMOGLOBIN C: TENDENCY TO CRYSTALLIZE AND INTERACTION WITH OTHER HEMOGLOBINS

In most instances, when concentrated solutions of purified hemoglobins are incubated in high-molarity phosphate buffer, hemoglobin crystals form.[236]

Gln-γ87 is largely responsible for the inhibitory effect of HbF and HbA$_2$ on HbC crystallization[237] as well as on that of HbF on HbS.[238] The Gln-γ87 has been recently used successfully in a vector construct for the gene therapy of transgenic mice with sickle cell disease.[239] The propensity of this site to inhibit polymerization was first detected in the study of *Hb D-Ibadan*.[240] In contrast, the mutant *Hb Quebec-Chori* (β87 [F3] Thr→Ile),[241] when found in a double heterozygote with HbS, *promotes* polymerization of HbS, most likely because isoleucine is more hydrophobic than threonine, and stabilizes this critical side-to-side contact in the polymer.

In contrast, *Hb Korle-Bu* (β73 [E17] Asp→Asn) accelerates HbC crystallization.[242] The double heterozygote for Hb Korle-Bu and HbC produces a mild microcytic hemolytic anemia and *in vitro* acceleration of crystal formation in which precrystal hemoglobin structures convert rapidly into cubic-like crystals as opposed to the typical tetragonal crystal structure found with CC and SC disease and HbC trait. *In vitro* crystallization studies led to the conclusion that β87 and β73 are contact sites of the oxy crystal.[237,238] Finally HbS also accelerates HbC crystallization.[243]

Of particular interest are the molecular interactions between Hb G-Philadelphia, HbC, and HbS, in an informative pedigree.[244] The tetramer $\alpha_2^{G\text{-Philadelphia}} \beta_2^C$ crystallizes faster than HbC; hence, position α68 is a contact site in the crystal of HbC. In addition, HbS enhances HbC crystallization (additive to the effect of $\alpha^{G\text{-Philadelphia}}$). The latter also inhibits polymerization of HbS. All of these findings help explain the phenotype of an individual simultaneously heterozygous for the β^S, β^C, and the $\alpha^{G\text{-Philadelphia}}$ genes (SC $\alpha^{G\text{-Philadelphia}}$ disease). This disease is characterized by a mild clinical course, abundant circulating intraerythrocytic crystals, and increased folded red cells. This phenotype is the result of increased crystallization and decreased polymerization brought about by the opposite effects of the gene product of the $\alpha^{G\text{-Philadelphia}}$ gene on the β^C and β^S gene products. Some of the intraerythrocytic crystals in this syndrome are unusually long and thin, resembling sugar canes, unlike those seen in SC disease. The mild clinical course associated with increased crystallization implies that, in SC disease, polymerization of HbS is pathogenically more important than the crystallization induced by β^C chains. SC α-G Philadelphia disease is an example of multiple hemoglobin chain interactions (epistatic effect among globin genes) creating a unique phenotype.

PROPERTIES OF HEMOGLOBIN C–CONTAINING ERYTHROCYTES

Erythrocytes in patients with HbC disease have microcytic and hyperchromic target cells, microspherocytes, and cells with crystalline inclusions.[232] Target cells, a diagnostically useful artifact, are presumably the consequence of the greater surface-to-volume ratio of HbC disease cells which, in turn, is the consequence of reduced water content (see later).

Red cell lifespan is shortened to approximately 40 days in HbC disease. However, this is at least three times as long as the lifespan of cells in sickle cell anemia.[245]

Scanning electron microscopic examination of cells isolated from density gradients showed intracellular HbC crystals.[246] Freeze-fracture preparations, followed by electron microscopy, also showed intracellular crystals.[247] Circulating crystals can be detected in unperturbed wet preparations from individuals with HbC disease, but they are rare. Together, these observations are consistent with early reports of an increase in intraerythrocytic crystals in patients with HbC disease after splenectomy.[248]

Why do red cells that contain HbC crystals not induce vaso-occlusion? The answer to this riddle is that crystal forms of oxy-HbC and deoxy-HbC differ. HbC crystals in the red cells of splenectomized patients with CC disease were found to be in the oxy state and melted after deoxygenation.[249] Also, when cells from venous and arterial blood were fixed and counted, there was a significant difference in the mean percentage of crystal-containing cells in the arterial circulation versus the venous circulation (1.6 ± 0.22 versus 1.1 ± 0.23 percent). Hence, the oxy-HbC crystals melt before they can do any damage to the microcirculation.

EFFECT OF HEMOGLOBIN C ON CELL DENSITY (MEAN CORPUSCULAR HEMOGLOBIN CONCENTRATION) BY MEMBRANE TRANSPORTERS

High mean corpuscular hemoglobin concentration (MCHC) and low intracellular water content are characteristics of HbC-containing cells.[232] Red cell density is directly related to the MCHC. Cells in both HbC trait and HbC disease are denser than normal.[232] Average MCHCs in CC disease, SC disease, HbC trait, and HbA cells were 38, 37, 34, and 33 g/dL, respectively. Cells in all four of these genotypes have a narrow density distribution so that the youngest and lightest cells differ from the oldest and most dense cells by only 3 to 4 g/dL. In contrast, cells in sickle cell anemia have a very wide density distribution. CC and SC disease and HbC trait reticulocytes are denser than normal reticulocytes. This implies either that these cells are denser than normal when they first enter the circulation or that their density changes within their first 24 hours in the circulation when they are still recognizable as reticulocytes.

Increased volume-regulated losses of red cell K$^+$ and water make the HbC-containing cell dehydrated and more dense than normal.[250] This single feature may be responsible for all of the abnormalities that have been detected in erythrocytes that contain high levels of this hemoglobin.

BINDING OF HEMOGLOBIN C TO CELL MEMBRANES

Like HbS, HbC interacts more strongly with the erythrocyte membrane than does HbA. This interaction has been studied by using changes in the fluorescence intensity of a membrane-embedded probe the fluorescence of which is quenched when it is approached by hemoglobin.[251–253] The cytoplasmic portion of band 3 was implicated as the binding site for both HbA and HbC. *Hb O-Arab* (has the same charge as HbC) is more strongly bound than HbS and is even more tightly membrane bound than HbC.[254] This suggests that both electrostatic charge and the protein conformation in the vicinity of the charged groups play a role in membrane binding.

All red cells from patients homozygous for Hb O-Arab were denser than normal red cells, as is observed for patients homozygous for HbC, and red cell density was strongly influenced by the presence of α-thalassemia, resulting in an average red cell density slightly greater than that of normal (Hb AA) red cells. Patients heterozygous for Hb O-Arab without α-thalassemia had denser red cells similar to those seen in patients with sickle cell disease with some cells of normal density but with most cells very dense.

Finally, double heterozygotes for HbS and Hb O-Arab had significant hemolytic anemia and red cells denser than normal with some as dense as the densest cells found in sickle cell anemia. Reticulocytes in patients homozygous for Hb O-Arab were found in the densest density fraction. Cation transport in patients homozygous for Hb O-Arab was abnormal, with K^+:Cl^- cotransport activity similar to that of Hb S-Oman and only somewhat lower than that in sickle cell anemia red cells. The activity of the Gardos channel was indistinguishable from that found in HbS, HbC, and Hb S-Oman cells. The data allow the conclusion that the erythrocytic pathogenesis of Hb O-Arab involves the dehydration of red cells due, at least in part, to the K^+:Cl^- cotransport system. The similarity of the charge and consequences of the presence of both HbC and Hb O-Arab, which are the products of mutations at opposite ends of the β chain, raises the possibility that this pathologic change is the result of a charge-dependent interaction of these hemoglobins with the red cell membrane or its cytoskeleton and that this abnormality is present early in red cell development.

In HbC, the substitution of a charged lysine residue for $β^6$ glutamic acid causes a very different pathophysiologic condition than does the hydrophobic $β^6$ valine present in HbS. While deoxy-HbS polymerizes, oxy-HbC has an increased tendency for intraerythrocytic crystallization, which, along with cell dehydration caused by the HbC-induced loss of K^+ and water, is the basis of the pathophysiology of HbC disease, particularly, the hemolytic process. Similar mechanisms contribute to the pathologic changes in Hb SC disease with the addition that here, the presence of intraerythrocytic HbC induces a reduction of volume by loss of water and K^+, increasing the tendency of HbS to polymerize.

HbC crystals are most likely to form in cells with low HbF content.[249] When the cells of individuals with CC disease are density fractionated, cells of highest density had the lowest Hb F content. In this dense cell fraction, no F cells contained HbC crystals. HbF inhibition of HbC crystallization might contribute to the potentially beneficial effects of hydroxyurea in Hb SC disease in those indi-

viduals who have an increase in Hb F in response to treatment with this drug (see later).

Vaso-occlusive episodes are not a feature of HbC disease despite the presence of intraerythrocytic HbC crystals, because, as mentioned earlier, oxy HbC crystals will melt when HbC cells approach the microcirculation in which the P_{O_2} is low.

Hb S-Oman has two mutations in the β chains. In addition to the classic $β^S$ mutation, it contains a second mutation in the same chain (β121 [GH4] Glu→Lys) as Hb O-Arab. An informative pedigree of heterozygous carriers of Hb S-Oman segregates into two types of patients; those expressing about 20 percent Hb S-Oman and concomitant –α/α α-thalassemia and those with about 14 percent of Hb S-Oman and concomitant –α/-α α-thalassemia.[25] The higher expressors of Hb S-Oman have a sickle cell anemia clinical syndrome of moderate intensity, whereas the lower expressors have no clinical syndrome. In addition, the higher expressors exhibit a unique form of irreversibly sickled cell shaped like a "yarn and knitting needle," in addition to folded and target cells. The C_{SAT} (solubility of the polymer) of Hb S-Oman is identical to that of Hb S-Antilles, another supersickling hemoglobin, whose carriers express the abnormal hemoglobin at 40 to 50 percent, with a clinical picture very similar to that of Hb S-Oman. Because the level of expression is so different and the clinical picture is so similar and on the basis of the C_{SAT} values of the hemolysates, it was concluded that Hb S-Oman produces pathologic changes beyond its sickling tendencies. A clue for the basis of this additional pathogenesis is found in those homozygous for Hb O-Arab: Hb O-Arab has the same second substitution as that found in Hb S-Oman and homozygotes have a moderately severe hemolytic anemia. When Hb O-Arab is combined with HbS, the phenotype of this double heterozygote is as severe as that of sickle cell anemia. Reticulocytes are much denser than normal (similar to those in SC and CC disease). A decrease in the K_m for Ca^{2+} needed to activate the Gardos channel (making this transporter more sensitive to Ca^{2+}) is seen. Returning to Hb S-Oman, there is increased association of Hb S-Oman with the red blood cell membrane, the presence of dense cells by isopyknic gradient, the presence of folded cells, and accelerated K^+:Cl^- cotransport in red cells expressing more than 20 percent Hb S-Oman. Hence, the pathologic effect of heterozygous Hb S-Oman is the product of the sickling properties of the Val-β6 mutation, which are enhanced by the second mutation at β121, but, in addition, further enhancement by a hemolytic anemia induced by the mutation at β121. It is likely that the additional hemolysis results from the abnormal association of the highly positively charged Hb S-Oman (three charges different from normal hemoglobin) with the red cell membrane.

PATHOPHYSIOLOGY OF THE INTERACTION BETWEEN HEMOGLOBIN S AND HEMOGLOBIN C DISEASE

The paradox here is that Hb SC disease is the product of double heterozygosity of two traits, each of which has minimal pathologic effects. Hence, why is the combination of HbS and HbC pathogenic?

Two hypotheses have been examined:

1. HbC increases the tendency of HbS to polymerize. Bookchin and associates[255] examined this issue and found no evidence of this effect.
2. The study of SC and CC cells by density gradients revealed that the presence of HbC dehydrated red cells makes them denser (having a high MCHC). Because the delay time of polymerization varies with the 32nd power of the initial Hb concentration, this explains why 50 percent of HbS can cause a sickle syndrome only moderately less severe that Hb SS disease.[250, 256]

In HbC, the substitution of a charged lysine residue for β^6 glutamic acid causes a very different pathophysiology than the hydrophobic β^6 valine present in HbS. Whereas deoxy-HbS polymerizes, oxy-HbC has an increased tendency for intraerythrocytic crystallization, which, along with cell dehydration caused by the HbC-induced loss of K^+ and water, is the basis of the pathophysiology of CC disease, particularly, the hemolytic process. Similar mechanisms contribute to the pathology of SC disease with the addition that here, the presence of intraerythrocytic HbC induces a reduction of volume by loss of water and K^+, increasing the tendency of HbS to polymerize.

HbC crystals are most likely to form in cells with low HbF content.[247] When the cells of individuals with HbC disease were density fractionated, cells with the highest density had the lowest HbF content. In this dense cell fraction, no F cells contained HbC crystals. HbF inhibition of HbC crystallization might contribute to the potentially beneficial effects of hydroxyurea in SC disease in those individuals who have an increase in HbF in response to treatment with this drug (see later).

Vaso-occlusive episodes are not a feature of CC disease despite the presence of intraerythrocytic HbC crystals, because, as mentioned earlier, oxy-HbC crystals will melt when HbC cells approach the microcirculation where the P_{O_2} is low.[247]

CELLULAR FACTORS ACCOUNTING FOR THE PATHOPHYSIOLOGY AND SEVERITY OF SC DISEASE

Crystals are observed in Wright's- and vital dye–stained smears and in wet preparations from finger-stick blood samples.[246] When α-thalassemia is present with SC disease, typical crystals are absent in some patients. Red cells of all patients with SC disease exhibit heavily stained conglomerations of hemoglobin that appear marginated with rounded edges compared with the straight-edged crystals. Such cells have been called "billiard ball" cells. Both crystals and billiard ball cells are found in the densest fraction of cells from individuals with SC disease and represent hemoglobin aggregation distinct from the polymerization of HbS.

Regardless of the α-globin gene haplotype, the blood of patients with SC disease has additional abnormally shaped cells that are strikingly apparent upon scanning electron microscopic examination. Typical are "folded cells," some of which have a single fold and resemble—to the gastronomically inclined—pita bread or a taco. These are most likely the cells what Diggs called "fat cells," because in Wright's-stained smears they appear as wide bipointed cells. Other misshapen cells are triconcave triangular cells with three dimples, very much like those seen in acute alcoholism that Bessis termed "knizocytes." One remarkable shape was the "triple-folded cells" that appeared as two pita breads stuck together. These bizarre shapes are the product of an increased surface-to-volume ratio, which provides an excess of surface for the cytosol volume. Excessive surface is resolved largely by membrane folding.

Not all cells in SC disease contain crystals. An enlarged, infarcted, and perhaps abnormally functioning spleen might fail intermittently in its pitting function, allowing hemoglobin crystals and aggregates to remain in the cell. HbS accelerates the crystallization of HbC *in vivo* as has been demonstrated *in vitro*.

CATION CONTENT

Cation content of SC disease red cells is intermediate between that of normal and that of CC disease cells.[257] Oxygenated SC disease cells exhibit a volume-stimulated potassium efflux similar to that observed in sickle cell anemia and CC disease.[258] This transporter appears to be chloride dependent, stimulated by *N*-ethylmaleimide,[259] and found in young cells of normal control subjects and individuals with sickle cell anemia and SC disease. It is inhibited by deoxygenation through cytosolic magnesium (Mg^{2+}) modulation.[260–262]

SC disease cells also exhibit a diminished change in cell volume in response to variations of the osmolarity of the suspending medium, which is likely to be due to the volume-regulated potassium efflux. Volume-regulated K^+ efflux should impact adversely the pathophysiology of disease because any increase of MCHC will aggravate HbS polymerization.

CORRECTION OF SC DISEASE

SC disease cells share the increased red cell density characteristics of all cells containing HbC. Because of the increased MCHC, the intracellular HbS concentration is raised to a level at which polymerization occurs under physiologic conditions. Reducing the MCHC in individuals with SC disease to normal levels of 33 g/dL by osmotically swelling SC cells results in normalization of many of the polymerization-dependent abnormal properties of these cells,[246] increased hemoglobin oxygen affinity (reduced in SC disease), reduction of viscosity of deoxygenated erythrocyte suspensions (increased in SC disease), a decrease in the rate of sickling (similar to that in sickle cell anemia), and reduction in the deoxygenation-induced K^+ leak (greater than that observed in sickle cell anemia). At osmolarity of 240 mOsmol/L, SC cells become biconcave disks. This is a welcome feature of the rehydration of SC disease cells, because the discoid shape is indispensable for normal deformation of red cells in the microcirculation.

This strategy is doomed to fail in patients with sickle cell anemia. Some cells are dehydrated, but the majority are normal discocytes with normal MCHC and mean cell hemoglobin. Rehydrating these cells will also decrease polymerization and produce cells that are no longer discocytes but become progressively spheroidal.

Better knowledge of the transport physiology and genetics of red cells could reveal interventions that can cure SC disease by changing the hydration status of SC cells.[256]

REFERENCES

1. Whitaker TL, Berry MB, Ho EL, et al: The D-helix in myoglobin and in the beta subunit of hemoglobin is required for the retention of heme. Biochemistry 1995; 34:8221.
2. Komiyama NH, Shih DT, Looker D, et al: Was the loss of the D helix in α-globin a functionally neutral mutation? Nature 1991; 352:349.
3. Perutz MF, Rossman MG, Cullis AF, et al: Structure of haemoglobin: A three-dimensional Fourier synthesis at 5.5 Å resolution, obtained by x-ray analysis. Nature 1960; 185:416.
4. Baldwin JM: The structure of human carbonmonoxy haemoglobin at 2.7 Å resolution. J Mol Biol 1980; 136:103.
5. Fermi G, Perutz MF, Shaanan B, et al: The crystal structure of human deoxyhaemoglobin at 1.7 Å resolution. J Mol Biol 1984; 175:159.
6. Chothia C, Wodak S, Janin J: Role of subunit interfaces in the allosteric mechanism of hemoglobin. Proc Natl Acad Sci USA 1976; 73:3793.
7. Monod J, Wyman J, Changeaux JP: On the nature of allosteric transition: A plausible model. J Mol Biol 1967; 12:88.
8. Perutz MF, Sanders JKM, Chenery DH, et al: Interactions between the quaternary structure of the globin and the spin state of the heme in ferric mixed spin derivatives of hemoglobin. Biochemistry 1978; 17:3640.
9. Perutz MF, Kilmartin JV, Nagai K, et al: Influence of globin structures on the state of the heme: Ferrous low spin derivatives. Biochemistry 1976; 15:378.
10. Baldwin J, Chothia C: Haemoglobin: The structural changes related to ligand binding and its allosteric mechanism. J Mol Biol 1979; 129:175.
11. Eaton WA, Henry ER, Hofrichter J, et al: Is cooperative oxygen binding by hemoglobin really understood? Nat Struct Biol 1999; 351–358.
12. Henry ER, Jones CM, Hofrichter J, et al: Can a two-state MWC allosteric model explain hemoglobin kinetics? Biochemistry 1997; 3:6511–6528.
13. Nagel RL, Ranney HM, Kucinskies LL: Tyrosine ionization in human CO and deoxyhemoglobin. Biochemistry 1966; 5:1934.
14. Perutz MF: Stereochemistry of the cooperative effects in haemoglobin. Nature 1970; 288:726.
15. Perutz MF, Gronenbom AM, Clore GM, et al: The pKa values of two histidine residues in human haemoglobin, the Bohr effect, and the dipole moments of α-helices. J Mol Biol 1985; 183:491.
16. Perutz MF: Molecular anatomy and physiology of hemoglobin. In Steinberg MH, Forget BG, Higgs, et al (eds): Disorders of Hemoglobin: Genetics, Pathophysiology, Clinical Management. New York, Cambridge University Press, 2000.
17. Perrella M, Kilmartin JV, Fogg J, et al: Identification of the high and low affinity CO_2 binding sites of human haemoglobin. Nature 1975; 256:759.
18. Kilmartin JV, Fogg JH, Perutz MF: Role of C-terminal histidine in the alkaline Bohr effect of human hemoglobin. Biochemistry 1980; 19:3189.
19. Nishikura K: Identification of histidine-122 in human haemoglobin as one of the unknown alkaline Bohr groups by hydrogen-tritium exchange. Biochem J 1978; 173:651.
20. Russu IM, Ho NT, Ho C: Role of the β146 histidyl residue in the alkaline Bohr effect of hemoglobin. Biochemistry 1980; 19:1043.
21. Fang TY, Zou M, Simplaceanu V, et al: Assessment of roles of surface histidyl residues in the molecular basis of the Bohr effect and of β143 histidine in the binding of 2,3-bisphosphoglycerate in human normal adult hemoglobin. Biochemistry 1999; 38:13423.
22. Benesch R, Benesch RE: The effect of organic phosphates from the human erythrocyte on the allosteric properties of hemoglobin. Biochem Biophys Res Commun 1967; 26:162.
23. Chanutin A, Curnish RR: Effect of organic and inorganic phosphates on the oxygen equilibrium of human erythrocytes. Arch Biochem Biophys 1967; 121:96.
24. Arnone A: X-ray diffraction study of binding of 2,3-diphosphoglycerate to human deoxyhaemoglobin. Nature 1972; 237:146.
25. Bonaventura J, Bonaventura C, Amiconi G, et al: Allosteric interactions in non-chains isolated from normal human hemoglobin, fetal hemoglobin, and hemoglobin Abruzzo [β^{143} (H21) His→Arg]. J Biol Chem 1975; 250:6278.
26. Rose ZB: The enzymology of 2,3-bisphosphoglycerate. Adv Enzymol 1980; 51:211.
27. Card R, Brain M: The "anemia" of childhood. N Engl J Med 1973; 288:388.
28. Purcell Y, Brozovic B: Red cell 2,3-diphosphoglycerate concentration in man decreases with age. Nature 1974; 251:511.
29. Ignarro LJ: A novel signal transduction mechanism for transcellular communication. Hypertension 1990. 16:477–483.
30. Head CA, Brugnara C, Martinez-Ruiz R, et al: Low concentrations of nitric oxide increase oxygen affinity of sickle erythrocytes in vitro and in vivo. J Clin Invest 1997; 100:1193–1198.
31. Gladwin MT, Schechter AN, Shelhamer JH, et al: Inhaled nitric oxide transport on sickle cell hemoglobin without affecting oxygen affinity. J Clin Invest 1999; 104:937–945.
32. Gow AJ, Stamler JS: Reactions between nitric oxide and haemoglobin under physiological conditions. Nature 1998, 391:169–173.
33. Patel RP, Hogg N, Spencer NY, et al: Biochemical characterization of human S-nitrosohemoglobin. Effects on oxygen binding and transnitrosation. J Biol Chem 1999; 274:15487–15492.
34. Yonetani T: Nitric oxide and hemoglobin. Nippon Yakurigaku Zasshi 1998; 112:155–160.
35. Holzmann A: Nitric oxide and sepsis. Respir Care Clin N Am 1997; 3:537–550.
36. Pabloski JR, Hess DT, Stamler JS: Export by red blood cells of nitric oxide bioactivity. Nature 2001; 409:622–626.
37. Korber E: Inaugural dissertation: Uber differenzen Blutfarbstoffes: Dorpat, 1866. In: Bischoff H. Z Exp Med 1926; 48:472.
38. Schroeder WA, Shelton JR, Shelton JB, et al: The amino acid sequence of the α-chain of human fetal hemoglobin. Biochemistry 1963; 2:992.
39. Schroeder WA, Huisman THJ, Efremov GD, et al: Further studies on the frequency and significance of the ^{T}α-chain of human fetal hemoglobin. J Clin Invest 1979; 63:268.
40. Slightom JL, Blechl AE, Smithies O: Human fetal ^{G}γ- and ^{A}γ-globin genes: Complete nucleotide sequences suggest that DNA can be exchanged between these duplicated genes. Cell 1980; 21:627.
41. Bouhassira EE, Lachman H, Krishnamoorthy R, et al: A gene conversion located 5′ to the ^{A}γ gene is in linkage disequilibrium with the Bantu haplotype in sickle cell anemia. J Clin Invest 1989; 83:2070.
42. Frier JA, Perutz M: Structure of human foetal deoxyhemoglobin. J Mol Biol 1977; 112:97.
43. Allen DW, Wyman J, Smith CA: The oxygen equilibrium of foetal and adult human hemoglobin. J Biol Chem 1953; 203:81.
44. Tyuma I, Shamizu K: Different response to organic phosphates of human fetal and adult hemoglobins. Arch Biochem Biophys 1969; 129:404.
45. Schroeder WA, Cua JT, Matsuda G, et al: Hemoglobin F$_1$, an acetyl-containing hemoglobin. Biochem Biophys Acta 1962; 63:532.
46. Poyart C, Burseaux E, Guesnon P, et al:. Chloride binding and Bohr effect of human fetal erythrocytes and HbF$_{II}$ solutions. Pfluegers Arch 1978; 37:169.
47. Gros G, Bauer C: High pK value of the N-terminal amino group of the γ chains causes low CO_2 binding of human fetal hemoglobin. Biochem Biophys Res Commun 1978; 80:56.
48. Burseaux E, Poyart C, Guesnon P, et al: Comparative effects of CO_2 on the affinity for O_2 of fetal and adult hemoglobins. Pfluegers Arch 1979; 378:197.
49. Charache S, Catalano P, Bums S, et al: Pregnancy in carriers of high-affinity hemoglobins. Blood 1985; 65:713.
50. Kleihauer E, Braun H, Betke K: Demonstration von fetalem Hamoglobin in den Erythrozyten eines Blutausstrichs. Klin Wochenschr 1957; 35:637.
51. Miyoshi K, Kaneto Y, Kawai H, et al: X-linked dominant control of F-cells in normal adult life: Characterization of the Swiss type as hereditary persistence of fetal hemoglobin regulated dominantly by gene(s) on X chromosome. Blood 1988; 72:1854.

52. Pembrey ME, Weatherall DJ, Clegg JB: Maternal synthesis of haemoglobin F in pregnancy. Lancet 1973; 16:1351.

53. Huehns ER, Hecht F, Keil JV, et al: Developmental hemoglobin anomalies in a chromosomal triplication: D_1 trisomy syndrome. Proc Natl Acad Sci USA 1964; 51:89.

54. Wood WG, Stamatoyannopoulos G, Lim G, et al: F-cells in the adult: Normal values and levels in individuals with hereditary and acquired elevations of Hb F. Blood 1975; 46:671.

55. Boyer SH, Belding TK, Margolet L, et al: Variations in the frequency of fetal hemoglobin-bearing erythrocytes (F-cells) in well adults, pregnant women, and adult leukemics. Johns Hopkins Med J 1975; 137:105.

56. Chang YC, Smith KD, Moore RD, et al: An analysis of fetal hemoglobin variation in sickle cell disease: The relative contributions of the X-linked factor, β-globin haplotypes, β-globin gene number, gender, and age. Blood 1995; 85:1111–1117.

57. Thein SL, Sampietro M, Rohde K, et al: Detection of a major gene for heterocellular hereditary persistence of fetal hemoglobin after accounting for genetic modifiers. Am J Hum Genet 1994; 54:214–228.

58. Thein SL, Craig JE: Genetics of Hb F/F cell variance in adults and heterocellular hereditary persistence of fetal hemoglobin. Hemoglobin 1998; 22:401–414.

59. Craig JE, Rochette J, Sampietro M, et al: Genetic heterogeneity in heterocellular hereditary persistence of fetal hemoglobin. Blood 1997; 90:428–434.

60. Garner C, Tatu T, Reittie J, et al: Twins en route to QTL mapping for heterocellular HPFH. Blood 1998; 92:694a.

61. Zon LI, Tsai SF, Burgess S, et al: The major human erythroid DNA-binding protein (GF-1): Primary sequence and localization of the gene to the X chromosome. Proc Natl Acad Sci USA 1990; 87:668–672.

62. Dover GJ, Boyer SH, Bell WR: Microscopic method for assaying F cell production: Illustrative changes during infancy and in aplastic anemia. Blood 1978; 52:664.

63. Dover GJ, Boyer SH, Pembrey ME: F cell production in sickle cell anemia: Regulation by genes linked to β-hemoglobin locus. Science 1981; 211:1441.

64. Dover GJ, Boyer SH, Charache S, et al: Individual variation in the production and survival of F-cells in sickle cell disease. N Engl J Med 1978; 299:1428.

65. Winters WP, Seale WR, Yodh J: Interaction of hemoglobin S with anionic polysaccharides. Am J Pediatr Hematol Oncol 1984; 6:77.

66. Newman DR, Pierre RV, Linman JW: Studies on the diagnostic significance of hemoglobin F levels. Mayo Clin Proc 1973; 48:199.

67. Lee-Potter JP, Deacon-Smith RA, Simpkiss MJ, et al: A new cause of haemolytic anemia in the newborn: A description of an unstable fetal haemoglobin—F Poole $\alpha_2{}^G\gamma_2$ 130 tryptophan→glycine. J Clin Pathol 1975; 28:317.

68. Hayashi A, Fujita T, Fujimura M, et al: A new fetal hemoglobin, HbF M Osaka ($\alpha_2\gamma_2$ 63 His→Leu): A mutant with high oxygen affinity and erythrocytosis. Am J Clin Pathol 1979; 72:1028.

69. Harano T, Harano K, Doi K, et al: HbF-Onoda or $\alpha_2\gamma_2{}^G$146(HC3) His→Tyr, a newly discovered fetal hemoglobin variant in a Japanese newborn. Hemoglobin 1990; 14:217.

70. Priest JR, Watterson J, Jones RT, et al: Mutant fetal hemoglobin causing cyanosis in a newborn. Pediatrics 1989; 83:734.

71. Glader BE: Hemoglobin FM-Fort Ripley: Another lesson from the neonate. Pediatrics 1989; 83:792.

72. Huisman THJ: The human fetal hemoglobins. Texas Rep Biol Med 1980–1981; 40:29–42.

73. Fischer S, Nagel RL, Bookchin RM, et al: The binding of hemoglobin to membranes of normal and sickle erythrocytes. Biochim Biophys Acta 1975; 375:422.

74. Codrington JF, Kutlar F, Harris HF, et al: Hb A_2-Wrens or $\alpha_2\gamma_2{}^G$ 98(FG5) Val→Met, an unstable chain variant identified by sequence analysis of amplified DNA. Biochim Biophys Acta 1989; 1009:87.

75. Garcia CR, Navarro JL, Lam H, et al: Hb A_2-Manzanares or $\alpha_2\gamma_2{}^G$ 121(GH4) Glu→Val, an unstable chain variant observed in a Spanish family. Hemoglobin 1983; 7:435.

76. Salkie ML, Gordon PA, Rigal WM, et al: Hb A_2-Canada or $\alpha_2\gamma_2{}^G$ 99(G1) Asp→Asn: A newly discovered chain variant with increased oxygen affinity occurring in *cis* to β-thalassemia. Hemoglobin 1982; 6:223.

77. Baglioni C: The fusion of two peptide chains in hemoglobin Lepore and its interpretation as a genetic deletion. Proc Natl Acad Sci USA 1962; 48:1880–1886.

78. Flavell RA, Kooter JM, De Boer E, et al: Analysis of the β-δ-globin gene loci in normal and Hb Lepore DNA: Direct determination of gene linkage and intergene distance. Cell 1987; 15:25–41.

79. Mears JG, Ramirez F, Leibowitz D, et al: Organization of human δ- and β-globin genes in cellular DNA and the presence of intragenic inserts. Cell 1978; 15:15–23.

80. Huehns ER, Dance N, Beaven GH, et al: Human embryonic hemoglobins. Cold Spring Harbor Symp Quant Biol 1964; 19:327–331.

81. Luo HY, Liang XL, Frye C, et al: Embryonic hemoglobins are expressed in definitive cells. Blood 1999; 94:359–361.

82. Stamatoyannopoulos G, Constantoulakis P, Brice M, et al: Coexpression of embryonic, fetal, and adult globins in erythroid cells of human embryos: Relevance to the cell-lineage models of globin switching. Dev Biol 1987; 123:191–197.

83. Leder A, Kuo A, Shen MM, et al: In situ hybridization reveals co-expression of embryonic and adult α globin genes in the earliest murine erythrocyte progenitors. Development 1992; 116:1041–1049.

84. Hoffmann OM, Brittain T, Wells RM: The control of oxygen affinity in the three human embryonic haemoglobins by respiration linked metabolites. Biochem Mol Biol Int 1997; 42:553–566.

85. Hoffmann OM, Brittain T: Ligand binding kinetics and dissociation of the human embryonic haemoglobins. Biochem J 1996; 315:65–70.

86. Perutz M, Fermi G, Poyart C, et al: A novel allosteric mechanism in haemoglobin. Structure of bovine deoxy-haemoglobin, absence of specific chloride-binding sites and origin of the chloride-linked Bohr effect in bovine and human haemoglobin. J Mol Biol 1993; 233:536–545.

87. Hoffman O, Currucan G, Robson N, et al: The chloride effect in the human embryonic haemoglobins. Biochem J 1995; 309:959–962.

88. Sutherland-Smith AJ, Baker HM, Hoffmann OM, et al: Crystal structure of human embryonic haemoglobin: The carbonmonoxide for Gower II ($\alpha_2\epsilon_2$) haemoglobin at 2.9 Å resolution. J Mol Biol 1998; 280:475–484.

89. He Z, Russell JE: Expression, purification, and characterization of human hemoglobins Gower-1 ($\zeta_2\epsilon_2$), Gower-2 ($\alpha_2\epsilon_2$), and Portland-2 ($\zeta_2\beta_2$) assembled in complex transgenic-knockout mice. Blood 2001; 97:1099–1105.

90. Ireland JH, Luo HY, Chui DH, et al: Detection of the (–SEA) double α-globin gene deletion by a simple immunologic assay for embryonic ζ-globin chains. Am J Hematol 1993; 44:22–28.

91. Charache S, Weatherall DJ, Clegg JB: Polycythemia associated with a hemoglobinopathy. J Clin Invest 1966; 45:813.

92. Clegg JB, Naughton MA, Weatherall DJ: Abnormal human haemoglobins: Separation and characterization of the α and β chains by chromatography, and the determination of two new variants, Hb Chesapeake and Hb J (Bangkok). J Mol Biol 1966; 19:91.

93. Nagel RL, Gibson QH, Charache S: Relation between structure and function in hemoglobin Chesapeake. Biochemistry 1967; 6:2395.

94. Shimasaki S: A new hemoglobin variant, hemoglobin Nunobiki [α 141 (HC3) Arg→Cys]: Notable influence of the carboxy-terminal cysteine upon various physico-chemical characteristics of hemoglobin. J Clin Invest 1985; 75:695.

95. Lacombe C, Craescu CT, Blouquit Y, et al: Structural and functional studies of hemoglobin Poissy $\alpha_2\beta_2$ 56 (D7) Gly→Arg and 86 (F2) Ala→Pro. Eur J Biochem 1985; 153:655.

96. Imai K: Oxygen-equilibrium characteristics of abnormal hemoglobin Hiroshima ($\alpha_2\beta_2$ 143 Asp). Arch Biochem Biophys 1968; 127:543.

97. Nagel RL, Gibson OH, Hamilton HB: Ligand kinetics in hemoglobin Hiroshima. J Clin Invest 1971; 50:1772.

98. Wajcman H, Kilmartin JV, Najman A, et al: Hemoglobin Cochin-Port-Royal: Consequences of the replacement of the β chain C-terminal by an arginine. Biochim Biophys Acta 1975 400:354.

99. Russu IM, Ho C: Assessment of role of β 146-histidyl and other histidyl residues in the Bohr effect of human normal adult hemoglobin. Biochemistry 1986; 25:1706.

100. Nute PE, Stamatoyannopoulos G, Hermodson MA, et al: Hemoglobinopathic erythrocytosis due to a new electrophoreti-

cally silent variant, hemoglobin San Diego (β 109 [Gil] Val→Met). J Clin Invest 1974; 53:320.

101. Maniatis A, Bousios T, Nagel RL, et al: Hemoglobin Crete (β 129 Ala→Pro): A new high-affinity variant interacting with β°- and delta β°-thalassemia. Blood 1979; 54:54.

102. Elder GE, Lappin TR, Horne AB, et al: Hemoglobin Old Dominion/Burton-upon-Trent, β 143 (H21) His→Tyr, codon 143 CAC→TAC—A variant with altered oxygen affinity that compromises measurement of glycated hemoglobin in diabetes mellitus: Structure, function, and DNA sequence. Mayo Clin Proc 1998;73:321–328.

103. Tondo CV, Bonaventura J, Bonaventura C, et al: Functional properties of hemoglobin Porto Alegre ($\alpha_2\beta_2$ 9 Ser→Cys) and the reactivity of its extra cysteinyl residue. Biochim Biophys Acta 1974; 342:15.

104. Bonaventura J, Riggs A: Polymerization of hemoglobins of mouse and man: Structural basis. Science 1967; 158:800.

105. Flatz G, Kinderlerer JL, Kilmartin JV, et al: Haemoglobin Tak: A variant with additional residues at the end of the β-chains. Lancet 1971; 10:732.

106. Imai K, Lehmann H: The oxygen affinity of haemoglobin Tak, a variant with elongated β-chain. Biochim Biophys Acta 1975; 412:288.

107. Vasseur C, Blouquit Y, Kister J, et al: Hemoglobin Thionville. An α-chain variant with a substitution of a glutamate for valine at NA-1 and having an acetylated methionine NH_2 terminus. J Biol Chem 1992; 267:12682–12691.

108. Kamel K, el-Najjar A, Webber BB, et al: Hb Doha or $\alpha_2\beta_2$[X-N-Met-1(NA1)Val→Glu]; a new β-chain abnormal hemoglobin observed in a Qatari female. Biochim Biophys Acta 1985; 831:257–260.

109. Boissel JP, Kasper TJ, Shah SC, et al: Amino-terminal processing of proteins: Hemoglobin South Florida, a variant with retention of initiator methionine and N α-acetylation. Proc Natl Acad Sci USA 1985; 82:8448–8452.

110. Prchal JT, Cashman DP, Kan YW: Hemoglobin Long Island is caused by a single mutation (adenine to cytosine) resulting in a failure to cleave amino-terminal methionine. Proc Natl Acad Sci USA 1986; 83:24–27.

111. White JM, Szur L, Gillies IDS, et al: Familial polycythaemia caused by a new haemoglobin variant: Hb Heathrow, β103 (G5) phenylalanine → leucine. Br Med J 1973; 3:665.

112. Rosa R, Prehu MO, Beuzard Y, Rosa J: The first case of a complete deficiency of diphosphoglycerate mutase in human erythrocytes. J Clin Invest 1978; 62:907.

113. Kales SN: Carbon monoxide intoxication. Am Fam Physician 1993; 48:1100.

114. Adamson JW: Familial polycythemia. Semin Hematol 1975; 12:383.

115. Sergeeva A, Gordeuk VR, Tokarev YN, et al: Congenital polycythemia in Chuvashia. Blood 1997; 89:2148–2154.

116. Vasserman NN, Karzakova LM, Tverskaya SM, et al: Localization of the gene responsible for familial benign polycythemia to chromosome 11q23. Hum Hered 1999 49:129–132.

117. Grace RJ, Gover PA, Treacher DF, et al: Venesection in haemoglobin Yakima, a high oxygen affinity haemoglobin. Clin Lab Haematol 1992; 14:1995.

118. Adamson JW, Finch CA: Erythropoietin and the polycythemias. Ann NY Acad Sci 1968; 149:560.

119. Adamson JW, Hayashi A, Stamatoyannopoulos G, et al: Erythrocyte function and marrow regulation in hemoglobin Bethesda (β 145 histidine). J Clin Invest 1972; 51:2883.

120. Adamson JW, Finch CA: Hemoglobin function, oxygen affinity and erythropoietin. Annu Rev Physiol 1975; 37:351.

121. Charache S, Achuff S, Winslow R, et al: Variability of the homeostatic response to altered p50. Blood 1978; 52:1156.

122. Butler WM, Spratling L, Kark JA, et al: Hemoglobin Osier: Report of a new family with exercise studies before and after phlebotomy. Am J Hematol 1982; 13:293.

123. Blouquit Y, Bardakdjian J, Lena-Russo D, et al: Hb Bruxelles: $\alpha_2\beta_2$ 41 or 42(C7 or CD1) Phe deleted. Hemoglobin 1989; 13:465.

124. Griffon N, Badens C, Lena-Russo D, et al: Hb Bruxelles, deletion of Phe β42, shows a low oxygen affinity and low cooperativity of ligand binding. J Biol Chem 1996; 271:25916.

125. Nagel RL, Lynfield J, Johnson J, et al: Hemoglobin Beth Israel: A mutant causing clinically apparent cyanosis. N Engl J Med 1976; 295:125.

126. Bonaventura C, Cashon R, Bonaventura J, et al: Involvement of the distal histidine in the low affinity exhibited by Hb Chico (Lys$^{\beta66}$→Thr) and its isolated β chains. J Biol Chem 1991; 266:23033–23040.

127. Marinucci M, Giuliani A, Maffi D, et al: Hemoglobin Bologna ($\alpha_2\beta_2$ 61(E5) Lys→Met), an abnormal human hemoglobin with low oxygen affinity. Biochim Biophys Acta 1981; 668:209.

128. Olson JS, Mathews AJ, Rohlfs RJ, et al: The role of the distal histidine in myoglobin and hemoglobin. Nature 1988; 336:265–266.

129. Imamura T, Fujita S, Ohta Y, et al: Hemoglobin Yoshizuka (G10 (108) β asparagine→aspartic acid): A new variant with a reduced oxygen affinity from a Japanese family. J Clin Invest 1969; 48:2341.

130. Moo-Penn WF, Wolff JA, Simon G, et al: Hemoglobin Presbyterian: βl08 (G10) asparagine→lysine—A hemoglobin variant with low oxygen affinity. FEBS Lett 1978; 92:53.

131. Horlein H, Weber G: Uber chronisch familiare Methamoglobinanue und eine neue Modifikation des Methamoglobins. Dtsch Med Wochenschr 1948; 73:476.

132. Gerald DS, Efron ML: Chemical studies of several varieties of Hb M. Proc Natl Acad Sci USA 1961; 47:1758.

133. Shibata S, Tanuira A, Iuchi I: Hemoglobin M_1 demonstration of a new abnormal hemoglobin in hereditary nigremia. Acta Haematol Jpn 1960; 23:96.

134. Greer J: Three dimension studies of abnormal human hemoglobins M Hyde Park and M Iwate. J Mol Biol 1971; 59:107.

135. Ranney HM, Nagel RL, Heller P, et al: Oxygen equilibrium of hemoglobin M-Hyde Park. Biochim Biophys Acta 1968; 160:112–115.

136. Brennan SO, Matthews JR: Hb Auckland [β87(F8) His→Asn]: A new mutation of the proximal histidine identified by electrospray mass spectrometry. Hemoglobin 1997. 21: 393–403.

137. Feher G, Isaacson RA, Scholes CP: Endor studies on normal and abnormal hemoglobins. Ann NY Acad Sci 1973; 222:86.

138. Peisach J, Gersonde K: Binding of CO to mutant chains of HbM Iwate: Evidence for distal imidazole ligation. Biochemistry 1977; 16:2539.

139. LaMar GR, Nagai K, Jue T, et al: Assignment of proximal histidyl imidazole exchangeable proton NMR resonances to individual subunits in HbA, Boston, Iwate and Milwaukee. Biochem Biophys Res Commun 1980; 96:1177.

140. Pulsinelli PD, Perutz MF, Nagel RL: Structure of hemoglobin M Boston, a variant with a five-coordinated ferric heme. Proc Natl Acad Sci USA 1973; 70:3870.

141. Perutz MF, Pulsinelli PD, Ranney HM: Structure and subunit interaction of haemoglobin M Milwaukee. Nature 1972; 237:259.

142. Lindstrom TR, Ho C, Pisciotta AV: Nuclear magnetic resonance studies of haemoglobin M Milwaukee. Nature 1972; 237:263.

143. Thillet J, Cohen-Solal M, Seligmann M, et al: Functional and physiochemical studies of hemoglobin St. Louis β 28 (B10) Leu→Gln. J Clin Invest 1976; 58:1098.

144. Wajcman H, Krishnamoorthy R, Gacon G, et al: A new hemoglobin variant involving the distal histidine: Hb Bicetre (β63 (E7) His→Pro). J Mol Med 1976; 1:187.

145. Rosa J, Labie D, Wajcman H, et al: Haemoglobin I Toulouse: β66 (E10) Lys→Glu: A new abnormal haemoglobin with a mutation localized on the E10 porphyrin surrounding zones. Nature 1969; 223:190.

146. Kurachi S, Hermodson M, Hornung S, et al: Structure of haemoglobin Seattle. Nature 1973; 243:275.

147. Shibata S, Mijaji T, Iuchi I: Methemoglobin M's of the Japanese. Bull Yamaguchi Med Sch 1967; 14:141.

148. Shibata S: Hemoglobinopathies in Japan. Hemoglobin 5:509, 1981.

149. Hayashi A, Suzuki T, Shimizu A, et al: Properties of hemoglobin M: Unequivalent nature of the α and β subunits in the hemoglobin molecule. Biochim Biophys Acta 1968; 168:262.

150. Ranney HM, Nagel RL, Heller P, et al: Oxygen equilibrium of hemoglobin M (Hyde Park). Biochim Biophys Acta 1968; 160:112.

151. Suzuki T, Hayashi A, Shimizu A, et al: The oxygen equilibrium of hemoglobin M Saskatoon. Biochim Biophys Acta 1966; 127:280.

152. Suzuki T, Hayashi A, Yamamura Y, et al: Functional abnormality of hemoglobin M. Biochem Biophys Res Commun 1965; 19:691.

153. Udem L, Ranney HM, Bunn HF, et al:. Some observations on the properties of hemoglobin M$_{Milwaukee}$. J Mol Biol 1970; 48:489.

154. Hayashi A, Suzuki T, Imai K, et al: Properties of hemoglobin M Milwaukee I variant and its unique characteristics. Biochem Biophys Acta 1969; 194:6.

155. Nagel RL, Bookchin RM: Human hemoglobin mutants with abnormal oxygen binding. Semin Hematol 1974; 11:385.

156. Moo-Penn WF, Bechtel KC, Schmidt RM, et al: Hemoglobin Raleigh (β1 valine→acetylamine). Biochemistry 1977; 16:4872.

157. Park CM, Nagel RL: Sulfhemoglobin: Clinical and molecular aspects. N Engl J Med 1984; 310:1579.

158. Park CM, Nagel RL, Blumberg WE, et al: Sulfhemoglobin: Properties of partially sulfurated tetramers. J Biol Chem 1986; 261:8805.

159. Beutler E: Hemoglobinopathies producing cyanosis. In: Williams J, Beutler E, Erslev AJ, et al (eds): Hematology. New York, McGraw-Hill, 1983.

160. Finch CA: Methemoglobinemia and sulfhemoglobinemia. N Engl J Med 1948; 239:470.

161. Pinkas J, Pjaldetti M, Joshua H, et al: Sulfhemoglobinemia and acute hemolytic anemia with Heinz bodies following contact with a fungicide-zinc ethylene bisthiocarbamate: In a subject with glucose-6-phosphate dehydrogenase deficiency and hypocatalassemia. Blood 1963; 21:484.

162. Bunn HF, Forget BG: Hemoglobin: Molecular, Genetic and Clinical Aspects. Philadelphia, WB Saunders, 1986.

163. Greenberg HB: Syncope and shock due to methemoglobinemia. Arch Environ Health 1964; 9:762.

164. Darling RC, Roughton FJW: The effect of methemoglobin on the equilibrium between oxygen and hemoglobin. Am J Physiol 1942; 137:56.

165. Cathie AB: Apparent idiopathic Heinz body anemia. Great Ormond St J 1952; 3:3.

166. Asakura T, Adachi K, Shapiro M, et al: Mechanical precipitation of hemoglobin Koln. Biochim Biophys Acta 1975; 412:197.

167. Roth EF Jr, Elbaum D, Bookchin RM, et al: The conformational requirements for the mechanical precipitation of hemoglobin S and other mutants. Blood 1976; 48:265.

168. Virshup DM, Zinkham WH, Sirota RL, et al: Unique sensitivity of Hb Zurich to oxidative injury by phenazopyridine: Reversal of the effects by elevating carboxyhemoglobin in vivo and in vitro. Am J Hematol 1983; 14:315.

169. Moo-Penn WF, Jue DL, Johnson MH, et al: Hemoglobin Brockton [β 138 (H16) Ala→Pro]: An unstable variant near the C-terminus of the β-subunits with normal oxygen-binding properties. Biochemistry 1988; 27:7614.

170. Wajcman H, Dahmane M, Prehu C, et al: Haemoglobin J-Biskra: A new mildly unstable α₁ gene variant with a deletion of eight residues (α50–57, α51–58 or α52–59) including the distal histidine. Br J Haematol 1998; 100.

171. Reider RF, Oski FA, Clegg JB: Hemoglobin Philly (β35 tyrosine→phenylalanine): Studies in the molecular pathology of hemoglobin. J Clin Invest 1969; 48:1627.

172. King MAR, Wiltshire BG, Lehmann H, et al: An unstable haemoglobin with reduced oxygen affinity: Haemoglobin Peterborough, β111 (G13) valine→phenylalanine, its interaction with normal haemoglobin and with haemoglobin Lepore. Br J Haematol 1972; 22:125.

173. Como PF, Wylie BR, Trent RJ, et al: A new unstable and low oxygen affinity hemoglobin variant: Hb Stanmore [β111(G13) Val→Ala]. Hemoglobin 1991; 15:53.

174. Martinez G, Lima F, Colombo B: Haemoglobin J Guantanamo (α₂β₂ 128 (H6) Ala→Asp). A new fast unstable haemoglobin found in a Cuban family. Biochim Biophys Acta 1977; 491:1.

175. Clegg JB, Weatherall DJ, Boon WH, et al:. Two new haemoglobin variants involving proline substitutions. Nature 1969; 22:379.

176. Brennan SO, Matthews JR: Hb Auckland [α 87(F8) His→Asn]: A new mutation of the proximal histidine identified by electrospray mass spectrometry. Hemoglobin 1997; 21:393–403.

177. Ohba Y: Unstable hemoglobins. Hemoglobin 1990; 14:353.

178. Ohba Y, Miyaji T, Matsouka M, et al: Hemoglobin Hirosaki [α43(CE1) Phe→Leu]: A new unstable variant. Biochim Biophys Acta 1975; 405:155.

179. Goossens M, Lee KY, Liebhaber SA, Kan YW: Globin structural mutant α125 Leu→Pro is a novel cause of α-thalassemia. Nature 1982; 296:864.

180. Argos P, Rossman MG, Grau UM, et al: Thermal stability and protein structure. Biochemistry 1979; 18:5698.

181. Rachmilewitz EA, Peisach J, Blumberg WE: Studies on the stability of oxyhemoglobin A and its constituent chains and their derivatives. J Biol Chem 1971; 246:3356.

182. Ohba Y, Yamamoto K, Hattori Y, et al: Hyperunstable hemoglobin Toyama α₂136 (H19) Leu→Arg β₂: Detection and identification by in vitro biosynthesis with radioactive amino acids. Hemoglobin 1987; 11:539.

183. Tatsis B, Dosik H, Rieder R, et al: Hemoblogin Hasharon: Severe hemolytic anemia and hypersplenism associated with a mildly unstable hemoglobin. Birth Defects 1972; 8:25.

184. Levine RL, Lincoln DR, Buchholz WM, et al: Hemoglobin Hasharon in a premature infant with hemolytic anemia. Pediatr Res 1975; 9:7.

185. Schmid R, Brecher G, Clemens T: Familial hemolytic anemia with erythrocyte inclusion bodies and a defect in pigment metabolism. Blood 1959; 14:991.

186. Eisinger J, Flores J, Tyson JA, et al: Fluorescent cytoplasm and Heinz bodies of Koln erythrocytes: Evidence for intracellular heme catabolism. Blood 1985; 65:886.

187. Koler RD, Jones RT, Bigley RH, et al: Hemoglobin Casper: β106 (G8) Leu→Pro, a contemporary mutation. Am J Med 1973; 55:549.

188. Nagel RL, Ranney HM: Drug-induced oxidative denaturation of hemoglobin. Semin Hematol 1973; 10:269.

187. Grimes AJ, Meisler A: Possible cause of Heinz bodies in congenital Heinz body anaemia. Nature 1962; 194:190.

188. Grimes AJ, Meisler A, Dacie JV: Congenital Heinz-body anaemia: Further evidence on the cause of Heinz-body production in red cells. Br Haematol 1964; 10:281.

189. Carrell RW, Kay R: A simple method for the detection of unstable hemoglobins. Br J Haematol 1972; 23:615.

190. Ohba Y, Hattori Y, Yoshinaka H, et al: Urea polyacrylamide gel electrophoresis of PCMB precipitate as a sensitive test for the detection of the unstable hemoglobin subunit Clin Chim Acta 1982; 119:179.

191. Asakura T, Adachi K, Shapiro M, et al: Mechanical precipitation of hemoglobin Koln. Biochim Biophys Acta 1975; 412:197.

192. Roth EF Jr, Elbaum D, Bookchin RM, Nagel RL: The conformational requirements for the mechanical precipitation of hemoglobin S and other mutants. Blood 1976; 48:265.

193. Perutz MF: Electrostatic effects in proteins. Science 1978; 201:1187.

194. Bigelow C: On the average hydrophobicity of proteins and the relation between it and protein structure. J Theor Biol 1967; 16:187.

195. Kauzmann W: Some factors in the interpretation of protein denaturation. Adv Protein Chem 1959; 14:1.

196. Argos P, Rossman MG, Grau UM, et al: Thermal stability and protein structure. Biochem 1979; 18:5698.

197. Perutz MF, Raidt H: Stereochemical bases of heat stability in bacterial ferredoxins and in hemoglobin A₂. Nature 1975; 255:256.

198. Bunn FH, Jandl JH: Exchange of heme among hemoglobins and between hemoglobin and albumin. J Biol Chem 1968; 243:465.

199. Jacob HS, Winterhalter KH: The role of hemoglobin heme loss in Heinz body formation: Studies with a partially heme-deficient hemoglobin and with genetically unstable hemoglobin. J Clin Invest 1970; 49:2008.

200. Jacob HS, Winterhalter KH: Unstable hemoglobins: The role of heme loss in Heinz body formation. Proc Natl Acad Sci USA 1970; 65:697.

201. Rachmilewitz EA, Peisach J, Blumberg WE. Studies on the stability of oxyhemoglobin A and its constituent chains and their derivatives. J Biol Chem 1971; 246:3356.

202. Rachmilewitz EA, Harari E: Intermediate hemichrome formation after oxidation of three unstable hemoglobins (Freiburg, Riverdale-Bronx and Koln). Haematol Bluttransfus 1972; 10:241.

203. Rachmilewitz EA, White JM: Haemichrome formation during the in vitro oxidation of haemoglobin Koln. Nature 1973; 241:115.

204. Rachmilewitz EA: Denaturation of the normal and abnormal hemoglobin molecule. Semin Hematol 1974; 11:441.

205. Peisach J, Blumberg WE, Rachmilewitz EA: The demonstration of ferrihemochrome intermediates in Heinz body formation following the reduction of oxyhemoglobin A by acetylphenylhydrazine. Biochem Biophys Acta 1975; 393:404.

206. Winterbourne CC, Carrell RW: Studies of hemoglobin denaturation and Heinz body formation in the unstable hemoglobins. J Clin Invest 1974; 54:678.

207. Winterbourne CC, McGrath BM, Carrell RW: Reactions involving superoxide and normal and unstable haemoglobins. Biochem J 1976; 155:503.

208. Rifkind RA: Heinz body anemia: An ultrastructural study. II: Red cell sequestration and destruction. Blood 1965; 26:433.

209. Schnitzer B, Rucknagel DL, Spencer HH, et al: Erythrocytes: Pits and vacuoles as seen with transmission and scanning electron microscopy. Science 1971; 173:251.

210. Winterbourne CC, Carrell RW: Characterization of Heinz bodies in unstable haemoglobin haemolytic anaemia. Nature 1972; 240:150.

211. Chan E, Desforges J: Role of disulfide bonds in Heinz body attachment to membranes. Blood 1974; 44:921.

212. Low P: Interaction of native and denatured hemoglobins with Band 3: Consequences for erythrocyte structure and function. In Agre P, Parker JC (eds): Red Blood Cell Membranes. New York, Marcel Dekker, 1989.

213. Low PS, Westfall MA, Allen DP, et al: Characterization of the reversible conformational equilibrium of the cytoplasmic domain of erythrocyte membrane band 3. J Biol Chem 1984; 259:13070.

214. Waugh SM, Low PS: Hemichrome binding to band 3: Nucleation of Heinz bodies on the erythrocyte membrane. Biochemistry 1985; 24:34.

215. Cho N, Song S, Asher SA: UV resonance Raman and excited-state relaxation rate studies of hemoglobin. Biochemistry 1994; 33:5932.

216. Fisher S, Nagel RL, Bookchin RM, et al: The binding of hemoglobin to membranes of normal and sickle erythrocytes. Biochim Biophys Acta 1975; 375:422.

217. Shaklai N, Sharma VS, Ranney HM: Interaction of sickle cell hemoglobin with erythrocyte membrane. Proc Natl Acad Sci USA 1981; 78:65.

218. Reiss GH, Ranney HM, Shaklai N: Association of Hb C with erythrocyte ghosts. J Clin Invest 1982; 70:946.

219. Walder JA, Chatterjee R, Steck T, et al: The interaction of hemoglobin with the cytoplasmic domain of band 3 of the human erythrocyte membrane. J Biol Chem 1984; 259:10238.

220. Jandl JH, Simmons RL, Castle WB: Red cell filtration and the pathogenesis of certain hemolytic anemias. Blood 1961; 18:133.

221. Miller DR, Weed RI, Stamatoyannopoulos G, et al: Hemoglobin Koln disease occurring as a fresh mutation: Erythrocyte metabolism and survival. Blood 1971; 38:715.

222. Chou AC, Fitch CD: Mechanism of hemolysis induced by ferriprotoporphyrin IX. J Clin Invest 1981; 68:672.

223. Allen DW, Burgoyne CF, Groat JD, et al: Comparison of hemoglobin Koln erythrocyte membranes with malondialdehyde-reacted normal erythrocyte membranes. Blood 1984; 64:1263.

224. Flynn TP, Allen DW, Johnson GJ, White JG: Oxidant damage of the lipids and proteins of the erythrocyte membranes in unstable hemoglobin disease: Evidence for the role of lipid peroxidation. J Clin Invest 1983; 71:1215.

225. Jacob HS, Brain MK, Dacie JV: Altered sulfhydryl reactivity of hemoglobins and red blood cell membranes in congenital Heinz body hemolytic anemia. J Clin Invest 1968; 47:2664.

226. DeFuria FG, Miller DR: Oxygen affinity in hemoglobin Koln disease. Blood 1972; 39:398.

227. Adams JG III, Boxer LA, Baehner RL, et al: Hemoglobin Indianapolis (β112 [G14] →arginine): An unstable β-chain variant producing the phenotype of severe β-thalassemia. J Clin Invest 1979; 63:931.

228. Adams JG, Steinberg MH, Boxer LA, et al: The structure of hemoglobin Indianapolis (β112 [G14] arginine): An unstable variant detectable only by isotopic labeling. J Biol Chem 1979; 254:3479.

229. Thein SL: Dominant β thalassaemia: Molecular basis and pathophysiology. Br J. Haematol 1992 80:273–277.

230. Kazazian HH Jr, Dowling CE, Hurwitz RL, et al: Dominant thalassemia-like phenotypes associated with mutations in exon 3 of the β-globin gene. Blood 1992; 79:3014–3018.

231. Traeger-Synodinos J, Papassotiriou I, Metaxotou-Mavrommati A, et al: Distinct phenotypic expression associated with a new hyperunstable α globin variant (Hb Heraklion, $\alpha_1$cd37(C2)Pro>0): Comparison to other α-thalassemic hemoglobinopathies. Blood Cells Mol Dis 2000; 26:276.

232. Nagel RL, Steinberg MH: HbSC and HbC disease. In Steinberg MH, Forget BG, Higgs DR, et al (eds): Disorders of Hemoglobin:

233. Modiano D, Luoni G, Sirima BS, et al: Haemoglobin C protects against clinical *Plasmodium falciparum* malaria. Nature 2001; 414:305–308.

234. Haldane JBS: The rate of mutation of human genes. Hereditas 1949; 35(Suppl):267–273.

235. Olson JA, Nagel RL: Synchronized cultures of *P. falciparum* in abnormal red cells: The mechanism of the inhibition of growth in HbCC cells. Blood 1987; 67:997–1000.

236. Adachi K, Asakura T: Kinetics of the polymerization of hemoglobin in high and low phosphate buffers. Blood Cells 1982; 8:213–224.

237. Adachi K, Asakura T: The solubility of sickle and non-sickle hemoglobins in concentrated phosphate buffer. J Biol Chem 1979; 254:4079–4084.

238. Hirsch RE, Lin MJ, Nagel RL: The inhibition of hemoglobin C crystallization by hemoglobin F. J Biol Chem 1988; 263:5936–5939.

239. Pawliuk R, Westerman KA, Fabry ME, et al: Correction of sickle cell disease in transgenic mouse models by gene therapy. Science 2001; 294:2368–2371.

240. Nagel RL, Bookchin RM, Johnson J, et al: The structural bases of the inhibitory effects of Hb F and Hb A_2 on the polymerization of Hb S. Proc Natl Acad Sci USA 1979; 76:670–672.

241. Witkowska, HE, Lubin BH, Beuzard Y, et al: Sickle cell disease in a patient with sickle cell trait compound heterozygosity for hemoglobin S and Hb Quebec-Chori. N Engl J Med 1991; 325: 1150.

242. Nagel RL, Lin MJ, Witkowska HE, et al: Compound heterozygosity for hemoglobin C and Korle-Bu: Moderate microcytic hemolytic anemia and acceleration of crystal formation [corrected]. Blood 1993; 82:1907–1912.

243. Lin MJ, Nagel RL, Hirsch RE: Acceleration of hemoglobin C crystallization by hemoglobin S. Blood 1989; 74:1823–1825.

244. Lawrence C, Hirsch RE, Fataliev NA, et al: Molecular interactions between Hb α-G Philadelphia, HbC, and HbS: Phenotypic implications for SC α-G Philadelphia disease. Blood 1997; 90:2819–2825.

245. Prindle KH Jr, McCurdy PR: Red cell lifespan in hemoglobin C disorders (with special reference to hemoglobin C trait). Blood 1970; 36:14–19.

246. Lawrence C, Fabry ME, Nagel RL: The unique red cell heterogeneity of SC disease: Crystal formation, dense reticulocytes, and unusual morphology. Blood 1991; 78:2104–2112.

247. Hirsch RE, Raventos-Suarez C, Olson JA, et al: Ligand state of intraerythrocytic circulating HbC crystals in hompzygote CC patients. Blood 1985; 66:775–777.

248. Nagel RL: Genetically Abnormal Red Cells. Boca Raton, FL, CRC Press, Vol 1, 1988.

249. Hirsch RE, Raventos-Suarez C, Olson JA, Nagel RL: Ligand state of intraerythrocytic circulating HbC crystals in homozygote CC patients. Blood 1985; 6:775–7.

250. Fabry ME, Kaul DK, Raventos C, et al: Some aspects of the pathophysiology of homozygous Hb CC erythrocytes. J Clin Invest 1981; 67:1284–1291.

251. Reiss GH, Ranney HM, Shaklai N: Association of HbC with erythocyte ghosts. J. Clin Invest 1982; 70:946–952.

252. Ballas SK, Embi K, Goshar D, et al: Binding of β S, β C and β O Arab globins to the erythrocyte membrane. Hemoglobin 1981; 5:501–505.

253. Nagel RL, Krishnamoorthy R, Fattoum S, et al: The erythrocyte effects of haemoglobin O(ARAB). Br J. Haematol 1999; 107:516–521.

254. Nagel RL, Daar S, Romero JR, et al: HbS-Oman heterozygote: A new dominant sickle syndrome. Blood 1998; 92:4375–4382.

255. Bookchin RM, Balazs T: Ionic strength dependence of the polymer solubilities of deoxyhemoglobin S + C and S + A mixtures. Blood 1986; 67:887–892.

256. Nagel RL, Lawrence C: The distinct pathobiology of sickle cell-hemoglobin C disease. Therapeutic implications [review]. Hematol Oncol Clin North Am 1991; 5:433–551.

257. Brugnara C, Kopin AS, Bunn HF, et al: Regulation of cation content and cell volume in hemoglobin erythrocytes from patients with homozygous hemoglobin C disease. J Clin Invest 1985; 75:1608–1617.

258. Brugnara C, Kopin AS, Bunn HF, et al: Electrolyte composition and equilibrium in hemoglobin CC red blood cells. Trans Assoc Am Physicians 1984; 97:104–112.

Genetics, Pathophysiology, Clinical Management. New York, Cambridge University Press, 2000.

259. Canessa M, Spalvins A, Nagel RL: Volume-dependent and NEM-stimulated K+,Cl⁻ transport is elevated in oxygenated SS, SC and CC human red cells. FEBS Lett 1986; 200:197–202.

260. Canessa M, Fabry ME, Blumenfeld N, Nagel RL: Volume-stimulated, Cl⁻dependent K⁺ efflux is highly expressed in young human red cells containing normal hemoglobin or HbS. J Membr Biol 1987; 97:97–105.

261. Canessa M, Fabry ME, Spalvins A, et al: Activation of a K:Cl cotransporter by cell swelling in HbAA and HbSS red cells. Prog Clin Biol Res 1987; 240:201–115.

262. Canessa M, Fabry ME, Nagel FL: Deoxygenation inhibit the volume-stimulated,Cl⁻ dependent K⁺ efflux in SS and young AA cells: A cytosolic Mg^{2+} modulation. Blood 1987; 70:1861.

19 | Sickle Cell Disease

George J. Dover • Orah S. Platt

HISTORY

Sickle cell anemia was first described in a West Indian student by Herrick in 1910.[1] Sydenstricker and associates[2] described the first occurrences in children, recognized the association with a hemolytic anemia, and introduced the term *crisis* to describe periodic acute episodes of pain. The pathologic basis of the disorder and its relationship to the hemoglobin molecule were defined in 1927 by Hahn and Gillespie.[3] Shortly after the application of moving-boundary electrophoresis to the separation of sickle from normal hemoglobin by Pauling and co-workers,[4] Neel[5] defined the genetics of the disorder and clearly distinguished sickle trait—the heterozygous condition (AS)—from sickle cell anemia—the homozygous state (SS). Further understanding of the molecular basis of the disorder was made possible by the finding that normal human hemoglobin is composed of two pairs of globin subunits: one pair that is invariant, the α chain; and another pair that is variable, the ε, ζ, γ, β, or δ chain. The relative ease with which sickle hemoglobin (HbS) could be isolated by chromatography or zone electrophoresis techniques led to Ingram's application of tryptic digestion, high-voltage electrophoresis, and paper chromatography to the isolated HbS, with the result that the amino acid substitution in HbS is now known to be a valine instead of a glutamic acid in position 6 of the β chain. The α chain is normal.[6] The chemical nomenclature for HbS is therefore $\alpha_2\beta_2 6Glu\zeta Val$. (See Fig. 19–1 for an overview of the pathophysiology of the β^S mutation.) Excellent reviews of the history of sickle cell anemia are available.[7]

ORIGINS OF MUTATION

The sickle gene is a common mutant that provides some protection to infants who might otherwise succumb to cerebral falciparum malaria, and its incidence parallels the incidence of malaria. The incidence of the sickle gene in a population parallels the historical incidence of malaria. Whereas the average incidence of the sickle gene among American blacks is approximately 8 percent,[8] the incidence is much higher in inhabitants of certain areas of Africa. Polymorphic sites around globin DNA and their

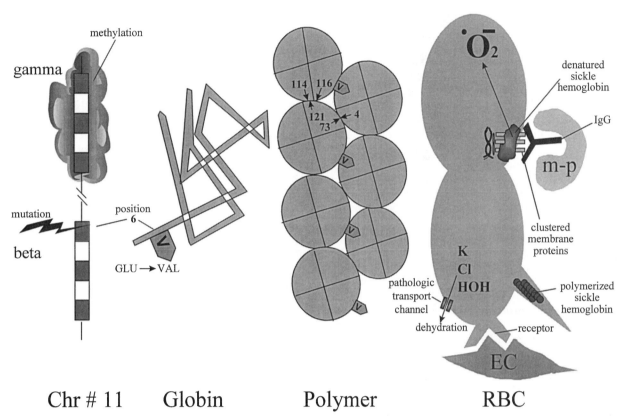

Chr # 11   Globin   Polymer   RBC

FIGURE 19–1. The pathophysiology of sickle cell disease chromosome 11 contains the genes for β and γ globin. Beyond fetal life, the γ gene is highly methylated and barely expressed. The $β^S$ gene contains an A→T mutation in the sixth codon, which results in an abnormal globin with valine instead of glutamic acid in the sixth position. That hydrophobic valine is exposed when the globin assumes the deoxy confirmation and tends to burrow within a hydrophobic pocket in neighboring β chains, forming a polymer. As indicated, other key residues at positions 4, 73, 114, 166, and 121 play roles in stabilizing the polymer. When this process takes place in red blood cells they become distorted and viscous and resist flow. The inherent unstable nature of sickle cell hemoglobin causes it to denature and produce oxidants. A variety of membrane abnormalities appear in the process. The red cells have a short survival, are young, and express receptors that promote adhesion to endothelial cells Membrane proteins (ankyrin and protein 3) cluster around deposits of denatured hemoglobin, promoting the deposition of immunoglobulin G (IgG), making the cells attractive targets (m-p). Pathologic transport channels (Gardos and K^+,Cl^- cotransport) are activated, leading to cation and water loss and cell dehydration. Chr #11 = chromosome 11; RBC = red blood cell; EC = endothelial cell; HOH = H_2O. (Adapted from Platt OS: Sickle cell paths converge on hydroxyurea. Nat Med 1995; 1:307.)

linkages to the $β^S$ gene indicate that this mutation may have developed independently and spontaneously at least five times.[9–12] However, analysis of nuclear and mitochondrial DNA from African populations suggests that a single mutation may have occurred 50,000 years ago.[13] In Africa, there are four major sickle haplotypes, each associated with a particular geographic region: "Senegal" (Atlantic West Africa), "Benin" (Central West Africa), "Bantu" (also called "CAR" for Central African Republic), and Cameroon.[11, 14] The Benin type is found not only in Benin but also in Ibadan,[15] Algeria,[11] Sicily,[16] Turkey,[17] Greece, Yemen, and southwest Saudi Arabia.[17] In Caribbean and North American patients of African heritage with sickle cell disease, 50 to 70 percent of chromosomes are Benin, 15 to 30 percent are Bantu-CAR, and 5 to 15 percent are Senegal.[18, 19] In Africa, virtually all patients in a region are homozygous for a given haplotype. Nagel and co-workers[20, 21] document the different hematologic characteristics of the different homozygote groups. The Benin and Senegalese patients have higher levels of fetal hemoglobin (HbF) and fewer dense cells compared with Bantu-CAR patients. The Senegalese patients have a high proportion of

$^Gγ$ HbF. In contrast to what is found among Africans in Africa, American Blacks are mainly heterozygotes. In Los Angeles, 38 percent of patients are Benin homozygotes (Benin/Benin), 25 percent are Benin/Bantu-CAR, 13 percent are Benin/Senegal, 5 percent are Bantu-CAR, and 3 percent are Bantu-CAR/Senegal.[18] Less common $β^S$ linked haplotypes are usually recombinations of the common haplotypes occurring 5′ to the β-globin gene.[22, 23] When patients identified in hospital-based clinics are studied, these haplotypes may be associated with overall clinical severity—the Bantu-CAR being the most severe and the Senegalese being the least severe.[24]

A different haplotype is found in India and parts of Saudi Arabia.[15] In the Eastern oases of Saudi Arabia, the African haplotypes are not seen, but a unique "Arabian-Indian" haplotype is found. This haplotype is also seen in patients from Orissa and Poona, India. Patients from these regions have long been recognized to have mild disease and elevated levels of HbF.[25–29] In contrast, in Riyadh, Saudi Arabia, all patients with sickle cell anemia are from Southwest Saudi Arabia and Yemen and are homozygous Benin.

MALARIA AND GLUCOSE-6-PHOSPHATE DEHYDROGENASE DEFICIENCY

The physiologic basis for the influence of malaria on the sickle gene (so-called "balanced polymorphism") is not well understood.[30] It has been suggested that HbS may be poorly metabolized by the parasite,[31] that infected cells are more easily sickled and removed from the circulation,[32, 33] that the intracellular potassium lost during sickling results in a hostile environment for the parasite,[34] and that increased membrane rigidity inhibits parasite invasion.[35] The recent discovery that transgenic mice expressing HbS are partially protected from malaria[36, 37] will permit a fuller exploration of the basis of the protective effect.

Glucose-6-phosphate dehydrogenase (G6PD) deficiency is another genetic variant common in black populations. Originally, because of the unexpectedly high incidence of G6PD deficiency among patients with sickle cell disease, it was concluded that G6PD deficiency conferred a protective effect on patients with sickle cell disease.[38, 39] Subsequent studies reveal no increased incidence of G6PD deficiency in the population with sickle cell disease.[40, 41] In a survey of 801 males with SS disease, G6PD deficiency did not cause more hemolysis or an increased number of anemic episodes.[41] Because the SS red cell is young, it is difficult to demonstrate the usual A⁻ variety of G6PD deficiency by conventional methods. Episodes of accelerated hemolysis of G6PD-deficient SS red cells have been described.[42] Because of the large population of very young G6PD-rich cells, this accelerated hemolysis is likely to be due to the enzyme abnormality only when the population is shifted toward the oldest cells, that is, during an aplastic episode.

MOLECULAR SICKLING

The Hemoglobin S Polymer

In 1927, Hahn and Gillespie[3] showed that sickling, the change from a biconcave disk to the sickle form, depended on deoxygenation. Harris[43] subsequently demonstrated that cellular sickling was associated with the formation of "tactoids" of HbS, which appeared as the hemoglobin became deoxygenated. Electron micrographs of sickled red cells[44–48] reveal long, thin bundles of HbS fibers that run parallel to the long axis of the cell or the abnormal protuberances. Details of the ultrastructure of these HbS fibers has been determined by electron microscopy and image reconstruction. These studies reveal a complex solid-core structure 21 nm in diameter, composed of 14 filaments arranged as 7 pairs of double filaments[49, 50]—an inner pair with 6 peripheral pairs.[51] Each filament pair is half-staggered along the fiber axis and has an inherent polarity. A model with three pairs of one polarity and four pairs of the other polarity is suggested by electron microscope evidence[52] and is compatible with x-ray diffraction analysis of HbS crystals.[53–55] The radii of the HbS fibers are polymorphic and are related to the helical pitch of the double filaments.[56]

Understanding of the fiber structure at the level of specific amino acid residues required additional evidence, obtained with optical dichroism,[57] x-ray diffraction,[58] and studies of mutant hemoglobins.[59–64] The detailed crystal structure suggested by Wishner and Love and colleagues[58, 65] shows several critical intermolecular contact sites: Asp-β73 and Glu-β121 (Fig. 19–1). In an elegant synthesis of several lines of evidence, Edelstein[66] proposed a topographic map of the HbS fiber, which describes three classes of intermolecular contacts: along the axis of a filament, lateral between filaments of a pair, and lateral between filaments (Fig. 19–2).

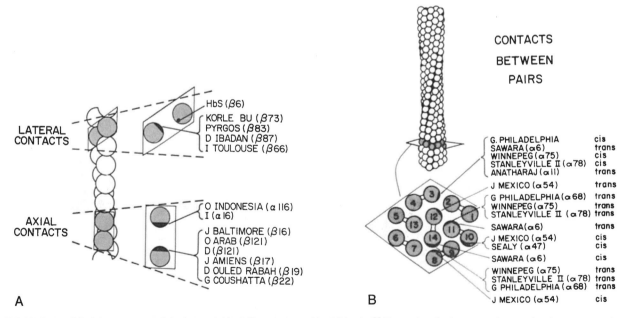

FIGURE 19–2. Model of the structure of the hemoglobin S fiber suggested by Edelstein,[66] illustrating the important intermolecular contact points and the associated hemoglobin variants. The notations *cis* and *trans* follow the convention where α_2 = *cis* and α_1 = *trans*, with the β6 valine involved in fiber formation in the β_2 subunit. (With thanks to Dr. Edelstein for his review.)

With resolution of the crystalline structure of HbS to 2.0 Å, this model has been confirmed.[67] The axial contacts are made through both α and β chains and include the following residues in which mutants affect fiber formation: β121 (O-Arab), β16 (J-Baltimore), β17 (J-Amiens), β19 (D-Ouled Rabah), β22 (G-Coushatta), α16 (I), and α116 (O-Indonesia). The lateral contacts between filaments of a pair are largely between β chains and include the primary sickle mutation—β6. For each hemoglobin tetramer, one chain contributes the β6 mutation whereas the other contributes a critical receptor region around the Phe-β85 residue. In this critical receptor region lie residues in which mutants affect fiber formation: β73 (Korle-Bu), β66 (I-Toulouse), β83 (Pyrgos), and β87 (D-Ibadan). The 2.0 Å model indicates that within the acceptor pocket the mutant valine closely contacts four different hydrophobic residues (β70, β73, β84, and β85) and in addition to the hydrophobic interaction, water molecules are present near the mutant valine, which form hydrophilic interactions in the lateral contact region.[67] The contacts between filament pairs are largely through α chains. α-Chain mutations that occur at sites critical for interpair associations influence fiber formation and include the following: J-Mexico (α54), Sealy (α47), Winnipeg (α75), Stanleyville-II (α78), Sawara (α6), Anantharaj (α11), and G-Philadelphia (α68).

Polymer Formation

The polymerization of deoxy-HbS is a highly complex process that results in the formation of gelled, aggregated HbS tetramers in equilibrium with hemoglobin tetramers in solution. Perturbations in oxygen levels,[68, 69] temperature,[70–72] pH,[73, 74] ionic strength,[75] 2,3-diphosphoglycerate (2,3-DPG),[74, 76] and carbon monoxide[77–79] affect the formation of HbS gels. This sol-gel transition of HbS is the basic feature that leads to the viscosity changes, distortion of cell morphology, sludging, and organ infarction that are identified as the clinical manifestations of sickle cell disease. The kinetics of HbS polymerization and the factors that modify this process have been studied with different techniques—light scattering and turbidimetry,[80, 81] sedimentation,[82, 83] optical birefringence,[57, 77, 84, 85] calorimetry,[57, 70] and nuclear magnetic resonance.[86–88] Although data obtained with the various techniques differ somewhat, a representative kinetic model was proposed by Hofrichter and colleagues[70, 77] and was expanded by Ferrone and associates[89] (Fig. 19–3).

The kinetics of HbS polymerization can be explained by a double nucleation mechanism. Gelation is initiated by a process called *homogeneous nucleation* in which single deoxy-HbS molecules aggregate. An aggregation of a few molecules is thermodynamically unstable, but once a certain number of molecules aggregate, termed the *critical*

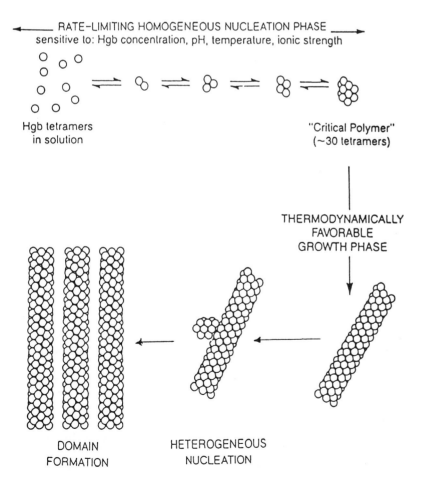

RATE–LIMITING HOMOGENEOUS NUCLEATION PHASE
sensitive to: Hgb concentration, pH, temperature, ionic strength

Hgb tetramers in solution

"Critical Polymer" (~30 tetramers)

THERMODYNAMICALLY FAVORABLE GROWTH PHASE

DOMAIN FORMATION

HETEROGENEOUS NUCLEATION

FIGURE 19–3. Model for the polymerization and alignment of deoxyhemoglobin S. Hgb = hemoglobin. (Adapted from Hofrichter J, Ross PD, Eaton WA: Supersaturation in sickle cell hemoglobin solutions. Proc Natl Acad Sci USA 1976; 73:3035–3039; and Ferrone FA, Hofrichter J, Eaton WA: Kinetics of sickle hemoglobin polymerization. II: A double nucleation mechanism. J Mol Biol 1985; 183:611–631.)

nucleus, addition of further molecules produces a more stable aggregate or polymer. Thus, homogeneous nucleation depends greatly on the concentration of deoxy-HbS molecules. The second nucleation phase, termed *heterogeneous nucleation,* takes place on the surface of a preexisting polymer. Recent data suggest that the same intermolecular contacts between the mutant valine and its receptor on the surface of the polymer are responsible for heterogeneous nucleation and cross-linking between strands.[90] As polymerization progresses, more surface area becomes available and therefore the reaction becomes autocatalytic. The result of this double nucleation mechanism is a measurable delay time between the initiation of polymerization and the exponential rise in polymer formation. The delay time varies as the 30th power of the hemoglobin concentration:

$$1/t_d = K\,(C/C_s)^n,$$

where t_d is delay time, C is hemoglobin concentration, C_s is hemoglobin solubility, and n is approximately equal to 30 (the number of hemoglobin tetramers in the "critical polymer"). Because n is so large, small changes in hemoglobin concentration have a profound effect on the delay time. For example, decreasing the mean corpuscular hemoglobin concentration (MCHC) from 32 to 30 g/dL will increase the delay time threefold.[91] Gelation is also exquisitely sensitive to changes in temperature and pH. A change from 38.5 to 37°C or an increase in intracellular pH of 0.03 unit would also double the delay time.

The phenomenon of delayed gelling of HbS in solution is also seen in cells containing HbS. Rampling and Sirs[92] studied cellular deformation after immediate deoxygenation and found a delay time of 30 seconds. Hahn and colleagues[93] observed changes in rheology and morphology of cells with partial deoxygenation and also demonstrated a delay time. Zarkowsky and Hochmuth[94] studied cell sickling at partial pressure of oxygen (O_2) (PO_2) of 0 and demonstrated a delay time that is sensitive to cell density, pH, osmolarity, and temperature. Coletta and coworkers[95] examined polymerization in single intact cells and demonstrated that polymerization kinetics of HbS in these cells was the same as the kinetics of HbS in solution. Furthermore, the distribution of observed delay times was consistent with the distribution of MCHC in cells from patients with sickle cell anemia. The double nucleation hypothesis provides for the formation of a network of polymers termed a *domain* that is nonuniformly distributed within the cell. Rapid deoxygenation leads to the formation of multiple small domains of polymer and little morphologic deformation of the cell. On the other hand, slow deoxygenation causes large, aligned polymers, which results in significant distortion of cell morphology.[96, 97]

A kinetic model of HbS gelation that incorporates the concept of a critical delay time led Eaton and his co-workers[98, 99] to propose that polymerization kinetics play an important role in the pathophysiology of SS disease. The oxygenation and deoxygenation of cells in the circulation take place in a time frame that is of the same order of magnitude as that of the sickling and unsickling of HbS *in vitro.* Cells exposed to the high PO_2 of the lungs are quickly "degelled," because HbS gels melt in less than 0.5 second when exposed to oxygen. The cells are then maintained in the unsickled state while they are in the oxygenated environment of the arterial circulation. As the cells enter the capillary circulation, the oxygen saturation decreases rapidly, as does the hemoglobin solubility. The red cell spends an average of 1 second in the capillary circulation, although this time is highly variable. If the delay time is less than 1 second, the cell will sickle and occlude the capillary. If the delay time is prolonged, sickling will not take place in the capillary and obstruction will not occur. If the transit time through the capillary is shortened and is less than the delay time, occlusion will not occur. This is presumably the situation in the myocardium, in which sickling and infarction do not occur, despite the high oxygen extraction, because the transit time is extremely short. Factors such as low pH, high hemoglobin concentration, and high ionic strength, which shorten the delay time *in vitro,* also affect *in vivo* sickling. Patients who become hypoxic, acidotic, dehydrated, and febrile are likely to experience vaso-occlusive episodes. The hypertonic renal medulla and the acidotic, high hematocrit environment of the spleen make these organs prime targets for sickling.

An alternative model relating HbS polymerization to the pathophysiology of SS disease was proposed by Noguchi and associates.[100] Using nuclear magnetic resonance techniques, they measured the quantity of HbS polymer in AS and SS red cells under various conditions related to MCHC and oxygenation.[101, 102] They found polymer formation and impaired erythrocyte deformability at oxygen saturations greater than the level at which cells appear to morphologically sickle.[103] They proposed that the amount of HbS polymer present at equilibrium in patients with SS trait is the major factor determining clinical severity.[104, 105]

Recent observations have not confirmed the relationship of mean HbS polymer fraction and clinical severity.[106] Important variables that affect the HbS polymer fraction (HbF, 2–3-DPG levels, oxygen saturation, and pH) are heterogeneously distributed within subsets of red cells, and these factors along with other factors (membrane abnormalities and red cell–endothelial cell interactions) are likely to play a role in the variable clinical severity of sickle cell disease. Indeed, the observation that increases in the level of HbF alone did not predict the decrease in painful crises seen in a controlled trial of hydroxyurea in adult patients with SS disease underlines the importance of multiple factors directly and indirectly related to HbS polymer formation in determining clinical severity and therapeutic responses in these patients.[107]

Interactions of Hemoglobin S with Hemoglobin A and Hemoglobin F

The study of the interaction of HbS with other hemoglobins supports a rational basis for the understanding of the clinical manifestations of the various sickle syndromes. Investigators have extensively studied mixtures of HbS and HbF or HbA to determine the effects on gelation[108–113] and solubility.[73, 114–116] In these studies, the nonideal behavior of concentrated hemoglobin solutions[71, 117] was considered—the bulky hemoglobin molecules take up much of the solution volume, making the *effective* concentration of the hemoglobin higher than the *measured* concentration. The kinetic data show that HbA

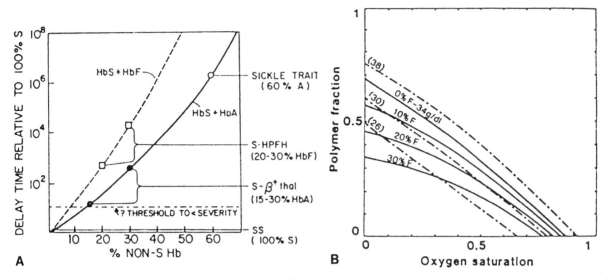

FIGURE 19–4. *A,* Effect of increasing concentrations of hemoglobin (Hb) F and HbA on delay time of polymerization of HbS. *B,* HbS polymer formation as a function of oxygen saturation for different levels of HbF and for different concentrations of pure HbS at concentrations of 26, 30, and 38 g/dL. S-HPFH = hemoglobin S and hereditary persistence of HbF; thal = thalassemia. (*A,* Based on the work of Sunshine HR, Hofrichter J, Eaton WA: Requirement for therapeutic inhibition of sickle haemoglobin gelation. Nature 1978; 275:238–240. *B,* Based on Noguchi CT, Torchia DA, Schechter AN: Intracellular polymerization of sickle hemoglobin. Effects of cell heterogeneity. J Clin Invest 1983; 72:846–852.)

and HbF have a profound, dose-related effect, increasing the delay time and decreasing HbS polymer content in cells (Fig. 19–4). The effect of HbF is considerably larger than the effect of HbA. Sunshine and colleagues[108] and Behe and Englander[110] demonstrated that, compared with pure HbS solutions (as seen in sickle cell anemia), mixtures with 15 to 30 percent HbA (as found in S-β^+-thalassemia) have delay times that are 10 to 10^2 longer, mixtures with 20 to 30 percent HbF (as found in HbS with hereditary persistence of HbF) have delay times that are 10^3 to 10^4 longer, and mixtures with 60 percent HbA (as found in sickle trait) have delay times that are 10^6 longer. HbA and HbF also increase the solubility of HbS, with HbF being more effective than HbA. Studies of the composition of the gels and supernatant of these mixtures demonstrate that asymmetric hybrids of HbS and HbA ($\alpha_2\beta^A\beta^S$) are readily incorporated into the gel. In mixtures of HbF and HbS in which the HbF concentration is less than 40 percent, very little, if any, HbF is incorporated into polymer, suggesting that asymmetric hybrids of HbS and HbF ($\alpha_2\beta^S\gamma$) and HbF ($\alpha_2\gamma_2$) are not incorporated into polymer under most physiologic conditions.[73, 109, 111, 115, 118] Compared with HbF, HbA has a lesser effect on HbS solubility because the asymmetric hybrids readily copolymerize with HbS.[118]

It is now possible to increase the level of HbF in patients with sickle cell anemia and therefore presumably to increase delay times and decrease polymer content within cells. Therefore, it will soon be possible to test the relationship between delay times or polymer content on the clinical severity of sickle cell anemia.

The effect of HbF on HbS polymer formation may have direct and indirect effects on other red cell characteristics. For example, it has been shown that the level of HbF as measured by the percentage of F cells does affect the red cell adhesive properties in patients with sickle cell disease.[119]

CELLULAR SICKLING

The oxygen-dependent gelation of HbS described in the previous section has profound effects on the morphology and rheology of the HbS-containing cell. The time course of cellular events associated with oxygenation and deoxygenation has been investigated by Hahn and colleagues,[93] who studied cells from patients with SS disease under physiologic time and oxygen conditions. They described two categories of cells—a fraction of dense cells (MCHC of 36 g/dL) that exhibited reversible polymerization and shape change (reversibly sickled cells [RSCs]) and a fraction of very dense cells (MCHC of 44 g/dL) that exhibited reversible polymerization but irreversible shape change (irreversibly sickled cells [ISCs]). Changes in the rheologic properties of the cells paralleled the appearance of polymers in the cytoplasm that occurred a considerable time before any detectable distortion of cell shape.

The RSCs have normal shape and normal viscosity when oxygenated. The vaso-occlusive complications of sickle cell disease may be due to the "Trojan horse performance" of these RSCs, which are able to slip into the microvasculature because of their normal rheologic properties when oxygenated and then become distorted and viscous as they become deoxygenated in the vessel.

The ISCs are the obvious, slender, elongated cells that are visible on an oxygenated peripheral blood smear in sickle cell disease (Fig. 19–5). In 1968, Dobler and Bertles[46] found unpolymerized hemoglobin in an oxygenated ISC: Numerous investigators have studied this bizarre cell, the membrane of which is frozen in its sickled form. In the studies of Hahn and colleagues,[93] ISCs underwent hemoglobin polymerization and depolymerization on deoxygenation and reoxygenation. Compared with the RSC fraction, however, the polymerization took place sooner, was much more highly aligned, and took longer to disappear on deoxygenation.

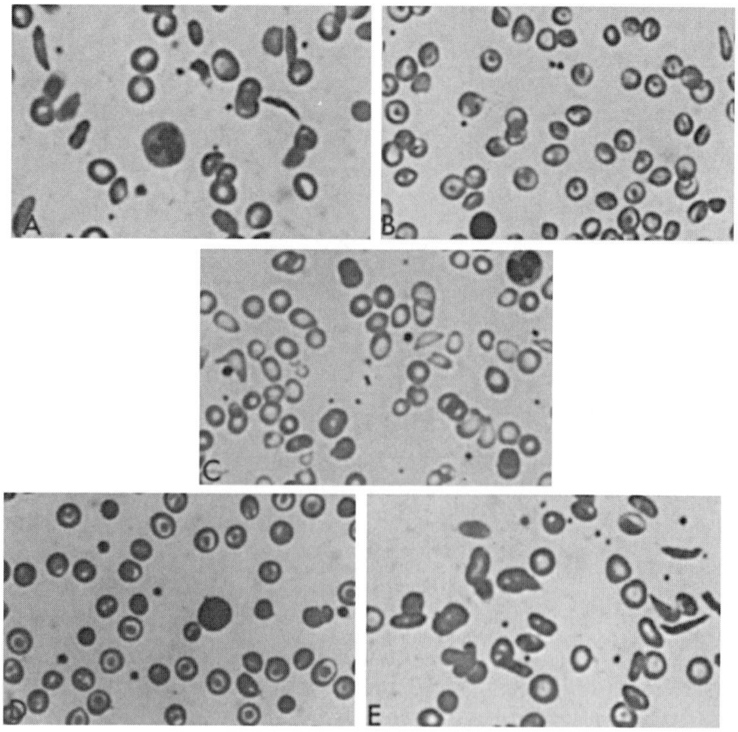

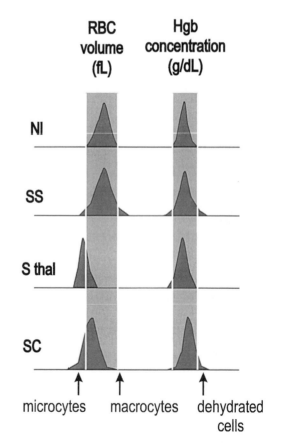

FIGURE 19–5. Oxygenated peripheral blood smears from individuals with sickle cell anemia *(A)*, hemoglobin SC disease *(B)*, sickle-β⁰ thalassemia *(C)*, homozygous hemoglobin C *(D)*, and hemoglobin SD disease *(E)*.

It is clear from electron microscopic observations and the data relating hemoglobin concentration to polymerization in solution[70] and in cells[95, 103] that the distribution of MCHC in the circulation should have profound clinical implications. A density profile of sickle red cells can be easily determined.[120] Individuals with sickle cell disease have more light cells (reticulocytes) and more dense cells (MCHC >37 mg/dL) than normal individuals. Because of the rigid abnormal shape of dense cells, the MCHC, as estimated electronically, is not accurate.[121] Laser light-scattering techniques accurately quantitate the red cell density profile but also tend to underestimate the hemoglobin concentration of very dense sickle cells.[122] The vaso-occlusive nature of these dense cells was reported by Kaul and colleagues,[123] who showed that cells separated by density (and therefore MCHC) from patients with sickle cell anemia obstruct flow in an artificially perfused capillary system in proportion to their MCHC. Although early reports suggested that the percentage of dense cells decreased during vaso-occlusive crises,[124] there is no correlation between the percentage of dense cells and the incidence or onset of crises.[125] In patients with sickle cell disease with α-thalassemia, there is less sickling-induced potassium loss, a more uniform distribution of red cell densities, and a decreased percentage of dense cells.[126, 127] Paradoxically, individuals with HbSC have milder clinical disease but more dense cells than individuals with homozygous sickle cell anemia (Fig. 19–6).[128]

The heterogeneity of red cell shape and density in sickle cell anemia may be due partially to the heterogeneous distribution of HbF. In normal individuals and individuals with sickle cell disease HbF is confined to a subset of red cells called *F cells*.[129] Because HbF interferes with HbS polymerization, F cells survive longer in the circulation than cells with no HbF,[130] and the relative proportions of F

FIGURE 19–6. Typical distribution patterns of cell volume and hemoglobin concentration in different sickle syndromes. Note that in SS disease, the cells fall below and above both the volume and concentration normal *(shaded)* range. The large (macrocytic) cells are the low-density reticulocytes. The dehydrated population is enriched in irreversibly sickled cells and low HbF. In S-thalassemia (S thal) syndromes, the entire volume curve is shifted toward the left, and few dense cells are seen. In SC disease, the microcytes are often spherocytic, very dehydrated cells. NI = normal.

cells in the densest cell fractions are very low.[126, 131] Even young reticulocytes poor in HbF can rapidly dehydrate and be found among the most dense cells in the circulation.[132]

RED CELL MEMBRANE ABNORMALITIES

The pathophysiologic basis of sickle cell anemia is the abnormal hemoglobin, which has the property of polymerizing when deoxygenated. As seen in other genetic diseases, however, secondary effects of the primary lesion may modulate the clinical expression of the disease. Alterations in the red cell membrane may be one of the important modulators of disease severity for several reasons (see Fig. 19–1). First, the membrane is the structure most intimately associated with the abnormal gene product and is therefore vulnerable to damage. Second, the membrane is largely responsible for maintaining the environment in which this abnormal product resides. Third, the membrane is the face with which the cell presents itself and is recognized by proteins in the plasma and cells in the circulation, along the vasculature, and in the reticuloendothelium.

Irreversibly Sickled Cells

The ISCs, which are easily identified and studied, have been a focus of attention in the study of the membrane lesion in sickle cell anemia. Bertles and Milner[131] showed that these cells are extremely dense, have little HbF to dilute their concentrated HbS, and survive in the circulation for only a few days. These cells provide the most graphic evidence of membrane damage in SS disease. Lux and co-workers[133] demonstrated that the abnormal shape of the ISC is maintained by the membrane (ghost) after hemolysis. Furthermore, when this membrane is treated with nonionic detergent (Triton X-100), all of its lipids and integral membrane are solubilized to maintain the

ISC shape (Fig. 19–7). As reviewed in detail in Chapter 15, the red cell skeleton plays a role not only in cell shape but also in permeability, lipid organization, deformability, and control of lateral mobility of integral proteins. ISCs can be formed *in vitro* by prolonged deoxygenation,[134] by incubation of red cells in high calcium buffer,[135] and by repeated oxygenation-deoxygenation cycles.[136] Horiuchi and associates[136] demonstrated that *in vitro* formation of ISCs is correlated with the maximal linear distortion of the red cell diameter under deoxygenated conditions, suggesting that the length of Hb S polymer fibers in SS cells contributes to irreversible membrane damage. As discussed in detail later, ISCs have different cation and water content, which is directly attributable to membrane-mediated events. ISCs vary widely from patient to patient and correspond well with hemolytic rate[137] and spleen size[138] but poorly with vaso-occlusive severity.

The Membrane and the Internal Milieu

Transport and Volume Control. As discussed earlier, the concentration of HbS in the cell has tremendous impact on the amount of polymer and the speed with which it forms at a given PO_2. The abnormal cation permeability of the sickle red cell allows it to become potassium depleted, calcium loaded, and pathologically dehydrated—enhancing the tendency to sickle. In 1952, Tosteson and colleagues[139, 140] showed that deoxygenation causes a reversible potassium loss and sodium gain in SS cells. Since then, the abnormal water and cation movements across the sickle cell membrane have been shown to be associated with a variety of pumps, channels, and leaks, involving water, potassium (K^+), sodium (Na^+), chloride (Cl^-), calcium (Ca^{2+}), and magnesium (Mg^{2+}). Although the pathogenesis of these pathways remains incompletely understood, they are undoubtedly related to the physical

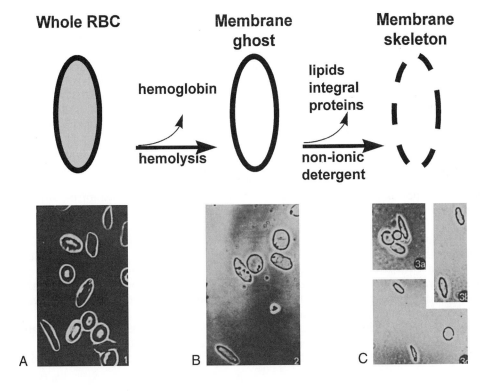

Whole RBC   hemoglobin   **Membrane ghost**   lipids integral proteins   **Membrane skeleton**

hemolysis   non-ionic detergent

A   B   C

FIGURE 19–7. *A*, Oxygenated intact red cells from a patient with SS disease showing typical round reversibly sickled cells (RSCs) and irreversibly sickled cells (ISCs). *B*, Same cells as in *A*, lysed to remove all intracellular material, leaving just membrane. Note the retained shape of the RSCs and ISCs. *C*, Same cells as in *B*, extracted with Triton X-100 to remove everything but the integral membrane proteins. Note the retained shape of the RSCs and ISCs. (Adapted from Lux SE, John KM, Karnovsky MJ: Irreversible deformation of the spectrin-actin lattice in irreversibly sickled cells. J Clin Invest 1976; 58:955–963.)

distortion associated with sickling,[141–148] young cell age,[149–152] oxidant damage,[153–157] and the hemoglobin mutation itself.[158–162] The two best characterized dehydrating pathways are the K^+, Cl^- cotransport pathway, and the Gardos channel (see Fig. 19–1). K^+,Cl^- cotransport is stimulated to lose K^+,Cl^- and water when (predominantly young) sickle cells are exposed to a low pH environment, as might occur in areas of poor perfusion.[163] The K^+,Cl^- cotransport pathway is inhibitable by magnesium *in vitro*.[151,164] The therapeutic potential of magnesium is confirmed by two important proof-of-principle studies that demonstrated the effectiveness of oral magnesium in the prevention of cellular dehydration in a mouse model of sickle cell disease[165] and in patients.[166, 167] Similarly, specific blockade of the Gardos channel—the pore that allows K^+ and water loss when stimulated by Ca^{2+}—would also be predicted to have beneficial effects. Clotrimazole, an imidazole antimycotic agent, is a potent inhibitor of this channel and is effective in preventing sickle red cell dehydration *in vitro*,[168] in the SAD mouse model for sickle cell disease *in vivo*,[169,170] and in a short-term study in patients with sickle cell disease.[171] Clinical studies of these potentially important antisickling agent are underway.

The Membrane and the Outside Surface

Membrane Deformability and Cytoskeletal Defects. There is no doubt that as sickle cells become deoxygenated and fill with polymerized hemoglobin they become less deformable.[172–175] However, even fully oxygenated cells have abnormal rheologic properties.[176] Using the ektacytometer, Clark and colleagues[177] studied the deformability of SS red cells and showed that decreased deformability was directly related to increased MCHC and that correcting the elevated MCHC restored normal deformability. By using a high shear/hemolysis assay, normalization of the tendency to hemolyze was noted when MCHC was corrected, except in the most dense fraction, in which normalization was incomplete.[178] This incomplete normalization suggests that severe cellular dehydration itself may contribute to the development of a membrane lesion. Membrane mechanical properties were measured with micropipette techniques in two studies.[179, 180] In both, it was found that MCHC is the major contributor to cell rigidity but that irreversible membrane changes accompany dehydration and result in increased membrane rigidity.

The clinical significance of membrane rigidity is not immediately obvious but is further evidence that a structural membrane lesion is present. The finding that the cytoskeleton of an ISC was permanently distorted led several investigators to analyze the various components. Abnormal ISC skeletal dissociation properties led to the observation that in sickle erythrocytes β-actin appears to have abnormally inaccessible cysteine residues, because of cross-linking or other post-translational modifications.[181] Maintaining the abnormal ISC shape probably requires that the cytoskeleton rearrange during a period of prolonged deformation under conditions that allow spectrin tetramers to dissociate into dimers and re-form with new spectrin partners.[182] The proteins involved in linking the cytoskeleton to the overlying membrane also behave abnormally. Protein 3 and glycophorin are clustered, with abnormal rotational and lateral mobility—especially in the most dehydrated cells (see Fig. 19–1).[183] This disordered mobility may relate to decreased binding of normal ankyrin to sickle protein 3[184] or to binding of normal spectrin to sickle ankyrin.[185]

Lipid Orientation. Although membrane lipid content and composition are relatively normal in SS red cells,[186–188] the organization of these lipids is quite unusual. Normally, the phospholipids of the red cell membrane are partitioned with amino phospholipids (phosphatidylserine [PS] and phosphatidylethanolamine [PE]) sequestered on the inner (cytoplasmic) surface and sphingomyelin and phosphatidylcholine (PC) exposed on the outer surface. This asymmetry is not unique to the red cell and probably reflects a general structural pattern that keeps the amino phospholipids from activating soluble coagulation factors. The asymmetry is maintained by the interaction of the spectrin[189] with the phospholipids and by a specific adenosine triphosphate (ATP)-dependent translocation process.[190] In RSCs, PS and PE flip back and forth from the inner leaflet to the outer leaflet during oxygenation and deoxygenation. Although early studies suggested that PS was permanently stuck to the outer leaflet in deoxygenated sickle cells,[191, 192] later studies suggested that small amounts of PS accumulate on the outer surface of subpopulations of sickle cells[193] where the lipid bilayer is uncoupled from the cytoskeleton and when the cell is ATP depleted.[194, 195] Exposure of PS or PE on the outer surface during sickling could accelerate blood coagulation or might alter the adhesiveness of red cells to other membranes.[196, 197] Alteration of the fatty acyl groups in PC results in changes in cell shape and deformability in SS cells, suggesting that the species composition of PC can affect membrane permeability and cellular deformability.[198]

Increased Adhesion to Endothelium. More than 15 years ago, investigators first discovered that sickle erythrocytes have an abnormal propensity to stick to vascular endothelial cells,[199, 200] an adhesive force resulting from numerous attachment sites[201] that can withstand detaching forces found in low shear vascular beds.[202, 203] This observation has taken on increased importance in conceptualizing the pathophysiology of sickle cell disease and has become a major research focus. As cells flow through vessels of critical dimension, an increased tendency to linger at the endothelial surface will increase the odds that polymerization and obstruction will occur (Fig. 19–8). Support for this hypothesis comes from studies that suggest a correlation between adhesiveness and clinical severity.[203, 204] Adhesive interactions are complex and undoubtedly involve a variety of ligands, receptors, and nonspecific interactions that vary depending on the age and density of the red cell, the type and health of endothelium, the amount of flow, and the composition of the plasma.

Young, light reticulocytes are particularly adherent, at least in part because they retain a variety of surface molecules such as very late antigen-4 (VLA-4)[205–207] and fibronectin receptors[208] that are characteristic of red cell precursors. As reticulocytes mature and shed these primitive receptors, they lose the ability to bind to ligands such as vascular cell adhesion molecule-1 (VCAM-1) and fibronectin that are either on or bridge endothelial cells. Older and denser sickle erythrocytes also adhere to endothelium,[201, 209] a difference that is highly dependent on experimental

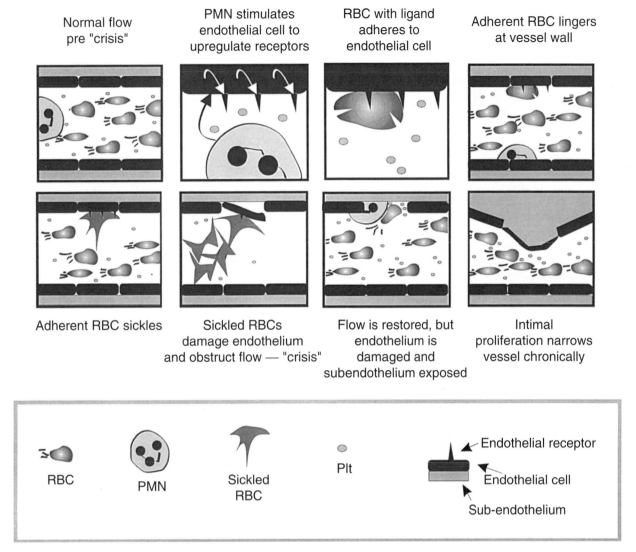

Normal flow
pre "crisis"

PMN stimulates
endothelial cell to
upregulate receptors

RBC with ligand
adheres to
endothelial cell

Adherent RBC lingers
at vessel wall

Adherent RBC sickles

Sickled RBCs
damage endothelium
and obstruct flow — "crisis"

Flow is restored, but
endothelium is
damaged and
subendothelium exposed

Intimal
proliferation narrows
vessel chronically

RBC

PMN

Sickled
RBC

Plt

Endothelial receptor
Endothelial cell
Sub-endothelium

FIGURE 19–8. Pathophysiology of vessel damage in sickle cell disease. RBCs = red blood cells; PNM = polymorphonuclear neutrophil leukocyte. (Adapted from Platt OS: Easing the suffering caused by sickle cell disease. N Engl J Med 1994; 330:783. Adapted, by permission, from *The New England Journal of Medicine.*)

conditions. Cells of various ages and densities[210] play different roles as they traverse different endothelial beds at different shear rates, oxygen tensions, and plasma compositions. Under some conditions, deoxygenation-induced erythrocyte-erythrocyte interactions may matter.[211]

The surface molecules of endothelial cells differ—for example, CD36 is expressed on microvascular but not large-vessel endothelium.[212] Endothelial cells also express differing amounts of surface molecules and become more or less adherent depending on environmental stimuli. Cytokines such as interleukin-18 and tumor necrosis factor[213] promote endothelial adherence, largely because of up-regulated VCAM-1 expression. Infected endothelial cells become adhesive by a variety of mechanisms. Herpesvirus-infected cells attract sickle red cells because of increased Fc receptor expression.[214] Endothelial cells exposed to Sendai viral double-stranded RNA become adhesive through up-regulated VCAM-1.[215]

The adhesion process can alter and even dislodge endothelial cells. Circulating endothelial cells from patients with sickle cell disease exhibit an activated phenotype displaying intracellular adhesion molecule-1 (ICAM-1), VCAM-1, E-selectin, P-selectin, and tissue factor.[216, 217] Such circulating cells may have left behind areas of exposed subendothelium. Subendothelial matrix proteins—laminin, thrombospondin, and fibronectin—provide adhesive surfaces for sickle erythrocytes. Two classes of binding sites for laminin have been identified on both normal and sickle red blood cells. An acidic lipid that binds both laminin and thrombospondin has been isolated.[218] The membrane protein B-CAM/LU (basal cell adhesion molecule/Lutheran) has been identified as the receptor for laminin.[219] The epitope on laminin that binds to red cells appears to lie within the α5 chain of the protein.[220]

Thrombospondin behaves differently depending on whether it is in solution or immobilized, as it would be in the subendothelium. In contrast to soluble thrombospondin, immobilized thrombospondin binds sickle red cells by an interaction that does not appear to involve red cell CD36.[221] This interaction is inhibited by von Willebrand factor even at concentrations found normally in plasma.[222] Sickle reticulo-cytes appear to bind fibronectin,[208, 223] although such binding is not consistently demonstrated in all assay systems.[221] Interestingly, neutrophils from patients with sickle cell disease are particularly adhesive to fibronectin, an interaction that correlates with plasma levels of interleukin-6.[223]

After exposure of endothelial cells to sickle erythrocytes, DNA synthesis is decreased in general,[224] but endothelin-1 expression is stimulated.[225]

Although over the years, an inconsistent profile of coagulation abnormalities has been described, particularly during crises, a growing body of evidence suggests that procoagulant and anticoagulant proteins and platelets play an important role in sickle vascular disease. This concept is particularly relevant to interactions at the endothelial surface, where von Willebrand factor,[226-230] platelets,[231] and thrombospondin[232, 233] increase adhesiveness. Recent evidence that platelet-activating factor increases sickle red cell adherence to endothelium, and that this interaction can be selectively blocked by an anti αVβ3 integrin antibody suggests a potential therapeutic strategy.[234]

Mechanism of Membrane Damage

Any pathophysiologically relevant damage to the SS red cell membrane must relate to the HbS concentrated on its inside surface. Even in normal cells, HbA has been shown to bind to membranes,[235, 236] at or near the cytoplasmic portion of band 3 protein[237-240] and with relatively low affinity to PS.[241] Hemoglobin at physiologic concentrations stabilizes the configuration of spectrin heterodimers.[242] HbS and β^S-globin bind to membranes more readily than does HbA.[243-247] Evans and Mohandas[248] demonstrated, using single-cell micropipette techniques, that membrane-associated sickle hemoglobin was a major determinant of erythrocyte rigidity. In these experiments, normal deformability was found when normal hemoglobin was reconstituted in sickle or normal membrane ghosts, but abnormal deformability was associated with reconstitution of sickle or normal red cell membranes with HbS. Deformability of ISC membranes also improved after the exchange of normal hemoglobin for HbS, although this process was not able to normalize the physical properties of the membrane. In one study, membrane rigidity was associated with the presence of a small amount of high-molecular-weight spectrin-hemoglobin complex in the membrane.[249]

HbS is inherently unstable[250, 251] and has an increased tendency to denature and form small aggregates—"micro-Heinz bodies" (see Fig. 19–1). These attach with high affinity to the cytoplasmic portion of band 3 protein at or near the HbA binding site.[252] This binding on the inside surface of the membrane is translated into changes on the outside surface, because both band 3 protein and glycophorin (the major bearers of the cell's antigens and charge) are found to be clustered above the micro-Heinz bodies.[253] The clustering of band 3 protein is associated with the deposition of specific anti-band 3 protein antibodies on the cell,[252, 254, 255] a process linked to normal cell senescence[256, 257] and perhaps contributing to the short life span of SS cells.[258] Ankyrin is also abnormally clustered around the denatured HbS, and, like band 3 protein, may be damaged in the process.[253] The hydrophobic

surface of the Heinz body also sequesters lipid, spectrin, band 3, ankyrin, and protein 4.1 inside the cell, and may contribute to the reduced surface area of such cells.[259]

HbS has an increased tendency to auto-oxidize and form methemoglobin, thereby generating superoxide and losing heme.[260] In fact, sickle cells generate twice the normal amounts of the potent oxidants superoxide, peroxide, and hydroxyl radical.[261] Hebbel[262] discusses several convincing lines of evidence suggesting that oxidation is a major contributor to the membrane abnormalities of sickle cells.[262] The increased amounts of membrane-associated hemoglobin, heme, and hemichrome[263-267] and nonheme iron[267] may target different vulnerable membrane components.[268-272]

APPROACHES TO ANTISICKLING THERAPY

Replacement of the Defective Gene. The most direct approach to reduction of HbS polymer is to replace the defective β-globin gene with a normal gene. Bone marrow transplants from siblings with sickle trait or normal siblings have been successful in a variety of transplant centers around the world.[273-278] After preparation for transplantation with various regimens and prophylactic treatment for graft-versus-host disease, more than 150 patients received bone marrow transplants, and a majority have done well. Overall, 80 to 85 percent of transplant recipients were reported to be alive and free of sickle cell disease–related symptoms, 6 to 8 percent had died, and 9 to 14 percent experienced graft failure. Newer, nonmyeloablative preparative regimens hold promise for reducing transplant morbidity and mortality. Major complications of transplantation have included central nervous system (CNS) hemorrhage (particularly in patients with a history of stroke),[279] graft rejection, and acute and chronic graft-versus-host disease. Prophylactic anticonvulsant treatment and maintenance of a high platelet count may result in reduced CNS morbidity. The restoration of splenic function in recipients of successful transplants holds out the hope that other chronic organ dysfunctions may improve with this approach.[280, 281] Selecting patients for this high-risk therapy is particularly problematic, however, because of the unpredictability of the clinical course, the paucity of sibling matches,[282] and parental concern.[283]

More specific "gene therapy" (i.e., inserting a normal β gene[284] or "correcting" the abnormal gene product[285, 286]) remains a long-term goal. In a clever and surprisingly effective experiment, Leboulch and colleagues[287] inserted a lentiviral vector bearing a mutant human β-globin gene into the stem cells of a mouse that had been engineered to express high levels of HbS. The mouse had clear-cut manifestations of sickle cell disease and exhibited long-term clinical improvement after the gene therapy. The specific mutation rendered in the therapeutic gene was β87 Thr:Gln, the mutation in Hb D-Ibaden that reduces fiber formation in HbS–Hb D-Ibaden mixtures.[287, 288]

Stimulation of Hemoglobin F Production. As was seen in the section on the interactions of HbS with HbF, increasing the amount of HbF will increase the delay time and solubility of HbS. In sickle cell disease, both 5-azacytidine[289-292] and hydroxyurea[293-296] have been used successfully to increase the level of HbF in individuals with SS disease. Recombinant human erythropoietin administered with hydroxyurea has inconsistently increased the level of HbF above levels obtained with hydroxyurea alone.[297, 298] Butyric acid analogs also increase HbF production in patients with sickle cell disease, in some patients with thalassemia, and in normal individuals.[299–301] Charache and colleagues[295] demonstrated that daily hydroxyurea treatment of adult patients with sickle cell disease increased HbF levels from pretreatment mean levels of 4 to 16 percent without clinically significant bone marrow toxicity. In addition to increasing the level of HbF, hydroxyurea has been noted to reduce the proportion of dense cells and increase the mean corpuscular volume (MCV) and mean corpuscular hemoglobin (MCH) of sickle cells.[289, 292–295] On the basis of epidemiologic data that increases in HbF from 4 to 16 percent could decrease the occurrence of vaso-occlusive crises by 50 percent,[302] a multicenter double-blind prospective clinical trial of daily hydroxyurea treatment of adults with sickle cell anemia was undertaken.[303] This trial was terminated early when it was obvious that the numbers of vaso-occlusive crisis, acute chest syndromes, and transfusions were reduced by almost 50 percent in the hydroxyurea-treated group compared with control subjects. The long-term follow-up of patients taking hydroxyurea reveals an impressive 40 percent reduction in mortality.[304] A number of small-scale trials of hydroxyurea therapy have been carried out in children with sickle cell anemia.[305–309] In general, the beneficial effects and toxicities in children appear to be similar to those observed in adults. However, an efficacy study has not yet been done, and the use of hydroxyurea in children should be considered investigational, particularly because of concerns regarding potential leukemogenesis, teratogenesis, and adverse effects on growth and development.

Decreased Cell Hemoglobin S Concentration. Because the polymerization of HbS is exquisitely concentration dependent, reduction of the MCHC by swelling the cell with water has been considered as a therapeutic maneuver. Two approaches have been tried: lowering plasma osmolarity and increasing intracellular cations. The first approach was used by Rosa and colleagues,[310] who successfully reduced the duration and incidence of painful crises by lowering the MCHC using dietary salt restriction and desmopressin. Subsequently, others have found this therapy too difficult to maintain, neurologically toxic, and ineffective.[311–313] The second approach has been used primarily *in vitro* and has focused on the property of various membrane-active agents to increase intracellular cations. Some of the interesting agents include the antibiotics monensin[314] and gramicidin[315]; calcium channel blockers nitrendipine, nifedipine, and verapamil[316]; and the peripheral vasodilator cetiedil.[317] As discussed earlier, preliminary evidence suggests that blockade of the Gardos channel with oral clotrimazole[171] and blockade of K^+,Cl^- cotransport with oral magnesium[166, 167] may decrease HbS concentrations by preventing dehydration and prove to be useful therapies.

Increased Hemoglobin S Solubility. The most straightforward approach to preventing the polymerization of HbS is to attack the β6 valine—the key to fiber formation. Unfortunately, this is an extremely unreactive residue, so that efforts to increase the solubility of HbS have hinged on the importance of the other intermolecular contacts. Reagents that increase deoxy-HbS solubility by noncovalent interactions with HbS have been recognized. Chang and colleagues[315] compared the effects of 15 antisickling agents on HbS solubility, oxygen affinity, and cell sickling. Urea is an effective agent but requires concentrations greater than 200 μmol/L, too high for *in vivo* use. The best studied covalent modifier is cyanate, but results of clinical trials have not been promising. Unfortunately, despite the encouraging clinical and *in vitro* data, this compound is not usable because of significant neurotoxicity[318] and cataract formation.[319] A major problem with covalent reagents is that they interact with a wide variety of functional groups found in many molecules other than hemoglobin.

Decreased Dwell Time of Cells in Narrow Vessels. Any manipulation that would allow a cell to traverse a vessel faster than its delay time will prevent occlusion of that vessel. Therapy aimed at reducing endothelial adherence may include altering the outer membrane lipids, surface charges, plasma proteins, platelets, white blood cells, or oxidants. An entirely different approach was suggested by the work of Rodgers and co-workers,[320] who showed that microcirculatory flow in patients with sickle cell disease has an unusual periodic pattern, indicating that it may be under vasomotor control and therefore possibly amenable to pharmacologic intervention.

DIAGNOSIS

The Fetus. The ability to perform prenatal diagnosis for sickle cell anemia has increased rapidly in the past two decades. In 1978, Kan and Dozy described DNA polymorphisms around the β-globin gene, which were in linkage disequilibrium with the β-S gene, thereby leading to the first DNA-based method for prenatal diagnosis. The A→T substitution in codon 6 responsible for the glutamic acid–valine change in β-globin can be detected by alteration of a site of a specific restriction enzyme by homologous synthetic oligonucleotides, which detect a single base substitution, and by polymerase chain reaction (PCR) amplification of DNA.[321–327] With the advent of PCR amplification of specific DNA sequences, sufficient DNA can be obtained from a very small number of fetal cells, thereby eliminating the necessity for culture of fetal fibroblasts.[328, 329] Chorionic villous biopsy offers an alternative to amniocentesis for obtaining fetal cells as early as 8 to 10 weeks' gestation.[330, 331] Preimplantation genetic diagnosis of single blastomeres using single-cell PCR followed by standard *in vitro* fertilization has led to the birth of unaffected twins to a couple who both had sickle trait.[332]

The Newborn. The newborn with sickle cell anemia is generally not anemic and is asymptomatic because of the protective effect of HbF. Results of the "sickle prep" and solubility tests are unreliable during the first few months of life. Because recognition of the disease in the newborn can lead to prevention of mortality and morbidity, it is now recommended that all newborns at risk be screened for sickle cell anemia. Screening combined with comprehensive follow-up care was first begun by Pearson in New Haven[333] and

Serjeant and associates in Jamaica[334] in the 1970s. Present screening methodologies include acid and alkaline electrophoresis, high-performance liquid chromatography, and isoelectric focusing. These tests can be performed on cord blood or on dried blood specimens blotted on filter paper. False-negative results using these methods have been reported in infants who received perinatal transfusions before screening.[335] Sickle cell anemia can also be diagnosed with PCR amplification of DNA extracted from filter paper.[336] Universal screening has been shown to identify more infants with disease, prevent more deaths, and be more cost effective in areas where sickle trait occurs in 7 to 15 infants per 1000 births compared with targeted screening of at-risk newborns.[337,338]

The Older Child. After the first few months of life, as β^S-globin production increases and the level of HbF declines, the clinical syndrome of sickle cell anemia emerges (Table 19–1). Although at 1 week of age the hemoglobin level of SS infants is statistically lower than that of AA infants, the overlap between the two groups is considerable and does not diverge much before the second month of life.[333] Anemia and a reticulocytosis is usually evident by 4 months of age. ISCs are often absent from the peripheral blood of young children, and the morphologic features are typical of those of normal newborns—target cells, fragments, and poikilocytes. By 3 years of age, the typical peripheral blood smear is seen, including ISCs, target cells, spherocytes, fragments, biconcave disks, Howell-Jolly bodies, and nucleated red cells. The amount of HbF decreases with age, as in normal children, but this occurs much more slowly.[333,339]

CLINICAL MANIFESTATIONS

The clinical manifestations of sickle cell disease are extremely varied. Some patients are entirely

TABLE 19–1. Hematology of Infants with SS Disease, SC Disease, and S-β⁺-Thalassemia

	Percentile	2–3	4–5	6–8	9–11	12–14	15–17	18–23	24–29	30–35	36–47	48–60
SS DISEASE												
Hemoglobin level (g/dL)	5	7.0	7.0	7.1	7.2	7.2	7.2	7.1	6.9	6.7	6.4	6.6
	50	9.3	9.2	9.2	9.2	9.1	9.0	8.9	8.6	8.3	8.1	8.3
	95	11.4	11.3	11.4	11.5	11.5	11.5	11.3	11.1	10.9	10.5	10.4
Mean corpuscular volume (fL)	5	72	69	68	67	67	67	67	68	69	71	72
	50	84	81	81	82	82	83	84	85	86	88	90
	95	96	94	94	95	96	96	96	97	97	98	100
Fetal hemoglobin level (%)	5	14.6	12.3	10.8	9.1	7.8	6.7	5.6	4.8	4.5	4.4	3.3
	50	43.5	34.1	29.1	24.3	20.6	17.7	14.8	12.8	12.4	12.4	9.0
	95	68.5	59.0	53.0	47.3	42.7	39.1	35.3	32.5	31.2	29.6	21.9
Reticulocyte count (%)	5	1.0	1.1	1.2	1.3	1.4	1.6	1.9	2.3	2.6	2.7	1.8
	50	4.0	5.1	5.9	6.7	7.4	8.0	8.7	9.3	9.8	10.4	11.8
	95	15.5	17.9	19.4	20.7	21.8	22.5	23.2	23.5	23.6	23.6	25.8
SC DISEASE												
Hemoglobin level (g/dL)	5	8.0	8.2	8.6	8.9	9.2	9.3	9.5	9.5	9.4	9.3	9.6
	50	9.7	9.8	10.1	10.3	10.5	10.6	10.7	10.8	10.7	10.6	10.6
	95	11.6	11.5	11.7	11.8	12.0	12.0	12.1	12.2	12.2	12.1	11.9
Mean corpuscular volume (fL)	5	68	65	64	64	63	63	63	63	64	66	69
	50	81	78	77	75	74	74	74	74	76	77	77
	95	91	88	86	85	84	84	84	84	86	88	87
Fetal hemoglobin level (%)	5	13.6	2.9	2.9	3.1	3.1	2.9	2.4	1.4	0.5	0.0	2.0
	50	31.6	17.9	14.5	11.6	9.3	7.4	5.5	4.2	3.9	4.4	4.2
	95	54.0	39.1	32.1	25.7	20.9	17.6	14.7	13.8	14.7	15.9	8.3
Reticulocyte count (%)	5	0.8	0.8	0.8	0.7	0.7	0.7	0.7	0.7	0.7	0.7	0.9
	50	2.8	2.8	2.7	2.6	2.5	2.5	2.5	2.6	2.7	2.9	2.8
	95	8.2	8.8	8.9	9.0	8.9	8.7	8.4	8.0	7.9	8.8	13.4
S-β⁺-THALASSEMIA												
Hemoglobin level (g/dL)	5	9.2	9.4	9.1	8.5	9.1	9.1	9.9	10.0	9.8	9.3	10.0
	50	10.8	10.9	11.0	10.8	10.6	11.2	10.9	11.0	10.7	10.6	10.8
	95	12.4	12.7	13.5	11.8	14.1	12.0	12.0	13.0	11.3	11.6	11.2
Mean corpuscular volume (fL)	5	70	64	61	61	63	82	63	61	66	64	66
	50	80	73	72	69	72	70	70	70	72	76	68
	95	88	83	84	75	84	73	77	79	76	76	76
Reticulocyte count (%)	5	1.1	0.0	1.1	0.9	0.8	0.9	0.7	1.5	1.2	1.0	3.0
	50	2.6	1.8	2.5	2.5	3.0	2.5	2.4	2.2	3.4	2.2	4.1
	95	8.5	6.4	2.5	4.6	5.9	7.4	5.1	6.2	7.4	7.6	5.7

Data from Brown AK, et al: Reference values and hematologic changes from birth to five years in patients with sickle cell disease. Arch Pediatr Adolesc Med 1994; 148:796.

asymptomatic, and the disease is detected only during population screening, whereas other patients are constantly plagued by painful episodes. The clinical picture in most patients falls between these extremes, and they have relatively long asymptomatic periods punctuated by occasional clinical crises. The complex nature of the clinical variability from patient to patient and from time to time in each patient has been prospectively studied on a large scale under the auspices of the Sickle Cell Disease Branch of the National Heart, Lung, and Blood Institute.[340, 341]

Sickle Cell Crisis

The term *sickle cell crisis* was defined by Diggs[342] as "any new syndrome that develops rapidly in patients with sickle cell disease due to the inherited abnormality." There are three categories of sickle crisis—vaso-occlusive, sequestration, and aplastic—and they are discussed individually in the next few sections. The best perspective on how these acute events occur in a typical group of children comes from a report by Gill and colleagues[343] describing

the experience of almost 700 infants followed up for 10 years as part of the Cooperative Study of Sickle Cell Disease. The age at the first event is displayed in Figure 19–9.

VASO-OCCLUSIVE SICKLE CRISES

Vaso-occlusive crises are acute, often painful episodes due to intravascular sickling and tissue infarction. In a prospective study of children with SS disease followed since birth in Jamaica, painful crisis was the first symptom in more than one fourth of the patients, and the symptom most commonly seen after age 2.[344] Painful episodes are such a prominent manifestation of the disease that African tribal names for sickle cell disease are onomatopoeic repetitive descriptions of pain, such as "chwechweechwa" (Ga tribe), "nwiiwii" (Fante tribe), "nucdudui" (Ewe tribe), and "ahotutuo" (Twi tribe). Tribal names translate as "beaten up," "body biting," and "body chewing."[345] Vaso-occlusive episodes are the major clinical manifestations of sickle cell disease and occur most commonly in

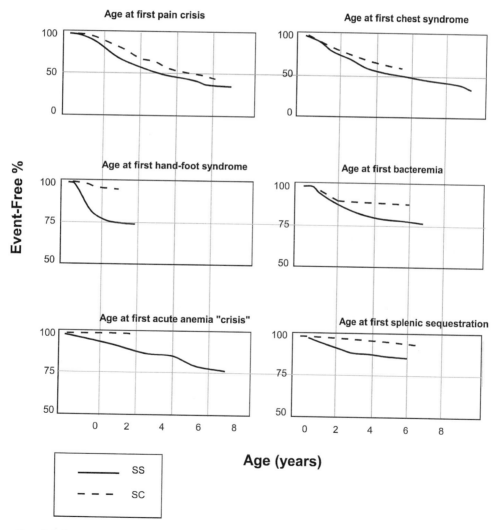

FIGURE 19–9. Age at first clinical event in patients with sickle cell disease, from birth to 10 years of age. *A,* Painful event. *B,* Acute chest syndrome. *C,* Hand-foot syndrome (dactylitis). *D,* Bacteremia. *E,* Acute anemic events not including splenic sequestration. *F,* Splenic sequestration. (Adapted from Gill FM, Sleeper LA, Weiner SJ, et al: Clinical events in the first decade in a cohort of infants with sickle cell disease. Cooperative Study of Sickle Cell Disease. Blood 1995; 86:776–783.)

the bones, lungs, liver, spleen, brain, and penis. Often the differential diagnosis is very difficult because there is no definitive objective hallmark of a vaso-occlusive crisis.

Painful Crisis. The most common acute vaso-occlusive crisis is acute pain. Virtually all patients with SS disease experience some degree of acute pain. For many, these episodes are mild and are handled entirely at home, school, or work. Little is known about the extent or nature of pain-coping activities that go on outside the medical environment, but diary studies suggest that it is enormous. The "tip" of the pain "iceberg" is represented by those episodes that drive patients to seek medical attention. These episodes vary widely among patients[302] (Fig. 19–10) and represent the most common reason for patients to visit outpatient offices and emergency departments and be admitted for inpatient care. Despite the fact that there is variation in how or why individual patients decide to seek attention for a given episode of pain, epidemiologic evidence strongly indicates that patients with higher rates of medical attention for pain have lower levels of HbF, higher steady-state levels of hemoglobins, and higher mortality.[302, 346] Some studies have suggested that infections, changes in climate,[347, 348] and psychologic factors may precipitate pain episodes, although commonly no precipitating factors can be identified. These patients typically are seen with rapid onset of deep, gnawing, throbbing pain, usually without any abnormal physical or laboratory findings but sometimes accompanied by local tenderness, erythema, warmth, and swelling. The underlying pathologic cause is bone marrow ischemia, sometimes leading to frank infarction with acute inflammatory infiltrate.[349–351] The areas involved most often are the lumbosacral spine, knee, shoulder, elbow, and femur. Less often, the sternum, ribs, clavicles, calcaneus, iliac crest, mandible, zygoma, and mandible are involved.[345] Joint effusions during acute episodes are particularly common in the knees and elbows. Typically, aspiration yields straw-colored fluid, usually with a "noninflammatory" profile. Rarely, sterile purulent exudates are found.[352] Given the range of marrow involvement and inflammatory response, it is not surprising that findings in patients with the most inflammation mimic those of osteomyelitis and those without findings are at risk of being considered malingerers.

Even in patients with measurable signs of inflammation, the diagnosis of infarction is favored over that of osteomyelitis. The results of one study suggest that acute long bone infarction is at least 50 times more common than osteomyelitis.[353] In this study of 41 patients with acute long bone infarcts, 38 percent affected the humerus, 23 percent affected the tibia, and 19 percent affected the femur. All patients experienced local tenderness, with swelling in 85 percent, joint findings in 68 percent, and local heat in 65 percent. Fourteen percent appeared "toxic," 21 percent had a temperature greater than 39°C, and 43 percent had a temperature less than 38°C. The total white blood cell count ranged between 7200 and 43,000 cells/mm^3, with a mean of 17,000 cells/mm^3. The mean sedimentation rate was 30.5 mm/hr, with a range of 3 to 66 mm/hr. Although various radionuclide scans have been suggested as a way of distinguishing between infarction and infection,[353–358] in many studies[359–361] such investigations were inconclusive. Magnetic resonance imaging (MRI) scans of patients with SS disease show decreased intensity of short relaxation time/echo time pulse sequence imaging, owing to hyperplastic marrow that converts to high intensity on long relaxation time/echo time images in painful crises,[351] but no definitive series compares infarction with infection. Except for positive results from blood or tissue culture, no laboratory test can differentiate acute infection from painful crisis.[350, 362] Needle aspiration and culture of the highly suspicious area are critical in isolating the organism and should be done before empirical antibiotic therapy is

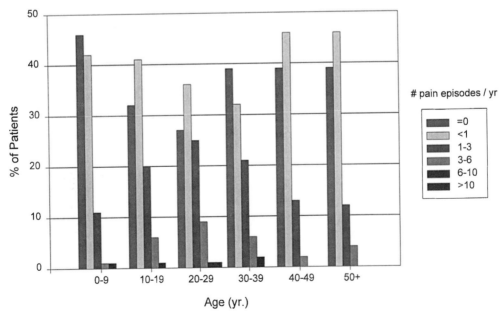

FIGURE 19–10. Distribution of pain rate among patients with SS disease. (Data from Platt OS, Thorington BD, Brambilla DJ, et al: Pain in sickle cell disease. Rates and risk factors. N Engl J Med 1991; 325:11–16.)

initiated. The aspirated fluid may be quite purulent even in the patients with sterile infarcts. In most series, the organism causing osteomyelitis most often is *Salmonella*.[363] *Staphylococcus* and *Streptococcus pneumoniae* are also commonly seen. Antibiotics effective against these organisms should be chosen initially. Treatment failures are seen when the most aggressive antibiotic regimens are not used.

As described earlier, episodes of acute bone pain and impressive signs of inflammation may be difficult to distinguish from osteomyelitis at the outset. More common and just as challenging are the evaluation and management of severely painful episodes in patients without signs of inflammation. Some of these patients will show laboratory evidence of acute inflammation such as elevated levels of C-reactive protein,[364] fibrinolysis such as elevated levels of D-dimers,[365, 366] or red cell trapping such as loss of dense cells.[367] These measurements are not helpful in the management of individual patients, nor should they be used as an attempt to "validate" an individual patient's report of symptoms. In a research setting, values for these measurements obtained from large numbers of patients with and without symptoms provide clues to potential innovative therapeutic interventions. For example, the common finding of elevated acute-phase reactants stimulated a trial of methylprednisolone for treating acute bone pain.[368] This preliminary work showed that a short course of high-dose corticosteroid decreased the duration of severe pain, and a larger-scale trial is underway to confirm the efficacy of this treatment. Similarly, despite the fact that results from earlier trials of aspirin therapy were not encouraging,[369] a renewed interest in the role of platelets, soluble procoagulants and anticoagulants, and endothelial cells in precipitation or propagation of vaso-occlusion will reopen interest in this potential line of treatment.

In children younger than 5 years of age, the small bones of the hands and feet are often affected, and in contrast to most episodes of bone pain in older children, physical findings are common. This painful *hand-foot syndrome* is typically the first clinical manifestation of sickle cell disease. The young child cries with pain refuses to bear weight, and has puffy, tender, and warm feet or hands or both. The child may appear to be acutely ill, be febrile, and have an impressive leukocytosis, ranging from 20,000 to 60,000 cells/mm³. At the onset of soft tissue swelling, there are usually no bony changes on radiographs. After 1 to 2 weeks, subperiosteal new bone, irregular areas of radiolucency, cortical thinning, or complete destruction of bones can be seen. All of the bone changes are usually reversible but may persist for as long as 8 months.[370, 371] Permanent shortening of the digits, a rare complication, has been reported after hand-foot syndrome.[372] General supportive care for a patient with an acute painful episode is described later in this chapter.

The age at which a child experiences the hand-foot syndrome is a strong predictor of overall severity (i.e., the risk of stroke, death, high pain rate, or recurrent acute chest syndrome) by 10 years of age. Those that have an episode before 1 year of age are at high risk of having a severe clinical course. The risk is further increased if the child also has experienced an episode in which the hemoglobin level dropped to less than 7 g/dL or the baseline white blood cell count was elevated.[373]

Acute Chest Syndrome. Episodes of acute lung injury with radiographic evidence of infiltrate are usually accompanied by chest pain, fever, cough, tachypnea, and hypoxia and are known as the *acute chest syndrome*. The vague terminology "chest syndrome" was originally used to indicate that the cause of any specific episode was usually unknown. Now that recent studies have identified the common causes, the imprecise terminology is still useful because it emphasizes the fact that in individual patients, knowing the specific cause is less critical for management than being able to assess the magnitude and pace of the lung injury.

The critical pathophysiologic features are that only deoxygenated HbS polymerizes and that reoxygenation eradicates the polymer. The lung is the critical organ that protects the arterial side of the circulation from the sludge of sickle polymers. When the lung is injured, underventilated, or inflamed, the protection is inadequate, and downstream tissues, including the injured lung itself, become increasingly susceptible to sickling and ischemia. In fact, when the flow is eventually restored, reperfusion injury may occur, as suggested by the study by Kaul and Hebbel[374] who found that cycles of oxygenation/deoxygenation caused classical P-selectin–inhibitable movement of inflammatory cells to tissue in a sickle mouse model.

The acute chest syndrome is a leading cause of morbidity and mortality in patients with sickle cell disease. It represents the second most common acute complication (pain episode is first) with a rate of 12.8 occurrences per 100 patient-years[375] and the most common condition at the time of death.[376] The highest incidence is in children aged 2 to 4 (25.3 occurrences per 100 patient-years), and the lowest incidence is in adults (8.8 occurrences 100 patient-years).[375] Patients who have not experienced an episode of acute chest syndrome have longer life expectancy than those who have, and those with a higher level of HbF and lower steady-state leukocyte count have a lower incidence of acute chest syndrome.[375] Hydroxyurea therapy lowers the incidence in adults by approximately 50 percent.[303]

Vichinsky and colleagues[377] prospectively studied 671 episodes of acute chest syndrome.[376] The most common etiologies were fat/bone marrow embolus and infection with *Chlamydia, Mycoplasma,* or a virus. In contrast to patients with infection, those with a bone marrow embolus were more likely to have an associated episode of bone pain, chest pain, abnormal neurologic symptoms, and a decrease in platelet count.[377]

Bacterial pneumonia was rarely seen overall, but was more common in children than adults. In children it was associated with bacteremia in 58 percent of patients with *S. pneumoniae* infection and 18 percent of patients with *Haemophilus influenzae* infection.[378] Regardless of cause, acute chest syndrome is always accompanied by some degree of localized sickling and lung ischemia; in 16 percent of patients no precipitating embolus or pathogen was identified. Overall, the prognosis is poor. Thirteen percent of patients required mechanical ventilation, 11 percent developed new abnormal neurologic findings, and 9 percent who were aged 20 or older died. In general, the death rate from acute chest syndrome is four times higher in adults than in children.[378]

Several important therapeutic principles emerged from the Vichinsky study. First of all, bronchodilator therapy was remarkably effective in 20 percent of patients with wheezing or pulmonary function tests indicating obstruction at presentation (61 percent of all the patients). This is consistent with the observation that measurable airway hyperactivity has been documented in as many as 73 percent of children with SS disease even without a history of asthma.[379] Secondly, red cell transfusion improved oxygenation. Simple transfusion was used in 68 percent of patients and appeared to be as effective as exchange transfusion, although the study was not designed to test this hypothesis. It may be that the efficacy of simple transfusions related to the fact that acute chest syndrome is typically associated with a 0.5 to 1.0 g/dL decrease in hemoglobin level at presentation. And third, the prominence of *Chlamydia* and *Mycoplasma* infections underscores the importance of including antibiotics effective against macrolides in the initial empiric therapy.

Although some patients, particularly adults, initially present with a full-blown picture of chest pain, hypoxia, and abnormal radiographic findings, often the diagnosis becomes clear only days into an event that starts as a fever without source, abdominal pain, or extremity pain. The diagnosis of acute chest syndrome can be very difficult to make. Children younger than 4 years of age often have few signs at presentation: 35 to 40 percent had a normal lung examination; 30 to 40 percent had no tachypnea; and 30 to 50 percent had no tachycardia.[378] Signs that are visible on radiographics often evolve slowly. In one series, only 36 percent of patients had an abnormal radiograph on presentation although all eventually developed abnormal radiographic findings.[380]

There were considerable changes in blood counts of patients with acute chest syndrome at the time of presentation. The hemoglobin level dropped an average of 0.7 g/dL, and white blood cell counts increased an average of 69 percent. The mean PO_2 was 71 mm Hg with one fifth of the patients having a PO_2 less than 60 mm Hg. Because the hemoglobin-oxygen dissociation curve varies among patients and because the shallow portion of the curve lies between a PO_2 of 50 and 100 mm Hg, transcutaneous oxygen saturation measurements are not sufficient to detect trends unless there are enough simultaneous direct measurements of arterial PO_2.[381] In one study, all children with SS disease and acute chest syndrome had transcutaneous saturation measurements less than 96 percent or only three points less than their steady-state values.[382] Given that it is not unusual for a transcutaneous measurement to vary as much as three points with slight differences in positioning in the probe, it is unwise to place too much reliance on a single measurement in isolation. Unfortunately, there are no clinical findings that reliably predict the degree of hypoxia.[378]

Although most patients recover from acute chest syndrome uneventfully, its course is unpredictable, and rapid, unexpected deterioration is common. Most series reporting on acute chest syndrome include a section on autopsy findings. Pulmonary postmortem findings typically include areas of alveolar wall necrosis and focal parenchymal scars.[383] In one autopsy, multiple large infarcts but no accompanying occluded vessels were found, suggesting that severe vasospasm may play a role in some instances.[384]

The optimal management of patients with acute chest syndrome requires vigilant monitoring and considered judgment. A few guidelines are presented here, but these should not substitute for consultation and collaboration with a clinician experienced in managing this complex problem. All patients with acute chest syndrome must be treated in the hospital, a setting in which vital signs and arterial blood gases can be regularly monitored. A PO_2 of less than 75 mm Hg (or a decrease of 25 percent from baseline, if the patient has chronic hypoxia) indicates a poor prognosis.[385] Oxygen therapy is critically important in hypoxic patients, and mechanical ventilation is sometimes required. Preliminary evidence suggests that inhaled nitric oxide may be of benefit in patients with severe hypoxia.[386] Antibiotics should be used empirically after careful culturing, keeping in mind the prevalence of infections from *Chlamydia*, *Mycoplasma*, *S. pneumoniae*, and *H. influenzae*. A trial of bronchodilator therapy should be used, especially in patients with a history of obstructive lung disease or those who have wheezing on examination. Transfusion is critical for patients with persistent hypoxia (PO_2 of less than 75 mm Hg or a decrease of 25 percent from baseline). Exchange transfusion is indicated if the hematocrit is high, if the patient is hypoxic, if the patient's condition is deteriorating rapidly, or if the patient's condition continues to deteriorate after simple red cell transfusion. Because the splinting and atelectasis associated with chest pain may exacerbate or even cause acute chest syndrome, analgesic therapy should not be withheld from patients with chest pain. Guidelines for analgesic usage are described later in this chapter. Analgesics should be used with extreme caution in patients with acute chest syndrome. These patients may hover on the brink of hypoventilation from either too little or too much analgesia. Regular monitoring of continuous oxygen saturation and respiratory rate and evaluation of pain are critical. Fluid overload with congestive heart failure occurs readily in patients with acute chest syndrome. After normal hydration is achieved, maintenance fluids should be given.

Acute Abdominal Pain. Severe acute abdominal pain is a common event that often poses a difficult problem of differential diagnosis. Its cause is unknown, although mesenteric sickling and vertebral disease with nerve root compression have been suggested. This type of crisis can be accompanied by symptoms of guarding, tenderness, rebound, fever, and leukocytosis that are indistinguishable from those associated with acute surgical abdomen. Often, the patient is the best judge and knows whether the pain is characteristic of a "crisis."

These patients should receive the general supportive measures described later in this chapter, with the omission of high-dose analgesics. Patients should be given nothing by mouth and followed closely by both medical and surgical personnel. Abdominal films, including upright views, may help to identify a perforated viscus. Usually, the condition of the patient with vaso-occlusive pain will remain stable or improve slightly with hydration and mild sedation. If the pain is extreme and the patient's clinical condition is deteriorating, emergency surgical exploration may be necessary. A simple or exchange transfusion should be done before surgery if possible.

Acute right upper quadrant pain with liver enlargement, tenderness, hyperbilirubinemia, and abnormal liver enzyme concentrations may be a result of intrahepatic sickling[387, 388] or acute cholecystitis. Abdominal ultrasonography is an excellent method for detecting the 50 percent of gallstones that are not radiopaque. Unfortunately, the presence of gallstones and a clinical syndrome characteristic of cholecystitis does not necessarily mean that the symptoms are due to the stones. Many patients and their physicians have been disappointed when their "cholecystitis" returned after cholecystectomy. In a retrospective study of acute abdomen in 28 patients with SS disease,[389] the presence of gallstones evident on ultrasound evaluation did not predict which patients could be managed without surgery. Biliary scans indicated obstruction in 13 patients, of whom 4 improved without surgery. Normal biliary scans were not found in any patient who needed immediate surgery. These patients with acute cholecystitis should be operated on after the gallbladder has had a chance to "cool down." Postoperative management of patients with sickle cell disease and acute cholecystitis can be fraught with complications.[390] Early experience indicates that laparoscopic cholecystectomy in patients with SS disease appears to be associated with fewer postoperative complications.

Acute Central Nervous System Event. Acute infarction of the brain can result in a devastating stroke, which occurs in approximately 7 percent of children with sickle cell disease.[391, 392] The incidence is estimated to be 0.7 percent per year during the first 20 years of life, with the highest rates in children 5 to 10 years of age.[393] This disaster may occur as an isolated event but also appears in the setting of evolving pneumonia, aplastic crisis, viral illness, painful crisis, priapism, or dehydration.[391–392] The most common underlying lesion is an intracranial arterial stenosis or obstruction, usually in the internal carotid artery but often in the proximal middle cerebral or anterior cerebral arteries.[395–397] On pathologic examination, these vessels, whose endothelium has presumably been chronically injured by sickle erythrocytes, show heaped-up intima with proliferation of fibroblasts and smooth muscle.[398] The lumen may be narrowed or completely obliterated by the vascular lesion, suggesting that *acute* sickling may simply be the "last straw," causing acute infarction in the setting of a chronically damaged vessel. Hemiparesis, speech defects, focal seizures, and gait dysfunction are the most common signs.

A careful discussion of the evaluation of the child with new neurologic symptoms is provided by Adams.[399] He suggests that the best initial diagnostic test is the computed tomographic (CT) scan, although it may not show positive evidence for infarction within the first 6 hours of the episode. Abnormalities are seen on MRI scans in 2 to 4 hours and are found in about 90 percent of patients with stroke.[400] The typical findings are infarcts associated with major vessel obstruction or distal obstruction of smaller vessels leading to infarction in the "border zone" area between the anterior cerebral and middle cerebral vessels.[401, 402] The intracranial and cervical artery vasculature can be well visualized using magnetic resonance angiography, and this

procedure is becoming increasingly useful in the early evaluation of the patient with new symptoms.

The standard approach to treating a patient with acute infarction is exchange transfusion (see section on transfusion for details). In untreated patients, the mortality rate is approximately 20 percent, with about 70 percent of patients experiencing a recurrence within 3 years. Of these untreated patients, more than 70 percent were left with permanent motor disabilities and a deficit in IQ.[391] Patients treated with exchange transfusion usually show marked improvement in motor function, although the prognosis is considerably worse for those with multiple infarcts. After the initial exchange, a maintenance transfusion program should be carried out (see section on transfusion). Prolonged transfusion has a profound influence on the morbidity and mortality of stroke.[394, 396, 403–405] A regular program designed to keep the amount of HbS at less than 30 percent lowers the recurrence rate of stroke to 10 percent, with only 30 percent of patients having residual motor abnormalities and 10 percent with IQ less than 70. Repeat arteriograms in patients maintained on transfusion generally, but not invariably, show stabilization and smoothing of intimal lesions, whereas patients who did not receive transfusions show progression of disease.[394] A study of 12 children with acute strokes revealed a 70 percent recurrence rate within 5 weeks to 11 months of ending a 1- to 2-year transfusion program.[396] In another follow-up study, recurrences were high even after 5 to 12 years of transfusion in an unusual group of patients with severe encephalomalacia.[406] In one informative series, 15 patients at the Children's Hospital of Philadelphia who had been receiving transfusions that kept the HbS level at less than 30 percent for 4 years had their regimen liberalized, allowing the pretransfusion amount of HbS to rise to 50 percent.[407] With a mean follow-up of 84 months, none had a recurrent infarction. Unfortunately, this program did not prevent hemorrhage—two patients died, one of intraventricular bleeding and one of subarachnoid bleeding. Although theoretically beneficial, indefinite maintenance transfusion regimens are associated with the risks of sensitization, hepatitis, and acquired immunodeficiency syndrome and the certain problem of iron overload. Bone marrow transplantation and use of hydroxyurea to increase the level of HbF have been tried in patients with strokes, but the data are insufficient to determine their relative efficacy compared to that of transfusions.[408, 409]

Application of newer techniques for noninvasive assessment of the brain and its vasculature has focused attention on two new areas—identifying children at high risk for stroke and identifying children with "asymptomatic" brain disease. Adams and associates[410] demonstrated that children with abnormally increased blood flow in their intracerebral arteries as measured by transcranial Doppler ultrasonography had a relative risk of stroke of 44 (95 percent confidence interval 5.5 to 346). A systematic study of MRI in asymptomatic children with sickle cell disease revealed that unanticipated infarcts are highly predictive of subsequent clinical stroke.[411] However, in older children (mean age 11 years) without evidence of prior CNS disease, abnormal transcranial Doppler ultrasonography and MRI results are often discordant, indicating that these tests may be measuring different aspects of CNS pathologic lesions in these subjects.[412] MRI scans have revealed that as many as 17 percent of children older than 6 years have evidence of silent infarcts[413] and in one study of 36 asymptomatic children 7 to 48 months old the incidence was 11 percent.[414] These silent infarcts are associated with impaired performance on psychometric tests that measure fine motor skills and cognitive ability.[415, 416] Older children (older than 6 years of age) with silent infarcts were more likely to have a history of seizures, low hemoglobin level, and high white blood cell count ($>11.8 \times 10^9$/L).[413] In a study of 392 children followed prospectively up to 10 years, elevated white blood cell counts, dactylitis, and low hemoglobin levels (<7 g/dL) before age 2 were associated with adverse outcomes including strokes.[370] In other studies low hematocrit,[417] acute chest syndrome,[418] and hypertension[419] have been associated with silent infarcts, clinical strokes, or both. In a multicenter prospective study of 130 asymptomatic children with increased Doppler flow measurements (>200 cm/sec), subjects were randomly assigned to receive transfusions or standard care. The study was terminated early when it was shown that only 1 of 63 children who received transfusions had strokes compared with 11 of 67 children who received standard care.[420] Subsequent to this study a Clinical Alert by the National Heart Lung and Blood Institute was issued suggesting that children between the ages of 2 and 16 should receive screening with Doppler ultrasonography and that treatment should be considered for those with abnormal results. These observations suggest that ultrasound or MRI should be used to screen older children with poor school performance or evidence of other risk factors. Under consideration are trials using transfusions, hydroxyurea,[309, 421] or bone marrow transplantation[422] in younger children who develop abnormal intracranial Doppler flow measurements or evidence on MRI scans of silent infarcts.

Not all acute focal neurologic events in patients with sickle cell anemia are infarcts. Intracranial hemorrhage is the other major category of sickle cell–related CNS events, although the incidence may be higher in adults than in children.[418] These events present as a sudden severe headache, sometimes with neck pain, vertigo, syncope, nystagmus, ptosis, meningismus, or photophobia. Many of these episodes are subarachnoid hemorrhages from small bleeding aneurysms that probably arise from intimal damage during childhood. Multiple aneurysms with extensive collateral vessels (similar to those seen in moyamoya disease) have been found incidentally during angiographic evaluation of children with stroke.[398] Although the mortality in some series approaches 50 percent,[391] other researchers describe more successful aggressive neurosurgical approaches to these bleeding lesions[423–425] and suggest that angiography should be done to identify patients with surgically amenable lesions.

Priapism. Priapism occurs in males of all ages. In a Jamaican study of 104 males aged 10 to 62 years, 42 percent reported at least one episode of priapism, with a median age of onset of 21 years.[426] Long-term follow-up of patients in Los Angeles indicated that approximately 7 percent of males with SS disease and approximately 2 percent of males with SC disease develop priapism, with a median age of onset of about 22 years.[24] A questionnaire

survey administered to 98 patients younger than age 20 in Dallas found the mean age at the initial episode to be 12 years, with an average number of episodes per patient of 15.7 and an average duration of 125 minutes.[427] Priapism most commonly occurred around 4:00 AM—during sleep or soon after waking. There was a surprisingly high prevalence of priapism in this age-group, with an 89 percent actuarial probability of patients experiencing priapism by age 20. Because early intervention and treatment may prevent irreversible penile fibrosis and impotence, patients and parents should be educated about this complication before it occurs.

Four clinical entities are described: stuttering priapism, with short (less than 2 to 3 hours), often multiple episodes; acute prolonged priapism (more than 24 hours), which can persist for weeks; chronic priapism, a painless induration that may last for years; and acute-on-chronic priapism, acute painful episodes complicating chronic induration. Sexual dysfunction was reported by 46 percent of patients with a history of priapism.[426] In general, young patients with brief episodes restricted to the corpora cavernosa ("bicorporal priapism") are less likely to experience sexual dysfunction,[428, 429] whereas adults with involvement of the corpora cavernosa and corpus spongiosa ("tricorporal priapism") tend to have prolonged episodes and a better than 50 percent chance of becoming impotent.[430] Urinary retention requiring catheterization may complicate such acute episodes.[430] Patients with tricorporal involvement are also particularly susceptible to acute severe neurologic complications and overall increased morbidity—even those treated with exchange transfusion.[431, 432] They should be monitored closely for early,[432] neurologic symptoms, especially headache.

Diagnostic studies such as scans with technetium, MRI scans, Doppler flow studies, and measurements of corporal pressures, hemoglobin electrophoresis, and blood gases are presently being used in a variety of settings to help define the anatomic and potential prognostic features of priapism. As yet, they have not had an impact on clinical decision making in individual patients.[433–435]

A consensus on treatment of priapism has not been reached; there are no controlled clinical trials to guide therapy. Short episodes of acute priapism usually occur on awakening and can be managed at home. Patients should be instructed to urinate often, do some vigorous exercise, increase fluid intake, and soak in a warm tub. If the episode does not resolve within a few hours, the patient should appear for medical treatment. In a small series of pediatric patients in Dallas, corporal aspiration and irrigation with dilute epinephrine were used successfully in an outpatient setting.[436] In general, treatment of acute priapism that has lasted more than a few hours should include analgesics, and preparation for possible transfusion should be made. Priapism may respond to simple red cell transfusion,[428] and this may be a reasonable temporary measure in the first 6 to 8 hours. Priapism in some patients begins to resolve within hours of exchange transfusion,[437, 438] although most patients do not show signs of detumescence for 24 to 48 hours, and in some no response at all is seen.[439] Use of intracorporal and oral α-adrenergic agents has been tried successfully in a small experimental group in Paris in patients with both acute and chronic priapism,[440] and in one group of patients with stuttering priapism in Jamaica, stilbestrol was helpful in preventing recurrence.[441]

Surgical shunting procedures should be considered for patients who have not shown any signs of detumescence 24 hours after exchange transfusion or corporal irrigation, particularly if they are postpubertal. Historically, these procedures have been associated with a high rate of complications with subsequent penile deformities and impotence. It is difficult to determine which of any observed adverse effects are related to the procedure and which to the priapism itself. The most conservative shunt is Winter's procedure or one of its modifications, whereby a needle or scalpel is inserted through the glans into one of the corpora and the viscous blood is aspirated. This allows for temporary drainage of cavernous blood into the systemic circulation and has been successfully used in patients with SS disease.[442] Intermittent compression with a blood pressure cuff is critical to limit refilling. Anecdotal evidence suggests that penile implants to correct impotence may be more easily done soon after an impotence-causing episode.[443, 444]

ACUTE SPLENIC SEQUESTRATION CRISIS

One of the leading causes of death in children with sickle cell anemia is the acute splenic sequestration crisis.[445] Children with SS disease who have not yet undergone autosplenectomy as well as older patients with SC disease or S-β-thalassemia[446] may have sudden, rapid, massive enlargement of the spleen with trapping of a considerable portion of the red cell mass. This complication has been described as early as 8 weeks of age.[447] Emond and associates[448] described the natural history of acute sequestration crisis in a cohort of 308 children with SS disease in Jamaica. Eighty-nine patients experienced 113 attacks, with 67 children having their first attack before age 2. There were 13 fatalities, 10 of which occurred before age 2. The most commonly associated clinical problems were upper respiratory tract infection and acute chest syndrome. Sixteen percent of the patients had positive blood culture results. Recurrences were seen in 49 percent of survivors of the first attack. A parental education program focused on teaching parents the technique of spleen palpation and the urgency of seeking medical attention for enlarged spleen and pallor led to an increase in occurrences (from 4.6 to 11.3 per 100 patient-years of observation) and a decrease in fatality rate (from 29.4 per 100 events to 3.1 per 100 events). Patients suddenly become weak and dyspneic, with rapidly distending abdomen, left-sided abdominal pain, vomiting, and shock. The tempo of this crisis may be so fast that the patient dies before reaching the hospital. On physical examination, there is profound hypotension with cardiac decompensation and massive splenomegaly. The hematocrit is half the patient's usual value, and there is usually a brisk reticulocytosis with increased nucleated red cells and moderate to severe thrombocytopenia.[449] Rao and Gooden[450] described a subacute form of sequestration in 11 patients, characterized by increased spleen size, 25 percent drop in hematocrit, less than 100,000 platelets/mm^3, and reticulocyte count elevation greater than the patient's baseline. In all patients a response to chronic transfusion programs was seen, but 7 patients had recurrent episodes after transfusions were stopped and eventually required splenectomy.

The review by Kinney and associates from Duke University of 23 patients with splenic sequestration strengthens the position of those who favor elective splenectomy for children who have had one episode of sequestration.[451] In this series of 23 patients, 4 underwent early splenectomy, 7 were observed carefully, and in 12 maintenance transfusion program was begun. Of those treated with transfusion, 2 are well and still receiving transfusions, 3 had recurrences while still receiving transfusions, 4 experienced recurrences within 3 months of the last transfusion, and only 3 remain well at 11 months (3.9 years after the last transfusion). Fourteen percent of children became alloimmunized, and 1 patient developed non-A, non-B hepatitis. Eventually 14 of the 23 patients underwent splenectomy. All were immunized against pneumococcus and were given penicillin for prophylaxis. None has experienced a life-threatening infection 65.6 patient-years later.

Therapy is the emergency restoration of intravascular volume and oxygen-carrying capacity by the immediate transfusion of packed red cells. Once normal cardiovascular status is restored, patients' conditions improve rapidly. The spleen usually shrinks within a few days, and the thrombocytopenia resolves. Sequestration may recur, usually within 4 months of the initial episode. To eliminate recurrence, some have recommended elective splenectomy after the first episode.[452] Others who are concerned with postsplenectomy sepsis have suggested splenectomy after two episodes of sequestration.[449] Serjeant and associates[453] demonstrated in a 22.5-year follow-up study that children in Jamaica do not have a greater risk of infection after splenectomy than a matched control group of patients with SS disease. Emergency splenectomy for acute sequestration is not indicated.

Sequestration may also take place in the liver. Liver enlargement and tenderness, with hyperbilirubinemia, increased anemia, and reticulocytosis are the usual clinical features.[387] Because the liver is not as distensible as the spleen, there is rarely pooling of red cells significant enough to cause cardiovascular collapse.

APLASTIC CRISIS

The clinical characteristics of the aplastic crisis of sickle cell disease have been well characterized.[454–456] In the normal steady state, the decreased red cell survival (15 to 50 days) in sickle cell anemia is compensated for by sixfold to eightfold increased bone marrow output. Temporary cessation of bone marrow activity due to suppression by intercurrent viral or bacterial infection causes the hematocrit value to fall as much as 10 to 15 percent per day with no compensatory reticulocytosis. The short-lived HbF-poor cells are the first to disappear from the circulation, whereas the high HbF-containing cells linger. This natural selection of HbF-containing cells accounts for the apparent increase in the percentage of HbF during aplastic episodes.

Spontaneous recovery is usually heralded by a markedly elevated nucleated red blood cell count, followed in 1 or 2 days by a brisk reticulocytosis. This recovery phase, with the characteristic anemia, nucleated red cells, reticulocytosis, and occasional hyperbilirubinemia, is probably responsible for most occurrences referred to as "hyperhemolytic crisis." Most aplastic episodes are short and mild and require no therapy. Occasionally, a transfusion is necessary if the marrow remains quiescent.

In 1981, Serjeant and colleagues[457] reported an outbreak of aplastic crises that was associated with an epidemic of parvovirus-like agent. Since then, the Jamaican group has documented the epidemiology and follow-up of parvovirus infection in a cohort of infants identified at birth—308 infants with sickle cell anemia and 239 control infants.[458, 459] They made a number of important observations: (1) the incidence of infection (about 40 percent) did not differ between sickle cell anemia and control groups; (2) 20 percent of infections in the sickle cell anemia group did *not* result in significant aplasia; (3) 100 percent of aplastic episodes were associated with parvovirus infection; (4) no patient had recurrent aplasia; and (5) 45 percent of infected patients had an elevated parvovirus-specific immunoglobulin G after 5 years. In a recent series of aplastic episodes, approximately 70 percent were associated with positive diagnostic tests for parvovirus.[460] Parvovirus has also been implicated as the etiologic agent in erythema infectiosum (fifth disease).[461, 462] An outbreak of both aplastic crisis and erythema infectiosum occurred in Ohio.[462, 463] All instances of aplastic crises occurred in individuals with hemolytic anemia (25 of 26 with sickle syndromes), and none of these patients had the classic rash of fifth disease. Since then, the relationship between parvovirus and erythropoiesis has been studied in detail. The virus specifically retards late erythroid precursor differentiation[464] and is responsible for temporary erythroid aplasia in a broad array of hemolytic anemias.[463]

Infections

Infection is the most common cause of death in children with sickle cell anemia.[445, 465] In one study, the risk of acquiring sepsis or meningitis was greater than 15 percent in children younger than 5 years of age, with an associated mortality of approximately 30 percent.[466] In young children, the risk of pneumococcal sepsis appears to be 400 times that of normal children, and *H. influenzae* sepsis appears two to four times as commonly.[467] In general, the organisms responsible for infection are not unusual pathogens (Table 19–2), but the infections that they cause in such patients are more common and severe.

The major risk factor for this increased vulnerability to infection is splenic dysfunction. The spleen normally serves two separate immunologic functions: (1) clearance of particles from the intravascular space and (2) antibody synthesis. Both functions are impaired in sickle cell anemia.

During the first year of life, *functional asplenia*, the inability to clear particulate matter from the blood, develops in patients with sickle cell anemia.[468] This is heralded by the appearance of red cells with Howell-Jolly bodies and irregular surface characteristics (pits). When the percentage of "pitted" red cells exceeds 3.5 percent, the spleen is generally nonfunctional.[469] Splenic dysfunction occurs early in life, with 50 percent of 2068 children with SS disease having greater than 3.5 percent pitted red cells by 2 years of age. Appearance of dysfunction was less rapid and less common in children with HbSC and S-β-thalassemia. Despite palpable splenomegaly, children with elevated numbers of pitted red blood cells have no splenic uptake of technetium-99m (^{99m}Tc) sulfur colloid and are susceptible to the most serious infectious complications of asplenia and pneumococcal sepsis.[470] Repeated infarction results in a nonpalpable, fibrotic, often calcified spleen that may be visualized on a ^{99m}Tc-diphosphonate bone scan.[471] Splenic infarction in young children with SS disease appears to be an insidious process—usually without many symptoms. In older children and adults, however, especially those with SC disease or sickle thalassemia, severe left upper quadrant pain often accompanies infarction. Transfusion,[472] hydroxyurea,[473] and bone marrow transplantation[280] can correct the splenic phagocytic defect, although these treatments are not indicated for splenic dysfunction per se.

TABLE 19–2. Bacteremias and Associated Acute Events in a Cohort of 694 Children with Sickle Cell Anemia (SS) and Hemoglobin SC Disease Followed Prospectively from Infancy

Organism	Patient	Total No. Cases	Isolated Bacteremia	Acute Chest Syndrome	Meningitis	Bone/Joint
Streptococcus pneumoniae	SS	62	39 (5 dead)	14 (1 dead)	8 (2 dead)	1
	SC	12	9	3	0	0
Haemophilus influenzae	SS	10	6 (2 dead)	3	1	0
	SC	4	2	2	1	0
Staphylococcus aureus	SS	5	2	2	0	1
	SC	1	1	0	0	0
Streptococcus viridans	SS	5	4	1	0	0
	SC	1	1	0	0	0
Escherichia coli	SS	5	3	1	0	1
	SC	2	0	1	0	1
Salmonella species	SS	3	2	0	0	1
	SC	2	1	0	0	1
Other	SS	2	1	1	0	0
	SC	0	0	0	0	0

Data from Gill FM, Sleeper LA, Weiner SJ, et al: Clinical events in the first decade in a cohort of infants with sickle cell disease. Blood 1995; 86:776.

Children with functional asplenia fail to respond to intravenously administered antigen,[474] even when the phagocytic function of the spleen has been restored by transfusion. As in other asplenic individuals, however, these children do normally show a response to intramuscularly administered antigen, such as pneumococcal vaccine.[475, 476]

Levels of serum immunoglobulins are normal or increased in children with sickle cell anemia.[476–478] However, the serum is deficient in heat-labile opsonizing activity[479] related to an abnormality of the properdin pathway,[480, 481] which is specific for the phagocytosis of pneumococci. There is an increased activation of complement via the alternate pathway[482] and no intrinsic defect in the complement system.[483] Opsonic activity can be reconstituted *in vitro* by addition of only the F(ab')$_2$ fragments of capsular antibodies to *S. pneumoniae*.[484] This abnormal opsonic activity and associated functional asplenia may partially explain the propensity for pneumococcal infections.

Boggs and co-workers[485] have demonstrated that the chronic leukocytosis of sickle cell disease is a reflection of a shift of granulocytes from the marginating to the circulating pool, with a high granulocyte turnover rate. Neutrophil chemotaxis is normal to slightly reduced, and no specific neutrophil abnormality has been found in patients with SS disease.[486–488] Epidemiologic studies have shown a positive correlation between chronic leukocytosis and early mortality[346, 375] and many episodes of acute chest syndromes.

Recurrent pneumococcal infections have been described in patients with sickle cell disease.[489] In one series, patients with serious invasive bacterial infections are 4.8 and 15.8 times more likely to have a second or third infection, suggesting that a subgroup of patients with SS disease have an increased susceptibility to infections.[490]

Treatment. Because of the increased incidence of serious bacterial infections in patients with sickle cell anemia, the index of suspicion for infection should always be high. In general, the higher the patient's temperature,[491] leukocyte count, and sedimentation rate,[492] the higher the probability of a serious bacterial infection. Unfortunately, however, the wide variability in the temperature and laboratory values of children with bacteremia does not permit an accurate prediction of whether an individual febrile child has bacteremia. The following are guidelines for empirical evaluation and treatment of the febrile child younger than age 12:

- Perform complete blood cell count, urinalysis, chest radiography, and cultures of blood, urine, and throat.
- "Toxic" children, or those with temperatures greater than 39.9°C, should be treated with parenteral antibiotics promptly, before radiographs are taken or the results of laboratory tests are available. These children should be admitted to the hospital.
- Lumbar puncture should be performed on toxic children and those with any signs of meningitis.
- Children with temperatures less than 40°C, but with infiltrate on a chest radiograph, a white blood cell count greater than 30,000/mm^3 or less than 500/mm^3, a platelet count less than 100,000/mm^3, a

hemoglobin level less than 5 g/dL, or a history of prior sepsis should be treated parenterally and admitted to the hospital.

- Children with temperatures less than 40°C, a normal chest radiograph, a normal leukocyte count, and reliable parents can be treated with a long-acting antibiotic (e.g., ceftriaxone, 50 to 75 mg/kg parenterally) observed over a period of hours and be discharged home for follow-up evaluation and repeated antibiotic dosing the next day.[493] Outpatient prophylaxis with long-acting cephalosporins, however, must be reevaluated with the emergence of penicillin- and cephalosporin-resistant *S. pneumoniae*.
- Antibiotics should be selected based on their ability to kill both pneumococci and *H. influenzae* and to penetrate the CNS: in areas in which β-lactamase–producing *H. influenzae* or penicillin- and cephalosporin-resistant pneumococci are regularly encountered, these issues should be considered when a drug is chosen.
- If children do well, and culture results remain negative after 48 to 72 hours, antibiotics can be discontinued.
- Documented sepsis should be treated parenterally for a minimum of 1 week.
- Bacterial meningitis should be treated for a minimum of 10 days parenterally or for at least 1 week after the cerebrospinal fluid has been sterilized.

Patients with infiltrate on the chest radiograph should have cultures of sputum, blood, and stool and be treated as described for acute chest syndrome. Because of the high incidence of pneumococcal, chlamydial, and mycoplasmal pneumonia, patients should be treated with an appropriate antipneumococcal agent and macrolide antibiotic. *Mycoplasma pneumoniae* infection may present as a lobar infiltrate,[494] and the presence of a positive cold agglutinin, albeit nonspecific, should be an indication for erythromycin. A stool culture positive for *Salmonella* may be the only evidence for pneumonia caused by *Salmonella*. In most instances, no confirmation of the bacteria will be available, and the patient should receive at least a 1-week course of antibiotics to cover for pneumococcal and *H. influenzae* infection.

Patients with clinical findings that are highly suggestive of osteomyelitis should have needle aspirate and culture of the lesion. After cultures are obtained, children who appear acutely ill should be given antibiotics. The antibiotics chosen should include agents effective against *Salmonella* and *Staphylococcus aureus*. Antibiotics should be discontinued or modified when culture reports are available.

Prevention. Attempts to prevent pneumococcal disease in patients with sickle cell anemia have focused on prophylactic antibiotics and vaccines. Prophylactic penicillin was first shown to be effective in the prevention of pneumococcal disease by John and associates,[495] who used monthly intramuscular injections of long-acting penicillin. However, if penicillin prophylaxis was terminated after age 3, an increase in pneumococcal infections was noted in the children who previously received penicillin. Gaston and co-workers,[496] in a blinded placebo-controlled clinical trial in the United States, showed that

84 percent of the pneumococcal infections in children younger than age 5 could be prevented with oral penicillin (125 mg twice a day). As a result of this landmark study, aggressive newborn screening programs have been organized throughout the United States, so that all children with sickle cell anemia can be identified and penicillin prophylaxis can be started by 8 weeks of age. In patients in whom penicillin is discontinued after 5 years no increased incidence in infections is seen compared with those who continue to receive prophylaxis,[497] and there are conflicting data regarding the increased risks of penicillin-resistant pneumococcal colonization while patients receive prophylaxis.[498, 499] Our approach to prophylaxis is as follows:

- Give prophylaxis to all newborns with SS disease, S-β[0]-thalassemia, and SC disease. (Some practitioners prefer not to treat infants with SC disease because their splenic dysfunction typically appears later in life.)
- Start as early as possible—optimally by 8 weeks of age.
- Prescribe penicillin, 125 mg orally, twice a day until age 3. At age 3, increase the dose to 250 mg orally, twice a day. Penicillin can be stopped after 5 years of age without resulting in an increased incidence of infection. Many practitioners stop penicillin at 5 to 6 years of age, with penicillin kept readily available at home, school, and daycare, while traveling, and so on, for prompt administration for fever.
- Prescribe erythromycin ethyl succinate, 10 mg/kg orally, twice a day for patients allergic to penicillin.
- Educate families about the importance of compliance and the early recognition of signs of infection.

Polyvalent pneumococcal vaccine has been shown to be effective in eliciting a normal antibody response, increasing pneumococcal opsonizing activity, and reducing the incidence of pneumococcal disease.[482, 500, 501] Both a heptavalent and a 24-valent pneumococcal vaccine are commercially available. The 24-valent vaccine represents 90 percent of the common serotypes of pathogenic pneumococci. The response of children younger than 2 years of age to this vaccine is relatively poor,[502] and the response of 2-year-old children to two common pneumococcal serotypes, 6A and 19, is also poor.[503] Revaccination after 4 years improved protective levels of antibody without serious adverse reactions in children.[504] The newer heptavalent vaccine, when given in repeated doses to children younger than 1 year of age, is effective in mounting antibody titers to the capsular antigens it includes and increases opsonizing activity; thus, it is recommended for all children including those with sickle cell disease.[501, 505, 506] *H. influenzae* vaccine is immunogenic in children with sickle cell disease and should be given on the same schedule used for normal infants.[507, 508]

Although prophylactic penicillin and new vaccines are clearly effective in preventing some overwhelming infections, several children who were vaccinated previously and who had been receiving oral penicillin have had fatal pneumococcal sepsis.[509] Although the incidence of penicillin-resistant pneumococcus was not demonstrated in patients receiving prophylaxis there appeared to be an emergence of multidrug-resistant pneumococcus in patients treated greater for longer than 5 years.[498] These examples underscore the need for physicians to emphasize the importance of compliance with drug regimens and to continue to have a high index of suspicion of sepsis in the febrile child with sickle cell disease.

Chronic Organ Damage

Cardiovascular System. Abnormal cardiac findings are present in most patients with sickle cell anemia[509–513] and are primarily the result of chronic anemia and the compensatory increased cardiac output.[514] On physical examination, the most common findings are systolic ejection murmur, S_3, split S_1, suprasternal notch thrill, and diastolic murmur.[511] Cardiac findings may closely resemble the findings in rheumatic valvular disease or congenital cardiac anomalies. Often, echocardiography is necessary to diagnose abnormal cardiac structure. Cardiomegaly is found in most patients, with electrocardiographic findings of left ventricular hypertrophy in about 50 percent of patients.[512]

In view of the fact that the hallmark of sickle cell disease is vaso-occlusion, it is remarkable that myocardial infarction is an extremely rare event.[512, 515] In one review of the postmortem literature in sickle cell disease including examination of 153 hearts, only four infarcts were reported.[515] Despite the high oxygen extraction in the coronary circulation, blood in the coronary sinus contains no more sickled forms than does blood in the general circulation,[516] presumably because of the short transit time through the coronary vessels.[514] Atherosclerosis is virtually absent in this population, seen in one study in none of the hearts of 100 patients (55 of whom were 16 to 47 years old, with a median age of 30) examined at autopsy.[515] This is in marked contrast to the Vietnam study,[517] in which atherosclerosis was found in 45 percent of 105 individuals who were battle casualties. When injected at autopsy, the heart from a patient with sickle cell disease has normal patent coronary arteries, often of larger caliber than that seen in normal hearts.[518] The cause of this apparent protective effect against atherosclerosis is unknown but may involve genetic or dietary factors or the anemia itself.

The most comprehensive prospective examination of cardiac function in an unselected population of patients with sickle cell anemia was done as part of the Cooperative Study of Sickle Cell Disease.[519] Echocardiography was performed on 191 patients aged 13 and older who had stable disease, and all of the measurements were done centrally by an investigator without access to other patient data. After appropriate adjustment for body surface area, left and right ventricles, aortic root, and left atrium were found to be larger than normal. Significant wall thickening was found only in the septum. The left ventricular dilatation correlated with hemoglobin and age, suggesting that the major cardiac findings are indeed related to the years of increased stroke volume in compensation for anemia and abnormal rheology. The finding of normal left and right ventricular function suggests that if a specific "sickle myocardiopathy" exists, it is rare. Pulmonary hypertension and right ventricular dysfunction are also rare, except in those with acute or chronic pulmonary disease.[520, 521] As discussed in the section on chronic lung disease, patients with cor pulmonale and right ventricular dysfunction have a high mortality rate.

Arrhythmias are rare under usual conditions, although in one study, during the first hour of treatment for painful crisis, 80 percent of patients had arrhythmias: 67 percent atrial and 60 percent ventricular. These were not clinically significant and probably represented response to pain.[522]

The blood pressure in patients with sickle cell anemia (and to a lesser extent SC disease) in stable condition is lower than in a race-, gender-, and age-matched normal population (Table 19-3).[419] This may be related to the tendency to lose sodium and water in the urine. This study demonstrates that high blood pressure is a risk factor for stroke and early mortality and that the diagnosis of high blood pressure depends on knowing the "normal values" for this population (Table 19-3). Blood pressures greater than the 90 percent percentile in this population overlap with the normal range in a normal population, and a steady-state blood pressure of 140/90 is an ominous sign. Such patients should be considered candidates for antihypertensive therapy.

Renal System. Hyposthenuria, hematuria, the nephrotic syndrome, and uremia are the major renal complications of sickle cell disease.[523] In addition, the production of erythropoietin in response to anemia may be lower in older patients with SS disease, possibly due to primary renal disease.[524]

Hyposthenuria[525, 526] develops early in childhood and, as with functional asplenia, may be temporarily reversed with a transfusion.[527, 528] The hypertonic environment of the renal medulla promotes sickling even at normal PO_2,[529] which leads to decreased medullary blood flow and derangement of the countercurrent multiplier. An abnormality of the countercurrent multiplier may be the mechanism for hyposthenuria, or, as suggested by Buckalew and Someren,[523] hyposthenuria may be due to decreased flow to nephrons with long loops of Henle and preservation of flow to nephrons with short loops. The obligatory water loss results in a tendency for dehydration and invalidates the use of urine volume or concentration as an indicator of the patient's state of hydration. Nocturia and enuresis are common complaints of these patients, who excrete large volumes of dilute urine.[529] Urinary sodium losses may be high and result in significant hyponatremia.[531] A renal tubular acidification defect,[532, 533] as well as hyporeninemic hypoaldosteronism[534] and impaired potassium excretion,[535] has been identified. In one review, de Jong and Statius van Eps[536] emphasized that renal vasodilating prostaglandins are increased in patients with sickle cell disease, leading to a compensatory increase in renal blood flow, glomerular filtration rate, and proximal tubular activity.

Although hematuria is usually mild, bleeding is occasionally severe enough to cause significant blood loss.[537] Papillary necrosis is usually the underlying anatomic defect.[538] Administration of ε-aminocaproic acid has been suggested to stop severe hematuria that is refractory to transfusion,[539] but this substance must be used cautiously because of the risk of ureteral or pelvic clotting and obstruction. In patients with long-standing hematuria, supplemental iron may be necessary to prevent iron deficiency. Hematuria may also be the presenting symptom of a renal tumor. A surprisingly high incidence of renal medullary carcinoma has been reported in adults and children with sickle cell anemia and sickle trait.[540-542]

Uremia is a rare complication in children with sickle cell disease that may follow a symptom complex of nephrotic syndrome[543] with glomerulonephritis. The nature of the glomerular lesion is unknown, and it may represent a response to iron deposition,[544] antigen-antibody complex,[547] or mesangial phagocytosis of fragmented sickled cells.[546, 547] Recently an association between parvovirus infection with or without an antecedent aplastic crises has been associated with acute glomerulonephritis.[548, 549] Microalbuminuria as manifested by a ratio of albumin to creatinine greater than 20 is seen in more than 40 percent of adults and in a similar percentage of children 10 to 18 years of age with sickle cell disease.[550] Recently a study of 442 children with sickle cell disease followed for 10 years showed that proteinuria occurred in 6.2 percent and the incidence increased to 12 percent in teenagers. Proteinuria was associated with lower hemoglobin levels, higher MCV, higher white cell counts, and more clinically severe disease.[551] A

TABLE 19-3. Blood Pressure in Patients with Sickle Cell Anemia

	Percentile	Age (yr)										
		2–3	4–5	6–7	8–9	10–11	12–13	14–15	16–17	18–24	25–34	35–44
FEMALES												
Systolic	50	90	95	96	96	104	106	110	110	110	110	110
	90	100	110	110	110	110	118	120	122	122	125	130
Diastolic	50	52	60	60	60	60	62	70	70	64	68	70
	90	62	70	70	70	74	74	80	78	80	80	84
MALES												
Systolic	50	90	95	100	100	100	110	108	112	112	114	110
	90	104	110	108	116	112	120	120	128	130	130	132
Diastolic	50	54	60	60	60	60	64	64	70	68	70	70
	90	66	68	68	70	70	72	78	80	80	80	84

Data from Pegelow CH, Colangelo L, Stunberg M, et al: Natural history of blood pressure in sickle cell disease. Am S Med 1997; 102:171–177.

study of 381 adults with sickle cell disease demonstrated that 7 percent had elevated serum creatinine levels and 26 percent had proteinuria.[552] Ten patients with proteinuria underwent renal biopsy, and the glomerular lesions showed perihilar focal segmental sclerosis and glomerular enlargement similar to findings in an animal model with glomerular hypertension and efferent arteriolar vasoconstriction. To test the animal analogy, these patients were treated with enalapril, an angiotensin-converting enzyme inhibitor that had been shown to decrease efferent arteriolar constriction. In all treated patients, the level of proteinuria fell during treatment and returned toward abnormal after discontinuation. Work is underway to determine whether early and chronic treatment of patients with proteinuria with enalapril can prevent the evolution to renal failure. Bakir and associates[547] estimated that 4 percent of adult patients with SS disease develop nephrosis and that two thirds of these patients then develop renal failure. Renal failure can be managed with peritoneal dialysis, hemodialysis, and transplantation.[553, 554]

Hepatobiliary System. Liver and biliary tract abnormalities are commonly seen in sickle cell disease[555, 556] and are the result of cholelithiasis, hepatic infarction, and transfusion-related hepatitis.

Bilirubin stones are also commonly seen.[557, 558] The incidence of gallstones as detected by ultrasound in children with SS disease has been studied in two large series.[559, 560] Of 226 patients aged 5 to 13 selected randomly from a group of children with SS disease identified at birth, 13 percent had gallstones,[555] a value lower than that found in a survey of clinic patients studied by Sarnaik and associates.[559] In this report, the incidence of gallstones was 12 percent by 2 to 4 years of age.[559] With advancing age, the incidence increased gradually, reaching 42 percent in the 15- to 18-year-old age-group. Fourteen of the 226 patients were noted to have "sludge" in the gallbladder and were followed with repeated ultrasonograms for up to 2 years. Four developed stones, 4 had no further evidence of sludge, and the conditions of 6 remained unchanged. Fourteen patients had symptoms of biliary tract disease. Ten had stones, 3 had sludge, and 1 had a normal gallbladder. The patients with stones had an average steady-state total bilirubin value (3.8 ± 0.3 mg/dL) that was higher than that of the patients without stones (2.6 ± 0.12 mg/dL). Total hemoglobin levels and reticulocyte counts did not differ between the two groups. Evidence indicates that children tolerate elective cholecystectomy with little morbidity if they are prepared properly for surgery.[561, 562] Laparoscopic cholecystectomy has been particularly effective for reducing the postoperative hospital stay in children with sickle cell disease.[563] In contrast, operating during the acute phase is associated with a significant risk of complication.[390]

Intrahepatic sickling can result in massive hyperbilirubinemia,[387] elevated liver enzyme values, and a painful syndrome mimicking acute cholecystitis[388] or viral hepatitis.[564] Fulminant hepatic failure with massive cholestasis and rapidly progressing hepatic encephalopathy and shock has been described as a rare, often fatal, complication of sickle cell disease that may resolve with exchange transfusion.[565–567]

A review of postmortem liver findings among 70 patients with sickle cell disease examined at Johns Hopkins Hospital[568] revealed evidence of unexplained hepatic injury. Hepatic necrosis, portal fibrosis, regenerative nodules, and cirrhosis were common features, thought to be a consequence of recurrent vascular obstruction and repair. In contrast, 19 liver biopsy specimens from symptomatic patients with SS disease failed to show necrosis and more often showed evidence of acute or subacute infection.[569]

Eyes. Tortuosity and sacculation of conjunctival vessels are seen in more than 90 percent of patients with sickle cell disease. These lesions are best seen in the lower temporal area, disappear after exchange transfusion, and are curiously related to the number of ISCs in the peripheral blood.[570] They have no deleterious effect on the eye.

Retinopathy is classified as either proliferative or nonproliferative. Nonproliferative retinopathy probably results from retinal arteriolar infarction with adjacent hemorrhage and requires no therapy. Depending on the age of the lesion and the layer and extension of the hemorrhage, the result can be a salmon patch, schism cavity, vitreous hemorrhage, or black sunburst.[571] In two patients with documented acute arteriolar occlusion, salmon patches developed in a matter of hours to days, with atrophic schism cavities evolving in 3 to 4 months.[572] In older patients, angioid streaks are common, but the cause is unknown.[573, 574]

The more serious complication is proliferative retinopathy, which has been classified by Goldberg[575] as follows: stage 1, peripheral arteriolar occlusions; stage 2, arteriolarvenular anastomoses; stage 3, neovascularization; stage 4, vitreous hemorrhages; and stage 5, retinal detachment. Because these lesions may eventually cause blindness, laser therapy to occlude feeding vessels of advanced proliferative lesions has been advocated. Unfortunately, photocoagulation is associated with the risks of neovascularization of the choroid[576] and retinal breaks,[577] complications that can result in blindness. The dilemma of choosing a therapy that can potentially cause blindness for a lesion that can potentially cause blindness is complicated by the observation that some proliferative lesions heal spontaneously by autoinfarction. In one study of untreated retinopathy in Jamaica, 567 eyes were observed for 8 years.[578] Proliferative retinopathy was initially present in 12 percent of the eyes; another 8 percent developed retinopathy during follow-up. Blindness was the result in 12 percent of the eyes with retinopathy. In the original group of eyes with retinopathy, 30 percent developed progressive retinopathy, 39 percent showed spontaneous regression, and the remaining 30 percent showed a mix of regression and progression. In another prospective Jamaican study, treatment of retinopathy was compared with no treatment.[579] No statistical difference in visual acuity between the two groups was reported. Macular ischemia and colorblindness have been reported to be prevalent in patients with SS disease without evidence on ophthalmologic examination of retinal lesions.[580, 581]

Rarely, acute painless loss of vision is the result of central retinal artery occlusion. Although such lesions may resolve spontaneously, exchange transfusion has been recommended for bilateral disease.[582]

Blunt trauma to the eye may result in hyphema (bleeding into the anterior chamber). Because the conditions in this chamber overwhelmingly favor sickling, any hemoglobin-containing red cell will sickle and may cause obstructive glaucoma and blindness. This blood should be evacuated as soon as possible to preserve vision.[583] This condition is one of the true ocular emergencies that occurs in patients with sickle trait as well as sickle cell disease.

Skin. Leg ulcers usually do not occur in childhood. In adolescence and adulthood, ulcers may be a crippling symptom. This skin lesion is seen with other chronic hemolytic anemias such as hereditary spherocytosis, thalassemia, elliptocytosis, and pyruvate kinase deficiency[584] and therefore may not represent vaso-occlusion. Ulceration may result from increased venous pressure in the legs caused by the expanded blood volume in the hypertrophied bone marrow.[585] In tropical areas in which shoes are not usually worn and insect bites are common, leg ulcers are often seen.[586] In Jamaica, leg ulcers typically start in the 10- to 20-year-old age-group and eventually appear in 75 percent of adults. Koshy and colleagues[587] have reported data from the Cooperative Study of Sickle Cell Disease regarding leg ulcers in patients with sickle cell disease. Leg ulcers appear to be less common in individuals with two α genes than in those with three or four α genes. In addition, low steady-state hemoglobin values were associated with a higher incidence of ulcer formation. The incidence of leg ulcers appears to decrease consistently with increases in HbF production.[587] There is decreased venous outflow in the lower extremities of patients with leg ulcers compared with that in patients without ulcers, suggesting that venous incompetence may contribute to the development of these lesions or their failure to heal.[588] Chronic lesions become a major source of morbidity and have a profound negative impact on educational achievement and employment.[589] Usually present over the medial surface of the lower tibia or just posterior to the medial malleolus, they begin as a small depression with central necrosis and, if unattended, widen to encircle the entire lower leg. Débridement, scrupulous hygiene, topical antibiotics, rest, and elevation of the leg are the mainstays of therapy. In some patients, protection of the ulcer by the application of a soft sponge-rubber doughnut and low-pressure elastic bandage seems to be beneficial. One report suggested that an RGD peptide matrix designed to mimic the normal matrix was beneficial.[590] Close attention to improved venous circulation by the use of above-the-knee elastic stockings may prevent ulceration. If ulcers persist despite optimal care, transfusion therapy may be used and consideration given to split-thickness skin grafts. Transfusion therapy is sometimes effective, but, in many patients, the ulcers either do not heal or recur after this therapy is discontinued. Oral administration of zinc sulfate may promote healing of leg ulcers,[591] and peripheral vasodilator therapy appears to be ineffective.[592]

Ears. Sensorineural hearing loss at both ends of the auditory spectrum was found in a substantial number of patients with sickle cell disease in Jamaica.[593, 594] In an American study, 12 percent of children with SS disease had high-frequency sensorineural hearing loss.[595]

Interestingly, although there was no increased otitis media or meningitis in the affected group, five of the six children with CNS disease had abnormal hearing. The pathologic change in the auditory apparatus appears to be sickling in the cochlear vasculature with destruction of hair cells.[596]

Skeleton. Skeletal changes in sickle cell disease are common[352, 597, 598] and are due to expansion of the marrow cavity and repeated bone infarction. The expanded marrow is best seen in radiographs of the thickened calvaria with a wide diploic space. Overgrowth of the anterior maxilla may lead to severe orthodontic and cosmetic problems. Vertebrae are generally flattened, with a characteristic biconcave deformity called "codfish vertebrae." In older patients, vertebral disease may cause chronic back pain. These individuals need to be treated as other patients who have chronic back disease—with appropriate exercises, braces, bed rest, muscle relaxants, and moral support. Another major chronic bone complication of sickle cell disease is aseptic necrosis. In children, the most common cause of aseptic necrosis of the femoral head is sickle cell disease. As shown in Figure 19–11 the incidence is relatively low in children and is remarkably increased in patients with SS disease and coexistent α-thalassemia.[599] The patients at highest risk of developing this complication were those with the highest rates of painful crises and those with the highest hematocrit values. Milner and colleagues,[599] reporting the findings of the Cooperative Study of Sickle Cell Disease, hypothesized that the pathophysiologic basis of this lesion is sludging in marrow sinusoids, marrow necrosis, healing with increased intramedullary pressure, bone resorption, and eventually collapse. The diagnosis is made radiographically; the classic spectrum of findings ranges from subepiphyseal lucency and widened joint space to flattening or fragmentation and scarring of the epiphysis. Although roughly one half of the patients in whom the diagnosis was made on the basis of screening radiographs were asymptomatic, significant chronic pain and limited joint mobility plagued the others. Treatment options are limited, and results are often disappointing. Strict bed rest is helpful in a minority of patients,[600] with little or no evidence to support the use of chronic transfusion therapy. Injection of cement[601] and core decompression[602] have been used successfully in some patients. It is possible that these procedures might be particularly helpful in patients with very early disease, perhaps those in whom the condition is diagnosed on the basis of MRI scans even before deformities are apparent on conventional films. A prospective study in a high-risk population such as young adults with SS disease and α-thalassemia would be helpful in determining the ultimate benefit of such treatment. Unfortunately, total hip replacement may be the only option for severely compromised patients. In the study of Milner and colleagues,[603] 17 percent of patients underwent hip replacement, 30 percent of replaced hips required surgical revision within 4.5 years, and more than 60 percent of patients continued to have pain and limited mobility postoperatively. Epidemiologic data for aseptic necrosis of the humeral head are virtually identical to those for the femur.[603] In general, however, the patients have fewer symptoms, and the use of shoulder arthroplasty was exceedingly rare.

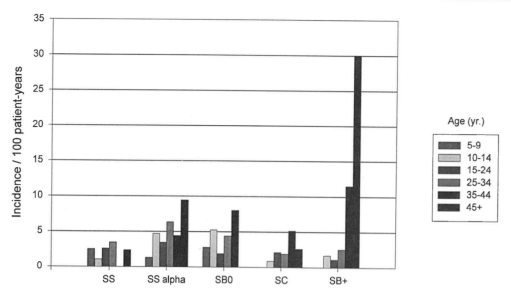

FIGURE 19–11. Incidence of osteonecrosis of the femoral head per 100 patient-years by genotype. (Data from Milner PF, Kraus AP, Sebes JI, et al: Sickle cell disease as a cause of osteonecrosis of the femoral head. N Engl J Med 1991; 325:1476–1481.)

Lungs. In contrast to the acute chest syndrome, chronic lung disease has been difficult to define and quantitate. In older children, lung volumes are reduced[604, 605] compared with those of the normal white population but are appropriate when compared with those of a black control population.[606] Resting arterial PO_2 in asymptomatic children with sickle cell disease is typically 65 to 85 mm Hg (normal >87 mm Hg). There are large alveolar-arterial PO_2 differences in room air (27 to 42 mm Hg; normal <16 mm Hg) and with 100 percent O_2 (186 to 246 mm Hg; normal <86 mm Hg). These values are consistent with increased pulmonary shunting of 12 to 16 percent (normal <7 percent).[606] The decreased membrane-diffusing capacity observed can be explained on the basis of anemia alone and does not suggest a substantial element of pulmonary vascular occlusion. Cor pulmonale has been described,[521] and in one survey of adults, fatal progressive pulmonary disease may have been related to a history of previous chest syndromes.[607] However, the relationship between episodes of acute chest syndrome and chronic lung disease has been difficult to establish reproducibly. Recently, an increase in obstructive lung disease was documented in adult patients who had two to four episodes of acute chest syndrome compared with patients with no history of acute chest syndrome.[608] In a Jamaican study that compared 20 patients with at least six episodes of acute chest syndrome to 20 patients without chest syndrome, no difference in pulmonary artery pressure was found using echocardiography and Doppler evaluation.[609] In another study, patients with SS disease were found to have abnormally small lungs, but this abnormality was not related to episodes of acute chest syndrome.[610] In a study of infants 3 to 30 months of age, restrictive lung disease was present in 3 of 12 infants and was not related to a history of acute chest syndrome.[611] These studies suggest that subtle subacute damage to the lungs proceeds even in the absence of acute disease. Hydroxyurea therapy[107] reduces the incidence of recurrent acute chest syndrome but does not lead to improved pulmonary function. In 24 patients with

a history of chest syndromes studied after bone marrow transplantation, 22 showed no improvement and 2 patients showed worse pulmonary function after the transplant.[278]

Central Nervous System. Abnormal neurologic findings in sickle cell disease were discussed earlier. Changes on CT and MRI scans may antedate neurologic dysfunction and represent subclinical infarcts.[400, 401, 403, 612] It is now clear that cognitive functioning and fine motor skills are impaired in patients with sickle cell disease with silent infarcts as diagnosed by an MRI scan.[613] Because abnormal Doppler or MRI studies can be seen in infants with decreased neurocognitive performance, these radiologic studies are being considered as screening tools to select very young patients for experimental therapies that may prevent further CNS damage.

Growth and Development. The birth weight of infants with sickle cell anemia is normal.[614] Subsequently, a pattern of delayed growth emerges. Detailed anthropomorphic measurements of Jamaican children revealed decreased limb length, sitting height, and skinfold thickness, with increased chest anteroposterior diameter[615] possibly related to cardiomegaly.[616] Height and weight growth curves (Fig. 19–12) for individuals with sickle cell disease in the United States were generated as part of the Cooperative Study of Sickle Cell Disease, sponsored by the Sickle Cell Disease Branch of the National Heart, Lung, and Blood Institute.[617] The important features of these curves are that they are different from those for normal black control subjects, that weight is more affected than height, and that patients with sickle cell anemia and S-β^0-thalassemia experience more delay in growth than patients with SC disease and S-β^+thalassemia. In general, by the end of adolescence, the patients with sickle cell disease have caught up with control subjects in height but not weight. The reason for this poor weight gain is not understood but is likely to represent increased caloric requirements in these anemic patients with increased bone marrow activity and cardiovascular compensation.[618] In a

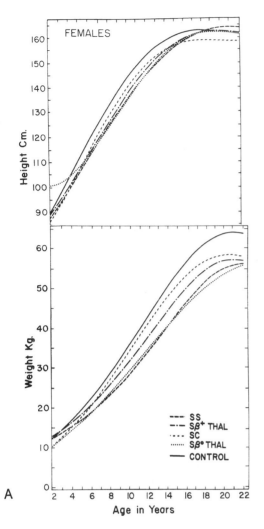

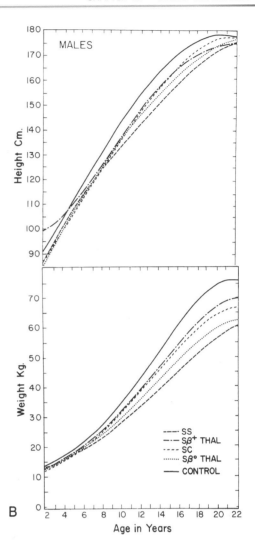

FIGURE 19–12. Height and weight growth curves for females *(A)* and males *(B)* 2 to 22 years of age, according to type of hemoglobinopathy. Shown are the 50 percent curves. (From Platt OS, Rosenstock W, Espeland MA: Influence of sickle hemoglobinopathies on growth and development. N Engl J Med 1984; 311:7–12. Reprinted, by permission, from *The New England Journal of Medicine.*)

second large prospective study in Jamaica, both height and weight were significantly lower than that of age- and sex-matched control subjects as early as 2 years of age.[619] Zinc deficiency has been suggested as a cause of poor growth in children with SS disease,[620, 621] but this suggestion has not been confirmed.[622] Growth hormone levels and growth hormone stimulation studies appear to be normal in children with SS disease who have impaired growth.[623] A review of nutritional studies in patients with SS disease is available,[624] and one study suggested that hyperalimentation may be useful in some patients.[625]

Sexual development is also delayed in patients with sickle cell disease.[617] This delay is found in both males and females and follows the same pattern as delays in height and weight in other hemoglobinopathies. The estimated median age of attainment of Tanner stage for each hemoglobinopathy is listed in Table 19–4. For females (regardless of hemoglobinopathy), menarche status is a function of age and weight. This normal relationship between menarche and weight suggests that in females, delayed sexual maturity is constitutional. This was confirmed in a careful analysis of female fertility in Jamaica, which revealed no difference in the interval between sexual exposure and pregnancy between patients and control subjects.[626] Most males do undergo delayed sexual maturation, also suggesting constitutional delay. However, among males there does seem to be evidence of decreased fertility, with abnormal sperm motility, morphologic characteristics, and number.[627] Transient primary hypogonadism[628] and hypothalamic hypogonadism responsive to clomiphene[629] also have been described.

Psychologic Aspects. As in any chronic disease, patients require strong, sympathetic support. Most patients with sickle cell anemia handle their illness very well. In one study,[630] patients did not differ from control subjects in personal, social, or total adjustment. Interestingly, patients showed less acute anxiety compared with control subjects, although the patients did demonstrate a lower self-concept. Another study points out the pitfalls in interpreting excessive fatigue as depression in these children.[631] Problems of particular concern to patients are coping with chronic pain, inability to keep up

TABLE 19–4. Estimated Median Age at Attainment of Tanner Stages, According to Hemoglobinopathy

Tanner Stage	Median Age			
	SS	SC	S-β⁺	S-β⁰
FEMALES				
Breasts 2	11.8	9.8	10.6	11.8
3	13.5	11.9	12.6	12.8
4	15	13.9	13.8	14.8
5	17.3	16	16.5	17.2
Public hair 2	12	10.1	10	11.5
3	13.5	11.8	11.2	12.8
4	15.2	14	13.8	14.2
5	19.2	17	17	20.8
MALES				
Penis 2	12	10.4	11.9	12.4
3	14.2	13	13	13.2
4	16	14.1	13.5	15.5
5	17.6	16.6	16.6	18.8
Public hair 2	13.2	11.5	12	13.2
3	14.8	13.2	13	13.9
4	16.2	14.2	13.9	16.2
5	17.9	16.6	17.1	18.5

Reprinted with permission from Platt OS, Rosenstock MSPH, Espeland MA: Influence of sickle hemoglobinopathies on growth and development. N Engl J Med 1984; 311:7.

with peers, fears of premature death, and delayed sexual maturity. Discussion of prenatal diagnosis and selective abortion, particularly in a patient's own family, increase doubts about self-worth. These issues need to be addressed openly and frankly and with appropriate psychologic support. Self-help groups for patients and families are gaining in effectiveness and popularity throughout the country.

TREATMENT

Routine Health Maintenance

Patients with sickle cell anemia should be followed on a routine basis (Table 19–5). Regular visits with routine laboratory studies when the patient is well help establish both the individual's steady-state normal values (e.g., hemoglobin, reticulocytes, white blood cells, differential, platelet count, erythrocyte sedimentation rate, chest film, and electrocardiogram) and baseline physical findings (e.g., icterus, cardiomegaly, murmurs, and organomegaly). These baseline data are extremely helpful in sorting out problems when the patient is ill.

Careful evaluation of the history of intervals between painful crises may provide insight into factors that provoke them. Continuing education of patients and families on how to avoid and treat painful episodes will reduce the morbidity and hospitalization rate and will promote the patient's sense of independence. Education should also include genetic counseling of the parents with the goal that they understand the risks of sickle cell disease occurring in children they may have in the future.

Careful attention should be paid to routine immunization schedules; all patients should receive pneumococcal *H. influenzae* and hepatitis B vaccines. Prophylactic penicillin should be given to all children younger than 5 years of age.[496] Most important, the patient and family should be educated about the importance of early detection and treatment of infection.

Although folic acid, 1 mg/day, is recommended for prevention of folate deficiency in adults, no definite advantage for this therapy has been seen in children.[632] Iron deficiency is extremely rare because of the hemolysis-induced increased absorption of gastrointestinal iron. Iron supplements are used only when iron deficiency is documented or when blood loss is chronic (e.g., with hematuria).

In many centers, transcranial Doppler ultrasonography is used to screen children with sickle cell anemia who are free of neurologic signs or symptoms to determine if they have an increased risk of stroke. Children with internal carotid or middle cerebral arterial blood flow of 200 cm/sec or higher have been shown to benefit from prophylactic maintenance transfusion to prevent stroke.[633] Special training of the ultrasonographer is needed to ensure that the results are valid in this clinical setting. The ideal age range for and timing of screening have not yet been determined.

Ophthalmologic examinations should be started at school age and repeated every few years unless retinopathy is discovered. For patients with retinopathy, regular follow-up and fluorescein angiographic examinations are necessary to establish the progression of the lesion and to determine appropriate therapy.

Regular dental care is critical to prevent intraoral lesions, such as mandibular osteomyelitis, that might predispose the patient to infections.[634]

Birth control options should be discussed as with any adolescent patient. Barrier methods of contraception and low-dose estrogen oral contraceptives can be used safely.[635]

The Painful Crisis

Most painful crises can be successfully treated at home with increased fluid intake and oral analgesics. If the pain is too severe to be relieved by oral analgesics or if the patient cannot maintain adequate fluid intake, the episode must be treated in the hospital. Hospital management of a painful crisis includes hydration and analgesia. In dehydrated patients, the intravenous fluid rate is usually one and one-half times maintenance (2250 mL/m²/day). In some patients, however, this expansion of intravascular volume may not be tolerated. Regular monitoring of vital signs during fluid administration is essential to prevent iatrogenic cardiac failure. Serum electrolyte levels must be checked early and intravenous solutions adjusted appropriately. Although theoretically sound, the use of intravenous bicarbonate has not been shown to be effective.[636] Administration of oxygen through a face mask has little therapeutic value unless the patient is hypoxic. Furthermore, Embury and colleagues[637] have shown that continuous oxygen inhalation can suppress erythropoiesis, with reticulocyte counts falling within days. In addition, a painful crisis may result from rebound marrow

TABLE 19–5. Routine Health Maintenance for Patients with Sickle Cell Anemia

	Age (yr)			
	<5	**5–10**	**10–20**	**20+**
ISSUES/ANTICIPATORY GUIDANCE				
Penicillin prophylaxi	⟶	→		
Splenic sequestration	⟶	→		
Fever or infection	⟶			→
Coping with pain	⟶			→
Dental care	⟶			→
Groups for parents	⟶		→	
Priapism		⟶		→
Smoking		⟶		→
Self-esteem, independence		⟶		→
Education		⟶		→
Recreation			⟶	→
Puberty, birth control, genetics			⟶	→
Leg ulcer			⟶	→
Career planning			⟶	→
Self-help groups			⟶	→
Family planning, fertility				⟶→
Prognosis				⟶→
LABORATORY				
Complete blood count	1–3/yr	1–2/yr	1–2/yr	1–2/yr
Red cell antigen typing	Once			
Liver function, renal function		Yearly	Yearly	Yearly
Urinalysis	Yearly	Yearly	Yearly	Yearly
SPECIAL STUDIES				
Pulmonary function		q 3–5 yr	q 3–5 yr	q 3–5 yr
Chest radiography		q 3–5 yr	q 2–3 yr	q 2–3 yr
Eye examination		q 3–5 yr	Yearly	Yearly
Transcranial Doppler	Age 2/Yearly	Yearly	Yearly	
TREATMENT				
Penicillin prophylaxis	⟶	→		
Folate				
Pneumococcal vaccine	2 mo	Boosters as recommended		
Haemophilus influenzae vaccine	Infant	Boosters as recommended		
Hepatitis B vaccine	Infant	Boosters as recommended		
Influenza vaccine	Yearly as recommended	⟶		→

activity after the abrupt discontinuation of oxygen therapy or cessation of transfusion programs.[638]

Analgesia must be sufficient to control the pain. "Standard doses" may not be enough for an individual patient. Although narcotic dependence or enhanced narcotic-seeking behavior may be a problem for rare patients, overestimation of the incidence of this unusual situation must not affect the decision to control severe pain.[639] It is unfortunate that subtle misconceptions interfere with provision of appropriate pain relief. In one study of a conceptual model of pain using standardized patient histories, results suggested that patients presenting with a chief complaint of pain with histories of frequent pain crises were given less narcotic by nurses than the identical patients whose histories included "occasional" pain episodes.[640]

When choosing narcotics, one should consider side effects, drug interactions, and serum half-lives. Changes in the route of administration (intravenous, intramuscular, or oral) require adjustments for equianalgesic dosages. Serial intramuscular injections can lead to the formation of sterile abscess and scarring and should be avoided in the treatment of prolonged painful episodes. At the onset of inpatient therapy for severe pain, regular dosage intervals should be used, not "as needed" dosages, thereby avoiding the recurrence of pain and anxiety before the next dose of medicine. High-dose meperidine may cause seizures, particularly if the patient has compromised renal function, which allows accumulation of toxic levels of normeperidine.[641] Hypoventilation is the most serious side effect and must be avoided by careful monitoring of oxygen saturation and the use of oxygen when the patient is hypoxic. Continuous intravenous narcotic therapy in children has been used successfully, but acute chest syndrome may be precipitated by respiratory depression.[642] In one study, epidural anesthesia was used successfully to alleviate pain and maintain or improve oxygenation.[643] The combination of continuous narcotic infusion with patient-controlled boluses is emerging as a particularly effective strategy. Constipation and urinary retention are common problems that should be remedied early.

Sometimes it is virtually impossible to make a patient entirely comfortable with safe doses of narcotics. This frustrating situation needs to be handled with care and sensitivity, with involvement of every member of the patient care team.[644, 645] The addition of nonsteroidal anti-inflammatory agents is helpful for some patients. Others have benefitted from adjuncts to therapy such as acupuncture,[646] biofeedback, and hypnosis.[647] For the rare patient who is incapacitated by recurrent episodes of pain and who spends more time in the hospital than out, chronic outpatient narcotic therapy may be useful.[648] A maintenance transfusion program can be used as a last resort. Although transfusion (even exchange transfusion) rarely works in acute situations, a maintenance program for a few months may be enough for the patient to finish the school year or to complete an important project at work.

Vasodilators have been studied as a possible treatment modality for painful crisis without conclusive results. Administration of cetiedil, a vasodilator that inhibits cell dehydration *in vitro*,[649, 650] in a blinded, controlled clinical trial reduced the mean duration of days in crisis from 4 to 3 days when given intravenously for the first 4 days of crisis.[651]

Several instances of acute gout that mimicked a painful crisis have been reported.[652] However, the increased renal clearance of urate usually prevents this complication.

Transfusion

Patients with sickle cell disease tolerate their chronic anemia well and require transfusions only under certain circumstances—sequestration crisis, CNS infarction, aplastic crisis, preparation for surgery, and hypoxia with acute chest syndrome. In sequestration crisis and aplastic crisis, a standard simple transfusion is necessary to restore a circulating red cell mass. In all other situations, some degree of exchange transfusion is probably preferable so that the increased viscosity due to the higher hematocrit is offset by a reduction in the number of circulating sickle cells. This concept is undergoing considerable scrutiny and debate. As discussed later in the preparation for surgery section, simple transfusion compares favorably with exchange transfusion in the preoperative setting. When rapid reduction of the level of HbS is necessary, as in CNS crisis, an exchange transfusion is preferable. At Johns Hopkins Hospital a routine for exchange transfusions in children with sickle cell disease has been developed. A 60 to 80 percent reduction in the number of circulating sickle cells can be accomplished in 6 to 12 hours by exchanging two times the red cell mass (2 × blood volume × hematocrit). In determining the total volume or the number of units of blood needed for the exchange one must take into consideration the packed red cell mass in a unit of blood (usually 40 percent of 500 mL of whole blood from a single donation). Initial exchanges can be done with packed red cells but when the hematocrit approaches 35 percent, packed cell units should be diluted with appropriate electrolyte solutions or plasma. Sickle trait blood should not be used. A similar procedure has been described by Charache.[653] In those centers in which an automated cell separator is available, a two-volume exchange transfusion can be efficiently accomplished in less than 90 minutes.[437, 438]

Maintenance transfusion programs are designed to suppress the patient's production of sickle cells. Indications for chronic transfusion include prevention of further strokes, chronic heart or pulmonary failure, prolonged hematuria, recurrent priapism, unremitting vaso-occlusive crises, and complicated pregnancy. The degree of suppression needed depends on the reason for the chronic transfusion and individual variability in the suppressive effect of the transfusions.[654] Transfusions that keep the percentage of HbS at less than 30 percent reduce the incidence of recurrent strokes from 70 to less than 10 percent and reduce the incidence of vaso-occlusive crises.[655] Iron overload is ultimately unavoidable but can be treated with desferrioxamine.[656, 657] As previously observed in patients with thalassemia major, the serum ferritin level is a poor predictor of liver iron burden and liver fibrosis; however, high levels of liver iron were not associated with as much liver disease as expected from similar data in patients with thalassemia.[658]

In children who have received multiple transfusions, the rate of alloimmunization is between 7 and 20 percent.[659–662] The likelihood of alloimmunization is related to the number of transfusions, the racial differences between donor and recipients, and as yet unknown genetic factors that control the responsiveness of the recipient to transfused antigens.[663] Ideally, patients with SS disease should receive antigen-matched red cells to reduce the hazard of sensitization. Such a strategy has been demonstrated to reduce sensitization,[664–666] although opinions still vary about the utility of preventing sensitization by using expensive antigen-matched cells compared with providing those cells after sensitization occurs.[667] Potential benefits from the prevention strategy include prevention of complications from the first delayed transfusion reaction and possibly the prevention of autoantibodies that appear in the same context. Clinically significant autoantibodies do occur in about 10 percent of patients with sickle cell disease, and the incidence appears to be higher in those with alloantibodies.[662, 665, 666] The most common antibody-provoking antigens are K, C, E, S, Fy[a], Fy[b], and Jk[b]. In 183 children the incidence of autoantibodies was 7.6 percent and, when associated with C3 on the red cells, their presence resulted in hemolysis.[668] Tahhan and colleagues[664] from North Carolina suggest a modest antibody-preventing strategy: match for K, C, E, and S in all patients; match for Fy[a] or Fy[b] in Fy (a–b+) or (a+b–) but not (a+b–) patients; and match for Jk[b] in Jk(a+b–) patients.

Preparation for Surgery

Children with sickle cell disease can be operated on safely if careful attention is paid to oxygenation, hydration, and acid-base balance during the procedure and in the postoperative period.[669–675] The choice of an anesthetic agent is not as critical as the care with which it is delivered.[671] Burrington and Smith[672] suggest some simple rules of procedure: Keep the operating room at 80 to 85°F, ventilate with 100 percent oxygen a few minutes before and after intubation or extubation, keep the patient warm in the recovery room (particularly if tremors are present), and take special care of intravenous infusion sites, casts, dressings and so on to ensure that circulation is maintained. In an analysis of more than 1000 surgical procedures from the Cooperative Study of Sickle Cell Disease, the overall mortality rate was 1.1 percent, but no deaths occurred in children younger than 14 years of age. Researchers in that same series found comparable complication rates in the SS and SC groups and suggested that patients undergoing regional anesthesia were at higher risk of complications than those undergoing general anesthesia.[675] That prospective "natural history" study did not definitively address the important question of the effectiveness of preoperative transfusion. In a review of records from Dallas Children's Hospital, pulmonary complications were particularly common among patients undergoing laparotomy, thoracotomy, or tonsillectomy and adenoidectomy who were not given preoperative transfusions (9 of 29), compared with those who were given transfusions for those procedures (0 of 8).[676] More recently, Vichinsky and collaborators in the Preoperative Transfusion in Sickle Cell Disease Study Group[677–679] reported the findings of a prospective, multi-institutional study in which more than 600 patients with Hb SS disease were randomly assigned preoperatively to receive either a simple transfusion designed to increase the total hemoglobin level to 10 g/dL or an exchange transfusion designed to decrease the level of HbS to less than 30 g/dL and increase the total hemoglobin level to 10 g/dL.[680, 681] Several key points emerged from that study:

- There was no significant difference between the two transfusion strategies in terms of complications; a high 30 percent postoperative complication rate was reported with both strategies. Transfusion-related complications were twice as common (14 percent) in the exchange transfusion arm compared with the simple transfusion arm (7 percent).
- The most common and serious complication was the acute chest syndrome, which occurred in 10 percent of procedures in both arms. The average time at onset was postoperative day 3, the average length of episode was 8 days, 11 percent of the patients required intubation, and two patients died.
- Patients in a higher surgical risk category and those with a history of pulmonary disease, previous incidence of acute chest syndrome, and multiple hospital admissions had a higher risk of complications.

These data suggest that, at least, a simple transfusion designed to raise the preoperative hemoglobin level to 10 g/dL should be given to all patients with Hb SS disease. The product of choice is probably antigen-matched, leukocyte-depleted packed red cells. All patients, especially those with prior occurrences of pulmonary dysfunction or a history of multiple hospital admissions, should receive a minimum of 12 hours of oxygen treatment and maintenance intravenous hydration and be monitored as high-risk patients, with emphasis on objective markers of oxygenation and regular measurement of input, output, and weight.

Management of Pregnancy

Although many women with sickle cell disease have normal pregnancies, pregnancy can be associated with serious problems for both the mother and fetus. Maternal complications may include increases in the occurrence and severity of painful crises, increases in the severity and occurrence of acute chest syndrome, exaggeration of the physiologic anemia of pregnancy, toxemia, and death.[682] Because of sickling in the placenta, fetal complications can include spontaneous abortion, prematurity, and intrauterine growth retardation. There has been a tremendous improvement in both maternal and fetal outcomes since the mid-1960s.[683–686] The older literature reports fetal and maternal mortality rates that approach 50 percent, with some authors suggesting voluntary sterilization of females with SS disease. Charache and colleagues[686] observed that with modern obstetric management, regular prenatal care, and better nutrition, maternal mortality has been reduced to less than 1 percent and perinatal deaths have declined to less than 15 percent.[687] Some authors have suggested that pregnancy outcome could be improved further if mothers are given prophylactic transfusions[688–691] using various transfusion techniques.[692, 693] Results in patients treated with this approach appear to be improved compared with those observed in historical control subjects, but benefits of this therapy are not as convincing in contemporary comparisons.[694] Koshy and colleagues[695] were unable to demonstrate any significant benefit of transfusions during pregnancy in the only prospective trial so far published. Hepatitis, alloimmunization, and hemolytic transfusion reactions[695, 696] have been reported in pregnant patients with sickle cell disease who have received transfusions. Pregnancies in patients with sickle cell disease should be considered "high risk." At the initial visit, complete red cell typing of both mother and father as well as antibody screening of the mother should be done. Both iron and folate should be given. The early stages of pregnancy should be carefully monitored with serial ultrasonographic studies. A maintenance transfusion program should be initiated if the mother shows increasing symptoms of either vaso-occlusive or anemia-related problems or if there is any sign of fetal distress or poor growth. Blood for transfusion should be carefully selected to be compatible in minor group antigens for which the mother is negative and the father positive. This approach minimizes the risk of maternal sensitization against fetal antigens.

DEATH

Leikin and his colleagues[697] from the Cooperative Study of Sickle Cell Disease examined mortality in children with sickle cell disease. They found that the peak incidence of death was between 1 and 3 years of age, and death was generally caused by infection. The overall mortality rate was 2.6 percent, and for patients with SS disease, the probability of surviving to age 29 was about 85 percent. For those with SC disease, the probability of surviving to age 20 was about 95 percent.

As shown in Figure 19–13, when the data on deaths of the children from the Cooperative Study of Sickle Cell

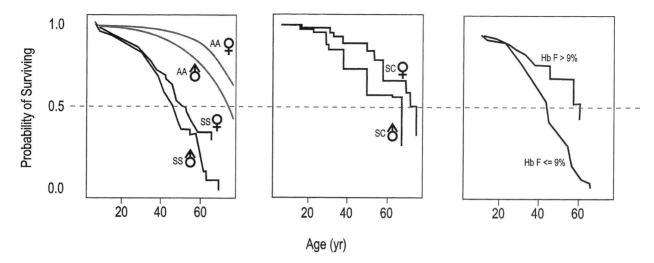

FIGURE 19–13. Survival of male and female patients with SS disease and SC disease, comparing those in the highest quartile (>9 percent) of HbF level with the others. African American (AA) controls are shown for comparison. (Adapted from Platt OS, Brambilla DJ, Rosse WF, et al: Mortality in sickle cell disease. Life expectancy and risk factors for early death. N Engl J Med 1994; 330:1639–1644. Adapted, by permission, from *The New England Journal of Medicine.*)

Disease are combined with the data from adults, it appears that the median age at death was 42 years for males with SS disease, 48 years for females with SS disease, 60 years for males with SC disease, and 68 years for females with SC disease.[346] Among the adults, those with the lowest levels of HbF, the highest steady-state white blood cell counts, and highest rates of pain and acute chest syndrome had the highest risk of dying at an early age. There is an age-related pattern in mortality rates: a peak in the patients younger than 5 years of age and a gradual increase starting in late adolescence. Younger patients die primarily of pneumococcal disease and less often of acute splenic sequestration, acute chest syndrome, or stroke.[445, 698] Older patients die of acute chest syndrome, during pain crises, of chronic organ system failure from cancer and other specific diseases of adults, and suddenly without obvious cause.[346] It is encouraging that the widespread use of prophylactic penicillin in young children, aggressive treatment of pulmonary disease and infection, careful selection of patients for transfusion therapy, and thoughtful comprehensive care have coincided with an improvement in survival.[699]

Much is known about the risk factors for early mortality in patients with sickle cell anemia. Those with a higher level of HbF have a longer life expectancy,[346] as do whose with: low rate of pain crisis,[346] low rate of acute chest syndrome,[375] no hand-foot syndrome before age 1 year,[370] no severe anemia before age 2,[346, 370] low baseline white blood cell count,[370] and low blood pressure.[419]

OTHER SICKLE SYNDROMES

Recently, it has been hypothesized that much of the diversity in clinical severity in sickle cell disease is due in part to modifier genes located throughout the genome.[700, 701] Two well-described examples of genetic modifiers that influence HbS polymerization are the coexistence of multiple forms of α-thalassemia among patients with sickle cell disease and the multiple genetic loci that influence

HbF levels (see sections on sickle syndromes with increased HbF and SS α-thalassemia later). Preliminary data suggest that a variety of other genes may play important roles in the development of strokes, acute chest syndrome, and renal disease in patients with SS disease. The completion of the Human Genome Project and the development of rapid screening techniques to determine the location of as yet unknown genetic modifiers will lead to the further identification of new genetic modifiers. It is likely that each child with SS disease will have a unique combination of genetic modifiers that will influence the clinical severity of the disease.

Sickle Cell Trait—$\alpha_2\beta_2$, $\alpha_2\beta_2^{6\ Val}$

Sickle cell trait is a benign condition that is not associated with increased morbidity or mortality.[702–706] There is no associated anemia, abnormal cell morphology, or decreased red cell survival. Most individuals have approximately 40 percent HbS and 60 percent HbA. A population with 28 to 35 percent HbS has been identified and shown to have accompanying α-thalassemia.[707] Decreased levels of HbS can also be seen in patients with iron[708] and folate[709] deficiencies. Growth, behavior, and educational achievement in children and pregnancy risks in women with sickle trait are entirely normal.[710–712] Black American professional football players have the same incidence of sickle trait as that in the general black population.[713] In a retrospective study of sudden death during physical training in the U.S. Armed Forces, Kark and colleagues[714] noted a 1 in 3200 incidence of sudden death among recruits with sickle trait, an incidence 27 times greater than that seen in control subjects with no HbS. All deaths were associated with strenuous physical exertion, and risks increased with age. After this report, modifications in basic training for all recruits have been recommended, but follow-up data are not yet available. A subsequent prospective study of 25 recruits with sickle trait and control subjects with no HbS revealed no difference in exercise tolerance or physical conditioning after 7 weeks of basic training.[715] Several authors have stressed that these data do not justify restriction of men with sickle trait from the armed services or organized sports.[716–718] Although anecdotal reports of various severe vaso-occlusive episodes in those with sickle trait appear in the literature, they are extremely rare and are not clearly due to sickle trait. Postmortem findings of intravascular sickling are not evidence that the sickling had occurred ante mortem. Under certain extreme conditions, however, sickling and even death may occur in individuals with sickle trait. These include severe pneumonia,[719] flying in unpressurized planes, and exercise at high altitudes.[720, 721] The risk of sickle trait in routine aviation has been overstated.[722] Carefully administered general anesthesia is not associated with a great risk for the individual with sickle trait,[723, 724] but tourniquet surgery[671] and deep hypothermia should be avoided. The most consistent abnormality found in sickle trait is the inability to concentrate urine.[725] Persistent hematuria in individuals with sickle trait has been associated with papillary necrosis of the kidney[726] and rarely with renal medullary carcinoma.[540] Traumatic hyphema in sickle trait is a medical emergency because in the hypoxic conditions of the anterior chamber of the eye Hb AS red cells will sickle, leading to increased intraocular pressure.[727] Women with sickle trait in one prospective study showed an increased risk of preeclampsia, and their infants showed a minimal decrease in gestational age at birth and birth weight but no increased mortality.[728] Prior retrospective and case-control studies have shown conflicting data regarding differences in birth weight or gestational age at birth.[729–732]

SC Disease—$\alpha_2\beta_2^{6\ Val}, \alpha_2\beta_2^{6\ Lys}$

Hb SC disease is a mild chronic hemolytic anemia associated with variable degrees of vaso-occlusive complications. As described in Table 19–1, the patient typically has a hemoglobin level of 10 to 12 g/dL, a reticulocyte count of 1 to 13 percent, and a relative microcytosis for the degree of reticulocytosis. The peripheral blood smear (see Fig. 19–5) is more characteristic of HbC than of HbS, showing impressive target cells and rare, if any, ISCs. The clinical course is quite variable: some patients are severely affected at an early age; others are entirely asymptomatic with disease identified during routine screening in adulthood. Hemolysis is less severe in SC disease than in SS disease,[733] resulting in a higher hematocrit in patients with SC disease.

The major complications of Hb SS disease—recurrent painful bone crises, painful abdominal crises, gallstones, pulmonary infarction, priapism, and CNS infarction—are not common in SC disease but have been reported.[734–737] As shown in Figure 19–9, the pattern of clinical events is different in SC disease, with most events occurring not only less often but also later in life. Certain complications appear to be more common in those with SC disease: eye disease,[575, 735, 738–740] aseptic necrosis of the femoral heads, renal papillary necrosis,[741] and pregnancy-related problems.[684] Splenomegaly is found in approximately 60 percent of patients with SC disease and has been associated with splenic infarction[742] and splenic sequestration,[743] particularly at high altitudes. Although infection is not as common in SC disease as in SS disease,[744] splenic hypofunction and an increased risk of pneumococcal and *H. influenzae* sepsis are found in SC disease.[745] Pneumococcal and *H. influenzae* vaccines are indicated in SC disease, and some recommend the use of prophylactic penicillin.

Patients with SC disease clearly have more sickling complications than do individuals with sickle trait, who are essentially free of sickling complications. One would therefore assume that mixtures of HbS and HbA are less likely to polymerize than mixtures of HbS and HbC. Interestingly, Bunn and associates[746] have shown that this is not the case, because the kinetic and equilibrium behaviors of mixtures of HbS and HbA are essentially identical with the behaviors of mixtures of HbS and HbC. One can resolve this apparent paradox by considering how the hemoglobin mixtures are packaged in SC and AS cells. There are two major factors that explain why SC cells sickle more readily than AS cells: (1) There is more HbS in an SC cell, and (2) the SC cell has a higher MCHC. Because of the differences in charge and affinity for α-globin between β-S-globin and β-C-globin, individuals with SC disease usually have 50 percent HbS and 50 percent HbC, whereas those with the sickle trait typically have 60 percent HbA and 40 percent HbS.[747] This increased HbS content of SC cells results in an approximately sevenfold increase in the rate of polymerization.[747] The increase in MCHC in SC disease, which is quite obvious on density separation of SC red cells[128, 746, 748] (see Fig. 19–6) and even C trait red cells,[747] is probably due to the activation by the positively charged HbC molecules of the K^+, Cl^- cotransport system.[161] The cellular dehydration and microcytosis associated with HbC has been well characterized by Brugnara and colleagues[749] and Ballas and associates.[748]

Hemoglobin SC and α-Thalassemia

One patient with HbSC and α-thalassemia trait has been described.[750] This 7-year-old child had the following laboratory values: hematocrit, 25.8 percent; Hb, 7.9 g/dL; MCV, 53 μm^3; MCH, 16.2 pg; MCHC, 30.6 g/dL; reticulocytes, 7.2 percent; HbS, 50.5 percent; HbC, 47.7 percent; and HbF, 1.8 percent. One parent had 27 percent HbS with an MCV of 71 μm^3; the other had 24 percent HbC with an MCV of 57 μm^3. This patient, like many patients with SC disease, was relatively asymptomatic. Of interest is the fact that her hematocrit level and reticulocyte count are compatible with a considerable degree of hemolysis.

Hemoglobin S O-Arab—$\alpha_2\beta_2^{6\ Val}, \alpha_2\beta_2^{121\ Lys}$

HbS O-Arab double heterozygotes are quite rare and have a relatively severe disorder with a chronic hemolytic anemia and vaso-occlusive episodes.[751] As seen in Figure 19–1, the O-Arab mutation lies within the area critical to the axial contact in the HbS fiber. Routine cellulose acetate electrophoresis at 8.6 does not distinguish between

HbC and Hb O-Arab. Citrate agar electrophoresis at pH 6 does separate HbC from HbO and should be done for patients who appear to have Hb SC disease on cellulose acetate electrophoretic examination but who have particularly severe symptoms.[752]

Hemoglobin SD—$\alpha_2\beta_2^{6\,Val}$, $\alpha_2\beta_2^{121\,Gln}$

SD double heterozygotes have a severe hemolytic anemia with a peripheral blood smear comparable to that seen in Hb SS disease (see Fig. 19–5). These rare patients have severe vaso-occlusive complications,[753–755] illustrating, as do those with Hb O-Arab, the critical nature of the β121 contact site. HbD migrates with HbS on cellulose acetate electrophoresis at alkaline pH and can be distinguished from HbS on citrate agar electrophoresis at acid pH. HbD is suspected when a hemoglobin appears to be HbS on cellulose acetate electrophoresis but gives a negative "sickle prep." The identification of a parent with HbD is important socially because it may become difficult to explain how a child has "SS disease" and only one parent has a positive sickle prep.

Hemoglobin S Korle-Bu—$\alpha_2\beta_2^{6\,Val}$, $\alpha_2\beta_2^{73\,Asn}$

Hb Korle-Bu is a rare hemoglobin mutant.[756] It is mentioned here only because it illustrates an important pathophysiologic point. Hb Korle-Bu participates poorly in sickling.[757] This mutation interferes with the lateral contact between HbS fibers by blocking the critical receptor area for the Val-β6. Hb S Korle-Bu double heterozygotes are entirely symptom free.

Hemoglobin C-Harlem (C-Georgetown)—$\alpha_2\beta_2^{6\,Val,\,73\,Asn}$

Hb C-Harlem (also known as C-Georgetown) has two substitutions on the β chain: the sickle mutation $\beta^{6\,Val}$ and the Korle-Bu mutation $\beta^{73\,Asn}$.[758] Patients with these mutations are asymptomatic. Patients doubly heterozygous for HbS and Hb C-Harlem have clinical crises resembling those in SS disease.[758, 759]

Hemoglobin S-Antilles—$\alpha_2\beta_2^{6\,Val,\,23\,Ile}$

Hb S-Antilles also has two substitutions on the β chain: the sickle mutation $\beta^{6\,Val}$ and a second mutation $\beta^{23\,Ile}$.[760] This mutation results in a low oxygen affinity hemoglobin that in heterozygotes for HbA and Hb S-Antilles results in a mild hemolytic anemia and the presence of 5 to 7 percent ISCs. A transgenic mouse with Hb S-Antilles and the Hb D (see earlier) mutations exhibits many of the clinical features of SS disease.[761]

Sickle Syndromes with Increased Fetal Hemoglobin

HbF levels in sickle cell anemia may vary over a 60-fold range from 0.5 to 30 percent. Because HbF is known to have an ameliorating effect by reducing HbS polymerization, the origin of this marked variability has been of great interest. Because HbF is heterogeneously distributed

among the red cells of individuals with SS disease, the percentage of HbF is the result of three independent processes: the number of cells containing HbF (F cells) produced, the amount of HbF produced per F cell, and the variable preferential survival of F cells compared with non-F cells in the circulation.[130]

Three broad categories of genetic mutations that increase HbF in association with HbS have been described.[762, 763] Large deletions of the β-globin gene region resulting in δ-β-thalassemia or pancellular hereditary persistence of fetal hemoglobin (HPFH) are rare in the general population with sickle cell disease (see Chapter 21 for more details on these deletions). The combination of HbS and pancellular HPFH represents a unique syndrome. Findings include between 24 and 34 percent of HbF distributed in all red cells, no anemia, minimal microcytosis (MCV of $78 \pm 8\ \mu m^3$), and no clinical disease.[764–767]

A second group of mutations in which HbF is increased in association with HbS are linked to the β-globin gene region and are termed *nondeletion HPFH*.[768–771] Some linked mutations may be associated with single nucleotide substitutions in the promoter regions of the γ genes, but these are quite rare among the general population with SS disease.[771, 772] HbF is usually distributed heterogeneously in these disorders, but a pancellular distribution is seen in some. Another type of linked nondeletion mutation that may increase HbF is the as-yet undefined mutation associated with the Senegal and Arab-Indian (Saudi) β-globin haplotypes.[20,25–28] These haplotypes are found commonly in genetic isolates in Western Africa, in Shiite Saudi Arabians, and in the Orissa region of India.[773–776] Among patients with sickle cell anemia in the United States, less than 10 percent have one chromosome with either of these haplotypes and less than 2 percent are homozygous for the Senegal haplotype.

Genetic disorders in the third group that influence HbF levels in patients with SS disease are not linked to the β-globin region.[777, 778] Boyer and associates[779] showed that approximately one third of full siblings, each with SS disease, have significantly different genetic programs for HbF production. Because both siblings inherited the same β-globin regions from their parents with sickle trait, the HbF program must be separate from the β-globin region. After Myoshi and co-workers[780] noted that HbF (defined by F-cell levels) in normal blood donors was inherited in an X-linked pattern, Dover and colleagues[781] showed that F-cell production in patients with sickle cell disease was inherited by a diallelic gene on the short arm of the X-chromosome, Xp22–23. They termed this gene the F-cell production (*FCP*) locus. Among the known forms of heterocellular HPFH, the *FCP* locus accounts for most of the variation in HbF levels in patients with sickle cell anemia.[781, 782] Thien and colleagues[784] localized another genetic locus that controls F-cell levels in normal whites to chromosome 6q22.3.[783, 784]

In addition to these disorders, it has been shown that α-thalassemia is associated with decreased HbF levels in SS disease.[785] Noguchi and associates[126] and Dover and co-workers[786] showed that the differences in HbF levels among patients with SS disease with or without α-thalassemia may be indirectly related to the lowered MCHC of the SS-α-thalassemia red cells. Preferential survival of F cells compared with non–F cells is less in SS-α-thalassemia because the non–F cells in α-thalassemia have less cation loss and a lower MCHC, which reduces HbS polymerization and results in a longer life span.

When all known factors responsible for elevated HbF levels in SS disease were studied in a random population including a cohort of patients with SS disease identified at birth, the following findings emerged. First, the X-linked *FCP* locus was responsible for almost 40 percent of the variation in HbF levels. Second, β-globin haplotypes, age, and sex together accounted for less than 10 percent of the variation. Third, approximately 50 percent of the variation remains undefined.[782] Early investigators suggested that different "threshold" levels of HbF (between 10 and 20 percent) were necessary to ameliorate the clinical severity of SS disease.[787, 788] In a natural history study, Platt and co-workers showed that any increment of HbF greater than 4 percent was associated with reduced pain crises[302] and HbF levels greater than 7 percent were associated with decreased mortality.[346]

Sickle β-Thalassemia

Patients heterozygous for HbS and β-thalassemia have clinically severe disease that depends on the output of the thalassemic β gene.[446, 737, 789, 790] If no HbA is produced (S-β^0-thalassemia), the clinical course is comparable (see Table 19–4 and Fig. 19–11) with that of homozygous sickle cell anemia. Electrophoretic analysis shows mostly HbS, with a slightly elevated amount of HbA_2 and variable amounts of HbF. Features that distinguish these patients from those with sickle cell anemia are that they may be of Mediterranean origin, have microcytosis, and often have splenomegaly. One parent will have classic sickle trait, whereas the other will have β-thalassemia trait. The hemolytic rate is lower, and the patients tend to have a slightly higher hematocrit and lower reticulocyte count. Peripheral blood morphologic findings include target cells, microcytosis, and generally fewer ISCs than in sickle cell anemia. If there is output from the β-thalassemia gene (S-β^+-thalassemia), the clinical course of the disease tends to be milder comparable with that in SC disease. Electrophoretic analysis shows predominantly HbS, elevated amounts of Hb-A^2, variable amounts of HbF, and HbA. The features that distinguish these individuals from those with sickle cell anemia are HbA, microcytosis, splenomegaly, and a relatively benign clinical course. The ameliorative effects of HbA (see Tables 19–1 and 19–4 and Fig. 19–11) are apparent. These patients can be distinguished from individuals with sickle trait because the level of HbS is greater than that of Hb A and microcytosis, hemolytic anemia, abnormal peripheral blood morphologic findings, and splenomegaly are seen. α-Thalassemia with Hb S-β^0-thalassemia results in higher hemoglobin levels, lower reticulocyte counts, and increases in the MCV and MCHC.[791]

SS α-Thalassemia

Homozygous Hb SS disease with accompanying α-thalassemia has been well described.[126, 785, 786, 792–800] The diagnosis is based on the following criteria: (1) hemoglobin electrophoretic analysis showing no HbA, normal HbA_2, and predominantly HbS; (2) microcytosis without iron deficiency; (3) both parents with S trait and one with the typical clinical findings of AS α-thalassemia (microcytosis and HbS concentration of less than 35 percent); (4) elevated level of Bart's Hb detectable in the cord blood; and (5) α gene mapping showing two or three genes. Approximately 30 percent of American blacks have three α genes, and approximately 2 percent have two α genes. α-Thalassemia in patients with SS disease in the United States is usually due to the α-thal-2 haplotype, a deletion of approximately 3.7 kb involving the entire α_2 gene.[799] There has been considerable interest in these patients because α-thalassemia has an effect on some of the hematologic features of sickle cell anemia and may provide insight into the pathophysiologic basis of the disease. The primary effect of α-thalassemia is to decrease the cellular HbS content. The MVC is also reduced, but not exactly in the same proportion as the hemoglobin content. The net effect is a slightly reduced MCHC and an increased surface-to-volume ratio. Patients with α-thalassemia tend to have smaller, lighter cells, with a higher hemoglobin level and fewer reticulocytes.[785, 791, 800, 801] Although the hematologic parameters of sickle cell anemia are clearly improved by coexisting α-thalassemia, the vaso-occlusive severity is not obviously different. One study[785] indicated that leg ulcers and acute chest syndrome was seen less often with α-thalassemia, but this finding was not confirmed by others.[796] Avascular necrosis of the femoral head was increased in sickle cell anemia with α-thalassemia (see Fig. 19–11).[802, 803] α-Thalassemia does not protect children with SS disease from strokes.[803] Mears and associates[805] suggested that α-thalassemia is associated with increased life expectancy. α-Thalassemia not only reduces the MCV and the MCHC, but it also reduces the percentage of dense cells and ISCs.[126, 806] The cells of patients with α-thalassemia and SS disease are more deformable and have less cation fluxes and a greater membrane surface area-to-volume ratio.[792] Differences in hemoglobin values among children with SS disease with four and two α genes is not apparent until after age 4,[807] but microcytosis and elevated red cell counts are present at birth.[808]

Hemoglobin C Disease—$\alpha_2\beta_2^{6\ Lys}$

Homozygous HbC disease is a mild disorder characterized by hemolytic anemia, microcytosis, and splenomegaly.[809–814] The tendency of HbC to aggregate and crystallize[815–817] is probably responsible for the characteristic target cell morphologic features of the stained and dried red cell in homozygous C disease and in HbC trait, although these crystals are not likely to be directly responsible for the hemolytic anemia. In HbC trait, target cell formation and mild microcytosis is the only manifestation of the anomaly. Hemolytic anemia is not present.

The basis of the aggregation and crystal formation of HbC cells is not precisely understood. It is thought that the substantial charge difference between HbC and HbA is in some way responsible for the tendency toward aggregation of C molecules, which leads to local increments of Hb concentration in excess of its solubility.[814] The structure of these crystals has been examined by x-ray diffraction analysis.[815–817]

The hemolytic anemia of homozygous HbC disease is probably due to the fact that these cells are dehydrated. Brugnara and colleagues[749] demonstrated that CC red cells have decreased water and cation content associated with a large potassium efflux. As discussed in the earlier section on membrane abnormalities, this volume-dependent potassium efflux is regulated by the K^+,Cl^- cotransport pathway.

REFERENCES

1. Herrick JB: Peculiar elongated and sickle-shaped red corpuscles in a case of severe anemia. Arch Intern Med 1910; 6:517.
2. Sydenstricker VP, Mulherin WA, Houseal RW: Sickle cell anemia: Report of two cases in children with necropsy in one case. Am J Dis Child 1923; 26:132.
3. Hahn EV, Gillespie EB: Sickle cell anemia: Report of a case greatly improved by splenectomy. Arch Intern Med 1927; 39:233.
4. Pauling L, Itano HA, Singer SJ, et al: Sickle cell anemia, a molecular disease. Science 1949; 110:543–546.
5. Neel JV: Inheritance of the sickling phenomenon with particular reference to sickle-cell disease. Blood 1951; 6:389.
6. Ingram VV: Gene mutations in human haemoglobin: The chemical difference between normal and sickle cell haemoglobin. Nature 1957; 180:326–328.
7. Conley CL: Sickle cell anemia: The first molecular disease. In Wintrobe MM (Ed.): Blood, Pure and Eloquent. New York, McGraw-Hill, 1980, pp 319–373.
8. Motulsky AG: Frequency of sickling disorders in U.S. blacks. N Engl J Med 1973; 288:31.
9. Kan YW, Dozy AM: Evolution of the hemoglobin S and C genes in world populations. Science 1980; 209:388–391.
10. Antonarakis SE, Boehm CD, Serjeant GR, et al: Origin of the β S-globin gene in blacks: The contribution of recurrent mutation or gene conversion or both. Proc Natl Acad Sci USA 1984; 81:853–856.
11. Pagnier J, Mears JG, Dunda-Belkhodja O, et al: Evidence for the multicentric origin of the sickle cell hemoglobin gene in Africa. Proc Natl Acad Sci USA 1984; 81:1771–1773.
12. Wainscoat JS, Bell JI, Thein SL, et al: Multiple origins of the sickle mutation: Evidence from β S globin gene cluster polymorphisms. Mol Biol Med 1983; 1:191–197.
13. Stine OC, Dover GJ, Zhu D, et al: The evolution of two West African populations. J Mol Evol 1992; 34:336–344.
14. Lapoumeroulie C, Dunda O, Ducrocq R, et al: A novel sickle cell mutation of yet another origin in Africa: The Cameroon type. Hum Genet 1992; 89:333–337.
15. Kulozik AE, Wainscoat JS, Serjeant GR, et al: Geographical survey of β S-globin gene haplotypes: Evidence for an independent Asian origin of the sickle-cell mutation. Am J Hum Genet 1986; 39:239–244.
16. Ragusa A, Lombardo M, Sortino G, et al: β S gene in Sicily is in linkage disequilibrium with the Benin haplotype: Implications for gene flow. Am J Hematol 1988; 27:139–141.
17. Aluoch JR, Kilinc Y, Aksoy M, et al: Sickle cell anaemia among Eti-Turks: Haematological, clinical and genetic observations. Br J Haematol 1986; 64:45–55.
18. Schroeder WA, Powars DR, Kay LM, et al: β-Cluster haplotypes, α-gene status, and hematological data from SS, SC, and S-β-thalassemia patients in southern California. Hemoglobin 1989; 13:325–353.
19. Hattori Y, Kutlar F, Kutlar A, et al: Haplotypes of β S chromosomes among patients with sickle cell anemia from Georgia. Hemoglobin 1986; 10:623–642.
20. Nagel RL, Fabry ME, Pagnier J, et al: Hematologically and genetically distinct forms of sickle cell anemia in Africa. The Senegal type and the Benin type. N Engl J Med 1985; 312:880–884.
21. Nagel RL, Rao SK, Dunda-Belkhodja O, et al: The hematologic characteristics of sickle cell anemia bearing the Bantu haplotype: The relationship between G gamma and HbF level. Blood 1987; 69:1026–1030.
22. Srinivas R, Dunda O, Krishnamoorthy R, et al: Atypical haplotypes linked to the β S gene in Africa are likely to be the product of recombination. Am J Hematol 1988; 29:60–62.
23. Antonarakis SE, Boehm CD, Giardina PJ, et al: Nonrandom association of polymorphic restriction sites in the β-globin gene cluster. Proc Natl Acad Sci USA 1982; 79:137–141.
24. Powars D, Chan LS, Schroeder WA: The variable expression of sickle cell disease is genetically determined. Semin Hematol 1990; 27:360–376.
25. Perrine RP, Brown MJ, Clegg JB, et al: Benign sickle-cell anaemia. Lancet 1972; 2:1163–1167.
26. Pembrey ME, Wood WG, Weatherall DJ, et al: Fetal haemoglobin production and the sickle gene in the oases of Eastern Saudi Arabia. Br J Haematol 1978; 40:415–429.
27. Perrine RP, Pembrey ME, John P, et al: Natural history of sickle cell anemia in Saudi Arabs. A study of 270 subjects. Ann Intern Med 1978; 88:1–6.
28. Ali SA: Milder variant of sickle-cell disease in Arabs in Kuwait associated with unusually high level of foetal haemoglobin. Br J Haematol 1970; 19:613–619.
29. Brittenham G, Lozoff B, Harris JW, et al: Sickle cell anemia and trait in southern India: Further studies. Am J Hematol 1979; 6:107–123.
30. Weatherall DJ: Common genetic disorders of the red cell and the 'malaria hypothesis.' Ann Trop Med Parasitol 1987; 81:539–548.
31. Allison AC: Protection afforded by sickle cell trait against subtertian malarial infection. Br Med J 1954; 1:290.
32. Luzzatto L, Nwachuku-Jarrett ES, Reddy S: Increased sickling of parasitised erythrocytes as mechanism of resistance against malaria in the sickle-cell trait. Lancet 1970; 1:319–321.
33. Roth EF Jr, Friedman M, Ueda Y, et al: Sickling rates of human AS red cells infected in vitro with Plasmodium falciparum malaria. Science 1978; 202:650–652.
34. Friedman MJ, Trager W: The biochemistry of resistance to malaria. Sci Am 1981; 244:154–155, 158–64.
35. Pasvol G, Weatherall DJ, Wilson RJ: Cellular mechanism for the protective effect of haemoglobin S against P. falciparum malaria. Nature 1978; 274:701–703.
36. Hood AT, Fabry ME, Costantini F, et al: Protection from lethal malaria in transgenic mice expressing sickle hemoglobin. Blood 1996; 87:1600–1603.
37. Shear HL, Roth EF Jr, Fabry ME, et al: Transgenic mice expressing human sickle hemoglobin are partially resistant to rodent malaria. Blood 1993; 81:222–226.
38. Lewis RA, Kay RW, Hathorn M: Sickle cell disease and glucose-6-phosphate dehydrogenase. Acta Haematol 1966; 36:399–411.
39. Piomelli S, Reindorf CA, Arzanian MT, et al: Clinical and biochemical interactions of glucose-6-phosphate dehydrogenase deficiency and sickle-cell anemia. N Engl J Med 1972; 287:213–217.
40. Beutler E, Johnson C, Powars D, et al: Prevalence of glucose-6-phosphate dehydrogenase deficiency in sickle-cell disease. N Engl J Med 1974; 290:826–828.
41. Steinberg MH, Dreiling BJ: Glucose-6-phosphate dehydrogenase deficiency in sickle-cell anemia. A study in adults. Ann Intern Med 1974; 80:217–220.
42. Smits HL, Oski FA, Brody JI: The hemolytic crisis of sickle cell disease: The role of glucose-6-phosphate dehydrogenase deficiency. J Pediatr 1969; 74:544–551.
43. Harris JW: Studies on the destruction of red blood cells. VIII. Molecular orientation in sickle cell hemoglobin solutions. Proc Soc Exp Biol Med 1950; 75:197.
44. Stetson CA Jr: The state of hemoglobin in sickled erythrocytes. J Exp Med 1966; 123:341–346.
45. White JG: The fine structure of sickled hemoglobin in situ. Blood 1968; 31:561–579.
46. Dobler J, Bertles JF: The physical state of hemoglobin in sickle-cell anemia erythrocytes in vivo. J Exp Med 1968; 127:711–714.
47. Lessin LS: Helicoidal polymerization of the hemoglobin molecules in sickle-shaped erythrocytes. Study by means of the frozen-etched method. C R Acad Sci Hebd Seances Acad Sci D 1968; 266:1806–1808.
48. Finch JT, Perutz MF, Bertles JF, et al: Structure of sickled erythrocytes and of sickle-cell hemoglobin fibers. Proc Natl Acad Sci USA 1973; 70:718–722.

49. Dykes G, Crepeau RH, Edelstein SJ: Three-dimensional reconstruction of the fibres of sickle cell haemoglobin. Nature 1978; 272:506–510.

50. Garrell RL, Crepeau RH, Edelstein SJ: Cross-sectional views of hemoglobin S fibers by electron microscopy and computer modeling. Proc Natl Acad Sci USA 1979; 76:1140–1144.

51. Dykes GW, Crepeau RH, Edelstein SJ: Three-dimensional reconstruction of the 14-filament fibers of hemoglobin S. J Mol Biol 1979; 130:451–472.

52. Edelstein SJ: Patterns in the quinary structures of proteins. Plasticity and inequivalence of individual molecules in helical arrays of sickle cell hemoglobin and tubulin. Biophys J 1980; 32:347–360.

53. Magdoff-Fairchild B, Chiu CC: X-ray diffraction studies of fibers and crystals of deoxygenated sickle cell hemoglobin. Proc Natl Acad Sci USA 1979; 76:223–226.

54. Rodgers DW, Crepeau RH, Edelstein SJ: Pairings and polarities of the 14 strands in sickle cell hemoglobin fibers. Proc Natl Acad Sci USA 1987; 84:6157–6161.

55. Carragher B, Bluemke DA, Becker M, et al: Structural analysis of polymers of sickle cell hemoglobin. III. Fibers within fascicles. J Mol Biol 1988; 199:383–388.

56. Makowski L, Magdoff-Fairchild B: Polymorphism of sickle cell hemoglobin aggregates: Structural basis for limited radial growth. Science 1986; 234:1228–1231.

57. Hofrichter J, Hendricker DG, Eaton WA: Structure of hemoglobin S fibers: Optical determination of the molecular orientation in sickled erythrocytes. Proc Natl Acad Sci USA 1973; 70:3604–3608.

58. Wishner BC, Ward KB, Lattman EE, et al: Crystal structure of sickle-cell deoxyhemoglobin at 5 A resolution. J Mol Biol 1975; 98:179–194.

59. Benesch RE, Yung S, Benesch R, et al: α-Chain contacts in the polymerisation of sickle haemogloblin. Nature 1976; 260:219–221.

60. Benesch RE, Kwong S, Benesch R, et al: Location and bond type of intermolecular contacts in the polymerisation of haemoglobin S. Nature 1977; 269:772–775.

61. Crepeau RH, Edelstein SJ, Szalay M, et al: Sickle cell hemoglobin fiber structure altered by α-chain mutation. Proc Natl Acad Sci USA 1981; 78:1406–1410.

62. Nagel RL, Johnson J, Bookchin RM, et al: β-Chain contact sites in the haemoglobin S polymer. Nature 1980; 283:832–834.

63. Benesch RE, Kwong S, Benesch R: The effects of α chain mutations *cis* and *trans* to the β6 mutation on the polymerization of sickle cell haemoglobin. Nature 1982; 299:231–234.

64. Rhoda MD, Martin J, Blouquit Y, et al: Sickle cell hemoglobin fiber formation strongly inhibited by the Stanleyville II mutation (α 78 Asn leads to Lys). Biochem Biophys Res Commun 1983; 111:8–13.

65. Padlan EA, Love WE: Refined crystal structure of deoxyhemoglobin S. II. Molecular interactions in the crystal. J Biol Chem 1985; 260:8280–8291.

66. Edelstein SJ: Molecular topology in crystals and fibers of hemoglobin S. J Mol Biol 1981; 150:557–575.

67. Harrington JP, Elbaum D, Bookchin RM, et al: Ligand kinetics of hemoglobin S containing erythrocytes. Proc Natl Acad Sci USA 1977; 74:203–206.

68. Gill SJ, Spokane R, Benedict RC, et al: Ligand-linked phase equilibria of sickle cell hemoglobin. J Mol Biol 1980; 140:299–312.

69. Sunshine HR, Hofrichter J, Ferrone FA, et al: Oxygen binding by sickle cell hemoglobin polymers. J Mol Biol 1982; 158:251–273.

70. Ross PD, Hofrichter J, Eaton WA: Calorimetric and optical characterization of sickle cell hemoglobin gelation. J Mol Biol 1975; 96:239–253.

71. Ross PD, Hofrichter J, Eaton WA: Thermodynamics of gelation of sickle cell deoxyhemoglobin. J Mol Biol 1977; 115:111–134.

72. Magdoff-Fairchild B, Poillon WN, Li T, et al: Thermodynamic studies of polymerization of deoxygenated sickle cell hemoglobin. Proc Natl Acad Sci USA 1976; 73:990–994.

73. Goldberg MA, Husson MA, Bunn HF: Participation of hemoglobins A and F in polymerization of sickle hemoglobin. J Biol Chem 1977; 252:3414–3421.

74. Briehl RW: Gelation of sickle cell hemoglobin. IV. Phase transitions in hemoglobin S gels: Separate measures of aggregation and solution–gel equilibrium. J Mol Biol 1978; 123:521–538.

75. Poillon WN, Bertles JF: Deoxygenated sickle hemoglobin. Effects of lyotropic salts on its solubility. J Biol Chem 1979; 254: 3462–3467.

76. Swerdlow PH, Bryan RA, Bertles JF, et al: Effect of 2, 3-diphosphoglycerate on the solubility of deoxy-sickle hemoglobin. Hemoglobin 1977; 1:527–537.

77. Hofrichter J, Ross PD, Eaton WA: Supersaturation in sickle cell hemoglobin solutions. Proc Natl Acad Sci USA 1976; 73:3035–3039.

78. Hofrichter J, Ross PD, Eaton WA: A physical description of hemoglobin S gelation. In Hercules JI, et al (Eds.): Proceedings of the Symposium on Molecular and Cellular Aspects of Sickle Cell Disease. Bethesda, National Institutes of Health, 1976, pp 185–223.

79. Hofrichter J: Ligand binding and the gelation of sickle cell hemoglobin. J Mol Biol 1979; 128:335–369.

80. Wilson WW, Luzzana MR, Penniston JT, et al: Pregelation aggregation of sickle cell hemoglobin. Proc Natl Acad Sci USA 1974; 71:1260–1263.

81. Moffat K, Gibson QH: The rates of polymerization and depolymerization of sickle cell hemoglobin. Biochem Biophys Res Commun 1974; 61:237–242.

82. Williams RC Jr: Concerted formation of the gel of hemoglobin S. Proc Natl Acad Sci USA 1973; 70:1506–1508.

83. Briehl RW, Ewert SM: Gelation of sickle cell haemoglobin. II. Methaemoglobin. J Mol Biol 1974; 89:759–766.

84. Mickols W, Maestre MF, Tinoco I Jr, et al: Visualization of oriented hemoglobin S in individual erythrocytes by differential extinction of polarized light. Proc Natl Acad Sci USA 1985; 82:6527–6531.

85. Beach DA, Bustamante C, Wells KS, et al: Differential polarization imaging. III. Theory confirmation. Patterns of polymerization of hemoglobin S in red blood sickle cells. Biophys J 1987; 52:947–954.

86. Zipp A, Kuntz ID, James TL: Hemoglobin-water interactions in normal and sickle erythrocytes by proton magnetic resonance T1ρ measurements. Arch Biochem Biophys 1977; 178:435–441.

87. Zipp A, James TL, Kuntz ID, et al: Water proton magnetic resonance studies of normal and sickle erythrocytes. Temperature and volume dependence. Biochim Biophys Acta 1976; 428:291–303.

88. Cottam GL, Valentine KM, Yamaoka K, et al: The gelation of deoxyhemoglobin S in erythrocytes as detected by transverse water proton relaxation measurements. Arch Biochem Biophys 1974; 162:487–492.

89. Ferrone FA, Hofrichter J, Eaton WA: Kinetics of sickle hemoglobin polymerization. II. A double nucleation mechanism. J Mol Biol 1985; 183:611–631.

90. Mirchev R, Ferrone FA: The structural link between polymerization and sickle cell disease. J Mol Biol 1997; 265:475–479.

91. Eaton WA, Hofrichter J: Hemoglobin S gelation and sickle cell disease. Blood 1987; 70:1245–1266.

92. Rampling MW, Sirs JA: The rate of sickling of cells containing sickle-cell haemoglobin. Clin Sci Mol Med 1973; 45:655–664.

93. Hahn JA, Messer MJ, Bradley TB: Ultrastructure of sickling and unsickling in time-lapse studies. Br J Haematol 1976; 34:559–565.

94. Zarkowsky HS, Hochmuth RM: Sickling times of individual erythrocytes at zero Po$_2$. J Clin Invest 1975; 56:1023–1034.

95. Coletta M, Hofrichter J, Ferrone FA, et al: Kinetics of sickle haemoglobin polymerization in single red cells. Nature 1982; 300:194–197.

96. Adachi K, Asakura T: Multiple nature of polymers of deoxyhemoglobin S prepared by different methods. J Biol Chem 1983; 258:3045–3050.

97. Asakura T, Mayberry J: Relationship between morphologic characteristics of sickle cells and method of deoxygenation. J Lab Clin Med 1984; 104:987–994.

98. Eaton WA, Hofrichter J, Ross PD: Editorial: Delay time of gelation: A possible determinant of clinical severity in sickle cell disease. Blood 1976; 47:621–627.

99. Mozzarelli A, Hofrichter J, Eaton WA: Delay time of hemoglobin S polymerization prevents most cells from sickling in vivo. Science 1987; 237:500–506.

100. Noguchi CT, Torchia DA, Schechter AN: Intracellular polymerization of sickle hemoglobin. Effects of cell heterogeneity. J Clin Invest 1983; 72:846–852.

101. Noguchi CT, Torchia DA, Schechter AN: Determination of deoxyhemoglobin S polymer in sickle erythrocytes upon deoxygenation. Proc Natl Acad Sci USA 1980; 77:5487–5491.

102. Noguchi CT, Schechter AN: The intracellular polymerization of sickle hemoglobin and its relevance to sickle cell disease. Blood 1981; 58:1057–1068.

103. Green MA, Noguchi CT, Keidan AJ, et al: Polymerization of sickle cell hemoglobin at arterial oxygen saturation impairs erythrocyte deformability. J Clin Invest 1988; 81:1669–1674.

104. Brittenham GM, Schechter AN, Noguchi CT: Hemoglobin S polymerization: Primary determinant of the hemolytic and clinical severity of the sickling syndromes. Blood 1985; 65:183–189.

105. Keidan AJ, Sowter MC, Johnson CS, et al: Effect of polymerization tendency on haematological, rheological and clinical parameters in sickle cell anaemia. Br J Haematol 1989; 71:551–557.

106. Poillon WN, Kim BC, Castro O: Intracellular hemoglobin S polymerization and the clinical severity of sickle cell anemia. Blood 1998; 91:1777–1783.

107. Charache S, Terrin ML, Moore RD, et al: Effect of hydroxyurea on the frequency of painful crises in sickle cell anemia. Investigators of the Multicenter Study of Hydroxyurea in Sickle Cell Anemia. N Engl J Med 1995; 332:1317–1322.

108. Sunshine HR, Hofrichter J, Eaton WA: Requirement for therapeutic inhibition of sickle haemoglobin gelation. Nature 1978; 275:238–240.

109. Sunshine HR, Hofrichter J, Eaton WA: Gelation of sickle cell hemoglobin in mixtures with normal adult and fetal hemoglobins. J Mol Biol 1979; 133:435–467.

110. Behe MJ, Englander SW: Mixed gelation theory. Kinetics, equilibrium and gel incorporation in sickle hemoglobin mixtures. J Mol Biol 1979; 133:137–160.

111. Adachi K, Segal R, Asakura T: Nucleation-controlled aggregation of deoxyhemoglobin S. Participation of hemoglobin F in the aggregation of deoxyhemoglobin S in concentrated phosphate buffer. J Biol Chem 1980; 255:7595–603.

112. Adachi K, Matarasso SL, Asakura T: Nucleation-controlled aggregation of deoxyhemoglobin S. Effect of organic phosphates on the kinetics of aggregation of deoxyhemoglobin S in concentrated phosphate buffer. Biochim Biophys Acta 1980; 624:372–377.

113. Adachi K, Ozguc M, Asakura T: Nucleation-controlled aggregation of deoxyhemoglobin S. Participation of hemoglobin A in the aggregation of deoxyhemoglobin S in concentrated phosphate buffer. J Biol Chem 1980; 255:3092–3099.

114. Cheetham RC, Huehns ER, Rosemeyer MA: Participation of haemoglobins A, F, A2 and C in polymerisation of haemoglobin S. J Mol Biol 1979; 129:45–61.

115. Benesch RE, Edalji R, Benesch R, et al: Solubilization of hemoglobin S by other hemoglobins. Proc Natl Acad Sci USA 1980; 77:5130–5134.

116. Jones MM, Steinhardt J: Evidence of the incorporation of normally nonaggregating hemoglobins into crystalline aggregates of deoxy hemoglobin S. J Biol Chem 1982; 257:1913–1920.

117. Minton AP: Non-ideality and the thermodynamics of sickle-cell hemoglobin gelation. J Mol Biol 1977; 110:89–103.

118. Sunshine HR: Effect of other hemoglobins on gelation of sickle cell hemoglobin. Tex Rep Biol Med 1980; 40:233–250.

119. Setty BN, Kulkarni S, Dampier CD, et al: Fetal hemoglobin in sickle cell anemia: Relationship to erythrocyte adhesion markers and adhesion. Blood 2001; 97:2568–2573.

120. Rodgers GP, Schechter AN, Noguchi CT: Cell heterogeneity in sickle cell disease: Quantitation of the erythrocyte density profile. J Lab Clin Med 1985; 106:30–37.

121. Mohandas N, Kim YR, Tycko DH, et al: Accurate and independent measurement of volume and hemoglobin concentration of individual red cells by laser light scattering. Blood 1986; 68:506–513.

122. Mohandas N, Johnson A, Wyatt J, et al: Automated quantitation of cell density distribution and hyperdense cell fraction in RBC disorders. Blood 1989; 74:442–447.

123. Kaul DK, Fabry ME, Windisch P, et al: Erythrocytes in sickle cell anemia are heterogeneous in their rheological and hemodynamic characteristics. J Clin Invest 1983; 72:22–31.

124. Billett HH, Fabry ME, Nagel RL: Hemoglobin distribution width: A rapid assessment of dense red cells in the steady state and during painful crisis in sickle cell anemia. J Lab Clin Med 1988; 112:339–344.

125. Billett HH, Kim K, Fabry ME, et al: The percentage of dense red cells does not predict incidence of sickle cell painful crisis. Blood 1986; 68:301–303.

126. Noguchi CT, Dover GJ, Rodgers GP, et al: Alpha thalassemia changes erythrocyte heterogeneity in sickle cell disease. J Clin Invest 1985; 75:1632–1637.

127. Baudin V, Pagnier J, Labie D, et al: Heterogeneity of sickle cell disease as shown by density profiles: Effects of fetal hemoglobin and α thalassemia. Haematologia 1986; 19:177–184.

128. Fabry ME, Kaul DK, Raventos-Suarez C, et al: SC erythrocytes have an abnormally high intracellular hemoglobin concentration. Pathophysiological consequences. J Clin Invest 1982; 70:1315–1319.

129. Boyer SH, Belding TK, Margolet L, et al: Fetal hemoglobin restriction to a few erythrocytes (F cells) in normal human adults. Science 1975; 188:361–363.

130. Dover GJ, Boyer SH, Charache S, et al: Individual variation in the production and survival of F cells in sickle-cell disease. N Engl J Med 1978; 299:1428–1435.

131. Bertles JF, Milner PF: Irreversibly sickled erythrocytes: A consequence of the heterogeneous distribution of hemoglobin types in sickle-cell anemia. J Clin Invest 1968; 47:1731–1741.

132. Franco RS, Barker-Gear R, Miller MA, et al: Fetal hemoglobin and potassium in isolated transferrin receptor-positive dense sickle reticulocytes. Blood 1994; 84:2013–2020.

133. Lux SE, John KM, Karnovsky MJ: Irreversible deformation of the spectrin-actin lattice in irreversibly sickled cells. J Clin Invest 1976; 58:955–963.

134. Jensen M, Shohet SB, Nathan DG: The role of red cell energy metabolism in the generation of irreversibly sickled cells in vitro. Blood 1973; 42:835–842.

135. Glader BE, Nathan DG: Cation permeability alterations during sickling: Relationship to cation composition and cellular hydration of irreversibly sickled cells. Blood 1978; 51:983–989.

136. Ohnishi ST, Horiuchi KY, Horiuchi K: The mechanism of in vitro formation of irreversibly sickled cells and modes of action of its inhibitors. Biochim Biophys Acta 1986; 886:119–129.

137. Serjeant GR, Serjeant BE, Milner PF: The irreversibly sickled cell; a determinant of haemolysis in sickle cell anaemia. Br J Haematol 1969; 17:527–533.

138. Serjeant GR: Irreversibly sickled cells and splenomegaly in sickle-cell anaemia. Br J Haematol 1970; 19:635–641.

139. Tosteson DC: The effects of sickling on ion transport. II. The effect of sickling on sodium and cesium transport. J Gen Physiol 1955; 39:55.

140. Tosteson DC, Carlsen E, Dunham ET: The effects of sickling on ion transport. I. Effect of sickling on potassium transport. J Gen Physiol 1955; 39:31.

141. Mohandas N, Rossi ME, Clark MR: Association between morphologic distortion of sickle cells and deoxygenation-induced cation permeability increase. Blood 1986; 68:450–454.

142. Joiner CH: Deoxygenation-induced cation fluxes in sickle cells: II. Inhibition by stilbene disulfonates. Blood 1990; 76:212–220.

143. Joiner CH, Dew A, Ge DL: Deoxygenation-induced cation fluxes in sickle cells: Relationship between net potassium efflux and net sodium influx. Blood Cells 1988; 13:339–358.

144. Clark MR, Rossi ME: Permeability characteristics of deoxygenated sickle cells. Blood 1990; 76:2139–2145.

145. Joiner CH, Morris CL, Cooper ES: Deoxygenation-induced cation fluxes in sickle cells. III. Cation selectivity and response to pH and membrane potential. Am J Physiol 1993; 264:C734–C744.

146. Johnson RM, Gannon SA: Erythrocyte cation permeability induced by mechanical stress: A model for sickle cell cation loss. Am J Physiol 1990; 259:C746–51.

147. Bookchin RM, Lew VL: Effects of a 'sickling pulse' on the calcium and potassium permeabilities of intact, sickle trait red cells. J Physiol (Lond) 1978; 284:93P–94P.

148. Etzion Z, Tiffert T, Bookchin RM, et al: Effects of deoxygenation on active and passive Ca^{2+} transport and on the cytoplasmic Ca^{2+} levels of sickle cell anemia red cells. J Clin Invest 1993; 92:2489–2498.

149. Bookchin RM, Ortiz OE, Lew VL: Evidence for a direct reticulocyte origin of dense red cells in sickle cell anemia. J Clin Invest 1991; 87:113–124.

150. Fabry ME, Romero JR, Buchanan ID, et al: Rapid increase in red blood cell density driven by K:Cl cotransport in a subset of sickle cell anemia reticulocytes and discocytes. Blood 1991; 78:217–225.

151. Canessa M, Fabry ME, Blumenfeld N, et al: Volume-stimulated, Cl⁻-dependent K⁺ efflux is highly expressed in young human red cells containing normal hemoglobin or HbS. J Membr Biol 1987; 97:97–105.

152. Sugihara T, Hebbel RP: Exaggerated cation leak from oxygenated sickle red blood cells during deformation: Evidence for a unique leak pathway. Blood 1992; 80:2374–2378.

153. Hebbel RP, Mohandas N: Reversible deformation-dependent erythrocyte cation leak. Extreme sensitivity conferred by minimal peroxidation. Biophys J 1991; 60:712–715.

154. Ney PA, Christopher MM, Hebbel RP: Synergistic effects of oxidation and deformation on erythrocyte monovalent cation leak. Blood 1990; 75:1192–1198.

155. Sugihara T, Rawicz W, Evans EA, et al: Lipid hydroperoxides permit deformation-dependent leak of monovalent cation from erythrocytes. Blood 1991; 77:2757–2763.

156. Hebbel RP, Shalev O, Foker W, et al: Inhibition of erythrocyte Ca²⁺-ATPase by activated oxygen through thiol- and lipid-dependent mechanisms. Biochim Biophys Acta 1986; 862:8–16.

157. Leclerc L, Girard F, Galacteros F, et al: The calmodulin-stimulated (Ca²⁺ + Mg²⁺)-ATPase in hemoglobin S erythrocyte membranes: Effects of sickling and oxidative agents. Biochim Biophys Acta 1987; 897:33–40.

158. Brugnara C, Bunn HF, Tosteson DC: Regulation of erythrocyte cation and water content in sickle cell anemia. Science 1986; 232:388–390.

159. Brugnara C, Bunn HF, Tosteson DC: Ion content and transport and the regulation of volume in sickle cells. Ann NY Acad Sci 1989; 565:96–103.

160. Olivieri O, Vitoux D, Galacteros F, et al: Hemoglobin variants and activity of the (K⁺Cl⁻) cotransport system in human erythrocytes. Blood 1992; 79:793–797.

161. Orringer EP, Brockenbrough JS, Whitney JA, et al: Okadaic acid inhibits activation of K-Cl cotransport in red blood cells containing hemoglobins S and C. Am J Physiol 1991; 261:C591–C593.

162. Canessa M, Spalvins A, Nagel RL: Volume-dependent and NEM-stimulated K⁺,Cl⁻ transport is elevated in oxygenated SS, SC and CC human red cells. FEBS Lett 1986; 200:197–202.

163. Brugnara C, Van Ha T, Tosteson DC: Acid pH induces formation of dense cells in sickle erythrocytes. Blood 1989; 74:487–495.

164. Brugnara C, Tosteson DC: Inhibition of K transport by divalent cations in sickle erythrocytes. Blood 1987; 70:1810–1815.

165. De Franceschi L, Beuzard Y, Jouault H, et al: Modulation of erythrocyte potassium chloride cotransport, potassium content, and density by dietary magnesium intake in transgenic SAD mouse. Blood 1996; 88:2738–2744.

166. De Franceschi L, Bachir D, Galacteros F, et al: Oral magnesium supplements reduce erythrocyte dehydration in patients with sickle cell disease. J Clin Invest 1997; 100:1847–1852.

167. De Franceschi L, Bachir D, Galacteros F, et al: Oral magnesium pidolate: Effects of long-term administration in patients with sickle cell disease. Br J Haematol 2000; 108:284–289.

168. Brugnara C, de Franceschi L, Alper SL: Inhibition of Ca²⁺-dependent K⁺ transport and cell dehydration in sickle erythrocytes by clotrimazole and other imidazole derivatives. J Clin Invest 1993; 92:520–526.

169. De Franceschi L, Saadane N, Trudel M, et al: Treatment with oral clotrimazole blocks Ca²⁺-activated K⁺ transport and reverses erythrocyte dehydration in transgenic SAD mice. A model for therapy of sickle cell disease. J Clin Invest 1994; 93:1670–1676.

170. De Franceschi L, Brugnara C, Rouyer-Fessard P, et al: Formation of dense erythrocytes in SAD mice exposed to chronic hypoxia: Evaluation of different therapeutic regimens and of a combination of oral clotrimazole and magnesium therapies. Blood 1999; 94:4307–4313.

171. Brugnara C, Gee B, Armsby CC, et al: Therapy with oral clotrimazole induces inhibition of the Gardos channel and reduction of erythrocyte dehydration in patients with sickle cell disease. J Clin Invest 1996; 97:1227–1234.

172. Itoh T, Chien S, Usami S: Deformability measurements on individual sickle cells using a new system with pO₂ and temperature control. Blood 1992; 79:2141–2147.

173. Mackie LH, Hochmuth RM: The influence of oxygen tension, temperature, and hemoglobin concentration on the rheologic properties of sickle erythrocytes. Blood 1990; 76:1256–1261.

174. Nash GB, Johnson CS, Meiselman HJ: Influence of oxygen tension on the viscoelastic behavior of red blood cells in sickle cell disease. Blood 1986; 67:110–118.

175. Sorette MP, Lavenant MG, Clark MR: Ektacytometric measurement of sickle cell deformability as a continuous function of oxygen tension. Blood 1987; 69:316–323.

176. Chien S, Usami S, Bertles JF: Abnormal rheology of oxygenated blood in sickle cell anemia. J Clin Invest 1970; 49:623–634.

177. Clark MR, Mohandas N, Shohet SB: Deformability of oxygenated irreversibly sickled cells. J Clin Invest 1980; 65:189–196.

178. Platt OS: Exercise-induced hemolysis in sickle cell anemia: Shear sensitivity and erythrocyte dehydration. Blood 1982; 59:1055–1060.

179. Evans E, Mohandas N, Leung A: Static and dynamic rigidities of normal and sickle erythrocytes. Major influence of cell hemoglobin concentration. J Clin Invest 1984; 73:477–488.

180. Nash GB, Johnson CS, Meiselman HJ: Mechanical properties of oxygenated red blood cells in sickle cell (HbSS) disease. Blood 1984; 63:73–82.

181. Shartava A, Monteiro CA, Bencsath FA, et al: A posttranslational modification of β-actin contributes to the slow dissociation of the spectrin-protein 4.1-actin complex of irreversibly sickled cells. J Cell Biol 1995; 128:805–818.

182. Liu SC, Derick LH, Palek J: Dependence of the permanent deformation of red blood cell membranes on spectrin dimer-tetramer equilibrium: Implication for permanent membrane deformation of irreversibly sickled cells. Blood 1993; 81:522–528.

183. Corbett JD, Golan DE: Band 3 and glycophorin are progressively aggregated in density-fractionated sickle and normal red blood cells. Evidence from rotational and lateral mobility studies. J Clin Invest 1993; 91:208–217.

184. Platt OS, Falcone JF: Membrane protein lesions in erythrocytes with Heinz bodies. J Clin Invest 1988; 82:1051–1058.

185. Platt OS, Falcone JF, Lux SE: Molecular defect in the sickle erythrocyte skeleton. Abnormal spectrin binding to sickle inside-our vesicles. J Clin Invest 1985; 75:266–271.

186. Clark MR, Unger RC, Shohet SB: Monovalent cation composition and ATP and lipid content of irreversibly sickled cells. Blood 1978; 51:1169–1178.

187. Westerman MP, Diloy-Puray M, Streczyn M: Membrane components in the red cells of patients with sickle cell anemia. Relationship to cell aging and to irreversibility of sickling. Biochim Biophys Acta 1979; 557:149–155.

188. Sasaki J, Waterman MR, Buchanan GR, et al: Plasma and erythrocyte lipids in sickle cell anaemia. Clin Lab Haematol 1983; 5:35–44.

189. Haest CW: Interactions between membrane skeleton proteins and the intrinsic domain of the erythrocyte membrane. Biochim Biophys Acta 1982; 694:331–352.

190. Seigneuret M, Devaux PF: ATP-dependent asymmetric distribution of spin-labeled phospholipids in the erythrocyte membrane: Relation to shape changes. Proc Natl Acad Sci USA 1984; 81:3751–3755.

191. Chiu D, Lubin B, Shohet SB: Erythrocyte membrane lipid reorganization during the sickling process. Br J Haematol 1979; 41:223–234.

192. Lubin B, Chiu D, Bastacky J, et al: Abnormalities in membrane phospholipid organization in sickled erythrocytes. J Clin Invest 1981; 67:1643–1649.

193. Kuypers FA, Lewis RA, Hua M, et al: Detection of altered membrane phospholipid asymmetry in subpopulations of human red blood cells using fluorescently labeled annexin V. Blood 1996; 87:1179–1187.

194. Franck PF, Bevers EM, Lubin BH, et al: Uncoupling of the membrane skeleton from the lipid bilayer. The cause of accelerated phospholipid flip-flop leading to an enhanced procoagulant activity of sickled cells. J Clin Invest 1985; 75:183–190.

195. Middelkoop E, Lubin BH, Bevers EM, et al: Studies on sickled erythrocytes provide evidence that the asymmetric distribution of phosphatidylserine in the red cell membrane is maintained by both ATP-dependent translocation and interaction with membrane skeletal proteins. Biochim Biophys Acta 1988; 937:281–288.

196. Chiu D, Lubin B, Roelofsen B, et al: Sickled erythrocytes accelerate clotting in vitro: An effect of abnormal membrane lipid asymmetry. Blood 1981; 58:398–401.

197. Schwartz RS, Duzgunes N, Chiu DT, et al: Interaction of phosphatidylserine-phosphatidylcholine liposomes with sickle erythrocytes. Evidence for altered membrane surface properties. J Clin Invest 1983; 71:1570–1580.

198. Kuypers FA, Chiu D, Mohandas N, et al: The molecular species composition of phosphatidylcholine affects cellular properties in normal and sickle erythrocytes. Blood 1987; 70:1111–1118.

199. Hoover R, Rubin R, Wise G, et al: Adhesion of normal and sickle erythrocytes to endothelial monolayer cultures. Blood 1979; 54:872–876.

200. Hebbel RP, Yamada O, Moldow CF, et al: Abnormal adherence of sickle erythrocytes to cultured vascular endothelium: Possible mechanism for microvascular occlusion in sickle cell disease. J Clin Invest 1980; 65:154–160.

201. Mohandas N, Evans E: Adherence of sickle erythrocytes to vascular endothelial cells: Requirement for both cell membrane changes and plasma factors. Blood 1984; 64:282–287.

202. Barabino GA, McIntire LV, Eskin SG, et al: Endothelial cell interactions with sickle cell, sickle trait, mechanically injured, and normal erythrocytes under controlled flow. Blood 1987; 70:152–157.

203. Smith BD, La Celle PL: Erythrocyte-endothelial cell adherence in sickle cell disorders. Blood 1986; 68:1050–1054.

204. Hebbel RP, Boogaerts MA, Eaton JW, et al: Erythrocyte adherence to endothelium in sickle-cell anemia. A possible determinant of disease severity. N Engl J Med 1980; 302:992–995.

205. Joneckis CC, Ackley RL, Orringer EP, et al: Integrin α4 β1 and glycoprotein IV (CD36) are expressed on circulating reticulocytes in sickle cell anemia. Blood 1993; 82:3548–3555.

206. Swerlick RA, Eckman JR, Kumar A, et al: α4 β1-Integrin expression on sickle reticulocytes: Vascular cell adhesion molecule-1-dependent binding to endothelium. Blood 1993; 82:1891–1899.

207. Gee BE, Platt OS: Sickle reticulocytes adhere to VCAM-1. Blood 1995; 85:268–274.

208. Patel VP, Ciechanover A, Platt O, et al: Mammalian reticulocytes lose adhesion to fibronectin during maturation to erythrocytes. Proc Natl Acad Sci USA 1985; 82:440–444.

209. Mohandas N, Evans E: Sickle erythrocyte adherence to vascular endothelium. Morphologic correlates and the requirement for divalent cations and collagen-binding plasma proteins. J Clin Invest 1985; 76:1605–1612.

210. Kaul DK, Chen D, Zhan J: Adhesion of sickle cells to vascular endothelium is critically dependent on changes in density and shape of the cells. Blood 1994; 83:3006–3017.

211. Morris CL, Rucknagel DL, Joiner CH: Deoxygenation-induced changes in sickle cell-sickle cell adhesion. Blood 1993; 81:3138–3145.

212. Swerlick RA, Lee KH, Wick TM, et al: Human dermal microvascular endothelial but not human umbilical vein endothelial cells express CD36 in vivo and in vitro. J Immunol 1992; 148:78–83.

213. Vordermeier S, Singh S, Biggerstaff J, et al: Red blood cells from patients with sickle cell disease exhibit an increased adherence to cultured endothelium pretreated with tumour necrosis factor (TNF). Br J Haematol 1992; 81:591–597.

214. Hebbel RP, Visser MR, Goodman JL, et al: Potentiated adherence of sickle erythrocytes to endothelium infected by virus. J Clin Invest 1987; 80:1503–1506.

215. Smolinski PA, Offermann MK, Eckman JR, et al: Double-stranded RNA induces sickle erythrocyte adherence to endothelium: A potential role for viral infection in vaso-occlusive pain episodes in sickle cell anemia. Blood 1995; 85:2945–2950.

216. Solovey A, Lin Y, Browne P, et al: Circulating activated endothelial cells in sickle cell anemia. N Engl J Med 1997; 337:1584–1590.

217. Solovey A, Gui L, Key NS, et al: Tissue factor expression by endothelial cells in sickle cell anemia. J Clin Invest 1998; 101:1899–904.

218. Hillery CA, Du MC, Montgomery RR, et al: Increased adhesion of erythrocytes to components of the extracellular matrix: Isolation and characterization of a red blood cell lipid that binds thrombospondin and laminin. Blood 1996; 87:4879–4886.

219. Udani M, Zen Q, Cottman M, et al: Basal cell adhesion molecule/Lutheran protein. The receptor critical for sickle cell adhesion to laminin. J Clin Invest 1998; 101:2550–2558.

220. Lee SP, Cunningham ML, Hines PC, et al: Sickle cell adhesion to laminin: Potential role for the α5 chain. Blood 1998; 92:2951–2958.

221. Joneckis CC, Shock DD, Cunningham ML, et al: Glycoprotein IV-independent adhesion of sickle red blood cells to immobilized thrombospondin under flow conditions. Blood 1996; 87: 4862–4870.

222. Barabino GA, Wise RJ, Woodbury VA, et al: Inhibition of sickle erythrocyte adhesion to immobilized thrombospondin by von Willebrand factor under dynamic flow conditions. Blood 1997; 89:2560–2567.

223. Kasschau MR, Barabino GA, Bridges KR, et al: Adhesion of sickle neutrophils and erythrocytes to fibronectin. Blood 1996; 87:771–780.

224. Weinstein R, Zhou MA, Bartlett-Pandite A, et al: Sickle erythrocytes inhibit human endothelial cell DNA synthesis. Blood 1990; 76:2146–2152.

225. Phelan M, Perrine SP, Brauer M, et al: Sickle erythrocytes, after sickling, regulate the expression of the endothelin-1 gene and protein in human endothelial cells in culture. J Clin Invest 1995; 96:1145–1151.

226. Wick TM, Moake JL, Udden MM, et al: Unusually large von Willebrand factor multimers preferentially promote young sickle and nonsickle erythrocyte adhesion to endothelial cells. Am J Hematol 1993; 42:284–292.

227. Brittain HA, Eckman JR, Wick TM: Sickle erythrocyte adherence to large vessel and microvascular endothelium under physiologic flow is qualitatively different. J Lab Clin Med 1992; 120:538–545.

228. Kaul DK, Nagel RL, Chen D, et al: Sickle erythrocyte-endothelial interactions in microcirculation: The role of von Willebrand factor and implications for vasoocclusion. Blood 1993; 81:2429–2438.

229. Fabry ME, Fine E, Rajanayagam V, et al: Demonstration of endothelial adhesion of sickle cells in vivo: A distinct role for deformable sickle cell discocytes. Blood 1992; 79:1602–1611.

230. Tsai HM, Sussman, II, Nagel RL, et al: Desmopressin induces adhesion of normal human erythrocytes to the endothelial surface of a perfused microvascular preparation. Blood 1990; 75:261–265.

231. Antonucci R, Walker R, Herion J, et al: Enhancement of sickle erythrocyte adherence to endothelium by autologous platelets. Am J Hematol 1990; 34:44–48.

232. Sugihara K, Sugihara T, Mohandas N, et al: Thrombospondin mediates adherence of CD36⁺ sickle reticulocytes to endothelial cells. Blood 1992; 80:2634–2642.

233. Brittain HA, Eckman JR, Swerlick RA, et al: Thrombospondin from activated platelets promotes sickle erythrocyte adherence to human microvascular endothelium under physiologic flow: A potential role for platelet activation in sickle cell vaso-occlusion. Blood 1993; 81:2137–2143.

234. Kaul DK, Tsai HM, Liu XD, et al: Monoclonal antibodies to αVβ3 (7E3 and LM609) inhibit sickle red blood cell-endothelium interactions induced by platelet-activating factor. Blood 2000; 95:368–374.

235. Shaklai N, Yguerabide J, Ranney HM: Classification and localization of hemoglobin binding sites on the red blood cell membrane. Biochemistry 1977; 16:5593–5597.

236. Shaklai N, Yguerabide J, Ranney HM: Interaction of hemoglobin with red blood cell membranes as shown by a fluorescent chromophore. Biochemistry 1977; 16:5585–5592.

237. Eisinger J, Flores J: Cytosol-membrane interface of human erythrocytes. A resonance energy transfer study. Biophys J 1983; 41:367–379.

238. Eisinger J, Flores J, Salhany JM: Association of cytosol hemoglobin with the membrane in intact erythrocytes. Proc Natl Acad Sci USA 1982; 79:408–412.

239. Cassoly R: Quantitative analysis of the association of human hemoglobin with the cytoplasmic fragment of band 3 protein. J Biol Chem 1983; 258:3859–3864.

240. Salhany JM, Cordes KA, Gaines ED: Light-scattering measurements of hemoglobin binding to the erythrocyte membrane. Evidence for transmembrane effects related to a disulfonic stilbene binding to band 3. Biochemistry 1980; 19:1447–1454.

241. Szundi I, Szelenyi JG, Breuer JH, et al: Interactions of haemoglobin with erythrocyte membrane phospholipids in monomolecular lipid layers. Biochim Biophys Acta 1980; 595:41–46.

242. Liu SC, Palek J: Hemoglobin enhances the self-association of spectrin heterodimers in human erythrocytes. J Biol Chem 1984; 259:11556–62.

243. Fischer S, Nagel RL, Bookchin RM, et al: The binding of hemoglobin to membranes of normal and sickle erythrocytes. Biochim Biophys Acta 1975; 375:422–433.

244. Klipstein FA, Ranney HM: Electrophoretic components of the hemoglobin of red cell membranes. J Clin Invest 1960; 39:1894.

245. Bank A, Mears G, Weiss R, et al: Preferential binding of β^s globin chains associated with stroma in sickle cell disorders. J Clin Invest 1974; 54:805–809.

246. Shaklai N, Ranney HM, Sharma V: Interactions of hemoglobin S with the red cell membrane. Prog Clin Biol Res 1981; 51:1–16.

247. Fung LW: Spin-label detection of hemoglobin-membrane interaction at physiological pH. Biochemistry 1981; 20:7162–7166.

248. Evans EA, Mohandas N: Membrane-associated sickle hemoglobin: A major determinant of sickle erythrocyte rigidity. Blood 1987; 70:1443–1449.

249. Fortier N, Snyder LM, Garver F, et al: The relationship between in vivo generated hemoglobin skeletal protein complex and increased red cell membrane rigidity. Blood 1988; 71:1427–1431.

250. Asakura T, Agarwal PL, Relman DA, et al: Mechanical instability of the oxy-form of sickle haemoglobin. Nature 1973; 244:437–438.

251. Asakura T, Minakata K, Adachi K, et al: Denatured hemoglobin in sickle erythrocytes. J Clin Invest 1977; 59:633–640.

252. Schluter K, Drenckhahn D: Co-clustering of denatured hemoglobin with band 3: Its role in binding of autoantibodies against band 3 to abnormal and aged erythrocytes. Proc Natl Acad Sci USA 1986; 83:6137–6141.

253. Waugh SM, Willardson BM, Kannan R, et al: Heinz bodies induce clustering of band 3, glycophorin, and ankyrin in sickle cell erythrocytes. J Clin Invest 1986; 78:1155–1160.

254. Green GA, Kalra VK: Sickling-induced binding of immunoglobulin to sickle erythrocytes. Blood 1988; 71:636–639.

255. Petz LD, Yam P, Wilkinson L, et al: Increased IgG molecules bound to the surface of red blood cells of patients with sickle cell anemia. Blood 1984; 64:301–304.

256. Kay MM: Mechanism of removal of senescent cells by human macrophages in situ. Proc Natl Acad Sci USA 1975; 72:3521–3525.

257. Kay MM, Sorensen K, Wong P, et al: Antigenicity, storage, and aging: Physiologic autoantibodies to cell membrane and serum proteins and the senescent cell antigen. Mol Cell Biochem 1982; 49:65–85.

258. Hebbel RP, Miller WJ: Phagocytosis of sickle erythrocytes: Immunologic and oxidative determinants of hemolytic anemia. Blood 1984; 64:733–741.

259. Liu SC, Yi SJ, Mehta JR, et al: Red cell membrane remodeling in sickle cell anemia. Sequestration of membrane lipids and proteins in Heinz bodies. J Clin Invest 1996; 97:29–36.

260. Hebbel RP, Morgan WT, Eaton JW, et al: Accelerated autoxidation and heme loss due to instability of sickle hemoglobin. Proc Natl Acad Sci USA 1988; 85:237–241.

261. Hebbel RP, Eaton JW, Balasingam M, et al: Spontaneous oxygen radical generation by sickle erythrocytes. J Clin Invest 1982; 70:1253–1259.

262. Hebbel RP: The sickle erythrocyte in double jeopardy: Autoxidation and iron decompartmentalization. Semin Hematol 1990; 27:51–69.

263. Schneider RG, Takeda I, Gustavson LP, et al: Intraerythrocytic precipitations of haemoglobins S and C. Nat New Biol 1972; 235:88–90.

264. Kim HC, Friedman S, Asakura T, et al: Inclusions in red blood cells containing Hb S or Hb C. Br J Haematol 1980; 44:547–554.

265. Liu SC, Zhai S, Palek J: Detection of hemin release during hemoglobin S denaturation. Blood 1988; 71:1755–1758.

266. Campwala HQ, Desforges JF: Membrane-bound hemichrome in density-separated cohorts of normal (AA) and sickled (SS) cells. J Lab Clin Med 1982; 99:25–28.

267. Kuross SA, Hebbel RP: Nonheme iron in sickle erythrocyte membranes: Association with phospholipids and potential role in lipid peroxidation. Blood 1988; 72:1278–1285.

268. Das SK, Nair RC: Superoxide dismutase, glutathione peroxidase, catalase and lipid peroxidation of normal and sickled erythrocytes. Br J Haematol 1980; 44:87–92.

269. Jain SK, Shohet SB: A novel phospholipid in irreversibly sickled cells: Evidence for in vivo peroxidative membrane damage in sickle cell disease. Blood 1984; 63:362–367.

270. Repka T, Shalev O, Reddy R, et al: Nonrandom association of free iron with membranes of sickle and β-thalassemic erythrocytes. Blood 1993; 82:3204–3210.

271. Sugihara T, Repka T, Hebbel RP: Detection, characterization, and bioavailability of membrane-associated iron in the intact sickle red cell. J Clin Invest 1992; 90:2327–2332.

272. Repka T, Hebbel RP: Hydroxyl radical formation by sickle erythrocyte membranes: Role of pathologic iron deposits and cytoplasmic reducing agents. Blood 1991; 78:2753–2758.

273. Johnson FL, Look AT, Gockerman J, et al: Bone-marrow transplantation in a patient with sickle-cell anemia. N Engl J Med 1984; 311:780–783.

274. Vermylen C, Cornu G: Bone marrow transplantation for sickle cell disease. The European experience. Am J Pediatr Hematol Oncol 1994; 16:18–21.

275. Johnson FL, Mentzer WC, Kalinyak KA, et al: Bone marrow transplantation for sickle cell disease. The United States experience. Am J Pediatr Hematol Oncol 1994; 16:22–26.

276. Walters MC, Patience M, Leisenring W, et al: Bone marrow transplantation for sickle cell disease. N Engl J Med 1996; 335:369–376.

277. Giardini C, Galimberti M, Lucarelli G, et al: Bone marrow transplantation in sickle-cell anemia in Pesaro. Bone Marrow Transplant 1993; 12:122–123.

278. Walters MC, Storb R, Patience M, et al: Impact of bone marrow transplantation for symptomatic sickle cell disease: An interim report. Multicenter investigation of bone marrow transplantation for sickle cell disease. Blood 2000; 95:1918–1924.

279. Walters MC, Sullivan KM, Bernaudin F, et al: Neurologic complications after allogeneic marrow transplantation for sickle cell anemia. Blood 1995; 85:879–884.

280. Abboud MR, Jackson SM, Barredo J, et al: Bone marrow transplantation for sickle cell anemia. Am J Pediatr Hematol Oncol 1994; 16:86–89.

281. Ferster A, Bujan W, Corazza F, et al: Bone marrow transplantation corrects the splenic reticuloendothelial dysfunction in sickle cell anemia. Blood 1993; 81:1102–1105.

282. Mentzer WC, Heller S, Pearle PR, et al: Availability of related donors for bone marrow transplantation in sickle cell anemia. Am J Pediatr Hematol Oncol 1994; 16:27–29.

283. Kodish E, Lantos J, Stocking C, et al: Bone marrow transplantation for sickle cell disease. A study of parents' decisions. N Engl J Med 1991; 325:1349–1353.

284. May C, Rivella S, Callegari J, et al: Therapeutic haemoglobin synthesis in β-thalassaemic mice expressing lentivirus-encoded human β-globin. Nature 2000; 406:82–86.

285. Cole-Strauss A, Yoon K, Xiang Y, et al: Correction of the mutation responsible for sickle cell anemia by an RNA-DNA oligonucleotide. Science 1996; 273:1386–1389.

286. Lan N, Howrey RP, Lee SW, et al: Ribozyme-mediated repair of sickle β-globin mRNAs in erythrocyte precursors. Science 1998; 280:1593–1596.

287. Pawliuk R, Westerman KA, Fabry ME, et al: Correction of sickle cell disease in transgenic mouse models by gene therapy. Science 2001; 294:2368.

288. Marshall E: Gene therapy. Gene *gemisch* cures sickle cell in mice. Science 2001; 294:2268.

289. Ley TJ, DeSimone J, Anagnou NP, et al: 5-Azacytidine selectively increases γ-globin synthesis in a patient with β^+ thalassemia. N Engl J Med 1982; 307:1469–1475.

290. Charache S, Dover G, Smith K, et al: Treatment of sickle cell anemia with 5-azacytidine results in increased fetal hemoglobin production and is associated with nonrandom hypomethylation of DNA around the $\gamma\delta\beta$-globin gene complex. Proc Natl Acad Sci USA 1983; 80:4842–4846.

291. Ley TJ, DeSimone J, Noguchi CT, et al: 5-Azacytidine increases γ-globin synthesis and reduces the proportion of dense cells in patients with sickle cell anemia. Blood 1983; 62:370–380.

292. Dover GJ, Charache SH, Boyer SH, et al: 5-Azacytidine increases fetal hemoglobin production in a patient with sickle cell disease. Prog Clin Biol Res 1983; 134:475–488.

293. Platt OS, Orkin SH, Dover G, et al: Hydroxyurea enhances fetal hemoglobin production in sickle cell anemia. J Clin Invest 1984; 74:652–656.

294. Dover GJ, Humphries RK, Moore JG, et al: Hydroxyurea induction of hemoglobin F production in sickle cell disease: Relationship

between cytotoxicity and F cell production. Blood 1986; 67:735–738.

295. Charache S, Dover GJ, Moyer MA, et al: Hydroxyurea-induced augmentation of fetal hemoglobin production in patients with sickle cell anemia. Blood 1987; 69:109–116.

296. Rodgers GP, Dover GJ, Noguchi CT, et al: Hematologic responses of patients with sickle cell disease to treatment with hydroxyurea. N Engl J Med 1990; 322:1037–1045.

297. Goldberg MA, Brugnara C, Dover GJ, et al: Treatment of sickle cell anemia with hydroxyurea and erythropoietin. N Engl J Med 1990; 323:366–372.

298. Rodgers GP, Dover GJ, Uyesaka N, et al: Augmentation by erythropoietin of the fetal-hemoglobin response to hydroxyurea in sickle cell disease. N Engl J Med 1993; 328:73–80.

299. Perrine SP, Ginder GD, Faller DV, et al: A short-term trial of butyrate to stimulate fetal-globin-gene expression in the β-globin disorders. N Engl J Med 1993; 328:81–86.

300. Dover GJ, Brusilow S, Charache S: Induction of fetal hemoglobin production in subjects with sickle cell anemia by oral sodium phenylbutyrate. Blood 1994; 84:339–343.

301. Sher GD, Olivieri NF: Rapid healing of chronic leg ulcers during arginine butyrate therapy in patients with sickle cell disease and thalassemia. Blood 1994; 84:2378–2380.

302. Platt OS, Thorington BD, Brambilla DJ, et al: Pain in sickle cell disease. Rates and risk factors. N Engl J Med 1991; 325:11–16.

303. Charache S, Terrin ML, Moore RD, et al: Effect of hydroxyurea on the frequency of painful crises in sickle cell anemia. Investigators of the Multicenter Study of Hydroxyurea in Sickle Cell Anemia. N Engl J Med 1995; 332:1317–1322.

304. Steinberg MH, Barton F, Castro O, et al: Hydroxyurea (HU) is associated with reduced mortality in adults with sickle cell anemia. Blood 2000; 96:485a.

305. Kinney TR, Helms RW, O'Branski EE, et al: Safety of hydroxyurea in children with sickle cell anemia: Results of the HUG-KIDS study, a phase I/II trial. Pediatric Hydroxyurea Group. Blood 1999; 94:1550–1554.

306. Scott JP, Hillery CA, Brown ER, et al: Hydroxyurea therapy in children severely affected with sickle cell disease. J Pediatr 1996; 128:820–828.

307. Jayabose S, Tugal O, Sandoval C, et al: Clinical and hematologic effects of hydroxyurea in children with sickle cell anemia. J Pediatr 1996; 129:559–565.

308. de Montalembert M, Begue P, Bernaudin F, et al: Preliminary report of a toxicity study of hydroxyurea in sickle cell disease. French Study Group on Sickle Cell Disease. Arch Dis Child 1999; 81:437–439.

309. Ware RE, Zimmerman SA, Schultz WH: Hydroxyurea as an alternative to blood transfusions for the prevention of recurrent stroke in children with sickle cell disease. Blood 1999; 94:3022–3026.

310. Rosa RM, Bierer BE, Thomas R, et al: A study of induced hyponatremia in the prevention and treatment of sickle-cell crisis. N Engl J Med 1980; 303:1138–1143.

311. Leary M, Abramson N: Induced hyponatremia for sickle-cell anemia. N Engl J Med 1981; 304:844–845.

312. Charache S, Walker WG: Failure of desmopressin to lower serum sodium or prevent crisis in patients with sickle cell anemia. Blood 1981; 58:892–896.

313. Charache S, Moyer MA, Walker WG: Treatment of acute sickle cell crises with a vasopressin analogue. Am J Hematol 1983; 15:315–319.

314. Clark MR, Mohandas N, Shohet SB: Hydration of sickle cells using the sodium ionophore monensin. A model for therapy. J Clin Invest 1982; 70:1074–1080.

315. Chang H, Ewert SM, Bookchin RM, et al: Comparative evaluation of fifteen anti-sickling agents. Blood 1983; 61:693–704.

316. Ohnishi ST, Horiuchi KY, Horiuchi K, et al: Nitrendipine, nifedipine and verapamil inhibit the in vitro formation of irreversibly sickled cells. Pharmacology 1986; 32:248–256.

317. Schmidt WFd, Asakura T, Schwartz E: Effect of cetiedil on cation and water movements in erythrocytes. J Clin Invest 1982; 69:589–594.

318. Peterson CM, Tsairis P, Onishi A, et al: Sodium cyanate induced polyneuropathy in patients with sickle-cell disease. Ann Intern Med 1974; 81:152–158.

319. Charache S, Duffy TP, Jander N, et al: Toxic-therapeutic ratio of sodium cyanate. Arch Intern Med 1975; 135:1043–1047.

320. Rodgers GP, Schechter AN, Noguchi CT, et al: Microcirculatory adaptations in sickle cell anemia: Reactive hyperemia response. Am J Physiol 1990; 258:H113–120.

321. Chang JC, Kan YW: A sensitive new prenatal test for sickle-cell anemia. N Engl J Med 1982; 307:30–32.

322. Orkin SH, Little PF, Kazazian HH Jr, et al: Improved detection of the sickle mutation by DNA analysis: Application to prenatal diagnosis. N Engl J Med 1982; 307:32–36.

323. Wallace RB, Johnson MJ, Hirose T, et al: The use of synthetic oligonucleotides as hybridization probes. II. Hybridization of oligonucleotides of mixed sequence to rabbit β-globin DNA. Nucleic Acids Res 1981; 9:879–894.

324. Conner BJ, Reyes AA, Morin C, et al: Detection of sickle cell β S-globin allele by hybridization with synthetic oligonucleotides. Proc Natl Acad Sci USA 1983; 80:278–282.

325. Pirastu M, Kan YW, Cao A, et al: Prenatal diagnosis of β-thalassemia. Detection of a single nucleotide mutation in DNA. N Engl J Med 1983; 309:284–287.

326. Saiki RK, Chang CA, Levenson CH, et al: Diagnosis of sickle cell anemia and β-thalassemia with enzymatically amplified DNA and nonradioactive allele-specific oligonucleotide probes. N Engl J Med 1988; 319:537–541.

327. Chehab FF, Kan YW: Detection of sickle cell anaemia mutation by colour DNA amplification. Lancet 1990; 335:15–17.

328. Saiki RK, Scharf S, Faloona F, et al: Enzymatic amplification of β-globin genomic sequences and restriction site analysis for diagnosis of sickle cell anemia. Science 1985; 230:1350–1354.

329. Embury SH, Scharf SJ, Saiki RK, et al: Rapid prenatal diagnosis of sickle cell anemia by a new method of DNA analysis. N Engl J Med 1987; 316:656–661.

330. Goossens M, Dumez Y, Kaplan L, et al: Prenatal diagnosis of sickle-cell anemia in the first trimester of pregnancy. N Engl J Med 1983; 309:831–833.

331. Old JM, Fitches A, Heath C, et al: First-trimester fetal diagnosis for haemoglobinopathies: Report on 200 cases. Lancet 1986; 2:763–767.

332. Xu K, Shi ZM, Veeck LL, et al: First unaffected pregnancy using preimplantation genetic diagnosis for sickle cell anemia. JAMA 1999; 281:1701–1706.

333. Pearson HA: A neonatal program for sickle cell anemia. Adv Pediatr 1986; 33:381–400.

334. Serjeant GR, Grandison Y, Lowrie Y, et al: The development of haematological changes in homozygous sickle cell disease: A cohort study from birth to 6 years. Br J Haematol 1981; 48:533–543.

335. Reed W, Lane PA, Lorey F, et al: Sickle-cell disease not identified by newborn screening because of prior transfusion. J Pediatr 2000; 136:248–250.

336. Jinks DC, Minter M, Tarver DA, et al: Molecular genetic diagnosis of sickle cell disease using dried blood specimens on blotters used for newborn screening. Hum Genet 1989; 81:363–366.

337. Panepinto JA, Magid D, Rewers MJ, et al: Universal versus targeted screening of infants for sickle cell disease: A cost-effectiveness analysis. J Pediatr 2000; 136:201–208.

338. Davies SC, Cronin E, Gill M, et al: Screening for sickle cell disease and thalassaemia: A systematic review with supplementary research. Health Technol Assess 2000; 4:1–99.

339. O'Brien RT, McIntosh S, Aspnes GT, et al: Prospective study of sickle cell anemia in infancy. J Pediatr 1976; 89:205–210.

340. Gaston M, Smith J, Gallagher D, et al: Recruitment in the Cooperative Study of Sickle Cell Disease (CSSCD). Control Clin Trials 1987; 8:131S-140S.

341. Gaston M, Rosse WF: The cooperative study of sickle cell disease: Review of study design and objectives. Am J Pediatr Hematol Oncol 1982; 4:197–201.

342. Diggs LW: Sickle cell crises. Am J Clin Pathol 1965; 44:1.

343. Gill FM, Sleeper LA, Weiner SJ, et al: Clinical events in the first decade in a cohort of infants with sickle cell disease. Cooperative Study of Sickle Cell Disease. Blood 1995; 86:776–783.

344. Bainbridge R, Higgs DR, Maude GH, et al: Clinical presentation of homozygous sickle cell disease. J Pediatr 1985; 106:881–885.

345. Konotey-Ahulu FI: The sickle cell diseases. Clinical manifestations including the "sickle crisis." Arch Intern Med 1974; 133:611–619.

346. Platt OS, Brambilla DJ, Rosse WF, et al: Mortality in sickle cell disease. Life expectancy and risk factors for early death. N Engl J Med 1994; 330:1639–1644.

347. Redwood AM, Williams EM, Desal P, et al: Climate and painful crisis of sickle-cell disease in Jamaica. Br Med J 1976; 1:66–68.

348. Ibrahim AS: Relationship between meteorological changes and occurrence of painful sickle cell crises in Kuwait. Trans R Soc Trop Med Hyg 1980; 74:159–161.

349. Milner PF, Brown M: Bone marrow infarction in sickle cell anemia: Correlation with hematologic profiles. Blood 1982; 60:1411–1419.

350. Charache S, Page DL: Infarction of bone marrow in the sickle cell disorders. Ann Intern Med 1967; 67:1195–200.

351. Mankad VN, Williams JP, Harpen MD, et al: Magnetic resonance imaging of bone marrow in sickle cell disease: Clinical, hematologic, and pathologic correlations. Blood 1990; 75:274–283.

352. Diggs LW: Bone and joint lesions in sickle-cell disease. Clin Orthop 1967; 52:119–143.

353. Keeley K, Buchanan GR: Acute infarction of long bones in children with sickle cell anemia. J Pediatr 1982; 101:170–175.

354. Sain A, Sham R, Silver L: Bone scan in sickle cell crisis. Clin Nucl Med 1978; 3:85–90.

355. Alavi A, Schumacher HR, Dorwart B, et al: Bone marrow scan evaluation of arthropathy in sickle cell disorders. Arch Intern Med 1976; 136:436–440.

356. Hammel CF, DeNardo SJ, DeNardo GL, et al: Bone marrow and bone mineral scintigraphic studies in sickle cell disease. Br J Haematol 1973; 25:593–598.

357. Lutzker LG, Alavi A: Bone and marrow imaging in sickle cell disease: Diagnosis of infarction. Semin Nucl Med 1976; 6:83–93.

358. Kahn CE Jr, Ryan JW, Hatfield MK, et al: Combined bone marrow and gallium imaging. Differentiation of osteomyelitis and infarction in sickle hemoglobinopathy. Clin Nucl Med 1988; 13:443–449.

359. Rao S, Solomon N, Miller S, et al: Scintigraphic differentiation of bone infarction from osteomyelitis in children with sickle cell disease. J Pediatr 1985; 107:685–688.

360. Kim HC, Alavi A, Russell MO, et al: Differentiation of bone and bone marrow infarcts from osteomyelitis in sickle cell disorders. Clin Nucl Med 1989; 14:249–254.

361. Guze BH, Hawkins RA, Marcus CS: Technetium-99m white blood cell imaging: False-negative result in *Salmonella* osteomyelitis associated with sickle cell disease. Clin Nucl Med 1989; 14:104–106.

362. Cole TB, Smith SJ, Buchanan GR: Hematologic alterations during acute infection in children with sickle cell disease. Pediatr Infect Dis J 1987; 6:454–457.

363. Syrogiannopoulos GA, McCracken GH Jr, Nelson JD: Osteoarticular infections in children with sickle cell disease. Pediatrics 1986; 78:1090–1096.

364. Stuart J, Stone PC, Akinola NO, et al: Monitoring the acute phase response to vaso-occlusive crisis in sickle cell disease. J Clin Pathol 1994; 47:166–169.

365. Devine DV, Kinney TR, Thomas PF, et al: Fragment D-dimer levels: An objective marker of vaso-occlusive crisis and other complications of sickle cell disease. Blood 1986; 68:317–319.

366. Francis RB Jr: Elevated fibrin D-dimer fragment in sickle cell anemia: Evidence for activation of coagulation during the steady state as well as in painful crisis. Haemostasis 1989; 19:105–111.

367. Ballas SK, Smith ED: Red blood cell changes during the evolution of the sickle cell painful crisis. Blood 1992; 79:2154–2163.

368. Griffin TC, McIntire D, Buchanan GR: High-dose intravenous methylprednisolone therapy for pain in children and adolescents with sickle cell disease. N Engl J Med 1994; 330:733–737.

369. Greenberg J, Ohene-Frempong K, Halus J, et al: Trial of low doses of aspirin as prophylaxis in sickle cell disease. J Pediatr 1983; 102:781–784.

370. Watson RJ, Burko H: The hand-foot syndrome in sickle cell disease in young children. Pediatrics 1963; 45:975.

371. Worrall VT, Butera V: Sickle-cell dactylitis. J Bone Joint Surg Am 1976; 58:1161–1163.

372. Serjeant GR, Ashcroft MT: Shortening of the digits in sickle cell anaemia: A sequela of the hand-foot syndrome. Trop Geogr Med 1971; 23:341–346.

373. Miller ST, Sleeper LA, Pegelow CH, et al: Prediction of adverse outcomes in children with sickle cell disease. N Engl J Med 2000; 342:83–89.

374. Kaul DK, Hebbel RP: Hypoxia/reoxygenation causes inflammatory response in transgenic sickle mice but not in normal mice. J Clin Invest 2000; 106:411–420.

375. Castro O, Brambilla DJ, Thorington B, et al: The acute chest syndrome in sickle cell disease: Incidence and risk factors. The Cooperative Study of Sickle Cell Disease. Blood 1994; 84:643–649.

376. Vichinsky EP, Neumayr LD, Earles AN, et al: Causes and outcomes of the acute chest syndrome in sickle cell disease. National Acute Chest Syndrome Study Group. N Engl J Med 2000; 342:1855–1865.

377. Vichinsky E, Williams R, Das M, et al: Pulmonary fat embolism: A distinct cause of severe acute chest syndrome in sickle cell anemia. Blood 1994; 83:3107–3112.

378. Vichinsky EP, Styles LA, Colangelo LH, et al: Acute chest syndrome in sickle cell disease: Clinical presentation and course. Cooperative Study of Sickle Cell Disease. Blood 1997; 89:1787–1792.

379. Leong MA, Dampier C, Varlotta L, et al: Airway hyperreactivity in children with sickle cell disease. J Pediatr 1997; 131:278–283.

380. Davies SC, Luce PJ, Win AA, et al: Acute chest syndrome in sickle-cell disease. Lancet 1984; 1:36–38.

381. Pianosi P, Charge TD, Esseltine DW, et al: Pulse oximetry in sickle cell disease. Arch Dis Child 1993; 68:735–738.

382. Rackoff WR, Kunkel N, Silber JH, et al: Pulse oximetry and factors associated with hemoglobin oxygen desaturation in children with sickle cell disease. Blood 1993; 81:3422–3427.

383. Haupt HM, Moore GW, Bauer TW, et al: The lung in sickle cell disease. Chest 1982; 81:332–337.

384. Athanasou NA, Hatton C, McGee JO, et al: Vascular occlusion and infarction in sickle cell crisis and the sickle chest syndrome. J Clin Pathol 1985; 38:659–664.

385. Charache S, Scott JC, Charache P: "Acute chest syndrome" in adults with sickle cell anemia. Microbiology, treatment, and prevention. Arch Intern Med 1979; 139:67–69.

386. Atz AM, Wessel DL: Inhaled nitric oxide in sickle cell disease with acute chest syndrome. Anesthesiology 1997; 87:988–990.

387. Buchanan GR, Glader BE: Benign course of extreme hyperbilirubinemia in sickle cell anemia: Analysis of six cases. J Pediatr 1977; 91:21–24.

388. Sheehy TW: Sickle cell hepatopathy. South Med J 1977; 70:533–538.

389. Serafini AN, Spoliansky G, Sfakianakis GN, et al: Diagnostic studies in patients with sickle cell anemia and acute abdominal pain. Arch Intern Med 1987; 147:1061–1062.

390. Stephens CG, Scott RB: Cholelithiasis in sickle cell anemia: Surgical or medical management. Arch Intern Med 1980; 140:648–651.

391. Powars D, Wilson B, Imbus C, et al: The natural history of stroke in sickle cell disease. Am J Med 1978; 65:461–471.

392. Balkaran B, Char G, Morris JS, et al: Stroke in a cohort of patients with homozygous sickle cell disease. J Pediatr 1992; 120:360–366.

393. Ohene-Frempong K: Stroke in sickle cell disease: Demographic, clinical, and therapeutic considerations. Semin Hematol 1991; 28:213–219.

394. Russell MO, Goldberg HI, Hodson A, et al: Effect of transfusion therapy on arteriographic abnormalities and on recurrence of stroke in sickle cell disease. Blood 1984; 63:162–169.

395. Stockman JA, Nigro MA, Mishkin MM, et al: Occlusion of large cerebral vessels in sickle-cell anemia. N Engl J Med 1972; 287:846–849.

396. Wilimas J, Goff JR, Anderson HR Jr, et al: Efficacy of transfusion therapy for one to two years in patients with sickle cell disease and cerebrovascular accidents. J Pediatr 1980; 96:205–208.

397. Boros L, Thomas C, Weiner WJ: Large cerebral vessel disease in sickle cell anaemia. J Neurol Neurosurg Psychiatry 1976; 39:1236–1239.

398. Merkel KH, Ginsberg PL, Parker JC Jr, et al: Cerebrovascular disease in sickle cell anemia: A clinical, pathological and radiological correlation. Stroke 1978; 9:45–52.

399. Adams RJ: Neurologic complications. In Embury SH, Hebbel RP, Mohandas N, et al (Eds.): Sickle Cell Disease: Basic Principles and Clinical Practice. New York: Raven Press, 1994, pp 599–621.

400. Pavlakis SG, Bello J, Prohovnik I, et al: Brain infarction in sickle cell anemia: Magnetic resonance imaging correlates. Ann Neurol 1988; 23:125–130.

401. Adams RJ, Nichols FT, McKie V, et al: Cerebral infarction in sickle cell anemia: Mechanism based on CT and MRI: Neurology 1988; 38:1012–1017.

402. Herold S, Brozovic M, Gibbs J, et al: Measurement of regional cerebral blood flow, blood volume and oxygen metabolism in patients with sickle cell disease using positron emission tomography. Stroke 1986; 17:692–698.

403. Russell MO, Goldberg HI, Reis L, et al: Transfusion therapy for cerebrovascular abnormalities in sickle cell disease. J Pediatr 1976; 88:382–387.

404. Lusher JM, Haghighat H, Khalifa AS: A prophylactic transfusion program for children with sickle cell anemia complicated by CNS infarction. Am J Hematol 1976; 1:265–273.

405. Seeler RA, Royal JE: Commentary: Sickle cell anemia, stroke, and transfusion. J Pediatr 1980; 96:243–244.

406. Wang WC, Kovnar EH, Tonkin IL, et al: High risk of recurrent stroke after discontinuance of five to twelve years of transfusion therapy in patients with sickle cell disease. J Pediatr 1991; 118:377–382.

407. Cohen AR, Martin MB, Silber JH, et al: A modified transfusion program for prevention of stroke in sickle cell disease. Blood 1992; 79:1657–1661.

408. Vichinsky EP, Lubin BH: A cautionary note regarding hydroxyurea in sickle cell disease. Blood 1994; 83:1124–1128.

409. Walters MC, Storb R, Patience M, et al: Impact of bone marrow transplantation for symptomatic sickle cell disease: An interim report. Blood 2000; 95:1918–1924.

410. Adams R, McKie V, Nichols F, et al: The use of transcranial ultrasonography to predict stroke in sickle cell disease. N Engl J Med 1992; 326:605–610.

411. Kugler S, Anderson B, Cross D, et al: Abnormal cranial magnetic resonance imaging scans in sickle-cell disease. Neurological correlates and clinical implications. Arch Neurol 1993; 50:629–635.

412. Wang WC, Gallagher DM, Pegelow CH, et al: Multicenter comparison of magnetic resonance imaging and transcranial Doppler ultrasonography in the evaluation of the central nervous system in children with sickle cell disease. J Pediatr Hematol Oncol 2000; 22:335–339.

413. Kinney TR, Sleeper LA, Wang WC, et al: Silent cerebral infarcts in sickle cell anemia: A risk factor analysis. The Cooperative Study of Sickle Cell Disease. Pediatrics 1999; 103:640–645.

414. Wang WC, Langston JW, Steen RG, et al: Abnormalities of the central nervous system in very young children with sickle cell anemia. J Pediatr 1998; 132:994–998.

415. Schatz J, Brown RT, Pascual JM, et al: Poor school and cognitive functioning with silent cerebral infarcts and sickle cell disease. Neurology 2001; 56:1109–1111.

416. Bernaudin F, Verlhac S, Freard F, et al: Multicenter prospective study of children with sickle cell disease: Radiographic and psychometric correlation. J Child Neurol 2000; 15:333–343.

417. Steen RG, Langston JW, Reddick WE, et al: Quantitative MR imaging of children with sickle cell disease: Striking T1 elevation in the thalamus. J Magn Reson Imaging 1996; 6:226–234.

418. Ohene-Frempong K, Weiner SJ, Sleeper LA, et al: Cerebrovascular accidents in sickle cell disease: Rates and risk factors. Blood 1998; 91:288–294.

419. Pegelow CH, Colangelo L, Steinberg M, et al: Natural history of blood pressure in sickle cell disease: Risks for stroke and death associated with relative hypertension in sickle cell anemia. Am J Med 1997; 102:171–177.

420. Adams RJ, McKie VC, Hsu L, et al: Prevention of a first stroke by transfusions in children with sickle cell anemia and abnormal results on transcranial Doppler ultrasonography. N Engl J Med 1998; 339:5–11.

421. Ferster A, Tahriri P, Vermylen C, et al: Five years of experience with hydroxyurea in children and young adults with sickle cell disease. Blood 2001; 97:3628–3632.

422. Hoppe CC, Walters MC: Bone marrow transplantation in sickle cell anemia. Curr Opin Oncol 2001; 13:85–90.

423. Oyesiku NM, Barrow DL, Eckman JR, et al: Intracranial aneurysms in sickle-cell anemia: Clinical features and pathogenesis. J Neurosurg 1991; 75:356–363.

424. Anson JA, Koshy M, Ferguson L, et al: Subarachnoid hemorrhage in sickle-cell disease. J Neurosurg 1991; 75:552–558.

425. Schmugge M, Frischknecht H, Yonekawa Y, et al: Stroke in hemoglobin (SD) sickle cell disease with moyamoya: Successful hydroxyurea treatment after cerebrovascular bypass surgery. Blood 2001; 97:2165–2167.

426. Emond AM, Holman R, Hayes RJ, et al: Priapism and impotence in homozygous sickle cell disease. Arch Intern Med 1980; 140:1434–1437.

427. Mantadakis E, Cavender JD, Rogers ZR, et al: Prevalence of priapism in children and adolescents with sickle cell anemia. J Pediatr Hematol Oncol 1999; 21:518–522.

428. Seeler RA: Priapism in children with sickle cell anemia. Clin Pediatr (Phila) 1971; 10:418–419.

429. Chakrabarty A, Upadhyay J, Dhabuwala CB, et al: Priapism associated with sickle cell hemoglobinopathy in children: Long-term effects on potency. J Urol 1996; 155:1419–1423.

430. Sharpsteen JR Jr, Powars D, Johnson C, et al: Multisystem damage associated with tricorporal priapism in sickle cell disease. Am J Med 1993; 94:289–295.

431. Grace DA, Winter CC: Priapism: An appraisal of management of twenty-three patients. J Urol 1968; 99:301–310.

432. Rackoff WR, Ohene-Frempong K, Month S, et al: Neurologic events after partial exchange transfusion for priapism in sickle cell disease. J Pediatr 1992; 120:882–885.

433. Dunn EK, Miller ST, Macchia RJ, et al: Penile scintigraphy for priapism in sickle cell disease. J Nucl Med 1995; 36:1404–1407.

434. Miller ST, Rao SP, Dunn EK, Glassberg KI: Priapism in children with sickle cell disease. J Urol 1995; 154:844–847.

435. Burnett AL, Allen RP, Tempany CM, et al: Evaluation of erectile function in men with sickle cell disease. Urology 1995; 45:657–663.

436. Mantadakis E, Ewalt DH, Cavender JD, et al: Outpatient penile aspiration and epinephrine irrigation for young patients with sickle cell anemia and prolonged priapism. Blood 2000; 95:78–82.

437. Rifkind S, Waisman J, Thompson R, et al: RBC exchange pheresis for priapism in sickle cell disease. JAMA 1979; 242:2317–2318.

438. Walker EM Jr, Mitchum EN, Rous SN, et al: Automated erythrocytopheresis for relief of priapism in sickle cell hemoglobinopathies. J Urol 1983; 130:912–916.

439. McCarthy LJ, Vattuone J, Weidner J, et al: Do automated red cell exchanges relieve priapism in patients with sickle cell anemia? Ther Apher 2000; 4:256–258.

440. Virag R, Bachir D, Lee K, et al: Preventive treatment of priapism in sickle cell disease with oral and self-administered intracavernous injection of etilefrine. Urology 1996; 47:777–781; discussion 781.

441. Serjeant GR, de Ceulaer K, Maude GH: Stilboestrol and stuttering priapism in homozygous sickle-cell disease. Lancet 1985; 2:1274–1276.

442. Noe HN, Wilimas J, Jerkins GR: Surgical management of priapism in children with sickle cell anemia. J Urol 1981; 126:770–771.

443. Douglas L, Fletcher H, Serjeant GR: Penile prostheses in the management of impotence in sickle cell disease. Br J Urol 1990; 65:533–535.

444. Upadhyay J, Shekarriz B, Dhabuwala CB: Penile implant for intractable priapism associated with sickle cell disease. Urology 1998; 51:638–639.

445. Seeler RA: Deaths in children with sickle cell anemia. A clinical analysis of 19 fatal instances in Chicago. Clin Pediatr (Phila) 1972; 11:634–637.

446. Pearson HA: Hemoglobin S-thalassemia syndrome in Negro children. Ann NY Acad Sci 1969; 165:83–92.

447. Pappo A, Buchanan GR: Acute splenic sequestration in a 2-month-old infant with sickle cell anemia. Pediatrics 1989; 84:578–579.

448. Emond AM, Collis R, Darvill D, et al: Acute splenic sequestration in homozygous sickle cell disease: Natural history and management. J Pediatr 1985; 107:201–206.

449. Seeler RA, Shwiaki MZ: Acute splenic sequestration crises (ASSC) in young children with sickle cell anemia. Clinical observations in 20 episodes in 14 children. Clin Pediatr (Phila) 1972; 11:701–704.

450. Rao S, Gooden S: Splenic sequestration in sickle cell disease: Role of transfusion therapy. Am J Pediatr Hematol Oncol 1985; 7:298–301.

451. Kinney TR, Ware RE, Schultz WH, et al: Long-term management of splenic sequestration in children with sickle cell disease. J Pediatr 1990; 117:194–199.

452. Jenkins ME, Scott RB: Studies in sickle cell anemia. XVI. Sudden death during sickle cell anemia crises in young children. J Pediatr 1960; 56:30.

453. Wright JG, Hambleton IR, Thomas PW, et al: Postsplenectomy course in homozygous sickle cell disease. J Pediatr 1999; 134:304–309.

454. MacIver JE, Parker-Williams EJ: Aplastic crisis in sickle cell anemia. J Lab Clin Med 1961; 35:721.

455. Singer K, Motulsky AG: Aplastic crisis in sickle cell anemia. J Lab Clin Med 1950; 35:721.

456. Leikin SL: The aplastic crisis of sickle cell disease: Occurrence in several members of families within a short period of time. Am J Dis Child 1957; 93:128.

457. Serjeant GR, Topley JM, Mason K, et al: Outbreak of aplastic crises in sickle cell anaemia associated with parvovirus-like agent. Lancet 1981; 2:595–597.

458. Goldstein AR, Anderson MJ, Serjeant GR: Parvovirus associated aplastic crisis in homozygous sickle cell disease. Arch Dis Child 1987; 62:585–588.

459. Serjeant GR, Serjeant BE, Thomas PW, et al: Human parvovirus infection in homozygous sickle cell disease. Lancet 1993; 341:1237–1240.

460. Rao SP, Desai N, Miller ST: B19 parvovirus infection and transient aplastic crisis in a child with sickle cell anemia. J Pediatr Hematol Oncol 1996; 18:175–177.

461. Plummer FA, Hammond GW, Forward K, et al: An erythema infectiosum-like illness caused by human parvovirus infection. N Engl J Med 1985; 313:74–79.

462. Chorba T, Coccia P, Holman RC, et al: The role of parvovirus B19 in aplastic crisis and erythema infectiosum (fifth disease). J Infect Dis 1986; 154:383–393.

463. Saarinen UM, Chorba TL, Tattersall P, et al: Human parvovirus B19-induced epidemic acute red cell aplasia in patients with hereditary hemolytic anemia. Blood 1986; 67:1411–1417.

464. Mortimer PP, Humphries RK, Moore JG, et al: A human parvovirus-like virus inhibits haematopoietic colony formation in vitro. Nature 1983; 302:426–429.

465. Barrett-Connor E: Bacterial infection and sickle cell anemia. An analysis of 250 infections in 166 patients and a review of the literature. Medicine (Baltimore) 1971; 50:97–112.

466. Overturf GD, Powars D, Baraff LJ: Bacterial meningitis and septicemia in sickle cell disease. Am J Dis Child 1977; 131:784–787.

467. Powars D, Overturf G, Turner E: Is there an increased risk of *Haemophilus influenzae* septicemia in children with sickle cell anemia? Pediatrics 1983; 71:927–931.

468. Pearson HA, Spencer RP, Cornelius EA: Functional asplenia in sickle-cell anemia. N Engl J Med 1969; 281:923–926.

469. Pearson HA, McIntosh S, Ritchey AK, et al: Developmental aspects of splenic function in sickle cell diseases. Blood 1979; 53:358–365.

470. Seeler RA, Reddi CU, Kittams D: *Diplococcus pneumoniae* osteomyelitis in an infant with sickle cell anemia. Clin Pediatr (Phila) 1974; 13:372–374.

471. Fischer KC, Shapiro S, Treves S: Visualization of the spleen with a bone-seeking radionuclide in a child with sickle-cell anemia. Radiology 1977; 122:398.

472. Pearson HA, Cornelius EA, Schwartz AD, et al: Transfusion-reversible functional asplenia in young children with sickle-cell anemia. N Engl J Med 1970; 283:334–337.

473. Claster S, Vichinsky E: First report of reversal of organ dysfunction in sickle cell anemia by the use of hydroxyurea: Splenic regeneration. Blood 1996; 88:1951–1953.

474. Schwartz AD, Pearson HA: Impaired antibody response to intravenous immunization in sickle cell anemia. Pediatr Res 1972; 6:145–149.

475. Ammann AJ, Addiego J, Wara DW, et al: Polyvalent pneumococcal-polysaccharide immunization of patients with sickle-cell anemia and patients with splenectomy. N Engl J Med 1977; 297:897–900.

476. Overturf GD, Rigau-Perez JG, Selzer J, et al: Pneumococcal polysaccharide immunization of children with sickle cell disease. I. Clinical reactions to immunization and relationship to preimmunization antibody. Am J Pediatr Hematol Oncol 1982; 4:19–23.

477. Evans HE, Reindorf C: Serum immunoglobulin levels in sickle cell disease and thalassemia major. Am J Dis Child 1968; 116:586–590.

478. De Ceulaer K, Forbes M, Maude GH, et al: Complement and immunoglobulin levels in early childhood in homozygous sickle cell disease. J Clin Lab Immunol 1986; 21:37–41.

479. Winkelstein JA, Drachman RH: Deficiency of pneumococcal serum opsonizing activity in sickle-cell disease. N Engl J Med 1968; 279:459–466.

480. Johnston RB Jr, Newman SL, Struth AG: An abnormality of the alternate pathway of complement activation in sickle-cell disease. N Engl J Med 1973; 288:803–808.

481. Wilson WA, Hughes GR, Lachmann PJ: Deficiency of factor B of the complement system in sickle cell anaemia. Br Med J 1976; 1:367–369.

482. Chudwin DS, Wara DW, Matthay KK, et al: Increased serum opsonic activity and antibody concentration in patients with sickle cell disease after pneumococcal polysaccharide immunization. J Pediatr 1983; 102:51–54.

483. Bjornson AB, Gaston MH, Zellner CL: Decreased opsonization for *Streptococcus pneumoniae* in sickle cell disease: Studies on selected complement components and immunoglobulins. J Pediatr 1977; 91:371–378.

484. Bjornson AB, Lobel JS: Lack of a requirement for the Fc region of IgG in restoring pneumococcal opsonization via the alternative complement pathway in sickle cell disease. J Infect Dis 1986; 154:760–769.

485. Boggs DR, Hyde F, Srodes C: An unusual pattern of neutrophil kinetics in sickle cell anemia. Blood 1973; 41:59–65.

486. Dimitrov NV, Douwes FR, Bartolotta B, et al: Metabolic activity of polymorphonuclear leukocytes in sickle cell anemia. Acta Haematol 1972; 47:283–291.

487. Strauss RG, Johnston RB Jr, Asbrock T, et al: Neutrophil oxidative metabolism in sickle cell disease. J Pediatr 1976; 89:391–394.

488. Boghossian SH, Wright G, Webster AD, et al: Investigations of host defence in patients with sickle cell disease. Br J Haematol 1985; 59:523–531.

489. Hongeng S, Wilimas JA, Harris S, et al: Recurrent *Streptococcus pneumoniae* sepsis in children with sickle cell disease. J Pediatr 1997; 130:814–816.

490. Magnus SA, Hambleton IR, Moosdeen F, et al: Recurrent infections in homozygous sickle cell disease. Arch Dis Child 1999; 80:537–541.

491. McIntosh S, Rooks Y, Ritchey AK, et al: Fever in young children with sickle cell disease. J Pediatr 1980; 96:199–204.

492. Buchanan GR, Glader BE: Leukocyte counts in children with sickle cell disease. Comparative values in the steady state, vaso-occlusive crisis, and bacterial infection. Am J Dis Child 1978; 132:396–398.

493. Wilimas JA, Flynn PM, Harris S, et al: A randomized study of outpatient treatment with ceftriaxone for selected febrile children with sickle cell disease. N Engl J Med 1993; 329:472–476.

494. Shulman ST, Bartlett J, Clyde WA Jr, et al: The unusual severity of mycoplasmal pneumonia in children with sickle-cell disease. N Engl J Med 1972; 287:164–167.

495. John AB, Ramlal A, Jackson H, et al: Prevention of pneumococcal infection in children with homozygous sickle cell disease. Br Med J (Clin Res Ed) 1984; 288:1567–1570.

496. Gaston MH, Verter JI, Woods G, et al: Prophylaxis with oral penicillin in children with sickle cell anemia. A randomized trial. N Engl J Med 1986; 314:1593–1599.

497. Falletta JM, Woods GM, Verter JI, et al: Discontinuing penicillin prophylaxis in children with sickle cell anemia. Prophylactic Penicillin Study II. J Pediatr 1995; 127:685–690.

498. Woods GM, Jorgensen JH, Waclawiw MA, et al: Influence of penicillin prophylaxis on antimicrobial resistance in nasopharyngeal *S. pneumoniae* among children with sickle cell anemia. The Ancillary Nasopharyngeal Culture Study of Prophylactic Penicillin Study II. J Pediatr Hematol Oncol 1997; 19:327–333.

499. Daw NC, Wilimas JA, Wang WC, et al: Nasopharyngeal carriage of penicillin-resistant *Streptococcus pneumoniae* in children with sickle cell disease. Pediatrics 1997; 99:E7.

500. Wong WY, Powars DR, Chan L, et al: Polysaccharide encapsulated bacterial infection in sickle cell anemia: A thirty year epidemiologic experience. Am J Hematol 1992; 39:176–182.

501. O'Brien KL, Swift AJ, Winkelstein JA, et al: Safety and immunogenicity of heptavalent pneumococcal vaccine conjugated to CRM_{197} among infants with sickle cell disease. Pneumococcal Conjugate Vaccine Study Group. Pediatrics 2000; 106:965–972.

502. Buchanan GR, Schiffman G: Antibody responses to polyvalent pneumococcal vaccine in infants with sickle cell anemia. J Pediatr 1980; 96:264–266.

503. Kaplan J, Frost H, Sarnaik S, et al: Type-specific antibodies in children with sickle cell anemia given polyvalent pneumococcal vaccine. J Pediatr 1982; 100:404–406.

504. Kaplan J, Sarnaik S, Schiffman G: Revaccination with polyvalent pneumococcal vaccine in children with sickle cell anemia. Am J Pediatr Hematol Oncol 1986; 8:80–82.

505. Nowak-Wegrzyn A, Winkelstein JA, Swift AJ, et al: Serum opsonic activity in infants with sickle-cell disease immunized with pneumococcal polysaccharide protein conjugate vaccine. The Pneumococcal Conjugate Vaccine Study Group. Clin Diagn Lab Immunol 2000; 7:788–793.

506. Overturf GD: American Academy of Pediatrics. Committee on Infectious Diseases. Technical report: Prevention of pneumococcal infections, including the use of pneumococcal conjugate and polysaccharide vaccines and antibiotic prophylaxis. Pediatrics 2000; 106:367–376.

507. Frank AL, Labotka RJ, Rao S, et al: *Haemophilus influenzae* type b immunization of children with sickle cell diseases. Pediatrics 1988; 82:571–575.

508. Gigliotti F, Feldman S, Wang WC, et al: Immunization of young infants with sickle cell disease with a *Haemophilus influenzae* type b saccharide-diphtheria CRM_{197} protein conjugate vaccine. J Pediatr 1989; 114:1006–1010.

509. Buchanan GR, Smith SJ: Pneumococcal septicemia despite pneumococcal vaccine and prescription of penicillin prophylaxis in children with sickle cell anemia. Am J Dis Child 1986; 140:428–432.

510. Ng ML, Liebman J, Anslovar J, et al: Cardiovascular findings in children with sickle cell anemia. Dis Chest 1967; 52:788–799.

511. Lindsay J Jr, Meshel JC, Patterson RH: The cardiovascular manifestations of sickle cell disease. Arch Intern Med 1974; 133:643–651.

512. Shubin H, Kaufman RE: Cardiovascular findings in children with sickle cell anemia. Am J Cardiol 1960; 6:875.

513. Chung EE, Dianzumba SB, Morais P, et al: Cardiac performance in children with homozygous sickle cell disease. J Am Coll Cardiol 1987; 9:1038–1042.

514. Finch CA: Pathophysiologic aspects of sickle cell anemia. Am J Med 1972; 53:1–6.

515. Barrett O Jr, Saunders DE Jr, McFarland DE, et al: Myocardial infarction in sickle cell anemia. Am J Hematol 1984; 16:139–147.

516. Jensen WN, Rucknagel DL, Taylor WJ: In vivo study of the sickle cell phenomenon. J Lab Clin Med 1960; 56:854.

517. McNamara JJ, Molot MA, Stremple JF, et al: Coronary artery disease in combat casualties in Vietnam. JAMA 1971; 216:1185–1187.

518. Gerry JL, Bulkley BH, Hutchins GM: Clinicopathologic analysis of cardiac dysfunction in 52 patients with sickle cell anemia. Am J Cardiol 1978; 42:211–216.

519. Covitz W, Espeland M, Gallagher D, et al: The heart in sickle cell anemia. The Cooperative Study of Sickle Cell Disease (CSSCD). Chest 1995; 108:1214–1219.

520. Manno BV, Burka ER, Hakki AH, et al: Biventricular function in sickle-cell anemia: Radionuclide angiographic and thallium-201 scintigraphic evaluation. Am J Cardiol 1983; 52:584–587.

521. Moser KM, Shea JC: The relationship between pulmonary infarction, cor pulmonale and the sickle states. Am J Med 1957; 22:561.

522. Maisel A, Friedman H, Flint L, et al: Continuous electrocardiographic monitoring in patients with sickle-cell anemia during pain crisis. Clin Cardiol 1983; 6:339–344.

523. Buckalew VM Jr, Someren A: Renal manifestations of sickle cell disease. Arch Intern Med 1974; 133:660–669.

524. Sherwood JB, Goldwasser E, Chilcote R, et al: Sickle cell anemia patients have low erythropoietin levels for their degree of anemia. Blood 1986; 67:46–49.

525. Whitten CF, Younes AA: Comparative study of renal concentrating ability in children with sickle cell anemia and in normal children. J Lab Clin Med 1960; 55:400.

526. Hatch FE, Culbertson JW, Diggs LW: Nature of the renal concentrating defect in sickle cell disease. J Clin Invest 1967; 46:336–345.

527. Statius van Eps LW, Schouten H, La Porte-Wijsman LW, et al: The influence of red blood cell transfusions on the hyposthenuria and renal hemodynamics of sickle cell anemia. Clin Chim Acta 1967; 17:449–461.

528. Statius van Eps LW, Pinedo-Veels C, Vries GHd, et al: Nature of concentrating defect in sickle-cell nephropathy. Microradioangiographic studies. Lancet 1970; 1:450–452.

529. Perillie PE, Epstein FH: Sickling phenomenon produced by hypertonic solutions: A possible explanation for the hyposthenuria of sicklemia. J Clin Invest 1963; 42:570.

530. Noll JB, Newman AJ, Gross S: Enuresis and nocturia in sickle cell disease. J Pediatr 1967; 70:965–967.

531. Radel EG, Kochen JA, Finberg L: Hyponatremia in sickle cell disease. A renal salt-losing state. J Pediatr 1976; 88:800–805.

532. Goossens JP, Statius van Eps LW, Schouten H, et al: Incomplete renal tubular acidosis in sickle cell disease. Clin Chim Acta 1972; 41:149–156.

533. Oster JR, Lee SM, Lespier LE, et al: Renal acidification in sickle cell trait. Arch Intern Med 1976; 136:30–35.

534. Yoshino M, Amerian R, Brautbar N: Hyporeninemic hypoaldosteronism in sickle cell disease. Nephron 1982; 31:242–244.

535. Oster JR, Lanier DC Jr, Vaamonde CA: Renal response to potassium loading in sickle cell trait. Arch Intern Med 1980; 140:534–536.

536. de Jong PE, Statius van Eps LW: Sickle cell nephropathy: New insights into its pathophysiology. Kidney Int 1985; 27:711–717.

537. Allen TD: Sickle cell disease and hematuria: A report of 29 cases. J Urol 1964; 91:177.

538. Diggs LW: Anatomic lesions in sickle cell disease. In Abramson H, Bertles JF (Eds.): Sickle Cell Disease, Diagnosis, Management, Education and Research. St Louis, Mosby, 1973.

539. Bilinsky RT, Kandel GL, Rabiner SF: ε-Aminocaproic acid therapy of hematuria due to heterozygous sickle cell diseases. J Urol 1969; 102:93–95.

540. Davis CJ Jr, Mostofi FK, Sesterhenn IA: Renal medullary carcinoma. The seventh sickle cell nephropathy. Am J Surg Pathol 1995; 19:1–11.

541. Wesche WA, Wilimas J, Khare V, et al: Renal medullary carcinoma: A potential sickle cell nephropathy of children and adolescents. Pediatr Pathol Lab Med 1998; 18:97–113.

542. Friedrichs P, Lassen P, Canby E, et al: Renal medullary carcinoma and sickle cell trait. J Urol 1997; 157:1349.

543. Nicholson GD, Amin UF, Alleyne GA: Proteinuria and the nephrotic syndrome in homozygous sickle cell anaemia. West Indian Med J 1980; 29:239–246.

544. McCoy RC: Ultrastructural alterations in the kidney of patients with sickle cell disease and the nephrotic syndrome. Lab Invest 1969; 21:85–95.

545. Pardo V, Strauss J, Kramer H, et al: Nephropathy associated with sickle cell anemia: An autologous immune complex nephritis. II. Clinicopathologic study of seven patients. Am J Med 1975; 59:650–659.

546. Elfenbein IB, Patchefsky A, Schwartz W, et al: Pathology of the glomerulus in sickle cell anemia with and without nephrotic syndrome. Am J Pathol 1974; 77:357–374.

547. Bakir AA, Hathiwala SC, Ainis H, et al: Prognosis of the nephrotic syndrome in sickle glomerulopathy. A retrospective study. Am J Nephrol 1987; 7:110–115.

548. Wierenga KJ, Pattison JR, Brink N, et al: Glomerulonephritis after human parvovirus infection in homozygous sickle-cell disease. Lancet 1995; 346:475–476.

549. Tolaymat A, Al Mousily F, MacWilliam K, et al: Parvovirus glomerulonephritis in a patient with sickle cell disease. Pediatr Nephrol 1999; 13:340–342.

550. Dharnidharka VR, Dabbagh S, Atiyeh B, et al: Prevalence of microalbuminuria in children with sickle cell disease. Pediatr Nephrol 1998; 12:475–478.

551. Wigfall DR, Ware RE, Burchinal MR, et al: Prevalence and clinical correlates of glomerulopathy in children with sickle cell disease. J Pediatr 2000; 136:749–753.

552. Falk RJ, Scheinman J, Phillips G, et al: Prevalence and pathologic features of sickle cell nephropathy and response to inhibition of angiotensin-converting enzyme. N Engl J Med 1992; 326:910–915.

553. Chatterjee SN: National study on natural history of renal allografts in sickle cell disease or trait. Nephron 1980; 25:199–201.

554. Gonzalez-Carrillo M, Rudge CJ, Parsons V, et al: Renal transplantation in sickle cell disease. Clin Nephrol 1982; 18:209–210.

555. Green TW, Conley CL: Liver in sickle cell anemia. Bull Johns Hopkins Hosp 1953; 92:99.

556. Bogosh A, Casselman WGB: Liver disease in sickle cell anemia: A correlation of clinical, biochemical and histochemical observations. Am J Med 1955; 19:583.

557. Barrett-Connor E: Cholelithiasis in sickle cell anemia. Am J Med 1968; 45:889–898.

558. Rennels MB, Dunne MG, Grossman NJ, et al: Cholelithiasis in patients with major sickle hemoglobinopathies. Am J Dis Child 1984; 138:66–67.

559. Sarnaik S, Slovis TL, Corbett DP, et al: Incidence of cholelithiasis in sickle cell anemia using the ultrasonic gray-scale technique. J Pediatr 1980; 96:1005–1008.

560. Webb DK, Darby JS, Dunn DT, et al: Gall stones in Jamaican children with homozygous sickle cell disease. Arch Dis Child 1989; 64:693–696.

561. Ware R, Filston HC, Schultz WH, et al: Elective cholecystectomy in children with sickle hemoglobinopathies. Successful outcome using a preoperative transfusion regimen. Ann Surg 1988; 208:17–22.

562. Malone BS, Werlin SL: Cholecystectomy and cholelithiasis in sickle cell anemia. Am J Dis Child 1988; 142:799–800.

563. Ware RE, Kinney TR, Casey JR, et al: Laparoscopic cholecystectomy in young patients with sickle hemoglobinopathies. J Pediatr 1992; 120:58–61.

564. Barrett-Connor E: Sickle cell disease and viral hepatitis. Ann Intern Med 1968; 69:517–527.

565. Sheehy TW, Law DE, Wade BH: Exchange transfusion for sickle cell intrahepatic cholestasis. Arch Intern Med 1980; 140:1364–1366.

566. Klion FM, Weiner MJ: Cholestasis in sickle cell anemia. Am J Med 1964; 37:829.

567. Schubert TT: Hepatobiliary system in sickle cell disease. Gastroenterology 1986; 90:2013–2021.

568. Bauer TW, Moore GW, Hutchins GM: The liver in sickle cell disease. A clinicopathologic study of 70 patients. Am J Med 1980; 69:833–837.

569. Omata M, Johnson CS, Tong M, et al: Pathological spectrum of liver diseases in sickle cell disease. Dig Dis Sci 1986; 31:247–256.

570. Armaly MF: Ocular manifestations in sickle cell disease. Arch Intern Med 1974; 133:670–679.

571. Asdourian G, Nagpal KC, Goldbaum M, et al: Evolution of the retinal black sunburst in sickling haemoglobinopathies. Br J Ophthalmol 1975; 59:710–716.

572. Jampol LM, Condon P, Dizon-Moore R, et al: Salmon-patch hemorrhages after central retinal artery occlusion in sickle cell disease. Arch Ophthalmol 1981; 99:237–240.

573. Condon PI, Serjeant GR: Ocular findings of elderly cases of homozygous sickle-cell disease in Jamaica. Br J Ophthalmol 1976; 60:361–364.

574. Hamilton AM, Pope FM, Condon PI, et al: Angioid streaks in Jamaican patients with homozygous sickle cell disease. Br J Ophthalmol 1981; 65:341–347.

575. Goldberg MF: Natural history of untreated proliferative sickle retinopathy. Arch Ophthalmol 1971; 85:428–437.

576. Dizon-Moore RV, Jampol LM, Goldberg MF: Chorioretinal and choriovitreal neovascularization. Their presence after photocoagulation of proliferative sickle cell retinopathy. Arch Ophthalmol 1981; 99:842–849.

577. Jampol LM, Goldberg MF: Retinal breaks after photocoagulation of proliferative sickle cell retinopathy. Arch Ophthalmol 1980; 98:676–679.

578. Condon PI, Sergeant GR: Behaviour of untreated proliferative sickle retinopathy. Br J Ophthalmol 1980; 64:404–411.

579. Condon PI, Serjeant GR: Photocoagulation in proliferative sickle retinopathy: Results of a 5-year study. Br J Ophthalmol 1980; 64:832–840.

580. Roy MS, Rodgers G, Gunkel R, et al: Color vision defects in sickle cell anemia. Arch Ophthalmol 1987; 105:1676–1678.

581. Lee CM, Charles HC, Smith RT, et al: Quantification of macular ischaemia in sickle cell retinopathy. Br J Ophthalmol 1987; 71:540–545.

582. Weissman H, Nadel AJ, Dunn M: Simultaneous bilateral retinal arterial occlusions treated by exchange transfusions. Arch Ophthalmol 1979; 97:2151–2153.

583. Goldberg MF, Dizon R, Raichand M, et al: Sickled erythrocytes, hyphema, and secondary glaucoma: III. Effects of sicle cell and normal human blood samples in rabbit anterior chambers. Ophthalmic Surg 1979; 10:52–61.

584. Peachey RD: Leg ulceration and haemolytic anaemia: An hypothesis. Br J Dermatol 1978; 98:245–249.

585. Thrall JH, Rucknagel DL: Increased bone marrow blood flow in sickle cell anemia demonstrated by thallium-201 and Tc-99m human albumin microspheres. Radiology 1978; 127:817–819.

586. Wolfort FG, Krizek TJ: Skin ulceration in sickle cell anemia. Plast Reconstr Surg 1969; 43:71–77.

587. Koshy M, Entsuah R, Koranda A, et al: Leg ulcers in patients with sickle cell disease. Blood 1989; 74:1403–1408.

588. Mohan JS, Vigilance JE, Marshall JM, et al: Abnormal venous function in patients with homozygous sickle cell (SS) disease and chronic leg ulcers. Clin Sci (Lond) 2000; 98:667–672.

589. Alleyne SI, Wint E, Serjeant GR: Social effects of leg ulceration in sickle cell anemia. South Med J 1977; 70:213–214.

590. Wethers DL, Ramirez GM, Koshy M, et al: Accelerated healing of chronic sickle-cell leg ulcers treated with RGD peptide matrix. RGD Study Group. Blood 1994; 84:1775–1779.

591. Serjeant GR, Galloway RE, Gueri MC: Oral zinc sulphate in sickle-cell ulcers. Lancet 1970; 2:891–892.

592. Serjeant GR, Howard C: Isoxsuprine hydrochloride in the therapy of sickle cell leg ulceration. West Indian Med J 1977; 26:164–166.

593. Todd GB, Serjeant GR, Larson MR: Sensori-neural hearing loss in Jamaicans with SS disease. Acta Otolaryngol 1973; 76:268–272.

594. Serjeant GR, Norman W, Todd GB: The internal auditory canal and sensori-neural hearing loss in homozygous sickle cell disease. J Laryngol Otol 1975; 89:453–455.

595. Friedman EM, Herer GR, Luban NL, et al: Sickle cell anemia and hearing. Ann Otol Rhinol Laryngol 1980; 89:342–347.

596. Morgenstein KM, Manace ED: Temporal bone histopathology in sickle cell disease. Laryngoscope 1969; 79:2172–2180.

597. Bohrer SP: Acute long bone diaphyseal infarcts in sickle cell disease. Br J Radiol 1970; 43:685–697.

598. Reynolds J: Radiologic manifestations of sickle cell hemoglobinopathy. JAMA 1977; 238:247–250.

599. Milner PF, Kraus AP, Sebes JI, et al: Sickle cell disease as a cause of osteonecrosis of the femoral head. N Engl J Med 1991; 325:1476–1481.

600. Washington ER, Root L: Conservative treatment of sickle cell avascular necrosis of the femoral head. J Pediatr Orthop 1985; 5:192–194.

601. Hernigou P, Bachir D, Galacteros F: Avascular necrosis of the femoral head in sickle-cell disease. Treatment of collapse by the injection of acrylic cement. J Bone Joint Surg Br 1993; 75:875–880.

602. Hungerford DS: Response: The role of core decompression in the treatment of ischemic necrosis of the femoral head. Arthritis Rheum 1989; 32:801–806.

603. Milner PF, Kraus AP, Sebes JI, et al: Osteonecrosis of the humeral head in sickle cell disease. Clin Orthop 1993:136–143.

604. Miller GJ, Serjeant GR: An assessment of lung volumes and gas transfer in sickle-cell anaemia. Thorax 1971; 26:309–315.

605. Femi-Pearse D, Gazioglu KM, Yu PN: Pulmonary function studies in sickle cell disease. J Appl Physiol 1970; 28:574–577.

606. Wall MA, Platt OS, Strieder DJ: Lung function in children with sickle cell anemia. Am Rev Respir Dis 1979; 120:210–214.

607. Powars D, Weidman JA, Odom-Maryon T, et al: Sickle cell chronic lung disease: Prior morbidity and the risk of pulmonary failure. Medicine (Baltimore) 1988; 67:66–76.

608. Santoli F, Zerah F, Vasile N, et al: Pulmonary function in sickle cell disease with or without acute chest syndrome. Eur Respir J 1998; 12:1124–1129.

609. Denbow CE, Chung EE, Serjeant GR: Pulmonary artery pressure and the acute chest syndrome in homozygous sickle cell disease. Br Heart J 1993; 69:536–538.

610. Pianosi P, D'Souza SJ, Charge TD, et al: Pulmonary function abnormalities in childhood sickle cell disease. J Pediatr 1993; 122:366–371.

611. Koumbourlis AC, Hurlet-Jensen A, Bye MR: Lung function in infants with sickle cell disease. Pediatr Pulmonol 1997; 24:277–281.

612. Wiznitzer M, Ruggieri PM, Masaryk TJ, et al: Diagnosis of cerebrovascular disease in sickle cell anemia by magnetic resonance angiography. J Pediatr 1990; 117:551–555.

613. Armstrong FD, Thompson RJ Jr, Wang W, et al: Cognitive functioning and brain magnetic resonance imaging in children with sickle cell disease. Neuropsychology Committee of the Cooperative Study of Sickle Cell Disease. Pediatrics 1996; 97:864–870.

614. Booker CR, Scott RB: Studies in sickle cell anemia. XXII. Clinical manifestations during the first two years of life. Clin Pediatr 1964; 3:111.

615. Stevens MC, Hayes RJ, Serjeant GR: Body shape in young children with homozygous sickle cell disease. Pediatrics 1983; 71:610–614.

616. Morais PV, Clarke WF, Hayes RJ, et al: Heart size and chest shape in homozygous sickle cell disease. West Indian Med J 1983; 32:157–160.

617. Platt OS, Rosenstock W, Espeland MA: Influence of sickle hemoglobinopathies on growth and development. N Engl J Med 1984; 311:7–12.

618. Singhal A, Davies P, Sahota A, et al: Resting metabolic rate in homozygous sickle cell disease. Am J Clin Nutr 1993; 57:32–34.

619. Stevens MC, Maude GH, Cupidore L, et al: Prepubertal growth and skeletal maturation in children with sickle cell disease. Pediatrics 1986; 78:124–132.

620. Prasad AS, Cossack ZT: Zinc supplementation and growth in sickle cell disease. Ann Intern Med 1984; 100:367–371.

621. Phebus CK, Maciak BJ, Gloninger MF, et al: Zinc status of children with sickle cell disease: Relationship to poor growth. Am J Hematol 1988; 29:67–73.

622. Abshire TC, English JL, Githens JH, et al: Zinc status in children and young adults with sickle cell disease. Am J Dis Child 1988; 142:1356–1359.

623. Oberfield SE, Wethers DL, Kirkland JL, et al: Growth hormone response to growth hormone releasing factor in sickle cell disease. Am J Pediatr Hematol Oncol 1987; 9:331–334.

624. Reed JD, Redding-Lallinger R, Orringer EP: Nutrition and sickle cell disease. Am J Hematol 1987; 24:441–455.

625. Heyman MB, Vichinsky E, Katz R, et al: Growth retardation in sickle-cell disease treated by nutritional support. Lancet 1985; 1:903–906.

626. Alleyne SI, Rauseo RD, Serjeant GR: Sexual development and fertility of Jamaican female patients with homozygous sickle cell disease. Arch Intern Med 1981; 141:1295–1297.

627. Osegbe DN, Akinyanju O, Amaku EO: Fertility in males with sickle cell disease. Lancet 1981; 2:275–276.

628. Olambiwonnu NO, Penny R, Frasier SD: Sexual maturation in subjects with sickle cell anemia: Studies of serum gonadotropin concentration, height, weight, and skeletal age. J Pediatr 1975; 87:459–464.

629. Landefeld CS, Schambelan M, Kaplan SL, et al: Clomiphene-responsive hypogonadism in sickle cell anemia. Ann Intern Med 1983; 99:480–483.

630. Kumar S, Powars D, Allen J, et al: Anxiety, self-concept, and personal and social adjustments in children with sickle cell anemia. J Pediatr 1976; 88:859–863.

631. Yang YM, Cepeda M, Price C, et al: Depression in children and adolescents with sickle-cell disease. Arch Pediatr Adolesc Med 1994; 148:457–460.

632. Rabb LM, Grandison Y, Mason K, et al: A trial of folate supplementation in children with homozygous sickle cell disease. Br J Haematol 1983; 54:589–594.

633. Adams RJ, McKie VC, Hsu L, et al: Prevention of a first stroke by transfusions in children with sickle cell anemia and abnormal results on transcranial Doppler ultrasonography. N Engl J Med 1998; 339:5–11.

634. Sanger RG, Greer RO Jr, Averbach RE: Differential diagnosis of some simple osseous lesions associated with sickle-cell anemia. Oral Surg Oral Med Oral Pathol 1977; 43:538–545.

635. Freie HM: Sickle cell diseases and hormonal contraception. Acta Obstet Gynecol Scand 1983; 62:211–217.

636. Treatment of sickle cell crisis with urea in invert sugar. A controlled trial. Cooperative Urea Trials Group. JAMA 1974; 228:1125–1128.

637. Embury SH, Garcia JF, Mohandas N, et al: Effects of oxygen inhalation on endogenous erythropoietin kinetics, erythropoiesis, and properties of blood cells in sickle-cell anemia. N Engl J Med 1984; 311:291–295.

638. Keidan AJ, Marwah SS, Vaughan GR, et al: Painful sickle cell crises precipitated by stopping prophylactic exchange transfusions. J Clin Pathol 1987; 40:505–507.

639. Shapiro BS, Benjamin LJ, Payne R, et al: Sickle cell-related pain: Perceptions of medical practitioners. J Pain Symptom Manage 1997; 14:168–174.

640. Armstrong FD, Pegelow CH, Gonzalez JC, et al: Impact of children's sickle cell history on nurse and physician ratings of pain and medication decisions. J Pediatr Psychol 1992; 17:651–664.

641. Szeto HH, Inturrisi CE, Houde R, et al: Accumulation of normeperidine, an active metabolite of meperidine, in patients with renal failure of cancer. Ann Intern Med 1977; 86:738–741.

642. Cole TB, Sprinkle RH, Smith SJ, et al: Intravenous narcotic therapy for children with severe sickle cell pain crisis. Am J Dis Child 1986; 140:1255–1259.

643. Yaster M, Tobin JR, Billett C, et al: Epidural analgesia in the management of severe vaso-occlusive sickle cell crisis. Pediatrics 1994; 93:310–315.

644. Vichinsky EP, Johnson R, Lubin BH: Multidisciplinary approach to pain management in sickle cell disease. Am J Pediatr Hematol Oncol 1982; 4:328–333.

645. Shapiro BS: The management of pain in sickle cell disease. Pediatr Clin North Am 1989; 36:1029–1045.

646. Co LL, Schmitz TH, Havdala H, et al: Acupuncture: An evaluation in the painful crises of sickle cell anaemia. Pain 1979; 7:181–185.

647. Zeltzer L, Dash J, Holland JP: Hypnotically induced pain control in sickle cell anemia. Pediatrics 1979; 64:533–536.

648. Portenoy RK: Chronic opioid therapy in nonmalignant pain. J Pain Symptom Manage 1990; 5:S46–62.

649. Berkowitz LR, Orringer EP: Effect of cetiedil, an in vitro antisickling agent, on erythrocyte membrane cation permeability. J Clin Invest 1981; 68:1215–1220.

650. Stuart J, Stone PC, Bilto YY, et al: Oxpentifylline and cetiedil citrate improve deformability of dehydrated sickle cells. J Clin Pathol 1987; 40:1182–1186.

651. Benjamin LJ, Berkowitz LR, Orringer E, et al: A collaborative, double-blind randomized study of cetiedil citrate in sickle cell crisis. Blood 1986; 67:1442–1447.

652. Leff RD, Aldo-Benson MA, Fife RS: Tophaceous gout in a patient with sickle cell-thalassemia: Case report and review of the literature. Arthritis Rheum 1983; 26:928–929.

653. Charache S: The treatment of sickle cell anemia. Arch Intern Med 1974; 133:698–705.

654. Quattlebaum TG, Pierce MM: Estimates of need for transfusions during hypertransfusion therapy in sickle cell disease. J Pediatr 1986; 109:456–459.

655. Styles LA, Vichinsky E: Effects of a long-term transfusion regimen on sickle cell-related illnesses. J Pediatr 1994; 125:909–911.

656. Cohen A, Schwartz E: Excretion of iron in response to deferoxamine in sickle cell anemia. J Pediatr 1978; 92:659–662.

657. Wang WC, Ahmed N, Hanna M: Non-transferrin-bound iron in long-term transfusion in children with congenital anemias. J Pediatr 1986; 108:552–557.

658. Harmatz P, Butensky E, Quirolo K, et al: Severity of iron overload in patients with sickle cell disease receiving chronic red blood cell transfusion therapy. Blood 2000; 96:76–79.

659. Davies SC, McWilliam AC, Hewitt PE, et al: Red cell alloimmunization in sickle cell disease. Br J Haematol 1986; 63:241–245.

660. Reisner EG, Kostyu DD, Phillips G, et al: Alloantibody responses in multiply transfused sickle cell patients. Tissue Antigens 1987; 30:161–166.

661. Sarnaik S, Schornack J, Lusher JM: The incidence of development of irregular red cell antibodies in patients with sickle cell anemia. Transfusion 1986; 26:249–252.

662. Vichinsky EP, Earles A, Johnson RA, et al: Alloimmunization in sickle cell anemia and transfusion of racially unmatched blood. N Engl J Med 1990; 322:1617–1621.

663. Rosse WF, Gallagher D, Kinney TR, et al: Transfusion and alloimmunization in sickle cell disease. The Cooperative Study of Sickle Cell Disease. Blood 1990; 76:1431–1437.

664. Tahhan HR, Holbrook CT, Braddy LR, et al: Antigen-matched donor blood in the transfusion management of patients with sickle cell disease. Transfusion 1994; 34:562–569.

665. Ambruso DR, Githens JH, Alcorn R, et al: Experience with donors matched for minor blood group antigens in patients with sickle cell anemia who are receiving chronic transfusion therapy. Transfusion 1987; 27:94–98.

666. Orlina AR, Unger PJ, Koshy M: Post-transfusion alloimmunization in patients with sickle cell disease. Am J Hematol 1978; 5:101–106.

667. Ness PM: To match or not to match: The question for chronically transfused patients with sickle cell anemia. Transfusion 1994; 34:558–560.

668. Castellino SM, Combs MR, Zimmerman SA, et al: Erythrocyte autoantibodies in paediatric patients with sickle cell disease receiving transfusion therapy: Frequency, characteristics and significance. Br J Haematol 1999; 104:189–194.

669. Spigelman A, Warden MJ: Surgery in patients with sickle cell disease. Arch Surg 1972; 104:761–764.

670. Howells TH, Huntsman RG: Anaesthesia in sickle cell states. Anaesthesia 1973; 28:339–341.

671. Searle JF: Anaesthesia and sickle-cell haemoglobin. Br J Anaesth 1972; 44:1335–1336.

672. Burrington JD, Smith MD: Elective and emergency surgery in children with sickle cell disease. Surg Clin North Am 1976; 56:55–71.

673. Janik JS, Seeler RA: Surgical procedures in children with sickle hemoglobinopathy. J Pediatr 1977; 91:505–506.

674. Bentley PG, Howard ER: Surgery in children with homozygous sickle cell anaemia. Ann R Coll Surg Engl 1979; 61:55–58.

675. Koshy M, Weiner SJ, Miller ST, et al: Surgery and anesthesia in sickle cell disease. Cooperative Study of Sickle Cell Diseases. Blood 1995; 86:3676–3684.

676. Griffin TC, Buchanan GR: Elective surgery in children with sickle cell disease without preoperative blood transfusion. J Pediatr Surg 1993; 28:681–685.

677. Vichinsky EP, Haberkern CM, Neumayr L, et al: A comparison of conservative and aggressive transfusion regimens in the perioperative management of sickle cell disease. The Preoperative Transfusion in Sickle Cell Disease Study Group. N Engl J Med 1995; 333:206–213.

678. Vichinsky EP, Neumayr LD, Haberkern C, et al: The perioperative complication rate of orthopedic surgery in sickle cell disease: Report of the National Sickle Cell Surgery Study Group. Am J Hematol 1999; 62:129–138.

679. Haberkern CM, Neumayr LD, Orringer EP, et al: Cholecystectomy in sickle cell anemia patients: Perioperative outcome of 364 cases from the National Preoperative Transfusion Study. Preoperative Transfusion in Sickle Cell Disease Study Group. Blood 1997; 89:1533–1542.

680. Neumayr L, Koshy M, Haberkern C, et al: Surgery in patients with hemoglobin SC disease. Preoperative Transfusion in Sickle Cell Disease Study Group. Am J Hematol 1998; 57:101–108.

681. Waldron P, Pegelow C, Neumayr L, et al: Tonsillectomy, adenoidectomy, and myringotomy in sickle cell disease: Perioperative morbidity. Preoperative Transfusion in Sickle Cell Disease Study Group. J Pediatr Hematol Oncol 1999; 21:129–135.

682. Freeman MG, Ruth GJ: SS disease, SC disease, and CC disease—Obstetric considerations and treatment. Clin Obstet Gynecol 1969; 12:134–156.

683. Morrison JC, Fort AT, Wiser WL, et al: The modern management of pregnant sickle cell patients: A preliminary report. South Med J 1972; 65:533–536.

684. Pritchard JA, Scott DE, Whalley PH, et al: The effects of maternal sickle cell hemoglobinopathies and sickle cell trait on reproductive performance. Am J Obstet Gynecol 1973; 117:662–670.

685. Milner PF, Jones BR, Dobler J: Outcome of pregnancy in sickle cell anemia and sickle cell-hemoglobin C disease. An analysis of 181 pregnancies in 98 patients, and a review of the literature. Am J Obstet Gynecol 1980; 138:239–245.

686. Charache S, Scott J, Niebyl J, et al: Management of sickle cell disease in pregnant patients. Obstet Gynecol 1980; 55:407–410.

687. Smith JA, Espeland M, Bellevue R, et al: Pregnancy in sickle cell disease: Experience of the Cooperative Study of Sickle Cell Disease. Obstet Gynecol 1996; 87:199–204.

688. Cunningham FG, Pritchard JA, Mason R: Pregnancy and sickle cell hemoglobinopathies: Results with and without prophylactic transfusions. Obstet Gynecol 1983; 62:419–424.

689. Cunningham FG, Pritchard JA, Mason R, et al: Prophylactic transfusions of normal red blood cells during pregnancies complicated by sickle cell hemoglobinopathies. Am J Obstet Gynecol 1979; 135:994–1003.

690. Morrison JC, Morrison FS: Prophylactic transfusions in pregnant patients with sickle cell disease. N Engl J Med 1989; 320:1286–1287.

691. Morrison JC, Wiser WL: The effect of maternal partial exchange transfusion on the infants of patients with sickle cell anemia. J Pediatr 1976; 89:286–289.

692. Nagey DA, Alawode NA, Pupkin MJ, et al: Isovolumetric partial exchange transfusion in the management of sickle cell disease in pregnancy. II. Simplified ambulatory technique. Am J Obstet Gynecol 1983; 147:693–696.

693. Key TC, Horger EOD, Walker EM Jr, et al: Automated erythrocytopheresis for sickle cell anemia during pregnancy. Am J Obstet Gynecol 1980; 138:731–737.

694. Miller JM Jr, Horger EOD, Key TC, et al: Management of sickle hemoglobinopathies in pregnant patients. Am J Obstet Gynecol 1981; 141:237–241.

695. Koshy M, Burd L, Wallace D, et al: Prophylactic red-cell transfusions in pregnant patients with sickle cell disease. A randomized cooperative study. N Engl J Med 1988; 319:1447–1452.

696. Brumfield CG, Huddleston JF, DuBois LB, et al: A delayed hemolytic transfusion reaction after partial exchange transfusion for sickle cell disease in pregnancy: A case report and review of the literature. Obstet Gynecol 1984; 63:13S–15S.

697. Leikin SL, Gallagher D, Kinney TR, et al: Mortality in children and adolescents with sickle cell disease. Cooperative Study of Sickle Cell Disease. Pediatrics 1989; 84:500–508.

698. Thomas AN, Pattison C, Serjeant GR: Causes of death in sickle-cell disease in Jamaica. Br Med J (Clin Res Ed) 1982; 285:633–635.

699. Davis H, Schoendorf KC, Gergen PJ, et al: National trends in the mortality of children with sickle cell disease, 1968 through 1992. Am J Public Health 1997; 87:1317–1322.

700. Chui DH, Dover GJ: Sickle cell disease: No longer a single gene disorder. Curr Opin Pediatr 2001; 13:22–27.

701. Nagel RL: Pleiotropic and epistatic effects in sickle cell anemia. Curr Opin Hematol 2001; 8:105–110.

702. Boyle E Jr, Thompson C, Tyroler HA: Prevalence of the sickle cell trait in adults of Charleston County, SC: An epidemiological study. Arch Environ Health 1968; 17:891–898.

703. Ashcroft MT, Miall WE, Milner PF: A comparison between the characteristics of Jamaican adults with normal hemoglobin and those with sickle cell trait. Am J Epidemiol 1969; 90:236–243.

704. Ashcroft MT, Desai P: Mortality and morbidity in Jamaican adults with sickle-cell trait and with normal haemoglobin followed up for twelve years. Lancet 1976; 2:784–786.

705. Sears DA: The morbidity of sickle cell trait: A review of the literature. Am J Med 1978; 64:1021–1036.

706. Kramer MS, Rooks Y, Pearson HA: Growth and development in children with sickle-cell trait. A prospective study of matched pairs. N Engl J Med 1978; 299:686–689.

707. Huisman TH: Trimodality in the percentages of β chain variants in heterozygotes: The effect of the number of active Hb-alpha structural loci. Hemoglobin 1977; 1:349–382.

708. Levere RD, Lichtman H: Effect of iron deficiency anaemia on the metabolism of the heterogenic haemoglobins in sickle trait. Nature 1964; 202:499.

709. Heller P, Yakulis V: Variation in the amount of hemoglobin S in a patient with sickle trait and megaloblastic anemia. Blood 1963; 21:479.

710. Ashcroft MT, Serjant GR: Growth, morbidity, and mortality in a cohort of Jamaican adolescents with homozygous sickle cell disease. West Indian Med J 1981; 30:197–201.

711. Kramer MS, Rooks Y, Pearson HA: Cord blood screening for sickle hemoglobins: Evidence for female preponderance of hemoglobin S. J Pediatr 1978; 93:998–1000.

712. Blattner P, Dar H, Nitowsky HM: Pregnancy outcome in women with sickle cell trait. JAMA 1977; 238:1392–1394.

713. Murphy JR: Sickle cell hemoglobin (Hb AS) in black football players. JAMA 1973; 225:981–982.

714. Kark JA, Posey DM, Schumacher HR, et al: Sickle-cell trait as a risk factor for sudden death in physical training. N Engl J Med 1987; 317:781–787.

715. Weisman IM, Zeballos RJ, Martin TW, et al: Effect of Army basic training in sickle-cell trait. Arch Intern Med 1988; 148:1140–1144.

716. Charache S: Sudden death in sickle trait. Am J Med 1988; 84:459–461.

717. Sullivan LW: The risks of sickle-cell trait: Caution and common sense. N Engl J Med 1987; 317:830–831.

718. Pearson HA: Sickle cell trait and competitive athletics: Is there a risk? Pediatrics 1989; 83:613–614.

719. Ober WB, Bruno MS: Fatal intravascular sickling in a patient with sickle cell trait. N Engl J Med 1960; 263:947.

720. Jones SR, Binder RA, Donowho EM Jr: Sudden death in sickle-cell trait. N Engl J Med 1970; 282:323–325.

721. O'Brien RT, Pearson HA, Godley JA, et al: Splenic infarct and sickle-(cell) trait. N Engl J Med 1972; 287:720.

722. Long ID: Sickle cell trait and aviation. Aviat Space Environ Med 1982; 53:1021–1029.

723. Atlas SA: The sickle cell trait and surgical complications. A matched-pair patient analysis. JAMA 1974; 229:1078–1080.

724. Metras D, Coulibaly AO, Ouattara K, et al: Open-heart surgery in sickle-cell haemoglobinopathies: Report of 15 cases. Thorax 1982; 37:486–491.

725. Schlitt LE, Keital HG: Renal manifestations of sickle cell disease: A review. Am J Med Sci 1960; 239:773.

726. Ataga KI, Orringer EP: Renal abnormalities in sickle cell disease. Am J Hematol 2000; 63:205–211.

727. Lai JC, Fekrat S, Barron Y, et al: Traumatic hyphema in children: Risk factors for complications. Arch Ophthalmol 2001; 119:64–70.

728. Larrabee KD, Monga M: Women with sickle cell trait are at increased risk for preeclampsia. Am J Obstet Gynecol 1997; 177:425–428.

729. Roopnarinesingh S, Ramsewak S: Decreased birth weight and femur length in fetuses of patients with the sickle-cell trait. Obstet Gynecol 1986; 68:46–48.

730. Anyaegbunam A, Langer O, Brustman L, et al: The application of uterine and umbilical artery velocimetry to the antenatal supervision of pregnancies complicated by maternal sickle hemoglobinopathies. Am J Obstet Gynecol 1988; 159:544–547.

731. Baill IC, Witter FR: Sickle trait and its association with birthweight and urinary tract infections in pregnancy. Int J Gynaecol Obstet 1990; 33:19–21.

732. Brown S, Merkow A, Wiener M, et al: Low birth weight in babies born to mothers with sickle cell trait. JAMA 1972; 221:1404–1405.

733. McCurdy PR: Erythrokinetics in abnormal hemoglobin syndromes. Blood 1962; 20:686.

734. Tuttle AH, Koch B: Clinical and hematological manifestations of hemoglobin CS disease in children. J Pediatr 1960; 56:331.

735. Serjeant GR, Ashcroft MT, Serjeant BE: The clinical features of haemoglobin SC disease in Jamaica. Br J Haematol 1973; 24:491–501.

736. Rowley PT, Enlander D: Hemoglobin S-C disease presenting as acute cor pulmonale. Am Rev Respir Dis 1968; 98:494–500.

737. Fabian RH, Peters BH: Neurological complications of hemoglobin SC disease. Arch Neurol 1984; 41:289–292.

738. Ryan SJ, Goldberg MF: Anterior segment ischemia following scleral buckling in sickle cell hemoglobinopathy. Am J Ophthalmol 1971; 72:35–50.

739. Goldberg MF: Treatment of proliferative sickle retinopathy. Trans Am Acad Ophthalmol Otolaryngol 1971; 75:532–556.

740. Barton CJ, Cockshott WP: Bone changes in hemoglobin SC disease. Am J Roentgenol Radium Ther Nucl Med 1962; 88:523.

741. Kay CJ, Rosenberg MA, Fleisher P, et al: Renal papillary necrosis in hemoglobin SC disease. Radiology 1968; 90:897–899.

742. Yeung KY, Lessin LS: Splenic infarction in sickle cell-hemoglobin C disease. Demonstration by selective splenic arteriogram and scintillation scan. Arch Intern Med 1976; 136:905–911.

743. Githens JH, Gross GP, Eife RF, et al: Splenic sequestration syndrome at mountain altitudes in sickle/hemoglobin C disease. J Pediatr 1977; 90:203–206.

744. Barrett-Connor E: Infection and sickle cell-C disease. Am J Med Sci 1971; 262:162–169.

745. Buchanan GR, Smith SJ, Holtkamp CA, et al: Bacterial infection and splenic reticuloendothelial function in children with hemoglobin SC disease. Pediatrics 1983; 72:93–98.

746. Bunn HF, Noguchi CT, Hofrichter J, et al: Molecular and cellular pathogenesis of hemoglobin SC disease. Proc Natl Acad Sci USA 1982; 79:7527–7531.

747. Bunn HF, McDonald MJ: Electrostatic interactions in the assembly of haemoglobin. Nature 1983; 306:498–500.

748. Ballas SK, Larner J, Smith ED, et al: The xerocytosis of Hb SC disease. Blood 1987; 69:124–130.

749. Brugnara C, Kopin AS, Bunn HF, et al: Regulation of cation content and cell volume in hemoglobin erythrocytes from patients with homozygous hemoglobin C disease. J Clin Invest 1985; 75:1608–1617.

750. Honig GR, Gunay U, Mason RG, et al: Sickle cell syndromes. I. Hemoglobin SC-alpha-thalassemia. Pediatr Res 1976; 10:613–620.

751. Milner PF, Miller C, Grey R, et al: Hemoglobin O Arab in four Negro families and its interaction with hemoglobin S and hemoglobin C. N Engl J Med 1970; 283:1417–1425.

752. Charache S, Zinkham WH, Dickerman JD, et al: Hemoglobin SC, SS/G$_{Philadelphia}$ and S$_{OArab}$ diseases: Diagnostic importance of an integrative analysis of clinical, hematologic and electrophoretic findings. Am J Med 1977; 62:439–446.

753. Sturgeon P, Itano HA: Clinical manifestations of inherited abnormal hemoglobins. I. The interaction of hemoglobin S with hemoglobin D. Blood 1955; 10:389.

754. Schneider RG, Ueda S, Alperin JB, et al: Hemoglobin D Los Angeles in two Caucasian families: Hemoglobin SD disease and hemoglobin D thalassemia. Blood 1968; 32:250–259.

755. Cawein MJ, Lappat EJ, Brangle RW, et al: Hemoglobin S-D disease. Ann Intern Med 1966; 64:62–70.

756. Konotey-Ahulu FI, Gallo E, Lehmann H, et al: Haemoglobin Korle-Bu (β 73 aspartic acid replaced by asparagine) showing one of the two amino acid substitutions of haemoglobin C Harlem. J Med Genet 1968; 5:107–111.

757. Bookchin RM, Nagel RL: Ligand-induced conformational dependence of hemoglobin in sickling interactios. J Mol Biol 1971; 60:263–270.

758. Bookchin RM, Nagel RL, Ranney HM: Structure and properties of hemoglobin C-Harlem, a human hemoglobin variant with amino acid substitutions in 2 residues of the β-polypeptide chain. J Biol Chem 1967; 242:248–255.

759. Moo-Penn W, Bechtel K, Jue D, et al: The presence of hemoglobin S and C Harlem in an individual in the United States. Blood 1975; 46:363–367.

760. Monplaisir N, Merault G, Poyart C, et al: Hemoglobin S Antilles: A variant with lower solubility than hemoglobin S and producing sickle cell disease in heterozygotes. Proc Natl Acad Sci USA 1986; 83:9363–9367.

761. Trudel M, De Paepe ME, Chretien N, et al: Sickle cell disease of transgenic SAD mice. Blood 1994; 84:3189–3197.

762. Boyer SH: The emerging complexity of genetic control of persistent fetal hemoglobin biosynthesis in adults. Ann NY Acad Sci 1989; 565:23–36.

763. Stamatoyannopoulos G, Nienhuis AW: Hemoglobin switching. In Stamatoyannopoulos G, Nienhuis A (Eds.): Molecular Basis of Blood Diseases. Philadelphia, WB Saunders, 1987.

764. Charache S, Conley CL: Hereditary persistence of fetal hemoglobin. Ann NY Acad Sci 1969; 165:37–41.

765. Bradley TB, Brawner JN: Further observations on an inherited anomaly characterized by persistence of fetal hemoglobin. Bull Johns Hopkins Hosp 1961; 108:242.

766. Jacob GR, Raper AB: Hereditary persistence of foetal haemoglobin production and its interaction with sickle trait. Br J Haematol 1958; 4:138.

767. Murray N, Serjeant BE, Serjeant GR: Sickle cell-hereditary persistence of fetal haemoglobin and its differentiation from other sickle cell syndromes. Br J Haematol 1988; 69:89–92.

768. Old JM, Ayyub H, Wood WG, et al: Linkage analysis of nondeletion hereditary persistence of fetal hemoglobin. Science 1982; 215:981–982.

769. Milner PF, Leibfarth JD, Ford J, et al: Increased HbF in sickle cell anemia is determined by a factor linked to the β S gene from one parent. Blood 1984; 63:64–72.

770. Stamatoyannopoulos G, Wood WG, Papayannopoulou T, et al: A new form of hereditary persistence of fetal hemoglobin in blacks and its association with sickle cell trait. Blood 1975; 46:683–692.

771. Makler MT, Berthrong M, Locke HR, et al: A new variant of sickle-cell disease with high levels of foetal haemoglobin homogeneously distributed within red cells. Br J Haematol 1974; 26:519–526.

772. Economou EP, Antonarakis SE, Kazazian HH Jr, et al: Variation in hemoglobin F production among normal and sickle cell adults is

not related to nucleotide substitutions in the γ promoter regions. Blood 1991; 77:174–177.

773. Miller BA, Salameh M, Ahmed M, et al: Analysis of hemoglobin F production in Saudi Arabian families with sickle cell anemia. Blood 1987; 70:716–720.

774. Kar BC, Satapathy RK, Kulozik AE, et al: Sickle cell disease in Orissa State, India. Lancet 1986; 2:1198–201.

775. Miller BA, Salameh M, Ahmed M, et al: High fetal hemoglobin production in sickle cell anemia in the eastern province of Saudi Arabia is genetically determined. Blood 1986; 67:1404–1410.

776. Kulozik AE, Kar BC, Satapathy RK, et al: Fetal hemoglobin levels and β^S globin haplotypes in an Indian populations with sickle cell disease. Blood 1987; 69:1742–1746.

777. Gianni AM, Bregni M, Cappellini MD, et al: A gene controlling fetal hemoglobin expression in adults is not linked to the non-α globin cluster. EMBO J 1983; 2:921–925.

778. Wood WG, Weatherall DJ, Clegg JB: Interaction of heterocellular hereditary persistence of foetal haemoglobin with β thalassaemia and sickle cell anaemia. Nature 1976; 264:247–249.

779. Boyer SH, Dover GJ, Serjeant GR, et al: Production of F cells in sickle cell anemia: Regulation by a genetic locus or loci separate from the β-globin gene cluster. Blood 1984; 64:1053–1058.

780. Miyoshi K, Kaneto Y, Kawai H, et al: X-linked dominant control of F-cells in normal adult life: Characterization of the Swiss type as hereditary persistence of fetal hemoglobin regulated dominantly by gene(s) on X chromosome. Blood 1988; 72:1854–1860.

781. Dover GJ, Smith KD, Chang YC, et al: Fetal hemoglobin levels in sickle cell disease and normal individuals are partially controlled by an X-linked gene located at Xp22.2. Blood 1992; 80:816–824.

782. Chang YC, Smith KD, Moore RD, et al: An analysis of fetal hemoglobin variation in sickle cell disease: The relative contributions of the X-linked factor, β-globin haplotypes, α-globin gene number, gender, and age. Blood 1995; 85:1111–1117.

783. Game L, Close J, Stephens P, et al: An integrated map of human 6q22.3-q24 including a 3-Mb high-resolution BAC/PAC contig encompassing a QTL for fetal hemoglobin. Genomics 2000; 64:264–276.

784. Thein SL, Craig JE: Genetics of Hb F/F cell variance in adults and heterocellular hereditary persistence of fetal hemoglobin. Hemoglobin 1998; 22:401–414.

785. Higgs DR, Aldridge BE, Lamb J, et al: The interaction of α-thalassemia and homozygous sickle-cell disease. N Engl J Med 1982; 306:1441–1446.

786. Dover GJ, Chang VT, Boyer SH, et al: The cellular basis for different fetal hemoglobin levels among sickle cell individuals with two, three, and four α-globin genes. Blood 1987; 69:341–344.

787. Powars DR, Schroeder WA, Weiss JN, et al: Lack of influence of fetal hemoglobin levels or erythrocyte indices on the severity of sickle cell anemia. J Clin Invest 1980; 65:732–740.

788. Powars DR, Weiss JN, Chan LS, et al: Is there a threshold level of fetal hemoglobin that ameliorates morbidity in sickle cell anemia? Blood 1984; 63:921–926.

789. Weatherall D: Biochemical phenotypes of thalassemia in the American Negro population. Ann NY Acad Sci 1964; 119:450.

790. Serjeant GR, Ashcroft MT, Serjeant BE, et al: The clinical features of sickle-cell-β thalassaemia in Jamaica. Br J Haematol 1973; 24:19–30.

791. Vyas P, Higgs DR, Weatherall DJ, et al: The interaction of α thalassaemia and sickle cell-β zero thalassaemia. Br J Haematol 1988; 70:449–454.

792. Embury SH, Dozy AM, Miller J, et al: Concurrent sickle-cell anemia and α-thalassemia: Effect on severity of anemia. N Engl J Med 1982; 306:270–274.

793. Honig GR, Koshy M, Mason RG, et al: Sickle cell syndromes. II. The sickle cell anemia-α-thalassemia syndrome. J Pediatr 1978; 92:556–561.

794. Serjeant BE, Mason KP, Kenny MW, et al: Effect of α thalassaemia on the rheology of homozygous sickle cell disease. Br J Haematol 1983; 55:479–486.

795. Higgs DR, Pressley L, Serjeant GR, et al: The genetics and molecular basis of alpha thalassaemia in association with Hb S in Jamaican Negroes. Br J Haematol 1981; 47:43–56.

796. Steinberg MH, Rosenstock W, Coleman MB, et al: Effects of thalassemia and microcytosis on the hematologic and vasoocclusive severity of sickle cell anemia. Blood 1984; 63:1353–1360.

797. de Ceulaer K, Higgs DR, Weatherall DJ, et al: α-Thalassemia reduces the hemolytic rate in homozygous sickle-cell disease. N Engl J Med 1983; 309:189–190.

798. Kulozik AE, Kar BC, Serjeant GR, et al: The molecular basis of α thalassemia in India. Its interaction with the sickle cell gene. Blood 1988; 71:467–472.

799. Steinberg MH, Embury SH: α-Thalassemia in blacks: Genetic and clinical aspects and interactions with the sickle hemoglobin gene. Blood 1986; 68:985–990.

800. Milner PF, Garbutt GJ, Nolan-Davis LV, et al: The effect of Hb F and α-thalassemia on the red cell indices in sickle cell anemia. Am J Hematol 1986; 21:383–395.

801. Embury SH: The interaction of coexistent α-thalassemia and sickle cell anemia: A model for the clinical and cellular results of diminished polymerization? Ann NY Acad Sci 1985; 445:37–44.

802. Steinberg MH, Embury SH: α-Thalassemia in blacks: Interactions with the sickle hemoglobin gene. Birth Defects Orig Artic Ser 1987; 23:43–48.

803. Hawker H, Neilson H, Hayes RJ, et al: Haematological factors associated with avascular necrosis of the femoral head in homozygous sickle cell disease. Br J Haematol 1982; 50:29–34.

804. Miller ST, Rieder RF, Rao SP, et al: Cerebrovascular accidents in children with sickle-cell disease and α-thalassemia. J Pediatr 1988; 113:847–849.

805. Mears JG, Lachman HM, Labie D, et al: α-Thalassemia is related to prolonged survival in sickle cell anemia. Blood 1983; 62:286–290.

806. Fabry ME, Mears JG, Patel P, et al: Dense cells in sickle cell anemia: The effects of gene interaction. Blood 1984; 64:1042–1046.

807. Felice AE, McKie KM, Cleek MP, et al: Effects of α-thalassemia-2 on the developmental changes of hematological values in children with sickle cell disease from Georgia. Am J Hematol 1987; 25:389–400.

808. Stevens MC, Maude GH, Beckford M, et al: α-Thalassemia and the hematology of homozygous sickle cell disease in childhood. Blood 1986; 67:411–414.

809. Itano HA: A third abnormal hemoglobin associated with hereditary hemolytic anemia. Proc Natl Acad Sci USA 1951; 37:775.

810. Thomas ED: Homozygous hemoglobin C disease. Am J Med 1955; 18:832.

811. Jensen WN: Clinical and necropsy findings in hemoglobin C disease. Blood 1957; 12:74.

812. Charache S, Conley CL, Waugh DF, et al: Pathogenesis of hemolytic anemia in homozygous hemoglobin C disease. J Clin Invest 1967; 46:1795–811.

813. Kraus AP, Diggs LW: In vitro crystallization of hemoglobin occurring in citrated blood from patients with hemoglobin C. J Clin Med 1965; 47:700.

814. Smith EW, Krevans JR: Clinical manifestations of hemoglobin C disorders. Bull Johns Hopkins Hosp 1959; 104:238.

815. Fitzgerald PM, Love WE: Structure of deoxy hemoglobin C (beta six Glu replaced by Lys) in two crystal forms. J Mol Biol 1979; 132:603–619.

816. Girling RL, Houston TE, Amma EL, et al: An X-ray determination of the molecular interactions in hemoglobin C: A disease characterized by intraerythrocytic crystals. Biochem Biophys Res Commun 1979; 88:768–773.

817. Houston TE, Girling RL, Amma EL, et al: Structure of human hemoglobin C: A disease with intraerythrocytic crystals. Biochim Biophys Acta 1979; 576:497–501.

20 | The Thalassemias

Stuart H. Orkin • David G. Nathan

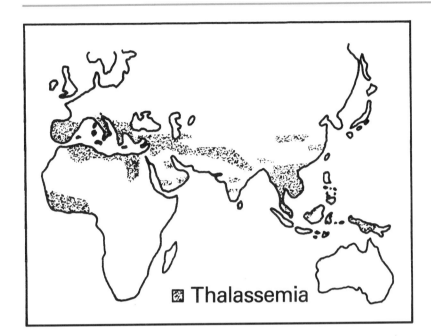

FIGURE 20–1. Geographic distribution of thalassemia.

The thalassemias are a heterogeneous group of inherited anemias caused by mutations affecting the synthesis of hemoglobin.[1-3] Milder forms are among the most commonly seen genetic disorders, whereas less often seen, severe forms lead to significant morbidity and mortality worldwide (Fig. 20–1).

A study of the thalassemias traces the history of the application of recombinant DNA methods to analysis of inherited diseases and underscores how naturally occurring mutations in humans illuminate genetic principles. Here the genetics of hemoglobin genes are reviewed as background for discussion of the molecular basis of the thalassemia syndromes, their clinical phenotypes, prenatal diagnosis, and current management.

HUMAN HEMOGLOBINS: COMPOSITION AND GENETICS

Normal hemoglobins are tetramers of two α-like and two β-like globin polypeptides. The predominant hemoglobin in normal adult red blood cells is hemoglobin A (HbA), $\alpha_2\beta_2$.[4,5] The α- and β-globins contain 141 and 146 amino acids, respectively. In addition to HbA, adult red cells normally contain two minor hemoglobins: HbA$_2$ ($\alpha_2\delta_2$) and fetal hemoglobin (HbF) ($\alpha_2\gamma_2$). The γ and δ polypeptides are related to β, but differ in their primary amino acid sequences; hence, they may be referred to as β-like globins. HbA$_2$ normally comprises 2 to 3.5 percent of total hemoglobin. Although a minor component in adult red cells, HbF is the predominant hemoglobin in fetal red cells during the latter two trimesters of gestation. Because it does not bind 2,3-diphosphoglycerate (2,3-DPG), its affinity for oxygen is higher than that of HbA.[6] As such, HbF enhances the fetus' ability to extract oxygen from the placenta. HbF constitutes a small fraction of the total hemoglobin in adult red cells (0.3 to 1.2 percent), in which it is largely restricted to a small subset of circulating erythrocytes (0.2 to 7 percent of total cells) referred to as F cells.[7,8] Production of HbF in normal adults appears

to be genetically controlled by several loci, including at least one on the X chromosome[9] and another on the long arm of chromosome 6.[10] During the first trimester *in utero*, embryonic hemoglobins with differing subunit composition are found in the yolk sac–derived macrocytic (or primitive) red cells.[1]

The genes that encode the globin polypeptides are organized into two small clusters.[2,4,5,11,12] The α-like genes are located near the telomere of the short arm of chromosome 16 (16p13.3), whereas the β-like genes reside on chromosome 11 at band 11p15.5.[13,14] A schematic diagram of the human globin genes and the compositions of the various hemoglobins are shown in Figure 20–2.

The α-globin gene cluster contains three functional genes, ζ, α_2, and α_1, oriented in the 5' to 3' direction along the chromosome.[2,12,15,16] ζ Globin, encoded by the ζ gene, is found in two embryonic hemoglobins, Hb Gower-1 ($\zeta_2\epsilon_2$) and Portland ($\zeta_2\gamma_2$).[17] The duplicated α-globin genes (α_1 and α_2) encode identical polypeptides. DNA sequence analysis has revealed three additional globin gene–like sequences in the cluster: pseudo-ζ (ζ_1), pseudo-α_1, and pseudo-α_2.[2,12] Although these resemble the functional genes, sequence differences in coding or critical regulatory regions render these genes inactive; hence, they are referred to as pseudogenes.

Five functional genes, ϵ, $^G\gamma$, $^A\gamma$, δ, and β, are present within the β-like cluster and are arranged 5' to 3' as they are expressed during development.[18-21] The product of the embryonic ϵ gene is found in the embryonic hemoglobins, Hb Gower-1 ($\zeta_2\epsilon_2$) and Hb Gower-2 ($\alpha_2\epsilon_2$). The fetal γ genes are duplicated, but encode globins differing only at amino acid 136; $^G\gamma$-globin and $^A\gamma$-globin contain a glycine or alanine residue, respectively. $^G\gamma$- and $^A\gamma$-globins are both found normally in HbF ($\alpha_2\gamma_2$). The δ-globin gene encodes a polypeptide differing in only 10 of 146 residues from β, and yet it is expressed at a very low level in adult red cells (<3 percent of β). The poor expression of

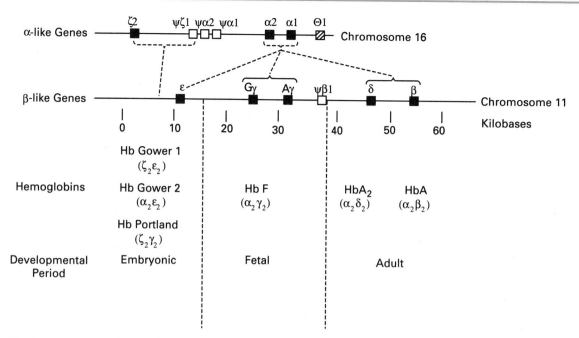

FIGURE 20–2. Chromosomal organization of the globin genes and their expression during development. The *solid boxes* indicate functional globin genes, whereas the *open boxes* indicate pseudogenes (see text). The scale of the depicted chromosomal segments is in kilobases of DNA. The switch from embryonic to fetal hemoglobin occurs between 6 and 10 weeks of gestation, and the switch from fetal to adult hemoglobin occurs at about the time of birth.

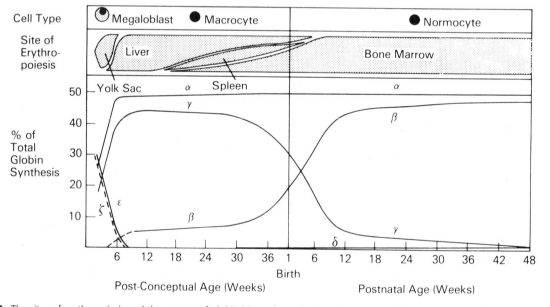

FIGURE 20–3. The sites of erythropoiesis and the pattern of globin biosynthesis during development. Nucleated megaloblasts are produced predominantly in the yolk sac. These are replaced by macrocytic fetal red cells produced in the liver and subsequently in the spleen and bone marrow. The height of the *shaded area* approximates the proportion of circulating red cells produced by each organ. Globin biosynthetic measurements were made to obtain the data shown in the lower part of the figure through incubation of intact cells in the presence of radioactive amino acids followed by globin chain separation. (From Weatherall DG, Clegg JB: The Thalassemia Syndromes. Oxford, England, Blackwell Scientific Publications, Inc., 1981, p 54.)

δ-globin is attributed to differences in critical regulatory sequences[22] within the gene, which appear to inhibit messenger RNA (mRNA) processing[23] and the inherent instability of δ mRNA.[24] Only a single functional β-globin gene is present in the cluster. β-Globin is the predominant β-like globin in adult red cells in which HbA ($\alpha_2\beta_2$) comprises more than 95 percent of the total hemoglobin.

The relative synthesis of individual globin chains and the major sites of erythropoiesis during development are depicted in Figure 20–3.[1, 4, 25–27] Embryonic hemoglobins are expressed nearly exclusively in primitive, nucleated red cells differentiating in the yolk sac blood islands. HbF is produced during the next wave of erythropoiesis in the fetal liver. Fetal liver-derived red cells lose their nuclei as terminal maturation occurs, whereas the primitive, yolk sac–derived cells remain nucleated. The transition from HbF to HbA coincides approximately with the switch from fetal liver to bone marrow erythropoiesis. Despite this correlation between the site of erythropoiesis and the hemoglobins expressed, careful analysis of tissues derived from experimental animals and human fetuses has shown that embryonic hemoglobins are synthesized in the liver as well as the yolk sac, and HbFs are produced in the bone marrow as well as in the liver. The developmental switches in hemoglobin expression are related to time of gestation rather than the anatomical site of erythropoiesis per se.

Globin Gene Structure

The globin genes were among the first eukaryotic genes to be isolated by recombinant DNA cloning methods in the late 1970s. Subsequent work has provided the entire DNA sequences of the human α- and β-globin gene clusters and extensive sequences of other vertebrate globin complexes.

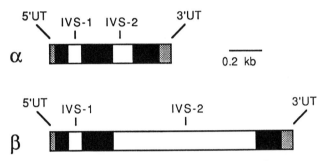

FIGURE 20–4. Structure of the human α- and β-globin genes. Untranslated regions, exon, and intervening sequences (introns) are depicted by *stippled, solid,* and *open boxes,* respectively.

These data have been invaluable for determining the mutations underlying thalassemia syndromes and for manipulating gene regulatory regions.

INTERVENING SEQUENCES OR INTRONS

A remarkable finding was made upon initial study of globin genes: the coding region, rather than organized in a single continuous unit, is interrupted by noncoding DNA, known as intervening sequences (IVS) or introns. The majority of eukaryotic genes contain one or more introns. As indicated in Figure 20–4, globin genes are interrupted at two positions. The discontinuous nature of the coding region of globin genes poses a formidable problem for the formation of mRNA that must be translated into globin polypeptides on cytoplasmic ribosomes. Transcription of a globin gene generates a precursor mRNA containing introns. Formation of mature mRNA is accomplished by post-transcriptional processing, termed *RNA splicing.* The pathway of RNA processing is depicted in Figure 20–5.

RNA splicing must be executed with exquisite precision for functional mRNA to be generated. Since translation of mRNA proceeds by the reading of triplets (codons), excision of introns needs to be accurate to the nucleotide; otherwise, shifts in the reading frame of the translated polypeptide will result. RNA processing is guided by specific sequences, known as splice site consensus sequences, located at the 5′ and 3′ boundaries of the introns. The donor site, which marks the 5′ end of the intron, generally conforms to the sequence 5′ (C/A)AG′GT (A/G)AGT, where the prime sign indicates the position of splicing and GT is an essentially invariant dinucleotide at the 5′ end of the intron. The acceptor site,

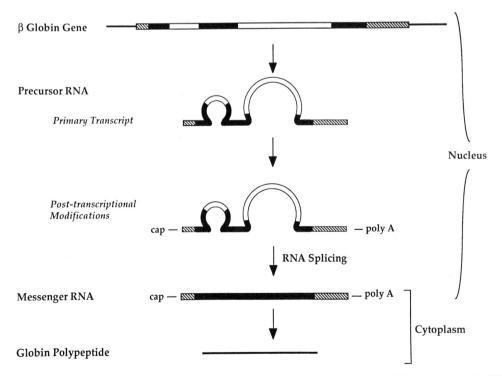

FIGURE 20–5. Expression of the β-globin gene. Transcription of the gene generates the precursor RNA, which is processed by RNA splicing to form messenger RNA.

which defines the 3′ end of the intron, usually fits the consensus 5′ $(T/C)_n N(C/T)\underline{AG}$′G, where n is greater than or equal to 11, N is any nucleotide, the prime sign indicates the site of splicing, and AG is an essentially invariant dinucleotide. Excision of introns generally occurs between the dinucleotides GT and AG, the GT-AG rule.

CONSERVED FEATURES OF MATURE GLOBIN mRNAS

Sequences of human globin genes represented in processed globin mRNAs include additional segments located before (5′) and after (3′) the coding region. These untranslated regions are depicted in Figure 20–5. In addition, the mature mRNA is modified at both termini. At the 5′ end a methylated guanylic acid (m^7G) cap structure is present. A variable number of adenylic acid residues are added at the 3′ end and constitute a poly(A) tail. The 5′-cap structure appears important for efficient initiation of mRNA translation, whereas the poly(A) tail contributes to mRNA stability.

Overlapping the beginning of the mRNA sequence in genomic DNA are sequences that aid in directing the initiation of transcription to the proper site. In some eukaryotic genes these sequences conform to an initiator (Inr) consensus element.[28] The human β-globin gene has been shown to possess an Inr element that is functional in transcription reactions performed *in vitro*.[29]

Polyadenylation at the 3′ end of mRNA precursors depends on a signal in the 3′-untranslated region, generally AAUAAA (AATAAA in genomic DNA). The mechanism of 3′ end modification is complex and involves not only polyadenylation but also cleavage of the precursor RNA, because the primary RNA transcript extends several hundreds nucleotides past what becomes the position at which the poly(A) tail is added.

Translation of mRNA into a polypeptide proceeds by the reading of triplets (codons) on cytoplasmic ribosomes. The first AUG codon (specifying methionine) present in the mRNA specifies the start site for translation of the mRNA into protein and is embedded in a sequence context (the Kozak consensus sequence, typically CC(A/G)CC$\underline{ATG}$G) that signals the binding of translation initiation factors and ribosomes to the RNA. Usually the amino-terminal methionine residue is removed from the growing polypeptide chain even before its synthesis is completed. Termination of polypeptide chain translation is directed by termination codons UAA, UAG, or UGA. Mutation of these codons allows for continued translation into the 3′-untranslated sequences of mRNA, as occurs in selected α-globin chain variants associated with α-thalassemia (see later).

As briefly reviewed earlier, information of functional mature mRNA demands extraordinary precision and depends on highly conserved sequence elements. As exemplified by the thalassemia syndromes, point (or other) mutations in these signals lead to reduced or absent polypeptide chain synthesis, the hallmark of thalassemia. Mutations causing thalassemia involve all phases of gene expression, including gene transcription, RNA splicing, integrity of the coding sequence, 3′ polyadenylation, and translation initiation (see later).

Regulation of Globin Gene Expression

Globin genes in all vertebrates are expressed in a tissue-specific and developmentally programmed manner. Their transcription is activated only within developing erythroid precursor cells. Moreover, individual globin genes are expressed at different developmental stages. Hence, within the genes of the β-cluster, globins are expressed at embryonic (ε), fetal (γ), or adult (β and δ) stages, whereas within the α-cluster, embryonic (ζ) and adult (α) chain expression is seen. A central problem posed by the organization of the globin gene clusters is how these patterns of tissue- and developmental-stage specificity are achieved. Current findings suggest that interactions between regulatory regions and their chromatin-bound proteins located near the genes (the proximal regulatory elements) and more distant control regions provide the means by which transcription is orchestrated in globin gene clusters.

PROXIMAL REGULATORY SEQUENCES AND TRANSCRIPTION FACTORS

Several conserved sequence elements (motifs) in the 5′-flanking sequences of globin genes comprise the promoter, a region required for accurate and efficient transcription of genes by RNA polymerase II.[30–33] Promoters of vertebrate globin genes are similar in overall configuration and subset of motifs present but differ in their detailed organization and sequences. Promoters generally cooperate with more distant regulatory elements termed *enhancers* to stimulate transcription.[34–36] As discussed later, globin gene promoters appear to interact in a synergistic fashion with very powerful distant elements, known as locus control regions (LCRs).

The TATA (or ATA) box is a motif seen in nearly all promoters, including those of the globin genes. The TATA box, typically located 20 to 30 base pairs (bp) upstream from the transcription start site, constitutes the binding site for a general transcription factor, the TATA-binding protein (TBP).[37–39] Binding of TBP to the TATA box is the first step in the assembly of a basal transcription complex (often termed TFIID) that includes many additional proteins (such as TFIIA, TFIIB, TFIIE/F, and TFIIH) and RNA polymerase II.[33] Mutations within the TATA box, as occur in some types of β-thalassemia,[40–46] decrease the binding of TBP to the promoter and decrease transcription.[37, 38, 47]

DNA sequence motifs located upstream of the TATA box bind proteins that interact with the general transcription machinery through protein-protein contacts with the TFIID complex and other associated proteins.[32, 34, 35, 39] These promoter-bound proteins may either increase (activate) or decrease (repress) the rate of transcription. A relatively small set of motifs is consistently present in globin gene promoters. These include CCAAT box, CACC box, and GATA consensus sequences. Each motif may be viewed as a potential binding site for one or multiple transcription factors, which are either tissue-restricted or ubiquitous in their cellular distribution.

Transcription factors are typically viewed as modular proteins made up of two domains that fulfill different functions: a DNA-binding domain responsible for sequence-specific DNA recognition and activation (or repression) domain(s) that interact with components of the basal complex to modulate transcription. It is currently believed that transcriptional specificity is achieved by functional cooperation and interaction between cell-restricted and general transcription factors. As background for understanding globin gene control, the presently characterized erythroid-enriched transcription factors are reviewed here. For additional discussion of these proteins, readers are referred elsewhere.[48]

The consensus motif (A/T)GATA(A/G), the GATA–motif, is found in the promoter region of most vertebrate globin genes and binds an abundant erythroid-restricted transcription factor GATA-1. GATA motifs have been identified in the regulatory elements of virtually all erythroid-expressed genes, consistent with the notion that GATA-1 should serve a critical role in erythroid gene expression. As noted later, multiple GATA sites are also present within distant regulatory elements. The essential role of GATA-1 in erythroid development was formally demonstrated through gene targeting experiments in mouse embryonic stem (ES) cells. Disruption of the single X chromosome GATA-1 gene in totipotent ES cells prevents their development into normal erythroid cells. The GATA-1 protein is a member of a small family of related "GATA factors," which are distinguished by a novel zinc-finger DNA-binding domain. In addition to merely specifying DNA recognition, this domain also mediates protein-protein interactions. Accordingly, GATA-1 is able to interact physically with other GATA-1 molecules or with other types of zinc-finger proteins, including the ubiquitous CACC- or GC-binding factor Sp1, the erythroid transcription factor EKLF, and a specific cofactor called FOG-1 (for friend of GATA-1)[49, 50] (see later). It is envisioned that through its multiple physical interactions GATA-1 cooperates with other transcription factors, perhaps bound to DNA at distant sites, to program erythroid-specific transcription.

CACC motifs, which are represented by diverse sequences within globin and other gene promoters, bind a variety of transcription factors. Many CACC sequences are recognized by Sp1, a ubiquitous zinc-finger, activator protein.[51] A particular CACC motif, CCACACCCT, is found in the adult β-globin gene promoter and is recognized with high affinity by the erythroid-specific protein, erythroid Krüppel-like factor (EKLF). The functional relevance of this binding site has been established through naturally occurring mutations that lead to β-thalassemia (see later). In addition, gene targeting (or knockout)

experiments in mice have formally established the requirement for EKLF for efficient β-globin transcription *in vivo*.[52]

A third erythroid transcription factor, known as NF-E2, binds to an extended motif—(T/C)TGCTGA(C/G)TCA(T/C)—that is found within some distant regulatory elements (see later) and a small subset of erythroid promoters but not within globin gene promoters. NF-E2 is a heterodimer of two polypeptides of the basic domain-leucine zipper (or b-zip) class of transcription factors.[53, 54] One subunit of NF-E2 is tissue-restricted, whereas the other is ubiquitous. Although NF-E2 is essential for globin gene expression in mouse erythroleukemia cells in tissue culture,[55, 56] its role *in vivo* appears to overlap with that of one or more unknown factors that may act through the same target sites in DNA.[57]

LOCUS CONTROL REGIONS AND CHROMATIN DOMAINS

How is globin gene transcription activated and developmentally controlled? Inspection of the DNA sequences of globin gene promoters in the early 1980s failed to provide substantive insights. Initial attempts to dissect control elements involved introducing globin genes into the germline of mice by oocyte injection but were plagued by low-level and erratic transgene expression. Nonetheless, it was possible to show that stage specificity was imparted by the human β- and γ-globin gene promoters. For example, when the human β-globin promoter is introduced into transgenic mice, it directs gene expression only in adult erythroid cells,[58–61] whereas the human γ-globin promoter is active only in embryonic erythroid cells (mice do not have an HbF stage).[61, 63]

These early globin gene regulation studies suggested that critical regulatory elements were missing from the immediate vicinity of the genes themselves. When sensitivity to digestion by the enzyme DNase I was used as an indicator of chromatin structure in the mid-1980s, regions of extreme sensitivity (hypersensitivity sites [HSs]) were identified far upstream (≈ 30 to 50 kilobases [kb]) of the adult human β-globin gene[64, 65] (Fig. 20–6). Four subregions were delimited; these are present in the chromatin of erythroid, but not nonerythroid, cells. An additional site located even further upstream was found in all tissues. In a formal test of their functional relevance, the HSs were linked to a human β-globin and introduced into the germline of mice. Remarkably, transgenic mice then expressed the human β-globin gene at a level equivalent to that of the endogenous mouse β gene.[66] Further studies

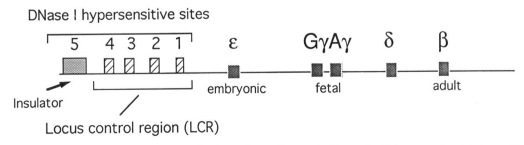

FIGURE 20–6. Schematic representation of the human β-globin gene locus. The *hatched boxes* depict the core DNase I hypersensitive subregions of the locus control region. The individual globin genes are indicated with their stage of expression.

showed that the transgene is expressed not only in a tissue-specific manner, but also in a copy number–dependent fashion independent of the chromosomal site of integration. These HSs comprise an essential distal regulatory domain, now referred to as the LCR (see reference 48 and 48a for more detailed history and discussion).

Other globin gene clusters also contain erythroid-specific DNase I hypersensitive sites. A segment of extreme DNase I hypersensitivity (known as HS-40) located far upstream of the human α-globin genes serves as an enhancer for the α-locus. HS-40, however, does not display the full properties of an LCR, as it does not direct copy number–dependent transgene expression.[67] Nonetheless, the in vivo relevance of both the β-LCR and HS-40 is underscored by the discovery of patients with thalassemia who have specific deletions in these regions (see later).

The human β-LCR, HS-40, and analogous regions studied in other species, are composed of cores, each encompassing a DNase I-hypersensitive site. Cores are approximately 200 to 300 bp in length. Remarkably, within the cores three major protein-binding sites are consistently found: GATA, AP-1 (NF-E2), and CACC sequences. The position-independent activity of the β-LCR correlates best with the presence of GATA and CACC motifs, particularly within the subregion known as HS-3. Enhancer activity of the LCR, particularly within subregion HS-2, requires the NF-E2 motif. The protein-binding motifs within the LCR are also found in globin and other erythroid-expressed gene promoters. To date, no protein-binding sites unique to LCR elements have been identified. Hence, the distinctive properties of the LCR (or HS-40) appear to reflect the synergistic interactions of more typical transcription factors, rather than the action of a new set of regulatory proteins.

The discovery of distant control elements, marked by DNase I hypersensitivity, emphasizes the relationship between chromatin structure and globin gene regulation, an association solidified by the unraveling of a rare syndrome, α-thalassemia with X-linked mental retardation.[68] This condition results from mutations in a gene designated *XH2* (or *ATR-X*) that encodes a member of the helicase superfamily.[69] Such proteins, which are often involved in DNA recombination and repair and in the regulation of transcription in *Drosophila* and yeast, appear to influence transcription in a global manner by altering chromatin structure.

REGULATION AT A DISTANCE: GLOBIN GENE SWITCHING

How do LCR sequences influence globin gene transcription over large distances (>50 kb)? How are the individual globin genes developmentally regulated? Two formal possibilities have been considered. On the one hand, the LCR might merely provide an environment conducive for activation of the downstream globin genes. The globin genes would be autonomously regulated; that is, the developmental profile of their expression would be intrinsic to the individual genes (and presumably determined by their promoters). The "influence" of the LCR is most simply viewed as reflecting physical association of the LCR with globin genes brought into apposition by chromosomal looping. On the other hand, sequential activation of the particular genes might depend (at least in part) on competition of each gene for the influence of LCR, such that only one gene-LCR interaction would be productive on a single chromosome at any time. The outcome of the competition would be dependent on the array of proteins bound not only at each promoter, but also at specific sites in the LCR. Data in favor of both autonomous and competitive mechanisms of regulation have been obtained (see reference 48 for a detailed discussion).

The human embryonic ζ- and ε-globin genes appear to be largely autonomously regulated. LCR-containing transgenes are expressed during embryonic erythropoiesis (the yolk sac stage) and then extinguished during the fetal liver stage. The information required for shut-off is contained near the globin genes and competition by adjacent globin genes is not required. Shut-off is hypothesized to reflect the action of repressors, or silencer proteins, that bind the gene promoters. Motifs within the human ε-globin promoter involved in silencing bind GATA-1 and a ubiquitous factor, YY1.[70]

The competitive model of gene regulation is based on experiments in chicken red blood cells, demonstrating competition between the chicken β- and ε-globin gene promoters for a single enhancer located between the genes.[71] In the chicken it has been proposed that an adult stage-specific factor (NF-E4) favors the interaction of the β-promoter with the enhancer to the exclusion of the ε-promoter. In an analogous fashion, data suggest that the human β-globin gene may be negatively regulated in a competitive fashion by the γ-globin gene. Whereas the γ gene is largely autonomously regulated, the β-globin gene is silenced in the embryonic and early fetal stage by a linked γ gene (a γ gene in *cis* to β). Shut-off of the γ gene, presumably due to repressors (or silencers), allows the adult β-globin to be expressed. It has been suggested that a protein complex, known as stage-selector protein (SSP), which binds to a site in the proximal γ-promoter, serves a function analogous to that proposed for chicken NF-E4 and tips the balance to γ-globin transcription at early stages.[72] Of interest, both NF-E4 and SSP complexes appear to contain the ubiquitous transcription factor CP2.[72] Although other models are theoretically possible, the capacity of the LCR to act at a distance in regulating activation of globin genes is most compatible with the formation of physical contacts between the LCR (or subregions thereof) and their associated proteins with regulatory elements neighboring the genes themselves. Stage-specific and competitive regulation would, therefore, reflect the engagement of the LCR with genes one at a time. LCR-gene interactions probably have intrinsic stabilities and off-rates, such that a single erythroid cell might express more than one globin over time, even from a single chromosome. Experiments examining nascent human globin RNAs along the β-gene complex tend to support such speculations and lend credence to the notion that chromosomal looping brings the LCR and individual genes in apposition. The dynamic interactions between the β-LCR and the γ- and β-globin genes appear to underlie the reciprocal expression of these genes in erythroid cells and provide hope that subtle alterations in the nuclear environment may facilitate reactivation of γ-globin genes in patients with hemoglobinopathies such as sickle cell anemia or with β-thalassemia.

CLASSIFICATION OF THE THALASSEMIAS

The hallmark of thalassemia syndromes is decreased (or absent) synthesis of one or more globin chains. α- and β-Thalassemias refer to deficits in α- and β-globin production, respectively. The α- and β-thalassemias include clinical syndromes of varying severity (Table 20–1). Knowledge of molecular genetics provides a framework in which to consider their clinical heterogeneity.

Because the structural gene for α-globin is duplicated on chromosome 16, each diploid cell contains four copies of the α-globin gene. The four α-thalassemia syndromes—silent carrier, α-thalassemia trait, HbH disease, and hydrops fetalis (Table 20–1)—reflect the inheritance of molecular defects affecting the output of 1, 2, 3, or 4 of the α-globin genes, respectively. More than 30 different mutations affecting one or both α-globin genes on a chromosome have been described. Some mutations abolish expression of an α-globin gene (α^0), whereas others reduce expression of the gene to a variable degree (α^+). Within the four general categories of α-thalassemia there is marked genetic and clinical heterogeneity. Heterogeneity arises because the syndrome in any given individual may represent the combination (or so-called interaction) of 2 of the 30 or more mutations that have been described.

The β-thalassemias also include four clinical syndromes of increasing severity—silent carrier, thalassemia trait, thalassemia intermedia, and thalassemia major (Table 20–1).[1, 3, 73, 74] In contrast to the α-thalassemias, the four classes of β-thalassemia are not correlated with the number of functioning genes. Because a single functional β-globin gene resides on each chromosome 11, a diploid cell normally has two β-globin genes. The clinical heterogeneity of the β-thalassemias represents the diversity of specific mutations that variably affect β-globin gene expression. Almost exclusively, these mutations involve the β-globin gene rather than an unlinked genetic determinant. Many mutations eliminate β-gene expression (β^0), whereas others cause a variable decrease in the level of β-gene expression (β^+).[3, 74] The capacity of individual patients to synthesize γ-globin modulates clinical severity. Such is the case because the severity of thalassemias is determined by the degree of globin chain imbalance rather than by the absolute level of either α- or β-globin synthesis per se.[75–79] Substantial synthesis of γ-globin in the marrow cells of individuals with β-thalassemia lessens the extent of chain imbalance and, therefore, improves red cell production.[80–82] Particular mutations of the β-globin gene in β-thalassemia mutations appear to affect γ-gene expression directly. However, some individuals with otherwise severe β-thalassemia may coinherit additional genetic determinants that enhance HbF synthesis. Coincident inheritance of an α-thalassemia mutation also reduces chain imbalance in patients with homozygous or heterozygous β-thalassemia.[83] Clinical severity in any individual patient represents the outcome of these complex genetic interactions.

Origin of Thalassemia Mutations: The Influence of Malaria

Mutations causing thalassemia have arisen spontaneously. The nearly exclusive distribution of lethal red blood cell disorders, such as thalassemia, sickle cell disease, and glucose-6-phosphate deficiency, in tropical and subtropical regions led Haldane in 1949 to propose that the heterozygous carrier state for these conditions confers a selective advantage where malaria is endemic.[84] The incidence of these genes in a population is determined by the balance between the premature death of the homozygote and the increased fitness of the heterozygote. The occurrence of β-thalassemia mutations is high (>0.01) in regions such as the Mediterranean basin, Northern Africa, Southeast Asia, India, and Indonesia, but are uncommon in Northern Europe, Korea, Japan, and Northern China.[3, 85, 86] The incidence of β-thalassemia trait may exceed 20 percent in some villages in Greece.[87] α-Thalassemia is perhaps the most common single gene disorder in the world.[2] The occurrence of α^+-thalassemia alleles ranges from 5 to 10 percent in the Mediterranean basin,[88] to 20 to 30 percent in portions of West Africa,[89] and to 68 percent in the Southwest Pacific.[90] The incidence of α-thalassemia is less than 0.01 in Britain, Iceland, and Japan.[91, 92] Although incidence of malaria and rate of occurrence of thalassemia are not always inversely correlated, the anomalies and inconsistencies seem to be the result of genetic drift, migration, and demographic changes that have occurred in the last 10,000 years.[93]

Additional epidemiologic studies have provided further evidence for the validity of the "malaria hypothesis" in both α-thalassemia and β-thalassemia.[90, 94–101] Siniscalco and associates[94] showed that β-thalassemia is uncommon in inhabitants of the mountainous areas of Sardinia, where malaria is rare, compared with the incidence in coastal populations. In Melanesia, α-thalassemia is correlated with malaria across both latitude and altitude.[90] β-Thalassemia in Melanesia also is associated with malarious coastal regions.[98]

The cellular mechanisms responsible for the selective advantage of thalassemia heterozygotes remain incompletely defined. Cultured erythrocytes containing high concentrations of HbF retard the growth and development of *Plasmodium falciparum*.[102] β-Thalassemia heterozygotes

TABLE 20–1. Clinical Classification of the Thalassemias

Silent carrier (α or β)	Hematologically normal
Thalassemia trait (α or β)	Mild anemia with microcytosis and hypochromia
HbH disease (α-thal)	Moderately severe hemolytic anemia, icterus, and splenomegaly
Hydrops fetalis (α-thal)	Death *in utero* caused by severe anemia
Severe β-thalassemia (Cooley anemia)	Severe anemia, growth retardation, hepatosplenomegaly, bone marrow expansion, and bone deformities
Thalassemia major	Transfusion dependent
Thalassemia intermedia	No regular transfusion requirement

thal=thalassemia trait.

have a delayed disappearance of HbF in the first year of life.[1] This might be protective from potentially fatal cerebral malaria early in life, as passive immunity acquired *in utero* wanes. Until recently, however, investigators were unable to document decreased invasion or growth of *P. falciparum* in red cells from thalassemia heterozygotes except under conditions of unusual oxidant stress.[86, 103] Using modified tissue culture conditions, Brockelman and associates[104] and more recently Pattanapanyasat and colleagues[105] demonstrated decreased parasite multiplication in red cells of β-thalassemia heterozygotes. They theorized that *P. falciparum* resistance was a consequence of the inability of the parasite to acquire sufficient nutrients from the digestion of hemoglobin in thalassemic red cells. In one study α- and β-thalassemia trait red cells bound greater levels of antibody than control cells. This could lead to greater removal of parasitized red cells and hence provide protection.[106] Erythrocytes from individuals with HbH disease also appear to inhibit *P. falciparum in vitro*,[104, 107] but a similar effect has not been found in erythrocytes from individuals with α-thalassemia trait. Recently, it has been suggested that rosette formation, the binding of uninfected red cells to *P. falciparum*-infected red cells, is decreased in thalassemia owing to reduced red cell size and may hinder the development of cerebral malaria by lessening sequestration.[108]

The difficulty in documenting the cellular mechanism of *P. falciparum* resistance in thalassemic erythrocytes *in vitro* suggests that the heterozygote advantage may be small. The high mortality associated with malaria in endemic regions is a powerful selective force that may be sufficient to amplify a small increase in fitness.

Classes of Mutations That Cause Thalassemia

Thalassemia is the consequence of mutations that diminish (or abolish) the production of either the α or β chain of hemoglobin. Molecular cloning, DNA sequencing, and functional analysis of cloned genes have provided the tools with which to dissect the thalassemia syndromes. This analysis has revealed remarkable heterogeneity in the specific alterations in DNA that lead to these clinical syndromes.

Typically single nucleotide mutations associated with thalassemia interfere with one of the critical steps in mRNA production (Fig. 20–7 and Table 20–2). Base substitutions alter promoter function, RNA processing, or mRNA translation or modify a codon into a "nonsense

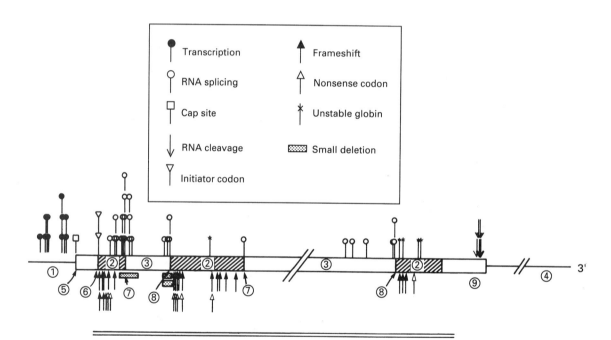

FIGURE 20–7. The location of various classes of point mutations that cause β-thalassemia, with respect to important structural elements present in the β-globin gene. (Adapted from Kazazian HH Jr, Boehm CD: Molecular basis and prenatal diagnosis of beta-thalassemia. Blood 1988; 72:1107.)

TABLE 20–2. Point Mutations That Cause Thalassemia

Gene	Position*		Mutation	Classification	Ethnic Group†	Detection‡	References
A. Transcription Mutations							
β:	1	−101	C-T	β⁺	Turkish		109
					Bulgarian		
					Italian		
	2	−92	C-T	β⁺	Mediterranean		3
	3	−88	C-T	β⁺	American black	(+) *Fok*I	110
					Asian Indian		
	4	−88	C-A	β⁺	Kurdish		111
	5	−87	C-G	β⁺	Mediterranean	(−) *Avr*II	112
	6	−86	C-G	β⁺	Lebanese		3
	7	−31	A-G	β⁺	Japanese		40
	8	−30	T-A	β⁺	Turkish		41
					Bulgarian		
	9	−30	T-C	β⁺	Chinese		42
	10	−29	A-G	β⁺	American black	(+) *Nla*III	43
					Chinese		44
	11	−28	A-C	β⁺	Kurdish		45
	12	−28	A-G	β⁺	Chinese		46
B. Cap Site Mutation							
β:	1	1	A-C	β⁺	Asian Indian		113
C. RNA Splicing Mutations							
1. Splice junction change in:							
a. 5′ donor site							
α2:	1	IVS-1 n. 2–6	5 bp deletion	α⁰	Mediterranean		114, 115
β:	1	IVS-1 n. 1	G-A	β⁰	Mediterranean	(−) *Bsp*M1	112
	2	IVS-1 n. 1	G-T	β⁰	Asian Indian	(−) *Bsp*M1	116
					Chinese		
	3	IVS-1 n. 2	T-G	β⁰	Tunisian		117
	4	IVs-1 n.2	T-C	β⁰	Black		118
	5	IVS-1 5′ end	44 bp deletion	β⁰	Mediterranean		119
	6	IVS-2 n. 1	G-A	β⁰	Mediterranean	(−) *Hph*I	120
					Tunisian		117
					American black		121
b. 3′ acceptor site							
β:	1	IVS-1 n. 130	G-C	β⁰	Italian		3
	2	IVS-1 n. 130	G-A	β⁰	Egyptian		3
	3	IVS-1 3′ end	17 bp deletion	β⁰	Kuwaiti		119
	4	IVS-1 3′ end	25 bp deletion	β⁰	Asian Indian		122
	5	IVS-2 n. 849	A-G	β⁰	American black		43
	6	IVS-2 n. 849	A-C	β⁰	American black		123
2. Splice consensus sequence change in:							
a. 5′ donor site							
β:	1	IVS-1 n. −3 (codon 29)	C-T	?	Lebanese		116
	2	IVS 1 n. −1 (codon 30)	G-C	Hb Monroe	Tunisian		117
					American black		124
	3	IVS 1 n. −1 (codon 30)	G-A	?	Bulgarian		125
	4	IVS-1 n. 5	G-C	β⁺	Asian Indian		116
					Chinese		126
	5	IVS-1 n. 5	G-T	β⁺	Melanesian		98
					Mediterranean		127
					American black		128
	6	IVS-1 n. 5	G-A	β⁺	Algerian	(+) *Eco*RV	129
					Mediterranean		
	7	IVS-1 n. 6	T-C	β⁺	Mediterranean	(+) *Sfa*NI	112
b. 3′ acceptor site							
β:	1	IVS-1 n. 128	T-G	β⁺	Saudi Arabian		130
	2	IVS-2 n. 843	T-G	β⁺	Algerian		131
	3	IVS-2 n. 848	C-A	β⁺	Iranian		130
					Egyption		
					American black		128

TABLE 20–2. Point Mutations That Cause Thalassemia (*Continued*)

Gene	Position*		Mutation	Classification	Ethnic Group†	Detection‡	References
3. Mutations within exons that affect processing							
β:	1	Codon 19 (Asn-Ser)	A-G	Hb Malay	Malaysian		132
	2	Codon 24 (silent)	T-A	β+	American black		133
	3	Codon 26 (Glu-Lys)	G-A	Hb E	Southeast Asian European	(−) *MnI*I	74, 134
	4	Codon 27 (Ala-Ser)	G-T	Hb Knossos	Mediterranean		135
4. Internal IVS change							
β:	1	IVS-1 n. 110	G-A	β+	Mediterranean		136, 137
	2	IVS-1 n. 116	T-G	β0	Mediterranean		138
	3	IVS-2 n. 654	C-T	β0	Chinese		126
	4	IVS-2 n. 705	T-G	β+	Mediterranean		139
	5	IVS-2 n. 745	C-G	β+	Mediterranean	(+) *Rsa*I	112
D. RNA Cleavage and Polyadenylation Mutations							
α_2:	1	Cleavage Signal	AATAAA-AATAAG	α+	Middle East Mediterranean		140, 141
β:	1	Cleavage Signal	AATAAA-AACAAA	β+	American black		142
	2	Cleavage Signal	AATAAA-AATAAG	β+	Kurdish		111
	3	Cleavage Signal	AATAAA-AATGAA	β+	Mediterranean		143
	4	Cleavage Signal	AATAAA-AATAGA	β+	Malaysian		143
	5	Cleavage Signal	AATAAA-A (-AATAA)	β+	Arab		3
E. Initiation Consensus Sequence Mutations							
α_2:	1	Initiation Codon	ATG-ACG	α0	Mediterranean	(−)*Nco*I	144
α_1:	2	Initiation Codon	ATG-GTG	α0	Mediterranean	(−)*Nco*I	145
−α:	3	Initiation Codon	ATG-GTG	α0	Black	(−)*Nco*I	146
$-\alpha^{3.7\text{II}}$:	4	Initiation Consensus	CCACCATGG- CC … CATGG	α+	Algerian Mediterranean		147 148
β:	1	Initiation Codon	ATG-AGG	β0	Chinese		3
	2	Initiation Codon	ATG-ACG	β0	Yugoslavian		143
	3	Initiation Codon	ATG-ATA	β0	Swedish		
F. Premature Termination Mutations							
1. Substitutions							
α_2:	1	Codon 116	GAC-TAG	α0	Black		149
B:	1	Codon 15	G-A	β0	Asian Indian		116
	2	Codon 17	A-T	β0	Chinese	(+)*Mae*I	150
	3	Codon 35	C-A	β0	Thai		151
	4	Codon 37	G-A	β0	Saudi Arabian		152
	5	Codon 39	C-T	β0	Mediterranean	(+) *Mae*I	153
	6	Codon 43	G-T	β0	European		154
	7	Codon 61	A-T	β0	Chinese Black	(−) *Hinf*I	155 128
2. Frameshifts							
−α:	1	Codons 30/31	− 2 bp (− AG)	α0	Black		156
β:	1	Codon 1	−1 bp (− G)	β0	Mediterranean		3
	2	Codon 5	− 2 bp (− CT)	β0	Mediterranean		157
	3	Codon 6	− 1 bp (−A)	β0	Mediterranean American black	(−) *Cvn*I	128 157
	4	Codon 8	− 2 bp (− AA)	β0	Turkish		158
	5	Codon 8/9	+ 1 bp (+ G)	β0	Asian Indian		116
	6	Codon 11	− 1 bp (−T)	β0	Mexican		3
	7	Codons 14/15	+ 1 bp (+ G)	β0	Chinese		159
	8	Codon 16	− 1 bp (− C)	β0	Asian Indian		116
	9	Codons 27/28	+ 1 bp (+ C)	β0	Chinese		3
	10	Codon 35	− 1 bp (− C)	β0	Indonesian		132
	11	Codons 36/37	− 1 bp (−T)	β0	Iranian		111
	12	Codon 37	− 1 bp (− G)	β0	Kurdish		111
	13	Codons 37–39	− 7 bp (− GACCCAG)	β0	Turkish		160

Continues

TABLE 20–2. Point Mutations That Cause Thalassemia (*Continued*)

Gene	Position*		Mutation	Classification	Ethnic Group[†]	Detection[‡]	References
	14	Codons 41/42		β^0	Asian Indian		116
			– 4 bp (– CTTT)		Chinese		161
	15	Codon 44	– 1 bp (– C)	β^0	Kurdish		162
	16	Codon 47	+ 1 bp (+ A)	β^0	Surinamese black		3
	17	Codon 64	– 1 bp (– G)	β^0	Swiss		163
	18	Codon 71	+ 1 bp (+ T)	β^0	Chinese		3
	19	Codons 71/72	+ 1 bp (+ A)	β^0	Chinese		126
	20	Codon 76	– 1 bp (– C)	β^0	Italian		164
	21	Codons 82/83	– 1 bp (– G)	β^0	Azerbaijani		3
	22	Codons 106/107	+ 1 bp (+ G)	β^0	American black		113
G. Termination Codon Mutations							
α_2:	1	Codon 142 (ter-Gin)	TAA-CAA	Hb Constant Spring	Chinese		165, 166
	2	Codon 142 (ter-Lys)	TAA-AAA	Hb lcaria	Mediterranean		167
	3	Codon 142 (ter-Ser)	TAA-TCA	Hb Koya Dora	Indian		168
	4	Codon 142 (ter-Glu)	TAA-GAA	Hb Seal Rock	Black		169
β:	1	Codon 147 (ter-Gin)		Hb Tak	Thai		170
H. Unstable Hemoglobin Chains							
1. Amino acid substitutions							
$-\alpha$:	1	Codon 14 (Trp-Arg)		Hb Evanston	Black		171
α_2:	2	Codon 109 (Leu-Arg)	T-G	Hb Suan Dok	Southeast Asian		172, 173
α:	3	Codon 110 (Ala-Asp)	T-C	Petah Tikvah	Middle Eastern		174
α_2:	4	Codon 125 (Leu-Pro)		Hb Quong Sze	Southeast Asian		175, 176
β:	1	Codon 60	T-A	β^+	Italian		177
	2	Codon 110 (Leu-Pro)	T-C	Hb Showa-Yakushiji	Japanese		178
	3	Codon 112 (Cys-Arg)		Hb Indianapolis	European		179
	4	Codon 127 (Gin-Pro)		Hb Houston	British		180
	5	Codons 127/128 (Gin, Ala-Pro)	–3 bp (– AGG)	β^+	Japanese		181
2. Frameshift, extended chain							
β:	1	Codon 94	+2 bp (+ TG)	Hb Agnana (inclusion body)	Italian		182
	2	Codons 109/110	–1 bp (– G)	Hb Manhattan	Lithuanian		3,180
	3	Codon 114	–2, +1 (–CT, + G)	Hb Geneva (Inclusion body)	French-Swiss		183
	4	Codons 128-135	Net -10 bp	β^+ (inclusion body)	Irish		184
3. Premature termination:							
β:	1	Codon 121	G-T	β^0 (inclusion body)	Greek-Polish French-Swiss British		184–186

*The position specifies the location in the gene at which the point mutation occurs. Positions are specified with reference to the start site for transcription (Cap site), the position within the intron (IVS), or the position of the codon.

[†]Where more than one ethnic group is indicated, the mutation has had more than one origin.

[‡]Loss (–) or gain (+) of a restriction enzyme site with mutation is indicated; the remainder of the mutations can be detected with allele-specific oligonucleotides (see section on direct detection of thalassemia mutations).

We are grateful to Drs. Halg Kazazian and to Titus Huisman and his colleagues for providing us with their detailed lists of β-thalassemia point mutations. (From Kazazian H: The thalassemia syndromes: Molecular basis and prenatal diagnosis in 1990. Semin Hematol 1990; 27:209, and from Huisman TH: Beta-thalassemia repository. Hemoglobin 1990; 14:661, by courtesy of Marcel Dekker, Inc.)

codon" that leads to premature termination of translation or in the substitution of an incorrect amino acid. Insertion or deletion mutations within the coding region of the mRNA create "frameshifts" that prevent the synthesis of a complete, normal globin polypeptide. Large deletions within the α- or β-globin clusters may remove one or more genes and alter the regulation of the remaining genes in the cluster. The phenotype that results from the diverse mutations found in thalassemia is determined by the degree of inactivation of the affected gene(s) and the extent of associated increases in expression of other genes within the cluster.

MUTATIONS AFFECTING GENE TRANSCRIPTION

Point mutations within promoter sequences recognized by transcription factors tend to reduce the affinity with which these proteins bind. Typically this leads to reduced gene transcription. Analysis of the promoter for the β-globin gene in patients with β-thalassemia has identified a variety of mutations clustered in the ATA and CACC-motifs (Table 20–2 and Fig. 20–8).[3, 40–46, 109–112] These mutations are associated with preservation of some β-globin expression and hence are customarily associated with the phenotype of thalassemia intermedia. The C→T substitution at position −101, which results in a particularly mild defect, is associated with the "silent carrier" phenotype in heterozygous carriers.[109, 187] Although the CCAAT box is highly conserved in globin genes, no mutations within this motif have been identified in thalassemia. At present, mutations in transcription factors that result in thalassemia have not been identified, although exceedingly rare families have been identified in which a thalassemia mutation is unlinked to the globin clusters (see section on mutations not linked to the globin gene clusters that alter globin gene expression).

Mutations of the ATA box presumably reduce binding of TBP and, therefore, lead to decreased transcription initiation. Substitutions in the CACC motifs decrease the affinity of binding by several transcription factors, including the erythroid-specific factor EKLF and the ubiquitous protein Sp1. Studies showing that mice engineered to lack EKLF suffer from lethal β-thalassemia at the fetal liver stage, establishing EKLF as a β-globin activator protein *in vivo*.[52, 188]

Human β-thalassemias resulting from mutation of a single CACC motif are presumably mild due to presence of one normal CACC motif within the promoter.

In addition to the protein-binding sites in the promoter, proper transcription depends on sequences surrounding the start site of transcription (known as +1). These sequences often display functional activity in *in vitro* assays, heralding the binding of specific protein complexes to this type of element, termed the *initiator* (Inr). Mild β-thalassemia has been associated with a base substitution (A→C) at +1. Recently this substitution has been shown to impair the β-globin Inr.[29] The proteins that mediate this effect are unknown.

RNA PROCESSING DEFECTS IN THALASSEMIA

The importance of RNA splicing for formation of functional mRNA cannot be overemphasized. As discussed earlier, removal of introns must be precise to the nucleotide for a continuous, translatable mRNA to be generated from an mRNA precursor. As soon as introns were discovered, it was hypothesized that mutations affecting RNA splicing would probably be involved in the thalassemia syndromes. Apart from its role in constructing a functional mRNA, RNA splicing also appears to be a determinant of mRNA stability[189, 190] and possibly coupled to RNA transport from nucleus to cytoplasm.[191]

MUTATIONS THAT ALTER SPLICE JUNCTIONS OR SPLICE CONSENSUS SEQUENCES

Mutations of the 5′ donor site (GT)[112, 114–121] or at the 3′ splice acceptor site (AG)[3, 43, 118, 119, 122, 123, 192] abolish proper splicing of the pre-mRNA transcript and result in α⁰- or β⁰-thalassemia (Table 20–2 and Fig. 20–9). Substitutions at other sites within the splice junction consensus sequence have varied effects; because some correctly spliced RNA, albeit a reduced amount, is produced, a β⁺-thalassemia phenotype ensues.★

Mutations within the splice site or the splice site consensus sequences favor improper processing of the mRNA precursor. These secondary splicing events, which are not seen under normal circumstances, occur at positions that resemble splice site consensus sequences.

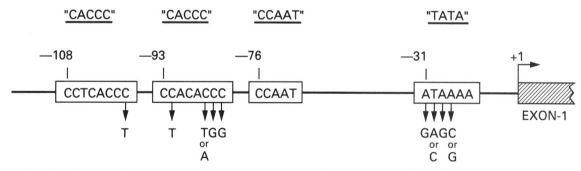

FIGURE 20–8. Point mutations in the β-globin gene promoter. The sequences of conserved motifs within the promoter and their distance from the transcription start site are indicated. Single base substitution at the indicated positions results in β⁺-thalassemia.

★References 98, 111, 112, 116, 117, 124–131, and 193.

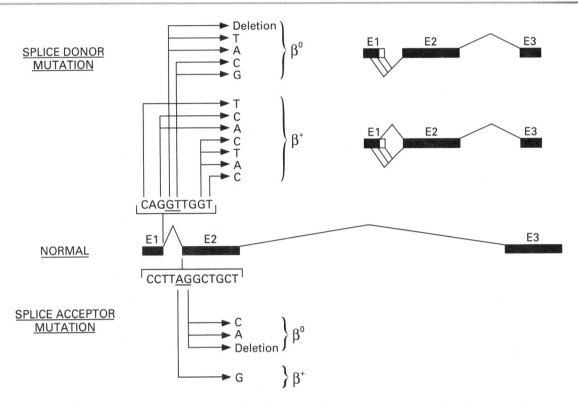

FIGURE 20–9. Examples of abnormal splicing that result from alterations in the splicing consensus sequences. The three β-globin gene exons are symbolized by *solid boxes,* the normal splicing pattern is illustrated by lines that project above the exons, and the splice donor and splice acceptor sequences of the first intron are shown. Mutations in the invariant GT dinucleotide of the splice donor site abolish normal splicing of the first intron and result in β⁰-thalassemia, whereas mutations elsewhere in the consensus sequence preserve some normal splicing and cause β⁺-thalassemia. Changes in the splice donor site are associated with abnormal splicing from three cryptic splice donors *(lines that project below the exons);* one site is within the first intron and results in the addition of intron sequences to exon 1 *(open box).* Similarly, changes in the invariant AG dinucleotide of the splice acceptor sequence are associated with β⁰-thalassemia, whereas a mutation in an adjacent nucleotide causes β⁺-thalassemia.

Splicing at these "cryptic" sites generates aberrantly processed, nonfunctional globin mRNAs (Fig. 20–9). Mutations within the β-globin IVS-1 splice donor site activate two cryptic donor sites in exon 1 and a third site in IVS-1,[112, 119, 194] whereas mutation in the IVS-2 splice donor activates a cryptic donor site in IVS-2.[120] Mutation of the IVS-2 splice acceptor site activates an upstream cryptic splice acceptor at position 579 in IVS-2.[43] These incorrectly spliced mRNAs suffer either insertions or deletions in the coding region and also shifts in the translational reading frame downstream of the cryptic splice site. The polypeptide synthesized beyond this point bears no resemblance to the globin chain and is often prematurely shortened by a termination codon encountered in the new reading frame.

MUTATIONS WITHIN EXONS THAT CREATE AN ALTERNATIVE SPLICE SITE

RNA from β-thalassemia genes with mutations in the IVS-1 donor splice site may be processed using a cryptic splice donor site GTG*GT*GAGG in exon 1 (codons 24 through 27). Four independent mutations have been identified that activate this cryptic site in the presence of a *normal* IVS-1 splice donor site (Table 20–2 and Fig. 20–10).[74, 133–135] These mutations appear to enhance the ability of the cryptic site to compete with the normal site for binding of the splicing complex. A T→A mutation at

codon 24 is "silent" at the translational level, yet approximately 80 percent of RNA transcripts are spliced at this incorrect site; hence, mild β⁺-thalassemia ensues. Two mutations—GAG→AAG in codon 26 and GCC→TCC in codon 27—lead to amino acid replacements that produce the hemoglobin variants HbE and Hb Knossos, respectively, in normally processed mRNA. Because a proportion of transcripts are aberrantly spliced, mild β⁺-thalassemia results. An analogous mutation in codon 19 produces β⁺-thalassemia with the hemoglobin variant Hb Malay.[132] These represent mutations that lead to thalassemic hemoglobinopathies.

MUTATIONS WITHIN INTRONS THAT CREATE AN ALTERNATE SPLICE SITE

Mutations within β-globin IVS-1 may create a new splice acceptor sequence (Table 20–2 and Fig. 20–11).[136–138] In the first of this class of mutations to be characterized, a G→A substitution at position 110 (19 nucleotides upstream of the normal intron/exon boundary), the majority of globin mRNA precursors are spliced at this alternate site.[136, 137, 195, 196] Because the incorrectly spliced mRNA contains 19 nucleotides from IVS-1, a shift in the reading frame leads to premature termination of translation. A T→G mutation at position 116 of IVS-1 creates a new acceptor site that is used exclusively, leading to little or no normal β mRNA production and β⁰-thalassemia.[138]

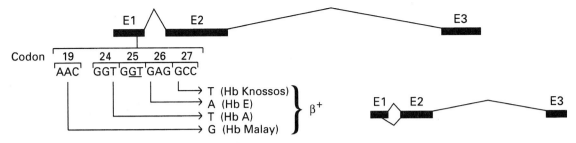

FIGURE 20–10. Mutations that create an alternate splice donor site in the first exon decrease but do not abolish the occurrence of normal splicing *(pattern that projects above the exons)* and are associated with splicing from the new site in the first exon *(pattern that projects below the exons).* Three of these mutations lead to the incorporation of a different amino acid into the β-globin chain derived from the decreased quantity of correctly spliced β-globin mRNA and generate variant hemoglobins.

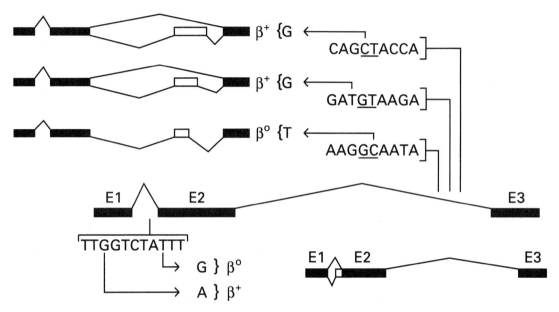

FIGURE 20–11. Mutations within introns that create a new splice site. Three mutations in the second intron create a new splice acceptor site (the invariant GT is underlined) and activate the identical cryptic splice donor site located just upstream. Abnormal splicing from these sites *(pattern that projects below the exons)* leads to the creation of a fourth exon *(open box)* derived from sequences within the second intron. Two mutations in the first intron create a new splice acceptor site with the conserved AG dinucleotide, and abnormal splicing from this site *(pattern that projects below the exons)* adds sequences from the first intron to the beginning of the second exon.

Three mutations in IVS-2 create new donor sites and activate an upstream cryptic donor site located 579 nucleotides from the exon 2-IVS-2 boundary (Table 20–2 and Fig. 20–11).[112, 126, 139] The consequence of these mutations is the insertion of a fourth "exon" derived from sequences within IVS-2. Although the normal donor and acceptor sites are unaffected, little or no correctly spliced β-globin mRNA may be produced.[112, 126, 139]

RNA CLEAVAGE AND POLYADENYLATION DEFECTS

Proper cleavage at the 3′ end of the pre-mRNA and subsequent poly(A) addition depend on the integrity of the AAUAAA signal in the 3′-untranslated region. The importance of the polyadenylation signal for the efficient production of globin mRNA was first demonstrated in α-thalassemia.[140, 141, 197] Mutation of AAUAAA→AAUAAG in the α_2 gene reduces the efficiency of cleavage-polyadenylation of precursors RNAs and leads to "run-on" transcripts that terminate downstream of the gene (see Fig. 20–13). Mutations in

the AAUAAA element have also been described in β-thalassemia,[111, 142, 143] in which the presence of the elongated *in vivo* transcripts has been demonstrated.[142] The transcripts appear to terminate at the next AAUAAA signal, which is present approximately 900 nucleotides downstream of the normal cleavage site. These mutations lead to a moderate reduction in the level of β-globin mRNA and a β+-phenotype.

MUTATIONS AFFECTING mRNA TRANSLATION INITIATION

Translation begins at an AUG codon that usually lies within a consensus sequence, (GCC)GCC(A/G)CCATGG.[198] Substitutions within the AUG codon abolish translation, whereas those in the other positions of the consensus often result in less efficient translation initiation.

Four mutations in α-globin genes alter the consensus sequence and impair translation (Table 20–2). Three of these affect the AUG initiator.[144–146] No globin polypeptide is produced, as the next downstream initiator is in a different reading frame. The fourth α-globin mutation in this class, found on a chromosome in which one α-globin gene was deleted, alters the consensus sequence by the deletion of 2 bp and reduces mRNA translation to 50 percent of normal.[147, 148] Two AUG initiator mutations of the β-globin gene have been described, and both are of the β[0] type (Table 20–2).[3, 143]

PREMATURE TERMINATION (NONSENSE) MUTATIONS

Nucleotide substitutions within the coding region are innocuous if they occur in the third position of a codon and do not alter the amino acid inserted during translation. Substitutions that alter codons from one amino acid to another lead to hemoglobin structural variants. Some substitutions change a triplet coding for an amino acid to a stop codon (UAG, UUA, or UGA). Such chain-termination (or

nonsense) mutations abort mRNA translation and lead to synthesis of a truncated polypeptide. Moreover, nonsense mutations also reduce the amount of stable mRNA generated, reflecting coupling between mRNA biogenesis and mRNA translation (Fig. 20–12).[199]

Chang and Kan[150] described the first nonsense mutation in β-thalassemia in which a lysine codon at amino acid position 17 was converted to a stop codon (AAG→UAG). Although no β-globin chains were produced *in vivo*, complete translation of the abnormal mRNA could be achieved in a cell-free extract capable of protein synthesis by the addition of a "suppressor" tRNA that inserts a serine at the UAG codon.[200] Several other nonsense mutations causing thalassemia have been described (Table 20–2 and Fig. 20–13).[116, 128, 151–155] In addition, single or dinucleotide insertions or deletions have been observed that alter the translational reading frame and introduce a premature stop codon as a

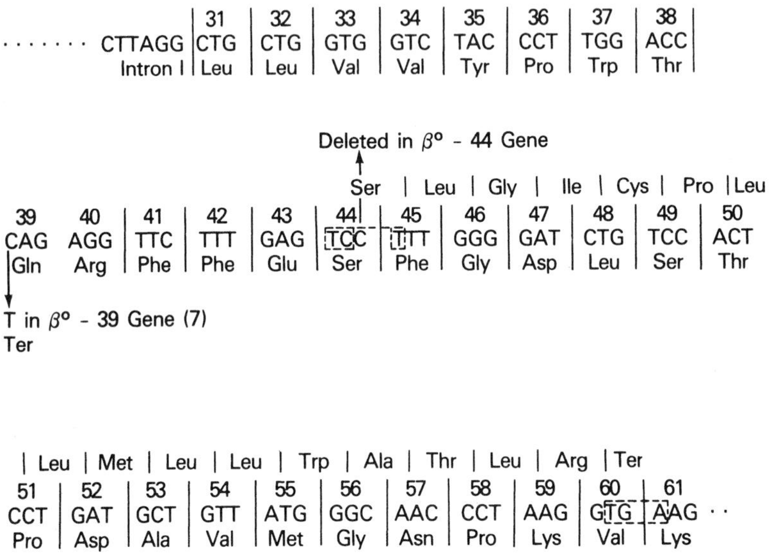

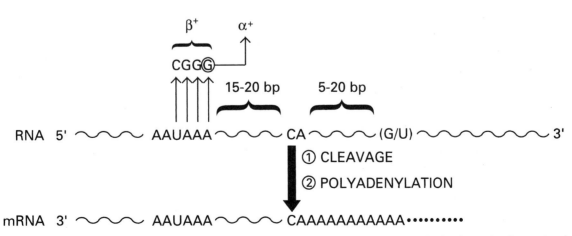

FIGURE 20–12. Two of the several thalassemia mutations that destroy gene function by introduction of a premature translation termination codon in β-globin mRNA. The numbers above the individual codons refer to position of the encoded amino acid in the β globin. Replacement of C with T in codon 39 introduces the terminator UAG in β-globin mRNA. Another β[0] gene has a deletion of the third nucleotide (C) in codon 41. This results in a shift in the reading frame of the mRNA; the new amino acid sequence is shown above the line. This new reading frame has an in-phase terminator (UGA) in a position corresponding to codon 60 to 61. (From Nienhuis AW, Anagnou NP, Ley TJ: Advances in thalassemia research. Blood 1984; 63:738.)

FIGURE 20–13. RNA cleavage and polyadenylation occurs 15 to 20 bp downstream from the AAUAAA polyadenylation signal. Mutational analysis in the rabbit β-globin gene has established that sequences located downstream from the polyadenylation site, called the G/U cluster, are also required for efficient cleavage and polyadenylation. Individual point mutations at one of several nucleotides within the AAUAAA polyadenylation signal result in β[+]-thalassemia. The same A to G mutation in the last position that causes β-thalassemia has been observed in the α₂-globin gene and results in α[+]-thalassemia.

consequence.* Two termination mutations have been described in the α-globin genes, one that introduces a stop codon[149] and the other a frameshift.[155] In addition, frameshift mutations have been described that result in abnormal elongation of globin chains (see section on unstable β-globin chains).

mRNAs with termination mutations often do not accumulate to a normal level *in vivo*.[197, 202] The extent of this effect is variable and depends on the specific mutations; deletion of the third nucleotide (C) from codon 41 (Fig. 20–14) leads to complete absence of globin mRNA,[203] whereas a single substitution in the β39 codon allows accumulation of roughly 5 to 10 percent of the normal amount of globin mRNA.[202] The basis for this quantitative deficiency of these mRNA species is of considerable interest. Speculation that abnormal mRNAs are unstable because impaired translation exposes such molecules to cytoplasmic nucleases has not been experimentally verified. Rather, data suggest that the such mutations lead to intranuclear degradation of abnormal globin RNA molecules and suggest a link between mRNA translation and nuclear RNA processing or nuclear to cytoplasmic transport of mRNA.[204, 205] Experimental studies in tissue culture systems have shown that the deficiency in β-globin mRNA accumulation is specific for nonsense mutations and is not observed with missense mutations[199]; a suppressor tRNA that allows the abnormal mRNA molecule to be translated completely will correct the quantitative deficiency in globin mRNA.[205] The specific mechanisms responsible for the defect in mRNA accumulation remain unclear.

TERMINATION CODON MUTATIONS

UAA is the normal termination codon for both α- and β-globin mRNA translation. The 3′-untranslated regions are 109 and 132 nucleotides for α- and β-mRNAs, respectively. A single nucleotide substitution in the termination codon could create either another stop codon (UAG) or permit incorporation of an amino acid at this position and the translation of the otherwise untranslated 3′ sequences until the next in-frame stop codon. Four termination codon mutations involving the α_2 gene have been reported (Table 20–2).[165–170] These mutants differ only

in the specific amino acid incorporated at the terminator codon position (Fig. 20–14). Translation terminates in each instance at a UAA codon in the polyadenylation signal (AAUAAA) downstream, producing a 172-amino acid polypeptide. The first of these elongated α chains to be described was found in Hb Constant Spring.[165, 166] The α chain in this hemoglobin has a glycine substituted at codon 142. Hb Constant Spring produces an associated thalassemia phenotype due to a marked reduction of α_2 globin mRNA stability.[206–208]

Mutations that give rise to elongated β-globin chains have also been described. Hb Tak is a 157-amino acid product of a β-globin mRNA molecule containing two inserted nucleotides in the terminator codon 147.[170] An analogous elongated β-globin with 157 amino acids found in Hb Cranston reflects a dinucleotide insertion in codon 147, but red cells containing Hb Cranston are morphologically normal.[209] The mechanism by which the β^{Tak} mutation causes thalassemia has not been elucidated.

MUTATIONS AFFECTING GLOBIN CHAIN STABILITY

Hemoglobin Assembly. Shortly after synthesis is completed, α- and β-globin chains bind a heme moiety and rapidly associate into $\alpha_1\beta_1$ dimers in a noncovalent reaction that is nearly irreversible under physiologic conditions.[210] The majority of the heme contact points are present in the portion of the globin chains encoded by exon 2, whereas most $\alpha_1\beta_1$ contacts are located within the exon 3 domain (Fig. 20–15).[6, 211] These dimers may then reversibly associate with other dimers to form the hemoglobin tetramer. The formation of the $\alpha_1\beta_1$ dimer, therefore, is the principal controlling step in the assembly of hemoglobin.

Hemoglobin assembly is an important determinant of the final hemoglobin composition of the erythrocyte.[210, 212, 213] The rate constant of dimer formation depends greatly on the surface electrostatic charge of the subunits.[210] α-Globin has a net positive surface charge, whereas β-globin has a net negative surface charge. The other normal β-like globin chains, γ-globin and δ-globin, dimerize with the α chain at a lower rate. δ-Globin has a lower net negative surface charge than β-globin, whereas the significant structural differences between

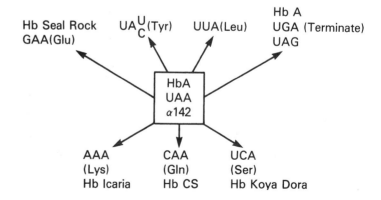

FIGURE 20–14. Point mutations in the terminator codon of the α-globin gene that lead to synthesis of elongated α globins. The normal terminator, UAA, of α-globin mRNA is shown in the center. Each of the nine possible single nucleotide substitutions is depicted; two would result in formation of another terminator codon, whereas the other seven would lead to insertion of an amino acid at this position and continued synthesis of the globin chain. Four such mutations have been described; the mutation that causes synthesis of Hb Constant Spring (CS) is the most common. (Adapted from Weatherall DJ, Clegg JB: The Thalassemia Syndromes. Oxford, England, Blackwell Scientific Publications, Inc., 1981, p 578.)

---

*References 3, 111, 126, 128, 132, 156–163, and 201.

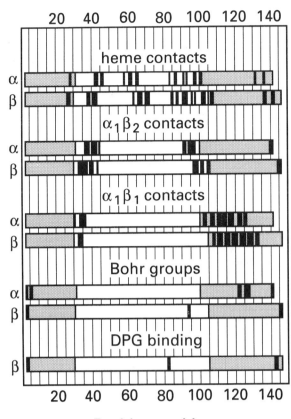

FIGURE 20–15. Schematic representation of the α- and β-globin chains, indicating the location of residues involved in different hemoglobin functions *(solid vertical bars)*. Heme contact sites and $\alpha_1\beta_2$ contacts are concentrated in the second exon *(unshaded)*, whereas $\alpha_1\beta_1$ contacts are principally located in the third exon *(shaded)*. DGP = diphosphoglycerate. (Adapted from Eaton WA: The relationship between coding sequences and function in haemoglobins. Nature 1980; 284:183. Reprinted by permission from Nature, copyright © 1980, Macmillan Magazines Limited.)

γ- and β-globin presumably account for the differing dimerization rates. Where β-globin chains are in limited supply (i.e., β-thalassemia), HbA_2 and HbF levels may rise because of enhanced dimerization with α chains, independent of changes in the production of δ and γ chains. In α-thalassemia or iron deficiency, HbA_2 and HbF levels will fall because competition with β chains for the limited number of α chains. Similarly, β-chain variants may have decreased (β^S and β^E) or increased ($\beta^{Baltimore}$) affinity for α chains based on their net surface charge. The net hemoglobin composition of the cell is determined by these simple rules of competition based on the relative affinity of hemoglobin subunits.

An efficient, energy-dependent proteolytic system is present in erythrocytes that rapidly degrades free globin chains, while leaving chains incorporated into dimers or tetramers unaffected.[210] Changes in globin chain structure that result from amino acid substitutions, premature chain termination, or chain elongation may slow or block the formation of stable $\alpha_1\beta_1$ dimers and lead to rapid degradation of the globin chain. In some instances, as discussed later, mutations may also enhance association of the free globin chain with the cell membrane, promoting oxidative damage to the membrane and shortened red cell survival.

Recently an erythroid-specific protein, called ASHP (for α hemoglobin stabilizing protein), has been identified that appears to act as a chaperone for free α-globin chains. In the absence of this protein mice exhibit a mild hemolytic anemia due to α-globin precipitation. It is possible that genetic variation in the structure or expression of this protein is a modifier of the severity of thalassemia phenotypes.[214]

UNSTABLE α-GLOBIN CHAINS

One such unstable variant was identified upon sequencing of a mutant α-globin gene (Table 20–2).[175] $\alpha^{Quong\ Sze}$, which contains a Leu→Pro substitution at position 125, is so unstable that the mutant globin chain cannot be detected by biosynthetic studies in intact cells or by conventional hemoglobin electrophoresis.[176] The $\alpha^{Quong\ Sze}$ chain appears to be stable once it is incorporated into the hemoglobin tetramer. Three other similar unstable α-globin chain mutations have been described (Table 20–2).[171–174]

UNSTABLE β-GLOBIN CHAINS

Several unstable β-globin chains have been associated with thalassemia (Table 20–2). Five mutations lead to amino acid substitutions in the β-globin chain.[177–181] Frameshift mutations in the third exon result in synthesis of an elongated β-globin chain with a novel carboxy terminus.[3, 180, 182–186] A premature termination mutation in exon 3 has also been described.[184–186] Many of the unstable β-globin chain mutations in exon 3 are associated with a dominantly inherited form of thalassemia (see section on dominant β-thalassemia).[180, 181] Thein and associates[184] proposed that alterations of β-globin structure in exon 3 interfere with $\alpha_1\beta_1$ dimer formation, yet may permit binding of heme to the mutant globin chain through contacts in the exon 2 domain. These free, heme-associated β chains may be more resistant to proteolysis and associate with the cell membrane, forming "inclusion bodies" and inducing oxidative damage.

THALASSEMIC HEMOGLOBINOPATHIES

The mutations described in this section, taken together with the RNA-processing mutants HbE, Hb Knossos, and Hb Malay and the termination mutant Hb Tak, comprise a distinctive set characterized by structural changes in the hemoglobin molecule *and* a thalassemia phenotype. These mutations are often referred to as "thalassemic hemoglobinopathies" (see section on thalassemic hemoglobinopathies)[215] and are characterized clinically by a syndrome of ineffective erythropoiesis. Other globin variants may be associated with mild hypochromia, microcytosis, and chronic hemolysis because of instability and degradation of hemoglobin tetramers and are discussed in detail in Chapter 18. Because thalassemia is the consequence of an imbalance in α- and β-globin chains, these variants are not considered part of the spectrum of thalassemia.

Identification, Characterization, and Ethnic Distribution of β-Thalassemia Mutations

The disorders of hemoglobin serve as a paradigm for the molecular analysis of genetic disease. The dissection of β-thalassemia was aided by the introduction of now widely used methods for identifying and characterizing mutant alleles. Accordingly, the identification of β-thalassemia mutations in many ethnic groups is nearly complete.[3, 119]

In this section, we briefly outline molecular techniques that have been applied to the characterization of β-thalassemia mutations. An understanding of these methods is important not only because of their broad use in the study of other genetic diseases but also because they are directly relevant to strategies for genetic screening and prenatal diagnosis of β-thalassemia.

HAPLOTYPE ANALYSIS

The first several β-thalassemia mutations were identified by the cloning and sequencing of β-globin genes isolated from individuals with β-thalassemia major.* Because certain mutations are extremely common, a nondirected strategy is inefficient: β genes with common mutations will be repeatedly studied. For example, 95 percent of the β-thalassemia alleles on the island of Sardinia contain the codon 39 nonsense mutation.[220]

To facilitate the search for new β-thalassemia mutations, Orkin, Kazazian, and their colleagues[112, 221, 222] introduced the concept of haplotype analysis to the study of thalassemia. Naturally occurring, genetically neutral, nonselected sequence differences among individuals constitute polymorphisms, which are estimated to occur roughly once every 100 bp.[223] These sequence differences are heritable, and those residing close to one another on a chromosome tend to be inherited together, a property known as *linkage*. A subset of polymorphisms will alter the cleavage site for a restriction enzyme or create a site where one did not exist. Therefore, when DNA from unrelated individuals is digested with a restriction enzyme and analyzed by Southern blotting, polymorphisms in the restriction enzyme digest pattern may be observed; these are referred to as restriction fragment length polymorphisms (RFLPs).[224] Within the 60 kb of the human β-globin cluster, more than such 20 RFLPs are known[5, 225]; at least 13 have been identified in the α cluster.[2, 226] The pattern of these RFLPs (each based on the presence [+] or absence [−] of a restriction enzyme cutting site) along the chromosome defines a haplotype of associated or linked polymorphisms. Seven RFLPs were used initially to define nine distinct haplotypes (I through IX) of the β-gene cluster in the analysis of thalassemia mutations in Greek and Italian populations from the Mediterranean basin (Fig. 20–16).[112]

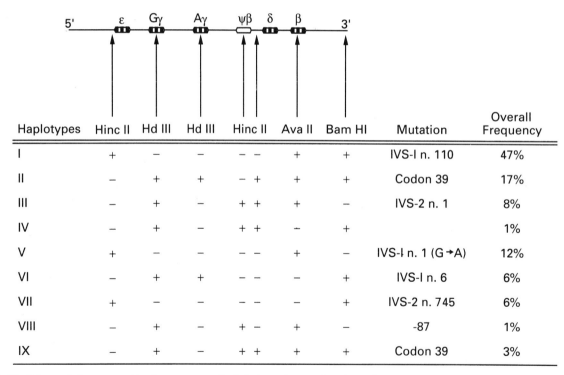

Haplotypes	Hinc II	Hd III	Hd III	Hinc II		Ava II	Bam HI	Mutation	Overall Frequency
I	+	−	−	−	−	+	+	IVS-I n. 110	47%
II	−	+	+	−	+	+	+	Codon 39	17%
III	−	+	−	+	+	+	−	IVS-2 n. 1	8%
IV	−	+	−	+	+	−	+		1%
V	+	−	−	−	−	+	−	IVS-I n. 1 (G→A)	12%
VI	−	+	+	−	−	−	+	IVS-I n. 6	6%
VII	+	−	−	−	−	−	+	IVS-2 n. 745	6%
VIII	−	+	−	+	−	+	−	-87	1%
IX	−	+	−	+	+	+	+	Codon 39	3%

FIGURE 20–16. Linkage of chromosomal haplotypes to specific β-thalassemia mutations in Mediterranean populations. A haplotype is defined by the sequential pattern of restriction enzyme sites (present "+" or absent "−") along a chromosome. In this example, seven restriction enzymes were used to classify nine haplotypes. Overall frequency refers to the prevalence of the specific haplotype as found in all individuals, with or without thalassemia. (Adapted from Orkin SH, Kazazian HH Jr, et al: Linkage of beta thalassemia mutations and beta-globin gene polymorphisms with DNA polymorphisms in the human beta-globin gene cluster. Nature 1982; 296:627. Reprinted by permission from Nature, copyright © 1982, Macmillan Magazines Limited.)

*References 113, 120, 136, 137, 150, 153, 201, and 216–219.

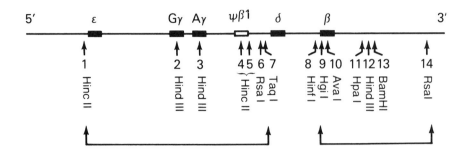

FIGURE 20–17. Restriction endonuclease sites for which restriction fragment length polymorphism (RFLP) have been identified in the β-globin gene cluster. A recombinational hot spot has been identified between the two brackets; the RFLP enclosed in each bracket must often remain associated during recombination (see text).

Close inspection of these haplotypes revealed a nonrandom association of restriction digest patterns within the β-gene cluster (Fig. 20–17).[221, 227] The pattern of restriction sites 5′ of the δ-globin gene is inherited as a group, whereas restriction sites downstream (including the β-globin gene) track as another set. In all populations only a few haplotypes predominate.[228] The full spectrum of haplotypes is derived from random association over evolutionary time between the 5′ and the 3′ subhaplotypes, presumably reflecting the presence of a recombination "hotspot" lying between these regions.[120, 227, 229, 230]

The generation of haplotypes appears to be an ancient event predating racial dispersion. Consequently, a specific haplotype may be found in diverse ethnic and racial groups from different geographical locations. The introduction of malaria as a selective pressure for certain random mutations is a more recent phenomena. A mutation leading to thalassemia would be under positive selection and amplified within a population; accordingly, the mutation would be expected to be found on the haplotype background in which it originated in that ethnic group. Several conclusions can be derived from the study of different racial groups.[74] Within a single population both normal and thalassemia β-globin genes are found on the same haplotype, but specific thalassemia mutations tend to be linked to a single haplotype. Individual thalassemia mutations are generally restricted to a single population (Table 20–2). In circumstances in which specific mutations are found in different populations, the identical thalassemia mutation may have occurred and been selected for independently and will be found on a different haplotype background.[44, 124, 231] This observation has provided a sound genetic basis for the belief that thalassemia has had multiple distinct origins throughout the world. In circumstances in which a specific mutation is found on more than one haplotype within a population, the 3′ subhaplotypes (where the β-globin gene resides) may be identical whereas the 5′ subhaplotypes differ because of recombination between the two subhaplotypes (for an example, see codon 39 mutation, Fig. 20–16). By this mechanism, specific mutations can be distributed to new haplotypes within an ethnic group and an independent origin of the mutation need not be invoked.

New thalassemia mutations were identified by cloning thalassemia β-globin genes from distinct haplotypes within a population, thereby avoiding the likelihood of repeated cloning of the same common mutation.[112] In this way, the great diversity of thalassemia mutations was elucidated.[122]

DIRECT DETECTION OF THALASSEMIA MUTATIONS

Restriction Enzyme Analysis. Several thalassemia mutations fortuitously result in the creation or destruction of a restriction enzyme cleavage site within the α- or β-globin gene. The change in the restriction digest pattern can be detected in a Southern blot of digested genomic DNA or can be visualized directly when the analysis is performed on DNA amplified by the polymerase chain reaction (PCR) (see later).[232–234] A list of mutations that alter restriction enzyme sites is provided in Table 20–2. Although approximately 50 percent of the common thalassemia mutations in Mediterranean populations may be detected in this manner, this approach is of less utility in other groups.[3, 122]

Allele Specific Oligonucleotide Hybridization and Polymerase Chain Reaction. Specific synthetic oligonucleotide probes approximately 19 nucleotides in length extend the capacity to detect specific thalassemia mutations directly in genomic DNA or DNA amplified by PCR.[234, 235] Single nucleotide mismatches between a probe of this length and a target DNA sequence destabilize hybridization.[236] To study a given mutation or allele, two probes are generally used, one identical in sequence to the normal gene and the other identical to the mutant sequence. To facilitate detection of a mutation, probes are generally designed to position the difference in the center of the probe. In Southern blots, such probes can be shown to be highly specific for cloned DNA fragments containing particular mutations (Fig. 20–18). When the target is DNA amplified by PCR, low specific activity probes or nonradioactive probes can be used to detect the presence or absence of the mutation.[237–240] Although there are many β-thalassemia mutations, relatively few predominate in each ethnic group (see section on ethnic distribution). Hence, a small panel of oligonucleotides can be used to identify the majority of potential mutations in any given population.[241, 242]

The introduction of the PCR in 1985[243] and the subsequent modification of the procedure with the use of thermostable *Taq* polymerase[244] have revolutionized molecular biology and the ease with which specific mutations can be identified in DNA.[245, 246] The application of PCR to the analysis of thalassemia facilitated the rapid identification of several new, and quite rare, mutations.[120] A schematic diagram of the PCR is provided in Figure 20–19. There are several features of the PCR method that are of particular relevance.[244–246] First, only minute quantities of relatively impure genomic DNA are required as starting material; in fact, the DNA of a single cell may be sufficient. Fragments ranging from 50 to several thousand

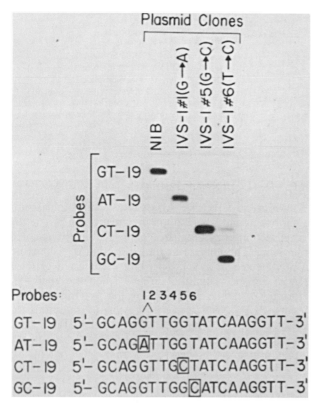

FIGURE 20–18. Detection of thalassemia point mutations using synthetic oligonucleotide probes. Southern blots of cloned DNA fragments were hybridized to a series of specific probes. The first probe shown below (GT-19) has the sequence of the normal β-globin gene at the exon 1–intron 1 boundary. The obligatory GT is indicated, above which appear the numbers that designate the first several nucleotides in intron 1. The three probes below, AT-19, CT-19, and GC-19, correspond to point mutations at the indicated positions that have been described in β-thalassemia genes. Cloned DNA fragments derived either from the normal gene or from a gene having one of the three point mutations underwent electrophoresis in agarose and were transferred to nitrocellulose by the Southern blotting method. The results show that each probe is nearly completely specific for the DNA fragment containing the corresponding point mutation. (From Orkin SH: Prenatal diagnosis of hemoglobin disorders by DNA analysis. Blood 1984; 63:249.)

base pairs can be rapidly amplified more than 10^6-fold *in vitro*. Second, the product of PCR, double-stranded DNA, can be readily subcloned, subjected to restriction enzyme analysis,[233, 234] hybridized to allele-specific probes,[237, 240] or directly sequenced.[113] As discussed earlier, the combination of PCR with restriction enzyme analysis or oligonucleotide hybridization lessens the need to work with high specific activity radioactive probes to detect mutations. Third, the technique is easily automated. Finally, the analysis, including DNA sequencing if required, can be completed within several days of obtaining tissue for DNA preparation.

Ethnic Distribution

Determining the incidence of specific β-thalassemia mutations in different ethnic groups is particularly relevant to strategies for prenatal diagnosis of thalassemia.[3] Nearly complete surveys of thalassemia mutations have been performed in Greek and Italian,[222] Asian Indian,[190, 247] American black,[43, 128] Sardinian,[220] Chinese,[248, 249]

Lebanese,[191] Turkish,[250] Spanish,[251] Sicilian,[164] Thai,[151] Kurdish Jewish,[111] and Japanese[181] populations. From these studies, several general conclusions can be drawn. First, in each ethnic group a small subset of mutations (as few as four or six) account for more than 90 percent of the mutant alleles. This is particularly striking on the island of Sardinia, where the codon 39 nonsense mutation accounts for 95 percent of the β-thalassemia genes, and a codon 6 frameshift represents another 4 percent.[220] Second, the remaining 5 to 10 percent of mutant alleles in an ethnic group are divided among a larger number of rarer alleles. For example, four alleles comprise 90 percent of the β-thalassemia genes in Chinese, and 11 rare alleles account for the remaining 10 percent.[3, 248] Third, several mutations appear to have originated independently in different ethnic groups and are present on different haplotype backgrounds as discussed earlier. For example, the IVS-2 number 1 (G→A) mutation is present in Mediterranean, Tunisian, and American black populations[117, 119, 121]; the IVS-1 number 5 (G→C) substitution is present in Asian Indians, Chinese, and Melanesians.[98, 116, 126] Finally, as a consequence of the large number of mutations present in each population, most individuals with severe β-thalassemia are genetic compound heterozygotes for two different thalassemia mutations.

Mutations That Affect β-Globin Gene Regulation

Deletions within the β-globin gene cluster often lead to thalassemia. Many of these are associated with a significant increase in the level of HbF, a finding that distinguishes them from the common varieties of β-thalassemia. Ordinarily, heterozygous carriers of β-thalassemia have an increase in the level of HbA_2 (to >3 percent of total Hb) and, at most, a slight increase in the level of HbF. Before detailed molecular analysis was available, these conditions were broadly grouped into two categories, hereditary persistence of fetal hemoglobin (HPFH) and δβ-thalassemia[4, 252, 253] (Table 20–3). HPFH heterozygotes have normocytic, normochromic red cells, whereas δβ-thalassemia heterozygotes have hypochromic and microcytic cells. Many HPFH heterozygotes have high levels of HbF (up to 30 percent) with a uniform or pancellular distribution in circulating erythrocytes, whereas in δβ-thalassemia heterozygotes, the amount of HbF is less abundant and is present in an uneven or

TABLE 20–3. Phenotypes of $^G\gamma^A\gamma$ Hereditary Persistence of Fetal Hemoglobin and $^G\gamma^A\gamma$ (δβ)^0-Thalassemia Heterozygotes

	HPFH	δβ-Thalassemia
Red cell morphology	Normal	Abnormal
MCH	Nearly normal	Decreased
Hematocrit	Normal	Slightly decreased
HbF (%)	15–30	1–15
HbF distribution in red cells	Pancellular	Heterocellular

HPFH-hereditary persistence of fetal hemoglobin; MCH-mean corpuscular hemoglobin.

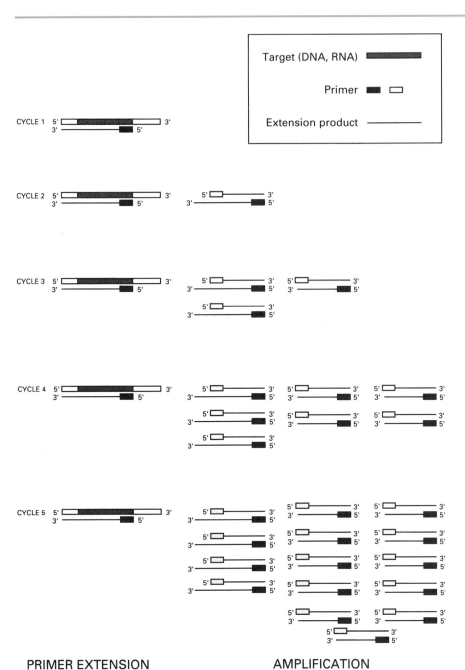

PRIMER EXTENSION

AMPLIFICATION

FIGURE 20–19. Polymerase chain reaction (PCR). The direct target for PCR is single-stranded DNA that can be derived from denaturation of double-stranded DNA or from RNA after reverse transcription. The amplification is carried out by hybridizing the target DNA with two short synthetic oligonucleotide "primers" that are complementary to sequences at either end of the segment of the target DNA to be amplified. The primers are "extended" by a DNA polymerase, in the presence of excess deoxynucleotide triphosphates, to the end of the molecule. After denaturation, these primer extension products become targets for hybridization and extension. After just several rounds of amplification, there is a dramatic accumulation of DNA products whose length and ends are delimited by the two oligonucleotide primers. Typical PCR protocols continue amplification for 25 to 40 cycles, in which each cycle encompasses one round of denaturation, hybridization, and extension.

heterocellular distribution among red cells. In rare individuals homozygous for either condition, only HbF is found. HPFH homozygotes have normal or slightly elevated total hemoglobin concentrations, their red cells are slightly hypochromic and microcytic, and globin synthesis is modestly imbalanced.[254, 255] Thus, these mutations are appropriately considered along with the thalassemia mutations.

Deletion mutations of the β-globin gene cluster represent *in vivo* experiments of nature useful in developing and validating experimental models of gene regulation. Multiple regulatory elements are present within the cluster, and the clinical phenotypes observed with specific deletions relate to removal of one or more such regulatory elements. More than 30 deletion mutations have been described (Table 20–4 and Fig. 20–20)[268]; these vary

greatly in size ranging from a few hundred base pairs of the β-globin gene to more than 100 kb with loss of the entire cluster. In addition to deletion mutations, significant elevations of HbF in adults may arise on account of single base substitutions within the γ-globin gene promoters (Table 20–5). Such mutations, also classified as non-deletion HPFH, appear to enable the γ-globin genes to "capture" the influence of the LCR at the adult stage. Individuals with these HPFH mutations have HbF values ranging from only slightly elevated to more than 20 percent, typically distributed in a heterocellular fashion.

The HPFH and δβ-thalassemia mutations are uncommon, and individuals who inherit these mutations are asymptomatic or have mild disease. Their importance relates to the insights they provide into globin gene

TABLE 20–4. Deletion Mutations of the β-Globin Gene Cluster

Type	Ethnic Group	Deletion Size (kb)	Deletion Coordinates	HbF Level in Heterozygotes (%)	Other Information	References
A. $A\gamma^0$:						
1		2.5	37.7–40.2	0.2	"Silent"	256
B. δ^0:						
1	Corfu	7.20	48.9–56.1	1.1–1.6	δ^0-Thalassemia	257, 258
C. β^0:						
1	Indian	0.619	63.?–64.0	Normal	β^0-Thalassemia	116, 218, 221, 259
2	American black	1.393	61.6–63.0	7.0–7.9	β^0-Thalassemia	260, 261
3	Dutch	12.6	59.7–72.3	4–11	β^0-Thalassemia	262, 263
4	Turkish	0.29	62.1–62.4	2.7–3.3	β^0-Thalassemia	264, 265
	Jordanian			9.4	β^0-Thalassemia	266
5	Czech	4.237	58.9–63.1	3.3–5.7	β^0-Thalassemia	267
	Canadian					
D. $(\delta\beta)^0$:						
1	Sicilian	13.377	56.0–69.4	5–15		268–270
2	Spanish	≈114	52.2–?	5–15		271–273
3	American black	12.0	52.3–64.1	25	Pancellular*	274
4	Japanese	>130	43.1–?	5–7		275, 276
5	Laotian	12.5	56.0–68.5	11.5		277
6	Macedonian	18–23	54–74	7–14		278
7	Mediterranean	7.4	55.3–62.7	1–5	Hb Lepore	279–281, 347
E. $G\gamma^+(A\gamma\delta\beta)^0$						
1	Indian	Total 8.3 kb	40.1–40.9	10–15		282, 283
	Iranian	Deleted	55.5–63.0			
	Kuwaiti	14.6 kb inverted	40.9–55.5			
2	American black	35.7	40.7–76.4	6–16		268, 284
3	Turkish	36.22	37.1–73.3	10–15		268, 285, 286
	American black					
4	Malaysian (1)	>27	37.0–?	Unknown		287
5	Malaysian (2)	>40	39.1–?	Unknown		288
6	Chinese	≈100	40.5–?	10–15		287, 289
7	German	53.0	37.6–90.6	9.9–12.5		290
8	Cantonese	>43	37.0–?	20		283
F. $(\gamma\delta\beta)^0$:						
1	Hispanic	39.5	−19.5–10.0			291
2	English	>100	?–35.9			292
3	Dutch	99.4	?–59.8			293–295
4	Anglo-Saxon	95.9	?–62.6			286, 294, 296
5	Mexican	>105	?–?			297
6	Scotch-Irish	>105	?–64–71			298
7	Yugoslavian	>148	?–?			299
8	Canadian	>185	?–?			299
H. HPFH:						
1	American black	≈106	51.2–?	20–30 (5% G)[†]	HPFH-1	273, 286, 300, 301
2	Black (Ghana)	≈105	47–?	20–30 (30% G)[†]	HPFH-2	256, 273, 300–304
3	Indian	48.5	45.0–93.5	22–23 (70% G)[†]	HPFH-3	273, 305, 306
4	Italian	40.0	50.0–90.0	14–30	HPFH-4	307
5	Italian	12.9	51.6–64.5	16–20 (15% G)[†]		308
6	Kenyan	22.8	40.0–62.8	5–8	Hb Kenya	309–311

*In a compound δβ-thalassemia/HbS heterozygote.

[†]Percentage $^G\gamma$ of total $\gamma(^G\gamma/^G\gamma + ^A\gamma)$. 40% $^G\gamma$ is the normal value for an adult.

regulation and the role of HbF in modulating disease severity in patients with severe β-thalassemia or sickle cell anemia.

Isolated point mutations of the δ-globin gene, similar to those in β-thalassemia, may lead to "δ-thalassemia." This is a benign condition with no clinical significance, which, when inherited with a β-thalassemia mutation, may lead to a normal or low HbA_2 thalassemia phenotype in heterozygotes.[344, 345]

CROSSOVER GLOBINS: HEMOGLOBIN LEPORE AND HEMOGLOBIN KENYA

Deletion mutations in the α- and β-globin gene clusters arise through unequal homologous recombination or through nonhomologous (illegitimate) recombination. In contrast to the α-globin cluster, in which there are blocks of tandem duplicated sequences (see later discussion), the only directly repeated homologous segments of DNA in the β cluster are the globin genes themselves. Hence,

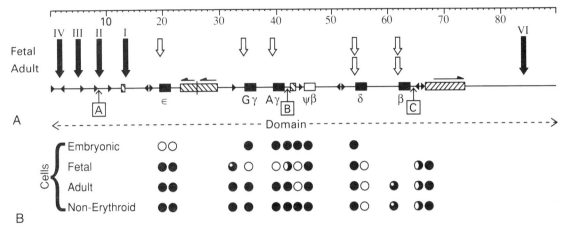

FIGURE 20–20. *A,* Organiztion and chromatin structure of the human β-globin cluster. The expressed genes are shown as *solid boxes,* and the single pseudogene in the cluster as an *open box.* The *arrowheads* in the line figure indicate the location and orientation of Alu repetitive DNA sequences, whereas the *hatched boxes* represent members of the L1 family of repetitive DNA. The *solid downward arrows* mark developmentally stable, erythroid-specific hypersensitive sites that constitute the locus-activating region (LAR), flanking the cluster. The true boundaries of the "active" chromatin domain established by these sites are unknown and extend beyond the cluster. Hypersensitive sites are also found over the promoters of the expressed genes *(open downward arrows).* The location of the three enhancers in the cluster are marked by letters: A = hypersensitive site II enhancer, B = 3′ $^A\gamma$ enhancer; C = 3′ β enhancer. *B,* The methylation pattern of the locus at different stages of ontogeny is depicted. *Open circles* show an unmethylated site, *closed circles* show a totally methylated site, and *partially filled circles* show the degree of site methylation. The coordinates refer to distance in kilobases. (Adapted from Stamatoyannopoulos G, Nienhuis AW: Hemoglobin switching. In Stamatoyannopoulos G, Nienhuis AW, et al (eds): The Molecular Basis of Blood Diseases. Philadelphia, WB Saunders, 1987, p 79.)

TABLE 20–5. Nondeletion Hereditary Persistence of Fetal Hemoglobin Mutations

	Molecular Defect	γGene	Ethnic Group	Percent HbF in Heterozygotes	Chains Gγ, Aγ	Distribution of HbF	References
1	C to G at −202	G	Black	15–20	G only	Pancellular	313, 314
2	C to T at −202	A	Black	2–3	93% A	Heterocellular	315
3	T to C at −198	A	British*	4–12	90% A	Heterocellular	316–318
4	C to T at −196	A	Chinese	10–15	90% A	Heterocellular†	319, 320
			Italian‡	10–20	95% A	Pancellular	321, 322
5	T to C at −175	G	Italian	20–30	90% G		323
			Black	30† §	G only	Pancellular	324
6	T to C at −175	A	Black	35–40	80% A	Pancellular	325
7	G to A at −161	G	Black	1–2		Heterocellular	326
8	G to T at −158¶	G	Saudi#	2–4	G > A	Heterocellular	327–333
9	G to A at −117	A	Mediterranean**	10–20	95% A	Pancellular	334–336
			Black	10–20	85% A	Pancellular	320
10	Deletion −114 to −102	A	Black	30† §	85% A††		337
11	X-Linked	G	"Swiss"‡‡	0.8–3.4		Heterocellular	338
12	Unknown‡	G	German	5–8	A and G	Heterocellular	339
13	Unknown	G	"Georgia"	2.6–6	G > A	Heterocellular	340, 341
14	Unknown	G	"Seattle"	3.7–7.8	G = A	Heterocellular	342, 343

*Also found in whites in North America.
†More than 80% of the red cells contain fetal hemoglobin.
‡Also found in *cis* to codon 39 mutation (Sardinian δβ-thalassemia).
§In a β-S heterozygote.
‖In a β-C heterozygote with the −158 T to C substitution in the $^G\gamma$ promoter.
¶This determinant appears to increase HbF only in patients with erythropoietic stress.
#Identified in Greek and Sardinian families.
**Also found in several other ethnic groups.
††Ratio varies in different families.
‡‡Found in all ethnic groups.
§§Associated with a translocation involving chromosome 11.

mutations arising from homologous, but unequal, crossing-over in the β-globin cluster are relatively uncommon and usually involve two globin genes directly (Fig. 20–21). Two crossover hemoglobins, Hb Lepore and Hb Kenya, are associated with thalassemia.

In 1958, Gerald and Diamond[346] identified a minor hemoglobin component by starch gel electrophoresis in the blood of parents of a patient with thalassemia major. Structural analysis revealed that the hemoglobin was composed of α globin and a heretofore undescribed globin,

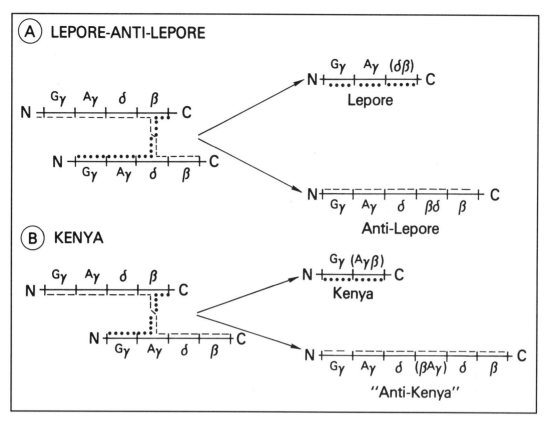

FIGURE 20–21. Schematic representation of the unequal crossover events that occurred during meiosis and resulted in formation of the Lepore and anti-Lepore *(A)* and Kenya *(B)* genes. (From Nienhuis AW, Benz EJ Jr: Regulation of hemoglobin synthesis during the development of the red cell. N Engl J Med 1977; 297:1318. Reprinted, by permission, from The New England Journal of Medicine.)

consisting of a fusion of the 80 to 100 amino-terminal amino acids of δ-globin with the carboxyl portion of β-globin.[279, 280, 347, 348] This "chimeric" globin polypeptide, named Lepore after the family in which it was first described, arose from an unequal, homologous recombination event between the δ-globin and β-globin genes (Fig. 20–21). It is poorly expressed because transcription of the fusion gene is under control of the γ-gene promoter. Other Lepore-type globins have been characterized in which the relative contribution of the δ and β genes to the fusion protein varies as a result of a different point of crossing-over. Homozygotes for Hb Lepore have 90 percent HbF and approximately 10 percent Hb Lepore, but no HbA or HbA$_2$, whereas heterozygotes have mainly HbA, 2 to 4 percent Hb Lepore, and 3 to 5 percent HbF.[349, 350] In heterozygotes, red cells have a very heterogeneous HbF content. Anti-Lepore globins having the amino-terminal sequence of β globin and the carboxyl sequence of δ globin have also been described (Fig. 20–21).[351–354] Individuals with anti-Lepore genes also have two normal δ- and two normal β-globin genes; hence, their red cells lack any stigmata of thalassemia. The anti-Lepore globins are produced in very low amounts, perhaps due to sequences within the large intron of the δ-globin gene that may reduce mRNA production.[23]

Hb Kenya, another important crossover hemoglobin, contains a non–α-globin comprised of amino sequences of γ globin and carboxyl sequences of β globin[309–311, 355] (Fig. 20–21). Molecular analysis demonstrated that the ^{A}γ-

globin gene was involved in the crossover. The crossover occurred approximately at the position of amino acid codon 100. Hb Kenya was first observed in an individual who was heterozygous for a β^S gene. This patient had an increased level of HbF (up to 6 percent) that was uniformly distributed in all his red cells. The HbF was entirely of the ^{G}γ type. Hb Kenya accounted for 17 to 20 percent of the total hemoglobin. Individuals who are heterozygous for Hb Kenya without HbS are clinically well. Approximately 10 percent Hb Kenya and 6 to 10 percent HbF of the ^{G}γ type are found homogenously distributed in their red cells, in contrast to the distribution of HbF with the Lepore type deletion.[312] It was originally hypothesized that the deletion removes a regulatory element that suppresses γ synthesis in adult life, leading to a pancellular or uniform increase of HbF in the red cells of individuals with the Kenya fusion gene.[356] Even before the discovery of the LCR and other regulatory elements within the β cluster, this hypothesis was disproved by analysis of several other deletion mutations (see later). Current models of hemoglobin switching posit that increased expression and pancellular distribution of the ^{A}γβ-fusion gene and the adjacent ^{G}γ gene result from deletion of the adult stage δ- and β-globin genes and their promoters, which serves to eliminate competition for the LCR. In addition, the deletion repositions an enhancer 3′ to the β-globin gene immediately downstream of the γ-globin genes and may also contribute to their increased expression.

SILENT DELETIONS

Deletions that eliminate a single γ-globin gene or the δ-globin gene are unlikely to result in a phenotype that would be detected in hematologic screening. Thus, few of these mutations have been detected and described. A clinically silent deletion of the $^{A}\gamma$-globin gene was identified through extensive molecular screening of chromosomes in Melanesians.[256] A 7.2-kb deletion involving the δ-globin gene but not the γ- or β-globin gene was reported in Corfu $(\delta\beta)^0$-thalassemia in *cis* to the G→A substitution at IVS-1 position 5.[257] Homozygotes for the IVS-1 position 5 mutation ordinarily exhibit a mild β^+-thalassemia intermedia phenotype with 10 to 20 percent Hb A,[129] but homozygotes for Corfu $(\delta\beta)^0$-thalassemia display the clinical phenotype of β^0-thalassemia intermedia with 100 percent HbF. This has been interpreted as evidence that sequences in the deleted region are important in activating the β-globin gene, and potentially in suppressing γ-gene expression. Subsequently, however, the identical deletion was identified in cis to a normal β-globin gene.[258] In this circumstance, the deletion leads to failure of δ-globin gene expression, but has no demonstrable effect on expression of the γ- and β-globin genes on the same chromosome. Hence, the basis for the lack of β-gene expression in Corfu $(\delta\beta)^0$-thalassemia remains unresolved.

β^0-THALASSEMIA DELETION MUTATIONS

Several deletions remove the β-globin gene and are associated with typical high HbA_2 β^0-thalassemia (see Table 20–4). Interestingly, deletions that remove the promoter region are associated with somewhat higher HbF levels than are usually seen in β^0-thalassemia heterozygotes (for example, see reference 357). The HbF is distributed in a heterocellular pattern. In contrast, a 0.6-kb deletion at the 3′ end of the β gene seen in Asian Indians, which spares the β-globin promoter, is not associated with an increased level of HbF in heterozygotes.[116, 216–218, 259] One explanation for the different phenotypes relates to the possibility that an intact β-gene promoter may interact productively with the LCR and thereby effectively compete with an incompletely silenced γ-globin gene at the adult stage. Removal of the promoter may alleviate competition and favor persistent γ-globin expression.

$\delta\beta$-THALASSEMIA

Individuals heterozygous for these deletions generally have 5 to 15 percent HbF, composed of both $^{G}\gamma$- and $^{A}\gamma$-globins, distributed in a heterocellular fashion (see Table 20–4). The erythrocytes are typically hypochromic and microcytic.[1] The level of HbA_2 is characteristically low compared with the modest elevations observed in most individuals with β-thalassemia trait. Homozygotes for these deletions produce only HbF, yet exhibit a mild β^0-thalassemia intermedia phenotype with hemoglobin levels of approximately 10 g/dL. The most common of these deletions is referred to as the Sicilian type.[260, 269, 270, 358] The deletion extends from within the δ-globin gene to just beyond the β-globin gene (see Table 20–4).

The 5′ breakpoint junctions of $\delta\beta$-thalassemia deletions generally lie between the pseudo-β gene and the δ-globin gene. Located within this region are moderately repetitive sequences, known as Alu sequences.[359] Although the function of such sequence elements is unknown, their preservation in $\delta\beta$-thalassemia deletions and their deletion in HPFH encouraged speculation that the Alu elements might be involved in modulating HbF production during development.[282, 356] Based on analysis of additional deletion mutations, this hypothesis seems unlikely (see Table 20–4). For example, the 7.2-kb Corfu deletion removes both Alu elements and the δ-globin gene, but it is not associated with increased γ-gene expression.[257, 258] Moreover, the Japanese type of deletion, which also removes the Alu elements, is associated with a heterocellular distribution of HbF and thalassemic red cell indices.[275, 276] The increase in HbF expression may be more appropriately explained by the deletion of local δ- and β-globin gene regulatory elements, leaving the γ-globin genes to interact with the LCR unopposed by competition from the adult genes.

$^{A}\gamma\delta\beta$-THALASSEMIA

The phenotype of these deletions in heterozygotes is identical to that of $\delta\beta$-thalassemia: hypochromic microcytic red cells with low levels of HbA_2 and moderately increased $^{G}\gamma$-HbF levels (5 to 15 percent) with a heterocellular distribution (see Table 20–4). Homozygotes have β^0-thalassemia intermedia with 100 percent $^{G}\gamma$-HbF. The 5′ breakpoints in these instances lie between the two γ genes or within the body of the $^{A}\gamma$ gene, thereby resulting in silencing of the $^{A}\gamma$ gene together with the δ and β genes.[282–286, 288–290, 360, 361] The 3′ endpoints of several of these deletions have been precisely mapped. Other deletions are very large and extend well beyond the boundary of the β-gene complex (see Table 20–4). One interesting mutation of this type, the Indian form (see Table 20–4), has two deletions, one involving the γ gene and the second involving a portion of the δ and β genes and intragenic DNA. The segment of DNA between the two deletions is inverted so that the 5′ ends of the γ and δ genes come to be adjacent but in an inverted orientation.[282, 283]

$\gamma\delta\beta$-THALASSEMIA

The diagnosis of $\gamma\delta\beta$-thalassemia should be considered in occurrences of hemolytic disease associated with hypochromic red cells in newborns. In adults, it is also a cause of normal HbA_2, normal HbF β-thalassemia trait. The syndrome was first identified in a newborn with a microcytic, hemolytic anemia.[362] Heterozygous β-thalassemia associated with normal levels of HbA_2, and HbF was identified in the father and many relatives. Decreased γ- and β-chain synthesis was demonstrated in the infant's reticulocytes. The anemia was self-limited; as the baby grew older, the hemolytic anemia disappeared and the child developed the phenotype of simple heterozygous β-thalassemia.

The syndrome of $\gamma\delta\beta$-thalassemia results from large deletions within the β-globin gene cluster (see Table 20–4). They can be divided into two categories: extremely large deletions that remove the entire β-globin gene cluster or all of the structural genes[297-299]; or deletions such as the Hispanic, English, Dutch, and Anglo-Saxon forms that leave structural genes intact, but remove LCR elements.[286, 291-296] The remaining genes on the chromosome are not expressed and are found in inactive chromatin that is methylated and resistant to nuclease digestion. Study of these deletions has provided the most convincing evidence that the LCR is required in normal erythroid cells for transcription of the β-like globin genes *in vivo*. Homozygous γδβ-thalassemia is expected to be incompatible with survival and has not been observed.

β-Thalassemia Mutants Unlinked to the β-Globin Complex

Until recently the mutations characterized in β-thalassemias resided within or near the β-globin gene itself or the β-globin locus. In principle, defects in *trans*-acting regulatory factors could lead to failure of proper β-globin gene expression. Two examples are now known.

Mutation of the *XPD* (xeroderma pigmentosum disease) helicase gene, which encodes a component of the general transcription factor TFIIH, results in β-thalassemia in association with trichothiodystrophy. Patients with specific mutations in *XPD* have typical features of β-thalassemia trait, including reduced levels of β-globin synthesis. Inadequate expression of diverse, highly expressed genes is presumed to be the direct consequence of an abnormality in TFIIH.[363]

Mild β-thalassemia trait in association with thrombocytopenia was reported as an X-linked trait in a rare family.[364] Linkage studies demonstrated that the gene mutated in this family resides on the short arm of the X chromosome, near the Wiskott-Aldrich Syndrome *(WAS)* gene and the erythroid/megakaryocytic transcription factor GATA-1 gene.[305] Subsequently, it was shown that the affected boys in this family have a specific amino acid substitution in the amino-zinc finger of GATA-1 that subtly alters its interaction with DNA and leaves its physical interaction with the cofactor FOG-1 intact.[306] How this change in the properties of GATA-1 leads to a slight imbalance in globin gene expression is unknown. Presumably interactions of the regulatory elements of the LCR and β-globin complex are affected by the manner by which GATA-1 binds to DNA.

Hereditary Persistence of Fetal Hemoglobin

Individuals heterozygous or homozygous for mutations that enhance HbF are asymptomatic. They are identified incidentally in routine screening programs or during investigation of family members with hematologic disease because of interaction of these variants with other mutations in the β-globin gene cluster. Homozygotes for deletion forms of HPFH have normal hemoglobin concentrations, but their red cells are slightly hypochromic and microcytic.[254, 255] Minimal globin chain biosynthetic imbalance may be seen. No symptoms or physiologic impairment has been associated with exclusive production of HbF, despite its high oxygen affinity.

HEREDITARY PERSISTENCE OF FETAL HEMOGLOBIN DELETION MUTATIONS

Several deletions produce the HPFH phenotype of increased levels of HbF in otherwise normal red cells (Table 20-5).* The 5′ breakpoints lie between the Aγ-globin gene and the δ-globin gene, and in all cases (with the exception of Hb Kenya) an enhancer 3′ to the Aγ gene is unaffected by the mutation. Two of the deletions (HPFH-1 and HPFH-2) are very large and extend beyond the 3′ end of the cluster (see Table 20-4). The Kenya mutation is also included in this category because of the pancellular distribution of HbF that is characteristic of this mutation.

Heterozygotes for these deletions produce up to 30 percent HbF, containing both Gγ and Aγ chains, in a pancellular distribution. Differences in the relative percentages of Gγ and Aγ chains can be detected between different types of HPFH deletions (see Table 20-4). Heterozygotes have normocytic red cells. The red cells of homozygotes contain HbF exclusively. The higher oxygen affinity of HbF may lead to slightly elevated hemoglobin levels in such individuals. Although homozygotes are clinically well, the α-to-γ-globin chain biosynthetic ratio may be slightly imbalanced, and mild microcytosis and hypochromia may be observed. This suggests that γ-chain synthesis occurs at levels below the output of the normal β-globin gene on these chromosomes.

Several hypotheses have been put forward to account for the increased expression and pancellular distribution of HbF in the deletion HPFH syndromes, particularly compared with the moderate increase and heterocellular distribution in δβ-thalassemia. Sequence analysis has confirmed that the γ-globin genes linked to the HPFH-1 deletion do not contain additional mutations responsible for the increased HbF expression.[367] As discussed earlier, deletion of postulated inhibitory sequences[272, 356] has not been substantiated by the effects of other mutations that remove similar elements. Because several mutations extend far beyond the 3′ end of the β-globin cluster, it has been suggested that introduction of a distant enhancer into the locus might lead to activation of the γ genes. Some evidence is consistent with this model. Sequences located immediately 3′ of the HPFH-1 deletion breakpoint, which are translocated into the cluster by the deletion event, display transient enhancer activity when tested in erythroid cell lines.[273] In addition, the DNA in the vicinity of this enhancer is hypomethylated and nuclease sensitive in normal erythroid cells and contains a long open reading frame,[273, 368] suggesting that the enhancer may belong to a distinct gene that is also transcribed in erythroid cells. RNA transcripts from this putative gene have been detected in erythroid cell lines.[369] In Spanish δβ-thalassemia, a deletion nearly identical to that in HPFH-1, the 3′ breakpoint is located approximately 9 kb downstream of

---

*References 268, 273, 286, 300-304, 306, 308-310, 312, 355, 365, and 366.

HPFH-1, and therefore the putative distant enhancer is not imported into the locus.[273]

In another type of deletion HPFH observed in an Italian family, a 12.9-kb deletion removes the δ- and β-globin genes and brings the enhancer 3′ of the β-globin gene closer to the γ-globin genes.[308] Analogous to the comparisons between HPFH-1 and Spanish δβ-thalassemia, deletions similar in size and location to the 12.9-kb Italian HPFH deletion that remove the 3′ β enhancer result in δβ-thalassemia rather than HPFH.[308] The Kenyan deletion also brings the 3′ β-globin gene enhancer closer to the γ-globin genes. Although distributed in a pancellular pattern, the level of HbF is lower in the Kenyan deletion than in the other HPFH syndromes. It is noteworthy that it is also the only deletion mutation that does not spare the 3′ ^{A}γ-globin enhancer.

NONDELETION HEREDITARY PERSISTENCE OF FETAL HEMOGLOBIN MUTATIONS

Individuals with these mutations exhibit elevated levels of HbF with normal red cell indices and are identified through hemoglobin screening programs or by study of families in which a segregating high HbF allele modulates severity of sickle cell disease or β-thalassemia.[80, 81] (The role of nondeletion HPFH mutations in modifying the course of sickle cell disease is discussed in more detail in Chapter 19.)[124] In many instances, single base changes have been discovered within the promoter region of either the ^{G}γ- or ^{A}γ-globin gene.[313–337, 370] These mutations are postulated to alter the binding of nuclear regulatory proteins and lead to a more favorable interaction of the promoter with the LCR at the adult stage.[334, 335, 371–376] Typically, only increased expression of the γ-globin gene in which the mutation is found occurs. In instances of the nondeletion HPFH syndrome, no mutation has been characterized. As discussed in a later section, the Swiss HPFH determinant may segregate with the X chromosome.[9]

The level of HbF observed in patients with this syndrome varies greatly and ranges from 1 to 4 percent in Swiss HPFH[9, 338] to 30 percent in the −175 T→C substitution found in either the ^{G}γ- or ^{A}γ-globin gene.[323–325]

Similar to the deletion forms of HPFH, the HbF may be found in either a heterocellular or pancellular distribution (Table 20–6 and Fig. 20–22). The −158 C→T substitution in the ^{G}γ-globin gene is associated with a normal level of HbF in otherwise normal heterozygotes, but with a high level of HbF in the presence of erythropoietic stress.[327–333] For example, in Saudi Arabia, patients with sickle cell anemia often have high HbF levels (25 percent or greater) and mild disease, whereas their parents with sickle cell trait have normal or only slightly elevated levels.[327] Identification of individuals with this mutation (or polymorphism) has been aided by the finding that it is linked to a rare subhaplotype.[328, 329] The −158 HPFH substitution also improves the clinical course of β-thalassemia. A Chinese individual homozygous for the −29 promoter mutation has transfusion-dependent β-thalassemia,[44] yet black patients homozygous for the same mutation who coinherit the −158 HPFH mutation in the ^{G}γ promoter have mild β-thalassemia.[43, 82]

The evidence that the base substitutions in the promoter region are the cause of increased γ-chain synthesis rather than associated random DNA polymorphisms is based on several lines of evidence (reviewed by Ottolenghi et al[377]). As mentioned earlier, they are generally associated with overexpression of the gene in which the mutation is found and typically represent the only sequence change. None of the mutations listed, with the exception of the −158 mutation, has been observed in individuals with normal HbF levels. Haplotype analyses in some pedigrees of patients with HPFH have demonstrated that the HPFH determinant is linked to the β-globin cluster. The British type of nondeletion HPFH is quite informative in this regard. The gene has been followed through three generations and three homozygous individuals have been observed.[316–318, 378] Haplotype analysis using restriction enzyme polymorphisms has established linkage of the British HPFH phenotype to the β-globin gene locus.[317] More than 90 percent of the γ chains are of the ^{G}γ type, whereas there is an associated mutation at −198 of the ^{G}γ gene.[317] Even the three homozygotes, with approximately 20 percent HbF, have heterogeneous distribution of the HbF among their red cells. Two homozygotes for the −117 ^{A}γ HPFH have also

TABLE 20–6. α-Thalassemia Syndromes

Syndrome	Clinical Features	Hemoglobin Pattern	α-Globin Genes Affected by Thalassemia Mutation
Silent carrier (α-thal-2)	No anemia, normal red cells	1–2% Hb Bart's ($γ_4$) at birth; may have 1–2% Hb Constant Spring; remainder HbA	1
Thalassemia trait (α-thal-1)	Mild anemia, hypochromic and microcytic red cells	5–10% Hb Bart's ($γ_4$) at birth; may have 1–2% Hb Constant Spring remainder HbA	2
HbH disease	Moderate anemia; fragmented, hypochromic, and microcytic red cells; inclusion bodies may be demonstrated	5–30% HbH ($β_4$); may have 1–2% Hb Constant Spring; remainder HbA	3
Hydrops fetalis	Death *in utero* caused by severe anemia	Mainly Hb Bart's, small amounts of HbH and Hb Portland also present	4

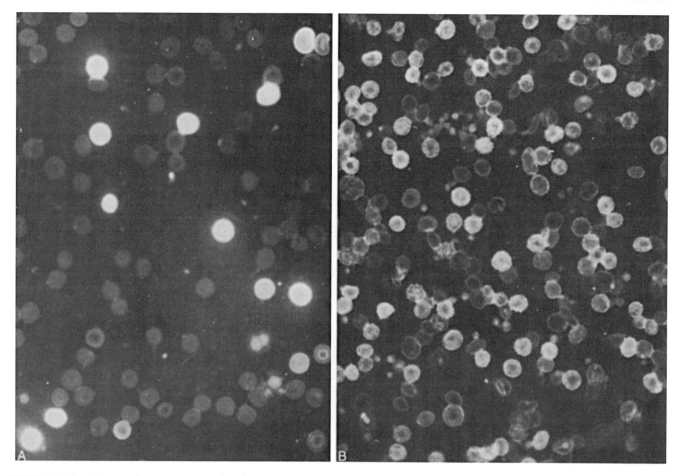

FIGURE 20–22. *A,* Immunofluorescence stain of erythrocytes with antibody directed against HbF shows distribution of HbF in a heterocellular pattern. *B,* Immunofluorescence stain of erythrocytes with HbF distributed in a pancellular pattern. (Courtesy of Dr. George Stamatoyannopoulos.)

been described, and they had 24 percent HbF in a pancellular pattern.[379] More recent transgenic experiments unequivocally demonstrate that single base substitutions seen in HPFH lead to enhanced γ globin expression into adult life.

An interesting aspect of this syndrome is a balanced α-to-non–α-globin chain synthetic ratio, even in homozygotes,[379] which implies that increased γ synthesis is offset by decreased β-globin synthesis.[336] Expression of the β gene in *cis* to the mutation may be reduced by 20 to 30 percent.[313, 324, 325, 337, 337, 380] It has also been observed that HbA$_2$ levels are uniformly low in the nondeletion HPFH syndromes and generally correlate inversely with HbF levels.[1] The reduction in δ- and β-globin gene expression in *cis* to the HPFH mutations is compatible with models of competitive regulation of β globin expression by the linked γ-globin gene.

Mutations That Alter α-Globin Gene Regulation

In contrast to the β-globin cluster, in which single nucleotide substitutions are the most common cause of thalassemia, large deletions within the α-globin cluster are the predominant basis of α-thalassemia. The overall impairment in α-globin chain synthesis that results from defects in the α-globin cluster is determined by the

number of genes inactivated (either by deletion or mutation), the type of lesion (deletion or mutation), and whether the lesion affects the α$_2$ or α$_1$ gene.

The α-globin cluster on chromosome 16[13, 381, 382] contains three functional genes (ζ, α$_2$, and α$_1$), an expressed gene of no apparent significance, and three pseudogenes[2, 12] (see Fig. 20–2). Transcription of the genes depends on the integrity of the distant regulatory element, HS-40. An α-thalassemia deletion mutation (αα^{RA}/) has been reported that removes a large segment of DNA upstream of the ζ$_2$ gene but spares the remainder of the cluster.[383] In heterozygotes, no expression of the ζ- or α-globin genes from this chromosome is detected in heterozygotes. This findings are formally analogous to those in Hispanic and English γδβ-thalassemias (see Table 20–4),[291, 292] in which upstream LCR elements of the β-globin cluster are deleted.

The two human α-globin genes are thought to have been generated through a gene duplication event that occurred approximately 60 million years ago.[384] The nucleotide sequences of the α$_2$ and α$_1$ genes have remained remarkably similar and represent an example of concerted evolution,[385–387] in which the two genes have exchanged genetic information through crossover fixation and gene conversion events. The coding regions of the two genes are virtually identical and encode identical polypeptides.[385–388] The genes differ only in minor respects within IVS-2, whereas the sequences diverge significantly in the 3′-untranslated region.

The α-globin genes are expressed in embryonic, fetal, and adult-stage erythroid cells. Initially, it was believed that the two α genes were expressed at similar levels, but subsequent RNA analysis relying on sequence differences in their 3′-untranslated regions revealed that the α_2 RNA predominates over α_1 RNA by a ratio of 3:1.[206, 389–391] Because two α-globin mRNAs have the same intrinsic stability, the higher level of α_2 RNA reflects increased transcription of the α_2 gene. "Transcriptional interference" of the α_1 gene by the upstream α_2 gene has been proposed as an explanation for this observation.[392] Ribosome-loading studies suggest that α_2 and α_1 transcripts are translated at equivalent rates.[393] The systematic characterization of the expression of α-globin structural variants at both the α_2 and α_1 locus confirmed that the α_2 gene has a predominant role in α-globin chain production.[391, 391] A direct prediction of this model is that mutations altering the α_2 gene would result in a greater deficiency in α-globin chain production than mutations of the α_1 gene. Clinical support for this prediction is provided by study of Sardinian patients with HbH disease who are heterozygous for one chromosome with a deletion of both α genes (–/) and a chromosome with a nondeletion mutation affecting the initiator codon of either the α_2 gene ($\alpha^T\alpha$/) or the α_1 gene ($\alpha\alpha^T$/).[145] Patients with the mutation in the α_2 gene (–/$\alpha^T\alpha$) have clinically more severe disease. Consistent with its predominance, the α_2 gene is involved in the majority of the reported mutations of the α-globin genes (see Table 20–2).

Deletion Mutations within the α-Globin Gene Cluster

MUTATIONS THAT REMOVE ONE α-GLOBIN GENE

The two α-globin genes are embedded in highly homologous, tandem repeated sequence blocks (called X, Y, and Z) that are separated by nonhomologous segments (Figure 20–23).[15] Unequal, homologous recombination through the X and the Z blocks generates a chromosome with a single α-globin gene and another with three α-globin genes. Recombination in the small Y box of homology has not been observed. The most common type of deletion in this class removes 3.7 kb as a result of misalignment of the Z boxes and is known as the "rightward deletion." The products of this crossover are the (–$\alpha^{3.7}$/)[394, 395] and ($\alpha\alpha\alpha^{anti3.7}$/) haplotypes.[396, 397] The –$\alpha^{3.7}$ products may be further subdivided into types I, II, and III by the precise location of recombination within the Z box.[387] Unequal crossover events through the X box leads to the "leftward deletion" of 4.2 kb of DNA and the –$\alpha^{4.2}$ chromosome[377] and its triplicated antitype.[398, 399] The incidence of the observed recombination products appears to reflect the size of the homologous target sequence within the boxes, because the –$\alpha^{3.7I}$ (1436 bp) is the most common, followed by –$\alpha^{4.2}$ (1339 bp), –$\alpha^{3.7II}$ (171 bp), and –$\alpha^{3.7III}$ (46 bp).[2, 385, 386, 400] Unequal α gene recombination through the X and Z boxes has been reproduced in both prokaryotic and eukaryotic experimental systems using episomal vectors.[15, 401, 402]

The –$\alpha^{3.7I}$ deletion is extremely common and is seen in all populations in which α-thalassemia is prevalent,

whereas the –$\alpha^{4.2}$ deletion is most common in Asian populations.[2, 12] Occurrences of up 80 to 90 percent for the single deletion chromosome have been reported in some populations.[90] The association of these mutations with a variety of α-globin cluster haplotypes and α-globin variants in different populations suggests that they have arisen through numerous independent mutational events.[90, 403]

Deletion of one α-globin gene does not affect expression of the ζ-globin gene[404] but has unanticipated consequences on expression of the remaining α-globin gene. The α_1 gene that remains on the –$\alpha^{3.7}$ chromosome is expressed approximately 1.8 times more often than the α_1 gene on a normal chromosome.[390] Individuals homozygous for the leftward deletion (–$\alpha^{4.2}$/–$\alpha^{4.2}$), who carry two copies of the α_1 gene, express more α-globin than the anticipated 25 percent of normal.[405] Homozygotes for the $\alpha^{3.7III}$ deletion (–$\alpha^{3.7III}$/–$\alpha^{3.7III}$), who carry two α_2 genes, express less than the anticipated 75 percent of normal.[405] The increased expression of the α_1 gene on the –$\alpha^{3.7}$ and –$\alpha^{4.2}$ chromosomes may be secondary to a release of transcriptional interference from the upstream α_2 gene,[392] whereas the lower expression of the α_2 gene in the –$\alpha^{3.7III}$ deletion remains to be explained. An important consequence of this observation however, is that the common mutations that delete the α_2 gene ($\alpha^{3.7I}$ and $\alpha^{4.2}$) may lead to increased expression of the remaining α_1 gene and to a less severe clinical phenotype than predicted from the expression studies of the native α-globin genes.[405] Single nucleotide substitutions that inactivate the α_2 gene do not affect α_1 expression and consequently lead to a more severe clinical phenotype than single gene deletions.[2, 12]

Triplicated α gene chromosomes are observed in populations in which the $\alpha^{3.7I}$ and $\alpha^{4.2}$ chromosomes are present. The third gene is expressed, leading to a slight increase in the α-to-β–chain ratio in homozygotes for the triplication, but this is generally of no clinical consequence.[406, 407] However, if a triplicated α gene chromosome is coinherited with a β-thalassemia gene, thalassemia intermedia may be seen.[408, 409]

MUTATIONS THAT REMOVE BOTH α-GLOBIN GENES

Illegitimate, nonhomologous recombination within the α-globin cluster results in the partial or complete deletion of both α-globin genes and generates an α^0 chromosome.[2, 383, 410–414] (Note that the term α^+ and α^0 may refer to the expression α-globin from a single gene or may refer to the presence or absence of an intact α-globin gene on a chromosome.) In some circumstances, the ζ-globin gene may also be encompassed by the deletion. The boundaries of many of the deletions that have been characterized are summarized in Figure 20–24. The geographic distribution of these lesions is more restricted than that of the α^+-thalassemia deletions, the most common being the $_–^{SEA}$ (Southeast Asia) and $_–^{MED}$ (Mediterranean) deletions, suggesting that they are rare genetic events. Theories concerning the mechanisms of these deletions are summarized elsewhere.[2]

Homozygotes for α^0 chromosomes (–/–) suffer from hydrops fetalis, whereas individuals heterozygous for an α^+ chromosome and an α^0 chromosome (–/–α or –/$\alpha^T\alpha$) exhibit HbH disease. Increased expression of minute

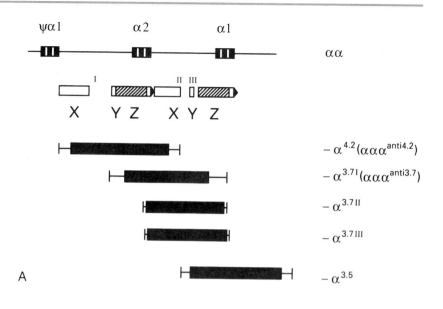

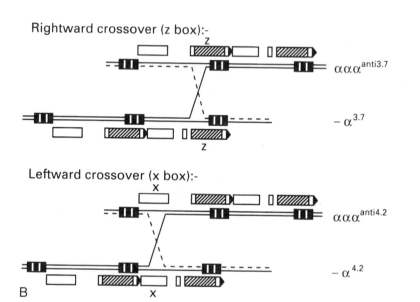

FIGURE 20–23. *A,* Deletion mutations that give rise to α-thalassemia. The two α-globin genes are embedded in a duplicated segment of DNA with homologous (X, Y, and Z boxes) and nonhomologous (I, II, and III) regions. The extent of specific mutations that delete a single α-globin gene are indicated by *solid boxes* and the limits of the breakpoints as *solid lines.* These deletions and the reciprocal chromosomes containing three functional α-globin genes result from misalignment and unequal recombination mediated by the homologous blocks. *B,* Unequal crossing over through the Z box deletes 3.7 kb of DNA and produces the $\alpha^{3.7}$ chromosome and its antitype, whereas recombination through the X box produces the $-\alpha^{4.2}$ chromosome and its antitype. The $-\alpha^{3.7}$ deletion can be further subdivided (I to III) by the exact location within the Z box where recombination occurs (see *A*). (From Higgs DR, Vickers MA, et al: A review of the molecular genetics of the human alpha-globin gene cluster. Blood 1989; 73:1081.)

quantities of ζ globin into adulthood may accompany some of the mutations in which the ζ gene is left intact by the deletion.[404] Sensitive radioimmunologic assays for the presence of ζ-globin chains in heterozygous adult carriers of these mutations have been devised,[415] and they may prove useful in areas such as Southeast Asia where the incidence of of the $-^{SEA}$ chromosome is as high as 3 percent.[416]

Mutations Not Linked to the Globin Gene Clusters That Alter Globin Gene Expression

ACQUIRED HEMOGLOBIN H DISEASE

A particularly severe, acquired form of HbH disease has been described in elderly men with clonal myeloproliferative disorders.[417–420] In this setting levels of HbH approaching 60 percent may be seen.[397] Extremely low α-to-β–chain synthesis ratios and low α-globin mRNA levels have been documented in bone marrow cells from affected individuals.[418, 419] Residual α mRNA expression may be derived from nonclonal erythroid cells. A bimorphic population of cells is present on examination of the peripheral blood smear. The manifestations of hemolytic disease caused by the HbH may increase and decrease with the clinical course of the myeloproliferative disorder.[418]

Available evidence suggests that the absence of a positive regulatory factor in the clonal population or the presence of an inhibitory factor is responsible for the lack of α-globin gene expression. Extensive molecular analysis of the α-globin gene cluster in patients with acquired HbH disease indicates that it is structurally intact and hypomethylated in these individuals.[418, 419] Human α-globin gene expression can be detected in somatic cell hybrids derived by fusion of bone marrow cells from patients with acquired HbH disease to murine erythroleukemia cells,[421] further suggesting that the

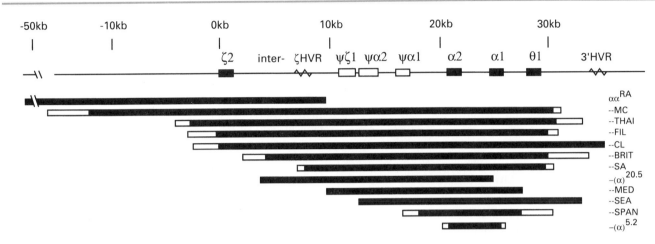

FIGURE 20–24. Deletion mutations that give rise to α⁰-thalassemia. The organization of the α-globin cluster is shown. Expressed genes are represented by *solid boxes*, whereas pseudogenes are shown as *open boxes*. Two hypervariable regions (HVR) are indicated as *zigzag lines*. Coordinates are in kilobase pairs (kb). The extent of each deletion is defined by a *solid box* and the uncertainty of the breakpoints by *open boxes*. The designation of the genotype is indicated to the *right* of each deletion. (From Higgs DR, Vickers MA, et al: A review of the molecular genetics of the human alpha-globin gene cluster. Blood 1989; 73:1081.)

transcriptional defect is not linked to the α-globin cluster. Further study of this unusual condition may provide important information about factors regulating the α-globin gene cluster.

X-LINKED α-THALASSEMIA ASSOCIATED WITH MENTAL RETARDATION SYNDROME

Rare instances of α-thalassemia occurring in individuals of Anglo-Saxon origin with phenotypically normal parents first drew attention to a new syndrome.[422] Further investigation revealed the commonly seen association of profound mental retardation, facial anomalies, and genital abnormalities.[68] Important recent studies demonstrated mutation of the *AH2* gene, a member of the DNA helicase superfamily and presumed global transcriptional regulator, as the underlying basis of this syndrome.[69]

SILENT β-THALASSEMIA

Hematologically normal "silent carriers" of β-thalassemia are identified through family studies.[1, 6, 423–426] Some instances of "silent" β-thalassemia may be attributed to mutations that cause a very modest reduction in β-globin gene expression—the –101 promoter mutation[109, 113] and the +1 cap site mutation)[116]—or to the inheritance of triplicated α-globin gene chromosomes.[408, 409] In an Albanian[363] family in which the father was a silent carrier, the mother had high HbA$_2$ β-thalassemia trait, and two children had β-thalassemia, the silent carrier determinant did not appear to segregate with either of the paternal β-globin gene clusters.[427–430] This family illustrates the rare circumstance in which determinants not linked to the β-globin gene cluster appear to regulate β-globin gene expression.

SWISS HPFH

Ordinarily, HbF constitutes less than 1 percent of the total hemoglobin in normal adult erythrocytes and is restricted to a subpopulation of erythrocytes (F cells) that represent between 3 and 7 percent of the total number of red cells.[7, 8] Both the percentage of F cells present in the circulation and the amount of HbF per F cell are under genetic control, and evidence suggests that the determinants are not linked to the β-globin gene cluster.[431]

In the Swiss type of nondeletion HPFH (Table 20–5), HbF is distributed in a heterocellular fashion with levels of HbF of 0.8 to 3.4 percent in heterozygotes.[1, 9, 80, 338, 431] The interpretation of earlier studies of Swiss HPFH was complicated by the small size of the pedigrees, overlap of HbF levels in heterozygotes and normal subjects, varying age of the research subjects (HbF levels tend to fall with age), and concomitant inheritance of β-globin gene alleles that can also influence HbF levels.

Several studies have been published in which linkage analysis clearly demonstrates that the HPFH determinant segregates independently from the β-globin gene cluster. In the first, a large Sardinian pedigree,[432, 433] and the second, a large Asian Indian pedigree,[434] nondeletion HPFH and β⁰-thalassemia genes were segregating in each family. Studies of normal individuals in Japan with Swiss HPFH, using the F-cell percentage to define HPFH rather than HbF levels, have demonstrated that the "high F-cell trait" segregates as an X-linked determinant.[9] A recent study has also localized a genetic determinant for HbF production to the long arm of chromosome 6 in a large HPFH pedigree.[10] Further mapping of these HPFH determinants may provide important insights into the mechanisms regulating hemoglobin switching.

CLINICAL HETEROGENEITY OF THALASSEMIA DUE TO DIVERSITY OF MUTATIONS

In the previous sections, the extraordinary array of mutations associated with the clinical syndrome of thalassemia has been described. In populations in which thalassemia is prevalent, different types of mutations, affecting genes of either the α-globin, β-globin, or both globin clusters, may coexist. Often patients are compound heterozygotes for these mutations. The relative degree to which globin chain synthesis is impaired reflects this genetic heterogeneity and determines the clinical phenotype. In the following clinical description of the thalassemia syndromes, we emphasize such genetic interrelationships.

α-Thalassemia

GENETICS OF α-THALASSEMIA

α-Thalassemias are divided into four clinical subsets that reflect the extent of impairment in α-globin chain production: silent carrier, α-thalassemia trait, HbH disease, and hydrops fetalis. Before the introduction of molecular analysis, these syndromes were classified on the basis of red blood cell parameters (hemoglobin level, mean corpuscular volume [MCV], mean corpuscular hemoglobin [MCH], globin biosynthetic ratio, presence of inclusions, and HbH (β_4) levels) as well as the manner in which they interacted genetically to produce different phenotypes. Much of this early work relied on the study of Asian populations in whom α-thalassemia is particularly common.[1] Thus, the silent carrier state for α-thalassemia in which a single α-globin gene on a chromosome was inactivated has traditionally been designated as α-thalassemia-2. Homozygosity for α-thalassemia-2 or heterozygosity for an allele causing more severe disease in which both α-globin genes were inactivated leads to α-thalassemia trait, also termed α-thalassemia-1. By the historical nomenclature, HbH disease reflects heterozygosity for α-thalassemia-2 and α-thalassemia-1, whereas hydrops fetalis results from heterozygosity for α-thalassemia-1.

Advances in the molecular characterization of the α-globin gene cluster clarified the genetic basis of these phenotypes. Weatherall and his colleagues proposed a more informative nomenclature for these mutations.[1, 2] Each chromosome may be designated as α^+ or α^0 to indicate the presence or absence of any α-globin chain production derived from that chromosome. This is referred to as a haplotype and should be distinguished from the usage of the term haplotype in describing the linkage of DNA polymorphisms on a chromosome. Haplotypes are further subdivided by the status of each α-globin gene on a chromosome. As discussed previously, mutations may be of the deletion or nondeletion type. Normal individuals are designated ($\alpha\alpha/\alpha\alpha$) to indicate the presence of four active α genes, two on each chromosome 16, where the first position corresponds to the α_2 gene and the second position to the α_1 gene. Deletion of a single α-globin gene on a chromosome is designated as ($-\alpha/$), while deletion of both genes is indicated as ($-/$). A further refinement of this nomenclature includes the designation of the specific mutation; for example ($-^{SEA}/$) signifies the α^0 deletion mutation that is common in the Southeastern Asian populations (Fig. 20–24), whereas ($-\alpha^{3.7}/$) symbolizes the α^+ rightward α gene deletion that is extremely common in the American black population (Fig. 20–24). Nondeletion mutations in a haplotype are designated in this scheme by a superscript T ($\alpha\alpha^T$), and can be more precisely described by symbols for the specific mutation and the gene affected. For example, ($\alpha^{CS}\alpha$) designates a chromosome bearing the Constant Spring chain

termination mutation affecting the α_2 gene (see Table 20–2), and ($\alpha^{QS}\alpha$) designates a chromosome bearing the α gene with a substitution in codon 125 that leads to synthesis of an unstable globin (see Table 20–2). This shorthand nomenclature is extremely useful when a patient's genotype is known in detail and has simplified the description of the many genotypes that interact to generate the heterogeneous clinical syndromes.

The silent carrier state, or α-thalassemia-2 defect, is due to the presence of a mutation affecting only one α-globin gene. Most often this occurs because of a deletion mutation ($-\alpha/\alpha\alpha$). Two genotypes, ($-/\alpha\alpha$) and ($-\alpha/-\alpha$), that reflect the inactivation of two α-globin genes are associated with α-thalassemia trait. Substitution mutations that affect the predominant α_2 gene ($\alpha^T\alpha/\alpha\alpha$) may also lead to α-thalassemia trait. The extent of the observed changes in red cell indices mirrors the reduction in α-globin production seen with each genotype with the ($-\alpha/-\alpha$) genotype being less affected than the ($-/\alpha\alpha$) genotype.

HbH disease occurs in individuals who have only a single fully functional α-globin gene. Genotypes leading to HbH disease are diverse.[2] Most common is heterozygosity for the single and double deletion chromosomes ($-/-\alpha$). As a result, HbH disease is observed most often in Southeast Asia ($-^{SEA}/-\alpha^{3.7}$) and the Mediterranean basin ($-^{MED}/-\alpha^{3.7}$) where the incidence of both the α^+ and α^0 haplotypes is significant. Nondeletion mutations may also interact to cause HbH disease. As discussed earlier, the α_2 genes are responsible for the production of approximately 75 percent of the total α-globin chains. Mutations that decrease expression from the α_2 gene ($\alpha^T\alpha/$) result in an α^+ haplotype that produces fewer α-globin chains than a deletion α^+ haplotype ($-\alpha/$). Thus, homozygosity for mutations in both α_2 genes ($\alpha^T\alpha/\alpha^T\alpha$) is phenotypically equivalent to deletion of three genes and is associated with HbH disease and not α-thalassemia trait.[2, 12] Consistent with this observation, nondeletion α^+-thalassemia haplotypes that are paired with α^0-thalassemia haplotypes ($-/\alpha^T\alpha$) lead to more severe HbH disease than does the interaction of the deletion α^+ haplotypes ($-/-\alpha$).

Homozygosity for the α^0 haplotype ($-/-$) leads to hydrops fetalis, a disorder that is particularly common in Southeast Asia where the α^0 haplotype is commonly seen. In rare infants from Greece and Southeast Asia, hydrops fetalis has been shown to result from the interaction of α^0 haplotypes with nondeletion α^+ haplotypes.[435–437]

At least 30 mutations that may inactivate one or both α-globin genes are known; thus, the different combinations of chromosomes bearing α-thalassemia mutations number more than 200. The number of occurrences of the different genotypes and haplotypes define the spectrum of disease observed in a given ethnic group. For example, severe forms of α-thalassemia (HbH disease and hydrops fetalis) are uncommon in blacks. In this group, the single deletion chromosome is very common,[438, 439] whereas chromosomes with two defective α genes are quite rare. In some circumstances, the phenotype of HbH disease is not readily related to genotype. Indeed, there is a significant spectrum of disease severity in individuals from the Southeast Asian area with the same genotype ($-\alpha^{3.7}/-^{SEA}$).[403] The observed phenotype may be further complicated by the inheritance of another hemoglobin

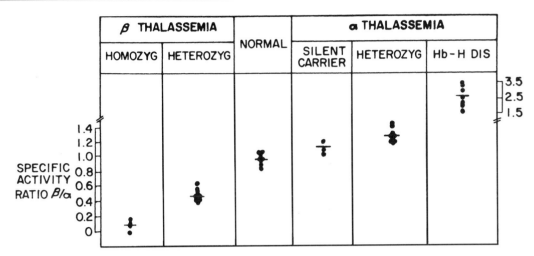

FIGURE 20–25. The α-to-β–globin biosynthetic ratio in various forms of thalassemia. Peripheral blood cells were incubated with [14C]leucine for 2 hours in autologous plasma. The globin chains were isolated by ion-exchange chromatography. The specific activity of the chains and the ratio of their radioactivities were then calculated. (From Nathan DG: Thalassemia. The New England Journal of Medicine 1972; 286:586. Copyright 1972, Massachusetts Medical Society.)

disorder (β-thalassemia) or the influence of environmental factors such as iron or other nutritional deficiency.

SILENT CARRIER

One parent of an individual with HbH disease (severe α-thalassemia) usually has the features of thalassemia trait, whereas the other has normal appearing red cells and no anemia (Table 20–6).[1] Offspring of individuals with HbH disease fall into two groups: those with thalassemia trait or those with nearly normal hemoglobin synthesis. These findings suggested that a silent carrier state for α-thalassemia existed. Patients who are silent carriers for α-thalassemia have three rather than four functional α-globin genes.[395, 440] Thus, impairment in α-globin synthesis is very mild. There is significant overlap of their globin biosynthetic ratio with both that of normal subjects and that of individuals having only two functional α-globin genes (Fig. 20–25). Similarly, the mean MCV of patients with three functional genes is slightly lower than that for normal subjects, but significant overlap between the two groups exists.[2] Despite these differences that become apparent on comparison of groups with different numbers of α-globin genes, there is no reliable way to diagnose silent carriers of α-thalassemia by hematologic criteria. Diagnosis has been reported by detection of small amounts of Hb Bart's in cord blood,[1] but additional studies indicate that this approach is unreliable in ascertaining the presence of the silent carrier state.[441, 442]

HEMOGLOBIN CONSTANT SPRING—ELONGATED α-GLOBINS

Some silent carriers for α-thalassemia produce small quantities of slowly migrating hemoglobins (Fig. 20–26), which contain elongated α-globin chain variants resulting from termination codon mutations (see Table 20–2 and Figure 20–14).[165–169] The original elongated α-chain variant, Hb Constant Spring, was named for the small Jamaican town in which the Chinese family in whom these

hemoglobins were first discovered resided.[166] The family had three children with HbH disease; each had a small amount of the abnormal hemoglobins. One parent had typical thalassemia trait, whereas the other had normal red cells but, in addition, had approximately 1 percent of the abnormal hemoglobin. Similar slowly migrating hemoglobins have been found in other racial groups in Thailand and Greece.[443] Individuals homozygous for the α^{CS} mutation ($\alpha^{CS}\alpha/\alpha^{CS}\alpha$) have a clinical syndrome similar to HbH disease, although their erythrocytes contain Hb Bart's (γ_4) rather than HbH, and the degree of anemia and the extent of abnormalities in red cell indices are milder than those in most patients with HbH disease.[444] Compound heterozygotes for α^0 and α^{CS} haplotypes ($-/\alpha^{CS}\alpha$) exhibit typical HbH disease.

α-THALASSEMIA TRAIT

α-Thalassemia trait is characterized by marked microcytosis and hypochromia of red cells in conjunction with mild anemia and erythrocytosis (Table 20–6). Levels of HbA$_2$ and HbF are generally normal or low. Diagnosis of this condition is typically made by family studies or by exclusion of iron deficiency and β-thalassemia trait. The incidence is particularly great among Asian populations and less among African, Mediterranean, and American black populations. Even in the neonatal period, the red cells appear hypochromic and microcytic. The amount of Hb Bart's may be up to 1 percent in the blood of normal newborns, but reaches levels of 4 to 6 percent in infants who are later shown to have α-thalassemia trait[1] (Table 20–6). Beyond the neonatal period, biochemical markers, such as HbA$_2$ and HbF in β-thalassemia, are not particularly helpful in confirming the diagnosis of α-thalassemia trait. The one exception occurs in circumstances in which the expression of ζ-globin is increased because of deletion of both α-globin genes on a chromosome.[404, 415, 445] In Southeast Asia, where the $-^{SEA}$ allele is common, a sensitive radioimmunoassay allows detection of ζ-globin chains in adult carriers of this mutation.

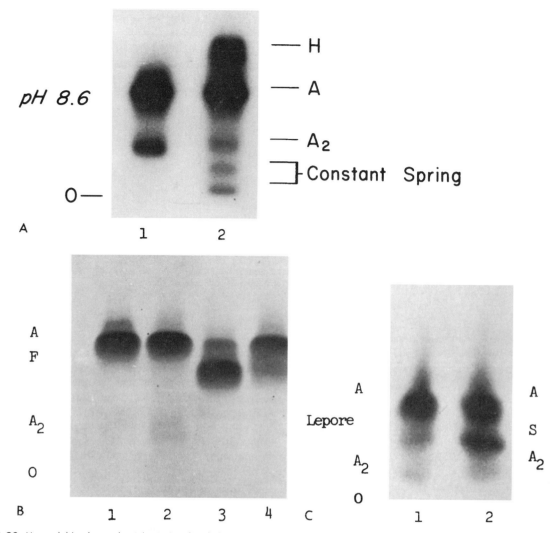

FIGURE 20–26. Hemoglobin electrophoresis. *A,* Starch gel electrophoresis at pH 8.6; 1, normal; 2, HbH disease with Hb Constant Spring. *B,* Agarose electrophoresis at pH 8.6; 1, normal; 2, β-thalassemia trait with increased HbA$_2$; 3 and 4, homozygous β-thalassemia with different relative amounts of HbA and HbF. *C,* Starch gel electrophoresis at pH 8.6; 1, Hb Lepore trait; 2, sickle cell trait. "O" indicates the origin. The anode is at the top of the page.

Measurement of the β-to-α biosynthetic ratio has little place in the routine diagnosis of α-thalassemia trait. Although detection of impaired α-globin synthesis has been reported,[446, 447] the measurement is technically difficult to obtain, because these individuals have a low reticulocyte count and the measured values overlap with those found in normal individuals (Table 20–6). Iron deficiency may raise the measured β-to-α biosynthetic ratio, further complicating interpretation.[448–451] Thus, in most patients, the diagnosis of α-thalassemia trait is established by red cell morphology and parameters, coupled with exclusion of β-thalassemia trait and iron deficiency. Gene deletions responsible for deficient α-globin production can be demonstrated by restriction endonuclease mapping; this technique may be applied when an accurate diagnosis is critical.

HEMOGLOBIN H DISEASE

Hemoglobin Pattern. Anemia of moderate severity characterized by hypochromia, microcytosis, striking red cell fragmentation (Fig. 20–27), and the presence of a

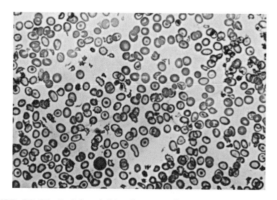

FIGURE 20–27. Peripheral blood smear from a patient with HbH disease.

fast migrating hemoglobin, HbH (β$_4$) on electrophoresis (see Fig. 20–26) may be shown to represent an α-thalassemia syndrome by measurement of the β-to-α biosynthetic ratio.[446, 452, 453] Incubation of peripheral blood reticulocytes with [³H]leucine and subsequent

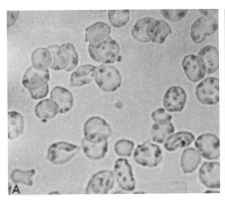 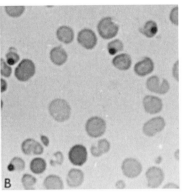

FIGURE 20–28. Red cell inclusions in HbH disease. *A*, Inclusions induced by incubation of peripheral blood in 1 percent brilliant cresyl blue and 0.4 percent citrate for 30 minutes at 37°C (patient not splenectomized). *B*, Preformed inclusions in peripheral blood of a splenectomized patient stained by new methylene blue reticulocyte stain.

chromatographic resolution of the globins indicate that such patients have a two- to fivefold excess of β chain synthesis (see Table 20–6 and Fig. 20–25). These excess β chains form HbH, which comprises 5 to 30 percent of the total hemoglobin in patients with HbH disease.[454] In approximately 50 percent of individuals with HbH disease in the Southeast Asia, small quantities of Hb Constant Spring are found (see Fig. 20–26). HbH disease may be suspected in anemic neonates in whom all the red cells are severely hypochromic. At birth, patients with HbH disease also have large amounts of Hb Bart's (γ_4). In patients with HbH disease with an intact spleen, incubation of the peripheral blood cells in brilliant cresyl blue produces many small inclusions in most red cells (Fig. 20–28). The dye induces precipitation of HbH by a redox reaction. In contrast, large and usually single preformed inclusions (Heinz bodies) may be visualized with methyl violet in red cells of splenectomized patients (Fig. 20–28).[78, 455] These inclusions are composed of precipitated β-globin, rendered insoluble by hemichrome formation or by interaction of the β-globin sulfhydryl groups with the red cell membrane.[78, 456]

Pathophysiology. HbH exhibits no Bohr effect or heme-heme interaction and thus is not effective for oxygen transport under physiologic conditions.[457] Consequently, patients with appreciable amounts of HbH have a more severe deficit in functional hemoglobin and oxygen-carrying capacity than the measured hemoglobin concentration might suggest. Red cells containing HbH are sensitive to oxidative stress, accounting for the enhanced red cell destruction that may occur on administration of oxidant drugs such as sulfonamides.[458] As erythrocytes age and lose their capacity to withstand oxidant stress, HbH precipitates, leading to premature destruction of circulating red cells.[78] Thus, HbH is primarily a hemolytic disorder.[455, 459] Inclusions of HbH are rarely seen in bone marrow cells,[460] and erythropoiesis is fairly effective.[459]

Clinical Features and Therapy. Typical patients with HbH disease live quite normally. Generally, anemia is moderate with a hemoglobin concentration of 7 to 10 g/dL, although occasional patients may have hemoglobin levels as low as 3 to 4 g/dL.[1] The complications of HbH disease are related to chronic hemolysis. Jaundice and hepatosplenomegaly are commonly present. Folic acid deficiency, pigment gallstones, leg ulcers, and increased susceptibility to infection are also observed. Hemolytic episodes may be precipitated by drugs or infection. Iron

overload is uncommon but may occur in patients receiving transfusions and those older than age 45.[461] Development of characteristic thalassemic facies, reflecting expansion of marrow space equivalent to that seen in patients with severe β-thalassemia, is rare. Usually only moderate bone marrow erythroid hyperplasia is evident.[451]

Consistent with the benign course of HbH disease, treatment is primarily supportive. Therapy includes supplementation with folic acid, avoidance of oxidant drugs and iron salts, prompt treatment of infectious episodes, and judicious use of transfusions. Splenectomy should be contemplated in patients with HbH disease only if hypersplenism is present as reflected by leukopenia, thrombocytopenia, and worsening anemia or development of a transfusion requirement in a patient whose condition was previously stable. In contrast to β-thalassemia, thrombocytosis after splenectomy may be complicated by a clotting diathesis and recurrent pulmonary emboli, particularly in patients with severe HbH disease and a fairly normal hematocrit.[461, 463] The use of measurements of red cell survival and splenic sequestration by ^{51}Cr labeling of red cells is controversial in making a clinical decision regarding splenectomy, because the label binds selectively to β-globin chains and may, by virtue of selective removal of HbH inclusions from red cells in the spleen, give a falsely high index of splenic destruction.[464] Other studies, however, suggest that results from the ^{51}Cr technique may be valid.[465]

Syndrome of α-Thalassemia with Mental Retardation. Patients with a syndrome characterized by mental retardation and a form of α-thalassemia that cannot be explained by simple Mendelian inheritance of an α-thalassemia gene have been described.[422, 466] In rare patients, the mutation arises as a *de novo* event in a paternal germ cell. These patients can be divided into two distinct syndromes (deletion and nondeletion) on the basis of their clinical features and the results of molecular analysis of their α-globin gene clusters.

Patients have been described with extensive deletions involving chromosome band 16p3.3 or, alternatively, with deletions resulting from unbalanced chromosome translocations that also led to aneuploidy in a second chromosome. Patients with deletion mutations exhibit mild to moderate mental retardation and a broad spectrum of dysmorphic features. Other rare patients are characterized by more severe mental retardation and a uniform pattern of dysmorphic features including genital abnormalities but no detectable deletions involving the α-globin gene cluster.[68]

Such patients fall into the category of the X-linked α-thalassemia with mental retardation syndrome. As noted earlier, the affected gene is a putative global regulator *(XH2)*.[69]

Although these disorders are seen rarely, they may be under-recognized. This is particularly true of ethnic groups in which α-thalassemia is uncommon, and the mild hematologic findings in patients who do not inherit a second α-thalassemia gene might be overlooked. Infants with uncharacterized mental retardation should be studied with techniques suitable for detection of a deficiency in α-globin synthesis.

Acquired Hemoglobin H Disease. HbH is also found rarely in the red cells of patients with erythroleukemia or a myeloproliferative syndrome.[417–419] The disorder may be clonal and displays a striking male predisposition (85 percent of confirmed instances).[422] The clinical features manifested by these patients are those of their primary disorder; the finding of HbH is incidental to the outcome of the disease, although striking red cell abnormalities and active hemolysis may be present. The genetic mechanism of this syndrome appears to involve abnormal regulation of α-gene expression because of a mutation affecting a distant genetic locus (see earlier).

Hydrops Fetalis. The birth of stillborn infants to parents with α-thalassemia trait reflects the most severe form of α-thalassemia.[467, 468] Infants are grossly edematous or hydropic resulting from congestive heart failure induced by severe anemia. Because of the inability to synthesize any α-globin, their blood contains only Hb Bart's (γ_4), HbH (β_4), and small amounts of Hb Portland ($\zeta_2\gamma_2$), within red cells displaying morphologic changes characteristic of severe thalassemia.[469, 470] The blood smear is characterized by large hypochromic macrocytes and numerous nucleated red cells. Although the hemoglobin concentration averages 6.2 g/dL, both HbH and Hb Bart's have high oxygen affinity and no subunit cooperativity. Therefore, the hydropic infant has very little functional hemoglobin. Viability *in utero* is maintained by the presence of small quantities of Hb Portland 1 and 2. Generally, affected infants are delivered stillborn at 30 to 40 weeks of gestation or die shortly after delivery at term.[416, 469] At autopsy, extensive extramedullary hematopoiesis and placental hypertrophy are seen.

A high incidence of toxemia of pregnancy and postpartum hemorrhage is observed in mothers of hydropic infants,[451, 471] presumably as a consequence of the massive placenta. Hence, early recognition of the disorder in at-risk pregnancies by prenatal diagnosis should lead to consideration of termination of the pregnancy. At least five infants born prematurely with hydrops fetalis have survived with the use of chronic transfusion regimens.[472, 473] Intrauterine transfusion of fetuses with hydrops fetalis should also be considered if treatment after delivery is contemplated.[474]

Mild β-Thalassemia

SILENT CARRIER

A silent carrier state for β-thalassemia was recognized through study of families in which affected children had a more severe β-thalassemia syndrome than a parent with

typical β-thalassemia trait.[1, 6, 423–426] A study of the "normal" parent often revealed mild microcytosis or a slight impairment in β-globin synthesis on radiolabeling of the globin chains in peripheral blood reticulocytes. Characteristically, silent carriers of β-thalassemia have normal levels of HbA₂. These silent carriers must be distinguished from individuals whose red cells have all the stigmata of β-thalassemia trait but have normal levels of HbA₂. Several patients who are homozygous for the silent carrier β-thalassemia gene have been described.[1] Anemia is moderate (hemoglobin concentration of 6 to 7.0 g/dL), and these patients rarely require transfusion. Hepatosplenomegaly may be significant. The HbF values range from 10 to 15 percent and the HbA₂ level is elevated to the range normally seen in individuals with thalassemia trait.

The silent carrier state of β-thalassemia appears to be a distinct clinical and biochemical entity. The underlying molecular defects cause only a modest reduction in β-globin synthesis. Two point mutations in the β-globin gene region have been linked to the silent carrier phenotype. The −101 promoter mutation appears to be a common cause of silent β-thalassemia in the Italian population[187] and has been observed in Bulgarian and Turkish individuals,[109] whereas the +1 cap site Inr mutation is associated with a silent carrier phenotype in an Indian family.[116] As noted above, rare instances of silent βthalassemia due to mutations unlinked to the β-gene cluster have been reported.

β-Thalassemia Trait

CLINICAL FEATURES

In 1925, Rietti[475] described Italian patients with mild anemia whose red cells exhibited increased resistance to osmotic lysis. A similar syndrome was later recognized in American patients of Italian descent by Wintrobe and co-workers,[476] who noted that both parents of a patient with Cooley anemia also had this syndrome. Detailed analysis of several pedigrees by Valentine and Neel[477] and others[478, 479] established the fact that this form of thalassemia occurs in individuals who are heterozygous for a mutation that affects β-globin synthesis.

Peripheral blood smears from patients with β-thalassemia trait are shown in Figure 20–29. Microcytosis, hypochromia, targeting, basophilic stippling, and elliptocytosis may be striking features, although in occasional patients the red cells may be nearly normal. The bone marrow is characterized by mild to moderate erythroid hyperplasia; red cell survival is modestly decreased, and slight ineffective erythropoiesis is present.[480] Inclusions in bone marrow cells and peripheral red cells are rare. Similar hematologic parameters appear to characterize Thai, Chinese, Greek, British, and Italian populations with β-thalassemia trait,[481–484] whereas American blacks appear to have a milder syndrome.[485] Hepatomegaly and splenomegaly have been reported in 10 to 19 percent of Italian and Greek patients but are less common in other groups.[483, 484] Iron or folic acid deficiency, pregnancy, or intercurrent illness may exacerbate the anemia in patients with thalassemia trait.

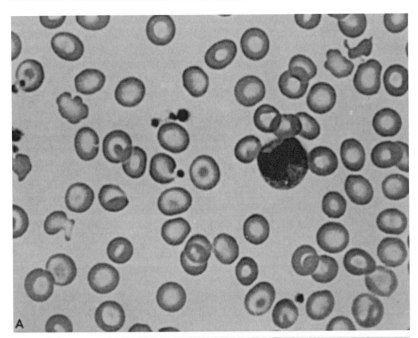

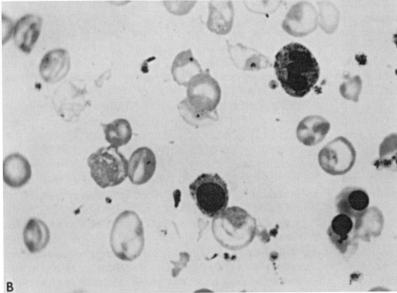

FIGURE 20–29. Peripheral blood smears in patients with heterozygous β-thalassemia *(A)* and homozygous β-thalassemia *(B)* after splenectomy.

Globin Biosynthetic Ratio. In peripheral blood reticulocytes, the measured β-to-α biosynthetic ratio varies from 0.5 to 0.7, as predicted for the inactivation of a single β gene (see Fig. 20–25). However, when bone marrow cells are incubated with [³H]leucine, the measured β-to-α biosynthetic ratio is often 1:1 in patients with heterozygous β-thalassemia.[486–490] The capacity of bone marrow cells to degrade free α-globin by proteolysis may explain why it is difficult to demonstrate unbalanced synthesis of β- and α-globin chains in the marrow cells of heterozygotes. The measured β-to-α ratio is approximately 0.5 in pulses of 10 to 20 minutes, but if the incubation of bone marrow cells is prolonged, proteolysis apparently destroys the excess newly synthesized α-globin.[491, 492] Fractionation of bone marrow cells after incubation in [³H]leucine demonstrated that proteolysis is most efficient in the earliest erythroid cels, namely proerythroblasts and basophilic erythroblasts.[492] The impairment in β-globin synthesis becomes easier to

detect as erythroid cells mature, accounting for the reduced β-to-α–globin biosynthetic ratio that is usually found in peripheral blood reticulocytes.

Classification and Genetics. Individuals with thalassemia trait are heterozygous for β-thalassemia. Expression of one β gene is impaired by mutation, whereas the other gene is normal. Characteristically, HbA₂ or HbF or both are elevated in patients with β-thalassemia trait, although occasionally normal levels are observed. The relative amounts of HbA₂ or HbF have been used to classify thalassemia trait that has relevance to the molecular lesion in certain instances and also to the severity of the disease in homozygous offspring.

δ-Globin Synthesis. Among inherited anemias, the elevation in HbA₂ level is unique to β-thalassemia. The absolute quantity of HbA₂ present in red cells is a complex function of the inherent capacity for δ-globin chain synthesis and factors regulating rates of hemoglobin dimer and tetramer assembly. As discussed earlier, δ-globin is normally expressed at a low level, approximately 2.5 percent that of β-globin. The level may be further reduced by mutations that affect δ-globin expression. Heterozygous[493, 494] and homozygous[495] states have been described. δ-Thalassemias reflect point mutations that completely silence the already defective δ-globin genes.[258, 344, 345, 426, 496–498]

In heterozygous β-thalassemia, the observed increase in HbA$_2$ represents an absolute increase in the quantity of HbA$_2$ per red cell from the normal level of 0.6 to 0.7 pg to 1.0 pg.[1] The increased amount of HbA$_2$ contains δ-globin chains derived from the δ gene adjacent to the mutant β gene as well as from the δ gene on the opposite chromosome. This has been inferred from the study of β-thalassemia heterozygotes who also have a variant δ chain.[499] The increase in the HbA$_2$ level can be accounted for by enhanced incorporation of δ-globin chains into hemoglobin dimers as a consequence of deficient β-globin chain production (see earlier discussion on hemoglobin assembly).[210]

Environmental factors also influence the absolute level of HbA$_2$. Iron deficiency leads to a decrease in the level of HbA$_2$, which may become normal in thalassemia heterozygotes and, therefore, mask the diagnosis of β-thalassemia trait. In such instances, the level of HbA$_2$ becomes elevated upon iron repletion.[500] An increase in the level of HbA$_2$ may be seen in acquired megaloblastic disorders associated with either folic acid or vitamin B$_{12}$ deficiency.[500]

High A$_2$ β-Thalassemia. This is the most common form of β-thalassemia trait. HbA$_2$ levels vary from 3.5 to 8.0 percent, whereas the HbF level varies from less than 1 to 5 percent.[1, 481–485] The vast majority of single base mutations leading to β-thalassemia (see Table 20–2) lead to typical high HbA$_2$ β-thalassemia trait. Although individual mutations variably reduce β-globin synthesis, efforts to differentiate the effect of specific mutations in heterozygous individuals have largely been unrewarding.[1, 483, 501, 502] In blacks, β^0 and β$^+$ mutations can often be distinguished in individual families owing to the rate of occurrence of double heterozygotes for a β-thalassemia mutation and the β^S mutation. In this population the mean MCV and MCH values are higher in β$^+$ heterozygotes than in β^0 heterozygotes, but the circulating hemoglobin concentrations are nearly equivalent.[485, 503] The common mutations found in American blacks, most notably residing in the ATA box of the promoter (see Table 20–2), only modestly impair β-globin gene expression,[43, 128] perhaps accounting for the relatively mild phenotype of many individuals with heterozygous or homozygous β$^+$-thalassemia in this population.

Homozygous offspring of two individuals with high HbA$_2$ β-thalassemia trait usually suffer from transfusion-dependent anemia, but may sometimes show a thalassemia intermedia phenotype. The precise nature of the mutation(s) in homozygous individuals is one factor in determining the clinical phenotype.

δβ-Thalassemia. Individuals heterozygous for these mutations have increased levels of HbF (5 to 15 percent) and low HbA$_2$ levels. This phenotype is most often generated by deletions that remove most or all of the coding sequences of the δ- and β-globin genes (see Table 20–4). The propensity of these deletion mutations for enhancement of the expression of the γ-globin genes contributes to a relatively mild phenotype in homozygous individuals or in those in whom a δβ-thalassemia deletion is inherited along with a thalassemia allele having a typical substitution mutation.

High A$_2$ High F β-Thalassemia. A distinct variant of β-thalassemia trait has been described in which the level of HbA$_2$ is elevated and the level of HbF is also elevated (5 to 20 percent).[262, 263, 504] This form of thalassemia trait is associated with deletions of the β-globin gene that leave the δ and γ genes intact (see Table 20–4).

Normal A$_2$ β-Thalassemia. This form of β-thalassemia trait should be distinguished from the silent carrier state. Although both are characterized by low or normal HbA$_2$ levels, the red cells in individuals with normal HbA$_2$ β-thalassemia are characteristically hypochromic and microcytic[425, 505] in contrast to silent carriers whose red cells appear near normal.[422, 424] Individuals who coinherit this type of β-thalassemia allele from one parent along with a high HbA$_2$ β-thalassemia allele from the other usually have severe transfusion-dependent β-thalassemia.

This phenotype is thought to represent coinheritance of mutations that decrease β and δ gene function. The mutations in the δ-globin gene may be present on the same chromosome or on the opposite chromosome from the β-thalassemia gene.[258, 344, 345, 426, 496–498]

Differential Diagnosis of Thalassemia Trait. In clinical practice thalassemia trait must be distinguished from iron deficiency (see Chapter 12 for additional discussion of the differential diagnosis of microcytosis and iron deficiency). Often the differential diagnosis may be suspected from red blood cell indices; mild erythrocytosis and marked microcytosis are characteristic of thalassemia trait (Table 20–7).[506–508] The red cell count is usually decreased in patients with iron deficiency, whereas the red cell volume may be normal or decreased, depending on whether the iron deficiency anemia is acute or chronic,[509–512] but the red cell volume is rarely as low as in thalassemia trait. The mean corpuscular hemoglobin concentration (MCHC) is usually normal in thalassemia trait and iron deficiency; in both syndromes the hypochromic appearance of the red cells reflects their small size, diminished hemoglobin content, and high surface-to-volume ratio. The red cell distribution width (RDW), a parameter available in modern automated cell counters, was originally believed to distinguish between iron deficiency and other causes of microcytosis.[513, 514] However, the RDW is also increased in the thalassemias and other hemoglobinopathies and is not a useful independent discriminator.[515–519] The absence of stainable iron in a bone marrow specimen is highly suggestive of iron deficiency, but the presence of iron does not necessarily exclude an iron-responsive anemia.

Several formulas have been developed to assist in the diagnosis of thalassemia trait during the assessment of microcytic hypochromic anemia (Table 20–8).[510, 520, 521] None of the discriminant functions is infallible. Nonetheless, the Mentzer index[510] is useful as an office screening test. More accuracy in separating thalassemia trait

TABLE 20–7. Hematologic Parameters in Thalassemia Trait and Iron Deficiency

Parameter	α-Thal	β-Thal	Iron Deficiency
Hemoglobin concentration (g/dL)	12.6 ± 1.1 (677)* 12 ± 0.7	†M—12.6 ± 1.4 (646–648, 652) F—10.8 ± 0.9 (646–648, 652) C—11.3 ± 1 (646–648, 652) Adults—12 ± 1.3	10.2 ± 1.6 (685)
Red cell count (× 10^6/µL)	5.6 ± 0.5	M—5.8 ± 0.6 (646–648, 652) F—5.1 ± 0.9 (646–648, 652) C—4.7 ± 0.6 (646–648, 652) Adults—6 ± 0.48	4.67 ± 0.43 (685)
Mean corpuscular volume (88.7 ± 5.3 (677) (4 m³/red cell)	72.2 ± 3.3 (677) 65.2 ± 3 (679)	64.7 ± 4.3 (677) 60.8 ± 5.6 (685)	67 ± 6.6 (685)
Mean corpuscular hemoglobin (pg/red cell)	23.2 ± 3.3 (677) 21 ± 1 (679)	20.3 ± 2.2 (677) 20.2 ± 1.9 (685)	21.8 ± 2.9 (685)
Hemoglobin A_2 (2–3.5%)	Normal or decreased	5.2 ± 0.8 (646–648, 652)	Normal or decreased
Hemoglobin F (<1%)	<1%	2.1 ± 1.2 (646–648, 652)	<1%

M = males; F = females; C = children.
*Numbers in parentheses are reference citations.

TABLE 20–8. Formulas for Differentiation of Thalassemia Trait from Iron Deficiency

	Thalassemia Trait	Iron Deficiency
Mentzer index (684)* MCV/RBC	<13	>13
Shine and Lal (694) (MCV) 2 × MCH	<1530	>1530
England and Fraser (696) MCV – RBC – (5 × Hb) – 8.4	Negative values	Positive values

MCV = mean corpuscular volume; RBC = red blood cell.
*Numbers in parentheses are reference citations.

from iron deficiency may be available from the England and Fraser function,[521–523] but when both conditions exist simultaneously all indices are subject to error. Additional discriminant functions and automated protocols have been proposed that may also prove useful.[524–526] The free erythrocyte protoporphyrin, often incorporated into the initial workup of hypochromic microcytic anemia in childhood to screen for lead exposure, is an additional useful test for patients suspected of having thalassemia trait.[527, 528] This technique has been especially useful in evaluating newly arrived Southeast Asian refugees to the United States.[529] Of course, measurement of transferrin saturation or ferritin may also be used to verify or exclude the diagnosis of iron deficiency.

In office practice the distinction between thalassemia trait and iron deficiency usually depends on examination of peripheral blood smears, evaluation of the color of serum (pale in iron deficiency), and above all the patient's clinical history. It is worth remembering that patients with thalassemia trait are not immune to iron deficiency. In these patients, iron deficiency may mask increases in the levels of HbA₂ and HbF that would otherwise suggest a diagnosis of β-thalassemia.

After iron deficiency is excluded, the differential diagnosis between α- and β-thalassemia trait depends on the measurement of HbA₂ and HbF levels (see Table 20–7)

and rarely on more sophisticated tests, such as the measurement of the α-to-β biosynthetic ratio in peripheral blood reticulocytes. In patients with microcytosis, hypochromia, and erythrocytosis but without evidence of iron deficiency or altered HbA₂ and HbF levels, α-thalassemia is the most probable diagnosis. When both α- and β-thalassemia coexist, changes in the levels of HbF and HbA₂ characteristic of β-thalassemia trait may not be present[83] (see later). Molecular genetic analysis and family studies are often necessary to define these complex interactions.

Severe β-Thalassemia

HISTORICAL PERSPECTIVE

It was not until Thomas Cooley, a Detroit pediatrician, first described the clinical entity that was to bear his name that thalassemia major was recognized as a distinct disease.[530, 531] Cooley recognized similarities in the appearance and clinical course in four children of Greek and Italian ancestry. These children exhibited severe anemia (hemoglobin concentrations of 3 to 7 g/dL), massive hepatosplenomegaly, and severe growth retardation. In addition, bony deformities, such as frontal bossing and maxillary prominence, gave the patients a characteristic facies. Deformities of the long bones of the legs were also commonly seen and thought to reflect severe osteoporosis. Thalassemia major, or "Cooley anemia," is far more common in Greece and Italy than in the United States, and descriptions of the disease in these countries soon followed Cooley original report.[532]

Autopsy studies revealed extraordinary expansion of bone marrow at the expense of the bony structures. Extramedullary hematopoiesis is often a striking feature, presenting either as isolated massive hepatosplenomegaly or as hepatosplenomegaly in association with intrathoracic or intra-abdominal masses.[531–533] Children were also noted to have significant iron deposition in almost all organs, the significance of which was not initially appreciated.[533] Before regular blood transfusion regimens were used, these changes progressed inexorably and were invariably fatal during the first few years of life. Patients died of the effects of their anemia: congestive heart failure, intercurrent infection, or complications resulting from all too commonly seen pathologic fractures.

Initial transfusion regimens were mainly palliative; transfusions were recommended only when anemia interfered significantly with a patient's ability to function on a daily basis. In defense of this regimen, we must realize that the pathophysiologic basis of the disease was not understood and that clinicians first attempted to minimize the transfusional iron administered because they feared that the iron, seen ubiquitously in these patients at autopsy, might itself be the cause of the disease.[533] Palliative transfusion therapy enabled affected individuals to live somewhat longer than patients not receiving transfusions, but the bony deformities and severe anemia forced them to lead markedly restricted lives.

In an attempt to improve the quality of life for these patients, trials using routine transfusion schedules to maintain hemoglobin levels greater than or equal to 8.5 g/dL were initiated.[534–536] The conditions of patients improved dramatically, with fewer overt side effects of anemia and more normal growth.[537, 538] Clinical improvement proved transient, however, as regular transfusions led to the complications of chronic iron overload, including growth retardation due to endocrine disturbances, diabetes mellitus, and delayed sexual maturation. Death invariably ensued in the second or early third decade of life, most often from cardiac arrhythmias or intractable congestive heart failure.[539]

PATHOPHYSIOLOGY

Imbalance in Globin Biosynthesis. That severe β-thalassemia was caused by impaired production of β-globin was established in the mid-1960s by direct measurement of globin biosynthesis in reticulocytes.[540–544] Soon thereafter impaired production of α chains was demonstrated in the α-thalassemia syndromes.[446] Decreased hemoglobin production is reflected in the peripheral blood smear by hypochromia, microcytosis, and target cells (that reflect the severe impairment in total hemoglobin production) and teardrops, fragments, and microspherocytes (Fig. 20–29). Red cell fragmentation is a direct consequence of unbalanced globin chain synthesis. Excess α chains, that have no complementary non–α chains with which to pair, form insoluble inclusions, demonstrable on methyl violet staining of the peripheral blood of asplenic patients with β-thalassemia (Fig. 20–30). In nonsplenectomized individuals, these inclusions are difficult to demonstrate, as they are efficiently removed during passage of red cells through the splenic sinusoids, generating fragments and teardrops (Fig. 20–31).

α-Globin inclusions in the erythrocytes and nucleated erythroid cells of patients with thalassemia major were first demonstrated by Fessas and associates[545–547] and by Nathan.[548] The incidence of the inclusions parallels the degree of impairment in β-globin synthesis. Inclusions have several deleterious effects on erythroid cells and are believed to lead to severe ineffective erythropoiesis.

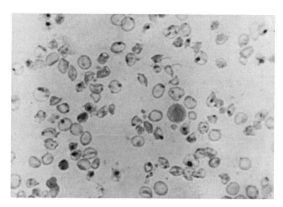

FIGURE 20–30. Supervital stain (methyl violet) of the peripheral blood cells from a patient with homozygous β-thalassemia after splenectomy.

Intranuclear α-globin inclusions, visualized using electron microscopy, have been hypothesized to interfere with cell division.[549, 550] Intracytoplasmic inclusions damage cell membranes, perturb the internal ionic environment, and thereby contribute to intramedullary death of erythroid cells. Moreover, α inclusions reduce red cell deformability and very likely interfere with egress from the bone marrow spaces. The combined effects of ineffective erythropoiesis and severe anemia account for the extraordinary marrow expansion seen in patients with thalassemia major. In fact, these individuals have a nonfunctional cell mass that approximates the 10^{12} tumor cells present in patients with fatal leukemia and is associated with a profound hypermetabolic state including fever, wasting, and hyperuricemia.[548]

The Red Cell Membrane. Numerous membrane abnormalities of thalassemic erythrocytes have been described.[456, 458, 551] Many are attributable to oxidative damage from excess globin chains and association of heme and iron with the cell membrane after degradation of precipitated hemoglobin chains.[456, 552] Other abnormalities may result from selective interaction of excess α or β chains with the membrane cytoskeleton. After oxidation, globin chains, as well as trace metals such as iron and copper, generate free oxygen radicals that foster oxidative injury of the membrane.[553] Peroxidation of lipids in the red cell membrane is reflected in altered membrane lipid composition and distribution; polymerization of membrane components caused by lipid peroxidation leads to cation loss and dehydration, decreased cell deformability, and increased rigidity of the phospholipid bilayer.[77, 78, 554] Similar changes are observed in normal red cells forced to engulf excess α chains.[555] Observed reductions in the level of serum and red cell vitamin E, a natural antioxidant, may result from accelerated consumption from oxidant stress. The abnormal lipid distribution may contribute to enhanced clearance by macrophages. Increased binding of autologous immunoglobulin G (IgG) with an α antigalactosyl specificity, originally proposed to reflect a decrease in sialic acid content of the membrane, may also promote clearance of thalassemic red cells from the circulation. Increased calcium content of thalassemic red cells is yet another manifestation of membrane damage.

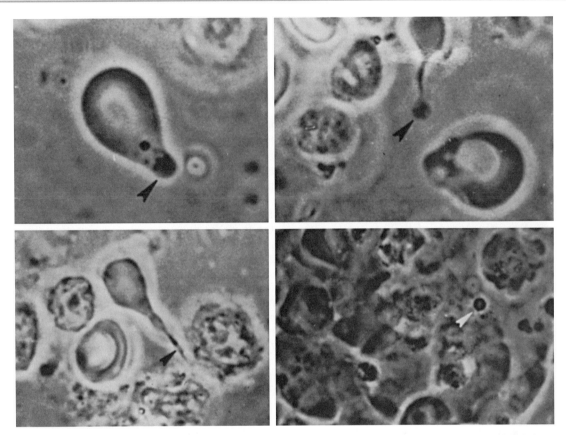

FIGURE 20–31. Phase-contrast microscopy of a wet preparation of scrapings from the spleen of a patient with homozygous β-thalassemia. Note the chain inclusion bodies *(black arrows)* within teardrop-shaped red cells, inclusions being pulled out, or "pitted," from the red cell by reticuloendothelial cell action *(lower left),* and inclusions free in the splenic pulp *(white arrow).*

Electrophoresis of red cell membrane proteins readily demonstrates increased association of globin chains with the red cell membranes (up to 11 percent of total protein), and similar findings can be reproduced in nonthalassemic erythrocytes by exposure to experimental oxidative stress.[556] α- and β-Globin chains interact differently with components of the cytoskeletal components.[557–559] The specificity of these interactions may contribute to the different phenotypic manifestations of the disorders. Membrane protein 4.1 of β-thalassemia erythrocytes has a diminished capacity to enhance binding of spectrin to actin. In HbH disease, protein 4.1 appears to be normal, but the binding of spectrin to inside out vesicles is decreased, potentially owing to oxidative damage of ankyrin promoted by binding of HbH to protein band 3 with which ankyrin interacts. Spectrin binding is normal in β-thalassemia erythrocytes.

Schrier and his colleagues[560] reported differences in the rheologic properties of erythrocytes obtained from patients with HbH disease and β-thalassemia intermedia. Erythrocytes from both groups had a normal surface area but decreased cellular volume and increased membrane rigidity that are manifested by decreased cellular deformability under conditions of hypertonic osmotic stress. Although HbH erythrocytes exhibit an increase in mechanical stability and a decrease in cell density, β-thalassemia erythrocytes are prone to cellular dehydration and have markedly decreased mechanical stability. In a murine model of β-thalassemia, these cellular abnormalities are correlated with the extent of α-globin association with the membrane; small increases in β-globin chain expression through the introduction of a β-globin transgene resulted in a marked decrease in membrane-associated globin and a significant reversal of rheologic abnormalities.[561] Thus, slight improvements in chain synthetic balance that accompany increased expression of γ-globin or decreased expression of α-globin may result in dramatic improvements in membrane integrity in patients with β-thalassemia. A more detailed understanding of the red cell membrane abnormalities in thalassemia may facilitate the development of novel therapies in the future.

Genetic Heterogeneity. In current hematologic parlance, the term *thalassemia major* refers to patients with severe β-thalassemia who require regular blood transfusions to sustain life. In the vast majority of such patients, both β-globin genes are affected by a thalassemia mutation; hence they have homozygous β-thalassemia. In other patients who also appear to be homozygous for β-thalassemia mutations, based on family studies, a hemoglobin concentration of 6 to 10 g/dL is maintained without blood transfusions except during periods of infection, surgery, or other stresses.[1, 562] Such patients are said to have thalassemia intermedia. *Thalassemia intermedia* is a clinical term that describes the transfusion status of the patient. The term *Cooley anemia* is still often used and applied somewhat indiscriminately to individual patients with either the major or the intermedia clinical syndromes.

Although other acquired and genetic modifiers exist, disease severity in the β-thalassemias is most directly related to the degree of imbalance between α- and total non–α-globin synthesis. Three major factors emerge as important determinants of the biosynthetic ratio in individual patients: the nature of the specific mutation or mutations, the presence of abnormalities in the α-globin cluster that increase or decrease α-globin expression, and the genetic capacity for HbF synthesis. Proteolysis of excess α chains, evident on comparison of the α-to-non–α biosynthetic ratio by short- and long-term incubations of bone marrow cells[486–490] (see earlier), is also likely to modulate disease severity, although no meaningful quantitative studies of this mechanism have yet appeared.

Nature of Specific Mutations. The capacity for production of β-globin chains in an individual with thalassemia is directly determined by the specific mutations involving the β-globin gene. Because several different mutations are commonly found in populations with a high incidence of β-thalassemia, most patients with clinical homozygous β-thalassemia are heterozygous for two different mutations. The effect of specific mutations may range from total loss to only a mild impairment in β-globin synthesis, and thus the potential interactions based on the many different mutations are extraordinary. Indeed, disease severity may be viewed as a continuum, the extremes of which have been shown to correlate with specific mutations.

The mutations in the IVS-1 splice donor site (see Table 20–2 and Figure 20–11) provide a particularly illustrative example of the variable consequences of specific mutations on β-chain synthesis. These mutations lead to either a complete block in correct splicing of β-globin mRNA or merely a reduction in the abundance of normal mRNA. Patients homozygous for a mutation in the conserved GT splice junction dinucleotide, who have not coinherited an α-thalassemia gene or a determinant that increases HbF synthesis, display severe transfusion-dependent β⁰-thalassemia.[112, 116–118] Substitutions of C or T at position 5 of the splice donor consensus sequence result in severe β⁺-thalassemia,[98, 116, 126–128] whereas substitution of A at the same position results in a more mild phenotype.[129] The T→C substitution at position 6 is also associated with a mild β⁺-thalassemia.[112]

Dominant β-Thalassemia. In rare circumstances, the heterozygous state of β-thalassemia may be associated with severe disease rather than typical thalassemia trait. Several pedigrees with severe heterozygous β-thalassemia characterized by splenomegaly, cholelithiasis, and leg ulcers have been described.[563, 564] A striking association has been noted between mutations involving exon 3 of the β-globin gene and these unusual cases of dominantly inherited β-thalassemia.[180, 184] Third exon mutations typically lead to the production of an unstable β-globin chain. A subset of third-exon β-thalassemia mutations are associated with the presence of inclusion bodies in the normoblasts of affected heterozygotes (see Table 20–2)[182–186] and were first reported as "inclusion-body β-thalassemia," originally defined as a dominantly inherited dyserythropoietic anemia.[565, 566] The inclusion bodies, which may contain both α-globin and β-globin, represent aggregation of precipitated α-globin and unstable β-globin chains with

the cell membrane, where they presumably potentiate oxidative damage. The dominantly inherited β-thalassemias are relatively rare and are found in ethnic groups from nonmalarious regions.[180, 184] Presumably there is little selective pressure for these mutations owing to the decreased fitness of heterozygous individuals.

Increased production of α-globin chains above normal levels may exacerbate chain imbalance in β-thalassemia heterozygotes; coinheritance of triplicated α-globin gene chromosomes is another potential cause of severe heterozygous β-thalassemia, usually with the phenotype of thalassemia intermedia.[408, 409, 567–569]

Interaction with Genetic Determinants That Increase Hemoglobin F Synthesis. Deletions within the β-globin gene cluster and mutations in the γ-globin promoters are sometimes associated with increased expression of γ-globin (see earlier discussion). Relatively small, genetically determined heterocellular increases in HbF ameliorate the clinical course of thalassemia,[80, 81, 317, 327, 432, 504] thereby raising the prospect that pharmacologic therapy augmentation of γ chain production may be of particular benefit in the management of thalassemia (see later).

Readily demonstrated in thalassemic patients is an apparent amplification of the capacity for HbF synthesis during erythroid maturation. In the earliest erythroid precursor cells, γ-globin may be synthesized at a level less than that of β-globin, and at only a few percent of that of α-globin, yet the final proportion of HbF in patients not receiving transfusions may be quite high.[1, 77] This occurs because the subset of cells expressing γ-globin have less overall globin chain imbalance and therefore preferentially survive in both bone marrow and peripheral blood. Hence, measurement of steady-state HbF levels provides an imperfect measure of the capacity for γ-globin synthesis in individual patients. A more accurate assessment of the HbF program is achieved by measurement of HbF accumulated in progenitor-derived erythroid colonies produced *in vitro*.[570]

Interaction of α- and β-Thalassemia Mutations. Because the clinical severity of α- and β-thalassemias correlates with the degree of imbalance in the production of α and non–α chains, coinheritance of α- and β-thalassemia mutations would be anticipated to yield syndromes of intermediate severity.[571–577] This principle has been validated by clinical experience.[83, 578, 579] One striking example is the influence of the number of functional α genes in individuals with β-thalassemia trait in Sardinia.[83] As shown in Table 20–9, the MCV and MCH improve in a stepwise fashion as α-globin production decreases and the α-globin-to-β-globin ratio approaches 1, but then deteriorates as the ratio decreases to less than 1. This analysis provides conclusive evidence that the degree of chain synthesis imbalance determines the red cell phenotype. Thus, a higher incidence of (gene deletions (–α/αα or –α/–α) has been found in those patients with thalassemia intermedia compared with those with thalassemia. Further evidence for the effect of α gene number on clinical phenotype is the occurrence of thalassemia intermedia in a subset of individuals doubly heterozygous for β-thalassemia and triplicated α genes (ααα/αα)[408, 509, 567–569] or severe β-thalassemia trait in individuals also heterozygous for

TABLE 20–9. Effect of Successive α-Globin Gene Deletion on Hematologic Parameters in a Homogeneous Population of β-Thalassemia Trait

Group/Genotype	Hb (g/dL)	MCV (µm³)	MCH (pg)	HbA₂ (%)	HbF (%)	Ratio
αα/αα ($n = 20$)	12.4 ± 1.2	66.2 ± 3.7	21.2 ± 1.2	4.8 ± 0.7	1.4 ± 1.3	2.2 ± 0.3
α −/αα ($n = 12$)	12.8 ± 1.3	67.3 ± 3.4	22.1 ± 1.1	5.2 ± 0.7	1 ± 0.3	1.3 ± 0.1
α −/α − ($n = 4$)	14.1 ± 1.1	76 + 3.4	24.8 ± 1.4	4.8 ± 0.6	1.3 ± 0.7	0.8 ± 0.1
α −/− − ($n = 4$)	11.7 ± 0.8	54.7 ± 2.5	18.4 ± 0.8	4.6 ± 0.2	—	0.5 ± 0.05

Adapted from Kanavakis E, Wainscoat JS, et al: The interaction of alpha thalassemia with beta thalassemia. Br J Haematol 1982; 52:465.

triplicated α genes.[558, 559, 580–586] Individuals heterozygous for β-thalassemia, but homozygous for triplicated α genes, invariably have thalassemia intermedia.

Clinical Features and Laboratory Values on Presentation. Severe β-thalassemia is most often diagnosed between 6 months and 2 years of age when the normal physiologic anemia of the newborn fails to improve. γ-Globin production is not impaired *in utero;* therefore, only when β-globin becomes the predominant β-like globin does anemia ensue. Occasionally, the disease is not recognized until 3 to 5 years of age because prolonged HbF synthesis compensates for the lack of HbA. On presentation, affected infants usually display pallor, poor growth, and abdominal enlargement from hepatosplenomegaly.

Children with severe β-thalassemia are readily distinguished from those with other congenital hemolytic anemias. At presentation, patients who have not had transfusions show 20 to 100 percent HbF, 2 to 7 percent HbA₂, and 0 to 80 percent HbA (see Fig. 20–26), depending on the precise genotype. Consistent with severe ineffective erythropoiesis and splenomegaly, the reticulocyte count is characteristically low (often <1 percent), whereas the nucleated red cell count is elevated. Erythrocytes are severely microcytic (MCV of 50 to 60 µm³) with a hemoglobin content as low as 12 to 18 pg/cell. HbF can be shown to be heterogenously distributed among the red cells either by the Betke-Kleihauer acid elution technique or by anti-HbF fluorescent staining (see Fig. 20–22).

Bone marrow examination reveals marked erythroid hyperplasia often with an erythroid-to-myeloid cell ratio of more than or equal to 20:1. Before the onset of hypersplenism, the accelerated rate of hematopoiesis may also be reflected in elevated white cell and platelet counts in peripheral blood. The serum iron value is markedly elevated, but the total iron-binding capacity is usually only slightly increased, resulting in a transferrin saturation of greater than or equal to 80 percent. Serum ferritin levels are generally elevated for age.

If laboratory parameters fail to establish the diagnosis of thalassemia on presentation, measurement of globin biosynthetic ratios in peripheral blood reticulocytes or bone marrow cells will unequivocally permit an accurate diagnosis. Unfortunately, this procedure is not routine and requires a well-equipped laboratory and experienced personnel. Most often, demonstration of a mild microcytic and hypochromic anemia, indicating the presence of thalassemia trait in both parents, will allow the diagnosis to be made with confidence.

Complications

RADIOLOGIC CHANGES

To appreciate the full spectrum of bony changes in severe β-thalassemia, one must examine patients who receive transfusions rarely.[530, 531] Bony disease in such patients is primarily related to erythroid expansion and not to iron overload or abnormalities in vitamin D metabolism.[587, 588] Maintenance of near-normal hemoglobin levels results in suppression of erythropoiesis and tends to reverse bony abnormalities,[558, 559, 580–586, 589–591] but osteoporosis is common even in patients who receive regular transfusions.[592–595] Some clinics report a high incidence of vertebral compression fractures.[594] Therapy with excessively high doses and sometimes even standard doses of deferoxamine may also lead to metaphyseal dysplasia.[596–598]

Radiologic abnormalities may be present during the first 6 months of life but are not usually marked until about 1 year of age.[599] In the small bones of the hands and feet the trabecular pattern is coarse, cystic abnormalities are present, and the bones are tubular in appearance. The long bones of the extremities exhibit thinning of the cortices and marked dilatation of the medullary cavities. Accordingly, they become extremely fragile and prone to pathologic fractures.[600] The skull is also classically involved with marked widening of the diploic space and arrangement of the trabeculae in vertical rows, tending to give a "hair on end" appearance to the skull radiograph (Fig. 20–32). Other radiologic abnormalities in the skull include failure of pneumatization of the maxillary sinuses and overgrowth of the maxilla. These changes lead to maxillary overbite, prominence of the upper incisors, and separation of the orbits—changes that contribute to the classic "thalassemic facies."

Other bony changes caused by the medullary overgrowth include widening of the ribs with notching and development of masses of extramedullary hematopoietic tissue, which may present as tumors in the chest and mediastinum. The vertebrae are square with coarse trabeculae. The aforementioned osteoporosis and associated bone pain may be relieved by calcitonin therapy,[601] but the role of vitamin D and calcium supplementation in the prevention of osteoporosis in thalassemia is not established nor is the potential value of bisphosphonate therapy known in this disorder.[602] Calcium bilirubinate gallstones due to excessive excretion of the products of heme catabolism are common in older patients.

Computed tomography (CT) has been used to demonstrate iron overload in patients with thalassemia by detection of increased density of the liver.[603–605] CT scans have

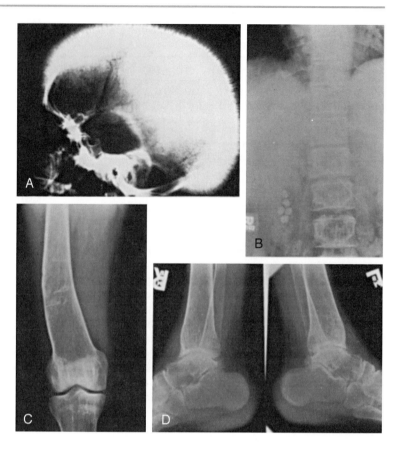

FIGURE 20–32. Radiologic abnormalities in a patient with homozygous β-thalassemia who receives blood transfusions rarely (thalassemia intermedia). *A,* Skull radiograph illustrates typical "hair-on-end" appearance of the diploë and failure of pneumatization of the frontal sinus. *B,* Abdominal film illustrates the coarse trabeculation and osteoporosis within the vertebrae. Multiple calcified gallstones also are seen. *C,* Severe osteoporosis, pseudofractures, thinning of the cortex, and bowing of the femur are illustrated. *D,* Degenerative arthritis affecting particularly the tibiotalar joint is reflected by loss of the cartilage space and sclerosis in the adjacent bone.

also shown increased density of the spleen, pancreas, adrenal glands, and lymph nodes in the abdomens of these patients,[606] while also offering another assessment of extramedullary hematopoiesis[607–609] and bony abnormalities.[609] Magnetic resonance imaging has also been used to evaluate these abnormalities.[610] More recently. hepatic magnetic susceptibility with a superconducting quantum interference devise (SQUID) has been proved to have excellent correlation with direct measurement of hepatic iron by biopsy.[611, 612] Measurement of hepatic iron stores by T_2-star magnetic resonance imaging, although having lower correlation with direct measurement of liver iron than SQUID, may prove to be equally useful in clinical assessment and in research.[613–615]

CLINICAL CONSEQUENCES OF IRON DEPOSITION

Mechanisms of Toxicity. The original pathologic description of thalassemia[533, 616] was concerned with conditions extant in the untreated state and is not relevant to conditions seen in patients today who receive transfusions chronically and thus become iron-overloaded. In countries where transfusion is widely available, patients demonstrate few of the stigmata that characterized the disease during the first few years of life in patients who do not receive transfusions. Depending on the level of hemoglobin maintained, most patients fortunately no longer have difficulty with the marked erythroid hyperplasia that causes extensive medullary expansion and its consequent pathologic changes.[534] However, patients are now confronted with consequences of chronic iron overload that accompany routine transfusion therapy.[617] In a study of

British Cypriot patients at autopsy, Modell[618] found evidence of marked iron deposition in the liver, pancreas, thyroid, parathyroid, adrenal zona glomerulosa, renal medulla, heart, bone marrow, and spleen. Such parenchymal iron loading and the accumulation of "free" or non–transferrin-bound iron in the blood remain the major causes of morbidity and mortality in patients with severe β-thalassemias.

Although the contribution of transfusional iron is easily appreciated, anemic thalassemic patients also have markedly enhanced gastrointestinal iron absorption.[619] This is particularly the case in patients with thalassemia intermedia such as those with HbE β-thalassemia.[620, 621] This seems paradoxical, because one might expect suppression of iron absorption in the presence of iron overload. In normal individuals a portion of dietary iron presented to the gut lumen is transported across the brush border of the gut epithelium and is available for transfer to the plasma iron transport protein, transferrin. The individual's iron status should then determine the amount of iron eventually presented to the serum pool.[622] The observation that anemic patients with thalassemia major have increased iron absorption remains an enigma. Elegant calculations by Modell and Berdoukas[623] suggested that the kinetic requirement of the expanded bone marrow for iron to make new red cells exceeds the rate at which the reticuloendothelial system is able to salvage iron from senescent red cells and replenish the erythron with iron. On this basis they argue that the bone marrow is relatively iron deficient on a kinetic basis leading to enhanced gastrointestinal absorption. Increased absorption is variable (range 2 to 40 percent)[619] and appears to be directly related to erythroid activity[624, 625] measured either by morphologic observation of patient bone marrow[626] or enumeration of nucleated red cells in the peripheral blood.[619] Experimental studies in animals suggest that hypoxia, even in the absence of increased erythropoiesis, may increase iron absorption.[627] Concomitant mutations in the *HFE* gene also increase iron overload in thalassemia.[628, 629]

With most modern transfusion regimens iron absorption is significantly decreased, but iron loading is increased as transfused red cells become senescent and their iron is deposited in the reticuloendothelial system. Reticuloendothelial cells relinquish iron directly to transferrin. Although the erythron usually claims most of this circulating iron, a certain amount is also delivered to other cells according to their individual needs. Cellular uptake may normally depend on the number of transferrin receptors on the cell membrane.[630] As iron accumulates in the body, individual tissues accelerate their production of apoferritin molecules to store the iron in a nontoxic form as ferritin or hemosiderin.[631, 632]

Apoferritin production can be monitored by measurement of serum ferritin concentration by radioimmunoassay. In patients receiving multiple transfusions[633] and in patients with increased gastrointestinal iron absorption who do not receive transfusions,[634] serum ferritin levels correlate well with total body iron stores during the first several years of iron loading, but less well later.[635] Serum ferritin is an acute-phase reactant as well as a product of hepatocellular damage. Infection, congestive heart failure, and hepatitis may elevate serum ferritin levels. Thus, in patients with marked iron overload, the serum ferritin level correlates poorly with liver iron concentration.

The human body is extremely conservative in its handling of iron (see Chapter 12). Under normal conditions, iron is always found in the presence of a chelating protein with a high affinity constant. Serum transferrin binds iron with an association constant of 10 to 20 mol/L.[636–638] When transferrin arrives at its surface receptor, the complex is transferred to the "labile iron pool"[639] by receptor-mediated endocytosis.[638, 640–642] This pool supplies iron to cytosolic proteins. The remaining iron is directed to apoferritin for storage as ferritin. When ferritin molecules accumulate, the protein moiety is apparently cleaved, leaving smaller hemosiderin granules but with greater iron concentrations.[643] Theoretically these storage forms of iron are inert and do not exert any pathologic damage. However, accumulated hemosiderin granules appear to cause release of hydrolytic enzymes from lysosomes that are toxic to the cell.[644, 645]

As iron stores increase both from transfusions and gastrointestinal absorption, transferrin becomes saturated to greater than 90 percent with iron. In parallel, a pool of non–transferrin-bound or free serum iron is found in iron-overloaded individuals.[646–651] Its source is uncertain, but presumably reflects an expansion of the intracellular labile iron pool, and it is thought to be particularly cardiotoxic.

Cell damage probably occurs as a result of iron-related catalysis leading to oxidation of membrane components.[652, 653] Unbound iron produces lipid peroxidation *in vitro*.[654–656] Peroxidation of mitochondrial membranes and hepatocyte microsomes has been demonstrated *in vivo* in rats overloaded with iron by parenteral or oral administration[657] and in the spleens of thalassemic patients.[658] Lysosomal leakage of hemosiderin and hydrolytic enzymes may also occur.[659, 660] Cultured rat myocardial cells have been used to study the effects of iron deposition.[661] Peroxidation of membrane lipids induces functional abnormalities in cultured myocardial cells that are exacerbated by ascorbic acid (see later) and corrected in part by the antioxidant, vitamin E, and markedly suppressed by deferoxamine.[662]

Further evidence in support of the free radical hypothesis stems from measurement of substances that defend against free-radical attack. Vitamin E, a potent antioxidant, is decreased in serum and red cells of iron-overloaded thalassemic patients.[456, 663] Both vitamin E levels[664] and serum total antioxidant activity bear strong inverse correlations to the degree of iron overload.[665] Perhaps, most intriguing is a correlation between superoxide production in resting neutrophils and serum ferritin in patients receiving multiple transfusions. The observed superoxide generation approaches five times normal in some patients.[666]

Indirect data also suggest that the route of accumulation (i.e., gastrointestinal absorption versus parenteral red cell transfusion) may be an important determinant of iron toxicity.[667, 668] Attention must be paid to the contribution of gastrointestinal iron absorption.[619, 626] Experiments in rats suggest that oral iron loading leads more global hepatocyte damage than parenteral loading.[657] Patients with hereditary hemochromatosis and thalassemia intermedia who do not receive transfusions sustain parenchymal damage entirely from gastrointestinal absorption.[626, 669, 670] On the other hand, extensive transfusion in patients with hypoplastic anemia is associated with a lower incidence of cirrhosis.[667] Nonetheless, the view that reticuloendothelial iron derived from transfused red cells is innocuous is overly simplistic. There are few reasons to believe that current transfusion protocols, designed to maintain a normal hemoglobin level and reduce gastrointestinal iron absorption, will be free of the complications of iron overload.

Assessment of Body Iron Burden. Most longitudinal studies of iron overload have used serum iron, iron-binding capacity, and ferritin as noninvasive measures of stored iron. As mentioned earlier, these parameters are easily perturbed by effects of other diseases (e.g., hepatitis) or are not highly quantitative (iron/iron-binding capacity), although some clinics still rely on the measurement of ferritin.[671] The relationship between serum ferritin and body iron stores as measured by quantitative assay of liver iron remains poor. In a recent study using SQUID technology, only 25 percent of the variance of body iron could be explained by the variance of serum ferritin.[672] This confirms the earlier studies of Brittenham and co-workers.[673] The poor correlation between serum ferritin and total body iron in thalassemic patients receiving many transfusions[674] can perhaps be improved somewhat by measuring the glycosylated form.[675] Grading of stainable iron in liver biopsies also offers a rough assessment of parenchymal iron stores, but it is clear that new treatment requires assessment by direct tissue measurement.

The study of iron loading in patients would be significantly advanced by the development of noninvasive methods for establishing parenchymal iron burden. CT has been suggested to be useful for longitudinal assessment of hepatic iron,[603, 605, 676] but it is not a reliable technique. The paramagnetic properties of iron have been used to make accurate measurements that correlate well with liver iron measured in biopsies by atomic absorption spectroscopy.[677] This is presently a research tool only. The aforementioned T_2-star magnetic resonance imaging may become a practical and clinically useful approach.

CARDIAC ABNORMALITIES

Patients with thalassemia major have traditionally died of the cardiac complications of iron overload.[539] Recurrent pericarditis distinguished by characteristic pain, fever, and a friction rub may be the initial manifestation of myocardial iron deposition and occasionally requires pericardectomy to relieve constriction. Ventricular tachycardia and fibrillation or severe refractory congestive heart failure often are fatal.[678]

Pathology. Cardiac iron deposition has been studied in autopsies of patients with transfusional hemosiderosis and idiopathic hemochromatosis.[679, 680] Patients whose history shows transfusions of more than 100 units of red cells without chronic blood loss generally exhibit significant cardiac iron deposition. Cardiac hemosiderosis is not observed unless significant iron accumulation has occurred in other organs. Cardiac iron deposits that are grossly visible at autopsy indicate that patients experienced cardiac dysfunction during life, but severe cardiac dysfunction may also occur in the absence of significant deposits of cardiac hemosiderin.[680, 681] Therefore, iron toxicity must be due to a small highly reactive intracellular iron pool or to the labile pool of non–transferrin-bound iron in plasma. Prevention of cardiac dysfunction, therefore, requires reduction of both iron load *and* the persistent presence of chelator in the blood. Cardiac disease in thalassemia intermedia is also unrelated to cardiac iron deposition but is instead due to pulmonary hypertension.[682] Gross anatomic cardiac changes include dilatation of the atrial and ventricular cavities and gross thickening of the muscle layer, resulting in a two- to threefold increase in heart weight. Microscopic evaluation suggests that iron is first deposited in the ventricular myocardium, and later in the conduction tissue.[679] Thus, intracavitary endomyocardial biopsy is not useful in these patients as a means to evaluate cardiac iron deposition.[683, 684] Supraventricular arrhythmias correlate well with the extent of iron deposition in the atrial myocardium but may occur in its relative absence. Cardiac abnormalities seem to be a function of both the quantity of iron deposited per fiber and the absolute number of fibers affected. Link and colleagues[685] have shown that myocardial cells in culture take up iron if there is no physiologic or pharmacologic chelator present. As iron loading takes place, peroxidation products accumulate and contractility and rhythm are disturbed.[662] This *in vitro* model parallels concepts developed from clinical findings.

Noninvasive Studies of Cardiac Function. Echocardiography, radionuclide cineangiography, and 24-hour recording of cardiac rhythm have been used to assess the effects of iron deposition in the heart and evaluate results of chelation therapy.[686] In general, echocardiography may reveal changes in cardiac anatomy but little change in cardiac function until clinically evident cardiomyopathy develops.[687–689] Low-dose dobutamine echocardiography is thought by some to be more helpful.[690] Radionuclide cineangiography offers the ability to observe dynamic cardiac function during exercise and may reveal changes in function before the appearance of clinical disease.[689, 691–693] Twenty-four-hour recordings of cardiac rhythm in patients with iron overload have demonstrated marked disturbances in most patients older than 12 years of age regardless of clinical symptoms.[686,] In one large series, Beirman and co-workers demonstrated abnormalities in more than 75 percent of patients, ranging from occasional premature beats to runs of ventricular tachycardia. Though a recent publication has claimed that magnetic resonance imaging may define cardiac iron content and ventricular function, the method is entirely unvalidated.[693a]

Table 20–10 summarizes the clinical course of patients before to the onset of aggressive chelation programs. The efficacy of future transfusion and chelation programs must be assessed in this context. Considerable data have recently demonstrated the benefits of chelation therapy, both for prophylaxis and treatment of cardiac disease in patients with iron overloading (see later).

TABLE 20–10. Cardiac Disease in Patients with Iron Overload

STAGE I (< 100 UNITS TRANSFUSION)

Asymptomatic
Echocardiogram: slight left ventricular wall thickening
Radionuclide cineangiogram: normal
24-hour ECG: normal

STAGE II (100–400 UNITS TRANSFUSION)

Asymptomatic or mild fatigue
Echocardiogram: left ventricular wall thickening; left ventricular dilatation but normal ejection fraction
Radionuclide cineangiogram: normal at rest but no increase or fall in ejection fracture with exercise
24-hour ECG: atrial and ventricular premature beats

STAGE III

Palpitations and/or congestive heart failure
Echocardiogram: decreased ejection fraction
Radionuclide cineangiogram: normal or decreased ejection fraction at rest but a fall in ejection fraction during exercise
24-hour ECG: atrial and ventricular premature beats, often in pairs or runs

ECG = electrocardiogram.
Adapted from Nienhuis AW, Griffith P, et al: Evaluation of cardiac function in patients with thalassemia major. Ann NY Acad Sci 1980; 344:384.

HEPATIC ABNORMALITIES

Liver enlargement, long viewed as a hallmark of thalassemia, is prominent with contemporary transfusion regimens only in patients older than 10 years of age. Hepatomegaly is due to progressive engorgement of hepatic parenchymal and phagocytic cells with hemosiderin deposits rather than to extramedullary hematopoiesis.[694] Hepatic iron stores correlate very well with total body iron stores.[695] In addition, iron deposition induces intralobular fibrosis.[696, 697] Intercurrent episodes of hepatitis may lead to marked liver dysfunction and contribute to development of fibrosis and cirrhosis.[698–700] Liver enzymes levels are rarely elevated in the absence of hepatitis. The concentration of total bilirubin in patients receiving adequate transfusion therapy is seldom greater than 2 mg/dL, of which 50 percent or less is typically indirect. Recent data clearly demonstrate that chelation therapy reduces liver iron concentration[695, 701–703] and forestalls iron-induced liver damage. Progressive liver disease in patients receiving appropriate therapy is often due to viral hepatitis.[704]

ENDOCRINE ABNORMALITIES

Endocrine disorders commonly associated with thalassemia in the United States today are generally thought to be caused by chronic iron loading.[617, 623, 705, 706] Most of the pathologic changes develop slowly and usually are not apparent until the second decade of life. In patients not receiving transfusions, these abnormalities develop more slowly.

Growth and Development. Growth retardation, historically considered a typical finding in thalassemia major,[705] is generally associated with moderate retardation in bone age. Patients undergoing chronic transfusion therapy may be spared growth retardation,[707] which is seen in more than 50 percent of patients and then not until the second decade of life.[623] Growth retardation is less evident in patients receiving chelation therapy,[707, 708] although excessive amounts of deferoxamine can also impair growth.[709, 710] Alternative causes should be sought in young thalassemic children who are receiving adequate transfusion therapy and still exhibit significant growth retardation.

Growth retardation may also be associated with evidence of endocrine dysfunction. Impaired growth hormone production has been reported in some patients[711–713] but not confirmed in earlier studies.[714] Treatment with growth hormone may accelerate growth rate but final height may not be changed.[715] A subset of patients with normal growth hormone production have low serum levels of somatomedin,[716] a factor produced by the liver in response to growth hormone that promotes cartilage growth. Failure of adrenal androgen production may also contribute to growth failure.[717] Thyroid deficiency is an additional factor that may potentially contribute (see later). A thorough search for endocrine dysfunction is warranted in patients with growth retardation, because a favorable response to specific replacement therapy may be anticipated.

Puberty. Puberty will occur normally in many patients with β-thalassemia who receive appropriate treatment and is typically seen in those with the least growth retardation. Sexual maturation is variably observed in other patients and is retarded in patients whose transfusion and chelation therapy is inadequate.[718] Failure of patients receiving transfusions to mature sexually may be the first indication of iron toxicity. Breast development in females tends to begin normally, but menarche is frequently delayed until the late teenage years. Eventually, many female patients who progress through puberty normally will develop secondary amenorrhea owing to progressive iron accumulation.

Failure of patients to develop sexually is usually not related to primary end-organ unresponsiveness.[719, 720] Although males tend to have low baseline testosterone levels, response to treatment with human chorionic gonadotropin is usually normal.[720] Moreover, spermatogenesis correlates directly with the stage of sexual maturation of the patient.[721] Gonadotropins, on the other hand, have been implicated in a number of studies as the primary cause of dysfunction in the hypothalamic-pituitary-gonadal axis.[720, 722–725] Although defective ovarian function has been described in some patients,[726] patients who fail to attain puberty or who have experienced regression of secondary sexual characteristics demonstrate blunted responses to luteinizing hormone–releasing factor (LHRF) and to follicle-stimulating hormone. Prolactin levels respond normally to thyroid-releasing factor stimulation. Failure of sexual maturation, therefore, appears most often to be related to hypothalamic-pituitary axis dysfunction.

Although one report suggested preservation of normal gonadotrophin production in young patients receiving large amounts of chelation therapy,[721] modification of transfusion schedules and chelation therapy has not yet been seen to preserve normal function in many patients. This is a problem of increasing severity as the long-term clinical prognosis for patients improves. In approaching such patients, Modell and Berdoukas[623] have likened the attainment of puberty as a trophy in a race between a patient's physical growth and iron overload. Patients with a constitution that favors tall stature and a rapid growth rate, whose transfusion programs and chelation regimens are adequate, are likely to attain puberty. Those who do not require transfusion in the first year of life may also have an advantage. Constitutionally short children and those whose transfusion and chelation regimens are inadequate often fail to "win the race."

For patients with delayed puberty, initial efforts should be devoted to assessment of nutritional status, general health (i.e., presence of hepatitis), and the adequacy of transfusion and chelation therapy. In addition, attention should be paid to the availability of calcium for growth (see later). For those receiving maximal therapy who have delayed puberty and also biochemical evidence of hypothalamic-pituitary axis dysfunction,[727, 728] pulsatile gonadotrophin-releasing hormone infusions have been used to artificially induce puberty and growth,[729,★] although this approach may or may not be successful.[724]

★Chaterjee B: personal communication.

More conventional treatment regimens include testosterone or estrogen supplementation after age 14 or 15 for those in whom puberty was not achieved or in whom secondary hypogonadism, either clinically or based on loss of response to LHRF, has developed.

Thyroid Gland. Even though iron deposition in thyroid parenchymal tissue is often extensive, dysfunction is usually limited to primary subclinical hypothyroidism.[730] In one large series in which simultaneous serum thyroxine and thyroid-stimulating hormone (TSH) levels were obtained in 31 thalassemic patients, mean thyroxine levels were significantly lower (6.2 μg/dL versus 9.5 μg/dL) and TSH levels were significantly higher (3.2 μunit/mL versus. 1.0 μunit/mL) than those in age-matched control subjects.[722] In a longitudinal study, serum thyroxine levels declined, whereas TSH secretion increased. Although the means were significantly different, individual patients with thalassemia could not be reliably distinguished from control subjects. Androgen replacement in males may correct abnormalities in thyroid function.[731]

Adrenal Gland. In the adrenal gland, pathologic changes in patients with thalassemia are historically characterized by iron deposition limited primarily to the zona glomerulosa,[616] the site of mineralocorticoid production. Iron deposition in the zona fasciculata may also occur.[623] In one series, normal aldosterone production in response to salt deprivation was achieved only at the expense of a marked increase in serum renin.[716] Basal morning adrenocorticotropin (ACTH) levels measured in prepubertal thalassemic patients were 3 to 10 times normal.[732] Basal glucocorticoid production and response to ACTH and insulin provocation are generally normal in younger patients, although older patients often demonstrate a blunted provocative response.

Pancreas. Diabetes mellitus is a common and often under-recognized complication of thalassemia, which is due both to pancreatic hypoproduction[733] and (at least in some patients) insulin resistance.[734] Even in patients between 5 and 10 years of age whose iron burden is approximately 5 to 20 g, fasting blood glucose levels are significantly elevated.[732] When glucose tolerance tests are performed, as many as 50 percent of thalassemic patients have "chemical diabetes," defined by glucose tolerance testing; the majority of these patients have normal or elevated circulating insulin levels.[734, 735] Insulin resistance may predate the onset of glucose intolerance, as revealed by the euglycemic clamp method.[736] In contrast, thalassemic patients who have not received transfusions display accelerated insulin clearance and normal tissue sensitivity.[737] As symptoms of diabetes become evident, insulin output decreases, as occurs in most patients with juvenile diabetes. Glucose intolerance generally correlates with the number of transfusions received, age of the patient, and genetic predispostion.[738]

Parathyroid Glands. Symptomatic parathyroid disease, presenting with classic tetany, hypocalcemia, and hyperphosphatemia, is said to be an uncommon complication of iron overload.[722, 733, 738–740] However, the prevalence was 10 percent in one recent study. The affected patients had severe iron overloading.[741] Subclinical deficiency of parathyroid function is difficult to diagnose. The provocative use of calcium chelates to identify subclinical deficiency of parathormone has been described.[742]

Patients with thalassemia major have been reported to show diminished response to a challenge. Although symptomatic parathyroid disease may be rare, more common defects may affect the mobilization of calcium for growth and the preservation of normal serum ionized calcium, which are important in patients with cardiomyopathy or arrhythmia. To complicate matters, deficiency of activated vitamin D may occur, perhaps partially as a consequence of parathormone deficiency. Symptoms of deficiency of 25-hydroxytachysterol, which are relieved either by iron chelation therapy or vitamin D supplementation, have been described in case reports.[743, 744] Therefore, careful attention should be paid to calcium, phosphate, and vitamin D intake in patients with growth disturbances and cardiac disease.

ARTERIAL HYPOXEMIA

In 1981, Fucharoen et al[745] reported significant arterial hypoxemia in patients with HbE β⁰-thalassemia, especially in those who had been splenectomized. These authors found circulating platelet aggregates in such patients, and successfully used aspirin and dipyridamole to improve oxygenation. Other groups have reported hypoxemia in thalassemia major[746–755] but have related it to changes in ventilatory mechanics, obstructive airway disease, or iron deposition in the lungs. Pulmonary hypertension, possibly associated with thrombocytosis and a general hypercoagulable state,[756] may contribute to right ventricular dysfunction in these patients.[757–762]

Therapy of β-Thalassemia[763–769]

TRANSFUSION

Choice of Transfusion Regimen. The mainstay of management of severe β-thalassemia remains blood transfusion.[763–767, 770] Transfusion programs have several aims. By increasing hemoglobin content, transfusions enhance the oxygen-carrying capacity of the blood and thereby decrease tissue hypoxia. The concomitant fall in erythropoietin levels blunts the massive erythroid expansion associated with the anemia. Furthermore, improved tissue oxygenation and the reversal of the hypercatabolic state promote more normal growth and development. Suppression of erythropoiesis is associated with decreased intestinal iron absorption. These benefits must be weighed against the prospects of excessive iron loading, particularly with more intensive transfusion protocols.

A major debate in the management of thalassemia centers on the optimal maintenance level of hemoglobin targeted by transfusion programs. Wolman and co-workers[534, 606] first recommended a pretransfusion hemoglobin level of 8.5 g/dL. This approach improved survival, but chronic illness, bone disease, and anemic cardiomyopathy persisted. To enhance quality of life Piomelli et al[538] suggested maintaining the hemoglobin level at greater than 10 g/dL with a mean of 12 g/dL. Such "hypertransfusion," if initiated in the first year of life, promotes normal initial growth and development, limits development of hepatosplenomegaly, prevents disfiguring bone abnormalities, reduces intestinal iron absorption, and decreases cardiac workload.[771–774]

In 1980, Propper et al[775] proposed that maintenance of a pretransfusion hemoglobin level greater than 12 g/dL with a mean of 14 g/dL would more effectively eliminate chronic tissue hypoxia. By continued suppression of endogenous erythropoiesis, this "supertransfusion" program was predicted to further decrease intestinal iron absorption, eliminate bone disease, and decrease hypercatabolism, thereby improving growth and development. Initial studies reported that the quantity of blood required to maintain a higher hemoglobin level was no greater than that required for maintenance of a lower level due to a decrease in intravascular volume.[775–777] Data from other centers, however, suggested that increasing the pretransfusion hemoglobin level may simply increase the quantity of transfused blood and thus increase iron loading.[623, 778] As a result of the conflicting clinical experience, supertransfusion has not been widely used in patient management. If it is to be implemented, iron balance parameters should be carefully monitored.[766]

Senescence in red cells is a function of cell age. Because the iron content of transfused erythrocytes is independent of cell age, attempts have been made to improve the "quality" of transfused blood by infusing the youngest third of red cells present in whole blood ("neocytes").[775, 779] Administration of these cells would be predicted to decrease the transfusion requirement. Neocytes can be readily prepared with automated cell separators,[780–784] but three or more units are required to prepare the equivalent of one unit of blood. Although prolonged survival of neocytes has been documented *in vivo,* the observed sparing in transfusions with such therapy has been disappointing.[785–788] Similarly, methods to remove "gerocytes" (old red cells) from the recipient's circulation at the time of transfusion, although technically feasible, have not been widely applied.[787, 789] These approaches should be considered experimental at present.

Although specific practices will differ among clinical centers, transfusion is indicated both to correct anemia and to suppress erythropoiesis.[763] After diagnosis, a period of observation should be initiated to determine if transfusion is required to maintain the hemoglobin level at greater than or equal to 7 g/dL. The condition of patients with thalassemia intermedia will be stable without transfusion. If the hemoglobin level falls to less than 7 g/dL, a transfusion program should be initiated to maintain the hemoglobin level at 9.5 to 11.5 g/dL. During the first decade of life, normal growth provides reassurance that the transfusion regimen is adequate. Because the rate of iron absorption parallels the number of nucleated red cells in the peripheral blood,[619] adequate transfusion should suppress the nucleated cell count to less than 5 of 100 white blood cells[763]; however, in older patients who received inadequate transfusion therapy early in life it may not be possible to achieve this level. During the teenage years, growth failure may reflect endocrine dysfunction rather than inadequate transfusions; laboratory investigation and appropriate replacement therapy are then indicated. After epiphyses are fused and growth is complete, a hemoglobin level of 8.0 of 9.0 g/dL may be well tolerated. If the transfusion requirement exceeds 200 mL of packed

red cells/kg/yr, splenectomy should be considered (see further discussion later).[763] Our current transfusion procedure is outlined in Table 20–11.

Complications of Blood Transfusion. The primary long-term complication of blood transfusion is iron loading and the resultant parenchymal organ toxicity, as discussed earlier. Febrile reactions to leukocyte antigenic determinants and allergic reactions to plasma components are commonly encountered in patients receiving transfusions chronically. Washing of red cells in saline or the use of microaggregate filtration to remove leukocytes can be beneficial.[790] Alternatively, frozen deglycerolized cells may be used in patients with severe sensitization but may be associated with an increase in transfusion requirements.[791] These strategies should be used only in patients with documented transfusion reactions.

Alloimmunization to minor blood group antigens occurs in 20 to 30 percent of patients[792–794] and may present as delayed hemolysis. In rare circumstances, this may be a potentially life-threatening complication in patients with transfusion-dependent β-thalassemia. Alloimmunization is often a less significant problem in patients in whom transfusion is initiated before the age 3.[792–794] The benefits of extended red cell phenotyping to minimize alloimmunization has been debated in the literature,[795, 796] but crossmatching for rhesus and Kell systems from the time of initial transfusion may decrease the incidence of alloimmunization.[793] Detailed red cell phenotyping should be performed

TABLE 20–11. Guidelines for Chronic Transfusions in Patients with Thalassemia

1. Determine the blood type of the patient completely to identify minor red cell antigens before first transfusion.
2. Keep the pretransfusion hemoglobin level between 9.5 and 11.5 mg/dL as needed for suppressing ineffective erythropoiesis and maintaining a reasonable sense of well-being.
3. Give 10 to 20 mL/kg of leukocyte-poor, washed, and filtered red blood cells with a maximum infusion rate of 10 mL/kg over 2 hours, transfusing more slowly in patients with heart disease.
4. Avoid raising the post-transfusion hemoglobin to >16 g/dL.
5. Choose a transfusion interval to maintain pretransfusion levels as outlined above (3–5 weeks depending on individual patient needs). (*Comment*: Some patients tolerate slightly lower pretransfusion hemoglobin levels and need 5 weeks between transfusions, whereas others feel best coming every 4 weeks. Some prefer getting fewer units and coming every 3 weeks. Some of the younger patients whose weights would require between 1 and 2 units receive a transfusion every 3 or 4 weeks and alternate between 1 and 2 units per transfusion.
6. Pretransfusion laboratory tests include a complete blood cell count, differential, crossmatch, and red cell antibody screen.
7. Height and weight are recorded at least every 3 months.
8. Liver function (AST, ALT, bilirubin, and LDH) is evaluated every 3 months and serum ferritin every 3 to 6 months. A deferoxamine (Desferal) challenge test is performed at irregular intervals to measure appropriate Desferal dosage and chelatable iron stores.

AST = aspartate transaminase; ALT = alanine transaminase; LDH = lactate dehydrogenase.

in all patients with newly diagnosed thalassemia before transfusion. The average transfusion regimen in most centers is 12 to 15 mL of leukocyte-poor red cells/kg/mo.

The transmission of viral infections by transfusion is a serious problem in patients receiving transfusions chronically. In one study, approximately 25 percent of transfusion-dependent patients with thalassemia had been exposed to hepatitis B, 80 percent of whom had clinical evidence of hepatitis.[797] Exposure to hepatitis C, with an incidence of approximately 6 percent per transfusion, was nearly inevitable in thalassemic patients receiving regular transfusion, and this agent may account for the active hepatitis seen in many older patients. The identification of the hepatitis C agent and the development of a serologic test to screen donors has greatly minimized this risk,[798, 799] but the infection can lead to fibrosis, cirrhosis, and hepatic carcinoma if untreated.[800-802] Treatment with interferon-α and ribavirin is indicated. Some studies have suggested that iron overload inhibits a therapeutic response,[803-806] but others have shown little or no such effect.[807, 808] A minority of patients with thalassemia have become infected with human immunodeficiency virus and the rate of progression to symptomatic acquired immunodeficiency syndrome has been proportionately lower than in most infected populations.[809] Although death and complications from these illnesses are uncommon in this patient population, it is prudent to exercise precautions. The most important consideration is the use of blood products screened for the presence of potential infectious agents. Patients should be immunized against hepatitis B upon diagnosis or if they have not acquired immunity. Where practical, exposure to multiple donors or units of blood should be minimized. In this regard, it is important to recognize that the use of washed or frozen red cells may lead to an increase in the number of transfused units.

Splenectomy. The role of the spleen must be considered in patients who are treated with transfusion, iron chelation programs, or both. The spleen serves both as a scavenger by increasing red cell destruction and iron redistribution and a storage depot by sequestration of the released iron in a potentially nontoxic pool. Unfortunately, splenic iron may equilibrate with other iron pools throughout the body. In one uncontrolled study, three splenectomized patients exhibited cirrhosis and massive iron deposition, whereas slightly younger patients with an intact spleen had only iron deposition.[810] Risdon and colleagues,[694] however, observed no difference between splenectomized and nonsplenectomized patients with regard to pathologic changes in the liver. If the spleen acts primarily as a storage depot for excess iron, premature removal could theoretically be detrimental. On the other hand, if the splenic pool is a particular target for deferoxamine, the beneficial effects of aggressive chelation therapy might be diminished by preferential removal of iron from this relatively innocuous pool. Perhaps most important is the feasibility of achievement of negative iron balance with conventional chelation regimens (see later). Eventually, an increased requirement for transfusion due to hypersplenism perturbs the balance and contributes to iron loading.[811]

Splenectomy is often indicated in the management of patients with severe β-thalassemia. Massive splenomegaly with hypersplenism causing leukopenia, thrombocytopenia, and an increasing transfusion requirement is often seen in young patients whose transfusion regimens are sporadic moderate. Early splenectomy is often required. The development of splenomegaly is delayed in patients who are receiving a high number of transfusions.[812] Several factors should be considered in the decision to remove the spleen. Modell[623, 813, 814] carefully documented the annual blood requirement for splenectomized patients with thalassemia major and suggested that the spleen be removed if the observed requirement exceeds that predicted by 50 percent. Data from other investigators suggest that the benefits of splenectomy on iron balance are realized if the transfusion requirement exceeds 200 to 250 mL of packed red cells/kg/yr with a minimum hemoglobin level of 10 g/dL.[811, 815] Because a huge spleen, irrespective of functional hypersplenism, may account for a large fraction of the total blood volume, its removal often leads to a marked, although transient, reduction in the patient's requirement for blood.[816, 817] Most patients show a moderate, but significant, reduction in their requirement for transfusion to the predicted 200 mL of packed red cells/kg/yr[813, 814] that remains stable over many years.[818]

The immediate surgical risk accompanying splenectomy is minimal for experienced practitioners. This is some evidence that iron overload itself may inhibit the immune response.[819, 820] The potential of overwhelming infection from *Diplococcus pneumoniae, Haemophilus influenzae,* or *Neisseria meningitidis*[821-823] should always be considered by the attending physician. Because removal of the spleen may blunt the primary immune response to encapsulated organisms, delay of splenectomy until after approximately 5 years of age is preferable. Patients should be immunized with polyvalent pneumococcal, meningococcal, and *H. influenzae* vaccines.[824-827] Supplemental prophylactic oral penicillin may also be used to prevent colonization by strains not covered by vaccines,[763] particularly in young children. Illnesses accompanied by high fever of uncertain cause should be aggressively treated with parenteral antibiotics until bacterial culture results are available. Patients in regions endemic for malaria should receive prophylactic treatment.[814] Infections appear to be significant causes of morbidity in HbE β-thalassemia.[828]

Red cell survival usually increases immediately after splenectomy.[816] The peripheral blood smear may reveal increased numbers of hypochromic, microcytic, and nucleated red cells. Platelet counts greater than 10^6 are often seen, although correction of anemia by transfusion usually results in suppression of platelet production.[462] White blood cell counts of 15,000 to 20,000 are common; the differential is usually normal.

As discussed in more detail later, arterial hypoxemia and evidence of pulmonary vascular disease have been reported in patients with thalassemia, and it has been suggested that splenectomy may exacerbate these problems.[745, 757] Accordingly, splenectomized patients should be examined carefully for these findings. Because thrombocytosis may be an inciting factor,[757, 829] prophylaxis with low-dose aspirin may be considered, although effective transfusion to correct anemia is probably the best form of preventive therapy.

CHELATION THERAPY

Progressive iron overload is the life-limiting complication of transfusion therapy. In the absence of adequate chelation, cardiac dysfunction ends the life of the thalassemic patient receiving transfusions during the teenage years. Regular chelation with the drug deferoxamine has proven remarkably effective in reducing the iron burden of patients receiving transfusions. Cardiac disease is delayed or prevented, susceptibility to infection is reduced,[830] and life expectancy is significantly extended; nonetheless, endocrine dysfunction may develop and persist. Unfortunately, effective use of deferoxamine requires strict compliance to subcutaneous administration via a mechanical pump. The lack of oral absorption of the drug and its short serum half-life dictate this cumbersome route of administration. An equally effective oral alternative has not yet been discovered, as discussed later.

Deferoxamine. Deferoxamine is a hexavalent hydroxylamine with a remarkable affinity for iron. Deferoxamine binds metal iron stoichiometrically with a weight ratio of deferoxamine to iron of approximately 11:1. Deferoxamine enters cells, chelates iron, and appears in serum and bile as the iron chelate product, feroxamine.[652] It is not absorbed from the gastrointestinal tract, and its removal from the plasma is extremely rapid.

Humans have no intrinsic mechanism for excreting excess iron. Iron available for chelation is thought to be derived from the "labile iron pool"[639]; the size of this pool is directly related to the total body iron burden.[831, 832] Non–transferrin-bound plasma iron should also be available for chelation.[647, 648] A fraction of reticuloendothelial iron salvaged from red cells may also be chelated,[833] perhaps only when stored as ferritin.[834] Urinary iron excretion appears to be proportional to marrow erythroid activity and is diminished by transfusion.[835] Net iron loss, however, is not compromised because the diminution of urinary iron excretion is balanced by an increased fecal excretion of iron.[834, 835] In patients with primary hemochromatosis in whom iron deposition is seen predominantly in parenchymal cells and erythropoiesis is normal, deferoxamine administration results primarily in enhanced fecal iron excretion.[652] Thus, the site of iron removal is influenced by the transfusion schedule, but there are no data available regarding the influence of the hemoglobin level on the prevention or removal of cardiac iron deposits.

Chelation Regimens. Deferoxamine is active when administered by the intramuscular, subcutaneous, or intravenous routes. After its introduction in 1962, the drug was given by the intramuscular route until the late 1970s. This regimen was only partially successful because iron removal was insufficient to achieve a negative net iron balance in most patients.[836] Supplemental oral ascorbic acid administration enhanced urinary excretion (see later),[837] but only 14 to 16 mg of iron could be removed per day even from patients with severe hemosiderosis. Adults receiving full transfusion support require removal of more than 35 mg/day to have negative net iron balance.[836] Furthermore, little iron excretion could be obtained by this regimen in patients whose iron stores were greater than 10 times normal.[838]

The efficacy of intramuscular injections is limited by the rapid clearance of deferoxamine from plasma via metabolism and biliary and urinary excretion.[652] Continuous intravenous infusion significantly enhances iron excretion,[836, 838] presumably because of exchange between deferoxamine and tissue iron pools. Significant plasma and tissue drug concentrations can be attained by continuous subcutaneous administration via a pump mechanism.[839] Iron excretion is markedly enhanced compared with the intramuscular route,[836, 839–841] and net negative iron balance can be achieved in most patients older than age 3 or 4 with an iron burden of 4 to 5 g.[771, 778, 839]

A typical regimen involves administration of 30 to 40 mg/kg of drug overnight (8 to 12 hours); thereby the patient avoids the need to carry the pump during the daytime hours. Patients are advised to use the drug at least 5 or 6 days per week. Obviously, such a program is a compromise in that optimal management demands drug infusion every hour of every day, a schedule met with poor compliance, particularly among teenagers. Data now show that regular use of deferoxamine, if started by age 3 or 4, forestalls significant iron overload. It also promotes elimination of excess iron in patients if started after a significant transfusional iron burden has already developed.[703, 842–846] There is general agreement that treatment should be initiated by age 5 in transfusion-dependent patients; some advocate treatment by age 3.[766, 778, 847–849] It has been argued that irreversible tissue damage, particularly to endocrine glands, occurs at a very low iron burden during the first years of life. However, the toxicity of deferoxamine is most significant in patients with a low iron burden (see later). Indeed, growth retardation and other toxic effects have been documented in children younger than age 3 who are given high doses of the drug.[617] A test infusion of deferoxamine may be used to determine if mobilizable iron is present.[763, 766]

Periodic intravenous administration of deferoxamine may also be used to accelerate the rate of iron removal in patients with symptoms of substantial iron burdens. Intravenous administration allows for use of higher doses (6 to 10 g/day); local reactions at the site of administration limit the tolerable subcutaneous dose to 2.0 to 2.5 g/day. By extending the time of infusion and increasing the drug dose, iron removal can be greatly enhanced over that achievable with conventional subcutaneous therapy. This approach is indicated in attempts to reverse established cardiac dysfunction in patients who have received many transfusions[850] (see later).

Efficacy of Chelation. Clinical experience has shown subcutaneous deferoxamine administration to be effective in preventing cardiac disease and prolonging the life of thalassemic patients receiving transfusions.[703, 845, 851–853] Life expectancy previously was approximately 16 years with rare patients surviving into their mid 20s.[539, 678, 854] Since the introduction of subcutaneous deferoxamine therapy, the projected life expectancy extends into the middle fourth decade.[855] Several studies have also documented sparing of cardiac disease in patients

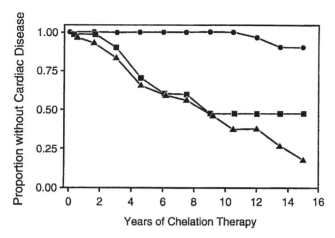

FIGURE 20–33. Cardiac disease–free survival of patients with respect to serum ferritin level. The *circles* depict cardiac disease–free survival assay patients with less than 33 percent of ferritin measurements greater than 2500 ng/mL; *squares,* patients with 33 to 67 percent greater than 2500 ng/mL; *triangles,* patients with more than 67 percent measurements greater than 2500 ng/mL. (From Olivieri NF, Nathan DG, et al: Survival in medically treated patients with homozygous beta-thalassemia. N Engl J Med 1994; 331:574. Copyright 1994, Massachusetts Medical Society.)

receiving adequate chelation therapy.[703, 845, 856, 857] Figure 20–33 shows a striking comparison between two groups of patients; one group received adequate chelation therapy, whereas the other group was poorly compliant. Onset of cardiac disease has been observed in the chelated group in whom negative iron balance was achieved,[856] but the dose of the drug used was relatively low.

Chelation with high drug doses by the intravenous route is capable of reversing established cardiac disease in some patients who continue to require transfusion.[692, 767, 858,*] This regimen must be instituted while the patient's heart is still compensating, either with or without cardiac medications. Individuals with refractory congestive heart failure or hypotension due to cardiac disease are poor candidates for intravenous deferoxamine.

Unfortunately, the cohort of patients in whom administration of subcutaneous deferoxamine was initiated in their late first decade of life after significant iron deposits had accumulated continue to exhibit endocrine dysfunction and growth retardation.[846] Glucose intolerance and diabetes are observed even in patients receiving adequate chelation therapy,[859] although the incidence is reduced.[703] There is scant evidence that deferoxamine can reverse established endocrine dysfunction. It remains to be determined whether patients in whom a regimen of subcutaneous deferoxamine is started at a very young age will fare better with respect to growth, sexual development, and endocrine function. Because this cohort of patients is just now entering their teenage years, information on this point may become available in the near future.

Toxicity of Deferoxamine. At high doses of deferoxamine, significant side effects are seen.[652, 763] Local erythema may occur at the site of infusion and contribute to an inflammatory response characterized by multiple subcutaneous nodules. These local reactions can be partially suppressed by inclusion of 5 to 10 mg of hydrocortisone in the deferoxamine solution.

Of particular concern is neurosensory toxicity observed at high doses. Several large series report a 30 to 40 percent incidence of high-frequency hearing loss, which may become symptomatic.[860–864] Reversal with discontinuation of the drug has been reported, although other patients have experienced persistent hearing loss. Ocular toxicity has also been reported.[860, 865] Progressive visual failure with night and color blindness and field loss are also described[866] but may be not be related to chelation therapy.[867] In fact, in one study iron dysfunction was thought to be related to failure to take dereroxamine.[868] Reversal after discontinuation of deferoxamine has also been reported.

The neurosensory complications of deferoxamine are dose related and inversely correlated with the body iron burden. Patients with heavy iron loading are relatively protected, but patients receiving aggressive chelation therapy with lower iron burdens may be more susceptible to these toxic effects.[863, 869, 870] Administration of deferoxamine to patients with rheumatoid arthritis with normal iron stores has induced neurologic deficits including confusion, nausea and vomiting, and coma.[869, 871] These findings suggest that the toxicity is caused by free drug, which may chelate other metal irons.[864] Alternatively, deferoxamine may reduce the concentration of iron in neurosensory cells below a threshold needed for normal function. These serious complications necessitate careful monitoring of patients receiving deferoxamine. Young children and individuals from whom the majority of iron has been removed by chelation are particularly susceptible to these effects. The occurrence of complications is most likely in patients receiving continuous intravenous infusions of more than 50 mg/kg/day. Formal audiometry and ophthalmologic examination should be performed at 6-month intervals. The use of a test infusion to assess the ability of deferoxamine to mobilize iron, as advocated by Fosburg and Nathan,[763] may help in avoiding toxicity.

Deferoxamine is normally used by microorganisms to facilitate iron uptake.[652, 872] *Yersina enterocolitica,* for example, uses deferoxamine in this manner.[813] Although it is associated with low virulence in humans, serious *Y. enterocolitica* infections have been reported in treated patients.[873, 874] Mucormycosis has also been reported in patients undergoing hemodialysis who receive deferoxamine.[875] Of interest is the observation that iron chelators have profound *in vitro* effects on T-lymphocyte function.[763, 876–881] Whether these effects can be put to practical use is not known.[880]

Additional rare complications have been associated with high-dose deferoxamine. Pulmonary infiltrates and respiratory insufficiency have been reported in eight patients[882, 883] and in iron-loaded mice.[884] Curiously, deferoxamine also protects the developing lung[885]; therefore, the view that deferoxamine causes pulmonary toxicity in the treatment of iron overload is controversial.[886]

---

*Nienhuis AW: Unpublished observations, 1990.

Indeed, iron overload is thought to contribute to pulmonary disease in thalassemia,[757] although the latter is complex and is probably also related to pulmonary vascular obstruction associated with chronic thrombocytosis.[758, 829] Acute and chronic renal decompensation has also been described.[758, 829, 887–889] Growth failure and skeletal changes have been reported.[890, 891]

The array of potential side effects should not obscure the finding that deferoxamine has proved to be very safe in the vast majority of patients. Many of the side effects have been seen only at higher intravenous doses. Although careful follow-up of patients is warranted, patients can be reassured that the deferoxamine therapy is both remarkably effective and generally quite safe. Indeed, methods have been designed to permit chronic intravenous infusion,[892–894] and a twice daily subcutaneous regimen that obviates use of a pump is being explored. The major limitation of deferoxamine use is compliance and the serious problems faced by patients and their families as they deal with this life-saving but inconvenient therapy.[895–897]

Deferiprone. The availability of effective oral chelators would be a major clinical advance. Of those examined thus far, only one, L-1-(1,2-dimethyl-3-hydroxy-pyridin-4-one, trade name Deferiprone), has been examined in multiple clinical trials. Deferiprone is a bivalent iron chelator initially synthesized by Hider and colleagues.[898] It was briefly licensed to CIBA-GEIGY (now Novartis), but abandoned by the company in 1993 because of its low therapeutic index in non–iron-overloaded animals, its poor stoichiometry (three molecules of drug are required for binding of each iron atom),[899] and its rapid removal from the circulation.[900, 901] The drug's efficacy is, therefore, critically dependent on its poorly maintained concentration in body fluids.

Deferoxamine was first investigated in uncontrolled clinical trials by a group at the Royal Free Hospital in London.[902] These were followed by two studies by Olivieri and Brittenham and their colleagues[903, 904] who measured iron stores by liver biopsy and SQUID in patients treated with deferoxamine. Their initial results, published in 1995, were encouraging.[905] The drug appeared to reduce or maintain liver iron levels in patients with thalassemia who were receiving many transfusions. Although an accompanying editorial warned that much more time would be required to determine its efficacy,[906] there were high expectations in the thalassemia community that deferoxamine would prove useful in the management of iron overload resulting from chronic transfusions. Deferoxamine-treated patients regularly exhibit a steady decline in hepatic iron levels if they comply with the therapy regimen. In a second study, hepatic iron levels were not reduced below their starting points or actually increased to a value substantially above their starting points in a substantial fraction of Deferiprone-treated patients.[904] In addition, some of the Deferiprone-treated patients but none of the deferoxamine-treated patients (who had much lower liver iron levels on average) appeared to have developed increased hepatic fibrosis.

The findings of Olivieri and Brittenham and their colleagues findings are controversial in part. Other studies confirmed that iron stores, measured by liver biopsy, are not effectively reduced by Deferiprone.[907, 908] The

influence of the drug on hepatic fibrosis remains uncertain.[907, 909, 909a] Recent published studies of Deferiprone have been based on the level of serum ferritin as an index of effectiveness, but such studies[910–912] are unreliable. Thus far, the drug has been inadequately assessed.[913] Further studies of Deferiprone are warranted. The drug may play a role in shuttling iron within membranes and within intracellular pools.[914, 915]

In addition to the issue of hepatic fibrosis, Deferiprone administration is associated with severe adverse side effects, including idiosyncratic agranulocytosis in nearly 2 percent of patients. Other complications include arthropathy, zinc deficiency, gastrointestinal symptoms, and abnormal liver function test results.[916, 917] Until the risk-to-benefit ratio of Deferiprone administration is established by additional clinical trials in which iron stores are measured, compliant patients should be advised to continue an effective deferoxamine chelation program.[650, 917, 918]

Other Oral Chelators. Many iron chelators have been developed, but only one, now known as ICL670, has produced promising results in early preclinical trials.[919] ICL670 is a tridentate chelator in a class of compounds known as 3,5-bis-(orthohydroxyphenyl)-1,2,4-triazoles. After an oral dose, the drug is promptly absorbed, persists in the blood with a half-time of 8 hours, and excretes iron largely in the feces. In short-term dose-finding clinical trials, the drug removes an amount of iron that would be expected to be delivered in a standard transfusion regimen. The long-term efficacy and toxicity of ICL670 are yet to be determined, but the drug appears to have high potential value.

VITAMIN SUPPLEMENTATION

Ascorbic Acid. The role of ascorbic acid in iron metabolism and chelation therapy is complex and controversial.[652,920] Patients with hemosiderosis often develop tissue deficiency of vitamin C due to accelerated catabolism; frank scurvy is documented in individuals with marginal dietary intake.[921–924] Administration of vitamin C significantly augments iron excretion in response to deferoxamine, particularly in patients who have a vitamin C deficiency. Serum iron and ferritin levels may also rise.[835, 924, 925] Ascorbic acid retards the rate of conversion of ferritin to hemosiderin[926, 927] and presumably allows more iron to remain in a chelatable form. Unfortunately, ascorbic acid also enhances iron-mediated peroxidation of membrane lipids[928, 929] and has been shown to enhance iron-induced membrane damage in cultured myocardial cells.[662] It has also been observed that patients with iron overloads who are receiving vitamin C may experience cardiac dysfunction that is reversed when supplementation is discontinued.[930, 931]

Some investigators have suggested giving low doses of ascorbic acid (3 mg/kg) at the start of each subcutaneous infusion of deferoxamine. The chelator should be able to block the deleterious effects of ascorbic acid on lipid peroxidation of cellular organelles *in vitro*. Others avoid using vitamin C in patients with iron overloads, arguing that iron depletion can be achieved without supplemental vitamin C. Patients with significant iron burdens should be cautioned against self-administration of substantial amounts of ascorbic acid, because abrupt cardiac deterioration has been observed in this setting.*

Vitamin E. Deficiency of vitamin E has been noted in many patients with thalassemia major receiving transfusions chronically.[664, 665, 838, 932, 933] It may contribute to hemolysis due to red cell membrane damage.[456, 663] α-Tocopherol has long been considered to be a potent antioxidant that protects membrane lipids from attack by free radicals, formed when excess iron is present. Deficiency in the neonatal period[934] or deficiency caused by malnutrition is associated with varying degrees of hemolysis. Hemolysis and the characteristic increased red cell susceptibility to *in vitro* hydrogen peroxide are readily reversed by administration of supplemental vitamin E. Of interest, supplemental iron administration increases the hemolytic rate, even among nonthalassemic patients with vitamin E deficiency.[934] In patients with iron overloads, supplemental vitamin E may lessen iron-mediated cellular toxicity. One study in experimental animals suggests that vitamin E may also inhibit deferoxamine-induced urinary iron excretion,[935] although this effect has not been demonstrated in humans.

Folic Acid. Megaloblastic anemia, which is almost invariably due to folic acid deficiency, may occur in patients with severe β-thalassemia.[936–938] In contrast, vitamin B_{12} deficiency is extremely rare in thalassemic patients.[938] Folic acid deficiency is thought to develop owing to decreased absorption, low dietary intake, and the enormous demand of bone marrow expansion. Most patients benefit from daily folic acid administration (1 mg), although patients receiving adequate transfusions probably do not require supplementation.

Trace Metals. Trace metal deficiency associated with thalassemia or aggressive chelation therapy is not commonly observed.[652, 939] An occurrence of zinc deficiency (acrodermatitis enteropathics) has been reported in a patient receiving diethylenetriamine pentaacetic acid for chelation.[940] The reversible toxic effects seen with high-dose deferoxamine chelation may reflect trace metal deficiency or intracellular chelation of a trace metal. Newer techniques to analyze trace metal concentrations may reveal subtle deficiencies.

ALLOGENEIC BONE MARROW TRANSPLANTATION

Successful cure of β-thalassemia by bone marrow transplantation was first reported by Thomas and associates in 1982.[941] Subsequently, a number of centers have explored use of this modality as definitive therapy for β-thalassemia. The most extensive published experience with bone marrow transplantation in β-thalassemia is that of Lucarelli and co-workers in Italy.[942–946] The results of their early attempts to use transplantation in this patient population were discouraging.[943] The preparative regimens used were often ineffective and associated with graft failure, toxicity, and high mortality. Their recent experience is considerably more promising.[946] In 222 patients (ages 1 to 15 years) who underwent transplantation between 1983 to 1988 with five different preparative regimens,

overall and event-free survival was 82 and 75 percent, respectively. The longest surviving patient was alive and disease-free 6 years after transplantation. Their current preparative protocol, which has been used in 116 patients since 1985, includes oral busulfan and intravenous cyclophosphamide. Patients were analyzed to identify clinically important variables predictive of transplant outcome. The probability of survival was decreased in the presence of poor chelation status, hepatomegaly (>2 cm), and portal fibrosis. The probability of event-free survival was reduced in the presence of hepatomegaly. The risk factors of hepatomegaly and portal fibrosis were used to divide the patients into three classes. Patients in class 1 (absence of both risk factors) had 3-year probabilities of survival, -free survival, and graft rejection of 94, 94, and 0 percent, respectively. In class 2 (one risk factor), the 3-year probabilities were 80, 77, and 9 percent; in class 3 (two risk factors) they were 61, 53, and 16 percent. However, such classification of patients may be difficult to reproduce (i.e., hepatomegaly of ≤2 cm and a history of adherence to chelation therapy). It is probably wise to consider the likely event-free survival to be closer to 75 percent, even though results from some small series can vary above or below that estimate.[947–949]

One of the major reasons for failure of bone marrow transplantation in patients with thalassemia may be the unpredictable pharmacologic effects of the busulphan used in most preparative regimens. Hyperabsorption of the drug is associated with hepatic veno-occlusive disease and hypoabsorption with recurrent thalassemia. Improved control of busulphan levels during induction may provide better clinical results.[950] Whatever the even-free survival estimates, bone marrow transplantation is the only viable option for patients who cannot or refuse to adhere to a well-administered transfusion and chelation program.[951]

On the basis of available data, bone marrow transplantation may be recommended to patients receiving adequate chelation without evidence of liver disease. Many of these patients can be cured. Although most such patients are very young, age does not appear to be a significant variable in determining outcome. Chronic graft-versus-host disease is still a potential long-term complication of successful allogeneic transplantation. A current limitation to the general applicability of this therapy is the availability of a related, HLA-matched donor. Only one in four siblings on average will be HLA identical. Improved management of graft-versus-host disease and the development of technologies for bone marrow transplantation from unrelated donors may expand the pool of potential donors in the near future. Some encouraging results have recently been reported.[952] The use of cord blood stem cells may also extend the donor pool.[953, 954]

Pharmacologic Manipulation of Hemoglobin F Synthesis

The interaction between β-thalassemia and genetic syndromes that increase γ-globin synthesis has illustrated how even small increases in γ-globin production lead to a

---

*Nienhuis AW: Unpublished observations, 1990.

significant improvement in the effectiveness of red blood cell production in patients with thalassemia. Although steady-state production of HbF is a genetically determined trait,[9] perturbations in erythropoiesis may be associated with increased capacity for HbF synthesis. Treatment of experimental animals or patients with a variety of cytoreductive agents, including 5-azacytidine, hydroxyurea, vinblastine, and cytosine arabinoside, leads to an increase in production of HbF.[955–965] Although the precise mechanism of action of these drugs remains incompletely defined, the increased capacity for γ-globin synthesis appears to be linked to rapid erythroid regeneration. Consistent with this hypothesis, hematopoietic growth factors that promote the expansion and maturation of the erythroid precursors have also been shown to enhance HbF synthesis in primate models; these include erythropoietin,[966–968] interleukin-3,[967–969] and granulocyte-macrophage colony-stimulating factor.[967] Of particular interest is the observation that infants delivered of diabetic mothers exhibit a delayed γ- to β-globin switch.[970] Levels of butyric acid derivatives are elevated in the serum of these mothers and their infants before birth. Similarly, patients with metabolic disorders associated with increased levels of short-chain fatty acids also have elevated HbF levels.[971] Infusions of sodium butyrate or α-aminobutyric acid into fetal sheep markedly delay the perinatal switch,[972] whereas infusions in primates lead to activation of the γ gene.[973, 974,*] It has been proposed that butyrate, propionate, or the metabolite acetate, promotes increased γ-globin expression by acetylation of histones and alteration of chromatin structure, but other mechanisms cannot be excluded.[975, 976] A flurry of articles described results of treatment of patients with sickle cell anemia with butyrate or its derivatives.[977–982] One patient[978] had a sustained increase in hemoglobin, and healing of leg ulcers without an increment in circulating hemoglobin has also been observed.[981] A recent report cited a sustained increase in HbF in sickle cell anemia.[983, 984] Caution must be exercised, however, because high doses of butyrate are associated with neurotoxicity in simians.[985]

The most extensive experience with pharmacologic manipulation of HbF synthesis in patients has involved administration of hydroxyurea to patients with sickle cell disease.[961, 986–990,†] In this population, the majority of patients appear to respond to the drug with a twofold or greater increase in HbF levels over their baseline. In many patients HbF levels between 10 and 15 percent of total hemoglobin are seen. This increase reflects both augmented production and enhanced survival of HbF-containing cells. The clinical results in patients with sickle cell anemia are impressive as described in Chapter 19. However, results in patients with thalassemia have been disappointing so far.[963]

In several patients with thalassemia a response to 5-azacytidine (5-Aza) has been seen[956, 991, 992] (Fig. 20–34). The dramatic increases in HbF levels associated with administration of this drug may result from a combination of cytotoxicity and inhibition of postsynthetic methylation of DNA.[992–996] After administration of 5-Aza, global demethylation of DNA, including the γ-globin gene, is observed. Despite its effectiveness, the use of 5-Aza in the treatment of the hemoglobinopathies has been limited by concerns about its known carcinogenic potential,[997–999] as well as the demonstrated effectiveness and safety of current treatment strategies involving transfusion and chelation. Because the response to the drug is short-lived, chronic therapy would be required.

Treatment of β-thalassemia with Myleran has been reported in two patients in China.[1000] Combinations of

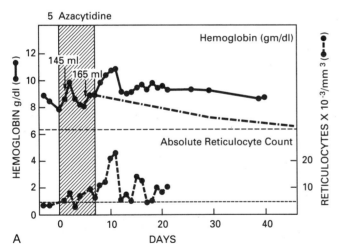
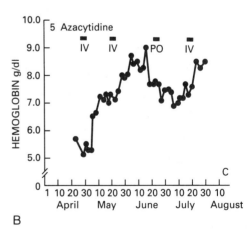

FIGURE 20–34. *A,* The effects of 5-azacytidine on erythropoiesis in a patient with severe homozygous β-thalassemia after a single administration of the drug by continuous infusion over 7 days. Two small blood transfusions were administered on days 2 and 5. The *dashed lines* indicate the projected hemoglobin concentration and reticulocyte count in this patient without treatment, based on clinical records. *B,* The effects of sequential courses of treatment with 5-azacytidine in a patient with β-thalassemia who had severe cardiomyopathy and alloimmunization. (*A* adapted from information appearing in Ley TJ, DeSimone J, et al: 5-Azacytidine selectively increases gamma-globin synthesis in a patient with beta thalassemia. N Engl J Med 1982; 307:1469. Reprinted by permission, from The New England Journal of Medicine. *B* from Dunbar C, Travis W, et al: 5-Azacytidine treatment in a beta[0]-thalassemic patient unable to be transfused due to multiple alloantibodies. Br J Haematol 1989; 72:467.)

---

*McDonagh KT, Bodine DM, Nienhuis AW: Unpublished observations.

†Dover GJ: Personal communication.

agents, notably erythropoietin and hydroxyurea, often enhance HbF production in experimental animals[968, 1001] and have shown promise in preliminary trials in sickle cell patients.* Undoubtedly, the response of individual patients to these medications will be influenced by their endogenous, genetically determined capabilities for γ- and β-chain synthesis.[1002, 1003]

Gene Therapy

As a result of advances in molecular biology, treatment of hematologic disease through the introduction of new genetic material into bone marrow stem cells is a goal for the foreseeable future.[1004–1007] Application of somatic gene therapy to the treatment of hematologic diseases requires improved efficiency of gene delivery, regulated and sustained expression of introduced genes, and biologic studies demonstrating expression of the foreign gene. Although active research is ongoing, experimental shortcomings in all these aspects presently preclude use of gene therapy in the management of thalassemia or sickle cell anemia.

Correction of thalassemia by gene transfer will necessitate introduction of a normal β-globin gene into pluripotent hematopoietic stem cells.[1004–1006] Experimental studies in mice have demonstrated that retroviral vectors are capable of transferring of foreign sequences to hematopoietic stem cells.[1008, 1009] Expression of transferred genes has been more problematic. The efficiency with which primate (or human) stem cells are infected by retroviral vectors appears to be lower than that observed with murine cells. Nonetheless, transfer of foreign sequences to long-term repopulating hematopoietic cells of primates and humans has been demonstrated.[1010]

For therapy of β-thalassemia (or sickle cell anemia), it will be necessary to express the transferred gene at high levels in erythroid cells. This has been a challenge in the field but recently vectors that incorporate elements of the LCR have been generated. Recently, lentiviral vectors containing such elements have been constructed. Indeed, it has become possible to achieve long-term correction of both sickle cell anemia and β-thalassemia in mouse models using these viruses.[1011–1013] During the next few years we may anticipate human gene therapy trials if vector safety can be demonstrated in preclinical studies.

Interaction of Thalassemia with Globin Structural Variants

In geographic areas where thalassemia mutations and structural variants of α- and β-globin genes are both commonly seen (such as Africa and Southeast Asia), compound heterozygotes with a thalassemia mutation and a structural variant are common.[1] In such double heterozygotes, disease may be more or less severe than that seen in individuals who are heterozygous for only the structural variant. For example, heterozygotes for a β[S] gene have 30 to 45 percent HbS and are usually clinically well, whereas patients with a β[S] gene and a β-thalassemia mutation (in the *trans* β gene) have 60 to 95 percent HbS and may have a severe sickling

disorder. Individuals with a β[S] gene and α-thalassemia trait generally have less HbS than those with sickle trait[1014, 1015] and are asymptomatic.[1016, 1017] The interaction of α- and β-thalassemia mutations and the HPFH mutations with the β[S] gene have been described in detail in Chapter 19.

Hemoglobin E β-Thalassemia

This syndrome is particularly common in Southeast Asia, where as many as 4000 to 5000 patients may reside in Thailand alone.[1018, 1019] As a result of immigration from Southeast Asia, HbE β-thalassemia is now a commonly encountered form of transfusion-dependent thalassemia in certain areas of the United States.[1020, 1021] Double heterozygotes not receiving transfusions have hemoglobin levels of 2.3 to 7 g/dL, depending primarily on the output of the β-thalassemia gene. Because α-thalassemia is common in Southeast Asia, more complex phenotypes may be observed.[1022] Nucleated red blood cells are found on the peripheral blood smear, whereas they are absent in patients homozygous for β[E]. HbE and HbA_2 account for 50 to 70 percent of total hemoglobin (5 percent HbA_2 by high performance liquid chromatography).[1021, 1023] Small quantities of HbA are found in association with a β[+]-thalassemia gene. Patients with HbE β-thalassemia are usually require transfusions and exhibit the clinical features of thalassemia major. In areas where intensive treatment is unavailable, the disease resembles classical thalassemia major with massive hepatosplenomegaly, hypersplenism, severe skeletal disease, and death from infection in childhood. Iron loading occurs either from transfusion or enhanced intestinal absorption.[1024] Proper treatment is the same as that recommended for thalassemia major or intermedia, depending on the requirement for regular blood transfusion.

Hemoglobin C β-Thalassemia

The β[C] gene, which encodes a variant β chain with a lysine-glutamic acid substitution at position 6,[1025] is common in blacks of West African origin. The only hematologic consequence of simple heterozygosity for the β[C] gene is increased target cells on the peripheral smear. Double heterozygotes with a β[C] gene and β-thalassemia genes exhibit a moderately severe hemolytic anemia with splenomegaly. The peripheral blood smear reveals hypochromia and microcytosis with many target cells. HbC comprises 65 to 95 percent of the total hemoglobin, depending on whether the thalassemia mutation is of the β[+] or β[0] variety. In the black population the disease is generally mild, reflecting the prevalence of mild β-thalassemia genes (see earlier),[485] whereas in Italian,[1026] North African,[1027] and Turkish patients[1028] the disease is more severe, particularly in those who have a β[0]-thalassemia mutation.

Thalassemic Hemoglobinopathies

As discussed in detail in earlier sections, several variant polypeptides can be described as thalassemic hemoglobinopathies. With the exception of HbE and the elongated

---

*Rodgers GP: Personal communication.

α-chain variants, these mutations are very uncommon. Interest in these mutations arises from the unique mechanisms by which they produce the thalassemia phenotype.[215, 1029] The most common thalassemic hemoglobinopathy is HbE disease.

Hemoglobin E Disease

As described earlier, the β^E mutation activates a cryptic splice site in exon-1 (see Fig. 20–10). Because the correct splice site is less efficiently utilized, decreased production of functional β-globin mRNA that codes for the variant ensues.[125] The incidence of the β^E gene is extraordinarily high in some populations ($\approx$ 30 percent in Laos, Cambodia, and Thailand).[1018, 1030] The occurrence of the gene observed in immigrants from Southeast Asia to the United States reflects these origins.[1021]

In the heterozygous form, patients are largely asymptomatic with a hemoglobin level greater than or equal to 12 g/dL, no reticulocytosis, an MCV of 74 ± 10.6 μ³ and an MCH of 25 ± 2.5 pg. The peripheral blood smear is distinguished by mild microcytosis and occasional target cells. Hemoglobin electrophoresis reveals HbE comigrating with HbA_2 in the range of 19 to 34 percent. The α-to-β biosynthetic ratio is usually greater than or equal to 0.8, hence, the mild nature of HbE trait.

Patients with homozygous HbE disease are also asymptomatic.[1019, 1023] The hemoglobin level is rarely less than 10 g/dL, and significant reticulocytosis is uncommon. The red cells, however, are markedly microcytic (of 50 to 66 μ³) and hypochromic (MCH of 20.1 pg). Targeting and occasional coarse stippling are evident on the smear. HbE comprises 90 percent or more of the total hemoglobin with varying levels of HbF.

The differential diagnosis of microcytic anemias in the Southeast Asian population initially requires exclusion of iron deficiency. When present, electrophoresis will identify HbE. However, its level may be diminished in the presence of α-thalassemia or iron deficiency, because the affinity of normal β chains for α- globin exceeds that of β^E

chains. The interaction of α-thalassemia mutations with the β^E gene is usually seen due to the high incidence of each in the Southeast Asian population.[1022]

Prenatal Diagnosis of Thalassemia

The morbidity and mortality associated with severe forms of thalassemia prompted efforts to develop effective prenatal diagnosis more than two decades ago. For the vast majority of β-thalassemias for which point mutations are usually responsible, early efforts focused on the determination of globin chain synthesis in fetal blood cells obtained by aspiration of placental vessels or direct visualization of fetal vessels.[1031–1033] The risk of fetal blood sampling at 18 to 20 weeks of gestation proved to be acceptably low when performed by experienced personnel (fetal loss rate of $\approx$3 percent; error rate of <0.5 percent), such that between 1975 and 1985 more than 7900 pregnancies were studied.[1034] As molecular methods and the knowledge of mutations leading to thalassemias improved, strategies for prenatal detection of these conditions evolved.

Successful prenatal diagnosis of α-thalassemia of the hydrops fetalis variety using solution hybridization methods to detect deficiency of α-globin genes in amniotic fluid cell DNA was first reported by Kan and associates in 1975.[1035] Southern blot analysis rapidly supplanted this approach for the detection of gene deletion in either the α- or β-thalassemias.[1036, 1037]

Detection of mutations in DNA rapidly became the preferred strategy for prenatal diagnosis as mutations became defined in β-thalassemias.[3] The introduction of PCR methods further facilitated detection of mutations and also permitted the use of nonradioactive tests.[1038] Coupled with chorionic villus biopsy, accurate and safe diagnoses can be accomplished within the first trimester of pregnancy.

Besides molecular biology, prenatal diagnosis of thalassemia has relied on identification of couples at risk, widespread public education, and genetic counseling. In

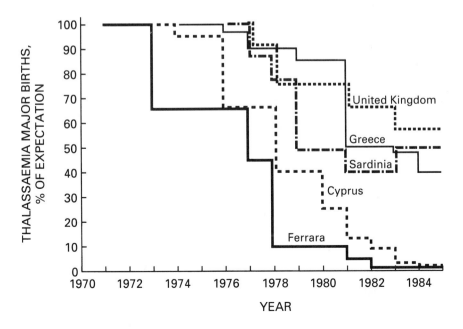

FIGURE 20–35. A decrease in the birth rate of infants with thalassemia major in Great Britain and several Mediterranean regions after the introduction of effective prenatal diagnosis. (Adapted from Modell B, Bulyzhenkov V: Distribution and control of some genetic disorders. World Health Stat Q 1988; 41:209. By permission of the World Health Organization.)

countries where the incidence of β-thalassemia is high and the burden of disease to the overall population great, such as on the island of Sardinia and in Greece, intensive prevention programs have been established and have proved to be extraordinarily successful. For example, the births of children with β-thalassemia in these area have been reduced by more than 90 percent in recent years[949, 1039–1043] (Fig. 20–35). These represent major achievements in the prevention of genetic disease and paradigms for other disorders.★

REFERENCES

1. Weatherall DJ, Clegg JB: The Thalassaemia Syndromes, 4th ed. Oxford, Blackwell Scientific Publications, 2001.
2. Higgs DR, Vickers MA, et al: A review of the molecular genetics of the human alpha-globin gene cluster. Blood 1989; 73:1081.
3. Kazazian HH Jr: The thalassemia syndromes: Molecular basis and prenatal diagnosis in 1990. Semin Hematol 1990; 27:209.
4. Karlsson S, Nienhuis AW: Developmental regulation of human globin genes. Annu Rev Biochem 1985; 54:1071.
5. Collins FS, Weissman SM: The molecular genetics of human hemoglobin. Prog Nucleic Acid Res Mol Biol 1984; 31:315.
6. Bunn HF, Forget BG: Hemoglobin: Molecular, Genetic and Clinical Aspects. Philadelphia, WB Saunders, 1986.
7. Boyer SH, Belding TK, et al: Fetal hemoglobin restricted to a few erythrocytes (F-cells) in normal human adults. Science 1975; 188:361.
8. Wood WG, Stamatoyannopoulos G, et al: F-cells in the adult: Normal values and levels in individuals with hereditary and acquired elevations of Hb F. Blood 1975; 46:671.
9. Miyoshi K, Kaneto Y, et al: X-linked dominant control of F-cells in normal adult life: Characterization of the Swiss type as hereditary persistence of fetal hemoglobin regulated dominantly by gene(s) on X chromosome. Blood 1988; 72:1854.
10. Craig JE, Rochette J, et al: Dissecting the loci controlling fetal haemoglobin production on chromosomes 11p and 6q by the regressive approach. Nat Genet 1996; 12:58.
11. Maniatis T, Fritsch EF, et al: The molecular genetics of human hemoglobins. Annu Rev Genet 1980; 14:145.
12. Liebhaber SA: Alpha thalassemia. Hemoglobin 1989; 13:685.
13. Deisseroth A, Nienhuis AW, et al: Localization of the human alpha-globin structural gene to chromosome 16 in somatic cell hybrids by molecular hybridization assay. Cell 1977; 12:205.
14. Deisseroth A, Nienhuis AW, et al: Chromosomal localization of the human beta-globin gene on chromosome 11 in somatic cell hybrids. Proc Natl Acad Sci USA 1978; 75:1459.
15. Lauer J, Shen CKJ, et al: The chromosomal arrangement of human alpha-like globin genes: Sequence homology and alpha-globin gene deletions. Cell 1980; 20:119.
16. Liebhaber SA, Goossens M, et al: Homology and concerted evolution at the alpha-l and alpha-2 loci of human alpha-globin. Nature 1981; 290:26.
17. Proudfoot NJ, Gil A, et al: The structure of the human zeta-globin gene and a closely linked, nearly identical pseudogene. Cell 1982; 31:553.
18. Fritsch EF, Lawn RM, et al: Molecular cloning and characterization of the human beta-like globin gene cluster. Cell 1980; 19:959.
19. Efstradiatis A, Posakony JW, et al: The structure and evolution of the human beta-globin gene family. Cell 1980; 21:653.
20. Slightom JL, Blechl AE, et al: Human fetal gamma and gamma globin genes: Complete nucleotide sequences suggest that DNA can be exchanged between these duplicated genes. Cell 1980; 21:627.
21. Baralle FE, Shoulders CC, et al: The primary structure of the human epsilon-globin gene. Cell 1980; 21:621.
22. Humphries RK, Ley T, et al: Differences in human alpha-, beta- and delta-globin gene expression in monkey kidney cells. Cell 1982; 30:173.
23. Kosche KA, Dobkin C, et al: DNA sequences regulating human beta globin gene expression. Nucleic Acids Res 1985; 13:7781.
24. Ross J, Pizarro A: Human beta and delta globin messenger RNAs turn over at different rates. J Mol Biol 1983; 167:607.
25. Pataryas HA, Stamatoyannopoulos G: Hemoglobins in human fetuses: Evidence for adult hemoglobin production after the 11th gestational week. Blood 1972; 39:688.
26. Henri A, Testa U, et al: Disappearance of the Hb F and i antigen during the first year of life. Am J Hematol 1980; 9:161.
27. Terrenato L, Bertilaccio C, et al: The switch from haemoglobin F to A: The time course of qualitative and quantitative variations of haemoglobins after birth. Br J Haematol 1981; 47:31.
28. Smale ST, Baltimore D: The "initiator" as a transcriptional control element. Cell 1989; 57:103.
29. Lewis BA, Orkin SH: A functional initiator element in the human β-globin promoter. J Biol Chem 1995; 270:28139.
30. Dynan WS, Tjian R: Control of eukaryotic messenger RNA synthesis by sequence-specific DNA-binding proteins. Nature 1985; 316:774.
31. McKnight S, Tjian R: Transcriptional selectivity of viral genes in mammalian cells. Cell 1986; 46:795.
32. Maniatis T, Goodbourn S, et al: Regulation of inducible and tissue-specific gene expression. Science 1987; 236:1237.
33. Saltzman AG, Weinmann R: Promoter specificity and modulation of RNA polymerase II transcription. FASEB J 1989; 3:1723.
34. Dynan WS: Modularity in promoters and enhancers. Cell 1989; 58:1.
35. Guarente L: UASs and enhancers: Common mechanism of transcriptional activation in yeast and mammals. Cell 1988; 52:303.
36. Muller MM, Gerster T, et al: Enhancer sequences and the regulation of gene transcription. Eur J Biochem 1988; 176:485.
37. Peterson MG, Tanese N, et al: Functional domains and upstream activation properties of cloned human TATA binding protein. Science 1990; 248:1625.
38. Kao CC, Lieberman PM, et al: Cloning of a transcriptionally active human TATA binding factor. Science 1990; 248:1646.
39. Lewin B: Commitment and activation at pol II promoters: A tail of protein-protein interactions. Cell 1990; 61:1161.
40. Takihara Y, Nakamura T, et al: A novel mutation in the TATA box in a Japanese patient with beta+-thalassemia. Blood 1986; 67:547.
41. Fei YJ, Stoming TA, et al: Beta-thalassemia due to a T→A mutation within the ATA box. Biochem Biophys Res Commun 1988; 153:741.
42. Cai SP, Zhang JZ, et al: A new TATA box mutation detected at prenatal diagnosis for beta-thalassemia. Am J Hum Genet 1989; 45:112.
43. Antonarakis SE, Irkin SH, et al: Beta thalassemia in American blacks: Novel mutations in the TATA box and an acceptor splice site. Proc Natl Acad Sci USA 1984; 81:1154.
44. Huang S-Z, Wong C, et al: The same TATA box beta thalassemia mutation in Chinese and U.S. blacks: Another example of independent origins of mutation. Hum Genet 1986; 74:152.
45. Poncz M, Ballantine M, et al: Beta thalassemia in a Kurdish Jew. J Biol Chem 1983; 257:5994.
46. Orkin SH, Sexton JP, et al: ATA box transcription mutation in beta-thalassemia. Nucleic Acids Res 1983; 11:4727.
47. Hoey T, Dynlacht BD, et al: Isolation and characterization of the *Drosophila* gene encoding the TATA box binding protein, TFIID. Cell 1990; 61:1179.
48. Orkin SH: Regulation of globin gene expression in erythroid cells. Eur J Biochem 1995; 231:271.
48a. Li Q, Peterson KR, Fang X, Stamatoyannopoulos G: Locus control regions. Blood 2002; 100:3077.
49. Tsang AP, Visvader JE, et al: FOG, a multitype zinc finger protein acts as a cofactor for transcription factor GATA-1 in erythroid and megakaryocytic differentiation. Cell 1997; 90:109.
50. Crispino JD, Lodish MB, et al: Use of altered specificity mutants to probe a specific protein-protein interaction in differentiation: The GATA-1:FOG complex. Mol Cell 1999; 3:219.
51. Kadonaga JT, Carner KR, et al: Isolation of cDNA encoding transcription factor Sp1 and functional analysis of the DNA binding domain. Cell 1987; 51:1079.

★References 256, 260, 261, 264–267, 271–274, 277, 278, 287, and 339–343.

52. Perkins AC, Sharpe AH, et al: Lethal β-thalassaemia in mice lacking the erythroid CACCC-transcription factor EKLF. Nature 1995; 375:318.

53. Andrews NC, Erdjument-Bromage H, et al: Erythroid transcription factor NF-E2 is a haematopoietic-specific basic-leucine zipper protein. Nature 1993; 362:722.

54. Andrews NC, Kotkow KJ, et al: The ubiquitous subunit of erythroid transcription factor NF-E2 is a small basic-leucine zipper protein related to the v-*maf* oncogene. Proc Natl Acad Sci USA 1993; 90:11488.

55. Lu SJ, Rowan S, et al: Retroviral integration within the Fli-2 locus results in inactivation of the erythroid transcription factor NF-E2 in Friend erythroleukemias: Evidence that NF-E2 is essential for globin expression. Proc Natl Acad Sci USA 1994; 91:8398.

56. Kotkow KJ, Orkin SH: Dependence of globin gene expression in mouse erythroleukemia cells on the NF-E2 heterodimer. Mol Cell Biol 1995; 15:4640.

57. Shivadasani RA, Orkin SH: Erythropoiesis and globin gene expression in mice lacking the transcription factor NF-E2. Proc Natl Acad Sci USA 1995; 92:8690.

58. Chada K, Magram J, et al: Specific expression of a foreign beta-globin gene in erythroid cells of transgenic mice. Nature 1985; 314:377.

59. Magram J, Chada K, et al: Developmental regulation of a cloned adult beta-globin gene in transgenic mice. Nature 1985; 315:338.

60. Townes TM, Lingrel JB, et al: Erythroid-specific expression of human beta-globin genes in transgenic mice. EMBO J 1985; 4:1715.

61. Costantini F, Radice G, et al: Developmental regulation of human globin genes in transgenic mice. Cold Spring Harbor Symp Quant Biol 1985; 50:361.

62. Chada K, Magram J, et al: An embryonic pattern of expression of a human fetal globin gene in transgenic mice. Nature 1986; 319:685.

63. Kollias G, Wrighton N, et al: Regulated expression of human ^{A}gamma-, beta-, and hybrid gamma beta-globin genes in transgenic mice: Manipulation of the developmental expression patterns. Cell 1986; 46:89.

64. Tuan D, Solomon W, et al: The "beta-like-globin" gene domain in human erythroid cells. Proc Natl Acad Sci USA 1985; 82:6384.

65. Tuan DY, Solomon WB, et al: An erythroid-specific, developmental-stage-independent enhancer far upstream of the human "beta-like globin" genes. Proc Natl Acad Sci USA 1989; 86:2554.

66. Grosveld F, van AG, et al: Position-independent, high-level expression of the human beta-globin gene in transgenic mice. Cell 1987; 51:975.

67. Higgs DR, Wood WG, et al: A major positive regulatory region is located far upstream of the human α-globin gene locus. Genes Dev 1990; 4:1588.

68. Gibbons RJ, Brueton L, et al: Clinical and hematologic aspects of the X-linked α-thalassemia/mental retardation syndrome (ATR-X). Am J Med Genet 1995; 55:288.

69. Gibbons RJ, Picketts DJ, et al: Mutations in a putative global transcriptional regulator cause X-linked mental retardation with alpha-thalassemia (ATR-X syndrome). Cell 1995; 80:837.

70. Raich N, Clegg CH, et al: GATA-1 and YY1 are developmental repressors of the human epsilon-globin gene. EMBO J 1995; 14:801.

71. Choi OR, Engel JD: Developmental regulation of beta-globin gene switching. Cell 1988; 55:17.

72. Jane SM, Ney PA, et al: Identification of a stage selector element in the human γ-globin gene promoter that fosters preferential interaction with the 5' HS2 enhancer when in competition with the β-promoter. EMBO J 1992; 11:2961.

73. Nienhuis AW, Anagnou NP, et al: Advances in thalassemia research. Blood 1984; 63:738.

74. Orkin SH, Kazazian HH Jr: Mutation and polymorphism of the human beta-globin gene and its surrounding DNA. Annu Rev Genet 1984; 18:131.

75. Benz EJ Jr, Nathan DG: Pathophysiology of the anemia in thalassemia. In Weatherall DJ (ed): Congenital Disorders of Erythropoiesis. Amsterdam, Elsevier, 1976, p 205.

76. Fessas P, Loukopoulos D: The beta-thalassemias. Clin Haematol 1974; 3:411.

77. Nathan DG, Gunn RB: Thalassemia: The consequences of unbalanced hemoglobin synthesis. Am J Med 1966; 41:815.

78. Nathan DG, Stossel TB, et al: Influence of hemoglobin precipitation on erythrocyte metabolism in alpha and beta thalassemia. J Clin Invest 1969; 48:33.

79. Nathan DG: Thalassemia. N Eng J Med 1972; 286:586.

80. Wood WG, Weatherall DJ, et al: Interaction of heterocellular hereditary persistence of fetal hemoglobin with beta thalassemia and sickle cell anemia. Nature 1976; 264:247.

81. Prchal J, Stamatoyannopoulos G: Two siblings with unusually mild homozygous beta thalassemia: A didactic example of nonallelic modifier gene on the expressivity of a monogenic disorder. Am J Med Genet 1981; 10:291.

82. Safaya S, Rieder RF, et al: Homozygous beta-thalassemia without anemia. Blood 1989; 73:324.

83. Kanavakis K, Wainscoat JS, et al: The interaction of alpha thalassemia with beta thalassemia. Br J Haematol 1982; 52:465.

84. Haldane JBS: The rate of mutation of human genes. In Proceedings of the VIII International Congress on Genetics and Heredity, 1949, p 267.

85. Livingstone FB: Frequency of Hemoglobin Variants. New York, Oxford University Press, 1985.

86. Weatherall DJ: Common genetic disorders of the red cell and the 'malaria hypothesis.' Ann Trop Med Parasitol 1987; 81:539.

87. Frazer GR, Kitsos C., et al.: Thalassemias, abnormal hemoglobins, and glucose-6-phosphate dehydrogenase deficiency in the Arta area of Greece: Diagnostic and genetic aspects of complete village studies. Ann NY Acad Sci 1964; 119:415.

88. Kanavakis E, Tzotzos S, et al: Molecular basis and prevalence of alpha-thalassemia in Greece. Birth Defects 1988; 23:377.

89. Falusi AG, Esan GJ, et al: Alpha-thalassaemia in Nigeria: Its interaction with sickle-cell disease. Eur J Haematol 1987; 38:370.

90. Flint J, Hill AV, et al: High frequencies of alpha-thalassaemia are the result of natural selection by malaria. Nature 1986; 321:744.

91. Flint J, Hill AV, et al: Alpha globin genotypes in two North European populations [letter]. Br J Haematol 1986; 63:796.

92. Shimizu K, Harano T, et al: Abnormal arrangements in the alpha- and gamma-globin gene clusters in a relatively large group of Japanese newborns. Am J Hum Genet 1986; 38:45.

93. Flint J, Harding RM, et al: The population genetics of the haemoglobinopathies. Bailieres Clin Haematol 1998; 11:1.

94. Siniscalco M, Bernini L, et al: Population genetics of haemoglobin variants, thalassemia and glucose-6-phosphate dehydrogenase deficiency, with particular reference to malaria hypothesis. Bull WHO 1966; 34:379.

95. Willcox M, Bjorkman A, et al: Falciparum malaria and beta-thalassaemia trait in northern Liberia. Ann Trop Med Parasitol 1983; 77:335.

96. Oppenheimer SJ, Higgs DR, et al: Alpha thalassaemia in Papua New Guinea. Lancet 1984; 1:424.

97. Teo CG, Wong HB: The innate resistance of thalassemia to malaria: A review of the evidence and possible mechanisms. Singapore Med J 1985; 26:504.

98. Hill AV, Bowden DK, et al: Beta thalassemia in Melanesia: Association with malaria and characterization of a common variant (IVS-1 nt 5 G→C). Blood 1988; 72:9.

99. Lell B, May J, et al: The role of red blood cell polymorphisms in resistance and susceptibility to malaria. Clin Infect Dis 1999; 28:794.

100. Sakai Y, Kobayashi S, et al: Molecular analysis of alpha-thalassemia in Nepal: Correlation with malaria endemicity. J Hum Genet 2000; 45:127.

101. Clegg JB, Weatherall DJ: Thalassemia and malaria: New insights into an old problem. Proc Assoc Am Physicians 1999; 111:278.

102. Pasvol G, Weatherall DJ, et al: Effects of foetal haemoglobin on susceptibility of red cells to *Plasmodium falciparum*. Nature 1977; 270:171.

103. Nagel RL, Roth EF: Malaria and red cell genetic defects. Blood 1989; 74:1213.

104. Brockelman CR, Wongsattayanont B, et al: Thalassemic erythrocytes inhibit in vitro growth of *Plasmodium falciparum*. J Clin Microbiol 1987; 25:56.

105. Pattanapanyasat K, Yongvanitchit K, et al: Impairment of *Plasmodium falciparum* growth in thalassemic red blood cells: Further evidence by using biotin labeling and flow cytometry. Blood 1999; 93:3116.

106. Luzzi GA, Merry AH, et al: Surface antigen expression on *Plasmodium falciparum*-infected erythrocytes is modified in alpha- and beta-thalassemia. J Exp Med 1991; 1991:785.

107. Ifediba TC, Stern A, et al: *Plasmodium falciparum* in vitro: Diminished growth in hemoglobin H disease erythrocytes. Blood 1985; 65:452.

108. Carlson J, Nash GB, et al: Natural protection against severe *Plasmodium falciparum* malaria due to impaired rosette formation. Blood 1994; 84:3909.

109. Gonzalez-Redondo JM, Stoming TA, et al: A C→T substitution at nt −101 in a conserved DNA sequence of the promotor region of the beta-globin gene is associated with "silent" beta-thalassemia. Blood 1989; 73:1705.

110. Orkin SH, Antonarakis SE, et al: Base substitution at position −88 in a beta-thalassemic globin gene. Further evidence for the role of distal promoter element ACACCC. J Biol Chem 1984; 259:8679.

111. Rund D, Filon D, et al: Molecular analysis of beta thalassemia in Kurdish Jews: Novel mutations and expression studies. Blood 1989; 74:821A.

112. Orkin SH, Kazazian HH Jr, et al: Linkage of beta thalassemia mutations and beta-globin gene polymorphisms with DNA polymorphisms in the human beta-globin gene cluster. Nature 1982; 296:627.

113. Wong C, Dowling CE, et al: Characterization of beta-thalassaemia mutations using direct genomic sequencing of amplified single copy DNA. Nature 1987; 330:384.

114. Orkin SH, Goff SC, et al: Mutation in an intervening sequence splice junction in man. Proc Natl Acad Sci USA 1981; 78:5041.

115. Felber BK, Orkin SH, et al: Abnormal RNA splicing causes one form of alpha thalassemia. Cell 1982; 29:895.

116. Kazazian HH Jr, Orkin SH, et al: Molecular characterization of seven beta-thalassemia mutations in Asian Indians. EMBO J 1984; 3:593.

117. Chibani J, Vidaud M, et al: The peculiar spectrum of beta-thalassemia genes in Tunisia. Hum Genet 1988; 78:190.

118. Gonzalez-Redondo JM, Stoming TA, et al: Severe Hb S-beta zero-thalassemia with a T→C substitution in the donor splice site of the first intron of the beta-globin gene. Br J Haematol 1989; 71:113.

119. Kazazian HH Jr, Boehm CD: Molecular basis and prenatal diagnosis of beta-thalassemia. Blood 1988; 72:1107.

120. Treisman R, Proudfoot NJ, et al: A single base change at a splice site in a beta thalassemia gene causes abnormal RNA splicing. Cell 1982; 29:903.

121. Wong C, Antonarakis SE, et al: On the origin and spread of beta-thalassemia: Recurrent observation of four mutations in different ethnic groups. Proc Natl Acad Sci USA 1986; 83:6529.

122. Orkin SH, Sexton JP, et al: Inactivation of an acceptor RNA splice site by a short deletion in beta-thalassemia. J Biol Chem 1983; 258:7249.

123. Atweh GF, Anagnou NP, et al: Beta-thalassemia resulting from a single nucleotide substitution in an acceptor splice site. Nucleic Acids Res 1985; 13:777.

124. Gonzalez-Redondo JM, Stoming TA, et al: Hb Monroe or alpha$_2$beta$_2$ 30(B12)Arg→Thr, a variant associated with beta-thalassemia due to A G→C substitution adjacent to the donor splice site of the first intron. Hemoglobin 1989; 13:67.

125. Kalydjieva L, Eigel A, et al: The molecular basis of thalassemia in Bulgaria. Presented at the 3rd International Conference on Thalassemia and the Hemoglobinopathies, Sardinia, 1989.

126. Cheng TC, Orkin SH, et al: Beta thalassemia in Chinese: Use of in vivo RNA analysis and oligonucleotide hybridization in systematic characterization of molecular defects. Proc Natl Acad Sci USA 1984; 81:2821.

127. Atweh GF, Wong C, et al: A new mutation in IVS-1 of the human beta globin gene causing beta thalassemia due to abnormal splicing. Blood 1987; 70:147.

128. Gonzalez-Redondo JM, Stoming TA, et al: Clinical and genetic heterogeneity in black patients with homozygous beta-thalassemia from the southeastern United States. Blood 1988; 72:1007.

129. Lapoumeroulie C, Pagnier J, et al: Beta thalassemia due to a novel mutation in IVS 1 sequence donor site consensus sequence creating a restriction site. Biochem Biophys Res Commun 1986; 139:709.

130. Wong C, Antonarakis SE, et al: Beta-thalassemia due to two novel nucleotide substitutions in consensus acceptor splice sequences of the beta-globin gene. Blood 1989; 73:914.

131. Beldjord C, Lapoumeroulie C, et al: A novel beta thalassemia gene with a single base mutation in the conserved polypyrimidine sequence at the 3′ end of IVS 2. Nucleic Acids Res 1988; 16:4927.

132. Yang KG, Kutlar F, et al: Molecular characterization of beta-globin gene mutations in Malay patients with Hb E-beta-thalassaemia and thalassaemia major. Br J Haematol 1989; 72:73.

133. Goldsmith ME, Humphries RK, et al: Silent nucleotide substitution in a beta$^+$-thalassemia globin gene activates splice site in coding sequence RNA. Proc Natl Acad Sci USA 1983; 80:2318.

134. Orkin SH, Kazazian HH Jr, et al: Abnormal RNA processing due to the exon mutation of the beta E globin gene. Nature 1982; 300:768.

135. Orkin SH, Antonarakis SE, et al: Abnormal processing of beta Knossos RNA. Blood 1984; 64:311.

136. Spritz RA, Jagadeeswaran P, et al: Base substitution in an intervening sequence of a beta$^+$ thalassemic human globin gene. Proc Natl Acad Sci USA 1981; 78:2455.

137. Westaway D, Williamson R: An intron nucleotide sequence variant in a cloned beta$^+$ thalassemia globin gene. Nucleic Acids Res 1981; 9:1777.

138. Metherall JE, Collins FS, et al: Beta zero thalassemia caused by a base substitution that creates an alternative splice acceptor site in an intron. EMBO J 1986; 5:2551.

139. Dobkin C, Pergolizzi RG, et al: Abnormal splice in a mutant human beta-globin gene not at the site of a mutation. Proc Natl Acad Sci USA 1983; 80:1184.

140. Higgs DR, Goodbourn SE, et al: Alpha-thalassaemia caused by a polyadenylation signal mutation. Nature 1983; 306:398.

141. Thein SL, Wallace RB, et al: The polyadenylation site mutation in the alpha-globin gene cluster. Blood 1988; 71:313.

142. Orkin SH, Cheng TC, et al: Thalassemia due to a mutation in the cleavage-polyadenylation signal of the human beta-globin gene. EMBO J 1985; 4:453.

143. Jankovic L, Efremov GD, et al: Three novel mutations leading to beta thalassemia. Blood 1989; 74:226A.

144. Pirastu M, Saglio G, et al: Initiation codon mutation as a cause of alpha thalassemia. J Biol Chem 1984; 259:12315.

145. Moi P, Cash FE, et al: An initiation codon mutation (AUG→GUG) of the human alpha 1-globin gene. Structural characterization and evidence for a mild thalassemic phenotype. J Clin Invest 1987; 80:1416.

146. Olivieri NF, Chang LS, et al: An alpha-globin gene initiation codon mutation in a black family with HbH disease. Blood 1987; 70:729.

147. Morle F, Starck J, et al: Alpha-thalassemia due to the deletion of nucleotides −2 and −3 preceding the AUG initiation codon affects translation efficiency both in vitro and in vivo. Nucleic Acids Res 1986; 14:3279.

148. Morle F, Lopez B, et al: Alpha thalassaemia associated with the deletion of two nucleotides at position −2 and −3 preceding the AUG codon. EMBO J 1985; 4:1245.

149. Liebhaber SA, Coleman MB, et al: Molecular basis for nondeletion alpha-thalassemia in American blacks: Alpha 2(116GAG→UAG). J Clin Invest 1987; 80:154.

150. Chang JC, Kan YW: Beta zero thalassemia, a nonsense mutation in man. Proc Natl Acad Sci USA 1979; 76:2886.

151. Fucharoen S, Fucharoen G, et al: A novel ochre mutation in the beta-thalassemia gene of a Thai. Identification by direct cloning of the entire β-globin gene amplified using polymerase chain reactions. J Biol Chem 1989; 264:7780.

152. Boehm CD, Dowling CE, et al: Use of oligonucleotide hybridization in the characterization of a beta zero-thalassemia gene (beta 37 TGG→TGA) in a Saudi Arabian family. Blood 1986; 67:1185. [Published erratum appears in Blood 1986;68:323.]

153. Trecartin RF, Liebhaber SA, et al: Beta zero thalassemia in Sardinia is caused by a nonsense mutation. J Clin Invest 1981; 68:1017.

154. Chehab FF, Honig GR, et al: Spontaneous mutation in beta-thalassaemia producing the same nucleotide substitution as that in a common hereditary form. Lancet 1986; 1:3.

155. Atweh GF, Brickner HE, et al: New amber mutation in a beta-thalassemic gene with nonmeasurable levels of mutant messenger RNA in vivo. J Clin Invest 1988; 82:557.

156. Safaya S, Rieder RF: Dysfunctional alpha-globin gene in hemoglobin H disease in blacks. A dinucleotide deletion produces a frameshift and a termination codon. J Biol Chem 1988; 263:4328.

157. Kollia P, Gonzalez-Redondo JM, et al: Frameshift codon 5 [Fsc-5 (−CT)] thalassemia; a novel mutation detected in a Greek patient. Hemoglobin 1989; 13:597.

158. Kazazian HH Jr, Orkin SH, et al: Beta thalassemia due to a deletion of the nucleotide which is substituted in the beta S-globin gene. Am J Hum Genet 1983; 35:1028.

159. Chan V, Chan TK, et al: A novel beta-thalassemia frameshift mutation (codon 14/15), detectable by direct visualization of abnormal restriction fragment in amplified genomic DNA. Blood 1988; 72:1420.

160. Schnee J, Griese EU, et al: Beta-thalassemia gene analysis in a Turkish family reveals a 7 BP deletion in the coding region [letter]. Blood 1989; 73:2224.

161. Kimura A, Matsunaga E, et al: Structural analysis of a beta-thalassemia gene found in Taiwan. J Biol Chem 1983; 258:2748.

162. Kinniburgh AJ, Maquat LE, et al: mRNA-deficient beta zero thalassemia results from a single nucleotide deletion. Nucleic Acids Res 1982; 10:5421.

163. Chehab FF, Winterhalter KH, et al: Characterization of a spontaneous mutation in beta-thalassemia associated with advanced paternal age. Blood 1989; 74:852.

164. DiMarzo R, Dowling CE, et al: The spectrum of beta-thalassaemia mutations in Sicily. Br J Haematol 1988; 69:393.

165. Clegg JB, Weatherall DJ, et al: Haemoglobin Constant Spring—A chain termination mutant? Nature 1971; 234:337.

166. Milner PF, Clegg JB, et al: Haemoglobin H disease due to a unique haemoglobin variant with an elongated alpha chain. Lancet 1971; 1:729.

167. Clegg JB, Weatherall DJ, et al: Haemoglobin Icaria, a new chain termination mutant which causes alpha thalassemia. Nature 1974; 251:245.

168. De Jong WW, Khan PM, et al: Hemoglobin Koya Dora: High frequency of a chain termination mutant. Am J Hum Genet 1975; 27:81.

169. Bradley TB, Wohl RC, et al: Elongation of the alpha globin chain in a black family: Interaction with Hb G Philadelphia. Clin Res 1975; 23:1314.

170. Lehmann H, Casey R, et al: Hemoglobin Tak: A beta chain elongation. Br J Haematol 1975; 31:119.

171. Honig GR, Shamsuddin M, et al: Hemoglobin Evanston (alpha 14 Trp→Arg): An unstable alpha-chain variant expressed as alpha-thalassemia. J Clin Invest 1984; 73:1740.

172. Sanguansermsri T, Matragoon S: Hemoglobin Suan-Dok (alpha 2 109(G16) Leu-Arg beta 2): An unstable variant associated with alpha thalassemia. Hemoglobin 1979; 3:161.

173. Steinberg MH, Coleman MB, et al: Thalassemic expression of an alpha-2 globin structural mutant. Blood 1987; 70:80A.

174. Honig GR, Shamsuddin M, et al: Hemoglobin Petah Tikvah (alpha110 Ala→Asp): A new unstable variant with alpha thalassemia like expression. Blood 1981; 57:705.

175. Goossens M, Lee KY, et al: Globin structural mutant alpha125 Leu→Pro is a novel cause of alpha thalassemia. Nature 1982; 296:864.

176. Liebhaber SA, Kan YW: Alpha thalassemia caused by an unstable alpha-globin mutant. J Clin Invest 1983; 71:461.

177. Podda A, Galanello R, et al: A new unstable hemoglobin variant producing a beta thalassemia like phenotype. Presented at the 3rd International Conference on Thalassemia and the Hemoglobinopathies, Sardinia, 1989.

178. Kobayashi Y, Fukumaki Y, et al: A novel globin structural mutant, Showa-Yakushiji (beta 110 Leu-Pro) causing a beta-thalassemia phenotype. Blood 1987; 70:1688.

179. Adams JG, Steinberg MH, et al: The structure of hemoglobin Indianapolis (β^{112}(G14) arginine): An unstable variant detectable only by isotopic labelling. J Biol Chem 1979; 254:3479.

180. Kazazian HH Jr, Dowling CE, et al: Thalassemia mutations in exon 3 of the beta globin gene often cause a dominant form of thalassemia and show no predilection for malarial-endemic regions of the world. Am J Hum Genet 1989; 45:A242.

181. Hattori Y, Yamane A, et al: Characterization of beta-thalassemia mutations among the Japanese. Hemoglobin 1989; 13:657.

182. Ristaldi MS, Pirastu M, et al: A spontaneous mutation produced a novel elongated beta-globin chain structural variant (Hb Agnana) with a thalassemia-like phenotype [letter]. Blood 1990; 75:1378.

183. Beris P, Miescher PA, et al: Inclusion body beta-thalassemia trait in a Swiss family is caused by an abnormal hemoglobin (Geneva) with an altered and extended beta chain carboxy-terminus due to a modification in codon beta 114. Blood 1988; 72:801.

184. Thein SL, Hesketh C, et al: Molecular basis for dominantly inherited inclusion body beta thalassemia. Proc Natl Acad Sci USA 1990; 87:3924.

185. Kazazian HH Jr, Orkin SH, et al: Characterization of a spontaneous mutation to a beta-thalassemia allele. Am J Hum Genet 1986; 38:860.

186. Fei YJ, Stoming TA, et al: One form of inclusion body beta-thalassemia is due to a GAA→TAA mutation at codon 121 of the beta chain [letter]. Blood 1989; 73:1075.

187. Ristaldi MS, Murru S, et al: The C-T substitution in the distal CACCC box of the beta-globin gene promoter is a common cause of silent beta thalassemia in the Italian population. Br J Haematol 1990; 74:480.

188. Nuez B, Michalovich D, et al: Defective haematopoiesis in fetal liver resulting from inactivation of the EKLF gene. Nature 1995; 375:316.

189. Brinster RL, Allen JM, et al: Introns increase transcriptional efficiency in transgenic mice. Proc Natl Acad Sci USA 1988; 85:836.

190. Buchman AR, Berg P: Comparison of intron-dependent and intron-independent gene expression. Mol Cell Biol 1988; 8:4395.

191. Chang DD, Sharp PA: Messenger RNA transport and HIV rev regulation. Science 1990; 249:614.

192. Padanilam BJ, Huisman TH: The beta zero-thalassemia in an American black family is due to a single nucleotide substitution in the acceptor splice junction of the second intervening sequence. Am J Hematol 1986; 22:259.

193. Chehab FF, Der KV, et al: The molecular basis of beta-thalassemia in Lebanon: Application to prenatal diagnosis. Blood 1987; 69:1141.

194. Treisman R, Orkin SH, et al: Specific transcription and RNA splicing defects in five cloned beta-thalassaemia genes. Nature 1983; 302:591.

195. Busslinger M, Moschonas N, et al: Beta-thalassemia: Aberrant splicing results from a single point mutation in an intron. Cell 1981; 27:289.

196. Fukumaki Y, Ghosh PK, et al Abnormally spliced messenger RNA in erythroid cells from patients with beta thalassemia and monkey kidney cells expressing a cloned beta-thalassemia gene. Cell 1982; 28:585.

197. Whitelaw E, Proudfoot N: Alpha-thalassaemia caused by a poly(A) site mutation reveals that transcriptional termination is linked to 3′ end processing in the human alpha 2 globin gene. EMBO J 1986; 5:2915.

198. Kozak M: An analysis of 5′-noncoding sequences from 699 vertebrate messenger RNAs. Nucleic Acids Res 1987; 15:8125.

199. Baserga SJ, Benz EJ: Nonsense mutations in the human beta-globin gene affect mRNA metabolism. Proc Natl Acad Sci USA 1988; 85:2056.

200. Chang JC, Temple GF, et al: Suppression of the nonsense mutation in homozygous beta thalassemia. Nature 1979; 281:602.

201. Orkin SH, Goff SC: Nonsense and frameshift mutations in β thalassemia detected in cloned β globin genes. J Biol Chem 1981; 256:9782.

202. Benz EJ Jr, Forget BG, et al: Variability in the amount of beta-globin mRNA in beta thalassemia. Cell 1978; 14:299.

203. Maquat LE, Kinniburgh AJ, et al: Unstable beta-globin mRNA in mRNA-deficient beta-thalassemia. Cell 1981; 27:543.

204. Humphries RK, Ley TJ, et al: Beta-39-thalassemia gene: A premature termination codon causes beta-mRNA deficiency without changing cytoplasmic beta-mRNA stability. Blood 1984; 23:64.

205. Takeshita K, Forget BG, et al: Intranuclear defect in beta-globin mRNA accumulation due to a premature translation termination codon. Blood 1984; 64:13.

206. Liebhaber SA, Kan YW: Differentiation of the mRNA transcripts originating from the alpha-1 and alpha-2 globin loci in normals and alpha thalassemics. J Clin Invest 1981; 68:439.

207. Hunt DM, Higgs DR, et al: Haemoglobin Constant Spring has an unstable alpha chain messenger RNA. Br J Haematol 1982; 51:405.

208. Derry S, Wood WG, et al: Hematologic and biosynthetic studies in homozygous hemoglobin Constant Spring. J Clin Invest 1984; 73:1673.

209. Bunn HF, Schmidt GJ, et al: Hemoglobin Cranston, an unstable variant having an elongated beta chain due to non-homologous cross over between two normal beta chain genes. Proc Natl Acad Sci USA 1975; 72:3609.

210. Bunn HF: Subunit assembly of hemoglobin: An important determinant of hematologic phenotype. Blood 1987; 69:1.

211. Eaton WA: The relationship between coding sequences and function in haemoglobins. Nature 1980; 284:183.

212. Adams JG, III, Coleman MB, et al: Modulation of fetal hemoglobin synthesis by iron deficiency. N Engl J Med 1985; 313:1402.

213. Chui DHK, Patterson M, et al: Hemoglobin Bart's disease in an Italian boy. N Engl J Med 1990; 323:179.

214. Kihm AJ, Kong Y et al: An abundant erythroid protein that stabilizes free alpha-haemoglobin. Nature 2002; 417:758.

215. Adams HGI, Coleman MB: Structural hemoglobin variants that produce the phenotype of thalassemia. Semin Hematol 1990; 27:229.

216. Flavell RA, Bernards R, et al: The structure of the human beta-globin gene in beta-thalassaemia. Nucleic Acids Res 1979; 6:2749.

217. Orkin SH, Old JM, et al: Partial deletion of beta-globin gene DNA in certain patients with beta-thalassemia. Proc Natl Acad Sci USA 1979; 76:2400.

218. Orkin SH, Kolodner R, et al: Cloning and direct examination of a structurally abnormal human beta-thalassemia globin gene. Proc Natl Acad Sci USA 1980; 77:3558.

219. Moschonas N, deBoer E, et al: Structure and expression of a cloned beta thalassemia globin gene. Nucleic Acids Res 1982; 9:4391.

220. Rosatelli C, Falchi AM, et al: Prenatal diagnosis of beta-thalassaemia with the synthetic-oligomer technique. Lancet 1985; 1:241.

221. Antonarakis SE, Boehm CD, et al: Nonrandom associations of polymorphic restriction sites in the beta-globin gene cluster. Proc Natl Acad Sci USA 1982; 79:137.

222. Kazazian HH Jr, Orkin SH, et al: Quantitation of the close association between DNA haplotypes and specific beta-thalassemia mutations in Mediterraneans. Nature 1984; 310:152.

223. Jeffreys AJ: DNA sequence variants in the ^{G}gamma-, ^{A}gamma-, delta, and beta-globin genes of man. Cell 1979; 18:1.

224. Kan YW, Dozy AM: Polymorphism of DNA sequence adjacent to human beta-globin structural gene: Relationship to sickle mutation. Proc Natl Acad Sci USA 1978; 75:5631.

225. Antonarakis SE, Kazazian HH Jr, et al: DNA polymorphism and molecular pathology of the human globin gene clusters. Hum Genet 1985; 69:1.

226. Higgs DR, Wainscoat JS, et al: Analysis of the human alpha-globin gene cluster reveals a highly informative genetic locus. Proc Natl Acad Sci USA 1986; 83:5165.

227. Chakravarti A, Buetow KH, et al: Nonuniform recombination within the human beta-globin gene cluster. Am J Hum Genet 1984; 36:1239.

228. Wainscoat JS, Hill AVS, et al: Evolutionary relationships of human populations from an analysis of nuclear DNA polymorphisms. Nature 1986; 319:491.

229. Gerhard DS, Kidd KK, et al: Identification of a recent recombination event within the human beta-globin gene cluster. Proc Natl Acad Sci USA 1984; 81:7875.

230. Old JM, Heath C, et al: Meiotic recombination between two polymorphic restriction sites within the beta globin gene cluster. J Med Genet 1986; 23:14.

231. Antonarakis SE, Orkin SH, et al: Evidence for multiple origins of the beta E-globin gene in Southeast Asia. Proc Natl Acad Sci USA 1982; 79:6608.

232. Chehab FF, Doherty M, et al: Detection of sickle cell anaemia and thalassaemias [letter]. Nature 1987; 329:293. [Published erratum appears in Nature 1987;329:678.]

233. Kulozik AE, Lyons J, et al: Rapid and non-radioactive prenatal diagnosis of beta thalassaemia and sickle cell disease: Application of the polymerase chain reaction (PCR). Br J Haematol 1988; 70:455.

234. Pirastu M, Ristaldi MS, et al: Prenatal diagnosis of beta thalassaemia based on restriction endonuclease analysis of amplified fetal DNA. J Med Genet 1989; 26:363.

235. Orkin SH, Markham AF, et al: Direct detection of the common Mediterranean beta-thalassemia gene with synthetic DNA probes. An alternative approach for prenatal diagnosis. J Clin Invest 1983; 71:775.

236. Wallace RB, Schold M, et al: Oligonucleotide directed mutagenesis of the human beta-globin gene: A general method for producing specific point mutations in cloned DNA. Nucleic Acids Res 1981; 9:3647.

237. Saiki RK, Chang CA, et al: Diagnosis of sickle cell anemia and beta-thalassemia with enzymatically amplified DNA and nonradioactive allele-specific oligonucleotide probes. N Engl J Med 1988; 319:537.

238. Cai SP, Zhang JZ, et al: A simple approach to prenatal diagnosis of beta-thalassemia in a geographic area where multiple mutations occur. Blood 1988; 71:1357.

239. Cai SP, Chang CA, et al: Rapid prenatal diagnosis of beta thalassemia using DNA amplification and nonradioactive probes. Blood 1989; 73:372.

240. Ristaldi MS, Pirastu M, et al: Prenatal diagnosis of beta-thalassaemia in Mediterranean populations by dot blot analysis with DNA amplification and allele specific oligonucleotide probes. Prenat Diagn 1989; 9:629.

241. Sutcharitchan P, Saiki R, et al: Reverse dot-blot detection of Thai beta-thalassaemia mutations. Br J Haematol 1995; 90:809.

242. Giambona A, Lo Gioco P, et al: The great heterogeneity of thalassemia molecular defects in Sicily. Hum Genet 1995; 95:526.

243. Saiki RK, Scharf S, et al: Enzymatic amplification of beta-globin genomic sequences and restriction site analysis for diagnosis of sickle cell anemia. Science 1985; 230:1350.

244. Saiki RK, Gelfand DH, et al: Primer-directed enzymatic amplification of DNA with a thermostable DNA polymerase. Science 1988; 239:487.

245. Erlich HA, Gelfand DH, et al: Specific DNA amplification. Nature 1988; 331:461.

246. Eisenstein BI: The polymerase chain reaction: A new method of using molecular genetics for medical diagnosis. N Engl J Med 1990; 322:178.

247. Thein SL, Hesketh C, et al: The molecular basis of thalassaemia major and thalassaemia intermedia in Asian Indians: Application to prenatal diagnosis. Br J Haematol 1988; 70:225.

248. Kazazian HH Jr, Dowling CE, et al: The spectrum of beta-thalassemia genes in China and Southeast Asia. Blood 1986; 68:964.

249. Zhang JZ, Cai SP, et al: Molecular basis of beta thalassemia in South China: Strategy for DNA analysis. Hum Genet 1988; 78:37.

250. Diaz-Chico JC, Yang KG, et al: Mild and severe beta-thalassemia among homozygotes from Turkey: Identification of the types by hybridization of amplified DNA with synthetic probes. Blood 1988; 71:248.

251. Amselem S, Nunes V, et al: Determination of the spectrum of beta-thalassemia genes in Spain by use of dot-blot analysis of amplified beta-globin DNA. Am J Hum Genet 1988; 43:95.

252. Weatherall DJ, Clegg JB: The Thalassemia Syndromes, 3rd ed. Oxford, Blackwell Scientific Publications, 1981.

253. Weatherall DJ, Wood WG, et al: The developmental genetics of human hemoglobin. In Stamatoyannopoulos G, Nienhuis AW (eds): Experimental Approaches for the Study of Hemoglobin Switching. New York, Alan R. Liss, 1985, p 3.

254. Charache S, Clegg JB, et al: The Negro variety of hereditary persistence of fetal hemoglobin is a model form of thalassemia. Br J Haematol 1976; 34:527.

255. Friedman S, Schwartz E, et al: Variation in globin chain synthesis in hereditary persistence of fetal hemoglobin. Br J Haematol 1976; 32:357.

256. Tate VE, Hill AV, et al: A silent deletion in the beta-globin gene cluster. Nucleic Acids Res 1986; 14:4743.

257. Kulozik AE, Yarwood N, et al: The Corfu delta beta zero thalassemia: A small deletion acts at a distance to selectively abolish beta globin gene expression. Blood 1988; 71:457. [Published erratum appears in Blood 1988;71:1509.]

258. Galanello R, Podda A, et al: Interaction between deletion delta-thalassemia and beta zero-thalassemia (codon 39 nonsense mutation) in a Sardinian family. Prog Clin Biol Res 1989; 316B:113.

259. Spritz RA, Orkin SH: Duplication followed by deletion accounts for the structure of an Indian deletion beta thalassemia. Nucleic Acids Res 1982; 10:8025.

260. Padanilam BJ, Felice AE, et al: Partial deletion of the 5′ beta-globin gene region causes beta zero-thalassemia in members of an American black family. Blood 1984; 64:941.

261. Anand R, Boehm CD, et al: Molecular characterization of a beta zero-thalassemia resulting from a 1.4 kilobase deletion. Blood 1988; 72:636.

262. Gilman JG, Huisman TH, et al: Dutch beta^0-thalassemia: A 10 kilobase DNA deletion associated with significant gamma-chain production. Br J Haematol 1984; 56:339.

263. Gilman JG: The 12.6 kilobase DNA deletion in Dutch beta zero-thalassaemia. Br J Haematol 1987; 67:369.

264. Diaz-Chico JC, Yang KG, et al: An approximately 300 bp deletion involving part of the 5′ beta-globin gene region is observed in members of a Turkish family with beta-thalassemia. Blood 1987; 70:583.

265. Spiegelberg R, Aulehla SC, et al: A beta-thalassemia gene caused by a 290-base pair deletion: Analysis by direct sequencing of enzymatically amplified DNA. Blood 1989; 73:1695.

266. Aulehla-Scholz C, Spiegelberg R, et al: A beta-thalassemia mutant caused by a 300-bp deletion in the human beta-globin gene. Hum Genet 1989; 81:298.

267. Popovich BW, Rosenblatt DS, et al: Molecular characterization of an atypical beta-thalassemia caused by a large deletion in the 5′ beta-globin gene region. Am J Hum Genet 1986; 39:797.

268. Henthorn PS, Smithies O, et al: Molecular analysis of deletions in the human beta-globin gene cluster: Deletion junctions and locations of breakpoints. Genomics 1990; 6:226.

269. Ottolenghi S, Giglioni B: Delta beta thalassemia is due to a gene deletion. Cell 1976; 9:71.

270. Bernards R, Kooter JM, et al: Physical mapping of the globin gene deletion in delta beta thalassemia. Gene 1979; 6:265.

271. Ottolenghi S, Giglioni B: The deletion in a type of delta beta thalassemia begins in an inverted Alu I repeat. Nature 1982; 300:770.

272. Ottolenghi S, Giglioni B, et al: Molecular comparison of delta beta thalassemia and hereditary persistence of fetal hemoglobin DNAs: Evidence of a regulatory area? Proc Natl Acad Sci USA 1982; 79:2347.

273. Feingold EA, Forget BG: The breakpoint of a large deletion causing hereditary persistence of fetal hemoglobin occurs within an erythroid DNA domain remote from the beta-globin gene cluster. Blood 1989; 74:2178.

274. Anagnou NP, Papayannopoulou T, et al: Structurally diverse molecular deletions in the beta-globin gene cluster exhibit an identical phenotype on interaction with the beta S-gene. Blood 1985; 65:1245.

275. Matsunaga E, Kimura A, et al: A novel deletion in delta beta-thalassemia found in Japan. Biochem Biophys Res Commun 1985; 126:185.

276. Shiokawa S, Yamada H, et al: Molecular analysis of Japanese delta beta-thalassemia. Blood 1988; 72:1771.

277. Zhang JW, Stamatoyannopoulos G, et al: Laotian (delta-beta)⁰-thalassemia: Molecular characterization of a novel deletion associated with increased production of fetal hemoglobin. Blood 1988; 72:983.

278. Efremov GD, Nikolov N, et al: The 18- to 23-kb deletion of the Macedonian delta beta-thalassemia includes the entire delta and beta globin genes. Blood 1986; 68:971.

279. Baglioni C: The fusion of two peptide chains in hemoglobin Lepore and its interpretation as a genetic deletion. Proc Natl Acad Sci USA 1962; 48:1880.

280. Flavell RA, Kooter JM, et al: Analysis of the beta delta globin gene loci in normal and Hb Lepore DNA: Direct determination of gene linkage and intergene distance. Cell 1978; 15:25.

281. Baird M, Driscoll C, et al: Localization of the site of recombination in formation of the Lepore Boston globin gene. J Clin Invest 1981; 68:560.

282. Jones RW, Old JM, et al: Major rearrangement in the human beta globin gene cluster. Nature 1981; 291:39.

283. Jennings MW, Jones RW, et al: Analysis of an inversion within the human beta globin gene cluster. Nucleic Acids Res 1985; 13:2897.

284. Henthorn PS, Smithies O, et al: (Agamma delta beta)-Thalassaemia in blacks is due to a deletion of 34 kbp of DNA. Br J Haematol 1985; 59:343.

285. Orkin AH, Alter B, et al: Deletion of the Agamma gene in Ggamma-delta-beta thalassemia. J Clin Invest 1979; 64:866.

286. Tuan D, Feingold E, et al: Different 3′ end points of deletions causing δβ-thalassemia and hereditary persistence of fetal hemoglobin: Implications for the control of γ-globin gene expression in man. Proc Natl Acad Sci USA 1983; 80:6937.

287. Jones RW, J.M. O, et al: Restriction mapping of a new deletion responsible for Ggamma(delta-beta) thalassemia. Nucleic Acids Res 1981; 9:6813.

288. George E, Faridah K, et al: Homozygosity for a new type of Ggamma (Agamma delta beta)⁰-thalassemia in a Malaysian male. Hemoglobin 1986; 10:353.

289. Mager DL, Henthorn PS, et al: A Chinese Ggamma⁺ (Agamma delta beta)⁰ thalassemia deletion: Comparison to other deletions in the human beta-globin gene cluster and sequence analysis of the breakpoints. Nucleic Acids Res 1985; 13:6559.

290. Anagnou NP, Papayannopoulou T, et al: Molecular characterization of a novel form of (Agamma delta beta)o-thalassemia deletion with a 3′ breakpoint close to those of HPFH-3 and HPFH-4: Insights for a common regulatory mechanism. Nucleic Acids Res 1988; 16:6057.

291. Driscoll MC, Dobkin CS, et al: Gamma delta beta-thalassemia due to a de novo mutation deleting the 5′ beta-globin gene activation-region hypersensitive sites. Proc Natl Acad Sci USA 1989; 86:7470.

292. Curtin P, Pirastu M, et al: A distant gene deletion affects beta-globin gene function in an atypical gamma delta beta-thalassemia. J Clin Invest 1985; 76:1554.

293. Kioussis D, Vanin E, et al: Beta-globin gene inactivation by DNA translocation in gamma beta-thalassaemia. Nature 1983; 306:662.

294. Vanin EF, Henthorn PS, et al: Unexpected relationships between four large deletions in the human beta-globin gene cluster. Cell 1983; 35:701.

295. Wright S, Taramelli R, et al: DNA sequences required for regulated expression of the human beta-globin gene. Prog Clin Biol Res 1985; 191:251.

296. Orkin SH, Goff SC, et al: Heterogeneity of the DNA deletion in gamma-delta-beta thalassemia. J Clin Invest 1981; 67:878.

297. Pirastu M, Kan YW, et al: Hemolytic disease of the newborn caused by a new deletion of the entire beta-globin cluster. J Clin Invest 1983; 72:602.

298. Fearon ER, Kazazian HJ, et al: The entire beta-globin gene cluster is deleted in a form of gamma delta beta-thalassemia. Blood 1983; 61:1269.

299. Diaz-Chico JC, Huang HJ, et al: Two new large deletions resulting in epsilon gamma delta beta-thalassemia. Acta Haematol (Basel) 1988; 80:79.

300. Fritsch EF, Lawn RM, et al: Characterization of deletions which affect the expression of fetal globin genes in man. Nature 1979; 279:598.

301. Tuan D, Murnane MJ, et al: Heterogeneity in the molecular basis of hereditary persistence of fetal hemoglobin. Nature 1980; 285:335.

302. Bernards R, Flavell RA: Physical mapping of the globin gene deletion in hereditary persistence of foetal hemoglobin (HPFH). Nucleic Acids Res 1980; 8:1521.

303. Jagadeeswaran P, Tuan D, et al: A gene deletion ending at the midpoint of a repetitive DNA sequence in one form of hereditary persistence of fetal hemoglobin. Nature 1982; 296:469.

304. Kutlar A, Gardiner MB, et al: Heterogeneity in the molecular basis of three types of hereditary persistence of fetal hemoglobin and the relative synthesis of the Ggamma and Agamma types of gamma chains. Biochem Genet 1984; 22:21.

305. Raskind W, Niakan KK, et al: Mapping of a syndrome of X-linked thrombocytopenia with thalassemia to band Xp11-12: Further evidence of genetic heterogeneity of X-linked thrombocytopenia. Blood 2000; 95:2262.

306. Yu C, Niakan KK, et al: X-linked thrombocytopenia with thalassemia from a mutation in the amino finger of GATA-1 affecting DNA binding rather than FOG-1 interaction. Blood 2002; 100:2040.

307. Saglio G, Camaschella C, et al: Italian type of deletional hereditary persistence of fetal hemoglobin. Blood 1986; 68:646.

308. Camaschella C, Serra A, et al: A new hereditary persistence of fetal hemoglobin deletion has the breakpoint within the 3′ beta-globin gene enhancer. Blood 1990; 75:1000.

309. Huisman THJ, Wrightstone RN, et al: Hemoglobin Kenya: The product of fusion of alpha- and beta-polypeptide chains. Arch Biochem Biophys 1972; 152:850.

310. Kendall AG, Ojwang PJ, et al: Hemoglobin Kenya, the product of a gamma-beta fusion gene: Studies of the family. Am J Hum Genet 1973; 25:548.

311. Huisman THJ, Shroeder WA, et al: Hemoglobin Kenya, the product of non-homologous crossing-over of gamma and beta genes. Blood 1972; 40:947.

312. Nute PE, Wood WG, et al: The Kenya form of hereditary persistence of fetal hemoglobin: Structural studies and evidence for homogeneous distribution of haemoglobin F using fluorescent anti-haemoglobin F antibodies. Br J Haematol 1976; 32:55.

313. Collins FS, Stoeckert CJJ, et al: ^{G}gamma beta$^+$ hereditary persistence of fetal hemoglobin: Cosmid cloning and identification of a specific mutation 5′ to the ^{G}gamma gene. Proc Natl Acad Sci USA 1984; 81:4894.

314. Collins FS, Boehm CD, et al: Concordance of a point mutation 5′ to the gamma globin gene with ^{G}gamma beta hereditary persistence of fetal hemoglobin in the black population. Blood 1984; 64:1292.

315. Gilman JG, Mishima Nea: Upstream promoter mutation associated with a modest elevation of fetal hemoglobin expression in human adults. Blood 1988; 72:78.

316. Weatherall DJ, Cartner R, et al: A form of hereditary persistence of fetal haemoglobin characterized by uneven cellular distribution of haemoglobin F and the production of haemoglobins A and A$_2$ in homozygotes. Br J Haematol 1975; 29:205.

317. Old JM, Ayyub H, et al: Linkage analysis of nondeletion hereditary persistence of fetal hemoglobin. Science 1982; 215:981.

318. Tate VE, Wood WG, et al: The British form of hereditary persistence of fetal hemoglobin results from a single base mutation adjacent to an S1 hypersensitive site 5′ to the ^{A}gamma globin gene. Blood 1986; 68:1389.

319. Farquhar M, Gelinas R, et al: Restriction endonuclease mapping of gamma-delta-beta-globin region in ^{G}gamma (beta)$^+$ HPFH and a Chinese ^{A}gamma HPFH variant. Am J Hum Genet 1983; 35:611.

320. Gelinas R, Bender M, et al: C to T at position −196 of the ^{A}gamma gene promoter. Blood 1986; 67:1777.

321. Giglioni B, Casini C, et al: A molecular study of a family with Greek hereditary persistence of fetal hemoglobin and beta-thalassemia. EMBO J 1984; 3:2641.

322. Ottolenghi S, Giglioni B, et al: Sardinian delta beta zero-thalassemia: A further example of a C to T substitution at position −196 of the ^{A}gamma globin gene promoter. Blood 1987; 69:1058.

323. Ottolenghi S, Nicolis S, et al: Sardinian ^{G}gamma-HPFH: A T→C substitution in a conserved "octamer" sequence in the ^{G}gamma-globin promoter. Blood 1988; 71:815.

324. Surrey S, Delgrosso K, et al: A single-base change at position −175 in the 5′-flanking region of the ^{G}gamma-globin gene from a black with ^{G}gamma-beta$^+$ HPFH. Blood 1988; 71:807.

325. Stoming TA, Stoming GS, et al: An ^{A}gamma type of nondeletional hereditary persistence of fetal hemoglobin with a T→C mutation at position −175 to the cap site of the ^{A}gamma globin gene. Blood 1989; 73:329.

326. Gilman JG, Kutlar F, et al: A G to A nucleotide substitution 161 base pairs 5′ of the ^{G}gamma globin gene cap site (−161) in a high ^{G}gamma non-anemic person. Prog Clin Biol Res 1987; 251:383.

327. Pembrey ME, Wood WG, et al: Fetal hemoglobin production and the sickle gene in the oases of Eastern Saudi Arabia. Br J Haematol 1978; 40:415.

328. Wainscoat JS, Thein SL, et al: A genetic marker for elevated levels of hemoglobin F in homozygous sickle cell disease? Br J Haematol 1985; 60:261.

329. Gilman JG, Huisman THJ: DNA sequence variation associated with elevated fetal ^{G}gamma globin production. Blood 1985; 66:783.

330. Labie D, Pagnier J, et al: Common haplotype dependency of high ^{G}gamma-globin gene expression and high Hb F levels in beta-thalassemia and sickle cell anemia patients. Proc Natl Acad Sci USA 1985; 82:2111.

331. Labie D, Dunda BO, et al: The −158 site 5′ to the ^{G}gamma gene and ^{G}gamma expression. Blood 1985; 66:1463.

332. Miller BA, Salameh M, et al: High fetal hemoglobin production in sickle cell anemia in the eastern province of Saudi Arabia is genetically determined. Blood 1986; 67:1404.

333. Miller BA, Olivieri N, et al: Molecular analysis of the high-hemoglobin-F phenotype in Saudi Arabian sickle cell anemia. N Engl J Med 1987; 316:244.

334. Collins FS, Metherall JE, et al: A point mutation in the ^{A}gamma-globin gene promoter in Greek hereditary persistence of fetal haemoglobin. Nature 1985; 313:325.

335. Gelinas R, Endlich B, et al: G to A substitution in the distal CCAAT box of the ^{A}gamma-globin gene in Greek hereditary persistence of fetal hemoglobin. Nature 1985; 313:323.

336. Ottolenghi S, Camaschella C, et al: A frequent ^{A}gamma-hereditary persistence of fetal hemoglobin in northern Sardinia: Its molecular basis and hematologic phenotype in heterozygotes and compound heterozygotes with beta-thalassemia. Hum Genet 1988; 79:13.

337. Gilman JG, Mishima N, et al: Distal CCAAT box deletion in the ^{A}gamma globin gene of two black adolescents with elevated fetal ^{A}gamma globin. Nucleic Acids Res 1988; 16:10635.

338. Marti HR: In Normale und Anormale Menschliche Hemoglobine. Berlin, Springer-Verlag, 1963, p 81.

339. Jensen M, Wirtz A, et al: Hereditary persistence of fetal haemoglobin (HPFH) in conjunction with a chromosomal translocation involving the haemoglobin beta locus. Br J Haematol 1984; 56:87.

340. Sukumaran PK, Huisman THJ, et al: A homozygote for the gamma type of fetal hemoglobin in India: A study of two Indians and four Negro families. Br J Haematol 1972; 23:403.

341. Boyer SH, Margolet L, et al: Inheritance of F cell frequency in heterocellular hereditary persistence of fetal hemoglobin: An example of allelic exclusion. Am J Hum Genet 1977; 29:256.

342. Stamatoyannopoulos G, Wood WG, et al: A new form of hereditary persistence of fetal hemoglobin in blacks and its association with sickle cell trait. Blood 1975; 46:683.

343. Gelinas RE, Rixon M, et al: Gamma gene promoter and enhancer structure in Seattle variant of hereditary persistence of fetal hemoglobin. Blood 1988; 71:1108.

344. Oggiano L, Pirastu M, et al: Molecular characterization of a normal Hb A$_2$ beta-thalassaemia determinant in a Sardinian family. Br J Haematol 1987; 67:225.

345. Moi P, Paglietti E, et al: Delineation of the molecular basis of delta- and normal HbA$_2$ beta-thalassemia. Blood 1988; 72:530.

346. Gerald PS, Diamond LK: The diagnosis of thalassemia trait by starch block electrophoresis of the hemoglobin. Blood 1958; 13:61.

347. Mavilio F, Giampaolo A, et al: The delta-beta crossover region in Lepore Boston hemoglobinopathy is restricted to a 59 base pair region around the 5′ splice junction of the large globin gene intervening sequence. Blood 1983; 62:230.

348. Mears JG, Ramirez F, et al: Changes in restricted human cellular DNA fragments containing globin gene sequences in thalassemia and related disorders. Proc Natl Acad Sci USA 1978; 75:1222.

349. Fessas P, Karaklis A: Two-dimensional paper-agar electrophoresis of hemoglobin. Clin Chim Acta 1962; 7:133.

350. Duma H, Efremov G, et al: Study of nine families with hemoglobin Lepore. Br J Haematol 1978; 15:161.

351. Lehmann H, Charlesworth D: Observations on hemoglobin P (Congo type). Biochem J 1970; 119:43.

352. Ohta Y, Yamaoka K, et al: Hemoglobin Miyada, a beta-delta fusion peptide (anti-Lepore) type discovered in a Japanese family. Nat (New Biol) 1971; 234:218.

353. Baird FM, Lorkin PA, et al: Hemoglobin P Nilotic containing a beta-delta chain. Nat (New Biol) 1973; 242:107.

354. Kimura A, Ohta Y, et al: A fusion gene in man: DNA sequence analysis of the abnormal globin gene of hemoglobin Miyada. Biochem Biophys Res Commun 1984; 119:968.

355. Ojwang PJ, Nakatsuji T, et al: Gene deletion as the molecular basis for the Kenya- gamma-HPFH condition. Hemoglobin 1983; 7:115.

356. Huisman THJ, Schroeder WA, et al: The present status of the heterogeneity of fetal hemoglobin in beta-thalassemia: An attempt to unify some observations in thalassemia and related conditions. Ann NY Acad Sci 1974; 232:107.

357. Oner C, Oner R, et al: A new Turkish type of beta-thalassemia major with homozygosity for two non-consecutive 7.6 kb deletions of the psi-beta and beta-genes and an intact delta gene. Br J Hematol 1995; 89:306.

358. Ramirez F, O'Donnell JV, et al: Abnormal or absent beta mRNA in beta Ferrara and gene deletion in delta beta thalassemia. Nature 1976; 263:471.

359. Schmid CW, Jelinek WR: The Alu family of dispersed repetitive sequences. Science 1982; 216:1065.

360. Trent RJ, Jones RW, et al: (^{A}gamma delta beta) thalassaemia: Similarity of phenotype in four different molecular defects, including one newly described. Br J Haematol 1984; 57:279.

361. Zeng YT, Huang SZ, et al: Hereditary persistence of fetal hemoglobin or (delta beta)^0-thalassemia: Three types observed in South-Chinese families. Blood 1985; 66:1430.

362. Kan YW, Forget BG, et al: Gamma-beta thalassemia: A cause of hemolytic disease of newborns. N Engl J Med 1972; 286:129.

363. Viprakasit V, Gibbons RJ, et al: Mutations in the general transcription factor TFIIH result in beta-thalassemia in individuals with trichothiodystrophy. Hum Mol Genet 2001; 10:2797.

364. Thompson AR, Wood WG, et al: X-linked syndrome of platelet dysfunction thrombocytopenia, and imbalanced globin chain synthesis with hemolysis. Blood 1977; 50:303.

365. Wainscoat JS, Old JM, et al: Characterization of an Indian (delta beta)^0 thalassaemia. Br J Haematol 1984; 58:353.

366. Henthorn PS, Mager D, et al: A gene deletion ending within a complex array of repeated sequences 3′ to the human beta-globin gene cluster. Proc Natl Acad Sci USA 1986; 83:5194.

367. Stolle CA, Penny LA, et al: Sequence analysis of the gamma-globin gene locus from a patient with the deletion form of hereditary persistence of fetal hemoglobin. Blood 1990; 75:499.

368. Elder JT, Forrester WC, et al: Translocation of an erythroid-specific hypersensitive site in deletion-type hereditary persistence of fetal hemoglobin. Mol Cell Biol 1990; 10:1382.

369. Feingold EA, Forget BG: The breakpoint of a large deletion causing hereditary persistence of fetal hemoglobin occurs within an erythroid DNA domain remote from the beta-globin gene cluster. Blood 1989; 74:2178.

370. Yang KG, Stoming TA, et al: Identification of base substitutions in the promoter regions of the ^{A}gamma- and ^{G}gamma-globin genes in ^{A}gamma- (or ^{G}gamma-) beta$^+$-HPFH heterozygotes using the DNA-amplification-synthetic oligonucleotide procedure. Blood 1988; 71:1414.

371. Gumucio DL, Rood KL, et al: Nuclear proteins that bind the human gamma-globin gene promoter: Alterations in binding produced by point mutations associated with hereditary persistence of fetal hemoglobin. Mol Cell Biol 1988; 8:5310.

372. Superti-Furga G, Barberis A, et al: The −117 mutation in Greek HPFH affects the binding of three nuclear factors to the CCAAT region of the gamma-globin gene. EMBO J 1988; 7:3099.

373. Martin DI, Tsai SF, et al: Increased gamma-globin expression in a nondeletion HPFH mediated by an erythroid-specific DNA-binding factor. Nature 1989; 338:435.

374. Mantovani R, Superti FG, et al: The deletion of the distal CCAAT box region of the ^{A}gamma-globin gene in black HPFH abolishes the binding of the erythroid specific protein NFE3 and of the CCAAT displacement protein. Nucleic Acids Res 1989; 17:6681.

375. Sykes K, Kaufman R: A naturally occurrin^{G}gamma globin gene mutation enhances SP1 binding activity. Mol Cell Biol 1990; 10:95.

376. Ronchi A, Nicolis S, et al: Increased Sp1 binding mediates erythroid-specific overexpression of a mutated (HPFH) gamma-globulin promoter. Nucleic Acids Res 1989; 17:10231.

377. Ottolenghi S, Mantovani R, et al: DNA sequences regulating human globin gene transcription in nondeletional hereditary persistence of fetal hemoglobin. Hemoglobin 1989; 13:523.

378. Wood WG, MacRae IA, et al: The British type of non-deletion HPFH: Characterization of developmental changes in vivo and erythroid growth in vitro. Br J Haematol 1982; 30:401.

379. Camaschella C, Oggiano L, et al: The homozygous state of G to A 117 ^{A}gamma hereditary persistence of fetal hemoglobin. Blood 1989; 73:1999.

380. Friedman S, Schwartz E: Hereditary persistence of foetal haemoglobin with beta-chain synthesis in *cis* position (^{G}gamma-beta$^+$-HPFH) in a Negro family. Nature 1976; 259:138.

381. Nicholls RD, Jonasson JA, et al: High resolution gene mapping of the human alpha globin locus. J Med Genet 1987; 24:39.

382. Simmers RN, Mulley JC, et al: Mapping the human alpha globin gene complex to 16p13.2-pter. J Med Genet 1987; 24:761.

383. Nicholls RD, Fischel-Ghodsian N, et al: Recombination at the human alpha-globin gene cluster: Sequence features and topological constraints. Cell 1987; 49:369.

384. Sawada I, Schmid CW: Primate evolution of the alpha-globin gene cluster and its Alu-like repeats. J Mol Biol 1986; 192:693.

385. Michelson AM, Orkin SH: Boundaries of gene conversion within the duplicated human alpha-globin genes. Concerted evolution by segmental recombination. J Biol Chem 1983; 258:15245.

386. Hess JF, Schmid CW, et al: A gradient of sequence divergence in the human adult alpha-globin duplication units. Science 1984; 226:67.

387. Higgs DR, Hill AV, et al: Independent recombination events between the duplicated human alpha globin genes; implications for their concerted evolution. Nucleic Acids Res 1984; 12:6965.

388. Foldi J, Cohen-Solal M, et al: The human alpha-globin gene. The protein products of the duplicated genes are identical. Eur J Biochem 1980; 109:463.

389. Orkin SH, Goff SC: The duplicated human alpha-globin genes: Their relative expression as measured by RNA analysis. Cell 1981; 24:345.

390. Liebhaber SA, Cash FE, et al: Compensatory increase in alpha 1-globin gene expression in individuals heterozygous for the alpha-thalassemia-2 deletion. J Clin Invest 1985; 76:1057.

391. Liebhaber SA, Cash FE, et al: Human alpha-globin gene expression. The dominant role of the alpha 2-locus in mRNA and protein synthesis. J Biol Chem 1986; 261:15327.

392. Proudfoot NJ: Transcriptional interference and termination between duplicated alpha-globin gene constructs suggests a novel mechanism for gene regulation. Nature 1986; 322:562.

393. Shakin SH, Liebhaber SA: Translational profiles of alpha 1−, alpha 2−, and beta-globin messenger ribonucleic acids in human reticulocytes. J Clin Invest 1986; 78:1125.

394. Orkin SH, Old J, et al: The molecular basis of alpha thalassemias: Frequent occurrence of dysfunctional alpha loci among non-Asians with Hb H disease. Cell 1979; 17:33.

395. Embury SH, Miller JA, et al: Two different molecular organizations account for the single alpha-globin gene of the alpha-thalassemia-2 genotype. J Clin Invest 1980; 66:1319.

396. Goossens M, Dozy AM, et al: Triplicated alpha-globin loci in humans. Proc Natl Acad Sci USA 1980; 77:518.

397. Higgs DR, Old JM, et al: A novel alpha-globin gene arrangement in man. Nature 1980; 284:632.

398. Lie-Injo LE, Herrera AR, et al: Two types of triplicated alpha-globin loci in humans. Nucleic Acids Res 1981; 9:3707.

399. Trent RJ, Higgs DR, et al: A new triplicated alpha-globin gene arrangement in man. Br J Haematol 1981; 49:149.

400. Hess JF, Fox M, et al: Molecular evolution of the human adult alpha-globin-like gene region: Insertion and deletion of Alu family repeats and non-Alu DNA sequences. Proc Natl Acad Sci USA 1983; 80:5970.

401. Hu WS, Shen CK: Reconstruction of human alpha thalassemia-2 genotypes in monkey cells. Nucleic Acids Res 1987; 15:2989.

402. Gomez-Pedrozo M, Hu WS, et al: Recombinational resolution in primate cells of two homologous human DNA segments with a gradient of sequence divergence. Nucleic Acids Res 1988; 16:11237.

403. Winichagoon P, Higgs DR, et al: The molecular basis of alpha-thalassaemia in Thailand. EMBO J 1984; 3:1813.

404. Chui DH, Wong SC, et al: Embryonic zeta-globin chains in adults: A marker for alpha-thalassemia-1 haplotype due to a greater than 17.5-kb deletion. N Engl J Med 1986; 314:76.

405. Bowden DK, Hill AV, et al: Different hematologic phenotypes are associated with the leftward (−alpha 4.2) and rightward (−alpha 3.7) alpha$^+$-thalassemia deletions. J Clin Invest 1987; 79:39.

406. Galanello R, Ruggeri R, et al: A family with segregating triplicated alpha globin loci and beta thalassemia. Blood 1983; 62:1035.

407. Trent RJ, Mickleson KN, et al: Alpha globin gene rearrangements in Polynesians are not associated with malaria. Am J Hematol 1985; 18:431.

408. Kulozik AE, Thein SL, et al: Thalassaemia intermedia: Interaction of the triple alpha-globin gene arrangement and heterozygous beta-thalassaemia. Br J Haematol 1987; 66:109.

409. Camaschella C, Bertero MT, et al: A benign form of thalassaemia intermedia may be determined by the interaction of triplicated alpha locus and heterozygous beta-thalassaemia. Br J Haematol 1987; 66:103.

410. Fischel-Ghodsian N, Vickers MA, et al: Characterization of two deletions that remove the entire human zeta-alpha globin gene complex (−/−THAI and −/−FIL). Br J Haematol 1988; 70:233.

411. Fortina P, Delgrosso K, et al: A large deletion encompassing the entire alpha-like globin gene cluster in a family of northern European extraction. Nucleic Acids Res 1988; 16:11223.

412. Drysdale HC, Higgs DR: Alpha-thalassaemia in an Asian Indian [letter]. Br J Haematol 1988; 68.

413. Gonzalez-Redondo JM, Diaz-Chico JC, et al: Characterization of a newly discovered alpha-thalassaemia-1 in two Spanish patients with Hb H disease. Br J Haematol 1988; 70:459.

414. Gonzalez-Redondo JM, Gilsanz F, et al: Characterization of a new alpha-thalassaemia-1 deletion in a Spanish family. Hemoglobin 1989; 13:103.

415. Luo HY, Clarke BJ, et al: A novel monoclonal antibody based diagnostic test for alpha-thalassemia-1 carriers due to the (−SEA/) deletion. Blood 1988; 72:1589.

416. Liang ST, Wong VC, et al: Homozygous alpha-thalassaemia: Clinical presentation, diagnosis and management. A review of 46 cases. Br J Obstet Gynaecol 1985; 92:680.

417. Keuh YK: Acute lymphoblastic leukemia with brilliant cresyl blue erythrocytic inclusions—Acquired hemoglobin H? N Engl J Med 1982; 307:193.

418. Higgs DR, Wood WG, et al: Clinical features and molecular analysis of acquired hemoglobin H disease. Am J Med 1983; 75:181.

419. Anagnou NP, Ley TJ, et al: Acquired alpha-thalassemia in preleukemia is due to decreased expression of all four alpha-globin genes. Proc Natl Acad Sci USA 1983; 80:6051.

420. Abbondanzo SL, Anagnou NP, et al: Myelodysplastic syndrome with acquired hemoglobin H disease. Evolution through megakaryoblastic transformation into myelofibrosis. Am J Clin Pathol 1988; 89:401.

421. Helder J, Deisseroth A: S1 nuclease analysis of alpha-globin gene expression in preleukemic patients with acquired hemoglobin H disease after transfer to mouse erythroleukemia cells. Proc Natl Acad Sci USA 1987; 84:2387.

422. Wilkie AO, Zeitlin HC, et al: Clinical features and molecular analysis of the alpha thalassemia/mental retardation syndromes. II. Cases without detectable abnormality of the alpha globin complex. Am J Hum Genet 1990; 46:1127.

423. Schwartz E: The silent carrier of beta thalassemia. N Engl J Med 1969; 281:1327.

424. Aksoy M, Dincol G, et al: Different types of beta-thalassemia intermedia. Acta Haematol (Basel) 1978; 59:178.

425. Kattamis C, Metaxotou-Mavromati A, et al: The heterogeneity of normal Hb A$_2$ beta thalassemia in Greece. Br J Haematol 1979; 42:109.

426. Kanavakis E, Metaxotou-Mavromati A, et al: Globin gene mapping in normal Hb A$_2$ types of beta thalassemia. Br J Haematol 1982; 51:59.

427. Semenza GL, Delgrosso K, et al: The silent carrier allele: Beta thalassemia without a mutation in the beta-globin gene or its immediate flanking regions. Cell 1984; 39:123.

428. Wong SC, Stoming TA, et al: High frequencies of a rearrangement (+ATA; −T) at −530 to the beta-globin gene in different populations indicate the absence of a correlation with a silent beta-thalassemia determinant. Hemoglobin 1989; 13:1.

429. Berg PE, Williams DM, et al: A common protein binds to two silencers 5′ to the human beta-globin gene. Nucleic Acids Res 1989; 17:8833.

430. Berg PE, Trabuchet G, et al: Is polymorphism 0.5 kb 5′ to the beta-globin gene relevant to beta S gene expression? Blood 1989; 74:143a.

431. Boyer SH: The emerging complexity of genetic control of persistent fetal hemoglobin biosynthesis in adults. Ann NY Acad Sci 1989; 565:23.

432. Cappellini MD, Fiorelli G, et al: Interaction between homozygous beta zero thalassemia and the Swiss type of hereditary persistence of fetal haemoglobin. Br J Haematol 1981; 48:561.

433. Gianni AM, Bregni M, et al: A gene controlling fetal hemoglobin expression in adults is not linked to the non-alpha globin cluster. EMBO J 1983; 2:921.

434. Thein SL, Weatherall DJ: A non-deletion hereditary persistence of fetal hemoglobin (HPFH) determinant not linked to the beta-globin gene complex. In Stamatoyannopoulos G, Nienhuis AW (eds): Hemoglobin Switching, Part B: Cellular and Molecular Mechanisms. New York, Alan R. Liss, 1989, p 97.

435. Sharma RS, Yu V, et al: Haemoglobin Bart's hydrops fetalis syndrome in an infant of Greek origin and prenatal diagnosis of alpha thalassemia. Med J Aust 1979; 2:433.

436. Trent RJ, Wilkinson T, et al: Molecular defects in 2 examples of severe Hb H disease. Scand J Haematol 1986; 36:272.

437. Chan V, Chan TK, et al: Hydrops fetalis due to an unusual form of Hb H disease. Blood 1985; 66:224.

438. Dozy AM, Kan YW, et al: Alpha-globin gene organization in blacks precludes the severe form of alpha-thalassemia. Nature 1979; 280:605.

439. Higgs DR, Pressley L, et al: Alpha thalassemia in black populations. Johns Hopkins Med J 1980; 146:300.

440. Phillips JAI, Vik TA, et al: Unequal crossing-over: A common basis of single alpha-globin genes in Asians and American blacks with hemoglobin-H disease. Blood 1980; 55:1066.

441. Galanello R, Maccioni L, et al: Alpha thalassaemia in Sardinian newborns. Br J Haematol 1984; 58:361.

442. Kanavakis E, Tzotzos S, et al: Frequency of alpha-thalassemia in Greece. Am J Hematol 1986; 22:225.

443. Weatherall DJ, Clegg JB: The alpha-chain-termination mutants and their relation to the alpha thalassemias. Philos Trans R Soc Lond 1975; 271:411.

444. Pootrakul P, Winichagoon P, et al: Homozygous haemoglobin Constant Spring: A need for revision of concept. Hum Genet 1981; 59:250.

445. Chui DH, Luo HY, et al: Potential application of a new screening test for alpha-thalassemia-1 carriers. Hemoglobin 1988; 12:459.

446. Kan YW, Schwartz E, et al: Globin chain synthesis in alpha-thalassemia syndromes. J Clin Invest 1968; 47:2515.

447. Pootrakul S, Sapprapa S, et al: Hemoglobin synthesis in 28 obligatory cases for alpha-thalassemia trait. Humangenetik 1975; 29:121.

448. Ben-Bassat I, Mozel M, et al: Globin synthesis in iron-deficiency anemia. Blood 1974; 44:451.

449. El-Hazmi MAF, Lehmann H: Interaction between iron deficiency and alpha thalassemia: The in vitro effect of haemin on alpha chain synthesis. Acta Haematol (Basel) 1978; 60:1.

450. Rigas DA, Koler RD, et al: New hemoglobin possessing a higher electrophoretic mobility than normal adult hemoglobin. Science 1955; 121:372.

451. Wasi P, Na-Nakorn S, et al: Alpha and beta-thalassemia in Thailand. Ann NY Acad Sci 1969; 165:60.

452. Clegg JB, Weatherall DJ: Hemoglobin synthesis in alpha-thalassemia (hemoglobin H disease). Nature 1967; 215:1241.

453. Benz EJ, Swerdlow PS, et al: Globin messenger RNA in Hb H disease. Blood 1973; 42:825.

454. Jones RT, Schroeder WA: Chemical characterization and subunit hybridization of human hemoglobin H and associated compounds. Biochemistry 1963; 2:1357.

455. Rigas DA, Koler RD: Decreased erythrocyte survival in hemoglobin H disease as a result of the abnormal properties of hemoglobin H: The benefit of splenectomy. Blood 1961; 18:1.

456. Rachmilewitz E, Shiner E, et al: Erythrocyte membrane alterations in beta-thalassemia. Clin Hematol 1985; 14:163.

457. Benesch RE, Ranney HM, et al: The chemistry of the Bohr effect: II. Some properties of hemoglobin H. J Biol Chem 1961; 236:2926.

458. Shinar E, Rachmilewitz EA: Oxidative denaturation of red blood cells in thalassemia. Semin Hematol 1990; 27:70.

459. Pearson HA, McFarland W: Erythrokinetics in thalassemia. II. Studies in Lepore trait and hemoglobin H disease. J Lab Clin Med 1962; 59:147.

460. Fessas P, Yataganas X: Intra-erythroblastic instability of hemoglobin beta (HbH). Blood 1968; 31:323.

461. Tso SC, Loh TT, et al: Iron overload in patients with haemoglobin H disease. Scand J Haematol 1984; 32:391.

462. Hirsh J, Dacie JV: Persistent post-splenectomy thrombocytosis and thromboembolism: A consequence of continuing anemia. Br J Haematol 1966; 12:45.

463. Tso SC, Chan TK, et al: Venous thrombosis in haemoglobin H disease after splenectomy. Aust NZ J Med 1982; 12:635.

464. Gabuzda TC, Nathan DG, et al: The metabolism of the individual C^{14} labeled hemoglobins in patients with H-thalassemia; with observations on radiochromate binding to the hemoglobins during red cell survival. J Clin Invest 1961; 44:315.

465. Tso SC: Red cell survival studies in hemoglobin H disease using [^{51}Cr]chromate and [^{32}P]di-isopropyl phosphofluoridate. Br J Haematol 1972; 23:621.

466. Wilkie AOM, Buckle VJ, et al: Clinical features and molecular analysis of the alpha thalassemia/mental retardation syndromes. I. Cases due to deletions involving chromosome band 16p13.3. Am J Hum Genet 1990; 46:1112.

467. Lie-Injo LE, Jo BH: A fast-moving hemoglobin in hydrops fetalis. Nature 1960; 185:698.

468. Kan YW, Allen A, et al: Hydrops fetalis with alpha thalassemia. N Engl J Med 1967; 276:18.

469. Weatherall DJ, Clegg JB, et al: The hemoglobin constitution of infants with haemoglobin Bart's hydrops foetalis syndrome. Br J Haematol 1970; 18:357.

470. Todd D, Lai MCS, et al: The abnormal hemoglobins in homozygous alpha thalassaemia. Br J Haematol 1970; 19:27.

471. Wasi P, Na-Nakorn S, et al: The alpha thalassemias. Clin Haematol 1974; 3:383.

472. Beaudry MA, Ferguson DJ, et al: Survival of a hydropic infant with homozygous alpha-thalassemia-1. J Pediatr 1986; 108:713.

473. Bianchi DW, Beyer EC, et al: Normal long-term survival with alpha-thalassemia. J Pediatr 1986; 108:716.

474. Carr S, Rubin L, et al: Intrauterine therapy for homozygous alpha-thalassemia. Obstet Gynecol 1995; 85:876.

475. Rietti F: Ittero emolitico primitivo. Atti Accad Sci Med Nat Ferrara 1925; 2:14.

476. Wintrobe MM, Mathews E, et al: Familial hemopoietic disorder in Italian adolescents and adults resembling Mediterranean disease (thalassemia). JAMA 1940; 114:1530.

477. Valentine WN, Neel JV: Hematologic and genetic study of transmission of thalassemia (Cooley's anemia: Mediterranean anemia). Arch Intern Med 1944; 74:185.

478. Smith CH: Detection of mild types of Mediterranean (Cooley's anemia). Am J Dis Child 1948; 75:505.

479. Silvestroni E, Bianco I: Microcytemia, constitutional microcytic anemia and Cooley's anemia. Am J Hum Genet 1949; l:83.

480. Pearson HA, McFarland W, et al: Erythrokinetic studies in thalassemia trait. J Lab Clin Med 1960; 56:866.

481. Mazza U, Saglio G, et al: Clinical and hematological data on 254 cases of beta-thalassemia trait in Italy. Br J Haematol 1976; 33:91.

482. Malamos B, Fessas P, et al: Types of thalassemia-trait carriers as revealed by a study of their incidence in Greece. Br J Haematol 1962; 8:5.

483. Pootrakul P, Wasi P, et al: Hematological data in 312 cases of beta-thalassemia trait in Thailand. Br J Haematol 1973; 24:703.

484. Knox-Macaulay, W.H.M., et al: Thalassaemia in the British. Br Med J 1973; 3:150.

485. Weatherall DJ: Biochemical phenotypes of thalassemia in the American Negro population. Ann NY Acad Sci 1964; 119:450.

486. Braverman AS, Bank A: Changing rates of globin chain synthesis during erythroid cell maturation in thalassemia. J Mol Biol 1969; 42:57.

487. Schwartz E: Heterozygous beta-thalassemia: Balanced globin synthesis in bone marrow cells. Science 1970; 167:1513.

488. Kan YW, Nathan DG, et al: Equal synthesis of alpha- and beta-globin chains in erythroid precursors in heterozygous beta-thalassemia. J Clin Invest 1972; 51:1906.

489. Freidman S, Oski FA, et al: Bone marrow and peripheral blood globin synthesis in an American black family with beta thalassemia. Blood 1972; 39:785.

490. Nienhuis AW, Canfield PH, et al: Hemoglobin messenger RNA from human bone marrow: Isolation and translation in homozygous and heterozygous beta thalassemia. J Clin Invest 1973; 52:1735.

491. Chalevelakis G, Clegg JB, et al: Imbalanced globin synthesis in heterozygous beta-thalassemia bone marrow. Proc Natl Acad Sci USA 1975; 72:3853.

492. Wood W, Stamatoyannopoulos G: Globin synthesis in fractionated normoblasts of beta thalassemia heterozygotes. J Clin Invest 1975; 55:567.

493. Fessas P, Stamatoyannopoulos G: Absence of haemoglobin A_2 in an adult. Nature 1962; 195:1215.

494. Thompson RB, Odom J, et al: Thalassemia with complete absence of hemoglobin A_2 in adult. Acta Haematol 1965; 33:186.

495. Ohta Y, Yamaoka K, et al: Homozygous delta-thalassemia first discovered in a Japanese family with hereditary persistence of fetal hemoglobin. Blood 1971; 37:706.

496. Kimura A, Matsunaga E, et al: Structure of cloned delta-globin genes from a normal subject and a patient with delta-thalassemia: Sequence polymorphisms found in the delta-globin gene region of Japanese individuals. Nucleic Acids Res 1982; 10:5725.

497. Taramelli R, Giglioni B, et al: Delta thalassemia: A non-deletion defect. Eur J Biochem 1983; 129:589.

498. Pirastu M, Galanello R, et al: Delta$^+$-thalassemia in Sardinia. Blood 1983; 62:341.

499. Huisman TJH, Punt K, et al: Thalassemia minor associated with hemoglobin B heterozygosity. A family report. Blood 1961; 17:747.

500. Alperin JB, Dow PA, et al: Hemoglobin A levels in health and various hematologic disorders. Am J Clin Pathol 1977; 67:219.

501. Pootrakul S, Assayamunkong S, et al: Beta-thalassemia trait: Hematologic and hemoglobin synthesis studies. Hemoglobin 1976; I:75.

502. Agraphiotis A, Fessas Pea: Hematological, biochemical and biosynthetic differences between beta and beta thalassemia heterozygotes. In Proceedings of the XVII Congress of the International Society of Hematology, Paris, 1978.

503. Millard DP, Mason K, et al: Comparison of hematological features of the beta and beta thalassemia traits in Jamaican Negroes. Br J Haematol 1977; 36:161.

504. Schokler RC, Went LN, et al: A new genetic variant of beta-thalassemia. Nature 1966; 209:44.

505. Kalpsoya-Tassopoulos A, Zoumbos N, et al: 'Silent' beta thalassemia and normal HbA$_2$ beta thalassemia. Br J Haematol 1980; 45:177.

506. Pearson HA, O'Brien RT, et al: Screening for thalassemia trait by electronic measurement of means corpuscular volume (MCV). N Engl J Med 1973; 288:351.

507. Torlontano G, Tata A, et al: A rapid screen test for thalassemia trait. Acta Haematol 1972; 48:234.

508. Hedge UM, White JM, et al: Diagnosis of alpha thalassemia trait from Coulter counter "S" indices. J Clin Pathol 1977; 30:884.

509. Conrad ME, Crosby WH: The natural history of iron deficiency induced by phlebotomy. Blood 1962; 20:173.

510. Mentzer WC: Differentiation of iron deficiency from thalassemia trait. Lancet 1973; I:882.

511. England JM, Fraser PM: Differentiation of iron deficiency from thalassemia trait by routine blood count. Lancet 1973; I:449.

512. England JM, Ward SM, et al: Microcytosis, anisocytosis, and the red cell indices in iron deficiency. Br J Haematol 1976; 34:589.

513. Bessman JB, Gilmer PR, et al: Improved classification of anemias by MCV and RDW. Am J Clin Pathol 1983; 80:322.

514. McClure S, Custer E, et al: Improved detection of early iron deficiency in nonanemic subjects. JAMA 1985; 253:1021.

515. Ghionni A, Miotti TC, et al: Differential erythrocyte parameters in thalassemia minor and hyposideremic syndromes. Minerva Med 1985; 76:1143.

516. Roberts GT, El-Badawi SB: Red blood cell distribution width in some hematologic diseases. Am J Clin Pathol 1985; 83:222.

517. Flynn MM, Reppun TS, et al: Limitations of red blood cell distribution width (RDW) in evaluation of microcytosis. Am J Clin Pathol 1986; 85:445.

518. Marti HR, Fischer S, et al: Can automated haematology analysers discriminate thalassaemia from iron deficiency? Acta Haematol (Basel) 1987; 78:180.

519. Miguel A, Linares M, et al: Red cell distribution width analysis in differentiation between iron deficiency and thalassemia minor. Acta Haematol (Basel) 1988; 80.

520. Shin I, Lal S: Strategy to detect beta thalassemia minor. Lancet 1977; I:692.

521. England JM, Fraser P: Discrimination between iron deficiency and heterozygous-thalassemia syndromes in the differential diagnosis of microcytosis. Lancet 1979; I:145.

522. Rowley PT: The diagnosis of beta thalassemia trait: A review. Am J Hematol 1976; l:129.

523. Chalevelakis G, Tsi Royannis K, et al: Screening for thalassemia and/or iron deficiency. Scand J Clin Lab Invest 1984; 44:1.

524. Bessman JD, McClure S, et al: Distinction of microcytic disorders: Comparison of expert, numerical-discriminant, and microcomputer analysis. Blood Cells 1989; 15:533.

525. Green R, King R: A new red cell discriminant incorporating volume dispersion for differentiating iron deficiency anemia from thalassemia minor. Blood Cells 1989; 15:481.

526. Makris PE: Utilization of a new index to distinguish heterozygous thalassemic syndromes: Comparison of its specificity to five other discriminants. Blood Cells 1989; 15:497.

527. Piomelli S, Brickman A, et al: Rapid diagnosis of iron deficiency by measurement of free erythrocyte porphyrins and hemoglobins: The FEP/hemoglobin ratio. Pediatrics 1976; 57:136.

528. Meloni T, Gallisai D, et al: Free erythrocyte porphyrin (REP) in the diagnosis of beta thalassemia trait and iron deficiency anemia. Haematologica 1982; 67:341.

529. Hurst D, Tittle B, et al: Anemia and hemoglobinopathies in Southeast Asian refugee children. J Pediat 1983; 102:692.

530. Cooley TB, Witwer ER, et al: Anemia in children with splenomegaly and peculiar changes in the bones. Report of cases. Am J Dis Child 1927; 34:347.

531. Cooley TB, Lee P: Series of cases of splenomegaly in children with anemia and peculiar bone changes. Trans Am Pediatr Soc 1925; 37:29.

532. Castagnari G: Intorno ad una particolare sindrome osteopatica diffusa in una caso di anemia eritroblastica dell'infanzia. Boll Sci Med (Bologna) 1933; 1:399.

533. Whipple GH, Bradford WL: Racial or familial anemia of children associated with fundamental disturbances of bone and pigment metabolism (Cooley-von Jaksch). Am J Dis Child 1932; 44:336.

534. Wolman LJ: Transfusion therapy in Cooley's anemia: Growth and health as related to long-range hemoglobin levels. A progress report. Ann NY Acad Sci 1964; 119:736.

535. Schorr JB, Radel E: Transfusion therapy and its complications in patients with Cooley's anemia. Ann NY Acad Sci 1964; 119:703.

536. Modell CB: High transfusion treatment of a case of thalassemia major. Trans R Soc Trop Med Hyg 1967; 61:1967.

537. Beard ME, Necheles TF, et al: Intensive transfusion therapy in thalassemia major. Pediatrics 1967; 40:911.

538. Piomelli S, Danoff SJ, et al: Prevention of bone malformation and cardiomegaly in Cooley's anemia by early hypertransfusion regimen. Ann NY Acad Sci 1969; 165:427.

539. Engle MA: Cardiac involvement in Cooley's anemia. Ann NY Acad Sci 1964; 119:694.

540. Heywood JD, Karon M, et al: Amino acid incorporation into alpha- and beta-chains of hemoglobin by normal and thalassemic reticulocytes. Science 1964; 146:530.

541. Heywood JD, Karon M, et al: Asymmetric incorporation of amino acids into alpha and beta chains of hemoglobin synthesized in thalassemic reticulocytes. J Lab Clin Med 1965; 66:476.

542. Weatherall DJ, Clegg JB, et al: Globin synthesis in thalassemia: An in vitro study. Nature 1965; 208:1061.

543. Bank A, Marks PA: Excess alpha chain synthesis relative to beta chain synthesis in thalassemia major and minor. Nature 1966; 212:1198.

544. Bargellesi A, Pontremoli S, et al: Absence of beta-globin synthesis in homozygous beta thalassemia. Eur J Biochem 1967; 1:73.

545. Fessas P: Inclusions of hemoglobin in erythroblasts and erythrocytes of thalassemia. Blood 1963; 21:21.

546. Fessas P, Loukopoulos D, et al: Absorption spectra of inclusion bodies in beta-thalassemia. Blood 1965; 25:105.

547. Fessas P, Loukopoulos D, et al: Peptide analysis of the inclusions of erythroid cells in beta thalassemia. Biochim Biophys Acta 1966; 124:430.

548. Nathan DG: Thalassemia as a proliferative disorder. Medicine (Baltimore) 1964; 43:779.

549. Polliack A, Yataganas P, et al: An electron-microscopic study of the nuclear abnormalities and erythroblasts in beta-thalassemia major. Br J Haematol 1974; 26:203.

550. Wichramsinghe SN: The morphology and kinetics of erythropoiesis in homozygous beta thalassemia. In Weatherall DJ (ed): Congenital Disorders of Erythropoiesis. Amsterdam, Elsevier, 1975, p 221.

551. Shinar E, Rachnilewitz EA: Haemoglobinopathies and red cell membrane function [review]. Baillieres Clin Haematol 1993; 6:357.

552. Schrier SL: Thalassemia: Pathophysiology of red cell changes. Annu Rev Med 1994; 45:211.

553. Yuan J, Bunyaratvej A, et al: The instability of the membrane skeleton in thalassemic red blood cells. Blood 1995; 86:3495.

554. Gaguzda TG, Nathan DG, et al: The metabolism of the individual C^{14}-labelled hemoglobins in patients with H-thalassemia, with observations on radiochromate binding to the hemoglobins during red cell survival. J Clin Invest 1965; 44:315.

555. Scott MD: Entrapment of purified alpha-hemoglobin chains in normal erythrocytes as a model for human beta thalassemia. Adv Exp Med Biol 1992; 326:139.

556. Shinar E, Shalev O, et al: Erythrocyte membrane skeleton abnormalities in severe beta-thalassemia. Blood 1987; 70:158.

557. Shinar E, Rachmilewitz EA, et al: Differing erythrocyte membrane skeletal protein defects in alpha and beta thalassemia. J Clin Invest 1989; 83:404.

558. Advani R, Rubin E, et al: Oxidative red blood cell membrane injury in the pathophysiology of severe mouse beta-thalassemia. Blood 1992; 79:1064.

559. Olivieri O, DeFranceschi L, et al: Oxidative damage and erythrocyte membrane transport abnormalities in thalassemias. Blood 1994; 84:315.

560. Schrier SL, Rachmilewitz E, et al: Cellular and membrane properties of alpha and beta thalassemic erythrocytes are different: Implication for differences in clinical manifestations. Blood 1989; 74:2194.

561. Sorensen S, Rubin E, et al: The role of membrane skeletal-associated alpha-globin in the pathophysiology of beta-thalassemia. Blood 1990; 75:1333.

562. Wainscoat JS, Thein SL, et al: Thalassaemia intermedia. Blood Rev 1987; 1:273.

563. McCarthy GM, Temperley IJ, et al: Thalassemia in an Irish family. Irish J Med Sci 1968; 1:303.

564. Friedman S, Ozsoylu S, et al: Heterozygous beta-thalassemia of unusual severity. Br J Haematol 1976; 32:65.

565. Weatherall DJ, Clegg JB, et al: A genetically determined disorder with features both of thalassemia and congenital dyserythropoietic anaemia. Br J Haematol 1973; 24:679.

566. Stamatoyannopoulos G, Woodson R, et al: Inclusion-body-beta-thalassemia trait. N Engl J Med 1974; 290:939.

567. Kanavakis E, Metaxotou MA, et al: The triplicated alpha gene locus and beta thalassaemia. Br J Haematol 1983; 54:201.

568. Sampietro M, Cazzola M, et al: The triplicated alpha-gene locus and heterozygous beta thalassaemia: A case of thalassaemia intermedia. Br J Haematol 1983; 55:709.

569. Thein SL, Al HI, et al: Thalassaemia intermedia: A new molecular basis. Br J Haematol 1984; 56:333.

570. Friedman AD, Linch DC, et al: Determination of the hemoglobin F program in human progenitor-derived erythroid cells. J Clin Invest 1985; 75:1359.

571. Pearson HA: Alpha-beta-thalassemia disease in a Negro family. N Engl J Med 1969; 281:1327.

572. Kan YW, Nathan DG: Mild thalassemia: The result of interactions of alpha and beta thalassemia genes. J Clin Invest 1970; 49:635.

573. Knox-McAulay HHM, Weatherall DJ, et al: The clinical and biosynthetic characterization of alpha beta-thalassemia. Br J Haematol 1972; 22:497.

574. Ozsoylu S, Hicsonmez C, et al: Hemoglobin H-beta-thalassemia. Acta Haematol 1973; 50:184.

575. Altay C, Say B, et al: Alpha-thalassemia and beta-thalassemia in a Turkish family. Am J Hematol 1977; 2:1.

576. Bate CM, Humphries G: Alpha-beta-thalassemia. Lancet 1977; 1:1031.

577. Furbetta M, Galanello R, et al: Interaction of alpha and beta thalassemia genes in two Sardinian families. Br J Haematol 1979; 41:203.

578. Wainscoat JS, Kanavakis E, et al: Thalassaemia intermedia in Cyprus: The interaction of alpha and beta thalassaemia. Br J Haematol 1983; 53:411.

579. Winichagoon P, Fucharoen S, et al: Concomitant inheritance of alpha-thalassemia in beta-thalassemia/Hb E disease. Am J Hematol 1985; 20:217.

580. Villegas A, Lopez Rubio M, et al: Primer caso de talasemia intermedia descrito en Espana debido a la interaccion de tres gene alpha con beta talasemia minor. Rev Clin Esp 1993; 192:268.

581. Camaschella C, Cappellini MD: Thalassemia intermedia. Haematologica 1995; 80:58.

582. Oron V, Filon D, et al: Severe thalassaemia intermedia caused by interaction of homozygosity for alpha-globin gene triplication with heterozygosity for beta zero-thalassemia. Br J Haematol 1994; 86:377.

583. Garewal G, Fearon CW, et al: The molecular basis of beta thalassaemia in Punjabi and Maharashtran Indians includes a multilocus aetiology involving triplicated alpha-globin loci. Brit J Haematol 1994; 86:372.

584. Oggiano L, Rimini E, et al: Haematological phenotypes in a family with triplicated alpha-globin gene, beta zero 39 and delta$^+$ 27 thalassaemia mutations. Clin Lab Haematol 1992; 14:289.

585. Villegas A, Perez-Clausell C, et al: A new case of thalassemia intermedia: Interaction of a triplicated alpha-globin locus and beta-thalassemia trait. Hemoglobin 1992; 16:99.

586. Leoni GG, Rosatelli C, et al: Molecular basis of beta-thalassemia intermedia in a southern Italian (Puglia). Acta Haematol 1991; 86:174.

587. Dandona P, Menon RK, et al: Serum 1,25 dihydroxyvitamin D and osteocalcin concentrations in thalassaemia major. Arch Dis Child 1987; 62:474.

588. Rioja L, Girot R, et al: Bone disease in children with homozygous beta-thalassemia. Bone Miner 1990; 8:69.

589. Lawson JP, Ablow RC, et al: The ribs in thalassemia. Radiology 1981; 140:663.

590. Williams BA, Morris LL, et al: Limb deformity and metaphyseal abnormalities in thalassaemia major. Am J Pediat Hematol Oncol 1992; 14:197.

591. Orvieto R, Leichter I, et al: Bone density, mineral content, and cortical index in patients with thalassemia major and the correlation to their bone fractures, blood transfusions, and treatment with desferrioxamine. Calcif Tissue Int 1992; 50:397.

592. Wonke B, A.V. H, et al: New approaches to the management of hepatitis and endocrine disorders in Cooley's anemia. Ann NY Acad Sci 1998; 850:232.

593. Jensen CE, et al: High incidence of osteoporosis in thalassemia major. J Pediatr Endocrinol Metab 1998; 3:975.

594. Giardina PJ, Schneider R, et al: Abnormal bone metabolism in thalassemia. In Ando S, Brancati C (eds): Endocrine Disorders in Thalassemia. Berlin, Springer-Verlag, 1995, p 39.

595. Lala R, Chiabotto P, et al: Bone density and metabolism in thalassemia. J Pediatr Endocrinol Metab 1998; 11:785.

596. Brill PW, P. W, et al: Deferoxamine-induced bone dysplasia in patients with thalassemia major. AJR Am J Roentgenol 1991; 156:561.

597. de Virgiliis S, Congia M, et al: Deferoxamine-induced growth retardation in patients with thalassemia major. J Pediatr 1988; 113:661.

598. Chan YL, Li CK, et al: Desferrioxamine-induced long bone changes in thalssaemic patients—Radiographic features, prevalence and relations with growth. Clin Radiol 2000; 55:610.

599. Baker DH: Roentgen manifestations of Cooley's anemia. Ann NY Acad Sci 1964; 119:641.

600. Michelson J, Cohen A: Incidence and treatment of fractures in thalassemia. J Orthop Trauma 1988; 2:29.

601. Canatan D, Akar N, et al: Effects of calcitonin therapy on osteoporosis in patients with thalassemia. Acta Haematol 1995; 93:20.

602. Shoemaker LR: Expanding role of bisphosphonate therapy in children. J Pediatr 1999; 134:264.

603. Mills SR, Doppman, J.L., et al: Computed tomography in the diagnosis of disorders of excessive iron storage of the liver. J Comput Assist Tomogr 1977; l:101.

604. Babiker MA, Patel PJ, et al: Comparison between serum ferritin and computed tomographic densities of liver, spleen, kidney and pancreas in beta-thalassaemia major. Scand J Clin Lab Invest 1987; 47:715.

605. Olivieri NF, Grisaru D, et al: Computed tomography scanning of the liver to determine efficacy of iron chelation therapy in thalassemia major. J Pediatr 1989; 114:427.

606. Long JA Jr, Doppmann JL, et al: Computed tomographic analysis of beta-thalassemic syndromes with hemochromatosis: Pathologic findings with clinical and laboratory correlations. J Comput Assist Tomogr 1980; 4:165.

607. Long JA Jr, Doppman JL, et al: Computed tomographic studies of thoracic extramedullary hematopoiesis. J Comput Assist Tomogr 1980; 4:67.

608. Papavasiliou C, Gouliamos A, et al: The marrow heterotopia in thalassemia. Eur J Radiol 1986; 6:92.

609. Singcharoen T: Unusual long bone changes in thalassaemia: Findings on plain radiography and computed tomography. Br J Radiol 1989; 62:168.

610. Papavasiliou C, Trakadas S, et al: Magnetic resonance imaging of marrow heterotopia in haemoglobinopathy. Eur J Radiol 1988; 8:50.

611. Brittenham G, Sheth S, et al: Noninvasive methods for quantitative assessment of transfusional iron overload in sickle cell disease. Semin Hematol 2001; 38:37.

612. Fischer R, Tiemann CD, et al: Assessment of iron stores in children with transfusion siderosis by biomagnetic liver susceptometry. Am J Hematol 1999; 60:289.

613. Wang ZJ, Haselgrove JC, et al: Evaluation of iron overload by single voxel MRS measurement of liver T2. J Magn Reson Imaging 2002; 15:395.

614. Anderson LJ, Holden S, et al: Cardiovascular T2-star (T2*) magnetic resonance for the early diagnosis of myocardial iron overload. Eur Heart J 2001; 22:2171.

615. Papakonstantinou O, Kostaridou S, et al: Quantification of liver iron overload by T2 quantitative magnetic resonance imaging in thalassemia: Impact of chronic hepatitis C on measurements. J Pediatr Hematol Oncol 1999; 21:142.

616. Ellis JT, Schulman I, et al: Generalized siderosis with fibrosis of liver and pancreas in Cooley's (Mediterranean) anemia with observations on the pathogenesis of the siderosis and fibrosis. Am J Pathol 1954; 30:287.

617. Fink H: Transfusion hemochromatosis in Cooley's anemia. Ann NY Acad Sci 1964; 119:680.

618. Modell B: A guide to the management of thalassemia. Presented at the EMBO Conference on Thalassemia, 1978.

619. de Alarcon PA, Donovan ME, et al: Iron absorption in the thalassemia syndromes and its inhibition by tea. N Engl J Med 1979; 300:5.

620. Olivieri NF, De Silva S, et al: Iron overload and iron-chelating therapy in hemoglobin E-beta thalassemia. J Pediatr Hematol Oncol 2000; 22:593.

621. Fucharoen S, Ketvichit P, et al: Clinical manifestation of beta-thalassemia/hemoglobin E disease. J Pediatr Hematol Oncol 2000; 22:552.

622. Worwood M: The clinical biochemistry of iron. Semin Hematol 1977; 14:30.

623. Modell B, Berdoukas V: The Clinical Approach to Thalassemia. New York, Grune & Stratton, 1984.

624. Cazzola M, Finch CA: Iron balance in thalassemia. Prog Clin Biol Res 1989; 309:93.

625. Cazzola M, Beguin Y, et al: Soluble transferrin receptor as a potential determinant of iron loading in congenital anaemias due to ineffective erythropoiesis. Br J Haematol 1999; 106:752.

626. Pippard MJ, Weatherall DJ: Iron absorption in non-transfused iron loading anemias: Prediction of risk for iron loading and response to iron chelation treatment in beta thalassemia intermedia and congenital sideroblastic anemias. Haematologica 1984; 17:17.

627. Peters TJ, Raja KB, et al: Mechanisms and regulation of intestinal iron absorption. Ann NY Acad Sci 1988; 526:141.

628. Melis M, A., Cau M, et al: H63D mutation in the *HFE* gene increases iron overload in beta-thalassemia carriers. Haematologica 2002; 87:242.

629. Piperno A, Mariani R, et al: Haemochromatosis in patients with beta-thalassaemia trait. Br J Haematol 2000; 111:908.

630. Bridges K, Cudkowicz A: Effect of iron chelators on the transferrin receptor in K562 cells. J Biol Chem 1984; 259:12970.

631. Harrison PM: Ferritin: An iron storage molecule. Semin Hematol 1977; 14:55.

632. Drysdale JW, Adelman TG, et al: Human isoferritins in normal and disease states. Semin Hematol 1977; 14:71.

633. Letsky EA, Miller F, et al: Serum ferritin in children with thalassemia regularly transfused. J Clin Pathol 1974; 27:652.

634. Logos P, Lagona E, et al: Serum ferritin in beta-thalassemia intermedia. Lancet 1980; 1:204.

635. Kaltwassen T, Werner E: Assessment of iron burden. Baillieres Clin Haematol 1989; 2:370.

636. Morgan EH: Transferrin biochemistry, physiology and clinical significance. Mol Aspects Med 1981; 4:1.

637. Aisen P: The role of transferrin in iron transport. Br J Haematol 1974; 26:159.

638. Huebers HA, Finch CA: Transferrin: Physiological behaviour and clinical implications. Blood 1984; 64:763.

639. Jacobs A: Low molecular weight intracellular iron transport compounds. Blood 1977; 50:433.

640. van Renswonde J, Bridges KR, et al: Receptor-mediated endocytosis of transferrin and the uptake of Fe in K562 cells: Identification of a nonlysosomal acidic compartment. Proc Natl Acad Sci USA 1982; 79:6186.

641. Dautry-Varsat A, Ciechanover A, et al: pH and the recycling of transferrin during receptor-mediated endocytosis. Proc Natl Acad Sci USA 1983; 80:2258.

642. Klausner RD, Ashwell G, et al: Binding of apo transferrin to K562 cells: Explanation of the transferrin cycle. Proc Natl Acad Sci USA 1983; 80:2263.

643. Seligman PA: The biochemistry of proteins involved in iron transport and storage. In Stamatoyannopoulos G, et al (eds): The Molecular Basis of Blood Diseases, Philadelphia, WB Saunders, 1987.

644. Seymour CA, Peters TJ: Organelle pathology in primary and secondary hemochromatosis with special reference to lysosomal changes. Br J Haematol 1978; 40:239.

645. Roifman CM, Eytan GD, et al: Ferritin-phospholipid interaction: A model system for intralysosomal ferritin segregation in iron-overloaded hepatocytes. J Ultrastruct Res 1982; 79:307.

646. Richter GW: The iron-loaded cell—The cytopathology of iron storage: A review. Am J Pathol 1978; 91:363.

647. Hershko C, Graham G, et al: Non-specific serum iron fraction of potential toxicity. Br J Haematol 1978; 40:255.

648. Anuwajanakulchai M, Pootrakul P, et al: Non-transferrin plasma iron in beta-thalassemia/Hb E and hemoglobin H diseases. Scand J Haematol 1984; 32:153.

649. Breuer W, Ronson A, et al: The assessment of serum nontransferrin-bound iron in chelation therapy and iron supplementation. Blood 2000; 95:2975.

650. Porter J: Practical management of iron overload. Br J Haematol 2001; 115:239.

651. Breuer W, Ermers MJ, et al: Desferrioxamine-chelatable iron, a component of serum non-transferrin-bound iron, used for assessing chelation therapy. Blood 2001; 97:792.

652. Hershko C, Weatherall DJ: Iron-chelating therapy. Crit Rev Clin Lab Sci 1988; 26:303.

653. Herbert V, Shaw S, et al: Most free-radical injury is iron-related: It is promoted by iron, hemin, holoferritin and vitamin C, and inhibited by desferoxamine and apoferritin. Stem Cells 1994; 12:289.

654. Willis ED: Effects of iron overload on lipid peroxide formation and oxidative demethylation by the liver endoplasmic reticulum. Biochem Pharmacol 1972; 21:239.

655. Tong Mak I, Weglicki WB: Characterization of iron-mediated peroxidative injury in isolated hepatic lysosomes. J Clin Invest 1985; 75:58.

656. Bacon BR, Park CH, et al: Hepatic mitochondrial oxidative metabolism in rats with chronic dietary iron overload. Hepatology 1985; 5:789.

657. Bacon BR, Tavill AS, et al: Hepatic lipid peroxidation in vivo in rats with chronic iron overload. J Clin Invest 1983; 71:429.

658. Heys AD, Dormandy TL: Lipid peroxidation in iron-overloaded spleens. Clin Sci 1981; 60:295.

659. Peters TJ, Seymour CA: Acid hydrolase activities and lysosomal integrity in liver biopsies from patients with iron overload. Clin Sci Mol Med 1978; 50:75.

660. O'Connell MJ, Ward RJ, et al: The role of iron in ferritin- and haemosiderin-mediated lipid peroxidation in liposomes. Biochem J 1985; 229:135.

661. Hershko C, Link G, et al: Modification of iron uptake and lipid peroxidation by hypoxia, ascorbic acid, and alpha-tocopherol in iron-loaded rat myocardial cell cultures. J Lab Clin Med 1987; 110:355.

662. Link G, Athias P, et al: Effect of iron loading on transmembrane potential, contraction, and automaticity of rat ventricular muscle cells in culture. J Lab Clin Med 1989; 113:103.

663. Rachmilewitz EA, Lubin BH, et al: Lipid membrane peroxidation in beta-thalassemia major. Blood 1976; 47:495.

664. Miniero R, Piga A, et al: Vitamin E and beta thalassemia. Haematologica 1983; 68:562.

665. Cranfield M, Gollan JL, et al: Serum antioxidant activity in normal and abnormal subjects. Ann Clin Biochem 1979; 16:299.

666. de Martino M, Rossi ME, et al: Change in superoxide anion production in neutrophils from multiply transfused beta thalassemia patients. Acta Haematol 1984; 71:289.

667. Bothwell TJ, and Finch CA: Iron Metabolism. Boston, Little, Brown, 1962.

668. Fawwaz RA, Winchell HS, et al: Hepatic iron deposition in humans. I. First-pass hepatic deposition of intestinally absorbed iron in patients with low plasma latent iron-binding capacity. Blood 1967; 30:417.

669. Buonanno G, Valente A, et al: Serum ferritin in beta thalassemia intermedia. Scand J Haematol 1984; 83:32.

670. Pippard MJ, Callender ST, et al: Iron absorption and loading in beta thalassemia intermedia. Lancet 1979; 2:819.

671. Telfar PT, Prestcott E, et al: Hepatic iron concentration combined with long-term monitoring of serum ferritin to predict complications of iron overload in thalassemia major. Br J Haematol 2000; 110:971.

672. Nielsen P, Gunther U, et al: Serum ferritin iron in iron overload and liver damage: Correlation to body iron stores and diagnostic relevance. J Lab Clin Med 2000; 135:413.

673. Brittenham GM, Cohen AR, et al: Hepatic iron stores and plasma ferritin concentration in patients with sickle cell anemia and thalassemia major. Am J Hematol 1993; 42:81.

674. de Virgiliis S, Sanna G, et al: Serum ferritin, liver iron stores, and liver histology in children with thalassemia. Arch Dis Child 1980; 55:43.

675. Worwood M, Cragg SJ, et al: Binding of serum ferritin to concanavalin A: Patients with homozygous beta thalassemia and transfusional iron overload. Br J Haematol 1980; 46:409.

676. Houang MTW, Skalicka A, et al: Correlation between computed tomographic values and liver iron content in thalassemia major with iron overload. Lancet 1979; l:1322.

677. Brittenham GM, Farrell DE, et al: Magnetic-susceptibility measurement of human iron stores. N Engl J Med 1982; 307:1671.

678. Engle MA, Erlandson M, et al: Late cardiac complications of chronic, severe, refractory anemia with hemochromatosis. Circulation 1964; 30:698.

679. Buja LM, Roberts WC: Iron in the heart. Etiology and clinical significance. Am J Med 1971; 51:209.

680. Sonakul D, Pacharee P, et al: Pathologic findings in 76 autopsy cases of thalassemia. Birth Defects Orig Artic Ser 1988; 23:157.

681. Finazzo M, Midiri M, et al: The heart of the patient with beta thalassemia major. Study with magnetic resonance [original article in Italian]. Radiol Med 1998; 96:462.

682. Aessopos A, Farmakis D, et al: Cardiac involvement in thalassemia intermedia: A multicenter study. Blood 2001; 97.

683. Lixi M, Montaldo P: Cardiological aspects and thalassemia syndrome in the past pediatric age: Instrumental findings, intracavitary cardiac biopsy reports and autopsy findings. Boll Soc Ital Cardiol 1979; 24:637.

684. Fitchett DH, Coltart DJ, et al: Cardiac involvement in secondary hemochromatosis: A catheter biopsy study and analysis of myocardium. Cardiovasc Res 1980; 14:719.

685. Link G, Pinson A, et al: Heart cells in culture: A model of myocardial iron overload and chelation. J Lab Clin Med 1985; 106:147.

686. Nienhuis AW, Griffith P, et al: Evaluation of cardiac function in patients with thalassemia major. Ann NY Acad Sci 1980; 80:384.

687. Henry WL, Nienhuis AW, et al: Echocardiographic abnormalities in patients with transfusion-dependent anemia and secondary myocardial iron deposition. Am J Med 1978; 64:547.

688. Valdez-Cruz LM, Reinecke C, et al: Preclinical abnormal segmental cardiac manifestations of thalassemia major in children on transfusion-chelation therapy: Echographic alterations of left ventricular posterior wall contraction and relaxation patterns. Am Heart J 1982; 103:505.

689. Kremastinos DT, Toutouzas PK, et al: Iron overload and left ventricular performance in beta thalassemia. Acta Cardiol 1984; 39:29.

690. Mariotti E, Agostini A, et al: Reduced left ventricular contractile reserve identified by low dose dobutamine echocardiography as an early marker of cardiac involvement in asymptomatic patients with thalassemia major. Echocardiography 1996; 13:463.

691. Leon MB, Borer JS, et al: Detection of early cardiac dysfunction in patients with severe beta-thalassemia and chronic iron overload. N Engl J Med 1979; 301:1143.

692. Freeman AP, Giles RW, et al: Early left ventricular dysfunction and chelation therapy in thalassemia major. Ann Intern Med 1983; 99:450.

693. Canale C, Terrachini V, et al: Thalassemic cardiomyopathy: Echocardiographic difference between major and intermediate thalassemia at rest and during isometric effort: Yearly follow-up. Clin Cardiol 1988; 11:563.

693a. Anderson LJ, Wonke B, Prescott E, et al: Comparison of effects of oral deferiprone and subcutaneous desferrioxamine on myocardial iron concentrations and ventricular function in beta-thalassemia. Lancet 2002; 360:516.

694. Risdon RA, Barry M, et al: Transfusional iron overload: The relationship between tissue iron concentration and hepatic fibrosis in thalassemia. J Pathol 1975; 116:83.

695. Angelucci E, Brittenham GM, et al: Hepatic iron concentration and total body iron stores in thalassemia major. N Engl J Med 2000; 343:327.

696. Iancu TL, Neustein HB: Ferritin in human liver cells of homozygous beta thalassemia: Ultrastructural observations. Br J Haematol 1977; 37:527.

697. Weintraub LR, Goral A, et al: Pathogenesis of hepatic fibrosis in experimental iron overload. Br J Haematol 1985; 59:321.

698. Masera G, Jean G, et al: Role of chronic hepatitis in development of thalassemic liver disease. Arch Dis Child 1976; 51:680.

699. Masera G, Jean G, et al: Sequential study of liver biopsy in thalassaemia. Arch Dis Child 1980; 55:800.

700. de Virgiliis S, Cornacchia G, et al: Chronic liver disease in transfusion-dependent thalassemia: Liver iron quantitation and distribution. Acta Haematol 1981; 65:32.

701. Barry M, Flynn DM, et al: Long-term chelation therapy in thalassemia major: Effect on liver iron concentration, liver histology, and clinical progress. Br Med J 1974; 2:16.

702. Cohen A: Current status of iron chelation therapy with deferoxamine. Semin Hematol 1990; 27:86.

703. Brittenham GM, Griffith PM, et al: Efficacy of deferoxamine in preventing complications or iron overload in patients with thalassemia major. N Engl J Med 1994; 331:567.

704. Aldouri MA, Wonke B, et al: Iron state and hepatic disease in patients with thalassaemia major, treated with long term subcutaneous desferrioxamine. J Clin Pathol 1987; 40:1353.

705. Wolman IJ, Ortalani M: Some clinical features of Cooley's anemia patients as related to transfusion schedules. Ann NY Acad Sci 1969; 105:407.

706. De Sanctis V, Vullo C, et al: Endocrine complications in thalassemia major. Prog Clin Biol Res 1989; 309:77.

707. Viprakasit V, Tanphaichitr VS, et al: Linear growth in homozygous beta-thalassemia and beta-thalassemia/hemoglobin E patients under different treatment regimens. J Med Assoc Thai 2001; 84:929.

708. Garcia-Mayor RV, Andrade Olivie A, et al: Linear growth in thalassemic children treated with intensive chelation therapy. A longitudinal study. Horm Res 1993; 40:189.

709. Benso L, Gambotto S, et al: Growth velocity monitoring of the efficacy of different therapeutic protocols in a group of thalassemic children. Eur J Pediatr 1995; 154:205.

710. Caruso-Nicoletti M, De Sanctis V, et al: Short stature and body proportion in thalassemia. J Pediatr Endocrinol Metab 1998; 3:81.

711. Pintor C, Cella SG, et al: Impaired growth hormone (GH) response to GH-releasing hormone in thalassemia major. J Clin Endocrinol Metab 1986; 62:263.

712. De Sanctis V, Stea S, et al: Growth hormone secretion and bone histomorphometric study in thalassaemic patients with acquired skeletal dysplasia secondary to desferrioxamine. J Pediatr Endocrinol Metab 1998; 3:827.

713. Chatterjee R, Katz M: Evaluation of gonadotrophin insufficiency in thalassemic boys with pubertal failure: Spontaneous versus provocative test. J Pediatr Endocrinol Metab 2001; 14:301.

714. Leheup BP, Cisternino M, et al: Growth hormone response following growth hormone releasing hormone injection in thalassemia major: Influence of pubertal development. J Endocrinol Invest 1991; 14:37.

715. Cavallo L, Gurrado R, et al: Short-term therapy with recombinant growth hormone in polytransfused thalassaemia major patients with growth deficiency. J Pediatr Endocrinol Metab 1998; 3:845.

716. Saenger D, Schwartz E, et al: Depressed serum somatomedin activity in beta-thalassemia. J Pediatr 1980; 96:214.

717. Sklar CA, Lew LQ, et al: Adrenal function in thalassemia major following long-term treatment with multiple transfusions and chelation therapy. Evidence for dissociation of cortisol and adrenal androgen secretion. Am J Dis Child 1987; 141:327.

718. George A, Bhaduri A, et al: Development of secondary sex characteristics in multitransfused thalassemic children. Indian J Pediatr 1997; 64:855.

719. Anoussakis CH, Alexiou D, et al: Endocrinological investigation of pituitary gonadal axis in thalassemia major. Acta Paediatr Scand 1977; 66:49.

720. Nienhuis AW, W. H, et al: Evaluation and treatment of chronic iron overload. In Zaino EC, Roberts RH (eds): Chelation Therapy in Chronic Iron Overload. Miami, Symposium Specialists, 1977, p 1.

721. Masala A, Melan T, et al: Endocrine functioning in multi-transfused prepubertal patients with homozygous beta thalassemia. J Clin Endocrinol Metab 1984; 58:667.

722. Flynn DM, Fairney A, et al: Hormonal changes in thalassaemia major. Arch Dis Child 1976; 51:828.

723. De Sanctis V, Vullo C, et al: Hypothalamic-pituitary-gonadal axis in thalassemic patients with secondary amenorrhea. Obstet Gynecol 1988; 72:643.

724. Wang C, Tso SC, et al: Hypogonadotropic hypogonadism in severe beta-thalassemia: Effect of chelation and pulsatile gonadotropin-releasing hormone therapy. J Clin Endocrinol Metab 1989; 68:511.

725. Valenti S, Giusti M, et al: Delayed puberty in males with beta-thalassemia major: Pulsatile gonadotropin-releasing hormone administration induced changes in gonadotropin isoform profiles and an increase in sex steroids. Eur J Endocrinol 1995; 133:48.

726. De Sanctis V, Vullo C, et al: Gonadal function in patients with beta thalassaemia major. J Clin Pathol 1988; 41:133.

727. Berkovitch M, Bistritzer T, et al: Iron deposition in the anterior pituitary in homozygous beta-thalassemia. J Pediatr Endocrinol Metab 2000; 13:179.

728. Argyropoulou MI, Metafratzi Z, et al: T2 relaxation rate as an index of pituitary iron overload in patients with beta-thalassemia major. AJR Am J Roentgenol 2000; 175:1567.

729. Chaterjee R, Katz M: Reversible hypogonadotrophic hypogonadism in sexually infantile male thalassaemic patients with transfusional iron overload. Clin Endocrinol 2000; 53:33.

730. Zervas A, Katopodi A, et al: Assessment of thyroid function in two hundred patients with beta-thalassemia major. Thyroid 2002; 12:151.

731. Spitz IM, Hirsch HJ, et al: TSH secretion in thalassemia. J Endocrinol Invest 1984; 7:495.

732. McIntosh N: Endocrinopathy in thalassemia major. Arch Dis Child 1976; 51:195.

733. Suadek CD, Hemm RM, et al: Abnormal glucose tolerance in beta-thalasaemia major. Metabolism 1977; 26:43.

734. Lassman MN, Genel M, et al: Carbohydrate homeostasis and pancreatic islet function in thalassemia. Ann Intern Med 1974; 80:65.

735. Chern JP, Lin KH, et al: Abnormal glucose tolerance in transfusion-dependent beta-thalassemic patients. Diabetes Care 2001; 24:850.

736. Merkel PA, Simonson DC, et al: Insulin resistance and hyperinsulinemia in patients with thalassemia major treated by hypertransfusion. N Engl J Med 1988; 318:809.

737. Brianda S, Maioli M, et al: The euglycemic clamp in patients with thalassaemia intermedia. Horm Metab Res 1987; 19:319.

738. Lassman MN, O'Brien RT, et al: Endocrine evaluation in thalassemia major. Ann NY Acad Sci 1974; 232:226.

739. Christenson RA, Pootrakul P, et al: Patients with thalassemia develop osteoporosis, osteomalacia, and hypoparathyroidism, all of which are corrected by transfusion. Birth Defects 1987; 23:409.

740. DeSanctis V, Vullo C, et al: Hypoparathyroidism in beta-thalassemia major. Acta Haem 1992; 88:105.

741. Chern JP, Lin KH: Hypoparathyroidism in transfusion-dependent patients with beta-thalassemia. J Pediatr Hematol Oncol 2002; 24:291.

742. Gerfner J, Boadus A, et al: Impaired parathyroid response to induced hypocalcemia in thalassemia major. J Pediat 1979; 95:210.

743. Mautalen CA, Kuicala R, et al: Hypoparathyroidism and iron storage disease. Am J Med Sci 1979; 276:363.

744. Aloia JF, Ostuni JA, et al: Combined vitamin D parathyroid defect in thalassemia major. Arch Intern Med 1982; 142:831.

745. Fucharoen S, Youngchaiyud P, et al: Hypoxaemia and the effect of aspirin in thalassemia. Southeast Asian J Med Public Health 1981; 12:90.

746. Keens T, O'Neal M, et al: Pulmonary function abnormalities in thalassemia patients on a hypertransfusion program. Pediatrics 1981; 65:1013.

747. Cooper D, Mangell A, et al: Low lung capacity and hypoxemia in children with thalassemia major. Am Rev Respir Dis 1980; 121:639.

748. Grant GP, Mansell AL, et al: The effect of transfusion on lung capacity, diffusing capacity, and arterial oxygen saturation in patients with thalassemia major. Pediatr Res 1986; 20:20.

749. Hoyt RW, Scarpa N, et al: Pulmonary function abnormalities in homozygous beta-thalassemia. J Pediatr 1986; 109:452.

750. Fung KP, Chow OK, et al: Pulmonary function in thalassemia major. J Pediatr 1987; 111:534.

751. Songkhla SN, Fucharoen S, et al: Lung perfusion in thalassemia. Birth Defects Orig Artic Ser 1987; 23:371.

752. Youngchaiyud P, Suthamsmai T, et al: Lung function tests in splenectomized beta-thalassemia/Hb E patients. Birth Defects Orig Artic Ser1987; 23:361.

753. Piatti G, Allegra L, et al: Beta-thalassemia and pulmonary function. Haematologica 1999; 84:804.

754. Filosa A, Esposito V, et al: Evidence of a restrictive spirometric pattern in older thalassemic patients. Respiration 2001; 68:273.

755. Zakynthinos E, Vassilakopoulos T, et al: Pulmonary hypertension, interstitial lung fibrosis, and lung iron deposition in thalassaemia major. Thorax 2001; 56:737.

756. Eldor A, Rachmilewitz EA: The hypercoagulable state in thalassemia. Blood 2002; 99:36.

757. Factor JM, Pottipati SR, et al: Pulmonary function abnormalities in thalassemia major and the role of iron overload. Am J Respir Crit Care Med 1994; 149:1570.

758. Eldor A, Maclouf J, et al: A chronic hypercoagulable state and life-long platelet activation in beta thalassemia major. Southeast Asian J Trop Med Public Health 1993; 24:92.

759. Koren A, Garty I, et al: Right ventricular cardiac dysfunction in beta-thalassemia major. Am J Dis Child 1987; 141:93.

760. Giardini C, Angelucci E, et al: Bone marrow transplantation for thalassemia. Experience in Pesaro, Italy. Am J Pediatr Hematol Oncol 1994; 16:6.

761. Giardini C, Galimberti M, et al: Bone marrow transplantation in thalassemia. Annu Rev Med 1995; 46:319.

762. Lucarelli G, Galimberti M, et al: Bone marrow transplantation in thalassemia. Hematol Oncol Clin North Am 1991; 5:549.

763. Fosburg MT, Nathan DG: Treatment of Cooley's anemia. Blood 1990; 76:435.

764. Giardina PJ, Hilgartner MW: Update on thalassemia. Pediatr Rev 1992; 13:55.

765. Dover GJ, Valle D: Therapy for beta-thalassemia—A paradigm for the treatment of genetic disorders. N Engl J Med 1994; 331:609.

766. Piomelli S, Loew T: Management of thalassemia major (Cooley's anemia). Hematol Oncol Clin North Am 1991; 5:557.

767. Olivieri NF: Thalassaemia: Clinical management. Baillieres Clin Haematol 1998; 11:147.

768. Olivieri NF: The beta-thalassemias. N Engl J Med 1999; 341:99.

769. Borgna-Pignatti C, Rugolotto S, et al: Survival and disease complications in thalassemia major. Ann NY Acad Sci 1998; 850:227.

770. Rebulla P, Modell B: Transfusion requirements and effects in patients with thalassaemia major. Lancet 1991; 337:277.

771. Weiner M, Kartpatkin M, et al: Cooley's anemia: High transfusion regimen and chelation therapy. Results and perspective. J Pediatr 1978; 92:653.

772. Necheles TF, Chang S, et al: Intensive transfusion therapy in thalassemia major: An eight year follow-up. Ann NY Acad Sci 1974; 232:179.

773. Brook CG, Thompson EN, et al: Growth in children with thalassemia major—An effect of two different transfusion regimens. Arch Dis Child 1969; 44:612.

774. Kattamis C, Touliatds N, et al: Growth of children with thalassemia: Effect of different transfusion regimens. Arch Dis Child 1970; 45:502.

775. Propper RD, Vutton LN, et al: New approaches to the transfusion management of thalassemia. Blood 1980; 55:55.

776. Masera G, Terzoli S, et al: Evaluation of the super-transfusion regimen in homozygous beta thalassemia children. Br J Haematol 1982; 52:11.

777. Gabutti V, Piga A, et al: Hemoglobin levels and blood requirement in thalassemia. Arch Dis Child 1982; 57:156.

778. Piomelli S, Graziano J, et al: Chelation therapy, transfusion requirement and iron balance in young thalassemia patients. Ann NY Acad Sci 1980; 344:409.

779. Piomelli S, Seamon C, et al: Separation of younger red cells with improved survival in vivo. An approach to chronic transfusion therapy. Proc Natl Acad Sci USA 1978; 75:3474.

780. Graziano JH, Piomelli S, et al: A simple technique for preparation of young red cells for transfusion from ordinary blood units. Blood 1982; 59:865.

781. Bracey AW, Klein HG, et al: Ex-vivo selective isolation of young red blood cells using the IBM-2991 cell washer. Blood 1983; 61:1068.

782. Hogan VA, Blanchette VS, et al: A simple method for preparing neocyte-enriched leukocyte poor blood for transfusion dependent patients. Transfusion 1986; 26:253.

783. Kevy SV, Jacobson MS, et al: A new approach to neocyte transfusion: Preliminary report. J Clin Apheresis 1988; 4:194.

784. Simon TL, Sohmer P, et al: Extended survival of neocytes produced by a new system. Transfusion 1989; 29:221.

785. Cohen AR, Schmidt JM, et al: Clinical trial of young red cell transfusions. J Pediatr 1984; 104:865.

786. Marcus RE, Wonke B, et al: A prospective trial of young red cells in 48 patients with transfusion-dependent thalassaemia. Br J Haematol 1985; 60:153.

787. Wolfe LC, Sallan D, et al: Current therapy and new approaches to the treatment of thalassemia major. Ann NY Acad Sci 1985; 45:248.

788. Piomelli S, Hart D, et al: Current strategies in the management of Cooley's anemia. Ann NY Acad Sci 1985; 445:256.

789. Propper RD: Neocytes and neocyte-gerocyte exchange. Prog Clin Biol Res 1982; 88:227.

790. Meryman HT, Hornblower M: The preparation of red cells depleted of leukocytes. Transfusion 1986; 26:101.

791. Piomelli S, Karpatkin MH, et al: Hypertransfusion regimen in patients with Cooley's anemia. Ann NY Acad Sci 1974; 232:186.

792. Coles SM, Klein HG, et al: Alloimmunization in two multitransfused patient populations. Transfusion 1981; 21:462.

793. Michail-Merianou V, Pamphili-Panousopoulou L, et al: Alloimmunization to red cell antigens in thalassemia: Comparative study of usual versus better-match transfusion programmes. Vox Sang 1987; 52:95.

794. Spanos T, Karageorga M, et al: Red cell alloantibodies in patients with thalassemia. Vox Sang 1990; 58:50.

795. Diamond WJ, Brown FL, et al: Delayed hemolytic transfusion reaction presenting a sickle cell crisis. Ann Intern Med 1980; 93:231.

796. Blumberg N, Ross K, et al: Should chronic transfusion be matched for antigens other than ABO and Rh(o)D? Vox Sang 1984; 47:205.

797. Moroni GA, Piacentini G, et al: Hepatitis B or non-A, non-B virus infection in multitransfused thalassaemic patients. Arch Dis Child 1984; 59:1127.

798. Choo Q, Kuo G, et al: Isolation of a cDNA clone derived from a blood-borne non-A non-B hepatitis genome. Science 1989; 244:359.

799. Kuo G, Choo Q, et al: An assay for circulating antibodies to a major etiologic virus of human non-A non-B hepatitis. Science 1989; 244:362.

800. Alter MJ: Epidemiology of hepatitis C. Hepatology 1997; 26(Suppl 1):62S.

801. Darby S, Ewart DW, et al: Mortality from liver cancer and liver disease in hemophiliac men and boys in UK given blood products contaminated with hepatitis C. Lancet 1997; 250:1425.

802. Jonas MM: Hepatitis C infection in children. N Engl J Med 1999; 341:912.

803. Barton AL, Banner BF, et al: Distribution of iron in the liver predicts the response of chronic hepatitis C infection to interferon therapy. Am J Clin Pathol 1995; 103:419. [Published erratum Am J Cln Pathol 1995; 104: 232.]

804. Fargion S, Fracanzani AL, et al: Liver iron influences the response to interferon alpha therapy in chronic hepatitis C. Eur J Gastroenterol Hepatol 1997; 9:497.

805. Haque S, B. C, et al: Iron overload in patients with chronic hepatitis C: A clinicopathologic study. Hum Pathol 1996; 27:1277.

806. Olynyk JK, Reddy KR, et al: Hepatic iron concentration as a predictor of response to interferon alfa therapy in chronic hepatitis C. Gastroenterology 1995; 108:1104.

807. Riggio O, Montagnese F, et al: Iron overload in patients with chronic viral hepatitis: How common is it? Am J Gastroenterol 1997; 92:1298.

808. Sievert W, Pianko S, et al: Hepatic iron overload does not prevent a sustained virological response to inferferon-alpha therapy: A long term follow-up study in hepatitis C-infected patients with beta thalassemia major. Am J Gastroenterol 2002; 97:982.

809. Manconi PE, Dessi C, et al: Human immunodeficiency virus infection in multi-transfused patients with thalassaemia major. Eur J Pediatr 1988; 147:304.

810. Okon E, Levij S, et al: Splenectomy, iron overload, and liver cirrhosis in beta-thalassemia major. Acta Haematol 1976; 56:142.

811. Graziano JH, Piomelli S, et al: Chelation therapy in beta-thalassemia major. III. The role of splenectomy in achieving iron balance. J Pediat 1981; 99:695.

812. al-Salem AH, al-Dabbous I, Bhamidibati P: The role of partial splenectomy in children with thalassemia. Eur J Pediatr Surg 1998; 8:334.

813. Modell B: Management of thalassemia major. Br Med Bull 1976; 32:270.

814. Modell CB: Total management of thalassaemia major. Arch Dis Child 1977; 52:489.

815. Cohen A, Markenson AL, et al: Transfusion requirements and splenectomy in thalassemia major. J Pediat 1980; 97:100.

816. Blendis LM, Modell CB, et al: Some effects of splenectomy in thalassemia major. Br J Haematol 1974; 28:77.

817. Engelhard D, Cividalli G, et al: Splenectomy in homozygous beta-thalassemia: A retrospective study of thirty patients. Br J Haematol 1975; 31:391.

818. Cohen A, Gayer R, et al: Long-term effect of splenectomy on transfusion requirements in thalassemia major. Am J Hematol 1989; 30:254.

819. Cunningham-Rundles S, Giardina PJ, et al: Effect of transfusional iron overload on immune response. J Infect Dis 2000; 182(Suppl 1):S115.

820. Walker EMJ, Walker SM: Effects of iron overload on the immune system. Ann Clin Lab Sci 2000; 30:354.

821. Eraklis AJ, Kevy SV, et al: Hazard of overwhelming infection after splenectomy in childhood. N Engl J Med 1967; 276:1225.

822. Erickson WD, Burgert EO, et al: The hazard of infection following splenectomy in children. Am J Dis Child 1968; 116:1.

823. Ein SH, Shandling V, et al: The morbidity and mortality of splenectomy in childhood. Ann Surg 1977; 185:307.

824. Aommann AJ, Addiego J, et al: Polyvalent pneumococcal polysaccharide immunization of patients with sickle cell anemia and patients with splenectomy. N Engl J Med 1977; 297:897.

825. Kafidi KT, Rotschafer JC: Bacterial vaccines for splenectomized patients. Drug Intell Clin Pharm 1988; 22:192.

826. Recommendations of the Advisory Committee on Immunization Practices (ACIP): Use of vaccines and immune globulins in persons with altered immunocompetence. MMWR Morbid Mortal Wkly Rep 1993; 42:1.

827. Ambrosino DM, Molrine DC: Critical appraisal of immunization strategies for prevention of infection in the immunocompromised host. Hematol Oncol Clin North Am 1993; 7:1027.

828. Wanachiwanawin W: Infections in E-beta thalassemia. J Pediatr Hematol Oncol 2000; 22:581.

829. Rostagno C, Prisco D, et al: Pulmonary hypertension associated with long-standing thrombocytosis. Chest 1991; 99:1303.

830. Green NS: *Yersinia* infections in patients with homozygous beta-thalassemia associated with iron overload and its treatment. Pediatr Hematol Oncol 1992; 9:247.

831. Karabus C, Fielding J: Desferroxamine chelatable iron in hemolytic, megaloblastic and sideroblastic anemia. Br J Haematol 1967; 13:924.

832. White GP, Bailey-Wood R, et al: The effect of chelating agents on cellular iron metabolism. Clin Sci Mol Med 1976; 50:152.

833. Hershko C, Rachmilewitz EA: Mechanism of desferrioxamine-induced iron excretion in thalassemia. Br J Haematol 1979; 42:125.

834. Bianco I, Graziani B, et al: A study of the mechanisms and sites of action of deferrioxamine in thalassemia major. Acta Haematol (Basel) 1984; 71:100.

835. Pippard M, Callendar ST, et al: Ferrioxamine excretion in iron-loaded man. Blood 1982; 60:288.

836. Propper RD, Shurin SB, et al: Reassessment of the use of desferrioxamine B in iron overload. N Engl J Med 1976; 294:1421.

837. O'Brien RT: Ascorbic acid enhancement of desferrioxamine-induced urinary iron excretion in thalassemia major. Ann NY Acad Sci 1974; 232:221.

838. Modell CB, Beck J: Long-term desferrioxamine therapy in thalassemia. Ann NY Acad Sci 1974; 232:201.

839. Propper RD, Cooper B, et al: Continuous subcutaneous administration of desferrioxamine in patients with iron overload. N Engl J Med 1977; 297:418.

840. Hussain MAM, Green N, et al: Subcutaneous infusion and intramuscular injection of desferrioxamine in patients with transfusional iron overload. Lancet 1976; 2:1278.

841. Graziano JH, Markenson A, et al: Chelation therapy in beta-thalassemia major. I. Intravenous and subcutaneous desferrioxamine. J Pediat 1978; 92:648.

842. Hoffbrand AV, Gorman A: Improvement in iron status and liver function in patients with transfusional iron overload with long-term subcutaneous desferrioxamine. Lancet 1979; I:947.

843. Cohen A, Martin M, et al: Response to long-term deferoxamine therapy in thalassemia. J Pediat 1981; 99:689.

844. Modell B, Letsky E, et al: Survival and desferrioxamine in thalassemia major. Br Med J 1982; 284:1081.

845. Wolfe L, Olivieri N, et al: Prevention of cardiac disease by subcutaneous deferoxamine in patients with thalassemia major. N Engl J Med 1985; 312:1600.

846. Maurer HS, Lloyd SJ, et al: A prospective evaluation of iron chelation therapy in children with severe beta-thalassemia. A six-year study. Am J Dis Child 1988; 142:287.

847. de Virgiliis S, Cossu P, et al: Effect of subcutaneous desferrioxamine on iron balance in young thalassemia patients. Am J Pediat Hematol Oncol 1983; 5:73.

848. Fargion S, Taddei MT, et al: Early iron overload in beta thalassemia major. When to start chelation therapy. Arch Dis Child 1982; 57:929.

849. Russo G, Romeo MA, et al: Early iron chelation therapy in thalassemia major. Haematologica 1983; 68:69.

850. Davis BA, Porter JB: Long-term outcome of continuous 24-hour deferoxamine infusion via indwelling intravenous catheters in high-risk beta-thalassemia. Blood 2000; 95:1229.

851. Freeman AP, Giles RW, et al: Sustained normalization of cardiac function by chelation therapy in thalassaemia major. Clin Lab Haematol 1989; 11:299.

852. Olivieri NF, Nathan DG, et al: Survival in medically treated patients with homozygous beta-thalassemia. N Engl J Med 1994; 331:574.

853. Ehlers KH, Giardina PJ, et al: Prolonged survival in patients with beta-thalassemia major treated with deferoxamine. J Pediatr 1991; 118:540.

854. Ehlers KH, Levin AR, et al: Longitudinal study of cardiac function in thalassemia major. Ann NY Acad Sci 1980; 344:397.

855. Matthew R, Brain M, et al: Thalassemia. In Current Therapy in Hematology/Oncology-3. Philadelphia, Decker, 1988, p 39.

856. Giardina PJ, Ehlers KH, et al: The effect of subcutaneous deferoxamine on the cardiac profile of thalassemia major: A five-year study. Ann NY Acad Sci 1985; 445:282.

857. Lerner N, Blei F, et al: Chelation therapy and cardiac status in older patients with thalassemia major. Am J Pediatr Hematol Oncol 1990; 12:56.

858. Marcus RE, Davies SC, et al: Desferrioxamine to improve cardiac function in iron overloaded patients with thalassemia major. Lancet 1984; I:392.

859. De Sanctis V, D'Ascola G, et al: The development of diabetes mellitus and chronic liver disease in long term chelated beta thalassaemic patients. Postgrad Med J 1986; 62:831.

860. Olivieri NF, Bunic JR, et al: Visual and auditory neurotoxicity in patients receiving subcutaneous deferoxamine infusions. N Engl J Med 1986; 314:869.

861. Barratt PS, Toogood IR: Hearing loss attributed to desferrioxamine in patients with beta-thalassaemia major. Med J Aust 1987; 147:177.

862. Albera R, Pia F, et al: Hearing loss and desferrioxamine in homozygous beta-thalassemia. Audiology 1988; 27:207.

863. Porter JB, Jaswon MS, et al: Desferrioxamine ototoxicity: Evaluation of risk factors in thalassaemic patients and guidelines for safe dosage. Br J Haematol 1989; 73:403.

864. de Virgiliis S, Congia M, et al: Depletion of trace elements and acute ocular toxicity induced by desferrioxamine in patients with thalassaemia. Arch Dis Child 1988; 63:250.

865. Davies SC, Marcus RE, et al: Ocular toxicity of high-dose intravenous desferrioxamine. Lancet 1983; 2:181.

866. Marciani MG, Cianciulli P, et al: Toxic effects of high-dose defer-oxamine treatment in patients with iron overload: An electrophysi-ological study of cerebral and visual function. Haematologica 1991; 76:131.

867. Rinaldi M, Della Corte M, et al: Ocular involvement correlated with age in patients affected by major and intermedia beta-thalassemia treatment or not with desferrioxamine. Metab Pediatr Syst Ophthalmol 1993; 16:23.

868. Jiang C, Hansen RM, et al: Rod and rod mediated function in patients with beta-thalassemia major. Doc Ophthalmol 1998; 96:333.

869. Polson RJ, Jawed A, et al: Treatment of rheumatoid arthritis with desferrioxamine: Relation between stores of iron before treatment and side effects. Br Med J 1985; 291:448.

870. Bentur Y, Koren G, et al: Comparison of deferoxamine phar-macokinetics between asymptomatic thalassemic children and those exhibiting severe neurotoxicity. Clin Pharmacol Ther 1990; 47:478.

871. Blake DR, Winyard P, et al: Cerebral and ocular toxicity induced by desferrioxamine. Q J Med 1985; 56:345.

872. Peto TEA, Hershko C: Iron and infection. Baillieres Clin Haematol 1989; 2:435.

873. Robins-Browne RM, Prpic JK: Effects of iron and desferrioxam-ine on infections with *Yersinia enterocolitica*. Infect Immun 1985; 47:774.

874. Gallant T, Freedman MH, et al: *Yersinia* sepsis in patients with iron overload treated with deferoxamine. N Engl J Med 1986; 314:1643.

875. Goodhill JJ, Abuelo JG: Mucormycosis—A new risk of deferoxam-ine therapy in dialysis patients with aluminum or iron overload? N Engl J Med 1987; 317:54.

876. Bowern N, Ramshaw IA, et al: Effect of an iron-chelating agent on lymphocyte proliferation. Aust J Exp Biol Med Sci 1984; 62(Part 6):743.

877. Bowern N, Ramshaw IA, et al: Inhibition of autoimmune neu-ropathological process by treatment with an iron-chelating agent. J Exp Med 1984; 160:1536.

878. Bierer BE, Nathan DG: The effect of desferrithiocin, an oral iron chelator, on T cell function. Blood 1990; 76:2052.

879. Carotenuto P, Pontesilli O, et al: Desferoxamine blocks IL 2 recep-tor on T lymphocytes. J Immunol 1986; 136:2342.

880. Estrov Z, Tawa A, et al: In vitro and in vivo effects of deferoxam-ine in neonatal acute leukemia. Blood 1987; 69:757.

881. Lederman HM, Cohen A, et al: Deferoxamine: A reversible S-phase inhibitor of human lymphocyte proliferation. Blood 1984; 64:748.

882. Freedman MH, Grisaru D, et al: Pulmonary syndrome in patients with thalassemia major receiving intravenous deferoxamine infu-sions. Am J Dis Child 1990; 144:565.

883. Tenenbein M, Kowalski S, et al: Pulmonary toxic effects of contin-uous desferrioxamine administration in acute iron poisoning. Lancet 1992; 339:699.

884. Adamson IY, Sienko A, et al: Pulmonary toxicity of deferoxamine in iron-poisoned mice. Toxicol Appl Pharmacol 1993; 120:13.

885. Frank L: Hyperoxic inhibition of newborn rat lung development: Protection by deferoxamine. Free Radic Biol Med 1991; 11:341.

886. Shannon M: Desferrioxamine in acute iron poisoning. Lancet 1992; 339:1601.

887. Koren G, Bentur Y, et al: Acute changes in renal function associ-ated with deferoxamine therapy. Am J Dis Child 1989; 143:1077.

888. Koren G, Kochavi-Atiya Y, et al: The effects of subcutaneous deferoxamine adminstration on renal function in thalassemia major. Int J Hematol 1991; 54:371.

889. Cianciulli P, Sollecito D, et al: Early detection of nephrotoxic effects in thalassemic patients receiving desferrioxamine therapy. Kidney Int 1994; 46:467.

890. Hartkamp MJ, Babyn PS, et al: Spinal deformities in deferoxam-ine-treated homozygous beta-thalassemia major patients. Pediatr Radiol 1993; 23:525.

891. Olivieri NF, Koren G, et al: Growth failure and bony changes induced by deferoxamine. Am J Pediatr Hematol Oncol 1992; 14:48.

892. Olivieri NF, Koren G, et al: Reduction of tissue iron stores and normalization of serum ferritin during treatment with the oral iron chelator L1 in thalassemia intermedia. Blood 1992; 79:2741.

892. Tamary H, Goshen J, et al: Long-term intravenous deferoxam-ine treatment for noncomplaint transfusion-dependent beta-thalassemia patients. Israel J Med Sci 1994; 30:658.

894. deMontalembert M, Jan D, et al: Intensification du traitement chelateur pu fer par la desferrioxamine a l'aide d'une chambre implantable d'acces veineux (Port-A-Cath). Arch Fr Pediatr 1992; 49:159.

895. Ward A, Caro JJ, et al: An international survey of patients with tha-lassemia major and their views about sustaining life-long desfer-rioxamine use. BMC Clin Phamacol 2002; 2:3.

896. Caro JJ, Ward A, et al: Impact of thalassemia major on patients and their families. Acta Haematol 2002; 107:150.

897. Treadwell MJ, Weissman L: Improving adherence with deferoxam-ine regimens for patients receiving chronic transfusion therapy. Semin Hematol 2001; 38:77.

898. Hider RC, Singh S, et al: The development of hydroxypyridin-4-ones as orally active iron chelators. Ann Clin Lab Sci 1990; 612:327.

899. Berdoukas V, Bentley P, et al: Toxicity of oral iron chelator L1 [let-ter to the editor]. Lancet 1993; 341:1088.

900. Singh S, Epemolu RO, et al: Urinary metabolic profiles in human and rat of 1,2-dimethyl- and 1,2-diethyl-substituted 3-hydrox-ypyridin-4-ones. Drug Metab Dispos 1992; 20:256.

901. Choudhury R, Singh S: Effect of iron overload on the metabolism and urinary recovery of 3-hydroxypyridin-4-one chelating agents in the rat. Drug Metab Dispos 1995; 23:314.

902. Kontoghiorghes GJ, Aldouri MA, et al: Effective chelation of iron in beta thalassemia with the oral chelator 1,2-dimethyl-3-hydrox-ypyrid-4-one. Br Med J 1987; 295:1509.

903. Olivieri NF, Brittenham GM, et al: Iron-chelation therapy with oral deferipronein patients with thalassemia major. N Engl J Med 1995; 332:918.

904. Olivieri NF, Brittenham GM, et al: Long-term safety and effec-tiveness of iron-chelation therapy with deferiprone for thalassemia major. N Engl J Med 1998; 339:47.

905. Olivieri NF, Brittenham GM, et al: Iron-chelation therapy and the treatment of thalassemia. Blood 1997; 89:739.

906. Nathan DG: An orally active iron chelator. N Engl J Med 1995; 332:953.

907. Töndury P, Zimmermann A, et al: Liver iron and fibrosis during long-term treatment with deferiprone in Swiss thalassaemic patients. Br J Haematol 1998; 101:413–415.

908. Del Vecchio GC, Crollo E, et al: Factors influencing effectiveness of defcriprone in a thalassaemia major clinical setting. Acta Haematol 2000; 104:99.

909. Kowdley KV, Kaplan MM: Iron-chelation therapy with oral deferiprone—Toxicity or lack of efficacy? [editorial] N Engl J Med 1998; 339:468.

909a. Wanless IR, Sweeney G, Dhillon AP, et al: Lack of progressive hepatic fibrosis during long-term therapy with deferiprone in sub-jects with transfusion-dependent beta-thalassemia. Blood 2002; 100:1566.

910. Taher A, Sheikh-Taha M, et al: Comparison between deferoxam-ine and deferiprone (L1) in iron loaded thalassemia patients. Eur Haematol 2001; 67:30.

911. Barman Balfour JA, Foster RH: Deferiprone: A review of its clini-cal potential in iron overload in beta-thalassemia major and other transfusion-dependent diseases. Drugs 1999; 58:553.

912. Taher A, Chamoun FM, et al: Efficacy and side effects of deferiprone (L1) in thalassemia patients not compliant with des-ferrioxamine. Acta Haematol 1999; 101:173.

913. Deferiprone: New preparation. Poorly assessed. Prescrire Int 2000; 9:131.

914. de Franceschi L, Shalev O, et al: Deferiprone therapy in homozy-gous human beta-thalassemia removes erythrocyte membrane free iron and reduces KCl cotransport activity. J Lab Clin Med 1999; 133:64.

915. Giardina PJ, Grady RW: Chelation therapy in beta-thalassemia: An optimistic update. Semin Hematol 2001; 38:360.

916. Hoffbrand AV: Oral iron chelation. Semin Hematol 1996; 33:1.

917. Pippard MJ, Weatherall DJ: Oral iron chelation therapy for tha-lassemia: An uncertain scene. Br J Haematol 2000; 111:2.

918. Naylor CD: The deferiprone controversy: Time to move on. Can Med Assoc J 2002; 166:452.

919. Nick HP, Acklin P, et al: A new, potent, orally active iron chelator. In Badman BR, Brittenham GM (eds): Iron Chelators: New

Development Strategies. Ponte Verde Beach, FL, Saratoga Group, 2000.

920. Roesner HP: The role of ascorbic acid in the turnover of storage iron. Semin Hematol 1983; 20:91.

921. Lynch SR, Seftel HC, et al: Accelerated oxidative catabolism of ascorbic acid in siderotic Bantu. Am J Clin Nutr 1967; 20:641.

922. Lipschitz DA, Bothwell TH, et al: The role of ascorbic acid in the metabolism of storage iron. Br J Haematol 1972; 20:155.

923. Wapnick AA, Bothwell TH, et al: The relationship between serum iron levels and ascorbic acid stores in siderotic Bantu. Br J Haematol 1970; 19:271.

924. Cohen A, Cohen IJ, et al: Scurvy and altered iron stores in thalassemia major. N Engl J Med 1981; 304:158.

925. Nienhuis AW, Delea C, et al: Evaluation of desferrioxamine and ascorbic acid for the treatment of chronic iron overload. In Bergsma D, Cerami, et al (eds): Birth Defects: Iron Metabolism and Thalassemia, New York, Alan R. Liss, 1976, p 177.

926. Bridges KR, Hoffman KE: The effects of ascorbic acid on the intracellular metabolism of iron and ferritin. J Biol Chem 1986; 261:14273.

927. Bridges KR: Ascorbic acid inhibits lysosomal autophagy of ferritin. J Biol Chem 1987; 262:14773.

928. Miller DM, Aust SD: Studies of ascorbate-dependent, iron-catalyzed lipid peroxidation. Arch Biochem Biophys 1989; 271:113.

929. Burkitt MJ, Gilbert BC: The control of iron-induced oxidative damage in isolated rat-liver mitochondria by respiration state and ascorbate. Free Radic Res Commun 1989; 5:333.

930. Henry W: Echocardiographic evaluation of the heart in thalassemia major. In Nienhuis, A.W., moderator: Thalassemia major: Molecular and clinical aspects. Ann Intern Med 1979; 91:883.

931. Nienhuis AW: Vitamin C and iron. N Engl J Med 1981; 304:170.

932. Hyman CB, Landing B, et al: *dl*-α-Tocopherol, iron, and lipofuscin in thalassemia. Ann NY Acad Sci 1974; 232:211.

933. Zannos-Mariolea L, Papagregoriou-Theodoridou M, et al: Relationship between tocopherols and serum lipid levels in children with beta-thalassemia major. Am J Clin Nutr 1978; 31:259.

934. Oski FA, Barnes LA: Vitamin E deficiency: A previously unrecognized cause of hemolytic anemia in the premature infant. J Pediatr 1967; 70:211.

935. Hershko C, Rachmilewitz EA: The inhibitory effect of vitamin E on desferrioxamine-induced iron excretion in rats. Proc Soc Exp Biol Med 1976; 152:249.

936. Lubhy AL, Cooperman JM, et al: Folic acid deficiency as a limiting factor in the anemia of thalassemia major. Blood 1961; 18:786.

937. Robinson MG, Watson RJ: Megaloblastic anemia complicating thalassemia major. Am J Dis Child 1963; 105:275.

938. Lubhy AL, Cooperman JM, et al: Vitamin B12 metabolism in thalassemia major. Ann NY Acad Sci 1969; 165:443.

939. Zaino E: Deferoxamine and trace metal excretion. In Zaino EC, Roberts RH (eds): Chelation Therapy in Chronic Iron Overload. Miami, Symposium Specialists, 1977, p 95.

940. Ridley CM: Zinc deficiency developing in treatment for thalassemia. J R Soc Med 1982; 75:38.

941. Thomas ED, Buckner CD, et al: Marrow transplantation for thalassaemia. Lancet 1982; 2:8292.

942. Lucarelli G, Polchi P, et al: Allogeneic marrow transplantation for thalassemia. Exp Hematol 1984; 12:676.

943. Piomelli S, Lerner N, et al: Bone marrow transplantation for thalassemia [correspondence]. N Engl J Med 1987; 317:964.

944. Lucarelli G, Polchi P, et al: Marrow transplantation for thalassaemia following busulphan and cyclophosphamide. Lancet 1985; 1:1355.

945. Lucarelli G, Galimberti M, et al: Marrow transplantation in patients with advanced thalassemia. N Engl J Med 1987; 316:1050.

946. Lucarelli G, Galimberti M, et al: Bone marrow transplantation in patients with thalassemia. N Engl J Med 1990; 322:417.

947. Walters MC, Sullivan KM, et al: Bone marrow transplantation for thalassemia. The USA experience. Am J Pediatr Hematol Oncol 1994; 16:11.

948. Vellodi A, Picton S, et al: Bone marrow transplantation for thalssaemia: Experience of two British centres. Bone Marrow Transplant 1994; 13:559.

949. Cao A, Galanello Renzo M, et al: Clinical experience of management of thalassemia: The Sardinian experience. Semin Hematol 1996; 33:66.

950. Shulman HM, Hinterberger W: Hepatic veno-occlusive disease-liver toxicity syndrome after bone marrow transplantation. Bone Marrow Transfus 1992; 10:197.

951. Apperley JF: Bone marrow transplant for the haemoglobinopathies: Past, present and future. Baillieres Clin Haematol 1993; 6:299.

952. La Nasa G, Giardini C, et al: Unrelated donor bone marrow transplantation for thalasemmia: The effect of extended haplotypes. Blood 2002; 99:4350.

953. Miniero R, Rocha V, et al: Cord blood transplantation in hemoglobinopathies. Bone Marrow Transplant 1999; 22:578.

954. Gluckman E, Rocha V, et al: Cord blood stem cell transplantation. Best Pract Res Clin Haematol 1999; 12:279.

955. DeSimone J, Heller P, et al: 5-Azacytidine stimulates fetal hemoglobin synthesis in anemia baboons. Proc Natl Acad Sci USA 1982; 79:4428.

956. Ley TJ, DeSimone J, et al: 5-Azacytidine selectively increases gamma-globin synthesis in a patient with beta thalassemia. N Engl J Med 1982; 307:1469.

957. Charache S, Dover G, et al: Treatment of sickle cell anemia with 5-azacytidine results in increased fetal hemoglobin production and is associated with nonrandom hypomethylation of DNA around the gamma-delta-beta-globin gene complex. Proc Natl Acad Sci USA 1983; 80:4842.

958. Ley TJ, DeSimone J, et al: 5-Azacytidine increases gamma-globin synthesis and reduces the proportion of dense cells in patients with sickle cell anemia. Blood 1983; 62:370.

959. Letvin NL, Linch DC, et al: Augmentation of fetal-hemoglobin production in anemic monkeys by hydroxyurea. N Engl J Med 1984; 310:869.

960. Papayannopoulou T, de Ron AT, et al: Arabinosylcytosine induces fetal hemoglobin in baboons by perturbing erythroid cell differentiation kinetics. Science 1984; 224:617.

961. Platt O, Orkin SH, et al: Hydroxyurea enhances fetal hemoglobin production in sickle cell anemia. J Clin Invest 1984; 74:652.

962. Lavelle D, DeSimone J, et al: Fetal hemoglobin reactivation in baboon and man: A short perspective. Am J Hematol 1993; 42:91.

963. Hajjar FM, Pearson HA: Pharmacologic treatment of thalassemia intermedia with hydroxyurea. J Pediatr 1994; 125:490.

964. Swank RA, Stamatoyannopoulos G: Fetal gene reactivation. Curr Opin Genet Dev 1998; 8:366.

965. Olivieri NF, Weatherall DJ: The therapeutic reactivation of fetal haemoglobin. Hum Mol Genet 1998; 7:1655.

966. Al-Khatti A, Veith RW, et al: Stimulation of fetal hemoglobin synthesis by erythropoietin in baboons. N Engl J Med 1987; 317:415.

967. McDonagh KT, Dover GJ, et al: Manipulation of HbF production with hematopoietic growth factors. In Stamatoyannopoulos G, Nienhuis AW (eds): Hemoglobin Switching, Part B: Cellular and Molecular Mechanisms. New York, Alan R. Liss, 1989, p 307.

968. McDonagh KT, Dover GJ, et al: Hydroxyurea-induced HbF production in anemic primates: Augmentation by erythropoietin, hematopoietic growth factors, and sodium butyrate. Exp Hematol 1992; 20:1156.

969. Umemura T, al KA, et al: Effects of interleukin-3 and erythropoietin on in vivo erythropoiesis and F-cell formation in primates. Blood 1989; 74:1571.

970. Perrine SP, Greene MF, et al: Delay in the fetal globin switch in infants of diabetic mothers. N Engl J Med 1985; 312:334.

971. Little JA, Dempsey NJ, et al: Metabolic persistance of fetal hemoglobin. Blood 1995; 75:1712.

972. Perrine SP, Rudolph A, et al: Butyrate infusions in the ovine fetus delay the biologic clock for globin gene switching. Proc Natl Acad Sci USA 1988; 85:8540.

973. Constantoulakis P, Papayannopoulou T, et al: alpha-Amino-N-butyric acid stimulates fetal hemoglobin in the adult. Blood 1988; 72:1961.

974. Constantoulakis P, Knitter G, et al: On the induction of fetal hemoglobin by butyrates: In vivo and in vitro studies with sodium butyrate and comparison of combination treatments with 5-AzaC and AraC. Blood 1989; 74:1963.

975. Burns LJ, Glauber JG, et al: Butyrate induces selective transcriptional activation of a hypomethylated embryonic globin gene in adult erythroid cells. Blood 1988; 72:1536.

976. Stamatoyannopoulos G, Blau CA, et al: Fetal hemoglobin induction by acetate, a product of butyrate catabolism. Blood 1994; 84:3198.

977. Dover GJ, Brusilow S, et al: Induction of fetal hemoglobin production in subjects with sickle cell anemia by oral sodium phenylbutyrate. Blood 1994; 84:339.

978. Perrine SP, Ginder GD, et al: A short-term trial of butyrate to stimulate fetal-globin-gene expression in the beta-globin disorders. N Engl J Med 1993; 328:81.

979. Perrine SP, Olivieri NF, et al: Butyrate derivatives. New agents for stimulating fetal globin production in the beta-globin disorders. Am J Pediatr Hematol Oncol 1994; 16:67.

980. Collins AF, Pearson HA, et al: Oral sodium phenylbutyrate therapy in homozygous beta thalassemia: A clinical trial. Blood 1995; 85:43.

981. Sher GD, Olivieri NF: Rapid healing of chronic leg ulcers during arginine butyrate therapy in patients with sickle cell disease and thalassemia. Blood 1994; 84:2378.

982. Sher GD, Ginder GD, et al: Extended therapy with intravenous arginine butyrate in patients with beta-hemoglobinopathies. N Engl J Med 1995; 332:1606.

983. Atweh GF, Sutton M, et al: Sustained induction of fetal hemoglobin by pulse butyrate therapy in sickle cell disease. Blood 1999; 93:1790.

984. Bunn HF: Induction of fetal hemoglobin in sickle cell disease. Blood 1999; 93:1787.

985. Blau CA, Constantoulakis P, et al: Fetal hemoglobin induction with butyric acid: Efficacy and toxicity. Blood 1993; 81:529.

986. Veith R, Galanello R, et al: Stimulation of F-cell production in patients with sickle-cell anemia treated with cytarabine or hydroxyurea. N Engl J Med 1985; 313:1571.

987. Dover GJ, Humphries RK, et al: Hydroxyurea induction of hemoglobin F production in sickle cell disease: Relationship between cytotoxicity and F-cell production. Blood 1986; 67:735.

988. Charache S, Dover GJ, et al: Hydroxyurea-induced augmentation of fetal hemoglobin production in patients with sickle cell anemia. Blood 1987; 69:109.

989. Rodgers GP, Dover GJ, et al: Hematologic responses of patients with sickle cell disease to treatment with hydroxyurea. N Engl J Med 1990; 322:1037.

990. Saxon BR, Rees D, et al: Regression of extramedullary haemopoiesis and augmentation of fetal haemoglobin concentration during hydroxyurea therapy in beta thalassaemia. Br J Haematol 1998; 101:416.

991. Dunbar C, Travis W, et al: 5-Azacytidine treatment in a beta zero-thalassaemic patient unable to be transfused due to multiple alloantibodies. Br J Haematol 1989; 72:467.

992. Lowrey CH, Nienhuis AW: Brief report: Treatment with azacytidine of patients with end-stage beta-thalassemia. N Engl J Med 1993; 329:845.

993. Riggs AD: 5-Methylcytosine, gene regulation, and cancer. Adv Cancer Res 1983; 40:1.

994. Santi DV, Garrett CE, et al: On the mechanism of inhibition of DNA-cytosine methyltransferases by cytosine analogs. Cell 1983; 33:9.

995. Cooper DN: Eukaryotic DNA methylation. Hum Genet 1983; 64:315.

996. Jones PA: Altering gene expression with 5-azacytidine. Cell 1985; 40:485.

997. Landolph JR, Jones PA: Mutageneticity of 5-azacytidine and related nucleosides in C3H/10T1/a clone 8 and V79 cells. Cancer Res 1982; 42:817.

998. Harrison JJ, Anisowicz A, et al: Azacytidine-induced tumorigenesis of CHEF/18 cells: Correlated DNA methylation and chromosome changes. Proc Natl Acad Sci USA 1983; 80:6606.

999. Darmon M, Nicolas J-F, et al: 5-Azacytidine is able to induce the conversion of teratocarcinoma-derived mesenchymal cells into epithelial cells. EMBO J 1984; 3:961.

1000. Liu DP, Liang CC, et al: Treatment of severe beta-thalassemia (patients) with Myleran. Am J Hematol 1990; 33:50.

1001. Al-Khatti A, Papayannopoulou T, et al: Cooperative enhancement of F-cell formation in baboons treated with erythropoietin and hydroxyurea. Blood 1988; 72:817.

1002. Stamatoyannopoulos JA: Future prospects for treatment of hemoglobinopathies. West J Med 1992; 157:631.

1003. Maragoudaki E, Kanavakis E, et al: Molecular, haematological and clinical studies of the −101 C→T substitution of the beta-globin gene promoter in 25 beta thalassaemia intermedia patients and 45 heterozygotes. Br J Haematol 1999; 108:699.

1004. Anderson WF: Prospects for human gene therapy. Science 1984; 226:401.

1005. Friedmann T: Progress toward human gene therapy. Science 1989; 244:1275.

1006. Cournoyer D, Caskey CT: Gene transfer into humans: A first step. N Engl J Med 1990; 323:601.

1007. Persons DA, Nienhuis AW: Gene therapy for the hemoglobin disorders: Past, present, and future. Proc Natl Acad Sci USA 2000; 97:5022.

1008. Nienhuis AW, McDonagh KT, et al: Gene transfer into hematopoietic stem cells. Cancer 1991; 67:2700.

1009. Friedmann T: The promise and overpromise of human gene therapy. Gene Ther 1994; 1:217.

1010. Brenner MK, Rill DR, et al: Gene-marking to trace origin of relapse after autologous bone-marrow transplantation. Lancet 1993; 341:85.

1011. May C, Rivella S, et al: Successful treatment of murine beta-thalassemia intermedia by transfer of the human beta-globin gene. Blood 2002; 99:1902.

1012. May C, Rivella MC, et al: Therapeutic haemoglobin synthesis in beta-thalassaemic mice expressing lentivirus-encoded human beta-globin. Nature 2000; 406:82.

1013. Pawliuk R, Westermark KA, et al: Correction of sickle cell disease in transgenic mouse models by gene therapy. Science 2001; 294:2368.

1014. Huisman THJ: Trimodality in the percentages of beta chain variants in heterozygotes. The effect of the number of active Hb alpha structural loci. Hemoglobin 1977; 1:239.

1015. Higgs DR, Pressley L, et al: The genetics and molecular basis of alpha thalassemia in association with HbS in Jamaican Negroes. Br J Haematol 1981; 47:43.

1016. Steinberg MH, Adams JG, et al: Alpha thalassemia in adults with sickle-cell trait. Br J Haematol 1975; 30:31.

1017. Shaeffer JR, DeSimone J, et al: Hemoglobin synthesis in a family with alpha-thalassemia trait and sickle cell trait. Biochem Genet 1975; 13:783.

1018. Wasi P: Hemoglobinopathies including thalassemia. Part I: Tropical Asia. Clin Haematol 1981; 10:707.

1019. Cunningham TM: Hemoglobin E in Indochinese refugees. West J Med 1982; 137:186.

1020. Monzon CM, Fairbanks VF, et al: Hereditary red cell disorders in Southeast Asian refugees and the effect on the prevalence of thalassemia disorders in the United States. Am J Med Sci 1986; 292:147.

1021. Anderson HM, Ranney HM: Southeast Asian Immigrants: The new thalassemias in Americans. Semin Hematol 1990; 27:239.

1022. Sicard D, Lieurzou Y, et al: High genetic polymorphism of hemoglobin disorders in Laos; complex phenotypes due to associated thalassemic syndromes. Hum Genet 1979; 50:327.

1023. Marsh WL, Rogers ZR, et al: Hematologic findings in Southeast Asian immigrants with particular reference to hemoglobin E. Ann Clin Lab Sci 1983; 13:299.

1024. Bhamarapravati N, Na-Nakorn S, et al: Pathology of abnormal hemoglobin diseases seen in Thailand: I. Pathology of beta-thalassemia hemoglobin E disease. Am J Clin Pathol 1967; 47:745.

1025. Itano HA: A new inherited abnormality of human hemoglobin. Proc Natl Acad Sci USA 1950; 36:613.

1026. Perosa L, Manganelli G, et al: Il primo caso di Hb C-thalassemia descritto in Tialia. Haematologica 1961; 46:211.

1027. Portier A, Traverse P, et al: L'hemoglobinose C-thalassemia. Presse Med 1960; 68:1760.

1028. Goksel V, Tartaroglu N: Haemoglobin-C-thalassemia bei zwei Geschwistern von Weisser Rasse. In Lehmann H, Betke K (eds): Haemoglobin Colloquium. Stuttgart, Georg Thieme Verlag, 1961, p 55.

1029. Steinberg MH, Adams JG: Thalassemic hemoglobinopathies. Am J Pathol 1983; 113:396.

1030. Flatz G: Hemoglobin E: Distribution and population genetics. Human Genet 1967; 3:189.

1031. Kan YW, Valenti C, et al: Fetal blood-sampling in utero. Lancet 1974; 1:79.

1032. Rodeck C: Fetoscopy guided by real-time ultrasound for pure fetal blood samples, fetal skin samples, and examination of the fetus in utero. Br J Obstet Gynaecol 1980; 87:449.

1033. Daffos F, Capella-Pavlovsky M, et al: Fetal blood sampling via the umbilical cord using a needle guided by ultrasound. Prenat Diagn 1983; 3:271.

1034. Alter BP: Prenatal diagnosis: General introduction, methodology, and review. Hemoglobin 1988; 12:763.

1035. Kan YW, Golbus MS, et al: Successful application of prenatal diagnosis in a pregnancy at risk for homozygous beta-thalassemia. N Engl J Med 1975; 292:1099.

1036. Orkin SH, Alter BP, et al: Application of endonuclease mapping to the analysis and prenatal diagnosis of thalassemias caused by globin-gene deletion. N Engl J Med 1978; 299:166.

1037. Dozy AM, Forman EN, et al: Prenatal diagnosis of homozygous alpha thalassemia. JAMA 1979; 241:1610.

1038. Saiki RK, Walsh PS, et al: Genetics analysis of amplified DNA with immobilized sequence-specific oligonucleotide probes. Proc Natl Acad Sci USA 1989; 86:6230.

1039. Modell B, Petrou M, et al: Effect of fetal diagnostic testing on birth-rate of thalassaemia major in Britain. Lancet 1984; 2:1383.

1040. Loukopoulos D: Prenatal diagnosis of thalassemia and of the hemoglobinopathies; a review. Hemoglobin 1985; 9:435.

1041. Modell B, Bulyzhenkov V: Distribution and control of some genetic disorders. World Health Stat Q 1988; 41:209.

1042. Cao A, Rosatelli C, et al: The prevention of thalassemia in Sardinia. Clin Genet 1989; 36:277.

1043. Loukopoulos D: Current status of thalassemia and the sickle cell syndromes in Greece. Semin Hematol 1996; 33:76.

VII The Phagocyte System

The Phagocyte System and Disorders of Granulopoiesis and Granulocyte Function

21 The Phagocyte System and Disorders of Granulopoiesis and Granulocyte Function

Mary C. Dinauer

DEFINITION AND CLASSIFICATION OF PHAGOCYTES

Phagocytic leukocytes are bone marrow-derived cells that have the capacity to engulf and digest particulate matter. Phagocytes are essential for the host response to infection and inflammation and are equipped with specialized machinery that enables them to seek out, ingest, and kill microorganisms. Other functions include the synthesis and secretion of cytokines, pyrogens, and other cellular mediators, as well as the digestion of senescent cells and debris.

The phagocyte system has two principal limbs: granulocytes (neutrophils, eosinophils, and basophils) and mononuclear phagocytes (monocytes and tissue macrophages). Neutrophils circulate in the bloodstream until they encounter specific chemotactic signals that promote adhesion to the vascular endothelium, diapedesis into tissues, and migration to sites of microbial invasion. In contrast, mononuclear phagocytes function primarily as resident cells in certain tissues, such as lung, liver, spleen, and peritoneum, in which they perform a surveillance role and also interact closely with lymphocytes to promote specific immune responses. Both groups of phagocytes dispose of appropriately opsonized targets by engulfment and sequestration within intracellular vacuoles, followed by the release of digestive lysosomal enzymes and bactericidal antibiotic proteins from storage granules and by the generation of highly reactive oxidants from the respiratory burst pathway.

This chapter is divided into three major sections. In the first, the distribution and functional properties of the granulocytic and mononuclear phagocytes are summarized. In the second section, clinical disorders associated with a deficiency or excess of phagocytic leukocytes in the circulation or tissues are reviewed. The third section is focused on disorders of phagocyte function, including those due to intrinsic phagocyte defects as well as those associated with other disease processes.

PHAGOCYTE MORPHOLOGY, DISTRIBUTION, AND STRUCTURE

Regulation of Myelopoiesis

Granulocytes and monocytes are produced in the bone marrow in a complex, highly regulated, and dynamic process that requires both specific hematopoietic growth factors and an appropriate bone marrow microenvironment. As reviewed in Chapter 6, multipotent, self-renewing hematopoietic stem cells produce lineage-restricted progenitor cells that divide and further differentiate in the bone marrow before their release into the intravascular compartment. Transcription factors of the PU.1 and myeloid transcription factor CCAAT/enhancer binding protein (C/EBP) families play prominent roles in normal myelopoiesis (Fig. 21–1). PU.1 is important for the development of early myeloid precursors and is absolutely essential for subsequent differentiation of the monocyte/macrophage lineage.[1] Early steps in the differentiation of granulocytes are dependent upon C/EBPα,[2] whereas C/EBPε activity is required for terminal matura-

tion beyond the metamyelocyte stage.[3] Cytokines that promote the proliferation and differentiation of neutrophils and monocytes from primitive precursor cells include interleukin (IL)-3, IL-6, granulocyte-macrophage colony-stimulating factor (GM-CSF), macrophage colony-stimulating factor (M-CSF), and granulocyte colony-stimulating factor (G-CSF).[4–6] The latter two cytokines are relatively specific for the monocyte and neutrophil lineages, respectively. During infections, activated macrophages release cytokines such as IL-1, IL-6, and tumor necrosis factor (TNF) that activate stromal cells and T lymphocytes to produce additional amounts of colony-stimulating factors and increase the production of myeloid cells. IL–5 plays an important role in inducing eosinophil differentiation[7–9] and IL-3 is the principal cytokine inducing human basophil growth and differentiation.[10] In addition to their regulatory role in hematopoiesis, hematopoietic growth factors can act on mature myeloid cells and stimulate their functional activities. For example, circulating phagocytes become "primed" to undergo an enhanced respiratory burst upon exposure to GM-CSF.[11]

Myeloid differentiation also appears to be modulated by retinoic acid through specific retinoic acid receptors,[12, 13] which are members of the nuclear hormone receptor superfamily.[14, 15] The participation of retinoic acid in myeloid development was originally surmised from its ability to induce differentiation of myeloid leukemia cell lines and, more recently, leukemic promyelocytes in patients with acute promyelocytic leukemia, which is distinguished by a t(15:17) translocation.[16] This rearrangement results in a fusion gene of the retinoic acid receptor and a putative transcription factor.[17, 18]

Granulocytes

NEUTROPHILS

The neutrophil life span is traditionally divided into the bone marrow, circulating, and tissue phases. Approximately 14 days are spent in the bone marrow, in which proliferation and the early stages of neutrophil differentiation are followed by the final stages of maturation and retention in a large, nonmitotic, storage pool that is many fold larger than the circulating and tissue neutrophil populations (Table 21–1).[19–22] Once released into the bloodstream, neutrophils have a half-life of 6 to 10 hours and move between circulating and marginated pools in a reversible fashion. Neutrophils then exit by diapedesis between endothelial cells into tissue sites of infection or inflammation. Once in the tissues, neutrophils are believed to live for another 1 to 2 days before undergoing apoptosis and engulfment by macrophages.[25–27] Myeloblasts are the earliest morphologically recognizable granulocyte precursors in the marrow and are identified by their relatively undifferentiated appearance with a large, oval nucleus, several prominent nucleoli, and few or no granules in a gray-blue cytoplasm using Wright's stain. This stage of neutrophil differentiation is followed by the promyelocyte and myelocyte stages, which are distinguished by the appearance of distinct neutrophil granule populations[28] (Table 21–2). Azurophilic, or primary, granules are formed during the

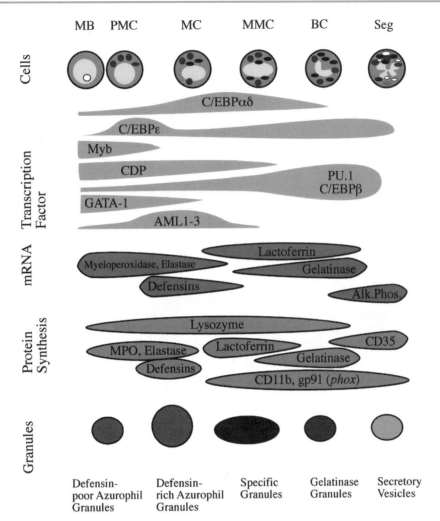

FIGURE 21–1. Neutrophil maturation. Neutrophil maturation and the control of granule protein biosynthesis are exerted by the sequential and combined action of specific transcription factors, including PU.1, the C/EBP and AML families, CDP, Myb, and GATA-1. The granules formed at any given stage of maturation will be composed of the granule proteins synthesized at that time. The different subsets of neutrophil granules are the result of differences in the biosynthetic windows during maturation and not the result of specific sorting between individual granule subsets. When the formation of granules ceases, it is believed that secretory vesicles will form. Because postranscriptional control cannot be ruled out, biosynthesis of proteins may not always be a precise reflection of the corresponding messenger RNA (mRNA) levels. MB = myeloblast; PMC = promyelocyte; MC = myelocyte; MMC = metamyelocyte; BC = band cell; Seg = segmented cell (mature neutrophil); MPO = myeloperoxidase; Alk.Phos. = alkaline phosphatase. (From Borregaard N, Cowland JB: Granules of the human neutrophilic polymorphonuclear leukocyte. Blood 1997; 89:3503–3521.)

promyelocyte stage and contain myeloperoxidase, bactericidal peptides, and lysosomal enzymes. The subsequent myelocyte stage is distinguished by the formation of peroxidase-negative specific, or secondary, granules containing lactoferrin. No further cell divisions occur after the myelocyte stage. The metamyelocyte, band, and mature neutrophil exhibit progressive nuclear condensation, accumulation of glycogen, and development of a third granule population that has a high content of gelatinase.[29]

In blood smears stained with Wright's stain, the mature neutrophil is 10 to 15 μm in size, with a multilobed, polymorphic nucleus with highly condensed chromatin and a yellow-pink cytoplasm containing numerous granules as well as clumps of glycogen. The mean lobe count is usually slightly less than three. Circulating neutrophils appear to be round with some cytoplasmic projections and surface ruffling. A scaffold of cytoskeletal filaments, composed largely of actin microfilaments and microtubules,

plays a key role in mediating neutrophil locomotion on surfaces, phagocytosis, and exocytosis.[30–32] Microtubules radiate from the centriole in the perinuclear cytoplasm near the Golgi region, whereas actin tends to be located more peripherally, where it forms an organelle-excluding meshwork. Actin is associated with a variety of actin-binding proteins that regulate the structure of this meshwork and link the actin cytoskeleton to the plasma membrane.

The morphologic changes seen with neutrophil differentiation are accompanied by temporally coordinated changes in gene expression and protein synthesis (Fig. 21–1).[33–35] Transcription and translation of messenger RNAs (mRNAs) for myeloperoxidase and cathepsin, which are both primary granule constituents, are restricted to myeloblasts and promyelocytes.[34, 36–38] In contrast, expression of the secondary granule proteins, such as lactoferrin and transcobalamin I, occurs in myelocytes and metamyelocytes.[36, 37] Gelatinase expres-

TABLE 21–1. Neutrophil and Monocyte Kinetics*

	Transit Time Range (hr)	Total Cells ($\times 10^9$/kg)
NEUTROPHILS		
Marrow mitotic compartment		
Myeloblast	23	0.14
Promyelocyte	26–78	0.51
Myelocyte	17–1266	1.95
Postmitotic marrow maturation and storage compartment		
Metamyelocyte	8–108	2.7
Band	12–96	3.6
Neutrophil	0–120	<u>2.5</u>
Total marrow storage		8.8
Vascular compartment		
Circulating neutrophils	4–10	0.3
Marginated neutrophils	4–10	<u>0.4</u>
Total blood neutrophils		0.7
Tissue compartments	0–3 days (?)	Not known
Neutrophil turnover rate	1.6×10^6/kg/day	
MONOCYTES		
Marrow mitotic compartment: promonocyte	~160	0.006
Postmitotic marrow compartment: monocyte	24	0.10
Vascular compartment	36–104	0.024
Tissue compartment	Days-months	Not known
Blood monocyte turnover rate	6×10^6/kg/day	

Based on references 19, 20, 22, 23, and 24.

TABLE 21–2. Content of Human Neutrophil Granules and Secretory Organelles

Primary: Azurophil Granules	Secondary: Specific Granules	Tertiary: Gelatinase Granules	Secretory Vesicles
MEMBRANES	**MEMBRANES**	**MEMBRANES**	**MEMBRANES**
CD63	CD15 antigens (Lewis X)	Mac-1 (CD11b/CD18)	Alkaline phosphatase
CD68	Cytochrome-b_{558}	Formyl peptide receptor	Cytochrome b_{558}
	Formyl peptide receptor	Diacylglycerol-deacylating enzyme	Formyl peptide receptor
			MAC-1 (CD11b/CD18)
MATRIX	**FIBRONECTIN RECEPTOR**	**MATRIX**	Uroplasminogen
Acid mucopolysaccharide	G-protein α-subunit	β_2-Microglobulin	activator-receptor
α_1-Antitrypsin	Laminin receptor	Gelatinase	FcγIIIR (CO16)
α-Mannosidase	Mac-1 (CD11b/CD18)	Acetyltransferase	
Azurocidin	Rap 1, Rap 2	Lysozyme	**MATRIX**
Bactericidal permeability–	Thrombospondin receptor		Plasma proteins
increasing protein	Tumor necrosis factor		
β-Glycerophosphatase	receptor		
β-Glucuronidase	Vitronectin		
Cathepsins			
Defensins	**MATRIX**		
Elastase	β_2-Microglobulin		
Heparin-binding protein	Collagenase		
Lysozyme	Gelatinase		
Myeloperoxidase	Histaminase		
N-Acetyl-β-glucosaminidase	Heparanase		
Proteinase-3	Lactoferrin		
Sialidase	Lysozyme		
	Plasminogen activator		
	Vitamin B_{12}–binding protein		
	(transcobalamin I)		

Adapted from Borregaard N, Lollike K, Kjeldsen L, et al: Human neutrophil granules and secretory vesicles. Eur J Haematol 1993, 51:187–198.

sion occurs even later in maturation and is first detected in bands and bone marrow neutrophils.[37] The leukocyte β-integrin subunit CD11b is first detectable in myelocytes and increases throughout the later stages of neutrophil differentiation.[34] The gp91^{phox} subunit of the respiratory burst oxidase complex is expressed relatively late in neutrophil maturation,[39] consistent with the observation that respiratory burst activity is not detected until the metamyelocyte stage.[40]

The mature neutrophil, previously thought of as an "end-stage" cell, retains the capacity for inducible gene expression and protein synthesis even after release from the marrow cavity. For example, expression of mRNA transcripts encoding respiratory burst oxidase components increases in response to inflammatory cytokines such as interferon-γ (IFN-γ).[41] Mature neutrophils can also synthesize and secrete a variety of cytokines, including IL-1, IL-6, TNF-α, GM-CSF, M-CSF, and IL-8, which may promote recruitment and activation of both phagocyte and lymphocyte populations in the inflammatory response.[42, 43]

Abnormalities in Neutrophil Morphology. Upon neutrophil activation by inflammatory signals, granule fusion can result in vacuolization and toxic granulation (prominent azurophilic granules). The degree of these changes in peripheral blood neutrophils can correlate with the presence of bacterial infection.[44] Large azurophilic granules are also seen in Alder-Reilly anomaly, an autosomal recessive trait, but neutrophil function does not appear to be affected. Inclusions referred to as Döhle bodies can be seen in infection. These represent strands of rough endoplasmic reticulum that are retained from a more immature stage and stain bluish due to their high content of ribosomes. Larger gray-blue cytoplasmic inclusions, made up of dense fibrils thought to be messenger RNA, are seen in both granulocytes and monocytes in May-Hegglin anomaly. Leukopenia, giant platelets, and variable thrombocytopenia characterize this autosomal dominant syndrome, which can be associated with hemorrhagic problems in approximately one third of patients. Neutrophil hypersegmentation can be a sign of vitamin B_{12} or folate deficiency. Hypersegmented neutrophils, with a mean of four lobes, also occur as a rare autosomal dominant trait that is not associated with disease. A hyposegmented nucleus is seen in Pelger-Huet anomaly, an autosomal dominant trait due to mutation of the lamin B receptor.[44a] Typically, the nucleus is bilobed (often described as "pince-nez"), but has mature, coarse, and densely clumped chromatin. The nucleus remains round in the rare homozygote. Pelger-Huet anomaly must be distinguished from neutrophil band forms and from the acquired or "pseudo" Pelger-Huet form that can be seen with malignant myeloproliferative disorders. Bilobed neutrophil nuclei are also seen in a rare disorder of neutrophil granule formation, specific granule deficiency, which is associated with recurrent pyogenic infections (see later). In this disorder, the pink-staining specific granules are absent in peripheral blood neutrophils. Giant granules representing fused azurophil and specific granules are seen in neutrophils of patients with Chédiak-Higashi syndrome (CHS), particularly in the bone marrow.

Neutrophil Granule Biosynthesis and Classification. The numerous intracellular granules and vesicles in the neutrophil cytoplasm function as storage pools for cell surface receptors and as reservoirs of sequestered digestive and microbicidal proteins. The older classification of granules as either peroxidase-positive (azurophilic or primary) and peroxidase-negative (specific or secondary) has proved to be too simplistic, on the basis of subcellular fractionation, immunoelectron microscopy, and biosynthetic studies.[29, 45] A current classification of neutrophil granules is shown in Table 21–2, which summarizes the composition of their membranes and luminal (matrix) contents.

Azurophilic (primary) granules are defined histochemically by their peroxidase positivity that is due to myeloperoxidase, an important enzyme in the respiratory burst–dependent killing pathway. Azurophilic granules also contain defensins and bactericidal/permeability-increasing (BPI) protein, cytotoxic polypeptides that participate in oxygen-independent killing of microbes. Other components of the azurophilic granule matrix include neutral serine proteases, such as cathepsin and elastase, and other digestive enzymes. Lactoferrin, an iron-binding protein believed to have bactericidal activity, is a marker for specific (secondary) granules, which are uniquely found in neutrophils. The membrane of the secondary granules contains a major store of the neutrophil's supply of flavocytochrome b_{558}, the electron carrier in the respiratory burst oxidase.[46, 47] Specific granule membranes also contain a pool of receptors for adhesive proteins, TNF, and chemotactic formyl peptides. Although specific granules contain some gelatinase, most of the store of this metalloproteinase in the neutrophil is localized to gelatinase (tertiary) granules. Gelatinase granules are formed relatively late in neutrophil differentiation and are smaller and more easily mobilized for exocytosis than secondary granules.[29] Secretory vesicles are other small granules that are formed in bands and mature neutrophils by endocytosis of the plasma membrane and serve as an important store of the adhesive protein Mac-1 (CD11b/CD18) and other membrane receptors.

The generation of different classes of granules at least in part reflects the sequential synthesis of granule proteins during granulopoiesis (Fig. 21–1). As mentioned earlier, expression of the primary or azurophilic granule proteins is restricted to myeloblasts and promyelocytes.[34, 36–38] Expression of specific and gelatinase granule matrix proteins occurs later in granulopoiesis and requires the transcription factor C/EBPε. Specific and gelatinase granules are absent in neutrophils from C/EBPε nullizygous mice generated by gene targeting.[3] The phenotype of C/EBPε nullizygous mice is similar to that seen in the rare inherited disorder, specific granule deficiency, and mutations in the C/EBPε coding sequence were reported in several affected patients (see later).[48, 49]

Neutrophil Cell Surface Receptors. The primary function of the mature neutrophil is to move rapidly into tissue sites to destroy invading microbes and clear inflammatory debris. To respond to inflammatory stimuli, the neutrophil is equipped with an array of cell surface receptors for adhesive ligands, chemoattractants, and cytokines that can be divided into groups on the basis of their structure and the major intracellular signaling pathway to which they are linked (Table 21–3). The signal transduction cascades triggered upon ligand binding to neutrophil receptors are complex and, in may cases, probably redundant.[50, 51] A common early event downstream of neutrophil receptor binding is activation of phospholipase C, which hydrolyzes the membrane phospholipid, phosphatidylinositol 4,5-bisphosphate (PIP_2) to generate two important second messengers, diacylglycerol and inositol 1,4,5-triphosphate (IP_3),[52, 53] which in turn cause release of calcium from intracellular stores and activate protein kinase C. Changes in intracellular calcium concentration are important for neutrophil degranulation and secretion and for phagolysosome fusion during phagocytosis.[51] Activation of phosphoinositide 3-kinase (PI 3-kinase) is another common early event, which catalyzes the phosphorylation of PIP_2 to generate a third important lipid messenger, phosphatidylinositol 3,4,5-trisphosphate (PIP_3). Neutrophil activation is also accompanied by alterations in the phosphorylation status of intracellular proteins, as regulated by protein kinase C, tyrosine kinases and phosphatases, and serine/threonine kinases of the mitogen-activated (MAP) kinase family.[51, 54–57] Guanine nucleotide–binding proteins play important roles in neutrophil signal transduction. These include the heterotrimeric guanosine triphosphate (GTP)–binding proteins that are coupled to the seven transmembrane-spanning domain (serpentine or heptahelical) receptors for chemokines and other chemoattractants[58–60] and the low molecular weight guanosine triphosphatases (GTPases) of the Ras superfamily.[61] The latter category includes p21Ras itself, which can be activated via chemoattractant receptors[62] and the Rho family GTPases Rho, Rac, and Cdc42, which are involved in the regulation of many neutrophil responses, including adhesion, the respiratory burst reduced nicotinamide adenine dinucleotide phosphate (NADPH)–oxidase, and actin remodeling during migration and phagocytosis.[63, 64] A dominant-negative form of the Rac2 GTPase was identified in an infant with recurrent deep-seated bacterial infections and leads to multiple defects in phagocyte function.[65, 66]

EOSINOPHILS

Like the neutrophil, the eosinophil is compartmentalized in the bone marrow into mitotic and storage pools that constitute up to no more than 0.3 percent of the nucleated bone marrow cells.[67] Eosinophils arise from a progenitor cell, the colony-forming cell–eosinophil, that is committed at a relatively early stage to differentiate into eosinophils instead of neutrophils and monocytes. Morphologic differentiation and maturation of the eosinophil parallel that of the neutrophil series, and the characteristic eosin-staining specific granules of this granulocyte lineage are prominent by the myelocyte stage. IL-5 plays a key role in regulating eosinophil proliferation, differentiation, and functional activation, and IL-5 levels can be elevated in patients with eosinophilia of diverse causes.[7–9, 68, 69] The mature eosinophil is slightly larger than the neutrophil, with a diameter of 12 to 17 μm. The nucleus is characteristically bilobed, although multiple lobes can be seen in patients with eosinophilia of diverse causes. The cytoplasm has prominent and morphologically distinctive granules that stain strongly with acid aniline dyes due to their high content of basic proteins.

Once released from the bone marrow, eosinophils have a half-life in the bloodstream similar to neutrophils.[70] After leaving the circulation, eosinophils typically localize

TABLE 21–3. Receptors in Neutrophils

Receptor Grouping	Examples	Structural Characteristics
G-protein linked	FMLP, C5a, PAF, LTB, IL-8, chemokines	Seven transmembrane spanning domains (serpentine); linked to heterotrimeric guanosine triphosphate binding proteins
Membrane tyrosine kinases	PDGF	Integral membrane protein, intrinsic tyrosine kinase activity; ligation leads to receptor dimerization and cross ("auto") phosphorylation.
Tyrosine kinase linked	FcγRIIA, GM-CSF	FcγRII is a member of the immunoglobulin family of receptors The GM-CSF receptor is an 84-kd transmembrane protein related to receptors of IL-2 and IL-6. Ligation of receptor activates cytosolic tyrosine kinases.
GPI linked	FcγRIIB, DAF	These receptors have no intracellular domain. FcγRIIIB may be linked to FcγRIIA.
Adhesion molecules	β₂ integrins, L-Selectin	β-integrins are heterodimers structured with relatively long cytoplasmic tails. L-Selectin has an extracellular lectin-binding domain and a very short cytoplasmic tail. Ligation results in potentiation of the oxidative burst and phagocytosis in adherent cells, calcium signalling, actin cytoskeletal changes, and upregulation of gene expression.
Ceramide linked	TNF	Two TNF receptors have been cloned; both are single membrane-spanning glycoproteins; ligation activates membrane-bound sphingomyelinase with generation of ceramide, which in turn activates a 96-kd protein kinase.

DAF = decay-accelerating factor; FMLP = N-formyl-methionyl-leucyl-phenylalanine; GM-CSF = granulocyte-macrophage colony-stimulating factor; GPI = glycosyl phosphatidylinositol; IL = interleukin; LTB = leukotriene B; PAF = platelet-activating factor; PDGF = platelet-derived growth factor; TNF = tumor necrosis factor.
   Adapted from Downey G: Signalling mechanisms in human neutrophils. Curr Opin Hematol, 1995; 2:76–88.

in areas exposed to the external environment, such as the tracheobronchial tree, gastrointestinal tract, mammary glands, and vagina and cervix.[71] They are also found in connective tissue immediately below the epithelial layer. As discussed in a later section, eosinophils have both immunoenhancing and immunosuppressive functions and play a role in helmintic infection, allergy, and the responses to certain tumors.[71–74] The majority of mature eosinophils reside in tissues, with a blood-to-tissue ratio estimated to be 1:300 to 1:500. The life span of tissue eosinophils is not known but may be several weeks.[71] The number of circulating eosinophils tends to be highest late at night, decreases during the morning, and begins to rise at mid-afternoon. These changes correlate with the diurnal variation in adrenal glucocorticoid levels, to which circulating eosinophils are very sensitive.[75]

Like the neutrophil, the mature eosinophil is endowed with the capacity for chemotaxis, phagocytosis, degranulation, and the synthesis of reactive oxidants and arachi-

donate metabolites[71, 76, 77] (Table 21–4). Eosinophil cell surface membranes have a variety of receptors for adhesive proteins, immunoglobulin and complement fragments, and numerous chemotactic molecules.[71] The latter includes the tetrapeptides that constitute the eosinophil chemotactic factor of anaphylaxis (ECFA),[78] which may be responsible for the accumulation of eosinophils at sites of anaphylactic allergies.[72–74]

Mature eosinophil granules are membrane-bound organelles, 0.15 to 1.5 μm in length and 0.3 to 1 μm in width, that contain a variety of enzymes and cytotoxic proteins (Table 21–4).[79] The small granules are round and homogeneous on electron microscopic examination. These include the primary granules, which develop early in eosinophilic maturation,[80] and a smaller population appearing in late eosinophils that contain arylsulfatase and other enzymes.[81] The more numerous eosin-staining secondary (specific) granules are large ovoid bodies that contain an electron-dense crystalloid core surrounded by

TABLE 21–4. Comparison of Eosinophils and Basophils

	Eosinophils	Basophils
CHEMOATTRACTANTS	C5a FMLP LTB_4 PAF Histamine IL-3 Eotaxin 1, 2 RANTES	ECFA C5a FMLP LTB_4 MCP-1 IL-8 Eotaxin 1, 2 RANTES
STIMULANTS FOR DEGRANULATION	LTB_4 ECFA RANTES TNF PAF IgG, IgA, IgE IL-3, IL-5 Histamine CSF-GM	IgE C3a, C5a RANTES MCP-1 IL-1, IL-5 Insect venoms Cold exposure Some drugs Some hormones CSF-GM
ARACHIDONIC ACID PRODUCTS PRODUCED BY CELLS	LTB_4 LTC_4	LTC_4 LTD_4 (slow-reaching substance of anaphylaxis) PAF
COLONY STIMULATING FACTORS FOR CELLS	IL-3 IL-5 GM-CSF	IL-1 IL-3 GM-CSF
GRANULE CONTENTS	Major basic protein (dense core) Eosinophil peroxidase (matrix) Eosinophil-derived neurotoxin Arginine-rich cationic proteins Acid phosphatase Aryl sulfatase Lysophospholipase	Histamine Kallikrein TAME-esterase Sulfated glycosaminoglycans (heparin, chondroitin sulfate) Trypsin Chymotrypsin
MEMBRANE	NADPH-dependent oxidase Fcα, Fcγ, Fcε	Fcε receptor Lysophospholipase

ECFA = eosinophil chemotactic factor of anaphylaxis; MCP-1 = monocyte chemoattractant protein 1; RANTES = regulated upon activation, normal T cell expressed and presumably secreted; TAME = *p*-tosyl-L-arginine methyl ester; NADPH = reduced nicotinamide adenine dinucleotide phosphate.

Adapted from Shurin S: Eosinophil and basophil structure and function. In Hoffman R, Benz EJ, et al (eds): Hematology: Basic Principles and Practice. New York, Churchill Livingston, 1995, pp 762–769.

a less dense matrix.[79] Hydrolytic enzymes, cathepsin, and an eosinophil-specific peroxidase are located in the matrix. The eosinophil peroxidase plays an important role in the antihelmintic function of eosinophils[82, 83] and utilizes bromate to generate hypobromous acid from hydrogen peroxide.[84] The specific granule matrix also contains eosinophilic cationic protein and eosinophil-derived neurotoxin, which are cationic proteins with ribonuclease activity.[71] The eosinophil major basic protein (MBP) makes up about 50 percent of the dense crystalloid core of the eosinophilic-specific granule, along with other basic proteins rich in lysine, arginine, and phospholipids.[72, 73, 85] MBP strongly absorbs to membranes, precipitates DNA, and neutralizes heparin. MBP is toxic to schistosomules of *Schistosoma mansoni* and larvae of *Trichinella spiralis*[72, 86] and induces histamine release from basophils and mast cells.[87]

Both eosinophils and basophils have a lysophospholipase in their plasma membranes and primary granules that can polymerize to form the bipyramidal hexagons known as Charcot-Leyden crystals (CLCs).[88, 89] CLCs are typically found in areas of eosinophil degeneration, such as the nasal mucus of patients with allergies, stools of patients with parasitic infections, and the pleural fluid of patients with pulmonary eosinophilic infiltrates. The CLC lysophospholipase, whose protein sequence is distinct from that of other eukaryotic or prokaryotic lysophospholipases,[74] catalyzes the hydrolysis and inactivation of lysophospholipids generated by phospholipase A_2, thus preventing the generation of pro-inflammatory arachidonic acid metabolites. The CLC protein composes about 5 percent of the total protein in eosinophils.[71]

BASOPHILS

Basophils, like other granulocytes, differentiate and mature in the bone marrow more than 7 days before their release into the bloodstream and are not normally found in the connective tissues.[90] Basophils account for 0.5 percent of the total circulating leukocytes and 0.3 percent of nucleated marrow cells.[91] Mature basophils have a bilobed nucleus and contain prominent metachromatic granules that stain purple or bluish with Wright's stain due to their high content of sulfated glycosaminoglycans. These granules are rich in heparin, chondroitin sulfate, histamine, and kallikrein but lack acid hydrolases, alkaline phosphatase, and peroxidase[92] (Table 21–4). The heparin of basophils appears to have poor anticoagulant activity. Basophil granules also contain small amounts of MBP as well as serine proteases. Receptors expressed on the plasma membrane for basophils include a high affinity receptor for the Fc portion of IgE, which is an important trigger for release of granule contents and production of arachidonic acid metabolites in anaphylactic degranulation[93] (Table 21–4). Hence, basophils are key effector cells in certain hypersensitivity reactions. Basophils can synthesize and secrete IL-4, which is the only known cytokine to be produced by human basophils.[94–96]

Basophils share certain morphologic and functional features with mast cells, which appear to be derived from a common marrow progenitor cell.[97] However, mast cells and basophils are distinct terminally differentiated cell lineages.[10, 98] Similar to basophils, mast cells contain histamine-laden metachromatic granules, express high-affinity IgE receptors and participate in immediate and cutaneous hypersensitivity.[99, 100] However, mast cells lack receptors for IL-2, IL-3, and CD11b/CD18 that are present on basophils.[10] Receptors for c-*kit* (stem cell factor) are present on mast cells but are absent on the majority of basophils.[100,101] Murine mast cells can secrete a wide variety of mitogenic or inflammatory cytokines, including many interleukins (1, 3, 4, 5, and 6), chemokines, GM-CSF, and TNF-α, that are likely to play an important role in leukocyte recruitment and inflammation.[100]

Mast cells are ordinarily distributed throughout normal connective tissue, in which they are often situated adjacent to blood and lymphatic vessels, near or within nerve sheaths, and beneath epithelial surfaces that are exposed to environmental antigens, such as the respiratory and gastrointestinal tracts.[99] Mast cells do not circulate in the blood and retain a limited proliferative capacity in the tissue compartment.[102] In contrast to monocytes and macrophages, a transformation between the circulating and tissue forms of basophils and mast cells has not been observed. The fate of the basophil in the tissues is unknown.

Mononuclear Phagocytes

The blood monocyte is derived from a bone marrow progenitor cell, the colony-forming unit granulocyte-macrophage, shared with the neutrophil, and undergoes similar stages of differentiation as monoblasts and promonocytes in the marrow cavity. However, the transit time in the marrow compartment is briefer, and the mature monocyte is released into the circulation only 24 hours after the last mitosis (see Table 21–1).[24, 103, 104] Consequently, a relative peripheral blood monocytosis commonly precedes the return of granulocytes during recovery from bone marrow aplasia or hypoplasia. The monocyte may spend several days in the intravascular compartment in either circulating or marginated pools.[105] Monocytes then migrate into tissues and body cavities to participate in inflammatory processes as exudate macrophages and to replenish the resident tissue population of macrophages, which have a relatively long life span. In patients receiving allogeneic bone marrow transplants, host tissue macrophages disappear gradually and are replaced by donor macrophages approximately 3 months after transplantation.[106]

The circulating monocyte in blood smears stained with Wright's stain is 10 to 18 μm in diameter with a convoluted surface, a gray-blue cytoplasm, and an indented or kidney-shaped, foamy nucleus. However, some monocytes can be as small as 7 μm in diameter[107] and can be difficult to distinguish morphologically from lymphocytes.[102] In contrast to neutrophils, monocytes contain a single class of granules with lysosomal characteristics.[108–110] After leaving the circulation, monocytes become larger and take on the appearance of tissue macrophages characteristic of the organ in which they reside. The macrophage nucleus is typically oval with more prominent nucleoli, and the cytoplasm stains blue because of an increase in RNA content. Monocytes and macrophages are distinguished by the presence of a fluoride-inhibitable nonspecific esterase, which can help in differentiating these cells from other mononuclear cells (e.g., lymphocytes) at inflammatory sites. Monoclonal antibodies specific for mononuclear phagocytes (e.g., the human CD14 antigen, a receptor for endotoxin)[111] are now also available.[105]

Monocytes and macrophages share many structural and functional features with neutrophils and are capable of sensing chemotactic gradients, migrating to inflamed sites, ingesting bacteria, and killing them using a variety of cytocidal products. However, compared with neutrophils, mononuclear phagocytes have a large and diverse developmental potential. In addition to their protective function as phagocytic cells in host defense, mononuclear phagocytes play a central role in the immune response by presenting antigens to lymphocytes, elaborate growth factors, and cytokines important for lymphocyte function, wound repair, and hematopoiesis, and participate in a variety of scavenger and homeostatic pathways.

Factors modifying the enzymatic, antigenic, and functional profile of mononuclear phagocytes are incompletely understood and involve a combination of tissue-specific signals as well as the release of inflammatory cytokines and toxins.[111–114] Mononuclear phagocytes at inflammatory sites become "activated," displaying morphologic alterations and a variety of enhanced functions. These include a more pronounced ruffling of the plasma membrane and pseudopod formation, an increased capacity for adherence and migration to chemotactic factors, increased microbicidal and tumoricidal activity, and enhanced ability to release cytokines.[112] IFN-γ is one of the principal macrophage-activating factors, and is secreted by T lymphocytes as well as by macrophages and neutrophils.[40, 110, 115, 116] INF-γ induces changes in macrophage gene expression through a pathway that is often referred to as the JAK-STAT pathway, whose general features are shared by many other cytokines, including IL-2, IL-6, and G-CSF.[31, 117, 118] Binding of IFN-γ to its cell surface receptor activates cytoplasmic protein tyrosine kinases of the Janus kinase (JAK) family, which then phosphorylate and activate a family of transcription factors known as STATs (for signal transducers and activators of transcription). Upon phosphorylation, STAT proteins translocate into the nucleus to bind to specific regulatory sequences in IFN-responsive genes. Endotoxin, the bacterial lipopolysaccharide derived from gram-negative bacteria, is another important trigger of macrophage activation.[111] Signals from the microenvironment in which tissue macrophages reside can also produce phenotypic changes. For example, although monocytes and macrophages are generally facultative anaerobes, pulmonary macrophages are entirely dependent on aerobic metabolism.[119]

In keeping with their broad range of activities, mononuclear phagocytes possess a variety of cell surface receptors not found in neutrophils. These include receptors for coagulation factors VII, VIIa, and thrombin[120, 121] and for low-density lipoproteins (LDLs) and very low-density lipoproteins (VLDLs).[122] Macrophages and monocytes are also active secretory cells and are capable of secreting more than 100 defined substances,[110] many

of which are listed in Table 21–5. These include molecules important in control of microbial pathogens, such as

TABLE 21–5. Products Secreted by Mononuclear Phagocytes

ENZYMES

Acid ceramidase, lipase, phosphatase, DNase, RNase
α-iduronidase, α-L-fucosidase, α-mannosidase, α-neuraminidase
α-naphthylesterase
Angiotensin-converting enzyme
Arginase
Aspartylglycosaminidase
β-glucuronidase, β-glucosidase, β-galactosidase
Cathepsins, collagenase, elastase
Leucine-2-naphthylaminidase
Lipoprotein lipase
Lysozyme
N-Acetyl-β-galactosaminidase, N-acetyl-β-glucosaminidase
Phospholipase A$_2$
Sphingomyelinase
Sulfatases

OXIDANTS

Hydroxyl radical, hydrogen peroxide, hypohalous acids, nitric oxide, peroxynitrate, and superoxide anion

BINDING PROTEINS

Avidin, apolipoprotein E, acidic isoferritins, gelsolin, haptoglobin, transcobalamin II, transferrin

COAGULATION SYSTEM PROTEINS

Factors V, VII, IX, X, XIII
Tissue factor/procoagulant activity, plasminogen activator, urokinase, thrombospondin, plasminogen activator inhibitors, plasmin inhibitors

LIPID METABOLITES

Prostaglandin (PG) E$_2$, PGF$_2$, PGI, thromboxane A$_2$; leukotrienes B, C, D, and E; malonyldialdehyde; mono-diHETEs; PAF

COMPLEMENT SYSTEM PROTEINS

C1, 2, 3, 4, 5; factors B, D, H; properdin; C3b inactivator

CYTOKINES AND GROWTH FACTORS

Interferon (INF)-α, INF-β, INF-γ
Interleukin-1α, IL-1β, IL-6, IL-8
TNF-α
Fibroblast growth factor, platelet-derived growth factor (PDGF), transforming growth factor-β
G-CSF, GM-CSF, M-CSF
Macrophage inflammatory proteins (MIP)-1α, MIP-1β, MIP-2
Monocyte chemoattractant proteins (MCP)-1, 2, 3
Thymosin B$_4$

MATRIX PROTEINS

Fibronectin, proteoglycans, thrombospondin

OTHER METABOLITES, PEPTIDES, AND PROTEINS

Glutathione, purines, pyrimidines
Sterol hormones, including 1α, 25-dihydroxyvitamin D$_3$

mono-diHETEs = mono- and dihydroxyeicosatetraenoic acids.
    Adapted from Nathan CF: Secretory products of macrophages. J Clin Invest 1987; 79:319, by copyright permission of the Society for Clinical Investigation.

lysozyme, neutral proteases, acid hydrolases and reactive oxidants, components of the complement cascade, and coagulation factors. Mononuclear phagocytes also secrete a large array of cytokines and hormones that regulate the proliferation and function of other cells that participate in the immune response, inflammation, wound repair, and hematopoiesis.

Monocytes and tissue macrophages are considered to make up a *mononuclear-phagocyte system*. This term has replaced *reticuloendothelial system*, which referred to the filtering function performed by mononuclear phagocytes in concert with nonspecific trapping mechanisms within lymphatics and blood vessels.[105] Resident tissue macrophages were formerly referred to as *histiocytes*, an imprecise and often loosely applied term than can be confusing. Tissue macrophages are widely distributed and are found both at portals of entry, such as the pulmonary alveoli, and in sterile sites, such as the bone marrow.

Spleen. Macrophages are distributed in all parts of the spleen, including the germinal centers in which they are associated with lymphocytes. Splenic macrophages located in the red pulp and sinuses serve a clearance function, where a sluggish blood circulation maximizes the interaction between blood elements and the macrophages lining the sinus walls.

Liver. The portal circulation percolates through a labyrinthine system, the spaces of Disse, before exiting via the hepatic venous system. This hepatic circulation, although less sluggish than that of the spleen, provides considerable contact between the blood and the resident liver macrophages, known as Kupffer cells, that reside within these vascular sinuses.

Lymph Nodes. As in the spleen, macrophages exist through all regions of peripheral lymph nodes. They are most abundant in the medullary zone close to efferent lymphatic and blood capillaries. This location is probably related to the important role macrophages play in the presentation of antigens to T lymphocytes.[123]

Lungs. Pulmonary macrophages reside both in the interstitium of alveolar sacs and free within the air spaces, where they participate in the clearance of inhaled microorganisms and particulate matter. The number of lung macrophages increases in many chronic pulmonary inflammatory disorders. Pulmonary macrophages are easily seen in lungs of smokers, in which black inclusions within macrophage vacuoles are noted.[124] Hemosiderin-laden alveolar macrophages can be indicative of recurrent pulmonary hemorrhage, such as that seen in idiopathic hemosiderosis or Goodpasture syndrome. Gastric aspiration to detect ingested iron-laden macrophages is a useful test for these disorders.

Bone Marrow. Macrophages are found throughout the bone marrow cavity. They are particularly abundant within hematopoietic islands and on the walls of the marrow sinuses. Bone marrow macrophages may have a clearance function in normal or pathologic states of ineffective hematopoiesis.[125] The clearance function of marrow macrophages is dramatically illustrated by the lysosomal storage diseases such as Gaucher disease.[126] Large inclusions build up within marrow macrophages (as well as hepatic and splenic macrophages), because of the inability of these cells to break down lysosomal contents. This can lead to a "myelophthisic" process with displacement of normal immature hematopoietic cells into the peripheral blood (leukoerythroblastosis) and, in Gaucher disease, a weakening of bone osteoid matrix.[112]

Other Sites. Mononuclear phagocytes associated with lymphoid cells reside throughout the alimentary tract, particularly in the submucosal tissues and small intestinal villi. They are present as microglial cells in the central nervous system (CNS), especially after injury if monocytes emigrate across the blood-brain barrier[127] and may contribute to the pathogenesis of the CNS manifestations of infection with the human immunodeficiency virus (HIV).[128] Mammary gland macrophages released into milk during lactation have been implicated as a potential source of postnatal transmission of HIV.[129]

Dendritic Cells. Dendritic cells are specialized antigen-presenting cells with long cytoplasmic processes that are located in tissues throughout the body, except for brain.[130, 131] These include the Langerhans cell of the epidermis, the veiled cells in lymph, and interdigitating cells in lymph nodes. Dendritic cells share some of the antigenic characteristics of mononuclear phagocytes and are derived from a common progenitor cell with granulocytes and monocyte/macrophages.[114, 130, 131] Monocytes can produce dendritic cells in various *in vitro* culture systems.[130, 132] Some dendritic cells also appear to be derived from the lymphoid lineage.[114, 133] Antigen presentation by dendritic cells, which have a high density of major histocompatability class (MHC) II molecules, is a particularly potent stimulus for naïve T lymphocytes and for inducing a primary immune response.[130, 131, 133]

Osteoclasts. Osteoclasts are large, multinucleated cells that resorb mineralized cartilage and bone and are closely related to mononuclear phagocytes.[134] Rodent transplantation studies have shown that osteoclasts can be derived from granulocyte-macrophage progenitor cells.[135] Defects in osteoclast function result in osteopetrosis, a genetically heterogeneous group of disorders characterized by progressive obliteration of the marrow space by the unchecked formation of new bone. The *op/op* osteopetrotic mouse mutant lacks M-CSF, which results in deficiencies of both osteoclasts and tissue macrophages.[136] M-CSF levels and osteoclast numbers are normal in human infantile ("malignant") osteopetrosis,[137] a disorder correctable by bone marrow transplantation.[138] Administration of IFN-γ, a major activator of macrophage function, can produce a clinically significant increase in bone resorption in children with infantile osteopetrosis.[139] Increases in both urinary hydroxyproline and urinary calcium excretion were observed during IFN-γ therapy, with associated decreases in trabecular-bone area, widening of cranial nerve foramina, and improvement in bone marrow function and peripheral blood counts.

FUNCTION OF PHAGOCYTES

Overview

Phagocytic leukocytes play a central role in the acute phases of the inflammatory response, during which they are rapidly mobilized into sites of tissue infection or injury and release an array of cytotoxic molecules to quickly but nonspecifically eliminate the offending substance or microbe. Phagocytes are also essential for normal repair of tissue injury, as evidenced by the impairment in wound healing in patients with deficits in leukocyte function or number.

The classic signs of the inflammatory response were described by the Roman writer, Celsus, as "rubor et tumor, cum calore et delore"—redness and swelling with heat and pain.[140] However, it was not until the late nineteenth century that the importance of the inflammatory process for host defense and wound healing was generally recognized.[141] The beneficial role of phagocytes in this process was championed by Metchnikov. Much of his work, for which he received a Nobel prize,[141, 142] involved studies on the wandering ameboid mesenchymal cells of marine organisms such as the larval starfish, for which he coined the term *phagocyte*, after the Greek word, *phagein*, "to eat."

In this section, the principal functions of granulocytes and mononuclear phagocytes in the inflammatory process are reviewed. Although these functions will be discussed as individual components, it is important to recognize that many occur either simultaneously or in rapid succession. Moreover, many of the cellular structures or secreted molecules participating in the inflammatory process have multiple functions. For example, phagocyte cell surface proteins that act as adhesive ligands for receptors on the vascular endothelium can also trigger phagocytosis and activation of the phagocyte respiratory burst.

Humoral Mediators of the Inflammatory Response

The inflammatory response reflects an ongoing collaboration between tissue macrophages and mast cells, vascular endothelial cells, and circulating phagocytes. The release of soluble inflammatory mediators plays a crucial role in activating and coordinating this process. These molecules can be generated from serum proteins (e.g., the complement-derived protein fragment C5a), secreted by endothelial cells or inflammatory leukocytes (e.g., lipid metabolites, histamine, or cytokines), or derived from invading microbes (e.g., endotoxin or formulated chemotactic peptides).

The pro-inflammatory cytokines, TNF-α and IL-1, have a broad range of activities in the acute inflammatory response.[143, 144] Both IL-1 and TNF can cause fever and muscle breakdown and are involved the cachexia associated with chronic infection and malignancy. The synthesis of acute phase reactants by the liver is induced by IL-6, whose synthesis and secretion are stimulated by IL-1. Pro-inflammatory cytokines also induce a pro-adhesive state on the surface of endothelium and increase the production of the chemotactic cytokines (chemokines). IFN-γ is another important pro-inflammatory mediator that enhances the responsiveness of phagocytes to inflammatory stimuli.[115, 116] Counterbalancing the activities of these polypeptides are IL-4, IL-10, and transforming growth factor-β, which tend to downregulate the acute inflammatory response.[145–147]

Vasodilation and increased vascular permeability are two early responses to an inflammatory insult that are elicited, in large part, by products secreted by granulocytes and mononuclear phagocytes. Activated basophils and tissue mast cells release histamine, which leads to vasodilation of tissue arterioles and microvascular beds through H_1-type receptors.[148–150] The lipid metabolite platelet-activating factor (PAF), which is secreted by activated macrophages, mast cells, and endothelial cells, induces platelet degranulation and the release of additional histamine and also serotonin, another vasoactive amine.[151, 152] Prostaglandin E and other arachidonic acid metabolites secreted by activated neutrophils and macrophages belong to another group of potent vasodilators.[153] Finally, vasodilation can be triggered by the release of nitric oxide from endothelial and smooth muscle cells as well as perhaps activated macrophages, which may be particularly important in the hypotension seen with gram-negative septicemia.[154, 155] The increased vascular permeability that produces the edema of acute inflammation allows plasma proteins such as immunoglobulins and complement to enter tissues to promote phagocyte activation and opsonize microbes. Agents that increase vascular permeability include histamine, serotonin, PAF, and leukotrienes (LTs) C_4, D_4, and E_4.[152, 156] Bradykinin, which is generated as the result of Hageman factor (factor XII) cleavage, also induces enhanced vascular permeability.

A wide variety of chemoattractants for neutrophils and other circulating phagocytes are generated at sites of inflammation (Table 21–6).[58, 157–160] These molecules are chemically diverse and are derived from many different sources in response to bacterial products and inflammatory mediators released as a result of tissue necrosis. This diversity provides a functional redundancy and ensures that leukocytes will be attracted to sites of injury or infection. In addition to molecules generated by the activation of complement (C5a) or bacteria themselves (formylated peptides), many are secreted by activated phagocytes, which act as a positive feedback loop for additional recruitment and activation of inflammatory cells. The phospholipid PAF, released by both activated phagocytes and endothelial cells, triggers platelet activation and granule release in addition to acting as a potent chemoattractant for neutrophils and eosinophils.[151, 152] Activation of phagocytes also stimulates the phospholipase A_2–mediated cleavage of membrane phospholipids to generate arachidonic acid, which is then converted into a variety of eicosanoid metabolites, including the chemoattractant LTB_4.[153]

Phagocyte chemoattractants include a family of small (8 to 10 kD) basic heparin-binding proteins known as chemokines (for their combined *chemo*tactic and cyto*kine* properties).[58, 150, 158, 159] Chemokines were first discovered in the late 1980s. These molecules interact relatively specifically with subsets of inflammatory leukocytes and therefore play an important role in mediating the sequential influx of neutrophils, monocytes, and finally lymphocytes into an inflamed tissue site. The heparin-binding sites on chemokines may bind to negatively charged proteoglycans on endothelial cells or in the subendothelial matrix to facilitate the production of locally high

TABLE 21–6. Granulocyte and Monocyte Chemoattractants in Humans

Chemoattractant	Source	Upregulators	Target Cells
LIPIDS			
PAF	N, E, B, P, M Endothelium (phosphatidyl choline metabolism)	Calcium ionophores	N, E
LTB$_4$	N, M (arachidonate metabolism)	Microbial pathogens, *N*-formyl peptides	N, M, E
CXC CHEMOKINES			
IL-8	M, N, endothelium, many other cells	LPS, IL-1, TNF, IL-3	N, B
GRO α, β, γ	M, endothelium, many other cells	IL-1, TNF	N
NAP-2	P★	Platelet activators	N
CC CHEMOKINES			
MCP-1 (MCAF)	M, endothelium, many other cells	IL-1, TNF, LPS, PDGF	M, B
RANTES	M, E	IL-1, TNF, anti-CD3	M, B
Eotaxin	M, endothelium, other	Allergens	E, B, Th2
OTHER			
N-formyl peptides	Bacteria Mitochondria	—	N, M, E, B
C5a	Complement activation	Complement activation	N, M, E, B

★Platelets, when activated, secrete platelet basic protein (PBP) and connective tissue–activating peptide-III (CTAP-III), which are cleaved to NAP-2 by cathepsin.

B = Basophil; E = eosinophil; F = fibroblast; GRO = growth-related gene; K = keratinocyte; LPS = lipopolysaccharide; M = monocyte; MCAF = monocyte chemotactic and activating factor; N = neutrophil; NAP-2 = neutrophil-activating peptide-2; P = platelet; RANTES = regulated upon activation, normal T cell expressed and presumably secreted; T = T lymphocyte.

Adapted from Curnutte JT, Orkin SH, Dinauer MC: Genetic disorders of phagocyte function. In Stamatoyannopoulos G, Nienhuis AW, et al (eds): The Molecular Basis of Blood Disease. 2nd ed. Philadelphia, W.B. Saunders Co., 1993, pp 493–522.

chemokine concentrations at an inflamed site.[161–163] As additional chemokines and their receptors have been identified, their function in lymphocyte homeostasis, the development of lymphoid and myeloid progenitors, and angiogenesis is also being recognized.[58, 159]

Members of the chemokine family, which have a conserved structure containing two cysteine pairs, have been divided into two groups on the basis of the disulfide sequence pattern. The CXC family, in which the first cysteine pair is separated by an intervening amino acid, includes IL-8, the growth-related gene (GRO) peptides, and neutrophil-activating peptide (NAP)-2, which are all potent neutrophil activators and, except for NAP-2, chemoattractants. NAP-2 is generated by the cleavage of platelet secretory proteins by cathepsin G released from monocytes and neutrophils,[164] whereas IL-8 and GRO are released from phagocytes and mesenchymal cells (including endothelial cells) in response to inflammatory mediators such as IL-1 and TNF.[150, 165] The other major family of chemokines is called the CC family, because the first two cysteines are adjacent to each other. CC chemokines include two important inducers of mononuclear phagocyte migration, monocyte chemoattractant protein 1 (MCP-1) and RANTES (*r*egulated upon *a*ctivation, *n*ormal *T* cell *e*xpressed and presumably *s*ecreted).[150, 165–168] MCP-1 is produced by a wide variety of cells, whereas RANTES is secreted by macrophages and eosinophils.[58] RANTES is chemotactic for eosinophils, basophils, memory T cells, and monocytes,[150, 167] and both MCP-1 and RANTES induce histamine release from basophils.[148, 149, 167]

Chemokine receptors are members of the seven transmembrane domain, G-protein–coupled receptor family, with five receptors for CXC chemokines and eight receptors for CC chemokines identified to date.[58, 159, 160] Most chemokines bind to more than one receptor, and most chemokine receptors, particularly those for CC chemokines, recognize more than one chemokine. Neutrophils, monocyte/macrophages, eosinophils, basophils, and T cells each express a distinctive subset of chemokine receptors. According to one model, specific receptors are used sequentially in successive gradients of chemoattractants, with some transmitting desensitizing rather than activating signals.[160] Of note, a number of chemokine receptors are co-receptors for HIV-1, including CCR5 and CCR3, whose ligands include RANTES, and CXCR4, a ligand for stromal cell–derived factor 1 (SDF-1), which is a chemoattractant for T lymphocytes and CD34$^+$ hematopoietic progenitor cells.[58]

In addition to their role as chemoattractants, the molecules listed in Table 21–6 induce the activation of many other phagocyte functions upon binding to their cognate cell surface receptors. These include the upregulation and increased affinity of integrin adhesion receptors to promote firm attachment to the endothelium, rearrangement of the actin cytoskeleton, degranulation, and activation of the phagocyte respiratory burst.[49, 58, 150, 153, 157, 159] These responses generally require higher ligand concentrations compared with those that elicit chemotaxis, which can be as low as 10^{-9} mol/L.[169]

Despite the diverse chemical structures of phagocyte chemoattractants listed in Table 21–6, all of the corresponding receptors that have been cloned to date belong to the seven transmembrane-spanning (7-TMS) family of receptors, also known as heptahelical or serpentine receptors.[57, 158, 170] The transduction of signals through serpentine receptors is mediated via heterotrimeric G-proteins, which bind to specific intracellular domains of the receptor.[171–174] Ligand binding to the receptor promotes the exchange of GTP for glucose diphosphate (GDP) bound to the G-protein α subunit, which in turns leads to the dissociation of the β-γ subunits and their interaction with downstream signaling effectors.[49] These include enzymes that catalyze the production of important phospholipid second messengers at the cell membrane.[51] Phospholipase C generates diacylglycerol and IP_3 from PIP_2, which then activate protein kinase C and induce release of intracellular calcium stores. PI 3-kinase is another key target of activated heterotrimeric G-proteins and catalyzes the phosphorylation of PIP_2 to form PIP_3. Binding of formylated peptides to neutrophils also activates the p21ras-MAP kinase pathway and the Rho GTPases, Cdc42 and Rac, with the latter being known to play important roles in regulating the actin cytoskeleton and oxidant production.[60–62, 175–178] Certain Gα subunits appear to be expressed preferentially in leukocytes and may be important in signaling through the phagocyte 7-TMS receptors.[179, 180]

Adhesion and Migration into Tissues

The discovery that leukocytes migrate from the bloodstream into extravascular sites of inflammation, described by Cohnheim in 1867, was a major milestone in the conceptualization of the inflammatory process.[141] Cohnheim, who used intravital microscopy to study the microvasculature in the frog tongue and mesentery after tissue injury, also proposed that inflammatory stimuli induce a molecular change in the blood vessel wall that promoted the increased adherence of leukocytes, a concept that was finally proved a century later.

To move from the bloodstream into inflamed sites, leukocytes must attach to the vascular endothelium, migrate between adjacent endothelial cells in a process referred to as diapedesis, and penetrate the basement membrane. The molecular mechanisms underlying these events have been the subject of intense study and involve a series of sequential adhesive interactions between chemoattractant-activated leukocytes and endothelial cells that are activated by inflammatory mediators (Fig. 21–2).[157, 181–183]

Leukocyte Adhesion. The initial step in emigration from postcapillary venules is a low-affinity interaction between the neutrophil and the endothelium that is often referred to as "rolling," on the basis of its appearance in intravital microscopy. This transient adherence, also called "tethering," is mediated by the upregulation of selectin expression on endothelial cells. The selectin family of adhesion molecules are membrane-spanning glycoproteins (Fig. 21–3) that bind to fucosylated structures such as Lewis X (Galβ1→4[Fucα1→3]GlcNac→R), sialyl Lewis X, and other specific carbohydrates.[184–187] P-selectin appears to be the most important substance for the initial steps of neutrophil adhesion to the endothelium and is stored in the Weibel-Palade bodies and α granules of endothelial cells and platelets, respectively.[182, 185] Upon activation of endothelial cells by histamine, thrombin, and other inflammatory molecules, these cytoplasmic storage granules fuse with the cell membrane to rapidly increase the surface expression of P-selectin. E-selectin is expressed on endothelial cells at low levels but is upregulated by transcriptional activation and *de novo* protein synthesis in response to inflammatory cytokines.[188] L-selectin is expressed constitutively on the surface of neutrophils, mononuclear phagocytes, and lymphocytes and is shed within minutes of leukocyte activation by a proteolytic cleavage event near the external membrane surface insertion site.[189, 190] Circulating L-selectin may modulate leukocyte adhesion during inflammation.[191]

FIGURE 21–2. Adhesive interactions during phagocyte emigration. Under conditions of flow within postcapillary venules, leukocytes are first observed to roll along the endothelium adjacent to the extravascular site of inflammation. Subsequently, some of the rolling leukocytes adhere firmly, diapedese between endothelial cells, and then migrate into subendothelial tissue. Studies *in vitro* and *in vivo* indicate that rolling is mediated by multiple low-affinity interactions between selectin receptors and carbohydrate counter-receptors, and firm adhesion and diapedesis largely depend on integrin and immunoglobulin (Ig)-like adhesion proteins. (From Carlos TM, Harlan JM: Leukocyte-endothelial adhesion molecules. Blood 1994; 84:2068.)

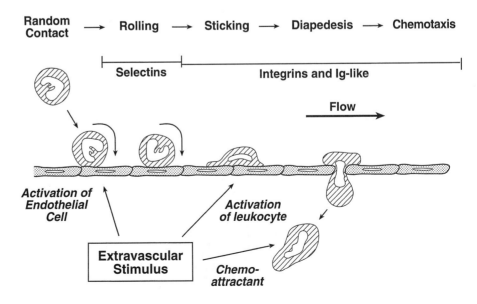

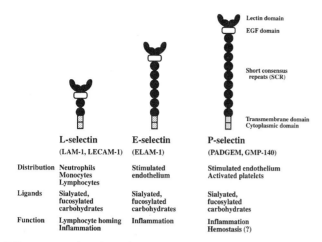

FIGURE 21–3. The selectin family of adhesion molecules. EGF = epidermal growth factor. (Adapted from Kishimoto TK, Rothlein R: Integrins, ICAMS, and selectins: Role and regulation of adhesion molecules in neutrophil recruitment to inflammatory sites, Adv Pharmacol 1994; 25:117.)

Rolling neutrophils can detach and return to the circulation. Others will come to a halt and, within seconds, adopt a flattened, adherent morphologic appearance and attach firmly to the vessel wall.[182] This firm attachment appears in large part to be mediated by leukocyte integrin

adhesion receptors binding to intracellular adhesion molecules (ICAMs) on the endothelium.[157,181,182] In addition, complement fragments are found on the endothelial surface at inflamed sites and may also function as integrin binding sites.[192] Leukocyte activation by chemoattractants is critical to the development of these strong adhesive interactions, because it leads to the up-regulation of the number and avidity of cell surface integrins. Exposure to locally high concentrations of chemoattractants may be enhanced by selectin-mediated tethering and by the retention of chemokines on extracellular matrix.[161–163]

The integrins are a large family of adhesion proteins that are glycosylated heterodimers of a noncovalently linked α and a β chain and are classified into subfamilies according to the type of β subunit.[184, 193–196] Many integrins mediate attachment to extracellular matrices by serving as receptors for matrix proteins. Others are involved in hemostasis, such as glycoprotein IIb/IIIa on platelets. The leukocyte β_2 integrins (Fig. 21–4) play a critical role in mediating adhesive interactions in inflammation, including the attachment of leukocytes to endothelial cells and are also opsonic receptors for complement fragment-coated particles.

There are four different leukocyte β_2 integrins, each having a common 95-kD β subunit (CD18) but different α subunits, CD11a (177 kD), CD11b (165 kD), CD11c

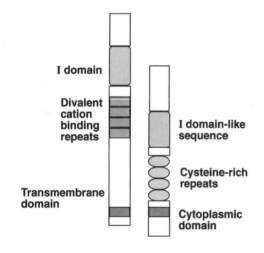

FIGURE 21–4. The β_2 (CD18) family of leukocyte integrins. LFA-1 = leukocyte function antigen 1; ICAM = intercellular adhesion molecule; LGL = large granular lymphocytes. See text for additional details and references.

	LFA 1	Mac-1 (CR3)	p150, 95	α_d β_2
α subunit	α_L (CDIIa)	α_m (CD11b)	α_x (CD11c)	α_d (CD11d)
β subunit	β_2 (CD18)	β_2 (CD18)	β_2 (CD18)	β_2 (CD18)
Ligands	ICAM-1 ICAM-2 ICAM-3	ICAM-1 C 3bi Fibringen Factor X other	C3bi? other	ICAM-3 other ?
Distribution	All leukocytes	Granulocytes Monocytes Macrophages LGL	Macrophages Monocytes Granulocytes LGL Some activated lymphocytes	Macrophages Monocytes Granulocytes T Lymphoctyes

(150 kD), and CD11d (160kD) (Fig. 21–4). CD11a/ CD11b (leukocyte function antigen 1 [LFA-1]) is expressed by all leukocytes, including lymphocytes. Mac-1 and p150,95 are expressed by granulocytes, mononuclear phagocytes, some activated T lymphocytes, and large granular lymphocytes.[182, 184] Mac-1 is the most prominent β_2 integrin on neutrophils, whereas $\alpha_d\beta_2$ is expressed particularly in tissue macrophages. Mutations in the common β subunit result in an inherited defect in phagocyte function, leukocyte adhesion deficiency type I (LAD I) as discussed in a later section. All β_2 integrins are absent in LAD I, indicating that the stability of each α subunit requires association with the β chain, which normally occurs in the Golgi compartment.[197] The β subunit has a large, glycosylated extracellular domain, a single transmembrane-spanning domain, and a short cytoplasmic tail.[198] The extracellular domain has two regions that are conserved among other β subunits.[182, 194, 197] There are four cysteine-rich tandem repeats that appear to be important for the tertiary structure of the β subunit. Another conserved region, located near the amino terminus, is critical for maintenance of the α/β heterodimer and may also bind divalent cations. Point mutations in these conserved regions were reported in LAD I.[182] The α subunit is also a glycosylated integral membrane protein with a single membrane-spanning segment and a short cytoplasmic tail. The external domain contains three divalent cation-binding motifs that must be occupied for ligand binding to occur.[193, 194] A second important extracellular domain, the I domain (for inserted or interactive domain), can coordinate divalent cations and is also thought to be involved in ligand binding. The intracellular domain of the α subunit includes a conserved sequence that is critical for the modulation of integrin avidity (see later).[199] The cytoplasmic tails of both the α and β integrin subunits also interact with the cytoskeletal proteins.[184, 200] The endoparasite hookworm, *Ancylostoma caninum*, produces a heavily glycosylated protein called NIF (for neutrophil inhibitory factor) that binds to CD11b/CD18 to inhibit neutrophil spreading and attachment to the endothelium.[201, 202]

Although β_2 integrins are constitutively expressed on the neutrophil cell surface, a large pool is also stored in intracellular secretory vesicles (see Table 21–2). These vesicles are rapidly mobilized upon neutrophil activation by chemoattractants and fuse with the membrane to increase the cell surface expression of β_2 integrins by about 10-fold.[27, 157, 203] Signaling through chemoattractant receptors also markedly increases the avidity of β_2 integrins for their ligands, which plays an even more important role in rapidly upregulating integrin activity and promoting firm attachment to the blood vessel wall.[194, 197] The increased adhesiveness of the β_2 integrins appears to involve a conformational change in integrin structure upon cellular activation.

The major counter-receptors for the β_2 integrins are the ICAMs (Fig. 21–5), which are members of the immunoglobulin superfamily.[181, 182, 197] These transmembrane proteins contain anywhere from two to six immunoglobulin domains and are present on endothelial cells, T cells, and a variety of other cell types. ICAM-1 and ICAM-2 are of particular importance in mediation of

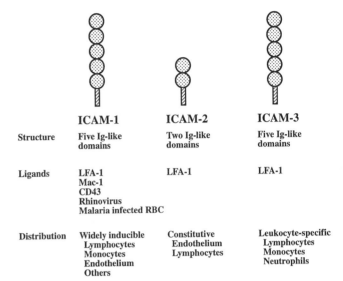

	ICAM-1	**ICAM-2**	**ICAM-3**
Structure	Five Ig-like domains	Two Ig-like domains	Five Ig-like domains
Ligands	LFA-1 Mac-1 CD43 Rhinovirus Malaria infected RBC	LFA-1	LFA-1
Distribution	Widely inducible Lymphocytes Monocytes Endothelium Others	Constitutive Endothelium Lymphocytes	Leukocyte-specific Lymphocytes Monocytes Neutrophils

FIGURE 21–5. The intercellular adhesion molecules (ICAMs). RBC = red blood cell (Adapted from Kishimoto TK, Rothlein R: Integrins, ICAMS, and selectins: Role and regulation of adhesion molecules in neutrophil recruitment to inflammatory sites. Adv Pharmacol 1994; 25:117.)

binding of neutrophils and other leukocytes to the endothelium. Endothelial cell expression of ICAM-1 increases in response to inflammatory cytokines, which promotes increased cell-cell interactions with leukocytes at inflamed sites. Vascular cell adhesion molecule 1 (VCAM-1) is another immunoglobulin superfamily member expressed on endothelial cells that is inducible by cytokines.[182] VCAM-1 is the counter-receptor for the β_1 integrin, very late activation antigen 4 (VLA-4), and appears to be important in promoting the adherence of monocytes and eosinophils during inflammation. The β_2 integrin Mac-1 (CD11b/CD18) also has an important role as an opsonic receptor for the complement fragment, C3bi, as discussed later.

In addition to their role in adhesion, β_2 integrins are now recognized to play an important role in leukocyte activation.[204, 205] Ligand binding to integrins results in their clustering and activation of tyrosine kinase and other signaling cascades, which provide costimulatory signals to enhance migration, respiratory burst, FcγIIR-mediated phagocytosis, and degranulation.[204–206] In neutrophils, Mac-1 must interact with the FcγRIII receptor (see later) for FcγRIII-mediated phagocytosis and activation of the respiratory burst.[207–209]

Although leukocyte β_2 integrin-mediated adhesion is clearly important for neutrophil recruitment from the systemic microvasculature into inflammatory sites, neutrophil emigration out of the pulmonary circulation can also be mediated by alternative pathways, depending on the inflammatory stimulus.[210, 211] Whether the alternative pathway in pulmonary capillaries involves selectins or other adhesion molecules remains to be defined. Neutrophil emigration from the bone marrow storage pool into the circulation is also a poorly understood process and appears to involve adhesion molecules distinct from the β_2 integrins and L-selectin.[212]

The final steps in emigration of neutrophils from the blood vessel lumen into inflamed tissue involves squeezing between adjacent endothelial cells (diapedesis) and penetrating the basement membrane (see Fig. 21–2). The presence of a chemotactic gradient is required to induce the directional migration of neutrophils.[161, 213, 214] Adhesive interactions between the β_2 integrins and ICAM-1 are essential for neutrophil diapedesis, whereas VCAM-1 and E-selectin can mediate the transmigration of monocytes and eosinophils.[182] Transendothelial migration of neutrophils also depends on homologous binding events between neutrophil and endothelial cell platelet-endothelial cell adhesion molecule 1 (PECAM-1) (CD31) adhesion receptors.[215, 216] PECAM-1, another member of the immunoglobulin superfamily, is expressed on leukocytes, platelets, and endothelial cells, where it is localized at the junctions between cells.[181] Migrating neutrophils may also induce an increase in endothelial intracellular calcium levels that facilitates the opening of spaces between endothelial cells via a still undefined mechanism.[217] Finally, chemoattractant-induced degranulation of neutrophil secretory vesicles results in the release of digestive enzymes, including collagenase, elastase, and gelatinase, which facilitate basement membrane penetration.[27, 218]

Chemotaxis. Chemotaxis is the directional movement of a cell along a concentration gradient.[30, 219, 220] Defects in neutrophil cellular motility or other steps in chemotaxis can result in decreased resistance to bacterial and fungal infections, as discussed later in this chapter. The neutrophil chemotactic response occurs at chemoattractant concentrations that approximate the dissociation constants of the chemotactic factors for their receptors, which are much lower than those that elicit degranulation and activation of the respiratory burst.[29, 169] Cells respond to a chemotactic gradient by sensing constantly across their surface, and bound chemotactic receptors are continuously internalized.[219] A migrating neutrophil has a polarized appearance, extending pseudopodia or lamellipodia, thin structures rich in actin filaments and lacking intracellular organelles, at the leading edge.[30] The pseudopods appear to glide forward, pulling the cell body behind them. The nucleus tends to remain at the posterior half of the moving leukocyte. Neutrophil movement requires reversible adhesion to the underlying substrate, and proteases localized at the neutrophil surface, such as urokinase-type plasminogen activator (uPA), may be involved in successive breaking of attachments to the extracellular matrix.[221–224] The glycosyl phosphatidylinositol (GPI)-linked receptor for uPA has also been shown to play a role in monocyte chemotaxis that is distinct from its role in localizing uPA-mediated proteolysis at the cell surface.[225]

Neutrophil movement depends on the dynamic assembly and disassembly of filamentous actin, which is coordinated by various actin-binding proteins whose activity is regulated by intracellular signaling molecules.[29, 30, 220, 226] Leukocyte motility is inhibited by the cytochalasins, which block actin assembly. Actin can exist as either a soluble monomer (globular actin) or in needle-like helical filaments (filamentous actin). Actin filaments align spontaneously in parallel bundles but in the cell are organized into a branching network due to the presence of actin filament cross-linkers such as actin-binding protein.[227] Another class of actin regulatory proteins sequesters actin

monomers and thus can control the availability of globular actin for filament formation. Prophyllin and thymosin B4 are two major actin monomer-binding proteins in neutrophils.[228] Other actin-binding proteins, such as gelsolin, cap the fast-growing barbed end of the actin filament or sever filamentous actin into shorter pieces.[29, 30]

Agonists acting via receptors on the cell membrane trigger the generation of second messengers, which interact with actin-binding proteins to control dynamic local cycles of filamentous actin assembly.[30] For example, increased local calcium concentrations activate gelsolin, promoting actin disassembly by cleaving actin filaments and capping its barbed ends. On the other hand, actin assembly is stimulated by the accumulation of phosphoinositols liberated from membrane phospholipids around an activated receptor. Phosphoinositols, such as PIP_2, interact both with actin-sequestering proteins to liberate actin monomers and with gelsolin to uncap the barbed ends of filamentous actin. The Rho GTPases, Cdc42 and Rac, are important regulators of actin remodeling and are activated by ligand binding to chemoattractant receptors.[59, 62, 176, 178, 220, 229] Cdc42 activates proteins of the Wiskott-Aldrich syndrome protein family, which then bind to a complex of seven proteins known as the Arp2/3 complex to nucleate assembly of new actin filaments at the leading edge of migrating cells.[220, 226, 230] Rac activation appears to be important both for de novo actin nucleation by the Arp2/3 complex and for stimulating the uncapping of existing actin filament barbed ends.[175]

During pseudopod extension in chemoattractant-activated neutrophils, new actin polymerization occurs at the site of membrane protrusion while the filamentous actin in the rear of the cell disassembles.[231–233] How actin assembly-disassembly results in membrane extension and formation of pseudopodia is not fully understood but may involve localized changes in osmotic pressure due to changes in actin polymerization.[29, 30] Membrane movement may also be mediated in part by contractile proteins such as myosin 1, but this mediation has not been well studied in leukocytes.

Opsonization and Phagocytosis

The ingestion and disposal of microbes, foreign particulate matter, and damaged cells constitute a major aspect of phagocyte function. To facilitate their recognition by phagocytes, these targets are coated with serum opsonins (from the Greek, "to prepare for dining"), which include proteolytic fragments derived from the complement cascade as well as specific immunoglobulins. Tissue macrophages, which are often the first cells to encounter invading microbes, also have receptors capable of recognizing ligands even in the absence of opsonins. These include the mannose receptor and the scavenger receptor.[234–237] The macrophage mannose receptor in the mouse, for example, recognizes *Pneumocystis carinii* and mediates its ingestion. The scavenger receptor has broad binding specificities and probably participates in the clearance of diverse foreign materials.[236]

The key humoral opsonins are the opsonic antibodies immunoglobin (Ig) M, IgG_1, and IgG_3 and the proteolytic cleavage products of C3 (C3b and C3bi). Targets are opsonized by the deposition of the IgG onto their surfaces via the specific (Fab) portion of the antibody or by deposition of C3b and C3bi. Antibacterial IgM antibodies, although not opsonic by themselves, play an important role in phagocytosis by activating complement. Opsonins are recognized by phagocyte cell surface glycoprotein receptors for immunoglobulin and C3 cleavage products (Table 21–7). Inherited deficiencies of either immunoglobulins or complement can result in increased susceptibility to bacterial infections, as discussed in a later section. In contrast, primary defects in phagocyte receptors for these opsonins appear to be an uncommon cause of recurrent infections.[238]

Immunoglobulin Receptors. Immunoglobulins are recognized by Fc receptors, which are members of the immunoglobulin gene superfamily. Fc receptors bind to the "constant domain" of the antibody molecule, which is specific to each class of immunoglobulins (IgA, IgE, IgG, and IgM).[238–242] The most important receptors from the standpoint of microbial opsonization are the Fc receptors that recognize IgG (Table 21–7). The Fcγ receptors include three distinct classes, FcγRI, FcγRII, and FcγRIII, which are encoded by at least eight genes that have evolved through gene duplication and alternative splicing, although not all yield detectable mRNA and/or protein.[239]

The low-affinity Fcγ receptor genes (FcγRII and FcγRIII families) and two of the genes for the high-affinity IgE receptor are clustered on chromosome 1q22. The high-affinity IgG Fc receptors map to other sites on chromosomal 1.

Except for FcγRIIIb, which is anchored in the membrane by a GPI moiety, the Fcγ receptor proteins have a single transmembrane domain. FcγRI and FcγRIIIa exist as oligomeric complexes with γ (in phagocytes) or ζ (in lymphocytes) chains that are important both for their stable expression and signaling functions.[239] These accessory chains contain YXXL immunoreceptor tyrosine activation motifs (ITAMs), which become tyrosine phosphorylated upon receptor cross-linking to initiate downstream signaling cascades.[238, 240, 241] The cytoplasmic tail of FcγRIIa receptors contains variant ITAMs, and hence this receptor does not require accessory chains for its function. There is no murine equivalent to FcγRIIa receptors.[240, 241] The GPI-linked FcγRIIIb receptors must be co-ligated to either FcγRIIa or CR3 receptors to initiate signaling functions upon ligation.[240, 241] FcγRIIb receptors, expressed on monocyte/macrophages, mast cells, and lymphocytes, contain immunoreceptor tyrosine inhibition motif sequences and instead inhibit cellular activation upon immunoglobulin cross-linking.[241, 242]

TABLE 21–7. Human Phagocyte Fcγ and Complement Receptors*

	FcγRIa (CD64)	FcγRIIa (CD32)	FcγRIIIa, b (CD16)	CR1 (CD35)	CR3 (CD11b/CD18)
Polymorphisms		131R/H	IIIa: 48L/R/H 158F/V IIIb: NA-1, NA-2		
Cell distribution	Monocytes Macrophages IFN-γ– or G-CSF–treated neutrophils IFN-γ–treated eosinophils	Monocytes Neutrophils Macrophages Eosinophils Basophils Platelets	IIIa: Macrophages Monocytes (some) T cells, NK cells IIIb: Neutrophils IFN-γ–treated eosinophils	Monocytes Macrophages Neutrophils Erythrocytes B lymphocytes	Neutrophils Macrophages Monocytes
Protein size and type	72 kD, transmembrane	40 kD, transmembrane	50–90 kD IIIa: transmembrane IIIb: GPI-anchored	160–250 kD transmembrane	Heterodimeric transmembrane protein
Associated proteins	FcRγ homodimer	—	IIIa: FcR γ homodimer (macrophage, monocyte) IIIb: co-ligation with FcγRIIa or CR3		
Ligands	Monomeric IgG $(G_1=G_3>G_4>>G_2)$	Complexed IgG $(G_1=G_3>>G_2,G_4)$ (FcγRIIA 131H-G_2)	Complexed IgG $(G_1=G_3>>G_2,G_4)$	C3b C4b	C3bi ICAM-1 ICAM-2
Affinity	High	Low	Low	Moderate	Moderate
Function	Phagocytosis Respiratory burst Endocytosis of IC ADCC Antigen presentation	Phagocytosis Respiratory burst Exocytosis Endocytosis of IC ADCC Antigen presentation	Phagocytosis Exocytosis Endocytosis of IC ADCC (IIIa) Antigen presentation (IIIa)	Phagocytosis	Phagocytosis Respiratory burst (neutrophils) Cell adhesion Activation

FcγR = Fc receptor for IgG; CR = complement receptor; NK = natural killer ICAM = intracellular adhesion molecule; IC = immune complexes; ADCC = antibody-dependent cellular cytotoxicity.
*See text for references.

Each Fcγ receptor is expressed at different levels, depending on the type of phagocytic cell (Table 21–7), and some FcγRII and FcγRIII family members are also expressed on lymphocytes, platelets, thymocytes, natural killer (NK) cells, and mast cells.[239, 241] The FcγRI class includes the products of three highly homologous genes, denoted A, B, and C, although the protein products of the latter two have not been detected *in vivo*. The FcγRIa receptors are expressed by monocytes and neutrophils or eosinophils stimulated by IFN-γ or G-CSF and have a high affinity for monomeric IgG.[238, 239, 241] Members of the FcγRII and FcγRIII families have a low affinity for monomeric IgG but a high affinity for clusters of IgG (e.g., several antibodies bound to the same particle) and immune complexes. Only neutrophils and IFN-γ–stimulated eosinophils appear to express FcγRIIIb, and polymorphisms in this receptor correspond to the serologically defined NA1/NA2 antigen system, which is a common antibody target in alloimmune and autoimmune neutropenia.[243] Other Fcγ receptor polymorphisms that have clinical significance include the FcγRIIa 131H allele, which is the only Fcγ receptor that mediates efficient phagocytosis of IgG$_2$-opsonized bacteria and has been linked to a lower incidence of infections with encapsulated bacteria.[238] Individuals homozygous for the FcγRIIIa 158F polymorphism are over-represented among patients with systemic lupus erythematosus and especially among those with nephritis.[244]

Cross-linking of Fcγ receptors can trigger a wide range of functional responses, including phagocytosis of IgG-coated microbes, blood cells, or tumor cells, ingestion of immune complexes, release of inflammatory mediators, activation of the respiratory burst, and antibody-dependent cellular cytotoxicity (ADCC). The relative roles of different phagocyte Fcγ receptor classes have not been clearly delineated, although all can function as receptors for opsonized particles or immune complexes. Binding of IgG to FcγRI and FcγRIIa receptors activates the respiratory burst, whereas secretion of granular contents is a prominent response upon binding to FcγRII and FcγRIIIb receptors.[238, 240–242] Although the ligand-binding domains of different Fcγ receptors all bind IgG, the specificity of the cellular response may be governed by the unique transmembrane and cytoplasmic domains of a particular Fc receptor subtype.[239]

Ligation and cross-linking of Fcγ receptors initiate a cascade of biochemical signals that are initiated by activation of nonreceptor protein tyrosine kinases of the Src family, which phosphorylate ITAM motifs in the Fc receptor γ chain and in FcγRIIa receptors to recruit and activate the Syk tyrosine kinase and further amplify ITAM phosphorylation.[240, 241] Subsequent activation of several parallel pathways, including activation of phospholipase C, PI 3–kinase, MAP kinase–related pathways, and targets involved in actin remodeling, leading to various cellular responses.

The opsonization of microbes with secretory IgA antibodies is likely to be important in the clearance of microbes from the mucosal surfaces of the respiratory, gastrointestinal, and urogenital tracts. Neutrophils and monocytes have an Fc receptor for IgA (Fcα receptor), which has close structural similarities with other members of the Fc receptor family.[245] Ligation of the phagocyte Fcα receptor can trigger phagocytosis, degranulation, and superoxide release.[246, 247] IgE antibodies can activate eosinophils and mast cells through the high-affinity FcεRI receptors.

Complement Receptors. The human phagocyte C3b receptor (CR1) is a high molecular weight, single-subunit glycoprotein that shows a substantial heterogeneity in size because of the presence of four distinct alleles in the human population that encode proteins ranging in size from 160 to 250 kD. CR1 is responsible for the binding of C3b-opsonized particles and for initiating their ingestion. The other major opsonic receptor, CR3, recognizes particles opsonized with C3bi. This receptor is the same as the β$_2$ integrin Mac-1 (CD11b/CD18) discussed in detail in an earlier section (see Fig. 21–4). Binding of C3bi-opsonized particles to CD11b/CD18 triggers both phagocytosis and the respiratory burst.

Phagocytosis. Engagement of any of the opsonic receptors initiates phagocytosis of an opsonized particle to form a phagocytic vacuole that encloses the particle. The molecular details of this process are incompletely understood but involve membrane remodeling and the regulated assembly and disassembly of the actin cytoskeleton, in a fashion analogous to the mechanisms that result in cell movement when chemotactic receptors are engaged. Fcγ receptor–mediated phagocytosis triggers the extension of long pseudopodia that attach in a zipper-like fashion around the particle, fusing to form the phagosome, which is then drawn into the cell.[248, 249] PI–3-kinase–dependent recruitment of endocytic vesicles to the nascent phagosome is important for pseudopod formation.[248] In contrast, complement-opsonized particles attach to the cell surface only at limited points and "sink" into the cytoplasm in the absence of any pseudopod extension.[249] These morphologic differences are associated with differences in the underlying biochemical pathways. Fc receptor–mediated phagocytosis is sensitive to inhibitors of tyrosine kinases and requires the Rac and Cdc42 GTPases, whereas CR3-mediated phagocytosis depends on protein kinase C and the Rho GTPase.[249]

Microorganisms can also enter phagocytes by nonopsonic routes that enable them to evade the cytocidal weapons that are otherwise activated upon phagocytosis. For example, after binding to the macrophage cell surface, *Salmonella typhimurium* induces extensive membrane ruffling that leads to internalization of the bacterium into a macropinosome or "spacious phagosome."[250] *Legionella pneumophila* attachment to macrophages induces the formation of a pseudopod that spirals around the bacterium to form a "coiling phagosome" that does not acidify or fuse with lysosomes.[250]

Cytocidal and Digestive Activity

The binding of ligands to phagocyte chemoattractant and opsonic receptors ultimately leads to the mobilization of phagocyte granules that contain cytotoxic and hydrolytic proteins and to the activation of enzymatic reactions that generate toxic oxygen metabolites. These complementary processes are designed to modify or destroy the inciting object and are often classified as oxygen-independent and oxygen-dependent pathways.

Neutrophil granules are secretory organelles that can be divided into four general classes, as discussed in an earlier section (see Table 21–2). Degranulation (also referred to as mobilization), the fusion of granule membranes with the plasma or phagosome membrane, results in the transfer of granule membrane constituents to a new membrane compartment and the discharge of the granule contents into the extracellular fluid or phagocytic vacuole. Microtubules and microfilaments are involved in granule translocation. Degranulation is triggered by increases in intracellular calcium concentration when neutrophils are activated through chemoattractant and other receptors. Marked differences are seen in the responsiveness of various granule classes to this signal. Thus, different granule classes are mobilized, depending on the calcium concentration, which, in turn, is in proportion to receptor occupancy.[27] Secretory vesicles, whose membranes are storage pools for β_2 integrin adhesion proteins and other receptors, are mobilized with relatively low concentrations of calcium. The degranulation of secretory vesicles provides rapid upregulating of the cell surface expression of these receptors. Gelatinase (tertiary) granules are also easily mobilized for exocytosis at the cell surface, and the release of gelatinase facilitates migration of neutrophils through the extracellular matrix.[218] In contrast, azurophil (primary) granules, which contain cytotoxic proteins and hydrolytic enzymes, are mobilized very slowly. Azurophil granules generally do not undergo exocytosis, fusing instead with phagocytic vacuoles to deliver their contents into a sequestered compartment.[251]

Certain microorganisms can become intracellular parasites because they have developed mechanisms to prevent granule fusion with the phagocytic vacuole or otherwise evade the phagocyte digestive and oxidative armamentarium. For example, although mycobacteria exist intracellularly within a phagosome, they produce compounds that inhibit their fusion of phagocyte granules.[252–254] *L. pneumophila* and *Toxoplasma* may inhibit acidification and lysosomal fusion.[250, 255, 256] Virulent strains of *Salmonella* engulfed by macrophages produce compounds that prevent translocation of the respiratory burst oxidase to the phagosomal membrane.[257] *Listeria monocytogenes* escapes from the phagocytic vacuole altogether to avoid attack by lysosomal products and can survive in the cytoplasm of relatively quiescent macrophages and hepatocytes.[258]

OXYGEN-INDEPENDENT TOXICITY

Phagocyte granules supply preformed cytotoxic and digestive compounds that play a key role in oxygen-independent killing and digestion of microbes, senescent cells, and particulate debris. Oxygen-independent pathways complement pathways that depend on the respiratory burst (see next section) and are also important for phagocyte antimicrobial activity under the adverse conditions of hypoxia and acidosis often encountered locally at the site of infection.

Numerous cationic antimicrobial proteins are contained within neutrophil azurophilic granules.[251, 259, 260]

Defensins are small (29 to 25 amino acid residues) basic peptides that constitute more than 5 percent of the total cellular protein of human neutrophils, although they are absent in murine neutrophils.[261] These peptides exhibit antimicrobial effects against a broad range of gram-positive and gram-negative organisms, fungi, mycobacteria, and some enveloped viruses. Defensins are also cytotoxic to mammalian cells. Defensins kill target cells by insertion into the cellular membrane and formation of voltage-regulated channels. Defensin-like peptides have also been found in small intestinal Paneth cells and in tracheal epithelium.[259] BPI is a 55-kD cationic protein that has potent cytotoxic effects toward gram-negative bacteria.[262] BPI binds avidly to lipopolysaccharide, leading to both bacterial killing by damaging the cell membrane and to the neutralization of endotoxin associated with the bacterial cell wall and in serum. Serpocidins are a family of 25- to 29-kD glycoproteins that are homologous to members of the serine protease superfamily and include azurocidin (CAP37) and three serine proteases (cathepsin G, elastase, and proteinase 3).[259] In human neutrophils, serpocidins are even more potent than the defensins in antimicrobial activity and have a broad spectrum of cytotoxicity, that is, with few exceptions, unrelated to proteolytic activity. Cathepsin G, elastase, and proteinase 3 are often referred to as neutral proteases because the pH optima for their proteolytic activity is approximately pH 7. The CAP37 protein has been shown to bind endotoxin, which appears to account for its activity for gram-negative bacteria.[263] CAP37 also is a potent chemoattractant for monocytes.[263] Exogenous administration of antimicrobial peptides is being studied as an alternative or adjunctive therapy to conventional antibiotics in a number of settings, including sepsis and topical use.[260]

Both azurophilic and specific granules contain lysozyme, which hydrolyzes the cell wall of saprophytic gram-positive organisms and may also assist in the nonlytic killing of other organisms.[251] Specific (secondary) granules contain the iron-binding glycoprotein lactoferrin, which has direct bacteriocidal activity both related and unrelated to the chelation of iron compounds required for bacterial metabolism.[264] Lactoferrin may also catalyze the nonenzymatic formation of hydroxyl radicals (OH•) during the respiratory burst (see next section). Vitamin B_{12} (cobalamin)–binding-protein has been proposed to bind the analogous family of compounds found in bacteria to exert an antimicrobial effect.[265]

Azurophilic granules contain a variety of hydrolases (see Table 21–2), which have a lower pH optimum (<6), consistent with the lysosomal character of these granules. Studies using indicator dyes and biochemical techniques suggest that after a transient rise, the pH of the phagocytic vacuole decreases to less than 6, which would enhance the activity of these enzymes upon their discharge into the vacuole.[266, 267] The acid hydrolases serve primarily a digestive function rather than a microbicidal function.[268] Azurophilic granules also contain myeloperoxidase, which is an important enzyme in microbicidal oxygen-dependent reactions that are described in the next section.

Inherited partial or complete deficiency of myeloperoxidase, which occurs in 0.05 percent of the population, can occasionally result in increased susceptibility to infection (see later). Deficiencies in other individual neutrophil granule proteins have not yet been described in humans, but gene-targeted mice lacking the neutrophil granule serine proteases elastase or cathepsin G have impaired host defense against gram-negative sepsis and fungal infections.[269, 270] Inherited mutations in neutrophil elastase have recently been identified in patients with cyclic neutropenia and severe congenital neutropenia.[271, 272] The mutant forms of elastase may have abnormal properties that exert a toxic effect on granulopoiesis. A few rare disorders involving defects in granule formation (specific granule deficiency) or degranulation (CHS) are associated with recurrent bacterial infections.

OXYGEN-DEPENDENT TOXICITY

The resting neutrophil relies primarily on glycolysis for energy and hence consumes relatively little oxygen.[273] However, within seconds after it contacts opsonized microbes or high concentrations of chemoattractants, its oxygen consumption increases dramatically, often by more than 100-fold. This "extra respiration of phagocytosis" was first observed in 1933,[274] but it was almost 30 years before this process was found to be insensitive to mitochondrial poisons and thus not related to increased energy demands.[275] The enzyme complex responsible for this phenomenon, referred to as the *NADPH or respiratory burst oxidase*, is associated with the plasma and phagolysosomal membranes and catalyzes the transfer of an electron from NADPH to molecular oxygen, thereby forming the superoxide radical (O_2^-) (Fig. 21–6).[276–278] Superoxide, although a relatively weak microbicidal agent, is the precursor to a family of potent oxidants that are essential for the killing of many microorganisms (Fig. 21–6).[276, 277, 279] The importance of the respiratory burst to normal host defense is underscored by the recurrent and often life-threatening infections seen in patients with chronic granulomatous disease (CGD), who have a genetic deficiency of respiratory burst oxidase activity.

The respiratory burst oxidase is a multisubunit enzyme complex assembled from membrane-bound and soluble proteins upon phagocyte activation (Fig. 21–7). The identification of the components of this enzyme has benefited greatly from the biochemical and molecular genetic analysis of patients with CGD. Four polypeptides, gp91^{phox}, p22^{phox}, p47^{phox}, and p67^{phox}, that are essential for respiratory burst function have been identified (Table 21–8), and mutations in the corresponding genes are responsible for the four different genetic subgroups of CGD. The oxidase subunits were given the designation *phox*, for *ph*agocyte *ox*idase. A fifth phox protein, p40^{phox}, exists in a complex with p47^{phox} and p67^{phox}, but its function in the NADPH oxidase remains to be determined.[280, 281]

An unusual *b*-type flavocytochrome, located in the plasma membranes and specific granules of resting neutrophils, mediates electron transfer in the oxidase complex. This flavocytochrome is a heterodimer that contains a 91-kD glycosylated protein, gp91^{phox}, and a nonglycosylated subunit, 22^{phox}.[282–285] The gene for gp91^{phox}, which is the site of mutations in the X-linked form of CGD, was one of the first to be identified by positional cloning.[285] The respiratory burst oxidase flavocytochrome has been referred to as flavocytochrome b_{558}, for its spectral peak of light absorbance at 558 nm or as flavocytochrome b_{-245} in reference to its midpoint potential of −245 mV, which is the lowest reported for any mammalian cytochrome.[286] gp91^{phox} is the redox center of the oxidase and contains two heme prosthetic groups embedded within the membrane in the hydrophobic amino terminus of the protein and a flavoprotein domain in the carboxy terminus with binding sites for flavin and NADPH binding.[278, 287–290] The p22^{phox} subunit is also an integral membrane protein and provides an important docking site for p47^{phox} during NADPH oxidase assembly.[291] Heterodimer formation with gp91^{phox} is essential for heme incorporation and intracellular stability of both flavocytochrome subunits.[290, 292]

The gp91^{phox} subunit is the first example of a new family of flavocytochromes with similar structural features. Proteins related to gp91^{phox} were subsequently identified in yeast[293] which act as a ferric iron reductase involved in transmembrane iron transport, and in plants,[294] which may be involved in generation of oxidative signals important for intracellular signaling and host defense.[295] Close mammalian homologs of gp91^{phox} have now recently been identified and are called the *NOX proteins* (for *N*ADPH *ox*idase).[296] One form is highly expressed in colon, and a

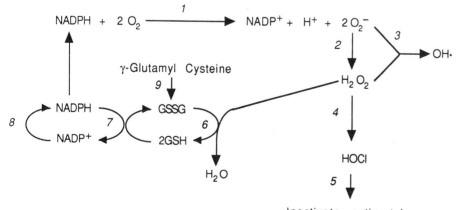

FIGURE 21–6. Reactions of the respiratory burst pathway. Reactions 1 to 9 are catalyzed as follows: (1) the respiratory burst oxidase (reduced nicotinamide adenine dinucleotide phosphate [NADPH] oxidase); (2) superoxide dismutase or spontaneous; (3) nonenzymatic, Fe^{2+}-catalyzed; (4) myeloperoxidase; (5) spontaneous; (6) glutathione peroxidase; (7) glutathione reductase; (8) glucose-6-phosphate dehydrogenase; and (9) glutathione synthetase. NADP = nicotinamide adenine dinucleotide phosphate; GSSG = oxidized glutathione; GSH = reduced glutathione; HOCl = hypochlorous acid; OH• = hydroxyl radical. (From Curnutte J, Orkin S, Dinauer M: Genetic disorders of phagocyte function. In Stamoyannopoulos G (ed): The Molecular Basis of Blood Diseases, 2nd ed. Philadelphia, WB Saunders, 1994, p 493.)

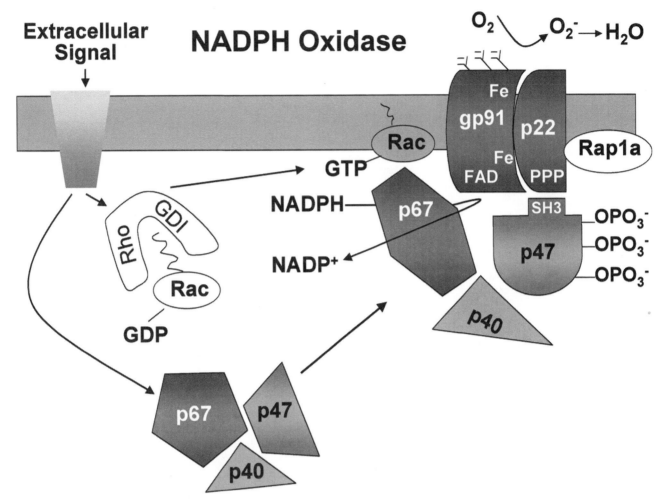

FIGURE 21–7. Model of NADPH oxidase activation. In unstimulated neutrophils, the subunits of the NADPH oxidase are separated in the cytoplasmic and membrane compartments. The plasma and specific granule membranes contain flavocytochrome *b* with its p22*phox* and glycosylated gp91*phox* subunits and the small guanosine triphosphatases (GTPase) Rap1a. The flavin and heme groups (Fe) that mediate the transfer of electrons from NADPH to molecular oxygen are localized in the gp91*phox* subunit. The cytosolic components p47*phox* and p67*phox* may exist as a preformed complex of 260 kDa, which also includes at least one additional protein, p40*phox*. The small GTPase Rac is also present in the cytosol in its inactive glucose diphosphate (GDP) bound state, in a complex with a GDP dissociation inhibitor (Rho-GDI). With neutrophil activation, the cytosolic phox subunits translocate to the membrane, which depends on phosphorylation of p47*phox* and exposure of an SH3 domain that binds to a proline-rich domain (PPP) in p22*phox*. Other binding sites between p47*phox* and gp91*phox* are also likely to be important. Neutrophil activation also triggers the conversion of Rac-GDP to Rac-GTP and dissociation from Rho-GDI. Rac-GTP is membrane-associated, interacting with p67*phox* and also probably flavocytochrome *b* in the oxidase complex. FAD = flavin adenine nucleotide. (From Dinauer MC, Lekstrom-Himes JA, Dale DC: Inherited neutrophil disorders: Molecular basis and new therapies. Hematology (Am Soc Hematol Educ Prog) 2000; 303–318.

second was identified in renal tubular epithelial cells. These gp91*phox* homologs have superoxide-generating activity (albeit at a much lower level compared with that of the phagocyte NADPH oxidase). Although their functions are currently unknown, it is proposed that superoxide anion–mediated intracellular signaling by these homologs may regulate gene expression, cell proliferation, and apoptosis in nonphagocytic cells.

On the basis of the redox properties of the flavocytochrome b_{558}, the following pathway has been proposed for transfer of electrons from NADPH to O_2 in the respiratory burst (reaction 1 in Fig. 21–6):

$$\text{NADPH} \xrightarrow[-330\text{ mV}]{} \text{flavin} \xrightarrow[-256\text{ mV}]{} \text{heme} \xrightarrow[-245\text{ mV}]{} O_2 \xrightarrow[-160\text{ mV}]{} O_2^-$$

The flavocytochrome spans membrane, so that NADPH is oxidized at the cytoplasmic surface and oxy-

gen is reduced to form O_2^- on the outer surface of the plasma membrane (or inner surface of the phagosomal membrane).[276]

The p47*phox* and p67*phox* subunits are believed to regulate NADPH binding and electron transfer in the flavocytochrome rather than being directly involved in these events. In resting neutrophils, p47*phox*, p67*phox*, and p40*phox*, are found in the cytosol as a complex that is stabilized by interactions between SH3 (Src homology domain 3) domains and proline-rich SH3 binding motifs within these proteins.[278] Phagocyte activation induces translocation of this complex to the membrane to form a catalytically active enzyme with the flavocytochrome, although p40*phox* is not necessary for enzyme function.[278, 289] Oxidase assembly requires the phosphorylation of p47*phox* at multiple serine residues and the binding of an SH3 domain in p47*phox* to a proline-rich target SH3–binding sequence in p22*phox*.[278, 289, 291] The p47*phox* and p40*phox*

TABLE 21–8. Properties of the Phagocyte Respiratory Burst Oxidase Components

	gp91^{phox}	p22^{phox}	p47^{phox}	p67^{phox}	p40^{phox}
Synonyms	β Chain	α Chain	NCF-1	NCF-2	NCF-4
	Heavy chain	Light chain	SOC II	SOC III	
Amino acids	570	195	390	526	339
Gene locus	*CYBB*	*CYBA*	*NCF1*	*NCF2*	*NCF4*
	Xp21.1	16q24	7q11.23	1q25	22q.13.1
Cellular location in resting neutrophil	Specific granule and secretory vesicle membranes; plasma membrane	Specific granule and secretory vesicle membranes; plasma membrane	Cytosol	Cytosol	Cytosol
Tissue specificity	Myeloid, B lymphocytes	mRNA in all cells tested; protein only in myeloid and B cells	Myeloid, B lymphocytes	Myeloid, B lymphocytes	Myeloid, other hematopoietic cells
Functional domains	Binding sites for heme and FAD and NADPH binding sites for cytosolic oxidase components	Proline-rich domain in carboxy terminus that binds p47^{phox}	9 potential serine phosphorylation sites; SH3 domains; proline-rich domains; PX domain	SH3 domains; proline-rich domains, TPR that bind Rac-GTP	SH3 domains; PX domain
Homologies	NOX protein family; ferredoxin-NADP$^+$ reductase; yeast ferric iron reductase	Polypeptide I of cytochrome *c* oxidase (weak homology)	—	—	NADP = nicotinamide adenine dinucleotide phosphate.

phox = *ph*agocyte *ox*idase component; NCF = neutrophil cytosol factor; SOC = soluble oxidase component; FAD = flavin adenine dinucleotide; NOX = *N*ADPH *ox*idase; NADP = nicotinamide adenine dinucleotide phosphate; SH3 = *src* homology domain 3; PX = *p*hox homology; TPR = tetratrico peptide repeats.

Modified from Curnutte JT: Molecular basis of the autosomal recessive forms of chronic granulomatous disease. Immunodef Rev 1992; 3:149.

subunits also contain a PX (for phox homology) domain for binding phosphorylated lipids that are generated during neutrophil activation.[297–299] The p47^{phox} subunit is necessary for translocation of p67^{phox} to the membrane of activated neutrophils on the basis of studies of p47^{phox}-deficient CGD neutrophils.[278, 300] However, substantial amounts of superoxide can be generated from neutrophil membranes *in vitro* in the absence of p47^{phox}, provided that high concentrations of p67^{phox} and Rac GTP are supplied.[278] Hence, p47^{phox} may function as an "adaptor" protein to mediate translocation of p67^{phox} and to position it correctly in the active NADPH oxidase complex. In addition to p47^{phox} and p67^{phox}, the active NADPH oxidase requires the Rho GTPase, Rac.[278, 289] Four α-helical tetratricopeptide repeat motifs in p67^{phox} create a binding site for Rac GTP.[301] The GTP-bound form of Rac also appears to interact with flavocytochrome *b* in the enzymatically active oxidase complex.[278, 302]

Oxidase assembly is triggered by receptor-mediated binding of many soluble chemoattractants (see Table 21–6), which requires higher concentrations of these molecules compared with the initiation of chemotaxis. The binding of opsonized microbes to Fcγ and complement receptors is another major physiologic trigger of the respiratory burst that is activated at sites of microbial contact.[303, 304] The specific pathways in the signal transduction cascade leading to oxidase assembly are still incompletely defined, but current evidence suggests that

two important regulatory events are the phosphorylation of p47^{phox} and the activation of Rac to its GTP-bound state.[278] The functional oxidase complex is assembled at the plasma membrane and is also incorporated into phagosomes during ingestion. Because release of O_2^- occurs largely at the extracellular side of the membrane, oxidants are released at sites of microbial contact or within the phagocytic vacuole, where they can interact with granule contents to potentiate their microbicidal effects. The degranulation and membrane fusion of specific granules, which contain the majority of flavocytochrome *b* in neutrophils,[27] may be important to maintain a sustained respiratory burst.

Once formed, the O_2^- radical is first converted, either spontaneously or by means of superoxide dismutase, into H_2O_2 (reaction 2 in Fig. 21–6). Myeloperoxidase (MPO), in the presence of halides, catalyzes the conversion of H_2O_2 to hypochlorous acid (HOCl), the active agent in household bleach (reaction 4 in Fig. 21–6). Hydrogen peroxide may also be converted into OH• in a nonenzymatic reaction with O_2^- catalyzed by either iron or copper ions (reaction 3 in Fig. 21–6). Hydrogen peroxide, HOCl, and OH• are all strong oxidants that participate in microbial killing within the phagocytic vacuole.[305] Reactive oxidants also regulate phagocyte proteolytic activity by activating latent phagocyte metalloproteinases (such as collagenase and gelatinase) and inactivating plasma antiproteinases.[218] Enhanced phagocyte proteolysis at localized sites may be important for facilitating cellular migration into inflamed tissues, destruction of microbes, and removal of cellular debris.

Other enzymatic pathways related to oxidant generation include the detoxification of H_2O_2 by glutathione peroxidase and reductase (reactions 6 and 7 in Fig. 21–6).[305] Glutathione is produced from γ-glutamyl cysteine by the enzyme glutathione synthetase (reaction 9 in Fig. 21–6). Other important antioxidant systems in phagocytes and other tissues include catalase, which catalyzes the conversion of H_2O_2 into oxygen and water; ascorbic acid; and α-tocopherol (vitamin E).[306] The generation of NADPH is important in providing a source of reducing equivalents for the glutathione detoxification pathway as well as the respiratory burst itself. NADPH is replenished from nicotinamide adenine dinucleotide phosphate ($NADP^+$) by leukocyte glucose-6-phosphate dehydrogenase (G6PD) (reaction 8 in Fig. 21–6) in the hexose monophosphate shunt.

A second oxygen-dependent pathway with antimicrobial effects, at least in the mouse, is the generation of nitric oxide (NO) from the oxidation of L-arginine to L-citrulline. This reaction is catalyzed by nitric oxide synthase (NOS), with molecular oxygen supplying the oxygen in NO.[155, 307, 308] There are three different nitric oxide synthases, two of which are constitutively expressed in a variety of tissues, including endothelium, brain, and neutrophils. Expression of a third NOS (iNOS) is inducible by inflammatory stimuli in a variety of cells, including macrophages and neutrophils, where it has a wide spectrum of antitumor and antimicrobial activity against bacteria, parasites, helminths, and viruses.[155, 307, 309] Mice with genetic absence of iNOS, generated by targeted disruption of the iNOS gene in murine embryonic stem cells, have increased susceptibility to infection with *L. monocytogenes*.[310] High levels of iNOS-catalyzed NO production are readily elicited in normal mouse macrophages by exposure, for example, to INF-γ and endotoxin. However, there has been some difficulty in documenting a similar phenomenon in human macrophages or neutrophils, casting doubt on a role for the inducible production of NO in human host defense. The expression of functional iNOS in human macrophages has been shown to be elicited with either the cross-linking of CD69, a member of the NK cell family of signal transducing receptors,[311] or with HIV-infected macrophages.[312] Cytokine-activated human neutrophils also exhibit inducible production of NO, which leads to nitration of ingested bacteria.[313]

Although the precise role of NO in host defense in humans remains to be fully defined, it is clear that in the mouse, NO cannot substitute for oxidants derived from the respiratory burst pathway. Gene targeting has been used to develop mouse models for both X-linked (gp91*phox* –/–) and an autosomal recessive (p47*phox* –/–) form of CGD.[314, 315] Affected mice exhibit delayed clearance of *Staphylococcus aureus* associated with abscess formation and have a marked increase in susceptibility to the opportunistic pathogens *Burkholderia (Pseudomonas) cepacia* and *Aspergillus fumigatus*.[315–318] These organisms are common causes of infections in patients with CGD, as discussed in a later section.

Specialized Functions of Mononuclear Phagocytes

Mononuclear phagocytes, particularly tissue macrophages, participate in a broad range of activities important for tissue homeostasis and repair as well as in the host defense against viruses, bacteria, fungi, and protozoa (Table 21–9).[116, 127, 319–323] From the standpoint of antimicrobial function, activated macrophages play a key role in the ingestion and killing of intracellular parasites, such as mycobacteria, *Listeria*, *Leishmania*, *Toxoplasma*, and some fungi.[324] Both oxygen-independent and oxygen-dependent systems are involved in this process, as described earlier. Activated macrophages also exhibit cytotoxicity against tumor cells, although the importance of this process *in vivo* remains to be determined. Tumor cell killing can be mediated by an antibody-dependent process (ADCC), which requires reactive oxygen intermediates for cytocidal effects.[113] Alternatively, macrophage tumoricidal activity can be mediated by an antibody-independent process, which involves the participation of TNF-α and a neutral serine protease secreted only by fully activated macrophages.[113]

Interactions of macrophages with T and B cells are essential for the development of cellular and humoral immunity.[123] Macrophages are involved in the processing of exogenous antigens, which are taken up by endocytosis and degraded by proteases in the endosomal or lysosomal compartments into small peptides.[123, 325] Some of these peptides bind to MHC II molecules and are transported to the plasma membrane for presentation to T lymphocytes, which stimulates inflammatory and antibody responses. Macrophages also produce IL-1, which supports B-cell proliferation and stimulates the production of IL-2 and other lymphokines by T cells.[143] Subsequent interactions between T and B cells result in the production of specific immunoglobulins.[123, 325]

Macrophages participate in many aspects of wound repair.[326–329] The early phases of this process are

TABLE 21–9. Functions of Mononuclear Phagocytes

TISSUE HOMEOSTASIS AND REPAIR

Wound repair
    Débridment and phagocytosis
    Secretion of growth factors for endothelial cells and
       fibroblasts
Hematopoiesis
    Secretion of growth factors
Participation in iron and lipid metabolism
Scavenger function
    Phagocytosis of debris
    Removal of senescent cells
    Detoxification

IMMUNE REGULATION

Antigen processing and presentation
Secretion of cytokines

INFLAMMATORY RESPONSE AND PATHOGEN CONTROL

Secretion of cytokines, ecosanoids, proteases, coagulation
    factors, and other products
Antimicrobial activity
Antiviral activity
Antitumor activity

dominated by an influx of neutrophils, followed by the migration of monocytes which differentiate into activated macrophages, and finally, the appearance of T lymphocytes. Proliferating fibroblasts secrete collage and other matrix proteins important for wound closure and tissue remodeling, and migrating keratinocytes regenerate the epithelial surface. Both neutrophils and macrophages protect against infection and dispose of phagocytosed debris. Mononuclear phagocytes also elaborate fibroblast, epithelial, and angiogenic growth factors (see Table 21–5), which stimulate the normal progression of tissue repair and neovascularization that characterize the later phases of wound healing.[110, 326, 330]

Resident tissue macrophages, including those lining the sinusoids of the spleen, ingest aged erythrocytes and other senescent cells. Mechanisms involved in the recognition of such cells are not fully defined. In the process of breaking down hemoglobin, iron is removed and incorporated into ferritin and hemosiderin, where it accounts for about two thirds of the body's store of reserve iron. Iron in this macrophage storage pool is constantly turning over and returned in a transferrin-bound form to the bone marrow for new red blood cell synthesis.[331, 332]

Monocytes and macrophages take up native VLDL as well as denatured (oxidized or otherwise modified) LDL by receptor-mediated endocytosis.[122, 333] The LDL enters the lysosomal compartments and free cholesterol is liberated and esterified in the cytoplasm. The scavenger receptor for denatured LDL is not subject to downregulation during uptake of high amounts of cholesterol, and cells exposed to sufficient quantities can acquire the appearance of foam cells, possibly contributing to atherogenesis.[122, 334, 335]

Specialized Functions of Eosinophils and Basophils

Although eosinophils and basophils share many of the functional characteristics of neutrophils and mononuclear phagocytes, they participate in distinctive aspects of the inflammatory response, and interact with each other in the context of certain allergic reactions. Eosinophils and mast cells are often situated beneath epithelial surfaces exposed to environmental antigens, such as the respiratory and gastrointestinal tracts, in which they may be actively involved in mucosal immune responses. However, the role of eosinophils, basophils, and mast cells are better known in pathologic settings than in normal homeostasis.

Eosinophils appear to have both immunoenhancing and immunosuppressive functions (Table 21–10).[69, 72, 336, 337] Although capable of ingesting and killing bacteria, eosinophils are not particularly efficient at this task. Rather, they possess an unusual ability to destroy invasive metazoan parasites, especially helminthic parasites. Eosinophils bind to the surface of both adult and larval helminths and inflict damage through release of cationic granule proteins and by the generation of reactive oxidants, including the eosinophil peroxidase-catalyzed formation of hypohalous acids via the action of the respiratory burst and eosinophil peroxidase (see Table 21–4).[72, 83, 338, 339]

Eosinophil production of the lipid inflammatory mediators, LTC4 and PAF, plays a role in the pathogenesis of allergic diseases.[71, 340] PAF and LTC_4 can induce smooth muscle contraction and promote the secretion of mucus, and PAF itself is a potent activator of eosinophils. The release of eosinophil granule contents may also contribute to localized tissue damage. Purified eosinophil major basic protein, for example, can cause cytopathic changes in tracheal epithelium *in vitro* that are similar to the changes observed in asthmatic patients.[341]

Eosinophils may also perform an immunosuppressive function in immediate hypersensitivity reactions (Table 21–10).[70, 71] IgE-activated basophils or mast cells release eosinophilic chemotactic factor of anaphylaxis, which recruit eosinophils to the site. Subsequent eosinophil degranulation releases products that can inactivate inflammatory mediators. For example, histaminase inactivates histamine, phospholipase B inactivates PAF, major basic protein inactivates mast cell heparin, and lysophospholipase prevents the generation of arachidonic acid metabolites.[72]

Basophils and mast cells are central participants in a variety of inflammatory and immunologic disorders, particularly immediate hypersensitivity diseases, and may also play a role in host defense against bacterial infections. Basophils and mast cells express plasma membrane receptors that specifically bind with high affinity the Fc portion of the IgE antibody (Fcε receptors).[239] After active or passive sensitization with IgE, exposure to specific multivalent antigen triggers an almost immediate release of granule contents (anaphylactic degranulation)

TABLE 21–10. Eosinophil Function

Function	Mechanism
Defense against helminths (both larval and adult forms)	1. Binding of eosinophils to surface 2. Peroxidation of larval surface mediated by eosinophil peroxidase 3. Toxicity to larval surface by released major basic protein
Immunosuppression of immediate hypersensitivity reactions	1. Engulfment of most cell granules 2. Release of prostaglandin E_1/E_2 to suppress basophil degranulation 3. Release of histaminase 4. Oxidation of slow-reacting substance of anaphylaxis 5. Release of phospholipase D to inactive mast cell platelet-activating factor 6. Release of major basic protein that binds mast cell heparin 7. Release of plasminogen to reduce local thrombus formation

and the synthesis and release of newly generated chemical mediators such as LTC_4, which stimulates smooth muscle contraction, mucus secretion, and vasoactive changes.[342] Degranulation can also be triggered in response to insect venoms, radiocontrast dye, and other nonspecific agents. Studies on mutant mice engineered by gene targeting to lack Fcγ or Fcε receptors have shown that mast cell FcγRIII receptors are essential in activating the inflammatory response to IgG immune complexes (Arthus reaction), heretofore an unrecognized role for the mast cell.[343] Mast cells can secrete numerous mitogenic or inflammatory cytokines, including many interleukins (1, 3, 4, 5, and 6), chemokines, GM-CSF, and TNF-α, which are also likely to regulate leukocyte recruitment and inflammation in IgE-dependent reactions and immune complex injury.[99, 344, 345] Inflammatory cytokines and leukotrienes released from tissue mast cells have been recognized to play an important role in neutrophil recruitment during the acute response to bacterial infection.[346–348]

Pathologic Consequences of Phagocyte Activation and Inflammatory Response

Although normally serving a protective function, the inflammatory response can also result in damage to host tissues. The release of proteases, oxygen radicals, and pro-inflammatory cytokines by activated phagocytes appears to play a major role in the generation of tissue injury in a wide variety of pathologic inflammatory processes (Table 21–11).[218, 349–353] For example, neutrophil elastase has been implicated in the pathogenesis of emphysema in both adult smokers and individuals with α_1-antitrypsin deficiency. Neutrophil granule proteases may contribute to joint destruction in rheumatoid arthritis and other chronic arthropathies.[354] Neutrophils are also believed to play a key role in the *systemic inflammatory response syndrome*, a term that was created to encompass the host response to both infectious (e.g., gram-negative sepsis) and noninfectious (e.g., pancreatitis or trauma) agents and can lead to organ dysfunction and tissue damage.[351] Sequestration of activated neutrophils in the pulmonary capillary bed and subsequent release of tissue-damaging agents is an important component in the development of adult respiratory distress syndrome.[235] Activation of the complement cascade by artificial membrane surfaces dur-

ing hemodialysis and cardiopulmonary bypass also can result in neutrophil activation, intrapulmonary sequestration, and lung injury. In addition to their cytotoxic effects, oxidative products released by activated phagocytes are also mutagenic, as documented by plasmid mutagenesis, sister chromatid exchange, and transformation of cells in culture.[353, 355] Hence, the increased risk of malignancy observed with certain chronic inflammatory states, such as ulcerative colitis or chronic hepatitis, has been postulated to be in part related to oxidant-induced carcinogenesis.

The development of anti-inflammatory interventions on the basis of agents that block leukocyte adhesion or inhibit the action of specific phagocyte products has been an area of intense interest. Protective effects of monoclonal antibodies directed against either β_2 integrins, ICAM-1, or selectins have been demonstrated in various animal models of inflammation, including ischemia-reperfusion injury, endotoxic shock, and acute arthritis.[184, 204] Furthermore, in a phase 1 trial in which anti–ICAM-1 monoclonal antibodies were given to renal allograft recipients improved function of cadaveric renal allografts and a reduced incidence of graft rejection were seen.[356] This approach may be less useful in other clinical settings in which the leukocyte-endothelial cell inflammatory cascade has already been activated. The contributions of nonphagocytic cells to inflammatory tissue injury must also be kept in mind. For example, the adult respiratory distress syndrome can occur in the presence of severe neutropenia.[357] Finally, despite the adverse consequences of the acute inflammatory process, these events are also important for normal healing. For example, the use of anti-inflammatory agents in myocardial infarction, which can decrease infarct size acutely, results in impaired healing of the myocardium and the formation of fragile scar tissue.[349, 358, 359]

QUANTITATIVE GRANULOCYTE DISORDERS

Overview

Abnormally high or low numbers of circulating granulocytes or monocytes are often seen in pediatric patients. In this section, the clinical disorders associated with disturbances in granulocyte numbers will be reviewed. Particular emphasis will be placed on those syndromes in which the granulocyte abnormality is a central feature. The clinical conditions discussed later, in general, are incompletely understood at the molecular level, and much of what is known about their pathophysiologic course is descriptive. This section of the chapter therefore will be organized along those lines.

Neutropenia

DEFINITION AND CLASSIFICATION

Neutropenia is defined as an absolute decrease in the number of circulating neutrophils in the blood. Normal neutrophil levels should be stratified for age, race, and other factors. For whites, the lower limit for normal neutrophil counts (neutrophils and band cells) is 1000 cells/μL in infants between 2 weeks and 1 year of age.

TABLE 21–11. Selected Pathologic Inflammatory Reactions Associated with Phagocyte-Induced Tissue Injury*

Arthus reaction
Systemic inflammatory response syndrome
Nephrotoxic and immune complex nephritis
Postischemic myocardial damage
Adult respiratory distress syndrome
Atherosclerosis
Bronchiectasis
Acute and chronic allograft rejection
Malignant transformation with chronic inflammation
Rheumatoid arthritis

*See text for references.

After infancy, the corresponding value is 1500 cells/μL. Blacks have somewhat lower neutrophil counts, and the lower limits of normal can tentatively be considered to be from 200 to 600 cells/μL less relative to counts in whites.[360–362] The basis for this observation is probably a relative decrease of neutrophils in the bone marrow storage compartment. Note that falsely low white blood cell counts can result when counts are done long after blood is drawn or after excessive leukocyte clumping in the presence of certain paraproteins.

Neutropenia can be due to disturbances in production, a shift of neutrophils from the circulating to marginated or tissue pools, increased peripheral utilization or destruction, or a combination of these causes. From the clinical standpoint, assays of leukokinetics and myelopoiesis are not routinely available. Classifications based on biochemical or functional studies are also difficult because of the paucity of neutrophils in the circulation of neutropenic patients. Therefore, the neutropenic syndromes discussed in this section are grouped according to whether the underlying cause of neutropenia is an intrinsic defect in the myeloid progenitors or whether neutropenia is acquired as a result of extrinsic factors, such as drugs, infections, or autoantibodies (Table 21–12).

Individual patients may be characterized as having mild neutropenia with neutrophil counts of 1000 to 1500 cells/μL, moderate neutropenia with counts of 500 to 1000 cells/μL, and severe neutropenia with counts of generally fewer than 500 cells/μL. This stratification is useful for predicting the risk of pyogenic infections, because only patients with severe neutropenia have increased susceptibility to life-threatening infections, particularly if the neutropenia persists for more than a few days. The diagnosis of chronic neutropenia is usually reserved for patients with neutropenia persisting for more than 6 months. Children with severe chronic neutropenia can be registered with the Severe Chronic Neutropenia International Registry.[363]

SYMPTOMS OF NEUTROPENIA

The hallmark of neutropenia is increased susceptibility to bacterial infection. The most types of pyogenic infections seen most often in patients with significant neutropenia are cutaneous cellulitis, superficial or deep cutaneous abscesses, furunculosis, pneumonia, and septicemia.[364–367] Stomatitis, gingivitis, and periodontitis are often chronic problems. Perirectal inflammation and otitis media (especially in children) occur as well. However, neutropenia in and of itself does not heighten susceptibility of patients to viral, fungal, and parasitic infections or to bacterial meningitis. Endogenous bacteria are the most common cause of infections, but colonization with a variety of organisms of nosocomial origin also occurs. The most commonly isolated organisms from neutropenic patients are *S. aureus* and gram-negative bacteria. The usual symptoms and signs of local infection—such as exudates, fluctuation, ulceration, and regional adenopathy—are much less evident in neutropenic patients than they are in non-neutropenic individuals.[368]

Susceptibility to bacterial infection, even in patients with severe neutropenia, can be quite variable, depending on the underlying etiology. For example, some patients with chronic neutropenia due to autoantibodies do not experience serious infections over a period of many years even with neutrophil counts as low as 200 cells/μL (or even lower), probably because these individuals have normocellular bone marrow. Many patients with chronic neutropenia also have normal to increased numbers of circulating monocytes.[364] However, the recruitment of monocytes to inflammatory sites is delayed relative to that of neutrophils, and monocytes are not as efficient as neutrophils in ingesting bacteria.[369, 370] Thus, monocytes appear to provide only marginal protection against pyogenic organisms in patients with severe neutropenia. It is likely that the humoral, cell-mediated, and tissue macrophage immune systems also play critical roles preventing infection in these individuals.

TABLE 21–12. Classification of Neutropenia

NEUTROPENIA CAUSED BY INTRINSIC DEFECTS IN GRANULOCYTES OR THEIR PROGENITORS

Reticular dysgenesis
Cyclic neutropenia
Severe congenital neutropenia (Kostmann disease)
Myelokathexis and WHIM syndrome
Shwachman-Diamond syndrome
Chédiak-Higashi syndrome
Familial benign neutropenia
Bone marrow failure syndromes (congenital and acquired)

NEUTROPENIA CAUSED BY EXTRINSIC FACTORS

Infection
Drug-induced neutropenia
Autoimmune neutropenia
Chronic benign neutropenia of childhood (autoimmune neutropenia of childhood)
Immune neonatal neutropenia
Neutropenia associated with immune dysfunction
Neutropenia associated with metabolic diseases
Nutritional deficiencies
Reticuloendothelial sequestration
Bone marrow infiltration
Chronic idiopathic neutropenia

NEUTROPENIA CAUSED BY INTRINSIC DEFECTS IN GRANULOCYTES OR THEIR PROGENITORS

Reticular Dysgenesis

The selective failure of stem cells committed to myeloid and lymphoid development leads to reticular dysgenesis.[371–376] Affected infants have severe neutropenia and moderate to severe lymphopenia associated with the absence of lymph nodes, tonsils, and Peyer patches and splenic follicles. Erythroid and megakaryocyte development is normal. Bilateral sensorineural deafness has also been associated with reticular dysgenesis.[377] Because of the combined effects of neutropenia, agammaglobulinemia, and lymphopenia, such infants are highly vulnerable to fatal bacterial or viral infections. Reticular dysgenesis may be an inherited disorder, and it was reported in both males (some who were siblings) and females. Bone marrow transplantation was used successfully to treat this disorder in at least two patients.[376, 378–380]

Cyclic Neutropenia

Cyclic neutropenia is a sporadic or autosomal dominant disorder characterized by regular periodic oscillations, approximately every 21 days, in the number of peripheral blood neutrophils, with a nadir of less than 200 cells/μL (Fig. 21–8).[381, 382] In most typical patients, reticulocytes, platelets, and other leukocytes also cycle. The rate of occurrence of cyclic neutropenia was estimated to be 0.5 to 1 per 1 million population.[363] In 1910, Leale[383] described recurrent furunculosis in an infant who showed a cyclical variation in peripheral blood counts; this is probably the first recorded report of human cyclic neutropenia. During the neutropenic period, the majority of patients suffer from malaise, fever, oral ulcers, gingivitis, and periodontitis, and pharyngitis associated with lymph node enlargement. Symptoms typically begin during the first year of life. More serious complications can occasionally occur, including mastoiditis, pneumonia, or recurrent ulcerations of vaginal or rectal mucosa. The severity of the infections tends to parallel the severity of the neutropenia, but some patients do not experience infections at all during the neutropenic period. In many patients symptoms lessen as they grow older. In these individuals, the cycles tend to become less noticeable as the hematologic picture begins to resemble that of chronic neutropenia. Although cyclic neutropenia is usually viewed as a benign condition, 10 percent of patients in historical reviews have died of infectious complications.[381, 384] Pneumonia and sepsis from peritonitis (*Clostridium perfringens* is a notable pathogen) have been the most common causes of death.[381, 382]

Oscillations in the rate of bone marrow production of neutrophils result in neutropenia with nadirs at intervals of 21 ± 3 days in the majority of patients, although the cycles can be as long as 28 to 36 days and as short as 14 days.[384] Neutrophil counts typically fall to 0 at some time during the nadir and remain at less than 200 cells/μL for at least 3 to 5 days. In some patients, monocytosis and eosinophilia occur when neutrophil counts are lowest. In the recovery phase, the neutrophil counts often remain at less than 1900 cells/μL, and cycles in which neutrophil counts do not increase to greater than 1000 cells/μL are seen in many patients. Oscillations are subtle in some individuals, who instead have a chronic neutropenia, a pattern that is also often seen in older patients. Oscillations in reticulocyte and platelet counts, when seen, parallel those seen for neutrophils, but range between normal and elevated counts.[381, 385] Marrow aspirates obtained during periods of neutropenia have shown either hypoplasia or an arrest at the myelocyte stage.

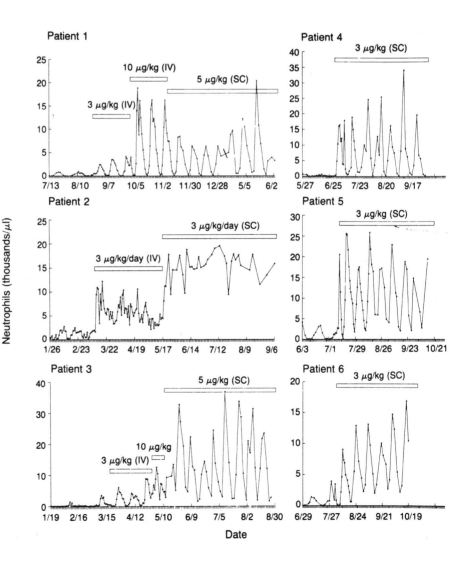

FIGURE 21–8. Cyclic neutropenia and the response to clinical administration of granulocyte colony-stimulating factor (G-CSF) in six patients. The cycling of neutrophil counts before and during therapy with various doses of G-CSF is shown. The *rectangles* represent the duration of G-CSF treatment, with the corresponding dose shown above each rectangle. Note the approximately 21-day cycle before therapy in patients 1, 5, and 6 that is characteristic of cyclic neutropenia. The cycle shortened to approximately 14 days during G-CSF therapy, whereas the peak neutrophil counts increased approximately 10-fold. IV = intravenous; SC = subcutaneous. (From Hammond WP IV, Price TH, et al: Treatment of cyclic neutropenia with granulocyte colony-stimulating factor. N Engl J Med 1989; 320:1307.)

A variety of studies suggest that cyclic neutropenia occurs because of a periodic disruption in cell production in the bone marrow.[382, 386] In collie dogs with autosomal recessive cyclic neutropenia, transplantation of marrow from normal dogs to affected animals abolished the blood count fluctuations, whereas in the converse experiment cyclic neutropenia was seen in previously normal animals.[382, 387] In both dogs and humans, oscillations of hematopoietic activity involving all hematopoietic lineages are seen. In humans, cyclic neutropenia was transferred by allogeneic bone marrow transplantation from a sibling with the disorder to another sibling undergoing treatment for leukemia.[387]

Patients with both sporadic and autosomal dominant forms of cyclic neutropenia have recently been shown to have coding sequence mutations of neutrophil elastase (ELA-2), a serine protease synthesized during the promyelocyte/myelocyte stage.[271, 272] This abnormality was discovered by linkage analysis of families with the autosomal dominant form.[272] How mutations in neutrophil elastase result in the cyclical production of neutrophils and other blood cells is currently not well understood. However, increased apoptosis of neutrophil precursors was documented in bone marrow samples from patients with cyclic neutropenia.[388] This may result from activation of the apoptotic process by mutant forms of ELA-2.

Cyclic neutropenia must be distinguished from cyclic fevers without neutropenia[389] and from other causes of neutropenia. To establish the diagnosis of cyclic neutropenia, neutrophil counts must be monitored at least two, and preferably three, times a week for 6 to 8 weeks.

The management of patients with cyclic neutropenia includes careful attention to the identification and treatment of infections acquired when these patents are neutropenic. In general, fevers, upper respiratory symptoms, and cervical lymphadenopathy occurring during neutropenic episodes require no specific therapy. However, the physician must remain alert to symptoms suggesting a specific infection or an acute abdomen. Careful attention to oral and dental hygiene is important to minimize periodontal disease and ameliorate the discomfort of mouth sores. To prevent the development of severe dental complications and because of the risk of life-threatening infections, prophylactic G-CSF therapy is now recommended for all patients with cyclic neutropenia. G-CSF therapy has been very effective in improving peripheral blood neutrophil counts in this disorder (see Fig. 21–7), along with the signs and symptoms associated with neutropenic nadirs.[363, 390] Some patients still experience neutropenic cycles but with decreased periodicity and increased neutrophil counts at the nadir. The dose of G-CSF required to maintain peripheral neutrophil counts in the normal range in most patients with cyclic neutropenia is usually 2 to 3 μg/kg/day, administered either daily or on alternate days.[390, 391] The occurrence of myelodysplastic syndrome (MDS) or leukemia has not been reported in patients with cyclic neutropenia, including those treated with G-CSF.[363, 390, 391]

Severe Congenital Neutropenia

Severe congenital neutropenia (SCN) was first described by Kostmann in 1956[392] as an autosomal recessive disorder associated with severe neutropenia that was identified in the population of an isolated northern parish in Sweden. Affected patients usually died of pyogenic infection during infancy and childhood. Other congenital neotropenias have since been identified that appear to be related to Kostmann disease, with either autosomal recessive or autosomal dominant, or in some instances, sporadic patterns of inheritance.[393–396] The incidence is estimated to be approximately 2 per 1 million population.[363] In affected patients an absolute neutrophil count (ANC) of fewer than 200 cells/μL is maintained chronically. This low ANC was documented on the first day of life in several patients.[392] Despite an accompanying monocytosis and moderate eosinophilia, these patients regularly have episodes of fever, skin infections (including omphalitis), stomatitis, pneumonia, and perirectal abscesses that typically appear during the first months of life. Infections often disseminate to the blood, meninges, and peritoneum, and are usually caused by *S. aureus*, *Escherichia coli*, and *Pseudomonas* species. Patients with SCN also have a significant risk for development of MDS and acute myelogenous leukemia (AML).[363, 397, 398]

Bone marrow examination in SCN typically shows normal neutrophil development up to the promyelocyte or myelocyte stage with a marked depletion of mature neutrophils.[392] Ultrastructural abnormalities in granules of neutrophilic cells have been observed in some patients.[393] The numbers of monocytes, eosinophils, macrophages, and reactive plasma cells are typically increased. Culture of bone marrow cells *in vitro* has generally demonstrated normal numbers of colony-forming granulocyte-monocyte progenitor cells that are capable of generating neutrophils in the presence of exogenous G-CSF.[393, 399–401] G-CSF[402, 403] and GM-CSF[404] production in patients with SCN appears to be normal, if not elevated.

The underlying etiology of SCN appears to be heterogeneous, but a recent study identified mutations in the neutrophil elastase gene *(ELA-2)* in 22 of 25 patients.[271] This series included five families with many affected members, whose inheritance was autosomal dominant. The same mutation was found in all of the affected members of each of these families, suggesting a germline rather than somatic mutation. These studies were originally prompted by linkage analysis in families with autosomal dominant cyclic neutropenia, which mapped this cyclic neutropenia to chromosome 19p13.3, and the subsequent identification of mutations in *ELA-2* in all patients with both autosomal dominant and sporadic cyclic neutropenia.[271, 272] The mutations in the *ELA-2* gene in SCN are more diverse than those identified in cyclic neutropenia, and some patients with SCN do not have *ELA-2* mutations. Similar to that seen in cyclic neutropenia, the bone marrow of patients with SCN shows evidence of accelerated apoptosis of neutrophil precursors.[396] How this finding relates to *ELA-2* mutations and the pathophysiologic basis of SCN or cyclic neutropenia remains to be established. It has been speculated that mutations in *ELA-2* may result in premature death of neutrophil precursors, leading to either cyclic myelopoiesis, when the rate of apoptosis is moderate or chronic, severe reductions of counts, as is seen in SCN.[396, 405]

Mutations in the G-CSF receptor itself are a rare cause of SCN. The G-CSF receptor is normal in almost all patients with SCN, including three Swedish patients with known familial disease.[386, 394, 406] As discussed in more detail later, therapy with G-CSF elicits an increase in neutrophil counts in almost all patients with SCN, suggesting that the defect in neutrophil production can be overcome by pharmacologic doses of this growth factor. In one of the rare patients with SCN who did not show a response to even very large doses of G-CSF, a point mutation in the extracellular domain of the G-CSF receptor was identified in both marrow and fibroblast cells, consistent with a germline event.[407] The patient was heterozygous for this mutation, which suggests that it has a dominant negative effect on the normal G-CSF receptor. The mutant G-CSF receptor was defective in both proliferation and survival signaling when expressed in myeloid cell lines. This study suggests that other patients with SCN who show hyporesponsiveness to G-CSF may have similar mutations in the G-CSF receptor.

A subset of patients with SCN are heterozygotes for acquired somatic mutations in the G-CSF receptor, which have been associated with the development of MDS/AML.[363] These mutations are present in myeloid cells only and are nonsense mutations that lead to truncation of the C-terminal cytoplasmic tail that is involved in intracellular receptor signaling.[363, 394, 406, 408] Additional studies in cell lines have suggested that the truncated G-CSF receptor interferes in a dominant negative manner with the function of wild-type G-CSF receptor to inhibit G-CSF induction of neutrophil maturation.[394, 406] It is not known if these mutations actually promote the evolution of SCN to MDS or AML.

G-CSF is now used as a standard treatment modality for SCN and has greatly improved both life span and quality of life.[363, 391, 401, 409] Before this cytokine was available in the 1980s, SCN would inevitably lead to fatal infections in the majority of patients, despite supportive care using prophylactic administration of trimethoprim-sulfamethoxazole, aggressive use of antibiotics at the time of documented infections, and scrupulous attention to oral hygiene. More than 95 percent of patients with SCN show a response to G-CSF treatment with an increase in ANC to greater than 1000 cells/μL and documented reduction in numbers of infections.[363, 391, 401, 409] There is often a delay of 7 to 10 days when treatment is first started before the peripheral blood neutrophil count increases. The median dose required for a complete response in patients with SCN who were enrolled in phase I/II/III studies of G-CSF use was 11.5 μg/kg/day.[363] The percentage of maturing neutrophils in the marrow increases with the administration of G-CSF, although morphologically abnormal promyelocytes with vacuolized and asynchronous nuclear-cytoplasmic maturation can still be present, and the number of eosinophils in marrow and peripheral blood may continue to be relatively high.[363] On the basis of data from the Severe Chronic Neutropenia Registry, a starting daily dose of G-CSF of 3 of 5 μg/kg/day is recommended. The dose should be increased gradually up to 100 μg/kg/day, generally in increments of

5-10 μg/kg/day, with at least 14 days at each dose level to achieve a neutrophil count of 1000 to 2000/μL.[410] Combination therapy with stem cell factor has been effective only occasionally, and the use of stem cell factor also leads to mast cell growth and activation with histamine release, thereby limiting its usefulness.[363] GM-CSF treatment results in large increases in eosinophils and monocytes, but not in neutrophils.[400] Side effects of G-CSF treatment are usually mild and include headache, bone pain, and rashes. Other findings noted in 44 patients treated for 4 or more years include splenomegaly (12 patients) and osteopenia (15 patients).[391] Unusual fractures or osteoporotic vertebral deformations can occur. Why bone demineralization develops in patients with SCN is unclear, and the degree of bone mineral loss does not seem to correlate with the dose of G-CSF, duration of treatment, or patients' age or sex.[411]

The development of MDS, AML, or both remains a serious potential complication of SCN. This predilection was recognized before the availability of G-CSF,[397, 398] but most affected children probably died from severe infections. At present, the relationship between G-CSF treatment and development of AML is unclear. However, a larger number of children with SCN who are receiving G-CSF therapy are developing MDS/AML. The general belief is that the prolonged survival associated with the treatment is the reason rather than the disorders being direct side effects. Of more than 350 patients with congenital neutropenia followed in the Severe Chronic Neutropenia Registry, 31 have developed MDS or AML (29 had SCN, and 2 had Shwachman-Diamond syndrome).[412] No relationship was found with the amount of G-CSF given or the duration of therapy or with age or sex. As mentioned earlier, the acquisition of somatic mutations in the G-CSF receptor was associated with progression to MDS and AML, in addition to monosomy 7 or other chromosomal abnormalities, and oncogene mutations (e.g., in *Ras*).[363] Time to progression has varied from months to years. Before G-CSF therapy is started, a bone marrow examination with cytogenetic analysis should be performed; how often subsequent studies should be undertaken in patients receiving G-CSF treatment is unclear at present. The Severe Chronic Neutropenia Registry currently recommends monitoring patients with SCN with regular blood count measurements and annual bone marrow examinations. Note that patients with either cyclic or idiopathic neutropenia are not at risk for the development of MDS/AML.

Hematopoietic stem cell transplantation should be considered in patients with SCN who require very high doses of G-CSF (>100 μg/kg/day) or whose SCN is refractory to G-CSF therapy or who show signs that suggest they have MDS or AML. In the small number of patients receiving transplants to date, survival is better in those without evidence of MDS/AML (9 of 12) compared with those who had MDS/AML (4 of 19).[410]

Myelokathexis and WHIM Syndrome

Myelokathexis is an uncommon form of moderate to severe chronic neutropenia characterized by granulocyte hyperplasia in the bone marrow, which contains degenerating neutrophils with cytoplasmic vacuoles, prominent granules, and nuclear hypersegmentation with very thin filaments connecting pyknotic-appearing nuclear lobes.[413, 414] Similar abnormalities can be seen in the majority of peripheral blood neutrophils. Eosinophils exhibit a similar abnormal morphologic appearance, but lymphocytes, monocytes, and basophils appear normal.[413] In addition to neutropenia, recurrent warts and hypogammaglobulinemia (low levels of IgG and occasionally low levels of IgM and IgA) have often been reported in patients with myelokathexis. Recurrent sinopulmonary infections are typical. Hence, the acronym *WHIM* was coined, referring to *w*arts, *h*ypogammaglobulinemia, *i*nfections, and *m*yelokathexis.[415] Relative lymphopenia has also been noted in some patients.[413] The recurrent bacterial infections in patients with WHIM syndrome probably reflect an increased susceptibility due to relative neutropenia and hypogammaglobulinemia. However, early deaths related to infection have not been reported, and affected patients are capable of mobilizing increased numbers of neutrophils into the peripheral blood during infectious episodes.[414] Neutrophil function has generally been reported to be normal.

Since the description of the first patient in 1964,[416, 417] more than 25 patients have been reported,[414, 418] including a kindred of 6 affected individuals in three generations[413] and dizygotic twin sisters.[419] The sex ratio among reported patients has a female predominance. The transmission of WHIM syndrome appears to be autosomal dominant, and there has been no male to male transmission. Search of the X-chromosome revealed no linkage, and an affected male has had an unaffected daughter.[413]

Myelokathexis has been suggested to result from retention of neutrophils in the marrow (*kathexis*, retention), where they undergo degenerative changes. Results of leukokinetic and morphologic studies are consistent with increased intramedullary destruction of neutrophils. However, recent studies have suggested that rather than an abnormal retention of cells, these findings reflect a disturbed balance between pro– and anti–apoptotic factors, leading to accelerated granulocyte apoptosis, which affects both precursors and mature granulocytes.[418] The expression of the anti–apoptotic factor *bcl-x* but not that of *bcl-2* was decreased in neutrophil precursors in the marrow.[418]

Patients with similar dysmyelopoietic features and chronic neutropenia but with additional findings have also been reported, which may reflect a different underlying cause. One patient with neutropenia had biploid- and tetraploid-nucleated neutrophils, band cells, and metamyelocytes in the marrow, but earlier neutrophil precursors were normal, as were the vast majority of peripheral blood neutrophils.[420] Chemotaxis of peripheral blood neutrophils was markedly decreased. In another patient with pseudoachondroplasia and short stature in addition to neutropenia and myelokathexis, decreased chemotaxis and respiratory burst activity were reported.[421]

The neutropenia and the accelerated granulocyte apoptosis are partially corrected by administration of either G-CSF or GM-CSF, and responses typically are seen within 4 to 8 hours of administration.[414, 418] Increased *bcl-x* expression was demonstrated in bone marrow granulocyte precursors from a patient treated with G-CSF.[418] Interestingly, immunoglobulin levels return to normal in patients treated with G-CSF.[414]

Shwachman-Diamond Syndrome

Shwachman-Diamond syndrome is a rare multiorgan disease of unknown cause that is inherited as an autosomal recessive trait.[422, 423] Neutropenia, progressive bone marrow failure, pancreatic exocrine insufficiency, short stature, and metaphyseal chondrodysplasia were noted.[424–429] Older patients are also at risk for development of MDS and AML. Dysmorphic features include cutaneous syndactyly, a bifid uvula, short soft palate, and hypertelorism. Diarrhea, weight loss, failure to thrive, eczema, otitis media, and pneumonia may occur in affected neonates. Skin infections, osteomyelitis, and sepsis can also be seen. Almost all infants develop malabsorption by 4 months of age. Growth failure and short stature are usually noted during the first or second year of life, and puberty is often delayed. Metaphyseal chondrodysplasia can occur in 25 percent of patients, and normal gait can become impaired because of secondary hip discomfort. The skeletal abnormalities can also result in pathologic fractures, coxa vara, kyphosis, and scoliosis.[430]

Virtually all patients with Shwachman-Diamond syndrome develop some degree of chronic neutropenia, and approximately two thirds of patients have a neutrophil count of less than 1000 cells/μL, with no reciprocal monocytosis. The neutropenia can be intermittent but is not cyclical. Some patients also have a moderately severe defect in chemotaxis that may contribute to the increased susceptibility to pyogenic infection.[428, 429] Anemia is also commonly seen, and one fourth of patients have mild to moderate thrombocytopenia.[429] Bone marrow studies have generally shown some degree of myeloid hypoplasia[424, 431] but are not diagnostic. Patients also have evidence of pancreatic exocrine insufficiency by laboratory testing. Histologic studies of the pancreas have shown acinar degeneration with fatty replacement. Skeletal radiologic findings can include "cup" deformation of the ribs, metaphyseal widening and hypoplasia of the iliac bones, and shortening of the extremities.[432, 433]

The underlying cause of the hemapoietic defect in Shwachman-Diamond syndrome has not been identified, but it appears to reflect a generalized bone marrow dysfunction. Recent *in vitro* studies have documented a marked reduction in the percentage of CD34+ cells in the marrow and *in vitro* colony formation, along with abnormalities in marrow stromal function, which were seen in patients without or with MDS.[434] Marrow cells from patients with Shwachman-Diamond syndrome also showed a higher tendency to undergo apoptosis, which was enhanced by activation of the Fas pathway, compared with normal marrow cells.[435] The gene locus affected in Shwachman-Diamond syndrome was mapped by linkage analysis to the centromeric region for chromosome 7.[436]

Treatment includes pancreatic enzyme replacement, which does not improve the neutropenia or dwarfism. Steatorrhea tends to diminish with time, although pancreatic insufficiency persists.[427] The occurrence of bacterial infections, which generally respond to appropriate antibiotics, can vary among patients. Administration of G-CSF increases the neutrophil count to the normal range[401, 437] and should be started as adjunctive therapy if the patient has a serious infection. Up to one fourth to one third of patients develop MDS, often with the acquisition of a structural chromosomal abnormality or aplastic anemia.[429] Hence, regular blood count measurements are recommended, and there may be a role for annual bone marrow examinations. As for other congenital bone marrow failure syndromes, there is a high risk of subsequent leukemic transformation if MDS develops.[425, 429]

Chédiak-Higashi Syndrome

CHS is a rare genetic disorder characterized by partial oculocutaneous albinism, giant lysosomes in many cell types, including granulocytes, and neuropathy.[438–441] Most patients have a moderate neutropenia, apparently due to ineffective granulopoiesis. This disorder is described in detail in a later section.

Familial Benign Neutropenia

Familial benign neutropenia is characterized by a mild neutropenia and no tendency for increased susceptibility to infection. An autosomal dominant transmission has been identified in some families.[442] Familial benign neutropenia has been described in Yemenite Jews,[443] American and African blacks,[444] and German, French, American, and South African individuals.[445]

Other Causes of Neutropenia Due to Intrinsic Defects in Myelopoiesis

Congenital or acquired bone marrow failure syndromes, including Fanconi anemia, dyskeratosis congenita, aplastic anemia, and MDS, occasionally present with isolated neutropenia. Fanconi anemia and dyskeratosis congenita should be easily recognized by other features associated with these disorders (see Chapter 8).[446]

NEUTROPENIA CAUSED BY EXTRINSIC FACTORS

Infection

The most common cause of transient neutropenia in childhood is viral infection. Viruses commonly causing neutropenia include hepatitis A and B, respiratory syncytial virus, influenza A and B, measles, rubella, and varicella.[109, 447–450] Neutropenia develops during the first 24 to 48 hours of the illness and may persist for 3 to 6 days. This time usually corresponds to the period of acute viremia and may relate to virus-induced redistribution of neutrophils from the circulating to the marginated granulocyte pool, sequestration, or increased neutrophil utilization after tissue damage by the viruses.[451, 452] Several human viruses, including measles and herpes simplex virus, were demonstrated to replicate in human endothelial cells, and lead to the expression of receptors on endothelium for immune complexes containing IgG and C3, which potentially might promote enhanced neutrophil adhesion to the endothelium.[453, 454] Acute transient neutropenia often occurs during the early stages of infectious mononucleosis.[455, 456] In most of these patients, the basis of the neutropenia is unknown, but in some it may be related to accelerated destruction of neutrophils

by anti-neutrophil antibodies.[457, 458] Parvovirus B19 can cause transient neutropenia and can also be associated with the development of prolonged neutropenia with or without the development of anti-neutrophil antibodies.[459–461]

Leukopenia is commonly seen in patients with the acquired immunodeficiency syndrome (AIDS).[462, 463] In pediatric patients with AIDS, neutropenia can be caused by antiviral drugs, vitamin B_{12} or folate deficiency, or cellular immune dysfunction.[464] Neutropenia in HIV infection can also be associated with hypersplenism and anti-neutrophil antibodies.[465, 466]

Significant neutropenia may occur during typhoid, paratyphoid, tuberculosis, brucellosis, tularemia, and rickettsial infections.[449, 450, 467–469] The mechanisms responsible for neutropenia in these conditions remain ill-defined. During periods of relapsing fever caused by acute vivax malaria, the apparent neutropenia may be associated with increased neutrophil margination in the intravascular compartment.[470]

Sepsis is one of the more serious causes of neutropenia. The neutropenia in patients with bacteremia and endotoxemia may result from excessive destruction of neutrophils. This can occur after phagocytosis of microbes, from the release of metabolites of arachidonic acid, or from activation of the complement system through either the alternate or classic pathway, leading to the generation of C5a. C5a, in turn, induces neutrophil aggregation and leads to the formation of leukoemboli in the pulmonary capillary bed, which adhere to endothelial surfaces. This process is probably accelerated as a result of "priming" of neutrophils by endotoxin and by TNF and IL-1 released by macrophages.[471] The adherent, activated neutrophils may release noxious substances that can cause acute cardiopulmonary complications. C5a neutropenia occurs transiently during hemodialysis, during continuous-flow leukapheresis, and after burn injury.[472–475]

Significant neutropenia can occur in neonatal bacterial sepsis. Newborns can exhaust their neutrophil reserves during overwhelming bacterial infection, because the neutrophil storage pool is small and neutrophil production is already near a maximum.[476] Newborns with sepsis may benefit from granulocyte transfusion[477–479] or G-CSF,[480–482] both of which are undergoing clinical investigation for this indication.

Drug-Induced Neutropenia

Drug-induced neutropenia is a disorder characterized by severe and selective reduction in the levels of circulating blood neutrophils (usually to levels of fewer than 200 cells/μL) and is due to an idiosyncratic reaction to the offending drug (Table 21–13).[483–496] This definition thus excludes disorders in which other cell lines are perturbed (such as aplastic anemia), those in which drug administration is not a feature, and the predictable neutropenias observed with anticancer therapy. Implicit in this definition is the unpredictability of the condition. Although the majority of patients will recover, drug-induced neutropenia is a serious disorder, with mortality rates reported to be as high as 32 percent in one series.[497]

Idiosyncratic reactions tend to develop more often in women than in men and more often in older than in younger persons.[489] Drugs reported to be associated with agranulocytosis have been extensively reviewed.[483, 484, 486, 493–495] These include antimicrobial agents, particularly sulfonamides and penicillins; antithyroid drugs; phenothiazines; antipyretics, including aspirin, acetaminophen, and phenylbutazone; antirheumatics, including gold, levamisole, and penicillamine; and sedatives, including barbiturates and benzodiazepines (Table 21–13).

Although the underlying mechanisms for most drug-induced neutropenias are unknown, studies with certain drugs have suggested at least three major mechanisms.[483, 485, 494, 495] First, differences in drug pharmacokinetics can lead to toxic levels of the drug or metabolites in the marrow microenvironment. An example is the neutropenia induced by sulfasalazine. Although neutropenia can be observed in any patient taking this drug, those individuals who are slow acetylators show much greater toxicity than

do those who are fast acetylators.[491] Second, myeloid precursors may be abnormally sensitive to typical drug concentrations. Phenothiazines and perhaps nitrous oxide induce neutropenia by this mechanism in that myeloid precursors in the marrow are particularly sensitive to these agents.[483, 494, 498] The toxic damage by phenothiazines manifests itself as a neutropenia that appears 20 to 40 days after the patient has received 10 to 12 g of the drug. Third, drugs can induce an immune-mediated neutropenia in two ways. In one way, the drug serves as a hapten in promoting the synthesis of antibodies that are capable of destroying mature neutrophils. Aminopyrine, penicillin, propylthiouracil, and gold can cause neutropenia by this mechanism.[483, 488, 492, 494] In the other way, the drug causes the formation of circulating immune complexes that presumably attach to the surface of the neutrophil and lead to its destruction, as in the case of quinidine. In addition, immunologic changes induced by drugs can suppress granulopoiesis. For example, activation of both cellular and humoral immune responses was reported to impair myelopoiesis after therapy with quinidine and phenytoin, respectively.[485, 494] Drug-induced immune neutropenia is characterized by its unpredictability. It usually begins abruptly 7 to 14 days after the first exposure to the drug or immediately after reexposure. Fever, chills, and severe prostration are common in these patients.

The duration of drug-induced neutropenia varies greatly. Acute idiosyncratic drug reactions may last only a few days, whereas chronic idiosyncratic reactions may last for months or years. In contrast, immune-mediated neutropenia usually lasts for 6 to 8 days. When neutropenia occurs, the most important therapeutic action is, of course, to withdraw all drugs that are not absolutely essential, particularly those suspected to be myelotoxic. During recovery from drug-induced neutropenia, a rebound leukocytosis can occur, accompanied by marrow and peripheral blasts.

Autoimmune Neutropenia

Autoimmune neutropenia (AIN) can be seen as an isolated phenomenon or in association with other autoimmune diseases. It is also associated with infection, drugs, or malignancy.[243, 499] Chronic idiopathic neutropenia in many children and adults is now recognized as being caused by autoimmune antibodies directed against neutrophils. In primary autoimmune neutropenia, low counts of circulating neutrophils are the only hematologic finding, and associated diseases or other factors that cause neutropenia are absent. The peak incidence of AIN is seen in infants and young children.[243] In these patients it is generally a benign disorder and spontaneous remission usually occurs, as discussed in the next section. Immune system–mediated neutropenias are also seen in association with other disorders (Table 21–14); these are often referred to as *secondary autoimmune neutropenias*.

Patients with AIN generally have neutrophil counts of 250 cells/µL or less, and neutrophils can be absent entirely. Monocytosis is common. Bone marrow examination shows normal to increased cellularity and decreased to normal numbers of mature neutrophils, although maturation arrest at earlier stages of neutrophil differentiation can also be seen.[243, 366, 500, 501] Mild splenomegaly is

TABLE 21–13. Partial List of Drugs Associated with Idiosyncratic Neutropenia*

Drug	Possible Mechanism		
	Direct Suppression	Metabolite Suppression	Immune Destruction
ANALGESICS/ ANTI-INFLAMMATORY AGENTS			
Aminopyrine			X
Ibuprofen			X
Indomethacin	X		
Phenylbutazone	X		
ANTIBIOTICS			
Chloramphenicol	X		
Penicillins	X		X
Sulfonamides	X		
ANTICONVULSANTS			
Phenytoin			X
Carbamazepine		X	
ANTITHYROID AGENTS			
Propylthiouracil			X
CARDIOVASCULAR AGENTS			
Hydralazine			X
Procainamide			X
Quinidine			X
HYPOGLYCEMIC AGENTS			
Chlorpropamide			X
TRANQUILIZERS			
Chlorpromazine	X		
Phenothiazines	X		
OTHER			
Cimetidine, ranitidine	X		
Levamisole			X

*The partial list of agents capable of causing idiosyncratic drug-induced neutropenia is summarized from references 484 through 495.

occasionally present. The incidence of pyogenic infection is not always related to the degree of neutropenia and is generally limited to cutaneous and respiratory infections. Serious infections are generally uncommon. Spontaneous remissions can occasionally occur, but are seen much less often than in younger patients (see next section).

Neutrophil-specific cell surface antigens are a commonly identified target of the autoantibodies identified in AIN, including NA1 and NA2, NB1, ND1, and NE1.[243] The NA1 and NA2 antigens are glycosylated isoforms of the neutrophil opsonic FcγRIIIb receptor (CD16) (see Table 21–7), and the NB1 antigen is a 58- to 64-kD GPI-anchored membrane glycoprotein on the plasma membrane and on secondary granules.[502] Mechanisms that trigger autoantibody production are unknown. In children, primary AIN is usually associated with NA allele–specific antibodies, but secondary AIN is associated with pan-FcγRIIIb antibodies.[503]

To detect antineutrophil antibodies, a combination of an indirect granulocyte immunofluorescence test and a granulocyte agglutination test appears to result in optimal sensitivity and specificity.[243, 499, 503–506] These assays detect IgG and IgM antibodies, both of which been identified in AIN.[243] In the granulocyte immunofluorescence test, a panel of heterologous donor granulocytes are incubated with serum or plasma from patients and control subjects, and bound immunoglobulins are detected by a fluorescent dye–labeled antihuman Ig antibody. The granulocyte agglutination test is less sensitive, but it is useful for detecting a subgroup of antibodies against antigens other than CD16, although these are not typical of AIN.[243, 506] Neutrophil-binding immune complexes may also give positive results in these assays and may be important in the pathogenesis of neutropenia in Felty syndrome.[499] Confirmatory testing of autoantibody specificity can be done using the monoclonal antibody immobilization of granulocyte antigens assay, in which binding of patient sera to a panel of donor neutrophils is compared with binding of monoclonal antibodies of defined specificity.[507] Sera containing HLA antibodies require preabsorption or other controls to determine whether there is specific antineutrophil activity. Several adult patients with AIN were found to have autoantibodies directed against the leukocyte adhesion β_2 integrin Mac-1 (CD11b/CD18).[508] Laboratory demonstration of antineutrophil antibodies may not always be necessary to make the diagnosis of AIN, and its utility depends on the specific clinical setting.

The neutropenia of AIN is presumed to be primarily due to the peripheral destruction of antibody-coated neutrophils, which may be also be augmented by the deposition of C3. Phagocytosis of neutrophils in the spleens of patients with AIN was observed.[509] In some patients, antineutrophil antibodies also appear to interfere with myelopoiesis.[243, 499, 510] Impairment of phagocytosis, respiratory burst activity, and adhesion by neutrophil-directed antibodies has also been observed, which may contribute to the risk of infection in patients with AIN.[243, 499, 508]

Treatment of patients with immune neutropenia includes the judicious use of appropriate antibiotics for bacterial infections and, in patients with occasional mouth sores or gingivitis, antibacterial mouthwashes and regular dental hygiene. Infections tend to be less common in patients with immune neutropenia than in those with the corresponding degree of neutropenia from other causes, probably because granulopoiesis is intact in most patients. Corticosteroid and intravenous γ-globulin administration can result in normalization of the neutrophil count, but efficacy is variable and often short-lived.[243, 499] Splenectomy appears to be of only transient benefit and further predisposes the patients to life-threatening bacterial infections. The daily administration of G-CSF in doses of 1 to 2 μg/kg has been successful in increasing the neutrophil count to the normal range or even higher within 2 weeks in patients with primary AIN, Evan syndrome, and Felty syndrome.[499] Hence, G-CSF therapy should be considered as part of the management of serious or recurrent infectious in patients with immune neutropenias. Prophylactic administration of trimethoprim/sulfamethoxazole may be also helpful for management of recurrent minor infections, although there are no controlled studies addressing the efficacy of this approach.

Chronic Benign Neutropenia and Autoimmune Neutropenia of Childhood

Most occurrences of what was termed *chronic benign neutropenia of infancy and childhood* are now believed to represent an AIN that has parallels to childhood idiopathic thrombocytopenic purpura and autoimmune hemolytic anemia.[243, 366, 511–514] The handful of occurrences reported as the "lazy leukocyte syndrome,"[515–517] characterized by profound neutropenia, normal-appearing bone marrow, and little increase in the peripheral blood neutrophil count in response to steroids or epinephrine, were also likely to have been AIN of childhood.

AIN of childhood occurs predominantly in children younger than 3 years of age (see Table 12–15). The median age of presentation is 8 to 11 months, with a range of 2 to 54 months.[243, 506, 511, 512] There is a slight female predominance. The mean ANC at presentation is 150 to 250 cells/μL and often is close to zero. A relative monocytosis or eosinophilia can occur. Transient increases in circulating neutrophil counts can occur in response to infection. Other peripheral blood cell counts are normal for age, although mild thrombocytopenia (≥100,000 cells/μl) was reported.[512] There is no family history of neutropenia.

Antineutrophil antibodies can be detected in almost all patients when a combination of immunofluorescent and agglutination assays are used, although repeated testing at intervals of 2 to 4 weeks is sometimes necessary.[506] However, absence of detectable antibody does not exclude the diagnosis. As with AIN in adults, antibodies are typically directed against neutrophil-specific antigens of the NA, NB, and ND loci. Antibody specificity to NA1, an allele of the neutrophil FcγRIII opsonin receptor, is seen in about one quarter of patients.[243, 511, 512] There is no correlation between the strength of the antibody and the severity of clinical manifestations; however, as neutropenia resolves, antibodies gradually become undetectable. Results of bone marrow examination generally show a normal to hypercellular marrow, with reduction in mature neutrophils and band cells, although a maturation arrest in earlier stages can occur.[243, 366, 512] Some, but not all, patients will manifest an increase in the peripheral neutrophil count in response to treatment with hydrocortisone or prednisone.

More bacterial infections are often seen during the neutropenic period, but they are usually mild (e.g., skin infections, upper respiratory infections, otitis media, and gingivitis) and respond to standard antibiotics.[243, 366, 511] Cellulitis involving the labia majora was seen in 23 percent of 26 girls with AIN in one series, often due to *Pseudomonas aeruginosa*.[366] Pneumonia, sepsis, and meningitis have been seen occasionally in infants with AIN.[243] Spontaneous remission occurs in almost all patients, with neutropenia persisting for a median duration of 20 months.[511] Children less than 9 months of age at time of diagnosis may recover normal peripheral neutrophil counts more rapidly.[512] With increasing age, spontaneous remission becomes less likely.

The diagnosis of autoimmune neutropenia of childhood is generally straightforward if the presentation occurs within the first 2 years of life, there is no history of serious infections over several months of observation, and neutrophil morphology and other peripheral counts are otherwise normal. Demonstration of an antineutrophil antibody is not necessary for diagnosis in the patient with the typical clinical features of childhood AIN (Table 21–15). Because of the association of AIN with immunodeficiency syndromes (see later in this section), evaluation of immunoglobulin levels should be performed to exclude hypogammaglobulinemias, and if lymphopenia or clinical signs of cell-mediated immunodeficiency are present, T-cell function should be studied. A bone marrow examination should always be performed if hematologic abnormalities other than neutropenia are present and if the child is either younger or older than the typical patient with AIN of childhood, particularly if a an unusual or deep-seated infection is present, which suggests poor marrow neutrophil reserve. In young infants, the characteristic promyelocytic arrest characteristic of SCN can be very helpful in making the distinction between this disease and AIN. Other laboratory tests to consider are discussed later in this section.

Febrile episodes should be managed conservatively in the first few months after the diagnosis of childhood AIN is suspected, and broad-spectrum parenteral antibiotics should be used. However, if during this initial observation period, the patient has either no infections or shows a prompt response to antibiotics, subsequent infectious illnesses can be managed as for any other child. Prophylactic administration of trimethoprim-sulfamethoxazole can be helpful in the child with recurrent otitis media. Administration of G-CSF results in an

TABLE 21–15. Summary of Autoimmune Neutropenia of Childhood

Incidence	Most common cause of chronic neutropenia in infancy and childhood; ≥ 1 per 100,0000 children per year
Clinical features	Median age of diagnosis is 8–11 months of age (range 3–38 months) with a slight female predominance (56% F; 44% M). Some patients have an increased incidence of relatively minor infections (otitis media, gingivitis, upper respiratory tract, skin), which respond well to antimicrobial therapy. Occasional patients have pneumonia or sepsis (usually infants).
Laboratory evaluation	Median ANC at time of diagnosis is ≈ 200 neutrophils/μL (range 0–500 cells/μL). Hemoglobin level and platelet count are generally normal. Antineutrophil antibodies can be detected in the majority of patients and are often directed to NA1 antigen (neutrophil FcγIII receptor). Bone marrow is normo- to hypercellular, often with a decrease in the number of mature neutrophils, although maturation arrest at earlier stages is noted occasionally.
Differential diagnosis	These include other causes of autoimmune neutropenia (e.g., Evan syndrome, drug reaction), transient post-infectious neutropenia, immunodeficiency syndromes, amino acidopathies, and intrinsic defects in myelopoiesis (e.g., severe congenital neutropenia, cyclic neutropenia, Shwachman-Diamond syndrome).
Therapy	Antibiotics for acute infection; prophylactic antibiotics may be helpful in some patients with recurrent otitis media. Consider use of G-CSF for serious infection.
Prognosis	Excellent. Although the ANC often remains below 500 cells/μL for 12 or more months, spontaneous remission occurs in almost all patients (median of 20 months, range 6–54 months).

ANC = absolute neutrophil count.

increased peripheral neutrophil count in childhood AIN[506, 518] and is the treatment of choice for the rare child with AIN who manifests severe or recurrent infections. G-CSF doses of 2 μg/k/day or less are usually effective, and responses are typically seen within days. Steroids and intravenous γ-globulin have also been used in the past but have limited efficacy.

Although AIN of childhood is the most common cause of chronic neutropenia in the pediatric age group, it is still a relatively uncommon diagnosis, with an incidence of approximately 1 in 100,000 children per year.[366, 513] However, this figure is probably an underestimate because of the generally benign course of this disorder.

Immune Neonatal Neutropenia

Neonatal alloimmune neutropenia is analogous to Rh hemolytic disease and results from maternal sensitization to fetal neutrophils bearing antigens that differ from the mother's. Maternal IgG antibodies cross the placenta and cause an immune-mediated neutropenia that can be severe and last for several weeks up to as long as 6 months.[519–521] During the neutropenic phase, the bone marrow demonstrates myeloid hyperplasia with depletion of mature neutrophil forms.

Neutrophil antibodies are found in the serum of the mother and the infant and are usually directed to the neutrophil-specific NA antigen system. The NA1 and NA2 antigens are two isotypes of the neutrophil FcγRIIIb receptor (see Table 21–7). Affected infants can be asymptomatic or develop omphalitis, other cutaneous infections, pneumonia, sepsis, and meningitis. Because neonatal sepsis can itself be associated with profound neutropenia, the underlying immune-mediated neutrophil destruction may not be recognized immediately in affected newborns who have sepsis.

The initial management of neonatal alloimmune neutropenia should include parenteral antibiotics even if signs of infection are absent, owing to the association of neutropenia with neonatal sepsis. Intravenous γ-globulin is not always effective in increasing neutrophil counts.[522, 523] However, the administration of three daily doses of G-CSF (5 μg/kg dose) resulted in normalization of the neutrophil count within 4 days in two infants with alloimmune neutropenia.[522] Thus, treatment with G-CSF should be considered when serious infections develop in infants with alloimmune neutropenia.

Neonatal immune neutropenia can also occur in infants whose mother has AIN. Transplacental passage of an IgG antineutrophil antibody can react with the infant's neutrophils bearing the inciting antigen and cause a profound neutropenia lasting for 2 to 4 weeks.[524] Leukoagglutinating antibodies have often been found in multiparous women, and these antibodies have been observed in their newborn children's sera without any corresponding neutropenia.[525, 526] The antibodies are directed against HLAs found on neutrophils and other tissues and are presumably absorbed by the placenta, various plasma antigens, and tissues in the fetus. As a result, serum concentrations of these antibodies are insufficient to induce neutropenia. It appears that only antibodies directed specifically against neutrophils can produce immune-mediated neonatal neutropenia.

Neutropenia Associated with Immune Disorders

Disorders of immunoglobulin production have been associated with neutropenic syndromes. One third of males with X-linked agammaglobulinemia have neutropenia at some time during the course of their disease.[527] Persistent or cyclic neutropenia is common in patients with the hyper-IgM immunodeficiency syndrome, which in many instances appears to be associated with the formation of autoantibodies.[528, 529] γ-Globulin abolished the neutropenia in some of these patients.[530] AIN and other autoimmune cytopenias can also be seen in common variable immunodeficiency and isolated IgA deficiency.[529, 531]

Cartilage hair hypoplasia, an autosomal recessive disorder often found in the Amish population, is characterized by short-limbed dwarfism, fine hair, moderate neutropenia (100 to 2000 cells/μL), and impaired cell-mediated immunity.[532, 533] Bone marrow transplantation has corrected both the immunologic defect and neutropenia.[534, 535]

Neutropenia can be seen with a variety of other disorders of the immune system. A syndrome of severe neutropenia associated with eczema, polyarthralgias, recurrent bacterial infections, eosinophilia, and depressed cellular immunity was reported in four siblings (three girls and a boy).[536] Serum IgA levels were markedly elevated, but antibody responses to tetanus and poliomyelitis vaccines were depressed. Severe granulocytic hypoplasia, which failed to improve with steroid treatment but responded to serial infusions of antithymocyte globulin, was reported in a girl with defects in T-cell function.[537] This patient had previously developed autoimmune thrombocytopenia and hemolytic anemia that showed positive results on a Coombs test, both of which responded to prednisone. Autoimmune disorders, such as systemic lupus erythematosus, can be associated with antibody or immune complex–mediated destruction of neutrophils and, in some instance, their precursors, as discussed earlier. Finally, neutropenia is common in patients with AIDS, in whom its causes can be multifactorial and include cellular immune dysfunction, ineffective hematopoiesis, antiviral drugs, antineutrophil antibodies, and hypersplenism.[462, 464–466]

Neutropenia Associated with Metabolic Diseases

Children suffering from hyperglycinemia, isovaleric acidemia, propionic acidemia, methylmalonic acidemia, and tyrosinemia may have significant neutropenia.[538–545] Significant neutropenia is also seen in Barth syndrome, a distinctive X-linked disorder also associated with dilated cardiomyopathy, growth retardation, and 3-methylglutaconic aciduria.[546–548] A relative monocytosis is common. Affected boys develop symptoms in infancy or childhood, and neutropenia can precede the development of cardiac abnormalities. The mechanisms underlying the neutropenia associated with disorders of organic acid metabolism are not known, although the finding that propionate and isovalerate impair the development of myeloid colonies *in vitro* suggests that altered levels of metabolites *in vivo* may suppress myelopoiesis.[549]

Neutropenia is common in glycogen storage disease type IB, and neutrophil counts of less than 500 cells/μL are not uncommon.[540, 541, 550, 551] Multiple abnormalities in neutrophil function are also common, including chemotaxis, respiratory burst activity, and bacterial killing.[540, 544] Recombinant G-CSF was used effectively to correct the neutropenia in patients with glycogen storage disease type IB, in association with reduction of serious infections.[550, 551] Decreased monocyte superoxide production and chemotaxis were reported in Gaucher disease, which may contribute to the infections occasionally seen in patients with this disease.[552, 553]

Nutritional Deficiencies

Ineffective granulopoiesis is part of the pathologic course of megaloblastic marrow observed in patients with nutritional deficiencies of vitamin B_{12} or folic acid.[554] As a reflection of the increased neutrophil turnover due to ineffective myelopoiesis, serum muramidase levels are often elevated.[554] Neutropenia also occurs with starvation in conditions such as anorexia nervosa[555] and marasmus in infants and occasionally in patients receiving parenteral feeding. Neutropenia and marrow megaloblastosis have also been observed in patients thought to have copper deficiency, because these patients have shown a prompt response to copper replacement.

Reticuloendothelial Sequestration

Splenic enlargement due to portal hypertension, intrinsic splenic disease, or splenic hyperplasia can lead to neutropenia. The usual clinical picture is moderate neutropenia that may be accompanied by a similar degree of thrombocytopenia and anemia. The reduced survival of neutrophils corresponds with the size of the spleen, and the extent of neutropenia is proportional to bone marrow compensatory mechanisms.[556] The neutropenia is usually mild and may be ameliorated by successful treatment of the underlying disease. Bed rest alone may lead to restoration of the neutrophil counts owing to a reduction in portal pressure. In selected patients, splenectomy may be necessary to restore the neutrophil count to normal. Malignant histiocyte disorders may also cause reticuloendothelial hyperplasia, leading to neutropenia and anemia associated with ingestion of neutrophils and red cells by the malignant cells.[486]

Bone Marrow Infiltration

Malignancies, such as leukemia or lymphoma, that infiltrate the bone marrow result in a myelophthisic picture, producing leukoerythroblastic peripheral blood smears. Tumor-induced myelofibrosis may further accentuate the neutropenia.[557] Myelofibrosis can also result from granulomatous infections, Gaucher disease, osteopetrosis, benzol drugs, fluoride, or exposure to X irradiation.[558–560]

Chronic Idiopathic Neutropenia

Chronic idiopathic neutropenia represents a group of disorders that, by definition, are poorly understood and cannot be placed in any of the categories discussed in the preceding sections.[364, 366, 367] Investigation of granulopoiesis has suggested that, in some patients, decreased or ineffective production of neutrophils may be the principal mechanism of neutropenia. The underlying cause of the defective myelopoiesis is not well characterized.[367, 561, 562]

Overall, the clinical features, bone marrow findings, and natural history of chronic idiopathic neutropenia are varied.[364, 366, 367] Many patients rarely have serious infections relative to their degree of neutropenia; it is likely that many of the patients described in older studies had antibody-mediated neutrophil destruction and normal bone marrow reserve.[563] Treatment should be based on the severity of symptoms. Corticosteroids, cytotoxic agents, and G-CSF have all been reported to be used successfully in individual patients.[367, 564]

EVALUATION OF THE PATIENT WITH NEUTROPENIA

The basic approach to a patient with neutropenia includes a history and physical examination with emphasis on (1) related phenotypic abnormalities, (2) determination of whether bacterial infection is present (including evaluation of gingiva and rectum), (3) evaluation of lymphadenopathy, hepatosplenomegaly, and any other signs of an underlying associated chronic illness and (4) history of recent infection and drug exposure. The rate of occurrence and duration of symptoms is important, and a history of periodontitis, dental abscesses, or tooth loss is particularly suspicious for significant chronic or recurrent neutropenia. The family history may reveal other individuals with recurrent infection. Unexplained deaths in children younger than 1 year of age and the race and ethnic group of each patient should be noted.

The duration and severity of the neutropenia and the presence or absence of other significant symptoms or physical findings greatly influence the speed and extent of laboratory evaluation. If the patient has isolated neutropenia, is asymptomatic, and has no other findings, clinical observation for several weeks is usually the best approach. Any medications known to be associated with neutropenia should be discontinued. If an acute bacterial infection is suspected, prompt evaluation and treatment should be initiated, including the use of intravenous antibiotics in the patient with moderate to severe neutropenia and fever.

In patients with persistent neutropenia white blood cell and differential counts should be obtained two to three times weekly for 6 to 8 weeks to evaluate periodicity suggestive of cyclic neutropenia. A Coombs test and measurement of serum immunoglobulin levels should also be performed to determine whether a red cell autoantibody or possible associated hypogammaglobulinemia syndrome is present, respectively. T-cell studies or HIV testing may also be indicated in certain patients. Bone marrow aspirate with cytogenetics and bone marrow biopsy should be performed on selected patients. If anemia, macrocytosis, or thrombocytopenia is present, these studies should be performed immediately. Other laboratory tests that should be considered, depending on the clinical situation, include investigation for antineutrophil antibodies, evaluation for collagen vascular disease and for metabolic and exocrine pancreatic disease, the acid hemolysis test, radiographic studies of long bones and chest, and measurement of vitamin B_{12}, folate, and copper levels. Assessing whether or not the peripheral neutrophil count increases in response to steroid or epinephrine therapy is of little clinical utility.

PRINCIPLES OF THERAPY FOR NEUTROPENIA

The management of neutropenia depends on the underlying cause and severity of the neutropenia. The major concern in neutropenic patients is the development of serious pyogenic infection. Patients with severe neutropenia (ANC ≤500 cells/μL) with poor marrow reserve caused by, for example, SCN, aplastic anemia, or chemotherapy, have the highest risk of developing progressive infection and septicemia. Fever may often be the only indication of infection, because the usual signs and symptoms of inflammation are often diminished in the presence of neutropenia. Organisms involved usually come from the skin or gastrointestinal tract. Thus, febrile patients with neutropenia due to poor marrow function should be treated promptly with broad-spectrum antimicrobials after blood and other appropriate culture results are obtained. If there is a defervescence response and blood cultures do not reveal any bacterial growth, the antibiotics should be continued for at least 3 days after the patient is afebrile. However, if the patient continues to have fevers up to 38°C or higher and blood culture results are negative, antimicrobial therapy should be continued. A large percentage of febrile patients with neutropenia who receive antibiotics for 7 days develop fungal infections, and empiric treatment with amphotericin B should be considered in this setting. Neutropenic patients with documented fungal or gram-negative bacterial sepsis who have shown a poor response to appropriate therapy are candidates for neutrophil transfusions.[565, 566]

Neutropenic patients with normal to increased marrow cellularity, for example, in the setting of AIN, often have a minimal history of pyogenic infection and show a more brisk response to appropriate antibiotics. A less aggressive course may be a reasonable approach to a febrile illness in such patients who clinically look well, even if the ANC is less than 500 cells/μL. A child in whom the diagnosis of AIN of childhood was established who develops fever or infection can generally be managed as an outpatient, unless the infection is severe.

An important component in management of all patients with chronic or cyclic neutropenia is close attention to oral hygiene. Chronic gingivitis and periodontitis can be a persistent source of morbidity and result in tooth loss. All patients should receive regular dental care, along with regular use of antibiotic mouthwash.

Therapy to increase the neutrophil count in patients with either intrinsic defects in myelopoiesis or with acquired neutropenia has included the use of steroids and intravenous γ-globulin. These treatments, in general, have been only variably successful. The use of recombinant G-CSF and other hematopoietic growth factors has revolutionized the therapy of neutropenias.[567] As discussed in earlier sections, G-CSF was successfully used to increase the neutrophil count in a wide variety of neutropenic conditions, including SCN, cyclic neutropenia, and immune-mediated neutropenias. In some situations, chronic prophylactic use of G-CSF is recommended, for example, in SCN, in which patients have poor marrow production of neutrophils and a high risk of developing serious infection. For other causes of neutropenia in which patients tend to have fewer problems with infection, for example, autoimmune neutropenia, G-CSF therapy should be reserved for specific clinical indications such as serious or progressive infection.

Neutrophilia

Neutrophilia refers to an alteration in the total number of blood neutrophils that is in excess of about 7500 cells/μL in adults (Table 21–16). During the first few days of life the upper limit of the normal neutrophil count ranges from 7000 to 13,000 cells/μL for neonates born prematurely and at term gestation, respectively.[568] A decrease to adult levels occurs within the first few weeks of life and is maintained thereafter. An increase in circulating neutrophils is the result of a disturbance of the normal equilibrium involving neutrophil bone marrow production, movement in and out of the marrow compartments into the circulation, and neutrophil destruction (Table 21–16). Three mechanisms, either alone or in combination, largely account for neutrophilia.[20, 569] First, increased numbers of neutrophils may be mobilized from either the bone marrow storage compartment or the peripheral marginating pools into the circulating pool. Second, there may be increased blood neutrophil survival owing to impaired neutrophil egress into tissue. Finally, there may be expansion of the circulating neutrophil pool as a result of (1) increased progenitor cell proliferation and terminal differentiation through the neutrophilic series, (2) increased mitotic activity of neutrophilic cell precursors, or (3) shortening of the cell mitotic cycle in neutrophil precursors.

TABLE 21–16. Classification of Neutrophilia*

INCREASED PRODUCTION

Chronic infection
Chronic inflammation
  Ulcerative colitis
  Rheumatoid arthritis
Tumors (perhaps with necrosis)
Postneutropenia rebound
Myeloproliferative disease
Drugs (lithium, occasionally ranitidine)
Chronic idiopathic neutrophilia
Familial cold urticaria
Leukemoid reactions

ENHANCED RELEASE FROM MARROW STORAGE POOL

Corticosteroids
Stress
Hypoxia
Acute infection
Endotoxin

DECREASED EGRESS FROM CIRCULATION

Corticosteroids
Splenectomy
Leukocyte adhesion deficiency

REDUCED MARGINATION

Stress
Infections
Exercise
Epinephrine

*See text for references.

Acute neutrophilia occurs rapidly within minutes in response to exercise- or epinephrine-induced reactions and has been attributed to mobilization of the marginating pool of neutrophils into the circulating pool.[570] It has been postulated that epinephrine stimulates β-receptors on endothelial cells to induce the release of cyclic adenosine monophosphate (cAMP), which affects the adhesive properties of neutrophils and might account for the release of neutrophils from the marginating pool.[571] Slower onset of acute neutrophilia can occur after glucocorticoid administration or with inflammation or infection associated with the generation of endotoxin, TNF, IL-1, and a cascade of growth factors.[5, 6, 572, 573] Maximal response usually occurs within 4 to 24 hours after exposure to these agents and is probably due to the release from the marrow storage compartment of neutrophils into the circulation. The mechanisms that underlie the release of neutrophils from the marrow pool are unknown, but they may involve neutrophil activation through chemoattractant or cytokine receptors.[212] Glucocorticoids may also slow the egress of neutrophils from the circulation into tissue.[574] Less well understood mechanisms leading to delayed-onset acute neutrophilia were reported after electric shock trauma, anesthesia, and surgery.[575–577]

Chronic neutrophilia usually is associated with continued stimulation of neutrophil production, possibly through perturbation of marrow feedback mechanisms. Chronic neutrophilia may follow the prolonged administration of glucocorticoids, persistent inflammatory reactions, infection, chronic blood loss, or chronic anxiety.[578–582] Most reactions of this type last for days or weeks, but some may persist for many months. Pyogenic microorganisms, leptospiral infection, and certain viruses (including herpes simplex, varicella, rabies, and poliomyelitis) all may produce neutrophilia.[583] Significant neutrophilic leukocytosis has also been reported with both Kawasaki disease and infectious mononucleosis.[584, 585] Occasionally, extreme neutrophilia has been observed in tuberculosis, usually in seriously ill patients with widespread necrotizing inflammatory disease.[586] Chronic inflammation is often responsible for persistent neutrophilia, especially in patients with juvenile rheumatoid arthritis.[587]

Sustained moderate neutrophilia invariably follows either surgical or functional asplenia.[588] It probably arises because of a failure to remove circulating neutrophils (a normal function of the spleen) rather than because of an increase in granulopoiesis.[21] Similarly, neutrophilia was reported in functional disorders of neutrophils associated with impaired adhesion or motility, such as that found in patients with leukocyte adhesion deficiency or actin dysfunction (see later).

There is an autosomal dominant form of hereditary neutrophilia in which the absolute granulocyte count is maintained between 14,000 and 164,000 cells/μL.[589] These patients have hepatosplenomegaly and increased alkaline phosphatase levels along with Gaucher-type histiocytes. Neutrophilia also occurs in familial cold urticaria, in which elevated neutrophil counts, fever, urticaria, and a rash characterized histologically by a neutrophil infiltrate occur about 7 hours after cold exposure.[590, 591]

LEUKEMOID REACTIONS

The elevation of total leukocyte counts to greater than 50×10^3 cells/μL is referred to as a *leukemoid reaction*. The peripheral blood often has increased numbers of immature myeloid cells, including occasional myeloblasts and promyelocytes. Chronic myelogenous leukemia can be differentiated from a leukemoid reaction by the usual finding of splenomegaly, a low leukocyte alkaline phosphatase score, and the presence of the Philadelphia chromosome on cytogenetic analysis of bone marrow. Basophils are almost always elevated in chronic myelogenous leukemia and are normal in reactive neutrophilia.[578] Juvenile myelogenous leukemias, which are seen in the first few years of life, are also generally distinguished from a leukemoid reaction by the findings of lymphadenopathy, skin rash, and thrombocytopenia. Leukemoid reactions can be triggered by pyogenic infections, especially those caused by *S. aureus* or *S. pneumoniae*. Tuberculosis, brucellosis, and toxoplasmosis have also been associated with leukemoid reactions.[592] Leukemoid reactions can also occur in inflammatory syndromes such as acute glomerulonephritis, acute rheumatoid arthritis, liver failure, and diabetic acidosis or after the administration of iron-containing complexes.[578, 593, 594] Tumor or granulomatous infiltration of bone marrow can also result in the appearance of immature myeloid cells in the peripheral circulation, along with teardrop-shaped erythrocytes and nucleated red blood cells (leukoerythroblastic response). Infants with Down syndrome may develop a transient myeloid leukemoid reaction that appears to arise from an intrinsic intracellular defect in the regulation of neutrophil proliferation and maturation within the bone marrow.[595] Large numbers of circulating blast cells can be present. Leukemoid reactions have also been identified in neonates in association with decreased numbers of megakaryocytes, thrombocytopenia, and congenital skeletal defects.[596]

Clinical States Associated with Alterations of Eosinophil Numbers

EOSINOPHILIA

Eosinophil stimulation most commonly occurs after repetitive or prolonged exposure to antigens, especially when they are deposited in the tissues and elicit hypersensitivity reactions, whether of the immediate (IgE-mediated) or delayed (T lymphocyte–mediated) type. Unlike neutrophilia, stimulation of eosinophilia is T lymphocyte–dependent and underlies the immune response to metazoan parasites.[69, 597]

There are differences between eosinophils obtained from normal individuals and those obtained from patients with eosinophilia.[69, 72, 598] "Resting" eosinophils from patients with eosinophilia and normal eosinophils stimulated *in vitro* both demonstrate a reduced cell surface charge, enhanced transport of glucose into the cell, and an activation of demonstrable acid phosphatase in the specific granules. Also, whereas oxidative metabolism of normal eosinophils is similar to that of normal neutrophils, both resting cells and cells stimulated during phagocytosis from patients with eosinophilia demonstrate a significant enhancement of oxidative metabolism. Thus, eosinophils from patients with eosinophilia appear to be significantly activated compared with normal eosinophils. A multilobulated eosinophil nucleus can be seen in patients with eosinophilia.

Allergy is the most common cause of eosinophilia in children in the United States[599] (Table 21–17). Acute allergic reactions may cause leukemoid eosinophilic responses, with eosinophil counts exceeding 20,000 cells/μL, whereas chronic allergy is rarely associated with eosinophil counts of more than 2000 cells/μL.[600] During an immediate hypersensitivity reaction, mast cells and basophils release ECFA, which is chemotactic for eosinophils[77] and may be related to the observation that tissues rich in mast cells, such as those found in the respiratory and gastrointestinal tracts, are particularly common

TABLE 21–17. Causes of Eosinophilia

ALLERGIC DISORDERS

Asthma
Hay fever
Acute urticaria
Drug reaction
Allergic bronchopulmonary aspergillosis

DEMATITIS

Pemphigus
Pemphigoid
Atopic dermatitis

PARASITIC AND OTHER INFECTIONS

Metazoan infection
Pneumocystis carinii infection
Toxoplasmosis
Amebiasis
Malaria
Scabies
Coccidioidomycosis

TUMORS

Brain tumors
Hodgkin and non-Hodgkin lymphoma
Myeloproliferative disorders

HEREDITARY DISORDERS

Hereditary eosinophilia

GASTROINTESTINAL DISORDERS

Radiation therapy of intra-abdominal neoplasms
Regional enteritis
Milk precipitin disease
Chronic active hepatitis

HYPEREOSINOPHILIC SYNDROMES

Löffler's syndrome
Eosinophilic leukemia
Polyarteritis nodosa

MISCELLANEOUS

Immunodeficiency disorders
Peritoneal dialysis
Thrombocytopenia with absent radius
Familial reticuloendotheliosis
Episodic angioedema associated with eosinophilia

sites for eosinophil tissue invasion. A variety of skin diseases have been associated with eosinophilia,[601, 602] the best documented being atopic dermatitis, eczema, pemphigus, acute urticaria, and toxic epidermal necrolysis. Gastrointestinal disorders may also be associated with eosinophilia,[601] including ulcerative colitis, which usually involves large numbers of tissue eosinophils associated with a slight elevation in the number of blood eosinophils. Crohn disease, during its symptomatic phases, is usually associated with a slight elevation in the number of blood eosinophils.[603] Both eosinophilic gastroenteritis and milk precipitin disease are associated with a modest elevation in the number of circulating eosinophils.[604] About one third of patients with chronic hepatitis have eosinophilia in excess of 5 percent. Nearly 40 percent of patients being treated for intra-abdominal neoplasms exhibit eosinophilia during the first few weeks after initiation of radiation therapy.

Eosinophilia is found in a significant proportion of most of the immunodeficiency syndromes, especially Wiskott-Aldrich syndrome.[604] Approximately 10 percent of patients with rheumatoid arthritis will develop a mild eosinophilia during the course of their disease. About one third of patients undergoing chronic hemodialysis develop blood eosinophilia without an apparent cause.[605] Similarly, chronic peritoneal dialysis may cause an eosinophilic peritoneal effusion and occasionally an elevated number of eosinophils in the blood.[606] Eosinophilia was described in a significant proportion of patients with congenital heart disease, usually in those types with stenotic lesions.[604] Eosinophilia is also usually present in the syndromes of thrombocytopenia with absent radii and familial reticuloendotheliosis with eosinophilia. A mild eosinophilia may accompany Hodgkin disease in 20 percent of patients; however, on occasion, marked eosinophilia with counts of up to 98 percent can occur.

In general, fungal diseases do not cause eosinophilia, but one dramatic exception is coccidioidomycosis.[604] Although not an invasive infection, allergic bronchopulmonary aspergillosis may be the most common disorder due to a fungal pathogen that causes eosinophilia. In contrast to viral exanthems, scarlet fever is often associated with modest degrees of eosinophilia. Eosinophilia is also observed in cytomegalovirus pneumonia of infancy, cat-scratch disease, infectious lymphocytosis, and occasionally, infectious mononucleosis. Many patients with acute pulmonary tuberculosis show decreased numbers of circulating eosinophils followed by an increase in eosinophil numbers during the convalescent phase.

Outside the United States, parasitic infections are the most common causes of eosinophilia.[607] Infestations by certain parasites, including helminths, induce greater degrees of eosinophilia than do protozoan infestations.[604] Although some parasite antigens appear to be potent immunogens, the eosinophilia resulting from parasitic infection is not due to some unique component of the parasites themselves but rather to a tissue granulomatous response requiring the participation of intact parasites. Other parasites, such as *Giardia lamblia*, *Enterobius vermicularis*, and *Trichuris trichiura*, fail to elicit an eosinophilic response, probably because they remain localized to the intestinal tract and do not enter the systemic circulation.

When parasites invade systemic organs, they may produce clinical symptoms and signs related to the involved organs, such as hepatomegaly and pulmonary infiltrates. These features are further associated with eosinophilic leukocytosis, anemia, and hyperglobulinemia, as are commonly seen in visceral larva migrans from *Toxocara canis*.[608, 609] The patient may be brought for medical attention because of fever, cough, and wheezing. Complications include seizures, encephalitis, myocarditis, retinal lesions (that are often difficult to distinguish from retinoblastoma), and skin nodules on the palms of the hands and soles of the feet. Leukocyte counts may exceed 100,000 cells/μL, with marked eosinophilia persisting from months to years after resolution of symptoms. Polyclonal hypergammaglobulinemia is commonly seen. Increased anti-A and anti-B titers are commonly observed because of cross-reactivity between red cell and parasitic antigens. No specific therapy is available to eradicate the invading parasites responsible for visceral larva migrans, but the condition generally subsides spontaneously within weeks to months. The broad-spectrum anthelminthic agent thiabendazole may relieve symptoms and shorten convalescence.[610]

An elevated blood eosinophil level was observed in several families with no specific association of illness or congenital abnormalities noted.[611] This disorder appears to be a benign one in which the normal regulation of eosinophil production is disturbed. Another syndrome associated with eosinophilia is episodic angioedema associated with eosinophilia.[336, 337] Affected patients have recurrent attacks of fever, urticaria, and angioedema with up to approximately 90,000 eosinophils/μL of blood. Symptoms generally respond to corticosteroid therapy.

HYPEREOSINOPHILIC SYNDROME

The term *hypereosinophilic syndrome* (HES) has been used to describe a broad continuum of illnesses varying from the self-resolving Loeffler pulmonary syndrome to severe chronic (and ultimately fatal) syndromes. HES is now defined as a persistent eosinophilia in patients that meets the following criteria: (1) eosinophilia as indicated by an eosinophil count of at least 1500 cells/μL for longer than 6 months (or death within 6 months), (2) lack of other diagnoses to explain the eosinophilia, and (3) signs and symptoms of organ involvement by infiltrating eosinophils.[612] HES probably represents a heterogeneous group of disorders, some of which have some resemblance to myeloproliferative states[612–614]; the relationship of HES to "eosinophilic leukemia" has been controversial, but the latter appears to be more appropriately considered a subgroup of acute myeloid leukemia[613] as discussed later.

The majority of patients with HES are male, with the greatest incidence occurring in the fourth decade of life, although there are rare reports of affected children.[612] The total leukocyte count is typically 10,000 to 30,000 cells/μL, of which 30 to 70 percent are eosinophils. Leukocyte alkaline phosphatase levels can be normal, decreased, or increased. The bone marrow is usually hypercellular with a predominance of eosinophils. Although dysplastic changes are occasionally seen, expansions of lineages other than eosinophils are rare, as is myelofibrosis. The presence of increased myeloblasts or numerous dysplastic cells suggests an alternative diagnosis, such as AML or a MDS. However, chromosomal abnormalities were reported in some patients with clinical features of HES.[615, 616] Clinical manifestations result from tissue infiltration by eosinophils and the release of eosinophil granule products that cause tissue damage. Symptoms include nonspecific findings of fever, weight loss, and fatigue. Hepatosplenomegaly can be seen. Cardiac damage is the major cause of morbidity and mortality in HES and includes endocardial fibrosis and formation of mural thrombi with infiltrating eosinophils. These findings can also be seen from eosinophilia from many other causes, including parasitic infection, drug reactions, or malignancies. Pulmonary and skin involvement with urticarial or nodular lesions is common. Neuropathies, encephalopathy, and central nervous system thromboemboli can also occur. Corticosteroids are used as first-line therapy for symptomatic patients, and hydroxyurea was beneficial in patients who do not show a response to steroids. Vinca alkaloids are also effective in HES and can cause a rapid decrease in blood eosinophil counts in 1 to 3 days.[613, 617]

The underlying causes of HES are unknown and are probably heterogeneous. Elevated levels of IL-5, which is considered to be the dominant cytokine that stimulates eosinophil production, were reported in HES and also in patients with eosinophilia from other causes.[613] Transgenic mice expressing high IL-5 levels exhibit chronic marked eosinophilia but do not have evidence of cardiac or other organ damage, suggesting that other factors are involved in producing the tissue injury seen in HES.[613]

The hypereosinophilic syndrome can generally be distinguished from the M4Eo variant of AML, which is characterized by myelomonocytic blasts with eosinophilia and was referred to in the past as "eosinophilic leukemia."[618] In acute leukemia, there is typically a marked increase in the number of immature eosinophils in the blood or bone marrow, tissue infiltration with immature cells of predominantly an eosinophilic type, and also anemia and thrombocytopenia. The eosinophils in M4Eo leukemia have an additional granule population that stains with periodic acid-Schiff and chloroacetate esterase and that is lacking in normal eosinophils. Almost all patients in the M4Eo leukemia subgroup have abnormalities in chromosome 16.[619]

EOSINOPENIA

Eosinopenia is not uncommon but is seldom recognized clinically, because its diagnosis requires an absolute eosinophil count.[620] The potential diagnostic usefulness of identification of eosinopenia is rarely recognized. Because it occurs in relatively limited circumstances, the finding of eosinopenia can be of value clinically. Eosinopenia may be produced by at least two mechanisms: (1) acute stress, with resultant stimulation of adrenal corticoids or release of epinephrine (or both), and (2) acute inflammatory states. The immediate eosinopenia after administration of glucocorticoids appears to be due to reversible sequestration of eosinophils at an unknown site, presumably in the marginating pool within the vascular compartment. The mechanism underlying this effect is unknown. Acute inflammation is associated with alterations in eosinophil distribution and production that resemble those observed after corticosteroid administration. Thus, there is an initial peripheral sequestration and an initial increase in marrow eosinophils, followed after 36 hours by a decrease in marrow production. At least part of this response occurs independently of adrenal corticoid release. Acute infections associated with a marked inflammatory response, including all invasive bacteria and most acute viral infections, are often associated with eosinopenia persisting during the period of the fever. Administration of appropriate antimicrobial therapy is followed by a return of the eosinophil count to normal levels. Persistent infections cause a less predictable eosinophil reaction.

Basophilia and Basophilopenia

Basophilia is commonly associated with hypersensitivity reactions of the immediate type[621] (Table 21–18). Basophil levels may be elevated in ulcerative colitis, juvenile rheumatoid arthritis, iron deficiency, and chronic renal failure and after radiation therapy.[622, 623, 630, 631] Basophil levels are often increased in chronic myeloproliferative disorders, particularly chronic myelogenous leukemia. In this disorder, basophils may appear abnormal both morphologically and ultrastructurally. Basophil counts exceeding 30 percent can occur during the course of chronic myelogenous leukemia; marked basophilia often heralds the terminal phase.[632] Occasionally, patients with chronic myelogenous leukemia may develop circulating basophil counts as high as 40 to 80 percent of the total leukocyte count at the beginning of the disease. Many of these patients will have developed symptoms attributed to the release of biogenic amines or heparin-like material from degranulated basophils.[633] Such individuals may benefit from the administration of antihistamines. Increased numbers of marrow basophils may occur in MDS and sideroblastic anemia when it appears to reflect disruption of normal maturational controls. Basophilopenia occurs in association with eosinophilopenia, for example, during acute infection or after the administration of glucocorticoids or epinephrine.[624, 625, 634] Also, basophil counts are diminished in thyrotoxicosis and after treatment with thyroid hormones, and conversely they may be increased in myxedema.[634]

Monocytosis and Monocytopenia

The average absolute blood monocyte count varies with the age of the patient, and this must be taken into account when monocytosis is assessed. During the first 2 weeks of life, the absolute monocyte count is more than 1000 cells/μL.[635] With increasing age, there is a gradual decline in the monocyte count until it reaches a plateau of 400 cells/μL in adulthood. Monocytosis may therefore be defined as a total monocyte count of more than 500 cells/μL. Given the widespread importance of monocytes, as discussed earlier, it is not surprising that many clinical disorders produce monocytosis (Table 21–19). Typically, monocytosis is associated with certain bacterial, protozoal, and rickettsial infections such as subacute bacterial endocarditis, tuberculosis, syphilis, Rocky Mountain spotted fever, and kala-azar.[636] In malignant disorders such as

preleukemia, AML, chronic myelogenous leukemia, and lymphomas, monocytosis can also be observed.[636, 637] Approximately 25 percent of all patients with Hodgkin disease have monocytosis, although its presence does not correlate with prognosis.[638] Monocytosis has also been noted in a wide variety of inflammatory and immune disorders, including collagen vascular diseases, sarcoidosis, and gastrointestinal disorders such as ulcerative colitis and regional enteritis.[636] Finally, monocytosis occurs in some forms of neutropenia and after splenectomy. As mentioned earlier, patients recovering from myelosuppressive chemotherapy exhibit monocytosis immediately before the return of their neutrophils.

Monocytopenia was observed after glucocorticoid administration and in infections associated with endotoxemia.[639, 640] In the latter case, systemic activation of complement occurs with the deposition of C5a on the surface of monocytes, leading to their aggregation and clearance. In contrast to the profound granulocytopenia and lymphopenia associated with irradiation or cytotoxic chemotherapy, noncirculating monocytes and tissue macrophages are relatively resistant to these agents.[641]

Besides the lysosomal storage diseases, there is one disorder, congenital osteopetrosis, in which an important qualitative abnormality in a specialized tissue macrophage has been described. Congenital osteopetrosis is an autosomal recessive disease seen in infants and is characterized by the progressive obliteration of the bone marrow space by the formation of new bone.[134] The disorder is caused by a failure of the osteoclast to resorb bone matrix. As discussed in an earlier section, human infantile osteopetrosis is associated with normal numbers of dysfunctional osteoclasts and not an absence of M-CSF as for the *op/op* osteopetrotic mouse. Recombinant human IFN-γ (rIFN-γ) was shown to increase bone resorption and improve hematopoietic marrow function in children with congenital osteopetrosis.[139]

DISORDERS OF GRANULOCYTE FUNCTION

Overview

Inherited and acquired clinical disorders have been identified that are caused by abnormalities in one or more steps of phagocyte function—adhesion, chemotaxis, ingestion, degranulation, and oxidative metabolism. Consistent with the critical role of phagocyte function in host defense, patients with these disorders often have recurrent, difficult-to-treat bacterial and fungal infections. This group of disorders can be classified according to a scheme on the basis of the phagocyte function primarily affected. As will be seen, in some of the disorders abnormalities in several phagocyte functions are seen. In these instances, the primary functional defect will be used to classify the disorder.

During the past 25 years, numerous articles have been published that describe abnormalities in phagocyte function, often associated with other diseases. In many of these reports, marginal abnormalities were noted using *in vitro* phagocyte assays, with little evidence that the observed defects were responsible for the clinical predisposition to infection. In this section, disorders in which good correlations exist between the phagocyte abnormality and the clinical condition will be emphasized. In several of these disorders, particularly LAD and CGD, the molecular basis for the functional abnormality is well understood. Because these conditions serve as prototypes for understanding the less well-characterized phagocyte disorders, the underlying biochemical and molecular genetic aspects of these conditions will be reviewed in some depth.

One final point should be emphasized. In clinical practice, most physicians encounter a large number of patients who suffer from recurrent bacterial infections. Although it is true that nearly all patients with well-characterized phagocyte abnormalities have recurrent infections, the converse is seldom true. Most patients with impressive histories of persistent and repeated infections do not have identifiable qualitative or quantitative phagocyte abnormalities. Therefore, the major disorders described in the following sections account for only a fraction of patients with recurrent infections. This point will be discussed further in the section describing the laboratory evaluation of phagocyte function.

Disorders of Adhesion

LEUKOCYTE ADHESION DEFICIENCY TYPE I

Leukocyte adhesion deficiency type I (LAD I) is a rare, autosomal recessive disorder in which phagocyte adhesion, chemotaxis, and ingestion of C3bi opsonized microbes are impaired owing to mutations in the gene for CD18 β subunit of the β_2 integrins. As a result, the expression of β_2 integrins on leukocyte cell surfaces is reduced or absent.[193, 642–645] More than 100 patients with this disorder have been described in the literature to date. The hallmark of LAD I is the occurrence of repeated, often severe bacterial and fungal infections without the accumulation of pus despite persistent granulocytosis (Table 21–20). The clinical syndrome is heterogeneous and is related to the severity of the reduction in β_2 integrin expression. A severe clinical phenotype is seen when fewer than 0.3 percent of the normal amount of β_2 integrins are present, whereas a more moderate phenotype is observed with levels of 2.5 to 11 percent of normal. Patients with the severe form of LAD I, which is the more common form of the disease, are generally seen in early infancy with omphalitis and delayed separation of the umbilical cord. Recurrent necrotic and indolent infections of skin, mucous membranes, and the gastrointestinal tract are also seen, including perirectal abscesses, which often heal poorly. An aggressive form of gingivitis and periodontitis is characteristic, and ulcerative lesions of the tongue and pharynx can be seen. Otitis media and pneumonia are also often encountered. The majority of infections are caused by *S. aureus* and gram-negative enteric bacteria. Fungal infections also occur, particularly from *Candida albicans* and *Aspergillus* species.

The molecular basis for LAD I was first suggested by Crowley and colleagues,[646] who found that neutrophils from a patient with this clinical syndrome lacked a high-molecular-weight membrane glycoprotein. Because the patient's neutrophils neither adhered to plastic surfaces nor underwent an oxidative burst when exposed to

TABLE 21–18. Disorders Associated with Basophilia and Basophilopenia*

BASOPHILIA

Hypersensitivity reactions
    Drug and food hypersensitivity
    Urticaria
Inflammation and infection
    Ulcerative colitis
    Rheumatoid arthritis
    Influenza
    Chickenpox
    Smallpox
    Tuberculosis
Myeloproliferative diseases
    Chronic myelogenous leukemia
    Myeloid metaplasia

BASOPHILOPENIA

Glucocorticoid administration
Thyrotoxicosis

*See references 621 through 629

TABLE 21–19. Disorders Associated with Monocytosis and Monocytopenia*

MONOCYTOSIS

Hematologic disorders and lymphomas
    Preleukemia
    Acute myelogenous leukemia
    Lymphoma (Hodgkin and non-Hodgkin)
    Chronic neutropenia
    Histocytic medullary reticulosis
Collagen vascular disease
    Systemic lupus erythematosus
    Rheumatoid arthritis
    Myositis
Granulomatous disease
    Ulcerative colitis
    Regional enteritis
    Sarcoidosis
Infection
    Subacute bacterial endocarditis
    Tuberculosis
    Syphilis
    Some protozoal and rickettsial infections (e.g., Rocky
    Mountain spotted fever, kala-azar)
    Fever of unknown origin
Malignant disease (usually carcinoma)
Miscellaneous disorders
    Postsplenectomy state
    Tetrachloroethane poisoning

MONOCYTOPENIA

Glucocorticoid administration
Infections associated with endotoxemia

*For review, see reference 636, as well as references 636 through 638.

serum-opsonized particles, it was hypothesized that the missing glycoprotein was responsible for both adhesion and cell particle interactions. A similar glycoprotein was also found to be missing in several other patients,[647, 648] which proved to be the α subunit (CD11b) of the Mac-1 β_2 integrin (CD11b/CD18).[649] It was subsequently rec-

TABLE 21–20. Clinical Presentations of Leukocyte Adhesion Deficiency, Type I*

Chronic Conditions	Acute Infections	Infecting Organisms	Other
Persistent granulocytosis (12,000–100,000 cells/μL)	Omphalitis	*Staphylococcus aureus*	Delayed umbilical cord separation
Gingivitis	Cutaneous abscesses and cellulitis (possibly invasive)	*Escherichia coli*	
Periodontitis	Perirectal abscesses and cellulitis (possibly invasive)	*Pseudomonas aeruginosa*	
Stomatitis	Facial cellulitis	*Pseudomonas* species	
Impaired wound healing	Sepsis	*Proteus*	
	Pneumonia	*Klebsiella*	
	Laryngotracheitis	*Candida albicans*	
	Peritonitis	*Aspergillus* species	
	Necrotizing enterocolitis	Viral (slightly increased risk)	
	Sinusitis		
	Esophagitis		
	Erosive gastritis		
	Appendicitis		
	Otitis media		

*Each list is arranged in approximate order of occurrence based on reviews summarizing various series of patients with leukocyte adhesion deficiency (see text for references).

ognized that the levels of the leukocyte β$_2$ integrins (see Fig. 21–4) were absent or severely deficient in LAD I.[193, 642–644] With deficient β$_2$ integrin expression a variety of leukocyte adhesion-dependent activities are impaired, with neutrophil function being the most significantly affected.[642–644, 646, 647, 650] In addition to their role in mediating adhesive interactions during neutrophil emigration and phagocytosis, signaling through β$_2$ integrins potentiates virtually all functional responses of adherent neutrophils, including production of reactive oxidants and degranulation.[205] Hence, neutrophils in LAD I have a profound defect in their ability to become fully activated.

One of the striking findings in LAD I is the failure of neutrophils to migrate to sites of inflammation. The initial phases of neutrophil adhesion to the endothelium (see Fig. 21–2), which is mediated by selectins and their sialylated counter-receptors, is normal in LAD. However, because of the absence or marked deficiency in Mac-1 (CD11b/CD18) expression, neutrophils in LAD I are neither able to attach firmly to the endothelium nor undergo transendothelial migration.[182, 651] Neutrophil intravascular survival is prolonged,[652] presumably related to deficient adhesion and migration. *In vitro* assays of neutrophil adhesion to glass or to cultured endothelial cells and of neutrophil chemotaxis also exhibit marked abnormalities. An exception to these observations is neutrophil adhesion and emigration in the pulmonary capillary bed, which can be mediated by CD11/CD18-independent mechanisms under some circumstances.[210] In autopsy tissue from a patient with severe LAD I, no neutrophils were observed in infected appendiceal and skin lesions, whereas many neutrophils were seen within the alveolar spaces.[210] In contrast to neutrophils, other leukocytes (monocytes, eosinophils, and lymphocytes) express the β$_1$ integrin, VLA-4 and are able to utilize this adhesion molecule to emigrate into inflammatory sites throughout the body.[182]

Another major defect in LAD I is the inability of neutrophils and monocytes to recognize microorganisms coated with the opsonic complement fragment C3bi,

since Mac-1 is the C3bi receptor.[642, 643, 646, 650, 653] The binding of C3bi normally triggers neutrophil degranulation, phagocytosis, and activation of the respiratory burst, but these responses are diminished or absent in neutrophils from patients with LAD I. Control experiments have consistently demonstrated, however, that these responses can be at least partially activated in LAD I neutrophils by opsonins (e.g., IgG and C3b) that have different cell surface receptors or by soluble agonists that bypass Mac-1.[205, 646]

Defects in lymphocyte functions dependent on LFA-1 (CD11a/CD18) have been observed in many patients with LAD I *in vitro*. These include proliferative responses to mitogens, NK cell function, and lymphocyte-mediated killing.[654–656] Nevertheless, most patients with LAD I manifest few, if any, problems related to lymphocyte dysfunction *in vivo*. Cutaneous hypersensitivity reactions are normal, and patients are generally not unusually susceptible to viral infections, including varicella. However, one patient has died of an overwhelming respiratory infection with picornavirus, and one or more episodes of aseptic meningitis were reported in three patients.[642]

Molecular Basis of Leukocyte Adhesion Deficiency

The fact that LAD I involves a deficiency of all leukocyte CD11/CD18 integrins focused attention on the common β$_2$ chain (CD18) of this integrin family as the site of the molecular defect. This hypothesis has proved to be correct. Expression of the leukocyte integrin α subunits is normal in LAD I, but these are not transported to the cell surface because the β$_2$ chain is absent or contains mutations that disrupt β$_2$ structure or its interaction with the α subunit.[657] Mutations in more than 20 patients with LAD I have now been characterized at the molecular genetic level, and all have been found in the β$_2$ gene, which is localized on chromosome 21q22.3. A heterogeneous group of mutations have been identified. Many patients are compound heterozygotes for two different mutant alleles, whereas others are homozygous for a single mutant allele. About one half of patients with LAD I in whom genetic defects were characterized have point mutations that result in single amino acid substitutions in CD18, which almost invariably reside between amino acids 111 and 361.[658–666] This protein domain is highly conserved among all β subunits and appears to be important for interaction with the α subunit. In this LAD I subgroup, approximately one half of patients exhibit a low level of CD11/CD18 cell surface expression and moderate disease, with the remainder having no expression and the severe phenotype. mRNA splicing abnormalities resulting in either deletion or insertion of amino acids in the conserved extracellular domain of CD18 have also been described in two kindreds.[665, 667] Finally, small deletions within the coding sequences of the CD18 gene disrupting the reading frame[663, 664, 668] or a nucleotide substitution resulting in a premature termination signal[668] have been reported.

There are several animal models of LAD I. These include the occurrences of a severe form of the disease in an Irish setter born of a mother-son mating[669, 670] and in Holstein cattle.[671–673] In the latter case, affected calves could be traced to a common sire and were shown to be homozygous for a point amino acid substitution in the conserved extracellular domain of CD18.[674] Finally, a CD18-deficient mouse with 2 to 6 percent of normal β₂ integrin expression was produced by gene targeting.[675]

Diagnosis and Treatment of Leukocyte Adhesion Deficiency Type I

The diagnosis of LAD I should be suspected in any infant or child who is seen with unusually severe or recurrent infections or periodontitis accompanied by persistently elevated peripheral blood neutrophil counts (Table 21–20). Although this laboratory finding may simply represent a leukemoid reaction in an otherwise immunologically normal infant, the diagnosis of LAD I should nonetheless be considered, particularly if a paucity of neutrophils at affected sites delayed separation of the umbilical cord is seen. The infant with delayed separation of the umbilical cord who is healthy and has normal blood counts is unlikely to have LAD I. Although the mean age of cord separation has been reported to be 7 to 15 days, 10 percent of healthy infants can have cord separation at 3 weeks of age or later.[676, 677] A rare cause of recurrent, deep-seated tissue infections in association with neutrophilia and poor formation of pus is a mutation in the Rac2 GTPase, which leads to neutrophil signaling defects affecting chemotaxis and adhesion (see section on disorders of chemotaxis).

The diagnosis of LAD I is established by flow cytometric analysis to assess cell surface expression of any of the β₂ integrin α (CD11) subunits or the shared CD18 subunit. Monoclonal antibodies to each are commercially available. Although they are not needed to establish the diagnosis of LAD I, *in vitro* functional assays of neutrophils obtained from these patients demonstrate striking defects in adherence, chemotaxis, and C3bi-mediated phagocytosis and respiratory burst activation. Carriers of LAD I can also generally be identified by flow cytometric analysis, whichtypically show expression of approximately 50 percent of the normal level of β₂ integrins on leukocyte cell surfaces.[642, 678] Prenatal diagnosis of LAD I can be made by one of two methods. In families with known mutations in the two CD18 alleles, chorionic villus or amniocyte DNA can be analyzed for the presence of the mutations. Alternatively, fetal blood granulocytes, which express Mac-1 by 20 weeks of gestation, can be assayed for expression of β₂ integrin using flow cytometric analysis.[645, 679]

Treatment of LAD I depends on the clinical severity of the disorder. In patients with the moderate clinical phenotype, who typically have some residual β₂ integrin expression, cutaneous and oral infections should be treated aggressively as they occur. The prophylactic use of trimethoprim-sulfamethoxazole appears to be beneficial. Aggressive prophylactic treatment for periodontal disease is also advisable in the form of regular cleaning of teeth by a dentist and the use of antimicrobial oral rinses such as chlorhexidine gluconate. The clinical management of patients with moderate LAD I should be guided by the fact that these patients are still at risk of dying of overwhelming infection, with 75 percent succumbing between the ages of 12 and 32.[645] The prognosis for patients with severe LAD I is even more grim, with a high incidence of death due to infection before age 2.[193, 643, 680] Bone marrow transplantation is recommended for these patients.[643, 645, 681, 682] The absence of LFA-1 may decrease the chance of graft rejection even with only partially compatible HLA matching.[682]

Because LAD I is caused by a defect in a single gene, transfer of a normal CD18 sequence into a patient's hematopoietic stem cells using retroviral or other vectors could, in principle, correct the defect. Preliminary *in vitro* studies using Epstein-Barr virus (EBV)–transformed B-lymphocyte cell lines from patients with LAD I and *in vivo* studies using a mouse system have shown the feasibility of this approach.[657, 683, 684] High-level expression of the transferred CD18 sequence may not be necessary to confer substantial clinical benefits, based on the milder course of the disease observed in patients with some residual β₂ integrin expression. At present, a major obstacle in applying this approach to clinical use is the development of techniques that achieve high-level gene transfer into human hematopoietic stem cells.[685, 686]

LEUKOCYTE ADHESION DEFICIENCY TYPE II

A clinical syndrome similar to LAD but associated with defective selectin-mediated adhesion was reported in three unrelated boys of Moslem Arab origin and one boy of Turkish origin and was termed *leukocyte adhesion deficiency type II* (LAD II).[687–689] The Arab patients were the offspring of consanguineous marriages, and the parents of the Turkish patient came from the same small village, suggesting an autosomal recessive inheritance. As in CD11/CD18-deficient LAD, these children suffered from periodontitis, recurrent cellulitis, otitis media, and pneumonia without the formation of pus despite peripheral leukocyte counts of 30,000 to 150,000 cells/μL. However, neutrophils had normal levels of CD18, and infectious symptoms were not as serious as in those in LAD I. Also, in contrast to persons with classic LAD I, these boys had short stature, a distinctive facial appearance with a flat face and depressed nasal bridge, and severe mental retardation.

Furthermore, all had the rare Bombay (hh) blood phenotype, in which red cells express a nonfucosylated variant of the H antigen. Red cells were also secretor negative and Lewis antigen negative. The Bombay and nonsecretor phenotypes are caused by deficient formation of Fucα1→2 Gal linkages in ABO blood group core antigens, whereas the Lewis antigen–negative phenotype is due to failure to synthesize Fucα1→4 *N*-acetylglucosamine (GlcNAc) and Fucα1→3 GlcNAc moieties. Neutrophils from both boys were found to lack immunoreactive sialyl-Lewis X structures, which also contain fucose and were unable to adhere to activated human umbilical cord endothelial cells that expressed E-selectin.[687]

Thus, the functional defect in neutrophils in LAD II appears to be caused by the absence of neutrophil sialyl Lewis X structures that serve as selectin counter-receptors. Intravital microscopic studies revealed a significant decrease in neutrophil rolling on activated endothelial cells *in vivo*,[651] consistent with the role of selectin-mediated adhesion in this process (see Fig. 21–2). However, chemoattractant-induced tight adhesion and emigration of neutrophils in LAD II are normal, both of which are severely impaired in LAD I.[651]

The defect in fucose metabolism in LAD II cells has recently been shown to insert from point mutations in the Golgi GDP-fucose transporter, which was cloned by complementation of cells derived from patients with LAD II.[690, 691] All of the Arab patients have the same nucleotide substitution in the Golgi GDP-fucose transporter mRNA, which alters an amino acid in a transmembrane domain, whereas the Turkish patient has a different nucleotide alteration that results in an amino acid substitution in a different transmembrane domain of the transporter.[690, 691] All patients were homozygous for their mutation, whereas their parents were heterozygous, consistent with autosomal recessive inheritance. The different mutations may explain why the Turkish patient had some response to oral fucose therapy, with increased expression of certain fucosylated ligands and improved clinical symptoms except mental retardation, but the Arab children did not.[692–694] It is speculated that the mutation in the Turkish child leads to a decrease in transport affinity for GDP-fucose, which can be overcome by higher concentrations of fucose, whereas the mutant protein in Arab children has normal affinity for GDP-fucose but decreased transport activity.[689]

ACQUIRED DISORDERS OF ADHERENCE

Neutrophils may exhibit decreased adhesiveness after exposure to a variety of drugs, the most common being corticosteroids and epinephrine.[571, 695, 696] Clinically, the diminished adhesiveness induced by these drugs is manifested by a dramatic increase in the total neutrophil count in the blood as cells from the marginated pool are quickly released into the circulating pool. Although the mechanism by which corticosteroids alter adherence is not known, epinephrine and other β-adrenergic agonists exert their effect indirectly by causing endothelial cells to release cAMP, which in turn impairs the ability of neutrophils to adhere.[571, 697]

The adhesiveness in neutrophils can be dramatically increased in a variety of clinical conditions that have in common the formation of biologically active complement fragments: gram-negative bacterial sepsis, severe thermal injury, pancreatitis, trauma, and exposure of neutrophils to artificial membrane surfaces during hemodialysis and cardiopulmonary bypass.[473, 474, 698–700] In these various conditions, the generation of complement fragments leads to activation of neutrophils and enhanced adhesiveness, possibly owing to enhanced expression of β₂ integrins. Under these conditions, neutrophils undergo increased aggregation with each other and become trapped within capillary beds, such as those in the lungs.[701] It is believed that the aggregated neutrophils then generate toxic oxygen radicals and release proteases that conspire to damage structural protein such as collagen and elastin.[218]

Amphotericin B has been associated with increased neutrophil aggregation, particularly when administered in conjunction with the transfusions of granulocytes that were harvested by filtration (rather than by centrifugation).[702, 703] It is possible that the enhanced aggregation is medicated by up-regulation of surface β₂ integrins induced both by the amphotericin B and by the filters used to harvest the cells.

Disorders of Chemotaxis

The directed migration into sites of infection and inflammation involves a complex series of events. As reviewed in the beginning of this chapter, the generation of chemotactic signals and their binding to specific receptors on the phagocyte surface lead to the generation of intracellular second messengers. These intracellular signals, in turn, trigger changes in adhesiveness and in the actin cytoskeleton that result in adhesion to the endothelium and chemotaxis into the inflamed tissue site. Given the numerous cellular functions involved in chemotaxis, it is perhaps not surprising that impaired phagocyte chemotaxis has been observed in a large number of clinical conditions.[704] Some of the more important syndromes are listed in Table 21–21. These disorders have been classified according to the mechanisms thought to be responsible for defective chemotaxis, which are related to either abnormalities in the production or inhibition of chemotactic factors or to defects in the phagocyte itself involving adhesiveness and locomotion. In some instances, abnormal chemotaxis is one component of a disorder that involves multiple defects.

In many of the reports describing defective *in vitro* chemotaxis of neutrophils from various clinical conditions, it is not clear whether the increased number of infections observed clinically is due to the observed chemotactic abnormality or to medical complications of the underlying disorder (such as malnutrition or exposure to nosocomial infection). Further complicating the interpretation of these reports is the fact that the *in vitro* assays for chemotaxis are subject to laboratory artifacts and may not accurately reflect the *in vivo* extracellular environment. These limitations apply to the micropore filter method developed by Boyden[705] and by Smith and colleagues[706] as well as to the under-agarose technique.[707] The former assay system consists of a chamber with a horizontal filter membrane separating two compartments. The upper compartment contains phagocytes that

TABLE 21–21. Clinical Conditions Associated with Impaired Neutrophil Chemotaxis

DEFECT IN GENERATION OF CHEMOTACTIC AGENTS

Familial deficiency of C1r, C2, C4
Familial deficiency of C3, C5
Other abnormalities of complement pathways (e.g., systemic lupus erythematosus, immature complement system in neonates, diabetes mellitus, C5 dysfunction, chronic hemodialysis, glomerulonephritis)

EXCESSIVE PRODUCTION OF NORMAL CHEMOTACTIC FACTOR INACTIVATORS

Hodgkin disease
Cirrhosis of the liver
Sarcoidosis
Lepromatous leprosy

INHIBITORS OF THE NEUTROPHIL RESPONSE TO CHEMOTACTIC FACTORS

Hyperimmunoglobulin E syndrome
Localized juvenile periodontitis
Immune complex diseases (rheumatoid arthritis)
IgA paraproteinemia states
Solid tumors
Bone marrow transplantation
Drugs (ethanol, antithymocyte globulin)

DEACTIVATION (DOWN-REGULATION) BY INCREASED LEVELS OF CHEMOTACTIC FACTORS

Wiskott-Aldrich syndrome
C5a generation in plasma (hemodialysis)
Bacterial sepsis

PHAGOCYTE DEFECTS

Neutrophil actin dysfunction
Localized juvenile periodontitis
Neonatal neutrophils
Leukocyte adhesion deficiency
Chédiak-Higashi syndrome
Specific granule deficiency

MISCELLANEOUS DEFECTS

Hypophosphatemia
Shwachman-Diamond syndrome
Burn patients

migrate through the micropore filter in response to chemotactic solutions that fill the lower compartment. The under-agarose assay uses a similar principle in that neutrophils in one agarose well migrate toward a chemoattractant in another. Phagocyte motility *in vivo* can be measured by the skin window technique of Rebuck and Crowley,[708] in which a superficial dermal abrasion is produced in the patient and the appearance of inflammatory cells in the lesion is monitored over a 24-hour period. Because of difficulties in standardizing the dermal lesion, variable results may be obtained with this method. Moreover, the assay can measure only the response of phagocytes to the chemotactic signals generated by this type of sterile injury.

As outlined in Table 21–21, several of the conditions associated with impaired neutrophil chemotaxis are due to complement deficiencies and other immunodeficiency syndromes (e.g., Wiskott-Aldrich syndrome). These disorders are discussed elsewhere in this text. In addition,

several disorders of phagocyte function (LAD, CHS, and specific granule deficiency) are reviewed in other sections of this chapter. This section focuses on clinical conditions in which there is evidence that a chemotactic defect plays a major contribution in decreased resistance to bacterial and fungal infections.

HYPERIMMUNOGLOBULIN E SYNDROME

The hyperimmunoglobulin E (hyper-IgE) syndrome (see also Chapter 23) is a relatively rare disorder characterized by markedly elevated serum levels of IgE (often greater than 2000 IU/mL), serious recurrent staphylococcal infections of the skin and lower respiratory tract, pneumatoceles, chronic pruritic dermatitis, and skeletal and dental abnormalities.[709–714] The key features of hyper-IgE syndrome are summarized in Table 21–22. Neutrophils from patients with this syndrome exhibit a variable, but at times severe, chemotactic defect.[709, 715–717] This syndrome was originally known as *Job syndrome* when it was first reported in 1966 in two red-haired, fair-skinned females who had hyperextensible joints and "cold" abscesses that lacked the usual characteristics of inflammation.[710] However, it is now known that only a small fraction of patients with hyper-IgE syndrome have red hair or hyperextensible joints, and thus, Job syndrome may be a variant subset of hyper-IgE syndrome. In larger series of patients the disease has been found in both males and females and also in other ethnic groups, including blacks and Asians. The mode of inheritance has not been firmly established, although familial patterns suggest an autosomal dominant inheritance with variable expressivity.[709, 711, 713, 714] Sporadic forms can also occur.

The clinical manifestations of the hyper-IgE syndrome are often severe and usually become apparent during infancy. Staphylococcal furuncles of the head and neck as well as chronic dermatitis are seen most often in younger patients. Chronic candidiasis of the mucosa and nail beds is also common and can occur in children. Recurrent staphylococcal pneumonia is a common problem as patients grow older and can be complicated by the formation of persistent pneumatoceles that can become superinfected with *Haemophilus influenzae*, gram-negative bacteria, or *Aspergillus*.[718] Chronic infections of the ears, sinuses, and eyes (keratoconjunctivitis) are seen, and septic arthritis and osteomyelitis have been observed. Dental and bone abnormalities are also common features of the hyper-IgE syndrome. A delay in shedding of or failure to shed primary teeth occurs in the majority of patients. Hyperextensible joints and scoliosis are often seen. Osteopenia of unknown etiology is observed in many patients, and there is also an increased risk of fractures of the long bones and the vertebral bodies, even in the absence of osteopenia.[713, 714] Coarse facial features characterized by a broad nasal bridge and a prominent nose are evident in the majority of patients by the time they reach the teenage years. Craniosynostosis can also occur.

The molecular basis of the hyper-IgE syndrome is unknown. The immunologic manifestations were proposed to reflect an underlying defect in T lymphocytes[719, 720] that is manifested, at least in part, by the greatly reduced production of IFN-γ and TNF.[721, 722]

TABLE 21–22. Summary of Hyperimmunoglobulin E Syndrome

Incidence	More than 200 patients reviewed in the literature
Inheritance	Autosomal dominant with variable expressivity; sporadic forms
Molecular defect	Unknown
Clinical manifestations	"Cold" cutaneous skin abscesses and furuncles
	Chronic eczematoid dermatitis
	Mucocutaneous candidiasis
	Staphylococcal pneumonia, pneumatoceles
	Fungal superinfection of lung cysts
	Coarse facies
	Delayed shedding of primary teeth
	Scoliosis
	Recurrent fractures
	Hyperextensible joints
Laboratory evaluation	Serum IgE > 2500 IU/mL
	Peripheral blood eosinophilia
Differential diagnosis	Atopic dermatitis
	Wiskott-Aldrich syndrome, DiGeorge syndrome
	Hypergammaglobulinemia
	Chronic granulomatous disease
Therapy	Prophylactic antibiotics for *Staphylococcus aureus*
	Aggressive treatment of acute infections with parenteral antibiotics
	Surgical drainage of deep infections and resection of lung cysts
	Monitoring for scoliosis and for fractures
Prognosis	Generally good if managed aggressively

This putative T-cell defect would then explain the hyperproduction of IgE (perhaps caused by the deficiency of IFN-γ) as well as the abnormal antibody responses that were documented in some patients in response to various vaccines.[723] This latter abnormality could directly contribute to the enhanced susceptibility of these patients to infection, whereas the former may reflect an imbalance in the production of various types of immunoglobulin. Patients with hyper-IgE syndrome produce excessive amounts of IgE directed against *S. aureus* at the expense of protective antistaphylococcal IgG.[195, 709] Finally, recurrent bacterial infections in patients with hyper-IgE syndrome may also be aggravated by the chemotactic defect that is periodically observed. How the immunologic abnormalities relate to the dental and skeletal defects that are the other hallmarks of this disorder is not certain.

The diagnosis of hyper-IgE syndrome should be considered in any child with the aforementioned clinical history. A markedly elevated polyclonal serum IgE level and peripheral blood eosinophilia are constant laboratory findings, although IgE levels can fluctuate over time and occasionally decrease to the normal range.[714] Despite the impressive elevations in the serum IgE level, this laboratory finding alone is not diagnostic, because comparably high serum levels of IgE can be seen in patients with atopic dermatitis.[709] Many patients with atopic dermatitis have superficial skin infections and eczema; thus, this disorder must be considered in the differential diagnosis of hyper-IgE syndrome. The two disorders can be distinguished from each other because of the severe and recurrent nature of the staphylococcal furuncles and occurrences of pneumonia seen in patients with hyper-IgE syndrome.

One of the mainstays of therapy for hyper-IgE syndrome is the use of prophylactic antibiotics, such as dicloxacillin or trimethoprim-sulfamethoxazole. These drugs can help prevent staphylococcal infections and should be prescribed at the time of diagnosis. Pneumonia and other deep-seated infections should be treated aggressively with parenteral antibiotics. Patients with hyper-IgE syndrome have an unusual predisposition to development of pneumatoceles as a result of staphylococcal lung infections. If these lesions persist, they should be surgically resected to prevent superinfection by fungal and gram-negative organisms. Delayed shedding of primary teeth may necessitate extraction. Patients should be carefully monitored for scoliosis, and skeletal fractures can occur even after minor trauma. If infections and their complications are managed aggressively, the prognosis for patients with hyper-IgE syndrome is good.

rIFN-γ was investigated as a therapeutic modality for hyper-IgE syndrome based on the observations that this cytokine can suppress IgE synthesis[724, 725] and that IFN-γ production by mononuclear leukocytes from patients with hyper-IgE syndrome is low or absent.[722, 726] In small uncontrolled studies, patients treated with rhIFN-γ (50 μg/m² subcutaneously three times per week) have reported feeling better, and neutrophil chemotaxis *in vitro* was improved.[115, 727] In another report, IgE production by peripheral blood mononuclear cells from patients with hyper-IgE syndrome was decreased by treatment with rhIFN-γ.[728] However, formal clinical trials have not yet been conducted to test the efficacy of IFN-γ in ameliorating the clinical manifestations of hyper-IgE syndrome. Studies on IFN-γ in the treatment of CGD suggest that this cytokine may reduce the rate of occurrence of infections by mechanisms that do not necessarily reverse the underlying defect in respiratory burst oxidase function.[729] IFN-γ administration may therefore have a general benefit in other immunodeficiencies, such as hyper-IgE syndrome.

NEUTROPHIL ACTIN DYSFUNCTION

Primary defects in neutrophil actin polymerization are exceedingly rare. The first such instance, described by Boxer and colleagues in 1974,[730] was in a male infant who suffered from recurrent skin infections due to *S. aureus* and a cutaneous-cecal fistula complicated by *Streptococcus faecalis* sepsis. Despite a marked neutrophilia, sites of infections were devoid of neutrophils and healed slowly. The patient's neutrophils showed markedly diminished chemotaxis and a decreased capacity to ingest serum-opsonized particles. He underwent a bone marrow transplant with transient engraftment of normally functioning neutrophils but died of infectious complications. The underlying defect in this patient appeared to involve neutrophil actin or an actin-binding protein. Neutrophils from his parents and a sibling had actin that polymerized *in vitro* one half as well as that of control subjects.[731] Neutrophils from family members also had intermediate levels of surface expression of the Mac-1 integrin (CD11b/CD18),[732] raising the question of whether the neutrophil actin dysfunction in the proband was due to a primary defect in the leukocyte β_2 integrins and hence represented a subgroup of LAD. However, actin filament assembly has been found to be normal in patients with LAD I.[732] Alternatively, a primary actin-associated defect might alter cell surface expression of the integrins, which have binding sites in their cytoplasmic domains for cytoskeletal proteins.[197]

Coates and co-workers[733] described a single male infant of Tongan descent who had severe skin and mucosal infections. At the age of 2 months, he was found to have hepatosplenomegaly, moderate thrombocytopenia, recurrent pulmonary infiltrates, and a lingual ulcer that grew *Candida tropicalis*. Two siblings had previously died in infancy with a similar clinical picture. Neutrophils from this patient, which had normal cell surface expression of CD11b, exhibited abnormalities in a wide range of motile behaviors, including chemotaxis, phagocytosis, and spreading on glass. Morphologically, the neutrophils displayed thin, filamentous projections of membrane with an underlying abnormal cytoskeletal structure. Biochemical studies revealed markedly defective actin polymerization, and a severe deficiency of an 89-kD protein, along with a markedly elevated level of a 47-kD protein. Hence, this disorder has been referred to as neutrophil actin dysfunction with 47- and 89-kD protein abnormalities (NAD 47/89). The 47-kD protein was identified as lymphocyte-specific protein 1 (LSP1),[734] which is an actin-binding protein present in normal neutrophils. Overexpression of LSP1 has been proposed to result in defective actin polymerization, cytoskeletal structure, and motility defects in neutrophils in NAD 47/89. The identity of the 89-kD protein and its relationship to LSP1 is presently unknown. Neutrophils from the patient's mother and father showed a partial defect in actin polymerization and intermediate abnormalities in the levels of LSP1 and the 89-kD protein. These observations, along with the history of previously affected siblings, suggest that NAD 47/89 is an autosomal recessive disorder. The patient received an allogeneic bone marrow transplant at the age of 7 months and no longer has thrombocytopenia or the neutrophil motility disorder.

Markedly impaired neutrophil chemotaxis has been associated with a heterozygous point mutation in β-actin, as reported by Nunoi and colleagues,[735] in a female patient with recurrent infections, stomatitis, photosensitivity, and mental retardation. The defect lies within a domain that binds to profilin and other actin-regulatory molecules, and heterozygous expression was postulated to interfere with normal actin function in a dominant-negative manner. Interestingly, formyl peptide–induced superoxide production was also decreased in patient neutrophils, suggesting that actin function is important for normal NADPH oxidase assembly.

LOCALIZED JUVENILE PERIODONTITIS

Localized juvenile periodontitis (LJP) is a group of disorders of unknown etiology characterized by severe alveolar bone loss localized to the first molars and incisors, with an onset around the time of puberty.[736–740] Defective neutrophil chemotaxis has been identified *in vitro* in approximately 70 percent of patients with LJP.[736, 739, 741–747] Many, but not all, patients with LJP exhibit abnormal chemotaxis, which may be due to the intrinsic variability in *in vitro* chemotaxis assays (see earlier) or to a fundamental heterogeneity in this disorder. Some support for the latter comes from studies showing that the spectrum of neutrophil defects may vary from patient to patient. For example, whereas most individuals with LJP showed defective chemotaxis in response to administration of both formyl peptides and C5a,[736, 743, 745] others may show an abnormality only with formyl peptides.[742] Further support for the heterogeneity of LJP is provided by studies showing that factors elaborated by periodontopathic bacteria may secondarily alter leukocyte function and depress chemotaxis (e.g., *Capnocytophaga* species, *Actinobacillus actinomycetemcomitans*, and *Bacteroides* species).[680, 748, 749] Whether these factors are the same as the chemotactic inhibitors identified in the sera from some patients with LJP remains to be determined.[743, 744] In one report, the serum chemotaxis inhibitor from 18 patients with LJP was partially neutralized by antibodies to TNF and IL-1.[744] In the subset of patients with LJP who have abnormal chemotaxis, phagocytosis has generally been found to be abnormal, whereas degranulation (of specific granules) and superoxide generation is unaltered.[745]

The observations that LJP tends to cluster in families and that the neutrophil chemotactic activity is not restored *in vitro* or after the patient is treated for periodontal infection lend support to the hypothesis that certain patients with LJP may have an inherited disorder affecting chemotactic receptors. A 40 to 50 percent decrease in the total number of receptors for formyl peptides and C5a has been reported for some patients with LJP.[736, 742] Preliminary studies have identified point mutations in the ligand-binding domain of the formyl peptide receptor in a few patients with LJP.[750] The diagnosis of LJP should be suspected in any adolescent in whom unusually severe and destructive alveolar bone loss involving the first molars and incisors is seen. From a diagnostic point of view, many qualitative and quantitative neutrophil disorders are associated with periodontal disease that, at times, may be severe.[737] Thus, the differential diagnosis should include LAD, CGD, CHS, leukemia, chronic neutropenia, and cyclic neutropenia.

NEONATAL NEUTROPHILS

Although most infants have the ability to successfully fight microbial challenges, they nonetheless have an increased risk for development of severe bacterial infections, particularly sepsis, pneumonia, and meningitis caused by group B streptococci.[751] The risk of infection and the rate of mortality from pyogenic infections are even greater in premature infants. As a result, phagocyte function in neonates has been the subject of intense investigation for many years.[751, 752] There is general agreement that neonates have defects in various aspects of specific immunity (immune cellular cytotoxic mechanisms and cytokine generation) as well as in nonspecific (phagocyte-mediated) immunity. In the latter category, defects in neutrophil adherence, chemotaxis, phagocytosis, and bacterial killing all were reported.[752] Compounding these functional defects in neonates is a deficiency of antibodies directed against organisms that typically infect infants. Furthermore, bone marrow reserves of granulocytes can be easily exhausted in neonates, and neutropenia develops in the midst of severe pyogenic infections, as discussed in the preceding section.

The most important of the functional defects, at least from a clinical point of view, appears to be the depressed chemotactic ability of neonatal neutrophils. Compared with that of adult cells, the directed migration of neonatal neutrophils toward a variety of chemotactic agents (C5a, formyl peptides, and bacterial extracts) is reduced by approximately 50 percent for the first several weeks of life.[752–756] The biochemical basis for the diminished chemotaxis does not appear to be abnormalities in the number or affinity of either the C5a or formyl peptide receptor.[752, 755] Instead, there appears to be a defect in the chemotaxis-induced upregulation of cell adhesion molecules. Baseline expression of the two subunits of the β_2 integrin Mac-1 (CD11b and CD18) was found to be normal in neonatal neutrophils but failed to increase normally after exposure to chemotactic concentrations of C5a and formyl peptides.[757, 758] Fetal, preterm, and term infant neutrophils expressed levels of Mac-1 in stimulated neutrophils that were only 40 to 60 percent of those seen in adult cells. This defect, in turn, appears to be due to diminished fusion of neutrophil granules with the plasma membrane after stimulation. Because the specific granule membranes serve as an intracellular pool for Mac-1 (see Table 21–3), abnormal mobilization of these granule populations could explain the diminished upregulation of Mac-1 seen in neonatal cells after stimulation. Another underlying biochemical defect that may contribute to the defect in chemotaxis is a diminished polymerization of F-actin in neonatal neutrophils after stimulation.[759] Finally, Hill[752] reported that in neonates the intracellular concentration of free calcium in neutrophils does not increase to normal levels in response to chemotactic factors. It is possible that this signal transduction defect could be responsible for both the diminished levels of Mac-1 upregulation and the F-actin polymerization.

OTHER DISORDERS OF NEUTROPHIL CHEMOTAXIS

A new syndrome of severe neutrophil dysfunction due to a dominant-negative mutation in the small GTPase, Rac2, was recently described in a male infant born to unrelated parents. This child was seen with recurrent rapidly progressive soft tissue infections, including perirectal abscesses and a necrotic periumbilical infection, associated with poor formation of pus and neutrophilia.[63, 64, 760] Although the clinical presentation suggested LAD, expression of β_2 integrins and fucosylated cell surface proteins was normal. However, marked abnormalities were seen in chemoattractant-induced neutrophil functions, including F-actin formation, chemotaxis, degranulation, and the respiratory burst, along with defects in phagocytosis and L-selectin–mediated adhesion.[63, 64] Responses to other agonists were normal, suggesting a selective defect in signal transduction. This constellation of functional abnormalities resembled those described for gene-targeted mice lacking the hematopoietic-specific GTPase, Rac2.[177, 178] Analysis of the *Rac2* gene in this patient identified a point mutation that affects the guanine nucleotide binding pocket. The patient was heterozygous for this mutation, which apparently exerts a dominant-negative effect on wild-type Rac2 to interfere with normal neutrophil signal transduction.[63, 64] Neither parent had the mutant *Rac2* allele. The patient was successfully treated by an HLA-matched bone marrow transplant from a sibling. The clinical history, neutrophilia, and functional neutrophil defects in this patient are very similar to those seen in another infant described in an earlier report.[761] That patient, a female, was the first child of nonconsanguineous healthy parents, both originating from India, and had chronic omphalitis and otitis media associated with *S. aureus*, buccal candidiasis, and an internal cecal fistula that ultimately lead to death from gram-negative sepsis at 8 months of age.

A study of 240 patients with a significant history of recurrent infection, generally requiring at least one hospitalization, identified 10 patients, all children, with a consistent marked reduction in chemotactic activity *in vitro* that was not associated with any other neutrophil abnormalities.[762] In 6 of these patients, a partial reduction in chemotactic activity was also seen in either the mother or a sibling. However, other than for the disorders discussed earlier, well-defined clinical entities in which defective neutrophil chemotaxis plays a predominant role in impaired host resistance to bacteria and fungi have not been established or the underlying mechanisms identified. In part, this is related to difficulties in performing and interpreting *in vitro* assays of adhesion and chemotaxis except in specialized research settings. Biochemical approaches to delineating a specific abnormality are also difficult due to the complex nature of the chemotactic response.

Disorders of Opsonization and Ingestion

Clinical disorders of recognition fall into two major categories: humoral and cellular. In the former, plasma-derived opsonins are deficient or absent and result in incomplete opsonization. In contrast, the cellular disorders are characterized by defective receptors for opsonins or by abnormalities in the actin cytoskeletal system responsible for microbial ingestion.

HUMORAL DISORDERS OF OPSONIZATION

Primary B-cell deficiencies result in the decreased or absent production of immunoglobulins, most commonly IgG. Patients with these antibody-deficiency syndromes have recurrent infections with pyogenic bacteria such as *S. aureus*, pneumococci, and *H. influenzae*. One of the major functional abnormalities in these disorders is the defective opsonization of pathogenic microorganisms. As a result, these microbes are not efficiently removed by the host phagocytic system. A variety of clinical disorders may lead to antibody deficiencies; these are discussed elsewhere in this text.

Complement deficiencies also can result in recurrent infections, particularly when they involve factors shared by both the classic and the alternative pathways. Therefore, patients with deficiencies of C1, C2, or C4 have relatively minor problems with infections, because the alternative pathway remains intact. In the case of C3, on the other hand, recurrent infections are much more common, because this is the protein that is the direct precursor of two major complement opsonins—C3b and C3bi. Two forms of C3 deficiency have been described, and both are rare. In one, there is a congenital deficiency of C3 inherited in an autosomal recessive manner.[763–766] Heterozygotes contain one half of the normal levels of C3 but do not experience infections. In at least one patients, the molecular genetic basis of the C3 deficiency has been identified.[764] This patient had an unusual RNA splicing abnormality that resulted in a 61-bp deletion in exon 18, with a premature stop codon 17 bp downstream from the abnormal splice site (the C3 gene is located on human chromosome 19 and consists of 41 exons that span approximately 41 kb). As a result of this splice mutation, the patient had no detectable levels of C3. A second type of C3 deficiency is caused by unchecked catabolism of C3 due to the absence of a C3 protease inhibitor.[767] In both types of C3 deficiencies, the majority of patients suffer from recurrent pyogenic infections caused by encapsulated bacteria such as pneumococci. Patients with deficiencies of the terminal complement components (C5, C6, C7, C8, or C9) are particularly susceptible to infections with meningococci or gonococci. Infections in complement-deficient individuals should be treated with the aggressive use of antibiotics, and immunization against *H. influenzae*, *S. pneumoniae*, and *Neisseria meningitidis* may be helpful.

Approximately 5 percent of the population have low serum levels of mannose binding protein (MBP), a serum lectin secreted by the liver that binds mannose sugars present on the surface of bacteria, fungi, and some viruses.[768] Bound MBP activates the complement cascade and hence functions as an opsonin of broad specificity. The incidence of MBP deficiency is higher in infants with frequent unexplained infections, chronic diarrhea, and otitis media, and it has been proposed that MBP is an important defense mechanism during the time when maternal antibody levels have waned and the infant's antibodies are still immature.[768] MBP deficiency is associated with autosomal dominant inheritance of point mutations in a collagen-like domain of the MBP polypeptide.[769–771] These mutations appear to interfere with the normal polymerization of MBP subunits to form an oligomeric structure required for complement activation. Clinical illness associated with MBP deficiency may not be limited to infants. In a recent report, MBP deficiency was the only identifiable immune defect in four adults with recurrent infections as well as in one patient who also had IgA deficiency.[772] The spectrum of illness included recurrent skin abscesses, chronic cryptosporidial diarrhea, meningococcal meningitis with recurrent herpes simplex, and fatal pneumonia due to *Klebsiella*. Three of the five adults were homozygotes for mutant MBP alleles.

CELLULAR DISORDERS OF INGESTION

Patients with LAD I show a marked abnormality in phagocytosis of C3bi-opsonized particles, because the Mac-1 β_2 integrin (CD11b/CD18) that is deficient in LAD I functions as the C3bi receptor (see Table 21–7 and Fig. 21–4). Patients with neutrophil actin dysfunction also show abnormal ingestion, because actin assembly plays a critical role in the formation of phagosomes.

A deficiency of FcγRIa has been described in four members of a Dutch family.[773] The monocytes from the affected family members did not bind IgG with high affinity. However, these individuals did not show an increased susceptibility to infection despite this receptor deficiency. The incidence is 4 in 3377 in the French population for the complete absence of FcγRIIIb, and neutrophils from affected individuals type as NA-null.[774] None of these individuals exhibit any increased incidence of infection, although infants of women with the NA-null phenotype can develop alloimmune neutropenia due to placental transmission of anti-FcγRIIIb antibodies. Similar findings were also reported in a study of 21 individuals from 14 families with FcγRIIIb deficiency in the Netherlands.[775] Complete absence of the FcγRIIIb gene was found in all kindreds studied. Three of the women who had multiple pregnancies lacked antineutrophil antibodies, suggesting that neonatal alloimmune neutropenia does not always develop in this setting. Marked deficiency in neutrophil FcγRIIIb has also been observed in patients with paroxysmal nocturnal hemoglobinuria (PNH),[776] an acquired stem cell disorder caused by a defect in the biosynthesis of GPI membrane anchors. Because neutrophil FcγRIIIb is linked to the plasma membrane by means of a GPI anchor,[777] this receptor is unable to insert in the cell membranes in patients with PNH. The membranes of patients with PNH are also deficient in decay-accelerating factor and acetylcholinesterase, because these two proteins are also anchored by GPI moieties. Neutrophils from patients with PNH undergo a normal oxidative burst in response to IgG-coated latex particles.[777] Thus, there appears to be sufficient redundancy in the function of Fc and complement receptors to permit normal phagocytic function in these instances of FcγRI and FcγRIIIb deficiencies.

Allelic polymorphisms in FcγRIIa (131H versus 131R) and in FcγRIIIb (NA1 versus NA2) may each contribute to a subtle defect in the host response to encapsulated microorganisms. The polymorphism in amino acid 131 in FcγRIIa affects binding to IgG$_2$, with "H" referring to "high" responder and the ability to bind to this IgG subclass. The 131H versus 131R polymorphism is seen in approximately equal numbers in the white population, but 131H and 131R are distributed in a 3:1 ratio in Japanese and Chinese populations.[238] The FcγRIIa *131H* allele is the only Fcγ receptor able to mediate efficient phagocytosis of IgG_2-opsonized bacteria, and the FcγRIIa *131H/131H* genotype in children was associated with a lower incidence of infections with encapsulated bacteria.[238] The NA1 polymorphism in the FcγRIIIb receptor, which affects receptor glycosylation, is associated with more efficient phagocytosis of IgG-opsonized particles compared with that for the *NA2* allele.[238, 241] The incidence of the *NA1* allele is approximately 0.33 compared with an incidence of approximately 0.64 for the *NA2* allele in whites, but this ratio is reversed in Japanese and Chinese populations. Patients who are homozygous for both the FcγRIIa *131R* and the FcγRIIIb *NA2* alleles appear to be at higher risk for the occurrence of meningococcal meningitis.[778]

Disorders of Degranulation

Phagocytes can kill microorganisms using a variety of cytotoxic compounds, as reviewed earlier in this chapter. These include a host of preformed antimicrobial polypeptides that are stored within intracellular granules and released into the phagocytic vacuole upon phagocytosis. The importance of granule contents in host defense is attested to by two clinical syndromes associated with disorders of degranulation—CHS and specific granule deficiency.

CHÉDIAK-HIGASHI SYNDROME

CHS is a rare, autosomal recessive, multiorgan disease resulting from defects in granule morphogenesis and is characterized by partial oculocutaneous albinism, repeated bacterial infections, giant lysosomes in granulocytes, and (in some patients) a mild bleeding diathesis as well as peripheral and cranial neuropathies associated with decussation defects at the optic chiasm[438–441] (Table

21–23). Ten types of oculocutaneous albinism have been described in humans, and CHS is one of the tyrosinase-positive forms that has been designated as type VIB.[441]

CHS is caused by a fundamental defect in granule morphogenesis that results in abnormally large granules in many tissues. The most extensively studied of the affected cells are the neutrophils. In the early stages of myelopoiesis, some of the normally sized azurophil granules coalesce to form giant granules that later fuse with some of the specific granules to form huge secondary lysosomes that contain constituents of both granule types.[779–782] In addition to this uncontrolled fusion of granules, CHS neutrophils are markedly deficient in neutral proteases,[783] including two azurophil granule enzymes, cathepsin G, and elastase.[784] In melanocytes, there are giant melanosomes that prevent the even distribution of melanin and result in hypopigmentation of the hair, skin, iris, and ocular fundus.[441] Giant granules are also seen in Schwann cells, leukocytes, and certain cells in the liver, spleen, pancreas, gastric mucosa, kidney, adrenal gland, and pituitary gland.[441] Disorders similar to human CHS have also been described in many mammalian species, including Aleutian mink, *beige* mice, blue foxes, cats, killer whales, and Hereford cattle.[440, 441, 785]

Mutations in a newly discovered gene, *CHS1*, appear to account for most, if not all, cases of CHS.[786–788] *CHS1* is homologous to the *bg* locus responsible for the granule defect in *beige* mice mapped to the proximal end of mouse chromosome 13, which is syntectic with human chromosome 1q.[789] The *beige* gene was positionally cloned and termed *LYST* for its presumed function as a lysosomal trafficking regulatory protein.[786, 788] The gene encodes a large (3801 amino acids) polypeptide, referred to as the CHS or LYST protein and is postulated to regulate organellar protein trafficking and lysosomal fission. Frameshift and nonsense mutations have been identified in the *CHS1* gene in patients with CHS, which result in truncated forms of the protein.[786–788, 790] Patients with

TABLE 21–23. Summary of Chédiak-Higashi Syndrome

Incidence	More than 200 patients described
Inheritance	Autosomal recessive
Molecular defect	Defect in granule morphogenesis in multiple tissues due to mutations in the *CHS1* gene, encoding a lysosomal trafficking protein
Pathogenesis	Giant coalesced azurophil/specific granules in neutrophils resulting in ineffective granulopoiesis and neutropenia, delayed and incomplete degranulation, and defective chemotaxis
Clinical manifestations	Partial oculocutaneous albinism
	Recurrent severe bacterial infections (usually *Staphylococcus aureus*)
	Gingivitis and periodontitis
	Cranial and peripheral neuropathies (muscle weakness, ataxia, sensory loss, nystagmus)
	Hepatosplenomegaly and complications of pancytopenia in the accelerated phase
Laboratory evaluation	Giant granules in peripheral blood granulocytes and in bone marrow myeloid progenitor cells
	Widespread lymphohistiocytic infiltrates in accelerated phase
Prenatal diagnosis	Demonstration of giant granules in fetal blood neutrophils or cultured amniotic cells.
Differential diagnosis	Other genetic forms of oculocutaneous albinism
	Giant granules can be seen in acute and chronic myelogenous leukemias
Therapy	Prophylactic trimethoprim-sulfamethoxazole
	Parenteral antibiotics for acute infections
	Ascorbic acid (200 mg/day for infants; 6 g/day for adults)
	Bone marrow transplantation before or at beginning of accelerated phase
Prognosis	Most patients die of infection or complications of the accelerated phase during the first or second decade of life unless transplanted. A few patients have survived into their thirties.

clinically typical CHS that do not appear to have mutations in CHS1 have been reported, suggesting that an additional genetic locus may sometimes be affected.[791]

Some of the most dramatic examples of the granule defect in CHS are manifested in the various blood cells and are summarized in Table 21–24. As discussed previously, a few to a large majority of circulating neutrophils contain giant coalesced azurophil-specific granules. These giant granules are often more prominent in the bone marrow than in the peripheral blood, because many of the abnormal myeloid precursors are destroyed before they ever leave the marrow. Extensive myeloid cell vacuolization, enhanced marrow cellularity, and elevated levels of serum lysozyme all reflect this process of intramedullary granulocyte destruction.[792] As a result, most patients with CHS have a moderate neutropenia, with ANCs ranging between 500 and 2000 cells/μL.[438, 439] Monocytes are also affected in CHS and have similar, but not identical, cytoplasmic inclusions that appear to be ring-shaped lysosomes.[793] Lymphocytes can also contain giant cytoplasmic granules that may contribute to abnormalities in specific immunity (see later). Finally, CHS platelets have a decreased number of dense granules and a storage pool deficiency of adenosine diphosphate and serotonin.[794–797] This abnormality leads to a defect in platelet aggregation and an increased bleeding time manifested clinically as easy bruising, intestinal bleeding, and epistaxis. Most patients with CHS do not have thrombocytopenia until they enter the accelerated phase of the disease (see later).

TABLE 21–24. Hematologic Manifestations of Chédiak-Higashi Syndrome

STABLE PHASE

Neutrophils
1. Giant, coalesced azurophil/specific granules
2. Vacuolization of marrow neutrophils (ineffective myelopoiesis)
3. Neutropenia (intramedullary destruction)
4. Decreased bactericidal activity
   a. Decreased chemotaxis *in vivo* and *in vitro*
   b. Delayed and incomplete degranulation

Monocytes/macrophages
1. Ring-shaped lysosomes
2. Decreased chemotaxis

Lymphocytes/natural killer cells
1. Giant cytoplasmic granules
2. Diminished natural killer function
3. Diminished antibody-dependent cell-mediated cytolysis of tumor cells

Platelets
1. Giant cytoplasmic granules may be seen
2. Normal platelet count
3. Increased bleeding time due to abnormal aggregation caused by storage pool deficiency of adenosine diphosphate and serotonin

ACCELERATED PHASE
1. Hepatosplenomegaly
2. Bone marrow infiltration
3. Hemophagocytosis by histiocytes
4. Worsening neutropenia, thrombocytopenia, and anemia due to 1, 2, and 3

The infections usually encountered with CHS involve the skin, respiratory tract, and mucous membranes and are caused by both gram-positive and gram-negative bacteria as well as by fungi. The most common organism is *S. aureus*. These infections are often recurrent and may result in death at any time. Gingivitis and periodontitis are common. The skin is also susceptible to severe sunburns, and photosensitivity in bright light is common.

The phagocytes are primarily responsible for the propensity to infection. In addition to moderate neutropenia, several defects in neutrophil function lead to impaired bactericidal activity. First, chemotaxis is markedly depressed, whether measured *in vivo* by the Rebuck skin window or *in vitro* by the method of Boyden.[439, 798] The large granules appear to interfere with the ability of neutrophils to travel through narrow passages, such as those between endothelial cells. Second, degranulation is delayed and incomplete in CHS neutrophils.[799–802] Third, the marked deficiency of antimicrobial proteins such as cathepsin G probably contributes to the diminished bactericidal potency of CHS neutrophils.[801] Finally, decreased expression of Mac-1 (CD11b/CD18) in CHS neutrophils may also play a role.[803]

Contributing to the enhanced susceptibility to infection are abnormalities in monocytes, lymphocytes, and NK cells. Monocytes, like neutrophils, exhibit decreased chemotaxis.[251] Peripheral blood CHS lymphocytes demonstrate diminished ADCC of tumor cells.[804] Perhaps most important, NK cell function is profoundly abnormal in CHS.[804–809] This defect not only contributes to the recurrent infection problem but also may be involved in the development of the accelerated phase of CHS.

Patients who survive the infectious and neurologic problems of the stable phase of CHS have a high risk of progression to the accelerated phase of the disease.[438] This transition generally occurs during the first or second decade of life.[438, 810] The accelerated phase is characterized pathologically by a diffuse lymphohistiocytic infiltration of the liver, spleen, lymph nodes, and bone marrow. This infiltration is not lymphomatous or neoplastic by histopathologic criteria, although the outcome for the patient is uniformly fatal if not treated.[810] The accelerated phase is heralded by hepatosplenomegaly, bone marrow infiltration, and hemophagocytosis lead to a worsening of the neutropenia and an ever-increasing risk of infection. Thrombocytopenia likewise develops and intensifies the bleeding disorder already present in the platelets.

The diagnosis of CHS should be suspected in any child who is seen one or more of the following findings: (1) recurrent bacterial infections of unknown etiology; (2) hypopigmentation of the hair, skin, and eyes; (3) the presence of giant peroxidase-positive lysosomal granules in granulocytes from peripheral blood or bone marrow; (4) mild to moderate neutropenia; (5) easy bruising or nose bleeds despite a normal platelet count; and (6) unexplained hepatosplenomegaly (associated with the accelerated phase of the disease). CHS usually manifests in infancy or early childhood but may be identified later when the disease is in the accelerated phase. In some patients, the disease may be suspected on the basis of neurologic abnormalities that include ataxia, muscle weakness, decreased deep tendon reflexes, sensory loss, a diffusely abnormal electroencephalogram, and abnormal visual and auditory evoked potentials.[811, 812] The physician should not be dissuaded from considering the diagnosis of CHS if the patient does not show clear-cut oculocutaneous albinism. Depending on the skin coloration in the family, the only manifestations of the albinism may be a metallic sheen in the hair (which can vary from blond to dark brown) and a lighter skin color than that seen in siblings. In younger patients, there is likely to be a cartwheel distribution of pigment in the iris and an abnormal red reflex.

The diagnosis of CHS is made on the basis of giant lysosomal granules found in blood or bone marrow myeloid cells. In some patients, relatively few abnormal granulocytes will be seen in the peripheral blood, presumably because of extensive intramedullary destruction of myeloid precursors. In these patients, a bone marrow aspirate may be necessary to identify the large lysosomes. Microscopic examination of the hair reveals giant melanin granules. An affected fetus with CHS diagnosed via fetal blood sampling, which showed large abnormal granules in neutrophils, was also found to have significantly larger than normal acid phosphatase lysosomes in cultured amniotic and chorionic villus cells.[813] This suggests that prenatal diagnosis of CHS might be accomplished using the latter techniques, which is less risky than fetal blood sampling. In the accelerated phase of the disease, biopsies of the liver, spleen, and lymph nodes reveal diffuse infiltrates of lymphohistiocytic cells.

The differential diagnosis for CHS includes other genetic forms of partial albinism.[441] These include Griscelli syndrome,[814] which is distinguished from CHS by the lack of giant cytoplasmic granules in neutrophils and the finding of large pigment clumps in hair shafts and accumulation of mature melanosomes in melanocytes. Patients with Griscelli syndrome typically develop a fatal lymphohistiocytic syndrome before the age of 10 that has some resemblance to the accelerated phase of CHS.[815] Hermansky-Pudlak syndrome is another disorder of partial albinism but is characterized by platelet function defects and an associated bleeding diathesis. Giant granules resembling those seen in CHS can be seen in both acute and chronic myelogenous leukemias[816–818] and should not be confused with those seen in CHS.

The management of the stable phase of CHS primarily involves treatment of infectious complications. The prophylactic administration of trimethoprim-sulfamethoxazole may be beneficial. Infections should be treated vigorously with appropriate intravenous antibiotics. Treatment with high doses of ascorbic acid (20 mg/kg/day) has been reported to cause clinical improvement as well as improved function of neutrophils *in vitro* (neutrophil chemotaxis and/or bactericidal function).[819, 820] Although there is some disagreement in the literature regarding the efficacy of ascorbic acid,[821] it seems reasonable to try this medication in all patients, given its safety in moderate doses. NK cell function appears to remain abnormal even after ascorbate therapy.

The treatment of the accelerated phase is extremely difficult. Administration of vincristine and corticosteroids has been effective in inducing remissions, albeit temporary.[438, 792, 810] The only curative therapy is bone marrow transplantation.[378, 727, 822–824] This procedure is ideally performed before the onset of the accelerated phase. The accelerated phase of CHS may possibly be prevented or delayed by vaccines against EBV[251] because it has been hypothesized that the accelerated phase may be triggered by the inability of patients with CHS to control this virus.[810, 825]

SPECIFIC GRANULE DEFICIENCY

Specific (secondary) granule deficiency (SGD) is an extremely rare congenital disorder of neutrophil function characterized by recurrent bacterial infections and multiple abnormalities in neutrophil structure and composition, including absent specific granules and bilobed nuclei.[826] Despite its rarity, SGD is an important part of the differential diagnosis in patients with suspected phagocyte immunodeficiencies and provides important insights into the transcriptional regulation of granule biogenesis and the functional roles of lactoferrin, vitamin B_{12}–binding protein, and other specific granule constituents in host defense. To date, five patients with specific granule deficiency have been described.[393, 784, 827–840] The occurrence of this disorder in both males and females, the parental consanguinity in one instance,[837, 838] and the death due to severe infection in a female sibling of one of the male patients[837] all suggest that this disorder is inherited in an autosomal recessive manner.

The key features of SGD are summarized in Table 21–25. Clinically, patients with this disorder suffer from indolent, smoldering cutaneous infections punctuated by episodes (sometimes prolonged) of severe infections involving the lungs, ears, lymph nodes, and the deeper structures of the skin. Lung abscesses and mastoiditis have been reported as complications of these infections. *S. aureus*, *P. aeruginosa*, *Proteus* species, other enteric gram-negative bacteria, and *C. albicans* appear to be the major pathogens. Further complicating the clinical course in some patients is the presence of neutropenia that is either intermittent and mild[827,829] or prolonged and severe.[393]

The clinical picture of SGD is consistent with the functional defects identified in neutrophils of patients. There is a marked abnormality in chemotaxis that is observed *in vivo* by the Rebuck skin window technique.[827, 829, 830, 838] The indolent nature of some infections in SGD may be attributable to this chemotactic defect. *In vitro* measurements of neutrophil killing of *E. coli* and *S. aureus* show a moderate impairment despite the presence of a normal respiratory burst.[827–830, 838, 840] Patient neutrophils adhere normally to plastic surfaces[828, 838] but exhibit slightly diminished sticking to nylon fibers and endothelial cells.[830] Degranulation of both azurophil and (to the extent that they are present) specific granules also appears to be normal.[828, 830, 838]

At least three cellular compartments are affected by the underlying molecular defect(s) in SGD: nucleus, specific granules, and azurophil granules. Approximately one half or more of the peripheral blood neutrophils in SGD have nuclei that resemble those seen in the Pelger-Huet anomaly. The nucleus has a kidney-shaped, bilobed configuration that is flawed by a series of microlobulations and clefts

TABLE 21–25. Summary of Neutrophil Specific Granule Deficiency

Incidence	Five patients reported
Inheritance	Autosomal recessive
Molecular defect	Protein deficiencies in azurophil granules (defensins), specific granules (lactoferrin, vitamin B_{12}–binding protein, gelatinase), and secretory vesicles (alkaline phosphatase) suggest a common defect in the regulation of the production of these proteins in myeloid cells. Eosinophil specific granules are also deficient in protein contents. Mutations in the myeloid transcription factor, C/EPBε, have been identified in several patients.
Pathogenesis	Recurrent infections result from the combined effect of deficiencies in microbicidal granule protein (e.g., defensins and lactoferrin) and abnormal chemotaxis, perhaps due to a failure to upregulate surface β_2 integrins and chemotactic peptide receptors from granule stores.
Clinical manifestations	Recurrent (sometimes indolent) pyogenic infections of the skin, ears, lungs and lymph nodes that may have diminished neutrophil infiltration; onset usually during infancy
Laboratory evaluation	Absent or empty specific granules vesicles in neutrophils by electron microscopy (by light microscopy, granules appear absent)
	Bilobed nuclei resembling the Pelger-Huet anomaly frequently seen in neutrophils
	Severe deficiency of neutrophil lactoferrin, vitamin B_{12}–binding protein, defensins, and alkaline phosphatase (by histochemical assay)
Differential diagnosis	Acquired specific granule deficiency (e.g., thermal burns or myeloproliferative syndromes)
Therapy	Prophylactic antibiotics
	Parenteral antibiotics for acute infections
	Surgical drainage or resection of refractory infections
Prognosis	With appropriate medical management, patients can survive into their adult years

apparent on electron microscopic examination.[829, 830, 838] As the name of the disorder indicates, neutrophils from these patients show a severe deficiency in normal specific granules.[829, 830] On a sample of peripheral blood stained with Wright's stain, neutrophils appear to be devoid of the pink-staining specific granules. By electron microscopic analysis, however, it is apparent that the specific granules are not actually absent but are instead present as empty, elongated vesicles that retain their characteristic trilamellar membrane structure and positive staining for complex carbohydrates.[829, 831, 833, 837] Results of biochemical measurements of specific granule contents parallel those of the morphologic studies. Lactoferrin, vitamin B_{12}–binding protein, and gelatinase[841] are present at levels that are only 3 to 10 percent of normal.[828, 830, 838] Thus, there appears to be an abortive and incomplete formation of normal specific granules. Azurophil (primary) granules in this disorder are also strikingly abnormal. Although they contain a normal (if not slightly elevated) amount of MPO and are present in normal numbers, they are severely deficient in defensins.[784] There is also a severe deficiency of alkaline phosphatase activity in peripheral blood neutrophils, as determined by standard histochemical techniques using naphthol AS phosphate as substrate.[827, 829, 838] This enzyme activity is localized to secretory vesicles, and its deficiency probably represents yet another organelle abnormality in this disorder.[833] Finally, granule formation also appears to be abnormal in eosinophils. These cells are deficient in three eosinophil-specific granule proteins (eosinophil cationic protein, major basic protein, and eosinophil-derived neurotoxin), although the corresponding mRNA transcripts are present.[842]

In view of the many deficits in granule matrix contents, it has been speculated that SGD is due to an abnormality in the transcriptional regulation of a series of granule (and probably nongranule) proteins. In one patient with SGD studied, lactoferrin mRNA was normal in size but its abundance in the nucleated marrow cells was greatly diminished, whereas the levels of lactoferrin and its transcript were normal in nasal glandular epithelia in the same patient.[836] It is also of interest that SGD involves a severe deficiency of defensins, which are stored in azurophilic granules. Defensins, in contrast to other azurophilic granule proteins that are synthesized at the promyelocyte stage, is produced during the subsequent myelocyte stage, along with the specific granule matrix proteins (see Fig. 21–1).

The hypothesis that SGD results from a defect in a myeloid specific, *trans*-acting factor that controls transcription of genes activated during granulocyte differentiation has recently been shown to be correct, at least in some patients, based on serendipitous observations from mice generated with a targeted deletion in the C/EBPε. Similar to characteristics seen in SGD patients, neutrophil secondary granules and their matrix proteins are not found in C/EBPε mice and bilobed neutrophil nuclei, impaired chemotaxis, and increased susceptibility to bacterial infection are seen.[3, 843, 844] Mutations in the C/EBPε gene have been identified in two patients to date. In one patient, a 5-bp deletion results in a truncated, nonfunctional protein,[46] whereas a second, unrelated patient was homozygous for a nucleotide insertion in the coding sequence that also leads to the synthesis of a truncated and nonfunctional form of C/EBPε.[47] However, DNA sequencing of the C/EBPε gene of several other patients with SGD has not revealed abnormalities, suggesting that SGD is a genetically heterogeneous disorder.[845]

The cellular defects described earlier can explain, at least in part, the observed clinical problems in SGD. The markedly abnormal specific granules and secretory vesicles, which contain intracellular stores of both β_2 integrins[846–848] and a chemotactic peptide receptor,[849] fail to support normal upregulation of these two types of receptors[835, 838] and may thereby contribute to the chemotactic defect. Furthermore, the severe deficiency of key bactericidal proteins such as lactoferrin and the defensins make the cell's killing of bacteria and *Candida* less efficient. Neutropenia, when it does occur, also impairs host defense and appears to be caused by intramedullary destruction of the abnormal neutrophils, as evidenced by their ingestion by marrow macrophages.[837]

The diagnosis of SGD can be made by light microscopic examination of peripheral blood neutrophils stained with Wright's stain. Electron microscopic studies can confirm the presence of empty specific granule vesicles. Bilobed nuclei and greatly diminished levels of alkaline phophatase by histochemical analysis also support the diagnosis. In conjunction with these morphologic studies, biochemical and immunologic measurements of lactoferrin, vitamin B_{12}–binding protein, and defensins can be made. As discussed earlier, all three of these granule proteins are severely deficient in this disorder. Acquired SGD is observed in myeloproliferative syndromes and after thermal burns.[826, 850] In these acquired disorders, however, at least a few intact specific granules are still observed microscopically, and the deficiencies of the various granule enzymes are less profound. As with other neutrophil disorders, prophylactic administration of antibiotics appears to be beneficial, based on anecdotal experience. Parenteral antibiotics should be used aggressively for acute infections. With appropriate medical management, patients can survive into their adult years. Malignant transformation of the dysmorphic myeloid cells in this disorder has not been reported.

Disorders of Oxidative Metabolism

The elimination of many pathogens requires oxygen-derived microbicidal compounds that are generated by the phagocyte respiratory burst pathway in response to inflammatory stimuli (see Fig. 21–6). Five clinically significant defects have been identified in this series of reactions. These include deficiencies in the NADPH oxidase (reaction 1 in Fig. 21–6), G6PD (reaction 8), MPO (reaction 4), glutathione reductase (reaction 7), and glutathione synthetase (reaction 9).

CHRONIC GRANULOMATOUS DISEASE

CGD is an inherited disorder of phagocyte function in which the generation of superoxide by the respiratory burst oxidase (see Fig. 21–7) in neutrophils, monocytes, macrophages, and eosinophils is absent or markedly deficient. The disorder occurs with an incidence of approximately 1 in 250,000 individuals, making it the most common clinically significant disorder of phagocyte function that is inherited.[851] CGD is due to mutations in any one of four essential subunits of the respiratory burst oxidase (see Tables 21–8 and 21–26). Although originally described as an X-linked recessive disorder affecting boys,[852–856] approximately one third of occurrences of CGD is inherited as an autosomal recessive trait[857, 858] (Table 21–26). In more than 90 percent of patients, superoxide production by activated phagocytes is undetectable. A respiratory burst of 1 to 10 percent of normal is observed in the remaining patients, who are often referred to as having "variant" CGD.[858, 860–862] Other

aspects of phagocyte function are normal in CGD, including adherence, ingestion, and degranulation.[863–865]

Clinical Manifestations

CGD is associated with a distinctive clinical syndrome that provides clear evidence for the importance of the phagocyte respiratory burst in host defense and the inflammatory response.[851, 866–873] Patients suffer from recurrent, often severe, purulent bacterial and fungal infections, which can be caused by organisms not ordinarily considered to be pathogens. The distinctive hallmark of this disorder is the propensity of patients to develop chronic inflammatory granulomas that can have widespread tissue distribution. The majority of patients with CGD manifest symptoms within the first year of life,[870] although some may remain relatively symptom-free until later in childhood or even adult life.[874–879]

Table 21–27 summarizes the types of infections and infecting organisms most often encountered in patients with CGD.[867, 868, 870–872, 880–882] The major sites of infection are those that come into contact with the external environment—lungs, skin, gastrointestinal tract, and the lymph nodes that drain these organs. Hematogenous seeding can lead to liver abscesses or osteomyelitis. The most common pathogens include *S. aureus*, *Aspergillus* species (most often *A. fumigatus* but occasionally *Aspergillus nidulans*),[882] and a variety of gram-negative bacilli, including *Serratia marcescens* and various *Salmonella* species. *B. cepacia* has been increasingly recognized as a potentially lethal pathogen in patients with CGD.[874, 883–885] In many patients, no organism can be identified despite extensive culturing. In these instances, it is important to look carefully for the presence of unusual microbes that can occasionally cause serious infections in CGD[875, 882, 890–893] (Table 21–27).

Pneumonia in patients with CGD is most often caused by *S. aureus*, *Aspergillus* species, and enteric bacteria. It is common for an organism not to be identified even in lung biopsy specimens. Complications of pneumonia include empyema or lung abscess. Suppurative lymphadenitis, usually involving the cervical nodes, is especially common in younger patients and is typically caused by *S. aureus* and enteric bacilli such as *Serratia* and *Klebsiella*. Staphylococcal skin infections are also common. Hepatic and perihepatic abscesses, usually caused by *S. aureus*, are surprisingly common and should suggest the diagnosis of CGD if it has not already been made.[894–896] Bone infections can be particularly problematic in patients with CGD and arise either from direct spread of infections from contiguous sites or from hematogenous spread from more distant locations.[897, 898] The former type of osteomyelitis is usually seen in ribs and vertebral bodies as a result of invasion by pulmonary *Aspergillus*.[897] The latter type is more often seen in peripheral long and small bones and is typically caused by *S. marcescens*, *Nocardia* species, and *S. aureus*.[897] Perirectal infections are extremely difficult to treat in patients with CGD and can lead to fistula formation.[894] The rare pathogen *Chromobacterium violaceum* is found in brackish waters and is an uncommon but potentially serious cause of soft tissue infection, pneumonia, or sepsis in CGD patients from the southern United States. *C. violaceum* infection

TABLE 21–26. Classification of Chronic Granulomatous Disease

Component Affected	Inheritance	Subtype*	Cytochrome b Spectrum	NBT Score (% Positive)	Incidence (% of Patients)	Immunoblot Levels†				Activity in Cell-Free System	
						gp91	p22	p47	p67	Membrane	Cytosol
gp91-*phox*	X	X91⁰	0	0	57	0	0-trace	N	N	0	N
		X91⁻	Low	80–100 (weak)	5	Low	Low	N	N	Trace	N
		X91⁻	Low	5–10	2	Low	Low	N	N	Trace	N
		X91⁺	0	0	2	N	N	N	N	0	N
p22-*phox*	A	A22⁰	0	0	5	0	0	N	N	0	N
		A22⁺	N	0	1	N	N	N	N	0	N
p47-*phox*	A	A47⁰	N	0	23	N	N	0	N	N	0
p67-*phox*	A	A67⁰	N	0	5	N	N	N	0	N	0

NTB = nitroblue tetrazolium; X = X-linked inheritance; A = autosomal recessive inheritance; N = normal level of protein; 0 = undetectable level of protein; N = normal level of protein activity.

*In this nomenclature, the first letter represents the mode of inheritance (X-linked [X] or autosomal recessive [A], and the number indicates the *phox* component that is genetically affected. The superscript symbols indicate whether the level of protein of the affected component is undetectable (⁰), diminished (⁻), or normal (⁺) as measured by immunoblot analysis.

†Defined by immunoblotting with component-specific antibodies.

Adapted from Curnutte JT: Molecular basis of the autosomal recessive forms of chronic granulomatous disease. Immunodef Rev 3:149, 1992; see also references 851, 854, and 859.

TABLE 21–27. Infections in Chronic Granulomatous Disease*

Infections	% of Infections	Infecting Organisms	% of Isolates
Pneumonia	70–80	*Staphylococcus aureus*	30–50
Lymphadenitis†	60–80	*Aspergillus* species	10–20
Cutaneous infections/impetigo†	60–70	*Escherichia coli*	5–10
Hepatic/perihepatic abscesses†	30–40	*Klebsiella* species	5–10
Osteomyelitis	20–30	*Salmonella* species	5–10
Perirectal abscesses/fistulae†	15–30	*Burkholderia cepacia*	5–10
Septicemia	10–20	*Serratia marcescens*	5–10
Otitis media†	≈20	*Staphylococcus epidermidis*	5
Conjunctivitis	≈15	*Streptococcus* species	4
Enteric infections	≈10	*Enterobacter* species	3
Urinary tract infections/pyelonephritis	5–15	*Proteus* species	3
Sinusitis	<10	*Candida albicans*	3
Renal/perinephric abscesses	<10	*Nocardia* species	2
Brain abscesses	<5	*Haemophilus influenzae*	1
Pericarditis	<5	*Pneumocystis carinii*	<1
Meningitis	<5	*Mycobacterium fortuitum*	<1
		Chromobacterium violaceum	<1
		Francisella philomiragia	<1
		Torulopsis glabrata	<1

CGD = chronic granulomatous disease.

*The relative rates of occurrence for different types of infections in patients with CGD are estimated from data pooled from several large series of patients in the United States, Europe, and Japan. See text for references. These series encompass approximately 550 patients with CGD after accounting for overlap between reports. The list of infecting organisms is also arranged according to the data in these reports and is not paired with the entries in the first column.

†Those infections seen most often at time of presentation.

has also been reported in northern areas. Other important but less commonly seen infections in CGD are summarized in Table 21–27. In a recent report based on a registry of United States residents with CGD, the most common causes of death were pneumonia or sepsis due to *Aspergillus* species or *B. cepacia*.[852]

Patients with CGD are particularly susceptible to organisms that contain catalase, which prevents the CGD phagocyte from scavenging microbe-generated H_2O_2 for phagosomal killing.[899] Another possible link among the organisms with increased virulence in CGD is that they are resistant to nonoxidative killing mechanisms of the phagocyte mediated by antibiotic proteins contained within the various granule compartments.[260, 900, 901]

Chronic conditions associated with CGD are responsible for many of the major complications seen with this disorder and are summarized in Table 21–28. These include the formation of granulomas, which are believed to reflect a chronic inflammatory response to inadequate phagocyte killing or digestion. These lesions contain a mixture of lymphocytes and inflammatory macrophages, some of which may have a foamy lipoid cytoplasm that has a characteristic yellow-brown color. Although not pathognomonic of CGD, the presence of such macrophages in granulomas or other tissue sites should suggest the diagnosis of CGD.[853, 854, 856, 902] Granuloma formation can lead to obstructive symptoms in the upper gastrointestinal tract, including gastric outlet obstruction that can be confused clinically with pyloric stenosis.[894, 896, 903–905] A chronic ileocolitis syndrome resembling Crohn disease is seen in approximately 5 to 10 percent of patients and can lead to a debilitating syndrome of diarrhea and malabsorption.[896, 906, 907] Chronic

inflammatory lesions have been identified in the urinary bladder walls of some patients and can cause chronic cystitis that can present as dysuria, penile pain, and decreased urine volume.[908–911] In one study of 60 patients with CDG, 11 instances of granulomatous inflammation of bladder wall lesions, ureters, or urethra were seen, accompanied by stricture formation in the latter two sites.[912] Hydronephrosis can occur as a complication of obstruction.

Other chronic inflammatory complications of CGD include lymphadenopathy, hepatosplenomegaly, and an eczematoid dermatitis,[868, 870, 913] along with hypergammaglobulinemia, anemia of chronic disease, and short stature (Table 21–28). Gingivitis and ulcerative stomatitis can be seen.[914] Chorioretinitis[915, 916] and destructive white matter lesions in the brain have also been described.[917, 918] Glomerulonephritis due to immune complex deposition has been reported.[919] Rarely, patients may develop either discoid or systemic lupus erythematosus[920–923] or juvenile rheumatoid arthritis.[924]

The severity and pattern of complications of CGD is heterogeneous, which may partly reflect the heterogeneity of molecular defects (see later) and whether any residual respiratory burst oxidase function is present. However, a severe clinical course can be seen in patients in the latter "variant" category that is indistinguishable from what is observed in patients with complete absence of phagocyte superoxide production.[862, 925] On the other hand, some individuals with undetectable levels of respiratory burst activity experience relatively few symptoms and have intervals of years between severe infections. Hence, polymorphisms in oxygen-independent antimicrobial systems or other components regulating the innate immune

TABLE 21–28. Chronic Conditions Associated with Chronic Granulomatous Disease*

Condition	% of Patients
Lymphadenopathy	98
Hypergammaglobulinemia	60–90
Hepatomegaly	50–90
Splenomegaly	60–80
Anemia of chronic disease	Common
Underweight	70
Chronic diarrhea	20–60
Short stature	50
Gingivitis	50
Dermatitis	35
Hydronephrosis	10–25
Ulcerative stomatitis	5–15
Pulmonary fibrosis	<10
Esophagitis	<10
Gastric antral narrowing	<10
Granulomatous ileocolitis	<10
Granulomatous cystitis	<10
Chorioretinitis	<10
Glomerulonephritis	<10
Discoid lupus erythematosus	<10

*The relative rates of occurrence of the chronic conditions associated with CGD were estimated from the series of reports listed in Table 21–27. See text for additional references.

response are likely to play an important role in modifying disease severity in CGD. Specific polymorphisms in the MPO, mannose-binding lectin, and FcγRIIa genes have recently been shown to be associated with a higher risk for granulomatous or autoimmune/rheumatologic complications in CGD.[926]

Heterozygous carriers of the CGD trait are generally asymptomatic, but there are several important exceptions. Carriers of the autosomal recessive forms of CGD have a normal phagocyte respiratory burst and are free from infection. Carriers of X-linked CGD, on the other hand, typically have two populations of circulating neutrophils and monocytes—some with normal respiratory burst activity and others with none[927–933]—due to random X chromosome inactivation.[934, 935] In most X-linked carriers, these two populations are approximately equal in number, but occasionally individuals have an unusually small percentage of either abnormal or normal cells. If the number of functioning neutrophils is less than 10 to 15 percent, the carrier often suffers from some of the infectious complications of CGD.[862, 876, 927, 936] Other clinical problems occasionally seen in female carriers of X-linked CGD are apthous ulcers or discoid lupus erythematosus. In a 1991 review of the literature,[922] 22 instances were summarized from 11 reports. Clinically, the carriers had discoid-like skin lesions (13 of 22 patients), photosensitivity (13 patients) and recurrent apthous stomatitis (12 patients). In a few, polyarthritis, arthralgia, and Raynaud phenomenon were also observed. Results of serologic testing for lupus were generally negative, as were results of immunofluorescence studies of biopsy specimens from lesions. Interestingly, all the reported patients were carriers of X-linked CGD. Discoid lupus-like lesions have also been reported in 5 patients with autosomal recessive

CGD.[920, 921, 937] Because the lupus-like skin lesions do not appear to develop unless there is at least a subpopulation of nonfunctioning phagocytes, it has been hypothesized that autoantibodies to antigens from incompletely destroyed microbes may be responsible for the syndrome.[222]

Molecular Basis of Chronic Granulomatous Disease

CGD is classified according to the respiratory burst oxidase subunit that is affected (see Table 21–26). Nomenclature has also been adopted for an abbreviated designation within each major genetic subgroup and includes the mode of inheritance and level of *phox* protein expression. The genes and corresponding complementary DNAs (cDNAs) of all four subunits have been cloned and their chromosomal locations have been mapped (see Table 21–8).[285, 626, 627, 938, 939] In two large studies of 140 pedigrees in the United States and Europe, defects in the X-linked gene for the gp91*phox* subunit of flavocytochrome *b* accounted for approximately two thirds of instances, with the remainder due to autosomal recessive inheritance of defects in p47*phox* (27 percent), p67*phox* (5 percent), and p22*phox* (6 percent).[857, 867] However, deficiency of p47*phox* has been reported to account for only 7 percent of instances of CGD in Japan.[628]

Mutations in Flavocytochrome *b*. More than two decades ago, it was reported that neutrophils obtained from the majority of patients with CGD lacked a low-potential cytochrome *b*.[629, 940, 941] This observation focused attention on the role of this cytochrome in the respiratory burst. It is known that the respiratory burst cytochrome is a flavocytochrome comprising two subunits and contains both flavin and heme groups that mediate the transfer of electrons from NADPH to molecular oxygen to generate superoxide.[942, 943] The cytochrome has two subunits, a 91-kD glycoprotein, gp91*phox*, that is the site of mutations in X-linked CGD, and a 22-kD polypeptide, p22*phox*, that is defective in a rare subgroup of patients with autosomal recessive inheritance of CGD. Formation of the gp91*phox*/p22*phox* heterodimer appears to be important to stabilize each subunit within the phagocyte, and no expression of both subunits is typically seen in both forms of cytochrome-negative CGD.[283, 944, 945]

The gene encoding gp91*phox* was mapped to Xp21.1 by its linkage to the X-linked form of CGD[946] and was the first human gene to be cloned on the basis of its chromosomal location,[285] an approach referred to as positional cloning or "reverse genetics." The gp91*phox* gene (termed *CYBB*) contains 13 exons and spans approximately 30 kb in the Xp21.1 region of the X chromosome.[285, 946, 947] Mechanisms that regulate the phagocyte-specific transcription of this gene include a repressor protein, CCAAT displacement protein (CDP), that binds to multiple sites upstream of the transcription start site in nonphagocytic or undifferentiated myeloid cells.[947] However, other regulatory elements appear to be located relatively long distances from the coding portion of the gp91*phox* gene.[947, 948]

Defects in the gene for gp91*phox* X-linked CGD have proved to be very heterogeneous[285, 878, 936, 946, 949–961] and, with few exceptions, are associated with absence of both the flavocytochrome heterodimer (X91[0]) and respiratory burst activity. Identification of the specific mutation in the gp91[phox] gene has been reported in more than 150 patients with X-linked CGD. An international registry compiling a large collection of identified mutations, X-CGDbase, is accessible at http://www.uta.fi/imt/bioinfo/CYBBbase/.[962] In general, each mutation is unique to a given kindred, although a few have been seen in several unrelated pedigrees. The overall heterogeneity of mutations and lack of any predominant genotype indicate that the incidence of CGD represents many different mutational events without any founder effect, as expected for a formerly lethal disorder. Approximately 10 to15 percent of X-linked CGD is caused by new germline mutations. In a small percentage of patients with X-linked CGD, a small amount of residual flavocytochrome b (X91⁻) associated with low levels of superoxide production is expressed. In addition, individuals have been reported who have normal levels of a dysfunctional flavocytochrome b (X91⁺).[878, 949, 959, 961]

Relatively large deletions in Xp21.1 involving *CYBB* and adjacent loci have been described in a few rare patients.[285, 946, 950–953] These individuals have complex phenotypes that include CGD and McLeod syndrome (a mild hemolytic anemia with acanthocytosis, associated with depressed levels of Kell antigens due to defects in the red cell antigen K_x), with or without concomitant Duchenne muscular dystrophy and retinitis pigmentosa. Patients with McLeod phenotype may develop anti-Kell antibodies when given transfusions of red blood cells, which can make future transfusion very difficult. Smaller deletions of the gp91[phox] gene have also been reported.[942, 958]

The majority of patients with X-linked CGD have mutations limited to only one or several nucleotides. These include missense mutations resulting in nonconservative amino acid substitutions, mutations of mRNA splicing sites, point deletions or insertions that disrupt the reading frame, and nonsense mutations that create a premature stop codon. Amino acid substitutions or in-frame insertions/deletions are generally associated with markedly reduced or absent expression of the gp91[phox] protein.[959, 960] Some of the mutations that result in normal levels of a dysfunctional flavocytochrome have involved gp91[phox] domains that appear to either participate in oxidase assembly[963, 964] or are involved in its redox function.[859, 937, 943, 959, 961, 965]

Mutations affecting the regulation of gp91[phox] transcription are rare and have been identified in two unusual phenotypes. In one type, described in two unrelated kindreds, affected males have two distinct populations of neutrophils.[925] In one population with normal respiratory burst activity, 5 to 15 percent of circulating phagocytes and myeloid progenitor cells were accounted for, whereas in the other population, who entirely lack a respiratory burst, the remainder of the cells were accounted for. Affected males had a severe clinical course.[925] Sequencing of the gp91[phox] gene identified a point mutation in the promoter sequence that was located 57 bp upstream of the normal transcription initiation site in one kindred, and 54 bp upstream in the other.[966] Another patient with X-linked CGD has been reported who had

normal levels of gp91[phox] expression and function in circulating eosinophils, but whose neutrophils, monocytes, and B lymphocytes had markedly reduced levels of gp91[phox].[957] Molecular analysis identified a mutation at 53 bp upstream of the transcription start site in this kindred.[967] These mutations disrupt the binding of several transcriptions important for normal expression of the *CYBB* gene,[967, 968] suggesting that gp91[phox] gene expression depends on this region of the promoter in all but a subset of granulocytes.

Mutations in the gene for the p22[phox] subunit of flavocytochrome *b*, designated *CYBA*, are an uncommon cause of autosomal recessive CGD (see Table 21–26). This locus has been mapped to 16q24 and contains six exons that span 8.5 kb.[938] The genetic defects that have been identified in this flavocytochrome subunit are also heterogeneous and range from a large interstitial gene deletion[938] to point mutations associated with missense, frameshift, or RNA splicing defects.[938, 955, 965, 969] The majority of the patients described are the offspring of consanguineous marriages. A single amino acid substitution (proline→glutamine) in a cytoplasmic domain of p22[phox] has been reported that is associated with normal levels of flavocytochrome *b* and a dysfunctional oxidase (A22⁺ CGD).[965] This mutation disrupts a proline-rich sequence in p22[phox] that normally interacts with a SH3 domain in p47[phox] during assembly of the active oxidase complex.[970–972] SH3 motifs, first described in the Src tyrosine kinase family, mediate protein-protein interactions via binding to proline-rich sequences in target proteins.[973] The proline substitution in p22[phox] is the second example of a genetic disease caused by disruption of protein-protein interactions mediated via SH3 domains. A kindred with X-linked agammaglobulinemia due to deletion of the SH3 region of Bruton tyrosine kinase has also been reported.[974]

Mutations in Cytosolic Factors. One of the key discoveries in unraveling the molecular basis of the different genetic subgroups in CGD was the observation that both the plasma membrane and the cytosol were required to reconstitute a catalytically active oxidase in a cell-free assay.[975–978] Complementation analysis using this assay identified two different subgroups of CGD in which the defect involved a cytosolic protein rather than the membrane-bound flavocytochrome *b*.[979, 980] Mutations in the gene encoding a cytosolic phosphoprotein, p47[phox], account for approximately one fourth of all instances of CGD, whereas inherited defects in the p67[phox] gene account for a small subgroup of patients with autosomal recessive CGD (see Table 21–26). Neither p47[phox] nor p67[phox] appears to participate directly in electron transfer, but they probably act in a regulatory role. The p47[phox] subunit may function as an "adaptor" protein important for efficient p67[phox] translocation to the flavocytochrome. *In vitro*, substantial amounts of superoxide can be generated from neutrophil membranes even in the absence of p47[phox], provided that high concentrations of p67[phox] and Rac GTP are supplied.[278]

The gene for p47[phox], termed *NCF1* (for neutrophil cytosolic factor 1), resides on chromosome 7,[981] and contains 9 exons spanning 18 kb.[982] In contrast to other forms of CGD, the majority of instances of p47[phox]-

deficient CGD are due to a single type of mutation, a GT deletion at the beginning of exon 2 that results in a frameshift and premature translational termination.[982, 983] Most patients appear to be homozygous for this mutation without any history of consanguinity, although a few compound heterozygotes have been described with a missense mutation accompanying the GT deletion. The high rate of occurrence of the GT deletion mutation appears to reflect the fact that humans have highly and closely linked conserved pseudogenes for p47^{phox} that contain the GT deletion.[984] Recombination or gene conversion events between the authentic p47^{phox} gene and its pseudogene(s) result in the creation of a mutant p47^{phox} alleles containing the GT deletion.[985] Neutrophils from p47^{phox} patients can generate very small but detectable amounts of superoxide, which may account for the overall milder course of disease for this genetic subgroup.[851, 986]

The gene for p67^{phox}, NCF2, which has been mapped to the long arm of chromosome 1,[987] spans 37 kb and contains 16 exons.[988] Mutations identified in p67^{phox}-deficient CGD have included missense mutations and splice junction mutations affecting mRNA processing.[955, 989] In one patient, in whom a triplet nucleotide deletion resulted in an in-frame deletion of lysine 58, a nonfunctional form of p67^{phox} was expressed, which failed to translocate and was unable to bind to Rac.[990–993]

Diagnosis

A diagnosis of CGD is suggested by characteristic clinical features (Tables 21–27 and 21–28) or by a family history of the disease. Because the severity and onset of the disease can vary considerably among different patients, CGD should still be considered in adolescents and adults who have an unusual site of infection or organism typical of CGD (see Table 21–27). The diagnosis of CGD is established by demonstration of an absent or greatly diminished neutrophil respiratory burst.

Many different methods have been used to monitor respiratory burst activity. These include assays using probes that exhibit either chemiluminescence or fluorescence when superoxide is released from activated phagocytes.[930, 931, 994, 995] One of the simplest and most accurate techniques is the nitro blue tetrazolium (NBT) test, in which neutrophils are stimulated to undergo a respiratory burst in the presence of NBT.[928, 929, 996, 997] When reduced by electrons donated from superoxide, the water-soluble, yellow tetrazolium dye is converted into deep blue, insoluble formazan deposits that precipitate on any cell that undergoes a respiratory burst. NBT reduction can be evaluated quantitatively using cells in suspension,[996] or, preferably, by examination of neutrophils and monocytes that have adhered to a microscope slide (the NBT slide test).[928, 929] As shown in the NBT slide test in Figure 21–9, there is a striking difference between resting neutrophils and monocytes (A) and those that have been stimulated (B), particularly if a strong respiratory burst agonist is used, such as phorbol myristate acetate. Cells from patients with X91^0, A22^0, A47^0, and A67^0 CGD fail to stain with NBT (cells from a patient with X91^0 CGD are shown in C), whereas patients with variant forms of the disease show light staining of all their neutrophils and monocytes (cells from a patient with X91$^-$ CGD are

shown in E). The NBT slide test is also very useful in diagnosing the carrier states of either X91^0 or X91$^-$ CGD, because a mixed population of NBT-positive and NBT-negative (or weakly stained with NBT) cells is observed (Fig. 21–10, D and F). Failure to detect a mixed population of formazan-staining cells does not necessarily rule out the X-linked carrier state, as nonrandom inactivation of cells with the mutant X chromosome can occur by chance. A normal maternal NBT test may also indicate that there has been a de novo mutation in the germ line of a parent[960, 981] or that the patient has one of the autosomal recessive forms of CGD. Intermediate levels of NBT reduction are not seen in phagocytes of autosomal recessive carriers. Flow cytometric assays of oxidase activity, such as those based on the conversion of dihydroxyrhodamine 123 to rhodamine 123,[994, 995] can also provide both quantitative measurements of peroxide generation and the cell-by-cell distribution of activity. In addition to X91$^-$ CGD neutrophils, weak staining in the NBT test and a small but measurable level of dihydroxyrhodamine 123 fluorescence can be seen in A47^0 cells, which reflects a small amount of residual oxidant production.

With the exception of classic X-linked disease in a male whose mother is a carrier, determining the specific oxidase gene affected in a given patient with CGD (see Table 21–26) requires techniques available only in research laboratories at present. These include immunoblot analysis of neutrophil extracts, flavocytochrome b spectroscopy, and functional analysis of membrane and cytosol fractions in the cell-free oxidase assay. In a male with no flavocytochrome b but without clear evidence for a maternal carrier, it is necessary to search for the mutation in both the gp91^{phox} and p22^{phox} genes by DNA sequencing or another method of analysis.

Identification of the specific genetic subgroup for a patient is useful primarily for purposes of genetic counseling and prenatal diagnosis, although it may also become increasingly important when successful approaches to somatic gene therapy are developed. In prenatal testing for suspected X-linked CGD, further analysis is not necessary if the fetus is determined to be a 46 XX female. In utero fetal blood sampling and NBT slide test analysis of fetal neutrophils can be used for prenatal diagnosis of CGD.[998–1001] However, even when the blood sample is successfully obtained, a low number of neutrophils adherent to the slide or contamination of the sample by maternal blood can complicate the interpretation of this test. DNA analysis of amniotic fluid cells or chorionic villus biopsy is an option for earlier prenatal diagnosis of CGD. Restriction fragment length polymorphisms have been identified for gp91^{phox}[954, 1002, 1003] and p67^{phox}[1004] and can be useful for diagnosis in informative families. The most specific approach to prenatal diagnosis is to first determine the family-specific mutation or mutations and then analyze fetal DNA for the presence of the mutant alleles using polymerase chain reaction–based technology.[1005] The latter techniques are presently available only in a few specialized research laboratories.

Prognosis and Treatment

The prognosis for patients with CGD has continued to improve since the disorder was first described in the

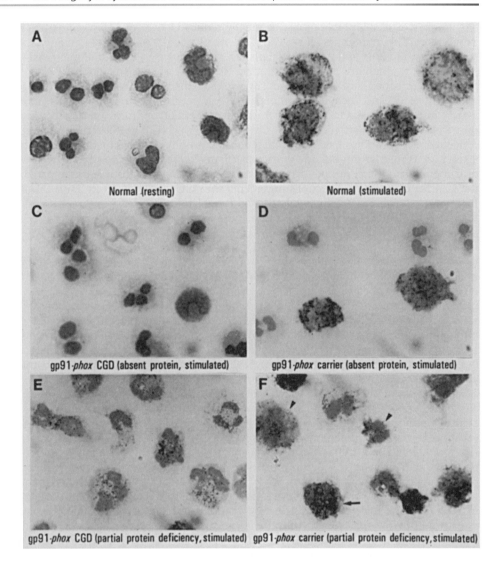

FIGURE 21–9. Evaluation of chronic granulomatous disease (CGD) using the nitro blue tetrazolium (NBT) test. Photomicrographs are shown of NBT tests performed on normal cells (at rest and after phorbol myristate acetate [PMA] stimulation) and on PMA-stimulated cells from patients with X91⁰ and X91⁻ CGD and their mothers (who are carriers). Dense formazan crystals are seen in all the normal phagocytes after stimulation (B) but are absent from resting cells (A). The patients with CGD are seen to have homogeneous populations of cells that either do not respond (X91⁰ [C]) or respond only minimally (X91⁻ [E]) to PMA. In contrast, the NBT tests on the CGD carriers show heterogeneous populations of cells that respond either normally or in a fashion similar to that of the abnormal cells from their offspring (D and F). For the maternal carrier shown in F, the cells with normal deposits of formazan (arrow) are intermixed with cells containing minimal amounts of formazan (arrowheads) identical to those seen in her affected male child (E). (From Smith RM, Curnutte JT: Molecular basis of chronic granulomatous disease. Blood 1991; 77:681.)

1950s, at which time almost all patients died in childhood.[852–854] In one retrospective review of 38 patients followed between 1964 and 1989, actuarial analysis showed 50 percent survival through the third decade of life.[873] In another retrospective study of 48 patients followed between 1969 and 1985 in Paris, the actuarial survival rate was 50 percent at 10 years of age, with a prolonged plateau thereafter.[871] Further refinements in treatment, coupled with the introduction of IFN-γ therapy, have continued to improve the prognosis for patients with CGD. Although there are no prospective data examining the long-term impact of these newer treatments, there is a general consensus that a majority of patients should survive well into their adult years. In one single institution study of 21 British children with CGD diagnosed since 1990, antibacterial and antifungal prophylaxis was routinely instituted at the time of diagnosis of CGD.[1006] No invasive or fungal infections occurred in the follow-up period (up to 10 years) nor were there any deaths. The overall mortality for all patients with CGD in the United States including adults has recently been estimated to be 5 percent per year for X-linked CGD and 2 percent per

year for autosomal recessive CGD.[851] As already noted, patients with a deficiency of p47^phox have often been noted to exhibit milder disease compared with those with flavocytochrome-negative CGD, possibly because of small amounts of residual superoxide produced.[826, 868, 986, 1007]

A multifaceted therapeutic approach has been responsible for the greatly improved prognosis in CGD. The cornerstones of current therapy include the following: (1) prevention and early treatment of infections; (2) use of prophylactic trimethoprim-sulfamethoxazole or dicloxacillin; (3) early use of parenteral antibiotics, including antifungal drugs, augmented by surgical drainage or resection of recalcitrant abscesses; (4) granulocyte transfusions for poorly responding infections; and (5) the use of prophylactic rIFN-γ.

Several approaches can be used to prevent infections. Patients with CGD should receive all routine immunizations (including live-virus vaccines) on schedule and an influenza vaccine yearly. Cuts and skin abrasions should be promptly cleansed with soap and water and rinsed with a 2 percent solution of hydrogen peroxide. The incidence and severity of rectal infections can be greatly reduced by avoiding constipation and soaking early lesions in warm, soapy water. Flossing and professional dental cleaning can help prevent gingivitis and periodontitis. The risk of *Aspergillus* infection can be decreased by avoiding marijuana smoke[1008] and decaying plant material (e.g., rotting wood, mulch, and hay), both of which often contain numerous *Aspergillus* spores.

Retrospective studies have shown that chronic prophylaxis with trimethoprim-sulfamethoxazole (5 mg/kg/day of trimethoprim given in one or two doses) can decrease the number of bacterial infections in patients with CGD. In one series of 36 patients followed at the National Institutes of Health, this regimen decreased the incidence of bacterial infections from 7.1 to 2.4/100 patient-months in patients with autosomal recessive CGD, and from 15.8 to 6.9 infections per 100 patients months in patients with X-linked CGD.[1007] Similar conclusions were reached in a review of 48 European patients.[871] The use of trimethoprim-sulfamethoxazole has not led to either increased rates of fungal infections or increased incidence of pathogens resistant to trimethoprim-sulfamethoxazole.[1007] Dicloxacillin (25 to 50 mg/kg/day) can be used in patients who are allergic to sulfa drugs, although there are relatively few data documenting its efficacy. Although administration of ketoconazole was found not to provide any protection against *Aspergillus* infections,[871] oral itraconazole may prove to be useful in this regard. A recent prospective study of 30 patients found an incidence of 3.4 *Aspergillus* infections (lung) per 100 patient years compared to 11.5 in a historical control group that did not receive any prophylaxis.[1009]

A frequent shortcoming in the treatment of patients with CGD is the failure to treat potentially serious infections promptly or long enough with the appropriate parenteral antibiotics. Patients with CGD do not always have typical symptoms and signs even with serious infections, and fever and leukocytosis can be absent, although an elevated sedimentation rate is often present.[880] Therapy should be directed initially at characteristic pathogens. In the absence of diagnostic culture results, a broad-spectrum antibiotic effective for gram-negative bacteria, including *B. cepacia*, should be administered in conjunction with a potent antistaphylococcal agent (e.g., a combination of nafcillin and ceftazidime). If the site of infection or offending pathogen is not known and if the patient is severely ill and a response to the initial therapy is not seen within 24 to 48 hours, an aggressive search for the underlying pathogen should be conducted. In these patients, therapy for fungi, *Nocardia* species, and *B. cepacia* may have to be given empirically. Even when appropriate antibiotics are used, infections often respond slowly, and some may require months of therapy, particularly *Aspergillus* infections and staphylococcal infections as well. Surgical drainage or resection can play a key role in the management of lymphadenitis, osteomyelitis, and abscesses of the liver, lungs, kidney, brain, and rectum[894, 1010] Finally, granulocyte transfusions may be helpful in the treatment of recalcitrant or life-threatening infections.[880, 1011]

rIFN-γ has recently been shown to be an effective and well-tolerated treatment that reduces the number of serious infections in patients with CGD.[1012,1013] IFN-γ enhances many aspects of normal phagocyte function, including microbial killing and rates of hydrogen peroxide production.[116, 1014] The latter appears, in part, to be related to increased levels of gp91^{phox} mRNA[1015] and prompted early attempts to use rIFN-γ to correct the functional defect in the respiratory burst in CGD. Initial studies showed that rIFN-γ improved both superoxide production and bacterial killing by CGD neutrophils both *in vitro* and *in vivo*.[1015–1017] This effect was most dramatic in some of the patients with variant X-linked CGD (X91⁻ CGD in Table 21–26). One site of action of rIFN-γ, at least in patients with X91⁻ CGD, appears to be granulocyte-monocyte precursor cells in the bone marrow. A single injection of rIFN-γ resulted in increased superoxide production by circulating phagocytes 2 weeks later, an effect that persisted for 28 days.[1016] Peripheral blood progenitor cells isolated 7 days after rIFN-γ injection and then cultured *in vitro* also yielded to NBT-positive colonies.[1018]

These encouraging results led to a double-blind, placebo-controlled phase III trial conducted over a 12-month period to evaluate whether rIFN-γ could have beneficial effects in CGD.[729] The findings in this study established this cytokine as an effective and well-tolerated treatment that reduces the infectious complications of CGD in all four genetic subgroups, a result that has continued to be supported by longer follow-up phase IV studies.[1013, 1019] The main conclusions of the original study are summarized in Table 21–29. Patients receiving rIFN-γ had a 70 percent reduction in the number of serious infections during the study period. These beneficial effects were independent of age, mode of inheritance, and concomitant use of prophylactic antibiotics. Patients younger than 10 years of age had the most pronounced reduction in infectious complications. Treatment (50 μg/m² three times a week subcutaneously) was well tolerated and easy to administer. The most common side effects were fever and headache. In contrast to what was observed in the initial studies of patients with variant CGD, there was no difference in neutrophil superoxide production and killing of *S. aureus* between the rIFN-γ and placebo groups.[729, 1020] Hence, the beneficial effect of rIFN-γ in most patients with CGD appears to be achieved by enhancing nonoxidative antimicrobial pathways. For example, administration of rIFN-γ to normal volunteers increases expression of FcγRI receptors and enhances phagocytosis.[1021]

Granulomatous inflammation in the esophagus, gastric antrum, and bladder can result in symptoms of obstruction and in the bowel wall a syndrome resembling inflammatory bowel disease. These complications can cause considerable morbidity in some patients with CGD and are generally treated with a combination of antibiotics and steroids.[905, 911, 1022–1025] Although the anti-inflammatory effects of steroids are often beneficial in this setting, their use should be carefully monitored because of the additional immunosuppression associated with their use. Cyclosporine was also used to successfully treat a patient with intractable gastrointestinal disease, although the patient did develop a serious fungal pneumonia caused by *Paecilomyces variotii* while receiving cyclosporine.[1026] IFN-γ has had no clear role in the management of the

TABLE 21–29. Summary of the Phase III Study Establishing the Efficacy of Recombinant Interferon-γ (rIFN-γ) for Infection Prophylaxis in Chronic Granulomatous Disease[*]

	Treatment Group		
Variable	Interferon	Placebo	P Value
Number of patients	63	65	
Age ± SD (yr)	14.3 ± 10.1	15.0 ± 9.6	
Number of patients with at least one serious infection (%)	14 (22%)	30 (46%)	0.0006
Total number of serious infections	20	56	<0.0001
Total hospital days	497	1493	0.02
Average hospital stay (days)	32	48	
	Percentage without Serious Infection[†]		
Age			
<10 yr (52 patients)	81	20	
≥ 10 yr (76 patients)	73	34	
Inheritance			
X-linked (86 patients)	79	33	
Autosomal (42 patients)	71	39	
Prophylactic antibiotics			
Yes (111 patients)	78	33	
No (17 patients)	69	28	

[*]The table shows a summary of the final results of a phase III randomized, double-blind, placebo-controlled study in which 128 patients with CGD received either recombinant IFN-γ (50 μg/m^2 per dose) or placebo by subcutaneous injections three times per week for an average duration of 8.9 months.[112] The major endpoints of the study were the time to the first serious infection and the number of such infections. A serious infection was defined as an event requiring hospitalization and parenteral antibiotics.

[†]The bottom portion of the table shows the Kaplan-Meler estimates of the cumulative proportion of patients free from serious infections of 12 months (after randomization) with adjustment for stratification factors.

chronic inflammatory complications of CGD, although anecdotal reports suggest that it may be beneficial in some patients.

Allogeneic bone marrow transplantation was used to successfully treat CGD in several patients.[378, 534, 1027, 1028] However, because of the risks associated with this procedure and the fact that an HLA-matched sibling is often lacking, conventional marrow transplantation is generally considered only for those patients who have recurrent and severe infections despite aggressive medical management. Recently developed nonmyeloablative conditioning regimens for allogeneic transplantation may be an alternative approach for bone marrow transplantation in CGD.[1029, 1030] In a phase I study targeted at high-risk patients with CGD who had a history of two or more serious infections and also had an HLA-identical sibling donor, patients were given conditioning with cyclophosphamide, fludarabine, and antithymocyte globulin before treatment and also received donor lymphocyte infusions after transplant.[1031] The transplant was generally well tolerated, and partial or complete chimerism was seen in 8 of 10 patients (5 children and 5 adults) at a median of 17 months of follow-up, with improvement of clinical symptoms of CGD. However, graft-versus-host disease was a significant problem in the adult patients and the cause of one death. One patient also died of pneumococcal pneumonia at 13 months post-transplant, reflecting the profound and prolonged immunosuppression associated with this transplant regimen, and in a third patient, who had previously received numerous granulocyte transfusions, the initial graft failed and the patient subsequently died of complications of a second transplant.

Because CGD results from single gene defects in proteins expressed in myeloid cells, this disorder is an excellent candidate for gene replacement therapy targeted at hematopoietic stem cells. Based on the lack of symptoms observed in female carriers of X-linked CGD with as few as 10 to 20 percent NBT-positive neutrophils, significant clinical benefit may result even if this fraction of the phagocyte population is successfully corrected. For the X-linked gene product, gp91^{phox}, it also appears that expression of even modest amounts of recombinant protein can lead to considerable reconstitution of superoxide-generating capacity.[1032, 1033] Mouse models of X-linked and A47^0 CGD recently developed by gene targeting have a phenotype that resembles human CGD, with increased susceptibility to serious infections due to *S. aureus*, *A. fumigatus*, and *B. cepacia* and abnormal inflammatory responses.[314–318] Studies using bone marrow transplantation and gene therapy in murine CGD have been useful in evaluating the level of correction required to prevent symptoms and have generally confirmed the clinical observations in female carriers of X-linked CGD and in variant X-linked CGD.[317, 318, 1033]

Numerous groups have reported using gene transfer technology to successfully reconstitute respiratory burst oxidase activity in EBV-transformed B lymphocytes or in bone marrow–derived myeloid progenitor cells from all four genetic subgroups of CGD.[1034] Both plasmid-based and retroviral vectors have been used. The major barriers to the future clinical use of gene replacement therapy for CGD relate to achieving efficient vector-mediated gene transfer into long-lived human hemapoietic stem cells[685, 686] and the ability of corrected cells to replace uncorrected cells in the marrow, because no selective growth advantage exists for NADPH oxidase-positive cells. Several phase I CGD gene therapy clinical trails using cytokine-mobilized peripheral blood CD34$^+$ cells have been conducted, all without prior bone marrow conditioning. In one trial involving five patients with the p47^{phox}-deficient form of CGD, oxidase-positive neutrophils were detected in peripheral blood of all five patients after infusion of trans-duced cells.[1035] Peak numbers of corrected neutrophils, ranging from 0.004 to 0.05 percent, were seen at 3 to 6 weeks, and lower neutrophil levels persisted in two patients for up to 6 months.

GLUCOSE-6–PHOSPHATE DEHYDROGENASE DEFICIENCY

The substrate for the respiratory burst oxidase, NADPH, is generated by the first two reactions of the hexose monophosphate shunt, G6PD (see Fig. 21–6, reaction 8) and 6-phosphogluconate dehydrogenase. Because G6PD is the first enzyme in this pathway, its absence results in greatly diminished shunt activity and thus a severe decrease in the availability of NADPH. As would be expected, severe G6PD deficiency in neutrophils results in attenuated respiratory burst and, in some patients, a clinical picture somewhat similar to that observed in CGD.[1036–1039] The key features of G6PD deficiency are summarized in Table 21–30. The organisms causing infection in patients with severe deficiency are similar to those observed in CGD and are predominately catalase-positive bacteria.

In light of the relatively high incidence of G6PD mutations in the American black and Mediterranean populations,[1040] as well as the fact that leukocyte and erythrocyte G6PD are encoded by the same gene,[1041] it might be expected that clinically significant neutrophil G6PD deficiency would occur more often than it does (less than 10 patients have been described in the literature). One of the reasons it does not is that neutrophils must have a severe deficiency of G6PD (less than 5 percent of normal) before respiratory burst function is adversely affected. Even low levels of G6PD are apparently sufficient to recycle NADP$^+$ back to NADPH at a rate that permits reasonable levels of respiratory burst activity. Furthermore, it is apparent from studies on patients with variant CGD that surprisingly low levels of respiratory burst activity (5 to 10 percent of normal) can still provide adequate protection against microbial infection (see earlier). Therefore, the rate at which these critically low levels of neutrophil G6PD are encountered is very low. In most types of G6PD deficiency, neutrophil levels are in the range of 20 to 75 percent of normal.[1042, 1043] Because most G6PD mutations cause the enzyme to decay over a period of days and weeks, levels in the short-lived neutrophil usually do not become critically low, even in some of the more unstable G6PD variants. Hence, it appears that only a rare (and poorly understood) group of mutations causes extremely low levels of G6PD in neutrophils.

The diagnosis of G6PD deficiency should be considered in any patient with congenital nonspherocytic hemolytic anemia in whom the erythrocyte G6PD level is unusually low or the incidence of infections is high. The diagnosis is established by measuring the level of G6PD activity in neutrophil homogenates. Although not necessary for the diagnosis, neutrophil function tests show a diminished respiratory burst (5 to 30 percent of normal).[1038, 1044] The treatment of neutrophil G6PD deficiency is similar to that of CGD except that the efficacy of rIFN-γ has not been demonstrated in the former. In general, the effects of G6PD deficiency appears to be somewhat milder than those of CGD, although recurrent episodes of pneumonia and a fatal infection with *C. violaceum* have been described.[1038, 1044]

MYELOPEROXIDASE DEFICIENCY

MPO deficiency is the most common inherited disorder of phagocytes. Although only 17 known instances had

TABLE 21–30. Summary of Neutrophil Glucose-6-Phosphate Dehydrogenase Deficiency

Incidence	Extremely rare
Inheritance	X-linked
Molecular defect	Poorly characterized family of mutations that cause CNSHA in erythrocytes and functional failure of G6PD in neutrophils (possibly kinetic mutants); other rare mutants may also be responsible
Pathogenesis	Severe functional failure of neutrophil G6PD (<5% of normal), leading to an extremely low steady-state concentration of NADPH, which serves as the substrate for NADPH oxidase
Clinical manifestations	CNSHA (hemolytic anemia that occurs even in the absence of redox stress)
	CGD-like syndrome with recurrent bacterial infections
Laboratory evaluation	Neutrophil G6PD activity <5% of normal
	Severely diminished respiratory burst and abnormal NTB test results
	Associated CNSHA with elevated reticulocyte count and diminished erythrocyte G6PD activity
Differential diagnosis	CGD
	Glutathione reductase or synthetase deficiency
Therapy	Prophylactic trimethoprim-sulfamethoxazole
	Aggressive use of parenteral antibiotics
	Transfusion support for severe anemia
Prognosis	Not clear, because too few patients have been reported
	May be as severe as CGD

CNSHA = chronic nonspherocytic hemolytic anemia; G6PD = glucose-6-phosphate dehydrogenase.
From Curnutte JT: Disorders of phagocyte function. In Hoffman R, Benz EF, et al (eds): Hematology: Basic Principles and Practice. New York, Churchill Livingstone, 1991, p 577.

been collected up to 1979, the diagnosis is now easily made with the widespread use of automated flow cytochemistry in clinical hematology laboratories to enumerate peripheral blood neutrophils using peroxidase activity. A complete deficiency is seen in approximately 1 in 4000 individuals, and partial deficiencies occur in 1 in 2000 people.[1045–1047] The enzymatic deficiency is seen in neutrophils and monocytes. Peroxidase levels in eosinophils, on the other hand, are normal, because eosinophil peroxidase is encoded by a different gene.[72]

MPO plays a pivotal role in amplifying the toxicity of hydrogen peroxide generated by the respiratory burst and catalyzes the formation of hypochlorous acid (HOCl) from chloride and hydrogen peroxide (Fig. 21–5, reaction 4).[218, 1048] HOCl, in turn, reacts with a variety of primary and secondary amines to form chloramines, some of which can be toxic.[218] Moreover, HOCl is capable of activating latent metalloproteinases.[218] On the basis of these considerations, one would expect that severe MPO deficiency should attenuate important antimicrobial reactions catalyzed by HOCl. Neutrophils from patients with MPO deficiency patients show markedly abnormal *in vitro* killing of *C. albicans* and hyphal forms of *A. fumigatus*.[1045, 1049, 1050] Curiously, however, these *in vitro* abnormalities are rarely reflected in an increased incidence of infection in patients except for rare individuals who also suffer from diabetes mellitus.[1045, 1047, 1049, 1051] In these individuals, disseminated candidiases can be seen (Table 21–31). Several studies have suggested that MPO deficiency may also be associated with an increased susceptibility to malignancy.[1045, 1047, 1052]

Congenital MPO deficiency is inherited in an autosomal recessive manner,[1046, 1051, 1052] and variable expression of the defect has been reported.[1052] The gene for MPO has been localized to the long arm of chromosome 17 at position q22-q23 near the breakpoint for the 15;17 translocation of promyelocytic leukemia.[1053, 1054] The primary translation product is a 80-kD protein that undergoes cotranslational glycosylation and subsequent proteolytic cleavage to heavy and light chains, which oligomerize to form a tetramer composed of two heavy and two light chains.[1046] The molecular basis of congenital MPO deficiency reflects defects affecting MPO processing.[1055–1057] Three different genotypes have been reported to date. One cause of complete absence of immunoreactive MPO is a point mutation that results in an arginine to tryptophan substitution at codon 569 (R569W), which was found in 6 of 12 patients with this phenotype.[1058, 1059] The R569W mutation results in a maturation arrest of the MPO apoprotein, which fails to incorporate heme.[1060] A second genotype involves a missense mutation in which tyrosine at codon 173 is replaced by a cysteine, and the mutant MPO is degraded rather than undergoing proteolytic maturation.[1061] The reported third genotype was a compound heterozygote in which one allele has a missense mutation with resultant replacement of methionine at codon 251 with threonine, and the second allele has a 14-bp deletion from exon 9.[1062]

In addition to inherited MPO deficiency, secondary or acquired MPO deficiency can occur. MPO-deficient cells can be seen in the M2, M3, and M4 forms of acute myeloid leukemia as well as in approximately 25 percent of patients with MDS and chronic myeloid leukemia.[1046, 1063, 1064] Other clinical situations in which secondary MPO deficiency can occur include pregnancy, iron deficiency, lead poisoning, ceroid lipofuscinosis, and Hodgkin disease.[1047]

There are several possible reasons for the surprisingly mild clinical phenotype of MPO deficiency. First, neutrophils contain such a large amount of MPO that appreciable levels may be left in the cell even in patients of severe deficiency. These residual stores, coupled with normal levels of eosinophil peroxidase, may provide at least some degree of peroxidative activity at sites of infection.

TABLE 21–31. Summary of Myeloperoxidase Deficiency

Incidence	1 in 2000 (partial deficiency)
	1 in 4000 (total deficiency)
Inheritance	Autosomal recessive with variable expression; MPO gene on chromosome 17 at q22-q23
Molecular defect	Defective post-translational processing of an abnormal MPO precursor polypeptide due to at least four genetic lesions; eosinophil peroxidase encoded by different gene and levels normal
Pathogenesis	Partial or complete MPO deficiency leads to diminished production of HOCl and HOCl-derived chloramines; MPO products are necessary for rapid killing of microbes (especially *Candida*) but not absolutely required
Clinical manifestations	Usually clinically silent
	Rarely disseminated candidiasis/fungal disease (usually in conjunction with diabetes mellitus)
	May be increased risk of malignancy in congenital MPO deficiency
Laboratory evaluation	Deficiency of neutrophil/monocyte peroxidase by histochemical analysis (eosinophil peroxidase normal)
	Delayed, but eventually normal, killing of bacteria *in vitro*
	Failure to kill *C. albicans* and hyphal forms of *Aspergillus fumigatus in vitro*
Differential diagnosis	Acquired partial MPO deficiency seen in acute myelogenous leukemia (M2, M3, and M4), myelodysplastic syndromes, iron deficiency, or pregnancy
Therapy	None in asymptomatic patients
	Aggressive treatment of fungal infections when they occur
	Control of blood glucose levels in diabetes
Prognosis	Usually excellent

HOCl = hypochlorous acid; MPO = myeloperoxidase; Modified from Curnutte JT: Disorders of phagocyte function. In Hoffman R, Benz EJ, et al (eds): Hematology: Basic Principles and Practice. New York, Churchill Livingstone, 1991, p 578.

Second, the respiratory burst in MPO-deficient neutrophils is substantially augmented in terms of velocity and duration.[1065, 1066] This may be due to the enhanced stability of the respiratory burst oxidase made possible by the absence of HOCl, which normally inactivates the oxidase.[1067] Finally, other oxidants produced by the respiratory burst may work together with the various granule antimicrobial proteins to provide sufficient protection against most microorganisms.

Given the mild clinical nature of MPO deficiency, no treatment is generally required. Infections, when they occur, are treated as are those in normal individuals. It is important for the clinician to be aware of the increased risk of *Candida* infections in patients with MPO deficiency and to treat them aggressively when they do occur.

DISORDERS OF GLUTATHIONE METABOLISM

As shown in Figure 21–6 (reaction 6), glutathione peroxidase protects neutrophil proteins (including NADPH oxidase) from the harmful effects of hydrogen peroxide generated in the course of the respiratory burst by degrading it to water. The reducing equivalents for this reaction are carried by the reduced form of glutathione (GSH), the intracellular levels of which are maintained by recycling oxidized glutathione back to GSH by means of glutathione reductase (see Fig. 21–6, reaction 7). Glutathione levels are also maintained through *de novo* synthesis catalyzed by glutathione synthetase (see Fig. 21–6, reaction 9). Severe deficiencies of glutathione reductase and glutathione synthetase in neutrophils have been reported and found to cause moderately severe abnormalities in the respiratory burst.[1068–1072] The key features of each of these extremely rare disorders are summarized in Table 21–32.

Glutathione reductase deficiency has been reported in one family in which three siblings were found to have a marked deficiency of this enzyme in their neutrophils (10 to 15 percent of normal).[1068, 1070] The inheritance appeared to be autosomal recessive, because the parents of the children were first cousins and their neutrophils contained 50 percent of the normal levels of glutathione reductase. The mutation responsible for the enzyme deficiency in this family has not been reported yet. It is known that the gene for glutathione reductase is located on chromosome 8 at position p21.1.[1073]

Clinically, none of the affected patients showed signs of increased infection. Their erythrocytes were also deficient in glutathione reductase and therefore were prone to hemolysis in the face of oxidant stress. Two siblings did suffer from juvenile cataracts and deafness. The structure and function of the neutrophil *in vitro* were normal except for a premature termination of the respiratory burst after about 5 minutes.[1068] The probable reason for this defect is that NADPH oxidase is inactivated by the products of the MPO reaction.[1067] If glutathione reductase is deficient, the neutrophils cannot maintain a level of GSH sufficient to detoxify hydrogen peroxide. After several minutes of the respiratory burst, toxic levels of hydrogen peroxide accumulate and lead to deactivation of the oxidase. This explanation is supported by experiments showing that glutathione reductase–deficient neutrophils pre-exposed to exogenous hydrogen peroxide fail to undergo even an abbreviated respiratory burst. One important insight gained from the study of these patients is that only a brief respiratory burst appears to be necessary for adequate microbial killing.

The diagnosis of glutathione reductase deficiency is made by measuring the levels of this enzyme in neutrophil homogenates. The finding of a truncated respiratory burst

TABLE 21–32. Disorders of Glutathione Metabolism

Disease Aspect	Glutathione Reductase Deficiency	Glutathione Synthetase Deficiency
Incidence	One family; three siblings	Several reported cases
Inheritance	Autosomal recessive	Autosomal recessive
Molecular defect	Diminished glutathione reductase levels in neutrophils (10%–15% of normal) and erythrocytes; mutation not known	Severe deficiency of glutathione synthetase activity (5%–10% of normal); mutation(s) not known
Pathogenesis	Brief respiratory burst truncated by toxic accumulation of H_2O_2 by glutathione	Same as with glutathione reductase deficiency except that the respiratory burst is normal; elevated 5-oxoproline levels due to lack of feedback inhibition by glutathione
Clinical manifestations	No history of repeated infection Hemolysis with oxidant stress	Metabolic acidosis due to elevated 5-oxoproline Otitis media Intermittent neutropenia Hemolysis with oxidant stress Severe decrease in glutathione synthetase level
Laboratory evaluation	Glutathione reductase level diminished Premature cessation of O_2 production by neutrophils	Normal respiratory burst
Differential diagnosis	CGD G6PD deficiency	Glutathione reductase deficiency
Therapy	None required	Vitamin E for hemolysis and infections Treatment of metabolic acidosis
Prognosis	Benign disorder	Relatively benign disorder

From Curnutte JT: Disorders of phagocyte function. In Hoffman R, Benz EJ, et al (eds): Hematology: Basic Principles and Practice. New York, Churchill Livingstone, 1991, p 578.

provides supporting evidence, although a similar abnormality can be seen in G6PD deficiency. No therapy is required, but avoiding foods and drugs containing potent oxidants will decrease the chance of depleting intracellular glutathione.

Several forms of congenital glutathione synthetase deficiency have been described, all of which are inherited in an autosomal recessive fashion. Specific mutations have not been reported. Only in those patients in whom glutathione synthetase activity is severely deficient in neutrophils (5 to 10 percent of normal) is a phagocytic abnormality

detected.[1069, 1071, 1072] In contrast to glutathione reductase deficiency, neutrophils deficient in glutathione synthetase have a normal respiratory burst.[1069, 1072] However, for reasons that are uncertain, *in vitro* bacterial killing is decreased. Despite this microbicidal defect, patients with glutathione synthetase deficiency have only a relatively mild problem resolving infections. They do suffer from a severe metabolic acidosis resulting from elevated levels of 5-oxoproline, a metabolite formed in one of the early steps in the pathway of glutathione synthesis. This acidosis may

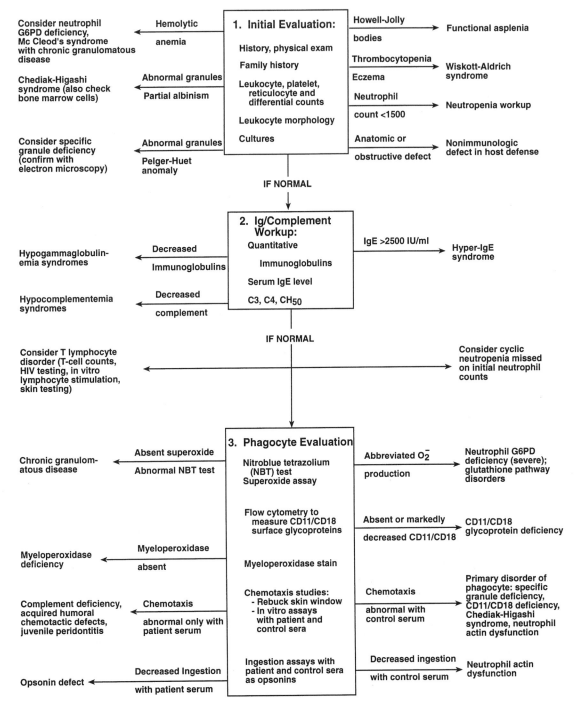

FIGURE 21–10. Algorithm for the workup of a patient with recurrent infections. The various tests are described in the appropriate sections of the chapter. G6PD = glucose-6-phosphate dehydrogenase; Ig = immunoglobulin; O_2^-, superoxide. The units for the neutrophil count (box 1) are neutrophils per cubic millimeter. (Adapted from Lehrer RI et al: Neutrophils and host defense. Ann Intern Med 1988; 109:127).

be responsible for the intermittent neutropenia observed in patients with glutathione synthetase deficiency.[1069] Because the erythrocytes in these patients are also deficient in glutathione synthetase, a hemolytic anemia brought on by oxidant stress is seen. Therapy with vitamin E (400 IU/day) was found to be beneficial in patients who suffer from hemolysis and infection.[1069]

Glutathione peroxidase (see Fig. 21–6, reaction 6) was found to be decreased to levels that were 25 percent of normal in three unrelated patients with a clinical syndrome resembling CGD.[1074, 1075] Although this enzyme plays an important role in removing hydrogen peroxide, whether the degree of deficiency seen in these patients is sufficient to cause functional abnormalities in neutrophils has not been established. Two of the affected kindreds have recently been restudied and a severe deficiency of the respiratory burst oxidase flavocytochrome *b* has been identified in affected members of each.[936] It thus appears that in at least two of these previously identified patients, CGD is the underlying problem, not glutathione peroxidase deficiency.

Evaluation of the Patient with Recurrent Infections

Diagnosis in the patient who is seen with recurrent infections can be a challenge. Many of the phagocyte disorders present with similar clinical manifestations, which can overlap those seen in inherited or acquired disorders of lymphocyte function. Furthermore, the majority of patients with recurrent infections do not have an identifiable granulocyte or monocyte defect. Given this low yield and the lack of ability to characterize many aspects of phagocyte function in routine laboratory studies, physicians are faced with the difficult question of which patients should have a complete evaluation. Those who have at least one of the following clinical features may have a phagocyte defect: (1) an unusually high incidence of bacterial and fungal infections; (2) the presence of an infection at an unusual site (e.g., a hepatic or brain abscess); (3) infections with atypical pathogens (e.g., *Aspergillus* pneumonia, disseminated candidiasis, or lymphadenitis due to *Serratia* or *Klebsiella*); (4) infections of exceptional severity, and (5) childhood periodontal disease. Certain other clinical findings can also be helpful. For example, a child with nystagmus, fair skin, and recurrent staphylococcal infections should be evaluated for CHS, whereas an infant with bacterial infections and delayed separation of the umbilical cord should be tested for LAD. Once the physician has decided that a phagocyte evaluation is warranted, the algorithm presented in Figure 21–10 may be helpful in organizing the workup. When coupled with a thorough clinical history and physical examination, the laboratory tests outlined in Figure 21–10 should allow the physician to establish the diagnosis and formulate an appropriate therapeutic plan.

REFERENCES

1. Tenen D: Myeloid: Transcription factors and development. In Zon L (ed): Hematopoiesis: A Developmental Approach. New York, Oxford University Press, 2001, p 417.
2. Zhang D-E, Zhang P, Wang N, et al: Absence of granulocyte colony-stimulating factor signaling and neutrophil development in CCAAT enhancer binding protein alpha-deficient mice. Proc Natl Acad Sci USA 1997; 94:569.
3. Yamanaka R, Barlow C, Lekstrom-Himes J, et al: Impaired granulopoiesis, myelodysplasia, and early lethality in CCAAT/enhancer binding protein epsilon-deficient mice. Proc Natl Acad Sci USA 1997; 94:13187.
4. Lieschke GJ, Burgess AW: Granulocyte colony-stimulating factor and granulocyte-macrophage colony-stimulating factor. Part II. N Engl J Med 1992; 327:99.
5. Metcalf D: The molecular control of cell division, differentiation commitment and maturation of hematopoietic stem cells. Blood 1989; 339:27.
6. Sieff CA: Hematopoietic growth factors. J Clin Invest 1987; 79:1549.
7. Clutterbuck EF, Hirst EM, Sanderson CG: Human interleukin-5 (IL-5) regulates the production of eosinophils in human bone marrow cultures: Comparison and interaction with IL-1, IL-3, IL-6, and GMCSF. Blood 1989; 73:1504.
8. Sanderson CJ: Interleukin-5, eosinophils, and disease. Blood 1992; 79:3101.
9. Warren DJ, Moore MA: Synergism among interleukin 1, interleukin 3, and interleukin 5 in the production of eosinophils from primitive hematopoietic stem cells. J Immunol 1988; 140:94.
10. Denburg JA: Basophil and mast cell lineages *in vitro* and *in vivo*. Blood 1992; 79:846.
11. Halett MB, Lloyds D: Neutrophil priming: The cellular signals that say 'amber' but not 'green.' Immunol Today 1995; 16:264.
12. Jacobsen SEW, Fahlman C, Blomhoff HK, et al: *All-trans-* and *9-cis-retinoic* acid: Potent direct inhibitors of primitive murine hematopoietic progenitors *in vitro*. J Exp Med 1994; 179:1665.
13. Tsai S, Collins SJ: A dominant negative retinoic acid receptor blocks neutrophil differentiation at the promyelocyte stage. Proc Natl Acad Sci USA 1993; 90:7153.
14. Mangelsdorf DJ, Evans RM: The RXR heterodimers and orphan receptors. Cell 1995; 83:841.
15. Mangelsdorf DJ, Thummel C, Beato M, et al: The nuclear receptor superfamily: The second decade. Cell 1995; 83:835.
16. Lo Coco F, Avvisati G, Diverio D, et al: Molecular evaluation of response to all-*trans* retinoic acid therapy in patients with acute promyelocytic leukemia. Blood 1991; 77:1657.
17. Borrow J, Goddard AD, Sheer D, et al: Molecular analysis of acute promyelocytic leukemia breakpoint cluster region on chromosome 17. Science 1990; 249:1577.
18. De The H, Lavau C, Marchio A, et al: The PML-RARa fusion mRNA generated by the t(15;17) translocation in acute promyelocytic leukemia encodes a functionally altered RAR. Cell 1991; 66:675.
19. Athens JW, Haab OP, Raab SO, et al: Leukokinetic studies. IV. The total blood, circulating and marginal granulocyte pools and the granulocyte turnover rate in normal subjects. J Clin Invest 1961; 40:989.
20. Cronkite EP: Kinetics of granulopoiesis. Clin Haematol 1979; 8:351.
21. Dancey JT, Deubelbeiss KA: Neutrophil kinetics in man. J Clin Invest 1976; 58:705.
22. Donohue DM, Reiff RH: Quantitative measurement of the erythrocytic and granulocytic cells of the marrow and blood. J Clin Invest 1958; 37:1571.
23. Klebanoff SJ, Durack DT: Functional studies on human peritoneal eosinophils. Infect Immun 1977; 17:167.
24. Van Furth R, Raeburn JA: Characteristics of human mononuclear phagocytes. Blood 1979; 54:485.
25. Fadok VA, Savill JS, Haslett C, et al: Different populations of macrophages use either the vitronectin receptor or the phosphatidylserine receptor to recognize and remove apoptotic cells. J Immunol 1992; 149:4029.
26. Savill J: Apoptosis in resolution of inflammation. J Leukoc Biol 1997; 61:375.
27. Savill JS, Wyllie AH, Henson JE, et al: Macrophage phagocytosis of aging neutrophils in inflammation. Programmed cell death in the neutrophil leads to recognition by macrophages. J Clin Invest 1989; 83:865.
28. Bainton DF: Neutrophilic leukocyte granules: From structure to function. Adv Exp Med Biol 1993; 336:17.

29. Borregaard N, Lollike K, Kjeldsen L, et al: Human neutrophil granules and secretory vesicles. Eur J Haematol 1993; 51:187.

30. Hoffstein S, Weissmann G: Microtubules in calcium ionophore induced secretion of lyosomal enzymes from human polymorphonuclear leukocytes. J Cell Biol 1978; 78:78.

31. Howard TH, Watts RG: Actin polymerization and leukocyte function. Curr Opin Hematol 1994; 1:61.

32. Stossel TP: On the crawling of animal cells. Science 1993; 260:1086.

33. Shapiro LH, Look AT: Transcriptional regulation in myeloid cell differentiation. Curr Sci 1995; 2:3.

34. Tenen D, Hromas R, Licht J, et al: Transcription factors, normal myeloid development, and leukemia. Blood 1997; 90:489.

35. Shivdasani R, Orkin S: The transcriptional control of hematopoiesis. Blood 1996; 87:4025.

36. Berliner N, Hsing A, Graubert T, et al: Granulocyte colony-stimulating factor induction of normal human bone marrow progenitors results in neutrophil-specific gene expression. Blood 1995; 85:799.

37. Borregaard N, Sehested M, Nielsen BS, et al: Biosynthesis of granule proteins in normal human bone marrow cells. Gelatinase Ia a marker of terminal neutrophil differentiation. Blood 1995; 85:812.

38. Grisolano JL, Sclar GM, Ley TJ: Early myeloid-specific expression of the human cathepsin G gene in transgenic mice. Proc Natl Acad Sci USA 1994; 91:8989.

39. Orkin SH: Molecular genetics of chronic granulomatous disease. Annu Rev Immunol 1989; 7:277.

40. Zakhireh B, Root R: Development of oxidase activity by human bone marrow granulocytes. Blood 1979; 54:429.

41. Newburger PE, Dai Q, Whitney C: *In vitro* regulation of human phagocyte cytochrome *b* heavy and light chain gene expression by bacterial lipopolysaccharide and recombinant human cytokines. J Biol Chem 1991; 266:16171.

42. Cassatella MA: The production of cytokines by polymorphonuclear neutrophils. Immunol Today 1995; 16:21.

43. Lloyd AR, Oppenheim JJ: Poly's lament: The neglected role of the polymorphonuclear neutrophil in the afferent limb of the immune response. Immunol Today 1992; 13:169.

44. Liu CH, Lehan C, Speer ME, et al: Degenerative changes in neutrophils: An indicator of bacterial infection. Pediatrics 1984; 74:823.

44a. Hoffman K, Dreger CK, Olins AL, et al: Mutations in the gene encoding the lamin B receptor produce an altered nuclear morphology in granulocytes (Pelger-Huet anomaly). Nat Genet 2002; 31:410.

45. Borregaard N, Kjeldsen L, Lollike K, et al: Granules and secretory vesicles of the human neutrophil. Int J Pediatr Hematol Oncol 1997; 3:307.

46. Jesaitis AJ, Buescher ES, Harrison D, et al: Ultrastructural localization of cytochrome *b* in the membranes of resting and phagocytosing human granulocytes. J Clin Invest 1990; 85:821.

47. Borregaard N, Tauber AI: Subcellular localization of the human neutrophils NADPH oxidase. *b*-Cytochrome and associated flavoprotein. J Biol Chem 1984; 259:47.

48. Lekstrom-Himes J, Dorman S, Kopar P, et al: Neutrophil-specific granule deficiency results from a novel mutation with loss of function of the transcription factor CCAAT/enhancer binding protein e. J Exp Med 1999; 189:1847.

49. Gombart AF, Shiohara M, Kwok SH, et al: Neutrophil-specific granule deficiency: Homozygous recessive inheritance of a frameshift mutation in the gene encoding transcription factor CCAAT/enhancer binding protein—epsilon. Blood 2001; 97:2561.

50. Bokoch GM: Chemoattractant signaling and leukocyte activation. Blood 1995; 86:1649.

51. Downey GP, Fukushima T, Fialkow L: Signaling mechanisms in human neutrophils. Curr Opin Hematol 1995; 2:76.

52. Thelen M, Wirthmueller U: Phospholipases and protein kinases during phagocyte activation. Curr Opin Immunol 1994; 6:106.

53. Wu D, Huang C, Jiang H: Roles of phospholipid signaling in chemoattractant-induced responses. J Cell Sci 2000; 113:2935.

54. Berkow RI, Dodson RW: Tyrosine-specific protein phosphorylation during activation of human neutrophils. Blood 1990; 75:2445.

55. Grinstein S, Furuya W, Butler JR, et al: Receptor-mediated activation of multiple serine/threonine kinases in human leukocytes. J Biol Chem 1993; 268:20223.

56. Herlaar E, Brown Z: p38 MAPK signalling cascades in inflammatory disease. Mol Med Today 1999; 5:439.

57. Rollet E, Caon AC, Roberge CJ, et al: Tyrosine phosphorylation in activated nehuman neutrophils: Comparison of the effects of differ-

58. Kunkel S, Lukacs N, Strieter R: Expression and biology of neutrophil and endothelial cell-derived chemokines. Cell Biol 1995; 6:327.

59. Perez HD: Chemoattractant receptors. Curr Opin Hematol 1994; 1:40.

60. Rollins B: Chemokines. Blood 1997; 90:909.

61. Bokoch GM, Knaus UG: Ras-related GTP-binding proteins and leukocyte signal transduction. Curr Opin Hematol 1994; 1:53.

62. Worthen GS, Avdi N, Buhl AM, et al: FMLP activates Ras and Raf in human neutrophils: Potential role in activation of MAP kinase. J Clin Invest 1994; 94:815.

63. Bernard V, Bohl BP, Bokoch GM: Characterization of rac and cdc42 activation in chemoattractant-stimulated human neutrophils using a novel assay for active GTPases. J Biol Chem 1999; 274:13198.

64. Bernard V, Bokoch GM, Diebold BA: Potential drug targets: Small GTPases that regulate leukocyte function. Trends Pharmacol Sci 1999; 20:365.

65. Williams DA, Tao W, Yang F, et al: Dominant negative mutation of the hematopoietic-specific Rho GTPase, Rac2, is associated with a human phagocyte immunodeficiency. Blood 2000; 96:1646.

66. Ambruso DR, Knall C, Abell AN, et al: Human neutrophil immunodeficiency syndrome is associated with an inhibitory Rac2 mutation. Proc Natl Acad Sci USA 2000; 97:4654.

67. Anderson V, Bro-Rasmussen F: Autoradiographic studies of eosinophil kinetics. Cell Tissue Kinet 1969; 2:139.

68. Carlson M, Peterson C, Venge P: The influence of IL-3, IL-5, and GM-CSF on normal human eosinophil and neutrophil C3b-induced degranulation. Allergy 1993; 48:437.

69. Enokihara H, Furusawa S, Nakakabo H, et al: T cells from eosinophilic patients produce interleukin-5 with interleukin-2 stimulation. Blood 1989; 73:1809.

70. Parwaresch MR, Walle AJ: The peripheral kinetics of human radio-labelled eosinophils. Virchows Arch 1976; 1321:57.

71. Weller PF: The immunobiology of eosinophils. N Engl J Med 1991; 324:1110.

72. Gleich G, Adolphson M, Leiferman K: The biology of the eosinophilic leukocyte. Annu Rev Med 1993; 44:85.

73. Rothenberg ME: Eosinophilia. N Engl J Med 1998; 338:1592.

74. Shurin SB: Pathologic states associated with activation of eosinophils and with eosinophilia. Hematol Oncol Clin North Am 1988; 2:171.

75. Thevathason OI, Gordon AS: Adrenocorticomedullary interactions on the blood eosinophils. Acta Haematol 1958; 19:162.

76. Baehner RL, Johnston RB Jr: Metabolic and bactericidal activities of human eosinophils. Br J Haematol 1971; 20:277.

77. Tauber AI, Goetzl EF, Babior BM: Unique characteristics of superoxide production by human eosinophils in eosinophilic states. Inflammation 1979; 3:261.

78. Goetzl EJ, Austin KF: Purification and synthesis of eosinophilotactic tetrapeptides of human lung tissue: Identification as eosinophil chemotactic factor of anaphylaxis. Proc Natl Acad Sci USA 1975; 72:4123.

79. Dvorak AM, Ackerman SJ, Weller PF: Subcellular morphology and biochemistry of eosinophils. In Harris JR (ed): Blood Cell Biochemistry. London: Plenum Publishing. 1990, Vol 2, p 237.

80. Bainton D, Farquhar MG: Segregation and packaging of granule enzymes in eosinophilic leukocytes. J Cell Biol 1970; 45.

81. Parmley RT, Spicer SS: Cytochemical and ultrastructural identification of a small type granule in human late eosinophils. Lab Invest 1974; 30:557.

82. Jong EC, Henderson WR, Klebanoff SR: Bactericidal activity of eosinophil peroxidase. J Immunol 1980; 124:1378.

83. Magler R, DeChatelet LR, Bass DA: Human eosinophil peroxidase: Role in bactericidal activity. Blood 1978; 51:445.

84. Weiss SJ, Test ST, Eckmann CM, et al: Brominating oxidants generated by human eosinophils. Science 1986; 234:200.

85. Olsson I, Venge P: Arginine-rich cationic proteins of human eosinophil granules. Comparison of the constituents of eosinophilic and neutrophilic leukocytes. Lab Invest 1977; 36:493.

86. Butterworth AE, Wassom DL, Gleich GJ, et al: Damage to schistosomula of *Schistosoma mansoni* induced indirectly by eosinophil major basic protein. J Immunol 1979; 122:221.

87. O'Donnell MC, Ackerman SJ, Gleich GJ, et al: Activation of basophil and mast cell histamine release by eosinophil major basic protein. J Exp Med 1983; 257:1981.

88. Dvorak AM, Letourneau L, Login GR, et al: Ultrastructural location of the Charcot-Leyden crystal proteins (lysophospholipase) to a distinct crystalloid-free granule population in mature human eosinophils. Blood 1988; 72:150.

89. Weller PF, Bach D, Austen KF: Human eosinophil lysophospholipase: The sole protein component of Charcot-Leyden crystals. J Immunol 1982; 128:1346.

90. Murakami I, Ogawa M, Amo H, et al: Studies on kinetics of human leukocytes *in vivo* with ^{3}H-thymidine autoradiography II. Eosinophils and basophils. Acta Haematol Jpn 1969; 32:384.

91. Juhlin L: Basophil leukocyte differential in blood and bone marrow. Acta Haematol 1963; 29:89.

92. Dvorak HF, Dvorak AM: Basophilic leukocytes: Structure, function, and role in disease. Clin Haematol 1975; 4:651.

93. Kinet J-P: The high-affinity receptor for IgE. Curr Opin Immunol 1989; 2:499.

94. Brunner T, Heusser CH, Dahinden CA: Human peripheral blood basophils primed by interleukin-3 (IL-3) produce IL-4 in response to immunoglobulin E receptor stimulation. J Exp Med 1993; 177:605.

95. Schroeder JT, MacGlashan DW, Kagey-Sobotka A, et al: Cytokine generation by human basophils. J Allergy Clin Immunol 1994; 94:1189.

96. Seder RA, Paul WE, Dvorak AM, et al: Mouse splenic and bone marrow cell populations that express high-affinity Fce receptors and produce interleukin-4 are highly enriched in basophils. Proc Natl Acad Sci USA 1991; 88:2835.

97. Hatanaka K, Kitamura Y, Nishimune Y: Local development of mast cells from bone marrow-derived precursors in the skin of mice. Blood 1979; 53:142.

98. Agis H, Fureder W, Bankl HC, et al: Comparative immunophenotypic analysis of human mast cells, blood basophils and monocytes. Immunology 1996; 87:535.

99. Galli S, Hammel I: Mast cell and basophil development. Curr Opin Hematol 1994; 1:33.

100. Galli SJ: New concepts about the mast cell. N Engl J Med 1993; 328:257.

101. Columbo M, Horowitz EM, Botana LM, et al: The human recombinant c-*kit* receptor ligand, rhSCF, induces mediator release from human cutaneous mast cells and enhances IgE-dependent mediator release from both skin mast cells and peripheral blood basophils. J Immunol 1992; 149:599.

102. Kuriu A, Sonoda S, Kanakura Y, et al: Proliferative potential of degranulated murine peritoneal mast cells. Blood 1989; 74:925.

103. Whitelaw DM: The intravascular lifespan of monocytes. Blood 1966; 28:445.

104. Whitelaw DM: Observations on human monocyte kinetics after pulse labeling. Cell Tissue Kinet 1972; 5:311.

105. Van Furth R: Development and distribution of mononuclear phagocytes. In Gallin JI, Goldstein IM, Snyderman R (eds): Inflammation: Basic Principles and Clinical Correlates. New York: Raven Press, 1992, p 325.

106. Thomas ED, Ramberg RE, Sale GE, et al: Direct evidence for a bone marrow origin of the alveolar macrophage in man. Science 1976; 192:1016.

107. Arenson EB, Epstein MB, Seeger RC: Monocyte subsets in neonates and children. Pediatrics 1979; 64:740.

108. Cohn ZA, Wiener E: The particulate hydrolases of macrophages. I. Comparative enzymology, isolation, and properties. J Exp Med 1963; 118:991.

109. Nagaraju M, Weitzman S, Baumann G: Viral hepatitis and agranulocytosis. Am J Dig Dis 1973; 18:247.

110. Nathan CF: Secretory products of macrophages. J Clin Invest 1987; 79:319.

111. Raetz CR, Ulevitch RJ, Wright SD, et al: Gram-negative endotoxin: An extraordinary lipid with profound effects on eukaryotic signal transduction. FASEB J 1991; 5:2652.

112. Johnston RB: Monocytes and macrophages. N Engl J Med 1988; 318:747.

113. Adams DO, Hamilton TA: Macrophages as destructive cells in host defense. In Gallin J, Goldstein I, Snyderman R (eds): Inflammation: Basic Principles and Clinical Correlates. New York, Raven Press, 1992, p 637.

114. Grage-Griebenow E, Flad H, Ernst M: Heterogeneity of human peripheral blood monocyte subsets. J Leukoc Biol 2001; 69:11.

115. Hill HR: Modulation of host defenses with interferon-γ in pediatrics. J Infect Dis 1993; 167:S23.

116. Murray HW: Interferon gamma: The activated macrophage, and host defense against microbial challenge. Ann Intern Med 1988; 108:595.

117. Darnell JE Jr, Kerr IM, Stark GR: Jak-STAT pathways and transcriptional activation in response to IFNs and other extracellular signaling proteins. Science 1994; 264:1415.

118. Ihle JN, Kerr IM: Jaks and Stats in signaling by the cytokine receptor superfamily. Trends Genet 1995; 11:69.

119. Simon LD, Robin ED, Phillips JR, et al: Enzymatic basis for bioenergetic differences of alveolar versus peritoneal macrophages and enzyme regulation by molecular oxygen. J Clin Invest 1977; 59:443.

120. Bar-Shavit R, Kahn A, Wilner GD, et al: Monocyte chemotaxis: Stimulation by specific exosite region in thrombin. Science 1983; 220:728.

121. Broze G: Binding of human factor VII and VIIa to monocytes. J Clin Invest 1982; 70:526.

122. Brown MS, Goldstein JL: Lipoprotein metabolism in the macrophage: Implications for cholesterol deposition in atherosclerosis. Annu Rev Biochem 1983; 52:223.

123. Unanue ER, Allen PM: The basis for the immunoregulatory role of macrophages and other accessory cells. Science 1987; 236:551.

124. Hocking WG, Golde DW: The pulmonary alveolar macrophage. N Engl J Med 1979; 301:580.

125. Tavassoli M: Intravascular phagocytosis in the rabbit bone marrow: A possible fate of normal senescent red cells. Br J Haematol 1977; 36:323.

126. Beutler E: Gaucher's disease. N Engl J Med 1991; 325:1354.

127. Gordon S: The macrophage. BioEssays 1995; 17:977.

128. Ho D, Pomerantz R, Kaplan JC: Pathogenesis of infection with human immunodeficiency virus. N Engl J Med 1987; 317:278.

129. Friedland GH, Klein RS: Transmission of the human immunodeficiency virus. N Engl J Med 1987; 317:1125.

130. Banchereau J, Steinman R: Dendritic cells and the control of immunity. Nature 1998; 392:245.

131. Hart D: Dendritic cells: Unique leukocyte populations which control the primary immune response. Blood 1997; 90:3245.

132. Randolph G, Beaulieu S, Lebecque S, et al: Differentiation of moncytes into dendritic cells in a model of transendothelial trafficking. Science 1998; 282:480.

133. Liu Y, Kanzler H, Soumelis V, et al: Dendritic cell lineage, plasticity and cross-regulation. Nat Immunol 2001; 2:585.

134. Marks SC: Osteoclast biology: Lessons from mammalian mutations. Am J Med Genet 1989; 34:43.

135. Schneider GB, Relfson M: The effects of transplantation of granulocyte-macrophage progenitors on bone resorption in *ia* osteopetrotic rats. J Bone Miner Res 1988; 3:225.

136. Suda T, Takahashi N, Martin T: Modulation of osteoclast differentiation. Endocrinol Rev 1992; 13:66.

137. Orchard PJ, Dahl N, Aukerman SL, et al: Circulating macrophage colony-stimulating factor is not reduced in malignant osteopetrosis. Exp Hematol 1992; 20:103.

138. Coccia PF, Krivit W, Cervenka J, et al: Successful bone-marrow transplantation for infantile malignant osteopetrosis. N Engl J Med 1980; 302:701.

139. Key LL, Rodriguiz RM, Willi SM, et al: Long-term treatment of osteopetrosis with recombinant human interferon gamma. N Engl J Med 1995; 332:1594.

140. Majino G: The Healing Hand: Man and Wound in the Ancient World. Cambridge, MA, Harvard University Press; 1975.

141. Craddock CG: Defenses of the body: The initiators of defense, the ready reserves, and the scavengers. In Wintrobe M (ed): Blood, Pure and Eloquent. New York, McGraw-Hill, 1980.

142. Metchnikov I: Immunity in Infective Diseases. In Starling FA, Starling EH (eds): New York, Dover, 1968.

143. Dinarello CA, Wolff SM: The role of interleukin-1 in disease. N Engl J Med 1993; 328:106.

144. Strieter RM, Kunkel SL: Acute lung injury: The role of cytokines in the elicitation of neutrophils. J Invest Med 1994; 42:640.

145. Kulkarni AB, Huh CG, Becker D, et al: Transforming growth factor beta-1 null mutation in mice causes excessive inflammatory response and early death. Proc Natl Acad Sci USA 1993; 90:770.

146. Moore KW, O'Garra A, de Waal Maalefyt R, et al: Interleukin-10. Annu Rev Immunol 1993; 11:165.

147. Wahl SM: Transforming growth factor beta: The good, the bad, and the ugly. J Exp Med 1994; 180:1587.

148. Alam R, Lett-Brown MA, Forsythe PA, et al: Monocyte chemotactic and activating factor is a potent histamine-releasing factor for basophils. J Clin Invest 1992; 89:723.

149. Kuna P, Reddigari SR, Schall TJ, et al: RANTES, a monocyte and T lymphocyte chemotactic cytokine releases histamine from human basophils. J Immunol 1992; 149:636.

150. Oppenheim JJ, Zachariae CO, Mukaida N, et al: Properties of the novel proinflammatory supergene "intercrine" cytokine family. Annu Rev Immunol 1991; 9:617.

151. Prescott SM, Zimmerman GA, McIntyre TM: Platelet-activating factor. J Biol Chem 1992; 120:17381.

152. Snyder F: Biochemistry of platelet-activating factor: A unique class of biologically active phospholipids. Proc Soc Exp Biol Med 1989; 190:125.

153. Serhan CN: Eicosanoids in leukocyte function. Curr Opin Hematol 1994; 1:69.

154. Lowenstein CJ, Snyder SH: Nitric oxide, a novel biologic messenger. Cell 1992; 70:705.

155. Nathan C: Nitric oxide as a secretory product of mammalian cells. FASEB J 1992; 6:3051.

156. Lewis RA, Austen KF, Soberman RJ: Leukotrienes and other products of the 5-lipoxygenase pathway. Biochemistry and relation to pathobiology in human disease. N Engl J Med 1990; 323:645.

157. Springer TA: Traffic signals for lymphocyte recirculation and leukocyte emigration: The multistep paradigm. Cell 1994; 76:310.

158. Murphy PM: The molecular biology of leukocyte chemoattractant receptors. Annu Rev Immunol 1994; 12:593.

159. Baggiolini M: Chemokines and leukocyte traffic. Nature 1998; 392:565.

160. Locati M, Murphy P: Chemokines and chemokine receptors: Biology and clinical relevance in inflammation and AIDS. Annu Rev Med 1999; 50:425.

161. Huber AR, Kunkel SL, Todd RF, et al: Regulation of transendothelial neutrophil migration by endogenous interleukin-8. Science 1991; 254:99.

162. Rot A: Endothelial cell binding of NAP-1/IL-8: Role in neutrophil emigration. Immunol Today 1992; 13:291.

163. Tanaka Y, Adams DH, Hubscher S, et al: T-cell adhesion induced by proteoglycan-immobilized cytokine MIp-1b. Nature 1993; 361:79.

164. Walz A, Baggiolini M: Generation of the neutrophil-activating peptide NAP-2 from platelet basic protein or connective tissue-activating peptide III through monocyte proteases. J Exp Med 1990; 171:449.

165. Baggiolini M, Walz A, Kunkel SL: Neutrophil-activating peptide-1/interleukin 8, a novel cytokine that activates neutrophils. J Clin Invest 1989; 84:1045.

166. Rollins BJ, Walz A, Baggiolini M: Recombinant human MCP-1/JE induces chemotaxis, calcium flux, and the respiratory burst in human monocytes. Blood 1991; 78:1112.

167. Schall TJ, Bacon K, Toy KJ, et al: Selective attraction of monocytes and T lymphocytes of the memory phenotype by cytokines RANTES. Nature 1990; 347:669.

168. Zachaiae CO, Anderson AO, Thompson HL, et al: Properties of monocyte chemotactic and activating factor (MCAF) purified from a human fibrosarcoma cell line. J Exp Med 1990; 171:2177.

169. Zigmond S: The ability of polymorphonuclear leukocytes to orient in gradients of chemotactic factors. J Cell Biol 1977; 117:606.

170. Gerard C, Gerard NP: The pro-inflammatory seven-transmembrane segment receptors of the leukocyte. Curr Opin Immunol 1994; 6:140.

171. Kaziro Y, Itoh H, Kozasa T, et al: Structure and function of signal-transducing GTP-binding proteins. Annu Rev Biochem 1991; 60:349.

172. Neer EJ: Heterotrimeric G proteins: Organizers of transmembrane signals. Cell 1995; 80:249.

173. Polakis PG, Uhing RJ, Snyderman R: The formylpeptide chemoattractant receptor copurifies with a GTP-binding protein containing a distinct 40 kDa pertussis toxin substrate. J Biol Chem 1988; 263:4969.

174. Wu D, LaRosa GJ, Simon MI: G protein-coupled signal transduction pathways for interleukin-8. Science 1993; 261:101.

175. Glogauer M, Hartwig J, Stossel T: Two pathways through Cdc42 couple the N-formyl receptor to actin nucleation in permeabilized human neutrophils. J Cell Biol 2000; 150:785.

176. Hall A: Rho GTPases and the actin cytoskeleton. Science 1998; 279:509.

177. Kim C, Dinauer M: Rac2 is an essential regulator of neutrophil NADPH oxidase activation in response to specific signaling pathways. J Immunol 2001; 166:1223.

178. Roberts A, Kim C, Zhen L, et al: Deficiency of the hematopoietic cell-specific Rho-family GTPase, Rac2, is characterized by abnormalities in neutrophil function and host defense. Immunity 1999; 10:183.

179. Amatruda TT, Steele DA, Slepak VZ, et al: Gα16, a G protein α subunit specifically expressed in hematopoietic cells. Proc Natl Acad Sci USA 1991; 88:5587.

180. Amatruda TT, Gerard NP, Gerard C, et al: Specific interactions of chemoattractant factor receptors with G-proteins. J Biol Chem 1993; 268:10139.

181. Albelda SM, Smith CW, Ward PA: Adhesion molecules and inflammatory injury. FASEB J 1994; 8:504.

182. Carlos TM, Harlan JM: Leukocyte-endothelial adhesion molecules. Blood 1994; 84:2068.

183. Lasky LA: Combinatorial mediators of inflammation? Curr Biol 1993; 3:366.

184. Kishimoto TK, Rothlein R: Integrins, ICAMS, and selectins: Role and regulation of adhesion molecules in neutrophil recruitment to inflammatory sites. Adv Pharmacol 1994; 25:117.

185. Lasky LA: Selectins: Interpreters of cell-specific carbohydrate information during inflammation. Science 1992; 258:964.

186. McEver RP: Selectins. Curr Opin Immunol 1994; 6:75.

187. Varki A: Selectin ligands. Proc Natl Acad Sci USA 1994; 91:7390.

188. Bevilacqua MP, Stengelin S, Gimbrone MA Jr, et al: Endothelial leukocyte adhesion molecule 1: An inducible receptor of neutrophils related to complement regulatory proteins and lectins. Science 1989; 243:1160.

189. Jung TM, Dailey MO: Rapid modulation of homing receptors (gp90MEL-14) induced by activators of protein kinase C: Receptor shedding due to accelerated proteolytic cleavage at the cell surface. J Immunol 1990; 144:3130.

190. Kishimoto TK, Jutila MA, Berg EL, et al: Neutrophil Mac-1 and MEL-14 adhesion proteins inversely regulated by chemotactic factors. Science 1989; 245:1238.

191. Gearing AJH, Newman W: Circulating adhesion molecules in disease. Immunol Today 1993; 14:506.

192. Jutila MA: Leukocyte traffic to sites of inflammation. Acta Pathol Microbiol Immunol Scand 1992; 100:191.

193. Arnaout MA: Structure and function of the leukocyte adhesion molecules CD11/CD18. Blood 1990; 75:1037.

194. Larson RS, Springer TA: Structure and function of leukocyte integrins. Immunol Rev 1990; 114:181.

195. Ruoslahti E: Integrins. J Clin Invest 1991; 87:1.

196. Kishimoto T, Baldwin E, Anderson D: The role of B2 integrins in inflammation. In Gallin JI, Snyderman R (eds): Inflammation: Basic Principles and Clinical Correlates, 3rd ed. Philadelphia: Lippincott Williams & Wilkins, 1999, p 537.

197. Springer TA: Adhesion receptors of the immune system. Nature 1990; 346:425.

198. Kishimoto TK, O'Connor K, Lee A, et al: Cloning of the β subunit of the leukocyte adhesion proteins: Homology to an extracellular matrix receptor defines a novel supergene family. Cell 1987; 48:681.

199. O'Toole TE, Katagiri Y, Faull RJ, et al: Integrin cytoplasmic domains mediate inside-out signal transduction. J Cell Biol 1994; 124:1047.

200. Clark EA, Brugge JS: Integrins and signal transduction pathways: The road taken. Science 1995; 268:233.

201. Moyle M, Foster DL, McGrath DE, et al: A hookworm glycoprotein that inhibits neutrophil gunction is a ligand of the integrin CD11b/CD18. J Biol Chem 1994; 269:10008.

202. Rieu P, Ueda T, Haruta I, et al: The A-domain of β2 integrin CR3 (CD11b/CD18) is a receptor for the hookworm-derived neutrophil adhesion inhibitor NIF. J Cell Biol 1994; 127:2081.

203. Sengelov H, Kjeldsen L, Diamond MS, et al: Subcellular localization and dynamics of Mac-1 (amb2) in human neutrophils. J Clin Invest 1993; 92:1467.

204. Brown E: Neutrophil adhesion and the therapy of inflammation. Semin Hematol 1997; 34:319.

205. Lowell CA, Berton G: Integrin signal transduction in myeloid leukocytes. J Leukoc Biol 1999; 65:313.

206. Mocsai A, Ligeti E, Lowell CA, et al: Adhesion-dependent degranulation of neutrophils requires the Src family kinases Fgr and Hck. J Immunol 1999; 162:1120.

207. Zhou M, Brown E: CR3 (Mac-1 aMb2, CD11b/CD18) and FcgRIII cooperate in generation of a neutrophil respiratory burst: Requirement for FcgRII and tyrosine phosphorylation. J Cell Biol 1994; 125:1407.

208. Krauss J, Xue W, Mayo-Bond L, et al: Reconstitution of antibody-dependent phagocytosis in fibroblasts expressing Fc gamma receptor IIIB and the complement receptor type 3. J Immunol 1994; 153:1769.

209. Gresham H, Graham I, Anderson D, et al: Leukocyte adhesion-deficient neutrophils fail to amplify phagocytic function in response to stimulation. Evidence for CD11b/CD18-dependent and-independent mechanisms of phagocytosis. J Clin Invest 1991; 88:588.

210. Doerschuk CM, Winn RK, Coxson HO, et al: CD18-dependent and independent mechanisms of neutrophil adherence in the pulmonary and systemic microbasculatrue of rabbits. J Immunol 1990; 144:2327.

211. Hogg JC, Doerschuk CM: Leukocyte traffic in the lung. Annu Rev Physiol 1995; 57:97.

212. Jagels MA, Hugli TE: Mechanisms and mediators of neutrophilic leukocytosis. Immunopharmacology 1994; 28:1.

213. Hechtman DH, Cybulsky MI, Fuchs HJ, et al: Intravascular IL-8: Inhibitor of polymorphonuclear leukocyte accumulation at sites of acute inflammation. J Immunol 1991; 147:883.

214. Rosengren S, Olofsson AM, von Andrian UH, et al: Leukotriene B$_4$-induced neutrophil-mediated endothelial leakage in vitro and in vivo. J Appl Physiol 1991; 71:1322.

215. Muller WA, Weigl SA, Deng X, et al: PECAM-1 is required for transendothelial migration of leukocytes. J Exp Med 1993; 178:449.

216. Vaporciyan AA, DeLisser HM, Yan HC, et al: Involvement of platelet-endothelial cell adhesion molecule-1 in neutrophil recruitment in vivo. Science 1993; 262:1580.

217. Huang AJ, Manning JE, Bandak TM, et al: Endothelial cell cytosolic free calcium regulates neutrophil migration across monolayers of endothelial cells. J Cell Biol 1993; 120:1371.

218. Weiss SJ: Tissue destruction by neutrophils. N Engl J Med 1989; 320:365.

219. Devreotes PN, Zigmond SH: Chemotaxis in eukaryotic cells: A focus on leukocytes and *Dictyostelium*. Annu Rev Cell Biol 1988; 4:649.

220. Jones GE: Cellular signaling in macrophage migration and chemotaxis. J Leukoc Biol 2000; 68:593.

221. Zigmond SH: Cell locomotion and chemotaxis. Curr Opin Cell Biol 1989; 1:80.

222. Estreicher A, Muhlhauser J, Carpentier J-L, et al: The receptor for urokinase type plasminogen activator polarizes expression of the protease to the leading edge of migrating monocytes and promotes degradation of enzyme inhibitor complexes. J Cell Biol 1990; 111:783.

223. Hebert C, Baker J: Linkage of extracellular plasminogen activator to the fibroblast cytoskeleton: Colocalization of cell surface urokinase with vincula. J Cell Biol 1988; 156:1241.

224. Pepper M, Vassalli JEA. Urokinase type plasminogen activatior is induced in migrating capillary endothelial cells. J Cell Biol 1987; 105:23.

225. Gyetko MR, Todd RF, Wilkinson CC, et al: The urokinase receptor is required for human monocyte chemotaxis in vitro. J Clin Invest 1994; 93:1380.

226. Bi E, Zigmond SH: Actin polymerization: Where the WASP stings. Curr Biol 1999; 9:R160.

227. Hartwing JH, Shevlin P: The architecture of actin filaments and the ultrastructural location of actin-binding protein in the periphery of lung macrophages. J Cell Biol 1986; 103:1007.

228. Cassimeris L, Safer D, Nachmias VT, et al: Thymosin B4 sequesters the majority of G-actin in resting human polymorphonuclear leukocytes. J Cell Biol 1992; 119:1261.

229. Ridley A, Hall A: The small GTP-binding protein Rac regulates growth factor-induced membrane ruffling. Cell 1992; 70:401.

230. Machesky L, Insall R: Signaling to actin dynamics. J Cell Biol 1999; 146:267.

231. Coates TD, Watts RG, Hartman R, et al: Relationship of F-actin distribution to development of polar shape in human polymorphonuclear neutrophils. J Cell Biol 1992; 117:765.

232. Cortese JD, Schwab B III, Frieden C, et al: Actin polymerization induces a shape change in actin-containing vesicles. Proc Natl Acad Sci USA 1989; 86:5773.

233. Tilney GL, DeRosier DJ, Tilney MS: How listeria exploits host cell actin to form its own cytoskeleton. I. Formation of a tail and how that tail might be involved in movement. J Cell Biology 1992; 118:71.

234. Ezekowitz RA, Sastry K, Bailly P, et al: Molecular characterization of the human macrophage mannose receptor: Demonstration of multiple carbohydrate recognition-like domain and phagocytosis of yeasts in Cos-I cells. J Exp Med 1990; 172:1785.

235. Ezekowitz RA, Williams DJ, Koziel H, et al: Uptake of *Pneumocystis carinii* is mediated by the macrophage mannose receptor. Nature 1991; 351:155.

236. Krieger M: Molecular flypaper and atherosclerosis: Structure of the macrophage scavenger receptor. Trends Biochem Sci 1992; 17:141.

237. Sastry K, Zahedi K, Lelias JM, et al: Molecular characterization of the mouse mannose-binding proteins. The mannose-binding protein A but not C is an acute phase reactant. J Immunol 1991; 147:692.

238. de Haas M, Vossebeld P, von dem Borne A, et al: Fcg receptors of phagocytes. J Lab Clin Med 1995; 126:330.

239. Ravetch JV. Fc receptors: Rubor redux. Cell 1994; 78:553.

240. McKenzie SE, Schreiber AD: Fc gamma receptors in phagocytes. Curr Opin Hematol 1998; 5:16.

241. Gessner JE, Heiken H, Tamm A, et al: The IgG Fc receptor family. Ann Hematol 1998; 76:231.

242. Ravetch JV, Clynes RA: Divergent roles for Fc receptors and complement in vivo. Annu Rev Immunol 1998; 16:421.

243. Bux J, Mueller-Eckhardt C: Autoimmune neutropenia. Semin Hematol 1992; 29:45.

244. Wu J, Edberg J, Redecha P, et al: A novel polymorphism of FcgRIIIa (CD16) alters receptor function and predisposes to autoimmune disease. J Clin Invest 1997; 100:1059.

245. Maliszewski CR, March CJ, Schoenborn MA, et al: Expression cloning of a human Fc receptor for IgA. J Exp Med 1990; 172:1665.

246. Albrechtsen M, Yeaman GR, Kerr MA: Characterization of the IgA receptor from human polymorphonuclear leucocytes. Immunology 1988; 64:201.

247. Kerr MA: The structure and function of human IgA. Biochem J 1990; 271:285.

248. Greenberg S: Modular components of phagocytosis. J Leukoc Biol 1999; 66:712.

249. Chimini G, Chavrier P: Function of Rho family proteins in actin dynamics during phagocytosis and engulfment. Nat Cell Biol 2000; 2:E191.

250. Aderem A, Underhill DM: Mechanisms of phagocytosis in macrophages. Annu Rev Immunol 1999; 17:593.

251. Boxer LA, Smolen JE: Neutrophil granule constituents and their release in health and disease. Hematol Oncol North Am 1988; 2:101.

252. D'Arcy Hart P, Young MR: Ammonium chloride, an inhibitor of phagosome-endosome fusion in macrophages, concurrently induces phagosome-endosome fusion and opens a novel pathway: Studies of a pathogenic mycobacterium and a nonpathogenic yeast. J Exp Med 1991; 174:881.

253. Goren MB, D'Arcy Hart P, Young MR, et al: Prevention of phagosome-lysosome fusion in cultured macrophages by sulfatides of *Mycobacterium tuberculosis*. Proc Natl Acad Sci USA 1976; 73:2510.

254. Sibley LD, Hunter SW, Brennan PJ, et al: Mycobacterial lipoarabinomannan inhibits gamma interferon-mediated action of macrophages. Infect Immunol 1988; 56:1232.

255. Horwitz MA, Maxfield FR: *Legionella pneumophila* inhibits acidification of its phagosome in human monocytes. J Cell Biol 1984; 99:1936.

256. Joiner KA, Fuhrman SA, Miettinen HM, et al: *Toxoplasma gondii*: Fusion competence of parasitophorous vacuoles in Fc receptor-transfected fibroblasts. Science 1990; 249:641.

257. Vazquez-Torres A, Xu Y, Jones-Carson J, et al: Salmonella pathogenicity island 2-dependent evasion of the phagocyte NADPH oxidase. Science 2000; 287:1655.

258. Kaufmann SHE: Immunity to intracellular bacteria. Annu Rev Immunol 1993; 11:129.

259. Weiss J: Leukocyte-derived antimicrobial proteins. Curr Opin Hematol 1994; 1:78.

260. Ganz T, Weiss J: Antimicrobial peptides of phagocytes and epithelia. Semin Hematol 1997; 34:343.

261. Kagan BL, Ganz T, Lehrer RI: Defensins: A family of antimicrobial and cytotoxic peptides. Toxicology 1994; 87:131.

262. Elsbach P, Weiss J: Oxygen-independent antimicrobial systems of phagocytes. In Gallin JI, Goldstein IM, Snyderman R (eds): Inflammation: Basic Principles and Clinical Correlates. New York: Raven Press, 1992, p 603.

263. Pereira HA: CAP37, a neutrophil-derived multifunctional inflammatory mediator. J Leukoc Biol 1995; 57:805.

264. Arnold RR, Cole MF, McGhee JR: A bactericidal effect for human lactoferrin. Science 1977; 197:263.

265. Murphy MF, Sourial NA, Burman JF, et al: Megaloblastic anemia due to vitamin B12 deficiency caused by small intestinal bacterial overgrowth: Possible role of vitamin B12 analogues. Br J Haematol 1986; 62:7.

266. Cech P, Lehrer RI: Phagolysosomal pH of human neutrophils. Blood 1984; 63:88.

267. Segal AW, Geisow M, Garcia R, et al: The respiratory burst of phagocytic cells is associated with a rise in vacuolar pH. Nature 1981; 290:406.

268. Welsh IRH, Spitznagel JK: Distribution of lysosomal enzymes, cationic proteins, and bactericidal substances and subcellular fractions of human polymorphonuclear leukocytes. Infect Immun 1971; 4:97.

269. Belaaouaj A, McCarthy R, Baumann M, et al: Mice lacking neutrophil elastase reveal impaired host defense against gram negative bacterial sepsis. Nat Med 1998; 4:615.

270. Tkalcevic J, Novelli M, Phylactides M, et al: Impaired immunity and enhanced resistance to endotoxin in the absence of neutrophil elastase and cathepsin G. Immunity 2000; 12:201.

271. Dale D, Person R, Bolyard A, et al: Mutations in the gene encoding neutrophil elastase in congenital and cyclic neutropenia. Blood 2000; 96:2317.

272. Horwitz M, Benson KF, Person RE, et al: Mutations in ELA2, encoding neutrophil elastase, define a 21-day biological clock in cyclic haematopoiesis. Nat Genet 1999; 23:433.

273. Babior BM: Oxygen-dependent microbial killing by phagocytes. N Engl J Med 1978; 298:659.

274. Baldridge CW, Gerard RW: The extra respiration of phagocytosis. Am J Physiol 1933; 103:235.

275. Sbarra AJ, Karnovsky ML: The biochemical basis of phagocytosis. I. Metabolic changes during the ingestion of particles by polymorphonuclear leukocytes. J Biol Chem 1959; 234:1355.

276. Cross AR, Jones OTG: Enzymic mechanisms of superoxide production. Biochim Biophys Acta 1991; 1057:281.

277. Babior BM, Kipnes RS, Curnutte JT: Biological defense mechanisms: The production by leukocytes of superoxide, a potential bactericidal agent. J Clin Invest 1973; 52:741.

278. Babior B: NADPH oxidase: An update. Blood 1999; 93:1464.

279. Segal A: The NADPH oxidase and chronic granulomatous disease. Mol Med Today 1996; 2:129.

280. Tsunawaki S, Mizunari H, Nagata M, et al: A novel cytosolic component, p40^{phox}, of respiratory burst oxidase associates with p67^{phox} and is absent in patients with chronic granulomatous disease who patients with chronic granulomatous disease who lack p67^{phox}. Biochem Biophys Res Commun 1994; 199:1378.

281. Wientjes FB, Hsuan JJ, Totty NF, et al: p40^{phox}, a third cytosolic component of the activation complex of the NADPH oxidase to contain src homology 3 domains. Biochem J 1993; 296:557.

282. Parkos CA, Allen RA, Cochrane CG, et al: Purified cytochrome *b* from human granulocyte plasma membrane is comprised of two polypeptides with relative molecular weights of 91,000 and 22,000. J Clin Invest 1987; 80:732.

283. Dinauer MC, Orkin SH, Brown R, et al: The glycoprotein encoded by the X-linked chronic granulomatous disease locus is a component of the neutrophil cytochrome *b* complex. Nature 1987; 327:717.

284. Teahan C, Rowe P, Parker P, et al: The X-linked chronic granulomatous disease gene codes for the beta-chain of cytochrome *b*-245. Nature 1987; 327:720.

285. Royer-Pokora B, Kunkel LM, Monaco AP, et al: Cloning the gene for an inherited human disorder—chronic granulomatous disease—on the basis of its chromosomal location. Nature 1986; 322:32.

286. Cross AR, Jones OTG, Harper AM, et al: Oxidation-reduction properties of the cytochrome *b* found in the plasma-membrane fraction of human neutrophils. Biochem J 1981; 194:599.

287. Segal A: Cytochrome *b*-245 is a flavocytochrome containing FAD and the NADPH-binding site of the microbicidal oxidase of phagocytes. Biochem J 1992; 284:781.

288. Rotrosen D, Yeung Cea. Cytochrome b_{558}: The flavin-binding component of the phagocyte NADPH oxidase. Science 1992; 256:1459.

289. DeLeo F, Quinn M: Assembly of the phagocyte NADPH oxidase: Molecular of oxidase proteins. J Leukoc Biol 1996; 60:677.

290. Yu L, Quinn M, Cross A, et al: Gp91^{phox} is the heme binding subunit of the superoxide-generating NADPH oxidase. Proc Natl Acad Sci USA 1998; 95:7993.

291. McPhail LC: SH3-dependent assembly of the phagocyte NADPH oxidase. J Exp Med 1994; 180:2011.

292. Parkos CA, Dinauer MC, Walker LE, et al: Primary structure and unique expression of the 22-kilodalton light chain of human neutrophil cytochrome *b*. Proc Natl Acad Sci USA 1988; 85:3319.

293. Shatwell K, Dancis A, Cross A, et al: The FRE1 ferric reductase of *Saccharomyces cerevisiae* is a cytochrome *b* similar to that of NADPH oxidase. J Biol Chem 1996; 271:14240.

294. Keller T, Damude H, Werner D, et al: A plant homolog of the neutrophil NADPH oxidase gp91^{phox} subunit gene encodes a plasma membrane protein with Ca^{2+} binding motifs. Plant Cell 1998; 10:255.

295. Lamb C: Plant disease resistance genes in signal perception and transduction. Cell 1994; 76:419.

296. Lambeth D: Novel homologs of gp91^{phox}. Trends Biochem Sci 2000; 25:459.

297. Wishart MJ, Taylor GS, Dixon JE: Phoxy lipids: Revealing PX domains as phosphoinositide binding modules. Cell 2001; 105:817.

298. Kanai F, Liu H, Field S, et al: The PX domains of p47phox and p40phox bind to lipid products of PI$_3$K. Nat Cell Biol 2001; 3:675.

299. Ellson C, Gobert-Gosse S, Anderson K, et al: PtdIns$_3$P regulates the neutrophil oxidase complex by binding to the PX domain of p40^{phox}. Nat Cell Biol 2001; 3:679.

300. Heyworth PG, Curnutte JT, Nauseef WM, et al: Neutrophil nicotinamide adenine dinucleotide phosphate oxidase assembly. Translocation of p47-*phox* and p67-*phox* requires interaction between p-47*phox* and cytochrome b_{558}. J Clin Invest 1991; 87:352.

301. Lapouge K, Smith SJ, Walker PA, et al: Structure of the TPR domain of p67phox in complex with Rac.GTP. Mol Cell 2000; 6:899.

302. Diebold B, Bokoch G: Molecular basis for Rac2 regulation of phagocyte NADPH oxidase. Nat Immunol 2001; 2:211.

303. Ohno YI, Hirai KI, Kanoh T, et al: Subcellular localization of hydrogen peroxide production in human polymorphonuclear leukocytes stimulated with lectins, phorbol myristate acetate, and digitonin: An electron microscope study using CeCl$_3$. Blood 1982; 60:1195.

304. Robinson JM, Badwey JA: The NADPH oxidase complex of phagocytic leukocytes: A biochemical and cytochemical view. Histochemistry 1995; 103:163.

305. Klebanoff SJ: Oxygen metabolites from phagocytes. In Gallin JI, Goldstein IM, Snyderman R (eds): Inflammation: Basic Principles and Clinical Correlates. New York: Raven Press, 1992, p 541.

306. Bast A, Haenen GRMM, Doelman CJA: Oxidants and antioxidants: State of the art. Am J Med 1991; 91(Suppl 3):2.

307. Marletta MA: Nitric oxide synthase: Aspects concerning structure and catalysis. Cell 1994; 78:927.

308. Prince R, Gunson D: Rising interest in nitric oxide synthase. Trends Biochem Sci 1993; 18:35.

309. Nathan C, Xie Q: Nitric oxide synthases: Roles, tolls and controls. Cell 1994; 78:915.

310. MacMicking J, Nathan C, et al: Altered responses to bacterial infection and endotoxic shock in mice lacking inducible nitric oxide synthase. Cell 1995; 81:641.

311. De Maria R, Cifone MG, Trotta R, et al: Triggering of human monocyte activation through CD69, a member of the NKC family of signal transducing receptors. J Exp Med 1994; 180.

312. Bukrinsky MI, Nottet HSLM, Schmidtmayerova N, et al: Regulation of nitric oxide synthase activity in HIV-1-infected monocytes: Implications for HIV-associated neurological disease. J Exp Med 1994; 180.

313. Evans T, Buttery L, Carpenter A, et al: Cytokine-treated human neutrophils contain inducible nitric oxide synthase that produces nitration of ingested bacteria. Proc Natl Acad Sci USA 1996; 93:9553.

314. Jackson SH, Gallin JI, Holland SM: The p47^{phox} mouse knock-out model of chronic granulomatous disease. J Expl Med 1995; 182:751.

315. Pollock J, Williams D, Gifford M, et al: Mouse Model of X-linked chronic granulomatous disease, an inherited defect in phagocyte superoxide production. Nat Genet 1995; 9:202.

316. Morgenstern D, Gifford M, Li L, et al: Absence of respiratory burst in x-linked chronic granulomatous disease mice leads to abnormalities in both host defense and inflammatory response to *Aspergillus fumigatus*. J Exp Med 1997; 185:207.

317. Mardiney M, Jackson S, Spratt S, et al: Enhanced host defense after gene transfer in the murine p47^{phox}-deficient model of chronic granulomatous disease. Blood 1997; 89:2268.

318. Dinauer M, Gifford M, Pech N, et al: Variable correction of host defense following gene transfer and bone marrow transplantation in murine X-linked chronic granulomatous disease. Blood 2001; 97:3738.

319. Nelson DS: Macrophages as effectors of cell-mediated immunity. In Laskin AI, LeChevalier H (eds): Macrophages and Cellular Immunity. Cleveland: CRC Press, 1972, p 45.

320. Nathan CF: Mechanisms of macrophage antimicrobial activity. Trans R Soc Trop Hyg 1983; 77:620.

321. Edelson PJ: Intracellular parasites and phagocytic cells: Cell biology and pathophysiology. Rev Infect Dis 1982; 4:124.

322. Lowrie DB, Andrew PW: Macrophage antimyocobacteial mechanisms. Br Med Bull 1988; 44:624.

323. Nacey CA, Green SJ, Leaby DA, et al: Macrophage, cytokines, and *Leishmania*. In Berenstein GL, Klostergaard J (eds): Mononuclear Phagocytes in Cell Biology. New York: CRC Press, 1993.

324. Sharma SD, Remington JS: Macrophage activation and resistance to intracellular infection. Lymphokines 1981; 3:181.

325. Perlmutter RM: Antigen processing and T-cell effector mechanisms. In Stamatoyannopoulos G, Nienhuis AW, Majerus PW, et al (eds): The Molecular Basis of Blood Diseases. Philadelphia, WB Saunders, 1994, p 463.

326. Barbul A: Immune aspects of wound repair. Clin Plastic Surg 1990; 17:433.

327. Cromack DT, Porras-Reyes B, Mustoe TA: Current concepts in wound healing: Growth factor and macrophage interaction. J Trauma 1990; 30:S129.

328. Knighton DR, Fiegel VD: Macrophage-derived growth factors in wound healing. Am Rev Respir Dis 1989; 140:1108.

329. Leibovich SK, Ross R: The role of the macrophage in wound repair: A study with hydrocortisone and antimacrophage serum. Am J Pathol 1975; 78:71.

330. Sunderkotter C, Goebler M, Schulze-Osthoff K, et al: Macrophage-derived angiogenesis factors. Pharmacol Ther 1991; 51:195.

331. Deiss A: Iron metabolism in reticuloendothelial cells. Semin Hematol 1983; 20:81.

332. Uchida T, Akitsuki T, Kimura H, et al: Relationship among plasma iron, plasma iron turnover, and reticuloendothelial iron release. Blood 1983; 61:799.

333. Kraemer FB, Chen YD, Lopez RD, et al: Characterization of the binding site on thioglycolate-stimulated mouse peritoneal macrophages that mediates uptake of very low density lipoproteins. J Biol Chem 1983; 258:12190.

334. Ross R: The pathogenesis of atherosclerosis: An update. N Engl J Med 1986; 314:488.

335. Steinberg D, Parthasrathy S, Carew TE, et al: Beyond cholesterol. Modifications of low-density lipoprotein that increase its atherogenicity. N Enlg J Med 1989; 320:915.

336. Abu-Ghazaleh RI, Kita H, Gleich GJ: Eosinophil Activation and Function in Health. Rochester MN, Mayo Clinic and Mayo Foundation, 1992.

337. Gleich GJ, Loegering DA: Immunobiology of eosinophils. Annu Rev Immunol 1984; 2:429.

338. Butterworth AE: Cell-mediated damage to helminths. Adv Parasitol 1984; 23:143.

339. Jong EC, Klebanoff SJ: Eosinophil-mediated mammalian tumor cell cytotoxicity: Role of the peroxidase system. J Immunol 1980; 124:1949.

340. Kay AB: Biological properties of eosinophils. Clin Exp Allergy 1991; 21:23.

341. Frigas E, Loegering DA: Cytotoxic effects of the guinea pig eosinophil major basic protein on tracheal epithelium. Lab Invest 1980; 42:35.

342. Marone G, Casolaro V, Cirillo R, et al: Pathophysiology of human basophils and mast cells in allergic disorders. Clin Immunol Immunopathol 1989; 50:524.

343. Sylvestre DL, Ravetch JV: Fc receptors initiate the Arthus reaction: Redefining the inflammatory cascade. Science 1994; 265:1095.

344. Ramos B, Qureshi R, Olsen K, et al: The importance of mast cells for the neutrophil influx in immune complex-induced peritonitis in mice. J Immunol 1999; 145:1868.

345. Ramos B, Zhang Y, Qureshi R, et al: Mast cells are critical for the production of leukotrienes responsible for neutrophil recruitment in immune complex-induced peritonitis in mice. J Immunol 1991; 147:1636.

346. Galli S, Wershil B: The two faces of the mast cell. Nature 1996; 381:21.

347. Malaviya R, Ikeda T, Ross E, et al: Mast cell modulation of neutrophil influx and bacterial clearance at sites of infection through TNF-α. Nature 1996; 381:77.

348. Echtenacher B, Mannel D, Hultner L: Critical protective role of mast cells in a model of acute septic peritonitis. Nature 1996; 381:75.

349. Lehr HA, Arfors KE: Mechanisms of tissue damage by leukocytes. Curr Opin Hematol 1994; 1:92.

350. Henson PM, Johnston RB: Tissue injury in inflammation. J Clin Invest 1987; 79:669.

351. American College of Chest Physicians/Society of Critical Care Medicine Consensus Conference: Definition for sepsis and organ failure and guidelines for the use of innovative therapies in sepsis. Crit Care Med 1992; 20:864.

352. Matzner Y: Acquired neutrophil dysfunction and diseases with an inflammatory component. Semin Hematol 1997; 34:291.

353. Jackson H, Cochrane C: Leukocyte-induced tissue injury. Hematol Oncol Clin North Am 1988; 2:317.

354. Brown KA: The polymorphonuclear cell in rheumatoid arthritis. Br J Rheumatol 1988; 27:150.

355. Weitzman SA, Gordon LI: Inflammation and cancer: Role of phagocyte-generated oxidants in carcinogenesis. Blood 1990; 76:655.

356. Haug CE, Colvin RB, Delmonico FL, et al: A phase I trial of immunosuppression with anti-ICAM-1 (CD54) mAb in renal allograft recipients. Transplantation 1993; 55:766.

357. Ognibene FP, Martin SE: Adult respiratory distress syndrome in patients with severe neutropenia. N Engl J Med 1986; 315:547.

358. Brown EJ, Kloner RA, Schoen FJ, et al: Scar thinning due to ibuprofen administration after experimental myocardial infarction. Am J Cardiol 1983; 51:877.

359. Bulkley BH, Roberts WC: Steroid therapy during acute myocardial infarction. A cause of delayed healing and of ventricular aneurysm. Am J Med 1974; 56:244.

360. Karayalcin G, Rosner F, Sawitsky A: Pseudoneutropenia in American Negroes. Lancet 1972; 1:387.

361. Reed WW, Diehl LF: Leukopenia, neutropenia, and reduced hemoglobin levels in healthy American blacks. Arch Intern Med 1991; 151:501.

362. Sadowitz PO, Oski FA: Differences in polymorphonuclear cell counts between healthy white and black infants: Response to meningitis. Pediatrics 1983; 72:405.

363. Welte K, Boxer L: Severe chronic neutropenia: Pathophysiology and therapy. Semin Hematol 1997; 34:267.

364. Pincus SH, Boxer LA, Stossel TP: Chronic neutropenia in childhood. Analysis of 16 cases and a review of the literature. Am J Med 1976; 61:849.

365. Howard MW, Strauss RG, Johnston RB: Infections in patients with neutropenia. Am J Dis Child 1977; 131:788.

366. Jonsson OG, Buchanan GR: Chronic neutropenia during childhood: A 13-year experience in a single institution. Am J Dis Child 1991; 145:232.

367. Dale DC, Guerry D, Wewerka JR, et al: Chronic neutropenia. Medicine (Baltimore) 1979; 58:128.

368. Sickles EA, Greene WH, Wiernik PH: Clinical presentation of infection in granulocytopenic patients. Arch Intern Med 1975; 135:715.

369. Greenwood MF, Jones EA Jr, Holland P: Monocyte functional capacity in chronic neutropenia. Am J Dis Child 1978; 132:131.

370. Baehner RL, Johnston RB Jr: Monocyte function in children with neutropenias and chronic infections. Blood 1972; 40:31.

371. De Vaal OM, Seynhaeve V: Reticular dysgenesia. Lancet 1959; 2:1123.

372. Gitlin D, Vawter G, Craig JM: Thymic alymphoplasia and congenital aleukocytosis. Pediatrics 1964; 33:184.

373. Ownby DR, Pizzo S, Blackmon L, et al: Severe combined immunodeficiency with leukopenia (reticular dysgenesis) in siblings: Immunologic and histopathologic findings. J Pediatr 1976; 89:382.

374. Roper M, Parmley RT, Crist WM, et al: Severe congenital leukopenia (reticular dysgenesis). Immunologic and morphologic characterizations of leukocytes. Am J Dis Child 1985; 139:832.

375. Alonso K, Dew JM, Starke WR: Thymic alymphoplasia and congenital aleukocytosis (reticular dysgenesia). Arch Pathol 1972; 94:179.

376. Levinsky RJ, Tiedeman K: Successful bone-marrow transplantation for reticular dysgenesis. Lancet 1983; 1:671.

377. Small T, Wall D, Kurtzberg J, et al: Association of reticular dysgenesis (thymic alymphoplasia and congenital aleukocytosis) with bilateral sensorineural deafness. J Pediatr 1999; 135:387.

378. Fischer A, Friedrich W, Levinsky R, et al: Bone-marrow transplantation for immunodeficiencies and osteopetrosis: European survey, 1968–1985. Lancet 1986; 1:1080.

379. Knutsen A, Wall D: Umbilical cord blood transplantation in severe T-cell immunodeficiency disorders: Two-year experience. J Clin Immunol 2000; 20:466.

380. De Santes K, Lai S, Cowan M: Haploidentical bone marrow transplants for two patients with reticular dysgenesis. Bone Marrow Transplant 1996; 17:1171.

381. Wright DG, Dale DC, Fauci AS, et al: Human cyclic neutropenia: Clinical review and long-term follow-up of patients. Medicine (Baltimore) 1981; 60:1.

382. Dale DC, Hammond WP: Cyclic neutropenia: A clinical review. Blood Rev 1988; 2:178.

383. Leale M: Recurrent furunculosis in an infant showing an unusual blood picture. JAMA 1910; 54:1845.

384. Lange RO: Cyclic hematopoiesis: Human cyclic neutropenia. Exp Hematol 1983; 11:435.

385. Engelhard D, Landreth KS, Kapoor N, et al: Cycling of peripheral blood and marrow lymphocytes in cyclic neutropenia. Proc Natl Acad Sci USA 1983; 80:5734.

386. Moore MAS: Clinical implications of positive and negative hematopoietic stem cell regulators. Blood 1991; 78:1.

387. Krance RA, Spruce WE, Forman SJ, et al: Human cyclic neutropenia transferred by allogeneic bone marrow grafting. Blood 1982; 60:1263.

388. Aprikyan A, Liles W, Rodger E, et al: Impaired survival of bone marrow hematopoietic progenitor cells in cyclic neutropenia. Blood 2001; 97:147.

389. Marshall G, Edwards K, Butler J, et al: Syndrome of periodic fever, pharyngitis, and aphthous stomatitis. J Pediatr 1987; 110:43.

390. Hammond WP, Price TH, Souza LM, et al: Treatment of cyclic neutropenia with granulocyte colony-stimulating factor. N Engl J Med 1989; 320:1306.

391. Bonilla MA, Dale D, Zeidler C, et al: Long-term safety of treatment with recombinant human granulocyte colony-stimulating factor (r-metHug-CSF) in patients with severe congenital neutropenias. Br J Haematol 1994; 88:723.

392. Kostmann R: Infantile genetic agranulocytosis. A review with presentation of ten new cases. Acta Paediatr Scand 1975; 64:362.

393. Parmley RT, Ogawa M, Darby CP Jr, et al: Congenital neutropenia: Neutrophil proliferation with abnormal maturation. Blood 1975; 56:723.

394. Dong F, Hoefsloot LH, Schelen AM, et al: Identification of a nonsense mutation in the granulocyte-colony-stimulating factor receptor in severe congenital neutropenia. Proc Natl Acad Sci USA 1994; 91:4480.

395. Parmley RT, Crist WM, Ragab AH, et al: Congenital dysgranulopoietic neutropenia: Clinical, serologic, ultrastructural, and *in vitro* proliferative characteristics. Blood 1980; 56:465.

396. Dinauer M, Lekstrom-Himes J, Dale D: Inherited neutrophil disorders: Molecular basis and new therapies. Hematology 2000:303.

397. Rosen RB, Kang SJ: Congenital agranulocytosis terminating in acute myelomonocytic leukemia. J Pediatr 1979; 94:406.

398. Gilman PA, Jackson DP, Guild HG: Congenital agranulocytosis: Prolonged survival and terminal acute leukemia. Blood 1970; 36:576.

399. Wriedt K, Kauder E, Mauer AM: Defective myelopoiesis in congenital neutropenia. N Engl J Med 1970; 283:1072.

400. Vadhan-Raj S, Jeha SS, Buescher S, et al: Stimulation of myelopoiesis in a patient with congenital neutropenia: Biology and nature of response to recombinant human granulocyte-macrophage colony-stimulating factor. Blood 1990; 75:858.

401. Bonilla MA, Gillio AP, Ruggeiro M, et al: Effects of recombinant human granulocyte colony-stimulating factor on neutropenia in patients with congenital agranulocytosis. N Engl J Med 1989; 320:1574.

402. Pietsch T, Buhrer C, Mempel K, et al: Blood mononuclear cells from patients with severe congenital neutropenia are capable of producing granulocyte colony-stimulating factor. Blood 1991; 77:1234.

403. Mempel K, Pietsch T, Menzel T, et al: Increased serum levels of granulocyte colony-stimulating factor in patients with severe congenital neutropenia. Blood 1991; 77:1919.

404. Glasser L, Duncan BR, Corrigan JJ Jr: Measurement of serum granulocyte colony-stimulating factor in a patient with congenital agranulocytosis (Kostmann's syndrome). Am J Dis Child 1991; 145:925.

405. Mackey MC: Unified hypothesis for the origin of aplastic anemia and periodic hematopoiesis. Blood 1978; 51:941.

406. Dong F, Brynes RK, Tidow N, et al: Mutations in the gene for the granulocyte colony-stimulating-factor receptor in patients with acute myeloid leukemia preceded by severe congenital neutropenia. N Engl J Med 1995; 333:487.

407. Ward AC, van Aesch YM, Gits J, et al: Novel point mutation in the extracellular domain of the granulocyte colony-stimulating factor (G-CSF) receptor in a case of severe congenital neutropenia hyporesponsive to G-CSF treatment. J Exp Med 1999; 190:497.

408. Guba SC, Sartor CA, Hutchinson R, et al: Granulocyte colony-stimulating factor (G-CSF) production and C-CSF receptor structure in patients with congenital neutropenia. Blood 1994; 83:1486.

409. Welte K, Zeidler C, Reiter A, et al: Differential effects of granulocyte-macrophage colony-stimulating factor and granulocyte colony-stimulating factor in children with severe congenital neutropenia. Blood 1990; 75:1056.

410. Bolyard M, Bonilla L, Boxer S, et al: Algorithm for the management of Kostmann's neutropenia based on data from the Severe Chronic Neutropenia International Registry. Blood 1999; 94:174b.

411. Yakisan E, Schirg E, Zeidler C, et al: High incidence of significant bone loss in patients with severe congenital neutropenia (Kostmann's syndrome). J Pediatr 1997; 131:592.

412. Freedman MH, Bonilla MA, Fier C, et al: Myelodysplasia syndrome and acute myeloid leukemia in patients with congenital neutropenia receiving G-CSF therapy. Blood 2000; 96:429.

413. Gorlin R, Gelb B, Diaz G, et al: WHIM syndrome, an autosomal dominant disorder: Clinical, hematological, and molecular studies. Am J Med Genet 2000; 91:368.

414. Hord J, Whitlock J, Gay J, et al: Clinical features of myelokathexis and treatment with hematopoietic cytokines: A case report of two patients and review of the literature. J Pediatr Hematol Oncol 1997; 19:443.

415. Wetzler M, Talpaz M, Kleinerman E, et al: A new familial immunodeficiency disorder characterized by severe neutropenia, a defective marrow release mechanism, and hypogammaglobulinemia. Am J Med 1990; 89:663.

416. Zuelzer W: Myelokathexis—A new form of chronic granulocytopenia: Report of a case. N Engl J Med 1964; 270:699.

417. Krill C, Smith H, Mauer A: Chronic idiopathic granulocytopenia. N Engl J Med 1964; 270:973.

418. Aprikyan A, Liles W, Park J, et al: Myelokathexis, a congenital disorder of severe neutropenia characterized by accelerated apoptosis and defective expression of *bcl-x* in neutrophil precursors. Blood 2000; 95:320.

419. Taniuchi S, Yamamoto A, Fujiwara T, et al: Dizygotic twin sisters with myelokathexis: Mechanism of its neutropenia. Am J Hematol 1999; 62:106.

420. Mamlok RJ, Juneja HS, Elder FFB, et al: Neutropenia and defective chemotaxis associated with binuclear, tetraploid myeloid-monocytic leukocytes. J Pediatr 1987; 111:555.

421. Plebani A, Cantu-Rajnoldi A, Collo G, et al: Myelokathexis associated with multiple congenital malformations: Immunological study on phagocytic cells and lymphocytes. Eur J Haematol 1988; 40:12.

422. Shwachman H, Diamond LK: The syndrome of pancreatic insufficiency and bone marrow dysfunction. J Pediatr 1964; 65:645.

423. Shmerling DH, Prader A, Hitzig WH, et al: The syndrome of exocrine pancreatic insufficiency, neutropenia, metaphyseal dysostosis and dwarfism. Helv Paediatr Acta 1969; 24:547.

424. Saunders EF, Gall G, Freedman MH: Granulopoiesis in Shwachman's syndrome (pancreatic insufficiency and bone marrow dysfunction). Pediatrics 1979; 64:515.

425. Huijgens PC, Van Der Veen EA, Muntinghe OG: Syndrome of Shwachman and leukaemia. Scand J Haematol 1977; 18:20.

426. Tada H, Yoshida TR, Ishimoto K, et al: A case of Shwachman syndrome with increased spontaneous chromosome breakage. Hum Genet 1987; 77:289.

427. Hill RE, Durie PR, Gaskin KJ, et al: Steatorrhea and pancreatic insufficiency in Shwachman syndrome. Gastroenterology 1982; 83:22.

428. Aggett PJ, Harries JT, Harvey BAM, et al: An inherited defect of neutrophil mobility in Shwachman's syndrome. J Pediatr 1979; 94:391.

429. Smith O, Hann I, Chessells J, et al: Haematological abnormalities in Shwachman-Diamond syndrome. Br J Haematol 1996; 94:278.

430. Bodian M, Sheldon W, Lightwood RI: Congenital hypoplasia of the exocrine pancreas. Acta Paediatr 1964; 53:282.

431. Aggett PJ, Cavanagh NPC, Matthew DJ, et al: Shwachman's syndrome. Arch Dis Child 1980; 55:331.

432. Berrocal T, Simon M, al-Assir I, et al: Shwachman-Diamond syndrome: Clinical, radiological and sonographic findings. Pediatr Radiol 1995; 25:356.

433. Berrocal T, Simon M, al-Assir I, et al: Shwachman-Diamond syndrome: Clinical, radiological and sonographic aspects. Pediatr Radiol 1995; 25:289.

434. Dror Y, Freedman M: Shwachman-Diamond syndrome: An inherited preleukemic bone marrow failure disorder with aberrant hematopoietic progenitors and faulty marrow microenvironment. Blood 1999; 94:3048.

435. Dror Y, Freedman M: Shwachman-Diamond syndrome marrow cells show abnormally increased apoptosis mediated through the Fas pathway. Blood 2001; 97:3011.

436. Goobie S, Popovic M, Morrison J, et al: Shwachman-Diamond syndrome with exocrine pancreatic dysfunction and bone marrow failure maps to the centromeric region of chromosome 7. Am J Hum Genet 2001; 68:1048.

437. Paley C, Murphy S, Karayalcin G, et al: Treatment of neutropenia in Shwachman diamond syndrome (SDS) with recombinant human granulocyte colony stimulating factor (RH-GCSF). Blood 1991; 78:3a.

438. Blume RS, Wolff SM: The Chediak-Higashi syndrome: Studies in four patients and a review of the literature. Medicine (Baltimore) 1972; 51:247.

439. Wolff SM, Dale DC, Clark RA, et al: The Chediak-Higashi syndrome: Studies of host defenses. Ann Intern Med 1972; 76:293.

440. Windhorst DB, Padgett G: The Chediak-Higashi syndrome and the homologous trait in animals. J Invest Dermatol 1973; 60:529.

441. Witkop CJ Jr, Quevedo WC Jr, Fitzpatrick TB, et al: Albinism. In Scriver CR, Beaudet AL, et al (eds): The Metabolic Basis of Inherited Disease. New York, McGraw-Hill, 1989.

442. Cutting HO, Lang JE: Familial benign chronic neutropenia. Ann Intern Med 1964; 61:876.

443. Mintz U, Sachs L: Normal granulocyte-forming cells in the bone marrow of Yemenite Jews with genetic neutropenia. Blood 1973; 41:745.

444. Shaper AG, Lewis P: Genetic neutropenia in people of African origin. Lancet 1971; 1:1021.

445. Jacobs P: Familial benign chronic neutropenia. S Afr Med J 1975; 49:692.

446. Sieff C, Nisbet-Brown E, Nathan D: Congenital bone marrow failure syndromes. Br J Haematol 2000; 111:30.

447. Benjamin B, Ward SM: Leukocytic responses to measles. Am J Dis Child 1932; 44:921.

448. Holbrook AA: The blood picture in chicken pox. Arch Intern Med 1941; 68:294.

449. Murdoch JM, Smith CC: Hematological aspects of systemic disease: Infection. Clin Haematol 1972; 1:619.

450. Horsfall FL, Tamm L: Viral and Rickettsial Infections of Man, 4th ed. Philadelphia, JB Lippincott, 1965.

451. Downie AW: Pathway of virus infection. In Smith E (ed): Mechanisms of Virus Infection. New York, Academic Press, 1963.

452. MacGregor RR, Friedman HM, Macarak EJ, et al: Virus infection of endothelial cells increased granulocyte adherence. J Clin Invest 1980; 65:1469.

453. Cines DB, Lyss AP, Bina M, et al: Fc and C3 receptors induced by herpes simplex virus on cultured human endothelial cells. J Clin Invest 1982; 69:123.

454. Ryan US, Schultz DR, Ruan JW: Fc and C3b receptors on pulmonary endothelial cells: Induction by injury. Science 1981; 214:557.

455. Hammond WP, Harlan JM, Steinberg SE: Severe neutropenia in infectious mononucleosis. West J Med 1979; 131:92.

456. Habib MA, Babka JC, Burningham RA: Profound granulocytopenia associated with infectious mononucleosis. Am J Med Sci 1973; 265:339.

457. Schooley RT, Densen P, Harmon D, et al: Antineutrophil antibodies in infectious mononucleosis. Am J Med 1984; 76:85.

458. Stevens DL, Everett ED, Boxer LA, et al: Infectious mononucleosis with severe neutropenia and opsonic antineutrophil activity. South Med J 1979; 72:519.

459. Scheurlen W, Ramasubbu K, Wachowski O, et al: Chronic autoimmune thrombopenia/neutropenia in a boy with persistent parvovirus B19 infection. J Clin Virol 2001; 20:173.

460. McClain K, Estrov Z, Chen H, et al: Chronic neutropenia of childhood: Frequent association with parvovirus infection and correlations with bone marrow culture studies [see comments]. Br J Haematol 1993; 85:57.

461. Mustafa MM, McClain KL: Diverse hematologic effects of parvovirus B19 infection. Pediatr Clin North Am 1996; 43:809.

462. Zon L, Groopman J: Hematologic manifestations of the human deficiency virus (HIV). Semin Hematol 1988; 25:208.

463. Moses A, Nelson J, Bagby G: The influence of human immunodeficiency virus-1 on hematopoiesis. Blood 1998; 91:1479.

464. Israel DS, Plaisance KI: Neutropenia in patients infected with human immunodeficiency virus. Clin Pharmacol 1991; 10:268.

465. Fronteira M, Myers A: Peripheral blood and bone marrow abnormalities in the acquired immunodeficiency syndrome. West J Med 1987; 147:157.

466. McCance-Katz E, Hoecker J, Vitale N: Severe neutropenia associated with anti-neutrophil antibody in a patient with acquired immunodeficiency syndrome-related complex. Pediatr Infect Dis 1987; 6:417.

467. Dietrich HS: Typhoid fever in children. A study of 60 cases. J Pediatr 1937; 10:191.

468. Ball K, Jones H: Acute tuberculosis septicemia with leukopenia. Br J Med 1951; 2:869.

469. Pullen RL, Stuart BM: Tularemia. JAMA 1945; 129:495.

470. Dale DC, Wolff SM: Studies of the neutropenia of acute malaria. Blood 1973; 41:197.

471. Nathan CF: Neutrophil activation on biological surfaces. J Clin Invest 1987; 80:1550.

472. Ivanovich P, Chenoweth DE, Schmidt R, et al: Symptoms of activation of granulocytes and complement with two dialysis membranes. Kidney Int 1983; 24:758.

473. Wolach B, Coates TD, Hugli TE, et al: Plasma lactoferrin reflects granulocyte activation via complement in burn patients. J Lab Clin Med 1984; 103:284.

474. Chenoweth DE, Cooper SW, Hugli TE, et al: Complement activation during cardiopulmonary bypass: Evidence for generation of C3a and C5a anaphylatoxins. N Engl J Med 1981; 304:497.

475. Craddock PR, Hammerschmidt DE, Moldow DF, et al: Granulocyte aggregation as a manifestation of membrane interactions with complement: Possible role in leukocyte margination, microvascular occlusion, and endothelial damage. Semin Hematol 1979; 16:140.

476. Strauss RG: Granulopoiesis and neutrophil function in the neonate. In Stockman JA, Pochedley (eds): Developmental and Neonatal Hematology. New York, Raven Press, 1988.

477. Cairo M: The use of granulocyte transfusions in neonatal sepsis. Trans Med Rev 1990; 4:14.

478. Christensen RD, Rothstein G, Anstall HB, et al: Granulocyte transfusions in neonates with bacterial infection, neutropenia, and depletion of mature marrow neutrophils. Pediatrics 1982; 70:1.

479. Christensen RD, Bradley PP, Rothstein G: The leukocyte left shift in clinical and experimental neonatal sepsis. J Pediatr 1981; 98:101.

480. Gillan E, Christensen R, Suen Y, et al: A randomized, placebo-controlled trial of recombinant human granulocyte colony-stimulating factor administration in newborn infants with presumed sepsis: Significant induction of peripheral and bone marrow neutrophilia. Blood 1994; 84:1427.

481. Cairo M: Review of G-CSF and GM-CSF. Effects on neonatal neutrophil kinetics. Am J Pediatr Hematol Oncol 1989; 11:238.

482. Roberts RL, Szelc CM, Scates SM, et al: Neutropenia in an extremely premature infant treated with recombinant human granulocyte colony-stimulating factor. Am J Dis Child 1991; 145:808.

483. Pisciotta AV: Drug induced agranulocytosis peripheral destruction of polymorphonuclear leukocytes and their marrow precursors. Blood Rev 1990; 4:226.

484. Vincent PC: Drug-induced aplastic anemia and agranulocytosis: Incidence and mechanisms. Drugs 1986; 31:52.

485. Salama A, Schutz B, Kiefel V, et al: Immune-mediated agranulocytosis related to drugs and their metabolites: Mode of sensitization and heterogeneity of antibodies. Br J Haematol 1989; 72:127.

486. Group TIAaAAS: Risks of agranulocytosis and aplastic anemia: A first report of their relation to drug use and special reference to analgesics. JAMA 1986; 256:1749.

487. Mamus SW, Burton JD, Groate JD, et al: Ibuprofen-associated pure white-cell aplasia. N Engl J Med 1986; 314:624.

488. Weitzman SA, Stossel TP: Drug-induced immunological neutropenia. Lancet 1978; 1:1068.

489. Pisciotta AV: Immune and toxic mechanisms in drug-induced agranulocytosis. Semin Hematol 1973; 10:291.

490. Heit WFW: Hematologic effects of antipyretic analgesics. Drug induced agranulocytosis. Am J Med 1983; 74:65.

491. Schroder H, Evans DAP: Acetylator phenotype and adverse effects of sulfasalazine in healthy subjects. Gut 1972; 13:278.

492. Murphy MF, Riordon T, Minchinton RM, et al: Demonstration of an immune-mediated mechanism of penicillin-induced neutropenia and thrombocytopenia. Br J Haematol 1983; 55:155.

493. Hartl PW: Drug-induced agranulocytosis. In Girdwood RH (ed): Blood Disorders Due to Drugs and Other Agents. Amsterdam, Excerpta Medica, 1973, p 147.

494. Young GA, Vincent PC: Drug-induced agranulocytosis. Clin Haematol 1980; 9:438.

495. Uetrecht J: Drug metabolism by leukocytes and its role in drug-induced lupus and other idiosyncratic drug reactions. CRC Crit Rev Toxicol 1990; 20:213.

496. van der Klauw M, Wilson J, Stricker B: Drug-associated agranulocytosis: 20 years of reporting in The Netherlands (1974–1994). Am J Hematol 1998; 57:206.

497. Bottiger LE, Furhoff AK, Holmberg L: Fatal reactions to drugs. A 10-year material from the Swedish Adverse Drug Reaction Committee. Acta Med Scand 1979; 205:451.

498. Anonymous. Editorial: Nitrous oxide and the bone-marrow. Lancet 1978; 2:613.

499. Shastri KA, Logue GL: Autoimmune neutropenia. Blood 1993; 81:1984.

500. Logue GL, Shimm DS: Autoimmune granulocytopenia. Annu Rev Med 1980; 31:191.

501. Currie MS, Weinberg JB, Rustagi PK, et al: Antibodies to granulocyte precursors in selective myeloid hypoplasia and other suspected autoimmune neutropenias: Use of HL-60 cells as targets. Blood 1987; 69:529.

502. Stroneck DF, Skubitz KM, Shanker RA, et al: Biochemical characterization of the neutrophil specific antigen NB1. Blood 1990; 75:744.

503. Bruin M, Kr von dem Borne A, Tamminga R, et al: Neutrophil antibody specificity in different types of childhood autoimmune neutropenia. Blood 1999; 94:1797.

504. Von Dem Borne AE: Neutrophil alloantigens nature and clinical relevance. Vox Sang 1994; 67:105.

505. Lucas GF, Carrington PA: Results of the First International Granulocyte Serology Workshop. Vox Sang 1990; 59:251.

506. Bux J, Behrens G, Jaeger G, et al: Diagnosis and clinical course of autoimmune neutropenia in infancy: Analysis of 240 cases. Blood 1998; 91:181.

507. Bux J, Kober B, Kiefel V, et al: Analysis of granulocyte-reactive antibodies using an immunoassay based upon monoclonal-antibody-specific immobilization of granulocyte antigens. Transfus Med 1993; 3:157.

508. Hartman KR, Wright DG: Identification of autoantibodies specific for the neutrophil adhesion glycoproteins CD11b/CD18 in patients with autoimmune neutropenia. Blood 1991; 78:1096.

509. Boxer LA, Greenberg MS, Boxer GJ, et al: Autoimmune neutropenia. N Engl J Med 1975; 293:748.

510. Duckham DJ, Rhyne RL Jr, Smith FE, et al: Retardation of colony growth of *in vitro* bone marrow culture using sera from patients with Felty's syndrome, disseminated lupus erythematosus (DLE), rheumatoid arthritis and other disease states. Arthritis Rheum 1975; 18:323.

511. Lalezari P, Khorshidi M, Petrosova M: Autoimmune neutropenia in infancy. J Pediatr 1986; 109:764.

512. Neglia JP, Watterson J, Clay M, et al: Autoimmune neutropenia of infancy and early childhood. Pediatr Hematol Oncol 1993; 10:369.

513. Lyall EGH, Lucas GF, Eden OB: Autoimmune neutropenia of infancy. J Clin Pathol 1992; 45:431.

514. Conway LT, Clay ME, Kline WE, et al: Natural history of primary autoimmune neutropenia in infancy. Pediatrics 1987; 79:728.

515. Miller ME, Oski FA, Harris MB: Lazy-leucocyte syndrome: A new disorder of neutrophil function. Lancet 1971; 1:665.

516. Aggarwal J, Khan AJ, Diamond S, et al: Lazy leukocyte syndrome in a black infant. J Natl Med Assoc 1985; 77:928.

517. Yoda S, Morosawa H, Komiyama A, et al: Transient `lazy-leukocyte' syndrome during infancy. Am J Dis Child 1980; 134:467.

518. Komiyama A, Ishigura A, Kubo T, et al: Increases in neutrophil counts by purified human urinary colon-stimulating factor in chronic neutropenia of childhood. Blood 1988; 71:41.

519. Boxer LA: Immune neutropenias. Clinical and biological implications. Am J Pediatr Hematol Oncol 1981; 3:89.

520. Lalezari P, Radel E: Neutrophil antigens: Immunology and clinical implications. Semin Hematol 1974; 11:231.

521. Levine D, Madyastha P: Isoimmune neonatal neutropenia. Am J Perinatol 1986; 3:231.

522. Gilmore M, Stroncek D, Korones D: Treatment of alloimmune neonatal neutropenia with granulocyte colony-stimulating factor. J Pediatr 1994; 125:948.

523. Cartron J, Tchernia G, Cleton J, et al: Alloimmune neonatal neutropenia. Am J Pediatr Hematol Oncol 1991; 13:21.

524. Van Leeuwen EF, Roord JJ, DeGast GC, et al: Neonatal neutropenia due to maternal autoantibodies against neutrophils. BMJ 1983; 287:94.

525. Payne R: Neonatal neutropenia and leukoagglutinins. Pediatrics 1964; 33:194.

526. Abilgaard H, Jensen KG: The influence of maternal leukocyte antibodies in infants. Scand J Haematol 1964; 1:47.

527. Buckley RH, Rowlands DJ: Agammaglobulinemia, neutropenia, fever and abdominal pain. J Allergy Clin Immunol 1973; 51:308.

528. Kozlowski C, Evans DI: Neutropenia associated with X-linked agammaglobulinaemia. J Clin Pathol 1991; 44:388.

529. Rosen FS, Cooper MD, Wedgwood RJP: The primary immunodeficiencies. N Engl J Med 1995; 333:431.

530. Rieger CHL, Moohr JW, Rothberg RM: Correction of neutropenia associated with dysgammaglobulinemia. Pediatrics 1974; 54:508.

531. Schaeffer FM, Monteiro RC, Volanakis JE, et al: IgA Deficiency. In Rosen FS, Seligmann M (eds): Immunodeficiencies. Chur, Harwood Academic, 1993, p 77.

532. McKusick VA, Eldridge R: Dwarfism in the Amish. II. Cartilage hair hypoplasia. Bull Johns Hopkins Hosp 1965; 116:285.

533. Lux SE, Johnston RB Jr, August CS, et al: Chronic neutropenia and abnormal cellular immunity in cartilage-hair hypoplasia. N Engl J Med 1970; 282:231.

534. O'Reilly RJ, Brochstein J, Dinsmore R, et al: Marrow transplantation for congenital disorders. Semin Hematol 1984; 21:188.

535. Amman AJ, Hang F: Disorders of T cell system. In Steinham RF, Fulginiti VA (eds): Immunological Disorders in Infants and Children. Philadelphia, WB Saunders, 1980, p 286.

536. Bjorksten B, Lundmark KM: Recurrent bacterial infections in four siblings with neutropenia, eosinophilia, hyperimmunoglobulinemia A, and defective neutrophil chemotaxis. J Infect Dis 1976; 133:63.

537. Chudwin DS, Cowan MJ, Greenberg PL, et al: Response of agranulocytosis to prolonged antithymocyte globulin therapy. J Pediatr 1983; 103:223.

538. Sweetman L: Branched chain organic acidurias. In Scriver CR, Beaudet AL, Sly WS, et al (eds): The Metabolic Basis of Inherited Disease. New York, McGraw-Hill, 1989, p 791.

539. Rosenberg LE, Fenton WA: Disorders of propionate and methylmalonate metabolism. In Scriver CR, Beaudet AL, Sly WS, et al (eds): The Metabolic Basis of Inherited Disease. New York, McGraw-Hill, 1989, p 821.

540. Beaudet AL, Anderson DC, Michels VV, et al: Neutropenia and impaired neutrophil migration in type 1B glycogen storage disease. J Pediatr 1980; 97:906.

541. Ambruso DR, McCabe ERB, Anderson D, et al: Infectious and bleeding complications in patients with glycogenosis Ib. Am J Dis Child 1985; 139:691.

542. Soriano JR, Taitz LS, Finberg L, et al: Hyperglycinemia with ketacidosis and leukopenia: Metabolic studies on the nature of the defect. Pediatrics 1967; 39:818.

543. Childs B, Nyhan W, Borden M, et al: Idiopathic hyperglycinemia and hyperglycinuria: A new disorder of amino acid metabolism. Pediatrics 1961; 27:522.

544. Couper R, Kapelushnik J, Griffiths AM: Neutrophil dysfunction in glycogen storage disease Ib: Association with Crohn's-like colitis. Gastroenterology 1991; 100:549.

545. Lindstedt S, Holme E, et al: Treatment of hereditary tyrosinaemia type I by inhibition of 4-hydroxyphenylpyruvate dioxygenase. Lancet 1992; 340:813.

546. Barth PG, Scholte HR, Berden JA, et al: An X-linked mitochondrial disease affecting cardiac muscle, skeletal muscle and neutrophil leucocytes. J Neurol Sci 1983; 62:327.

547. Ades LC, Gedeon AK, Wilson MJ, et al: Barth syndrome: Clinical features and confirmation of gene localisation to distal Xq28. Am J Med Genet 1993; 45:327.

548. Kelley RI, Cheatham JP, Clark BJ, et al: X-linked dilated cardiomyopathy with neutropenia, growth retardation, and 3-methylglutaconic aciduria. J Pediatr 1991; 119:738.

549. Hutchinson RJ, Bunnell K, Thoene JG: Suppression of granulopoietic progenitor cell proliferation by metabolites of the branched chain amino acids. J Pediatr 1985; 106:62.

550. Wang WC, Crist WM, Ihle JN, et al: Granulocyte colony-stimulating factor corrects the neutropenia associated with glycogen storage disease type. Leukemia 1991; 5:347.

551. Schroten H, Wendel U, Burdach S, et al: Colony-stimulating factors for neutropenia in glycogen storage disease Ib. Lancet 1991; 337:736.

552. Liel Y, Rudich A, Nagauker-Shriker O, et al: Monocyte dysfunction in patients with Gaucher disease: Evidence for interference of glucocerebroside with superoxide generation. Blood 1994; 83:2646.

553. Aker M, Zimran A, Abrahamov A, et al: Abnormal neutrophil chemotaxis in Gaucher disease. Br J Haematol 1993; 83:187.

554. Perillie PE, Kaplan SS, Finch SC: Significance of changes in serum muramidase activity in megaloblastic anemia. N Engl J Med 1967; 277:10.

555. Pearson HA: Marrow hypoplasia in anorexia nervosa. J Pediatr 1967; 71:211.

556. Natelson EA, Lynch EC, Hettig RA, et al: Histiocytic medullary reticulosis: The role of phagocytosis in pancytopenia. Arch Intern Med 1968; 122:223.

557. Boxer LA, Camitta BM, Berenberg W, et al: Myelofibrosis-myeloid metaplasia in childhood. Pediatrics 1975; 55:861.

558. Crail HW, Alt HL, Nadler WH: Myelofibrosis associated with tuberculosis—A report of four cases. Blood 1948; 3:1426.

559. Erf LA, Herbut PA: Primary and secondary myelofibrosis: A clinical and pathological study of thirteen cases of fibrosis of the bone marrow. Ann Intern Med 1945; 21:863.

560. Ward H, Block MH: The natural history of agnogenic myeloid metaplasia and a critical evaluation of its relationship with the myeloproliferative syndrome. Medicine (Baltimore) 1971; 50:357.

561. Price TH, Lee MY, Dale DC, et al: Neutrophil kinetics in chronic neutropenia. Blood 1979; 54:581.

562. Greenburg PL, Mara B, Steed S, et al: The chronic idiopathic neutropenic syndrome: Correlation of clinical features with in vitro parameters of granulocytopoiesis. Blood 1980; 55:915.

563. Logue GL, Shastri KA, Laughlin M, et al: Idiopathic neutropenia: Antineutrophil antibodies and clinical correlations. Am J Med 1991; 90:211.

564. Jakabowski AA, Souza L, Kelly F, et al: Effects of human granulocyte colony-stimulating factor in a patient with idiopathic neutropenia. N Engl J Med 1989; 320:38.

565. Huestis DW, Glasser L: Neutrophil in transfusion medicine. Transfusion 1994; 34:630.

566. Strauss RG: Therapeutic granulocyte transfusions in 1993. Blood 1993; 31:1675.

567. Dale DC: Potential role of colony-stimulating factors in the prevention and treatment of infectious diseases. Clin Infect Dis 1994; 18:S180.

568. Coulombel L, Dehan M, Tchernia G, et al: The number of polymorphonuclear leukocytes in relation to gestational age in the newborn. Acta Paediatr Scand 1979; 68:709.

569. Cartwright GE, Athens JW: Blood granulocyte kinetics in conditions associated with granulocytosis. Ann NY Acad Sci 1964; 113:963.

570. Athens JW: Leukocyte physiology. JAMA 1966; 198:38.

571. Boxer LA, Allen JM, Baehner RL: Diminished polymorphonuclear leukocyte adherence. Function dependent on release of cyclic AMP by endothelial cells after stimulation of beta-receptors by epinephrine. J Clin Invest 1980; 66:268.

572. Ostlund RE, Bishop CR, Athens JW: Evaluation of non-steady-state neutrophil kinetics during endotoxin-induced granulocytosis. Proc Soc Exp Biol Med 1968; 137:461.

573. Dale DC, Fauci AS, Guerry D IV, et al: Comparison of agents producing a neutrophilic leukocytosis in man. J Clin Invest 1975; 56:808.

574. Bishop CR, Athens JW, Boggs DR, et al: Leukokinetic studies. XIII. A non-steady-state evaluation of the mechanism of cortisone-induced granulocytosis. J Clin Invest 1968; 47:249.

575. Rey JJ, Wolf PL: Extreme leukocytosis in accidental electric shock. Lancet 1968; I:18.

576. Watkins J, Ward AM: Changes in peripheral blood leukocytes following I.V. anaesthesia and surgery. Br J Anaesthesiol 1977; 49:953.

577. Ryhanen P: Effects of anesthesia and operative surgery on the immune response of patients of different ages. Ann Clin Res 1977; 9(Suppl):19.

578. Peterson LA, Hrisinko MA: Benign lymphocytosis and reactive neutrophilia. Clin Lab Med 1993; 13:863.

579. Shoenfeld Y, Gurewich Y: Prednisone-induced leukocytosis. Influence of dosage, method, and duration of administration on the degree of leukocytosis. Am J Med 1981; 71:773.

580. Craddock CG, Perry S: Dynamics of leukopoiesis and leukocytosis, as studied by leukapheresis and isotopic techniques. J Clin Invest 1956; 35:285.

581. Milhout AT, Small SM: Leukocytosis during various emotional states. Arch Neurol Psychiatr 1942; 47:779.

582. Walker RI, Willemze R: Neutrophil kinetics and the regulation of granulopoiesis. Rev Infect Dis 1980; 2:282.

583. Holland P, Mauer AM: Myeloid leukemoid reactions in children. Am J Dis Child 1963; 105:568.

584. Calabro JJ, Williamson P: Kawasaki syndrome. N Engl J Med 1982; 306:237.

585. Finch SC: Laboratory findings in infectious mononucleosis. In Carter RL, Penman HG (eds): Infectious Mononucleosis. Oxford, Blackwell Scientific Publications, 1969, p 57.

586. Skarberg KO: Leukaemia, leukaemoid reaction and tuberculosis. Acta Med Scand 1967; 182:427.

587. Schaller J, Wedgewood R: Juvenile rheumatoid arthritis: A review. Pediatrics 1970; 50:940.

588. McBride JA, Dacie JV: The effect of splenectomy on the leukocyte count. Br J Haematol 1968; 14:225.

589. Herring WB, Smith LB, Walker RI, et al: Hereditary neutrophilia. Am J Med 1974; 56:729.

590. Tindall JP, Beeker SK, Rosse WF: Familial cold urticaria. A generalized reaction involving leukocytosis. Arch Intern Med 1969; 124:129.

591. Hendrik M, Doeglas M, Bleumink E: Familial cold urticaria. Clinical findings. Arch Dermatol 1974; 110:382.

592. MacDougall LG, Strickwold B: Myeloid leukemoid reactions in South African blacks. S Afr Med J 1978; 53:14.

593. Nettleship A: Leukocytosis associated with acute inflammation. Am J Clin Pathol 1938; 8:398.

594. Tullis JL: A cause of leukocytosis in diabetic acidosis: Effects of experimental hypertonia on circulating leukocytes. J Clin Invest 1947; 26:1098.

595. Engel RR, Hammond D: Transient congenital leukemia in seven children with mongolism. J Pediatr 1964; 65:303.

596. Dignan PS, Mauer AM, Frantz C: Phocomelia with congenital hypoplastic thrombocytopenia and myeloid leukemoid reactions. J Pediatr 1967; 70:561.

597. Basten A, Beeson PB: Mechanisms of eosinophilia: II. Role of the lymphocyte. J Exp Med 1970; 131:1288.

598. Bass DA, Lewis JC: Biochemistry and metabolism of human eosinophils. Trans R Soc Trop Med Hyg 1980; 74(Suppl):11.

599. Stickney JM, Heck FJ: The clinical occurrence of eosinophilia. Med Clin North Am 1944; 28:914.

600. Lowell FC: Clinical aspects of eosinophilia in atopic diseases. JAMA 1967; 202:109.

601. Lecka HI, Kravis L: The allergist and the eosinophil. Pediatr Clin North Am 1969; 16:125.

602. Donohugh DL: Eosinophils and eosinophilia. Calif Med 1966; 104:421.

603. Haeberle MG, Griffen WO Jr: Eosinophilia and regional enteritis. A possible diagnostic aid. Am J Dig Dis 1972; 17:200.

604. Beeson PB, Bass DA: The Eosinophil. Philadelphia, WB Saunders, 1977.

605. Hoy WE, Castero RVM: Eosinophilia in maintenance hemodialysis patients. J Dial 1979; 3:73.

606. Lee S, Schoen I: Eosinophilia and peritoneal fluid and peripheral blood associated with chronic peritoneal dialysis. Am J Clin Pathol 1967; 47:638.

607. Conrad ME: Hematologic manifestations of parasitic infections. Semin Hematol 1971; 8:267.

608. Huntley CC, Costas MD, Lyerly A: Visceral larvae migrans syndrome. Clinical characteristics in immunologic studies in 51 patients. Pediatrics 1965; 36:523.

609. Mok CH: Visceral larvae migrans: A discussion based on review of the literature. Clin Pediatr 1968; 7:565.

610. Aur JA, Pratt CB, Johnson WW: Thiabendazole and visceral larvae migrans. Am J Dis Child 1971; 121:226.

611. Naiman JL, Oski FA, Allen FH Jr, et al: Hereditary eosinophilia. Report on a family and review of literature. Am J Hum Genet 1971; 16:195.

612. Chusid MJ, Dale DC, West BC, et al: The hypereosinophilic syndrome: Analysis of fourteen cases with review of the literature. Medicine (Baltimore) 1975; 54:1.

613. Weller PF, Bubley GJ: The idiopathic hypereosinophilic syndrome. Blood 1994; 83:2759.

614. Spry CJ: The hypereosinophilic syndrome: Clinical features, laboratory findings and treatment. Allergy 1982; 37:539.

615. Fauci AS, Harley JB, Roberts WC, et al: NIH Conference: The idiopathic hypereosinophilic syndrome. Clinical, pathophysiologic, and therapeutic considerations. Ann Intern Med 1982; 97:78.

616. da Silva MAP, Heerema N, Schwenk GRJ, et al: Evidence for the clonal nature of hypereosinophilic syndrome. Cancer Genet Cytogenet 1988; 32:109.

617. Bain BJ: Hypereosinophilia. Curr Opin Hematol 2000; 7:21.

618. Bennett J, Catovsky D, Daniel M: Proposed revised criteria for the classification of acute myeloid leukemia. A report of the French-American-British cooperative group. Ann Intern Med 1985; 103:626.

619. Liu PP, Hajra A, Wijmenga C, et al: Molecular pathogenesis of the chromosome 16 inversion in the M4Eo subtype of acute myeloid leukemia. Blood 1995; 85:2289.

620. Bass DA: Eosinopenia. In Mahmoud AAF, Austen KF (eds): The Eosinophil in Health and Disease. New York, Grune & Stratton, 1980, p 275.

621. Shelley WB, Parnes HM: The absolute basophil count. JAMA 1965; 192:108.

622. May ME, Waddell CC: Basophils in peripheral blood and bone marrow. A retrospective review. Am J Med 1984; 76:509.

623. Athreya BH, Moser G, Raghaven TES: Increased circulating basophils in juvenile rheumatoid arthritis. Am J Dis Child 1975; 129:935.

624. Galli SJ, Colvin RB, Orenstein NS, et al: Patients without basophils. Lancet 1977; 2:409.

625. Juhlin L, Michaelsson G: A new syndrome characterized by absence of eosinophils and basophils. Lancet 1977; I:1233.

626. Volpp BD, Nauseef WM, Donelson JE, et al: Cloning of the cDNA and functional expression of the 47-kilodalton cytosolic component of the human neutrophil respiratory burst oxidase. Proc Natl Acad Sci USA 1989; 86:7195.

627. Leto TL, Lomax KJ, Volpp BD, et al: Cloning of a 67-kDa neutrophil oxidase factor with similarity to a non-catalytic region of p60^{c-src}. Science 1990; 248:727.

628. Iwata M, Nunoi H, Yamazaki H, et al: Homologous dinucleotide (GT or TG) deletion in Japanese patients with chronic granulomatous disesae with p47-phox deficiency. Biochem Biophys Res Commun 1994; 199:1372.

629. Segal AW, Jones OTG, Webster D, et al: Absence of a newly described cytochrome *b* from neutrophils of patients with chronic granulomatous disease. Lancet 1978; 2:446.

630. Fredericks RE, Maloney WC: The basophilic granulocyte. Blood 1959; 14:571.

631. Juhlin L: Basophil leukocytes in ulcerative colitis. Acta Med Scand 1963; 173:351.

632. Lennert K, Koster E, et al: Uber die Mastzellen-leukaemie. Acta Haematol 1956; 16:255.

633. Rosenthal S, Schwartz JH, Canellos GP: Basophilic chronic granulocytic leukemia with hyperhistaminemia. Br J Haematol 1977; 36:367.

634. Juhlin L: Basophil and eosinophil leukocytes in various internal disorders. Acta Med Scand 1963; 174:249.

635. Kato K: Leukocytes in infancy and childhood: A statistical analysis of 1,081 total and differential counts from birth to fifteen years. J Pediatr 1935; 7:7.

636. Maldonado JE, Hanlon DG: Monocytosis: A current appraisal. Mayo Clin Proc 1965; 40:248.

637. Koeffler HP, Golde DW: Human preleukemia. Ann Intern Med 1980; 93:347.

638. Ultmann JE: Clinical features and diagnosis of Hodgkin's disease. Cancer 1966; 9:297.

639. Scully FJ: The reaction after intravenous injections of foreign protein. JAMA 1917; 69:20.

640. Thompson J, Van Furth R: The effect of glucocorticoids on the proliferation and kinetics of promonocytes and monocytes of the bone marrow. J Exp Med 1973; 137:10.

641. Valkmann A, Gowans JL: The production of macrophages in the rat. Br J Exp Pathol 1965; 46:50.

642. Anderson DC, Schmalsteig FC, Finegold MJ, et al: The severe and moderate phenotypes of heritable Mac-1, LFA-1 deficiency: Their quantitative definition and relation to leukocyte dysfunction and clinical features. J Infect Dis 1985; 152:668.

643. Todd RF III, Freyer DR: The CD11/CD18 leukocyte glycoprotein deficiency. Hematol Oncol Clin North Am 1988; 2:13.

644. Anderson DC, Springer TA: Leukocyte adhesion deficiency: An inherited defect in the Mac-1, LFA-1 and p150,95 glycoproteins. Annu Rev Med 1987; 38:175.

645. Fischer A, Lisowska-Grospierre B, Anderson DC, et al: Leukocyte adhesion deficiency: Molecular basis and functional consequences. Immunodef Rev 1988; 1:39.

646. Crowley CA, Curnutte JT, Rosin RE, et al: An inherited abnormality of neutrophil adhesion: Its genetic transmission and its association with a missing protein. N Engl J Med 1980; 302:1163.

647. Arnaout MA, Pitt J, Cohen HJ, et al: Deficiency of a granulocyte-membrane glycoprotein (gp150) in a boy with recurrent bacterial infections. N Engl J Med 1982; 306:693.

648. Bowen TJ, Ochs HD, Altman LC, et al: Severe recurrent bacterial infections associated with defective adherence and chemotaxis in two patients with neutrophils deficient in a cell-associated glycoprotein. J Pediatr 1982; 101:932.

649. Dana N, Todd RF III, Pitt J, et al: Deficiency of a surface membrane glycoprotein (Mo1) in man. J Clin Invest 1984; 73:153.

650. Arnaout MA: Leukocyte adhesion molecules deficiency: Its structural basis, pathophysiology and implications for modulating the inflammatory response. Immunol Rev 1990; 114:145.

651. von Andrian UH, Berger EM, Ramezani L, et al: In vivo behavior of neutrophils from two patients with distinct inherited leukocyte adhesion deficiency syndromes. J Clin Invest 1993; 91:2893.

652. Davies KA, Toothill VJ, Savill J, et al: A 19-year-old man with leukocyte adhesion deficiency. *In vitro* and *in vivo* studies of leucocyte function. Clin Exp Immunol 1991; 84:223.

653. Beller DI, Springer TA, Schreiber RD: Anti-Mac 1 selectively inhibits the mouse and human type three complement receptor. J Exp Med 1982; 156:1000.

654. Kohl S, Springer TA, Schmalstieg FC, et al: Defective natural killer cytotoxicity and polymorphonuclear leukocyte antibody-dependent cellular cytotoxicity in patients with LFA-1/OKM-1 deficiency. J Immunol 1984; 133:2972.

655. Kohl S, Loo LS, Schmalstieg FC, et al: The genetic deficiency of leukocyte surface glycoprotein Mac-1, LFA-1, p150,95 in humans is associated with defective antibody-dependent cellular cytotoxicity *in vitro* and defective protection against herpes simplex virus infection *in vivo*. J Immunol 1986; 137:1688.

656. Krensky AM, Sanchez-Madrid F, Robbins E, et al: The functional significance, distribution, and structure of LFA-1, LFA-2, LFA-3: Cell surface antigens associated with CTL-target interactions. J Immunol 1983; 131:611.

657. Hibbs ML, Wardlaw AJ, Stacker SA, et al: Transfection of cells from patients with leukocyte adhesion deficiency with an integrin β subunit (CD18) restores lymphocyte function-associated antigen-1 expression and function. J Clin Invest 1990; 85:674.

658. Arnaout MA, Dana N, Gupta SK, et al: Point mutations impairing cell surface expression of the common β subunit (CD18) in a patient with leukocyte adhesion molecule (Leu-CAM) deficiency. J Clin Invest 1990; 85:977.

659. Wardlaw AJ, Hibbs ML, Stacker SA, et al: Distinct mutations in two patients with leukocyte adhesion deficiency and their functional correlates. J Exp Med 1990; 172:335.

660. Ohashi Y, Yambe T, Tsuchiya S, et al: Familial genetic defect in a case of leukocyte adhesion deficiency. Hum Mutat 1993; 2:458.

661. Back AL, Kerkering M, Baker D, et al: A point mutation associated with leukocyte adhesion deficiency type 1 of moderate severity. Biochem Biophys Res Commun 1993; 193:912.

662. Corbi AL, Vara A, Ursa A, et al: Molecular basis for a severe case of leukocyte adhesion deficiency. Eur J Immunol 1992; 22:1877.

663. Sligh JE Jr, Hurwitz MY, Zhu C, et al: An initiation codon mutation in CD18 in association with the moderate phenotype of leukocyte adhesion deficiency. J Biol Chem 1992; 267:714.

664. Back AL, Hickstein DD: Two different CD18 mutations in a child with severe leukocyte adhesion deficiency (LAD) [abstract]. Blood 1990; 76:176a.

665. Nelson C, Rabb H, Arnaout MA: Genetic cause of leukocyte adhesion molecule deficiency. Abnormal splicing and a missense mutation in a conserved region of CD18 impair cell surface expression of β2 integrins. J Biol Chem 1992; 267:3351.

666. Wright AH, Douglass WA, Taylor GM, et al: Molecular characterization of leukocyte adhesion deficiency in six patients. Eur J Immunol 1995; 25:717.

667. Kishimoto TK, O'Connor K, Springer TA: Leukocyte adhesion deficiency: Aberrant splicing of a conserved integrin sequence causes a moderate deficiency phenotype. J Biol Chem 1989; 264:3588.

668. Lopez RC, Nueda A, Grospierre B, et al: Characterization of two new CD18 alleles causing severe leukocyte adhesion deficiency. Eur J Immunol 1993; 23:2792.

669. Giger U, Boxer LA, Simpson PJ, et al: Deficiency of leukocyte surface glycoproteins Mo1, LFA-1, and Leu M5 in a dog with recurrent bacterial infections: An animal model. Blood 1987; 69:1622.

670. Renshaw HW, Davis WC: Canine granulocytopathy syndrome: An inherited disorder of leukocyte function. Am J Pathol 1979; 95:731.

671. Hagemoser WA, Roth JA, Lofstedt J, et al: Granulocytopathy in a Holstein heifer. J Am Vet Med Assoc 1983; 183:1093.

672. Kehrli ME, Schmalstieg FC, Anderson DC, et al: Molecular definition of the bovine granulocytopathy syndrome: Identification of deficiency of the Mac-1 (CD11b/CD18) glycoprotein. Am J Vet Res 1990; 51:1826.

673. Kehrli ME, Ackermann MR, Shuster DE, et al: Animal model of human disease. Bovine leukocyte adhesion deficiency. β2 integrin deficiency in young Holstein cattle. Am J Pathol 1992; 140:1489.

674. Shuster D, Kehrli M, Ackermann M, et al: Identification and prevalence of a genetic defect that causes leukocyte adhesion deficiency in Holstein cattle. Proc Natl Acad Sci USA 1992; 89:9225.

675. Wilson RW, Ballantyne CM, Smith CW, et al: Gene targeting yields a CD18-mutant mouse for study of inflammation. J Immunol 1993; 151:1571.

676. Oudesluys-Murphy A, Eilers G, de Groot C: The time separation for the umbilical cord. Eur J Pediatr 1987; 146:387.

677. Wilson C, Ochs H, Almquist J, et al: When is umbilical cord separation delayed? J Pediatr 1985; 107:292.

678. Arnaout MA, Spits H, Terhorst C, et al: Deficiency of a leukocyte surface glycoprotein (LFA-1) in two patients with Mo1 deficiency. Effects of cell activation on Mo1/LFA-1 surface expression in normal and deficient leukocytes. J Clin Invest 1984; 74:1291.

679. Weisman SJ, Mahoney MJ, Anderson DC, et al: Prenatal diagnosis for Mo1 (CDw18) deficiency [abstract]. Clin Res 1987; 35:435a.

680. Anderson DC, Smith CW, Springer TA: Leukocyte adhesion deficiency and other disorders of leukocyte motility. In Scriver CR, Beaudet AL (eds): The Metabolic Basis of Inherited Disease. New York, McGraw-Hill, 1989, p 2751.

681. Fischer A, Descamps-Latscha B, Gerota I, et al: Bone marrow transplantation for inborn error of phagocytic cells associated with defective adherence, chemotaxis and oxidative response during opsonized particle phagocytosis. Lancet 1983; 2:473.

682. Fischer A, Landais P, Friedrich W, et al: Bone marrow transplantation (BMT) in Europe for primary immunodeficiencies other than severe combined immunodeficiency: A report from the European Group for BMT and the European Group for Immunodeficiency. Blood 1994; 83:1149.

683. Wilson JM, Ping AJ, Krauss JC, et al: Correction of CD18-deficient lymphocytes by retrovirus-mediated gene transfer. Science 1990; 248:1413.

684. Back AL, Kwok WW, Adam M, et al: Retroviral-mediated gene transfer of the leukocyte integrin CD18 subunit. Biochem Biophys Res Commun 1990; 171:787.

685. Kohn D: Gene therapy using hematopoietic stem cells. Curr Opin Mol Ther 1999; 1:437.

686. Dunbar C: Gene transfer to hematopoietic stem cells: Implications for gene therapy of human disease. Annu Rev Med 1996; 47:11.

687. Etzioni A, Frydman M, Pollack S, et al: A syndrome of leukocyte adhesion deficiency (LAD II) due to deficiency of sialyl-Lewis-X, a ligand for selectins. N Engl J Med 1992; 327:1789.

688. Marquardt T, Brune T, Luhn K, et al: Leukocyte adhesion deficiency II syndrome, a generalized defect in fucose metabolism. J Pediatr 1999; 134:681.

689. Hirschberg CB: Golgi nucleotide sugar transport and leukocyte adhesion deficiency II. J Clin Invest 2001; 108:3.

690. Lubke T, Marquardt T, Etzioni A, et al: Complementation cloning identifies CDG-IIc, a new type of congenital disorders of glycosylation, as a GDP-fucose transporter deficiency. Nat Genet 2001; 28:73.

691. Luhn K, Wild MK, Eckhardt M, et al: The gene defective in leukocyte adhesion deficiency II encodes a putative GDP-fucose transporter. Nat Genet 2001; 28:69.

692. Sturla L, Puglielli L, Tonetti M, et al: Impairment of the Golgi GDP-L-fucose transport and unresponsiveness to fucose replacement therapy in LAD II patients. Pediatr Res 2001; 49:537.

693. Marquardt T, Luhn K, Srikrishna G, et al: Correction of leukocyte adhesion deficiency type II with oral fucose. Blood 1999; 94:3976.

694. Etzioni A, Tonetti M: Fucose supplementation in leukocyte adhesion deficiency type II. Blood 2000; 95:3641.

695. Oseas RS, Allen J, Yang HH, et al: Mechanism of dexamethasone inhibition of chemotactic factor-induced granulocyte aggregation. Blood 1982; 59:265.

696. Skubitz KM, Craddock PR, Hammerschmidt DE, et al: Corticosteroids block binding of chemotactic peptide to the receptor on granulocytes and cause disaggregation of granulocyte aggregates *in vitro*. J Clin Invest 1981; 68:13.

697. Bryant RE, Sutcliff MC: The effect of 3′,5′-adenosine monophosphate on granulocyte adhesion. J Clin Invest 1974; 54:1241.

698. Craddock PR, Fehr J, Brigham KL, et al: Complement- and leukocyte-mediated pulmonary dysfunction in hemodialysis. N Engl J Med 1977; 196:769.

699. Heflin AC Jr, Brigham KL: Prevention by granulocyte depletion of increased vascular permeability of sheep lung following endotoxemia. J Clin Invest 1981; 68:1253.

700. Craddock PR, Hammerschmidt D, White JG: Complement (C5a)-induced granulocyte aggregation *in vitro*: A possible mechanism of complement-mediated leukostasis and leukopenia. J Clin Invest 1977; 60:260.

701. Tate RM, Repine JE: Neutrophils and the adult respiratory distress syndrome. Am Rev Respir Dis 1983; 128:552.

702. Wright DG, Robiechaud KJ, Pizzo PA, et al: Lethal pulmonary reactions associated with the combined use of amphotericin B and leukocyte transfusions. N Engl J Med 1981; 304:1185.

703. Boxer LA, Ingraham LM, Allen J, et al: Amphotericin B promotes leukocyte aggregation of nylon wool fiber-treated polymorphonuclear leukocytes. Blood 1981; 58:518.

704. Brown CC, Gallin JI: Chemotactic disorders. Hematol Oncol Clin North Am 1988; 2:61.

705. Boyden S: The chemotactic effect of mixtures of antibody and antigen on polymorphonuclear leukocytes. J Exp Med 1962; 115:453.

706. Smith CW, Hollers JC, Patrick RA, et al: Motility and adhesiveness in human neutrophils: Effects of chemotactic factors. J Clin Invest 1979; 63:221.

707. Nelson RD, Quie PG, Simmons RL: Chemotaxis under agarose: A new and simple method for measuring chemotaxis and spontaneous migration of human polymorphonuclear leukocytes and monocytes. J Immunol 1975; 115:1650.

708. Rebuck JW, Crowley JH: A method of studying leukocytic functions. Ann NY Acad Sci 1955; 59:757.

709. Leung DYM, Geha RS: Clinical and immunologic aspects of the hyperimmunoglobulin E syndrome. Hematol Oncol Clin North Am 1988; 2:81.

710. Davis SD, Schaller J, Wedgwood RJ: Job's syndrome: Reccurent, "cold," staphylococcal abscesses. Lancet 1966; 1:1013.

711. Donabedian H, Gallin JI: The hyperimmunoglobulin E recurrent-infection (Job's) syndrome. A review of the NIH experience and the literature. Medicine (Baltimore) 1983; 62:195.

712. Buckley RH, Wray BB, Belmaker EZ: Extreme hyperimmunoglobulinemia E and undue susceptibility to infection. Pediatrics 1972; 49:59.

713. Buckley RH: Immunodeficiency, hyper IgE type. In Buyse ML (ed): Birth Defects Encyclopedia. Cambridge, Blackwell Scientific Publications, 1990, p 953.

714. Grimbacher B, Holland SM, Gallin JI, et al: Hyper-IgE syndrome with recurrent infections—An autosomal dominant multisystem disorder [see comments]. N Engl J Med 1999; 340:692.

715. Hill HR, Estensen RD, Hogan NA, et al: Severe staphylococcal disease associated with allergic manifestation, hyperimmunoglobulinemia E, and defective neutrophil chemotaxis. J Lab Clin Med 1976; 88:796.

716. Hill HR, Ochs HD, Qioe PG, et al: Defect in neutrophil granulocyte chemotaxis in Job's syndrome of recurrent "cold" staphylococcal abscesses. Lancet 1974; 2:617.

717. Mawhinney H, Killen M, Fleming WA, et al: The hyperimmunoglobulin E syndrome: A neutrophil chemotactic defect reversible by histamine H2 receptor blockade? Clin Immunol Immunopathol 1980; 17:483.

718. Merten DF, Buckley RH, Pratt PC, et al: Hyperimmunoglobulinemia E syndrome: Radiographic observations. Radiology 1979; 132:71.

719. Buckley RH, Becker WG: Abnormalities in the regulation of human IgE synthesis. Immunol Rev 1978; 41:288.

720. Geha RS, Reinherz E, Leung D, et al: Deficiency of suppressor T cells in hyperimmunoglobulin E syndrome. J Clin Invest 1981; 68:783.

721. Martricardi PM, Capobianchi MR: Interferon production in primary immunodeficiencies. J Clin Immunol 1984; 4:388.

722. Del Prete G, Tiri A, Maggi E, et al: Defective *in vitro* production of gamma interferon and tumor necrosis factor-alpha by circulating T cells from patients with the hyper-immunoglobulin E syndrome. J Clin Invest 1989; 84:1830.

723. Sheerin KA, Buckley RH: Antibody responses to protein, polysaccharide, and φ X174 antigens in the hyperimmunoglobulinemia E (hyper-IgE) syndrome. J Allergy Clin Immunol 1991; 87:803.

724. Snapper CM, Paul WE: Interferon-gamma and B cell stimulatory factor-1 reciprocally regulate Ig isotype production. Science 1987; 236:944.

725. Coffman RL, Carty J: A T-cell activity that enhances polyclonal IgE production and its inhibition by interferon-γ. J Immunol 1986; 136:949.

726. Matricardi PM, Capobianchi MR, Paganelli R, et al: Interferon production in primary immunodeficiencies. J Clin Immunol 1984; 4:388.

727. Kazmierowski JA, Elin RJ, Reynolds HY, et al: Chédiak-Higashi syndrome: Reversal of susceptibility to infection by bone marrow transplantation. Blood 1976; 47:555.

728. King CL, Gallin JI, Malech HL, et al: Regulation of immunoglobulin production in hyperimmunoglobulin E recurrent-infection syndrome of interferon gamma. Proc Natl Acad Sci USA 1989; 86:10085.

729. A controlled trial of interferon gamma to prevent infection in chronic granulomatous disease. The International Chronic Granulomatous Disease Cooperative Study Group. N Engl J Med 1991; 324:509.

730. Boxer LA, Hedley-Whyte ET, Stossel TP: Neutrophil actin dysfunction and abnormal neutrophil behavior. N Engl J Med 1974; 291:1093.

731. Southwick FS, Dabiri GA, Stossel TP: Neutrophil actin dysfunction is a genetic disorder associated with partial impairment of neutrophil actin assembly in three family members. J Clin Invest 1988; 82:1525.

732. Southwick FS, Howard TH, Holbrook T, et al: The relationship between CR3 deficiency and neutrophil actin assembly. Blood 1989; 73:1973.

733. Coates TD, Torkildson JC, Torres M, et al: An inherited defect of neutrophil motility and microfilamentous cytoskeleton associated with abnormalities in 47-Kd and 89-Kd proteins. Blood 1991; 78:1338.

734. Howard T, Li Y, Torres M, et al: The 47-kD protein increased in neutrophil actin dysfunction with 47- and 89-kD protein abnormalities is lymphocyte-specific protein. Blood 1994; 83:231.

735. Nunoi H, Yamazaki T, Tsuchiya H, et al: A heterozygous mutation of β-actin associated with neutrophil dysfunction and recurrent infection. Proc Natl Acad Sci USA 1999; 96:8693.

736. Van Dyke TE: Role of the neutrophil in oral disease: Receptor deficiency in leukocytes from patients with juvenile periodontitis. Rev Infect Dis 1985; 7:419.

737. Van Dyke TE, Hoop GA: Neutrophil function and oral disease. CRC Oral Biol Med 1990; 1:117.

738. Van Dyke TE, Vaikuntam J: Neutrophil function and dysfunction in periodontal disease. Curr Opin Periodontol 1994:19.

739. Van Dyke TE, Schweinebraten M, Cianciola LJ, et al: Neutrophil chemotaxis in families with localized juvenile periodontitis. J Periodontol Res 1985; 20:503.

740. Donly KJ, Ashkenazi M: Juvenile periodontitis: A review of pathogenesis, diagnosis and treatment. J Clin Pediat Dent 1992; 16:73.

741. Cianciola LJ, Genco RJ, Patters MR, et al: Defective polymorphonuclear leukocyte function in a human periodontal disease. Nature 1977; 265:445.

742. Perez HD, Kelly E, Elfman F, et al: Defective polymorphonuclear leukocyte formyl peptide receptor(s) in juvenile periodontitis. J Clin Invest 1991; 87:971.

743. Clark RA, Page RC, Wilde G: Defective neutrophil chemotaxis in juvenile periodontitis. Infect Immun 1977; 18:694.

744. Agarwal S, Suzuki JB: Altered neutrophil function in localized juvenile periodontis: Intrinsic cellular defect or effect of immune mediators? J. Periodontol Res 1991; 26:276.

745. Van Dyke TE, Zinney W, Winkel K, et al: Neutrophil function in localized juvenile periodontitis. Phagocytosis, superoxide production and specific granule release. J Periodontol 1986; 57:703.

746. Van Dyke TE, Horoszewicz HU, Cianiola LJ, et al: Neutrophil chemotaxis dysfunction in human periodontitis. Infect Immun 1980; 27:124.

747. Suzuki JB, Colison C, Falker WF, et al: Immunologic profile of juvenile periodontitis. II. Neutrophil chemotaxis, phagocytosis and spore germination. J Periodontal 1984; 55:461.

748. Shurin SB, Socransky SS, Sweeney E, et al: A neutrophil disorder induced by capnocytophaga, a dental micro-organism. N Engl J Med 1979; 301:849.

749. Tsai C-C, McArthur WP, Baehni PC, et al: Extraction and partial characterization of a leukotoxin from a plaque-derived gram-negative microorganism. Infect Immun 1979; 25:427.

750. De Nardin E: The molecular basis for neutrophil dysfunction in early-onset periodontitis. J Periodontal 1996; 67:345.

751. Wilson CB: Immunologic basis for increased susceptibility of the neonate to infection. J Pediatr 1986; 108:1.

752. Hill HR: Biochemical, structural, and functional abnormalities of polymorphonuclear leukocytes in the neonate. Pediatr Res 1987; 22:375.

753. Hill HR, Augustin NH, Jaffe HS: Human recombinant interferon gamma enhances neonatal polymorphonuclear leukocyte activation and movement, and increases free intracellular calcium. J Exp Med 1991; 173:767.

754. Klein RB, Fischer TJ, Gard SE, et al: Decreased mononuclear and polymorphonuclear chemotaxis in human newborns, infants, and young children. Pediatrics 1977; 60:467.

755. Anderson DC, Hughes BJ, Smith CW: Abnormal motility of neonatal polymorphonuclear leukocytes: Relationship to impaired redistribution of surface adhesion sites by chemotactic factor or colchicine. J Clin Invest 1981; 68:863.

756. Anderson DC, Hughes BJ, Wible LJ, et al: Impaired motility of neonatal PMN leukocytes: Relationship to abnormalities of cell orientation and assembly of microtubules in chemotactic gradients. J Leukoc Biol 1984; 36:1.

757. Anderson DC, Becker Freeman KL, Heerdt B, et al: Abnormal stimulated adherence of neonatal granulocytes: Impaired induction of surface MAC-1 by chemotactic factors or secretagogues. Blood 1987; 70:740.

758. Smith JB, Campbell DE, Ludomirsky A, et al: Expression of the complement receptors CR1 and CR3 and the type III Fc-γ receptor on neutrophils from newborn infants and from fetuses with Rh disease. Pediatr Res 1990; 28:120.

759. Sacchi F, Rondini G, Mingrat G, et al: Clinical and laboratory observations: Different maturation of neutrophil chemotaxis in term and preterm newborn infants. J Pediatr 1982; 101:273.

760. Kurkchubasche AG, Panepinto JA, Tracy TF Jr, et al: Clinical features of a human Rac2 mutation: A complex neutrophil dysfunction disease. J Pediatr 2001; 139:141.

761. Roos D, Kuijpers TW, Mascart-Lemone F, et al: A novel syndrome of severe neutrophil dysfunction: Unresponsiveness confined to chemotaxin-induced functions. Blood 1993; 81:2735.

762. Brenneis H, Schmidt A, Blaas-Mautner P, et al: Chemotaxis of polymorphonuclear neutrophils (PMN) in patients suffering from recurrent infection. Eur J Clin Invest 1993; 23:693.

763. Alper CA, Colten HR, Rosen FS, et al: Homozygous deficiency of C3 in a patient with repeated infections. Lancet 1972; 2:1179.

764. Botto M, Fong KY, So AK, et al: Molecular basis of hereditary C3 deficiency. J Clin Invest 1990; 86:1158.

765. Roord JJ, Daha M, Kuis W, et al: Inherited deficiency of the third component of complement associated with recurrent pyogenic infections, circulating immune complexes, and vasculitis in a Dutch family. N Engl J Med 1983; 71:81.

766. Borzy MS, Gewurz A, Wolff L, et al: Inherited C3 deficiency with recurrent infections and glomerulonephritis. Am J Dis Child 1988; 142:79.

767. Alper CA, Abramson N, Johnston RB Jr, et al: Studies *in vivo* and *in vitro* on an abnormality in the metabolism of C3 in a patient with increased susceptibility to infection. J Clin Invest 1970; 49:1975.

768. Super M, Thiel S, Lu J, et al: Association of low levels of mannan-binding protein with a common defect of opsonisation. Lancet 1989; 2:1236.

769. Sumiya M, Super M, Tabona P, et al: Molecular basis of opsonic defect in immunodeficient children. Lancet 1991; 337:1569.

770. Turner MW, Lipscombe RJ, Levinsky RJ, et al: Mutations in the human mannose binding protein gene: Their frequencies in three distinct populations and relationship to serum levels of the protein. Immunodeficiency 1993; 4:285.

771. Madsen HO, Garred P, Kurtzhals JA, et al: A new frequent allele is the missing link in the structural polymorphism of the human mannan-binding protein. Immunogenetics 1994; 40:37.

772. Summerfield JA, Ryder S, Sumiya M, et al: Mannose binding protein gene mutations associated with unusual and severe infections in adults. Lancet 1995; 345:886.

773. Ceuppens JL, Bloemmen FJ, Van Wauwe JP: T-cell unresponsiveness to the mitogenic activity of OKT3 antibody results from a deficiency of the monocyte Fc-γ receptors for murine IgG2a and inability to cross-link the T3-Ti complex. J Immunol 1985; 135:165.

774. Fromont P, Bettaib A, Skouri H, et al: Frequency of the polymorphonuclear neutrophil Fc-γ receptor III deficiency in the French population and its involvement in the development of neonatal alloimmune neutropenia. Blood 1992; 79:2131.

775. de Haas M, Kleijer M, van Zwieten R, et al: Neutrophil FcγRIIIb deficiency, nature, and clinical consequences: A study of 21 individuals from 14 families. Blood 1995; 86:2403.

776. Selvaraj P, Rosse WF, Silber R, et al: The major Fc receptor in blood has a phosphatidylinositol anchor and is deficient in paroxysmal nocturnal haemoglobinuria. Nature 1988; 333:565.

777. Huizinga TW, van der Schoot CE, Jost C, et al: The PI-linked receptor FcR III is released on stimulation of neutrophils. Nature 1988; 333:667.

778. Van De Winkel JGJ, Capel PJA: Human IgG Fc receptor heterogeneity: Molecular aspects and clinical implications. Immunol Today 1993; 14:215.

779. White JG, Clawson CC: The Chédiak-Higashi syndrome: The nature of the giant neutrophil granules and their interactions with cytoplasm and foreign particulates. I. Progressive enlargement of the massive inclusions in mature neutrophils. II. Manifestations of cytoplasmic injury and sequestration. III. Interactions between giant organelles and foreign particulates. Am J Pathol 1980; 98:151.

780. Rausch PG, Pryzwansky KB, Spitznagel JK: Immunocytochemical identification of azurophilic and specific granule markers in the giant granules of Chédiak-Higashi neutrophils. N Engl J Med 1978; 298:693.

781. Davis WC, Douglas SD: Defective granule formation and function in the Chédiak-Higashi syndrome in man and animals. Semin Hematol 1972; 9:431.

782. Davis WC, Spicer SS, Greene WB, et al: Ultrastructure of cells in bone marrow and peripheral blood of normal mink and mink with the homologue of the Chédiak-Higashi trait of humans. II. Cytoplasmic granules in eosinophils, basophils, mononuclear cells and platelets. Am J Pathol 1971; 63:411.

783. Vassali JD, Piperno-Granelli A, Griscelli C, et al: Specific protease deficiency in polymorphonuclear leukocytes of Chédiak-Higashi syndrome and beige mice. J Exp Mice 1978; 149:1285.

784. Ganz T, Metcalf JA, Gallin JI, et al: Microbicidal/cytotoxic proteins of neutrophils are deficient in two disorders: Chédiak-Higashi syndrome and "specific" granule deficiency. J Clin Invest 1988; 82:552.

785. Sjaastad OV, Blom AK, Stormorken H, et al: Adenine nucleotides, serotonin and aggregation properties of the platelets of blue foxes *(Alopex lagopus)* with the Chédiak-Higashi syndrome. Am J Med Genet 1990; 35:373.

786. Barbosa M, Nguyen Q, Tchernev V, et al: Identification of the homologous beige and Chédiak-Higashi syndrome genes. Nature 1996; 382:262.

787. Nagle DL, Karim MA, Woolf EA, et al: Identification and mutation analysis of the complete gene for Chédiak-Higashi syndrome. Nat Genet 1996; 14:307.

788. Perou CM, Moore KJ, Nagle DL, et al: Identification of the murine beige gene by YAC complementation and positional cloning. Nat Genet 1996; 13:303.

789. Jenkins NA, Justice MJ, Gilbert DJ, et al: Nidogen/entactin *(Nid)* maps to the proximal end of mouse chromosome 13 linked to beige *(bg)* and identifies a new region of homology between mouse and human chromosomes. Genomics 1991; 9:401.

790. Certain S, Barrat F, Pastural E, et al: Protein truncation test of LYST reveals heterogenous mutations in patients with Chédiak-Higashi syndrome. Blood 2000; 95:979.

791. Fukai K, Oh J, Karim MA, et al: Homozygosity mapping of the gene for Chédiak-Higashi syndrome to chromosome 1q42-q44 in a segment of conserved synteny that includes the mouse beige locus *(bg)*. Am J Hum Genet 1996; 59:620.

792. Blume RS, Bennett JM, Yankee RA, et al: Defective granulocyte regulation in the Chédiak-Higashi syndrome. N Engl J Med 1968; 279:1009.

793. White JG, Clawson CC: The Chédiak-Higashi syndrome. Ring-shaped lysosomes in circulating monocytes. Am J Pathol 1979; 96:781.

794. Buchanan GB, Handin RI: Platelet function in the Chédiak-Higashi syndrome. Blood 1976; 47:941.

795. Boxer GJ, Holmsen H, Robkin L, et al: Abnormal platelet functions in Chédiak-Higashi syndrome. Br J Haematol 1977; 35:521.

796. Novak EK, McGarry MP, Swank RT: Correction of symptoms of platelet storage pool deficiency in animal models for Chédiak-Higashi syndrome and Hermansky-Pudlak syndrome. Blood 1985; 66:1196.

797. Bell TG, Meyers KM, Prieur DJ, et al: Decreased nucleotide and serotonin storage associates with defective function in Chédiak-Higashi syndrome cattle and human platelets. Blood 1976; 48:175.

798. Clark RA, Kimball HR: Defective granulocyte chemotaxis in the Chédiak-Higashi syndrome. J Clin Invest 1971; 50:2645.

799. Clawson CC, Repine JE, White JG: Chédiak-Higashi syndrome: Quantitative defect in bactericidal capacity. Blood 1971; 38:814.

800. Clawson CC, Repine JE, White JG: The Chédiak-Higashi syndrome. Quantitation of a deficiency in maximal bactericidal capacity. Am J Pathol 1979; 94:539.

801. Root RK, Rosenthal AS, Balestra DJ: Abnormal bactericidal, metabolic, and lysosomal functions of Chédiak-Higashi syndrome leukocytes. J Clin Invest 1972; 51:649.

802. Clawson CC, Repine JE, White JG: Quantitation of bactericidal capacity in normal and abnormal human neutrophils. Pediatr Res 1972; 6:367.

803. Cairo MS, Vandeven C, Toy C, et al: Fluorescent cytometric analysis of polymorphonuclear leucocytes in Chédiak-Higashi syndrome: Diminished C3bi receptor expression (OKM-1) with normal granular cell density. Pediatr Res 1988; 24:673.

804. Klein M, Roder J, Haliotis T, et al: Chédiak-Higashi gene in humans. II. The selectivity of the defect in natural-killer and antibody dependent cell-mediated cytotoxicity function. J Exp Med 1980; 151:1049.

805. Targan SR, Oseas R: The "lazy" NK cells of Chédiak-Higashi syndrome. J Immunol 1983; 130:2671.

806. Nair MPN, Gray RH, Boxer LA, et al: Deficiency of inducible suppressor cell activity in the Chédiak-Higashi syndrome. Am J Hematol 1987; 26:55.

807. Abo T, Roder JC, Abo W, et al: Natural killer (HNK-1⁺) cells in Chédiak-Higashi patients are present in normal numbers but are abnormal in function and morphology. J Clin Invest 1982; 70:193.

808. Haliotis T, Roder J, Klein M, et al: Chédiak-Higashi gene in humans. I. Impairment of natural-killer function. J Exp Med 1980; 151:1039.

809. Merino F, Klein GO, Henle W, et al: Elevated antibody titers to Epstein-Barr virus and low natural killer cell activity in patients with Chédiak-Higashi syndrome. Clin Immunol Immunopathol 1983; 27:326.

810. Rubin CM, Burke BA, McKenna RW, et al: The accelerated phase of Chédiak-Higashi syndrome. An expression of the virus-associated hemophagocytic syndrome? Cancer 1985; 56:524.

811. Pettit RE, Berdal KG: Chédiak-Higashi syndrome: Neurologic appearance. Arch Neurol 1984; 41:1001.

812. Creel D, Boxer LA, Fauci AS: Visual and auditory anomalies in Chédiak-Higashi syndrome. Electroencephalogr Clin Neurophysiol 1983; 55:252.

813. Diukman R, Tanigawara S, Cowan MJ, et al: Prenatal diagnosis of Chédiak-Higashi syndrome. Prenat Diagn 1992; 12:877.

814. Griscelli C, Durandy A, Guy-Grand D, et al: A syndrome associating partial albinism and immunodeficiency. Am J Med 1978; 65:691.

815. Kumar M, Sackey K, Schmalstieg F, et al: Griscelli syndrome: Rare neonatal syndrome of recurrent hemophagocytosis. Am J Pediatr Hematol Oncol 2001; 23:464.

816. Van Slyck E, Rebuck JW: Pseudo-Chédiak-Higashi anomaly in acute leukemia. Am J Clin Pathol 1974; 62:673.

817. Gorman AM, O'Connell LG: Letter to the editor. Pseudo-Chédiak-Higashi anomaly in acute leukemia. Am J Clin Pathol 1976; 65:1030.

818. Tulliez M, Vernant JP, Brenton-Gorius J, et al: Pseudo-Chédiak-Higashi anomaly in a case of acute myeloid leukemia: Electron microscopic studies. Blood 1979; 54:863.

819. Weening RS, Schoorel EP, Roos D, et al: Effect of ascorbate on abnormal neutrophil, platelet, and lymphocyte function in a patient with the Chédiak-Higashi syndrome. Blood 1981; 57:856.

820. Boxer LA, Watanabe AM, Rister M, et al: Correction of leukocyte function in Chédiak-Higashi syndrome by ascorbate. N Engl J Med 1976; 295:1041.

821. Gallin JI, Elin RJ, Hubert RT, et al: Efficacy of ascorbic acid in Chédiak-Higashi syndrome (CHS): Studies in humans and mice. Blood 1979; 53:226.

822. Virelizier JL, Lagrue A, Durandy A, et al: Reversal of natural killer defect in a patient with Chédiak-Higashi syndrome after bone-marrow transplantation. N Engl J Med 1981; 306:1055.

823. Colgan SP, Hull-Thrall MA, Gasper PW, et al: Restoration of neutrophil and platelet function in feline Chédiak-Higashi syndrome by bone marrow transplantation. Bone Marrow Transplant 1991; 7:365.

824. Griscelli C, Virelizier J-L: Bone marrow transplantation in a patient with Chédiak-Higashi syndrome. In Wedgwood RJ, Rosen F, et al (eds): Primary Immunodeficiency Diseases. New York, Alan R. Liss, 1983, p 333.

825. Merino F, Henle W, Ramirez Duque P: Chronic active Epstein-Barr virus infection in patients with Chédiak-Higashi syndrome. J Clin Immunol 1986; 6:299.

826. Gallin JI: Neutrophil specific granule deficiency. Annu Rev Med 1985; 36:263.

827. Komiyama A, Morosawa H, Nakahata T, et al: Abnormal neutrophil maturation in a neutrophil defect with morphologic abnormality and impaired function. J Pediatr 1979; 94:19.

828. Ambruso DR, Sasada M, Nishiyama H, et al: Defective bactericidal activity and absence of specific granules in neutrophils from a patient with recurrent bacterial infections. J Clin Immunol 1984; 4:23.

829. Strauss RG, Bove KE, Jones JF, et al: An anomaly of neutrophil morphology with impaired function. N Engl J Med 1974; 290:278.

830. Boxer LA, Coates TD, Haak RA, et al: Lactoferrin deficiency associated with altered granulocyte function. N Engl J Med 1982; 307:404.

831. Parmley RT, Tzeng DY, Baehner RL, et al: Abnormal distribution of complex carbohydrates in neutrophils of a patient with lactoferrin deficiency. Blood 1983; 62:538.

832. Borregaard N, Boxer LA, Smolen JE, et al: Anomalous neutrophil granule distribution in a patient with lactoferrin deficiency: Pertinence to the respiratory burst. Am J Hematol 1985; 18:255.

833. Parmley RT, Gilbert CS, Boxer LA: Abnormal peroxidase-positive granules in "specific granule" deficiency. Blood 1989; 73:838.

834. Lomax KJ, Leto TL, Nunoi H, et al: Recombinant 47-kD cytosol factor restores NADPH oxidase in chronic granulomatous disease. Science 1989; 245:409.

835. Petty HR, Francis JW, Todd RF III, et al: Neutrophil C3bi receptors: Formation of membrane clusters during cell triggering requires intracellular granules. J Cell Physiol 1987; 133:235.

836. Lomax KJ, Gallin JI, Rotrosen D, et al: Selective defect in myeloid cell lactoferrin gene expression in neutrophil specific granule deficiency. J Clin Invest 1989; 83:514.

837. Breton-Gorius J, Mason DY, Buriot D, et al: Lactoferrin deficiency as a consequence of a lack of specific granules in neutrophils from a patient with recurrent infections. Detection by immunoperoxidase staining for lactoferrin and cytochemical electron microscopy. Am J Pathol 1980; 99:413.

838. Gallin JI, Fletcher MP, Seligmann BE, et al: Human neutrophil-specific granule deficiency: A model to assess the role of neutrophil-specific granules in the evolution of the inflammatory response. Blood 1982; 59:1317.

839. O'Shea JJ, Brown EJ, Seligmann BE, et al: Evidence for distinct intracellular pools of receptors for C3b and C3bi in human neutrophils. J Immunol 1985; 134:2580.

840. Spitznagel JK, Cooper MR, McCall AE, et al: Selective deficiency of granules associated with lysozyme and lactoferrin in human polymorphs (PMN) with reduced microbicidal capacity. J Clin Invest 1972; 51:92a.

841. Hibbs MS, Bainton DF: Human neutrophil gelatinase is a component of specific granules. J Clin Invest 1989; 84:1395.

842. Rosenberg HF, Galin JI: Neutrophil-specific granule deficiency includes eosinophils. Blood 1993; 82:268.

843. Lekstrom-Himes J, Xanthopoulos KG: CCAAT/enhancer binding protein ε is critical for effective neutrophil-mediated response to inflammatory challenge. Blood 1999; 93:3096.

844. Verbeek W, Lekstrom-Himes J, Park DJ, et al: Myeloid transcription factor C/EBPc is involved in the positive regulation of lactoferrin gene expression in neutrophils. Blood 1999; 94:3141.

845. Khanna-Gupta A, Zibello T, Sun H, et al: C/EBP ε mediates myeloid differentiation and is regulated by the CCAAT displacement protein (CDP/cut). Proc Natl Acad Sci USA 2001; 98:8000.

846. Todd RF III, Arnaout MA, Rosin RE, et al: Subcellular localization of the large subunit of Mo1 (Mo1; formerly gp110), a surface glycoprotein associated with adhesion. J Clin Invest 1984; 74:1280.

847. Miller LJ, Bainton DF: Stimulated mobilization of monocyte Mac-1 and p150,95 adhesion proteins from an intracellular vesicular compartment to the cell surface. J Clin Invest 1987; 80:535.

848. Petrequin PR, Todd RF III, Devall LJ, et al: Association between gelatinase release and increased plasma membrane expression of the Mo1 glycoprotein. Blood 1987; 69:605.

849. Fletcher MP, Gallin JI: Human neutrophils contain an intracellular pool of putative receptors for the chemoattractant N-formyl-methionyl-leucyl-phenylalanine. Blood 1983; 62:792.

850. Kuriyama K, Tomonaga M, Matsuo T, et al: Diagnostic significance of detecting pseudo-Pelger-Huet anomalies and micromegakaryocytes in myelodysplastic syndrome. Br J Haematol 1986; 63:665.

851. Winkelstein JA, Marino MC, Johnston RB Jr, et al: Chronic granulomatous disease. Report on a national registry of 368 patients. Medicine (Baltimore) 2000; 79:155.

852. Berendes H, Bridges RA, Good RA: Fatal granulomatosis of childhood: Clinical study of new syndrome. Minn Med 1957; 40:309.

853. Landing BH, Shirkey HS: Syndrome of recurrent infection and infiltration of viscera by pigmented lipid histiocytes. Pediatrics 1957; 20:431.

854. Bridges RA, Berendes H, Good RA: A fatal granulomatous disease of childhood. The clinical, pathological, and laboratory features of a new syndrome. Am J Dis Child 1959; 97:387.

855. Windhorst DB, Holmes B, Good RA: A newly defined X-linked trait in man with demonstration of the Lyon effect in carrier females. Lancet 1967; 1:737.

856. Johnston RB, McMurry JS: Chronic familial granulomatosis: Report of five cases and the literature. Am J Dis Child 1967; 114:370.

857. Clark RA, Malech HL, Gallin JI, et al: Genetic variants of chronic granulomatous disease: Prevalence of deficiencies of two cytosolic components of the NADPH oxidase system. N Engl J Med 1989; 321:647.

858. Casimir C, Chetty M, Bohler M-C, et al: Identification of the defective NADPH-oxidase component in chronic granulomatous disease: A study of 57 European families. Eur J Clin Invest 1992; 22:403.

859. Cross A, Heyworth P, Rae J, et al: A variant X-linked chronic granulomatous disease patient (X91⁺) with partially functional cytochrome b*. J Biol Chem 1995; 270:8194.

860. Curnutte JT: Molecular basis of the autosomal recessive forms of chronic granulomatous disease. Immunodef Rev 1992; 3:149.

861. Newburger PE, Luscinskas FW, Ryan T, et al: Variant chronic granulomatous disease: Modulation of the neutrophil by severe infection. Blood 1986; 68:914.

862. Roos D, de Boer M, Borregaard N, et al: Chronic granulomatous disease with partial deficiency of cytochrome b_{558} and incomplete respiratory burst: Variants of the X-linked, cytochrome b_{558}-negative form of the disease. J Leukoc Biol 1992; 51:164.

863. Stossel TP, Root RK: Phagocytosis in chronic granulomatous disease and the Chédiak-Higashi syndrome. N Engl J Med 1972; 286:120.

864. Gaither TA, Medley SR, Gallin JI, et al: Studies of phagocytosis in chronic granulomatous disease. Inflammation 1987; 11:211.

865. Hasui M, Hirabayashi Y, Hattori K, et al: Increased phagocytic activity of polymorphonuclear leukocytes of chronic granulomatous disease as determined with flow cytometric assay. J Lab Clin Med 1991; 117:291.

866. Bohler MC, Seger RA, Mouy R, et al: A study of 25 patients with chronic granulomatous disease: A new classification by correlating respiratory burst, cytochrome b, and flavoprotein. J Clin Immunol 1986; 6:136.

867. Tauber AI, Borregaard N, Simons E, et al: Chronic granulomatous disease: A syndrome of phagocyte oxidase deficiencies. Medicine (Baltimore) 1983; 62:286.

868. Forrest CB, Forehand JR, Axtell RA, et al: Clinical features and current management of chronic granulomatous disease. Hematol Oncol Clin North Am 1988; 2:253.

869. Babior BM, Woodman RC: Chronic granulomatous disease. Semin Hematol 1990; 27:247.

870. Johnston RB Jr, Newman SL: Chronic granulomatous disease. Pediatr Clin North Am 1977; 24:365.

871. Mouy R, Fischer A, Vilmer E, et al: Incidence, severity, and prevention of infections in chronic granulomatous disease. J Pediatr 1989; 114:555.

872. Hayakawa H, Kobayashi N, Yata J: Chronic granulomatous disease in Japan: A summary of the clinical features of 84 registered patients. Acta Paediatr Jpn 1985; 27:501.

873. Finn A, Hadzic N, Morgan G, et al: Prognosis of chronic granulomatous disease. Arch Dis Child 1990; 65:942.

874. Styrt B, Klempner MS: Late-presenting variant of chronic granulomatous disease. Pediatr Infect Dis 1984; 3:556.

875. Chusid MJ, Parrillo JE, Fauci AS: Chronic granulomatous disease: Diagnosis in a 27-year-old man with Mycobacterium fortuitum. JAMA 1975; 233:1295.

876. Cazzola M, Sacchi F, Pagani A, et al: X-linked chronic granulomatous disease in an adult woman. Evidence for a cell selection favoring neutrophils expressing the mutant allele. Haematologica 1985; 70:291.

877. Dilworth JA, Mandell GL: Adults with chronic granulomatous disease of "childhood." Am J Med 1977; 63:233.

878. Schapiro BL, Newburger PE, Klempner MS, et al: Chronic granulomatous disease presenting in a 69-year-old man. N Engl J Med 1991; 325:1786.

879. Liese J, Jendrossek V, Jansson A, et al: Chronic granulomatous disease in adults. Lancet 1996; 347:220.

880. Gallin JI, Buescher ES, Seligmann BE, et al: Recent advances in chronic granulomatous disease. Ann Intern Med 1983; 99:657.

881. Hitzig WH, Seger RA: Chronic granulomatous disease, a heterogeneous syndrome. Hum Genet 1983; 64:207.

882. Cohen MS, Isturiz RE, Malech HL, et al: Fungal infection in chronic granulomatous disease. Am J Med 1981; 71:59.

883. Speert DP, Bond M, Woodman RC, et al: Infection with Pseudomonas-cepacia in chronic granulomatous disease—Role of nonoxidative killing by neutrophils in host defense. J Infect Dis 1994; 170:1524.

884. O'Neil KM, Herman JH: Pseudomonas cepacia: An emerging pathogen in chronic granulomatous diseae. J Pediatr 1986; 108:940.

885. Clegg HW, Ephros M, Newburger PE: Pseudomonas cepacia pneumonia in chronic granulomatous disease. Pediatr Infect Dis 1986; 5:111.

886. Phillips P, Forbes JC, Speert DP: Disseminated infection with Pseudallescheria boydii in a patient with chronic granulomatous disease: Response to γ-interferon plus antifungal chemotherapy. Pediatr Infect Dis 1991; 10:536.

887. Schwartz DA: Sporothrix tenosynovitis—Differential diagnosis of granulomatous inflammatory disease of the joints. J Rheumatol 1989; 16:550.

888. Sorensen RU, Jacobs MR, Shurin SB: Chromobacterium violaceum adenitis acquired in the northern United States as a complication of chronic granulomatous disease. Pediatr Infect Dis 1985; 4:701.

889. Macher AM, Casale TB, Fauci AS: Chronic granulomatous disease of childhood and Chromobacterium violaceum infections in the southeastern United States. Ann Intern Med 1982; 97:51.

890. Wenger JD, Hollis DG, Weaver RE, et al: Infection caused by Francisella philomiragia (formerly Yersinia philomiragia). A newly recognized human pathogen. Ann Intern Med 1990; 110:888.

891. Kenney RT, Kwon-Chung KJ, Witebsky FG, et al: Invasive infection with Sarcinosporon inkin in a patient with chronic granulomatous disease. Am J Clin Pathol 1990; 94:344.

892. Pedersen FK, Johansen KS, Rosenkvist J, et al: Refractory Pneumocytis carini infection in chronic granulomatous disease: Successful treatment with granulocytes. Pediatrics 1979; 64:935.

893. Adinoff AD, Johnston RB Jr, Dolen J, et al: Chronic granulomatous disease and Pneumocytis carinii pneumonia. Pediatrics 1982; 69:133.

894. Mulholland MW, Delaney JP, Simmons RL: Gastrointestinal complications of chronic granulomatous disease of childhood: Surgical implications. Surgery 1983; 94:569.

895. Garel LA, Pariente DM, Nezelof C, et al: Liver involvement in chronic granulomatous disease: The role of ultrasound in diagnosis and treatment. Radiology 1984; 153:117.

896. Barton L, Moussa S, Villar R, et al: Gastrointestinal complications of chronic granulomatous disease: Case report and literature review. Clin Pediatrics 1998; 37:231.

897. Sponseller PD, Malech HL, McCarthy EF Jr, et al: Skeletal involvement in children who have chronic granulomatous disease. J Bone Joint Surg 1991; 73a:37.

898. Wolfson JJ, Kane WJ, Laxdal SD, et al: Bone findings in chronic granulomatous disease of childhood: A genetic abnormality of leukocyte function. Surgery 1969; 51:1573.

899. Mandell GL, Hook EW: Leukocyte bactericidal activity in chronic granulomatous disease: Correlation of bacterial hydrogen peroxide production and susceptibility in intracellular killing. J Bacteriol 1969; 100:531.

900. Gabay JE, Scott RW, Campanelli D, et al: Antibiotic proteins of human polymorphonuclear leukocytes. Proc Natl Acad Sci. USA 1989; 86:5610.

901. Odell EW, Segal AW: Killing of pathogens associated with chronic granulomatous disease by the non-oxidative microbicidal mechanisms of human neutrophils. J Med Microbiol 1991; 34:129.

902. Johnston RB Jr, Baehner RL: Chronic granulomatous disease: Correlation between pathogenesis and clinical findings. Pediatrics 1971; 48:730.

903. Renner WR, Johnson JF, Lichtenstein JE, et al: Esophageal inflammation and stricture: Complication of chronic granulomatous disease of childhood. Radiology 1991; 178:189.

904. Griscom NT, Kirkpatrick JA Jr, Girdany BR, et al: Gastric antral narrowing in chronic granulomatous disease of childhood. Pediatrics 1974; 54:456.

905. Hiller N, Fisher D, Abrahamov A, et al: Esophageal involvement in chronic granulomatous disease. Pediatr Radiol 1995; 25:308.

906. Ament ME, Ochs HD: Gastrointestinal manifestations of chronic granulomatous disease. N Engl J Med 1973; 288:382.

907. Isaacs D, Wright VM, Shaw DG, et al: Case report: Chronic granulomatous disease mimicking Crohn's disease. J Pediatr Gastroenterol Nutr 1985; 4:498.

908. Aliabadi H, Gonzalez R, Quie PG: Urinary tract disorders in patients with chronic granulomatous disease. N Engl J Med 1989; 321:706.

909. Bauer SB, Kogan SJ: Vesical manifestations of chronic granulomatous disease in children. Its relation to eosinophilic cystitis. Urology 1991; 37:463.

910. Cyr WL, Johnson H, Balfour J: Granulomatous cystitis as a manifestation of chronic granulomatous disease of childhood. J Urol 1973; 110:357.

911. Southwick FS, Van der Meer JWM: Recurrent cystitis and bladder mass in two adults with chronic granulomatous disease. Ann Intern Med 1988; 109:118.

912. Walther M, Malech H, Berman A, et al: The urological manifestations of chronic granulomatous disease. J Urol 1992; 147:1314.

913. Windhorst DB, Good RA: Dermatologic manifestations of fatal granulomatous disease of childhood. Arch Dermatol 1971; 103:351.

914. Cohen MS, Leong PA, Simpson DM: Phagocytic cells in periodontal defense: Periodontal status of patients with chronic granulomatous disease of childhood. J Periodontol 1985; 56:611.

915. Martyn LJ, Lischner HW, Pileggi AJ, et al: Chorioretinal lesions in familial chronic granulomatous disease of childhood. Am J Ophthalmol 1972; 73:403.

916. Valluri S, Chu FC, Smith ME: Ocular pathologic findings of chronic granulomatous disease of childhood. Am J Ophthalmol 1995; 120:120.

917. Hadfield MG, Ghatak NR, Laine FJ, et al: Brain lesions in chronic granulomatous disease. Acta Neuropathol 1991; 81:467.

918. Walker DH, Okiye G: Chronic granulomatous disease involving the central nervous system. Pediatr Pathol 1983; 1:159.

919. Van Rhenen DJ, Koolen MI, Feltkamp-Vroom TM, et al: Immune complex glomerulonephritis in chronic granulomatous disease. Acta Med Scand 1979; 206:233.

920. Stalder JF, Dreno B, Bureau B, et al: Discoid lupus erythematosus-like lesions in an autosomal form of chronic granulomatous disease. Br J Dermatol 1986; 114:251.

921. Smitt JHS, Bos JD, Weening RS, et al: Discoid lupus erythematosus-like skin changes in patients with autosomal recessive chronic granulomatous disease. Arch Dermatol 1990; 126:1656.

922. Manzi S, Urbach AH, McCune AB, et al: Systemic lupus erythematosus in a boy with chronic granulomatous disease: Case report and review of the literature. Arthritis Rheum 1991; 34:101.

923. Schmitt CP, Scharer K, Waldherr R, et al: Glomerulonephritis associated with chronic granulomatous disease and systemic lupus erythematosus. Nephrol Dial Transplant 1995; 10:891.

924. Lee BW, Yap HK: Poly arthritis resembling juvenile rheumatoid arthritis in a girl with chronic granulomatous disease. Arthritis Rheum 1994; 37:773.

925. Woodman RC, Newburger PE, Anklesaria P, et al: A new X-linked variant of chronic granulomatous disease characterized by the existence of a normal clone of respiratory burst-competent phagocytic cells. Blood 1995; 85:231.

926. Foster C, Lehrnbecher T, Mol F, et al: Host defense molecule polymorphisms influence the risk for immune-mediated complications in chronic granulomatous disease. J Clin Invest 1998; 102:2146.

927. Johnston RB, Harbecker RJ, Johnston RB Jr: Recurrent severe infections in a girl with apparently variable expression of mosaicism for chronic granulomatous disease. J Pediatr 1985; 106:50.

928. Ochs HD, Igo RP: The NBT slide test: A simple screening method for detecting chronic granulomatous disease and female carriers. J Pediatr 1973; 83:77.

929. Meerhof LJ, Roos D: Heterogeneity in chronic granulomatous disease detected with an improved nitroblue tetrazolium slide test. J Leukoc Biol 1986; 39:699.

930. Roesler J, Hecht M, Freihorst J, et al: Diagnosis of chronic granulomatous disease and of its mode of inheritance by dihydrorhodamine 123 and flow microcytofluorometry. Eur J Pediatr 1991; 150:161.

931. Rothe G, Emmendorffer A, Oser A, et al: Flow cytometric measurements of the respiratory burst activity of phagocytes using dihydrorhodamine 123. J Immunol Methods 1991; 138:133.

932. Hassan NF, Campbell DE, Douglas SD: Phorbol myristate acetate induced oxidation of $2',7'$-dichlorofluorescein by neutrophils from patients with chronic granulomatous disease. J Leukoc Biol 1988; 43:317.

933. Windhorst DB, Page AR, Holmes B, et al: The pattern of genetic transmission of the leukocyte defect in fatal granulomatous disease of childhood. J Clin Invest 1968; 47:1026.

934. Lyon MF: Sex chromatin and gene action in the mammalian X-chromosome. Am J Hum Genet 1962; 14:135.

935. Beutler E, Yeh M, Fairbans VF: The normal human female as a mosaic of X-chromosome activity: Studies using the gene for G-6-PD deficiency as a marker. Proc Natl Acad Sci USA 1962; 48:9.

936. Newburger PE, Malawista SE, Dinauer MC, et al: Chronic granulomatous disease and glutathione peroxidase deficiency, revisited. Blood 1994; 84:3861.

937. Strate M, Brandup F, Wang P: Discoid lupus erythematosus-like skin lesions in a patient with autosomal recessive chronic granulomatous disease. Clin Genet 1986; 30:184.

938. Dinauer MC, Pierce EA, Bruns GAP, et al: Human neutrophil cytochrome b light chain (p22-*phox*): Gene structure, chromosomal location, and mutations in cytochrome-negative autosomal recessive chronic granulomatous disease. J Clin Invest 1990; 86:1729.

939. Segal BH, Leto TL, Gallin JI, et al: Genetic, biochemical, and clinical features of chronic granulomatous disease. Medicine (Baltimore) 2000; 79:170.

940. Borregaard N, Staehr-Johansen K, Taudorff E, et al: Cytochrome *b* is present in neutrophils from patients with chronic granulomatous disease. Lancet 1979; 1:949.

941. Segal AW, Cross AR, Garcia RC, et al: Absence of cytochrome *b*-245 in chronic granulomatous disease: A multicenter European evaluation of its incidence and relevance. N Engl J Med 1983; 308:245.

942. Dinauer M: The respiratory burst oxidase and the molecular genetics of chronic granulomatous disease. Crit Rev Clin Lab Sci 1993; 30:329.

943. Thrasher A, Keep N, et al: Review: Chronic granulomatous disease. Biochim Biophys Acta 1994; 1227:1.

944. Segal AW: Absence of both cytochrome b_{245} subunits from neutrophils in X-linked chronic granulomatous disease. Nature 1987; 326:88.

945. Parkos CA, Dinauer MC, Jesaitis AJ, et al: Absence of both the 91-kD and 22-kD subunits of human neutrophil cytochrome *b* in two

genetic forms of chronic granulomatous disease. Blood 1989; 73:1416.

946. Baehner RL, Kunkel LM, Monaco AP, et al: DNA linkage analysis of X chromosome-linked chronic granulomatous disease. Proc Natl Sci Acad U.S.A 1986; 83:3398.

947. Skalnik DG, Strauss EC, Orkin SH: CCAAT displacement protein as a repressor of the myelomonocytic-specific gp91-*phox* gene promoter. J Biol Chem 1991; 266:16736.

948. Lien LL, Lee Y, Orkin SH: Regulation of the myeloid-cell-expressed human gp91-phox gene as studied by transfer of yeast artificial chromosome clones into embryonic stem cells: suppression of a variegated cellular pattern of expression requires a full complement of distant cis elements. Mol Cell Biol 1997; 17:2279.

949. Dinauer MC, Curnutte JT, Rosen H, et al: A missense mutation in the neutrophil cytochrome *b* heavy chain in cytochrome-positive X-linked chronic granulomatous disease. J Clin Invest 1989; 84:2012.

950. Francke U, Ochs HD, DeMartinville B, et al: Minor Xp21 chromosome deletion in a male associated with expression of Duchenne muscular dystrophy, chronic granulomatous disease, retinitis pigmentosa, and McLeod syndrome. Am J Hum Genet 1985; 37:250.

951. Kousseff B: Linkage between chronic granulomatous disease and Duchenne's muscular dystrophy. Am J Dis Child 1981; 135:1149.

952. Frey D, Machler M, Seger R, et al: Gene deletion in a patient with chronic granulomatous disease and McLeod syndrome: Fine mapping of the Xk gene locus. Blood 1988; 71:252.

953. De Saint-Basile G, Bohler MC, Fischer A, et al: Xp21 DNA microdeletion in a patient with chronic granulomatous disease, retinitis pigmentosa, and McLeod phenotype. Hum Genet 1988; 80:85.

954. Pelham A, O'Reilly MAJ, Malcolm S, et al: RFLP and deletion analysis for X-linked chronic granulomatous disease using the cDNA probe: Potential for improved prenatal diagnosis and carrier determination. Blood 1990; 76:820.

955. De Boer M, Bolscher BGJM: Splice site mutations are a common cause of X-linked chronic granulomatous disease. Blood 1992; 80:1553.

956. Bolscher BGJM, De Boer M, De Klein A, et al: Point mutations in the β-subunit of cytochrome *b*₅₅₈ leading to X-linked chronic granulomatous disease. Blood 1991; 7:2482.

957. Kuribayashi F, Kumatori A, Suzuki S, et al: Human peripheral eosinophils have a specific mechanism to express gp91-*phox*, the large subunit of cytochrome *b*₅₅₈. Biochem Biophys Res Commun 1995; 2009:146.

958. Ariga T, Sakiyama Y, Matsumoto S: A 15-base pair (bp) palindromic insertion associated with a 3-bp deletion in exon 10 of the gp91-*phox* gene, detected in two patients with X-linked chronic granulomatous disease. Hum Genet 1995; 96:6.

959. Roos D, de Boer M, Kuribayashi F, et al: Mutations in the X-linked and autosomal recessive forms of chronic granulomatous disease. Blood 1996; 87:1663.

960. Rae J, Newburger P, Dinauer M, et al: X-linked chronic granulomatous disease: Mutations in the CYBB gene encoding the gp91*phox* component of respiratory-burst oxidase. Am J Hum Genet 1998; 62:1320.

961. Heyworth PG, Curnutte JT, Rae J, et al: Hematologically important mutations: X-linked chronic granulomatous disease (second update). Blood Cells Mol Dis 2001; 27:16.

962. Roos D, Curnutte J, Hossle J, et al: X-CGDbase: A database of X-CGD-causing mutations. Immunol Today 1996; 17:517.

963. Azuma H, Oomi H, Sasaki K, et al: A new mutation on exon 12 of the gp91-*phox* gene leading to cytochrome *b*-positive X-linked chronic granulomatous disease. Blood 1995; 85:3274.

964. Leusen J, de Boer M, Bolscher B, et al: A point mutation in gp91-*phox* of cytochrome *b*₅₅₈ of the human NADPH oxidase leading to defective translocation of the cytosolic proteins p47-phox and p67-phox. J Clin Invest 1994; 93:2120.

965. Dinauer MC, Pierce EA, Erickson RW, et al: Point mutation in the cytoplasmic domain of the neutrophil p22-*phox* cytochrome *b* subunit is associated with a nonfunctional NADPH oxidase and chronic granulomatous disease. Proc Natl Acad Sci USA 1991; 88:11231.

966. Newburger P, Skalnik D, Hopkins P, et al: Mutations in the promoter region of the gene gp91-*phox* in X-linked chronic granulomatous disease with decreased expression of cytochrome *b*₅₅₈. J Clin Invest 1994; 94:1205.

967. Suzuki S, Kumatori A, Haagen I, et al: PU.1 as an essential activator for the expression of gp91phox gene in human peripheral neutrophils, monocytes, and B lymphocytes. Proc Natl Acad Sci USA 1998; 95:6085.

968. Eklund E, Skalnik D: Characterization of a gp91-phox promoter element that is required for interferon γ-induced transcription. J Biol Chem 1995; 270:8267.

969. Rae J, Noack D, Heyworth PG, et al: Molecular analysis of 9 new families with chronic granulomatous disease caused by mutations in CYBA, the gene encoding p22phox. Blood 2000; 96:1106.

970. Leusen JHW, Bolscher GJM, Hilarius PM, et al: 156Pror→Gln substitution in the light chain of cytochrome. J Exp Med 1994; 180:2011.

971. Sumimoto H, Kage Yea. Role of Src homology 3 domains in assembly and activation of the phagocyte NADPH oxidase. Proc Natl Acad Sci USA 1994; 91:5345.

972. Leto T, Adams A, DeMendez I: Assembly of the phagocyte NADPH oxidase: Binding of Src homology 3 domains to proline-rich targets. Proc Natl Acad Sci USA 1994; 91:10650.

973. Ren R, Mayer BJ, Cicchetti P, et al: Identification of a 10-amino acid proline-rich SH3 binding site. Science 1993; 259:1157.

974. Zhu Q, Zhang M, Rawlings DJ, et al: Detection within the Src homology domain 3 of Bruton's tyrosine kinase resulting in X-linked agammaglobulinemia (XLA). J Exp Med 1994; 180:461.

975. Bromberg Y, Pick E: Unsaturated fatty acids stimulate NADPH-dependent superoxide production by cell-free system derived from macrophages. Cell Immunol 1984; 88:213.

976. Heyneman RA, Vercauteren RE: Activation of a NADPH oxidase from horse polymorphonuclear leukocytes in a cell-free system. J Leukoc Biol 1984; 36:751.

977. Curnutte JT: Activation of human neutrophil nicotinamide adenine dinucleotide phosphate, reduced (triphosphopyridine nucleotide, reduced) oxidase by arachidonic acid in a cell-free system. J Clin Invest 1985; 75:1740.

978. McPhail LC, Shirley PS, Clayton CC, et al: Activation of the respiratory burst enzyme from human neutrophils in a cell-free system. J Clin Invest 1985; 75:1735.

979. Nunoi H, Rotrosen D, Gallin JI, et al: Two forms of autosomal chronic granulomatous disease lack distinct neutrophil cytosol factors. Science 1988; 242:1298.

980. Curnutte JT, Scott PJ, Mayo LA: Cytosolic components of the respiratory burst oxidase: Resolution of four components, two of which are missing in complementing types of chronic granulomatous disease. Proc Natl Acad Sci USA 1989; 86:825.

981. Francke U, Ochs HD, Darras BT, et al: Origin of mutations in two families with X-linked chronic granulomatous disease. Blood 1990; 76:602.

982. Chanock SJ, Barrett DM, Curnutte JT, et al: Gene structure of the cytosolic component, phox-47 and mutations in autosomal recessive chronic granulomatous disease. Blood 1991; 78:165a.

983. Casimir CM, Bu-Ghanim HN, Rodaway ARF, et al: Autosomal recessive chronic granulomatous disease caused by deletion at a dinucleotide repeat. Proc Natl Acad Sci USA 1991; 88:2753.

984. Gorlach A, Lee P, Roesler J, et al: A p47*phox* pseudogene carries the most common mutation causing p47*phox*-deficient chronic granulomatous disease. J Clin Invest 1997; 100:1907.

985. Roesler J, Curnutte JT, Rae J, et al: Recombination events between the p47*phox* gene and its highly homologous pseudogenes are the main cause of autosomal recessive chronic granulomatous disease. Blood 2000; 95:2150.

986. Weening RS, Corbeel L, De Boer M, et al: Cytochrome *b* deficiency in an autosomal form of chronic granulomatous disease. A third form of chronic granulomatous disease recognized by monocyte hybridization. J Clin Invest 1985; 75:915.

987. Francke U, Hsieh CL, Foellmer BE, et al: Genes for two autosomal recessive forms of chronic granulomatous disease assigned to 1q25 (NCF2) and 7q11.23 (NCF1). Am J Hum Genet 1990; 47:483.

988. Kenney RT, Malech HL, Leto TL: Structural characterization of the p67-*phox* gene [abstract]. Clin Res 1992; 40:261a.

989. Tanugi-Cholley LC, Issartel JP, Lunardi J, et al: A mutation located at the 5′ splice junction sequence of intron 3 in the p67phox gene causes the lack of p67phox mRNA in a patient with chronic granulomatous disease. Blood 1995; 85:242.

990. Leusen J, de Klein A, Hilarius P, et al: Disturbed interaction of p21-rac with mutated p67*phox* causes chronic granulomatous disease. J Exp Med 1996; 184:1243.

991. Noack D, Rae J, Cross AR, et al: Autosomal recessive chronic granulomatous disease caused by novel mutations in NCF-2, the gene encoding the p67-phox component of phagocyte NADPH oxidase. Hum Genet 1999; 105:460.

992. Bonizzato A, Russo M, Donini M, et al: Identification of a double mutation (D160V-K161E) in the p67phox gene of a chronic granulomatous disease patient. Biochem Biophys Res Comm 1997; 231:861.

993. Noack D, Rae J, Cross AR, et al: Autosomal recessive chronic granulomatous disease caused by defects in NCF-1, the gene encoding the phagocyte p47-phox: Mutations not arising in the NCF-1 pseudogenes. Blood 2001; 97:305.

994. Vowells S, Sekhsaria S, Malech H, et al: Flow cytometric analysis of the granulocyte respiratory burst: A comparison study of fluorescent probes. J Immunol Methods 1995; 178:89.

995. Vowells S, Fleisher T, Sekhsaria S, et al: Genotype-dependent variability in flow cytometric evaluation of reduced nicotinamide adenine dinucleotide phosphate oxidase function in patients with chronic granulomatous disease. J Pediatr 1996; 128:104.

996. Baehner RL, Nathan DG: Quantitative nitroblue tetrazolium test in chronic granulomatous disease. N Engl J Med 1968; 278:971.

997. Segal AW: Nitroblue-tetrazolium tests. Lancet 1974; 2:1248.

998. Matthay KK, Golbus MS, Wara DW, et al: Prenatal diagnosis of chronic granulomatous disease. Am J Med Genet 1984; 17:731.

999. Huu TP, Dumez Y, Marquetty C, et al: Prenatal diagnosis of chronic granulomatous disease (CGD) in four high risk male fetuses. Prenat Diagn 1987; 7:253.

1000. Borregaard N, Bang J, Berthelesen JG, et al: Prenatal diagnosis of chronic granulomatous disease. Lancet 1982; 1:114.

1001. Newburger PE, Cohen HJ, Rothchild SB, et al: Prenatal diagnosis of chronic granulomatous disease. N Engl J Med 1979; 300:178.

1002. Battat L, Francke U: *NsiI* RFLP at the X-linked chronic granulomatous disease locus (CYBB). Nucleic Acids Res 1989; 18:4966.

1003. Muhlebach TJ, Robinson W, Seger RA, et al: A second *NsiI* RFLP at the CYBB locus. Nucleic Acids Res 1990; 18:4966.

1004. Kenney R, Leto T: A *Hind*III polymorphism in the human NCF2 gene. Nucleic Acids Res 1990; 18:7193.

1005. Hopkins PJ, Bemiller LS, Curnutte JT: Chronic granulomatous disease: Diagnosis and classification at the molecular level. Clin Lab Med 1992; 12:277.

1006. Cale CM, Jones AM, Goldblatt D: Follow up of patients with chronic granulomatous disease diagnosed since 1990. Clin Exp Immunol 2000; 120:351.

1007. Margolis DM, Melnic DA, Alling DW, et al: Trimethoprim-sulfamethoxazole prophylaxis in the management of chronic granulomatous disease. J Infect Dis 1990; 162:723.

1008. Chusid MJ, Gelfand JA, Nutter C, et al: Pulmonary aspergillosis, inhalation of contaminated marijuana smoke, chronic granulomatous disease. Ann Intern Med 1975; 82:682.

1009. Mouy R, Veber F, Blanche S, et al: Long-term itraconazole prophylaxis against *Aspergillus* infections in thirty-two patients with chronic granulomatous disease. J Pediatr 1994; 125:998.

1010. Roback SA, Weintraub WH, Good RA, et al: Chronic granulomatous disease of childhood: Surgical considerations. J Pediatr Surg 1971; 6:601.

1011. Emmerndorffer A, Lohmann-Mathes ML, Roesler J: Kinetics of transfused neutrophils in peripheral blood and BAL fluid of a patient with variant X-linked chronic granulomatous disease. Eur J Haematol 1991; 47:246.

1012. Gallin JI, Malech HL, Weening RS, et al: A controlled trial of interferon gamma to prevent infection in chronic granulomatous disease. N Engl J Med 1991; 324:509.

1013. Weening RS, Leitz GJ, Seger RA: Recombinant human interferon-gamma in patients with chronic granulomatous disease-European follow up study. Eur J Pediatr 1995; 154:295.

1014. Nathan CF, Murray HW, Wiebe ME, et al: Identification of interferon gamma as the lymphokine that activates human macrophage oxidative metabolism and antimicrobial activity. J Exp Med 1983; 158:670.

1015. Ezekowitz RAB, Orkin SH, Newburger PE: Recombinant interferon gamma augments phagocyte superoxide production and X-chronic granulomatous disease gene expression in X-linked variant chronic granulomatous disease. J Clin Invest 1987; 80:1009.

1016. Ezekowitz RB, Dinauer MC, Jaffe HS, et al: Partial correction of the phagocyte defect in patients with X-linked chronic granulomatous disease by subcutaneous interferon gamma. N Engl J Med 1988; 319:146.

1017. Sechler JMG, Malech HL, White CJ, et al: Recombinant human interferon-gamma reconstitutes defective phagocyte function in patients with chronic granulomatous disease. Proc Natl Acad Sci USA 1988; 85:4374.

1018. Ezekowitz RAB, Sieff CA, Dinauer MC, et al: Restoration of phagocyte function by interferon-gamma in X-linked chronic granulomatous disease occurs at the level of a progenitor cell. Blood 1990; 76:2443.

1019. Bemiller L, Roberts D, Starko K, et al: Safety and effectiveness of long-term interferon gamma therapy in patients with chronic granulomatous disease. Blood Cells Mol Dis 1995; 21:239.

1020. Woodman RC, Erickson RW, Rae J, et al: Prolonged recombinant interferon-gamma therapy in chronic granulomatous disease: Evidence against enhanced neutrophil oxidase activity. Blood 1992; 79:1558.

1021. Schiff D, Rae J, Martin T, et al: Increased phagocyte FcγRI expression and improved Fcγ-receptor-mediated phagocytosis after in vivo recombinant human interferon-γ treatment of normal human subjects. Blood 1997; 90:3187.

1022. Chin TW, Stiehm ER, Falloon J, et al: Corticosteroids in treatment of obstructive lesions of chronic granulomatous disease. J Pediatr 1987; 111:349.

1023. Quie PG, Belani KK: Corticosteroids for chronic granulomatous disease. J Pediatr 1987; 111:393.

1024. Fischer A, Segal AW, Weening RS: The management of chronic granulomatous disease. Eur J Pediatr 1993; 152:896.

1025. Danziger RN, Goren AT, Becker J, et al: Outpatient management with oral corticosteroid therapy for obstructive conditions in chronic granulomatous disease. J Pediatr 1993; 122:303.

1026. Rosh JR, Tang HB, Mayer L, et al: Treatment of intractable gastrointestinal manifestations of chronic granulomatous disease with cyclosporine. J Pediatr 1995; 126:143.

1027. Schettini F, De Mattia D, Manzionna MM, et al: Bone marrow transplantation for chronic granulomatous disease associated with cytochrome *b* deficiency [letter to the editor]. Pediatr Hematol Oncol 1987; 4:277.

1028. Kamani N, August CS, Campbell DE, et al: Marrow transplantation in chronic granulomatous disease: An update, with 6-year follow-up. J Pediatr 1988; 113:697.

1029. Storb R, Yu C, Barnett T, et al: Stable mixed hematopoietic chimerism in dog leukocyte antigen-identical littermate dogs given lymph node irradiation before and pharmacologic immunosuppression after marrow transplantation. Blood 1999; 94:1131.

1030. Slavin S, Nagler A, Naparstek E, et al: Nonmyeloablative stem cell transplantation and cell therapy as an alternative to conventional bone marrow transplantation with lethal cytoreduction for the treatment of malignant and nonmalignant hematologic diseases. Blood 1998; 91:756.

1031. Horwitz M, Barrett A, Brown M, et al: Treatment of chronic granulomatous disease with nonmyeloablative conditioning and a T-cell-depleted hematopoietic allograft. N Engl J Med 2001; 344:881.

1032. Kume A, Dinauer MC: Retrovirus-mediated reconstitution of respiratory burst activity in X-linked chronic granulomatous disease cells. Blood 1994; 84:331.

1033. Bjorgvinsdottir H, Ding C, Pech N, et al: Retroviral-mediated gene transfer of gp91^{phox} into bone marrow cells rescues in host defense against *Aspergillus fumigatus* in murine X-linked chronic granulomatous disease. Blood 1997; 89:41.

1034. Kume A, Dinauer M: Gene therapy for chronic granulomatous disease. J Lab Clin Med 1999; 135:122.

1035. Malech H, Maples P, Whiting-Theobald N, et al: Prolonged production of NADPH oxidase-corrected granulocytes after gene therapy of chronic granulomatous disease. Proc Natl Acad Sci USA 1997; 94:12133.

1036. Gray GR, Stamatoyannopoulos G, Naiman SC, et al: Neutrophil dysfunction, chronic granulomatous disease, and non-spherocytic haemolytic anaemia caused by complete deficiency of glucose-6-phosphate dehydrogenase. Lancet 1973; 2:530.

1037. Baehner RL, Johnston RB, Nathan DG: Comparative study of the metabolic and bactericidal characteristics of severely glucose-6-phosphate dehydrogenase deficient polymorphonuclear leukocytes and leukocytes from children with chronic granulomatous disease. J Reticuloendothel Soc 1972; 12:150.

1038. Vives Corrons JL, Feliu E, Pujades MA, et al: Severe glucose-6-phosphate dehydrogenase (G6PD) deficiency associated with chronic hemolytic anemia, granulocyte dysfunction, and increased susceptibility to infections: Description of a new molecular variant (G6PD Barcelona). Blood 1982; 59:428.

1039. Cooper MR, Dechatelet LR, McCall CE, et al: Leukocyte G-6-PD deficiency. Lancet 1970; 2:110.

1040. Beutler E: G6PD Deficiency. Blood 1994; 84:3613.

1041. Yoshida A, Stamatoyannopoulos G, Motulsky A: Biochemical genetics of glucose-6-phosphate dehydrogenase variation. Ann NY Acad Sci 1968; 155:868.

1042. Justice P, Shih L-Y, Gordon J, et al: Characterization of leukocyte glucose-6-phosphate dehydrogenase in normal and mutant human subjects. J Lab Clin Med 1966; 68:552.

1043. Ramot B, Fisher S, Szeinberg A, et al: A study of subjects with erythrocyte glucose-6-phosphate dehydrogenase deficiency. II. Investigation of leukocyte enzymes. J Clin Invest 1959; 38:2234.

1044. Mamlok RJ, Mamlok V, Mills GC, et al: Glucose-6-phosphate dehydrogenase deficiency, neutrophil dysfunction and *Chromobacterium violaceum* sepsis. J Pediatr 1987; 111:852.

1045. Parry MF, Root RK, Metcalf JA, et al: Myeloperoxidase deficiency: Prevalence and clinical significance. Ann Intern Med 1981; 95:293.

1046. Nauseef WM: Myeloperoxidase deficiency. Hematol Oncol Clin North Am 1988; 2:135.

1047. Lanza F: Clinical manifestation of myeloperoxidase deficiency. J Mol Med 1998; 76:676.

1048. Nauseef WM, Metcalf JA, Root RK: Role of myeloperoxidase in the respiratory burst of human neutrophils. Blood 1983; 61:483.

1049. Lehrer RI, Cline MJ: Leukocyte myeloperoxidase deficiency and disseminated candidiasis: The role of myeloperoxidase in resistance to *Candida* infection. J Clin Invest 1969; 48:1478.

1050. Diamond RD, Clark RA, Haudenschild CC: Damage to *Candida albicans* hyphae and pseudohypae by the myeloperoxidase system and oxidative products of neutrophil matabolism *in vitro*. J Clin Invest 1980; 66:908.

1051. Cech P, Stalder H, Widmann JJ, et al: Leukocyte myeloperoxidase deficiency and diabetes mellitus associated with *Candida albicans* liver abscess. Am J Med 1979; 66:149.

1052. Kitahara M, Eyre HJ, Simonian Y, et al: Hereditary myeloperoxidase deficiency. Blood 1981; 57:888.

1053. Chang KS, Schroeder W, Siciliano MJ, et al: The localization of the human myeloperoxidase gene is in close proximity to the translocation breakpoint in acute promyelocytic leukemia. Leukemia 1987; 1:458.

1054. Van Tuinen P, Johnson KR, Ledbetter SA, et al: Localization of myeloperoxidase to the long arm of human chromosome 17: Relationship to the 15,17 translocation of acute promyelocytic leukemia. Oncogene 1987; 1:319.

1055. Nauseef WM: Aberrant restriction endonuclease digests of DNA from subjects with hereditary myeloperoxidase deficiency. Blood 1989; 73:290.

1056. Tobler A, Selsted ME, Miller CW, et al: Evidence for a pretranslational defect in hereditary and acquired myeloperoxidase deficiency. Blood 1989; 73:1980.

1057. Selsted ME, Miller CW, Novotny MJ, et al: Molecular analysis of myeloperoxidase deficiency shows heterogeneous patterns of the complete deficiency state manifested at the genomic, mRNA, and protein levels. Blood 1993; 82:1317.

1058. Kizaki M, Miller CW, Selsted ME, et al: Myeloperoxidase (MPO) gene mutation in hereditary MPO deficiency. Blood 1994; 83:1935.

1059. Nauseef WM, Brigham S, Cogley M: Hereditary myeloperoxidase deficiency due to a missense mutation of arginine 569 to tryptophan. J Biol Chem 1994; 269:1212.

1060. Nauseef WM, Cogley M, McCormick S: Effect of the R569W missense mutation on the biosynthesis of myeloperoxidase. J Biol Chem 1996; 271:9546.

1061. DeLeo F, Renee J, McCormick S, et al: Neutrophils exposed to bacterial lipopolysaccharide upregulate NADPH oxidase assembly. J Clin Invest 1998; 101:455.

1062. Romano M, Dri P, Dadalt L, et al: Biochemical and molecular characterization of hereditary myeloperoxidase deficiency. Blood 1997; 90:4126.

1063. Bendix-Hansen K, Kerndrup G: Myeloperoxidase-deficient polymorphonuclear leukocytes. V: Relation to FAB classification and neutrophil alkaline phosphatase activity in primary myelodysplastic syndromes. Scand J Haematol 1985; 35:197.

1064. Bendix-Hansen K, Kerndrup G, Pedersen B: Myeloperoxidase-deficient polymorphonuclear leukocytes. VI: Relation to cytogenetic abnormalities in primary myelodysplastic syndromes. Scand J Haematol 1986; 36:3.

1065. Stendahl O, Coble B-I, Dahlgren C, et al: Myeloperoxidase modulates the phagocytic activity of polymorphonuclear leukocytes. Studies with cells from a myeloperoxidase-deficient patient. J Clin Invest 1984; 73:366.

1066. Rosen H, Klebanoff SJ: Chemiluminescence and superoxide production by myeloperoxidase-deficient leukocytes. J Clin Invest 1976; 58:50.

1067. Jandl RC, Andre-Schwartz J, Borges-Dubois L, et al: Termination of the respiratory burst in human neutrophils. J Clin Invest 1978; 61:1176.

1068. Roos D, Weening RS, Voetman AA, et al: Protection of phagocytic leukocytes by endogenous glutathione: Studies in a family with glutathione reductase deficiency. Blood 1979; 53:851.

1069. Boxer LA, Oliver JM, Spielberg SP, et al: Protection of granulocytes by vitamin E in glutathione synthetase deficiency. N Engl J Med 1979; 301:901.

1070. Loos H, Roos D, Weening RS, et al: Familial deficiency of glutathione reductase in human blood cells. Blood 1976; 48:53.

1071. Spielberg SP, Kramer LI, Goodman SI, et al: S-Oxoprolinuria: Biochemical observations and case report. J Pediatr 1977; 91:237.

1072. Spielberg SP, Boxer LA, Oliver JM, et al: Oxidative damage to neutrophils in glutathione synthetase deficiency. Br J Haematol 1979; 42:215.

1073. Nevin NC, Morrison PJ, Jones J, et al: Inverted tandem duplication of 8p12-p23.1 in a child with increased activity of glutathione reductase. J Med Genet 1990; 27:135.

1074. Holmes B, Park BH, Malawista SE, et al: Chronic granulomatous disease in females: A deficiency of leukocyte glutathione peroxidase. N Engl J Med 1970; 283:217.

1075. Matsuda I, Oka Y, Taniguchi N, et al: Leukocyte gluatathione peroxidase deficiency in a male patient with chronic granulomatous disease. J Pediatr 1976; 88:581.

Index

Page numbers in *italics* denote illustrations; those followed by "t" denote tables